Davis's

DRUG GUIDE for Nurses

Third Edition

Davis's DRUG GUIDE for Nurses

Third Edition

JUDITH HOPFER DEGLIN, PharmD
University of Connecticut
Schools of Pharmacy and Nursing
Storrs, Connecticut

Consultant Pharmacist
Hospice of Norwich
Norwich, Connecticut

APRIL HAZARD VALLERAND, MSN, RN
University of Pennsylvania
School of Nursing
Philadelphia, Pennsylvania

University of Medicine and Dentistry
of New Jersey
Department of Nursing Education and Services
Newark, New Jersey

F. A. DAVIS COMPANY • Philadelphia

Printed in the United States of America

Last digit indicates print number 10 9 8 7 6 5 4 3 2 1

NOTE: As new scientific information becomes available through basic and clinical research, recommended treatments and drug therapies undergo changes. The author(s) and publisher have done everything possible to make this book accurate, up-to-date, and in accord with accepted standards at the time of publication. However, the reader is advised always to check product information (package inserts) for changes and new information regarding dose and contraindications before administering any drug. Caution is especially urged when using new or infrequently ordered drugs.

Library of Congress Cataloging-in-Publication Data

Deglin, Judith Hopfer, 1950–
Davis's drug guide for nurses / Judith Hopfer Deglin, April Hazard Vallerand.—3rd ed.
p. cm.
Includes bibliographical references and index.
ISBN 0-8036-2457-3 (hardbound : alk. paper)
1. Drugs—Handbooks, manuals, etc. 2. Nursing—Handbooks, manuals, etc. I. Vallerand, April Hazard. II. Title. III. Title: Drug guide for nurses.
[DNLM: 1. Drugs—handbooks. 2. Drugs—nurses' instruction. QV 39 D318d]
RM301.12.D44 1992
615'.1'024613—dc20
DNLM/DLC
for Library of Congress 92-4588
CIP

To my husband and best friend, Stuart, whose continued patience, support, and love has made my participation in this project possible.

JHD

To my father, Keith Randall Hazard, whose constant support and belief in my accomplishments is always there when I need it.

To my mother, Vivian Hazard Warner, who taught me to look for the positive in everything and whose presence is always with me.

To my grandmother, Lora B. Ellis, whose dream of becoming a nurse has helped mine come true.

AHV

CONSULTANTS

Diane Cline, RN
Victor Valley College
Victorville, California

Laurel A. Eisenhauer, RN, PhD
Boston University
Boston, Massachusetts

Gary G. Ferguson, PharmD
School of Pharmacy
Northeast Louisiana University
Monroe, Louisiana

Milly Gustkoski, RN
College of Nursing
Montana State University
Bozeman, Montana

Nancy Harms, RN, MSN
Division of Nursing
Midland Lutheran College
Fremont, Nebraska

Kathleen E. Mahan, RN, MSN, CCRN
Clinical Nurse Specialist
Sarasota Memorial Hospital
Sarasota, Florida

Anita Lee Malen, PharmD
University of Portland
School of Nursing
Portland, Oregon

Patricia Neafsey, MS, RD, PhD
University of Connecticut
School of Nursing
Storrs, Connecticut

Steven O. Price, PharmD
Medical University of South Carolina
Charleston, South Carolina

Mildred M. Russin, MSN, RN
Shands Hospital at the
University of Florida
Gainesville, Florida

Kathleen Herman Scanlon, RN, MSN, MA
Elmhurst College
Elmhurst, Illinois

M. Jeanne Van Tyle, PharmD
Butler University
College of Pharmacy
Indianapolis, Indiana

Lloyd Yee Young, PharmD
Department of Pharmacy
Washington State University
Spokane, Washington

With special acknowledgment to Kirsten Hoen.

ACKNOWLEDGMENTS

We offer our thanks and gratitude to our families, whose support and patience with our endless computer time and phone calls gave us the time and strength to complete this manuscript.

To those at F.A. Davis, especially Bob Martone, Ruth De George, and Art Ofner, who saw our projects through to completion.

Judi and April

WHAT'S NEW IN THE THIRD EDITION

In keeping with the fine tradition of earlier editions of *Davis's Drug Guide for Nurses,* this third edition strives to set new standards for nursing drug references by providing the most comprehensive, up-to-date, efficient, and practical information available to nurses. While there certainly are other technical resources available, no other forum concisely makes available to the nurse only the most relevant information required for the safe and effective administration and monitoring of drug therapy. The distillation of information into a uniform, easily followed format ensures that once the nurse is familiar with the layout of drug monographs, finding specific facts for individual drugs becomes a very efficient process.

The third edition reflects the authors' commitment to providing the most up-to-date material available. At least 75 new pharmacologic entities have been added. Included are three new calcium channel blockers, four new angiotensin converting enzyme (ACE) inhibitors, two new agents approved for managing AIDS patients, several new antiarrhythmic and antineoplastic agents, as well as a variety of other recently introduced drugs. These new agents have been added to the Classifications Section as well, so that the nurse may appreciate the place of the new agents with respect to similar drugs already on the market. Newly written monographs on hormonal contraceptives and topical glucocorticoids have also been put into place.

In addition to adding new drugs, all of the existing monographs have been revised to reflect updated information and additional clinical "pearls." Newly approved indications have been added, as well as unlabeled uses. Drug–drug interactions have been updated to reflect interactions with new agents and recently reported significant interactions with traditional drugs.

The most recently released drugs which may rapidly become clinically significant are highlighted in a new Appendix P: Recent Drug Release Update. Another new appendix, Appendix N, profiles Routine Pediatric and Adult Immunizations.

Nursing implications have been streamlined to afford better accessibility to data; IV administration information has been more clearly delineated to facilitate rapid retrieval.

The dosage recommendations in the text are those ranges recommended by manufacturers and approved by the FDA. The reader is reminded that special dosing considerations are to be borne in mind depending upon the age, size, condition, and tolerance of the patient. The book's information on contraindications, precautions, adverse reactions, interactions, and side effects is condensed to a level essential to responsible clinical practice.

This reference not only provides the pharmacologic profile on what each drug does, and how it works, but also links essential nursing data such as what parameters to assess in the patient taking the drug; how to administer the medication; and how to evaluate the drug's effectiveness while incorporating the nursing diagnoses applicable to its administration. In addition, the necessary information to provide appropriate patient and family teaching is covered.

It is hoped that the third edition of *Davis's Drug Guide for Nurses* will fill the drug information needs of every student and practicing nurse and facilitate the safe and efficacious use of medications.

No other drug reference presents such depth of pharmacologic content within the framework of the nursing process, and does it in such a convenient size and format. The authors are to be congratulated once again for breathing life into the nursing process as it relates to pharmacologic principles and practice.

FROM THE PUBLISHER

TABLE OF CONTENTS

Recent Drug Release Update

GENERIC NAME (BRAND NAME)	CLASSIFICATION	USE(S)	FDA APPROVAL STATUS
amlodipine (Norvasc)	Calcium channel blocker	Hypertension, angina pectoris	Recommended for FDA approval 6/91
azithromycin (Zithromax)	Anti-infective —macrolide	Respiratory tract infections, skin infections, chlamydia	Approved by FDA 11/91
butorphanol intranasal (Stadol NS)	Narcotic analgesic —agonist/ antagonist	Analgesia	Approved by FDA
cefprozil (Cefzil)	Anti-infective —cephalosporin	Respiratory tract, skin and skin structure infections	Approved by FDA
chickenpox vaccine (Varivax)	Vaccine	Prevention of chickenpox	UK
diltiazem IV (Cardizem)	Calcium channel blocker	Atrial fibrillation, atrial flutter, conversion of PSVT	Approved by FDA 12/91
enoxacin (Penetrex)	Anti-infective —fluoroquinolone	Skin, genitourinary, and respiratory tract infections	Recommended for FDA approval 12/90
finasteride (Proscar)	Enzyme inhibitor	Benign prostatic hypertrophy	Recommended for FDA approval 2/92
flumazenil (Mazicon)	Benzodiazepine antagonist	Reversal of benzodiazepine effects	Approved by FDA
isosorbide mononitrate (Ismo)	Vasodilator—nitrate	Management of angina pectoris	Approved by FDA
ketorolac oral (Toradol)	Non-narcotic analgesic —nonsteroidal anti-inflammatory agent	Analgesia (short-term)	Approved by FDA
loracarbef (Lorabid)	Anti-infective —cephalosporin	Skin, urinary and respiratory tract infections	Approved by FDA
MAb (Xomazyme CD5 Plus)	Monoclonal antibody	Graft versus host disease	UK
nabumetone (Relafen)	Nonsteroidal anti-inflammatory agent	Rheumatoid arthritis, osteoarthritis	Approved by FDA
nedocromil (Tilade)	Mast cell stabilizer	Reversible airway disease	Recommended for FDA approval 6/90
nicotine transdermal (Habitrol, Nicoderm, Prostep)	Smoking deterrent	Cessation therapy for smokers	Approved by FDA 1/92
pamidronate (Aredia)	Electrolyte modifier —hypocalcemic	Hypercalcemia of malignancy	Approved by FDA 10/91
sertraline (Zoloft)	Antidepressant	Depression	Recommended for approval 9/91
simvastatin (Zocor)	Lipid-lowering agent	Hyperlipidemia	UK
sumatriptan (Sumatrex)	Serotonin agonist	Migraine and cluster headache	UK
temafloxacin (Omniflox)	Anti-infective —fluoroquinolone	Respiratory and urinary tract infections	UK

HOW TO USE *DAVIS'S DRUG GUIDE FOR NURSES*

The purpose of *Davis's Drug Guide for Nurses* is to provide readily accessible, easy to understand drug information for the most commonly prescribed drugs for clinical use. The sections below describe the organization of the book and the information provided for each drug.

Special Dosing Considerations

In many clinical situations, the average dosing range can be inappropriate. This section presents general guidelines for conditions in which special considerations must be made to assure optimum therapeutic outcome.

Classifications

Brief summaries of the major therapeutic classifications are provided along with a listing of those drugs included in *Davis's Drug Guide for Nurses* and the page numbers on which those monographs may be found.

Drug Monographs

The following information appears for each drug:

Generic/Trade Name: The generic name appears first, with a pronunciation key. This is followed by an alphabetical listing of trade names. The generic name is the official name of the drug assigned by the United States Adopted Names (USAN) Council in the United States and by the World Health Organization (WHO) in other countries. In many institutions, drugs are labeled generically. Canadian trade names appear in brackets. Common names, abbreviations, and selected foreign names are also included. For users who do not know the generic name, there is a color-coded Comprehensive Drug and Agent Index which contains entries for both trade names and generic names, as well as classifications—and provides this information quickly and easily.

Classification: The most common classification is listed first followed by other classification(s) according to the use(s) of the drug. For example, phenytoin (Dilantin) is classified first as an anticonvulsant but is also used as an antiarrhythmic. For a better explanation of drug classifications, refer to the Classifications section of the book (pages C1–C79), which provides brief summaries of the classifications, lists the drugs contained in each classification, and identifies the page numbers on which the drugs can be found.

Controlled Substance Schedule: If a drug is a controlled substance, its legal status or schedule will be listed. This information alerts the reader to observe the necessary regulations when handling these drugs and should help instruct the patient regarding refill allotments. (See Appendix C for a description of the Schedule of Controlled Substances and a list of controlled substances included in *Davis's Drug Guide for Nurses.*)

Pregnancy Category: If the Food and Drug Administration (FDA) assigned pregnancy category is known, it will be listed in this part of the monograph. A more detailed explanation of these categories (A, B, C, D, and X) is found in Appendix E. These categories allow for some assessment of risk to the fetus when a drug is used in the pregnant patient or in the patient who may be trying to conceive while receiving the drug.

Indications: The most common Food and Drug Administration (FDA) uses of the drug are listed. Significant unlabeled uses are also included.

Action: This section contains a concise description of how a drug is known or believed to act in producing the desired therapeutic effect.

Pharmacokinetics: This information describes what happens to a drug following administration and includes an analysis of the absorption, distribution, metabolism, excretion, and half-life (amount of time for drug level to decrease by 50%).

Absorption: Absorption describes the process of drug administration and its delivery to systemic circulation. If only a small fraction is absorbed following oral administration (diminished bioavailability), then the oral dose will be much larger than the parenteral dose. Absorption into systemic circulation also follows other routes of administration such as topical, transdermal, intramuscular, subcutaneous, rectal, and ophthalmic routes. Drugs administered intravenously are usually 100% bioavailable.

Distribution: Following absorption, drugs are distributed, sometimes selectively, to various body tissues and fluids. These factors become important in choosing one drug over another, as in selecting antibiotics that may need to penetrate the central nervous system in the treatment of meningitis, or avoiding drugs which cross the placenta in pregnancy or concentrate in breast milk during lactation. During distribution many drugs interact with specific receptors and exert their pharmacologic effect. Bonding to proteins, including albumin, occurs as well. Only the free or unbound portion of drug is available for activity at receptor sites.

Metabolism and Excretion: Following their intended action, drugs leave the body by either being converted to inactive compounds by the liver (metabolism or biotransformation) which are then excreted by the kidneys, or by renal elimination of unchanged drug. In addition, some drugs may be eliminated by other pathways such as biliary excretion, sweat, feces, and breath. If drugs are extensively liver-metabolized, then patients with severe liver disease may require dosage reduction. If the kidney is the major organ of elimination, then dosage adjustment may be necessary in the face of renal impairment. The very young (premature infants and neonates) and the elderly (over 60 years old) have diminished renal excretory and hepatic metabolic capacity. These patients may require dosage reduction or increased dosing intervals.

Half-Life: The half-life of a drug is useful to know in planning effective regimens, since it correlates roughly with the duration of action. Half-lives are given for patients with normal renal or hepatic function. Other conditions which may alter the half-life are noted.

Contraindications and Precautions: Situations where drug use should be avoided or alternatives strongly considered are listed as contraindications. In general, most drugs are contraindicated in pregnancy or lactation, unless the potential benefits outweigh the possible risks to the mother or baby (for example, anticonvulsants and antihypertensives). Contraindications may be absolute (i.e., the drug in question should be avoided completely) or relative where certain clinical situations may allow cautious use of the drug. The precautions portion includes disease states or clinical situations where drug use involves particular risks or dosage modification may be necessary.

Adverse Reactions and Side Effects: In order to simplify long lists of possible reactions, a systems approach to side effects and adverse reactions has been taken. The order is such that these reactions have been listed in head-to-toe order for systems amenable to noting in this manner (CNS, EENT, Resp, CV, GI, GU). Other systems follow in alphabetical order (Endo, F and E, Hemat, Metab, Local, Neuro), ending with a miscellaneous section. While it is not possible to include all reported reactions, an effort has been made to include major side effects. Life-threatening adverse reactions or side effects will be CAPITALIZED, while the most commonly encountered problems will be underlined. The following abbreviations will be used for body systems.

CNS: central nervous system
EENT: eye, ear, nose, and throat
Resp: respiratory
CV: cardiovascular
GI: gastrointestinal
GU: genitourinary
Derm: dermatologic
Endo: endocrinologic
F and E: fluid and electrolyte
Hemat: hematologic
Local: local
Metab: metabolic
MS: musculoskeletal
Neuro: neurologic
Misc: miscellaneous

Interactions: As the number of medications a patient receives increases, so does the likelihood of experiencing a drug–drug interaction. The most important drug–drug interactions and their results are explained. Significant drug–food interactions are also noted.

Route and Dosage: The usual routes of administration are grouped together and include recommended dosages for adults, children, and other more specific age groups if available. Dosage units are given in the terms in which they will most likely be prescribed. (For example, Penicillin G dosage is given in units rather than milligrams.) Dosing intervals are also mentioned in the manner in which they are most likely to be ordered. While antibiotics and antiarrhythmics should be given at regular intervals around the clock, it is neither necessary nor practical to give other medications, such as oral antihypertensives, in this manner. In situations where dosage or interval is different from that commonly encountered, these indications will be listed separately for clarification.

Pharmacodynamics: This information is provided so that at the onset of drug action, its peak effect and duration of activity can be anticipated and considered in planning dosage schedules. The pharmacodynamics of each route of administration has been tabulated so that the reader may appreciate differences achieved by choosing one route over another. Durations of action of anti-infective agents have generally not been included. Most regimens for these agents are designed to avoid toxicity while ensuring high peak levels necessary for anti-infective action. Because of this, duration of action and blood level information are not necessarily comparable.

Nursing Implications

This section has been developed to help the nurse apply the nursing process to pharmacotherapeutics. It is divided into subsections which give the nurse a step-by-step guide to the nursing process as it is related to medication administration.

Assessment: This subsection includes parameters for patient history and physical data that should be assessed before and during drug therapy. The **General Info** section describes assessment that is pertinent to all patients taking the medication. Other sections are also identified to specify assessments based on the drug's various indications. **Lab Test Considerations** provides the nurse with information regarding which laboratory tests to monitor and how the results may be effected by the medication. **Toxicity and Overdose** discusses therapeutic serum drug levels and signs and symptoms of toxicity. The antidote and treatment for toxicity or overdose of appropriate medications are also included.

Potential Nursing Diagnoses: The nursing diagnoses approved through the Ninth National Conference of the North American Nursing Diagnosis Association (NANDA) are used. The three most pertinent diagnoses that apply to a patient receiving the medication are listed. Following each diagnosis, the location of the information from which the diagnosis has been developed is listed in parentheses to provide a reference for the nursing diagnosis—for example, Infection, high risk for (indications, side effects). All of the NANDA diagnostic labels are listed in Appendix O.

Implementation: Guidelines specific for medication administration are discussed in this subsection. The information listed under the **General Info** heading applies to all routes of administration and includes the forms and combinations the drug is available in, timing of administration, and details for patient care. Other headings in this section provide data regarding routes of administration. **PO** describes when and how to administer the drug, whether tablets may be crushed or capsules opened, and when to administer the medication in relation to food. **IV** provides details for reconstitution and dilution. **Direct IV** (IV Push), **Intermittent Infusion,** and **Continuous Infusion** specify amount and type of further dilution. *Rate* includes infusion time for each type of administration. **Syringe Compatibility/Incompatibility** identifies the medications each drug is compatible or incompatible with when mixed in a syringe. This type of compatibility is usually limited to 15 minutes after mixing. **Y-Site Compatibility/Incompatibility** identifies those medications that are compatible or incompatible with each drug when administered via Y-injection site or 3-way stopcock in IV tubing. **Additive Compatibility/Incompatibility** identifies those medications that are compatible or incompatible when admixed in solution. This type of compatiblity is usually limited to 24 hours.

Patient/Family Teaching: This subsection includes material which should be taught to patients and/or families of patients. Side effects which should be reported, information on how to minimize side effects, details on administration, and follow-up requirements are presented. The nurse should also refer to the "Adverse Reactions and Side Effects" and "Interactions" sections for additional data to complete the patient/family teaching plan.

Evaluation: Outcome criteria for determination of the effectiveness of the medication are provided.

SPECIAL DOSING CONSIDERATIONS

For almost every drug there is an average dosing range. There are many common situations, however, when this average range can be either toxic or ineffective. The purpose of this section is to describe situations in which special dosing considerations must be made to ensure a successful therapeutic outcome. The guidelines presented are general but should lead to a finer appreciation of individual dosing parameters. When these clinical situations are encountered, the doses of drugs ordered should be reviewed and the necessary adjustments made.

The Pediatric Patient

The most obvious reason for adjusting dosages in pediatric patients is size. Most drug dosages for this population are given on a mg/kg basis, or even more specifically on the basis of body surface area (BSA). Body surface area is determined by using a Body Surface Area Nomogram (see Appendix G).

The neonate and the premature infant require additional adjustments besides those made on the basis of size. In this population, absorption following oral administration may be incomplete or altered due to changes in gastric pH or GI motility; distribution may be altered due to varying amounts of total body water; and metabolism and excretion may be delayed because liver and kidney function have not yet matured. Hepatic and renal function maturation may necessitate frequent dosage adjustments during the course of therapy to reflect improved drug handling in the premature infant or neonate. Rapid weight changes in this age group require that additional adjustments be made.

In addition to pharmacokinetic variables, other nursing considerations should be addressed. The route of administration chosen in pediatric patients often reflects the seriousness of the illness. The nurse should consider the child's developmental level and ability to understand the situation. Medications that must be administered intravenously or by intramuscular injection may seem frightening to a young child or cause concern to the parents. The nurse should allay these fears by educating the parents and comforting the child. Intramuscular or subcutaneous injection sites should be carefully chosen in this age group to prevent possible nerve or tissue damage.

The Geriatric Patient

In patients over 60 years of age, the pharmacokinetic behavior of drugs changes. Drug absorption may be delayed secondary to diminished GI motility (from age or other drugs) or passive congestion of abdominal blood vessels as seen in congestive heart failure. Distribution may be altered because of low plasma proteins, particularly in malnourished patients. Because plasma proteins are decreased, a larger proportion of free or unbound drug will result in an increase in drug action. The result may be a patient becoming toxic while receiving a standard dose of a drug. Metabolism performed by the liver and excretion handled by the kidneys are both slowed as part of the aging process and may result in prolonged and exaggerated drug action. Body composition also changes with age. There is an increase in fatty tissue, and a decrease in skeletal muscle and total body water. Height and weight also usually decrease. A dosage of medication that was acceptable for the robust 50-year-old patient may be excessive in the same patient 20 years later.

An additional concern is that most elderly patients are receiving numerous drugs. With increasing numbers of drugs being used, there is an increased risk of one drug negating, potentiating, or otherwise altering the effects of another drug (drug–drug interaction). In general, doses of most medications should be decreased in the geriatric population. Drugs to be specifically concerned about are the cardiac glycosides (digoxin and digitoxin), sedatives/hypnotics, oral anticoagulants, and antihypertensives.

Dosing regimens should be kept simple in this patient population, since many of these patients are taking multiple drugs. Doses should be scheduled so that the patient's day is not interrupted multiple times to take medications. The use of fixed-dose combination drugs may help to simplify dosing regimens. However, some of these combinations are more expensive than the individual components.

In explaining medication regimens to elderly patients, the nurse should remember that hearing deficits are common in this group. Patients may find it embarrassing to disclose this information and full compliance may be hindered.

The Obstetrical Patient

During pregnancy both the mother and the fetus must be considered. The placenta, once thought to be a protective barrier, is simply a membrane that is capable only of protecting the fetus from extremely large molecules. Transfer of drugs through the placenta to the fetus occurs by both passive and active processes. The fetus is particularly vulnerable during two of the three stages of pregnancy, the first trimester and the last trimester. During the first trimester, the vital organs are being formed. Ingestion of drugs that cause harm (potential teratogens) during this stage of pregnancy may lead to fetal malformation or cause miscarrage. Unfortunately, this is the time when a woman is least likely to know that she is pregnant. Therefore, it is wise to inform all patients of childbearing age of potential harm to an unborn child. In the third trimester the major concern is that drugs that are administered to the mother and transferred to the fetus may not be safely metabolized and excreted by the fetus. This is especially true of drugs administered near term. After the infant is delivered, he/she no longer has the placenta available to help with drug excretion. If drugs administered before delivery are allowed to accumulate, toxicity may result.

The possibility of medications altering sperm quality and quantity in potential fathers is also becoming an area of increasing concern. Male patients should be informed of this risk when taking any medications known to have this potential.

There are situations where, for the sake of the mother's health and to protect the fetus, drug administration is required throughout pregnancy. Two examples of this are the epileptic patient and the hypertensive patient. In these circumstances, the safest drug in the smallest effective dose is chosen. Because of changes in the behavior of drugs which may occur throughout pregnancy, dosage adjustments may be required during the progression of pregnancy and after delivery. A special situation related to drug behavior in pregnancy is the mother who abuses drugs. Infants born to mothers addicted to alcohol, sedatives (including benzodiazepines), heroin, and cocaine may be of low birth weight, may experience drug withdrawal after birth, and may display developmental delay. A careful history should alert the nurse to these possibilites.

Kidney Disease

The kidneys are the major organ of drug elimination. Some drugs are excreted only after being metabolized or biotransformed by the liver. Others may be eliminated unchanged by the kidneys. The premature infant has immature renal function. Elderly patients have an age-related decrease in renal function. In order to make dosage adjustments in patients with renal dysfunction, assessment of the degree of renal impairment in the individual patient and the percentage of drug which is eliminated by the kidneys must be made. The degree of renal function can be measured by laboratory testing, most commonly by the creatinine clearance. The percentage of each drug excreted by the kidneys can be determined from references on pharmacokinetics. In addition, the dosage can frequently be optimized by measuring blood levels of the drug in the individual patient and making any further necessary changes. Two types of drugs for which this type of dosage adjustment are commonly used are digoxin and the aminoglycoside antibiotics (amikacin, gentamicin, and tobramycin).

Liver Disease

The liver is the major organ for metabolism of drugs. For most drugs this is an inactivation step. The inactive metabolites are subsequently excreted by the kidneys. The conversion process usually changes the drug from a relatively lipid or fat-soluble compound to a more water-soluble substance. Liver function is not as easily quantified as renal function; therefore, it is difficult to predict the correct dosage for a patient with liver dysfunction based on laboratory tests alone. In addition, it appears that only a minimal level of liver function may be required for complete drug metabolism.

A patient who is severely jaundiced or has very low serum proteins (particularly albumin) may be expected to have some problems metabolizing drugs. Chronic alcoholic patients are at risk of developing this type of situation. In advanced liver disease, drug absorption may also be impaired secondary to portal vascular congestion. Examples of drugs which should be carefully dosed in patients with liver disease include theophylline and sedatives which are liver-metabolized. Some drugs require the liver for activation (such as sulindac or cyclophosphamide) and should be avoided in patients with severely compromised liver function.

Congestive Heart Failure

Patients with congestive heart failure also require dosage modifications. In these patients, drug absorption may be impaired due to passive congestion of blood vessels feeding the GI tract. This same passive congestion slows drug delivery to the liver and delays metabolism. In addition, renal function may be compromised, leading to delayed elimination and prolonged drug action. Many patients who have congestive heart failure are already in a special dosing category because of their age. Dosages of drugs that are mainly metabolized by the liver or mainly excreted by the kidneys should be decreased in patients with apparent congestive heart failure.

Body Size

In most situations, drug dosing is based on total body weight. Some drugs selectively penetrate fatty tissues. If the drug is known not to penetrate fatty tissues and the patient is obese, dosage should be determined by ideal body weight or estimated lean body mass (for example, digoxin, gentamicin). These quantities may be determined from tables of desirable weights or may be estimated using formulas for lean body mass when the patient's height and weight are known. If this type of adjustment is not made, considerable toxicity may result.

Delivery to Sites of Action

In order to have a successful therapeutic outcome, the drug must reach its intended site of action. Under the most desirable of conditions, the drug will have only a minimal effect on other tissues or body systems. A good example is drugs that are applied topically for skin conditions and are only minimally absorbed. In many diseases this arrangement is neither achievable nor practical. Often unusual routes of administration must be used to guarantee the presence of drug at the intended site of response. In patients with bacterial meningitis, administering drugs parenterally may not produce high enough levels in the cerebrospinal fluid. Intrathecal administration may be required in addition to parenteral therapy, as is the case with the aminoglycoside antibiotics (amikacin, gentamicin, and tobramycin). The eye represents another barrier which is relatively impermeable to many drugs. To overcome this barrier, local instillation or injection may be required.

In some cases local absorption may not occur and the desired systemic effect will not happen. Drugs may not be absorbed into systemic circulation from subcutaneous sites in patients with shock or poor tissue perfusion due to other causes.

When considering the route of administration identify the site at which the drug is intended to have its primary action. In order to achieve its maximal effect it must be delivered to its intended site of action.

Drug Interactions

The presence of additional drugs may also necessitate dosage adjustments. Drugs which are highly bound to plasma proteins such as warfarin and phenytoin may be displaced by other highly protein bound drugs. When this phenomenon occurs, the drug that has been displaced exhibits an increase in its activity since it is the free or unbound drug which is active.

Some agents decrease the ability of the liver to metabolize other drugs. Drugs which are capable of doing this include cimetidine and chloramphenicol. Concurrently administered drugs that are highly metabolized by the liver may need to be administered in decreased dosages. Other agents, such as phenobarbital, other barbiturates, and rifampin are capable of stimulating (inducing) the liver to metabolize drugs more rapidly, requiring larger doses to be administered.

Drugs that significantly alter urine pH can affect excretion of other drugs for which the excretory process is pH dependent. Alkalinizing the urine will hasten the excretion of acidic drugs. Acidification of the urine will enhance reabsorption of acidic drugs, prolonging and enhancing drug action. In the reverse situation, drugs that acidify the urine will hasten the excretion of alkaline drugs. An example of this is administering sodium bicarbonate in cases of aspirin overdose. Alkalinizing the urine promotes renal excretion of aspirin.

Some drugs compete for enzyme systems with other drugs. Allopurinol inhibits the enzyme which is involved in uric acid production, but it also inhibits the metabolism (inactivation) of 6-mercaptopurine, greatly increasing its toxicity. The dosage of mercaptopurine needs to be significantly reduced when coadministered with allopurinol.

Dosage Forms

The nurse will frequently encounter problems that relate to the dosage form itself. Some medications may not be commercially available in liquid or chewable dosage forms. The pharmacist may have to compound such dosage forms for an individual patient. It may be necessary to disguise the taste or appearance of a medication in food or a beverage in order for the patient to fully comply with a given regimen. Finally, some dosage forms such as aerosol inhalers may not be suitable for very young patients because their use requires cooperation beyond the patient's developmental level.

Before altering dosage forms (crushing tablets or opening capsules) check to be sure that the effect of the drug will not be altered by doing so. In general, extended- or sustained-release dosage forms should not be crushed, nor should capsules containing beads of medication be opened. Altering these dosage forms may shorten and intensify their intended action. Enteric-coated tablets, which may appear to be sugar-coated or candy-coated, should also not be crushed. This coating may be designed to protect the stomach from the irritating effects of these drugs. Crushing the tablets will expose the stomach lining to these agents and increase GI irritation. If a dosage form needs to be crushed, it should be ingested right away. A glass of water should be taken before administration of powders or crushed tablets to wet the esophagus and prevent the material from sticking to upper GI mucosal surfaces.

Environmental Factors

Cigarette smoke is capable of inducing liver enzymes to metabolize drugs more rapidly. Patients who smoke may need larger doses of liver-metabolized drugs to compensate for this. Patients who are passively exposed to cigarette smoke may also exhibit otherwise unexplained needs for larger doses of medications. The effect of smoking on drug metabolism may persist for months.

Nutritional Factors

Certain foods can alter the dosing requirement for some medications. Dietary calcium found in high concentrations in dairy products combines (chelates) with tetracycline and prevents its absorption. Many antibiotics are absorbed better if taken when the stomach is empty. Foods which are high in pyridoxine (vitamin B_6) content can negate the antiparkinson effect of levodopa (this is counteracted with coadministration of carbidopa). Foods which are capable of altering urine pH may effect the excretion patterns of medications, enhancing or diminishing their effectiveness. There are no general guidelines for nutritional factors. It is prudent to check if these problems exist or if they may explain therapeutic failures and to make the necessary dosage adjustments.

Summary

The average dosing range for drugs is intended for an average patient. However, every patient is an individual with specific drug-handling capabilities. Taking into account these special dosing considerations allows the planning of an individualized drug regimen that will result in a desired therapeutic outcome while minimizing the risk of toxicity.

KEY TO COMMONLY USED ABBREVIATIONS

ABGs	arterial blood gases
ac	before meals
ACE	angiotensin converting enzyme
AD	right ear
ADD	attention deficit disorder
AIDS	acquired immune deficiency syndrome
ANC	absolute neutrophil count
AS	left ear
AU	both ears
bid	two times a day
BP	blood pressure
c̄	with
cap	capsule
CBC	complete blood count
CNS	central nervous system
COPD	chronic obstructive pulmonary disease
CR	controlled-release
CSF	colony-stimulating factor; cerebrospinal fluid
CV	cardiovascular
CVP	central venous pressure
D5/LR	5% dextrose and lactated Ringer's solution
D5/0.9% NaCl	5% dextrose and 0.9% NaCl; 5% dextrose and normal saline
D5/0.25% NaCl	5% dextrose and 0.25% NaCl; 5% dextrose and quarter normal saline
D5/0.45% NaCl	5% dextrose and 0.45% NaCl; 5% dextrose and half normal saline
D5W	5% dextrose in water
D10W	10% dextrose in water
Derm	dermatologic
dl	deciliter
DNA	deoxyribonucleic acid
ECG	electrocardiogram
EENT	eye, ear, nose, and throat
Endo	endocrinologic
ER	extended-release
F and E	fluid and electrolyte
g	gram(s)
GERD	gastroesophageal reflux disease
GI	gastrointestinal
gr	grain(s)
G6-PD	glucose-6-phosphate dehydrogenase
gtt	drop(s)
GU	genitourinary
hr(s)	hour(s)

HDL	high-density lipoproteins
Hemat	hematologic
HIV	human immunodeficiency virus
hs	hour of sleep (bed time)
IA	intra-articular
IL	intralesional
IM	intramuscular
in	inch(es)
Inhaln	inhalation
IPPB	intermittent positive pressure breathing
IS	intrasynovial
IT	intrathecal
IV	intravenous
IU	international unit
K	potassium
KCl	potassium chloride
kg	kilogram
L	liter
LDL	low-density lipoproteins
LR	lactated Ringer's solution
m	minim
MAO	monoamine oxidase
Metab	metabolic
mcg	microgram(s)
mg	milligram(s)
min(s)	minute(s)
Misc	miscellaneous
ml	milliliter(s)
mon(s)	month(s)
MS	musculoskeletal; morphine sulfate
Na	sodium
NaCl	sodium chloride
0.9% NaCl	0.9% sodium chloride, normal saline
Neuro	neurologic
ng	nanogram(s)
NS	sodium chloride, normal saline (0.9% NaCl)
NSAIAs (or NSAIDs)	nonsteroidal anti-inflammatory agents/drugs
OD	right eye
OCD	obsessive-compulsive disorder
Oint	ointment
Ophth	ophthalmic
OS	left eye
OTC	over-the-counter
OU	both eyes
oz	ounce(s)
pc	after meals
PCA	patient-controlled analgesia
PO	by mouth, orally
prn	as needed
q	every
qd	every day
qh	every hour
qid	four times a day

qod .... every other day
qwk .... every week
q 2 h .... every 2 hours
q 3 h .... every 3 hours
q 4 h .... every 4 hours
RBC .... red blood cell count
Rect .... rectally or rectal
REM .... rapid eye movement
Resp .... respiratory
RNA .... ribonucleic acid
s̄ .... without
SC .... subcutaneous
sec(s) .... second(s)
SL .... sublingual
soln(s) .... solution(s)
SR .... sustained-release
$\overline{ss}$ .... one half
stat .... immediately
supp .... suppository
tab .... tablet
tbs .... tablespoon(s)
tid .... three times a day
Top .... topically or topical
tsp .... teaspoon(s)
UK .... unknown
Vag .... vaginal
VLDL .... very low-density lipoproteins
WBC .... white blood cell count
wk(s) .... week(s)
yr(s) .... year(s)

CLASSIFICATIONS

▪ ALPHA-ADRENERGIC BLOCKING AGENTS

Pharmacologic Profile

General Use: Used in situations of adrenergic (sympathetic) excess such as pheochromocytoma or hypertensive crises associated with excessive sympathomimetic amines (interaction between monoamine oxidase [MAO] inhibitors and foods containing tyramine).

General Action and Information: Alpha-adrenergic blocking agents noncompetitively block alpha-adrenergic receptors, inhibiting the normal excitatory response to epinephrine and norepinephrine. Receptors primarily affected are located in vascular smooth muscle and exocrine glands.

Contraindications: Conditions where a precipitous fall in blood pressure could be dangerous.

Precautions: Cardiovascular effects may be severe and require intervention and supportive treatment. Use cautiously in patients with history of peptic ulcer.

Interactions: Any drugs that stimulate alpha-adrenergic receptors will be antagonized. Alpha-adrenergic and beta-adrenergic amines in combination with alpha blockers will result in exaggerated hypotension and arrhythmias.

Nursing Implications

Assessment
- Monitor blood pressure and pulse frequently during initial or IV administration and periodically throughout therapy.

Potential Nursing Diagnoses
- Tissue perfusion, altered (indications).
- Injury, high risk for (side effects).
- Knowledge deficit related to medication regimen (patient/family teaching).

Implementation
- **PO:** May be administered with meals or milk if GI irritation becomes a problem.
- **IV:** Patient should remain supine throughout parenteral administration.

Patient/Family Teaching
- Advise patient to make position changes slowly to minimize orthostatic hypotension.

Evaluation
Effectiveness of therapy can be demonstrated by: ▪ Decrease in blood pressure.

Alpha-adrenergic Blockers Included in *Davis's Drug Guide for Nurses*

phenoxybenzamine, 920
phentolamine, 921

▪ ANESTHETICS/GENERAL AND LOCAL

Pharmacologic Profile

General Use: Ketamine and thiopental are used as intravenous general anesthetic agents. Other agents which have been used alone or as adjuncts include diazepam, midazolam, propofol, and droperidol/fentanyl. Benzocaine, dibucaine, and lidocaine are available in a variety of dosage forms for local use.

General Action and Information: General anesthetics provide sufficient CNS depression to allow invasive procedures and are frequently used with sedative/hypnotics, narcotic analgesics, and neuromuscular blocking agents. Local anesthetics produce limited and brief effects by decreasing nerve transmission only in the area of injection or application; used in situations when generalized CNS depression is not warranted.

Contraindications: Hypersensitivity.

Precautions: General anesthesia requires skilled personnel and facilities to support respiration. Choose agents and doses carefully in pediatric, geriatric, cardiac, and obstetrical patients. Cross-sensitivity may exist for local anesthetics.

Interactions: Many general anesthetics increase cardiac irritability. Risk of arrhythmias may be increased by concurrent cardiac glycoside, beta blocker, or antiarrhythmic therapy. Degree of respiratory depression may be increased by concurrent use of sedative/hypnotics, narcotic analgesics, antihistamines, or antidepressants. Concurrent injection of epinephrine with local anesthetics helps to localize and prolong effects.

Nursing Implications—General Anesthetics

Assessment
- Assess level of consciousness frequently throughout therapy.
- Monitor blood pressure, ECG, and respiratory status frequently throughout therapy.

Potential Nursing Diagnoses
- Injury, high risk for (side effects).
- Knowledge deficit related to medication regimen (patient/family teaching).

Implementation
- Administer on an empty stomach to prevent vomiting and aspiration.

Patient/Family Teaching
- Psychomotor impairment may last for 24 hr following anesthesia. Caution patient to avoid driving or other activities requiring alertness until response to medication is known.
- Advise patient to avoid alcohol or other CNS depressants for 24 hr following anesthesia.

Evaluation
Effectiveness of therapy can be demonstrated by: ▪ General anesthesia.

Nursing Implications—Local Anesthetics

Assessment
- Assess type, location, and intensity of pain or feeling prior to and a few minutes following administration.
- Assess integrity of involved skin and mucous membranes prior to and periodically throughout course of therapy.

Potential Nursing Diagnoses
- Comfort, altered: pain (indications).
- Knowledge deficit related to medication regimen (patient/family teaching).

Implementation
- **Throat Spray:** Ensure gag reflex is intact before allowing patient to eat or drink.
- **Infiltration:** Lidocaine may be combined with epinephrine to minimize systemic absorption and prolong local anesthesia.

Patient/Family Teaching
- Instruct patient on correct application technique. Emphasize the need to avoid contact with the eyes.
- Advise patient to discontinue use if erythema, rash, or irritation at site of administration occurs.

Evaluation
Effectiveness of therapy can be demonstrated by: ▪ Temporary relief of discomfort associated with minor irritations of the skin or mucous membranes ▪ Local anesthesia.

Anesthetics Included in *Davis's Drug Guide for Nurses*

general anesthetics/adjuncts

diazepam, 348
droperidol/fentanyl, 415
ketamine, 641
midazolam, 775
propofol, 1004
thiopental, 1122

local anesthetics

benzocaine, 108
dibucaine, 353
lidocaine, 667

▪ ANTACIDS

Pharmacologic Profile

General Use: Antacids are used as adjunctive therapy in the treatment of peptic ulcers. They are also useful in the treatment of other types of gastric hyperacidity, indigestion, and gastroesophageal reflux disease (GERD).

General Action and Information: Antacids are capable of partially neutralizing gastric acid. They do not coat the stomach lining. The most commonly used antacids contain a mixture of aluminum and magnesium salts formulated to minimize GI side effects (aluminum causes constipation; magnesium causes diarrhea). In addition, many contain simethicone, an antiflatulent.

Contraindications: Abdominal pain of unknown cause especially if accompanied by fever.

Precautions: Antacids containing magnesium should be used cautiously in patients with renal insufficiency.

Interactions: Antacids may alter the absorption of drugs administered concurrently. Antacids decrease the absorption of tetracyclines (except doxycycline and minocycline), fluoroquinolones, mexiletine, isoniazid, and digoxin. If sufficient antacid is ingested to alkalinize the urine, the excretion of quinidine, flecainide, or amphetamines is markedly reduced and may lead to toxicity.

Nursing Implications

Assessment
- Assess for heartburn and indigestion as well as the location, duration, character, and precipitating factors of gastric pain.

Potential Nursing Diagnoses
- Comfort, altered: pain (indications).
- Knowledge deficit related to medication regimen (patient/family teaching).

Implementation
- Antacids cause premature dissolution and absorption of enteric-coated tablets and may interfere with absorption of other oral medications. Separate administration of antacids and other oral medications by at least 1 hr.
- Shake liquid preparations well before pouring. Follow administration with water to assure passage to stomach. Liquid and powder dosage forms are considered to be more effective than tablets.
- Chewable tablets must be chewed thoroughly before swallowing. Follow with ½ glass of water.
- Administer 1 and 3 hr after meals and at bedtime for maximum antacid effect.

Patient/Family Teaching
- Caution patient to consult physician before taking antacids for more than 2 wk or if problem is recurring. Advise patient to consult physician if relief is not obtained or if symptoms of gastric bleeding (black, tarry stools, coffee-ground emesis) occur.

Evaluation
Effectiveness of therapy can be demonstrated by: ▪ Decrease in GI pain and irritation ▪ Increase in the pH of gastric secretions.

Antacids Included in *Davis's Drug Guide for Nurses*

aluminum hydroxide, 30
calcium carbonate, 150
magaldrate, 689
magnesium hydroxide, 692
magnesium hydroxide/aluminum hydroxide, 693
sodium bicarbonate, 1056

▪ ANTIANEMICS

Pharmacologic Profile

General Uses: Prevention and treatment of anemias.

General Action and Information: Iron (ferrous fumarate, ferrous gluconate, ferrous sulfate, iron dextran) is required for production of hemoglobin, which is necessary for oxygen transport to cells. Cyanocobalamin (vitamin B_{12}) and folic acid (vitamin B_9) are water-soluble vitamins that are required for red blood cell production.

Contraindications: Undiagnosed anemias. Hemochromatosis, hemosiderosis, hemolytic anemia (iron).

Precautions: Use parenteral iron cautiously in patients with a history of allergy or hypersensitivity reactions.

Interactions: Iron can decrease the absorption of tetracycline, fluoroquinolones, or penicillamine. Vitamin E may impair the therapeutic response to iron. Phenytoin and other anticonvulsants may decrease the absorption of folic acid.

Nursing Implications

Assessment
- Assess patient's nutritional status and dietary history to determine possible cause of anemia and need for patient teaching.
- **Lab Test Considerations:** Monitor hemoglobin, hematocrit, reticulocyte, and indices values before and periodically throughout therapy.

Potential Nursing Diagnoses
- Activity intolerance (indications).
- Nutrition, altered: less than body requirement (indications).
- Knowledge deficit related to medication regimen (patient/family teaching).

Implementation
- Available in combination with many vitamins and minerals (see Appendix A).

Patient/Family Teaching
- Encourage patients to comply with diet recommendations of physician. Explain that the best source of vitamins and minerals is a well-balanced diet with foods from the 4 basic food groups.
- Patients self-medicating with vitamin and mineral supplements should be cautioned not to exceed RDA (see Appendix L). The effectiveness of megadoses for treatment of various medical conditions is unproven and may cause side effects.

Evaluation
Clinical response is indicated by: ▪ Resolution of anemia.

Antianemics Included in *Davis's Drug Guide for Nurses*

▪ ANTIANGINALS

Pharmacologic Profile

General Uses: Nitrates are used to treat and prevent attacks of angina. Only nitrates (sublingual, lingual spray, or intravenous) may be used in the acute treatment of attacks of angina pectoris. Calcium channel blockers and beta-adrenergic blockers are used prophylactically in long-term management of angina.

General Action and Information: Several different groups of medications are used in the treatment of angina pectoris. The nitrates (isosorbide dinitrate and nitroglycerin) are available as a lingual spray, sublingual tablets, parenterals, transdermal systems, and sustained-release oral dosage forms. Nitrates dilate coronary arteries and cause systemic vasodilation (decreased preload). Calcium channel blockers dilate coronary arteries. Beta-adrenergic blocking agents decrease myocardial oxygen consumption via a decrease in heart rate. Therapy may be combined if selection is designed to minimize side effects or adverse reactions.

Contraindications: Hypersensitivity. Avoid use of beta blockers or calcium channel blockers in advanced heart block, cardiogenic shock, or untreated congestive heart failure.

Precautions: Beta-adrenergic blockers should be used cautiously in patients with diabetes mellitus, pulmonary disease, or hypothyroidism.

Interactions: Nitrates, calcium channel blockers, and beta-adrenergic blockers may cause hypotension with other antihypertensive agents or acute ingestion of alcohol. Verapamil, diltiazem, and beta-adrenergic blockers may have additive myocardial depressant effects when used with other agents which affect cardiac function.

Nursing Implications

Assessment
- Assess location, duration, intensity, and precipitating factors of patient's anginal pain.
- Monitor blood pressure and pulse periodically throughout therapy.

Potential Nursing Diagnoses
- Comfort, altered: pain (indications).
- Tissue perfusion, altered (indications).
- Knowledge deficit related to medication regimen (patient/family teaching).

Implementation
- Available in various dose forms. See specific drugs for information on administration.

Patient/Family Teaching
- Instruct patient on concurrent nitrate therapy and prophylactic antianginal agents to continue taking both medications as ordered and using SL nitroglycerin as needed for anginal attacks.
- Advise patient to contact physician immediately if chest pain does not improve, worsens after therapy, or is accompanied by diaphoresis or shortness of breath, or if severe, persistent headache occurs.
- Caution patient to make position changes slowly to minimize orthostatic hypotension.
- Advise patient to avoid concurrent use of alcohol with these medications.

Evaluation
Effectiveness of therapy can be demonstrated by: ▪ Decrease in frequency and severity of anginal attacks ▪ Increase in activity tolerance.

Antianginals Included in *Davis's Drug Guide for Nurses*

▪ ANTIARRHYTHMICS

Pharmacologic Profile

General Use: Suppression of cardiac arrhythmias.

General Action and Information: Correct cardiac arrhythmias by a variety of mechanisms, depending on the group used. The therapeutic goal is decreased symtomatology and increased hemodynamic performance. Choice of agent depends on etiology of arrhythmia and individual patient characteristics. Treatable causes of arrhythmias should be corrected before therapy is initiated (e.g., electrolyte disturbances). Major antiarrhythmics are generally classified by their effects on cardiac conduction tissue (see Table below). Adenosine, atropine, cardiac glycosides (digitoxin, digoxin), edrophonium, and isoproterenol are also used as antiarrhythmics.

MECHANISM OF ACTION OF MAJOR ANTIARRHYTHMIC DRUGS

TYPE/CLASS	DRUGS	MECHANISM
I	moricizine	Shares properties of IA, IB and IC agents
IA	quinidine, procainamide, disopyramide	Depress Na conductance, increase APD and ERP, decrease membrane responsiveness
IB	tocainide, lidocaine, phenytoin, mexiletine	Increase K conductance, decrease APD and ERP
IC	flecainide, propafenone	Profound slowing of conduction, markedly depress phase O
II	acebutolol, esmolol, propranolol	Interfere with Na conductance, depress cell membrane, decrease automaticity and increase ERP of the AV node, block excess sympathetic activity
III	amiodarone, bretylium	Interfere with norepinephrine, increase APD and ERP
IV	diltiazem, verapamil	Increase AV nodal ERP, Ca channel blocker

Na = sodium; K = potassium; Ca = calcium; ERP = effective refractory period; APD = action-potential duration.

Contraindications: Differ greatly among various agents. See individual drugs.

Precautions: Differ greatly among agents used. Appropriate dosage adjustments should be made in the elderly and those with renal or hepatic impairment, depending on agent chosen. See individual drugs.

Interactions: Differ greatly among agents used. See individual drugs.

Nursing Implications

Assessment
- Monitor ECG, pulse, and blood pressure continuously throughout IV administration and periodically throughout oral administration.

Potential Nursing Diagnoses
- Cardiac output, decreased (indications).
- Knowledge deficit related to medication regimen (patient/family teaching).

Implementation
- Take apical pulse before administration of oral doses. Withhold dose and notify physician if heart rate is <50 bpm.
- Administer oral doses with a full glass of water. Sustained-release preparations should be swallowed whole. Do not crush, break, or chew tablets or open capsules.

Patient/Family Teaching
- Instruct patient to take oral doses around the clock, as directed, even if feeling better.
- Instruct patient or family member on how to take pulse. Advise patient to report changes in pulse rate or rhythm to physician.
- Caution patient to avoid taking over-the-counter medications without consulting physician or pharmacist.
- Advise patient to carry identification describing disease process and medication regimen at all times.
- Emphasize the importance of follow-up examinations to monitor progress.

Evaluation
Effectiveness of therapy can be demonstrated by: ▪ Resolution of cardiac arrhythmias without detrimental side effects.

Antiarrhythmics Included in *Davis's Drug Guide for Nurses*

▪ ANTICHOLINERGICS

Pharmacologic Profile

General Uses: Atropine—Bradyarrhythmias. **Scopolamine**—Nausea and vomiting related to motion sickness and vertigo. **Propantheline and glycopyrrolate**—Decreasing gastric secretory activity and increasing esophageal sphincter tone. **Benztropine and trihexyphenidyl**—Management of dyskinesias, including the Parkinsonian syndrome. Atropine, scopolamine, and cyclopentolate are also used as ophthalmic mydriatics.

General Action and Information: Competitively inhibit the action of acetylcholine. In addition, atropine, glycopyrrolate, propantheline, and scopolamine are antimuscarinic in that they inhibit the action of acetylcholine at sites innervated by postganglionic cholinergic nerves.

Contraindications: Hypersensitivity, narrow-angle glaucoma, severe hemorrhage, tachycardia (due to thyrotoxicosis or cardiac insufficiency), or myasthenia gravis.

Precautions: Elderly and pediatric patients are more susceptible to adverse effects. Use cautiously in patients with urinary tract pathology, those at risk for GI obstruction, and those with chronic renal, hepatic, pulmonary, or cardiac disease.

Interactions: Additive anticholinergic effects (dry mouth, dry eyes, blurred vision, constipation) with other agents possessing anticholinergic activity, including antihistamines, antidepressants, quinidine, and disopyramide. May alter GI absorption of other drugs by inhibiting GI motility and increasing transit time. Antacids may decrease absorption of anticholinergics.

Nursing Implications

Assessment

- Assess vital signs and ECG tracings frequently during the course of IV drug therapy. Report any significant changes in heart rate or blood pressure, or increased ventricular ectopy or angina to physician promptly.
- Monitor intake and output ratios in elderly or surgical patients; may cause urinary retention.
- Assess patient regularly for abdominal distension and auscultate for bowel sounds. Constipation may become a problem. Increasing fluids and adding bulk to the diet may help alleviate constipation.

Potential Nursing Diagnosis

- Cardiac output, decreased (indications).
- Oral mucous membrance, altered (side effects).
- Bowel elimination, altered: constipation (side effects).

Implementation

- **PO:** Administer oral doses of atropine, glycopyrrolate, propantheline, or scopolamine 30 min before meals. Benztropine and trihexyphenidyl should be administered with or immediately after meals.

Patient/Family Teaching

- **General Info:** Instruct patient that frequent rinses, sugarless gum or candy, and good oral hygiene may help relieve dry mouth.
- May cause drowsiness. Caution patient to avoid driving or other activities requiring alertness until response to medication is known.
- **Ophth:** Advise patients that ophthalmic preparations may temporarily blur vision and impair ability to judge distances. Dark glasses may be needed to protect eyes from bright light.

Evaluation

Effectiveness of therapy can be demonstrated by: ▪ Increase in heart rate ▪ Decrease in nausea and vomiting related to motion sickness or vertigo ▪ Dryness of mouth ▪ Dilation of pupils ▪ Decrease in GI motility ▪ Resolution of signs and symptoms of Parkinson's disease.

Anticholinergics included in *Davis's Drug Guide for Nurses*

atropine, 86
benztropine, 111
cyclopentolate (ophth only), 305
glycopyrrolate, 543
propantheline, 1002
scopolamine, 1047
trihexyphenidyl, 1169

▪ ANTICOAGULANTS/ANTIPLATELET AGENTS

Pharmacologic Profile

General Uses: Prevention and treatment of thromboembolic disorders including deep vein thrombosis, pulmonary embolism, and atrial fibrillation with embolization. Antiplatelet agents are used in a variety of settings to prevent thromboembolic events including stroke and myocardial infarction. Aspirin is used to prevent strokes and myocardial infarction. Dipyridamole is commonly used after cardiac surgery. Ticlopidine is used to prevent thrombotic strokes.

General Action and Information: Anticoagulants are used to prevent clot extension and formation. They do not dissolve clots. The two types of anticoagulants in common use are parenteral heparin and oral warfarin. Therapy is usually initiated with heparin because of its rapid onset of action, while maintenance therapy consists of warfarin. Warfarin takes several days to produce therapeutic anticoagulation. In serious or severe thromboembolic events, heparin therapy may be preceded by thrombolytic therapy (alteplase, anistreplase, streptokinase, or urokinase). Other agents, including aspirin, dipyridamole, and ticlopidine may be considered as anticoagulants because of their antiplatelet activity.

Contraindications: Underlying coagulation disorders, ulcer disease, malignancy, recent surgery, or active bleeding.

Precautions: Anticoagulation should be undertaken cautiously in any patient with a potential site for bleeding. Pregnant or lactating patients should not receive warfarin. Heparin does not cross the placenta.

Interactions: Oral anticoagulants are highly protein-bound and may displace or be displaced by other highly protein-bound drugs. The resultant interactions depend on which drug is displaced. Bleeding may be potentiated by aspirin or large doses of penicillins or penicillin-like drugs, cefamandole, cefotetan, cefoperazone, moxalactam, plicamycin, or valproic acid.

Nursing Implications

Assessment

- Assess patient for signs of bleeding and hemorrhage (bleeding gums, nose bleed, unusual bruising; tarry, black stools, hematuria, fall in hematocrit or blood pressure; guaiac-positive stools, urine, or nasogastric aspirate).
- Assess patient for evidence of additional or increased thrombosis. Symptoms will depend on area of involvement.
- **Lab Test Considerations:** Monitor activated partial thromboplastin time (aPTT) with heparin therapy, prothrombin time (PT) with warfarin therapy, and hematocrit and other clotting factors frequently during therapy.
- **Toxicity and Overdose:** If overdose occurs or anticoagulation needs to be immediately reversed, the antidote for heparin is protamine sulfate; for warfarin the antidote is vitamin K [phytonadione (AquaMEPHYTON)]. Administration of whole blood or plasma may also be required in severe bleeding due to warfarin because of the delayed onset of vitamin K.

Potential Nursing Diagnoses

- Tissue perfusion, altered (indications).
- Injury, high risk for (side effects).
- Knowledge deficit related to medication regimen (patient/family teaching).

Implementation

- Inform all personnel caring for patient of anticoagulant therapy. Venipunctures and injection sites require application of pressure to prevent bleeding or hematoma formation.
- Use an infusion pump with continuous infusions to ensure accurate dosage.

Patient/Family Teaching

- Caution patient to avoid activities leading to injury, to use a soft tooth brush and electric razor, and to report any symptoms of unusual bleeding or bruising to physician immediately.
- Instruct patient not to take over-the-counter medications, especially those containing aspirin, or alcohol without advice of physician or pharmacist.
- Review foods high in vitamin K (see Appendix K) with patients on warfarin. Patient should have consistent limited intake of these foods as vitamin K is the antidote for warfarin and alternating intake of these foods will cause PT levels to fluctuate.
- Emphasize the importance of frequent lab tests to monitor coagulation factors.
- Instruct patient to carry identification describing medication regimen at all times and to inform all health care personnel caring for patient of anticoagulant therapy before laboratory tests, treatment, or surgery.

Evaluation

Clinical response can be evaluated by: ▪ Prevention of undesired clotting without signs of hemorrhage.

Anticoagulants Included in *Davis's Drug Guide for Nurses*

anticoagulants	***antiplatelet agents***
heparin, 565	aspirin, 79
warfarin, 1203	ticlopidine, 1138

▪ ANTICONVULSANTS

Pharmacologic Profile

General Uses: See Table below.

General Action and Information: Anticonvulsants include a variety of agents, all capable of depressing abnormal neuronal discharges in the CNS that may result in seizures. They may work by preventing the spread of seizure activity, depressing the motor cortex, raising seizure threshold, or altering levels of neurotransmitters, depending on the group. See individual drugs.

MAJOR ANTICONVULSANT CLASSES, DRUGS, AND MOST COMMON USES

CLASS	DRUGS	TYPE OF SEIZURE CONTROLLED
Barbiturates	amobarbital	status epilepticus
	phenobarbital	Tonic-clonic seizures, partial seizures, prophylaxis of febrile seizures
	primidone	Prophylaxis of partial seizures with complex symptomatology
Benzodiazepines	clonazepam	Absence seizures, akinetic seizures, myoclonic seizures
	clorazepate	Partial seizures
	diazepam (IV)	Status epilepticus, tonic-clonic seizures
Hydantoins	phenytoin	Tonic-clonic seizures, partial seizures with complex symptomatology
Succinimides	ethosuximide	Absence seizures
Miscellaneous	acetazolamide	Refractory seizures
	carbamazepine	Tonic-clonic seizures, complex partial seizures, mixed seizures
	magnesium sulfate	Eclamptic seizures
	valproates	Simple and complex partial seizures

Contraindications: Previous hypersensitivity.

Precautions: Use cautiously in patients with severe hepatic or renal disease; dosage adjustment may be required. Choose agents carefully in pregnant and lactating women. Fetal hydantoin syndrome may occur in offspring of patients who receive phenytoin during pregnancy.

Interactions: Barbiturates stimulate the metabolism of other drugs that are metabolized by the liver, decreasing their effectiveness. Hydantoins are highly protein-bound and may displace or be displaced by other highly protein-bound drugs. For more specific interactions, see individual drugs. Many drugs are capable of lowering seizure threshold and may decrease the effectiveness of anticonvulsants, including tricyclic antidepressants and phenothiazines.

Nursing Implications

Assessment

- Assess location, duration, and characteristics of seizure activity.
- **Toxicity and Overdose:** Monitor serum drug levels routinely throughout anticonvulsant therapy.

Potential Nursing Diagnoses

- Injury, high risk for (indications, side effects).
- Knowledge deficit related to medication regimen (patient/family teaching).

Implementation

- Administer anticonvulsants around-the-clock. Abrupt discontinuation may precipitate status epilepticus.
- Implement seizure precautions.

Patient/Family Teaching

- Instruct patient to take medication every day, exactly as directed.
- May cause drowiness. Caution patient to avoid driving or other activities requiring alertness until response to medication is known. Do not resume driving until physician gives clearance based on control of seizures.
- Advise patient to avoid taking alcohol or other CNS depressants concurrently with these medications.
- Advise patient to carry identification describing disease process and medication regimen at all times.

Evaluation

Effectiveness of therapy can be demonstrated by: ▪ Decrease or cessation of seizures without excessive sedation.

Anticonvulsants Included in *Davis's Drug Guide for Nurses*

barbiturates

amobarbital, 50
phenobarbital, 915
primidone, 980
thiopental, 1122

benzodiazepines

clonazepam, 267
clorazepate, 271
diazepam, 348

hydantoins

phenytoin, 927

succinamides

ethosuximide, 460

valproates

valproic acid, 1181
divalproex sodium, 1181

miscellaneous

acetazolamide, 4
carbamazepine, 164
magnesium sulfate, 695

▪ ANTIDEPRESSANTS

Pharmacologic Profile

General Uses: Used in the treatment of various forms of endogenous depression, often in conjunction with psychotherapy. Other uses include: ▫ Treatment of anxiety (doxepin) ▫ Enuresis (imipramine) ▫ Chronic pain syndromes (amitriptyline, doxepin, imipramine, and nortriptyline).

General Action and Information: Antidepressant activity most likely due to preventing the reuptake of dopamine, norepinephrine, and serotonin by presynaptic neurons resulting in accumulation of these neurotransmitters. Most possess significant anticholinergic and sedative properties, which explain many of their side effects (except bupropion and fluoxetine).

Contraindications: Hypersensitivity. Should not be used in narrow-angle glaucoma. Should not be used in pregnancy or lactation, or immediately after myocardial infarction.

Precautions: Use cautiously in older patients and those with pre-existing cardiovascular disease. Elderly males with prostatic enlargement may be more susceptible to urinary retention. Anticholinergic side effects (dry eyes, dry mouth, blurred vision, and constipation) may require dosage modification or drug discontinuation. Dosage requires slow titration; onset of therapeutic response may be 2–4 wk. May decrease seizure threshold, especially bupropion.

Interactions: Tricyclic antidepressants—May cause hypertension, tachycardia, and convulsions when used with monoamine oxidase (MAO) inhibitors. May prevent therapeutic response to some antihypertensives. Additive CNS depression with other CNS depressants. Sympathomimetic activity may be enhanced when used with other sympathomimetics. Additive anticholinergic effects with other drugs possessing anticholinergic properties. **MAO inhibitors**—Hypertensive crisis may occur with concurrent use of MAO inhibitors and amphetamines, methyldopa, levodopa, dopamine, epinephrine, norepinephrine, desipramine, imipramine, guanethidine, reserpine, vasoconstrictors, or ingestion of tyramine-containing foods. Hypertension or hypotension, coma, convulsions, and death may occur with meperidine or other narcotic analgesics and MAO inhibitors. Additive hypotension with antihypertensives or spinal anesthesia and MAO inhibitors. Additive hypoglycemia with insulin or oral hypoglycemic agents and MAO inhibitors. Neither fluoxetine nor bupropion should be used in combination with MAO inhibitors.

Nursing Implications

Assessment

- Monitor mental status and affect. Assess for suicidal tendencies, especially during early therapy. Restrict amount of drug available to patient.
- **Toxicity and Overdose:** Concurrent ingestion of monamine oxidase inhibitors and tyramine-containing foods may lead to hypertensive crisis. Symptoms include chest pain, severe headache, nuchal rigidity, nausea and vomiting, photosensitivity, and enlarged pupils. Treatment includes IV phentolamine.

Potential Nursing Diagnoses

- Coping, ineffective individual (indications).
- Injury, high risk for (side effects).
- Knowledge deficit related to medication regimen (patient/family teaching).

Implementation

- Administer drugs which are sedating at bedtime to avoid excessive drowsiness during waking hours and drugs which cause insomnia (fluoxetine, monamine oxidase inhibitors) in the morning. Bupropion must be given in divided doses.

Patient/Family Teaching

- Caution patient to avoid alcohol and other CNS depressants. Patients receiving monamine oxidase inhibitors should also avoid over-the-counter drugs, and foods or beverages containing tyramine (see Appendix K for foods included) during and for at least 2 wk after therapy has been discontinued, as they may precipitate a hypertensive crisis. Physician should be contacted immediately if symptoms of hypertensive crisis develop.
- Inform patient that dizziness or drowiness may occur. Caution patient to avoid driving and other activities requiring alertness until response to the drug is known.
- Caution patient to make position changes slowly to minimize orthostatic hypotension.
- Advise patient to notify physician if dry mouth, urinary retention, or constipation occurs. Frequent rinses, good oral hygiene, and sugarless candy or gum

may diminish dry mouth. An increase in fluid intake, fiber, and exercise may prevent constipation.

- Advise patient to notify physician or dentist of medication regimen before treatment or surgery. Monamine oxidase inhibitor therapy usually needs to be withdrawn at least 2 wk before use of anesthetic agents.
- Emphasize the importance of participation in psychotherapy and follow-up examinations to evaluate progress.

EVALUATION

Effectiveness of therapy can be demonstrated by: ▪ Resolution of depression ▪ Decrease in anxiety ▪ Control of bedwetting in children over 6 yrs of age ▪ Management of chronic neurogenic pain.

Antidepressants Included in *Davis's Drug Guide for Nurses*

tricyclic antidepressants	***miscellaneous antidepressants***	***monoamine oxidase (MAO) inhibitors***
amitriptyline, 48	bupropion, 137	isocarboxazid, 793
amoxapine, 52	fluoxetine, 509	phenelzine, 793
doxepin, 404	maprotiline, 699	tranylcypromine, 793
imipramine, 603	trazadone, 1158	
nortriptyline, 851		

▪ ANTIDIABETIC AGENTS

Pharmacologic Profile

General Use: Insulin is used in the management of insulin-dependent diabetes mellitus (IDDM, type I, juvenile-onset, ketosis-prone). It may also be used in adult-onset noninsulin-dependent diabetes mellitus (NIDDM, type II, adult-onset, nonketosis-prone) when diet and/or oral hypoglycemic therapy fails to adequately control blood sugar. The choice of insulin preparation (rapid-acting, intermediate-acting, long-acting) and source (beef, beef/pork, pork, semisynthetic, human-recombinant DNA) depend upon the degree of control desired, daily blood sugar fluctuations, and history of previous reactions. Oral hypoglycemics can only be used in adult-onset noninsulin-dependent diabetes mellitus (NIDDM, type II, adult-onset, nonketosis-prone). Oral agents are used when diet therapy alone fails to control blood sugar or symptoms.

General Action and Information: Insulin, a hormone produced by the pancreas, lowers blood glucose by increasing transport of glucose into cells and promotes the conversion of glucose to glycogen. It also promotes the conversion of amino acids to proteins in muscle, stimulates triglyceride formation, and inhibits the release of free fatty acids. Oral hypoglycemic agents lower blood sugar by stimulating endogenous insulin secretion by beta cells of the pancreas, and by increasing sensitivity to insulin at intracellular receptor sites. Intact pancreatic function is required for oral agents. Chemically, oral hypoglycemics are referred to as sulfonylureas.

Contraindications: Insulin—Hypoglycemia. **Oral hypoglycemic agents**—Hypersensitivity. Hypoglycemia. Cross-sensitivity with other sulfonylureas and sulfonamides may exist. Contraindicated in insulin-dependent diabetes mellitus (IDDM, type I, juvenile-onset, brittle, ketosis-prone). Avoid use in patients with severe kidney, liver, thyroid, and other endocrine dysfunction. Should not be used in pregnancy or lactation.

Precautions: Insulin—Infection, stress, or changes in diet may alter requirements. **Oral hypoglycemic agents**—Use cautiously in the elderly—dosage reduction may be necessary. Infection, stress, or changes in diet may alter requirements. Use with caution in patients with a history of cardiovascular disease.

Interactions: Insulin—Additive hypoglycemic effects with oral hypoglycemic agents. **Oral hypoglycemic agents**—Ingestion of alcohol may result in disulfiram-like reaction. Alcohol, glucocorticoids, rifampin, glucagon, and thiazide diuretics may decrease effectiveness. Anabolic steroids, chloramphenicol, clofibrate, MAO inhibitors, nonsteroidal anti-inflammatory agents, salicylates, sulfonamides, and oral anticoagulants may increase hypoglycemic effect. Beta-adrenergic blocking agents may produce hypoglycemia and mask signs and symptoms.

Nursing Implications

Assessment
- Observe patient for signs and symptoms of hypoglycemic reactions.

Potential Nursing Diagnoses
- Nutrition, altered: more than body requirements (indications).
- Knowledge deficit related to medication regimen (patient/family teaching).
- Noncompliance (patient/family teaching).

Implementation
- **General Info:** Patients stabilized on a diabetic regimen who are exposed to stress, fever, trauma, infection, or surgery may require sliding scale insulin.
- Patients switching from daily insulin dose may require gradual conversion to oral hypoglycemics.
- **Insulin:** Available in different types and strengths and from different species. Check type, species' source, dose, and expiration date with another licensed nurse. Do not interchange insulins without physician's order. Use only insulin syringes to draw-up dose.

Patient/Family Teaching
- **General Info:** Explain to patient that medication controls hyperglycemia but does not cure diabetes. Therapy is long term.
- Review signs of hypoglycemia and hyperglycemia with patient. If hypoglycemia occurs, advise patient to take a glass of orange juice or 2–3 tsp of sugar, honey, or corn syrup dissolved in water, and notify physician.
- Encourage patient to follow prescribed diet, medication, and exercise regimen to prevent hypoglycemic or hyperglycemic episodes.
- Instruct patient in proper testing of serum glucose or urine glucose and ketones.
- Advise patient to notify physician if nausea, vomiting, or fever develops; if unable to eat usual diet; or if blood sugar levels are not controlled.
- Advise patient to carry sugar and identification describing medication regimen at all times.
- **Insulin:** Instruct patient on proper technique for administration; include type of insulin, equipment (syringe and cartridge pens), storage, and where to discard syringes. Discuss the importance of not changing brands of insulin or syringes, selection and rotation of injection sites, and compliance with therapeutic regimen.

- **Oral Hypoglycemic Agents:** Advise patient that concurrent use of alcohol may cause a disulfiram-like reaction (abdominal cramps, nausea, flushing, headaches, and hypoglycemia).

EVALUATION

Effectiveness of therapy can be demonstrated by: ▪ Control of blood glucose levels without the appearance of hypoglycemic or hyperglycemic episodes.

Antidiabetic Agents Included in *Davis's Drug Guide for Nurses*

oral hypoglycemic agents
- chlorpropamide, 238
- glipizide, 534
- glyburide, 540
- tolazamide, 1147
- tolbutamide, 1151

insulins, 613

rapid-acting insulin
- regular insulin
- prompt zinc suspension

intermediate-acting insulin
- isophane suspension, NPH insulin
- zinc suspension, lente insulin

long-acting insulin
- protamine zinc suspension
- extended zinc suspension, ultra lente insulin

insulin mixture
- regular plus NPH insulin

▪ ANTIDIARRHEALS

Pharmacologic Profile

General Use: For the control and symptomatic relief of acute and chronic nonspecific diarrhea.

General Action and Information: Diphenoxylate/atropine, difenoxin/atropine, loperamide, and paregoric slow intestinal motility and propulsion. Kaolin/pectin and bismuth subsalicylate affect fluid content of the stool. Polycarbophil acts as an antidiarrheal by taking on water within the bowel lumen to create a formed stool. Octreotide is used specifically for diarrhea associated with gastrointestinal endocrine tumors.

Contraindications: Previous hypersensitivity. Severe abdominal pain of unknown cause, especially when associated with fever.

Precautions: Use cautiously in patients with severe liver disease or inflammatory bowel disease. Safety in pregnancy and lactation not established (diphenoxylate/atropine and loperamide). Octreotide may aggravate gall bladder disease.

Interactions: Kaolin may decrease absorption of digoxin. Polycarbophil decreases the absorption of tetracycline. Octreotide may alter the response to insulin or oral hypoglycemic agents.

Nursing Implications

ASSESSMENT
- Assess the frequency and consistency of stools and bowel sounds before and throughout course of therapy.
- Assess patient's fluid and electrolyte status and skin turgor for dehydration.

Potential Nursing Diagnoses
- Bowel elimination, altered: diarrhea (indications).
- Bowel elimination, altered: constipation (side effects).
- Knowledge deficit related to medication regimen (patient/family teaching).

Implementation
- Shake liquid preparations before administration.

Patient/Family Teaching
- Instruct patient to notify physician if diarrhea persists; or if fever, abdominal pain, or palpitations occur.

Evaluation
Effectiveness of therapy can be demonstrated by: ▪ Decrease in diarrhea.

Antidiarrheals Included in *Davis's Drug Guide for Nurses*

▪ ANTIDOTES

Pharmacologic Profile

General Use: See Table below.

General Action and Information: Antidotes are employed in accidental and intentional overdoses of medications or toxic substances. The goal of antidotal therapy is to decrease systemic complications of the overdosage while supporting vital functions. Obtaining a precise history will determine aggressiveness of therapy, choice, and dose of agent. Some antidotes are designed to aid removal of the offending agent before systemic absorption occurs, or speed elimination (activated charcoal). Other agents are more specific and require more detailed history as to type and amount of agent ingested.

POISONS AND SPECIFIC ANTIDOTES

POISON	ANTIDOTE
acetaminophen	acetylcysteine
anticholinesterases	atropine, pralidoxime
cyanide	amyl nitrite, sodium nitrite, sodium thiosulfate
digoxin, digitoxin	digoxin immune Fab
ethylene glycol, methanol	ethanol
heparin	protamine sulfate
iron	deferoxamine
lead	edetate calcium disodium, dimercaprol, succimer
methotrexate	leucovorin calcium
narcotic analgesics, heroin	naloxone
tricyclic antidepressants	physostigmine
warfarin	phytonadione (vitamin K_1)

Contraindications: See individual drugs.

Precautions: See individual drugs.

Interactions: See individual drugs.

Nursing Implications

Assessment

- Inquire as to the type of drug or poison and time of ingestion.
- Consult reference, poison control center, or physician for symptoms of toxicity of ingested agent(s) and antidote. Monitor vital signs, affected systems, and serum levels closely.
- Monitor for suicidal ideation; institute suicide precautions as necessary.

Potential Nursing Diagnosis

- Ineffective coping, individual (indications).
- Injury, high risk for: poisoning (patient/family teaching).
- Knowledge deficit related to medication regimen (patient/family teaching).

Implementation

- May be used in conjunction with induction of emesis or gastric aspiration and lavage, cathartics, agents to modify urine pH, and supportive measures for respiratory and cardiac effects of overdose or poisoning.

Patient/Family Teaching

- When counseling about poisoning in the home, discuss methods of prevention and the need to confer with poison control center, physician, or emergency department prior to administering syrup of ipecac, and the need to bring ingested substance to the hospital for identification. Reinforce need to keep all medications and hazardous substances out of the reach of children.

Evaluation

Effectiveness of therapy is demonstrated by: ▪ Prevention or resolution of toxic side effects of ingested agent.

Antidotes Included in *Davis's Drug Guide for Nurses*

▪ ANTIEMETICS

Pharmacologic Profile

General Use: Phenothiazines, benzquinamide, and metoclopramide are used to manage nausea and vomiting of many etiologies, including surgery, anesthesia, and antineoplastic therapy. Dimenhydrinate, scopolamine, and meclizine are used almost exclusively to prevent motion sickness. Dronabinol and ondansetron are used exclusively for short-term management of nausea and vomiting associated with antineoplastics.

General Action and Information: Agents used in the management of glaucoma decrease intraocular pressure by either decreasing the formation of aqueous humor or increasing the outflow of aqueous humor. Ophthalmic beta blockers and orally administered carbonic anhydrase inhibitors decrease the production of aqueous humor. Direct-acting miotics, cholinesterase inhibitors, and sympathomimetics increase aqueous humor outflow.

Contraindications: Previous hypersensitivity.

Precautions: Use phenothiazines cautiously in children who may have viral illnesses. Choose agents carefully in pregnant patients (no agents are approved for safe use).

Interactions: Additive CNS depression with other CNS depressants including antidepressants, antihistamines, narcotic analgesics, and sedative/hypnotics. Phenothiazines may produce hypotension when used with antihypertensives, nitrates, or acute ingestion of alcohol.

Nursing Implications

Assessment

- Assess nausea, vomiting, bowel sounds, and abdominal pain before and following administration.
- Monitor hydration status and intake and output. Patients with severe nausea and vomiting may require IV fluids in addition to antiemetics.

Potential Nursing Diagnoses

- Fluid volume deficit (indications).
- Nutrition, altered: less than body requirements (indications).
- Injury, high risk for (side effects).

Implementation

- For prophylactic administration, follow directions for specific drugs so that peak effect corresponds to time of anticipated nausea.

Patient/Family Teaching

- Advise patient and family to use general measures to decrease nausea (begin with sips of liquids and small nongreasy meals, provide oral hygiene, and remove noxious stimuli from environment).
- May cause drowiness. Advise patient to call for assistance when ambulating and to avoid driving or other activities requiring alertness until response to medication is known.
- Advise patient to make position changes slowly to minimize orthostatic hypotension.

Evaluation

Effectiveness of therapy can be demonstrated by: ▪ Prevention of, or decrease in, nausea and vomiting.

Antimetics Included in *Davis's Drug Guide for Nurses*

anticholinergic

scopolamine, 1047

antihistamines

cyclizine, 302
dimenhydrinate, 378
meclizine, 705

phenothiazines

chlorpromazine, 235
perphenazine, 911
prochlorperazine, 990
promethazine, 998
thiethylperazine, 1119
trifluoperazine, 1165

miscellaneous

benzquinamide, 109
dronabinol, 411
metoclopramide, 759
ondansetron, 860
trimethobenzamide, 1173

▪ ANTIFUNGALS

Pharmacologic Profile

General Use: Treatment of fungal infections. Infections of skin or mucous membranes may be treated with topical preparations. Deep seated or systemic infections require oral or parenteral therapy.

General Action and Information: Kill (fungicidal) or stop growth of (fungistatic) susceptible fungi by affecting the permeability of the fungal cell membrane or protein synthesis within the fungal cell itself.

Contraindications: Previous hypersensitivity.

Precautions: Since most systemic antifungals may have adverse effects on bone marrow function, use cautiously in patients with depressed bone marrow reserve. Amphotericin B commonly causes renal impairment. Flucytosine and fluconazole require dosage adjustment in the presence of renal impairment. Adverse reactions to fluconazole may be more severe in HIV-positive patients.

Interactions: Differ greatly among various agents. See individual drugs.

Nursing Implications

Assessment

- Assess patient for signs of infection and assess involved areas of skin and mucous membranes before and throughout therapy.

Potential Nursing Diagnoses

- Infection, high risk for (indications).
- Skin integrity, impairment of (indications).
- Knowledge deficit related to medication regimen (patient/family teaching).

Implementation

- **General Info:** Available in various dosage forms. Refer to specific drugs for directions for administration.
- **Top:** Consult physician for cleansing technique before applying medication. Wear gloves during application. Do not use occlusive dressings unless specified by physician.

Patient/Family Teaching

- Instruct patient on proper use of medication form.
- Advise patient to report increased skin irritation or lack of therapeutic response to physician.

Evaluation

Effectiveness of therapy can be demonstrated by: ▪ Resolution of signs and symptoms of infection. Length of time for complete resolution depends on organism and site of infection. Deep seated fungal infections may require prolonged therapy (wks–mons).

Antifungals Included in *Davis's Drug Guide for Nurses*

systemic antifungals

amphotericin B, 60
fluconazole, 496
flucytosine, 498
griseofulvin, 551
ketoconazole, 463
miconazole, 773

topical antifungals

clotrimazole, 273
econazole, 421
ketoconazole, 463
miconazole, 773
naftifine, 812
natamycin, 822
nystatin, 853
oxiconazole, 865
terconazole, 1106
tioconazole, 1142

▪ ANTIGLAUCOMA AGENTS

Pharmacologic Profile

General Use: Management of glaucoma. Open-angle glaucoma is usually treated with medications. Other forms of glaucoma may require surgery.

General Action and Information: Agents used in the management of glaucoma decrease intraocular pressure by either decreasing the formation of aqueous humor or increasing the outflow of aqueous humor. Ophthalmic beta blockers and orally administered carbonic anhydrase inhibitors decrease the production of aqueous humor. Direct-acting miotics, cholinesterase inhibitors, and sympathomimetics increase aqueous humor outflow.

Contraindications: Avoid use in patients with hypersensitivity to medications themselves, additives, or preservatives. Miotics should be avoided in patients with narrow-angle glaucoma.

Precautions: Use cautiously in patients with underlying cardiovascular disease, diabetes mellitus, or severe pulmonary disease.

Interactions: Beta blockers and carbonic anhydrase inhibitors have additive effects on intraocular pressure with other agents. Miotics and sympathomimetics also have additive effects and are frequently used together. Cholinesterase inhibitors may prolong the action of neuromuscular blocking agents.

Nursing Implications

Assessment

- Monitor patient for changes in vision, eye irritation, and peristent headache.
- Monitor patient for signs of systemic side effects. Notify physician if these signs occur.

Potential Nursing Diagnoses
- Sensory-perceptual alteration: visual (indications, side effects).
- Knowledge deficit related to medication regimen (patient/family teaching).

Implementation
- When instilling eyedrops, have patient tilt head back, pull down on the lower lid, and instill drops into the conjunctival sac. Apply pressure to the inner canthus for one minute following instillation to prevent systemic absorption.

Patient/Family Teaching
- Instruct patient to take as directed and not to discontinue without physician's approval. Lifelong therapy may be required.
- Instruct patient on correct technique for administration of ophthalmic medication. Emphasize the importance of not touching tip of container to eye, finger, or any other surface, and of preventing systemic absorption by placing pressure on the inner canthus.
- Explain to patient that temporary stinging and blurring of vision may occur. Physician should be notified if blurred vision or brow ache persist.
- Caution patient that night vision may be impaired. Advise patient not to drive at night until response to medication is known. To prevent injury at night, patient should use a night-light and keep environment uncluttered.
- Advise patient of the need for regular eye examinations to monitor intraocular pressure and visual fields.

Evaluation
Effectiveness of therapy can be demonstrated by: ▪ Control of elevated intraocular pressure.

Antiglaucoma Agents Included in *Davis's Drug Guide for Nurses*

beta blockers (ophthalmic)
betaxolol, 117
levobunolol, 658
metipranolol, 757
timolol, 1139

carbonic anhydrase inhibitors
acetazolamide, 4
methazolamide, 734

miotic (cholinesterase inhibitors)
demecarium, 330
echothiophate, 419
physostigmine, 932

miotics (direct-acting)
carbachol, 163
pilocarpine, 936

sympathomimetics
apraclonidine, 73
epinephrine, 430

miscellaneous
glycerin, 542

▪ ANTIGOUT AGENTS

Pharmacologic Profile

General Use: In the treatment of active gout (colchicine) and prevention of recurrent attacks (allopurinol, probenecid). Allopurinol and probenecid are also used to treat secondary hyperuricemia.

General Action and Information: Reduce the inflammatory response (colchicine), or lower serum uric acid either by enhancing its renal excretion (probenecid, sulfinpyrazone) or decreasing its production (allopurinol). Sulfinpyarazone also has antiplatelet activity.

Contraindications: Hypersensitivity. Allopurinol should be avoided during acute attacks of gout.

Precautions: Akalinizing the urine enhances uricosuric effects. Rapid lowering of uric acid may cause precipitation of urate cystals in soft tissue.

Interactions: Probenecid promotes reabsorption of many drugs including penicillins and cephalosporins. This interaction may be used to produce higher and more sustained blood levels of these drugs. Allopurinol increases toxicity from several antineoplastic agents (6-mercaptopurine, azathioprine). When allopurinol and ampicillin are used concurrently, the incidence of skin rash is greatly increased. Small doses of aspirin (<2 g/day) elevate serum uric acid and may interfere with the management of gout. Sulfinopyrazone may increase the risk of bleeding with other agents that affect hemostasis (aspirin, anticoagulants).

Nursing Implications

Assessment

- Assess for joint pain and swelling throughout therapy.
- Monitor intake and output ratios. Ensure that patient maintains adequate fluid intake (minimum 2500–3000 ml/day) to minimize risk of kidney stone formation.

Potential Nursing Diagnoses

- Comfort, altered: pain (indications).
- Knowledge deficit related to medication regimen (patient/family teaching).

Implementation

- Administer with or after meals to minimize gastric irritation.

Patient/Family Teaching

- Inform patient of the need for increased fluid intake.
- Advise patient to follow physician's recommendations regarding weight loss, diet, and alcohol consumption.

Evaluation

Effectiveness of therapy can be demonstrated by: ▪ Prevention or treatment of gout.

Antigout Agents Included in *Davis's Drug Guide for Nurses*

allopurinol, 20	probenecid, 982
colchicine, 280	sulfinpyrazone, 1091

▪ ANTIHISTAMINES

Pharmacologic Profile

General Uses: Relief of symptoms associated with allergies, including rhinitis, urticaria, and angioedema, and as adjunctive therapy in anaphylactic reactions. Some antihistamines are used to treat motion sickness (dimenhydrinate and meclizine), insomnia (diphenhydramine), and other nonallergic conditions.

General Action and Information: Antihistamines block the effects of histamine at the H_1 receptor. They do not block histamine release, antibody production, or antigen-antibody reactions. Most antihistamines have anticholinergic properties and may cause constipation, dry eyes, dry mouth, and blurred vision. In addition, many antihistamines cause sedation. Some phenothiazines have strong antihistaminic properties (hydroxyzine and promethazine).

Contraindications: Hypersensitivity and narrow-angle glaucoma. Should not be used in premature or newborn infants.

Precautions: Elderly patients may be more susceptible to adverse anticholinergic effects of antihistamines. Use cautiously in patients with pyloric obstruction, prostatic hypertrophy, hyperthyroidism, cardiovascular disease, or severe liver disease. Use cautiously in pregnancy and lactation.

Interactions: Additive sedation when used with other CNS depressants, including alcohol, antidepressants, narcotic analgesics, and sedative/hypnotics. MAO inhibitors prolong and intensify the anticholinergic properties of antihistamines.

Nursing Implications

Assessment

- **General Info:** Assess allergy symptoms (rhinitis, conjunctivitis, and hives) before and periodically throughout course of therapy.
- Monitor pulse and blood pressure before initiating and throughout IV therapy.
- Assess lung sounds and character of bronchial secretions. Maintain fluid intake of 1500–2000 ml/day to decrease viscosity of secretions.
- **Nausea and Vomiting:** Assess degree of nausea and frequency and amount of emesis when administering for nausea and vomiting.
- **Anxiety:** Assess mental status, mood, and behavior when administering for anxiety.
- **Pruritus:** Observe the character, location, and size of affected area when administering for pruritic skin conditions.

Potential Nursing Diagnoses

- Airway clearance, ineffective (indications).
- Injury, high risk for (adverse reactions).
- Knowledge deficit related to medication regimen (patient/family teaching).

Implementation

- When used for prophylaxis of motion sickness administer at least 30 min and preferably 1–2 hr before exposure to conditions that may precipitate motion sickness.
- When administering concurrently with narcotic analgesics (hydroxyzine, promethazine) supervise ambulation closely to prevent injury secondary to increased sedation.

Patient/Family Teaching

- Inform patient that drowiness may occur. Avoid driving or other activities requiring alertness until response to drug is known.
- Drowsiness is less likely to occur with astemizole and terfenadine.
- Caution patient to avoid using concurrent alcohol or CNS depressants.
- Advise patient that good oral hygiene, frequent rinsing of mouth with water, and sugarless gum or candy may help relieve dryness of mouth.
- Instruct patient to contact physician if symptoms persist.

Evaluation

Effectiveness of therapy can be demonstrated by: ▪ Decrease in allergic symptoms ▪ Prevention or decreased severity of nausea and vomiting ▪ Decrease in anxiety ▪ Relief of pruritus ▪ Sedation when used as a sedative/hypnotic.

Antihistamines Included in *Davis's Drug Guide for Nurses*

▪ ANTIHYPERTENSIVE AGENTS

Pharmacologic Profile

General Use: Treatment of hypertension of many causes; most commonly essential hypertension. Parenteral products are used in the treatment of hypertensive emergencies. Oral treatment should be initiated as soon as possible and individualized to assure compliance for long-term therapy. Therapy is initiated with agents having minimal side effects. When such therapy fails, more potent drugs with different side effects are added in an effort to control blood pressure while causing minimal patient discomfort.

General Action and Information: As a group, the antihypertensives are used to lower blood pressure to a normal level (<90 mmHg diastolic) or to the lowest level tolerated. Antihypertensives are classified into groups according to their site of action. These include peripherally acting antiadrenergics, centrally acting alpha adrenergics, beta-adrenergic blockers, vasodilators, angiotensin converting enzyme (ACE) inhibitors, calcium channel blockers, diuretics, and indapamide, a diuretic with vasodilatory properties. Hypertensive emergencies may be managed with parenteral vasodilators such as diazoxide or nitroprusside, or enalaprilat.

Contraindications: Hypersensitivity to individual agents.

Precautions: Choose agents carefully in pregnancy, lactation, or patients receiving cardiac glycosides. Alpha-adrenergic agonists and beta-adrenergic blockers should be used only in patients who will comply with regimen since abrupt discontinuation of these agents may result in rapid and excessive rise in blood pressure (rebound phenomenon). Thiazide diuretics may increase the requirement for insulin, diet therapy, or oral hypoglycemic agents in diabetic patients. Vasodilators may cause tachycardia if used alone and are commonly used in combination with beta-adrenergic blocking agents. Most antihypertensives (except for beta-adrenergic blockers, angiotensin converting enzyme [ACE] inhibitors, and calcium channel blockers) cause sodium and water retention and are usually combined with a diuretic.

Interactions: Many drugs can negate the therapeutic effectiveness of antihypertensives, including antihistamines, nonsteroidal anti-inflammatory agents, sympathomimetic bronchodilators, decongestants, appetite suppressants, antidepressants, and MAO inhibitors. Hypokalemia from diuretics may increase the risk of cardiac glycoside toxicity. Potassium supplements and potassium-sparing diuretics may cause hyperkalemia when used with angiotensin coverting enzyme (ACE) inhibitors.

Nursing Implications

Assessment

- Monitor blood pressure and pulse frequently during dosage adjustment and periodically throughout therapy.
- Monitor intake and output ratios and daily weight.

Potential Nursing Diagnoses

- Tissue perfusion, altered (indications).
- Knowledge deficit related to medication regimen (patient/family teaching).
- Noncompliance (patient/family teaching).

Implementation

- Many antihypertensive agents are available as combination products to enhance compliance (see Appendix A).

Patient/Family Teaching

- Instruct patient to continue taking medication, even if feeling well. Abrupt withdrawal may cause rebound hypertension. Medication controls but does not cure hypertension.
- Encourage patient to comply with additional interventions for hypertension (weight reduction, low-sodium diet, regular exercise, discontinuation of smoking, moderation of alcohol consumption, and stress management).
- Instruct patient and family on proper technique for monitoring blood pressure. Advise them to check blood pressure weekly and report significant changes to physician.
- Caution patient to make position changes slowly to minimize orthostatic hypotension. Advise patient that exercising or hot weather may enhance hypotensive effects.
- Advise patient to consult physician or pharmacist before taking any over-the-counter medications, especially cold remedies. Patients should also avoid excessive amounts of tea, coffee, or cola.
- Advise patient to inform physician or dentist of medication regimen before treatment or surgery.
- Emphasize the importance of follow-up examinations to monitor progress.

EVALUATION

Effectiveness of therapy can be demonstrated by: ▪ Decrease in blood pressure.

Antihypertensive Agents Included in *Davis's Drug Guide for Nurses*

▪ ANTI-INFECTIVES

Pharmacologic Profile

General Use: Treatment and prophylaxis of various bacterial infections. See specific drugs for spectrum and indications. Some infections may require additional surgical intervention and supportive therapy.

General Action and Information: Kill (bactericidal) or inhibit the growth of (bacteriostatic) susceptible pathogenic bacteria. Not active against viruses or fungi. Anti-infectives are subdivided into categories depending on chemical similarities and antimicrobial spectrum.

Contraindications: Known hypersensitivity to individual agents. Cross-sensitivity among related agents may occur.

Precautions: Culture and susceptibility testing is desirable to optimize therapy. Dosage modification may be required in patients with hepatic or renal insufficiency. Use cautiously in pregnant and lactating women. Prolonged inappropriate use of broad spectrum anti-infectives may lead to superinfection with fungi or resistant bacteria.

Interactions: Penicillins and aminoglycosides chemically inactivate each other and should not be physically admixed. Erythromycins may decrease hepatic metabolism of other drugs. Probenecid increases serum levels of penicillins and related compounds. Highly protein-bound anti-infectives such as sulfonamides may displace or be displaced by other highly bound drugs. See individual drugs. Extended-spectrum penicillins (mezlocillin, ticarcillin, piperacillin) and some cephalosporins (cefamandole, cefoperazone, cefotetan, and moxalactam) may increase the risk of bleeding with anticoagulants, antiplatelet agents, or nonsteroidal anti-inflammatory agents.

Nursing Implications

Assessment
- Assess patient for signs and symptoms of infection prior to and throughout course of therapy.
- Determine previous hypersensitivities in patients receiving penicillins or cephalosporins.
- Obtain specimens for culture and sensitivity prior to initiating therapy. First dose may be given before receiving results.

Potential Nursing Diagnoses
- Infection, high risk for (indications).
- Knowledge deficit related to medication regimen (patient/family teaching).
- Noncompliance (patient/family teaching).

Implementation
- Most anti-infectives should be administered around the clock to maintain therapeutic serum drug levels.

Patient/Family Teaching
- Instruct patient to continue taking medication around the clock until finished completely, even if feeling better.
- Advise patient to report the signs of superinfection (black, furry overgrowth on the tongue, vaginal itching or discharge, loose or foul-smelling stools) and allergy to physician.
- Instruct patient to notify physician if fever and diarrhea develop, especially if stool contains pus, blood, or mucus. Advise patient not to treat diarrhea without consulting physician or pharmacist.
- Instruct patient to notify physician if symptoms do not improve.

Evaluation
Effectiveness of therapy can be demonstrated by: ▪ Resolution of the signs and symptoms of infection. Length of time for complete resolution depends on organism and site of infection.

Anti-Infectives Included in *Davis's Drug Guide for Nurses*

▪ ANTIMANIC AGENTS

Pharmacologic Profile

General Use: Lithium is used in the treatment of a variety of psychiatric disorders. Particularly useful in the treatment of bipolar affective disorders, in which lithium is used both to treat acute manic episodes and as prophylaxis against their recurrence.

General Action and Information: Lithium alters cation transport in nerve and muscle cells by competing with other cations such as sodium and potassium. May also increase the re-uptake of neurotransmitters and alter levels of cAMP (cyclic adenosine monphosphate). Has antimanic and antidepressant properties.

Contraindications: Hypersensitivity. Generally should be avoided in patients with severe cardiovascular or renal disease; dehydrated or debilitated patients. Should only be used where therapy (particularly blood levels) may be closely monitored. Avoid use during lactation.

Precautions: Use cautiously in elderly patients or patients with any degree of cardiac, renal or thyroid disease, or diabetes mellitus. Should only be used during pregnancy when benefits outweigh risks to fetus; malformations may occur. Safety in children not established.

Interactions: May prolong neuromuscular blockade. Encephalopathic syndrome may occur with haloperidol. Diuretics, methyldopa, probenecid, indomethacin, and other nonsteroidal anti-inflammatory agents may increase the risk of toxocity. Aminophylline, phenothiazines, sodium bicarbonate, and sodium chloride may hasten excretion and lead to decreased effect. Lithium may decrease the effectiveness of phenothiazines. Hypothyroid effects may be additive with potassium iodide. Phenothiazines may mask signs of lithium toxicity.

Nursing Implications

Assessment

- Assess mood, ideation, and behaviors frequently. Initiate suicide precautions if indicated.
- Monitor intake and output ratios. Notify physician of significant changes in totals. Unless contraindicated, fluid intake of at least 2000–3000 ml/day should be maintained.
- **Toxicity and Overdose:** Serum lithium levels should be monitored twice weekly during initiation of therapy and every 2–3 mon during chronic therapy. Blood samples should be drawn in the morning immediately prior to next dose. Therapeutic levels range from 0.5–1.5 mEq/liter.
- Assess patient for signs and symptoms of lithium toxicity (vomiting, diarrhea, slurred speech, decreased coordination, drowsiness, muscle weakness, or twitching). If these occur, inform physician prior to administering next dose.

Potential Nursing Diagnoses

- Thought processes, altered (indications).
- Violence, high risk for: self-directed or directed at others (indications).
- Knowledge deficit related to medication regimen (patient/family teaching).

Implementation

- Administer with food or milk to minimize GI irritation. Extended-release preparations should be swallowed whole; do not break, crush, or chew.

Patient/Family Teaching

- Medication may cause dizziness or drowsiness. Caution patient to avoid driving or other activities requiring alertness until response to medication is known.
- Low sodium levels may predispose patient to toxicity. Advise patient to drink 2000–3000 ml of fluid each day and eat a diet with liberal sodium intake. Excessive amounts of coffee, tea, and cola should be avoided because of diuretic effect. Avoid activities that cause excess sodium loss (heavy exertion, exercise in hot weather, and saunas). Notify physician of vomiting and diarrhea, which also cause sodium loss.
- Advise patient that weight gain may occur. Review principles of a low-calorie diet.
- Instruct patient to consult physician or pharmacist before taking over-the-counter medications concurrently with this therapy.
- Advise patient to use contraception and to consult physician if pregnancy is suspected.
- Review side effects and symptoms of toxicity with patient. Inform patient of the importance of reporting adverse effects to physician promptly.
- Emphasize the importance of periodic laboratory tests to monitor for lithium toxicity.

Evaluation

Effectiveness of therapy can be demonstrated by: ▪ Resolution of the symptoms of mania ▪ Decreased incidence of mood swings in bipolar disorders ▪ Improved affect in unipolar disorders.

Antimanic Agents Included in *Davis's Drug Guide for Nurses*

lithium, 677

▪ ANTINEOPLASTICS

Pharmacologic Profile

General Use: Used in the treatment of various solid tumors, lymphomas, and leukemias. Also used in some autoimmune disorders such as rheumatoid arthritis (cyclophosamide, methotrexate). Often used in combinations to minimize individual toxicities and increase response. Chemotherapy may be combined with other treatment modalities such as surgery and radiation therapy. Dosages vary greatly depending on extent of disease, other agents used, and patient's condition.

General Action and Information: Act by many different mechanisms (see Table below). Most commonly affect DNA synthesis or function. Action may not be limited to neoplastic cells.

MECHANISM OF ACTION OF VARIOUS ANTINEOPLASTIC AGENTS

MECHANISM OF ACTION	AGENT	EFFECTS ON CELL CYCLE
ALKYLATING AGENTS cause cross-linking of DNA	busulfan carboplatin chlorambucil cisplatin cyclophosphamide dacarbazine estramustine ifosfamide mechlorethamine melphelan procarbazine thiotepa	Cell cycle—nonspecific
ANTHRACYCLINES interfere with DNA and RNA synthesis	daunorubicin doxorubicin idarubicin	Cell cycle—nonspecific
ANTITUMOR ANTIBIOTICS interfere with DNA and RNA synthesis	bleomycin dactinomycin mitomycin mitoxantrone plicamycin streptozocin	Cell cycle—nonspecific (except bleomycin)
ANTIMETABOLITES take the place of normal proteins	cytarabine fludarabine fluorouracil hydroxyurea mercaptopurine methotrexate thioguanine	Cell cycle—specific, work mostly in S phase (DNA synthesis)
ENZYME (depletes asparagine)	asparaginase	Cell cycle—phase specific
HORMONAL AGENTS alter hormonal status in tumors which are sensitive	diethylstilbestrol (estrogens) estramustine flutamide leuprolide megestrol tamoxifen testosterone (androgens)	Unknown
PODOPHYLLOTOXIN DERIVATIVE (damages DNA before mitosis)	etoposide	Cell cycle—phase specific
VINCA ALKALOIDS interfere with mitosis	vinblastine vincristine	Cell cycle—specific, work during M phase (mitosis)
ANTIPROLIFERATIVE	interferon alfa-2A interferon alfa-2B	Unknown
ADRENAL SUPPRESSANT	mitotane	Unknown
IMMUNE MODULATOR	BCG levamisole	Unknown Unknown
MISCELLANEOUS	altretamine pentostatin	Unknown Unknown

Contraindications: Previous bone marrow depression or hypersensitivity. Contraindicated in pregnancy and lactation.

Precautions: Use cautiously in patients with active infections, decreased bone marrow reserve, radiation therapy, or other debilitating illnesses. Use cautiously in patients with childbearing potential.

Interactions: Allopurinol decreases metabolism of mercaptopurine. Toxicity from methotrexate may be increased by other nephrotoxic drugs or larger doses of aspirin or nonsteroidal anti-inflammatory agents. Bone marrow depression is additive. See individual drugs.

Nursing Implications

Assessment

- Assess for fever, chills, sore throat, and signs of infection. Notify physician if these symptoms occur.
- Monitor platelet count throughout therapy. Assess for bleeding (bleeding gums, bruising, petichiae; guaiac stools, urine, and emesis). If thrombocytopenia occurs, avoid IM injections, rectal temperatures, and apply pressure to venipuncture sites for 10 min.
- Monitor intake and output ratios, appetite, and nutritional intake. Confer with physician regarding administration of an antiemetic. Adjusting diet as tolerated may help maintain fluid and electrolyte balance and nutritional status.
- Anemia may occur. Monitor for increased fatigue, dyspnea, and orthostatic hypotension.
- Monitor IV site carefully and ensure patency. Discontinue infusion immediately if discomfort, erythema along vein, or infiltration occurs. Tissue ulceration and necrosis may result from infiltration. Notify physician.
- Monitor for symptoms of gout (increased uric acid, joint pain, and edema). Encourage patient to drink at least 2 liters of fluid each day. Allopurinol may be given to decrease uric acid levels. Alkalinization of urine may be ordered to increase excretion of uric acid.

Potential Nursing Diagnoses

- Infection, high risk for (side effects).
- Nutrition, altered: less than body requirements (adverse reactions).
- Knowledge deficit related to medication regimen (patient/family teaching).

Implementation

- Solutions for injection should be prepared in a biologic cabinet. Wear gloves, gown, and mask while handling medication. Discard equipment in designated containers (see Appendix I for guidelines for safe handling).

Patient/Family Teaching

- Caution patient to avoid crowds and persons with known infections. Physician should be informed immediately if symptoms of infection occur.
- Instruct patient to report unusual bleeding. Advise patient of thrombocytopenia precautions.
- These drugs may cause gonadal suppression; however, patient should still practice birth control, as most are teratogenic. Advise patient to inform physician immediately if pregnancy is suspected.
- Discuss with patient the possibility of hair loss. Explore methods of coping.
- Instruct patient to inspect oral mucosa for erythema and ulceration. If ulceration occurs advise patient to use sponge brush, rinse mouth with water after eating and drinking, and confer with physician if mouth pain interferes with eating.
- Instruct patient not to receive any vaccinations without advice of physician.
- Advise patient of need for medical follow-up and frequent lab tests.

EVALUATION

Effectiveness of therapy can be demonstrated by: ▪ Decrease in size and spread of tumor ▪ Improvement in hematologic status in patients with leukemia.

Antineoplastics Included in *Davis's Drug Guide for Nurses*

▪ ANTIPARKINSON AGENTS

Pharmacologic Profile

General Use: Used in the treatment of parkinsonism of various causes: degenerative, toxic, infective, neoplastic, or drug-induced.

General Action and Information: Drugs used in the treatment of the Parkinsonian syndrome and other dyskinesias are aimed at restoring the natural balance of two major neurotransmitters in the CNS: acetylcholine and dopamine. The imbalance is a deficiency in dopamine which results in excessive cholinergic activity. Drugs used are either anticholinergics (benztropine, biperiden, orphenadrine, and trihexyphenidyl) or dopaminergic agonists (amantadine, bromocriptine, levodopa, and pergolide). Selegiline inhibits the enzyme which degrades dopamine, augmenting its effects.

Contraindications: Anticholinergics should be avoided in patients with narrow-angle glaucoma.

Precautions: Use cautiously in patients with severe cardiac disease, pyloric obstruction, or prostatic enlargement.

Interactions: Pyridoxine, MAO inhibitors, benzodiazepines, phenytoin, phenothiazines, and haloperidol may antagonize the effects of levodopa. Concurrent use of selegiline with narcotic analgesics may result in two potentially fatal reactions (excitation, sweating, rigidity, and hypertension; or hypotension and coma). Doses of selegiline >10 mg/day may produce reactions with tyramine-containing foods.

Nursing Implications

Assessment

- Assess parkinsonian and extrapyramidal symptoms (akinesia, rigidity, tremors, pill rolling, mask facies, shuffling gait, muscle spasms, twisting motions, and drooling) before and throughout course of therapy. On-off phenomena may cause symptoms to appear or improve suddenly.
- Monitor blood pressure frequently during therapy. Instruct patient to remain supine during and for several hrs after first dose of bromocryptine, as severe hypotension may occur.

Potential Nursing Diagnoses

- Mobility, impaired physical (indications).
- Injury, high risk for (indications).
- Knowledge deficit related to medication regimen (patient/family teaching).

Implementation

- In the carbidopa/levodopa combination the number following the drug name represents the mg of each respective drug.

Patient/Family Teaching

- May cause drowiness or dizziness. Advise patient to avoid driving or other activities that require alertness until response to medication is known.
- Caution patient to make position changes slowly to minimize orthostatic hypotension.
- Instruct patient that frequent rinsing of mouth, good oral hygiene, and sugarless gum or candy may decrease dry mouth. Patient should notify physician if dryness persists (saliva substitutes may be used). Also notify the dentist if dryness interferes with use of dentures.
- Advise patient to confer with physician or pharmacist before taking over-the-counter medications, especially cold remedies, or drinking alcoholic beverages. Patients receiving levodopa should avoid multivitamins. Vitamin B_6 (pyridoxine) may interfere with levodopa's action.
- Caution patient that decreased perspiration may occur. Overheating may occur during hot weather. Patients should remain indoors in an air-conditioned environment during hot weather.
- Advise patient to increase activity, bulk, and fluid in diet to minimize constipating effects of medication.
- Advise patient to notify physician if confusion, rash, urinary retention, severe constipation, visual changes, or worsening of Parkinson's disease symptoms occur.

Evaluation

Effectiveness of therapy can be demonstrated by: ■ Resolution of parkinsonian signs and symptoms ■ Resolution of drug-induced extrapyramidal symptoms.

Antiparkinson Agents Included in *Davis's Drug Guide for Nurses*

anticholinergics
- benztropine, 111
- biperiden, 121
- trihexyphenidyl, 1169

dopamine agonist
- amantadine, 32
- bromocriptine, 130
- carbidopa/levodopa, 168
- levodopa, 661
- pergolide, 908

monoamine oxidase type B inhibitor
- selegiline, 1051

■ ANTIPSYCHOTICS

Pharmacologic Profile

General Use: Treatment of acute and chronic psychoses, particularly when accompanied by increased psychomotor activity. Clomipramine is only used for obsessive-compulsive disorder (OCD). Use of clozapine is limited to schizophrenia unresponsive to conventional therapy. Selected agents are also used as antihistamines or antiemetics. Chlorpromazine is also used in the treatment of intractable hiccups.

General Action and Information: Block dopamine receptors in the brain, also alter dopamine release and turnover. Peripheral effects include anticholinergic properties and alpha-adrenergic blockade. Most antipsychotics are phenothiazines except for haloperidol, which is a butyrophenone; molidone, which resembles a phenothiazine in its action; clomipramine, which resembles tricyclic antidepressants; and loxapine and clozapine, which are miscellaneous compounds. Phenothiazines differ in their ability to produce sedation (greatest with chlorpromazine, promazine, thioridazine, and thiothixine), extrapyramidal reactions (greatest with fluphenazine, perphenazine, prochlorperazine, and trifluoperazine), and anticholinergic effects (greatest with chlorpromazine, promazine).

Contraindications: Hypersensitivity. Cross-sensitivity may exist among phenothiazines. Should not be used in narrow-angle glaucoma. Should not be used in patients who have CNS depression.

Precautions: Safety in pregnancy and lactation not established. Use cautiously in patients with symptomatic cardiac disease. Avoid exposure to extremes in temperature. Use cautiously in severely ill or debilitated patients, diabetics, and patients with respiratory insufficiency, prostatic hypertrophy, or intestinal obstruction. May lower seizure threshold. Clozapine may cause agranulocytosis. Most agents are capable of causing neuroleptic malignant syndrome.

Interactions: Additive hypotension with acute ingestion of alcohol, antihypertensives, or nitrates. Antacids may decrease absorption. Phenobarbital may increase metabolism and decrease effectiveness. Additive CNS depression with other CNS depressants, including alcohol, antihistamines, antidepressants, narcotic analgesics, or sedative/hypnotics. Lithium may decrease blood levels and effectiveness of phenothiazines. May decrease the therapeutic response to levodopa. May increase the risk of agranulocytosis with antithyroid agents.

Nursing Implications

Assessment

- Assess patient's mental status (orientation, mood, behavior) before and periodically throughout therapy.
- Monitor blood pressure (sitting, standing, lying), pulse, and respiratory rate before and frequently during the period of dosage adjustment.
- Observe patient carefully when administering medication to ensure medication is actually taken and not hoarded.
- Observe patient carefully for extrapyramidal symptoms (pill-rolling motions, drooling, tremors, rigidity, and shuffling gait), tardive dyskinesia (uncontrolled movements of face, mouth, tongue, or jaw, and involuntary movements of extremities), and neuroleptic malignant syndrome (pale skin, hyperthermia, skeletal muscle rigidity, autonomic dysfunction, altered consciousness, leukocytosis, elevated liver function tests, and elevated CPK). Notify physician immediately at the onset of these symptoms.

Potential Nursing Diagnoses

- Thought processes, altered (indications).
- Knowledge deficit related to medication regimen (patient/family teaching).
- Noncompliance (patient/family teaching).

Implementation

- **General Info:** Keep patient recumbent for at least 30 min following parenteral administration to minimize hypotensive effects.
- To prevent contact dermatitis avoid getting soln on hands.
- Phenothiazines should be discontinued 48 hr before and not resumed for 24 hr following metrizamide myelography, as they lower the seizure threshold.
- **PO:** Administer with food, milk, or a full glass of water to minimize gastric irritation.
- Dilute most concentrates in 120 ml of distilled or acidified tap water, or fruit juice just before administration.

Patient/Family Teaching

- Advise patient to take medication exactly as directed and not to skip doses or double up on missed doses. Abrupt withdrawal may lead to gastritis, nausea, vomiting, dizziness, headache, tachycardia, and insomnia.
- Advise patient to make position changes slowly to minimize orthostatic hypotension.
- Medication may cause drowsiness. Caution patient to avoid driving or other activities requiring alertness until response to the medication is known.
- Caution patient to avoid taking alcohol or other CNS depressants concurrently with this medication.
- Advise patient to use sunscreen and protective clothing when exposed to the sun to prevent photosensitivity reactions. Extremes of temperature should also be avoided, as these drugs impair body temperature regulation.
- Advise patient that increasing activity, bulk, and fluids in the diet help minimize the constipating effects of this medication.

- Instruct patient to use frequent mouth rinses, good oral hygiene, and sugarless gum or candy to minimize dry mouth.
- Advise patient to notify physician or dentist of medication regimen before treatment or surgery.
- Emphasize the importance of routine follow-up examinations and continued participation in psychotherapy as indicated.

Evaluation

Effectiveness of therapy can be demonstrated by: ▪ Decrease in excitable, paranoic, or withdrawn behavior ▪ Relief of nausea and vomiting.

Antipsychotics Included in *Davis's Drug Guide for Nurses*

phenothiazines

butyrophenone

miscellaneous

▪ ANTIPYRETICS

Pharmacologic Profile

General Use: Used to lower fever of many causes (infection, inflammation, and neoplasms).

General Action and Information: Antipyretics lower fever by affecting thermoregulation in the CNS and by inhibiting the action of prostagladins peripherally.

Contraindications: Avoid aspirin or ibuprofen in patients with bleeding disorder (risk of bleeding is less with other salicylates). Aspirin and other salicylates should be avoided in children and adolescents.

Precautions: Use aspirin or ibuprofen cautiously in patients with ulcer disease. Avoid chronic use of large doses of acetaminophen.

Interactions: Large doses of aspirin may displace other highly protein-bound drugs. Additive GI irritation with ibuprofen, aspirin, and other nonsteroidal anti-inflammatory agents or glucocorticoids. Aspirin or ibuprofen may increase the risk of bleeding with other agents affecting hemostasis (anticoagulants, thrombolytics, antineoplastics, and certain anti-infectives).

Nursing Implications

Assessment

- Assess fever; note presence of associated symptoms (diaphoresis, tachycardia, and malaise).

Potential Nursing Diagnoses

- Body temperature, altered, high risk for (indications).
- Knowledge deficit related to medication regimen (patient/family teaching).

Implementation

- Administration with food or antacids may minimize GI irriation (aspirin and ibuprofen).
- Available in oral and rectal dosage forms, and in combination with other drugs.

Patient/Family Teaching

- Advise patient to consult physician if fever is not relieved by routine doses or if greater than 39.5°C (103°F) or lasts longer than 3 days.
- Centers for Disease Control warn against giving aspirin to children or adolscents with varicella (chickenpox), or influenza-like or viral illnesses because of a possible association with Reye's syndrome.

Evaluation

Effectiveness of therapy can be demonstrated by: ▪ Reduction of fever.

Antipyretics Included in *Davis's Drug Guide for Nurses*

acetaminophen, 2
aspirin, 79
choline magnesium trisalicylate, 244
choline salicylate, 246
ibuprofen, 594
salsalate, 1044

▪ ANTITHYROID AGENTS

Pharmacologic Profile

General Use: Used in the treatment of hyperthyroidism of various causes (Graves' disease, multinodular goiter, thyroiditis, and thyrotoxic crisis) in children, pregnant women, and other patients in whom hyperthyroidism is not expected to be permanent. These agents are also used to prepare patients for thyroidectomy or those in whom thryoidectomy is contraindicated. Beta-adrenergic blockers (propranolol) are sometimes used in conjunction with antithyroid agents to control symptoms (tachycardia and tremor), but have no effect on thyroid status. Iodine and iodides are also used as radiation protectants.

General Action and Information: Inhibit thyroid hormone formation (iodine) or inhibit oxidation of iodine (methimazole and propylthiouracil).

Contraindications: Hypersensitivity. Previous bone marrow depression.

Precautions: Use methimazole cautiously in patients with decreased bone marrow reserve.

Interactions: Lithium may cause thyroid abnormalities and interfere with the response to antithyroid therapy. Phenothiazines may increase the risk of agranulocytosis.

Nursing Implications

Assessment

- **General Info:** Monitor response of symptoms of hyperthyroidism or thyrotoxicosis (tachycardia, palpitations, nervousness, insomnia, fever, diaphoresis, heat intolerance, tremors, weight loss, diarrhea).
- Assess patient for development of hypothyroidism (intolerance to cold, constipation, dry skin, headache, listlessness, tiredness, or weakness). Dosage adjustment may be required.
- Assess patient for skin rash or swelling of cervical lymph nodes. Treatment may be discontinued if this occurs.
- Monitor thyroid function studies before and periodically throughout therapy.
- **Iodides:** Assess for signs and symptoms of iodism (metallic taste, stomatitis, skin lesions, cold symptoms, severe GI upset) or anaphylaxis. Report these symptoms promptly to physician.

Potential Nursing Diagnoses

- Knowledge deficit related to medication regimen (patient/family teaching).

Implementation

- Mix iodide solutions in a full glass of fruit juice, water, or milk. Administer after meals to minimize GI irritation.

Patient/Family Teaching

- Instruct patient to take medication exactly as directed. Missing doses may precipitate hyperthyroidism.
- Advise patient to consult physician regarding dietary sources of iodine (iodized salt, shellfish, cabbage, kale, turnips).
- Advise patient to carry identification describing medication regimen at all times and to notify physician or dentist of medical regimen before treatment or surgery.
- Emphasize the importance of routine examinations to monitor progress and check for side effects.

Evaluation

Effectiveness of therapy can be demonstrated by: ▪ Decrease in severity of symptoms of hyperthyroidism ▪ Decrease in vascularity and friability of the thyroid gland before preparation for surgery ▪ Protection of the thyroid gland during radiation emergencies.

Antithyroid Agents Included in *Davis's Drug Guide for Nurses*

methimazole, 737
potassium iodide, 964
propylthiouracil, 1011
strong iodine solution, 1077

▪ ANTITUBERCULARS

Pharmacologic Profile

General Use: Used in the treatment and prevention of tuberculosis and other diseases caused by mycobacterium. Combinations are used in the treatment of active disease to rapidly decrease the infectious state and delay or prevent the emergence of resistance strains. In selected situations, intermittent (twice weekly) regimens may be employed. Streptomycin is also used as an antitubercular.

General Action and Information: Kill (tuberculocidal) or inhibit the growth of (tuberculostatic) mycobacterium responsible for causing tuberculosis. Combination therapy with two or more agents is required, unless used as prophylaxis (isoniazid alone).

Contraindications: Hypersensitivity. Severe liver disease.

Precautions: Use cautiously in patients with a history of liver disease; elderly or debilitated patients. Ethambutol requires ophthalmologic follow-up. Safety in pregnancy and lactation not established, although selected agents have been used without adverse effects on the fetus. Compliance is required for optimal response.

Interactions: Isoniazid inhibits the metabolism of phenytoin. Rifampin stimulates hepatic drug-metabolizing enzymes and may decrease the effects of drugs that are metabolized by the liver.

Nursing Implications

Assessment

- Mycobacterial studies and susceptibility tests should be performed prior to and periodically throughout therapy to detect possible resistance.

Potential Nursing Diagnoses

- Infection, high risk for (indications).
- Knowledge deficit related to medication regimen (patient/family teaching).
- Noncompliance (patient/family teaching).

Implementation

- Most medications can be administered with food or antacids if GI irritation occurs.

Patient/Family Teaching

- Advise patient of the importance of continuing therapy even after symptoms have subsided.
- Emphasize the importance of regular follow-up examinations to monitor progress and check for side effects.

Evaluation

Effectiveness of therapy can be demonstrated by: ▪ Resolution of the signs and symptoms of tuberculosis ▪ Negative sputum cultures.

Antituberculars Included in *Davis's Drug Guide for Nurses*

ethambutol, 457
isoniazid, 628
pyrazinamide, 1017
rifampin, 1041
streptomycin, 1073

▪ ANTITUSSIVES/EXPECTORANTS

Pharmacologic Profile

General Use: Used for the symptomatic relief of cough due to various causes including viral upper respiratory infections. Not intended for chronic use.

General Action and Information: Antitussives (codeine, dextromethorphan, diphenhydramine, hydrocodone, and hydromorphone) suppress cough by central mechanisms. Benzonatate suppresses cough locally in the respiratory tract. Expectorants (acetylcysteine and guaifenesin) aid in mobilizing pulmonary secretions. Productive cough should not be suppressed unless it interferes with sleeping or other activities of daily living. Increasing fluid intake probably serves as the best expectorant, decreasing the viscosity of secretions so that they may be more easily mobilized.

Contraindications: Hypersensitivity.

Precautions: Use cautiously in children. Should not be used for prolonged periods unless under the advice of a physician.

Interactions: Centrally acting antitussives may have additive CNS depression with other CNS depressants.

Nursing Implications

Assessment

- Assess frequency and nature of cough, lung sounds, and amount and type of sputum produced.

Potential Nursing Diagnoses

- Airway clearance, ineffective (indications).
- Knowledge deficit related to medication regimen (patient/family teaching).

Implementation

- Unless contraindicated, maintain fluid intake of 1500–2000 ml to decrease viscosity of bronchial secretions.

Patient/Family Teaching

- Instruct patient to cough effectively, sit upright and take several deep breaths before attempting to cough.
- Advise patient to minimize cough by avoiding irritants (cigarette smoke, fumes, dust). Humidification of environmental air, frequent sips of water, and sugarless hard candy may also decrease the frequency of dry, irritating cough.
- Caution patient to avoid taking concurrent alcohol or CNS depressants.
- May cause dizziness or drowsiness. Caution patient to avoid driving or other activities requiring alertness until response to medication is known.
- Advise patient that any cough lasting over 1 wk or accompanied by fever, chest pain, persistent headache, or skin rash warrants medical attention.

Evaluation

Effectiveness of therapy can be demonstrated by: ▪ Decrease in frequency and intensity of cough without eliminating patient's cough reflex.

Antitussives Included in *Davis's Drug Guide for Nurses*

Expectorants Included in *Davis's Drug Guide for Nurses*

▪ ANTIVIRALS

Pharmacologic Profile

General Uses: Acyclovir and vidarabine are used in the management of serious herpes virus infections. Amantadine is used primarily in the prevention of influenza A viral infections. Zidovudine and didanosine slow the progression of AIDS. Idoxuridine and trifluridine are used for ophthalmic viral infections. Ribavirin is used in the management of respiratory syncitial virus (RSV). Ganciclovir and foscarnet are used in the treatment of cytomegalovirus (CMV) retinitis.

General Action and Information: Acyclovir, didanosine, foscarnet, ganciclovir, idoxuridine, ribavirin, trifluridine, vidarabine, and zidovudine inhibit viral replication. Amantadine prevents penetration of the virus into host cells.

Contraindications: Previous hypersensitivity.

Precautions: All require dosage adjustment in renal impairment. Acyclovir may cause renal impairment. Acyclovir and amantadine may cause CNS toxicity. Vidarabine commonly causes GI adverse reactions. Zidovudine should be used cautiously in patients with bone marrow depression. Didanosine and foscarnet increase risk of seizures.

Interactions: Acyclovir may have additive CNS and nephrotoxicity with drugs causing similar adverse reactions. Amantadine may have additive anticholinergic properties with other drugs causing anticholinergic side effects. Adverse reactions to vidarabine may be potentiated by concurrent allopurinol. Chronic high-dose acetaminophen may increase zidovudine toxicity. Food significantly decreases absorption of didanosine.

Nursing Implications

Assessment

- **General Info:** Assess patient for signs and symptoms of infection before and throughout course of therapy.
- **Ophth:** Assess eye lesions before and daily during therapy.
- **Top:** Assess lesions before and daily during therapy.

Potential Nursing Diagnoses

- Infection, high risk for (indications).
- Skin Integrity, impairment of (indications).
- Knowledge deficit related to medication regimen (patient/family teaching).

Implementation

- Most systemic antiviral agents should be administered around the clock to maintain therapeutic serum drug levels.

Patient/Family Teaching

- Instruct patient to continue taking medication around the clock for full course of therapy, even if feeling better.
- Instruct patient in correct technique for topical or ophthalmic preparations.
- Instruct patient to notify physician if symptoms do not improve.

Evaluation

Effectiveness of therapy can be demonstrated by: ▪ Prevention or resolution of the signs and symptoms of viral infection. Length of time for complete resolution depends on organism and site of infection.

Antivirals Included in *Davis's Drug Guide for Nurses*

▪ BETA-ADRENERGIC BLOCKING AGENTS

Pharmacologic Profile

General Uses: Used in the management of hypertension, angina pectoris, tachyarrhythmias, hypertrophic subaortic stenosis, migraine headache (prophylaxis), myocardial infarction (prevention), glaucoma (betaxolol, levobunolol, metipranalol, and timolol), pheochromocytoma, tremors (propranolol only), and hyperthyroidism (management of symptoms only).

General Action and Information: Beta-adrenergic receptor blocking agents compete with adrenergic (sympathetic) neurotransmitters (epinephrine and norepinephrine) for beta-adrenergic receptor sites. Beta$_1$-adrenergic receptor sites are located chiefly in the heart, where stimulation results in increased heart rate, contractility, and AV conduction. Beta$_2$-adrenergic receptors are found mainly in bronchial and vascular smooth muscle and the uterus. Stimulation of beta$_2$-adrenergic receptors produces vasodilation, bronchodilation, and uterine relaxation. Blockade of these receptors antagonizes the effect of the neurotransmitters. Beta blockers may be relatively *selective* for beta$_1$-adrenergic receptors (acebutolol, atenolol, betaxolol, esmolol, and metoprolol) or *nonselective* (carteolol, labetalol, levobunolol, nadolol, penbutolol, pindolol, propranolol, and timolol) blocking both beta$_1$- and beta$_2$-adrenergic receptors. Labetalol has additional alpha-adrenergic blocking action. Acebutolol, carteolol, penbutolol, and pindolol possess *intrinsic sympathomimetic action (ISA)* which may result in less bradycardia than other agents.

Contraindications: Congestive heart failure, acute bronchospasm, some forms of valvular heart disease, bradyarrhythmias, and heart block.

Precautions: Use cautiously in pregnant and lactating females (may cause fetal bradycardia and hypoglycemia). Use cautiously in any form of lung disease,

C L A S S I F I C A T I O N S

bradyarrhythmias, or underlying compensated congestive heart failure. Use cautiously in diabetics and patients with severe liver disease. Beta-adrenergic blockers should not be discontinued abruptly in patients with cardiovascular disease.

Interactions: May cause additive myocardial depression and bradycardia when used with other agents having this effect (cardiac glycosides and selected antiarrhythmics). May antagonize the therepeutic effect of bronchodilators. May alter insulin dosage requirements. Cimetidine may decrease metabolism and increase the effect of certain beta blockers.

Nursing Implications

Assessment

- **General Info:** Monitor blood pressure and pulse frequently during dosage adjustment and periodically throughout therapy.
- Monitor intake and output ratios and daily weight. Assess patient routinely for signs and symptoms of congestive heart failure (dyspnea, rales/crackles, weight gain, peripheral edema, and jugular venous distension).
- **Angina:** Assess frequency and severity of episodes of chest pain periodically throughout therapy.
- **Migraine Prophylaxis:** Assess frequency and severity of migraine headaches periodically throughout therapy.

Potential Nursing Diagnoses

- Tissue perfusion, altered (indications).
- Knowledge deficit related to medication regimen (patient/family teaching).
- Noncompliance (patient/family teaching).

Implementation

- Take apical pulse before administering. If heart rate is <50 bpm or if arrhythmias occur hold medication and notify physician.
- Many beta-adrenergic blockers are available as combination products to enhance compliance (see Appendix A).

Patient/Family Teaching

- **General Info:** Instruct patient to continue taking medication, even if feeling well. Abrupt withdrawal may cause life-threatening arrhythmias, hypertension, or myocardial ischemia. Medication controls but does not cure hypertension.
- Encourage patient to comply with additional interventions for hypertension (weight reduction, low-sodium diet, regular exercise, discontinuation of smoking, moderation of alcohol consumption, and stress management).
- Instruct patient and family on proper technique for monitoring blood pressure. Advise them to check blood pressure weekly and report significant changes to physician.
- Caution patient to make position changes slowly to minimize orthostatic hypotension. Advise patient that exercising or hot weather may enhance hypotensive effects.
- Advise patient to consult physician or pharmacist before taking any over-the-counter medication, especially cold remedies. Patients should also avoid excessive amounts of tea, coffee, or cola.

- Caution patient that these medications may cause increased sensitivity to cold.
- Diabetics should monitor blood sugar closely, especially if weakness, malaise, irritability, or fatigue occur.
- Advise patient to inform physician or dentist of medication regimen before treatment or surgery.
- Advise patient to carry identification describing disease process and medication regimen at all times.
- Emphasize the importance of follow-up examinations to monitor progress.
- **Ophth:** Instruct patient in correct technique for administration of ophthalmic preparations.

Evaluation

Effectiveness of therapy can be demonstrated by: ▪ Decrease in blood pressure ▪ Decrease in frequency and severity of anginal attacks ▪ Control of arrhythmias ▪ Prevention of myocardial reinfarction ▪ Prevention of migraine headaches ▪ Decrease in tremors ▪ Lowering of intraocular pressure.

Beta-Adrenergic Blocking Agents Included in *Davis's Drug Guide for Nurses*

nonselective beta-adrenergic blockers

selective beta-adrenergic blockers

▪ BRONCHODILATORS

Pharmacologic Profile

General Uses: Used in the treatment of reversible airway obstruction due to asthma or COPD.

General Action and Information: Beta-adrenergic agonists (albuterol, epinephrine, isoproterenol, metaproterenol, and terbutaline) produce bronchodilation by stimulating the production of cyclic adenosine monophosphate (cAMP). Newer agents (albuterol, metaproterenol, pirbuterol, and terbutaline) are relatively selective for pulmonary ($beta_1$) receptors, while older agents produce cardiac stimulation ($beta_2$-adrenergic effects) in addition to bronchodilation. Ephedrine also has alpha-adrenergic effects. Phosphodiesterase inhibitors (aminophylline, dyphylline, oxtriphylline, and theophylline) inhibit the breakdown of cAMP. Ipratropium is an anticholinergic compound that produces bronchodilation by blocking the action of acetylcholine in the respiratory tract.

Contraindications: Hypersensitivity to agents, preservatives (bisulfites), or propellants used in their formulation. Avoid use in uncontrolled cardiac arrhythmias.

Precautions: Use cautiously in patients with diabetes, cardiovascular disease, or hyperthyroidism.

Interactions: Therapeutic effectivness may be antagonized by concurrent use of beta-adrenergic blocking agents. Additive sympathomimetic effects with other adrenergic (sympathetic) drugs, including vasopressors and decongestants. Cardiovascular effects may be potentiated by antidepressants and MAO inhibitors.

Nursing Implications

Assessment

- Assess blood pressure, pulse, respiration, lung sounds, and character of secretions before and throughout therapy.
- Patients with a history of cardiovascular problems should be monitored for ECG changes and chest pain.

Potential Nursing Diagnoses

- Airway clearance, ineffective (indications).
- Activity intolerance (indications).
- Knowledge deficit related to medication regimen (patient/family teaching).

Implementation

- Administer around the clock to maintain therapeutic plasma levels.

Patient/Family Teaching

- Emphasize the importance of taking only the prescribed dose at the prescribed time intervals.
- Encourage the patient to drink adequate liquids (2000 ml/day minimum) to decrease the viscosity of the airway secretions.
- Advise patient to avoid over-the-counter cough, cold, or breathing preparations without consulting physician or pharmacist, and minimize intake of xanthine-containing foods or beverages (colas, coffee, and chocolate), as these may increase side effects and cause arrhythmias.
- Caution patient to avoid smoking and other respiratory irritants.
- Instruct patient on proper use of metered-dose inhaler.
- Advise patient to contact physician promptly if the usual dose of medication fails to produce the desired results, symptoms worsen after treatment, or toxic effects occur.
- Patients using other inhalation medications and bronchodilators should be advised to use bronchodilator first and allow 5 min to elapse before administering the other medication, unless otherwise directed by physician.

Evaluation

Effectiveness of therapy can be demonstrated by: ■ Decreased bronchospasm ■ Increased ease of breathing.

Bronchodilators Included in *Davis's Drug Guide for Nurses*

alpha- and beta-adrenergic agonists
ephedrine, 428

beta-adrenergic agonists
albuterol, 16
epinephrine, 430
isoproterenol, 630
metaproterenol, 728
pirbuterol, 944
terbutaline, 1104

phosphodiesterase inhibitors
aminophylline, 43
dyphylline, 417
oxtriphylline, 866
theophylline, 1114

anticholinergic agents
ipratropium, 625

▪ CALCIUM CHANNEL BLOCKERS

Pharmacologic Profile

General Uses: Used in the treatment of hypertension (diltiazem SR, felodipine, isradipine, nicardipine, nifedipine, verapamil), treatment and prophylaxis of angina pectoris or coronary artery spasm (bepridil, diltiazem, nicardipine, verapamil). Verapamil and diltiazem are also used for control of arrhythmias. Nimodipine is used to prevent neurologic damage due to certain types of cerebral vasospasm.

General Action and Information: Block calcium entry into cells of vascular smooth muscle and myocardium. Dilate coronary arteries in both normal and ischemic myocardium and inhibit coronary artery spasm. Decrease AV conduction (verapamil and diltiazem). Nimodipine appears to have a relatively selective effect on cerebral blood vessels.

Contraindications: Hypersensitivity. Contraindicated in bradycardia, second and third degree heart block, or uncompensated congestive heart failure (bepridil, verapamil).

Precautions: Safety in pregnancy and lactation not established. Use cautiously in patients with liver disease or uncontrolled arrhythmias. Bepridil has been associated with serious arrythmias and agranulocytosis.

Interactions: Additive myocardial depression with beta-adrenergic blocking agents and disopyramide (verapamil and diltiazem). Effectiveness may be decreased by phenobarbital or phenytoin; increased by propranolol or cimetidine. Verapamil and diltiazem may increase serum digoxin levels and cause toxicity.

Nursing Implications

Assessment

- **General Info:** Monitor blood pressure and pulse before and periodically during therapy.
- Monitor intake and output ratios and daily weight. Assess patient routinely for signs and symptoms of congestive heart failure (dyspnea, rales/crackles, weight gain, peripheral edema, jugular venous distension).
- **Angina:** Assess frequency and severity of episodes of chest pain periodically throughout therapy.

- **Arrhythmias:** ECG should be monitored continuously during IV therapy and periodically during long-term therapy with verapamil.
- **Cerebral Vasospasm:** Assess patient's neurologic status (level of consciousness, movement) before and periodically during therapy with nimodipine.
- **Lab Test Considerations:** Patients receiving cardiac glycosides concurrently with verapamil or diltiazem should have routine serum digitalis levels and be monitored for signs and symptoms of cardiac glycoside toxicity.

Potential Nursing Diagnoses

- Tissue perfusion, altered (indications).
- Comfort, altered: pain (indications).
- Knowledge deficit related to medication regimen (patient/family teaching).

Implementation

- Do not crush, brush, chew, or open sustained-release tablets or capsules.

Patient/Family Teaching

- **General Info:** Caution patient to make position changes slowly to minimize orthostatic hypotension.
- May cause dizziness or drowsiness. Caution patient to avoid driving or other activities requiring alertness until response to medication is known.
- Instruct patient to avoid concurrent use of alcohol or over-the-counter medications without consulting physician or pharmacist.
- Advise patient to inform physician or dentist of medication regimen before treatment or surgery.
- Advise patient to carry identification describing disease process and medication regimen at all times.
- Emphasize the importance of follow-up examinations to monitor progress.
- **Angina:** Instruct patients on concurrent nitrate therapy to continue taking both medications as ordered and using SL nitroglycerin as needed for anginal attacks.
- Advise patient to contact physician if chest pain worsens or does not improve after therapy, or is accompanied by diaphoresis, or shortness of breath, or if severe, persistent headache occurs.
- Advise patient to discuss activity limitations with physician.
- **Hypertension:** Encourage patient to comply with additional interventions for hypertension (weight reduction, low-sodium diet, regular exercise, discontinuation of smoking, moderation of alcohol consumption, stress management). Medication controls but does not cure hypertension.
- Instruct patient and family on proper technique for monitoring blood pressure. Advise them to check blood pressure weekly and report significant changes to physician.

Evaluation

Effectiveness of therapy can be demonstrated by: ▪ Decreased frequency and severity of anginal attacks ▪ Decreased need for nitrate therapy ▪ Increase in activity tolerance and sense of well-being ▪ Decreased blood pressure ▪ Resolution and prevention of supraventricular tachyarrhythmias ▪ Improvement in neurologic deficits due to vasospasm which may follow subarachnoid hemorrhage due to ruptured intracranial aneurysms.

Calcium Channel Blockers Included in *Davis's Drug Guide for Nurses*

bepridil, 113
diltiazem, 376
felodipine, 476
isradipine, 637
nicardipine, 832
nifedipine, 835
nimodipine, 837
verapamil, 1189

▪ CENTRAL NERVOUS SYSTEM STIMULANTS

Pharmacologic Profile

General Use: Used in the the treatment of narcolepsy and as adjunctive treatment in the management of attention deficit disorder (ADD).

General Action and Information: Produce CNS stimulation by increasing levels of neurotransmitters in the CNS. Produce CNS and respiratory stimulation, dilated pupils, increased motor activity and mental alertness, diminished sense of fatigue, and brighter spirits. In children with attention deficit disorder (ADD) these agents decrease restlessness and increase attention span.

Contraindications: Hypersensitivity. Should not be used in pregnant or lactating women. Should not be used in hyperexcitable states. Avoid use in patients with psychotic personalities or suicidal or homicidal tendencies. Contraindicated in glaucoma and severe cardiovascular disease.

Precautions: Use cautiously in patients with a history of cardiovascular disease, hypertension, or diabetes mellitus, or in elderly or debilitated patients. Continual use may result in psychological dependence or addiction.

Interactions: Additive sympathomimetic effects. Use with MAO inhibitors can result in hypertensive crisis. Alkalinizing the urine (sodium bicarbonate and acetazolamide) decreases excretion and enhances effect of amphetamines. Acidification of urine (ammonium chloride and ascorbic acid) decreases effect of amphetamines. Phenothiazines may also decrease effect. Methylphenidate may decrease the metabolism of other drugs.

Nursing Implications

Assessment

- **General Info:** Monitor blood pressure, pulse, and respiration before administering and periodically throughout course of therapy.
- Monitor weight biweekly and inform physician of significant loss.
- Monitor height periodically in children; inform physician if growth inhibition occurs.
- May produce a false sense of euphoria and well-being. Provide frequent rest periods and observe patient for rebound depression after the effects of the medication have worn off.
- **Attention Deficit Disorders:** Assess attention span, impulse control, and interactions with others in children. Therapy may be interrupted at intervals to determine if symptoms are sufficient to warrant continued therapy.
- **Narcolepsy:** Observe and document frequency of episodes.

Potential Nursing Diagnoses
- Thought processes, altered (side effects).
- Knowledge deficit related to medication regimen (patient/family teaching).

Implementation
- Medication should be administered at least 6 hr before bedtime to minimize sleep disturbances.

Patient/Family Teaching
- **General Info:** Instruct patient not to alter dose without consulting physician. These medications have a high dependence and abuse potential. Abrupt cessation with high doses may cause extreme fatigue and mental depression.
- Inform patient that the effects of drug-induced dry mouth can be minimized by rinsing frequently with water or chewing sugarless gum or candies.
- Advise patient to avoid the intake of large amounts of caffeine.
- Medication may impair judgment. Advise patients to use caution when driving or during other activities requiring alertness until response to medication is known.
- Inform patient that physician may order periodic holidays from the drug to assess progress and decrease dependence.

Evaluation

Effectiveness of therapy can be demonstrated by: ▪ Decreased frequency of narcoleptic episodes ▪ Improved attention span and social interactions.

Central Nervous System Stimulants
Included in *Davis's Drug Guide for Nurses*

▪ CHOLINERGICS

Pharmacologic Profile

General Use: Used in the treatment of nonobstructive urinary retention (bethanechol), and the diagnosis (edrophonium) and treatment (neostigmine and pyridostigmine) of myasthenia gravis. Physostigmine is used in the diagnosis and management of cholinergic excess, which occurs following antidepressant overdosage. Cholinesterase inhibitors may be used to reverse nondepolarizing neuromuscular blocking agents. Edrophonium has been used in the treatment of supraventricular tachyarrhythmias. Acetylcholine is administered as an eye drop to produce miosis during ophthalmic surgery.

General Action and Information: Cholinergics intensify and prolong the action of acetylcholine by either mimicking its effects at cholinergic receptor sites (bethanecol) or preventing the breakdown of acetylcholine by inhibiting cholinesterases (edrophonium, neostigmine, physostigmine, and pyridostigmine). Effects include increased tone in GU and skeletal muscle, decreased intraocular pressure, increased secretions, and decreased bladder capacity.

Contraindications: Hypersensitivity. Avoid use in patients with possible obstruction of the GI or GU tract.

Precautions: Use with extreme caution in patients with a history of asthma, peptic ulcer disease, cardiovascular disease, epilepsy, or hyperthyroidism. Safety in pregnancy and lactation not established. Atropine should be available to treat excessive dosage.

Interactions: Additive cholinergic effects. Do not use with depolarizing neuromuscular blocking agents. Use with ganglionic blocking agents may result in severe hypotension.

Nursing Implications

Assessment

- **General Info:** Monitor pulse, respiratory rate, and blood pressure frequency throughout parenteral administration.
- **Myasthenia Gravis:** Assess neuromuscular status (ptosis, diplopia, vital capacity, ability to swallow, and extremity strength) before and at time of peak effect.
- Assess patient for overdosage and underdosage or resistance. Both have similar symptoms (muscle weakness, dyspnea, and dysphagia), but symptoms of overdosage usually occur within 1 hr of administration, while underdosage symptoms occur 3 or more hrs after administration. A Tensilon test (edrophonium chloride) may be used to distinguish between overdosage and underdosage.
- **Antidote to Nondepolarizing Neuromuscular Blocking Agents:** Monitor reversal of effects of neuromuscular blocking agents with a peripheral nerve stimulator.
- **Urinary Retention:** Monitor intake and output ratios. Palpate abdomen for bladder distention. Physician may order catheterization to assess post-void residual.
- **Glaucoma:** Monitor patient for changes in vision, eye irritation, and persistent headache.
- **Toxicity and Overdose:** Atropine is the specific antidote.

Potential Nursing Diagnoses

- Urinary elimination, altered (indications).
- Breathing pattern, ineffective (indications).
- Knowledge deficit related to medication regimen (patient/family teaching).

Implementation

- **Myasthenia Gravis:** For patients who have difficulty chewing, medication may be administered 30 min before meals.

Patient/Family Teaching

- **General Info:** Instruct patients with myasthenia gravis to take medication exactly as ordered. Taking the dose late may result in myasthenic crisis. Taking the dose early may result in a cholinergic crisis. This regimen must be continued as a lifelong therapy.
- **Ophth:** Instruct patient on correct method of application of drops or ointment (see Appendix H).
- Explain to patient that pupil constriction and temporary stinging and blurring of vision is expected. Physician should be notified if blurred vision and brow ache persist.
- Caution patient that night vision may be impaired.

CLASSIFICATIONS

- Advise patient of the need for regular eye examinations to monitor intraocular pressure and visual fields.

EVALUATION

Effectiveness of therapy can be demonstrated by: ▪ Reversal of CNS symptoms secondary to anticholinergic excess resulting from drug overdosage or ingestion of poisonous plants ▪ Control of elevated intraocular pressure ▪ Increase in bladder function and tone ▪ Decrease in abdominal distention ▪ Relief of myasthenic symptoms ▪ Differentiation of myasthenic from cholinergic crisis ▪ Reversal of paralysis after anesthesia ▪ Resolution of supraventricular tachycardia.

Cholinergic Agents Included in *Davis's Drug Guide for Nurses*

▪ DIURETICS

Pharmacologic Profile

General Use: Thiazide and loop diuretics are used alone or in combination in the treatment of hypertension or edema due to congestive heart failure or other causes. Potassium-sparing diuretics have weak diuretic and antihypertensive properties and are used mainly to conserve potassium in patients receiving thiazide or loop diuretics. Carbonic anhydrase inhibitors are used mainly in the treatment of glaucoma. Osmotic diuretics are often used in the management of cerebral edema.

General Action and Information: Enhance the selective excretion of various electrolytes and water by affecting renal mechanism for tubular secretion and reabsorption. Groups commonly used are thiazide diuretics and thiazide-like diuretics (chlorothiazide, chlorthalidone, hydrochlorothiazide, indapamide, and metolazone), loop diuretics (bumetanide, ethacrynic acid, and furosemide), potassium-sparing diuretics (amiloride, spironolactone, and triamterene), osmotic diuretics (mannitol), and carbonic anhydrase inhibitors (acetazolamide). Mechanisms vary depending on agent.

Contraindications: Hypersensitivity. Thiazide diuretics may exhibit cross-sensitivity with other sulfonamides.

Precautions: Use with caution in patients with renal or hepatic disease. Safety in pregnancy and lactation not established.

Interactions: Additive hypokalemia with glucocorticoids, amphotericin B, mezlocillin, piperacillin, or ticarcillin. Hypokalemia enhances cardiac glycoside toxicity. Potassium-losing diuretics decrease lithium excretion and may cause toxicity. Additive hypotension with other antihypertensives or nitrates. Potassium-sparing diuretics may cause hyperkalemia when used with potassium supplements or angiotensin converting enzyme (ACE) inhibitors.

Nursing Implications

Assessment
- **General Info:** Assess fluid status throughout therapy. Monitor daily weight, intake and output ratios, amount and location of edema, lung sounds, skin turgor, and mucous membranes.
- Assess patient for anorexia, muscle weakness, numbness, tingling, paresthesia, confusion, and excessive thirst. Notify physician promptly if these signs of electrolyte imbalance occur.
- **Increased Intracranial Pressure:** Monitor neurologic status and intracranial pressure readings in patients receiving osmotic diuretics to decrease cerebral edema.
- **Increased Intraocular Pressure:** Monitor for persistent or increased eye pain or decreased visual acuity.
- **Lab Test Considerations:** Monitor electrolytes (especially potassium), blood glucose, BUN, and serum uric acid levels before and periodically throughout course of therapy.
- Thiazide diuretics may cause increased serum cholesterol, low-density lipoprotein (LDL), and triglyceride concentrations.

Potential Nursing Diagnoses
- Fluid volume excess (indications).
- Knowledge deficit related to medication regimen (patient/family teaching).

Implementation
- Administer oral diuretics in the morning to prevent disruption of sleep cycle.
- Many diuretics are available in combination with antihypertensives or potassium-sparing diuretics.

Patient/Family Teaching
- **General Info:** Caution patient to make position changes slowly to minimize orthostatic hypotension. Caution patient that the use of alcohol, exercise during hot weather, or standing for long periods during therapy may enhance orthostatic hypotension.
- Instruct patient to consult physician regarding dietary potassium guidelines.
- Instruct patient to monitor weight weekly and notify physician of significant changes. Instruct patients with hypertension in the correct technique for monitoring weekly blood pressure.
- Caution patient to use sunscreen and protective clothing to prevent photosensitivity reactions.
- Advise patient to consult physician or pharmacist before taking over-the-counter medication concurrently with this therapy.
- Instruct patient to notify physician or dentist of medication regimen before treatment or surgery.
- Advise patient to contact physician immediately if muscle weakness, cramps, nausea, dizziness, or numbness or tingling of extremities occur.
- Emphasize the importance of routine follow-up.
- **Hypertension:** Reinforce the need to continue additional therapies for hypertension (weight loss, regular exercise, restricted sodium intake, stress reduction, moderation of alcohol consumption, and cessation of smoking).

EVALUATION

Effectiveness of therapy can be demonstrated by: ▪ Decreased blood pressure ▪ Increased urine output ▪ Decreased edema ▪ Reduced intracranial pressure ▪ Reduced intraocular pressure ▪ Prevention of hypokalemia in patients taking diuretics ▪ Treatment of hyperaldosteronism.

Diuretics Included in *Davis's Drug Guide for Nurses*

▪ ELECTROLYTES/ELECTROLYTE MODIFIERS

Pharmacologic Profile

General Use: Use to prevent or treat deficiencies or excesses of electrolytes. Acidifiers and alkalinizers are used to increase solubility and promote renal excretion of substances which accumulate in certain disease states (kidney stones and uric acid).

General Action and Information: Electrolytes are essential for homeostasis. Maintenance of electrolyte levels within normal levels is required for many physiologic processes such as cardiac, nerve, and muscle function; bone growth and stability; and other processes. Electrolytes may also serve as catalysts in many enzymatic reactions.

Contraindications: Contraindicated in situations where replacement would cause excess or where risk factors for retention are present.

Precautions: Use cautiously in disease states where electrolyte imbalances are common, such as hepatic or renal disease, adrenal disorders, pituitary disorders, and diabetes mellitus.

Interactions: Depend on individual agents. Akalinizers and acidifiers can alter excretion of drugs whose renal elimination is pH-dependent. See specific entries.

Nursing Implications

ASSESSMENT

- Observe patient carefully for evidence of electrolyte excess or insufficiency. Monitor lab values before and periodically throughout therapy.

POTENTIAL NURSING DIAGNOSES

- Nutrition, altered: less than body requirements (indications).

- Knowledge deficit related to medication and dietary regimens (patient/family teaching).

IMPLEMENTATION

- **Potassium chloride:** Do not administer parenteral potassium chloride undiluted.

PATIENT/FAMILY TEACHING

- Review diet modifications with patients with chronic electrolyte disturbances.

EVALUATION

Effectiveness of therapy can be demonstrated by: ▪ Return to normal serum electrolyte concentrations and resolution of clinical symptoms of electrolyte imbalance ▪ Changes in pH or composition of urine which prevent formation of renal calculi.

Electrolytes/Electrolyte Modifiers
Included in *Davis's Drug Guide for Nurses*

alkalinizing agents
sodium bicarbonate, 1056

calcium salts
calcium carbonate, 150
calcium chloride, 152
calcium gluceptate, 154
calcium gluconate, 155
calcium lactate, 158

hypocalcemic agent
calcitonin, 146
etidronate, 462
gallium nitrate, 527
plicamycin, 949

hypophosphatemic
aluminum hydroxide, 30

magnesium salts
magnesium citrate, 691
magnesium sulfate, 695

phosphates
monobasic potassium phosphate, 966
potassium and sodium phosphates, 956
potassium phosphate, 966
sodium phosphate, 1063

potassium exhange resin
sodium polystyrene sulfonate, 1064

potassium salts
potassium bicarbonate, 958
potassium chloride, 960
potassium gluconate, 962

replacement solutions
sodium chloride, 1059

urinary acidifier
potassium and sodium phosphate, 956
monobasic potassium phosphate, 966

urinary alkalinizer
sodium citrate and citric acid, 1061

▪ GLUCOCORTICOIDS

Pharmacologic Profile

General Use: Used in replacement doses (20 mg of hydrocortisone or equivalent) to treat adrenocortical insufficiency. Larger doses are usually used for their anti-inflammatory, immunosuppressive, or antineoplastic activity. Used adjunctively in many other situations including hypercalcemia and autoimmune diseases.

General Action and Information: Produce profound and varied metabolic effects in addition to modifying the normal immune response and suppressing inflammation. Available in a variety of dosage forms including oral, injectable, topical, and inhalation.

Contraindications: Serious infections (except for certain forms of meningitis). Do not administer live vaccines to patients on larger doses.

Precautions: Chronic treatment will result in adrenal suppression. Do not discontinue abruptly. Additional doses may be needed during stress (surgery and infection). Safety in pregnancy and lactation not established. Chronic use in children will result in decreased growth. May mask signs of infection. Use lowest dose possible for shortest time possible. Alternate day therapy is preferable during chronic treatment.

Interactions: Additive hypokalemia with amphotericin B, potassium-losing diuretics, mezlocillin, piperacillin, and ticarcillin. Hypokalemia may increase the risk of cardiac glycoside toxicity. May increase requirements for insulin or oral hypoglycemic agents. Phenytoin, phenobarbital, and rifampin stimulate metabolism and may decrease effectiveness. Oral contraceptives may block metabolism. Cholestyramine, colestipol may decrease absorption.

Nursing Implications

Assessment

- These drugs are indicated for many conditions. Assess involved systems before and periodically throughout course of therapy.
- Assess patient for signs of adrenal insufficiency (hypotension, weight loss, weakness, nausea, vomiting, anorexia, lethargy, confusion, restlessness) prior to and periodically throughout course of therapy.
- Children should also have periodic evaluations of growth.

Potential Nursing Diagnoses

- Infection, high risk for (side effects).
- Knowledge deficit related to medication regimen (patient/family teaching).
- Body image disturbance (side effects).

Implementation

- **General Info:** If dose is ordered daily or every other day, administer in the morning to coincide with the body's normal secretion of cortisol.
- **PO:** Administer with meals to minimize gastric irritation.

Patient/Family Teaching

- Emphasize need to take medication exactly as directed. Review symptoms of adrenal insufficiency which may occur upon stopping the medication and may be life-threatening.
- Encourage patients on long-term therapy to eat a diet high in protein, calcium, and potassium and low in sodium and carbohydrates.
- These drugs cause immunosuppression and may mask symptoms of infection. Instruct patient to avoid people with known contagious illnesses and to

report possible infections. Advise patient to consult physician before receiving any vaccinations.
- Discuss possible effects on body image. Explore coping mechanisms.
- Advise patient to carry identification in the event of an emergency in which patient cannot relate medical history.

EVALUATION

Effectiveness of therapy can be demonstrated by: ▪ Suppression of the inflammatory and immune responses in autoimmune disorders, allergic reactions, and organ transplants ▪ Replacement therapy in adrenal insufficiency.

Glucocorticoids Included in *Davis's Drug Guide for Nurses*

topical glucocorticoids, 1155

short-acting glucocorticoids
- cortisone, 293
- hydrocortisone, 579

intermediate-acting glucocorticoids
- methylprednisolone, 753
- prednisolone, 975
- prednisone, 978
- triamcinolone, 1160

long-acting glucocorticoids
- beclomethasone, 104
- betamethasone, 114
- dexamethasone, 338
- flunisolide, 503

▪ HISTAMINE H_2 ANTAGONISTS

Pharmacologic Profile

General Uses: Treatment and prophylaxis of peptic ulcer, gastric hypersecretory conditions such as Zollinger-Ellison syndrome, and gastroesophageal reflux disease (GERD).

General Action and Information: Competitively inhibit the action of histamine at the H_2 receptor, located primarily in gastric parietal cells. Result is the inhibition of gastric acid secretion.

Contraindications: Hypersensitivity.

Precautions: Dosage reduction recommended in renal impairment and the elderly. Safety in pregnancy, lactation, and children not established.

Interactions: Cimetidine inhibits the ability of the liver to metabolize several drugs which may increase the risk of toxicity from oral anticoagulants, theophylline, tricyclic antidepressants, metoprolol, phenytoin, propranolol, or lidocaine. All agents will decrease the absorption of ketoconazole.

Nursing Implications

ASSESSMENT
- Assess patient routinely for epigastric or abdominal pain and frank or occult blood in the stool, emesis, or gastric aspirate.
- Assess elderly and severely ill patients for confusion routinely. Notify physician promptly should this occur.
- **Lab Test Considerations:** Antagonizes the effects of pentagastrin and histamine during gastric acid secretion test. Avoid administration during the 24 hr preceding the test.

- May cause false-negative results in skin tests using allergen extracts. These drugs should be discontinued 24 hr prior to the test.

POTENTIAL NURSING DIAGNOSES
- Comfort, altered in: pain (indications).
- Knowledge deficit related to medication regimen (patient/family teaching).

IMPLEMENTATION
- If administering oral doses concurrently with antacids, give at least 1 hr apart.

PATIENT/FAMILY TEACHING
- Instruct patient to take medication as prescribed for the full course of therapy, even if feeling better. If a dose is missed, it should be taken as soon as remembered, but not if almost time for next dose. Do not double doses.
- Inform patient that smoking interferes with the action of some of these drugs. Encourage patient to quit smoking or at least not to smoke after last dose of the day.
- Advise patient to avoid alcohol, products containing aspirin, and foods that may cause an increase in GI irritation.
- Advise patient to report onset of black, tarry stools, diarrhea, dizziness, rash, or confusion to the physician promptly.

EVALUATION
Effectiveness of therapy can be demonstrated by: ▪ Decreased abdominal pain ▪ Prevention of gastric irritation and bleeding. Healing of duodenal ulcers can be seen by x-rays or endoscopy. Therapy is continued for at least 6 wk after initial episode.

Histamine H_2 Antagonists Included in *Davis's Drug Guide for Nurses*

cimetidine, 248	nizatidine, 846
famotidine, 472	ranitidine, 1032

▪ HORMONES

Pharmacologic Profile

General Use: Used in the treatment of deficiency states including diabetes (insulin), diabetes insipidus (desmopressin), hypothyroidism (thyroid hormone), and menopause (estrogens). Combinations of hormones (estrogens and progestins) are used as oral contraceptive agents. Hormones may be used to treat hormonally sensitive tumors (androgens and estrogens) and in other selected situations. See individual drugs.

General Action and Information: Natural or synthetic substances which have a specific effect on target tissue. Differ greatly in their effects, depending on individual agent and function of target tissue.

Contraindications: Differ greatly among agents. See individual entries.

Precautions: Use cautiously in patients with severe cardiac, hepatic, or renal disease. When used in deficiency states appropriate laboratory monitoring is necessary to adjust dosages and monitor progress.

Interactions: Differ greatly among agents. See individual entries.

Nursing Implications

Assessment

- **General Info:** Monitor patient for symptoms of hormonal excess or insufficiency.
- **Sex hormones:** Blood pressure and hepatic function tests should be monitored periodically throughout therapy.
- **Epoetin Alpha:** Monitor blood pressure, hematocrit, hemoglobin, reticulocyte count, and RBC, as well as symptoms of anemia throughout therapy. Uncontrolled hypertension is contraindicated.

Potential Nursing Diagnoses

- Sexual dysfunction (indications).
- Body image disturbance (indications, side effects).
- Knowledge deficit related to medication regimen (patient/family teaching).

Implementation

- **Sex hormones:** Continue to administer according to schedule followed prior to hospitalization.

Patient/Family Teaching

- **General Info:** Explain dosage schedule (and withdrawal bleeding with female sex hormones).
- Emphasize importance of follow-up examinations to monitor effectiveness of therapy and to ensure proper development of children and early detection of possible side effects.
- **Female sex hormones:** Advise patient to report signs and symptoms of fluid retention, thromboembolic disorders, mental depression, or hepatic dysfunction to physician.

Evaluation

Effectiveness of therapy can be demonstrated by: ▪ Resolution of clinical symptoms of hormone imbalance including menopausal symptoms and effective contraception ▪ Correction of fluid and electrolyte imbalances ▪ Control of the spread of advanced metastatic breast or prostate cancer ▪ Slowed progression of postmenopausal osteoporosis ▪ Increase in hematocrit.

Hormones Included in *Davis's Drug Guide for Nurses*

hormonal contraceptives, 287

anabolic steroid

nandrolone, 817

adrenocorticotropic

corticotropin, 290
cosyntropin, 295

androgens

danazol, 321
testosterone, 1108

antidiuretic

desmopressin, 336
vasopressin, 1185

estrogens

chlorotrianisene, 231
dienestrol, 360
diethylstilbestrol, 362
estrogens, conjugated, 452
estropipate, 455

gastrointestinal

octreotide, 855

gonadotripin-releasing hormone

nafarelin, 809

continued

gonadotropins
menotropins, 715

growth hormone
somatrem, 1066
somatropin, 1066

ovulation inducer
clomiphene, 263

oxytocic
oxytocin, 873

progestin
medroxyprogesterone, 708
progesterone, 994

thyroid
levothyroxine, 665
liothyronine, 671
liotrix, 673
thyroid, 1132

miscellaneous
calcitonin, 146
epoetin alfa, 434
glucagon, 536
insulin, 613

▪ IMMUNOSUPPRESSANTS

Pharmacologic Profile

General Use: Azathioprine and cyclosporine are used with glucocorticoids in the prevention of transplantation rejection reactions. Muromonab-CD3 is used to manage rejection reactions not controlled by other agents. Azathioprine, cyclophosphamide, and methotrexate are used in the management of selected autoimmune diseases (nephrotic syndrome of childhood and severe rheumatoid arthritis).

General Action and Information: Inhibit cell-mediated immune responses by different mechanisms. In addition to azathioprine and cyclosporine, which are used primarily for their immunomodulating properties, cyclophosphamide and methotrexate are used to suppress the immune responses in certain disease states (nephrotic syndrome of childhood and severe rheumatoid arthritis). Muromonab-CD3 is a recombinant immunoglobulin antibody which alters T cell function.

Contraindications: Hypersensitivity to drug or vehicle.

Precautions: Use cautiously in patients with infections. Safety in pregnancy and lactation not established.

Interactions: Allopurinol inhibits the metabolism of azathioprine. Drugs which alter liver metabolizing processes may change the effect of cyclosporine. The risk of toxicity of methotrexate may be increased by other nephrotoxic drugs, large doses of aspirin, or nonsteroidal anti-inflammatory agents. Muromonab-CD3 has additive immunosuppressive properties; concurrent immunosuppressive doses should be decreased or eliminated.

Nursing Implications

ASSESSMENT

- **General Info:** Monitor for infection (vital signs, sputum, urine, stool, WBC). Notify physician immediately if symptoms occur.
- **Organ Transplant:** Assess for symptoms of organ rejection throughout therapy.

- **Lab Test Considerations:** Monitor CBC and differential throughout course of therapy.

Potential Nursing Diagnoses
- Infection, high risk for (side effects).
- Knowledge deficit related to medication regimen (patient/family teaching).

Implementation
- Protect transplant patients from staff and visitors who may carry infection.
- Maintain protective isolation as indicated.

Patient/Family Teaching
- Reinforce the need for lifelong therapy to prevent transplant rejection. Review symptoms of rejection for transplanted organ and stress need to notify physician immediately if they occur.
- Advise patient to avoid contact with contagious persons and those who have recently taken oral poliovirus vaccine. Patients should not receive vaccinations without first consulting with physician.
- Emphasize the importance of follow-up examinations and lab tests.

Evaluation
Effectiveness of therapy can be demonstrated by: ▪ Prevention or reversal of rejection of organ transplants or decrease in symptoms of autoimmune disorders.

Immunosuppressants Included in *Davis's Drug Guide for Nurses*

cyclophosphamide, 306
cyclosporine, 309
methotrexate, 743
muromonab-CD3, 805

▪ INOTROPIC AGENTS

Pharmacologic Profile

General Use: Management of congestive heart failure or cardiac decompensation unresponsive to conventional therapy with cardiac glycosides, diuretics, or vasodilators. Also used during cardiac surgery.

General Action and Information: Increase cardiac output mainly by direct myocardial effects and some peripheral vascular effects. Cardiac glycosides (deslanoside, digoxin, and digitoxin) act by direct effects on the myocardium.

Contraindications: Hypersensitivity. Avoid use in patients with idiopathic hypertrophic subaortic stenosis.

Precautions: Safety in pregnancy and lactation not established.

Interactions: Beta-adrenergic blockers may negate the effects of dobutamine or dopamine. Several drugs may increase the arrhythmogenic and hypertensive effects of dobutamine or dopamine. Amrinone may produce excessive hypotension when given with disopyramide. Agents which cause hypokalemia, hypomagnesemia, or hypercalcemia increase the risk of cardiac glycoside toxicity. Bradycardia from beta blockers may be additive with cardiac glycosides. Quinidine increases serum digoxin levels.

Nursing Implications

Assessment

- Monitor pulse, blood pressure, ECG, and hemodynamic parameters frequently during parenteral administration and periodically throughout oral administration.
- Monitor intake and output ratios and daily weights. Assess patient for signs and symptoms of congestive heart failure (peripheral edema, rales/crackles, dyspnea, weight gain, and jugular venous distension) throughout therapy.
- Before administering initial loading dose, determine if patient has taken any cardiac glycoside preparations in the preceding 2–3 wk.
- **Lab Test Considerations:** Serum electrolyte levels, especially potassium, magnesium, and calcium, and renal and hepatic function should be evaluated periodically during course of therapy.
- **Toxicity and Overdose:** Patients taking cardiac glycosides should have serum levels measured regularly.

Potential Nursing Diagnoses

- Cardiac output, decreased (indications).
- Knowledge deficit related to medication regimen (patient/family teaching).

Implementation

- Hypokalemia should be corrected before administration of amrinone, deslanoside, digoxin, or digitoxin.
- Hypovolemia should be corrected with volume expanders before administration.

Patient/Family Teaching

- Advise patient to notify physician if symptoms are not relieved or worsen.
- Instruct patient to notify nurse immediately if pain or discomfort at the insertion site occurs during IV administration.

Evaluation

Effectiveness of therapy can be demonstrated by: ▪ Increased cardiac output ▪ Decrease in severity of congestive heart failure ▪ Increased urine output.

Inotropic Agents Included in *Davis's Drug Guide for Nurses*

▪ LAXATIVES

Pharmacologic Profile

General Uses: Used to treat or prevent constipation or to prepare the bowel for radiologic or endoscopic procedures.

General Action and Information: Induce one or more bowel movements per day. Groups include stimulants (bisacodyl, cascara and its dervatives, phenolphthalein, and senna), saline laxatives (magnesium salts and phosphates), stool softeners (docusate), bulk-forming agents (polycarbophil and psyllium), lubricants (mineral oil), and osmotic cathartics (glycerin, lactulose, polyethylene glycol/electrolyte). Increasing fluid intake, exercise, and adding more dietary fiber are also useful in the management of chronic constipation.

Contraindications: Hypersensitivity. Contraindicated in persistant abdominal pain, nausea, or vomiting of unknown etiology, especially if accompanied by fever or other signs of an acute abdomen.

Precautions: Excessive or prolonged use may lead to dependence. Should not be used in children unless advised by a physician.

Interactions: Theoretically may decrease the absorption of other orally administered drugs by decreasing transit time.

Nursing Implications

Assessment

- Assess patient for abdominal distention, presence of bowel sounds, and usual pattern of bowel function.
- Assess color, consistency, and amount of stool produced.

Potential Nursing Diagnoses

- Bowel elimination, altered: constipation (indications).
- Knowledge deficit related to medication regimen (patient/family teaching).

Implementation

- Many laxatives may be administered at bedtime for morning results.
- Taking oral doses on an empty stomach will usually produce more rapid results.
- Do not crush or chew enteric-coated tablets. Take with a full glass of water or juice.
- Stool softeners and bulk laxatives may take several days for results.

Patient/Family Teaching

- Advise patients, other than those with spinal cord injuries, that laxatives should be used only for short-term therapy. Long-term therapy may cause electrolyte imbalance and dependence.
- Advise patient to increase fluid intake to a minimum of 1500–2000 ml/day during therapy to prevent dehydration.
- Encourage patients to utilize other forms of bowel regulation: increasing bulk in the diet, increasing fluid intake, and increasing mobility. Normal bowel habits are individualized and may vary from 3 times/day to 3 times/wk.
- Instruct patients with cardiac disease to avoid straining during bowel movements (Valsalva maneuver).
- Advise patient that laxatives should not be used when constipation is accompanied by abdominal pain, fever, nausea, or vomiting.

Evaluation

Effectiveness of therapy can be demonstrated by: ▪ The patient having a soft, formed bowel movement ▪ Evacuation of the colon.

Laxatives Included in *Davis's Drug Guide for Nurses*

▪ LIPID-LOWERING AGENTS

Pharmacologic Profile

General Use: Used as a part of a total plan including diet and exercise to reduce blood lipids in an effort to reduce the morbidity and mortality of atherosclerotic cardiovascular disease.

General Action and Information: Lower cholesterol and/or triglycerides by a variety of mechanisms. See individual drugs.

Contraindications: Hypersensitivity.

Precautions: Safety in pregnancy, lactation, and children not established. See individual drugs. Dietary therapy should be given a 2–3 mon trial before drug therapy is initiated.

Interactions: Bile acid sequestrants (cholestyramine and colestipol) may bind lipid-soluble vitamins (A, D, E, and K) and other concurrently administered drugs in the GI tract.

Nursing Implications

Assessment

- Obtain a diet history, especially in regard to fat and alcohol consumption.
- **Lab Test Considerations:** Serum cholesterol and triglyceride levels should be evaluated before initiating and periodically throughout course of therapy. Medication should be discontinued if paradoxical increase in cholesterol level occurs.
- Liver function tests should be assessed before and periodically throughout therapy. May cause an increase in levels.

Potential Nursing Diagnoses

- Knowledge deficit related to medication regimen (patient/family teaching).
- Noncompliance (patient/family teaching).

Implementation

- See specific medications to determine timing of doses in relation to meals.

Patient/Family Teaching

- Advise patient that these medications should be used in conjunction with diet restrictions (fat, cholesterol, carbohydrates, and alcohol), exercise, and cessation of smoking.

Evaluation

Effectiveness of therapy can be demonstrated by: ▪ Decreased serum triglyceride and low-density lipoprotein (LDL) cholesterol levels and improved high-density lipoprotein (HDL) cholesterol ratios. Therapy is usually discontinued if the clinical response is not evident after 3 mon of therapy.

Lipid-Lowering Agents Included in *Davis's Drug Guide for Nurses*

bile acid sequestrants

cholestyramine, 242
colestipol, 282

miscellaneous agents

clofibrate, 262
gemfibrozil, 530
lovastatin, 684
niacin, nicotinic acid, 830
pravastatin, 970
probucol, 984

▪ NARCOTIC ANALGESICS

Pharmacologic Profile

General Uses: Management of moderate to severe pain. Some agents used as general anesthetic adjuncts (alfentanil, fentanyl, and sufentanil).

General Action and Information: Narcotics bind to opiate receptors in the CNS, where they act as agonists of endogenously occurring opioid peptides (eukephalins and endorphins). The result is alteration to the perception of and response to pain.

Contraindications: Hypersensitivity to individual agents.

Precautions: Use cautiously in patients with undiagnosed abdominal pain, head trauma or pathology, liver disease, or history of addiction to narcotics. Use smaller doses initially in the elderly and those with respiratory diseases. Chronic use may result in tolerance and the need for larger doses to relieve pain. Psychological or physical dependence may occur.

Interactions: Increases the CNS depressant properties of other drugs, including alcohol, antihistamines, antidepressants, sedative/hypnotics, phenothiazines, and MAO inhibitors. Use of partial-antagonist narcotic analgesics (buprenorphine, butorphanol, dezocine, nalbuphine, and pentazocine) may precipitate narcotic withdrawal in physically dependent patients. Use with MAO inhibitors or procarbazine may result in severe paradoxical reactions (especially with meperidine). Nalbuphine or pentazocine may decrease the analgesic effects of other concurrently administered narcotic analgesics.

Nursing Implications

Assessment

- Assess type, location, and intensity of pain prior to and at peak following administration.
- Assess blood pressure, pulse, and respiratory rate before and periodically during administration.
- Prolonged use may lead to physical and psychological dependence and tolerance. This should not prevent patient from receiving adequate analgesia. Most patients who receive narcotic analgesics for medical reasons do not develop psychological dependency. Progressively higher doses may be required to relieve pain with long-term therapy.
- Assess bowel function routinely. Increased intake of fluids and bulk, stool softeners, and laxatives may minimize constipating effects.
- Monitor intake and output ratios. If significant discrepancies occur, assess for urinary retention and inform physician.
- **Toxicity and Overdose:** If overdosage occurs, naloxone (Narcan) is the antidote. Monitor patient closely; dose may need to be repeated or may need to be administered as an infusion.

Potential Nursing Diagnoses

- Comfort, altered: pain (indications).
- Sensory-perceptual alteration: visual, auditory (side effects).
- Injury, high risk for (side effects).
- Knowledge deficit related to medication regimen (patient/family teaching).

Implementation

- Explain therapeutic value of medication before administration to enhance the analgesic effect.
- Regularly administered doses may be more effective than prn administration. Analgesic is more effective if given before pain becomes severe.
- Coadministration with non-narcotic analgesics may have additive analgesic effects and may permit lower doses.
- Medication should be discontinued gradually after long-term use to prevent withdrawal symptoms.

Patient/Family Teaching

- Instruct patient on how and when to ask for prn pain medication.
- Medication may cause drowsiness or dizziness. Caution patient to call for assistance when ambulating or smoking and to avoid driving or other activities requiring alertness until response to medication is known.
- Advise patient to make position changes slowly to minimize orthostatic hypotension.
- Caution patient to avoid concurrent use of alcohol or other CNS depressants with this medication.
- Encourage patient to turn, cough, and breathe deeply every 2 hr to prevent atelectasis.

Evaluation

Effectiveness of therapy can be demonstrated by: ▪ Decreased severity of pain without a significant alteration in level of consciousness, respiratory status, or blood pressure.

Narcotic Analgesics Included in *Davis's Drug Guide for Nurses*

▪ NEUROMUSCULAR BLOCKING AGENTS

Pharmacologic Profile

General Use: Used to facilitate mechanical ventilation or as adjuncts with general anesthesia to allow skeletal muscle paralysis which may be required during surgical procedures.

General Action and Information: Paralyze muscular function by inhibiting neuromuscular transmission. These agents act as agonists of acetylcholine, producing initial fasciculation then neuromuscular blockade. Blockade from depolarizing agents resists the action of cholinesterase and is more prolonged than that of nondepolarizing agents. Neuromuscular blocking agents have no analgesic properties.

Contraindications: Products may contain iodides, bromides, parabens, or sulfites. Select agents carefully in patients with known hypersensitivity. Avoid use of succinylcholine in patients with a history of malignant hyperthermia or fractures.

Precautions: Use with caution in the very young or elderly patients (increased sensitivity). Provide adequate analgesia/anesthesia as required. Use cautiously in patients with cardiovascular or pulmonary disease.

Interactions: Additive respiratory depression with narcotic analgesics and other CNS depressants. Increased risk of adverse cardiovascular reactions with antihypertensives, cardiac glycosides, or antiarrhythmics. Neuromuscular blockade may be enhanced by nonpenicillin anti-infectives, diuretics, antiarrhythmics, anticholinesterases, or local anesthetics. Avoid concurrent use of succinylcholine with any agents which may act as cholinesterase inhibitors (results in prolonged neuromuscular blockade).

Nursing Implications

Assessment

- Assess respiratory status continuously throughout therapy. Neuromuscular blocking agents should be used only for intubated patients. Assess patient for increased respiratory secretions; suction as necessary.
- Neuromuscular response to these medications should be monitored with a peripheral nerve stimulator intraoperatively. Monitor deep tendon reflexes

during prolonged administration. Paralysis is initially selective and usually occurs consecutively in the following muscles: levator muscles of eyelids, muscles of mastication, limb muscles, abdominal muscles, muscles of the glottis, intercostal muscles, and the diaphragm. Recovery of muscle function usually occurs in reverse order.

- Monitor heart rate, ECG, and blood pressure periodically throughout therapy. May cause a slight increase in heart rate and blood pressure.
- Observe the patient for residual muscle weakness and respiratory distress during the recovery period.
- **Toxicity and Overdose:** If overdose occurs, use peripheral nerve stimulator to determine the degree of neuromuscular blockade. Maintain airway patency and ventilation until recovery of normal respirations occurs.
- Administration of anticholinesterase agents (edrophonium, neostigmine, and pyridostigmine) may be used to antagonize the action of nondepolarizing neuromuscular blocking agents. Atropine is usually administered before or concurrently with anticholinesterase agents.

Potential Nursing Diagnoses

- Breathing pattern, ineffective (indications).
- Communication, impaired: verbal (side effects).
- Fear (patient/family teaching).

Implementation

- Neuromuscular blocking agents have no effect on consciousness or the pain threshold. Adequate anesthesia should *always* be used when these agents are used as an adjunct to surgical procedures or when painful procedures are performed. Benzodiazepines and/or analgesics should be administered concurrently when prolonged therapy is used for ventilator patients; patient is awake and able to feel all sensations.
- If eyes remain open throughout prolonged adminstration, protect corneas with artificial tears.

Patient/Family Teaching

- Explain all procedures to patient receiving neuromuscular-blocking agents without anesthesia; consciousness is not affected by these agents alone. Provide emotional support.
- Reassure patient that communication abilities will return as the medication wears off.

Evaluation

Effectiveness of therapy can be demonstrated by: ▪ Adequate suppression of the twitch response when tested with peripheral nerve stimulation and subsequent muscle paralysis.

Neuromuscular Blocking Agents Included in *Davis's Drug Guide for Nurses*

depolarizing

succinylcholine, 1080

nondepolarizing

atracurium, 84
doxacurium, 399
gallamine, 525
metocurine, 761
pancuronium, 877
pipecuronium, 940
tubocurarine, 1177
vecuronium, 1187

▪ NON-NARCOTIC ANALGESICS/NONSTEROIDAL ANTI-INFLAMMATORY AGENTS

Pharmacologic Profile

General Use: Most agents in this group are used to control mild to moderate pain, fever, and various inflammatory conditions, such as rheumatoid arthritis and osteoarthritis. Acetaminophen has analgesic and antipyretic properties but is not effective as an anti-inflammatory agent. Phenazopyridine is used as a urinary tract analgesic only. Methotrimeprazine is a phenothiazine with analgesic properties; however, excessive hypotension precludes routine use.

General Action and Information: The largest group of non-narcotic analgesics are the nonsteroidal anti-inflammatory agents (NSAIAs, NSAIDs). Although not labelled for all actions, NSAIAs and salicylates have analgesic, antipyretic, and anti-inflammatory properties. Phenylbutazone is also an NSAIA, but its toxicity is too great to allow routine use. The mechanism for analgesia is probably due to inhibition of prostaglandin synthesis. Antipyretic action is due to prostaglandin synthesis inhibition in the CNS and vasodilation. Prostaglandin synthesis inhibition also explains the ability to suppress inflammation. Acetaminophen possesses antipyretic and analgesic action but has no anti-inflammatory properties.

Contraindications: Hypersensitivity to aspirin is a contraindication for the whole class of NSAIAs. Only acetaminophen is safe for occasional use in pregnancy or lactation.

Precautions: Use NSAIAs cautiously in patients with a history of bleeding disorders or gastrointestinal bleeding (effect may be less with nonaspirin salicylates), and in severe hepatic, renal, or cardiovascular disease. Safety of NSAIAs in pregnancy is not established.

Interactions: NSAIAs prolong bleeding time and potentiate the effect of anticoagulants, thrombolytic agents, plicamycin, some cephalosporins, and valproic acid. Chronic use of NSAIAs with aspirin may result in increased GI side effects and decreased effectiveness. NSAIAs may decrease the response to diuretics or antihypertensive therapy. Chronic use of acetaminophen with NSAIAs may increase the rick of adverse renal reactions. Toxicity of zidovudine may be increased by chronic use of acetaminophen. Methotrimeprazine will produce additive hypotension with other agents that lower blood pressure.

Nursing Implications

Assessment

- **General Info:** Patients who have asthma, aspirin-induced allergy, and nasal polyps are at increased risk for developing hypersensitivity reactions. Assess for rhinitis, asthma, and urticaria.
- **Arthritis:** Assess pain and range of motion before and 1–2 hr following administration.
- **Pain:** Assess pain (note type, location, and intensity) before and 1–2 hr following administration.
- **Fever:** Monitor temperature; note signs associated with fever (diaphoresis, tachycardia, and malaise).
- **Lab Test Considerations:** May cause prolonged bleeding time which may persist following discontinuation of therapy.

Potential Nursing Diagnoses

- Comfort, altered: pain (indications).
- Mobility, impaired physical (indications).
- Knowledge deficit related to medication regimen (patient/family teaching).

Implementation

- **General Info:** Coadminstration with narcotic analgesics may have additive analgesic effects and may permit lower narcotic doses.
- **PO:** For rapid initial effect, administer 30 min before or 2 hr after meals. May be administered with food, milk, or antacids to decrease GI irritation. Food slows but does not reduce the extent of absorption.
- **Dysmenorrhea:** Administer as soon as possible after the onset of menses. Prophylactic treatment has not been shown to be effective.

Patient/Family Teaching

- Advise patients to take these medications with a full glass of water and to remain in an upright position for 15–30 min after administration.
- These medications may occasionally cause drowsiness or dizziness. Advise patient to avoid driving or other activities requiring alertness until response to medication is known.
- Caution patient to avoid the concurrent use of alcohol, aspirin, acetaminophen, or other over-the-counter medications without consultation with physician or pharmacist.
- Advise patient to inform physician or dentist of medication regimen before treatment or surgery.

Evaluation

Effectiveness of therapy can be demonstrated by: ▪ Improved joint mobility ▪ Relief of moderate pain ▪ Reduction in fever. Patients who do not respond to one nonsteroidal anti-inflammatory agent may respond to another.

Non-Narcotic Analgesics/Nonsteroidal Anti-inflammatory Agents Included in *Davis's Drug Guide for Nurses*

nonsteroidal anti-inflammatory agents

aspirin, 79
choline magnesium trisalicylate, 244
choline salicylate, 246
diclofenac, 355
etodolac, 465
fenoprofen, 478
flurbiprofen, 515
indomethacin, 610
ibuprofen, 594
ketoprofen, 645
ketorelac, 647
meclofenamate, 707
naproxen, 820
piroxicam, 946
salsalate, 1044
sulindac, 1095
tolmetin, 1153

non-narcotic analgesics

acetaminophen, 2
etodolac, 465
fenoprofen, 478
ibuprofen, 594
ketoprofen, 645
ketorelac, 647
meclofenamate, 707
methotrimeprazine, 746
naproxen, 820
phenazopyridine, 914

salicylates

aspirin, 79
choline magnesium trisalicylate, 244
choline salicylate, 246
salsalate, 1044

▪ SEDATIVE/HYPNOTICS

Pharmacologic Profile

General Use: Sedatives are used in the treatment of various anxiety states. Hypnotics are used to treat insomnia. Selected agents are useful as anticonvulsants (clorazepate, diazepam, and phenobarbital), as skeletal muscle relaxants (diazepam), as adjuncts in the treatment of the alcohol withdrawal syndrome (chlordiazepoxide, clorazepate, diazepam, and oxazepam), and as general anesthetic adjunts or amnesics. Some phenothiazines are also used as sedatives.

General Action and Information: Cause generalized CNS depression. May produce tolerance with chronic use and the potential for psychological or physical dependance. These agents have no analgesic properties.

Contraindications: Hypersensitivity. Should not be used in comatose patients or those with pre-existing CNS depression. Should not be used in patients with uncontrolled severe pain. Avoid use during pregnancy or lactation.

Precautions: Use cautiously in patients with hepatic dysfunction, severe renal impairment, or severe underlying pulmonary disease. Use with caution in patients who may be suicidal or who may have been addicted to drugs previously. Hypnotic use should be short-term. Elderly patients may be more sensitive to CNS depressants effects: dosage reduction may be required.

Interactions: Additive CNS depression with alcohol, antihistamines, antidepressants, narcotic analgesics, or phenothiazines. Barbiturates induce hepatic drug-metabolizing enzymes and can decrease the effectiveness of drugs metabolized by the liver. Should not be used with MAO inhibitors.

Nursing Implications

Assessment

- **General Info:** Monitor blood pressure, pulse, and respiratory status frequently throughout IV administration.
- Prolonged high-dose therapy may lead to psychological or physical dependence. Restrict the amount of drug available to patient, especially if patient is depressed, suicidal, or has a history of addiction.
- **Insomnia:** Assess sleep patterns before and periodically throughout course of therapy.
- **Anxiety:** Assess degree of anxiety and level of sedation (ataxia, dizziness, and slurred speech) before and periodically throughout therapy.
- **Seizures:** Observe and record intensity, duration, and characterisitics of seizure activity. Institute seizure precautions.
- **Muscle Spasms:** Assess muscle spasms, associated pain, and limitation of movement before and throughout therapy.
- **Alcohol Withdrawal:** Assess patient experiencing alcohol withdrawal for tremors, agitation, delirium, and hallucinations. Protect patient from injury.

Potential Nursing Diagnoses

- Sleep pattern disturbance (indications).
- Injury, high risk for (side effects).
- Knowledge deficit related to medication regimen (patient/family teaching).

Implementation

- Supervise ambulation and transfer of patients following administration of hypnotic doses. Remove cigarettes. Side rails should be raised and call bell within reach at all times. Keep bed in low position.

Patient/Family Teaching

- Discuss the importance of preparing environment for sleep (dark room, quiet, avoidance of nicotine and caffeine). If less effective after a few wks, consult physician; do not increase dose. Gradual withdrawal may be required to prevent reactions following prolonged therapy.
- May cause daytime drowsiness. Caution patient to avoid driving or other activities requiring alertness until response to medication is known.
- Advise patient to avoid the use of alchol and other CNS depressants concurrently with these medications.
- Advise patient to inform physician if pregnancy is planned or suspected.

Evaluation

Effectiveness of therapy can be demonstrated by: ▪ Improvement in sleep patterns ▪ Decrease in anxiety level ▪ Control of seizures ▪ Decrease in muscle spasm ▪ Decreased tremulousness ▪ More rational ideation when used for alcohol withdrawal.

Sedative/Hypnotics Included in *Davis's Drug Guide for Nurses*

▪ SKELETAL MUSCLE RELAXANTS

Pharmacologic Profile

General Use: Two major uses are spasticity associated with spinal cord diseases or lesions (baclofen and dantrolene) or adjunctive therapy in the symptomatic relief of acute painful musculoskeletal conditions (cyclobenzaprine, diazepam, and methocarbamol). IV dantrolene is also used to treat and prevent malignant hyperthermia.

General Action and Information: Act either centrally (baclofen, carisoprodol, cyclobenzaprine, diazepam, and methocarbamol) or directly (dantrolene).

Contraindications: Baclofen and oral dantrolene should not be used in patients in whom spasticity is used to maintain posture and balance.

Precautions: Safety in pregnancy and lactation not established. Use cautiously in patients with a previous history of liver disease.

Interactions: Additive CNS depression with other CNS depressants, including alcohol, antihistamines, antidepressants, narcotic analgesics, and sedative/hypnotics.

Nursing Implication

Assessment
- Assess patient for pain, muscle stiffness, and range of motion before and periodically throughout therapy.

Potential Nursing Diagnoses
- Comfort, altered (indications).
- Mobility, impaired physical (indications).
- Injury, high risk for (side effects).

Implementation
- Provide safety measures as indicated. Supervise ambulation and transfer of patients.

Patient/Family Teaching
- Encourage patient to comply with additional therapies prescribed for muscle spasm (rest, physical therapy, heat).
- Medication may cause drowsiness. Caution patient to avoid driving or other activities requiring alertness until response to drug is known.
- Advise patient to avoid concurrent use of alcohol or other CNS depressants with these medications.

Evaluation
Effectiveness of therapy can be demonstrated by: ▪ Decreased musculoskeletal pain ▪ Decreased muscle spasticity ▪ Increased range of motion.

Skeletal Muscle Relaxants Included in *Davis's Drug Guide for Nurses*

centrally acting

direct-acting

▪ THROMBOLYTIC AGENTS

Pharmacologic Profile

General Use: Used in the treatment of acute massive pulmonary emboli and deep vein thromboses. Also used to lyse coronary artery thrombi following myocardial infarction and arterial thrombi, and to clear IV catheters and arteriovenous cannulae.

General Action and Information: Activate plasminogen by converting it to plasmin, which subsequently degrades fibrin clots, fibrinogen, and other plasma proteins. Alteplase stimulates the conversion to plasmin by binding to fibrin. Anistreplase produces local fibrinolysis at the site of new thrombus.

Contraindications: Hypersensitivity. Recent streptococcal infection (streptokinase only). Contraindicated in active internal bleeding, recent cerebrovascular accident, surgery, or intracranial neoplasm.

Precautions: Safety in pregnancy, lactation, and children not established. Use cautiously in patients who have risk of left heart thrombus, had recent minor trauma, cerebrovascular disease, or diabetic hemorrhagic retinopathy.

Interactions: Concurrent use with other anticoagulants, including aspirin and other antiplatelet agents, some cephalosporins, plicamycin, or valproic acid may increase the risk of bleeding.

Nursing Implications

Assessment

- **General Info:** Assess patients for signs of bleeding and hemorrhage. Monitor all previous puncture sites. May cause internal bleeding including intracranial hemorrhage. Guaiac all body fluids and stools. Monitor neurologic status. Assess peripheral pulses.
- **Coronary Thrombosis:** Monitor ECG continuously. Notify physician if significant arrhythmias or chest pain occur. Cardiac enzymes should be monitored.
- **Cannula/Catheter Occulsion:** Monitor ability to aspirate blood as indicator of patency. Ensure patient exhales and holds breath when connecting and disconnecting IV syringe to prevent air embolism.
- **Toxicity and Overdose:** Aminocaproic acid (Amicar) may be used as an antidote.

Potential Nursing Diagnoses

- Tissue perfusion, altered (indications).
- Injury, high risk for (side effects).

Implementation

- These medications should only be used in settings where hematologic function and clinical response can be adequately monitored.
- Invasive procedures, such as IM injections or arterial punctures, should be avoided with this therapy.
- Obtain type and cross-match and have blood available at all times in case of hemorrhage.
- Systemic anticoagulation with heparin is usually begun several hrs after the completion of thrombolytic therapy.

Patient/Family Teaching

- Explain purpose of the medication. Instruct patient to report hypersensitivity reactions (rash, dyspnea) or bleeding or bruising.
- Explain need for bed rest and minimal handling during therapy to avoid injury.

Evaluation

Effectiveness of therapy can be demonstrated by: ▪ Lysis of thrombi or emboli ▪ Restoration of blood flow ▪ Cannula or catheter patency.

Thrombolytic Agents Included in *Davis's Drug Guide for Nurses*

alteplase, 25
anistreplase, 69
streptokinase, 1071
urokinase, 1179

▪ VASOPRESSORS

Pharmacologic Profile

General Use: Used to correct the hemodynamic imbalances which may persist despite adequate fluid replacement in the treatment of shock. Phenylephrine is also used as a topical decongestant and mydriatic. Isoproterenol is used as a bronchodilator.

General Action and Information: Stimulate adrenergic receptors, resulting in vasoconstriction (alpha-adrenergic effects) and/or myocardial stimulation (beta-adrenergic effects).

Contraindications: Contraindicated in occlusive vascular diseases, uncorrected arrhythmias, or hypotension secondary to fluid deficit.

Precautions: Use cautiously in patients with underlying cardiovascular disease. Safety in pregnancy and lactation not established.

Interactions: Use with MAO inhibitors may result in severe hypertension. Beta-adrenergic blockers may block therapeutic effectiveness.

Nursing Implications

Assessment

- Monitor blood pressure, pulse, respiration, ECG, and hemodynamic parameters every 5–15 min during and after administration. Notify physician if significant changes in vital signs or arrhythmias occur. Consult physician for parameters for pulse, blood pressure, or ECG changes for adjusting dosage or discontinuing medication.
- Monitor urine output frequently throughout administration. Notify physician promptly if urine output decreases.
- Assess IV site frequently throughout infusion. Administer into a large vein to minimize the risk of extravasation. Extravasation of dopamine, epinephrine, or phenylephrine may cause severe irritation, necrosis, and sloughing of tissue. If extravasation occurs, affected area should be infiltrated with 10–15 ml of 0.9% NaCl containing 5–10 mg of phentolamine.

Potential Nursing Diagnoses

- Cardiac output, decreased (indications).
- Tissue perfusion, altered (indications).

Implementation

- Hypovolemia should be corrected before administration of vasopressors.
- Infusions must be administered via infusion pump to ensure precise amount

delivered. Rate of administration is titrated according to patient response (blood pressure, heart rate, urine flow, peripheral perfusion, presence of ectopic activity, and cardiac output).

PATIENT/FAMILY TEACHING
- Instruct patient to inform nurse immediately if chest pain, dyspnea, or pain at infusion site occurs.

EVALUATION
Effectiveness of therapy can be demonstrated by: ▪ Increase in blood pressure ▪ Increase in peripheral circulation ▪ Increase in urine output.

Vasopressors Included in *Davis's Drug Guide for Nurses*

dopamine, 397	metaraminol, 729
ephedrine, 428	norepinephrine, 847
isoproterenol, 630	phenylephrine, 923

▪ VITAMINS

Pharmacologic Profile

General Use: Used in the prevention and treatment of vitamin deficiencies and as supplements in various metabolic disorders.

General Action and Information: Serve as components of enzyme systems which catalyze numerous varied metabolic reactions. Necessary for homeostasis. Water-soluble vitamins (B-vitamins, vitamin C, and pantothenic acid) rarely cause toxicity. Fat-soluble vitamins (vitamins A, D, E, and K) may accumulate and cause toxicity.

Contraindications: Hypersensitivity to additives, preservatives, or colorants.

Precautions: Dosage should be adjusted to avoid toxicity, especially for fat-soluble vitamins.

Interactions: Pyridoxine in large amounts may interfere with the effectiveness of levodopa. Cholestyramine, colestipol, and mineral oil decrease absorption of fat-soluble vitamins.

Nursing Implications

ASSESSMENT
- Assess patient for signs of vitamin deficiency before and periodically throughout therapy.
- Assess nutritional status through 24 hr diet recall. Determine frequency of consumption of vitamin-rich foods.

POTENTIAL NURSING DIAGNOSES
- Nutrition, altered: less than body requirements (indications).
- Knowledge deficit related to medication regimen (patient/family teaching).

IMPLEMENTATION
- Because of infrequency of single vitamin deficiencies, combinations are commonly administered.

Patient/Family Teaching

- Encourage patients to comply with diet recommendations of physician. Explain that the best source of vitamins is a well-balanced diet with foods from the 4 basic food groups.
- Patients self-medicating with vitamin supplements should be cautioned not to exceed RDA (see Appendix L). The effectiveness of megadoses for treatment of various medical conditions is unproven and may cause side effects and toxicity.

Evaluation

Effectiveness of therapy may be demonstrated by: ▪ Prevention of or decrease in the symptoms of vitamin deficiencies.

Vitamins Included in *Davis's Drug Guide for Nurses*

A

ACEBUTOLOL
(ace-**but**-toe-lole)
Sectral

CLASSIFICATION(S):
Antihypertensive, Beta-adrenergic blocker—selective, Antiarrhythmic—type II
Pregnancy Category B

INDICATIONS

■ Treatment of hypertension (single agent or in combination with other antihypertensives) ■ Treatment of ventricular tachyarrhythmias. **Unlabeled Uses:** ■ Prophylaxis of myocardial infarction, treatment of angina pectoris, anxiety, tremors, thyrotoxicosis, mitral valve prolapse, idiopathic hypertrophic subaortic stenosis.

ACTION

■ Blocks stimulation of $beta_1$ (myocardial) adrenergic receptors. Does not usually effect $beta_2$ (pulmonary, vascular, or uterine) receptor sites. **Therapeutic Effects:** ■ Decreased heart rate ■ Decreased AV conduction ■ Decreased blood pressure.

PHARMACOKINETICS

Absorption: Well absorbed following oral administration.
Distribution: Minimal penetration of the CNS. Crosses the placenta and enters breast milk.
Metabolism and Excretion: Most acebutolol is converted by the liver to diacetolol, which is also a beta blocker.
Half-life: 3–4 hr (8–13 hr for diacetolol).

CONTRAINDICATIONS AND PRECAUTIONS

Contraindicated in: ■ Uncompensated congestive heart failure ■ Pulmonary edema ■ Cardiogenic shock ■ Bradycardia or heart block.
Use Cautiously in: ■ Renal impairment (dosage reduction necessary) ■ Elderly patients (increased sensitivity to the effects of beta-adrenergic blockers) ■ Thyrotoxicosis (may mask symptoms) ■ Diabetes mellitus (may mask symptoms of hypoglycemia) ■ Pregnancy, lactation, or children (safety not established).

ADVERSE REACTIONS AND SIDE EFFECTS*

CNS: fatigue, weakness, dizziness, depression, insomnia, memory loss, mental changes, nightmares, anxiety, nervousness, drowsiness.
EENT: blurred vision, stuffy nose.
CV: BRADYCARDIA, CONGESTIVE HEART FAILURE, PULMONARY EDEMA, peripheral vasoconstriction, hypotension.
Resp: bronchospasm, wheezing.
GI: constipation, diarrhea, nausea, vomiting.
GU: impotence, diminished libido, urinary frequency.
Derm: rashes.
Endo: hyperglycemia, hypoglycemia.
MS: joint pain, athralgia.

INTERACTIONS

Drug-Drug: ■ **General anesthesia, IV phenytoin,** and **verapamil** may cause additive myocardial depression ■ Concurrent use with **cardiac glycosides** may produce additive bradycardia ■ **Antihypertensive agents,** acute ingestion of **alcohol,** or **nitrates** may cause additive hypotension ■ Use with **epinephrine** may result in unapposed alpha-adrenergic stimulation ■ Concurrent **thyroid** administration may decrease effectiveness ■ Use with **insulin** may result in prolonged hypoglycemia.

ROUTE AND DOSAGE

- **PO (Adults):** 400–800 mg/day—single dose or twice daily (up to 1200 mg/day).

PHARMACODYNAMICS

	ONSET	PEAK	DURATION
Antihypertensive effect			
PO	1–1.5 hr	2–8 hr	12–24 hr
Antiarrhythmic effect			
PO	1 hr	4–6 hr	up to 10 hr

*Underlines indicate most frequent; **CAPITALS** indicate life-threatening.

NURSING IMPLICATIONS

Assessment

- Monitor blood pressure, ECG, and pulse frequently during dosage adjustment period and periodically throughout therapy.
- Monitor intake and output ratios and daily weights. Assess routinely for signs and symptoms of congestive heart failure (dyspnea, rales/crackles, weight gain, peripheral edema, jugular venous distension).
- **Lab Test Considerations:** May cause increased serum lipoproteins, potassium, triglyceride, and uric acid concentrations.

Potential Nursing Diagnoses

- Cardiac output, decreased (side effects).
- Knowledge deficit related to medication regimen (patient/family teaching).
- Noncompliance related to medication regimen (patient/family teaching).

Implementation

- **PO:** Take apical pulse prior to administering. If <50 bpm or if arrhythmia occurs, withhold medication and notify physician.
- May be administered with food or on an empty stomach.

Patient/Family Teaching

- Instruct patient to take medication exactly as prescribed even if feeling well; do not skip or double up on missed doses. If a dose is missed, it should be taken as soon as remembered up to 4 hr before next dose. Abrupt withdrawal may precipitate life-threatening arrhythmias, hypertension, or myocardial ischemia.
- Teach patient and family how to check pulse and blood pressure. Instruct them to check pulse daily and blood pressure biweekly and to report significant changes to physician.
- May occasionally cause drowsiness. Caution patients to avoid driving or other activities that require alertness until response to the drug is known.
- Reinforce the need to continue additional therapies for hypertension (weight loss, exercise, restricted sodium intake, stress reduction, regular exercise, moderation of alcohol consumption, and cessation of smoking). Acebutolol controls but does not cure hypertension.
- Caution patient that this medication may cause increased sensitivity to cold.
- Instruct patient to consult physician or pharmacist before taking any over-the-counter medications concurrently with this medication.
- Diabetics should closely monitor blood sugar, especially if weakness, malaise, irritability, or fatigue occur.
- Advise patient to notify physician if slow pulse, dizziness, lightheadedness, confusion, or depression occurs.
- Instruct patient to inform physician or dentist of medication regimen prior to treatment or surgery.
- Advise patient to carry identification describing disease process and medication regimen at all times.

Evaluation

Effectiveness of therapy can be demonstrated by: ▪ Decrease in blood pressure ▪ Control of arrhythmias without appearance of detrimental side effects.

ACETAMINOPHEN

(a-seat-a-**mee**-noe-fen)
Acephen, Anacin-3, Anuphen, APAP, {Atasaol}, Banesin, {Campain}, Datril, Dolanex, Genapap, Halenol, Liquiprin, Myapap, N-acetyl-P-aminophenol, Neopan, Panadol, Panex, paracetamol, {Robigesic}, {Rounox}, St. Joseph's Aspirin-Free, Suppap, Tempra, Tenol, Tylenol, Typap, Ty-tabs

CLASSIFICATION(S):
Nonnarcotic analgesic —miscellaneous, Antipyretic
Pregnancy Category B

{} = Available in Canada only.

INDICATIONS

▪ Mild to moderate pain ▪ Fever.

ACTION

▪ Inhibits the synthesis of prostaglandins that may serve as mediators of pain and fever. **Therapeutic Effects:** ▪ Analgesia, which may be due to peripheral prostaglandin inhibition ▪ Antipyresis (lowers fever), which may be due to inhibition of prostaglandins in the CNS (hypothalmus) ▪ No significant anti-inflammatory properties.

PHARMACOKINETICS

Absorption: Well absorbed following oral administration. Rectal absorption is variable.
Distribution: Widely distributed. Crosses the placenta and enters breast milk.
Metabolism and Excretion: 85–95% metabolized by the liver. Metabolites may be toxic in overdose situation. Metabolites excreted by the kidneys.
Half-life: 1–4 hr.

CONTRAINDICATIONS AND PRECAUTIONS

Contraindicated in: ▪ Previous hypersensitivity ▪ Products containing alcohol, aspartame, saccharin, sugar, or tartrazine (FDC yellow dye #5) should be avoided in patients who have hypersensitivity or intolerance to these compounds.
Use Cautiously in: ▪ Severe hepatic disease ▪ Renal disease ▪ Chronic alcohol abuse ▪ Malnutrition ▪ Pregnancy and lactation ▪ Self-medication for longer than 10 days in adults or 5 days in children.

ADVERSE REACTIONS AND SIDE EFFECTS*

GI: HEPATIC NECROSIS (overdose).
Derm: rash, urticaria.

INTERACTIONS

Drug-Drug: ▪ **Antipyretics** may cause severe hypothermia when used with phenothiazine antipsychotics ▪ Hepatotoxicity may be additive with other **hepatotoxic substances** including **alcohol.** ▪ **Phenobarbital** may increase liver toxicity in acetaminophen overdosage ▪ **Cholestyramine** and **colestipol** decrease absorption and may decrease effectiveness.

ROUTE AND DOSAGE

Note: Children 12 yr and under should not receive more than 5 doses/24 hr without notifying physician.

- **PO (Adults and Children >12 yr):** 325–1000 mg q 4–6 hr as needed (not to exceed 4 g/day, or 2.6 g/day chronically)
- **PO (Children 11–12 yr):** 480 mg q 4–6 hr as needed.
- **PO (Children 9–11 yr):** 400 mg q 4–6 hr as needed.
- **PO (Children 6–9 yr):** 320 mg q 4–6 hr as needed.
- **PO (Children 4–6 yr):** 240 mg q 4–6 hr as needed.
- **PO (Children 2–4 yr):** 160 mg q 4–6 hr as needed.
- **PO (Children 1–2 yr):** 120 mg q 4–6 hr as needed.
- **PO (Children 4–12 mon):** 80 mg q 4–6 hr as needed.
- **PO (Children <3 mon):** 40 mg q 4–6 hr as needed.
- **Rect (Adults and Children >12 yr):** 325–650 mg q 4 hr as needed.
- **Rect (Children 11–12 yr):** 480 mg q 4–6 hr as needed.
- **Rect (Children 9–11 yr):** 400 mg q 4–6 hr as needed.
- **Rect (Children 6–9 yr):** 320 mg q 4–6 hr as needed.
- **Rect (Children 4–6 yr):** 240 mg q 4–6 hr as needed.
- **Rect (Children 2–4 yr):** 160 mg q 4–6 hr as needed.

PHARMACODYNAMICS (analgesia and antipyresis)

	ONSET	PEAK	DURATION
PO	0.5–1 hr	1–3 hr	3–4 hr
Rect	0.5–1 hr	1–3 hr	3–4 hr

*Underlines indicate most frequent; CAPITALS indicate life-threatening.

NURSING IMPLICATIONS

Assessment

- **General Info:** Assess overall health status and alcohol usage before administering acetaminophen. Malnourished patients or chronic alcohol abusers are at higher risk of developing hepatotoxicity with chronic use of usual doses of this drug.
- **Pain:** Assess type, location, and intensity prior to and 30–60 min following administration.
- **Fever:** Assess fever; note presence of associated signs (diaphoresis, tachycardia, and malaise).
- **Lab Test Considerations:** Hepatic, hematologic, and renal function should be evaluated periodically throughout prolonged, high-dose therapy.
- □ Increased serum bilirubin, LDH, SGOT (AST), SGPT (ALT), and prothrombin time may indicate hepatotoxicity.
- **Toxicity and Overdose:** If overdose occurs, acetylcysteine (Mucomyst) is the antidote.

Potential Nursing Diagnoses

- Comfort, altered: pain (indications).
- Body temperature, altered (indications).
- Knowledge deficit related to medication regimen (patient/family teaching).

Implementation

- **General Info:** Available forms include tablets, chewable tablets, caplets, drops, elixir, syrup, oral soln and suspension, and rectal suppositories. Concentrations of pediatric forms vary. Sugar-free and alcohol-free solns are available.
- □ Available in combination with many other drugs (see Appendix A).
- **PO:** Administer with a full glass of water.
- □ May be taken with food or on an empty stomach.

Patient/Family Teaching

- □ Advise patient to take medication exactly as directed and not to take more than the recommended amount. Severe and permanent liver damage may result from prolonged use or high doses of acetaminophen. Adults should not take acetaminophen longer than 10 days and children longer than 5 days unless directed by physician.
- □ Advise patient to consult the physician if discomfort or fever is not relieved by routine dosages of this drug or if fever is greater than 39.5°C (103°F) or lasts longer than 3 days.

Evaluation

Effectiveness of therapy can be demonstrated by: ▪ Relief of mild to moderate discomfort ▪ Reduction of fever.

ACETAZOLAMIDE

(a-set-a-**zole**-a-mide)
AK-zol, Cetazol, Diamox, Hydrazol

CLASSIFICATION(S):
Diuretic—carbonic anhydrase inhibitor, Anticonvulsant, Antiurolithic
Pregnancy Category C

INDICATIONS

▪ Lowers intraocular pressure in the treatment of glaucoma ▪ Adjunct treatment of refractory seizures ▪ Acute altitude sickness. **Unlabeled Uses:** ▪ Prevention of renal calculi composed of uric acid or cystine.

ACTION

▪ Inhibition of carbonic anhydrase in the eye decreases the secretion of aqueous humor ▪ Inhibits renal carbonic anhydrase, resulting in self-limiting urinary excretion of sodium, potassium, bicarbonate, and water ▪ CNS inhibition of carbonic anhydrase and resultant diuresis may decrease abnormal neuronal firing ▪ Alkaline diuresis also prevents precipitation of uric acid or cystine in the urinary tract. **Therapeutic Effects:** ▪ Reduction of intraocular pressure ▪ Diuresis ▪ Control of certain types of seizures ▪ Prevention and treatment

A

of acute altitude sickness ▪ Prevention of uric acid or cystine renal calculi.

PHARMACOKINETICS

Absorption: Well absorbed following oral administration.
Distribution: Widely distributed. Crosses the placenta.
Metabolism and Excretion: Excreted mainly unchanged in the urine.
Half-life: 2.4–5.8 hr.

CONTRAINDICATIONS AND PRECAUTIONS

Contraindicated in: ▪ Hypersensitivity to acetazolamide or other sulfonamides.
Use Cautiously in: ▪ Chronic respiratory disease ▪ Electrolyte abnormalities ▪ Diabetes mellitus ▪ Pregnancy and lactation (safety not established).

ADVERSE REACTIONS AND SIDE EFFECTS*

CNS: drowsiness, paresthesias.
EENT: transient myopia.
GI: nausea, vomiting, anorexia.
GU: crytalluria, renal calculi.
Derm: rash.
Endo: hyperglycemia.
F and E: hyperchloremic acidosis, hypokalemia.
Hemat: **APLASTIC ANEMIA, HEMOLYTIC ANEMIA, LEUKOPENIA.**
Metab: hyperuricemia.
Misc: allergic reactions.

INTERACTIONS

Drug-Drug: ▪ Excretion of **barbiturates, aspirin,** and **lithium** is increased and may lead to decreased effectiveness ▪ Excretion of **amphetamines, quinidine, procainamide,** and possibly **tricyclic antidepressants** is decreased and may lead to toxicity.

ROUTE AND DOSAGE

Glaucoma

- **PO (Adults):** 250-100 mg in 1–4 divided doses or 500 mg extended-release capsules twice daily.
- **PO (Children):** 8–30 mg/kg/day in divided doses.
- **IM, IV (Adults):** 250–500 mg; may repeat in 2–4 hr.
- **IM, IV (Children):** 5–10 mg/kg q 6 hr.

Epilepsy

- **PO (Adults and Children):** 8–30 mg/kg in 1–4 divided doses.

Altitude Sickness

- **PO (Adults):** 250 mg 2–4 times daily.

Antiurolithic

- **PO (Adults):** 250 mg at bedtime.

PHARMACODYNAMICS (effect on intraocular pressure)

	ONSET	PEAK	DURATION
PO	1 hr	2–4 hr	8–12 hr
PO–ER	2 hr	8–18 hr	18–24 hr
IV	2 min	0.25 hr	4–5 hr

NURSING IMPLICATIONS

Assessment

- **General Info:** Observe patient for signs of hypokalemia (muscle weakness, malaise, fatigue, ECG changes, vomiting).
- □ Assess for allergy to sulfonamides.
- **Intraocular Pressure:** Assess for eye discomfort or decrease in visual acuity.
- **Seizures:** Monitor neurologic status in patients receiving acetazolamide for seizures. Initiate seizure precautions.
- **Altitude Sickness:** Monitor for decrease in severity of symptoms (headache, nausea, vomiting, fatigue, dizziness, drowsiness, shortness of breath). Notify physician immediately if neurologic symptoms worsen or patient becomes more dyspneic and rales/crackles develop.
- **Lab Test Considerations:** Serum electrolytes and complete blood counts should be evaluated initially and periodically throughout prolonged therapy. May cause decreased potassium, bicarbonate, WBCs, and RBCs. May cause increased serum chloride.
- □ May cause increase in serum glucose;

*Underlines indicate most frequent; **CAPITALS** indicate life-threatening.

monitor serum and urine glucose carefully in diabetic patients.

- May cause false-positive results for urine protein and 17-hydroxysteroid tests.
- May cause increased blood ammonia, bilirubin, uric acid, and increased urine urobilinogen and calcium. May decrease urine citrate.

Potential Nursing Diagnoses

- Sensory-perceptual alteration: visual (indications).
- Knowledge deficit related to medication regimen (patient/family teaching).

Implementation

- **General Info:** Encourage fluids to 2000–3000 ml per day, unless contraindicated, to prevent crystalluria and stone formation.
- **PO:** Give with food to minimize GI irritation. Tablets may be crushed and mixed with fruit-flavored syrup to minimize bitter taste for patients with difficulty swallowing. Long-acting capsules (Diamox Sequels) may be opened and sprinkled on soft food, but do not crush, chew, or swallow contents dry.
- **IM:** Extremely painful; avoid if possible.
- **IV:** Dilute 500 mg in at least 5 ml of sterile water for injection. Use reconstituted soln within 24 hr.
- **Direct IV:** Administer over at least 1 min.
- **Intermittent Infusion:** Further dilute in D5W, D10W, 0.45% NaCl, 0.9%, NaCl, Ringer's or lactated Ringer's soln, or combinations of dextrose and saline or dextrose and Ringer's soln.
  - *Rate:* Infuse over 4–8 hr.
- **Additive Compatibility:** cimetidine.
- **Additive Incompatibility:** multiple vitamins.

Patient/Family Teaching

- **General Info:** Instruct patient to take exactly as directed. If a dose is missed, take as soon as remembered unless almost time for next dose. Do not double doses. Patients on anticonvulsant therapy may need to gradually reduce dosage prior to discontinuation.
  - Advise patient to report numbness or tingling of extremities, weakness, rash, sore throat, unusual bleeding, or fever to the physician.
  - May occasionally cause drowsiness. Caution patient to avoid driving and other activities that require alertness until response to the drug is known.
- **Intraocular Pressure:** Advise patient of the need for periodic ophthalmologic examinations; loss of vision may be gradual and painless.

Evaluation

Effectiveness of therapy can be demonstrated by: ▪ Decrease in intraocular pressure when used for glaucoma ▪ Decrease in the frequency of seizures ▪ Prevention of altitude sickness ▪ Prevention of uric acid or cystine stones in the urinary tract.

ACETYLCYSTEINE

(a-se-til-**sis**-tay-een)
{Airbron}, Mucomyst, Mucosol, Parrolex

CLASSIFICATION(S):
Antidote—specific for acetaminophen, Mucolytic
Pregnancy Category B

INDICATIONS

- **PO:** Overdosage of acetaminophen
- **Inhaln:** Mucolytic.

ACTION

▪ **PO:** Decreases the build-up of a hepatotoxic metabolite in acetaminophen overdosage ▪ **Inhaln:** Degrades mucus, allowing easier mobilization and expectoration. **Therapeutic Effects:** ▪ ***PO:*** Prevention of liver damage following acetaminophen overdose by decreasing the build-up of a hepatotoxic metabolite ▪ ***Inhaln:*** Lowers the viscosity of mucus.

{} = Available in Canada only.

PHARMACOKINETICS

Absorption: Absorbed from the GI tract following oral administration. Action is local following inhalation; remainder may be absorbed from pulmonary epithelium.
Distribution: Not known.
Metabolism and Excretion: Metabolized by the liver.
Half-life: UK.

CONTRAINDICATIONS AND PRECAUTIONS

Contraindicated in: ▪ Hypersensitivity.
Use Cautiously in: ▪ Severe respiratory insufficiency or asthma ▪ Elderly or debilitated patients ▪ Pregnancy or lactation (safety not established).

ADVERSE REACTION AND SIDE EFFECTS*

CNS: drowsiness.
EENT: rhinorrhea, stomatitis.
Resp: increased secretions.
GI: nausea, vomiting.
Derm: urticaria.
Misc: fever, chills.

INTERACTIONS

Drug–Drug: ▪ **Activated charcoal** may absorb acetylcysteine and decrease its effectiveness as an antidote.

ROUTE AND DOSAGE

Acetaminophen Overdose

- **PO (Adults and Children):** 140 mg/kg initially followed by 70 mg/kg q 4 hr for 17 additional doses.

Mucolytic

- **Inhaln (Adults and Children):** 1–10 ml of 20% soln or 2–20 ml of 10% soln q 2–6 hr.

PHARMACODYNAMICS

	ONSET	PEAK	DURATION
PO (antidote)	UK	UK	4 hr
Inhaln (mucolytic)	1 min	5–10 min	short

NURSING IMPLICATIONS

Assessment

- **Antidote in Acetaminophen Overdose:** Monitor SGOT (AST), SGPT (ALT), bilirubin, prothrombin time, creatinine, BUN, serum glucose, electrolytes, and acetaminophen levels. Initial serum levels are drawn 4 hr after ingestion of acetaminophen. Do not wait for results to administer dose.
- ▫ Assess patient for nausea, vomiting, and urticaria. Notify physician if these occur. Maintain fluid and electrolyte balance.
- **Mucolytic:** Assess respiratory function (lung sounds, dyspnea) and color, amount, and consistency of secretions before and immediately following treatment to determine effectiveness of therapy.

Potential Nursing Diagnoses

- Coping, ineffective individual (indications).
- Airway clearance, ineffective (indications).
- Knowledge deficit related to medication regimen (patient/family teaching).

Implementation

- **General Info:** After opening, may turn light purple; does not alter potency. Refrigerate open vials and discard after 96 hr.
- ▫ Drug reacts with rubber and metals (iron, nickel, copper); avoid contact with these substances.
- **PO: Acetaminophen Overdose**—first empty stomach contents by inducing emesis or lavage. Dilute 20% soln with cola, water, or juice to a final concentration of 1:3 to increase palatability for oral administration. May be administered by duodenal tube if patient unable to swallow. If patient vomits loading dose or maintenance doses within 1 hr of administration, readminister dose.
- **Inhaln: Mucolytic**—encourage adequate fluid intake (2000–3000 ml/

*Underlines indicate most frequent; **CAPITALS** indicate life-threatening.

day) to decrease viscosity of secretions.

- For aerosol use, the 20% soln may be diluted with 0.9% NaCl for injection or inhalation or sterile water for injection or inhalation. May use 10% soln undiluted. May be administered by nebulization, or 1–2 ml may be instilled directly into airway. During administration, when 25% of medication remains in nebulizer, dilute with equal amount of 0.9% NaCl or sterile water.
- An increased volume of liquified bronchial secretions may occur following administration. Have suction equipment available for patients unable to effectively clear airways.
- If bronchospasm occurs during treatment, discontinue and consult physician regarding possible addition of bronchodilator to therapy.
- Rinse patient's mouth and wash face following treatment as drug leaves a sticky residue on surfaces.

Patient/Family Teaching

- **Inhaln:** Instruct patient to clear airway by coughing deeply before taking aerosol treatment.
- Inform patient that unpleasant odor of this drug becomes less noticeable as treatment progresses.

Evaluation

Effectiveness of therapy can be demonstrated by: ▪ Decreased acetaminophen levels and no further increase in hepatic damage during acetaminophen overdose therapy ▪ Decreased dyspnea and clearing of lung sounds when used as a mucolytic.

ACTIVATED CHARCOAL

Acta-Char, Acta-Char Liquid-A, Actidose-Aqua, Arm-a-Char, {Aqueous Charcodote}, Charcocaps, Insta-Char, Insta-Char Aqueous Suspension, Liqui-Char, SuperChar, SuperChar Aqueous

CLASSIFICATION(S):
Antidote—adsorbent, Antiflatulant, Antidiarrheal—adsorbent
Pregnancy Category C

INDICATIONS

▪ Acute management of many oral poisonings following emesis/lavage ▪ Relief of excess flatulance (efficacy not demonstrated) ▪ Treatment of diarrhea (efficacy not demonstrated).

ACTION

▪ Binds drugs and chemicals within the GI tract ▪ May decrease the volume of intestinal gas and absorb various toxins capable of causing diarrhea. **Therapeutic Effect:** ▪ Decreased intestinal absorption of drugs or chemicals in the overdose situation, thereby preventing toxicity.

PHARMACOKINETICS

Absorption: None.
Distribution: None.
Metabolism and Excretion: Excreted unchanged in the feces.
Half-life: UK.

CONTRAINDICATIONS AND PRECAUTIONS

Contraindicated in: ▪ No known contraindications.
Use Cautiously in: ▪ Poisonings due to cyanide, corrosives, ethanol, methanol, petroleum distillates, organic solvents, mineral acids, or iron ▪ Endoscopic examination (observation will be obscured).

ADVERSE REACTIONS AND SIDE EFFECTS*

GI: vomiting, constipation, diarrhea, black stools.

INTERACTIONS

Drug-Drug: ▪ **Other drugs** including **ipecac** and **laxatives** will be adsorbed by charcoal and not be systemically absorbed from the GI tract.

{} = Available in Canada only.
*Underlines indicate most frequent; **CAPITALS** indicate life-threatening.

Drug–Food: ▪ **Milk, ice cream,** and **sherbet** will decrease the ability of charcoal to absorb other agents.

ROUTE AND DOSAGE

Antidote

- **PO (Adults or Children):** 30–100 g or 1 g/kg or 5–20 times the amount of poison ingested.

Antiflatulant, Antidiarrheal

- **PO (Adults):** 520–975 mg 3 times daily after meals (not to exceed 4.16 g/day).

PHARMACODYNAMICS (antidote)

	ONSET	PEAK	DURATION
PO	within min	UK	4–12 hr

NURSING IMPLICATIONS

Assessment

- **General Info:** Assess neurologic status; administer only if patient is alert (unless airway is protected).
  - Consult reference, poison control center, or physician for symptoms of toxicity of ingested agent(s).
  - Monitor blood pressure, pulse, respiratory and neurologic status, and urine output as indicated by toxicity of agent(s). Notify physician if symptoms persist or worsen.
- **Poisoning:** Inquire as to the type of drug or poison and time of ingestion.
- **Flatulence:** Assess abdomen periodically throughout therapy. Note distention, bowel sounds, tympany, and discomfort level.
- **Diarrhea:** Monitor amount, frequency, and consistency of bowel movements.
- **Lab Test Considerations:** Chronic use may impair absorption of essential nutrients. This may result in decreased mineral or electrolyte levels.

Potential Nursing Diagnoses

- Coping, ineffective individual (indications).
- Injury, high risk for (indications).
- Bowel elimination, altered: diarrhea (indications, side effects).

Implementation

- **General Info:** Available in tablets, capsules, powder, and slurry (premixed in water or sorbitol and sweetened to increase palatability).
- **Treatment of Poisoning:** Activated charcoal is most effective if administered within 30 min of ingestion of drug or poison. Dosage may be repeated for drugs subjected to enterohepatic elimination to minimize further absorption.
  - Administer syrup of ipecac first and wait until emesis occurs before administering activated charcoal.
  - Powder is the most effective form and should be the form used. Tablets and capsules should not be used in the treatment of poisoning.
- **PO:** Mix dose in 6–8 oz of water, administer as a slurry. May be flavored with juice, cocoa, or chocolate powder to make more palatable. Do not administer with milk products (milk, ice cream, or sherbet). May need to be diluted with additional water to be thin enough to administer through a nasogastric tube.
  - Rapid ingestion may cause vomiting. If vomiting occurs shortly after administering dose, confer with physician about repeating dose.
  - Do not administer other oral drugs for 2 hr before or after administering activated charcoal.
  - Slurry is constipating; physician may order a laxative to speed removal of the drug. Sorbitol or magnesium citrate are commonly used for this purpose and may cause diarrhea. Some products contain sorbitol.

Patient/Family Teaching

- **General Info:** Inform patient that stools will turn black.
- **Poisoning:** When counseling, discuss methods of prevention, need to confer with poison control center, physician, or emergency department prior to administering, and need to bring ingested substance to emergency room for identification.
- **Flatulence:** Instruct patient to notify physician if symptoms persist more than 1 wk.

- **Diarrhea:** Instruct patient to inform physician if diarrhea persists more than 2 days or is accompanied by fever.

EVALUATION

Effectiveness of therapy can be demonstrated by: ▪ Prevention or resolution of toxic side effects of ingested agent ▪ Flatulence should improve within 1 wk ▪ Diarrhea should resolve within 2 days of starting therapy.

ACYCLOVIR
(ay-sye-kloe-veer)
Zovirax

CLASSIFICATION(S):
Antiviral
Pregnancy Category C

INDICATIONS

▪ **PO:** Treatment of initial and prophylaxis of recurrent genital herpes infections ▪ **PO:** Treatment of localized cutaneous herpes zoster infections ▪ **IV:** Used in the treatment of severe initial episodes of genital herpes in nonimmunosuppressed patients ▪ **IV:** Management of initial or recurrent mucosal or cutaneous herpes simplex infections in immunosuppressed patients ▪ **IV:** Treatment of herpes simplex encephalitis in patients > 6 mon ▪ **Top:** Treatment of herpes genitalis infections.

ACTION

▪ Interferes with viral DNA synthesis. **Therapeutic Effect:** ▪ Inhibition of viral replication, decreased viral shedding, and reduced time to healing of lesions.

PHARMACOKINETICS

Absorption: Oral absorption is poor (15–30%), although therapeutic blood levels are achieved.
Distribution: Widely distributed. CSF concentrations are 50% of plasma. Crosses the placenta.
Metabolism and Excretion: >90% eliminated unchanged by the kidneys; remainder metabolized by the liver.
Half-life: 2.1–3.5 hr (increased in renal failure).

CONTRAINDICATIONS AND PRECAUTIONS

Contraindicated in: ▪ Hypersensitivity.
Use Cautiously in: ▪ Pre-existing serious neurologic, hepatic, pulmonary, or fluid and electrolyte abnormalities ▪ Renal impairment (dosage reduction required) ▪ Pregnancy and lactation (safety not established).

ADVERSE REACTIONS AND SIDE EFFECTS*

CNS: dizziness, headache, hallucinations, trembling, SEIZURES.
EENT: gingival hyperplasia.
GI: diarrhea, nausea, vomiting, anorexia, abdominal pain.
GU: RENAL FAILURE, hematuria, crystalluria.
Derm: acne, unusual sweating, skin rashes, hives.
Endo: changes in menstrual cycle.
Local: pain, phlebitis.
MS: joint pain.
Misc: polydypsia.

INTERACTIONS

▪ **Probenecid** increases blood levels of acyclovir ▪ Concurrent use of other **nephrotoxic drugs** increases the risk of adverse renal effects ▪ Intrathecal **methotrexate** increases the risk of CNS side effects.

ROUTE AND DOSAGE

Note: Dosage should be decreased in renal impairment.

Initial Genital Herpes

- **PO (Adults):** 200 mg q 4 hr while awake (5 times a day) for 10 days.
- **IV (Adults):** 5 mg/kg q 8 hr for 5 days.

Chronic Suppressive Therapy for Recurrent Genital Herpes

- **PO (Adults):** 400 mg twice daily for up to 12 mon.

*Underlines indicate most frequent; **CAPITALS** indicate life-threatening.

A

Intermittent Therapy for Recurrent Genital Herpes
- **PO (Adults):** 200 mg q 4 hr while awake (5 times a day) for 5 days, initiated at first sign of symptoms.

Acute Treatment of Herpes Zoster
- **PO (Adults):** 800 mg q 4 hr while awake (5 times a day) for 7–10 days.

Mucosal and Cutaneous Herpes Simplex Infections in Immunosuppressed Patients
- **IV (Adults and Children >12 yr):** 5 mg/kg q 8 hr for 7 days.
- **IV (Children <12 yr):** 250 mg/m^2 q 8 hr for 7 days.
- **Top (Adults):** ½ in ribbon of 5% ointment for every 4 square in area q 3 hr 6 times/day for 7 days.

Herpes Simplex Encephalitis
- **IV (Adults):** 10 mg/kg q 8 hr for 10 days.
- **IV (Children <12 yrs):** 500 mg/m^2 q 8 hr for 10 days.

Varicella Zoster Infections in Immunosuppressed Patients
- **IV (Adults):** 10 mg/kg q 8 hr for 7 days.
- **IV (Children <12 yr):** 500 mg/m^2 q 8 hr for 7 days.

PHARMACODYNAMICS (antiviral blood levels)

	ONSET	PEAK
PO	UK	1.5–2.5 hr
IV	prompt	end of infusion

NURSING IMPLICATIONS

Assessment
- Assess lesions prior to and daily during therapy.
- Monitor neuro status in patients with herpes encephalitis.
- **Lab Test Considerations:** Monitor BUN, serum creatinine, and creatinine clearance before and during therapy. Increased BUN and serum creatinine levels or decreased creatinine clearance may indicate renal failure.

Potential Nursing Diagnoses
- Protection altered; tissue integrity, impaired (indications).
- Infection transmission, high risk for (indications, patient/family teaching).
- Knowledge deficit related to medication regimen (patient/family teaching).

Implementation
- **General Info:** Acyclovir treatment should be started as soon as possible after herpes symptoms appear.
- Available in tablets, capsules, oral suspension, ointment, and parenteral soln.
- **PO:** Acyclovir capsules may be administered with food or on an empty stomach.
- **IV:** Maintain adequate hydration (2000–3000 ml/day), especially during first 2 hr following IV infusion, to prevent crystalluria.
- Observe infusion site for phlebitis. Rotate infusion site to prevent phlebitis.
- Acyclovir sodium should not be administered topically, IM, SC, PO, or in the eye.
- **Intermittent Infusion:** Reconstitute 500 mg with 10 ml of sterile or bacteriostatic water without parabens for injection for a concentration of 50 mg/ml. Do not reconstitute with bacteriostatic water with benzyl alcohol when used for neonates. Shake well to dissolve completely. Dilute in D5W, D5/0.25% NaCl, D5/0.45% NaCl, D5/0.9% NaCl, 0.9% NaCl, or lactated Ringer's soln for a concentration not to exceed 7 mg/ml. Use reconstituted soln within 12 hr. Once diluted for infusion, should be used within 24 hr. Refrigeration results in precipitation, which dissolves at room temperature.
- *Rate:* Administer slowly, via infusion pump, over at least 1 hr to minimize renal tubular damage.
- **Y-Site Compatibility:** amikacin, ampicillin, cefamandole, cefazolin, cefonicid, cefoperazone, ceforanide, cefotaxime, cefoxitin, ceftazidime, ceftizoxime, ceftriaxone, cefuroxime,

cephapirin, chloramphenicol, cimetidine, clindamycin, co-trimoxazole, dexamethasone sodium phosphate, dimenhydrinate, diphenhydramine, erythromycin lactobionate, gentamicin, heparin, hydrocortisone sodium succinate, hydromorphone, imipenem/cilastatin, lorazepam, magnesium sulfate, meperidine, methylprednisolone sodium succinate, metoclopramide, metronidazole, morphine, multivitamin infusion, nafcillin, oxacillin, penicillin G potassium, pentobarbital, perphenazine, piperacillin, potassium chloride, ranitidine, sodium bicarbonate, tetracycline, theophylline, ticarcillin, tobramycin, or vancomycin.

- **Y-Site Incompatibility:** dobutamine, dopamine, ondansetron, or verapamil.
- **Additive Incompatibility:** blood products, protein-containing solutions, dobutamine, or dopamine.
- **Top:** Apply to skin lesions only; do not use in the eye.

Patient/Family Teaching

- **General Info:** Advise patient to take medication exactly as directed for the full course of therapy. If a dose is missed take as soon as remembered but not just before next dose is due; do not double doses. Acyclovir should not be used more frequently or longer than prescribed.
- □ Advise patients that the additional use of over-the-counter creams, lotions, and ointments can delay healing and may cause spreading of lesions.
- □ Inform patient that acyclovir is not a cure, as the virus lays dormant in the ganglia, and will not prevent the spread of infection to others.
- □ Advise patient that condoms should be used during sexual contact and that no sexual contact should be made while lesions are present.
- □ Instruct patient on the importance of maintaining good dental hygiene and seeing a dentist for teeth cleaning regularly to prevent tenderness, bleeding, and gingival hyperplasia.
- □ Patient should consult the physician if symptoms are not relieved following 7 days of topical therapy or if oral acyclovir does not decrease the frequency and severity of recurrences.
- □ Instruct women with genital herpes to have yearly Pap smears because they may be more likely to develop cervical cancer.
- **Top:** Instruct patient to apply ointment in sufficient quantity to cover all lesions every 3 hr, 6 times/day for 7 days. One ½-in ribbon of ointment covers approximately 4 square in. Use a finger cot or glove when applying to prevent autoinoculation of other body parts or spread of virus to other people. Affected areas should be kept clean and dry. Loose fitting clothing should be worn to prevent irritation.
- □ Avoid drug contact in or around eyes. Report any unexplained eye symptoms to the physician immediately, as ocular herpetic infection can lead to blindness.

Evaluation

Effectiveness of therapy can be demonstrated by: ▪ Crusting over and healing of skin lesions ▪ Decrease in frequency and severity of recurrences ▪ Shortening of time to complete healing and cessation of pain in herpes zoster.

ADENOSINE

(a-**den**-oh-seen)
Adenocard

CLASSIFICATION(S):
Antiarrhythmic—miscellaneous
Pregnancy Category C

INDICATIONS

▪ Conversion of paroxysmal supraventricular tachycardia to normal sinus rhythm when vagal manuevers have been unsuccessful.

ACTION

▪ Restores normal sinus rhythm by interrupting re-entrant pathways in the AV node ▪ Slows conduction time

A

through the AV node. **Therapeutic Effect:** ▪ Restoration of normal sinus rhythm.

PHARMACOKINETICS

Absorption: Following IV administration absorption is essentially complete.
Distribution: Taken up by erythrocytes and vascular endothelium.
Metabolism and Excretion: Rapidly cleared by conversion to inosine and adenosine monophosphate.
Half-life: < 10 sec.

CONTRAINDICATIONS AND PRECAUTIONS

Contraindicated in: ▪ Hypersensitivity ▪ 2nd- or 3rd-degree AV block or sick sinus syndrome, unless a functional artificial pacemaker is present.
Use Cautiously in: ▪ Patients with a history of asthma (may induce bronchospasm) ▪ Pregnancy, lactation, or children (safety not established).

ADVERSE REACTIONS AND SIDE EFFECTS*

CNS: headache, lightheadedness, dizziness, apprehension, head pressure.
EENT: blurred vision, throat tightness.
Resp: shortness of breath, chest pressure, hyperventilation.
CV: facial flushing, transient arrhythmias, palpitations, chest pain, hypotension.
GI: nausea, metallic taste.
Derm: sweating, burning sensation, facial flushing.
MS: neck and back pain.
Neuro: tingling, numbness.
Misc: pressure sensation in groin, heaviness in arms.

INTERACTIONS

Drug–Drug: ▪ **Carbamazepine** may increase the likelihood of progressive heart block ▪ **Dipyridamole** potentiates the effects of adenosine (dosage reduction of adenosine recommended) ▪ Effects of adenosine may be decreased by **theophylline** or **caffeine** (larger doses of adenosine may be required) ▪ **Nicotine** (in cigarette smoke or nicotine gum) may increase risk of tachycardia.

ROUTE AND DOSAGE

- **IV (Adults):** 6 mg by rapid IV bolus, if no results repeat 1–2 min later as 12 mg rapid bolus. This dose may be repeated. (Single dose not to exceed 12 mg).

PHARMACODYNAMICS

	ONSET	PEAK	DURATION
IV	3–4 sec	UK	1–2 min

NURSING IMPLICATIONS

Assessment

- Monitor heart rate frequently (every 15–30 sec) and ECG continuously throughout therapy. Once conversion to normal sinus rhythm is achieved, transient arrhythmias (premature ventricular contractions, atrial premature contractions, sinus tachycardia, sinus bradycardia, skipped beats, AV nodal block) may occur, but generally last a few secs.
- Monitor blood pressure during therapy.
- Assess respiratory status (breath sounds, rate) following administration. Patients with history of asthma may experience bronchospasm.

Potential Nursing Diagnoses

- Cardiac output, decreased (indications).
- Knowledge deficit related to medication regimen (patient/family teaching).

Implementation

- **General Info:** Crystals may occur if adenosine is refrigerated. Warm to room temperature to dissolve crystals. Soln must be clear before use. Discard unused portions.
- **Direct IV:** Administer undiluted over 1–2 sec via direct IV or into proximal IV line. Follow with rapid saline flush to ensure injection reaches systemic circulation. Slow administration may

*Underlines indicate most frequent; **CAPITALS** indicate life-threatening.

cause increased heart rate in response to vasodilation.

PATIENT/FAMILY TEACHING

- Caution patient to make position changes slowly to minimize orthostatic hypotension. Doses >12 mg decrease blood pressure by decreasing peripheral vascular resistance.
- Instruct patient to report facial flushing, shortness of breath, or dizziness.

EVALUATION

Effectiveness of therapy can be demonstrated by: ▪ Conversion of supraventricular tachycardia to normal sinus rhythm.

ALBUMIN

(al-**byoo**-min)
Albuminar, Albumisol, Albutein, Buminate, Normal Human Serum Albumin, Plasbumin

CLASSIFICATION(S):
Blood derivative
Pregnancy Category C

INDICATIONS

▪ Expansion of plasma volume and maintenance of cardiac output in situations associated with fluid volume deficit including shock, hemorrhage and burns ▪ Temporary replacement of albumin in diseases associated with low levels of plasma proteins such as nephrotic syndrome or end stage liver disease resulting in relief or reduction of associated edema.

ACTION

▪ Provides colloidal oncotic pressure, which serves to mobilize fluid from extravascular tissues back into the intravascular space ▪ Major constituent of plasma proteins ▪ Able to bind drugs and other substances such as bilirubin.
Therapeutic Effect: ▪ Mobilization of fluid from extravascular tissue into intravascular space.

PHARMACOKINETICS

Absorption: Following IV administration absorption is essentially complete.
Distribution: Confined to the intravascular space, unless capillary permeability is increased.
Metabolism and Excretion: Normally produced by the liver, also probably degraded by the liver.
Half-life: UK.

CONTRAINDICATIONS AND PRECAUTIONS

Contraindicated in: ▪ Allergic reactions to albumin ▪ Severe anemia ▪ Congestive heart failure ▪ Normal or increased intravascular volume.
Use Cautiously in: ▪ Severe hepatic or renal disease ▪ Dehydration (additional fluids may be required).

ADVERSE REACTIONS AND SIDE EFFECTS*

CNS: headache.
CV: hypertension, hypotension, fluid overload, PULMONARY EDEMA, tachycardia.
GI: nausea, vomiting, increased salivation.
Derm: urticaria, rash.
MS: back pain.
Misc: fever, chills, flushing.

INTERACTIONS

Drug–Drug: ▪ None significant.

ROUTE AND DOSAGE

Note: Available as 5% and 25% soln. Dose is highly individualized and depends on condition being treated.

- **IV (Adults):** 25 g, may be repeated in 15–30 min, not to exceed 125 g in 24 hr or 250 g in 48 hr.
- **IV (Children):** 25 g or 25–50% of the adult dose.
- **IV (Premature Infants):** 1 g/kg as 25% soln administered prior to necessary transfusion.

*Underlines indicate most frequent; **CAPITALS** indicate life-threatening.

PHARMACODYNAMICS (oncotic effect)

	ONSET	PEAK	DURATION
IV	15–30 min	UK	UK

NURSING IMPLICATIONS

Assessment

- **General Info:** Monitor vital signs, CVP, and intake and output prior to and frequently throughout therapy. If fever, tachycardia, or hypotension occur, stop infusion and notify physician immediately. Antihistamines may be required to suppress this hypersensitivity response. Hypotension may also result from infusing too rapidly.
- □ Assess for signs of vascular overload (elevated CVP, rales/crackles, dyspnea, hypertension, jugular venous distention) during and following administration.
- **Surgical Patients:** Assess for increased bleeding following administration caused by increased blood pressure and circulating blood volume. Albumin does not contain clotting factors.
- **Lab Test Considerations:** Serum protein levels should increase with albumin therapy.
- □ Monitor serum sodium; may cause increased concentrations.
- □ Infusions of normal serum albumin may cause false elevation of alkaline phosphatase levels.
- **Hemorrhage:** Monitor hemoglobin and hematocrit. These values may decrease due to hemodilution.

Potential Nursing Diagnoses

- Cardiac output, decreased (indications).
- Fluid volume deficit, actual (indications).
- Fluid volume excess (side effects).

Implementation

- **General Info:** Follow manufacturer's recommendations for administration and use set provided. Administer through a large gauge (at least 20-g) needle or catheter.
- □ Soln should be clear amber; do not administer cloudy soln or one containing a precipitate. Store at room temperature.
- □ There is no danger of serum hepatitis or HIV infection from normal serum albumin. Crossmatching is not required.
- □ Twenty-five grams of normal serum albumin are osmotically equivalent to 2 units of fresh frozen plasma; 100 ml of normal serum albumin 25% provides the plasma protein of 500 ml plasma or 2 pt of whole blood. Normal serum albumin 5% is isotonic and osmotically equivalent to an equal amount of plasma. The 25% albumin soln is equal to 5 times the osmotic value of plasma. Each liter of normal serum albumin contains 130–160 mEq of sodium and are thus no longer labeled "salt-poor" albumin.
- □ Administration of large quantities of normal serum albumin may need to be supplemented with whole blood to prevent anemia. If more than 1000 ml of 5% normal serum albumin are given or if hemorrhage has occurred, the administration of whole blood or packed red blood cells may be needed. Hydration status should be monitored and maintained with additional fluids.
- **Continuous Infusion:** Administer 5% normal serum albumin undiluted. Normal serum albumin 25% may be administered undiluted or diluted in 0.9% NaCl or D5W. Infusion must be completed within 4 hr.
- □ *Rate:* Rate of administration is determined by concentration of soln, blood volume, indication, and patient response. In patients with normal blood volume 5% normal serum albumin should be administered at 2–4 ml/min and 25% normal serum albumin at a rate of 1 ml/min. The rate for children is usually one fourth to one half the adult rate.
- □ *Shock with Associated Hypovolemia:* 5% or 25% normal serum al-

bumin may be administered as rapidly as tolerated and repeated in 15–30 min if necessary.

- *Burns:* Rate after the first 24 hr should be set to maintain a plasma albumin level of 2.5 g/100 ml or a total serum protein level of 5.2 g/100 ml.
- *Hypoproteinemia:* Normal serum albumin 25% is the preferred soln due to the increased concentration of protein. The rate should not exceed 3 ml/min of 25% or 5–10 ml/min of 5% soln to prevent circulatory overload and pulmonary edema. This treatment provides a temporary rise in plasma protein until the hypoproteinemia is corrected.

■ **Additive Compatibility:** Normal serum albumin is compatible with 0.9%, NaCl, D5W, D5/0.9% NaCl, D5/0.45% NaCl, D5/LR, and lactated Ringer's soln.

Patient/Family Teaching

- Explain the purpose of this soln to the patient.
- Instruct patient to report signs and symptoms of hypersensitivity reaction.

Evaluation

Effectiveness of therapy can be demonstrated by: ■ Increase in blood pressure and blood volume when used to treat shock and burns ■ Increased urinary output reflects the mobilization of fluid from extravascular tissues ■ Elevated serum plasma protein in patients with hypoproteinemia.

ALBUTEROL

(al-**byoo**-ter-ole)
Proventil, Ventolin

CLASSIFICATION(S):
Bronchodilator—beta-adrenergic agonist
Pregnancy Category C

INDICATIONS

■ **PO, Inhaln:** Used as a bronchodilator in reversible airway obstruction due to asthma or COPD ■ **Inhaln:** Prevention of exercise-induced bronchospasm.

ACTION

■ Results in the accumulation of cyclic adenosine monophosphate (cAMP) at beta-adrenergic receptors ■ Produces bronchodilation, CNS and cardiac stimulation, diuresis, and gastric acid secretion ■ Relatively selective for $beta_2$ (pulmonary) receptors. **Therapeutic Effect:** ■ Bronchodilation.

PHARMACOKINETICS

Absorption: Well absorbed following oral administration, but rapidly undergoes extensive metabolism.

Distribution: Not well known. Small amounts appear in breast milk.

Metabolism and Excretion: Extensively metabolized by the liver and other tissues.

Half-life: 3.8 hr.

CONTRAINDICATIONS AND PRECAUTIONS

Contraindicated in: ■ Hypersensitivity to adrenergic amines. ■ Hypersensitivity to fluorocarbons (inhaler) or benzalkonium chloride (soln for nebulization).

Use Cautiously in: ■ Cardiac disease ■ Hypertension ■ Hyperthyroidism ■ Diabetes ■ Glaucoma ■ Elderly patients (more susceptible to adverse reactions; may require dosage reduction) ■ Pregnancy (near term), lactation, and children <5 yr (safety not established) ■ Excessive use may lead to tolerance and paradoxical bronchospasm (inhaler).

ADVERSE REACTIONS AND SIDE EFFECTS*

CNS: nervousness, restlessness, insomnia, tremor, headache.
CV: hypertension, arrhythmias, angina.
Endo: hyperglycemia.
GI: nausea, vomiting.

INTERACTIONS

Drug-Drug: ■ Concurrent use with other **adrenergic (sympathomimetic)**

*Underlines indicate most frequent; CAPITALS indicate life-threatening.

agents will have additive adrenergic side effects ▪ Use with **MAO inhibitors** may lead to hypertensive crisis ▪ **Beta-adrenergic blockers** may negate therapeutic effect.

ROUTE AND DOSAGE

- **PO (Adults and Children ≥12 yr):** 2–4 mg 3–4 times daily (not to exceed 32 mg/day) or 4–8 mg of extended-release tablets (Proventil Repetabs) twice daily.
- **PO (Children 6–14 yr):** 2 mg 3–4 times daily. May be carefully increased as needed (not to exceed 24 mg/day).
- **PO (Children 2–6 yr):** 0.1 mg/kg 3 times daily (not to exceed 2 mg 3 times daily initially), may be carefully increased to 0.2 mg/kg 3 times daily (not to exceed 4 mg 3 times daily).
- **Inhaln (Adults and Children ≥12 yr):** via metered-dose inhaler—2 inhalations q 4–6 hr or 2 inhalations 15 min prior to exercise (90 mcg/spray).
- **Inhaln (Adults and Children >5 yr):** via nebulization or IPPB—1.25–5 mg 3–4 times daily.

PHARMACODYNAMICS (bronchodilation)

	ONSET	PEAK	DURATION
PO	30 min	2–3 hr	6 hr or more
PO–ER	30 min	2–3 hr	12 hr
Inhaln	5–15 min	60–90 min	4–6 hr

NURSING IMPLICATIONS

Assessment

- Assess lung sounds, pulse, and blood pressure before administration and during peak of medication.
- Monitor pulmonary function tests before initiating therapy and periodically throughout course to determine effectiveness of medication.
- Observe for paradoxical bronchospasm (wheezing). If condition occurs, withhold medication and notify physician immediately.

Potential Nursing Diagnoses

- Airway clearance, ineffective (indications).
- Knowledge deficit related to medication regimen (patient/family teaching).

Implementation

- **General Info:** Available in tablets, syrup, inhalation aerosol (metered-dose inhaler), and inhalation soln for nebulization.
- **PO:** Administer oral medication with meals to minimize gastric irritation.
- **Inhaln:** Allow at least 1 min between inhalations of aerosol medication.

Patient/Family Teaching

- Instruct patient to take albuterol exactly as directed. If on a scheduled dosing regimen, take a missed dose as soon as remembered, spacing remaining doses at regular intervals. Do not double doses. Caution patient not to exceed recommended dose; may cause adverse effects, paradoxical bronchospasm, or loss of effectiveness of medication.
- Instruct patient in the proper use of the metered-dose inhaler. Shake well, exhale, close lips firmly around mouth piece, administer during second half of inhalation and hold breath as long as possible after treatment to ensure deep instillation of medication. Do not take more than 2 inhalations at one time; allow 1–2 min between inhalations. Wash inhalation assembly at least daily in warm running water.
- Advise patients to use albuterol first if using other inhalant medications, and allow 5 min to elapse before administering other inhalant medications, unless otherwise directed by physician.
- Instruct patient to contact physician immediately if shortness of breath is not relieved by medication or is accompanied by diaphoresis, dizziness, palpitations, or chest pain.
- Advise patient to rinse mouth with water after each inhalation dose to minimize dry mouth.
- Advise patient to consult physician or pharmacist before taking any over-the-counter medications or alcoholic

beverages concurrently with this therapy. Caution patient to also avoid smoking and other respiratory irritants.

Evaluation

Effectiveness of therapy can be demonstrated by: ▪ Prevention or relief of bronchospasm.

ALFENTANIL

(al-**fen**-ta-nil)

Alfenta, {Rapifen}

CLASSIFICATION(S):

Narcotic analgesic—agonist

Schedule II

Pregnancy Category C

INDICATIONS

▪ Analgesic adjunct when given in increasing doses in the maintenance of anesthesia with barbiturate/nitrous oxide/oxygen ▪ Analgesic when administered by continuous IV infusion with nitrous oxide/oxygen while maintaining general anesthesia ▪ Primary induction of anesthesia when endotracheal intubation and mechanical ventilation are required.

ACTION

▪ Binds to opiate receptors in the CNS, altering the response to and perception of pain and causing generalized CNS depression. **Therapeutic Effects:** ▪ Relief of moderate to severe pain ▪ Anesthesia.

PHARMACOKINETICS

Absorption: Following IV administration absorption is essentially complete.
Distribution: Does not readily penetrate adipose tissue. Crosses the placenta, enters breast milk.
Metabolism and Excretion: >95% metabolized by the liver.
Half-life: 60–130 min.

CONTRAINDICATIONS AND PRECAUTIONS

Contraindicated in: ▪ Hypersensitivity ▪ Known intolerance.
Use Cautiously in: ▪ Elderly patients ▪ Debilitated or severely ill patients ▪ Diabetics ▪ Severe pulmonary or hepatic disease ▪ CNS tumors ▪ Increased intracranial pressure ▪ Head trauma ▪ Adrenal insufficiency ▪ Undiagnosed abdominal pain ▪ Hypothyroidism ▪ Alcoholism ▪ Cardiac disease (arrhythmias) ▪ Pregnancy, lactation, and children <12 yr (safety not established).

ADVERSE REACTIONS AND SIDE EFFECTS*

CNS: dizziness, sleepiness.
EENT: blurred vision.
CV: <u>bradycardia</u>, <u>tachycardia</u>, <u>hypotension</u>, <u>hypertension</u>, arrhythmias.
Resp: apnea.
GI: <u>nausea</u>, <u>vomiting</u>.
MS: <u>thoracic muscle rigidity</u>, skeletal muscle rigidity.

INTERACTIONS

Drug-Drug: ▪ **Alcohol, antihistamines, antidepressants,** and other **sedative/hypnotics**—concurrent use results in additive CNS depression ▪ **MAO inhibitors** should be avoided for 14 days prior to use ▪ **Cimetidine** or **erythromycin** may prolong duration of recovery ▪ Concurrent use with **benzodiazepines** may increase the risk of hypotension ▪ **Nalbuphine** or **pentazocine** may decrease analgesia.

ROUTE AND DOSAGE

Incremental Injection (Duration of anesthesia <30 min)

Induction Period

▪ **IV (Adults):** 8–20 mcg/kg.

Maintenance Period

▪ **IV (Adults):** 3–5 mcg/kg increments or 0.5–1.0 mcg/kg/min (total dose 8–40 mcg/kg).

{} = Available in Canada only.

*<u>Underlines</u> indicate most frequent; **CAPITALS** indicate life-threatening.

A

Incremental Injection (Duration of anesthesia 30–60 min)

Induction Period

- **IV (Adults):** 20–50 mcg/kg.

Maintenance Period

- **IV (Adults):** 5–15 mcg/kg increments (up to total dose of 75 mg/kg).

Continuous Infusion (Duration of anesthesia >45 min)

Induction

- **IV (Adults):** 50–75 mcg/kg.

Maintenance

- **IV (Adults):** 0.5–3.0 mcg/kg/min (average infusion rate 1–1.5 mcg/kg/min). Infusion rate should be decreased by 30–50% after first hr of maintenance. If lightening occurs, infusion rate may be increased up to 4 mcg/kg/min or boluses of 7 mg/kg may be administered.

Anesthetic Induction (Duration of anesthesia >45 min)

- **IV (Adults):** 130–245 mcg/kg followed by 0.5–1.5 mcg/kg/min or general anesthesia.

PHARMACODYNAMICS (analgesia and respiratory depression)

	ONSET	PEAK	DURATION
IV	immediate	1–1.5 min	5–10 min

NURSING IMPLICATIONS

Assessment

- Assess vital signs, especially respiratory status and ECG, frequently throughout and following administration. Notify physician immediately of significant changes.
- **Lab Test Considerations:** May cause elevated serum amylase and lipase concentrations.
- **Toxicity and Overdose:** Symptoms of toxicity include respiratory depression, hypotension, arrhythmias, bradycardia, and asystole. Respiratory depression may be reversed with naloxone. Bradycardia may be treated with atropine. Narcotic antagonist, oxygen, and resuscitative equipment should be readily available during the administration of alfentanil.

Potential Nursing Diagnoses

- Comfort, altered: pain (indications).
- Sensory–perceptual alteration: visual, auditory (side effects).
- Breathing pattern, ineffective (side effects).

Implementation

- **General Info:** Benzodiazepines may be administered prior to administration of alfentanil to reduce the induction dose requirements and decrease the time to loss of consciousness. This combination may also increase the risk of hypotension.
- Alfentanil's duration of action is short, therefore postoperative pain may require treatment relatively early in the recovery period.
- **Direct IV:** Administer small volumes for direct IV use via tuberculin syringe for accuracy.
- *Rate:* Injections should be administered slowly over 90 sec to 3 min. Slow IV administration may reduce the incidence and severity of muscle rigidity, bradycardia, or hypotension. Neuromuscular blocking agents may be administered concurrently to decrease muscle rigidity.
- **Continuous Infusion:** For continuous IV infusion dilute to a concentration of 25–80 mcg/ml (20 ml of alfentanil in 230 ml of diluent provides a 40 mcg/ml soln) with 0.9% NaCl, D5W, D5/0.9% NaCl, or lactated Ringer's soln.
- IV infusion should be discontinued at least 10–15 min prior to the end of surgery.

Patient/Family Teaching

- Discuss the use of anesthetic agents and the sensations to expect with the patient prior to surgery.
- Alfentanil may cause drowsiness and dizziness. Advise patient to call for assistance when ambulating or smoking.
- Advise patient to make position changes slowly to minimize orthostatic hypotension.

□ Following outpatient surgery instruct patients to avoid alcohol or other CNS depressants for 24 hr after the administration of alfentanil.

Evaluation

Effectiveness of therapy can be demonstrated by: ▪ General quiescence □ Reduced motor activity ▪ Pronounced analgesia.

ALLOPURINOL
(al-oh-**pure**-i-nole)
Lopurin, Zyloprim

CLASSIFICATION(S):
Antigout agent—xanthene oxidase inhibitor
Pregnancy Category C

INDICATIONS

▪ Prevention of attack of gouty arthritis and nephropathy ▪ Treatment of secondary hyperuricemia, which may occur during treatment of tumors or leukemias.

ACTION

▪ Inhibits the production of uric acid. **Therapeutic Effect:** ▪ Lowering of serum uric acid levels.

PHARMACOKINETICS

Absorption: Well absorbed (80%) following oral administration.
Distribution: Widely distributed in tissue water.
Metabolism and Excretion: Metabolized to oxypurinol, an active compound with a long half-life. Both allopurinol and oxypurinol are excreted mainly by the kidneys.
Half-life: 2–3 hr (oxypurinol 24 hr).

CONTRAINDICATIONS AND PRECAUTIONS

Contraindicated in: ▪ Hypersensitivity ▪ Pregnancy or lactation.
Use Cautiously in: ▪ Acute attacks of gout ▪ Renal insufficiency (dosage reduction required) ▪ Dehydration (adequate hydration necessary).

ADVERSE REACTIONS AND SIDE EFFECTS*

Derm: rash, urticaria.
GI: nausea, vomiting, diarrhea, hepatitis.
GU: renal failure.
Hemat: bone marrow depression.
Misc: hypersensitivity reactions.

INTERACTIONS

Drug-Drug: ▪ Use with **mercaptopurine** and **azathioprine** increases bone marrow depressant properties—dosages of these drugs should be reduced ▪ Use with **ampicillin** increases the risk of rash ▪ Use with **oral hypoglycemics** and **oral anticoagulants** increases the effects of these drugs ▪ Use with **thiazide diuretics** increases the risk of hypersensitivity reactions.

ROUTE AND DOSAGE

▪ **PO (Adults):** 200–800 mg/day (doses >300 mg should be divided and given twice a day).
▪ **PO (Children 6–10 yr):** 300 mg/day.
▪ **PO (Children <6 yr):** 150 mg/day.

PHARMACODYNAMICS (hypouricemic effect)

	ONSET	PEAK	DURATION*
PO	2 days	1–3 wk	1–2 wk

*Duration after discontinuation of allopurinol.

NURSING IMPLICATIONS

Assessment

□ Monitor for joint pain and swelling. Addition of colchicine or nonsteroidal anti-inflammatory agents may be necessary for acute attacks. The incidence of acute attacks may increase during the initial months of therapy.
□ Monitor intake and output ratios. Decreased kidney function can cause drug accumulation and toxic effects. Ensure that patient maintains adequate fluid intake (minimum 2500–

*Underlines indicate most frequent; **CAPITALS** indicate life-threatening.

3000 ml/day) to minimize risk of kidney stone formation.

- **Lab Test Considerations:** Serum and urine uric acid levels usually begin to decrease 2–3 days after initiation of therapy.
- □ Monitor blood glucose in patients receiving oral hypoglycemic agents. May cause hypoglycemia.
- □ Hematologic, renal, and liver function tests should be monitored prior to and periodically throughout course of therapy. May cause elevation of serum alkaline phosphatase, SGOT (AST), and SGPT (ALT) levels. Decreased CBC and platelets may indicate bone marrow depression. Elevated BUN, serum creatinine, and creatinine clearance may indicate nephrotoxicity. These are usually reversed with discontinuation of therapy.

Potential Nursing Diagnoses

- Comfort, altered: pain (indications).
- Knowledge deficit related to medication regimen (patient/family teaching).

Implementation

- **PO:** Allopurinol may be administered after meals to minimize gastric irritation. May be crushed and given with fluid or mixed with food for patients who have difficulty swallowing.

Patient/Family Teaching

- □ Instruct patient to take allopurinol exactly as directed. If a dose is missed, take as soon as remembered. If dosing schedule is once daily, do not take if remembered the next day. If dosing schedule is more than once a day, take up to 300 mg for the next dose.
- □ Alkaline diet may be ordered. Urinary acidification with large doses of vitamin C or other acids may increase kidney stone formation (see Appendix K). Advise patient of need for increased fluid intake.
- □ Instruct patient to report itching, skin rash, chills, fever, nausea, or vomiting to physician promptly.
- □ Advise patient that large amounts of alcohol increase uric acid concentrations and may decrease the effectiveness of allopurinol.
- □ Emphasize the importance of follow-up examinations to monitor effectiveness and side effects.

Evaluation

Effectiveness of therapy can be determined by: ▪ Decreased serum and urinary uric acid levels. May take 2 days to 3 wk to observe improvement.

ALPHA$_1$-PROTEINASE INHIBITOR

alpha$_1$-antitrypsin, Prolastin

CLASSIFICATION(S):
Enzyme inhibitor
Pregnancy Category C

INDICATIONS

▪ Replacement therapy (chronic) in patients with demonstrated panacinar emphysema associated with alpha-antitrypsin deficiency.

ACTION

▪ Prevents the destructive action of elastase on alveolar tissue in patients who have alpha$_1$-antitrypsin deficiency. **Therapeutic Effect:** ▪ Slowing of the destructive process on long tissue.

PHARMACOKINETICS

Absorption: Following IV administration absorption is essentially complete.
Distribution: Achieves high concentration in epithelial fluid of lungs.
Metabolism and Excretion: Broken down in the intravascular space.
Half-life: 4.5–5.2 days.

CONTRAINDICATIONS AND PRECAUTIONS

Contraindicated in: ▪ Hypersensitivity to polyethylene glycol ▪ Emphysema associated with alpha$_1$-antitrypsin deficiency where risk of panacinar emphysema is small (PiMZ and PiMS phenotype).
Use Cautiously in: ▪ Patients with irreversible destruction of lung tissue sec-

ondary to $alpha_1$-antitrypsin deficiency ▪ Pregnancy, lactation, and children (safety not established).

ADVERSE REACTIONS AND SIDE EFFECTS*

CNS: lightheadedness, dizziness.
Hemat: transient leukocytosis.
Misc: delayed fever.

INTERACTIONS

Drug–Drug: ▪ None known.

ROUTE AND DOSAGE

▪ **IV (Adults):** 60 mg/kg once weekly.

PHARMACODYNAMICS (increased serum levels of $alpha_1$-proteinase inhibitor)

	ONSET	PEAK	DURATION
IV	2–6 days	several wks	UK

NURSING IMPLICATIONS

Assessment

- Monitor respiratory status (rate, lung sounds, dyspnea) prior to and weekly throughout course of therapy.
- **Lab Test Considerations:** Monitor serum $alpha_1$-proteinase inhibitor levels to determine response to therapy. Minimum serum concentration should be 80 mg/100 ml.
- May cause transient mild increase in leukocytes.

Potential Nursing Diagnoses

- Gas exchange, impaired (indications).
- Knowledge deficit related to medication regimen (patient/family teaching). ing).

Implementation

- **Direct IV:** Bring bottles to room temperature. Reconstitute with provided sterile water for injection to yield a concentration of 20 mg/ml. May be diluted in 0.9% NaCl if necessary. Do not refrigerate after reconstitution. Use within 3 hr.
- *Rate:* Administer direct IV at a rate of 0.8 ml/kg/min or greater.

Patient/Family Teaching

- Explain purpose of medication and need for chronic weekly therapy to patient. Patient should avoid smoking and notify physician of any changes in breathing pattern or sputum production.
- Advise patient of need for periodic pulmonary function tests to determine progression of disease and response to therapy.
- Explain purpose of vaccination with hepatitis B vaccine prior to beginning therapy. A small risk of hepatitis is caused by the manufacturing process and vaccination is recommended to ensure prevention of hepatitis.

Evaluation

Effectiveness of therapy can be demonstrated by: ▪ Slowing of the destructive process on lung tissue as measured by increased serum $alpha_1$-proteinase inhibitor levels.

ALPRAZOLAM

(al-**pray**-zoe-lam)
Xanax

CLASSIFICATION(S):
Sedative/hypnotic—benzodiazepine
Schedule IV
Pregnancy Category D

INDICATIONS

▪ Treatment of anxiety ▪ Adjunct in the treatment of depression ▪ Management of panic attacks.

ACTION

▪ Acts at many levels in the CNS to produce anxiolytic effect ▪ Depresses the CNS, probably by potentiating gamma aminobutyric acid (GABA), an inhibitory neurotransmitter. **Therapeutic Effect:** ▪ Relief of anxiety.

PHARMACOKINETICS

Absorption: Slowly but completely absorbed from the GI tract.

*Underlines indicate most frequent; **CAPITALS** indicate life-threatening.

Distribution: Widely distributed, crosses blood–brain barrier. Probably crosses the placenta and enters breast milk.
Metabolism and Excretion: Metabolized by the liver to an active compound that is subsequently rapidly metabolized.
Half-life: 12–15 hr.

CONTRAINDICATIONS AND PRECAUTIONS

Contraindicated in: ▪ Hypersensitivity ▪ Cross-sensitivity with other benzodiazepines may exist ▪ Patients with pre-existing CNS depression ▪ Severe uncontrolled pain ▪ Narrow-angle glaucoma ▪ Pregnancy and lactation.
Use Cautiously in: ▪ Hepatic dysfunction (dosage reduction required) ▪ Patients who may be suicidal or have been addicted to drugs previously ▪ Elderly or debilitated patients (dosage reduction required).

ADVERSE REACTIONS AND SIDE EFFECTS*

CNS: dizziness, drowsiness, lethargy, hangover, paradoxical excitation, confusion, mental depression, headache.
EENT: blurred vision.
GI: nausea, vomiting, diarrhea, constipation.
Derm: rashes.
Misc: tolerance, psychological dependence, physical dependence.

INTERACTIONS

Drug-Drug: ▪ **Alcohol, antidepressants, antihistamines,** and **narcotic analgesics**—concurrent use results in additive CNS depression ▪ **Cimetidine, oral contraceptives, disulfiram, fluoxetine, isoniazid, ketoconazole, metoprolol, propoxyphene, propranolol,** or **valproic acid** may decrease the metabolism of alprazolam, enhancing its actions ▪ May decrease efficacy of **levodopa** ▪ **Rifampin** or **barbiturates** may increase the metabolism and decrease effectiveness of alprazolam ▪ Sedative effects may be decreased by **theophylline.**

ROUTE AND DOSAGE

- **PO (Adults):** 0.25–0.5 mg 2–3 times daily (not to exceed 4 mg/day).

PHARMACODYNAMICS (sedation)

	ONSET	PEAK	DURATION
PO	1–2 hr	1–2 hr	up to 24 hr

NURSING IMPLICATIONS

Assessment

- Assess degree and manifestations of anxiety and mental status prior to and periodically throughout therapy.
- Assess patient for drowsiness, lightheadedness, and dizziness. These symptoms usually disappear as therapy progresses. Dosage should be reduced if these symptoms persist.
- Prolonged high-dose therapy may lead to psychological or physical dependence. Restrict the amount of drug available to patient.

Potential Nursing Diagnoses

- Anxiety (indications).
- Injury, high risk for (side effects).
- Knowledge deficit related to medication regimen (patient/family teaching).

Implementation

- **PO:** Tablets may be crushed and taken with food or fluids if patient has difficulty swallowing.

Patient/Family Teaching

- Instruct patient to take medication exactly as prescribed; do not skip or double up on missed doses. If a dose is missed it can be taken within 1 hr, otherwise skip the dose and return to the regular schedule. If medication is less effective after a few wks, check with physician; do not increase dose. Abrupt withdrawal of alprazolam may cause sweating, vomiting, muscle cramps, tremors, and convulsions.
- Alprazolam may cause drowsiness or dizziness. Caution patient to avoid driving and other activities requiring alertness until response to the medication is known.

*Underlines indicate most frequent; **CAPITALS** indicate life-threatening.

- ▫ Advise patient to avoid the use of alcohol or other CNS depressants concurrently with this medication. Instruct patient to consult physician or pharmacist before taking over-the-counter medications concurrently with this medication.

EVALUATION

Effectiveness of therapy can be demonstrated by: ▪ Decreased sense of anxiety and an increased ability to cope. Treatment with this medication should not exceed 4 mon without re-evaluation of the patient's need for the drug.

ALPROSTADIL

(al-**pros**-ta-dil)
prostaglandin E_1, Prostin VR Pediatric

CLASSIFICATION(S):
Hormone—prostaglandin
Pregnancy Category UK

INDICATIONS

▪ Temporary maintenance of patent ductus arteriosus in neonates who depend on patency until surgery can be performed.

ACTION

▪ Directly relaxes smooth muscle of the ductus arteriosus ▪ Other effects include: ▫ Vasodilation ▫ Inhibition of platelet aggregation ▫ Stimulation of intestinal and uterine smooth muscle. **Therapeutic Effect:** ▪ Short-term maintenance of patent ductus arteriosus in neonates born with congenital heart defects who require patency to maintain blood oxygenation and perfusion of the lower body.

PHARMACOKINETICS

Absorption: Following IV administration absorption is essentially complete.
Distribution: UK.
Metabolism and Excretion: Up to 80% rapidly metabolized in the lungs.
Half-life: 5–10 min.

CONTRAINDICATIONS AND PRECAUTIONS

Contraindicated in: ▪ Respiratory distress syndrome.
Use Cautiously in: ▪ Neonates with bleeding tendencies.

ADVERSE REACTIONS AND SIDE EFFECTS*

CNS: SEIZURES, cerebral bleeding, irritability, jitteriness, lethargy.
CV: bradycardia, hypotension.
Resp: APNEA, wheezing, hypercapnea, respiratory depression, altered respiratory rate (slow and fast).
GI: diarrhea, gastric regurgitation, hyperbilirubinemia.
GU: anuria, hematuria.
Derm: flushing.
F and E: hypokalemia.
Hemat: disseminated intravascular coagulation, anemia thrombocytopenia, bleeding.
Metab: hypoglycemia.
MS: neck hyperextension, stiffness.
Misc: fever, hypothermia, sepsis, peritonitis.

INTERACTIONS

Drug-Drug: ▪ None known.

ROUTE AND DOSAGE

▪ **IV, Intra-Arterial, or Intra-Aortic (Neonates):** 0.1 mcg/kg/min initially until satisfactory response is obtained, then decrease to maintenance dose of 1/100–1/10 of initial dose. (Initial dose may be increased up to 0.4 mcg/kg if no response is obtained).

PHARMACODYNAMICS (improvement in blood gases, pulmonary blood flow)

	ONSET	PEAK	DURATION
IV (achd)*	1.5–3 hr	1.5–3 hr	duration of infusion
IV (cghd)†	15–30 min	30 min	duration of infusion

*Acyanotic congenital heart disease.
†Cyanotic congenital heart disease.

*Underlines indicate most frequent; CAPITALS indicate life-threatening.

A

NURSING IMPLICATIONS

Assessment

- Monitor rectal temperature, respiratory rate, pulse, blood pressure, and ECG continuously during therapy.
- In neonates with aortic arch anomalies also monitor pulmonary artery and descending aorta pressures, and urinary output. Palpate femoral pulse frequently to assess circulation to lower extremities. Blood pressure may be monitored in a lower and upper extremity simultaneously.
- Assess lung sounds and heart sounds frequently. Monitor neurologic status closely. Neonates less than 2 kg are at higher risk of developing respiratory, cardiovascular, and neurologic side effects. A ventilator should be readily available. Monitor for the development of congestive heart failure. Observe for seizure activity.
- During intra-aortic and intra-arterial administration, assess frequently for facial or arm flushing, which may indicate catheter displacement and necessitate repositioning of the catheter.
- **Lab Test Considerations:** Monitor arterial blood gases prior to and periodically throughout therapy. In cyanotic defects, PaO_2 should increase within 30 min. In noncyanotic defects, correction of metabolic acidosis should occur within 4–11 hr.
- May rarely cause decreased serum glucose, or increased serum bilirubin levels. May increase or decrease serum potassium levels.
- **Toxicity and Overdose:** Symptoms of overdose include flushing, hypotension, bradycardia, fever, and decreased respiratory rate or apnea. Infusion should be discontinued if apnea or bradycardia occurs.

Potential Nursing Diagnoses

- Cardiac output, decreased (indications).
- Tissue perfusion, altered: (indications).

Implementation

- **General Info:** May be administered intravenously through a peripheral or central line; intra-arterially through an umbilical artery catheter or pulmonary artery catheter; or by intra-aortic infusion.
- Duration of therapy is usually limited to 24–48 hr. Closure of the ductus arteriosus usually begins within 1 or 2 hr after discontinuing therapy.
- Notify physician if fever or hypotension occur. These side effects may resolve with a decrease in infusion rate.
- **Continuous Infusion:** Available in soln at concentration of 500 mcg/ml. Dilute further in 0.9% NaCl or D5W. Diluting 1 ml (500 mcg) of alprostadil in 250 ml of IV fluid will yield a final concentration of 2 mcg/ml; in 100 ml of IV fluid will yield 5 mcg/ml; in 50 ml of IV fluid will yield 10 mcg/ml; in 25 ml of IV fluid will yield 20 mcg/ml. Do not use soln containing benzyl alcohol as a diluent. Stable for 24 hr at room temperature.
- Infusion must be administered via infusion pump to ensure precise dose delivered.
- Do not admix.

Patient/Family Teaching

- Explain the purpose of alprostadil and the need for continuous monitoring to the parents.

Evaluation

Effectiveness of therapy in the neonate with congenital heart disease may be demonstrated by: ▪ Maintained patency of the ductus arteriosus as evidenced by improved oxygenation in cyanotic disorders ▪ Improved circulation to the lower extremities ▫ Correction of metabolic acidosis ▫ Improved urine output in noncyanotic disorders.

ALTEPLASE

(**al**-te-plase)

Activase, {Activase rt-PA}, tissue plasminogen activator, t-PA

{} = Available in Canada only.

CLASSIFICATION(S):
Thrombolytic
Pregnancy Category C

INDICATIONS

▪ Acute (within 4–6 hr from onset of chest pain) management of myocardial infarction ▪ Management of acute massive pulmonary embolism associated with obstructed pulmonary blood flow or unstable hemodynamics.

ACTION

▪ Stimulates the conversion of plasminogen trapped in thrombi to plasmin by binding to fibrin. **Therapeutic Effects:** ▪ Lysis of coronary thrombi and subsequent limitation of infarct size ▪ Lysis of life-threatening pulmonary emboli.

PHARMACOKINETICS

Absorption: Following IV administration absorption is essentially complete.
Distribution: Not known.
Metabolism and Excretion: >80% rapidly metabolized by the liver.
Half-life: 35 min.

CONTRAINDICATIONS AND PRECAUTIONS

Contraindicated in: ▪ Active internal bleeding ▪ History of cerebrovascular accident ▪ Recent (within 2 mon) intracranial or intraspinal trauma or surgery ▪ Intracranial neoplasm ▪ Severe uncontrolled hypertension ▪ Arteriovenous malformation ▪ Known bleeding tendencies.
Use Cautiously in: ▪ Recent (within 10 days) major surgery, trauma, GI or GU bleeding ▪ Cerebrovascular disease ▪ Uncontrolled hypertension ▪ Left heart thrombus ▪ Severe hepatic or renal disease ▪ Hemorrhagic ophthalmic conditions ▪ Septic phlebitis ▪ Elderly patients (>75 yr) ▪ Children, pregnancy, or lactation (safety not established).
Extreme Caution in: ▪ Early postpartum period (10 days) ▪ Patients receiving oral anticoagulant therapy.

ADVERSE REACTIONS AND SIDE EFFECTS*

CNS: INTRACRANIAL BLEEDING, headache.
CV: arrhythmias (due to reperfusion), hypotension.
EENT: epistaxis, gingival bleeding.
GI: GASTROINTESTINAL BLEEDING, RETROPERITONEAL BLEEDING, nausea, vomiting.
GU: GENITOURINARY TRACT BLEEDING.
Derm: ecchymoses, urticaria, itching, flushing.
Hemat: BLEEDING.
MS: musculoskeletal pain.
Misc: fever, hypersensitivity reactions.

INTERACTIONS

Drug-Drug: ▪ **Aspirin, oral anticoagulants, heparin, nonsteroidal anti-inflammatory agents,** or **dipyridamole**—concurrent use may increase the risk of bleeding, although these agents are frequently used together or in sequence.

ROUTE AND DOSAGE

Acute Myocardial Infarction

Note: See infusion rate chart in Appendix D. Doses greater than 150 mg have been associated with an increased risk of intracranial bleeding.

- **IV (Adults >65 kg):** 60 mg over the first hr (6–10 mg of this given as a bolus over the first 1–2 min), 20 mg over the second hr and 20 mg over the third hr for a total of 100 mg.
- **IV (Adults <65 kg):** 1.25 mg/kg total dose over 3 hr given as 0.75 mg/kg over the first hr (0.075–0.125 mg/kg of this given as a bolus over the first 1–2 min), 0.25 mg/kg over the second hr and 0.25 mg/kg over the third hr.

Pulmonary Embolism

- **IV (Adults):** 100 mg over 2 hr. Follow with heparin therapy.

*Underlines indicate most frequent; **CAPITALS** indicate life-threatening.

PHARMACODYNAMICS (reperfusion of occluded coronary arteries)

	ONSET	PEAK	DURATION
IV	UK	20 min–2 hr (45 min avg)	UK

NURSING IMPLICATIONS

Assessment

- ▫ Monitor vital signs every 15 min until stable then every hr. Notify physician if systolic BP >180 mmHg or diastolic BP >110 mmHg. Alteplase should not be given if hypertension is uncontrolled. Inform physician if hypotension occurs. Hypotension may result from the drug, hemorrhage, or cardiogenic shock.
- ▫ Monitor ECG continuously. Document changes in ST segment. Notify physician if arrhythmias occur. Accelerated idioventricular rhythm, bradycardia, asystole, and ventricular arrhythmias due to reperfusion have been reported. Prophylactic antiarrhythmic therapy may be ordered concurrently and following alteplase administration.
- ▫ Assess intensity, character, location, and radiation of chest pain. Note presence of associated symptoms (nausea, vomiting, diaphoresis). Administer analgesics as ordered by physician. Notify physician if chest pain is unrelieved or recurs.
- ▫ Monitor heart sounds and breath sounds frequently. Inform physician if signs of congestive heart failure occur (rales/crackles, dyspnea, S_3 heart sound, jugular venous distension, elevated CVP).
- ▫ Assess patients for signs of bleeding and hemorrhage. Monitor all previous puncture sites every 15 min. May cause internal bleeding including intracranial hemorrhage. Guaiac all body fluids and stools. Monitor neurologic status. Assess peripheral pulses.
- ▫ Assess patient for development of urticaria, which may indicate hypersensitivity reaction. Inform physician promptly if this occurs.
- ▪ **Lab Test Considerations:** Monitor prothrombin time, partial thromboplastin time, fibrinogen, fibrin degradation products, CBC and platelets, and CPK-MB to assess effectiveness of therapy and prevent hemorrhage. CPK-MB may rise from washout of reperfused area. Confer with physician about type and crossmatch of blood in the event of hemorrhage.
- ▪ **Toxicity and Overdose:** Alteplase is rapidly cleared from the body; discontinue immediately if serious bleeding occurs.

Potential Nursing Diagnoses

- ▪ Comfort, altered: pain, acute (indications).
- ▪ Tissue perfusion, altered (indications).
- ▪ Injury, high risk for (side effects).

Implementation

- ▪ **General Info:** Avoid IM injections prior to and throughout period of anticoagulation. Avoid unnecessary venipunctures. Apply pressure to all arterial and venous punctures for at least 30 min. Avoid venipunctures at all noncompressable sites (e.g., jugular and subclavian sites).
- ▫ Maintain patient on bedrest. Avoid all unnecessary procedures such as shaving and vigorous toothbrushing for 24 hr.
- ▫ Heparin and/or aspirin therapy may be ordered concurrently and following alteplase administration.
- ▪ **IV:** Prior to therapy start two IV lines: one for alteplase, the other for any additional IV infusions.
- ▫ Vials are packaged with sterile water for injection (without preservatives) to be used as diluent. Do not use bacteriostatic water for injection. Reconstitute 20-mg vials with 20 ml and 50-mg vials with 50 ml using 18-g needle. Avoid excess agitation during dilution; swirl or invert gently to mix. Soln may foam upon reconstitution. Bubbles will resolve upon standing a

few mins. Soln will be clear to pale yellow. Stable for 8 hr at room temperature.

- **Intermittent Infusion:** May be administered as reconstituted (1 mg/ml) or may be further diluted immediately prior to use in equal amount of 0.9% NaCl or D5W. Do not admix.
- ☐ *Myocardial Infarction:* Standard dose is given over 3 hr. Infuse 60% of the total dose via infusion pump for the first hr. Infuse 20% of the total dose over the second hr and 20% over the third hr. Flush line with 25–30 ml of saline at completion of infusion to ensure entire dose is received.
- ☐ *Pulmonary Emboli:* Administer over 2 hr.
- **Y-Site Compatibility:** lidocaine.
- **Y-Site Incompatibility:** dobutamine, dopamine, heparin, or nitroglycerin.

Patient/Family Education

- ☐ Explain purpose of alteplase and the need for close monitoring to patient and family.
- ☐ Instruct patient to report signs of hypersensitivity and bleeding promptly.

Evaluation

Effectiveness of therapy can be demonstrated by: ▪ Restoration of coronary perfusion as demonstrated by cardiac catherization ☐ Clinically, by improved ventricular function ▪ Decreased incidence of congestive heart failure without the occurrence of bleeding ▪ Lysis of pulmonary emboli with improvement of hemodynamic status.

ALTRETAMINE

(al-**tret**-a-meen)
hexamethylmelamine, Hexalen

CLASSIFICATION(S):
Antineoplastic agent—miscellaneous
Pregnancy Category D

INDICATIONS

▪ Management of persistent or recurrent ovarian cancer unresponsive to treatment with first line agents (cisplatin or alkylating agent combination).

ACTION

▪ Mechanism unknown, but appears to disrupt DNA synthesis. **Therapeutic Effect:** ▪ Death of rapidly replicating cells, particularly malignant ones.

PHARMACOKINETICS

Absorption: Well absorbed following oral administration. Rapidly converted by the liver to compounds with antineoplastic activity.
Distribution: Reaches high concentrations in liver, kidney, and small intestine. Poor penetration into brain.
Metabolism and Excretion: Mostly metabolized by the liver (99%).
Half-life: 4.7–10.2 hr.

CONTRAINDICATIONS AND PRECAUTIONS

Contraindicated in: ▪ Hypersensitivity ▪ Pregnancy or lactation.
Use Cautiously in: ▪ Children (safety not established) ▪ Pre-existing neurologic diseases ▪ Patients with child-bearing potential ▪ Infections ▪ Decreased bone marrow reserve ▪ Other chronic debilitating illnesses.

ADVERSE REACTIONS AND SIDE EFFECTS*

CNS: SEIZURES, fatigue.
GI: <u>nausea</u>, <u>vomiting</u>, anorexia, hepatic toxicity.
GU: renal toxicity, gonadal suppression.
Derm: alopecia (<1%), skin rash, pruritus.
Endo: gonadal suppression.
Hemat: <u>anemia</u>, leukopenia, thrombocytopenia.
Neuro: <u>peripheral neuropathy</u>.

INTERACTIONS

Drug-Drug: ▪ Concurrent use with **MAO inhibitors** may produce orthostatic hypotension.

*<u>Underlines</u> indicate most frequent; **CAPITALS** indicate life-threatening.

A

ROUTE AND DOSAGE

- **PO (Adults):** 260 mg/m^2/day in 4 divided doses for 14 or 21 days of each 28-day cycle. Dosage reduction to 200 mg/m^2/day in 4 divided doses after meals and at bedtime recommended after 14 or more day rest for any of the following: GI intolerance, severe bone marrow depression, or progressive neurologic toxicity.

PHARMACODYNAMICS (effects on blood counts when given as 14–21 day course)

	ONSET	PEAK	DURATION
PO	UK	3–4 wk	6 wk

NURSING IMPLICATIONS

Assessment

- Nausea and vomiting of gradual onset frequently occurs. Tolerance may develop after several wks of therapy. Treatment includes antiemetics or dosage reduction, and rarely discontinuation. Monitor amount of emesis of notify physician if emesis exceeds guidelines to prevent dehydration.
- Assess for signs of anemia (increased fatigue, dyspnea, orthostatic hypotension) throughout therapy.
- Assess for fever, chills, sore throat, and signs of infection. Notify physician if these symptoms occur.
- Assess for signs of bleeding (bleeding gums, bruising, petechiae; guaiac stools, urine, and emesis). Avoid IM injections and rectal temperatures. Apply pressure to venipuncture sites for 10 min.
- Assess patient for signs of peripheral neuropathy (numbness, tingling, paresthesia) prior to initiation of each course and routinely throughout therapy. Pyridoxine may be used concurrently to minimize peripheral neuropathy. Peripheral neuropathy is usually reversible on discontinuation of medication.
- **Lab Test Considerations:** Monitor CBC and platelets prior to each course of therapy, monthly, and as clinically indicated. The nadir of leukopenia and thrombocytopenia occur in 3–4 wk with 21-day therapy and recover in 6 wk, and occur in 6–8 wk with continuous therapy. Dose should be held for 14 or more days and resumed at 200 mg/m^2/day in 4 divided doses for any of the following: GI intolerance unresponsive to conventional therapy, WBC <2000 mm^3, granulocytes <1000 mm^3, platelet count $<75{,}000$ mm^3, or progressive neurologic toxicity.

Potential Nursing Diagnoses

- Infection, high risk for (adverse reactions).
- Injury, high risk for (side effects).
- Knowledge deficit related to medication regimen (patient/family teaching).

Implementation

- **PO:** Administer doses after meals and at bedtime.

Patient/Family Teaching

- Instruct patient to notify physician promptly if fever, sore throat, signs of infection, bleeding gums, bruising, petechiae; blood in stools, urine, or emesis; increased fatigue, dyspnea, or orthostatic hypotension occur. Caution patient to avoid crowds and persons with known infections. Instruct patient to use soft toothbrush and electric razor and to avoid falls. Caution patient not to drink alcoholic beverages or take medications containing aspirin, as these may precipitate gastric bleeding.
- Instruct patient to report promptly any numbness or tingling in extremities.
- Instruct patient not to receive any vaccinations without advice of physician.
- Advise patient of the need for contraception.
- Emphasize the need for periodic lab tests to monitor for side effects.

Evaluation

Effectiveness of therapy can be demonstrated by: ▪ Decrease in size or spread of malignancy.

ALUMINUM ACETATE
Bluboro, Burow's Solution, Modified Burow's Solution, Domeboro, Pedi-Boro

CLASSIFICATION(S):
Astringent—topical
Pregnancy Category C

INDICATIONS
■ Symptomatic relief of minor inflammation of skin.

ACTION
■ Acts as an astringent; soothing effect results from cooling and vasoconstriction. **Therapeutic Effect:** ■ Relief of painful inflammation of the skin.

PHARMACOKINETICS
Absorption: Small amounts may be systemically absorbed.
Distribution: UK.
Metabolism and Excretion: UK.
Half-life: UK.

CONTRAINDICATIONS AND PRECAUTIONS
Contraindicated in: ■ Hypersensitivity to aluminum or aluminum acetate ■ Use in or near eyes ■ For external use only.
Use Cautiously in: ■ Skin conditions in which irritation continues to spread.

ADVERSE REACTIONS AND SIDE EFFECTS*
Misc: hypersensitivity.

INTERACTIONS
Drug-Drug: ■ May inactivate concurrently applied **collagenase**.

ROUTE AND DOSAGE
- **Top (Adults and Children):** 1:20 or 1:40 soln as a soak every 15–30 min for 4–8 hr.

PHARMACODYNAMICS (relief of inflammation)

	ONSET	PEAK	DURATION
Top	upon application	UK	during application

NURSING IMPLICATIONS
Assessment
□ Inspect skin for erythema, excoriation, vesicles, maceration, and drainage.

Potential Nursing Diagnoses
- Comfort, altered: pain (indications).
- Infection, high risk for (indications).
- Knowledge deficit related to medication regimen (patient/family teaching).

Implementation
- **Topical:** Prepare soln by mixing one packet in 1 pt lukewarm water (or per manufacturer's directions). Use only clear portion. Do not apply precipitate to skin.

□ Soothing effect results from cooling and vasoconstriction. Do not apply occlusive dressing or this will hinder evaporation and may cause maceration.
□ To prevent chilling and hypothermia, do not apply to more than one third of the body at one time. Position patient away from drafts.
□ Clear, unprecipitated soln is stable for 7 days at room temperature.

Patient/Family Teaching
□ Instruct patient on preparation of soln and application of soaks.
□ Instruct patient not to apply soln near eyes or to mucous membranes.
□ Advise patient to notify physician if area of skin irritation spreads or worsens.

Evaluation
Effectiveness of therapy can be demonstrated by: ■ Resolution of skin irritation.

ALUMINUM HYDROXIDE
AlternaGEL, Alucap, {Alugel}, Aluminet, Alu-tab, Amphojel, Basalgel, Dialume, Nephrox

CLASSIFICATION(S):
Antacid, Electrolyte modifier—hypophosphatemic
Pregnancy Category UK

*Underlines indicate most frequent; **CAPITALS** indicate life-threatening.
{} = Available in Canada only.

A

INDICATIONS

▪ Lowering of phosphate levels in patients with chronic renal failure ▪ Adjunctive therapy in the treatment of peptic, duodenal, and gastric ulcers ▪ Hyperacidity, indigestion, reflux esophagitis.

ACTION

▪ Binds phosphate in the GI tract ▪ Neutralizes gastric acid and inactivates pepsin. **Therapeutic Effects:** ▪ Lowering of serum phosphate levels ▪ Healing of ulcers and diminution of pain associated with ulcers or gastric hyperacidity ▪ High incidence of constipation limits use alone in the treatment of ulcer disease ▪ Frequently found in combination antacids with magnesium-containing compounds.

PHARMACOKINETICS

Absorption: With chronic use, small amounts of aluminum are systemically absorbed.
Distribution: Small amounts of aluminum absorbed are widely distributed, cross the placenta, and enter breast milk. With chronic use, aluminum concentrates in the CNS.
Metabolism and Excretion: Most aluminum hydroxide binds phosphate in the GI tract and is excreted in feces. Small amounts absorbed are excreted by the kidneys in patients with normal renal function.
Half-life: UK.

CONTRAINDICATIONS AND PRECAUTIONS

Contraindicated in: ▪ Severe abdominal pain of unknown cause.
Use Cautiously in: ▪ Hypercalcemia ▪ Hypophosphatemia ▪ Pregnancy (generally considered safe; chronic high-dose therapy should be avoided).

ADVERSE REACTIONS AND SIDE EFFECTS*

GI: constipation.
F and E: hypophosphatemia.

INTERACTIONS

Drug–Drug: ▪ Absorption of **tetracyclines, chlorpromazines, iron salts, isoniazid,** or **fluoroquinolones** may be decreased ▪ **Salicylate** blood levels may be decreased ▪ **Quinidine, mexiletine,** and **amphetamine** levels may be increased if enough antacid is ingested such that urine pH is increased.

ROUTE AND DOSAGE

Hypophosphatemic

- **PO (Adults):** 1.9–4.8 g 3–4 times daily.
- **PO (Children):** 50–150 mg/kg/24 hr—titrate to normal serum phosphate levels.

Antacid

- **PO (Adults):** 500–1800 mg (5–30 ml) 3–6 times daily.

PHARMACODYNAMICS

	ONSET	PEAK	DURATION
PO (hypophosphate)	hr–days	days–wks	days
PO (antacid)	15–30 min	30 min	30 min–3 hr

NURSING IMPLICATIONS

Assessment

- Assess location, duration, character, and precipitating factors of gastric pain.
- **Lab Test Considerations:** Monitor serum phosphate and calcium levels periodically during chronic use of aluminum hydroxide.
- May cause increased serum gastrin and decreased serum phosphate concentrations.
- In treatment of severe ulcer disease, guaiac stools and emesis and monitor pH of gastric secretions.

Potential Nursing Diagnoses

- Comfort, altered: pain (indications).
- Bowel elimination, altered: constipation (side effects).
- Knowledge deficit related to medication regimen (patient/family teaching).

*Underlines indicate most frequent; **CAPITALS** indicate life-threatening.

Implementation

- **General Info:** Antacids cause premature dissolution and absorption of enteric-coated tablets and may interfere with absorption of other oral medications. Separate administration of aluminum hydroxide and oral medications by at least 1 hr.
  - Tablets must be chewed thoroughly before swallowing to prevent entering small intestine in undissolved form. Follow with ½ glass of water.
  - Shake liquid preparations well before pouring. Follow administration with water to assure passage into stomach.
  - Liquid and powder dosage forms are considered to be more effective than tablets.
- **Hypophosphatemic:** For phosphate lowering, follow dose with full glass of water or fruit juice.
- **Antacid:** May be given in conjunction with magnesium-containing antacids to minimize constipation, except in patients with renal failure. Administer 1 and 3 hr after meals and at bedtime for maximum antacid effect.
  - For treatment of peptic ulcer aluminum hydroxide may be administered every 1–2 hr while awake or diluted with two to three parts of milk or water and administered intragastrically every 30 min for 12 or more hrs per day. Physician may order nasogastric tube clamped following administration.

Patient/Family Teaching

- **General Info:** Instruct patient to take aluminum hydroxide exactly as directed. If on a regular dosing schedule and a dose is missed, take as soon as remembered if not almost time for next dose; do not double doses.
  - Advise patients to check label for sodium content. Patients with congestive heart failure, hypertension, or those on a sodium restriction should use low-sodium preparations.
  - Inform patients of potential for constipating effects of aluminum hydroxide.
- **Hypophosphatemic:** Patients taking aluminum hydroxide for hyperphosphatemia should be taught the importance of a low-phosphate diet.
- **Antacid:** Caution patient to consult physician before taking antacids for more than 2 wk or if problem is recurring. Advise patient to consult physician if relief is not obtained or if symptoms of gastric bleeding (black tarry stools, coffee ground emesis) occur.

Evaluation

Effectiveness of therapy can be demonstrated by: ▪ Decrease in serum phosphate levels ▪ Decrease in GI pain and irritation and an increase in the pH of gastric secretions. In treatment of peptic ulcer, antacid therapy should be continued for at least 4–6 wk after all symptoms have disappeared, since there is no correlation between disappearance of symptoms and healing of ulcers.

AMANTADINE

(a-**man**-ta-deen)
Symmetrel, Symadine

CLASSIFICATION(S):
Antiparkinson agent, Antiviral
Pregnancy Category C

INDICATIONS

▪ Symptomatic initial and adjunct treatment of Parkinson's disease ▪ Prophylaxis and treatment of influenza A viral infections.

ACTION

▪ Potentiates the action of dopamine in the CNS ▪ Prevents penetration of influenza A virus into host cell. **Therapeutic Effects:** ▪ Alleviation of Parkinsonian symptoms ▪ Prevention and decreased symptoms of influenza virus A infection.

PHARMACOKINETICS

Absorption: Well absorbed from the GI tract.

Distribution: Distributed to various body tissues and fluids. Crosses blood–brain barrier and enters breast milk.
Metabolism and Excretion: Excreted unchanged in the urine.
Half-life: 24 hr.

CONTRAINDICATIONS AND PRECAUTIONS

Contraindicated in: ▪ Hypersensitivity.
Use Cautiously in: ▪ History of seizure disorders ▪ Liver disease ▪ Psychiatric problems ▪ Cardiac disease ▪ Renal impairment (dosage reduction required) ▪ May increase susceptibility to rubella infections ▪ Pregnancy and lactation (safety not established).

ADVERSE REACTIONS AND SIDE EFFECTS*

CNS: <u>dizziness</u>, <u>ataxia</u>, <u>insomnia</u>, depression, psychosis, anxiety, drowsiness, confusion.
CV: <u>hypotension</u>, congestive heart failure, edema.
EENT: dry mouth, blurred vision.
GU: urinary retention.
Derm: rashes, <u>mottling</u>.
Hemat: leukopenia, neutropenia.
Resp: dyspnea.

INTERACTIONS

Drug–Drug: ▪ Concurrent use of **antihistamines, phenothiazines, quinidine, disopyramide,** and **tricyclic antidepressants** may result in additive anticholinergic effects (dry mouth, blurred vision, constipation).

ROUTE AND DOSAGE

Parkinson's Disease

- **PO (Adults):** 100 mg twice daily.

Influenza A Viral Infection

- **PO (Adults and Children >9 yr):** 100 mg twice daily.
- **PO (Children 1–9 yr):** 4.4–8.8 mg/kg/day up to 150 mg/day as a single daily dose or 2 divided doses.

PHARMACODYNAMICS (antiparkinson effect)

	ONSET	PEAK	DURATION
PO	10–15 min	1–4 hr	12–24 hr

NURSING IMPLICATIONS

Assessment

- **General Info:** Monitor blood pressure periodically. Assess patient for drug-induced orthostatic hypotension.
- □ Monitor intake and output closely in the elderly. May cause urinary retention. Notify physician if significant discrepancy or bladder distention occurs.
- □ Monitor vital signs and mental status periodically during first few days of dosage adjustment in patients receiving more than 200 mg daily, as side effects are more likely.
- □ Assess for congestive heart failure (peripheral edema, weight gain, dyspnea, rales/crackles, jugular venous distension) especially in patients with chronic therapy or history of congestive heart failure.
- □ Assess patient for confusion, hallucinations, and mood changes. Notify physician if these signs of toxicity occur.
- □ Assess patient for the appearance of a diffuse red mottling of the skin (livedo reticularis), especially in the lower extremities or on exposure to cold. This common side effect disappears with continued therapy but may not completely resolve until several wks after therapy has been discontinued.
- **Parkinson's Disease:** Assess akinesia, rigidity, tremors, and gait disturbances prior to and throughout course of therapy.
- **Influenza Prophylaxis or Treatment:** Monitor respiratory status (rate, breath sounds, sputum) and temperature periodically. Supportive treatment is indicated if symptoms occur.

*<u>Underlines</u> indicate most frequent; **CAPITALS** indicate life-threatening.

- **Toxicity and Overdose:** Symptoms of toxicity include CNS stimulation (confusion, mood changes, tremors, seizures, arrhythmias, and hypotension). There is no specific antidote, although physostigmine has been used to reverse CNS effects.

POTENTIAL NURSING DIAGNOSES

- Mobility, impaired physical (indications).
- Infection, high risk for (indications).
- Knowledge deficit related to medication regimen (patient/family teaching).

IMPLEMENTATION

- **PO:** Do not administer last dose of medication near bedtime, as this drug may produce insomnia in some patients.
  - Administering amantadine in divided doses may decrease CNS side effects.
  - The contents of capsules may be mixed with food or fluids if the patient has difficulty swallowing pills. Also available as a syrup.

PATIENT/FAMILY TEACHING

- **General Info:** Advise patient to take medication around the clock as directed and not to skip doses or double up on missed doses. If a dose is missed, do not take within 4 hr of the next dose.
  - Amantadine may cause dizziness or blurred vision. Advise patient to avoid driving or other activities that require alertness until response to the drug is known.
  - Advise patient to make position changes slowly to minimize orthostatic hypotension.
  - Inform patient that frequent mouth rinses, good oral hygiene, and sugarless gum or candy may decrease dry mouth.
  - Advise patient to confer with physician or pharmacist prior to taking over-the-counter medications, especially cold remedies, or drinking alcoholic beverages.
  - Instruct patient and family to notify physician if influenza symptoms occur (when used as prophylaxis) or if confusion, mood changes, difficulty with urination, edema and shortness of breath, or worsening of Parkinson's disease symptoms occur.
- **Parkinson's Disease:** Amantadine should be tapered off gradually, abrupt withdrawal may precipitate a parkinsonian crisis.

EVALUATION

Effectiveness of therapy can be demonstrated by: ▪ Decrease in akinesia and rigidity. Full therapeutic effects may require 2 wk of therapy ▪ Absence or reduction of influenza A symptoms.

AMIKACIN

(am-i-**kay**-sin)
Amikin

CLASSIFICATION(S):
Anti-infective—aminoglycoside
Pregnancy Category D

INDICATIONS

▪ Treatment of serious gram-negative bacillary infections and infections due to staphylococci when penicillins or other less toxic drugs are contraindicated.

ACTION

▪ Inhibits protein synthesis in bacteria at the level of the 30S ribosome. **Therapeutic Effect:** ▪ Bactericidal action against susceptible bacteria. **Spectrum:** ▪ Notable for activity against: ▫ *Pseudomonas aeruginosa* ▫ *Klebsiella pneumoniae* ▫ *Escherichia coli* ▫ *Proteus* ▫ *Serratia* and *Acenitobacter* where resistance to gentamicin or tobramycin has occurred ▪ In the treatment of enterococcal infections, synergy with a penicillin is required.

PHARMACOKINETICS

Absorption: Well absorbed after IM administration.
Distribution: Widely distributed throughout extracellular fluid. Crosses the placenta. Poor penetration into CSF.
Metabolism and Excretion: Excretion

is mainly (>90%) renal. Dosage adjustments are required for any decrease in renal function. Minimal amounts metabolized by the liver.
Half-life: 2–3 hr (increased in renal impairment).

CONTRAINDICATIONS AND PRECAUTIONS

Contraindicated in: ▪ Hypersensitivity ▪ Cross-sensitivity with other aminoglycosides may exist.
Use Cautiously in: ▪ Renal impairment of any kind (dosage adjustments necessary—blood level monitoring useful in preventing ototoxicity and nephrotoxicity) ▪ Pregnancy, lactation, infants, and neonates (safety not established) ▪ Neuromuscular diseases such as myasthenia gravis.

ADVERSE REACTIONS AND SIDE EFFECTS*

EENT: ototoxicity (vestibular and cochlear).
GU: nephrotoxicity.
Neuro: enhanced neuromuscular blockade.
Misc: hypersensitivity reactions.

INTERACTIONS

Drug-Drug: ▪ Inactivated by **penicillins** when coadministered to patients with renal insufficiency ▪ Possible respiratory paralysis after **inhalation anesthetics (ether, cyclopropane, halothane, nitrous oxide)** or **neuromuscular blockers (tubocurarine, succinylcholine)** ▪ Increased incidence of ototoxicity with **loop diuretics (ethacrynic acid, furosemide)** ▪ Increased incidence of nephrotoxicity with other **nephrotoxic drugs (cisplatin).**

ROUTE AND DOSAGE

- **IM, IV (Adults, Children, and Older Infants):** 15 mg/kg/day in divided doses every 8–12 hr.
- **IM, IV (Children):** 15 mg/kg/day in divided doses every 8–12 hr.
- **IM, IV (Younger Infants and Neonates):** 10 mg/kg initially, 7.5 mg/kg every 12 hr.

PHARMACODYNAMICS (peak blood levels)

	ONSET	PEAK
IM	rapid	0.75–1.5 hr
IV	rapid	end of infusion

NURSING IMPLICATIONS

Assessment

- ▫ Assess patient for infection (vital signs; wound appearance, sputum, urine, and stool; WBC) at beginning and throughout course of therapy.
- ▫ Obtain specimens for culture and sensitivity prior to initiating therapy. First dose may be given before receiving results.
- ▫ Evaluate eighth cranial nerve function by audiometry prior to and throughout course of therapy. Hearing loss is usually in the high-frequency range. Prompt recognition and intervention is essential in preventing permanent damage. Also monitor for vestibular dysfunction (vertigo, ataxia, nausea, vomiting). Eighth cranial nerve dysfunction is associated with persistently elevated peak amikacin levels.
- ▫ Monitor intake and output and daily weight to assess hydration status and renal function.
- ▫ Assess patient for signs of superinfection (fever, upper respiratory infection, vaginal itching or discharge, increasing malaise, diarrhea). Report to physician.
- ▪ **Lab Test Considerations:** Monitor renal function by urinalysis, specific gravity, BUN, creatinine, and creatinine clearance prior to and throughout therapy.
- ▫ May cause increased BUN, SGOT (AST), SGPT (ALT), serum alkaline phosphatase, bilirubin, creatinine, and LDH concentrations.
- ▫ May cause decreased serum calcium,

*Underlines indicate most frequent; **CAPITALS** indicate life-threatening.

magnesium, potassium, and sodium concentrations.

- **Toxicity and Overdose:** Therapeutic blood levels should be monitored periodically during therapy. Timing of blood levels is important in interpreting results. Draw blood for peak levels 1 hr after IM injection and 15–30 min after IV infusion is completed. Trough levels should be drawn just prior to next dose. Acceptable peak level is 30–35 mcg/ml; trough level should not exceed 5–10 mcg/ml.

Potential Nursing Diagnoses

- Infection, high risk for (indications).
- Sensory-perceptual alteration: auditory (side effects).

Implementation

- **General Info:** Keep patient well hydrated (1500–2000 ml/day) during therapy.
- **Intermittent Infusion:** Dilute 500 mg of amikacin in 100–200 ml of D5W, D10W, 0.9% NaCl, D5/0.9% NaCl, D5/0.45% NaCl, D5/0.25% NaCl, or lactated Ringer's soln. Soln may be pale yellow without decreased potency. Stable for 24 hr at room temperature. Flush IV line with D5W or 0.9% NaCl following administration.
  - *Rate:* Infuse over 30–60 min (over 1–2 hr for infants).
  - Administer separately; do not admix. Give aminoglycosides and penicillins at least 1 hr apart to prevent inactivation.
- **Syringe Incompatibility:** heparin.
- **Y-Site Compatibility:** enalaprilat, furosemide, magnesium sulfate, morphine, or ondansetron.
- **Y-Site Incompatibility:** hetastarch.
- **Additive Compatibility:** amobarbital, ascorbic acid, bleomycin, calcium chloride, calcium gluconate, cefoxitin, chloramphenicol, chlorpheniramine, cimetidine, clindamycin, dimenhydrinate, diphenhydramine, epinephrine, ergonovine, hydrocortisone, metronidazole, norepinephrine, pentobarbital, phenobarbital, phytonadione, polymyxin B, prochlorperazine, promethazine, secobarbital, sodium bicarbonate, succinylcholine, vancomycin, or verapamil.
- **Additive Incompatibility:** amphotericin B, ampicillin, cefazolin, cephalothin, cephapirin, chlorothiazide, heparin, methicillin, phenytoin, sulfadiazine, or thiopental.

Patient/Family Teaching

- Instruct patient to report signs of hypersensitivity, tinnitus, vertigo, or hearing loss.

Evaluation

Clinical response can be evaluated by:
- Resolution of the signs and symptoms of infection. If no response is seen within 3–5 days, new cultures should be taken.

AMILORIDE
(a-**mill**-oh-ride)
Midamor

CLASSIFICATION(S):
Diuretic—potassium-sparing
Pregnancy Category B

INDICATIONS

- Counteracts potassium loss induced by other diuretics - Commonly used in combination with other agents to treat: ▫ Edema ▫ Hypertension ▫ Hyperaldosteronism.

ACTION

- Causes excretion of sodium bicarbonate and calcium while conserving potassium and hydrogen ions. **Therapeutic Effects:** - Weak diuretic and antihypertensive response when compared to other diuretics - Conservation of potassium.

PHARMACOKINETICS

Absorption: Variable absorption from the GI tract (15–50%).

Distribution: Not known, appears to distribute widely into extravascular space.

Metabolism and Excretion: 50% eliminated unchanged by the kidneys, 40%

excreted in the feces (unabsorbed drug).
Half-life: 6–9 hr.

CONTRAINDICATIONS AND PRECAUTIONS

Contraindicated in: ▪ Hypersensitivity ▪ Renal insufficiency.
Use Cautiously in: ▪ Hepatic dysfunction ▪ Elderly patients ▪ Debilitated patients ▪ Pregnancy, lactation, or children (safety not established).

ADVERSE REACTIONS AND SIDE EFFECTS*

CNS: headache, dizziness.
CV: arrhythmias.
GI: nausea, vomiting, anorexia, diarrhea, cramps, constipation, flatulence.
GU: impotence.
F and E: hyperkalemia, hyponatremia, hypochloremia.
Hemat: dyscrasias, megaloblastic anemia.
MS: muscle cramps.

INTERACTIONS

Drug-Drug: ▪ Additive hypotension with acute ingestion of **alcohol,** other **antihypertensive agents,** or **nitrates** ▪ Use with **angiotensin converting enzyme (ACE) inhibitors** or **potassium supplements** may lead to hyperkalemia. ▪ Decreases **lithium** excretion; may lead to toxicity.

ROUTE AND DOSAGE

- **PO (Adults):** 5–10 mg/day (up to 20 mg).

PHARMACODYNAMICS (effects on electrolyte excretion)

	ONSET	PEAK	DURATION
PO	2 hr	6–10 hr	24 hr

NURSING IMPLICATIONS

Assessment

- Monitor intake and output ratios and daily weight throughout therapy.
- If medication is given as an adjunct to antihypertensive therapy, blood pressure should be evaluated before administering.
- Periodic ECGs are recommended in patients receiving prolonged therapy.
- Assess patient frequently for signs of hyperkalemia (fatigue, muscle weakness, paresthesia, flaccid paralysis, cardiac arrhythmias). Patients who have diabetes mellitus, kidney disease, or who are elderly are at an increased risk of developing these symptoms.
- **Lab Test Considerations:** Monitor serum electrolytes, glucose, BUN, and creatinine periodically throughout therapy. Withhold drug and notify physician if patient becomes hyperkalemic. Patients with elevated BUN and creatinine may be at an increased risk for developing hyperkalemia. May cause elevated magnesium and uric acid levels. May cause decreased serum sodium and chloride levels.
- May cause increased serum glucose in patients with diabetes. Discontinue amiloride 3 days prior to a glucose tolerance test.

Potential Nursing Diagnoses

- Fluid volume excess (indications).
- Knowledge deficit related to medication regimen (patient/family teaching).

Implementation

- **General Info:** Available in combination with hydrochlorothiazide (Moduretic); see appendix A.
- **PO:** Administer in AM to avoid interrupting sleep pattern.
- Administer with food or milk to minimize gastric irritation.

Patient/Family Teaching

- Instruct patient to take medication exactly as directed, even if feeling well. If dose is missed, take as soon as remembered unless almost time for next dose; do not double doses.
- Teach patients on antihypertensive therapy how to check blood pressure weekly.
- Caution patients to avoid salt

*Underlines indicate most frequent; **CAPITALS** indicate life-threatening.

tutes and foods that contain high levels of potassium unless physician specifically prescribes them (see Appendix K).

□ Reinforce need to continue additional therapies for hypertension (weight loss, restricted sodium intake, stress reduction, regular exercise, moderation of alcohol consumption, and cessation of smoking). Amiloride controls but does not cure hypertension.

□ Advise patient to consult with physician or pharmacist before taking any over-the-counter decongestants, cough or cold preparations, or appetite suppressants concurrently with this medication because of potential for increased blood pressure.

□ May cause dizziness. Caution patient to avoid driving or other activities requiring alertness until effects of medication are known.

□ Instruct patient to notify physician or dentist of medication regimen prior to treatment or surgery.

□ Advise patient to notify physician if muscle weakness or cramps, fatigue, or weakness occur.

EVALUATION

Effectiveness of therapy can be demonstrated by: ▪ Lowering of blood pressure and increase in diuresis while maintaining serum potassium levels in acceptable ranges.

AMINO ACIDS

Aminess, Aminosyn, Branch-Amin, FreAmine, HepatAmine, NeprAmine, Novamine, ProcalAmine, RenAmin, Travasol, Trophamine

CLASSIFICATION(S):
Caloric agent—protein source
Pregnancy Category C

INDICATIONS

▪ Provides protein to patients who are unable to ingest enough protein by mouth to maintain positive nitrogen balance. □ Used perioperatively in patients who are unable to ingest protein, as in GI disorders, or to provide an extra source of protein in patients with large requirements who are unable to ingest enough, as seen in extensive burns, severe trauma, or overwhelming sepsis. □ Usually used with a carbohydrate source (dextrose) and a fat source as part of a total parenteral nutrition (TPN, hyperalimentation) program or protein-sparing regimen. Electrolytes, minerals, trace elements, and vitamins are also included. **Treatment must be individualized for each patient and requires facilities and personnel skilled in its use.**

ACTION

▪ Promotes protein synthesis by acting as a protein calorie source, decreases rate of protein breakdown (catabolism). **Therapeutic Effect:** ▪ Maintenance of positive nitrogen balance.

PHARMACOKINETICS

Absorption: Following IV administration absorption is essentially complete.
Distribution: Widely distributed.
Metabolism and Excretion: Metabolized as part of anabolic processes, then excreted in urine as urea nitrogen.
Half-life: UK.

CONTRAINDICATIONS AND PRECAUTIONS

Contraindicated in: ▪ No known contraindications.
Use Cautiously in: ▪ Uncontrolled sepsis ▪ Advanced cardiac, renal, and hepatic disease (specific formulations may be required).

ADVERSE REACTIONS AND SIDE EFFECTS*

CNS: headache, confusion.
CV: congestive heart failure, hypotension, hypertension.
GI: nausea, vomiting.
F and E: hypervolemia, hypovolemia, electrolyte disturbances.
Metab: hyperglycemia, hypoglycemia,

*Underlines indicate most frequent; **CAPITALS** indicate life-threatening.

azotemia, fatty acid deficiency, hyperammonemia.
Misc: INFECTION.

INTERACTIONS

Drug–Drug: ▪ **Glucocorticoids, diuretics,** or **tetracyclines** may exaggerate negative nitrogen balance.

ROUTE AND DOSAGE

Note: Doses must be carefully individualized and titrated to meet metabolic needs. If amino acids are part of total parenteral nutrition (hyperalimentation), then additional calories (as dextrose and lipid emulsions) must be provided along with electrolytes, vitamins, trace minerals and other necessary micronutrients.

- **IV (Adults):** 1–2 g protein/kg/day.
- **IV (Children):** 2–3 g protein/kg/day.
- **IV (Neonates):** 2–3 g protein/kg/day.

PHARMACODYNAMICS

	ONSET	PEAK	DURATION
IV	Not Available		

NURSING IMPLICATIONS

Assessment

- ▫ Nutritional status must be assessed prior to and periodically throughout therapy because amino acids are most commonly used as a component of total parenteral nutrition. Parameters to assess include height, weight, skinfold thickness, arm circumference, total protein, serum albumin, CBC, electrolytes, nitrogen balance, function of gastrointestinal tract, and caloric need.
- ▫ Monitor intake and output; assess for fluid overload (rales/crackles, dyspnea, peripheral edema).
- ▫ Monitor for infection (fever, chills, diaphoresis). If sepsis occurs, physician may order changing site, culturing catheter tip, hanging new solution and tubing, and obtaining blood cultures.
- ▪ **Lab Test Considerations:** May cause increased BUN. A 10–15% increase for 3 consecutive days may necessitate discontinuing therapy or altering formulation.
- ▫ May cause increased ammonia and ketone levels.

Potential Nursing Diagnoses

- ▪ Nutrition, altered: less than body requirements (indications).
- ▪ Infection, high risk for (side effects).
- ▪ Knowledge deficit related to medication regimen (patient/family teaching).

Implementation

- ▪ **General Info:** Component of total parenteral nutrition. Usually given in conjunction with hypertonic dextrose. Trace elements, vitamins, electrolytes, and insulin are usually incorporated into formulation.
- ▫ Special formulas available for patients with hepatic or renal dysfunction, patients under extreme stress (trauma, sepsis), and children.
- ▪ **IV:** Do not add anything to soln without conferring with pharmacist. Total parenteral nutrition solns should be prepared aseptically in a biologic cabinet.
- ▫ Soln should be clear. Addition of multivitamins will result in bright yellow color.
- ▫ Infuse through 0.22-micron filter unless mixed with dextrose and fat emulsion in a 3-in-1 admixture. Control infusion rate with pump or controller.
- ▫ If administered peripherally, change peripheral site every 48–72 hr or according to institutional policy. Monitor for thrombophlebitis. Avoid infiltration; may cause tissue necrosis.
- ▫ Peripheral line may be used to administer protein-sparing regimen using dilute amino acid soln (3.5%) with or without D5W or D10W and fat emulsion. Central line must be used to administer more concentrated soln when mixed with hypertonic glucose.
- ▫ Fat emulsion may be piggybacked with amino acids.
- ▫ Use aseptic technique with c line. Change dressing every

according to institutional policy. Auscultate breath sounds and assess site for erythema, edema, and leakage.

Patient/Family Teaching

- ▫ If used as a component of total parenteral nutrition, assure patient that solution is capable of fulfilling all nutritional needs.
- ▫ Instruct patient to report fever, chills, or swelling, pain, and leakage at infusion site immediately.
- ▫ Patients receiving total parenteral nutrition at home may receive infusion only at night. Prior to discharge the patient and family must understand rationale for therapy, procedures, and symptoms to report to physician. Patients must correctly demonstrate aseptic technique in caring for site, spiking bag, and priming tubing, and regulating infusion pump. Discharge planning should be coordinated with home care agency that will provide equipment, solns, and professional support to the patient and family.

Evaluation

Effectiveness of therapy can be demonstrated by: ▪ Increased weight ▫ Improvement of nutritional parameters ▫ Improved healing.

AMINOCAPROIC ACID

(a-mee-noe-ka-**proe**-ik)

Amicar, episilon aminocaproic acid

CLASSIFICATION(S):
Hemostatic

Pregnancy Category UK

INDICATIONS

▪ Management of acute, life-threatening hemorrhage due to systemic hyperfibrinolysis or urinary fibrinolysis. **Unlabeled Use:** ▪ Prevention of recurrent subarachnoid hemorrhage.

ACTION

▪ Inhibits activation of plasminogen. **Therapeutic Effects:** ▪ Inhibition of fibrinolysis ▪ Stabilization of clot formation.

PHARMACOKINETICS

Absorption: Rapidly and completely absorbed following oral administration.

Distribution: Widely distributed.

Metabolism and Excretion: Mostly eliminated unchanged by the kidneys.

Half-life: UK.

CONTRAINDICATIONS AND PRECAUTIONS

Contraindicated in: ▪ Active intravascular clotting.

Use Cautiously in: ▪ Hematuria originating in the upper urinary tract ▪ Patients with cardiac, renal, or liver disease (dosage reduction may be required) ▪ Pregnancy and lactation (safety not established) ▪ Disseminated intravascular coagulation (DIC)—should be used concurrently with heparin.

ADVERSE REACTIONS AND SIDE EFFECTS*

CNS: dizziness, malaise.

CV: arrhythmias, hypotension (IV only).

EENT: tinnitus, nasal stuffiness.

GI: nausea, cramping, diarrhea, anorexia, bloating.

GU: diuresis, renal failure.

MS: myopathy.

INTERACTIONS

Drug-Drug: ▪ None significant.

ROUTE AND DOSAGE

Acute Bleeding Syndromes due to Elevated Fibrinolytic Activity

- **PO (Adults):** 4–5 g first hr, followed by 1–1.25 g q hr for 8 hr or until hemorrhage is controlled.
- **IV (Adults):** 4–5 g over first hr, followed by 1 g/hr for 8 hr or until hemorrhage is controlled (not to exceed 30 g/day).
- **IV (Children):** 100 mg/kg or 3 g/m^2 over first hr, followed by continuous

*Underlines indicate most frequent; **CAPITALS** indicate life-threatening.

infusion of 33.3 mg/kg/hr or 1 g/m^2/hr; (total dosage not to exceed 18 g/m^2/24 hr).

Chronic Bleeding Tendency

- **PO (Adults):** 5–30 g/day given at 3–6 hr intervals.

PHARMACODYNAMICS (peak blood levels)

	ONSET	PEAK
PO	UK	2 hr
IV	UK	2 hr

NURSING IMPLICATIONS

Assessment

- Monitor blood pressure, pulse, and respiratory status as indicated by severity of bleeding.
- Monitor for overt bleeding every 15–30 min.
- Monitor neurologic status (pupils, level of consciousness, motor activity) in patients with subarachnoid hemorrhage.
- Monitor intake and output ratios frequently; notify physician if significant discrepancies occur.
- Assess for thromboembolic complications (especially in patients with previous history). Notify physician if positive Homans' sign, leg pain and edema, hemoptysis, dyspnea, or chest pain occurs.
- **Lab Test Considerations:** Monitor platelet count and clotting factors prior to and periodically throughout therapy in patients with systemic fibrinolysis.
- Increased CPK, SGOT (ALT), and serum aldolase may indicate myopathy.
- May cause an elevated serum potassium level.

Potential Nursing Diagnoses

- Tissue perfusion, altered (indications).
- Injury, high risk for (indications, side effects).
- Knowledge deficit related to medication regimen (patient/family teaching).

Implementation

- **PO:** Available as tablet and syrup for patients able to take oral medications.
- **IV:** Stabilize IV catheter to minimize thrombophlebitis. Monitor site closely.
- **Intermittent Infusion:** Do not administer undiluted. Dilute initial 4–5 g dose in 250 ml of sterile water, 0.9% NaCl, D5W, or lactated Ringer's soln. Do not dilute with sterile water in patients with subarachnoid hemorrhage.
- *Rate:* Administer over 1 hr.
- **Continuous Infusion:** Initial dose may be followed by a continuous infusion of 1 g/hr.
- Administer IV soln using infusion pump to ensure accurate dose. Administer via slow IV infusion. Rapid infusion rate may cause hypotension, bradycardia, or other arrhythmias.
- Do not admix with other medications.

Patient/Family Teaching

- **General Info:** Instruct patient to notify the nurse immediately if bleeding recurs, or if thromboembolic symptoms develop.
- **IV:** Caution patient to make position changes slowly to avoid orthostatic hypotension.

Evaluation

Effectiveness of therapy can be demonstrated by: ▪ Cessation of bleeding ▪ Prevention of rebleeding in subarachnoid hemorrhage, without occurrence of undesired clotting.

AMINOGLUTETHIMIDE

(a-meen-oh-gloo-**teth**-i-mide)
Cytadren

CLASSIFICATION(S):
Antineoplastic agent—miscellaneous
Pregnancy Category D

INDICATIONS

■ Short-term suppression of adrenal function in patients with Cushing's syndrome. **Unlabeled Uses:** ■ Advanced metastatic postmenopausal breast or prostate cancer.

ACTION

■ Inhibits the synthesis of adrenal hormones including glucocorticoids, mineralocorticoids, estrogens, and androgens ■ Decreases spread of hormonally sensitive tumors including breast and prostate cancer. **Therapeutic Effects:** ■ Decreased production of adrenal hormones in Cushing's disease ■ Decreased spread of postmenopausal breast or prostate cancer.

PHARMACOKINETICS

Absorption: Well absorbed following oral administration.
Distribution: Distribution not known.
Metabolism and Excretion: 50% metabolized by the liver. 50% excreted unchanged by the kidneys.
Half-life: 11–16 hr initially, drops to 2–9 hr after 2 wk of therapy.

CONTRAINDICATIONS AND PRECAUTIONS

Contraindicated in: ■ Hypersensitivity to glutethimide or aminoglutethimide.
Use Cautiously in: ■ Pregnancy (although normal pregnancies have occurred, may cause fetal harm) ■ Lactation or children (safety not established) ■ Stress including trauma, surgery, or acute illness (additional mineralocorticoid and hydrocortisone may be required).

ADVERSE REACTIONS AND SIDE EFFECTS*

CNS: drowsiness, headache, dizziness, weakness.
CV: hypotension.
GI: nausea, anorexia, vomiting, drug-induced hepatitis.
Derm: morbilliform rash, pruritus, urticaria.
Endo: adrenal suppression, adrenal insufficiency, hypothyroidism, masculinization in females, hirsutism in females.
MS: myalgia.
Misc: fever.

INTERACTIONS

Drug-Drug: ■ Increases metabolism and decreases effectiveness of **dexamethasone** ■ Decreases the effects of **warfarin, theophylline, digitoxin,** and **medroxyprogesterone** ■ **Alcohol** potentiates the effects of aminoglutethimide.

ROUTE AND DOSAGE

- **PO (Adults):** 250 mg qid (at 6 hr intervals), may be increased by 250 mg/day at 1–2 wk intervals, up to a daily total of 2 g.

PHARMACODYNAMICS (adrenal suppression)

	ONSET	PEAK	DURATION
PO	3–5 days	UK	36–72 hr*

*Recovery of adrenal function following discontinuation of short-term therapy; may take longer (up to 1 yr) after chronic therapy.

NURSING IMPLICATIONS

Assessment

- □ Monitor patient for changes in signs of Cushing's syndrome (moon face, buffalo hump, hypertension, fragility, hirsutism, mood swings, increased susceptibility to infections) throughout therapy.
- □ Monitor blood pressure periodically throughout therapy.
- □ Assess patient for rash throughout therapy. Dose reduction or temporary discontinuation may be required if severe skin rash occurs.
- ■ **Lab Test Considerations:** Monitor plasma cortisol levels throughout therapy. Dose may be titrated according to levels.
- □ May cause hypothyroidism. Monitor thyroid function tests periodically during therapy.
- □ May cause elevated SGOT (AST), alkaline phosphatase, and bilirubin concentrations.

*Underlines indicate most frequent; **CAPITALS** indicate life-threatening.

□ Monitor CBC and serum electrolytes periodically during therapy.

Potential Nursing Diagnoses

■ Injury, high risk for (side effects).

■ Knowledge deficit related to medication regimen (patient/family teaching).

Implementation

■ **General Info:** Therapy should be initiated in a hospital setting until a stable dosing regimen has been achieved.

□ Mineralocorticoid replacement (fludrocortisone) or glucocorticoid replacement (hydrocortisone) may be necessary.

■ **PO:** Administer around the clock, every 6 hr.

Patient/Family Teaching

□ May cause drowsiness or dizziness. Caution patient to avoid driving or other activities requiring alertness until response to medication is known.

□ Instruct patient to notify physician if rash, fainting, weakness, or headache become pronounced.

□ Advise patient that nausea and loss of appetite may occur during first 2 wk of therapy. Physician should be notified if these persist or become pronounced.

□ Advise patient to avoid concurrent use of alcohol while taking aminoglutethimide.

Evaluation

Effectiveness of therapy can be demonstrated by: ■ Suppression of adrenal function in patients with Cushing's syndrome ■ Decreased spread of malignancy in advanced postmenopausal or prostate cancer.

AMINOPHYLLINE

(am-in-**off**-i-lin)

Aminophyllin, Amoline, {Corophyllin}, {Palaron}, Phyllocontin, Somophyllin, Truphylline

CLASSIFICATION(S):
Bronchodilator—phosphodiesterase inhibitor
Pregnancy Category C

INDICATIONS

■ Bronchodilator in reversible airway obstruction due to asthma or COPD. **Unlabeled Use:** ■ Respiratory and myocardial stimulant in apnea of infancy.

ACTION

■ Inhibits phosphodiesterase, producing increased tissue concentrations of cyclic adenosine monophosphate (cAMP). Increased levels of cAMP result in: □ Bronchodilation □ CNS stimulation □ Positive inotropic and chronotropic effects □ Diuresis □ Gastric acid secretion. Aminophylline is a salt of theophylline and releases free theophylline following administration. **Therapeutic Effect:** ■ Bronchodilation.

PHARMACOKINETICS

Absorption: Well absorbed from oral dosage forms. Absorption from extended-release dosage forms is slow but complete. Absorption from rectal suppositories is erratic and unreliable. Absorption from rectal soln is rapid and reliable if soln is retained.

Distribution: Widely distributed as theophylline. Crosses the placenta. Breast milk concentrations 70% of plasma levels.

Metabolism and Excretion: Metabolized by the liver to caffeine, which may accumulate in neonates. Metabolites are renally excreted.

Half-life: 3–13 hr (theophylline). Increased in the elderly (>60 yr), neonates, and in patients with congestive heart failure or liver disease. Shortened in cigarette smokers and children.

CONTRAINDICATIONS AND PRECAUTIONS

Contraindicated in: ■ Uncontrolled arrhythmias ■ Hyperthyroidism.

Use Cautiously in: ■ Elderly patients

{} = Available in Canada only.

(>60 yr), CHF, or liver disease (dosage reduction required) ▪ Has been used safely in pregnancy.

ADVERSE REACTIONS AND SIDE EFFECTS*

CNS: nervousness, anxiety, headache, insomnia, SEIZURES.
CV: tachycardia, palpitations, arrhythmias, angina pectoris.
GI: nausea, vomiting, anorexia, cramps.
Neuro: tremor.

INTERACTIONS

Drug-Drug: ▪ Additive CV and CNS side effects with **adrenergic (sympathomimetic) agents** ▪ May decrease the therapeutic effect of **lithium** ▪ **Smoking, adrenergic agents, barbiturates, phenytoin, ketoconazole,** and **rifampin** may increase metabolism and may decrease effectiveness ▪ **Erythromycin, beta blockers, cimetidine, influenza vaccination, oral contraceptives, glucocorticoids, disulfiram, interferon, mexiletine, thiabendazol, flouroquinolones,** and large doses of **allopurinol** decrease metabolism and may lead to toxicity ▪ Increased risk of arrhythmias with **halothane** ▪ **Isoniazid, carbamazepine,** and **loop diuretics** may increase or decrease theophylline levels.
Drug-Food: ▪ Excessive regular intake of **charcoal-broiled foods** may decrease effectiveness ▪ Excessive intake of **xanthine-containing foods** or **beverages (colas, coffee, chocolate)** may increase the risk of CV and CNS side effects.

ROUTE AND DOSAGE

Note: Dosage should be determined by theophylline serum level monitoring. Loading dose should be decreased or eliminated if theophylline preparation has been used in preceding 24 hr. Aminophylline is 85% theophylline.

- **PO (Adults):** Loading dose—500 mg, followed by 250–500 mg q 6–8 hr.
- **PO (Children):** Loading dose—7.5 mg/kg, followed by 3–6 mg/kg q 6–8 hr.
- **Rect (Adults):** 500 mg retention enema every 6–8 hr.
- **IV (Adults):** Loading dose—5.6 mg/kg infused over 30 min, followed by 0.2–0.9 mg/kg/hr continuous infusion.
- **IV (Children):** Loading dose—5.6 mg/kg, followed by 1 mg/kg/hr continuous infusion.
- **IV, PO (Neonates >8 wk):** Initial dose—1 mg/kg (theophylline) for each 2 mcg/ml increase in plasma level desired, then 1–3 mg/kg (theophylline) q 6 hr.
- **IV, PO (Neonates 4–8 wk):** Initial dose—1 mg/kg (theophylline) for each 2 mcg/ml increase in plasma level desired, then 1–2 mg/kg (theophylline) q 8 hr.
- **IV, PO (Term Neonates <4 wk):** Initial dose—1 mg/kg (theophylline) for each 2 mcg/ml increase in plasma level desired, then 1–2 mg/kg (theophylline) q 12 hr.
- **IV, PO (Premature Neonates):** Initial dose—1 mg/kg (theophylline) for each 2 mcg/ml increase in plasma level desired, then 1 mg/kg (theophylline) q 12 hr.

PHARMACODYNAMICS (bronchodilation)

	ONSET	PEAK*	DURATION
PO	15–60 min	1–2 hr	6–8 hr
PO-ER	UK	4–7 hr	8–12 hr
IV	rapid	end of infusion	6–8 hr
Rect	rapid	1–2 hr	6–8 hr

*Peak plasma levels.

NURSING IMPLICATIONS

ASSESSMENT

- **General Info:** Assess blood pressure, pulse, respiration, and lung sounds before administering medication and throughout therapy.
- ▫ Patients with a history of cardiovascular problems should be monitored for chest pain and ECG changes (PACs, supraventricular tachycardia, PVCs, ventricular tachycardia). Re-

*Underlines indicate most frequent; **CAPITALS** indicate life-threatening.

suscitative equipment should be readily available.
- Monitor intake and output ratios for an increase in diuresis.
- **Rectal Administration:** Monitor for complaints of rectal burning or discomfort.
- **Respiratory Stimulant:** Monitor neonate for apnea, bradycardia, and cyanosis.
- **Toxicity and Overdose:** Monitor drug levels routinely. Therapeutic plasma levels range from 10 to 20 mcg/ml. Drug levels in excess of 20 mcg/ml are associated with toxicity.
- Observe patient closely for symptoms of drug toxicity (anorexia, nausea, vomiting, restlessness, insomnia, tachycardia, arrhythmias, seizures). Notify physician immediately if these occur.

Potential Nursing Diagnoses
- Airway clearance, ineffective (indications).
- Activity intolerance (indications).
- Knowledge deficit related to medication regimen (patient/family teaching).

Implementation
- **General Info:** Administer around the clock to maintain therapeutic plasma levels.
- Determine if patient has had any form of theophylline within 24 hr prior to administering loading dose.
- Wait at least 4 hr after discontinuing IV therapy to begin immediate-release oral dosage; for extended-release oral dosage form, administer first oral dose at time of IV discontinuation.
- Available in tablet, enteric-coated tablet, extended-release tablet, oral soln, enema, and injectable forms.
- **PO:** Administer oral preparations with food or a full glass of water to minimize GI irritation. Food slows but does not reduce the extent of absorption. Once-a-day tablets should be given in the morning, after fasting overnight, and 1 hr before eating. Do not crush, break, or chew enteric-coated or extended-release tablets.
- **Rect:** Encourage patient to retain for 20–30 min.
- If enema soln has crystallized, dissolve by placing container in warm water and shaking. Discard if crystals do not dissolve.
- **IM:** Avoid IM route, because it is painful and may cause tissue damage.
- **IV:** May be diluted in D5W, D10W, D20W, 0.9% NaCl, 0.45% NaCl, D5/0.9% NaCl, D5/0.45% NaCl, D5/0.25% NaCl, or lactated Ringer's soln. Mixture is stable for 24 hr if refrigerated.
- Do not administer discolored or precipitated soln. Flush main IV line prior to administration. Admixing infusion is not recommended due to many incompatibilities.
- If extravasation occurs, local injection of 1% procaine and application of heat may relieve pain and promote vasodilation.
- *Rate:* Do not exceed 25 mg/min. Administer via infusion pump to ensure accurate dosage. Rapid administration may cause hypotension, arrhythmias, syncope, and death.
- **Direct IV:** Do not administer at a rate faster than 25 mg/min.
- **Intermittent Infusion:** Dilute in 100–200 ml of compatible IV soln.
- **Continuous Infusion:** Usually given as a loading dose in a small volume followed by continuous infusion in larger volume.
- **Syringe Compatibility:** heparin, metoclopramide, pentobarbital, or thiopental.
- **Y-Site Compatibility:** amrinone, atracurium, cimetidine, enalaprilat, foscarnet, heparin sodium with hydrocortisone sodium succinate, morphine, neticmicin, pancuronium, potassium chloride, ranitidine, tolazoline, or vecuronium.
- **Y-Site Incompatibility:** dobutamine, hydralazine, or ondansetron.
- **Additive Compatibility:** amobarbital, bretylium, calcium gluconate, chloramphenicol, dexamethasone, diphen-

hydramine, dopamine, erythromycin lactobionate, esmolol, heparin, hydrocortisone, lidocaine, methyldopate, metronidazole, pentobarbital, potassium chloride, ranitidine, secobarbital, sodium bicarbonate, sodium iodide, terbutaline, or verapamil.

- **Additive Incompatibility:** ascorbic acid, bleomycin, cephalothin, cefotaxime, chlorpromazine, cimetidine, clindamycin, codeine, dimenhydrinate, dobutamine, doxorubicin, doxycycline, epinephrine, erythromycin gluceptate, hydralazine, hydroxyzine, insulin, isoproterenol, meperidine, methicillin, morphine, nafcillin, nitroprusside, norepinephrine, oxytetracycline, papaverine, penicillin G, pentazocine, phenobarbital, phenytoin, prochlorperazine, promazine, promethazine, sulfisoxazole, tetracycline, or vancomycin.

Patient/Family Teaching

- Emphasize the importance of taking only the prescribed dose at the prescribed time intervals. Missed doses should be taken as soon as remembered or omitted if close to next dose.
- Encourage the patient to drink adequate liquids (2000 ml/day minimum) to decrease the viscosity of the airway secretions.
- Advise patient to avoid over-the-counter cough, cold, or breathing preparations without consulting physician or pharmacist. These medications may increase side effects and cause arrhythmias.
- Encourage patients not to smoke. A change in smoking habits may necessitate a change in dosage.
- Advise patient to minimize intake of xanthine-containing foods or beverages (colas, coffee, chocolate) and not to eat charcoal-broiled foods daily.
- Instruct patient not to change brands or dosage forms without consulting physician.
- Advise patient to contact physician promptly if the usual dose of medication fails to produce the desired results, symptoms worsen after treatment, or toxic effects occur.
- Emphasize the importance of having serum levels routinely tested every 6–12 mon.

Evaluation

Effectiveness of therapy can be demonstrated by: ▪ Increased ease in breathing and clearing of lung fields on auscultation ▪ Respiratory and myocardial stimulation in apnea of infancy.

AMIODARONE

(am-ee-**oh**-da-rone)
Cordarone

CLASSIFICATION(S):
Antiarrhythmic—type III
Pregnancy Category C

INDICATIONS

▪ Management and prophylaxis of life-threatening ventricular arrhythmias unresponsive to conventional therapy with less toxic agents.

ACTION

▪ Prolongs the action potential and refractory period in myocardial tissue ▪ Inhibits adrenergic stimulation ▪ Slows the sinus rate, increases PR and QT intervals, and decreases peripheral vascular resistance. **Therapeutic Effect:** ▪ Suppression of ventricular arrhythmias.

PHARMACOKINETICS

Absorption: Slowly and variably absorbed from the GI tract (35–65%).
Distribution: Distributed to and accumulates slowly in many body tissues. Crosses the placenta and enters breast milk.
Metabolism and Excretion: Metabolized by the liver, excreted into bile. Minimal renal excretion.
Half-life: 13–107 days.

CONTRAINDICATIONS AND PRECAUTIONS

Contraindicated in: ▪ Severe sinus node dysfunction ▪ 2nd- and 3rd-degree

AV block ▪ Bradycardia (has caused syncope unless a pacemaker is in place) ▪ Pregnancy and lactation.
Use Cautiously in: ▪ Thyroid disorders ▪ Severe pulmonary or liver disease ▪ Children (safety not established).

ADVERSE REACTIONS AND SIDE EFFECTS*

CNS: malaise, fatigue, dizziness, insomnia, headache.
Resp: PULMONARY FIBROSIS.
CV: congestive heart failure, bradycardia, WORSENING OF ARRHYTHMIAS.
Derm: photosensitivity.
EENT: corneal microdeposits, photophobia, dry eyes, abnormal taste, abnormal smell.
Endo: hypothyroidism, hyperthyroidism.
GI: nausea, vomiting, constipation, anorexia, LIVER DAMAGE, abdominal pain.
GU: decreased libido.
Neuro: tremor, involuntary movement, poor coordination, peripheral neuropathy, paresthesia.

INTERACTIONS

Drug–Drug: ▪ Increases blood levels and may lead to toxicity from **digoxin** (decrease dose by 50%), ▪ Increases blood levels and may lead to toxicity from other **class I antiarrhthymics** (**quinidine, procainamide, mexiletine,** or **flecainide**—decrease doses by 30–50%) ▪ Increases blood levels of **phenytoin** ▪ Increases the activity of **warfarin** (decrease dose by 33–50%) ▪ Increased risk of bradyarrhythmias, sinus arrest, or AV heart block with **beta blockers** or **calcium channel blockers** ▪ Concentrated **oxygen** administered postoperatively may increase the risk of pulmonary fibrosis.

ROUTE AND DOSAGE

- **PO (Adults):** 800–1600 mg/day in 1–2 doses for 1–3 wk, then 600–800 mg/day in 1–2 doses for 1 mon, then 400 mg/day maintenance dose.

PHARMACODYNAMICS (suppression of ventricular arrhythmias)

	ONSET	PEAK	DURATION
PO	1–3 wk	UK	wks–mons

NURSING IMPLICATIONS

Assessment

- ECG should be monitored continuously during initiation of therapy. Monitor heart rate and rhythm throughout therapy. PR prolongation, slight QRS widening, T-wave amplitude reduction with T-wave widening and bifurcation, and U-wave development may occur. QT prolongation may be associated with worsening of arrhythmias. Report bradycardia or increase in arrhythmias to physician promptly.
- Assess patient for signs of pulmonary toxicity (rales/crackles, decreased breath sounds, pleuritic friction rub, fatigue, dyspnea, cough, pleuritic pain, fever). May need to discontinue therapy.
- Ophthalmic examinations should be performed prior to therapy and if visual changes (photophobia, halos around lights, decreased acuity) occur.
- Assess patient for signs of thyroid dysfunction, especially during initial therapy. Lethargy, edema of the hands, feet, and periorbital region and cool, pale skin suggest hypothyroidism and may require decrease in dosage or discontinuation of therapy and supplementation of thyroid hormone. Tachycardia, weight loss, and warm, flushed, moist skin suggest hyperthyroidism and may require discontinuation of therapy and treatment with antithyroid agents.
- **Lab Test Considerations:** Monitor liver, lung, thyroid, and neurologic functions prior to and periodically throughout therapy. Long elimination half-life causes persistent drug ef-

*Underlines indicate most frequent; **CAPITALS** indicate life-threatening.

fects long after adjustment or discontinuation.

- May cause increased SGOT (AST), SGPT (ALT), and serum alkaline phosphatase concentrations.

Potential Nursing Diagnoses

- Cardiac output, decreased (indications).
- Gas exchange, impaired (side effects).
- Knowledge deficit related to medication regimen (patient/family teaching).

Implementation

- **General Info:** Patients should be hospitalized and monitored closely during the initiation of amiodarone therapy.
- Hypokalemia may decrease effectiveness of amiodarone or may cause additional arrhythmias and should be corrected prior to initiation of therapy.
- Assist patient during ambulation to prevent falls from neurologic deficits. Peripheral neuropathy (proximal muscle weakness, tingling, numbness), tremors, and abnormal gait are common side effects during initial therapy.
- **PO:** May be administered with meals and in divided doses if GI intolerance occurs.

Patient/Family Teaching

- Instruct patient to take this medication exactly as directed. If a dose is missed, do not take at all. Consult physician if more than two doses are missed.
- Teach patients to monitor pulse daily and report abnormalities to physician.
- Advise patients that photosensitivity reactions may occur through window glass, thin clothing, and with sun screens. Protective clothing and sun block are recommended during and for 4 mon following therapy.
- Inform patients that bluish discoloration of the face, neck, and arms is a possible side effect of this drug following prolonged use. This is usually reversible and will fade over several mons. Notify physician if this occurs.
- Instruct patient to notify physician or dentist of medication regimen prior to treatment or surgery.
- Emphasize the importance of follow-up examinations, including chest x-ray and pulmonary function tests every 3–6 mon and ophthalmic examinations after 6 mon of therapy, and then annually.

Evaluation

Effectiveness of therapy can be demonstrated by: ▪ Cessation of life-threatening ventricular arrhythmias. Pharmacologic effects may not be seen for 1–3 wk. Adverse effects may take up to 4 mon to resolve.

AMITRIPTYLINE

(a-mee-**trip**-ti-leen)
Amitril, {Apo-Amitriptyline}, Elavil, Emitrip, Endep, Enovil, {Levate}, {Meravil}, {Novotriptyn}

CLASSIFICATION(S):
Antidepressant—tricyclic

INDICATIONS

▪ Treatment of various forms of depression, often in conjunction with psychotherapy. **Unlabeled Use:** ▪ Management of chronic pain syndromes.

ACTION

▪ Potentiates the effect of serotonin and norepinephrine in the CNS ▪ Also has significant anticholinergic properties. **Therapeutic Effect:** ▪ Antidepressant action that may only develop over several wks.

PHARMACOKINETICS

Absorption: Well absorbed from the GI tract.
Distribution: Widely distributed.
Metabolism and Excretion: Extensively metabolized by the liver. Some

A

metabolites are pharmacologically active. Undergoes enterohepatic recirculation and secretion into gastric juices. Appears to cross the placenta and enter breast milk.
Half-life: 10–50 hr.

CONTRAINDICATIONS AND PRECAUTIONS

Contraindicated in: ▪ Narrow-angle glaucoma ▪ Pregnancy and lactation.
Use Cautiously in: ▪ Elderly patients ▪ Patients with pre-existing cardiovascular disease ▪ Elderly men with prostatic hypertrophy (increased susceptibility to urinary retention) ▪ History of seizures (threshold may be lowered).

ADVERSE REACTIONS AND SIDE EFFECTS*

CNS: drowsiness. sedation, lethargy, fatigue.
EENT: dry mouth, dry eyes, blurred vision.
CV: hypotension, ECG changes, ARRHYTHMIAS.
Derm: photosensitivity.
Endo: gynecomastia, changes in blood glucose.
GI: constipation, paralytic ileus, hepatitis.
GU: urinary retention.
Hemat: blood dyscrasias.

INTERACTIONS

Drug-Drug: ▪ May cause hypotension, tachycardia, and potentially fatal reactions when used with **MAO inhibitors** (avoid concurrent use—discontinue 2 wk prior to amitriptyline) ▪ May prevent the therapeutic response to most **antihypertensives** ▪ May cause severe hypertension when used with **clonidine** (avoid concurrent use) ▪ Additive CNS depression with other **CNS depressants** including **alcohol, antihistamines, narcotic analgesics,** and **sedative/hypnotics** ▪ **Adrenergic** and **anticholinergic** side effects may be additive with other **agents having these properties** ▪ **Cimetidine, fluoxetine, phenothiazines,** or **oral contraceptives** increase levels and may cause toxicity ▪ May produce organic brain syndrome with **disulfiram** ▪ **Smoking** may increase metabolism and decrease effectiveness.

ROUTE AND DOSAGE

- **PO (Adults):** 30–100 mg/day single bedtime dose or divided doses. Dose may be gradually increased up to 300 mg/day.
- **IM (Adults):** 20–30 mg 4 times daily.

PHARMACODYNAMICS (antidepressant effect)

	ONSET	PEAK	DURATION
PO	2–3 wk	2–6 wk	days–wks
IM	2–3 wk	2–6 wk	days–wks

NURSING IMPLICATIONS

Assessment

- Monitor mental status and affect. Assess for suicidal tendencies, especially during early therapy. Restrict amount of drug available to patient.
- Monitor blood pressure and pulse prior to and during initial therapy. Notify physician of significant decreases in blood pressure (10–20 mmHg) or a sudden increase in pulse rate.
- **Lab Test Considerations:** Assess leukocyte and differential blood counts, liver function, and serum glucose periodically. May cause an elevated serum bilirubin and alkaline phosphatase. May cause bone marrow depression. Serum glucose may be increased or decreased.

Potential Nursing Diagnoses

- Coping, ineffective individual (indications).
- Injury, high risk for (side effects).
- Knowledge deficit related to medication regimen (patient/family teaching).

Implementation

- **General Info:** Dose increases should be made at bedtime because of sedation. Dose titration is a slow process;

*Underlines indicate most frequent; **CAPITALS** indicate life-threatening.

may take wks to mons. May give entire dose at bedtime.

- **PO:** Administer medication with or immediately following a meal to minimize gastric irritation. Tablet may be crushed and administered with food or fluids.
- **IM:** For short-term IM administration only. Do not administer IV

PATIENT/FAMILY TEACHING

- Instruct patient to take medication exactly as prescribed. Advise patient that drug effects may not be noticed for at least 2 wk. Abrupt discontinuation may cause nausea, headache, and malaise.
- May cause drowsiness and blurred vision. Caution patient to avoid driving and other activities requiring alertness until response to drug is known.
- Orthostatic hypotension, sedation, and confusion are common during early therapy, especially in the elderly. Protect patient from falls and advise patient to make position changes slowly.
- Advise patient to avoid alcohol or other CNS depressant drugs during and for 3–7 days after therapy has been discontinued.
- Instruct patient to notify physician if urinary retention occurs or if dry mouth or constipation persist. Sugarless candy or gum may diminish dry mouth and an increase in fluid intake or bulk may prevent constipation. If these symptoms persist, dosage reduction or discontinuation may be necessary.
- Caution patient to use sunscreen and protective clothing to prevent photosensitivity reactions.
- Inform patient of need to monitor dietary intake, because possible increase in appetite may lead to undesired weight gain.
- Inform patient that urine may turn a blue-green color.
- Advise patient to notify physician or dentist of medication regimen prior to treatment or surgery.
- Therapy for depression is usually prolonged. Emphasize the importance of follow-up examinations to monitor effectiveness and side effects.

EVALUATION

Effectiveness of therapy can be demonstrated by: ▪ Increased sense of well-being ▫ Renewed interest in surroundings ▫ Increased appetite ▫ Improved energy level ▫ Improved sleep ▪ Decrease in chronic pain symptoms. Full therapeutic effects may be seen 2 wk to 1 mon after initiating therapy.

AMOBARBITAL

(ah-mo-**bar**-bi-tal)
Amytal

CLASSIFICATION(S):
Sedative/hypnotic—barbiturate, Anticonvulsant
Schedule II
Pregnancy Category D

INDICATIONS

▪ Preoperative sedative and in other situations where sedation may be required ▪ Hypnotic ▪ Anticonvulsant ▪ Narcoanalysis and narcotherapy.

ACTION

▪ Produces all levels of CNS depression: ▫ Depresses sensory cortex ▫ Decreases motor activity ▫ Alters cerebral function ▪ Inhibits transmission in the CNS and raises seizure threshold. **Therapeutic Effects:** ▪ Anticonvulsant action ▪ Sedation.

PHARMACOKINETICS

Absorption: Well absorbed following oral or IM administration.

Distribution: Rapidly and widely distributed, concentrates in brain, liver, and kidneys. Readily crosses placenta, small amounts enter breast milk.

Metabolism and Excretion: Mostly metabolized by the liver.

Half-life: 16–40 hr.

A

CONTRAINDICATIONS AND PRECAUTIONS

Contraindicated in: ▪ Hypersensitivity ▪ Comatose patients ▪ Pre-existing CNS depression ▪ Severe uncontrolled pain ▪ Pregnancy and lactation.

Use Cautiously in: ▪ Hepatic dysfunction ▪ Severe renal impairment ▪ Suicidal patients ▪ Patients previously addicted to barbiturates ▪ Elderly patients (dosage should be reduced) ▪ Hypnotic use (should be short-term only).

ADVERSE REACTIONS AND SIDE EFFECTS*

CNS: drowsiness, lethargy, vertigo, depression, hangover, excitation, delerium, syncope.

Resp: respiratory depression, LARYNGOSPASM (IV ONLY), BRONCHOSPASM (IV ONLY).

CV: hypotension, bradycardia.

GI: nausea, vomiting, diarrhea, constipation.

Derm: rashes, urticaria, photosensitivity, exfoliative dermatitis.

Local: phlebitis at IV site, pain at IM site.

Misc: hypersensitivity reactions including STEVENS JOHNSON SYNDROME.

MS: mylagia, arthralgia.

INTERACTIONS

Drug-Drug: ▪ Additive CNS depression with other **CNS depressants** including **alcohol, antidepressants, antihistamines, narcotics,** and **other sedative/hypnotics** ▪ Sedation may be prolonged with **MAO inhibitors** ▪ Induces hepatic enzymes that metabolize other drugs, thereby decreasing their effectiveness, including **oral contraceptives, chloramphenicol, acebutolol, propranolol, metoprolol, timolol, doxycycline, glucocorticoids, tricyclic antidepressants, phenothiazines,** and **quinidine**.

ROUTE AND DOSAGE

Daytime Sedation

- **PO (Adults):** 15–120 mg 2–4 times daily.
- **PO (Children):** 2 mg/kg/day or 70 $mg/m^2/day$ in 4 divided doses.

Hypnotic

- **PO (Adults):** 65–200 mg.
- **IM (Adults):** 65–200 mg (not to exceed 500 mg).
- **IM (Children):** 2–3 mg/kg.

Preanesthetic Sedation

- **PO (Adults):** 200 mg 1–2 hr prior to procedure.

Anticonvulsant

- **IM, IV (Children <6 yr):** 3–5 mg/kg or 125 mg/m^2 per dose.
- **IV (Adults and Children >6 yr):** 65–500 mg (not to exceed 1 g).

PHARMACODYNAMICS (sedation)

	ONSET	PEAK	DURATION
PO	45–60 min	UK	6–8 hr
IM	30–45 min	UK	6–8 hr
IV	several mins	UK	6–8 hr

NURSING IMPLICATIONS

Assessment

- **General Info:** Monitor respiratory status, pulse, and blood pressure frequently in patients receiving amobarbital IV.
- ▫ Prolonged therapy may lead to psychological or physical dependence. Restrict amount of drug available to patient, especially if depressed, suicidal, or having a history of addiction.
- **Hypnotic:** Assess sleep patterns prior to and periodically throughout therapy. Hypnotic doses of amobarbital suppress REM sleep. Patient may experience an increase in dreaming upon discontinuation of medication.
- **Seizures:** Assess location, duration, and characteristics of seizure activity. Institute seizure precautions.

Potential Nursing Diagnoses

- Sleep pattern disturbance (indications).
- Injury, high risk for (side effects).

*Underlines indicate most frequent; CAPITALS indicate life-threatening.

- Knowledge deficit related to medication regimen (patient/family teaching).

Implementation

- **General Info:** Remove cigarettes and monitor ambulation following administration.
- **PO:** Rate of absorption is increased if taken on an empty stomach.
- **IM/IV:** Reconstitute with sterile water for injection for a concentration of 100 mg/ml. Rotate vial to mix; do not shake. May be further diluted in D5W, D10W, D20W, D5/0.9% NaCl, D5/LR, 0.9% NaCl, 3% NaCl, or lactated Ringer's injection. Soln should be used within 30 min of reconstitution. Do not use if soln does not become absolutely clear within 5 min following reconstitution or if precipitate forms after the soln clears.
- **IM:** Do not administer SC. IM injections should be given deep into the gluteal muscle to minimize tissue irritation. Do not inject more than 5 ml into any one site because of tissue irritation.
- **Direct IV:** Use the largest vein possible to prevent thrombosis. Soln is highly alkaline; avoid extravasation, which may cause tissue damage and necrosis. If extravasation occurs, infiltration of 5% procaine soln into affected area and application of moist heat may be ordered.
- □ *Rate:* Administer at a rate of 100 mg over at least 1 min for adults or 60 mg/m^2/min for children. Titrate slowly for desired response. Rapid administration may result in respiratory depression, apnea, laryngospasm, bronchospasm, or hypotension. Equipment for resuscitation and artificial ventilation should be readily available.
- **Additive Compatibility:** amikacin, aminophylline, or sodium bicarbonate.
- **Additive Incompatibility:** cefazolin, cephalothin, cimetidine, chlorpromazine, clindamycin, codeine, diphenhydramine, droperidol, hydroxyzine, regular insulin, levorphanol, meperidine, methadone, morphine, norepinephrine, pentazocine, procaine, streptomycin, tetracycline, or vancomycin.

Patient/Family Teaching

- □ Advise patient to take medication exactly as prescribed. Do not increase the dose of the drug without consulting physician. Advise patients on prolonged therapy not to discontinue medication without consulting physician. May need to be gradually discontinued over 5–6 days to prevent withdrawal symptoms.
- □ Discuss the importance of preparing environment for sleep (dark room, quiet, avoidance of nicotine and caffeine).
- □ Medication may cause daytime drowsiness. Caution patient to avoid driving and other activities requiring alertness until response to medication is known.
- □ Advise patient to make position changes slowly to minimize orthostatic hypotension.
- □ Caution patients to avoid taking alcohol or other CNS depressants concurrently with this medication.
- □ Instruct patient to contact physician immediately if pregnancy is suspected or if sore throat, fever, mouth sores, unusual bleeding or bruising, or petechiae occur.

Evaluation

Effectiveness of therapy can be demonstrated by: ▪ Improvement in sleep pattern without excessive daytime sedation. May take 2 days for effects to become evident. Therapy is usually limited to a 2 wk period ▪ Sedation ▪ Control of seizures.

AMOXAPINE

(a-**mox**-a-peen)
Asendin

CLASSIFICATION(S):
Antidepressant—tricyclic
Pregnancy Category C

INDICATIONS

▪ Treatment of various forms of depression accompanied by anxiety, often in conjunction with psychotherapy.

ACTION

▪ Potentiates the effects of serotonin and norepinephrine in the CNS ▪ Has significant anticholinergic properties ▪ Also has antianxiety effect related to sedative properties. **Therapeutic Effect:** ▪ Antidepressant action that may only develop slowly over several wks.

PHARMACOKINETICS

Absorption: Well absorbed following oral administration.

Distribution: Widely distributed. High concentrations in brain, lungs, spleen, and heart. Enters breast milk.

Metabolism and Excretion: Extensively metabolized by the liver. At least two metabolites have antidepressant activity—8-hydroxyamoxapine and 7-hydroxyamoxapine.

Half-life: Amoxapine—8 hr; 8-hydroxyamoxapine—30 hr; 7-hydroxyamoxapine—6.5 hr.

CONTRAINDICATIONS AND PRECAUTIONS

Contraindicated in: ▪ Narrow-angle glaucoma ▪ Pregnancy and lactation.

Use Cautiously in: ▪ Elderly patients (dosage reduction required) ▪ Patients with pre-existing cardiovascular disease ▪ Elderly men (increased susceptibility to urinary retention) ▪ History of seizures (threshold may be lowered) ▪ Children <16 yr (safety not established).

ADVERSE REACTIONS AND SIDE EFFECTS*

CNS: drowsiness, lethargy, sedation, fatigue, extrapyramidal reactions, tardive dyskinesia.

CV: hypotension, ECG changes, ARRHYTHMIAS.

EENT: dry mouth, dry eyes, blurred vision.

GI: constipation, paralytic ileus.

GU: urinary retention, testicular swelling.

Derm: photosensitivity, rash.

Endo: gynecomastia, sexual dysfunction.

Hemat: blood dyscrasias.

Misc: fever, weight gain.

INTERACTIONS

Drug-Drug: ▪ May cause hypotension, tachycardia, and potentially fatal reactions when used with **MAO inhibitors** (avoid concurrent use—discontinue 2 wk prior to amoxepine) ▪ May prevent the therapeutic response to most **antihypertensives** ▪ May cause severe hypertension when used with **clonidine** (avoid concurrent use) ▪ Additive CNS depression with other **CNS depressants** including **alcohol, antihistamines, narcotic analgesics,** and **sedative/hypnotics** ▪ **Adrenergic** and **anticholinergic** side effects may be additive with other **agents having these properties** ▪ **Cimetidine, fluoxetine, phenothiazines,** or **oral contraceptives** increase levels and may cause toxicity ▪ May produce organic brain syndrome with **disulfiram** ▪ **Smoking** may increase metabolism and decrease effectiveness.

ROUTE AND DOSAGE

▪ **PO (Adults):** 100–150 mg daily initially in divided doses, increase to 200–300 mg daily by end of first wk (not to exceed 400 mg daily in outpatients, 600 mg in hospitalized patients). Once optimal dose is achieved, may be given as a single bedtime dose; no single dose to exceed 300 mg.

PHARMACODYNAMICS (antidepressant effect)

	ONSET	PEAK	DURATION
PO	1–2 wk	2–6 wk	days–wks

NURSING IMPLICATIONS

Assessment

□ Monitor mental status and affect. Assess for suicidal tendencies, espe-

*Underlines indicate most frequent; **CAPITALS** indicate life-threatening.

cially during early therapy. Restrict amount of drug available to patient.

- □ Observe for onset of extrapyramidal side effects (pill-rolling motions, drooling, tremors, rigidity, mask facies, shuffling gait, restlessness, muscle spasms, twisting motions) and for tardive dyskinesia (uncontrolled movements of the face, mouth, tongue, or jaw, and involuntary movements of extremities). Notify physician immediately if these symptoms occur. Dosage reduction or discontinuation may be necessary. Physician may order antiparkinsonian agents to control extrapyramidal effects. Tardive dyskinesia may be irreversible.
- □ Monitor for drug rash or fever. Notify physician if these symptoms of hypersensitivity reaction occur.
- ■ **Lab Test Considerations:** May cause elevated serum prolactin levels.
- □ Monitor CBC and differential during chronic therapy. May rarely cause bone marrow suppression.
- □ In chronic therapy periodically monitor hepatic, pancreatic, and renal function.

POTENTIAL NURSING DIAGNOSES

- ■ Coping, ineffective individual (indications).
- ■ Injury, high risk for (side effects).
- ■ Knowledge deficit related to medication regimen (patient/family teaching).

IMPLEMENTATION

- ■ **General Info:** Dose increases should be made at bedtime because of sedation. Dosage titration is a slow process; may take wks to mons. May give entire dose at bedtime.
- ■ **PO:** Administer medication with or immediately following a meal to minimize gastric irritation.

PATIENT/FAMILY TEACHING

- □ Instruct patient to take medication exactly as prescribed. Abrupt discontinuation may cause nausea, headache, and malaise.
- □ May cause drowsiness and blurred vision. Caution patient to avoid driving and other activities requiring alertness until response to drug is known.
- □ Advise patient to avoid alcohol or other CNS depressant drugs during course of therapy and for 3–7 days after cessation of therapy.
- □ Instruct patient to notify physician if dry mouth or constipation persists or if urinary retention, uncontrolled movements, or rigidity occur. Sugarless candy or gum may diminish dry mouth, and an increase in fluid intake or bulk may prevent constipation. If these symptoms persist, dosage reduction or discontinuation may be necessary.
- □ Advise patient to inform physician if breast enlargement or sexual dysfunction occurs.
- □ Caution patient to use sunscreen and protective clothing to prevent photosensitivity reactions.
- □ Inform patient of need to monitor dietary intake, because possible increase in appetite may lead to undesired weight gain.
- □ Advise patient to notify physician or dentist of medication regimen prior to treatment or surgery.
- □ Therapy for depression is usually prolonged. Emphasize the importance of follow-up examinations to monitor effectiveness and side effects.

EVALUATION

Effectiveness of therapy can be demonstrated by: ■ Increased sense of well-being □ Renewed interest in surroundings □ Increased appetite □ Improved energy level □ Improved sleep □ Decreased anxiety. Initial response may be noted in 4–7 days in some patients. Most patients respond within 2 wk after initiating therapy.

AMOXICILLIN

(a-mox-i-**sill**-in)

Amoxil, {Apo-Amoxi}, {Novamoxin}, Polymox, Sumox, Trimox

CLASSIFICATION(S):
Anti-infective—extended-spectrum penicillin
Pregnancy Category B

INDICATIONS

▪ Treatment of a variety of infections including: ▫ Skin and skin structure infections ▫ Otitis media ▫ Sinusitis ▫ Respiratory tract infections ▫ Genitourinary tract infections ▫ Meningitis ▫ Septicemia ▪ Endocarditis prophylaxis.

ACTION

▪ Binds to bacterial cell wall, causing cell death. **Therapeutic Effect:** ▪ Bactericidal action against susceptible bacteria. Resists action of beta-lactamase, an enzyme produced by bacteria that is capable of inactivating some penicillins. **Spectrum:** ▪ Active against: ▫ Streptococci ▫ Pneumococci ▫ Enterococci ▫ *Hemophilus influenzae* ▫ *Escherichia coli* ▫ *Proteus mirabilis* ▫ *Neisseria menigitidis* ▫ *Neisseria gonorrhea* ▫ *Shigella* ▫ *Salmonella.*

PHARMACOKINETICS

Absorption: Well absorbed from the duodenum (75–90%). More resistant to acid inactivation than other penicillins.
Distribution: Diffuses readily into most body tissues and fluids. CSF penetration is increased in the presence of inflamed meninges. Crosses the placenta and enters breast milk in small amounts.
Metabolism and Excretion: 70% excreted unchanged in the urine. 30% metabolized by the liver.
Half-life: 1–1.3 hr.

CONTRAINDICATIONS AND PRECAUTIONS

Contraindicated in: ▪ Hypersensitivity to penicillins.
Use Cautiously in: ▪ Severe renal insufficiency (dosage reduction necessary) ▪ Has been used during pregnancy and lactation ▪ Infectious mononucleosis (increased incidence of rash).

ADVERSE REACTIONS AND SIDE EFFECTS*

CNS: SEIZURES (high doses).
Derm: <u>rashes</u>, urticaria.
GI: nausea, vomiting, <u>diarrhea</u>.
Hemat: blood dyscrasias.
Misc: superinfection, allergic reactions including serum sickness.

INTERACTIONS

Drug-Drug: ▪ **Probenecid** decreases renal excretion and increases blood levels of amoxicillin—therapy may be combined for this purpose ▪ May potentiate the effect of **oral anticoagulants** ▪ May decrease the effectiveness of **oral contraceptive agents.**

ROUTE AND DOSAGE

- **PO (Adults and Children >20 kg):** 250–500 mg q 8 hr.
- **PO (Children 8–20 kg):** 6.7–13.3 mg/kg q 8 hr.
- **PO (Children 6–8 kg):** 50–100 mg q 8 hr.
- **PO (Children <6 kg):** 25–50 mg q 8 hr.

Gonorrhea

- **PO (Adults):** 3 g plus 1 g probenecid single dose.
- **PO (Children >2 yr):** 50 mg/kg plus 25 mg/kg probenecid single dose.

PHARMACODYNAMICS (peak blood levels)

	ONSET	PEAK
PO	30 min	1–2 hr

NURSING IMPLICATIONS

Assessment

▫ Assess patient for infection (vital signs; appearance of wound, sputum, urine, and stool; WBC) at beginning and throughout course of therapy.
▫ Obtain a history before initiating therapy to determine previous use of and reactions to penicillins or cephalosporins. Persons with a negative history of penicillin sensitivity may still have an allergic response.

*<u>Underlines</u> indicate most frequent; **CAPITALS** indicate life-threatening.

- □ Observe patient for signs and symptoms of anaphylaxis (rash, pruritus, laryngeal edema, wheezing). Notify the physician immediately if these occur.
- □ Obtain specimens for culture and sensitivity prior to initiating therapy. First dose may be given before receiving results.
- ■ **Lab Test Considerations:** May cause false-positive reactions with copper sulfate urine glucose tests (Clinitest). Use Clinistix or Tes-Tape to monitor urine glucose.
- □ May cause increased SGOT (AST) and SGPT (ALT) concentrations.

POTENTIAL NURSING DIAGNOSES

- ■ Infection, high risk for (indications, side effects).
- ■ Knowledge deficit related to medication regimen (patient/family teaching).
- ■ Noncompliance related to medication regimen (patient/family teaching).

IMPLEMENTATION

- ■ **PO:** Administer around the clock. May be given without regard to meals. May be given with meals to decrease GI side effects. Capsule contents may be emptied and swallowed with liquids. Chewable tablets should be crushed or chewed before swallowing with liquids. Available as a powder for reconstitution to an oral suspension. Refrigerated reconstituted suspension should be discarded after 14 days.

PATIENT/FAMILY TEACHING

- □ Instruct patients to take medication around the clock and to finish the drug completely as directed, even if feeling better. Advise patients that sharing of this medication may be dangerous.
- □ Advise patient to report the signs of superinfection (furry overgrowth on the tongue, vaginal itching or discharge, loose or foul-smelling stools) and allergy.
- □ Instruct the patient to notify the physician if symptoms do not improve or if nausea or diarrhea persist when drug is administered with food.
- □ Patients with a history of rheumatic heart disease or valve replacement need to be taught the importance of using antimicrobial prophylaxis before invasive medical or dental procedures.

EVALUATION

Clinical response can be evaluated by:
■ Resolution of the signs and symptoms of infection. Length of time for complete resolution depends on the organism and site of infection ■ Endocarditis prophylaxis.

AMOXICILLIN/ CLAVULANATE

(a-mox-i-**sill**-in/klav-yoo-**lan**-ate)
Augmentin

CLASSIFICATION(S):
Anti-infective—extended-spectrum penicillin
Pregnancy Category B

INDICATIONS

■ Treatment of a variety of infections including: □ Skin and skin structure infections □ Otitis media □ Sinusitis □ Respiratory tract infections □ Genitourinary tract infections □ Meningitis □ Septicemia.

ACTION

■ Binds to bacterial cell wall, causing cell death. Resists action of beta-lactamase, an enzyme produced by bacteria that is capable of inactivating some penicillins. Combination with clavulanate enhances this resistance. **Therapeutic Effect:** ■ Bactericidal action against susceptible bacteria. **Spectrum:** ■ Active against: □ Streptococci □ Pneumococci □ Enterococci □ *Hemophilus influenzae* □ *Escherichia coli* □ *Proteus mirabilis* □ *Neisseria menigitidis* □ *Neisseri gonorrhea* □ *Shigella* □ *Salmonella*.

A

PHARMACOKINETICS

Absorption: Well absorbed from the duodenum (75–90%). More resistant to acid inactivation than other penicillins.
Distribution: Diffuses readily into most body tissues and fluids. CSF penetration is increased in the presence of inflammed meninges. Crosses the placenta and enters breast milk in small amounts.
Metabolism and Excretion: 70% excreted unchanged in the urine. 30% metabolized by the liver.
Half-life: 1–1.3 hr.

CONTRAINDICATIONS AND PRECAUTIONS

Contraindicated in: ▪ Hypersensitivity to penicillins ▪ Hypersensitivity to clavulanate.
Use Cautiously in: ▪ Severe renal insufficiency (dosage reduction necessary) ▪ Infectious mononucleosis (increased incidence of rash).

ADVERSE REACTIONS AND SIDE EFFECTS*

CNS: SEIZURES (high doses).
Derm: rashes, urticaria.
GI: nausea, vomiting, diarrhea.
Hemat: blood dyscrasias.
Misc: superinfection, allergic reactions including serum sickness.

INTERACTIONS

Drug–Drug: ▪ **Probenecid** decreases renal excretion and increases blood levels of amoxicillin—therapy may be combined for this purpose ▪ May potentiate the effect of **oral anticoagulants**. ▪ Concurrent **allopurinol** therapy increases risk of rash ▪ May decrease the effectiveness of **oral contraceptive agents**.

ROUTE AND DOSAGE

Note: Two 250 mg tablets are not equivalent to one 500 tablet, because both have the same amount of clavulanate.

- **PO (Adults):** 250–500 mg amoxicillin with 125 mg clavulanate q 8 hr.
- **PO (Children ≤40 kg):** 6.7–13.3 mg/kg amoxicillin equivalent q 8 hr.

PHARMACODYNAMICS (peak blood levels)

	ONSET	PEAK
PO	30 min	1–2 hr

NURSING IMPLICATIONS

Assessment

- □ Assess patient for infection (vital signs; appearance of wound, sputum, urine, and stool; WBC) at beginning and throughout course of therapy.
- □ Obtain a history before initiating therapy to determine previous use of and reactions to penicillins or cephalosporins. Persons with a negative history of penicillin sensitivity may still have an allergic response.
- □ Observe patient for signs and symptoms of anaphylaxis (rash, pruritus, laryngeal edema, wheezing). Notify the physician immediately if these occur.
- □ Obtain specimens for culture and sensitivity prior to initiating therapy. First dose may be given before receiving results.
- ▪ **Lab Test Considerations:** May cause false-positive reactions with copper sulfate urine glucose tests (Clinitest). Use Clinistix or Tes-Tape to monitor urine glucose.
- □ May cause increased SGOT (AST) and SGPT (ALT) concentrations.

Potential Nursing Diagnoses

- ▪ Infection, high risk for (indications, side effects).
- ▪ Knowledge deficit related to medication regimen (patient/family teaching).
- ▪ Noncompliance related to medication regimen (patient/family teaching).

Implementation

- ▪ **PO:** Administer around the clock. May be given without regard to meals. May be given with meals to decrease GI side effects. Capsule contents may be

*Underlines indicate most frequent; **CAPITALS** indicate life-threatening.

emptied and swallowed with liquids. Chewable tablets should be crushed or chewed before swallowing with liquids. Available as a powder for reconstitution to an oral suspension. Refrigerated reconstituted suspension should be discarded after 14 days.

Patient/Family Teaching

- □ Instruct patients to take medication around the clock and to finish the drug completely as directed, even if feeling better. Advise patients that sharing of this medication may be dangerous.
- □ Advise patient to report the signs of superinfection (furry overgrowth on the tongue, vaginal itching or discharge, loose or foul-smelling stools) and allergy.
- □ Instruct the patient to notify the physician if symptoms do not improve or if nausea or diarrhea persist when drug is administered with food.

Evaluation

Clinical response can be evaluated by: ▪ Resolution of the signs and symptoms of infection. Length of time for complete resolution depends on the organism and site of infection.

AMPHETAMINE

(am-fet-a-meen)

CLASSIFICATION(S):
CNS stimulant
Schedule II
Pregnancy Category C

INDICATIONS

▪ Treatment of narcolepsy ▪ Adjunct in the management of attention deficit disorder (ADD).

ACTION

▪ Produces CNS stimulation by releasing norepinephrine from nerve endings. Pharmacologic effects are: □ CNS and respiratory stimulation □ Vasoconstriction □ Mydriasis (pupillary dilation) □ Contraction of the urinary bladder sphincter. **Therapeutic Effects:** ▪ Increased motor activity, mental alertness, and decreased fatigue in narcoleptic patients ▪ Increased attention span in attention deficit disorder.

PHARMACOKINETICS

Absorption: Well absorbed following oral administration.

Distribution: Widely distributed throughout body tissues with high concentrations in the brain and CSF. Crosses the placenta and enters breast milk. Potentially embryotoxic.

Metabolism and Excretion: Some metabolism by the liver. Urinary excretion is pH dependent. Alkaline urine promotes reabsorption and prolongs action.

Half-life: Amphetamine, 10–30 hr (depending on pH of urine).

CONTRAINDICATIONS AND PRECAUTIONS

Contraindicated in: ▪ Pregnancy or lactation ▪ Hyperexcitable states including hyperthyroidism ▪ Psychotic personalities ▪ Suicidal or homicidal tendencies ▪ Chemical dependence ▪ Glaucoma.

Use Cautiously in: ▪ Cardiovascular disease ▪ Hypertension ▪ Diabetes mellitus ▪ Elderly or debilitated patients ▪ Continual use (may result in psychological dependence or addiction).

ADVERSE REACTIONS AND SIDE EFFECTS*

CNS: restlessness, tremor, hyperactivity, insomnia, irritability, dizziness, headache.

CV: tachycardia, palpitations, hypertension, hypotension.

Derm: urticaria.

GI: nausea, vomiting, anorexia, dry mouth, cramps, diarrhea, constipation, metallic taste.

GU: impotence, increased libido.

Misc: psychological dependence, addiction.

*Underlines indicate most frequent; **CAPITALS** indicate life-threatening.

A

INTERACTIONS

Drug–Drug: ▪ Additive adrenergic effects with other **adrenergic (sympathomimetic) agents** ▪ Use with **MAO inhibitors** can result in hypertensive crisis ▪ **Alkalinizing the urine (sodium bicarbonate, acetazolamide)** decreases excretion, enhances effect ▪ **Acidification of urine (ammonium chloride,** large doses of **ascorbic acid)** decreases effect ▪ **Phenothiazines** may decrease effect ▪ May antagonize **antihypertensives** ▪ **Tricyclic antidepressants** may enhance the effect of amphetamine.

Drug–Food: Foods that acidify the urine (cranberry juice) can enhance the effect of amphetamine.

ROUTE AND DOSAGE

Narcolepsy

- **PO (Adult):** 5–60 mg/day in divided doses.
- **PO (Children >12 yr):** 10 mg/day, increase by 10 mg at weekly intervals.
- **PO (Children 6–12 yr):** 5 mg/day, increase by 5 mg at weekly intervals.

Attention Deficit Disorder

- **PO (Children >6 yr):** 5 mg/day, increase by 5 mg at weekly intervals.
- **PO (Children 3–5 yr):** 2.5 mg/day, increase by 2.5 mg at weekly intervals.

PHARMACODYNAMICS (CNS stimulation)

	ONSET	PEAK	DURATION
PO	1–2 hr	UK	4–10 hr

NURSING IMPLICATIONS

Assessment

- □ Monitor blood pressure, pulse, and respiration before administering and periodically throughout course of therapy.
- □ Monitor weight biweekly and inform physician of significant loss. Monitor height periodically in children; inform physician if growth inhibition occurs.
- □ Observe and document frequency of narcoleptic episodes.
- □ Assess attention span, impulse control, and interactions with others in children with attention-deficit disorders.
- □ May produce a false sense of euphoria and well-being. Provide frequent rest periods and observe patient for rebound depression after the effects of the medication have worn off.
- □ Has high dependence and abuse potential. Tolerance to medication occurs rapidly; do not increase dose.

Potential Nursing Diagnoses

- ▪ Thought processes, altered (side effects).
- ▪ Knowledge deficit related to medication regimen (patient/family teaching).

Implementation

- ▪ **General Info:** Therapy should utilize the lowest effective dose.
- ▪ **PO:** Extended-release capsules should be swallowed whole; do not break, crush, or chew.
- □ Available in tablets, capsules, and elixir preparations.

Patient/Family Teaching

- □ Instruct patient to take medication at least 6 hr before bedtime to avoid sleep disturbances. Missed doses should be taken as soon as remembered up to 6 hr before bedtime. Do not double doses. Instruct patient not to alter dosage without consulting physician. Abrupt cessation with high doses may cause extreme fatigue and mental depression.
- □ Inform patient that the effects of drug-induced dry mouth can be minimized by rinsing frequently with water or chewing sugarless gum or candies.
- □ Advise patient to avoid the intake of large amounts of caffeine.
- □ Medication may impair judgement. Advise patients to use caution when driving or during other activities requiring alertness.
- □ Inform patient that physician may order periodic holidays from the drug to assess progress and decrease dependence.
- □ Advise patient to notify physician if nervousness, restlessness, insomnia,

dizziness, anorexia, or dry mouth becomes severe.

EVALUATION

Effectiveness of therapy can be demonstrated by: ▪ Decrease in narcoleptic symptoms ▪ Improved attention span.

AMPHOTERICIN B
(am-foe-**ter**-i-sin)
Fungizone

CLASSIFICATION(S):
Antifungal
Pregnancy Category UK

INDICATIONS

▪ Treatment of active, progressive, potentially fatal fungal infections.

ACTION

▪ Binds to fungal cell membrane, allowing leakage of cellular contents. **Therapeutic Effect:** ▪ Fungistatic action against susceptible organisms. **Spectrum:** ▪ Active against: ▫ Aspergillosis ▫ Blastomycosis ▫ Disseminated Candidiasis ▫ Coccidioidomycosis ▫ Histoplasmosis ▫ Mucormycosis.

PHARMACOKINETICS

Absorption: Not active orally. Topical preparations are not significantly absorbed.

Distribution: Following intravenous administration, distributed to body tissues and fluids. Poor penetration into CSF.

Metabolism and Excretion: Elimination is very prolonged. Detectable in urine up to 7 wk after discontinuation.

Half-life: Biphasic—initial phase, 24–48 hr; terminal phase, 15 days.

CONTRAINDICATIONS AND PRECAUTIONS

Contraindicated in: ▪ Hypersensitivity.

Use Cautiously in: ▪ Renal impairment ▪ Electrolyte abnormalities ▪ Pregnancy and lactation (safety not established).

ADVERSE REACTIONS AND SIDE EFFECTS*

CNS: headache.
CV: hypotension, arrhythmias.
F and E: hypokalemia.
GI: nausea, vomiting, diarrhea.
GU: nephrotoxicity, hematuria.
Hemat: anemia, dyscrasias.
Local: phlebitis.
Misc: fever, chills, HYPERSENSITIVITY REACTIONS.
MS: mylagia, arthralgia.
Neuro: peripheral neuropathy.
Resp: dyspnea, wheezing.

INTERACTIONS

Drug-Drug: ▪ Increased risk of nephrotoxicity with **aminoglycosides** and other **nephrotoxic agents** ▪ **Diuretics, glucorticoids, mezlocillin, piperacillin,** or **ticarcillin** may potentiate hypokalemia.

ROUTE AND DOSAGE

- **IV (Adults):** Give test dose of 1–5 mg, then initial dose of 0.25 mg/kg, slowly over 6 hr; increase daily doses slowly to 0.5 mg/kg (can give up to 1 mg/kg/day or 1.5 mg/kg every other day).
- **IV (Children):** 0.25 mg/kg infused over 6 hr initially; increase by 0.25 mg/kg every other day to maximum of 1 mg/kg/day.
- **IT (Adults):** 25–100 mcg (0.025–0.1 mg) q 48–72 hr; increase to 500 mcg (0.5 mg) as tolerated to maximum total dose of 15 mg (unlabeled route).
- **Top:** 3% cream, lotion, or ointment—apply 2–4 times daily.
- **Bladder Irrigation (Adults):** 50 mcg/ml instilled intermittently or continuously (unlabeled route).

PHARMACODYNAMICS (blood levels)

	ONSET	PEAK
IV	rapid	end of infusion

*Underlines indicate most frequent; CAPITALS indicate life-threatening.

A

NURSING IMPLICATIONS

Assessment

- □ This drug should be administered IV only to hospitalized patients or those under close medical supervision. Diagnosis should be confirmed with cultures prior to administration.
- □ Monitor patient closely during test dose and the first 1–2 hr of each dose for fever, chills, headache, anorexia, nausea, or vomiting. Premedication with aspirin, corticosteroids, antihistamines, and antiemetics, and maintaining sodium balance may decrease these reactions. Febrile reaction usually subsides within 4 hr after the infusion is completed.
- □ Assess injection site frequently for thrombophlebitis or leakage. Drug is extremely irritating to tissues. The addition of heparin to IV soln may decrease the likelihood of thrombophlebitis.
- □ Monitor pulse and blood pressure every 15–30 min during test dose and initial therapy. Assess respiratory status (lung sounds, dyspnea) daily. Notify physician of changes.
- □ Monitor intake and output and weigh daily. Adequate hydration (2000–3000 ml/day) may minimize nephrotoxicity.
- ▪ **Lab Test Considerations:** Monitor weekly hemoglobin and hematocrit, magnesium, BUN, and serum creatinine and biweekly potassium levels. Life-threatening hypokalemia may occur following each dose. If BUN exceeds 40 mg/100 ml or serum creatinine exceeds 3 mg/100 ml, dosage should be decreased or discontinued until renal function improves. May cause decreased hemoglobin, hematocrit, and magnesium levels.
- □ Liver function tests should be monitored periodically throughout therapy. Elevated bromsulphalein, alkaline phosphatase, and bilirubin may require discontinuation of therapy.

Potential Nursing Diagnoses

- ▪ Infection, high risk for (indications).
- ▪ Knowledge deficit related to medication regimen (patient/family teaching).

Implementation

- ▪ **IV:** Reconstitute 50-mg vial with 10 ml of sterile water without bacteriostatic agent. Concentration equals 5 mg/ml. Shake until clear. Further dilute each 1 mg with at least 10 ml of D5W (pH>4.2) for a concentration of 100 mcg/ml. Do not use other diluents. Avoid use of precipitated soln. Use 20-gauge needle; change for each step of dilution. Wear gloves while handling.
- □ Store in dark area. Reconstituted soln is stable for 24 hr at room temperature and 1 wk if refrigerated.
- ▪ **Test Dose:** Administer 1 mg in 20 ml of D5W over 10–30 min to determine patient tolerance. If medication is withheld for 7 days, restart at lowest dose level.
- ▪ **Intermittent Infusion:** Administer preferably through central line. If peripheral site is used, change site with each dose to prevent phlebitis. If an in-line filter is used, the mean pore diameter should be no less than 1 micron. Agitate hanging soln to mix every half hr. Short-term exposure to light (8–24 hr) does not appreciably alter potency.
- □ Administer separately, do not admix or piggyback with antibiotics. Avoid extravasation.
- □ *Rate:* Administer slowly via infusion pump over 6 hr.
- ▪ **Syringe Compatibility:** heparin.
- ▪ **Y-Site Incompatibility:** foscarnet or ondansetron.
- ▪ **Additive Compatibility:** heparin, hydrocortisone, methylprednisolone, or sodium bicarbonate.
- ▪ **Additive Incompatibility:** amikacin, calcium chloride, calcium disodium edetate, calcium gluconate, chlorpromazine, cimetidine, diphenydramine, dopamine, gentamicin, kanamycin, methyldopate, oxytetracycline, penicillin G, polymyxin B, potassium chloride, prochlorperazine, saline solutions, tetracycline, or verapamil.

- **Bladder Irrigation:** May be administered as a continuous bladder irrigation through a catheter for fungal infections of the bladder.
- **Top:** While wearing gloves, apply topical preparations liberally and rub in well. Do not use occlusive dressings. Discontinue if lesions worsen or signs of hypersensitivity develop.

Patient/Family Teaching

- **General Info:** Explain need for long duration of IV or topical therapy.
- **IV:** Inform patient of potential side effects and discomfort at IV site.
- **Top:** Advise patient that topical preparations may stain clothing. Cream or lotion may be removed with soap and warm water; ointment may be removed with cleaning fluid.

Evaluation

Effectiveness of therapy may be determined by: ▪ Resolution of signs and symptoms of infection. Several wks to mons of therapy may be required to prevent relapse.

AMPICILLIN

(am-pi-**sill**-in)

{Ampicin}, {Ampilean}, {Apo-Amp}, NaMPICIL, {Novoampicillin}, Omnipen, Penbritin, Principen, Polycillin, Supen, Totacillin

CLASSIFICATION(S):
Anti-infective—penicillin
Pregnancy Category B

INDICATIONS

▪ Treatment of a variety of skin and skin structure infections, soft tissue infections including: ▫ Otitis media ▫ Sinusitis ▫ Respiratory tract infections ▫ Genitourinary tract infections ▫ Meningitis ▫ Septicemia ▪ Endocarditis prophylaxis.

ACTION

▪ Binds to bacterial cell wall, resulting in cell death. **Therapeutic Effect:** ▪ Bactericidal action against susceptible bacteria. Resists action of beta-lactamase, an enzyme produced by bacteria that is capable of inactivating some penicillins. **Spectrum:** ▪ Active against: ▫ Streptococci ▫ Pneumococci ▫ Enterococci ▫ *Hemophilus influenzae* ▫ *Escherichia coli* ▫ *Proteus mirabilis* ▫ *Neisseria menigitidis* ▫ *Neisseria gonorrhea* ▫ *Shigella* ▫ *Salmonella*.

PHARMACOKINETICS

Absorption: Moderately absorbed from the duodenum (30–50%).
Distribution: Diffuses readily into most body tissues and fluids. CSF penetration is increased in the presence of inflammed meninges. Crosses the placenta and enters breast milk in small amounts.
Metabolism and Excretion: Variably metabolized by the liver (12–50%). Renal excretion of unchanged drug also variable, depending on route of administration (25–60% after oral dosing; 50–85% following IM administration).
Half-life: 1–1.5 hr.

CONTRAINDICATIONS AND PRECAUTIONS

Contraindicated in: ▪ Hypersensitivity to penicillins.
Use Cautiously in: ▪ Severe renal insufficiency (dosage reduction required) ▪ Has been used during pregnancy and lactation ▪ Infectious mononucleosis (increased incidence of rash).

ADVERSE REACTIONS AND SIDE EFFECTS*

CNS: SEIZURES (high doses).
Derm: <u>rashes</u>, urticaria.
GI: nausea, vomiting, <u>diarrhea</u>.
Hemat: blood dyscrasias.
Misc: superinfection, allergic reactions including ANAPHYLAXIS and serum sickness.

INTERACTIONS

Drug–Drug: ▪ **Probenecid** decreases renal excretion and increases blood lev-

{} = Available in Canada only.
*<u>Underlines</u> indicate most frequent; **CAPITALS** indicate life-threatening.

els of ampicillin—therapy may be combined for this purpose ▪ May potentiate the effect of **oral anticoagulants** ▪ Incidence of rash increases with concurrent **allopurinol** therapy ▪ May decrease the effectiveness of **oral contraceptive agents**.

ROUTE AND DOSAGE

- **PO (Adults and Children >20 kg):** 250–500 mg q 6 hr.
- **PO (Children <20 kg):** 50–100 mg/kg/day in divided doses q 6–8 hr.
- **IM, IV (Adults and Children >40 kg):** 8–12 g/day in divided doses q 3–4 hr.
- **IM, IV (Children <40 kg):** 25–50 mg/kg/day in divided doses q 6–8 hr (up to 100–200 mg/kg/day).
- **IM, IV (Neonates 7–28 days):** 50–100 mg/kg/day in divided doses q 8 hr (up to 200–300 mg/kg/day).
- **IM, IV (Neonates <7 days):** 5–100 mg/kg/day in divided doses q 12 hr (up to 200 mg/kg/day).

PHARMACODYNAMICS (blood levels)

	ONSET	PEAK
PO	rapid	1.5–2 hr
IM	rapid	1 hr
IV	rapid	end of infusion

NURSING IMPLICATIONS

Assessment

- □ Assess patient for infection (vital signs; wound appearance, sputum, urine, and stool; WBC) at beginning and throughout course of therapy.
- □ Obtain a history before initiating therapy to determine previous use and reactions to penicillins or cephalosporins. Persons with a negative history of penicillin sensitivity may still have an allergic response.
- □ Obtain specimens for culture and sensitivity prior to initiating therapy. First dose may be given before receiving results.
- □ Observe patient for signs and symptoms of anaphylaxis (rash, pruritus, laryngeal edema, wheezing). Discontinue the drug and notify the physician immediately if these occur. Keep epinephrine, an antihistamine, and resuscitation equipment close by in the event of an anaphylactic reaction.
- □ Assess skin daily for "ampicillin rash," a nonallergic, dull red, macular or maculopapular, and mildly pruritic rash.
- ▪ **Lab Test Considerations:** May cause false-positive copper sulfate urine glucose tests (Clinitest); test urine with glucose oxidase method (Keto-diastix or Tes-Tape).
- □ May cause increased SGOT (AST) and SGPT (ALT).

Potential Nursing Diagnoses

- Infection, high risk for (indications, side effects).
- Knowledge deficit related to medication regimen (patient/family teaching).
- Noncompliance related to medication regimen (patient/family teaching).

Implementation

- **General Info:** Available in combination with probenicid (see Appendix A).
- **PO:** Administer the oral form of the drug around the clock on an empty stomach at least 1 hr before or 2 hr after meals with a full glass of water. Tablets may be crushed and capsules may be opened and mixed with water. Reconstituted oral suspensions retain potency for 7 days at room temperature and 14 days if refrigerated. Combination with probenicid should be used immediately after reconstitution.
- **IM/IV:** Reconstitute ampicillin for IM or IV use by adding sterile water 0.9–1.2 ml to the 125-mg vial, 0.9–1.9 ml to the 250-mg vial, 1.2–1.8 ml to the 500-mg vial, 2.4–7.4 ml to the 1-g vial and 6.8 ml to the 2-g vial.
- **Direct IV:** May be administered over 3–5 min (125–500 mg) or over 10–15 min (1–2 g) within 1 hr of reconstitution. More rapid administration may cause seizures.
- **Intermittent Infusion:** Dilute for infu-

sion in 50 ml or more of 0.9% NaCl, D5W, D5/0.45% NaCl, or lactated Ringer's soln for a concentration of no more than 30 mg/ml, and administer within 4 hr.

- **Syringe Compatibility:** chloramphenicol, colistimethate, heparin, or procaine.
- **Syringe Incompatibility:** erythromycin, gentimicin, kanamycin, lincomycin, oxytetracycline, streptomycin, or tetracycline.
- **Y-Site Compatibility:** enalaprilat, foscarnet, heparin with hydrocortisone sodium succinate, hydromorphone, magnesium sulfate, meperidine, morphine, phytonadione, potassium chloride, or tolazoline.
- **Y-Site Incompatibility:** epinephrine, hydralazine, or ondansetron.
- **Additive Compatibility:** heparin or verapamil.
- **Additive Incompatibility:** amikacin, aminophylline, amphotericin B, calcium gluconate, chlorpromazine, clindamycin, dopamine, erythromycin, gentamicin, hydralazine, hydrocortisone, kanamycin, lidocaine, methicillin, nafcillin, norepinephrine, oxacillin, penicillin, prochlorperazine, tetracycline, or ticarcillin. Incompatible with aminoglycosides; do not admix. Administer at least 1 hr apart to prevent inactivation.

Patient/Family Teaching

- **General Info:** Instruct patient to take medication around the clock and to finish the drug completely as directed, even if feeling better. Advise patients that sharing of this medication can be dangerous.
  - Advise patient to report the signs of superinfection (furry overgrowth on the tongue, vaginal itching or discharge, loose or foul-smelling stools) and allergy.
  - Advise patient to use a nonhormonal method of contraception while taking ampicillin.
  - Instruct the patient to notify the physician if symptoms do not improve.
  - Patients with a history of rheumatic heart disease or valve replacement need to be taught the importance of using antimicrobial prophylaxis before invasive medical or dental procedures.

Evaluation

Clinical response can be evaluated by:
▪ Resolution of the signs and symptoms of infection. Length of time for complete resolution depends on the organism and site of infection ▪ Endocarditis prophylaxis.

AMPICILLIN/SULBACTAM

(am-pi-**sill**-in/sul-**bak**-tam)
Unasyn

CLASSIFICATION(S):
Anti-infective—penicillin
Pregnancy Category B (Ampicillin)

INDICATIONS

▪ Treatment of a variety of skin and skin structure infections, soft tissue infections including: ▫ Otitis media ▫ Sinusitis ▫ Respiratory tract infections ▫ Genitourinary tract infections ▫ Meningitis ▫ Septicemia.

ACTION

▪ Binds to bacterial cell wall, resulting in cell death. Addition of sulbactam increases resistance to beta-lactamases, enzymes produced by bacteria that may inactivate ampicillin. **Therapeutic Effect:** ▪ Bactericidal action against susceptible bacteria. **Spectrum:** ▪ Active against: ▫ Streptococci ▫ Pneumococci ▫ Enterococci ▫ *Hemophilus influenzae* ▫ *Escherichia coli* ▫ *Proteus mirabilis* ▫ *Neisseria menigitidis* ▫ *Neisseria gonorrhea* ▫ *Shigella* ▫ *Salmonella* ▪ Use should be reserved for infections caused by beta-lactamase producing strains.

PHARMACOKINETICS

Absorption: Well absorbed from IM sites.

Distribution: Ampicillin diffuses readily into most body tissues and fluids. CSF penetration is increased in the presence of inflammed meninges. Crosses the placenta and enters breast milk in small amounts.
Metabolism and Excretion: Ampicillin is variably metabolized by the liver (12–50%). Renal excretion of unchanged drug is also variable, depending on route of administration (25–60% after oral dosing; 50–85% following IM administration).
Half-life: 1.5 hr (ampicillin).

CONTRAINDICATIONS AND PRECAUTIONS

Contraindicated in: ▪ Hypersensitivity to penicillins or sulbactam.
Use Cautiously in: ▪ Severe renal insufficiency (dosage reduction required) ▪ Has been used during pregnancy and lactation (ampicillin) ▪ Infectious mononucleosis (increased incidence of rash) ▪ Children <12 yr (safety not established).

ADVERSE REACTIONS AND SIDE EFFECTS*

CNS: SEIZURES (high doses).
Derm: rashes, urticaria.
GI: nausea, vomiting, diarrhea.
Hemat: blood dyscrasias.
Local: pain at IM site, pain at IV site.
Misc: superinfection, allergic reactions including ANAPHYLAXIS and serum sickness.

INTERACTIONS

Drug-Drug: ▪ **Probenecid** decreases renal excretion and increases blood levels of ampicillin—therapy may be combined for this purpose ▪ May potentiate the effect of **oral anticoagulants** ▪ Concurrent **allopurinol** therapy (increased incidence of rash) ▪ May decrease the effectiveness of **oral contraceptive agents**.

ROUTE AND DOSAGE

▪ **IM, IV (Adults):** 1.5–3 g (1 g ampicillin plus 0.5 g sulbactam–2 g ampicillin plus 1 g sulbactam) q 6 hr (not to exceed 4 g sulbactam/day).

PHARMACODYNAMICS (blood levels)

	ONSET	PEAK
IM	rapid	1 hr
IV	immediate	end of infusion

NURSING IMPLICATIONS

Assessment

- Assess patient for infection (vital signs; wound appearance, sputum, urine, and stool; WBC) at beginning and throughout course of therapy.
- Obtain a history before initiating therapy to determine previous use and reactions to penicillins or cephalosporins. Persons with a negative history of penicillin sensitivity may still have an allergic response.
- Obtain specimens for culture and sensitivity prior to initiating therapy. First dose may be given before receiving results.
- Observe patient for signs and symptoms of anaphylaxis (rash, pruritus, laryngeal edema, wheezing). Discontinue the drug and notify the physician immediately if these occur. Keep epinephrine, an antihistamine, and resuscitation equipment close by in the event of an anaphylactic reaction.
- **Lab Test Considerations:** May cause false-positive copper sulfate urine glucose tests (Clinitest); test urine with glucose oxidase method (Keto-diastix or Tes-Tape).
- May cause increased SGOT (AST), SGPT (ALT), LDH, alkaline phosphatase, monocytes, basophils, eosinophils, BUN, and creatinine. May also cause presence of RBCs and hyaline casts in the urine.
- May cause decreased hemoglobin, hematocrit, RBC, WBC, neutrophils, lymphocytes, platelets, serum albumin, and total proteins.

Potential Nursing Diagnoses

- Infection, high risk for (indications, side effects).

*Underlines indicate most frequent; CAPITALS indicate life-threatening.

- Knowledge deficit related to medication regimen (patient/family teaching).

Implementation

- **IM:** Reconstitute for IM use by adding 3.2 ml of sterile water or 0.5% or 2% lidocaine HCl to the 1.5-g vial or 6.4 ml to the 3-g vial. Administer within 1 hr of preparation, deep IM into well-developed muscle.
- **IV:** For IV use reconstitute each 1.5 g with at least 4 ml of sterile water for a concentration of 375 mg/ml (250 mg ampicillin/125 mg sulbactam). Foaming should dissipate upon standing. Administer only clear solns.
- **Direct IV:** May be administered over 10–15 min (1–2 g) within 1 hr of reconstitution. More rapid administration may cause seizures.
- **Intermittent Infusion:** Dilute immediately for infusion in 50–100 ml or more of 0.9% NaCl, D5W, D5/0.45% NaCl, or lactated Ringer's soln. Stability of soln varies from 2–8 hr at room temperature or 3–72 hr if refrigerated, depending on concentration and diluent.
- □ *Rate:* Administer over 15–30 min.
- **Y-Site Compatibility:** enalaprilat, meperidine, or morphine.
- **Y-Site Incompatibility:** ondansetron.
- **Additive Incompatibilities:** Incompatible with aminoglycosides; do not admix. Administer at least 1 hr apart to prevent inactivation.

Patient/Family Teaching

- □ Advise patient to report the signs of superinfection (furry overgrowth on the tongue, vaginal itching or discharge, loose or foul-smelling stools) and allergy.
- □ Advise patient to use a nonhormonal method of contraception while taking ampicillin/sulbactam.
- □ Instruct the patient to notify the physician if symptoms do not improve.

Evaluation

Clinical response can be evaluated by:

- Resolution of the signs and symptoms of infection. Length of time for complete resolution depends on the organism and site of infection.

AMRINONE
(am-ri-none)
Inocor

CLASSIFICATION(S):
Inotropic agent
Pregnancy Category C

INDICATIONS

- Short-term treatment of congestive heart failure unresponsive to conventional therapy with cardiac glycosides, diuretics, and vasodilators.

ACTION

- Increases myocardial contractility
- Decreases preload and afterload by a direct dilating effect on vascular smooth muscle. **Therapeutic Effect:**
- Increased cardiac output (inotropic effect).

PHARMACOKINETICS

Absorption: Administered IV only, resulting in complete bioavailability.
Distribution: Distribution not known.
Metabolism and Excretion: 50% metabolized by the liver. 10–40% excreted unchanged by the kidneys.
Half-life: 3.6–5.8 hr (increased in congestive heart failure).

CONTRAINDICATIONS AND PRECAUTIONS

Contraindicated in: ▪ Hypersensitivity to amrinone or bisulfites ▪ Idiopathic hypertrophic subaortic stenosis.
Use Cautiously in: ▪ Atrial fibrillation or flutter (may increase ventricular response; pretreatment with cardiac glycosides may be necessary) ▪ Children <18 yr (safety not established).

ADVERSE REACTIONS AND SIDE EFFECTS*

CV: arrhythmias, hypotension.
Resp: dyspnea.

*Underlines indicate most frequent; **CAPITALS** indicate life-threatening.

A

GI: nausea, vomiting, diarrhea, hepatotoxicity.
F and E: hypokalemia.
Hemat: thrombocytopenia.
Misc: hypersensitivity reactions, fever.

INTERACTIONS

Drug–Drug: ▪ Inotropic effects may be additive with **cardiac glycosides** ▪ Hypotension may be exaggerated by **disopyramide**.

ROUTE AND DOSAGE

Note: See infusion rate chart in Appendix D.

- **IV (Adults):** 0.75 mg/kg loading dose; may be repeated in 30 min if necessary, then 5–10 mcg/kg/min infusion (total daily dose should not exceed 10 mg/kg).

PHARMACODYNAMICS (inotropic effect)

	ONSET	PEAK	DURATION*
IV	2–5 min	10 min	0.5–2 hr

*After infusion is discontinued.

NURSING IMPLICATIONS

Assessment

- Monitor blood pressure, pulse, ECG, respiratory rate, cardiac index, pulmonary capillary wedge pressure, and central venous pressure frequently during the administration of this medication. Notify physician promptly if drug-induced hypotension occurs.
- Monitor intake and output and weigh daily. Assess patient for resolution of signs and symptoms of congestive heart failure (peripheral edema, dyspnea, rales/crackles, weight gain). Fluid intake may need to be increased cautiously to ensure adequate cardiac filling pressure.
- Observe the patient for the appearance of hypersensitivity reactions (pleuritis, pericarditis, ascites). Withhold drug and notify physician immediately if a reaction occurs.
- **Lab Test Considerations:** Platelet counts, serum electrolytes, liver enzymes, and renal function should be evaluated periodically throughout the course of therapy. If platelet count is $<150,000/mm^3$ notify physician promptly. Increased liver enzymes may indicate hepatotoxicity. May cause decreased potassium levels.

Potential Nursing Diagnoses

- Cardiac output, decreased (indications).
- Activity intolerance (indications).
- Fluid volume excess (indications).

Implementation

- **General Info:** Hypokalemia should be corrected prior to administration.
- Patients with atrial fibrillation/flutter may require digitalis glycoside therapy prior to treatment, because amrinone enhances atrioventricular conduction.
- **Direct IV:** Loading dose should be administered over 2–3 min. An additional loading dose may be given in 30 min.
- **Continuous Infusion:** Dilute amrinone with 0.9% NaCl or 0.45% NaCl only, for a concentration of 1–3 mg/ml. Dilution with dextrose products may lead to decomposition of amrinone, but may be administered through Y-tubing or directly into tubing of a running dextrose soln. Administer via infusion pump to ensure accurate dosage. Change tubing whenever concentration of soln is changed. Soln should be clear yellow. Use reconstituted soln within 24 hr of preparation.
- *Rate:* Rate is titrated according to patient response.
- **Y-Site Compatibility:** aminophylline, atropine, bretylium, calcium chloride, cimetidine, dobutamine, dopamine, epinephrine, hydrocortisone sodium succinate, isoproterenol, lidocaine, metaraminol bitartrate, methylprednisolone sodium succinate, nitroglycerin, nitroprusside, norepinephrine,

phenylephrine, potassium chloride, procainamide, or verapamil.

- **Y-Site Incompatibility:** furosemide or sodium bicarbonate.

PATIENT/FAMILY TEACHING

- Advise patient to report an increase in dyspnea or chest pain, or the onset of hypersensitivity reactions promptly.
- Advise patient to make position changes slowly to minimize any drug-induced postural hypotension.

EVALUATION

Effectiveness of therapy may be determined by: ▪ Increase in cardiac index and diuresis ▫ Decrease in pulmonary capillary wedge pressure, dyspnea, and edema.

AMYL NITRITE
(am-il-nye-trite)

CLASSIFICATION(S):
Antianginal, Antidote—cyanide poisoning
Pregnancy Category X

INDICATIONS

▪ Acute treatment of angina pectoris. **Unlabeled Uses:** ▪ Acute management of cyanide poisoning ▪ Diagnosis of cardiac murmurs.

ACTION

▪ Reduces systemic arterial pressure (reduces afterload) ▪ Forms methemoglobin, which combines with cyanide, forming a nontoxic compound (cyanmethemoglobin). **Therapeutic Effects:** ▪ Relief of angina pectoris ▪ Prevention of fatal outcome in cyanide poisoning.

PHARMACOKINETICS

Absorption: Amyl nitrite is well absorbed through nasal mucosa.
Distribution: Widely distributed.
Metabolism and Excretion: Combines to form methemoglobin.
Half-life: UK.

CONTRAINDICATIONS AND PRECAUTIONS

Contraindicated in: ▪ Hypersensitivity ▪ Increased intracranial pressure ▪ Severe anemia ▪ No contraindications in cyanide poisoning.
Use Cautiously in: ▪ Hypotension ▪ Hypovolemia ▪ Constrictive pericarditis or cardiac tamponade ▪ Glaucoma ▪ Hyperthyroidism ▪ Recent head trauma ▪ Cerebral hemorrhage ▪ Recent myocardial infarction ▪ Cyanide poisoning in children (titrate doses based on methemoglobin levels).

ADVERSE REACTIONS AND SIDE EFFECTS*

CNS: headache, dizziness, fainting, weakness.
Resp: shortness of breath.
CV: hypotension, tachycardia.
Derm: cyanosis of lips, fingernail, or palms (indicates methemoglobinemia).

INTERACTIONS

Drug-Drug: ▪ Additive hypotension with **antihypertensive agents** ▪ Decreases the effects of **histamine, acetylcholine,** and **norepinephrine** ▪ Antianginal activity decreased by **adrenergic (sympathomimetic) agents** including **epinephrine, ephedrine,** and **phenylephrine** ▪ Blocks the alpha-adrenergic effects of **epinephrine,** resulting in hypotension and tachycardia.

ROUTE AND DOSAGE

Antianginal

- **Inhaln (Adults):** 1 ampule (aspirol, vaporole) crushed and inhaled, may be repeated in 3–5 min.

Cyanide Poisoning

- **Inhaln (Adults and Children):** Inhale for 15–30 sec of each min until sodium nitrite is prepared.

PHARMACODYNAMICS (antianginal)

	ONSET	PEAK	DURATION
Inhaln	30 sec	UK	3–5 min

*Underlines indicate most frequent; **CAPITALS** indicate life-threatening.

NURSING IMPLICATIONS

Assessment

- **General Info:** Assess heart rate and blood pressure prior to and periodically throughout therapy.
- **Angina:** Assess patient for location, duration, intensity, and precipitating factors of chest pains prior to and following administration.
- **Cyanide Poisoning:** Determine source of cyanide and assess patient for signs of cyanide poisoning (tachycardia, headache, drowsiness, hypotension, coma, convulsions).
- **Heart Murmurs:** Assess heart rate prior to and throughout administration.

Potential Nursing Diagnoses

- Comfort, altered: pain (indications).
- Injury, high risk for (side effects).
- Knowledge deficit related to medication regimen (patient/family teaching).

Implementation

- **General Info:** Ampule is wrapped in woven, absorbent covering. Do not remove covering. Crush ampule between fingers and hold to patient's nostrils for inhalation. Patient should be sitting during and immediately after administration.
- **Angina:** Titrate dose according to patient's response.
- **Cyanide Poisoning:** Begin treatment at the first sign of toxicity if cyanide exposure is known or strongly suspected.
  - *For Adults or Children*—Crush a 0.3 ml ampule every min and have the patient inhale the vapors for 15–30 sec until IV sodium nitrate infusion is available.
- **Heart Murmurs:** Amyl nitrate should be inhaled until reflex tachycardia begins and then discontinued immediately.

Patient/Family Teaching

- Explain purpose and procedure for therapy to patient.
- Caution patient to change positions slowly to minimize orthostatic hypotension.

Evaluation

Effectiveness of therapy can be demonstrated by: ▪ Relief of angina pectoris ▪ Relief of signs and symptoms of cyanide poisoning ▪ Change in intensity of heart murmurs.

ANISTREPLASE

(an-**eye**-strep-lase)
aniosoylated plasminogen—streptokinase activator complex, APSAC, Eminase

CLASSIFICATION(S):
Thrombolytic agent
Pregnancy Category C

INDICATIONS

- Acute management of myocardial infarction, in order to lyse thrombi in coronary arteries and thereby preserve ventricular function.

ACTION

- Consists of an inactive complex of plasminogen and streptokinase. Following administration, controlled activation of the complex occurs, allowing the conversion of plasminogen to plasmin and subsequent fibrinolysis. **Therapeutic Effect:** ▪ Lysis of thrombi in coronary arteries with preservation of ventricular function.

PHARMACOKINETICS

Absorption: Following IV administration absorption is essentially complete.
Distribution: Distribution not known.
Metabolism and Excretion: Inactivated by binding to plasmin inactivators.
Half-life: 70–120 min.

CONTRAINDICATIONS AND PRECAUTIONS

Contraindicated in: ▪ Active internal bleeding ▪ History of cerebrovascular accident ▪ Recent (within 2 mon) intracranial or intraspinal trauma ▪ Intracranial neoplasm ▪ Severe uncontrolled hypertension ▪ Arteriovenous malformation ▪ Known bleeding tendencies ▪ Hypersensitivity to anistreplase or streptokinase

Use Cautiously in: ▪ Recent (within 10 days) major surgery, trauma, GI or GU bleeding ▪ Uncontrolled hypertension ▪ Left heart thrombus ▪ Severe hepatic or renal disease ▪ Hemorrhagic ophthalmic conditions ▪ Septic phlebitis ▪ Elderly patients (>75yr) ▪ Pregnancy, lactation, or children (safety not established) ▪ Recent streptococcal infection or previous therapy with anistreplase or streptokinase (from 5 days–6 mon)—may produce resistance due to antibody formation; increased dosage requirements may be encountered.

Extreme Caution in: Early postpartum period (10 days) ▪ Patients receiving oral anticoagulant therapy.

ADVERSE REACTIONS AND SIDE EFFECTS*

CNS: INTRACRANIAL HEMORRHAGE.
EENT: epistaxis, gingival bleeding.
RESP: hemoptysis.
CV: arrhythmias, hypotension.
GI: GASTROINTESTINAL BLEEDING, RETROPERITONEAL BLEEDING.
GU: GENITOURINARY TRACT BLEEDING.
Hemat: BLEEDING.
Misc: allergic reactions including ANAPHYLAXIS, fever.

INTERACTIONS

Drug-Drug: ▪ **Aspirin, nonsteroidal anti-inflammatory agents, oral anticoagulants, heparin,** or **dipyridamole**—concurrent use may increase the risk of bleeding, although these agents are frequently used together or in sequence.

ROUTE AND DOSAGE

▪ **IV (Adults):** 30 units over 2–5 min.

PHARMACODYNAMICS (fibrinolysis)

	ONSET	PEAK	DURATION
IV	UK	45 min	6 hr*

*Systemic hyperfibrinolytic state may persist for 2 days.

NURSING IMPLICATIONS

Assessment

▪ **General Info:** Therapy should be administered as soon as possible after the onset of symptoms.
□ Monitor vital signs, including temperature, closely following therapy.
□ Assess patient carefully for bleeding. Frank bleeding may occur from invasive sites or body orifices. Internal bleeding may also occur (decreased neurologic status, abdominal pain with coffee ground emesis or black tarry stools, joint pain). If bleeding occurs, stop medication and notify physician immediately.
□ Inquire about previous reaction to anistreplase or streptokinase therapy. Assess patient for hypersensitivity reaction (changes in facial skin color, rash, dyspnea, swelling around eyes, wheezing). If these occur, inform physician promptly. Keep epinephrine, an antihistamine, and resuscitation equipment close by in the event of an anaphylactic reaction.
□ Inquire about recent streptococcal infection. Anistreplase may not be effective if administered within 5 days to 6 mon of a streptococcal infection.

▪ **Coronary Thrombosis:** Monitor ECG continuously. Notify physician if significant arrhythmias occur. Cardiac enzymes should be monitored. Radionucleotide myocardial scanning and/or coronary angiography may be ordered 7–10 days following therapy.

▪ **Lab Test Considerations:** Hematocrit, hemoglobin, platelet count, prothrombin time, thrombin time, bleeding time, and activated partial thromboplastin time should be evaluated prior to and frequently throughout course of therapy. Fibrinogen degradation products (FDP) may also be monitored prior to and following therapy.
□ Obtain type and crossmatch and have blood available at all times in case of hemorrhage.

▪ **Toxicity and Overdose:** If local bleed-

*Underlines indicate most frequent; **CAPITALS** indicate life-threatening.

ing occurs, apply pressure to site. If severe or internal bleeding occurs, clotting factors and/or blood volume may be restored through infusions of whole blood, packed red blood cells, fresh frozen plasma, cryoprecipitate, platelets, and/or desmopressin. Do not administer dextran as it has antiplatelet activity. If heparin is being administered, discontinue and consider administration of protamine. Aminocaproic acid (Amicar) may be used as an antidote.

Potential Nursing Diagnoses

- Tissue perfusion, altered (indications).
- Injury, high risk for (side effects).
- Knowledge deficit related to medication regimen (patient/family teaching).

Implementation

- **General Info:** Invasive procedures, such as IM injections or arterial punctures, should be avoided with this therapy. If such procedures must be performed, apply pressure to IV puncture sites for at least 15 min and to arterial puncture sites for at least 30 min.
- □ Systemic anticoagulation with heparin is usually begun several hrs after the completion of thrombolytic therapy. Aspirin may also be used to inhibit platelet aggregation.
- □ Acetaminophen may be ordered to control fever.
- **Direct IV:** Reconstitute with 5 ml of sterile water (direct to sides of vial) and swirl gently; do not shake to minimize foaming. Do not dilute further. Use reconstituted soln within 30 min of preparation.
- □ *Rate:* Administer via IV line or vein over 2–5 min.
- **Y-Site/Additive Incompatibility:** Do not admix or administer via Y-site injection with any other medication.

Patient/Family Teaching

- □ Explain purpose of the medication. Instruct patient to report hypersensitivity reactions (rash, dyspnea), bleeding, or bruising.
- □ Explain need for bedrest and minimal handling during therapy to avoid injury.

Evaluation

Effectiveness of therapy may be determined by: ▪ Lysis of thrombi ▪ Restoration of coronary blood flow.

ANTIHEMOPHILIC FACTOR

AHF, AHG, Factor VIII, Hemofil M, Humate-P, Koate-HS, Koate HT, Monoclate, Profilate-HP

CLASSIFICATION(S):
Hemostatic, Blood derivative
Pregnancy Category C

INDICATIONS

- Management of hemophilia A associated with a deficiency of factor VIII.

ACTION

- An essential clotting factor required for the conversion of prothrombin to thrombin. **Therapeutic Effect:** ▪ Correction of deficiency states with resultant control of excessive bleeding.

PHARMACOKINETICS

Absorption: Following IV administration absorption is essentially complete.
Distribution: Rapidly cleared from plasma. Does not cross the placenta.
Metabolism and Excretion: Used up in the clotting process.
Half-life: 4–24 hr (12 hr average).

CONTRAINDICATIONS AND PRECAUTIONS

Contraindicated in: ▪ Hypersensitivity to mouse protein (monoclonal antibody-derived products only).
Use Cautiously in: ▪ Pregnancy (safety not established).

ADVERSE REACTIONS AND SIDE EFFECTS*

CNS: headache, somnolence, lethargy, loss of consciousness.

*Underlines indicate most frequent; **CAPITALS** indicate life-threatening.

EENT: visual disturbances.
CV: tachycardia, hypotension, chest tightness.
GI: nausea, vomiting.
Hemat: intravascular hemolysis.
Derm: flushing, urticaria.
MS: back pain.
Neuro: paresthesia.
Misc: rigor, jaundice, allergic reactions, hepatitis B or HIV virus infection (small risk from frequent use of large amounts).

INTERACTIONS

Drug–Drug: ▪ None significant.

ROUTE AND DOSAGE

Note: Dosage should be determined by levels of circulating antihemophilic factor.

Joint Hemorrhage

- **IV (Adults and Children):** 5–10 units/kg q 8–12 hr for 1 or more days.

Minor Hemorrhage into Nonvital Areas

- **IV (Adults and Children):** 8–10 units/kg q 24 hr for 2–3 days or 8 units/kg q 12 hr for 2 days, then q 24 hr for 2 more days.

Hemorrhage into Muscles near Vital Organs

- **IV (Adults and Children):** 15 units/kg initially, then 8 units/kg q 8 hr for 48 hr, then 4 units/kg q 8 hr for 48 hr.

Overt Bleeding

- **IV (Adults and Children):** 15–25 units/kg initially, then 8–15 units/kg q 8–12 hr for 3–4 days.

Hemorrhage from Massive Wounds or Vital Organs

- **IV (Adults and Children):** 40–50 units/kg initially, then 20–25 units/kg q 8–12 hr.

Major Surgical Procedures

- **IV (Adults and Children):** 26–30 units/kg before surgery, then 15 units/kg q 5–8 hr postoperatively.

Prophylaxis of Hemophilia A

- **IV (Patients >50 kg):** 500 units daily.
- **IV (Patients <50 kg):** 250 units daily.

PHARMACODYNAMICS (levels of factor VIII)

	ONSET	PEAK	DURATION
IV	rapid	UK	8–12 hr

NURSING IMPLICATIONS

Assessment

- □ Monitor blood pressure, pulse, and respirations. If tachycardia occurs, slow or stop infusion rate and notify physician.
- □ Obtain history of current trauma; estimate amount of blood loss.
- □ Monitor for renewed bleeding every 15–30 min. Immobilize and apply ice to affected joints.
- □ Monitor intake and output ratios; note color of urine. Notify physician if significant discrepancy occurs or urine becomes red or orange. Patients with types A, B, and AB blood are particularly at risk for hemolytic reaction.
- □ Assess for allergic reaction (wheezing, tachycardia, urticaria, hives, chest tightness, stinging at IV site, nausea and vomiting, lethargy). Stop infusion, notify physician.
- ▪ **Lab Test Considerations:** Obtain baseline and periodic CBC, direct Coombs', urinalysis, partial thromboplastin time (PTT), thromboplastin generation test, and prothrombin generation test. Decreased hematocrit and increased Coombs' test may indicate hemolytic anemia.
- □ Monitor coagulation studies before, during, and after therapy to assess effectiveness of therapy.
- □ Patients with increased inhibitor levels may not respond or may require increased doses.

Potential Nursing Diagnoses

- Tissue perfusion, altered (indications).
- Injury, high risk for (indications).
- Knowledge deficit related to medication regimen (patient/family teaching).

A

IMPLEMENTATION

- **General Info:** Inform all personnel of bleeding tendency to prevent further trauma. Apply pressure to all venipuncture sites for at least 5 min; avoid all IM injections.
- Physician may order premedication with diphenhydramine (Benadryl) to prevent acute reactions.
- Dosage varies with degree of clotting factor deficit, desired level of clotting factors, and weight.
- Obtain type and crossmatch of blood in case a transfusion is necessary.
- To prevent spontaneous bleeding at least 5% of the normal Factor VIII level must be present. To control moderate bleeding or prior to minor surgery 30–50% must be present. For severe bleeding associated with trauma, or patient undergoing major surgery 80–100% of the normal Factor VIII level must be present.
- The first dose of antihemophilic factor is given 1 hr before surgery. The second dose (half of the first dose) is given 5–8 hr postoperatively. Factor VIII level must be maintained at 30% of the normal level for 10–14 days postoperatively.
- **IV:** Administer IV only. Refrigerate concentrate until just prior to reconstitution. Warm concentrate and diluent (provided by manufacturer) to room temperature before reconstituting. Use plastic syringe for preparation and administration. Use an additional needle as an air vent to the vial when reconstituting. After adding diluent rotate vial gently until completely dissolved. Soln may vary in color from light yellow to clear with a bluish tint. Do not refrigerate after reconstitution; use within 3 hr. Preparations should be filtered prior to administration.
- **Direct IV:** May be administered by slow IV push (see Intermittent Infusion for rates).
- **Intermittent Infusion:** Administration rate is based on antihemophilic factor (AHF) units/ml. Concentration of more than 34 AHF units/ml (Hemofil) should be administered no faster than 2 ml/min. Concentrations of less than 34 AHF units/ml (Profilate) may be administered at a rate of 10–20 ml over 3 min. Infusion rate should not exceed 10 ml/min.
- Do not admix.

PATIENT/FAMILY TEACHING

- Instruct patient to notify nurse immediately if bleeding recurs.
- Advise patient to observe for bleeding of gums, skin, urine, stool, or emesis.
- Advise patient to carry identification describing disease process at all times.
- Caution patient to avoid aspirin-containing products as they may further impair clotting.
- Review methods of preventing bleeding with patient (use of soft toothbrush, avoid IM and SC injections, avoid potentially traumatic activities).
- Advise patient that the risk of hepatitis or AIDS transmission may be diminished by the use of heat-treated or monoclonal antibody preparations. Current screening programs should decrease the risk.

EVALUATION

Effectiveness of therapy can be demonstrated by: ▪ Prevention of spontaneous bleeding ▪ Cessation of bleeding.

APRACLONIDINE

(ap-ra-**kloe**-ni-deen)
aplonidine, lopidine

CLASSIFICATION(S):
Ophthalmic—alpha-adrenergic agonist
Pregnancy Category C

INDICATIONS

- Management of elevated intraocular pressure in patients who have undergone argon laser ocular surgical procedures (trabeculoplasty, iridotomy).

ACTION

■ Reduces the formation of aqueous humor as a result of stimulating alpha-adrenergic receptors in the eye. **Therapeutic Effect:** ■ Lowering of elevated intraocular pressure.

PHARMACOKINETICS

Absorption: Some systemic absorption follows ophthalmic application.
Distribution: Distribution not known.
Metabolism and Excretion: Metabolism and excretion not known.
Half-life: UK.

CONTRAINDICATIONS AND PRECAUTIONS

Contraindicated in: ■ Hypersensitivity to apraclonidine, clonidine, or benzalkonium chloride.
Use Cautiously in: ■ Pregnancy, lactation, or children <21 (safety not established).

ADVERSE REACTIONS AND SIDE EFFECTS*

EENT: upper lid elevation, conjunctival blanching, mydriasis, ocular irritation.

INTERACTIONS

Drug-Drug: ■ **Ophthalmic beta-adrenergic blockers**—intraocular pressure lowering effect may be additive.

ROUTE AND DOSAGE

■ **Ophth (Adults):** 1 drop in eye 1 hr prior to surgery, repeat when surgery is completed.

PHARMACODYNAMICS (lowering of intraocular pressure)

	ONSET	PEAK	DURATION
Ophth	1 hr	3–5 hr	12 hr

NURSING IMPLICATIONS

Assessment

□ Monitor pulse and blood pressure. Systemic absorption may cause slight decrease in pulse or blood pressure.

Potential Nursing Diagnoses

■ Knowledge deficit related to medication regimen (patient/family teaching).

Implementation

■ **General Info:** Administer ophthalmic soln by having patient tilt head back and look up, gently depress lower lid with index finger until conjunctival sac is exposed and instill medication. After instillation, maintain gentle pressure on the inner canthus for 1 min to avoid systemic absorption of the drug. Wait at least 5 min before administering other types of eyedrops.

Patient/Family Teaching

□ Instruct patient to report involuntary elevation of upper eyelid or ocular irritation.

Evaluation

Effectiveness of therapy can be demonstrated by: ■ Prevention of increased intraocular pressure during and after ocular laser surgery.

ASCORBIC ACID

(as-**kor**-bik **as**-id)
{Apo-C}, Arco-Cee, Ascorbicap, Cecon, Cemill, Cetane, Cevalin, Ce-Vi-Bid, Ce-Vi-Sol, Flavorcee, {Redoxon}, Vitamin C

CLASSIFICATION(S):
Vitamin—water-soluble
Pregnancy Category C

INDICATIONS

■ Treatment and prevention of vitamin C deficiency (scurvy) in conjunction with dietary supplementation ■ Supplemental therapy in some GI diseases, during long-term parenteral nutrition or chronic hemodialysis ■ States of increased requirements such as: □ Pregnancy □ Lactation □ Stress □ Hyperthyroidism □ Trauma □ Burns □ Infancy. **Unlabeled Uses:** ■ Urinary acidification ■ Prevention of the common cold.

*Underlines indicate most frequent; **CAPITALS** indicate life-threatening.

{} = Available in Canada only.

ACTION

▪ Necessary for collagen formation and tissue repair ▪ Involved in oxidation-reduction reactions, tyrosine, folic acid, iron and carbohydrate metabolism, lipid and protein synthesis, cellular respiration, and resisting infection. **Therapeutic Effect:** ▪ Replacement in deficiency states.

PHARMACOKINETICS

Absorption: Actively absorbed following oral administration by a saturable process.
Distribution: Widely distributed. Crosses the placenta and enters breast milk.
Metabolism and Excretion: Oxidized to inactive compounds that are excreted by the kidneys. When serum levels are high, unchanged ascorbic acid is excreted by the kidneys.
Half-life: UK.

CONTRAINDICATIONS AND PRECAUTIONS

Contraindicated in: ▪ No known contraindications ▪ Tartrazine hypersensitivity (some products contain tartrazine—FDC yellow dye #5).
Use Cautiously in: ▪ Recurrent kidney stones ▪ Avoid chronic use of large doses in pregnant women.

ADVERSE REACTIONS AND SIDE EFFECTS*

CNS: fatigue, headache, insomnia, drowsiness.
GI: nausea, vomiting, heartburn, cramps, diarrhea.
GU: kidney stones.
Derm: flushing.
Hemat: deep vein thrombosis, sickle cell crises, hemolysis (in G6-PD deficiency).
Local: pain at SC or IM sites.

INTERACTIONS

Drug-Drug: ▪ If urinary acidification occurs, may increase excretion and decrease effects of **mexiletine, amphetamines,** or **tricyclic antidepressants** ▪ May decrease response to **oral anticoagulants** (large doses only) ▪ **Smoking, salicylates,** and **primidone** may increase requirements for ascorbic acid ▪ Increases iron toxicity when given concurrently with **deferoxamine.**

ROUTE AND DOSAGE

Scurvy

- **PO, IV, IM, SC (Adults):** 100–250 mg 1–2 times daily.
- **PO, IV, IM, SC (Children):** 100–300 mg/day in divided doses.

Supplementation

- **PO (Adults):** 45–60 mg/day.

Chronic Hemodialysis

- **PO (Adults):** 100–200 mg/day.

Pregnancy and Lactation

- **PO (Adults):** 60–80 mg/day.

Other States of Increased Requirements

- **PO (Adults):** 150–500 mg/day.

PHARMACODYNAMICS (response to skeletal and hemorrhagic changes in scurvy)

	ONSET	PEAK	DURATION
PO, IM, IV, SC	2 days–3 wk	UK	UK

NURSING IMPLICATIONS

Assessment

- **Vitamin C Deficiency:** Assess patient for signs of vitamin C deficiency (faulty bone and tooth development, gingivitis, bleeding gums, and loosened teeth) prior to and throughout therapy. Vitamin C deficiency is also called scurvy.
- □ Megadoses of ascorbic acid (>10 times the RDA requirement) may cause false-negative results for occult blood in the stool, false-positive urine glucose test results with copper sulfate method (Clinitest), and false-negative urine glucose test results with glucose oxidase method (Tes-Tape).

*Underlines indicate most frequent; **CAPITALS** indicate life-threatening.

- May cause decreased serum bilirubin and increased urine oxalate, urate, and cysteine levels.
- **Lab Test Considerations:** *Urinary Acidification*—Monitor the urinary pH of patients receiving ascorbic acid for urinary acidification periodically throughout therapy.

Potential Nursing Diagnoses

- Nutrition, altered: less than body requirements (indications).
- Knowledge deficit related to medication regimen (patient/family teaching).

Implementation

- **General Info:** Often ordered as a part of multivitamin supplementation, because inadequate diet often results in multiple-vitamin deficiency.
- **PO:** Extended-release tablets and capsules should be swallowed whole without crushing, breaking, or chewing; contents of capsules may be mixed with jelly or jam. Chewable tablets should be chewed well or crushed before swallowing. Effervescent tablets should be dissolved in a glass of water immediately before swallowing. Oral soln may be mixed with fruit juice, cereal, or other food.
- Available in combination with other vitamins and iron (see Appendix A).
- **IM:** May be preferred route due to increased absorption and utilization.
- **Direct IV:** Ascorbic acid may be administered IV undiluted at a rate of 100 mg over at least 1 min. Rapid IV administration may result in temporary dizziness and fainting.
- **Intermittent Infusion:** Dilute with D5W, D10W, 0.9% NaCl, 0.45% NaCl, lactated Ringer's or Ringer's soln, dextrose/saline or dextrose/Ringer's combinations. At room temperature, pressure in ampules may increase; wrap with protective cover before breaking.
- **Syringe Compatibility:** metoclopramide.
- **Syringe Incompatibility:** cefazolin or doxapram.
- **Additive Compatibility:** amikacin, calcium chloride, calcium gluceptate, calcium gluconate, cephalothin, chloramphenicol, chlorpromazine, colistimethate, cyanocobalamin, diphenhydramine, heparin, kanamycin, methicillin, methyldopate, penicillin G potassium, polymyxin B, prednisolone, procaine, prochlorperazine, promethazine, tetracycline, or verapamil.
- **Additive Incompatibility:** bleomycin, cephapirin, nafcillin, sodium bicarbonate, or warfarin.

Patient/Family Teaching

- **General Info:** Advise patient to take this medication as directed and not to exceed dose prescribed. Excess dosage may lead to urinary stone formation. If a dose is missed, skip dose and return to dosage schedule.
- **Vitamin C Deficiency:** Encourage patient to comply with physician's diet recommendations. Explain that the best source of vitamins is a well-balanced diet with foods from the 4 basic food groups.
- Foods high in ascorbic acid include citrus fruits, tomatoes, strawberries, cantaloupe, and raw peppers. Gradual loss of ascorbic acid occurs when fresh food is stored, but not when frozen. Rapid loss is caused by drying, salting, and cooking.
- Patients self-medicating with vitamin supplements should be cautioned not to exceed RDA (see Appendix L). The effectiveness of megadoses of vitamins for treatment of various medical conditions is unproven and may cause side effects. Abrupt withdrawal of megadoses of ascorbic acid may cause rebound deficiency.
- **Urinary Acidification:** Teach patients taking vitamin C for urinary acidification how to check urine pH.

Evaluation

Effectiveness of therapy may be determined by: ▪ Decrease in the symptoms of ascorbic acid deficiency ▪ Acidification of the urine.

A

ASPARAGINASE
(a-**spare**-a-gin-ase)
Colaspase, Elspar, {Kidrolase}

CLASSIFICATION(S):
Antineoplastic—enzyme
Pregnancy Category C

INDICATIONS
▪ Part of combination chemotherapy in the treatment of acute lymphocytic leukemia (ALL) unresponsive to first line agents.

ACTION
▪ Catalyst in the conversion of asparagine (an amino acid) to aspartic acid and ammonia ▪ Depletes asparagine in leukemic cells. **Therapeutic Effect:** ▪ Death of leukemic cells.

PHARMACOKINETICS
Absorption: Not absorbed from the GI tract. Is absorbed from IM sites.
Distribution: Mostly remains in the intravascular space. Poor penetration into the CSF.
Metabolism and Excretion: Slowly sequestered in the reticuloendothelial system.
Half-life: IV, 8–30 hr; IM, 39–49 hr.

CONTRAINDICATIONS AND PRECAUTIONS
Contraindicated in: ▪ Previous hypersensitivity.
Use Cautiously in: ▪ History of hypersensitivity reactions ▪ Severe liver disease ▪ Renal disease ▪ Pancreatric disease ▪ CNS depression ▪ Clotting abnormalities ▪ Patients with childbearing potential ▪ Chronic debilitating illnesses.

ADVERSE REACTIONS AND SIDE EFFECTS*
CNS: depression, somnolence, fatigue, SEIZURES, coma, headache, confusion, irritability, agitation, dizziness, hallucinations.
GI: <u>nausea</u>, <u>vomiting</u>, anorexia, cramps, weight loss, pancreatitis, hepatotoxicity.
Derm: rashes, urticaria.
Endo: hyperglycemia.
Hemat: coagulation abnormalities, transient bone marrow depression.
Metab: hyperuricemia, hyperammonemia.
Misc: hypersensitivity reactions including ANAPHYLAXIS.

INTERACTIONS
Drug-Drug: ▪ May negate the antineoplastic activity of **methotrexate** ▪ May enhance the hepatotoxicity of other **hepatotoxic drugs** ▪ Additive hyperglycemia with **glucocorticoids** ▪ Concurrent IV use with or immediately preceding **vincristine** may result in increased neurotoxicity.

ROUTE AND DOSAGE
Note: Various other regimens may be used.

Multiple Agent Induction Regimen (in combination with vincristine and prednisone)
- **IV (Children):** 1000 IU/kg/day for 10 successive days beginning on day 22 of regimen.

Single-Agent Therapy for Acute Lymphocytic Leukemia
- **IV (Adults and Children):** 200 IU/kg daily for 28 days.

Desensitization Regimen
- **IV (Adults and Children):** Administer 1 IU then double dose every 10 min until total dose for that day has been given or reaction occurs.

Test Dose
- **Intradermal (Adults and Children):** 2 IU

PHARMACODYNAMICS (depletion of asparagine)

	ONSET	PEAK*	DURATION
IM	immediate	14–24 hr	23–33 days
IV	immediate	UK	23–33 days

*Plasma levels of asparaginase.

{} = Available in Canada only.
*<u>Underlines</u> indicate most frequent; **CAPITALS** indicate life-threatening.

NURSING IMPLICATIONS

Assessment

- Monitor vital signs prior to and frequently during therapy. Inform physician if fever or chills occur.
- Monitor intake and output. Notify physician if significant discrepancies occur. Encourage patient to drink 2000–3000 ml/day to promote excretion of uric acid. Allopurinol and alkalinization of the urine may be ordered to help prevent urate stone formation.
- Monitor for hypersensitivity reaction (urticaria, diaphoresis, facial swelling, joint pain, hypotension, bronchospasm). Epinephrine and resuscitation equipment should be readily available. Reaction may occur up to 2 hr after administration.
- Assess nausea, vomiting, and appetite. Weigh weekly. Confer with physician regarding an antiemetic prior to administration.
- Monitor affect and neurologic status. Notify physician if depression, drowsiness, or hallucinations occur. Symptoms usually resolve 2–3 days after drug is discontinued.
- **Lab Test Considerations:** Monitor CBC prior to and periodically throughout therapy. May alter coagulation studies. Platelets, PT, PTT, and thrombin time may be increased. May cause elevated BUN.
- Hepatotoxity may be manifested by increased SGOT (AST), SGPT (ALT), alkaline phosphatase, bilirubin, or cholesterol. Liver function tests usually return to normal after therapy. May cause pancreatitis; monitor for elevated amylase or glucose.
- May cause decreased serum calcium.
- May cause elevated serum and urine uric acid concentrations.
- May interfere with thyroid function tests.

Potential Nursing Diagnoses

- Injury, high risk for (side effects).
- Infection, high risk for (side effects).
- Knowledge deficit related to medication regimen (patient/family teaching).

Implementation

- **General Info:** Soln should be prepared in a biologic cabinet. Wear gloves, gown, and mask while handling medication. Discard equipment in specially designated containers (see Appendix I).
- If coagulopathy develops, apply pressure to venipuncture sites; avoid IM injections.
- **Test Dose:** Intradermal test dose must be performed prior to initial dose, and doses must be separated by more than 1 wk. Reconstitute vial with 5 ml of sterile water or 0.9% NaCl for injection (without preservatives). Add 0.1 ml of this 2000 IU/ml soln to 9.9 ml additional diluent to yield a 20 IU/ml soln. Inject 0.1 ml (2 IU) intradermally. Observe site for 1 hr for formation of wheal. Wheal is indicative of a positive reaction; physician may order desensitization therapy.
- **Desensitization Therapy:** Begin desensitization therapy by administering 1 IU every 10 min IV. Double dose every 10 min if hypersensitivity does not occur until full daily dose is administered.
- **IM:** Prepare for IM dose by adding 2 ml of 0.9% NaCl for injection (without preservatives) to the 10,000-IU vial. Shake vial gently. Administer no more than 2 ml per injection site.
- **Direct IV:** Prepare IV dose by diluting 10,000-IU vial with 5 ml of sterile water or 0.9% NaCl (without preservatives). If gelatinous fibers are present, administration through a 5-micron filter will not alter potency. Administration through a 0.2-micron filter may cause loss of potency. Soln should be clear after reconstitution. Discard if cloudy. Stable for 8 hr if refrigerated.
- *Rate:* Administer through Y-site of rapidly flowing IV of D5W or 0.9% NaCl over at least 30 min. Maintain IV infusion for 2 hr after dose.

A

PATIENT/FAMILY TEACHING

- ▫ Instruct patient to notify physician if abdominal pain, severe nausea and vomiting, jaundice, fever, chills, sore throat, bleeding or bruising, excess thirst or urination, or mouth sores occur. Caution patient to avoid crowds and persons with known infections. Instruct patient to use soft toothbrush, electric razor, and to avoid falls. Patients should also be cautioned not to drink alcoholic beverages or take medication containing aspirin, because these may precipitate gastric bleeding.
- ▫ Advise patient of the need for contraception.
- ▫ Instruct patient not to receive any vaccinations without advice of physician. Advise parents that this may alter immunization schedule.
- ▫ Emphasize need for periodic lab test to monitor for side effects.

EVALUATION

Effectiveness of therapy can be demonstrated by: ▪ Improvement of hematologic status in patients with leukemia.

ASPIRIN

(**as**-pir-in)

acetylsalicylic acid, ASA, {Arthrinol}, Artria, Aspergum, {Astrin}, Bayer Aspirin, {Coryphen}, Easprin, Ecotrin, {Entrophen}, Halfprin, Measurin, {Novasen}, {Riphen}, {Sal-Adult}, {Sal-Infant}, {Supasa}, {Triaphen}, ZORprin

CLASSIFICATION(S):
Non-narcotic analgesic, Nonsteroidal anti-inflammatory agent, Antipyretic, Antiplatelet agent
Pregnancy Category D

INDICATIONS

▪ Management of inflammatory disorders including: ▫ Rheumatoid arthritis ▫ Osteoarthritis ▪ Treatment of mild to moderate pain ▪ Treatment of fever due to a variety of causes ▪ Prophylaxis of transient ischemic attacks ▪ Prophylaxis of myocardial infarction.

ACTION

▪ Produces analgesia and reduces inflammation and fever by inhibiting the production of prostaglandins. ▪ Decreases platelet aggregation. **Therapeutic Effects:** ▪ Analgesia ▪ Reduction of inflammation ▪ Reduction of fever ▪ Decreased incidence of transient ischemic attacks and myocardial infarction

PHARMACOKINETICS

Absorption: Well absorbed from the upper small intestine. Absorption from enteric coated preparations may be unreliable. Rectal absorption is slow and variable.

Distribution: Rapidly and widely distributed. Crosses the placenta and enters breast milk.

Metabolism and Excretion: Extensively metabolized by the liver. Inactive metabolites excreted by the kidneys.

Half-life: 2–3 hr for low doses. For larger doses half-life may increase up to 15–30 hr due to saturation of liver metabolism.

CONTRAINDICATIONS AND PRECAUTIONS

Contraindicated in: ▪ Hypersensitivity to aspirin, tartrazine (FDC yellow dye #5), or other salicylates ▪ Cross-sensitivity with other nonsteroidal anti-inflammatory agents may exist ▪ Bleeding disorders or thrombocytopenia.

Use Cautiously in: ▪ History of GI bleeding or ulcer disease ▪ Severe renal or hepatic disease ▪ Pregnancy (may have adverse effects on fetus and mother) ▪ Lactation (safety not established) ▪ Self-medication for more than 10 days in adults or 5 days in children without medical supervision.

ADVERSE REACTIONS AND SIDE EFFECTS*

EENT: tinnitus, hearing loss.
GI: dyspepsia, heartburn, epigastric distress, nausea, vomiting, anorexia, abdominal pain, GI bleeding, hepatotoxicity.
Hemat: anemia, hemolysis.
Misc: noncardiogenic pulmonary edema, allergic reactions including ANAPHYLAXIS and LARYNGEAL EDEMA.

INTERACTIONS

Drug–Drug: ▪ May potentiate **oral anticoagulants, heparin,** or **thrombolytic agents** ▪ May enhance the activity of **penicillins, phenytoin, methotrexate, valproic acid, oral hypoglycemic agents,** and **sulfonamides** ▪ May antagonize the beneficial effects of **probenecid** or **sulfinpyrazone** ▪ **Glucocorticoids** may decrease serum salicylate levels ▪ **Urinary acidification** enhances reabsorption and may increase serum salicylate levels ▪ **Alkalinization of the urine** or the ingestion of large amounts of **antacids** promotes excretion and decreases serum salicylate levels ▪ May blunt the therapeutic response to **diuretics, antihypertensives,** or **nonsteroidal anti-inflammatory agents** ▪ May increase the risk of bleeding with **cefamandole, cefoperazone, cefotetan, moxalactam, valproic acid,** or **plicamycin** ▪ Increased risk of gastrointestinal irritation with **nonsteroidal anti-inflammatory agents** ▪ Increased risk of ototoxicity with **vancomycin.**
Drug–Food: ▪ **Foods capable of acidifying the urine** (see Appendix K) may enhance reabsorption and increase serum salicylate levels.

ROUTE AND DOSAGE

Analgesia and Antipyresis

- **PO, Rect (Adults):** 325–1000 mg q 4–6 hr as needed (not to exceed 4 g/day).
- **PO, Rect (Children 2–11 yr):** 65 mg/kg/day in 4–6 divided doses.

Anti-Inflammatory

- **PO (Adults):** 2.6–5.2 g/day in divided doses.
- **PO (Children):** 90–130 mg/kg/day in divided doses.

Prevention of Transient Ischemic Attacks

- **PO (Adults):** 1.3 g daily in 2–4 divided doses.

Prevention of Myocardial Infarction

- **PO (Adults):** 325 mg/day (smaller doses have been used).

PHARMACODYNAMICS

	ONSET	PEAK	DURATION
PO	5–30 min	1–3 hr	3–6 hr
Rect	1–2 hr	4–5 hr	7 hr

NURSING IMPLICATIONS

Assessment

- **General Info:** Patients who have asthma, allergies, and nasal polyps or who are allergic to tartrazine are at an increased risk for developing hypersensitivity reactions.
- **Pain:** Assess pain and limitation of movement; note type, location, and intensity prior to and 30–60 min following administration.
- **Fever:** Assess fever and note associated signs (diaphoresis, tachycardia, malaise, chills).
- **Lab Test Considerations:** Aspirin prolongs bleeding time for 4–7 days and, in large doses, may cause prolonged prothrombin time, false-negative urine glucose test results with glucose oxidase method (Clinistix, Tes-Tape), and false-positive urine glucose test results with copper sulfate method (Clinitest).
- **Toxicity and Overdose:** Observe patient for the onset of tinnitus, hyperventilation, agitation, mental confusion, lethargy, diarrhea, and sweating. If these symptoms appear, withhold medication and notify physician immediately.

*Underlines indicate most frequent; **CAPITALS** indicate life-threatening.

Potential Nursing Diagnoses

- Comfort, altered: pain (indications).
- Mobility, impaired physical (indications).
- Knowledge deficit related to medication regimen (patient/family teaching).

Implementation

- **General Info:** Available in a variety of forms (tablets, caplets, chewable tablets, gum, enteric-coated tablets, effervescent tablets, and buffered aspirin).
  - Available in combination with many other drugs (see Appendix A).
- **PO:** Administer aspirin after meals or with food or an antacid to minimize gastric irritation. Food slows but will not alter the total amount absorbed.
  - Do not crush or chew enteric-coated tablets (Ecotrin). Do not take antacids within 1–2 hr of enteric-coated tablets. Chewable tablets may be chewed, dissolved in liquid, or swallowed whole. Some extended-release tablets may be broken or crumbled but must not be ground up before swallowing. See manufacturer's prescribing information for individual products.

Patient/Family Teaching

- **General Info:** Instruct patient to take aspirin with a full glass of water and to remain in an upright position for 15–30 min after administration.
  - Advise patient to report tinnitus, unusual bleeding of gums, bruising, black, tarry stools, or fever lasting longer than 3 days.
  - Caution patient to avoid concurrent use of alcohol with this medication to minimize possible gastric irritation.
  - Patients on a sodium restricted diet should be taught to avoid effervescent tablets or buffered aspirin preparations.
  - Tablets with an acetic (vinegar-like) odor should be discarded.
  - Advise patients on long-term therapy to inform physician or dentist of medication regimen prior to surgery. Aspirin may need to be withheld for 1 wk prior to surgery.
  - Centers for Disease Control warn against giving aspirin to children or adolescents with varicella (chickenpox), influenza-like or viral illnesses because of a possible association with Reye's syndrome.
- **Transient Ischemic Attacks or Myocardial Infarction:** Advise patients receiving aspirin prophylactically to take only prescribed dosage. Increasing the dosage has not been found to provide additional benefits.

Evaluation

Effectiveness of therapy can be demonstrated by: ▪ The relief of mild to moderate discomfort ▪ Increased ease of joint movement ▪ Reduction of fever ▪ Prevention of transient ischemic attacks ▪ Prevention of myocardial infarction.

ASTEMIZOLE

(a-**stem**-mi-zole)
Hismanyl

CLASSIFICATION(S):
Antihistamine
Pregnancy Category C

INDICATIONS

▪ Symptomatic relief of allergic symptoms caused by histamine release. ▪ Conditions in which it is most useful include seasonal allergic rhinitis and chronic idiopathic urticaria ▪ May be less sedating than other antihistamines.

ACTION

▪ Blocks the following effects of histamine: ▫ Vasodilation ▫ Increased GI tract secretions ▫ Increased heart rate ▫ Hypotension. **Therapeutic Effect:** ▪ Relief of symptoms associated with histamine excess usually seen in allergic conditions. Does not block the release of histamine.

PHARMACOKINETICS

Absorption: Well absorbed following oral administration.
Distribution: Distribution not known.
Metabolism and Excretion: Extensively metabolized by the liver, partially converted to desmethylastemizole, which has antihistaminic activity.
Half-life: 100 hr—astemizole; 12 days—desmethylastemizole.

CONTRAINDICATIONS AND PRECAUTIONS

Contraindicated in: ▪ Hypersensitivity ▪ Acute attacks of asthma ▪ Lactation (avoid use).
Use Cautiously in: ▪ Narrow-angle glaucoma ▪ Liver disease ▪ Elderly patients (more susceptible to adverse reactions) ▪ Pregnancy or children <12 yr (safety not established).

ADVERSE REACTIONS AND SIDE EFFECTS*

CNS: drowsiness, ataxia, dizziness, inability to concentrate, headache, fatigue, stimulation.
EENT: conjunctivitis, pharyngitis.
Resp: cough.
GI: dry mouth, nausea, diarrhea, abdominal pain, flatulence.
Derm: rash, eczema.
MS: joint pain.
Misc: weight gain.

INTERACTIONS

Drug-Drug: ▪ Additive CNS depression with other **CNS depressants** including **alcohol, narcotics,** and **sedative/hypnotics** ▪ **MAO inhibitors** intensify and prolong the anticholinergic effects of antihistamines.
Drug-Food: ▪ **Food** decreases the absorption of astemizole.

ROUTE AND DOSAGE

- **PO (Adults):** 10 mg/day. More rapid effect may be achieved by giving 30 mg on day 1, 20 mg on day 2, then 10 mg/day thereafter.

PHARMACODYNAMICS (antihistaminic effects)

	ONSET	PEAK	DURATION
PO	2–3 days	UK	up to several wks

NURSING IMPLICATIONS

Assessment

- □ Assess allergy symptoms (rhinitis, conjunctivitis, hives) prior to and periodically throughout course of therapy.
- □ Assess lung sounds and character of bronchial secretions. Maintain fluid intake of 1500–2000 ml/day to decrease viscosity of secretions.
- ▪ **Lab Test Considerations:** May cause false-negative allergy skin testing.

Potential Nursing Diagnoses

- ▪ Airway clearance, ineffective (indications).
- ▪ Injury, high risk for (adverse reactions).
- ▪ Knowledge deficit related to medication regimen (patient/family teaching).

Implementation

- ▪ **PO:** Administer oral doses on empty stomach.

Patient/Family Teaching

- □ Instruct patient to take medication 1 hr before or 2 hr after eating.
- □ May cause drowsiness. Caution patient to avoid driving or other activities requiring alertness until response to medication is known.
- □ Discuss possibility of increased appetite. Patients on chronic therapy may need to limit caloric intake and increase activity to avoid undesired weight gain.
- □ Advise patient that good oral hygiene, frequent rinsing of mouth with water, and sugarless gum or candy may help relieve dry mouth. Patient should notify dentist if dry mouth persists >2 wk.
- □ Instruct patient to contact physician if symptoms persist.

*Underlines indicate most frequent; **CAPITALS** indicate life-threatening.

A

Evaluation

Effectiveness of therapy may be determined by: ▪ Decrease in allergic symptoms.

ATENOLOL

(a-**ten**-oh-lole)
Tenormin

CLASSIFICATION(S):
Antihypertensive—beta-adrenergic blocker, Beta-adrenergic blocker—selective, Antianginal
Pregnancy Category C

INDICATIONS

▪ **PO:** Treatment of hypertension, alone or in combination with other agents ▪ **PO:** Management of angina pectoris ▪ **PO, IV:** Prevention of myocardial infarction. **Unlabeled Uses:** ▪ Management of arrhythmias, hypertrophic cardiomyopathy, mitral valve prolapse, pheochromocytoma, vascular headache, tremors, thyrotoxicosis.

ACTION

▪ Blocks stimulation of $beta_1$ (myocardial) adrenergic receptors. In therapeutic doses does not usually effect $beta_2$ (pulmonary, vascular, or uterine) receptor sites. **Therapeutic Effects:** ▪ Decreased heart rate ▪ Decreased blood pressure ▪ Prevention of myocardial infarction.

PHARMACOKINETICS

Absorption: Incompletely absorbed from the GI tract (50–60%).
Distribution: Does not significantly cross the blood–brain barrier. Crosses the placenta and enters breast milk.
Metabolism and Excretion: 40–50% excreted unchanged by the kidneys. Remainder excreted in the feces as unabsorbed drug.
Half-life: 6–9 hr.

CONTRAINDICATIONS AND PRECAUTIONS

Contraindicated in: ▪ Uncompensated congestive heart failure ▪ Pulmonary edema ▪ Cardiogenic shock ▪ Bradycardia ▪ Heart block ▪ Lactation.
Use Cautiously in: ▪ Thyroxcicosis (may mask symptoms) ▪ Diabetes mellitus (may mask symptoms of hypoglycemia) ▪ Renal impairment (dosage reduction required) ▪ Pregnancy and children (safety not established).

ADVERSE REACTIONS AND SIDE EFFECTS*

CNS: fatigue, weakness, dizziness, depression, memory loss, mental changes, nightmares, drowsiness.
EENT: dry eyes, blurred vision.
Resp: bronchospasm, wheezing.
CV: **BRADYCARDIA, CONGESTIVE HEART FAILURE, PULMONARY EDEMA,** peripheral vasoconstriction, hypotension.
GI: constipation, diarrhea, nausea.
GU: impotence, diminished libido.
Endo: hyperglycemia.

INTERACTIONS

Drug-Drug: ▪ **General anesthesia, IV phenytoin,** and **verapamil** may cause additive myocardial depression ▪ Additive bradycardia may occur with concurrent use of **cardiac glycosides** ▪ Additive hypotension may occur with other **antihypertensive agents** or **nitrates** ▪ Use with **epinephrine** may result in unopposed alpha-adrenergic stimulation ▪ Concurrent **thyroid** administration may decrease effectiveness.

ROUTE AND DOSAGE

▪ **PO (Adults):** 50–150 mg once daily.
▪ **IV (Adults):** 5 mg over 5 min initially, wait 10 min then give another 5 mg.

PHARMACODYNAMICS (antihypertensive response)

	ONSET	PEAK	DURATION
PO	60 min	2–4 hr	24 hr

*Underlines indicate most frequent; **CAPITALS** indicate life-threatening.

NURSING IMPLICATIONS

Assessment

- □ Monitor blood pressure and pulse frequently during dosage adjustment and periodically throughout therapy.
- □ Monitor intake and output ratios and weigh daily. Assess patient routinely for signs and symptoms of fluid overload (peripheral edema, dyspnea, rales/crackles, weight gain, jugular venous distension).
- ■ **Lab Test Considerations:** May cause elevated serum uric acid, BUN, lipoproteins, and triglyceride concentrations.

Potential Nursing Diagnoses

- ■ Activity intolerance (indications).
- ■ Cardiac output, decreased (adverse reactions).
- ■ Knowledge deficit related to medication regimen (patient/family teaching).

Implementation

- ■ **General Info:** Take apical pulse prior to administration. If <50 bpm, withhold medication and notify physician.
- □ Available in combination with chlorthalidone (Tenoretic); see Appendix A.
- ■ **PO:** Atenolol may be administered without regard to meals. Tablets may be crushed and mixed with fluids if the patient has difficulty swallowing.

Patient/Family Teaching

- □ Instruct patient to take medication exactly as directed, even if feeling well; do not skip or double up on missed doses. A missed dose may be taken as soon as remembered up to 8 hr before next dose. Abrupt withdrawal may precipitate life-threatening arrhythmias, hypertension, or myocardial ischemia.
- □ Teach patient and family how to check pulse and blood pressure. Advise them to take pulse daily and blood pressure weekly, and to report any significant changes to physician.
- □ May occasionally cause drowsiness. Caution patient to avoid driving or other activities that require alertness until response to drug is known.
- □ Advise patients to make position changes slowly to minimize orthostatic hypotension.
- □ Reinforce need to continue additional therapies for hypertension (weight loss, restricted sodium intake, stress reduction, regular exercise, moderation of alcohol consumption, and cessation of smoking). Atenolol controls but does not cure hypertension.
- □ Caution patient that atenolol may cause increased sensitivity to cold.
- □ Advise patient to consult physician or pharmacist before taking any over-the-counter drugs concurrently with this medication.
- □ Diabetics should closely monitor blood sugar, especially if weakness, malaise, irritability, or fatigue occur.
- □ Instruct patient to inform physician or dentist of this therapy prior to treatment or surgery.
- □ Advise patients to carry identification describing disease process and medication regimen at all times.
- □ Instruct patient to notify physician if symptoms of fluid overload, slow pulse rate, dizziness, confusion, depression, skin rash, fever, sore throat, or unusual bleeding or bruising occur.

Evaluation

Effectiveness of therapy can be demonstrated by: ■ Decrease in blood pressure ■ Decrease in anginal attacks and an increase in activity tolerance.

ATRACURIUM

(a-tra-**cure**-ee-um)
Tracrium

CLASSIFICATION(S):
Neuromuscular blocking agent—nondepolarizing
Pregnancy Category C

INDICATIONS

- ■ Production of skeletal muscle paralysis, after induction of anesthesia.

A

ACTION

▪ Prevents neuromuscular transmission by blocking the effect of acetylcholine at the myoneural junction. **Therapeutic Effect:** ▪ Skeletal muscle paralysis.

PHARMACOKINETICS

Absorption: Following IV administration absorption is essentially complete.
Distribution: Distributes into extracellular space. Crosses the placenta.
Metabolism and Excretion: Metabolized in plasma.
Half-life: 20 min.

CONTRAINDICATIONS AND PRECAUTIONS

Contraindicated in: ▪ Hypersensitivity to atracurium, benzenesulfonic acid, or benzyl alcohol.
Use Cautiously in: ▪ History of pulmonary disease ▪ Renal or liver impairment ▪ Elderly or debilitated patients ▪ Electrolyte disturbances ▪ Digitalized patients ▪ Myasthenia gravis or myasthenic syndromes (extreme caution) ▪ Has been used in pregnant women undergoing cesarian section.

ADVERSE REACTIONS AND SIDE EFFECTS*

CV: bradycardia, hypotension.
Resp: wheezing, increased bronchial secretions.
Derm: skin flush, erythema, pruritus, urticaria.
Misc: allergic reactions, including ANAPHYLAXIS.

INTERACTIONS

Drug-Drug: ▪ Intensity and duration of paralysis may be prolonged by pretreatment with **succinylcholine, general anesthesia, aminoglycoside antibiotics, polymyxin B, colistin, clindamycin, lidocaine, quinidine, procainamide, beta-adrenergic blocking agents, potassium-losing diuretics**, or **magnesium**.

ROUTE AND DOSAGE

- **IV (Adults and Children >2 yr):** 0.4–0.5 mg/kg initially (0.25–0.35 mg/kg if administered after steady state anesthesia with enflurane or isoflurane or 0.3–0.4 mg/kg following succinylcholine), then 0.08–0.1 mg/kg as necessary or 5–9 mcg/kg/min by continuous infusion (range 2–15 mcg/kg/min).
- **IV (Children 1 mon–2 yr):** 0.3–0.4 mg/kg initially (while under halothane anesthesia).

PHARMACODYNAMICS (neuromuscular blockade)

	ONSET	PEAK	DURATION
IV	2–2.5 min	5 min	30–40 min

NURSING IMPLICATIONS

Assessment

- □ Assess respiratory status continuously throughout atracurium therapy. Atracurium should be used only by individuals experienced in endotracheal intubation, and equipment for this procedure should be readily available.
- □ Neuromuscular response to atracurium should be monitored with a peripheral nerve stimulator intraoperatively. Paralysis is initially selective and usually occurs sequentially in the following muscles: levator muscles of eyelids, muscles of mastication, limb muscles, abdominal muscles, muscles of the glottis, intercostal muscles, and the diaphragm. Recovery of muscle function usually occurs in reverse order.
- □ Observe the patient for residual muscle weakness and respiratory distress during the recovery period.
- ▪ **Toxicity and Overdose:** If overdose occurs use peripheral nerve stimulator to determine the degree of neuromuscular blockade. Maintain airway patency and ventilation until recovery of normal respirations occur.

*Underlines indicate most frequent; **CAPITALS** indicate life-threatening.

- ▫ Administration of anticholinesterase agents (edrophonium, neostigmine, pyridostigmine) may be used to antagonize the action of atracurium. Atropine is usually administered prior to or concurrently with anticholinesterase agents to counteract the muscarinic effects.
- ▫ Administration of fluids and vasopressors may be necessary to treat severe hypotension or shock.

Potential Nursing Diagnoses

- ▪ Breathing pattern, ineffective (indications).
- ▪ Communication, impaired: verbal (side effects).
- ▪ Fear (side effects).

Implementation

- ▪ **General Info:** Dose is titrated to patient response.
- ▫ Atracurium has no effect on consciousness or the pain threshold. Adequate anesthesia should always be used when atracurium is used as an adjunct to surgical procedures.
- ▫ Store in refrigerator.
- ▪ **IM:** Avoid IM route; may cause tissue irritation.
- ▪ **Direct IV:** Administer initial IV dose as a bolus over 1 min.
- ▪ **Intermittent Infusion:** Maintenance dose is usually required 20–45 min following initial dose
- ▫ Dilute further in D5W, 0.9% NaCl, or D5/0.9% NaCl and administer every 15–25 min or by continuous infusion.
- ▪ **Continuous Infusion:** Maintenance dose is administered by infusion. Titrate according to patient response.
- ▪ **Y-Site Compatibility:** aminophylline, cefazolin, cefuroxime, cimetidine, co-trimoxazole, dobutamine, dopamine, epinephrine, esmolol, fentanyl, gentamicin, heparin, hydrocortisone sodium succinate, isoproterenol, lorazepam, midazolam, morphine, nitroglycerin, ranitidine, sodium nitroprusside, or vancomycin.
- ▪ **Y-Site Incompatibility:** diazepam.
- ▪ **Additive Incompatibility:** Incompatible with most barbiturates and sodium bicarbonate; do not administer in the same syringe or through the same needle during infusion.

Patient/Family Teaching

- ▫ Explain all procedures to patient receiving atracurium therapy without general anesthesia, because consciousness is not affected by atracurium alone.
- ▫ Reassure patient that communication abilities will return as the medication wears off.

Evaluation

Effectiveness of atracurium can be demonstrated by: ▪ Adequate suppression of the twitch response when tested with peripheral nerve stimulation and subsequent muscle paralysis.

ATROPINE
(at-ro-peen)

CLASSIFICATION(S):
Anticholinergic—antimuscarinic, Antiarrhythmic—miscellaneous, Ophthalmic—mydriatic
Pregnancy Category C

INDICATIONS

▪ **IM:** Preoperative medication to inhibit salivation and excessive respiratory secretions ▪ **IV:** Treatment of sinus bradycardia ▪ **PO:** Adjunctive therapy in the management of peptic ulcer and the irritable bowel syndrome ▪ **Ophth:** Produces mydriasis, allows cycloplegic refraction, and used in the treatment of certain inflammatory conditions of the iris and uvea ▪ **Inhaln:** Short-term treatment of bronchospasm ▪ **IV:** Reversal of adverse muscarinic effects of anticholinesterase agents (neostigmine, physostigmine, or pyridostigmine) ▪ **IM, IV:** Treatment of anticholinesterase (organophosphate pesticide) poisoning.

ACTION

▪ Inhibits the action of acetylcholine at postganglionic sites located in: ▫ Smooth muscle ▫ Secretory glands

▫ CNS (antimuscarinic activity). ▪ Low doses decrease: ▫ Sweating ▫ Salivation ▫ Respiratory secretions. ▪ Intermediate doses result in: ▫ Mydriasis (pupillary dilation) ▫ Cycloplegia (loss of visual accommodation) ▫ Increased heart rate ▪ GI and GU tract motility are decreased at larger doses ▪ Produces selective bronchodilation when administered by inhalation. **Therapeutic Effects:** ▪ Increased heart rate ▪ Decreased GI and respiratory secretions ▪ Reversal of muscarinic effects ▪ Bronchodilation ▪ May have a spasmolytic action on the biliary and genitourinary tract.

PHARMACOKINETICS

Absorption: Well absorbed following oral, SC, or IM administration.
Distribution: Well distributed. Readily crosses the blood–brain barrier. Crosses the placenta and enters breast milk.
Metabolism and Excretion: Mostly metabolized by the liver; 30–50% excreted unchanged by the kidneys.
Half-life: 13–38 hr.

CONTRAINDICATIONS AND PRECAUTIONS

Contraindicated in: ▪ Hypersensitivity ▪ Narrow-angle glaucoma ▪ Acute hemorrhage ▪ Tachycardia secondary to cardiac insufficiency or thyrotoxicosis.
Use Cautiously in: ▪ Elderly and the very young (increased susceptibility to adverse reactions) ▪ Intra-abdominal infections ▪ Prostatic hypertrophy ▪ Chronic renal, hepatic, pulmonary, or cardiac disease ▪ Pregnancy and lactation (safety not established).

ADVERSE REACTIONS AND SIDE EFFECTS*

CNS: <u>drowsiness</u>, confusion.
EENT: dry eyes, <u>blurred vision</u>, mydriasis, cycloplegia.
CV: palpitations, <u>tachycardia</u>.
GI: <u>dry mouth</u>, constipation.
GU: <u>urinary hesitancy</u>, retention.
Misc: decreased sweating.

INTERACTIONS

Drug–Drug: ▪ Additive anticholinergic effects with other **anticholinergic compounds**, including **antihistamines, tricyclic antidepressants, quinidine**, and **disopyramide** ▪ Anticholinergics may alter the absorption of other **orally administered drugs** by slowing motility of the GI tract ▪ **Antacids** decrease the absorption of anticholinergics ▪ May increase GI mucosal lesions in patients taking **oral potassium chloride tablets**.

ROUTE AND DOSAGE

Preanesthesia

- **IM, SC (Adults and Children >40 kg):** 0.4–0.6 mg 30–60 min preop.
- **IM, SC (Children 30–40 kg):** 0.4 mg 30–60 min preop.
- **IM, SC (Children 18–30 kg):** 0.3 mg 30–60 min preop.
- **IM, SC (Children 11–18 kg):** 0.2 mg 30–60 min preop.
- **IM, SC (Children 8–11 kg):** 0.15 mg 30–60 min preop.
- **IM, SC (Children 3–7 kg):** 0.1 mg 30–60 min preop.

Bradycardia

- **IV (Adults):** 0.5–1.0 mg; may repeat as needed q 5 min to a total of 2 mg (total vagolytic dose).
- **IV (Children):** 0.01 mg/kg (maximum dose 0.4 mg); repeat as needed q 4–6 hr.

Adjunctive Therapy of GI Disorders

- **PO (Adults):** 0.3–1.2 mg q 4–6 hr (antimuscarinic dose).

Cycloplegic Refraction

- **Ophth (Adults):** 1–2 drops of 1% soln 1 hr before examination.
- **Ophth (Children):** 1–2 drops of 0.5% soln 2–3 times/day for 1–3 days before and 1 hr after examination.

Bronchospasm

- **Inhaln (Adults):** 0.025 mg/kg 3–4 times daily (total dose not to exceed 2.5 mg).
- **Inhaln (Children):** 0.05 mg/kg 3–4 times daily.

*<u>Underlines</u> indicate most frequent; **CAPITALS** indicate life-threatening.

Reversal of Adverse Muscarinic Effects of Anticholinesterases

- **IV (Adults):** 0.6–1.2 mg for each 0.5–2.5 mg of neostigmine methylsulfate or 10–20 mg of pyridostigmine bromide concurrently with anticholinesterase.

Organophosphate Poisoning

- **IM, IV (Adults):** 1–2 mg initially, then 2 mg q 5–60 min as needed. In severe cases 2–6 mg may be used initially and repeated every 5–60 min as needed.
- **IM, IV (Children):** 0.05 mg/kg q 10–30 min as needed.

PHARMACODYNAMICS (PO, IM, SC, IV = inhibition of salivation, Inhaln = bronchodilation, Ophth = mydriasis)

	ONSET	PEAK	DURATION
PO	30 min	30–60 min	4–6 hr
IM, SC	rapid	15–50 min	4–6 hr
IV	immediate	2–4 min	4–6 hr
Inhaln	15 min	15 min–1.5 hr	UK
Ophth	30–40 min	up to 24 hr	1–2 wk

NURSING IMPLICATIONS

Assessment

- **General Info:** Assess vital signs and ECG tracings frequently during the course of IV drug therapy. Report any significant changes in heart rate or blood pressure, or increased ventricular ectopy or angina to physician promptly.
  - Monitor intake and output ratios in elderly or surgical patients because atropine may cause urinary retention.
  - Assess patients routinely for abdominal distention and auscultate for bowel sounds. If constipation becomes a problem, increasing fluids and adding bulk to the diet may help alleviate the constipating effects of the drug.
- **Bronchodilator:** Assess respiratory rate and lung sounds when used to prevent or treat bronchospasm.
- **Toxicity and Overdose:** If overdose occurs, physostigmine is the antidote.

Potential Nursing Diagnoses

- Cardiac output, decreased (indications).
- Oral mucous membranes, altered (side effects).
- Bowel elimination, altered: constipation (side effects).

Implementation

- **General Info:** Available in combination with barbiturates and narcotics (see Appendix A).
- **PO:** Oral doses of atropine are usually given 30 min before meals.
- **IM:** Intense flushing of the face and trunk may occur 15–20 min following IM administration. In children, this response is called "atropine flush" and is not harmful.
- **Direct IV:** Give IV undiluted or dilute in 10 ml of sterile water.
  - *Rate:* Administer at a rate of 0.6 mg over 1 min. Do not add to IV soln. Inject through Y-tubing or 3-way stopcock. When given IV in doses less than 0.4 mg or over more than 1 min, atropine may cause paradoxical bradycardia, which usually resolves in approximately 2 min.
- **Syringe Compatibility:** benzquinamide, butorphanol, chlorpromazine, cimetidine, dimenhydrinate, diphenhydramine, droperidol, fentanyl, glycopyrrolate, heparin, hydromorphone, hydroxyzine, meperidine, metoclopramide, midazolam, morphine, nalbuphine, pentazocine, perphenazine, prochlorperazine, promazine, promethazine, propiomazine, ranitidine, or scopolamine.
- **Y-Site Compatibility:** amrinone, famotidine, heparin, hydrocortisone sodium succinate, nafcillin, or potassium chloride.
- **Additive Compatibility:** dobutamine, netilmicin, sodium bicarbonate, or verapamil.
- **Ophth:** Ophth soln can be instilled by having patient tilt head back and look up, gently depress lower lid with index finger until conjunctival sac is exposed, and instill medication. After instillation, maintain gentle pressure

on inner canthus for 1 min to avoid systemic absorption of the drug. Wait at least 5 min before instilling other types of eyedrops.

- **Inhaln:** Dilute dose with 3–5 ml of 0.45% NaCl or 0.9% NaCl for administration via nebulizer. Administer atropine first if using other inhalation medications, and allow 5 min to elapse before administering other medications, unless directed by physician.

Patient/Family Teaching

- **General Info:** Instruct patient to take exactly as directed. If a dose is missed, take as soon as remembered unless almost time for next dose. Do not double doses.
- □ May cause drowsiness. Caution patients to avoid driving or other activities requiring alertness until response to medication is known.
- □ Instruct patient that oral rinses, sugarless gum or candy, and frequent oral hygiene may help relieve dry mouth.
- □ Caution patients that atropine impairs heat regulation. Strenuous activity in a hot environment may cause heat stroke.
- □ Instruct patient to consult physician or pharmacist before taking any over-the-counter medications concurrently with this medication.
- □ Inform male patients with benign prostatic hypertrophy that atropine may cause urinary hesitancy and retention. Changes in urinary stream should be reported to the physician.
- **Ophth:** Advise patients that ophthalmic preparations may temporarily blur vision and impair ability to judge distances. Dark glasses may be needed to protect eyes from bright light.

Evaluation

Effectiveness of therapy can be demonstrated by: ▪ Increase in heart rate ▪ Dryness of mouth ▪ Dilation of pupils ▪ Decrease in GI motility ▪ Reversal of muscarinic effects ▪ Bronchodilation.

AURANOFIN

(au-**rane**-oh-fin)
Ridaura

CLASSIFICATION(S):
Anti-inflammatory agent—gold compound
Pregnancy Category C

INDICATIONS

▪ Treatment of progressive rheumatoid arthritis resistant to conventional therapy.

ACTION

▪ Inhibits the inflammatory process ▪ Has immunomodulating properties. **Therapeutic Effects:** ▪ Relief of pain and inflammation ▪ Slowing of the disease process in rheumatoid arthritis.

PHARMACOKINETICS

Absorption: 20–25% absorbed from the GI tract.
Distribution: Widely distributed. Appears to concentrate in arthritic joints. Enters breast milk.
Metabolism and Excretion: 60–90% slowly excreted by the kidneys (up to 15 mon). 10–40% excreted in the feces.
Half-life: Gold—26 days in blood, 40–128 days in tissue.

CONTRAINDICATIONS AND PRECAUTIONS

Contraindicated in: ▪ Hypersensitivity ▪ Severe hepatic or renal dysfunction ▪ Previous heavy metal toxicity ▪ Previous adverse reaction to gold therapy ▪ History of colitis or exfoliative dermatitis ▪ Uncontrolled diabetes mellitus ▪ Tuberculosis ▪ Congestive heart failure ▪ Systemic lupus erythematosus ▪ Recent radiation therapy ▪ Pregnancy or lactation ▪ Debilitated patients.
Use Cautiously in: ▪ History of blood dyscrasias ▪ Hypertension ▪ Rashes ▪ Discontinue at first sign of toxicity, skin rash, proteinuria, or stomatitis.

ADVERSE REACTIONS AND SIDE EFFECTS*

EENT: corneal gold deposition, corneal ulcerations.
CNS: dizziness, syncope, headache.
CV: bradycardia.
Resp: pneumonitis.
GI: metallic taste, stomatitis, diarrhea.
GU: proteinuria, nephrotoxicity.
Derm: rash, dermatitis, pruritus, photosensitivity reactions.
Hemat: thrombocytopenia, **APLASTIC ANEMIA, AGRANULOCYTOSIS,** leukopenia, eosinophilia.
Misc: allergic reactions including anaphylaxis, angioneurotic edema, nitritoid reactions.

INTERACTIONS

Drug–Drug: ▪ Bone marrow toxicity may be additive with other **agents causing bone marrow depression (antineoplastics, radiation therapy)**.

ROUTE AND DOSAGE

- **PO (Adults):** 6 mg/day in 1–2 doses; up to 9 mg/day in 3 divided doses.

PHARMACODYNAMICS (anti-inflammatory activity)

	ONSET	PEAK	DURATION
PO	3–6 mon	UK	mons

NURSING IMPLICATIONS

Assessment

- Assess patient's range of motion and degree of swelling and pain in affected joints prior to and periodically throughout therapy.
- **Lab Test Considerations:** Monitor renal, hepatic, and hematologic function and urinalysis prior to and monthly throughout therapy. Notify physician immediately if WBC $<4000/mm^3$, eosinophils $>5\%$, granulocytes $<1500/mm^3$, or platelets $<100,000/mm^3$. These values may indicate severe hypersensitivity reactions and should improve upon discontinuation. Proteinuria or hematuria may necessitate discontinuation of therapy.
- May cause false-positive tuberculin skin test.
- **Toxicity and Overdose:** If signs of overdose occur, glucocorticoids are usually used to reverse effects. A chelating agent dimercaprol (BAL) may be given to enhance gold excretion when glucocorticoids are ineffective.

Potential Nursing Diagnoses

- Mobility, impaired physical (indications).
- Bowel elimination, altered: diarrhea (adverse effects).
- Knowledge deficit related to medication regimen (patient/family teaching).

Implementation

- **PO:** Administer oral doses with meals to minimize gastric irritation.

Patient/Family Teaching

- Instruct patient to take medication exactly as prescribed, do not skip or double doses. Take missed dose as soon as remembered except if next dose almost due. Concurrent therapy with salicylates or other nonsteroidal anti-inflammatory agents or adrenocorticoids is usually necessary, especially during the first few mons of gold therapy. Patients should continue physical therapy and ensure adequate rest. Explain that joint damage will not be reversed; the goal is to slow or stop disease process.
- Emphasize the importance of good oral hygiene to reduce the incidence of stomatitis.
- Caution patient to use sunscreen and protective clothing to prevent photosensitivity reactions.
- Instruct patient to report symptoms of leukopenia (fever, sore throat, signs of infection) or thrombocytopenia (bleeding gums, bruising, petechiae, blood in stools, urine, or emesis) immediately to physician.
- Discuss the need for contraception while receiving this medication. Ad-

*Underlines indicate most frequent; **CAPITALS** indicate life-threatening.

vise patient to notify physician promptly if pregnancy is suspected.
- □ Instruct patient to notify physician immediately if symptoms of gold toxicity (pruritus, skin rash, metallic taste in mouth, stomatitis, diarrhea) occur. Diarrhea may be resolved by decreasing the dose.
- □ Emphasize the importance of regular visits to physician to monitor progress and evaluate blood and urine tests for side effects.

EVALUATION

Effectiveness of therapy can be demonstrated by: ▪ Decrease in swelling, pain, and stiffness of joints □ Increase in mobility. Continuous therapy for 3–6 mon may be required before therapeutic effects are seen.

AUROTHIOGLUCOSE

(aur-oh-thye-oh-**gloo**-kose)
Solganol

CLASSIFICATION(S):
Anti-inflammatory agent—gold compound
Pregnancy Category C

INDICATIONS

▪ Treatment of progressive rheumatoid arthritis resistant to conventional therapy.

ACTION

▪ Inhibits the inflammatory process. ▪ Has immunomodulating properties. **Therapeutic Effects:** ▪ Relief of pain and inflammation ▪ Slowing of the destructive process in rheumatoid arthritis.

PHARMACOKINETICS

Absorption: Slowly and irregularly absorbed following IM administration.
Distribution: Widely distributed. Appears to concentrate in arthritic joints. Enters breast milk.
Metabolism and Excretion: 60–90% slowly excreted by the kidneys (up to 15 mon); 10–40% excreted in the feces.
Half-life: Gold—26 days in blood, 40–128 days in tissue.

CONTRAINDICATIONS AND PRECAUTIONS

Contraindicated in: ▪ Hypersensitivity ▪ Severe hepatic or renal dysfunction ▪ Previous heavy metal toxicity ▪ Previous adverse reaction to gold therapy ▪ History of colitis ▪ History of exfoliative dermatitis ▪ Uncontrolled diabetes mellitus ▪ Tuberculosis ▪ Congestive heart failure ▪ Systemic lupus erythematosus ▪ Recent radiation therapy ▪ Pregnancy or lactation ▪ Debilitated patients.
Use Cautiously in: ▪ History of blood dyscrasias ▪ Hypertension ▪ Rashes ▪ Discontinue at first sign of toxicity, skin rash, proteinuria, or stomatitis ▪ Children <6 yr (safety not established).

ADVERSE REACTIONS AND SIDE EFFECTS*

CNS: dizziness, syncope, headache.
EENT: corneal gold deposition, corneal ulcerations.
CV: bradycardia.
Resp: pneumonitis.
GI: metallic taste, difficulty swallowing, stomatitis, nausea, vomiting, diarrhea, abdominal pain, cramping, anorexia, dyspepsia, flatulence, hepatitis.
GU: proteinuria, nephrotoxicity.
Derm: rash, dermatitis, pruritus, photosensitivity reactions.
Hemat: thrombocytopenia, **APLASTIC ANEMIA, AGRANULOCYTOSIS,** leukopenia, eosinophilia.
Neuro: neuropathy.
Misc: allergic reactions including **ANAPHYLAXIS,** angioneurotic edema, nitritoid reaction.

INTERACTIONS

Drug-Drug: ▪ Bone marrow toxicity may be additive with other **agents causing bone marrow depression (antineoplastics, radiation therapy)**.

*Underlines indicate most frequent; **CAPITALS** indicate life-threatening.

ROUTE AND DOSAGE

- **IM (Adults):** 10 mg first wk, 25 mg second and third wk, then 25–50 mg weekly until 800 mg–1 g has been given; then maintenance dose of 25–50 mg q wk for 2–20 wk, then 25–50 mg q 3–4 wk.
- **IM (Children 6–12 yr):** 2.5 mg first wk, 6.25 mg second and third wk, then 12.5 mg weekly until 200–250 mg has been given; then maintenance dose of 6.25–12.5 mg q 3–4 wk or 1 mg/kg/wk for 20 wk.

PHARMACODYNAMICS (anti-inflammatory effect)

	ONSET	PEAK	DURATION
IM	6–8 wk	UK	mons

NURSING IMPLICATIONS

Assessment

- Assess patient's range of motion and degree of swelling and pain in affected joints prior to and periodically throughout therapy.
- Monitor patient for nitritoid reaction (flushing, fainting, dizziness, sweating, nausea, vomiting, headache, blurred vision, weakness, malaise) that may occur immediately to 10 min following injection. Reaction is transient and does not usually require discontinuation of therapy.
- **Lab Test Considerations:** Monitor renal, hepatic, and hematologic function and urinalysis prior to and periodically throughout therapy. Obtain urinalysis prior to each injection. Proteinuria or hematuria may necessitate discontinuation of therapy. Monitor CBC and platelets prior to every other injection or every 2–4 wk. Notify physician immediately if WBC $<4000/mm^3$, eosinophils $>5\%$, granulocytes $<1500/mm^3$, or platelets $<100,000/mm^3$. These values may indicate severe hypersensitivity reactions and should improve upon discontinuation.
- May interfere with determination of serum protein-bound iodine by the chloric method.
- **Toxicity and Overdose:** If signs of overdose occur, glucocorticoids are usually used to reverse effects. A chelating agent dimercaprol (BAL) may be given to enhance gold excretion when glucocorticoids are ineffective.

Potential Nursing Diagnoses

- Mobility, impaired physical (indications).
- Bowel elimination, altered: diarrhea (adverse effects).
- Knowledge deficit related to medication regimen (patient/family teaching).

Implementation

- **IM:** Immerse vial in warm water bath and shake suspension well for ease of withdrawal. Use 1½–2 in, 20-gauge needle. Administer into the gluteal muscle only. Do not administer IV. Patient should remain supine for 10 min after injection and should be closely monitored for development of nitritoid reaction for 15 min.

Patient/Family Teaching

- Discuss need for continued therapy. Initially injections are given weekly. Later injections are spaced 3–4 wk apart. Concurrent therapy with salicylates, nonsteroidal anti-inflammatory agents, or glucocorticoids may be necessary. Patient should continue physical therapy and ensure adequate rest. Explain that joint damage will not be reversed; the goal is to slow or stop disease process.
- Emphasize the importance of good oral hygiene to reduce the incidence of stomatitis.
- Caution patient to use sunscreen and protective clothing to prevent photosensitivity reactions.
- Instruct patient to report symptoms of leukopenia (fever, sore throat, signs of infection) or thrombocytopenia (bleeding gums, bruising, petechiae, blood in stools, urine, or emesis) immediately to physician.
- Discuss the need for contraception while receiving this medication. Ad-

vise patient to notify physician promptly if pregnancy is suspected.

- Instruct patient to notify physician immediately if symptoms of gold toxicity (pruritus, skin rash, metallic taste in mouth, stomatitis, diarrhea) occur.
- Emphasize the importance of regular visits to physician to monitor progress and evaluate blood and urine tests for side effects.

EVALUATION

Effectiveness of therapy can be demonstrated by: ▪ Decrease in swelling, pain, and stiffness of joints ▫ Increase in mobility. Continuous therapy for 3–6 mon may be required before therapeutic effects are seen.

AZATADINE
(a-**za**-ta-deen)
Optimine

CLASSIFICATION(S):
Antihistamine
Pregnancy Category B

INDICATIONS

▪ Symptomatic relief of allergic symptoms caused by histamine release. Conditions in which it is most useful include nasal allergies and allergic dermatoses.

ACTION

▪ Blocks the following effects of histamine: ▫ Vasodilation ▫ Increased GI tract secretions ▫ Increased heart rate ▫ Hypotension ▪ Also has antiserotonin properties. **Therapeutic Effect:** ▪ Relief of symptoms associated with histamine excess usually seen in allergic conditions. Does not block the release of histamine.

PHARMACOKINETICS

Absorption: Well absorbed following oral administration.
Distribution: Probably crosses the placenta.
Metabolism and Excretion: Extensively metabolized by the liver; 20% excreted unchanged by the kidneys.
Half-life: 12 hr.

CONTRAINDICATIONS AND PRECAUTIONS

Contraindicated in: ▪ Hypersensitivity ▪ Acute attacks of asthma ▪ Lactation (avoid use).
Use Cautiously in: ▪ Narrow-angle glaucoma ▪ Liver disease ▪ Elderly patients (more susceptible to adverse reactions) ▪ Pregnancy or children <12 yr (safety not established) ▪ Hyperthyroidism ▪ Hypertension.

ADVERSE REACTIONS AND SIDE EFFECTS*

CNS: drowsiness, sedation, dizziness, headache, excitation, seizures.
CV: hypotension, hypertension, palpitations, arrhythmias, tachycardia, chest tightness.
EENT: blurred vision, tinnitus, nasal stuffiness.
Resp: thickened bronchial secretions, wheezing.
GI: dry mouth, vomiting, diarrhea, constipation, epigastric distress, anorexia.
GU: urinary hesitancy, retention, early menses.
Hemat: anemia, thrombocytopenia, agranulocytosis.
Derm: sweating.

INTERACTIONS

Drug–Drug: ▪ Additive CNS depression with other **CNS depressants** including **alcohol, narcotic analgesics,** and **sedative/hypnotics** ▪ **MAO inhibitors** intensify and prolong the anticholinergic effects of antihistamines.

ROUTE AND DOSAGE

▪ **PO (Adults and Children >12 yr):** 1–2 mg twice daily.

PHARMACODYNAMICS (antihistaminic effects)

	ONSET	PEAK	DURATION
PO	15–60 min	UK	12 hr

*Underlines indicate most frequent; **CAPITALS** indicate life-threatening.

NURSING IMPLICATIONS

Assessment

- ▫ Assess allergy symptoms (rhinitis, conjunctivitis, hives) prior to and periodically throughout course of therapy.
- ▫ Assess lung sounds and character of bronchial secretions. Maintain fluid intake of 1500–2000 ml/day to decrease viscosity of secretions.
- ▪ **Lab Test Considerations:** May cause false-negative allergy skin testing. Discontinue antihistamines at least 72 hr before testing.

Potential Nursing Diagnoses

- ▪ Airway clearance, ineffective (indications).
- ▪ Injury, high risk for (adverse reactions).
- ▪ Knowledge deficit related to medication regimen (patient/family teaching).

Implementation

- ▪ **General Info:** Available in combination with pseudoephedrine (see Appendix A).
- ▪ **PO:** Administer oral doses with food or milk to decrease GI irritation.

Patient/Family Teaching

- ▫ Instruct patient to take azatadine exactly as directed.
- ▫ May cause drowsiness. Caution patient to avoid driving or other activities requiring alertness until effects of the medication are known.
- ▫ Advise patient to avoid taking alcohol or other CNS depressants concurrently with this drug.
- ▫ Advise patient that good oral hygiene, frequent rinsing of mouth with water, and sugarless gum or candy may help relieve dry mouth. Patient should notify dentist if dry mouth persists >2 wk.
- ▫ Elderly patients are at risk for orthostatic hypotension. Advise patient to make position changes slowly.
- ▫ Instruct patient to contact physician if symptoms persist.

Evaluation

Effectiveness of therapy may be determined by: ▪ Decrease in allergic symptoms.

AZATHIOPRINE

(ay-za-**thye**-oh-preen)
Imuran

CLASSIFICATION(S):
Immunosuppressant
Pregnancy Category UK

INDICATIONS

▪ Adjunct with corticosteroids, local radiations, or other cytotoxic agents in the prevention of renal transplant rejection ▪ Treatment of severe, active, erosive rheumatoid arthritis unresponsive to more conventional therapy with or without disease-modifying agents such as gold salts.

ACTION

▪ Antagonizes purine metabolism with subsequent inhibition of DNA and RNA synthesis. **Therapeutic Effects:** ▪ Suppression of cell-mediated immunity and altered antibody formation.

PHARMACOKINETICS

Absorption: Readily absorbed following oral administration.
Distribution: Rapidly cleared. Crosses the placenta.
Metabolism and Excretion: Metabolized to mercaptopurine, which is subsequently further metabolized. Minimal renal excretion of unchanged drug.
Half-life: 3 hr.

CONTRAINDICATIONS AND PRECAUTIONS

Contraindicated in: ▪ Hypersensitivity ▪ Pregnancy or lactation.
Use Cautiously in: ▪ Infections ▪ Malignancies ▪ Decreased bone marrow reserve ▪ Previous or concurrent radiation therapy ▪ Other chronic debilitating ill-

nesses ▪ Patients with childbearing potential.

ADVERSE REACTIONS AND SIDE EFFECTS*

EENT: retinopathy.
GI: nausea, vomiting, diarrhea, anorexia, mucositis, hepatotoxicity, pancreatitis.
Derm: rash, alopecia.
Hemat: leukopenia, anemia, pancytopenia, thrombocytopenia.
MS: arthralgia.
Resp: pulmonary edema.
Misc: fever, chills, serum sickness, retinopathy, Raynaud's phenomenon.

INTERACTIONS

Drug-Drug: ▪ Additive myelosuppression with **antineoplastics** and **myelosuppressive agents** ▪ **Allopurinol** inhibits the metabolism of azathioprine increasing toxicity. Dosage of azathioprine should be decreased by 25–33% with concurrent allopurinol.

ROUTE AND DOSAGE

Renal Allograft Rejection Prevention

- **PO, IV (Adults and Children):** 3–5 mg/kg/day initially; maintenance dose 1–3 mg/kg/day.

Rheumatoid Arthritis

- **PO (Adults):** 1 mg/kg/day for 6–8 wk, increase by 0.5 mg/kg q 4 wk until response or up to 2.5 mg/kg/day.

PHARMACODYNAMICS

	ONSET	PEAK	DURATION
PO (anti-inflammatory)	6–8 wk	12 wk	UK
IV (immunosuppression)	days–wks	UK	days–wks

NURSING IMPLICATIONS

Assessment

- **General Info:** Assess for infection (vital signs; sputum, urine, stool, WBC) throughout therapy.
  - Monitor intake and output and daily weight. Decreased urine output may lead to toxicity with this medication.
- **Rheumatoid Arthritis:** Assess range of motion, degree of swelling, pain and strength in affected joints, and ability to perform activities of daily living prior to and periodically throughout therapy.
- **Lab Test Considerations:** Renal, hepatic, and hematologic functions should be monitored prior to beginning the course of therapy, weekly during the first mon, bimonthly for the next 2–3 mon, and monthly thereafter during the course of therapy.
  - Notify physician if leukocyte count is <3000 or platelet count is <100,000/mm^3; these may necessitate a reduction in dosage.
  - A decrease in hemoglobin may indicate bone marrow suppression.
  - Hepatotoxicity may be manifested by increased alkaline phosphatase, bilirubin, SGOT (AST), SGPT (ALT), and amylase.
  - May decrease serum and urine acid and plasma albumin.

Potential Nursing Diagnoses

- Infection, high risk for (indications).
- Knowledge deficit related to medication regimen (patient/family teaching).

Implementation

- **General Info:** Protect transplant patients from staff and visitors who may carry infection. Maintain protective isolation as indicated.
- **PO:** May be administered with or after meals or in divided dose to minimize nausea.
- **IV:** Reconstitute each 100 mg with 10 ml of sterile water for injection. Swirl the vial gently until completely dissolved. Reconstituted soln may be administered for up to 24 hr after preparation.
- **Intermittent Infusion:** Soln may be further diluted in 50 ml of 0.9% NaCl, 0.45% NaCl, or D5W. Do not admix.
  - *Rate:* Each single dose should be infused over at least 30 min.

*Underlines indicate most frequent; **CAPITALS** indicate life-threatening.

PATIENT/FAMILY TEACHING

- **General Info:** Instruct patient to take azathioprine exactly as directed. If a dose is missed on a once-daily regimen, skip the dose; if on several-times-a-day dosing, take as soon as remembered or double next dose. Consult physician if more than one dose is missed or if vomiting occurs shortly after dose taken. Do not discontinue therapy without consulting physician.
  - Advise patient to report the onset of infection, bleeding gums, bruising, or signs and symptoms of hepatic dysfunction (abdominal pain, pruritus, clay-colored stools) or transplant rejection to the physician immediately.
  - Reinforce the need for life-long therapy to prevent transplant rejection.
  - Instruct the patient to consult with physician or pharmacist before taking any over-the-counter medications or receiving any vaccinations while taking this medication.
  - Advise patient to avoid contact with contagious persons and those who have recently taken oral poliovirus vaccine.
  - This drug may have teratogenic properties. Advise patient to practice contraception during therapy and for at least 4 mon after therapy has been completed.
  - Emphasize the importance of follow-up examination and lab tests.
- **Rheumatoid Arthritis:** Concurrent therapy with salicylates, nonsteroidal anti-inflammatory agents, or glucocorticoids may be necessary. Patient should continue physical therapy and ensure adequate rest. Explain that joint damage will not be reversed; goal is to slow or stop disease process.

EVALUATION

Effectiveness of therapy may be determined by: ▪ Prevention of transplant rejection ▪ Decreased stiffness, pain, and swelling in affected joints in 6–8 wk in rheumatoid arthritis. Therapy is discontinued if there is no improvement in 12 wk.

AZTREONAM
(az-**tree**-oh-nam)
Azactam

CLASSIFICATION(S):
Anti-infective—monobactam
Pregnancy Category B

INDICATIONS

▪ Treatment of serious gram-negative infections including: ▫ Bone and joint infections ▫ Septicemia ▫ Skin and skin structure infections ▫ Intra-abdominal infections ▫ Gynecologic infections ▫ Respiratory tract infections ▫ Urinary tract infections.

ACTION

▪ Binds to the bacterial cell wall membrane, causing cell death. **Therapeutic Effect:** ▪ Bactericidal action against susceptible bacteria. **Spectrum:** ▪ Displays significant activity against gram-negative aerobic organisms only: ▫ *Escherichia coli* ▫ *Serratia* ▫ *Klebsiella* ▫ *Enterobacter* ▫ *Shigella* ▫ *Providencia* ▫ *Salmonella* ▫ *Neisseria gonorrhea* ▫ *Haemophilus influenzae* ▪ Has good activity against *Pseudomonas aeruginosa,* including strains resistant to other drugs ▪ Not active against: ▫ *Staphylococcus aureus* ▫ *Enterococcus* ▫ *Bacteroides fragilis.*

PHARMACOKINETICS

Absorption: Well absorbed following IM administration.

Distribution: Widely distributed. Crosses the placenta and enters breast milk in low concentrations.

Metabolism and Excretion: 65–75% excreted unchanged by the kidneys. Small amounts metabolized by the liver.

Half-life: 1.5–2.2 hr (increased in renal impairment).

CONTRAINDICATIONS AND PRECAUTIONS

Contraindicated in: ▪ Hypersensitivity ▪ Possible cross-sensitivity with penicillins or cephalosporins.

A

Use Cautiously in: ▪ Renal impairment (dosage reduction required) ▪ Pregnancy, lactation, and young children (safety not established).

ADVERSE REACTIONS AND SIDE EFFECTS*

CNS: SEIZURES.

GI: altered taste (IV only), diarrhea, nausea, vomiting.

Derm: rashes.

Local: phlebitis at IV site, pain at IM site.

Misc: superinfection, allergic reactions including ANAPHYLAXIS.

INTERACTIONS

Drug–Drug: ▪ May have synergistic or antagonistic effects when combined with other **anti-infectives**.

ROUTE AND DOSAGE

- **IM, IV (Adults):** 0.5–2.0 g q 6–12 hr.

PHARMACODYNAMICS (blood levels)

	ONSET	PEAK
IM	rapid	60 min
IV	rapid	end of infusion

NURSING IMPLICATIONS

Assessment

- **General Info:** Assess patient for infection (vital signs; wound appearance, sputum, urine, and stool; WBC) at beginning and throughout therapy.
  - Obtain a history before initiating therapy to determine previous use of and reactions to penicillins and cephalosporins. Patients allergic to these drugs may exhibit hypersensitivity reactions to aztreonam.
  - Obtain specimens for culture and sensitivity prior to initiating therapy. First dose may be given before receiving results.
- **Lab Test Considerations:** May cause elevations in SGOT (AST), SGPT (ALT), alkaline phosphatase, LDH, and serum creatinine. May cause increased prothrombin and partial thromboplastin times, eosinophilia, and positive Coombs' test.

Potential Nursing Diagnoses

- Infection, high risk for (indications).
- Knowledge deficit related to medication regimen (patient/family teaching).

Implementation

- **General Info:** After adding diluent to vial, shake immediately and vigorously. Not for multi-dose use; discard unused soln.
- **IM:** For IM administration use 15-ml vial and dilute each g of aztreonam with at least 3 ml of 0.9% NaCl, sterile water, or bacteriostatic water for injection. Stable at room temperature for 48 hr or 7 days if refrigerated.
  - Administer into large, well-developed muscle.
- **Direct IV:** For direct IV use add 6–10 ml of sterile water to each 15-ml vial.
  - *Rate:* Administer slowly over 3–5 min by direct injection or into tubing of a compatible soln.
- **Intermittent Infusion:** Dilute 15-ml vial with at least 3 ml of sterile water for each g aztreonam. Dilute further with 50–100 ml of 0.9% NaCl, Ringer's or lactated Ringer's soln, D5W, D10W, D5/0.9% NaCl, D5/0.45% NaCl, D5/0.25% NaCl, sodium lactate, 5% or 10% Mannitol. Final concentration should not exceed 20 mg/ml. Soln is stable for 48 hr at room temperature and 7 days if refrigerated. Solns range from colorless to light, straw yellow, or may develop a pink tint upon standing; this does not affect potency.
  - *Rate:* Infuse over 20–60 min.
- **Syringe Compatibility:** clindamycin.
- **Y-Site Compatibility:** ciprofloxacin, enalaprilat, foscarnet, ondansetron, or zidovudine.
- **Y-Site Incompatibility:** vancomycin.
- **Additive Compatibility:** cefazolin, ciprofloxacin, clindamycin, gentamicin, or tobramycin. Admixture is stable for 48 hr at room temperature and 7 days if refrigerated.

*Underlines indicate most frequent; **CAPITALS** indicate life-threatening.

- □ May be admixed with ampicillin in 0.9% NaCl; stable for 24 hr at room temperature and 48 hr if refrigerated. May also be admixed with ampicillin in D5W; stable for 2 hr at room temperature and 8 hr if refrigerated.
- ■ **Additive Incompatibility:** nafcillin, cephradine, or metronidazole.

PATIENT/FAMILY TEACHING

- □ Warn patient that IV infusion may cause mild taste alteration.
- □ Advise patient to report the signs of superinfection (furry overgrowth on the tongue, vaginal itching or discharge, loose or foul-smelling stools) and allergy.

EVALUATION

Effectiveness of therapy can be demonstrated by: ■ Resolution of signs and symptoms of infection. Length of time for complete resolution depends on the organism and site of infection.

BACITRACIN

(ba-si-**tray**-sin)
Ak-tracin, Baci-guent, Baci-IM, Baci-Rx, Ocu-tracin, Ziba-Rx

CLASSIFICATION(S):
Anti-infective—miscellaneous
Pregnancy Category UK

INDICATIONS

■ **IM:** Treatment of staphylococcal pneumonia or empyema in infants ■ **Ophth:** Treatment of conjunctivitis due to susceptible organisms ■ **Top:** Treatment of minor skin infections and prevention of superficial skin infections associated with abrasion. **Unlabeled Use:** ■ ***PO:*** Treatment of antibiotic associated colitis.

ACTION

■ Inhibits bacterial cell wall synthesis. **Therapeutic Effect:** ■ Bacteristatic or bactericidal action against susceptible bacteria (depends on concentration). **Spectrum:** ■ Active against many gram-positive organisms including: □ Streptococci □ Staphylococci □ Anaerobic cocci □ Corynebacteria □ Clostridia ■ Also active against: □ Gonococci □ Meningococci □ Fusobactera □ *Actinomyces israelii* □ *Treponema pallidum.*

PHARMACOKINETICS

Absorption: Well absorbed following IM administration. Minimally absorbed following oral, ophthalmic, and topical administration.
Distribution: Widely distributed. Does not enter the CNS.
Metabolism and Excretion: 10–40% excreted unchanged by the kidneys. Following oral administration, most bacitracin is excreted in the feces.
Half-life: UK.

CONTRAINDICATIONS AND PRECAUTIONS

Contraindicated in: ■ Hypersensitivity ■ Pregnancy ■ Renal impairment.
Use Cautiously in: ■ History of renal disease ■ Myasthenia gravis (may potentiate neuromuscular blockade).

ADVERSE REACTIONS AND SIDE EFFECTS*

EENT: Ophth—ocular irritation, stinging, burning.
GI: anorexia, nausea, vomiting, diarrhea.
GU: renal tubular necrosis, glomerular necrosis, proteinuria, oliguria, renal failure.
Derm: rashes.
Hemat: blood dycrasias, eosinophilia.
Local: pain, induration at IM site.
Misc: fever, anaphylactoid reactions, superinfection.

INTERACTIONS

Drug-Drug: ■ Additive nephrotoxic effects with other potentially **nephrotoxic agents** ■ Additive neuromuscular blockade with **neuromuscular blocking agents** and **anesthetics**.

*Underlines indicate most frequent; **CAPITALS** indicate life-threatening.

ROUTE AND DOSAGE

- **IM (Infants <2.5 kg):** 900 units/kg/day in 2–3 divided doses (course of therapy should not exceed 12 days).
- **IM (Infants >2.5 kg):** 1000 units/kg/day in 2–3 divided doses (course of therapy should not exceed 12 days).
- **PO:** 20,000–25,000 units q 6 hr for 7–10 days.
- **Ophth (Adults and Children):** ½–1 in ribbon q 3–24 hr.
- **Top (Adults and Children):** Apply 1–3 times daily.

PHARMACODYNAMICS

	ONSET	PEAK	DURATION
IM	rapid	1–2 hr	UK

NURSING IMPLICATIONS

Assessment

- □ Assess patient for infection (vital signs; wound appearance, sputum, urine, and stool; WBC) at beginning and throughout course of therapy.
- □ Obtain specimens for culture and sensitivity prior to initiating therapy. First dose may be given before receiving results.
- □ Observe patient for signs and symptoms of anaphylaxis (rash, pruritus, laryngeal edema, wheezing). Discontinue the drug and notify the physician immediately if these occur. Keep epinephrine, an antihistamine, and resuscitation equipment close by in the event of an anaphylactic reaction.
- □ Note frequency and character of stools. Inform physician if diarrhea or vomiting occurs, because dehydration increases risk of renal toxicity.
- □ Assess for allergy to neomycin. Patients allergic to neomycin may be cross-sensitive to bacitracin.
- □ Monitor for development of superinfection (furry overgrowth on the tongue, vaginal itching or discharge, loose or foul-smelling stools) in patients receiving IM bacitracin.
- **Lab Test Considerations:** Monitor renal function and urinalysis prior to and periodically throughout IM therapy. Albumuria, hematuria, and cylindruria may indicate renal tubular or glomerular necrosis. BUN should be checked daily.
- □ Monitor urine pH. Sodium bicarbonate may be ordered to maintain alkaline pH (>6) to reduce risk of renal toxicity.

Potential Nursing Diagnoses

- Skin integrity, impaired (indications).
- Infection, high risk for (indications, patient/family teaching).
- Knowledge deficit related to medication regimen (patient/family teaching).

Implementation

- **IM:** Reconstitute 10,000-unit vial with 2 ml of 0.9% NaCl with 2.0% procaine hydrochloride to yield concentration of 5000 units/ml. Vial containing 50,000 units may be reconstituted with either 9.8 ml of 0.9% NaCl with 2.0% procaine hydrochloride to yield concentration of 5000 units/ml or 50 ml of 0.9% NaCl to yield a concentration of 1000 units/ml (an equal volume of procaine hydrochloride 2.0% can then be added for a final concentration of 500 units/ml). Soln is stable for 1 wk when refrigerated.
- □ IM therapy is limited to 12 days because of adverse renal effects.
- □ Administer in large, well-developed muscle mass. Rotate sites. Avoid IV administration; may cause phlebitis.
- **Ophth:** Administer ophthalmic soln by having patient tilt head back and look up, gently depress lower lid with index finger until conjunctival sac is exposed, and instill medication. Wait at least 5 min before administering other types of eyedrops.
- **Top:** Available without prescription for topical application. Wash lesions and pat dry before applying medication in a thin layer.

Patient/Family Teaching

- **Ophth:** Instruct patient in proper technique for instillation of ophthalmic medications. Advise patient to use medication for the full course of therapy. Emphasize the importance of not touching the applicator tip to any surface. Discuss methods to prevent spread of infection: separate wash cloth, good handwashing, and avoiding rubbing infected eye. Demonstrate how to wipe from inner to outer canthus. Patient should notify physician if itching, burning, or irritation of eyes occurs. Advise patients that sharing of this medication may be dangerous.

- **Top:** Instruct patient in proper method of cleaning wound or skin lesion and applying medication in a thin layer. The physician should be notified if symptoms do not improve.

EVALUATION

Clinical response to therapy can be evaluated by: ▪ Resolution of the signs and symptoms of infection. Length of time for complete resolution depends on the organism and site of infection.

BACLOFEN

(**bak**-loe-fen)
Lioresal

CLASSIFICATION(S):
Skeletal muscle relaxant—centrally acting
Pregnancy Category UK

INDICATIONS

▪ Treatment of reversible spasticity associated with multiple sclerosis or spinal cord lesions. **Unlabeled Use:** ▪ Management of pain in trigeminal neuralgia.

ACTION

▪ Inhibits reflexes at the spinal level. **Therapeutic Effect:** ▪ Relief of muscle spasticity; bowel and bladder function may also be improved.

PHARMACOKINETICS

Absorption: Rapidly and almost completely absorbed following oral administration.
Distribution: Widely distributed, crosses the placenta.
Metabolism and Excretion: 70–80% eliminated unchanged by the kidneys.
Half-life: 2.5–4 hr.

CONTRAINDICATIONS AND PRECAUTIONS

Contraindicated in: ▪ Hypersensitivity.
Use Cautiously in: ▪ Patients in whom spasticity is used to maintain posture and balance ▪ Pregnancy, lactation, and children (safety not established) ▪ Epileptics (may lower seizure threshold) ▪ Elderly (increased susceptibility to CNS side effects) ▪ Renal impairment (dosage reduction may be required).

ADVERSE REACTIONS AND SIDE EFFECTS*

CNS: <u>drowsiness</u>, <u>dizziness</u>, <u>weakness</u>, <u>fatigue</u>, headache, confusion, insomnia, ataxia, depression.
EENT: nasal congestion, tinnitus.
CV: hypotension, edema.
GI: <u>nausea</u>, constipation.
GU: frequency.
Derm: rash, pruritus.
Metab: hyperglycemia, weight gain.
Misc: hypersensitivity reactions, sweating.

INTERACTIONS

Drug-Drug: ▪ Additive CNS depression with other **CNS depressants** including **alcohol, antihistamines, narcotic analgesics,** and **sedative/hypnotics** ▪ Use with **MAO inhibitors** may lead to increased CNS depression or hypotension.

ROUTE AND DOSAGE

- **PO (Adults):** 5 mg 3 times daily. May increase q 3 days by 5 mg/dose to maximum of 80 mg/day (total daily

*<u>Underlines</u> indicate most frequent; **CAPITALS** indicate life-threatening.

dose may also be given in divided doses 4 times daily).

PHARMACODYNAMICS (effects on spasticity)

	ONSET	PEAK	DURATION
PO	hrs–wks	UK	UK

NURSING IMPLICATIONS

Assessment

- Assess muscle spasticity prior to and periodically throughout course of therapy.
- Observe patient for drowsiness, dizziness, or ataxia. If these occur, notify physician; a change in dosage may alleviate these problems.
- **Lab Test Considerations:** May cause increase in serum glucose, alkaline, phosphatase, SGOT (AST), and SGPT (ALT) levels.

Potential Nursing Diagnoses

- Mobility, impaired physical (indications).
- Injury, high risk for (adverse reactions).
- Knowledge deficit related to medication regimen (patient/family teaching).

Implementation

- **PO:** May be administered with milk or food to minimize gastric irritation.

Patient/Family Teaching

- Instruct patient to take baclofen exactly as directed. If a dose is missed, take within 1 hr; do not double doses. Caution patient to avoid abrupt withdrawal of this medication as it may precipitate an acute withdrawal reaction (hallucinations, increased spasticity, seizures, mental changes, restlessness).
- May cause dizziness and drowsiness. Advise patient to avoid driving or other activities requiring alertness until response to drug is known.
- Instruct patient to make position changes slowly to minimize orthostatic hypotension.
- Advise patient to avoid concurrent use of alcohol or other CNS depressants while taking this medication.
- Instruct patient to notify physician if frequent urge to urinate or painful urination, constipation, nausea, headache, insomnia, tinnitus, depression, or confusion persist. Advise patient to report signs and symptoms of hypersensitivity (rash, itching) to physician promptly.

Evaluation

Effectiveness of therapy can be demonstrated by: ▪ Decrease in muscle spasticity and associated musculoskeletal pain with an increased ability to perform activities of daily living ▪ Decreased pain in patients with trigeminal neuralgia. May take wks to obtain optimal effect.

BCG (Bacillus Calmette-Guerin)

(bee-see-gee)

{ImmuCyst}, TheraCys (live preparation), TICE BCG (percutaneous vaccine); BCG vaccine, intradermal

CLASSIFICATION(S):

Antineoplastic—immune modulator

Pregnancy Category C

INDICATIONS

▪ **Intravesical:** Instilled in the bladder in the management of *in situ* carcinoma of the bladder in patients who are not candidates for radical surgery ▪ **Intradermal** and **Percutaneous:** Induction of immunity in patients not previously exposed who expect to be heavily exposed to active tuberculosis.

ACTION

▪ Consists of freeze-dried attenuated strain of *Mycobacterium bovis* ▪ Produces local inflammatory response in lining of urinary bladder, which re-

duces or eliminates local cancerous lesions (Intravesical) ▪ Percutaneous or intradermal vaccination stimulates the reticuloendothelial system to produce macrophages that decrease the multiplication of virulent mycobacteria.
Therapeutic Effects: ▪ ***Intravesical:*** Elimination of residual tumor cells and prevention of recurrence ▪ ***Intradermal*** or ***Percutaneous:*** Provision of immunity to tuberculosis and a decrease in serious complications from primary tuberculosis in children.

PHARMACOKINETICS

Absorption: Systemic absorption following bladder instillation not known. Systemic absorption follows intradermal or percutaneous administration.
Distribution: Systemic distribution not known.
Metabolism and Excretion: Metabolism and excretion not known.
Half-life: UK.

CONTRAINDICATIONS AND PRECAUTIONS

Contraindicated in: ▪ Immunosuppression due to underlying disease or medications such as antineoplastic agents, immunotherapy, or glucocorticoids ▪ Fever ▪ Untreated infection ▪ Positive TB test (Mantoux) or active tuberculosis (TICE BCG or intradermal product) ▪ TheraCys and ImmuCyst not to be used to immunize against TB.
Use Cautiously in: ▪ Pregnancy, lactation, and children (safety not established) ▪ Current anti-infective therapy ▪ Small bladder capacity (increased irritation with bladder instillation) ▪ Previous (1–2 wk) transurethral resection (increased risk of disseminated infection).

ADVERSE REACTIONS AND SIDE EFFECTS*

Bladder Instillation

CNS: malaise, fatigue.
CV: hypotension.
GI: nausea, vomiting, hepatitis, abdominal pain.
GU: dysuria, hematura, frequency, urgency, infection, genital pain, renal toxicity, granulomatous prostatitis, incontinence, urethritis, genital inflammation, nocturia, decreased bladder capacity.
Hemat: anemia, leukopenia, coagulopathy.
MS: myalgia, arthralgia, athritis.
Misc: fever, chills, flu-like syndrome, infection including **SEPSIS** and **DISSEMINATED BCG INFECTION**.

Intradermal and Percutaneous

Note: Adverse reactions are much less frequent following percutaneous administration.
Misc: granuloma at intradermal site, prolonged irritation or necrosis at site, lymphadenopathy, osteomyelitis, lymphadenitis, **DISSEMINATED BCG INFECTION**.

INTERACTIONS

Drug–Drug ▪ **Immunosuppressive agents** or **radiation therapy** will decrease the proper immune response to intradermal or percutaneous BCG and increase the risk of disseminated BCG infection with all routes of administration ▪ May impair immune response to other **live vaccines** ▪ Decreases metabolism of **theophylline,** increases the risk for **theophylline** toxicity ▪ Decreases effectiveness of concurrently administered **rifampin, isoniazid,** or **streptomycin.**

ROUTE AND DOSAGE

Treatment and Prevention of Bladder Cancer

- **Intravesical (Adults):** TheraCys or ImmuCyst—81mg (three 27-mg vials) weekly for 6 wk. TICE BCG—50 mg once weekly for 6 wk.

Active Immunization Against Tuberculosis

- **Intradermal (Adults and Children >3 mon):** 0.1 ml.

*Underlines indicate most frequent; **CAPITALS** indicate life-threatening.

- **Intradermal (Children <3 mon):** 0.05 ml.
- **Percutaneous (Adults):** 0.2–0.3 ml applied with multipuncture disc.

PHARMACODYNAMICS

	ONSET	PEAK	DURATION
Intravasical*	rapid	UK	UK
Intradermal†	rapid	UK	prolonged (yrs)
Percutaneous†	rapid	UK	prolonged (yrs)

*Antineoplastic effect.
†Antibody response.

NURSING IMPLICATIONS

Assessment

- **Bladder Instillation:** Assess urinary tract symptoms frequently throughout therapy. If patient's symptoms persist or increase or if hematuria, urinary frequency, or dysuria occur, notify physician.
- □ Monitor patient for systemic BCG infection (fever, severe malaise). Notify physician if these symptoms occur.
- □ Periodically assess patient for cough following administration of BCG. Cough may indicate a life-threatening BCG systemic infection.
- **Intradermal/Percutaneous:** Assess injection site. Initial skin lesion appears in 7–10 days following intradermal and 10–14 days following percutaneous administration. Repeat tuberculin test in 2–3 mon; revaccinate if negative.
- **Intradermal:** Site has small red papule reaching maximum diameter of 8 mm in 5 wk. Top scales and dries. Lesion shrinks to smooth or scaly pink or bluish scar 3 mon after vaccination and to smooth or pitted white scar in 6 mon.
- **Percutaneous:** Site has papules that reach maximum 3 mm size in 4–6 wk, then scale and slowly subside. Usually no visible sign of vaccination remains at 6 mon.

Potential Nursing Diagnoses

- Urinary elimination, altered (indications).
- Infection, high risk for (adverse reactions).
- Knowledge deficit related to medication regimen (patient/family teaching).

Implementation

- **Bladder Instillation:** Patient should be NPO for 4 hr prior to instillation and should void immediately prior to instillation.
- □ Refrigerate BCG and diluent. Do not use after expiration date on vial; may be inactive. Use immediately after reconstitution; do not use after 2 hr. Do not use soln with flocculant or clumps not dispersed by gentle shaking. Do not expose to sunlight; minimize exposure to artificial light.
- □ Immediately following instillation, all equipment that may have come in contact with BCG should be placed in plastic bags marked "Infectious Waste" and disposed of accordingly as biohazardous waste.
- □ Use aseptic technique throughout catheter insertion and instillation and use caution not to unduly traumatize the urinary mucosa.
- □ During the first hr following instillation, patient should lie prone, supine, and on each side for 15 min in each position. After the first hr, patient is allowed to get up but should retain the soln for another hr (2 hr total). If patient is unable to retain soln for full 2 hr, allow to void in a seated position. At the end of 2 hr patient should be instructed to void in a seated position.
- □ Maintain adequate hydration throughout procedure.
- □ Following instillation, all urine voided for 6 hr should be disinfected with equal volume of 5% hypochlorite soln (undiluted household bleach) and allowed to stand for 15 min before flushing.
- □ *TheraCys:* Do not remove rubber stopper from the vial. Prepare immediately before use. Use mask and gloves when handling TheraCys. Reconstitute *only* with diluent provided to ensure proper dispersion of organisms.
- □ Further dilute the reconstituted soln

from 3 vials (1 dose) in 50 ml of sterile preservative-free saline for a final volume of 53 ml.

- *TICE BCG:* Use 3-ml syringe to draw up 1 ml of sterile, preservative-free saline and add to 1 ampule of TICE BCG. Draw the mixture into the syringe and gently expel back into the ampule 3 times to ensure mixing and minimize clumping of the mycobacteria. Soln is cloudy; add to top end of a catheter-tipped syringe containing 49 ml of saline diluent for a total volume of 50 ml. Rotate syringe gently. Do not filter.

- **Intradermal/Percutaneous:** Do not administer other live vaccines within 3 wk of BCG. Vaccines containing toxoids or other killed organisms may be administered 7 days before or 10 days after BCG. Diphtheria/tetanus may be given at same time as BCG but in the other arm.
- **Intradermal:** Add 1 ml of sterile water to each ampule and allow to stand for 1 min. Do not shake; withdrawal from ampule mixes soln. Refrigerate prior to use. Sterilize unused portion by autoclave or formalin soln.
- **Percutaneous:** Add 1 ml of preservative-free sterile water for injection to each ampule of vaccine. Draw mixture into syringe and expel into ampule 3 times to ensure mixing of soln. Refrigerate soln and protect from light. Use *TICE BCG* within 2 hr and *BCG vaccine* within 8 hr of reconstitution.

Patient/Family Teaching

- Advise patient to notify physician if symptoms increase or persist after a number of treatments, or if blood in the urine, fever and chills, frequent urge to urinate, increased frequency of urination, joint pain, nausea and vomiting, painful urination, cough, or skin rash occur.
- Instruct patient to sit to void following instillation of solution.

Evaluation

Effectiveness of therapy may be determined by: ▪ Elimination of residual tumor cells and prevention of recurrence ▪ Immunity to tuberculosis and decrease in serious complications from primary tuberculosis in children.

BECLOMETHASONE

(be-kloe-**meth**-a-sone)
Beclovent, Beconase, Vanceril, Vancernase

CLASSIFICATION(S):
Glucocorticoid—long-acting
Pregnancy Category C

INDICATIONS

▪ **Inhaln:** Anti-inflammatory and immunosuppressant in the treatment of chronic steroid-dependent asthma. May decrease requirement for or avoid use of systemic glucocorticoids ▪ **Intranasal:** Used in the management of allergic rhinitis and other chronic nasal inflammatory conditions, including nasal polyps.

ACTION

▪ Potent, locally acting anti-inflammatory and immune modifier. **Therapeutic Effects:** ▪ Decrease in symptoms of chronic asthma and allergic rhinitis.

PHARMACOKINETICS

Absorption: Action is mostly local. Additional drug may be swallowed, but systemic absorption is minimal at recommended doses.
Distribution: Action is local; 10–25% of inhaled dose is deposited at sites of action in respiratory tract.
Metabolism and Excretion: Elimination is mainly fecal; remainder is rapidly metabolized. Crosses the placenta.
Half-life: 15 hr.

CONTRAINDICATIONS AND PRECAUTIONS

Contraindicated in: ▪ Allergy to fluorocarbon propellants.
Use Cautiously in: ▪ Chronic treatment at higher than recommended doses may lead to adrenal suppression ▪ Systemic glucocorticoid therapy

(should not be abruptly discontinued when inhalable or intranasal therapy is started).

ADVERSE REACTIONS AND SIDE EFFECTS*

EENT: nasal burning, nasal irritation, nasal bleeding, sneezing attacks (following intranasal administration), oropharyngeal fungal infections (following inhalation).

Resp: wheezing, bronchospasm (following inhalation).

INTERACTIONS

Drug-Drug: ▪ None significant at recommended doses.

ROUTE AND DOSAGE

Note: Each spray/inhalation contains 42 mcg.

- **Inhaln (Adults):** 2–4 inhalations 3–4 times daily (not to exceed 20 inhalations/day).
- **Inhaln (Children 6–11 yr):** 1–2 inhalations 3–4 times daily (not to exceed 10 inhalations/day).
- **Intranasal (Adults):** 1 spray in each nostril 2–4 times daily.
- **Intranasal (Children 6–11 yr):** 1 spray in each nostril 3 times daily.

PHARMACODYNAMICS (anti-inflammatory activity)

	ONSET	PEAK	DURATION
Inhaln	days–wks	1–4 wk	UK
Intranasal	days–wks	1–4 wk	UK

NURSING IMPLICATIONS

Assessment

- **General Info:** When changing from oral systemic steroids or discontinuing beclomethasone, monitor patient for signs of steroid withdrawal (muscle and joint pain, fatigue, dizziness, hypotension). Notify physician immediately should these symptoms occur.
- **Inhaln:** Assess respiratory status, (rate, ease of breathing, lung sounds) periodically throughout therapy. Inspect oral membranes frequently for signs of candida infection (white patches; red, sore mucous membranes). Report sore throat, hoarseness, and cough to physician.
- **Nasal:** Assess degree of nasal stuffiness and character of discharge. Nasal burning and irritation may follow administration.

Potential Nursing Diagnoses

- Airway clearance, ineffective (indications).
- Oral mucous membranes, altered (side effects).
- Knowledge deficit related to medication regimen (patient/family teaching).

Implementation

- **Inhaln:** Inhalation bronchodilators, if used, should be administered several mins before beclomethasone in order to open airways and allow delivery of steroid to site of action. Wait 5 min before using other inhalation medications.
- **Nasal Spray:** Decongestant or antihistamine may be ordered prior to installation of nasal spray if secretions are present.

Patient/Family Teaching

- **General Info:** Advise patient to carry identification describing disease process and medication regimen at all times.
- □ Instruct patient to notify physician immediately if symptoms of oral or nasal infection occur, because therapy may need to be discontinued.
- **Inhaln:** Instruct patient in the proper use of the metered-dose inhaler. Shake well, exhale, close lips firmly around mouth piece, administer during second half of inhalation, and hold breath as long as possible after treatment to ensure deep instillation of medication. Instruct patient to wait at least 1 min between inhalations. Wash inhalation assembly at least daily in warm running water.
- □ Caution patient not to use higher than recommended doses or to increase frequency. Maximum of 20 inhal-

*Underlines indicate most frequent; **CAPITALS** indicate life-threatening.

ations/day for adults, 10/day for children aged 6–12. Notify physician if prescribed dose is ineffective. Doses >1600 mcg/day may result in adrenal insufficiency.

- Caution patient that medication is for prophylactic use only. During an acute asthma attack supplemental systemic steroids may be needed.
- Rinsing mouth and gargling with warm water or mouthwash may reduce dry mouth and hoarseness.
- **Nasal:** Instruct patient to gently clear nose first, then to position self with head tilted back. Patient places spray nozzle in one nostril, and gently presses on other nostril, then depresses activator while inhaling through nostril. Patient exhales through mouth.

Evaluation

Effectiveness of therapy can be demonstrated by: ▪ Improved pulmonary function in chronic bronchial asthma ▪ Relief of symptoms of seasonal or perennial rhinitis ▪ Prevention of recurrence of nasal polyps. One to 4 wk may be required before effects are seen in patients not receiving systemic steroids.

BENAZAPRIL

(ben-**az**-a-pril)

Lotensin

CLASSIFICATION(S):

Antihypertensive—angiotensin converting enzyme (ACE) inhibitor

Pregnancy Category D

INDICATIONS

▪ Alone or in combination with thiazide diuretics in the management of hypertension.

ACTION

▪ Prevents the production of angiotensin II, a potent vasoconstrictor that stimulates the production of aldosterone by blocking its conversion to the active form—result is systemic vasodilation. **Therapeutic Effect:** ▪ Lowering of blood pressure in hypertensive patients.

PHARMACOKINETICS

Absorption: 37% absorbed following oral administration.

Distribution: Much of the distribution not known. Crosses the placenta. Trace amounts enter breast milk.

Metabolism and Excretion: Metabolized by the liver to the benazaprilate, its active metabolite.

Half-life: 10–11 hr (benzaprilate); increased in renal impairment.

CONTRAINDICATIONS AND PRECAUTIONS

Contraindicated in: ▪ Hypersensitivity ▪ Cross-sensitivity with other ACE inhibitors may exist.

Use Cautiously in: ▪ Renal impairment, hypovolemia, hyponatremia, elderly patients (dosage reduction required) ▪ Aortic stenosis ▪ Collagen vascular disorders (increased risk of adverse renal effects) ▪ Cerebrovascular or cardiac insufficiency ▪ Pregnancy (may cause fetal malformation; hypotension, oliguria, or hypokalemia may occur in newborn) ▪ Lactation and children (safety not established) ▪ Surgery/anesthesia (hypotension may be exaggerated).

Extreme Caution in: Family history of hereditary angioedema.

ADVERSE REACTIONS AND SIDE EFFECTS*

CNS: dizziness, headache, fatigue.

Resp: cough.

CV: hypotension, tachycardia, angina pectoris.

GI: anorexia, loss of taste, nausea.

GU: proteinuria, renal failure.

Derm: rashes, pruritus.

F and E: hyperkalemia.

*Underlines indicate most frequent; **CAPITALS** indicate life-threatening.

Hemat: LEUKOPENIA, AGRANULOCYTOSIS.
Misc: fever, edema of face or lips.

INTERACTIONS

Drug–Drug: ▪ Additive hypotension with other **antihypertensives, nitrates, phenothiazides,** and acute ingestion of **alcohol** ▪ Hyperkalemia may result from concurrent use of **potassium supplements** or **potassium-sparing diuretics** ▪ Antihypertensive response may be blunted by **nonsteroidal anti-inflammatory agents** ▪ May increase serum **digoxin** levels ▪ May increase the risk of **lithium** toxicity ▪ Increased risk of hypersensitivity reactions with **allopurinal**.

ROUTE AND DOSAGE

Hypertension

- **PO (Adults):** 5–10 mg once daily initially, increased gradually to maintenance dose of 20–40 mg/day as a single dose or 2 divided doses.

PHARMACODYNAMICS (effect on blood pressure*)

	ONSET	PEAK	DURATION
PO	1 hr	2–4 hr	12–24 hr

*Full effects may not be noted until several wks of therapy.

NURSING IMPLICATIONS

Assessment

- Monitor blood pressure and pulse frequently during initial dosage adjustment and periodically throughout course of therapy. Notify physician of significant changes.
- **Lab Test Considerations:** Monitor BUN, creatinine, and electrolyte levels periodically. Serum potassium may be increased and BUN and creatinine transiently increased while sodium levels may be decreased.

Potential Nursing Diagnoses

- Cardiac output, decreased (indications, side effects).
- Knowledge deficit related to medication regimen (patient/family teaching).
- Noncompliance (patient/family teaching).

Implementation

- **PO:** Precipitous drop in blood pressure following first dose may occur. Discontinuing diuretic therapy 2–3 days prior to initiation of benazapril may decrease risk of hypotension. Resume diuretics if blood pressure is not controlled with benazapril.

Patient/Family Teaching

- Instruct patient to take benazapril exactly as directed, even if feeling better. Missed doses should be taken as soon as remembered but not if almost time for next dose. Do not double doses. Medication controls but does not cure hypertension. Warn patients not to discontinue benazapril therapy unless directed by the physician.
- Encourage patients to comply with additional interventions for hypertension (weight reduction, discontinuation of smoking, moderation of alcohol consumption, regular exercise, and stress management).
- Instruct patient and family on proper technique for blood pressure monitoring. Advise them to check blood pressure at least weekly and report significantly changes to physician.
- Caution patient to avoid salt substitutes or foods containing high levels of potassium or sodium unless directed by physician (see Appendix K).
- Caution patient to change positions slowly to minimize orthostatic hypotension, particularly after initial dose. Patients should also be advised that exercising or hot weather may increase hypotensive effects.
- Advise patients to consult physician or pharmacist before taking any over-the-counter medications, especially cold remedies. Patients should also avoid excessive amounts of tea, coffee, or cola.
- May cause dizziness. Caution patient to avoid driving and other activities

requiring alertness until response to medication is known.

- Advise patient to inform physician or dentist of medication regimen prior to treatment or surgery.
- Instruct patient to notify physician if rash, mouth sores, sore throat, fever, swelling of hands or feet, irregular heart beat, chest pain, dry cough, swelling of face, eyes, lips, or tongue, or difficulty breathing occurs or if taste impairment persists.
- Emphasize the importance of follow-up examinations to monitor progress.

EVALUATION

Effectiveness of therapy can be demonstrated by: ■ Decrease in blood pressure without appearance of side effects.

BENZOCAINE

(**ben**-zoe-kane)

Aerocaine, Aerotherm, Americaine, Anbesol, Benzocol, BiCozine, Cepacol, Chiggerex, Children's Chloraseptic, Colrex, Dermacoat, Dermoplast, ethylaminobenzoate, Foille, Hurricaine, Oracin, Orajel, Rhulicaine, Rid-a-Pain, Semets, Solarcaine, Spec-T, T-Caine, Tyrobenz

CLASSIFICATION(S):

Anesthetic—topical

Pregnancy Category C

INDICATIONS

■ **Skin and Local:** Relief of pruritus or pain associated with minor burns, fungal infections, and rashes including: □ Chickenpox □ Prickly heat □ Diaper rash □ Abrasions □ Bruises □ Small wounds or incisions including episiotomy □ Sunburn □ Poison ivy, oak, or sumac □ Insect bites □ Eczema ■ **Mucous Membranes:** Temporary relief of minor throat or mouth pain ■ **Male Genital Desensitizer:** Prevention of premature ejaculation.

ACTION

■ Inhibits conduction of sensory nerve impulses. **Therapeutic Effects:** ■ Local anesthesia with subsequent relief of pain and/or pruritus ■ Prevention of premature ejaculation.

PHARMACOKINETICS

Absorption: Poorly absorbed through intact skin; absorption increases with surface area and abrasions.

Distribution: Distribution not known.

Metabolism and Excretion: Small amounts that may be absorbed are primarily metabolized in plasma.

Half-life: UK.

CONTRAINDICATIONS AND PRECAUTIONS

Contraindicated in: ■ Hypersensitivity ■ Cross-sensitivity with other local anesthetics may exist ■ Hypersensitivity to any components of preparations including stabilizers, colorants, or bases ■ Active, untreated infection of affected area ■ Not to be used in the eye.

Use Cautiously in: ■ Extensive abrasion of skin or mucous membrane ■ Prolonged use (not recommended) ■ Gag reflex may be diminished following oral or nasotracheal application ■ Elderly patients, debilitated patients, and children (use smaller doses) ■ Children <2 yr (safety not established).

ADVERSE REACTIONS AND SIDE EFFECTS*

EENT: diminished gag reflex, decreased taste sensation.

Derm: contact dermatitis, urticaria, edema, burning stinging, tenderness, irritation.

Misc: allergic reactions including **ANAPHYLAXIS.**

INTERACTIONS

Drug-Drug: ■ Risk of systemic toxicity increased by concurrent administration of **cholinesterase inhibitors**.

*Underlines indicate most frequent; **CAPITALS** indicate life-threatening.

B

ROUTE AND DOSAGE

Local Anesthetic

- **Top or Mucous Membrane (Adults and Children):** Apply 5–20% preparation or use 3–10 mg lozenge 3–4 times daily as needed.

Male Genital Desensitizer

- **Top (Adults):** Apply 3–7.5% preparation in water-soluble base prior to intercourse.

PHARMACODYNAMICS (anesthetic effect following application to mucous membranes)

	ONSET	PEAK	DURATION
Top	within 1 min	1 min	30–60 min

NURSING IMPLICATIONS

Assessment

- □ Assess type, location, and intensity of pain prior to and a few mins after administration of benzocaine.
- □ Assess integrity of involved skin and mucous membranes prior to and periodically throughout course of therapy. Notify physician if signs of infection or irritation develop.

Potential Nursing Diagnoses

- Comfort, altered: pain (indications).
- Knowledge deficit related to medication regimen (patient/family teaching).

Implementation

- **General Info:** Available as gel, lozenge, soln, spray, and lotion.
- **Top:** Alcohol-free preparation available for teething pain in babies. Apply to gums by rubbing gel on with fingers or cotton swab.
- **Throat Spray:** Ensure gag reflex intact before allowing patient to drink or eat.
- **Otic:** Ensure tympanic membrane intact prior to administration of ear drops.

Patient/Family Teaching

- **General Info:** Instruct patient on correct application technique. Emphasize need to avoid contact with eyes.
- □ Advise patient to discontinue use if erythema, rash, or irritation at site of administration occurs.
- □ Advise adults using liquid form around the mouth to avoid smoking until soln is dry.
- **Teething Gel:** Instruct parents to notify pediatrician if pain is excessive or prolonged. Advise parents to avoid feeding immediately after application to prevent choking from diminished gag reflex.
- **Lozenge:** Instruct patient to suck on lozenge and allow it to slowly dissolve. Consult physician if throat pain persists more than 2 days. Avoid use in young children because of danger of choking.
- **Male Genital Desensitizer:** Discuss need to question partner regarding allergies to local anesthetics, sulfonamides, hair dye, and sunscreen to prevent possible sensitivity response.
- □ Explain that benzocaine should not impair partners' response. Instruct male to apply benzocaine to head and shaft of penis prior to intercourse and to wash penis after intercourse to remove remaining medication.

Evaluation

Effectiveness of therapy can be demonstrated by: ▪ Temporary relief of discomfort associated with minor irritations of skin or mucous membranes ▪ Prevention of premature ejaculation.

BENZQUINAMIDE

(benz-**kwin**-a-mide)
Emete-con

CLASSIFICATION(S):
Antiemetic
Pregnancy Category UK

INDICATIONS

- Prevention and treatment of nausea and vomiting associated with anesthesia and surgery.

ACTION

- Depresses the chemoreceptor trigger zone in the CNS. **Therapeutic Effect:** ▪ Relief of nausea and vomiting.

PHARMACOKINETICS

Absorption: Rapidly absorbed following IM administration.
Distribution: Widely distributed.
Metabolism and Excretion: Mostly metabolized by the liver. Minimal amounts excreted unchanged in the urine.
Half-life: 30–40 min.

CONTRAINDICATIONS AND PRECAUTIONS

Contraindicated in: ▪ Hypersensitivity ▪ Pregnancy (avoid use).
Use Cautiously in: ▪ History of cardiovascular disease ▪ Lactation and children (safety not established).

ADVERSE REACTIONS AND SIDE EFFECTS*

CNS: drowsiness, insomnia, restlessness, tremor.
EENT: blurred vision, increased salivation, dry mouth.
CV: hypotension, hypertension, arrhythmias.
GI: nausea, vomiting, cramps.

INTERACTIONS

Drug-Drug: ▪ Additive CNS depression with other **CNS depressants** including **alcohol, antihistamines, narcotic analgesics,** and **sedative/hypnotics** ▪ May cause hypertension in patients **receiving vasopressors** or **epinephrine**.

ROUTE AND DOSAGE

- **IM (Adults):** 50 mg (0.5–1.0 mg/kg), may be repeated in 1 hr, then q 3–4 hr as needed.
- **IV (Adults):** 25 mg (0.2–0.4 mg/kg).

PHARMACODYNAMICS (antiemetic effect)

	ONSET	PEAK	DURATION
IM	15 min	30 min	3–4 hr
IV	15 min	UK	3–4 hr

NURSING IMPLICATIONS

Assessment

- □ Assess nausea, vomiting, bowel sounds, and abdominal pain prior to and following administration. Benzquinamide may mask the signs of an acute abdomen.
- □ Monitor hydration status and intake and output. Patients with severe nausea and vomiting may require IV fluids in addition to antiemetics.
- □ Following IV administration, monitor patient for arrhythmias and changes in blood pressure.

Potential Nursing Diagnoses

- ▪ Fluid volume deficit (indications).
- ▪ Nutrition, altered: less than body requirements (indications).
- ▪ Injury, high risk for (side effects).

Implementation

- ▪ **General Info:** This drug may be administered prophylactically at least 15 min prior to emergence from anesthesia.
- □ Reconstitute with 2.2 ml of sterile or bacteriostatic water for injection. Results in 2 ml soln with concentration of 25 mg/ml. Do not use 0.9% NaCl for reconstitution as soln may form a precipitate. Reconstituted soln is stable at room temperature for 14 days if protected from light. Do not refrigerate.
- ▪ **IM:** IM injection should be made deep into muscle mass. Use deltoid site only if well developed. IM route is preferred because of arrhythmias resulting from IV administration. Aspirate carefully to prevent inadvertent IV administration.
- ▪ **Direct IV:** Do not administer through an IV line containing saline.
- □ *Rate:* Administer slowly, 1 ml (25 mg) over 30–60 sec, through Y-tubing or 3-way stopcock.
- ▪ **Syringe Compatibility:** atropine, droperidol/fentanyl, glycopyrrolate, hydroxyzine, ketamine, meperidine, midazolam, morphine, naloxone, pentazocine, propranolol, or scopolamine.

*Underlines indicate most frequent; **CAPITALS** indicate life-threatening.

B

- **Syringe Incompatibility:** chlordiazepoxide, diazepam, pentobarbital, phenobarbital, secobarbital, sodium chloride, or thiopental.
- **Y-Site Compatibility:** foscarnet.

PATIENT/FAMILY TEACHING

- Advise patient to call for assistance when ambulating, because this drug may cause drowsiness and sedation.
- Instruct patient to make position changes slowly to minimize orthostatic hypotension.
- Inform patient that this drug may cause dry mouth. Frequent oral rinses, good oral hygiene, and sugarless gum or candy may minimize this effect.
- Advise patient and family to use general measures to decrease nausea (begin with sips of liquids, small non-greasy meals, provide oral hygiene, remove noxious stimuli from environment).

EVALUATION

Effectiveness of therapy may be determined by: ▪ Decreased nausea and vomiting within 15–30 min following administration.

BENZTROPINE

(**benz**-troe-peen)
{Apo-benztropin}, {Bensylate}, benzatropine, Cogentin

CLASSIFICATION(S):
Anticholinergic—miscellaneous, Antiparkinson agent—anticholinergic
Pregnancy Category C

INDICATIONS

▪ Adjunctive treatment of all forms of Parkinson's disease, including drug-induced extrapyramidal effects and acute dystonic reactions.

ACTION

▪ Blocks cholinergic activity in the CNS, which is partially responsible for the symptoms of Parkinson's disease ▪ Restores the natural balance of neurotransmitters in the CNS. **Therapeutic Effect:** ▪ Reduction of rigidity and tremors.

PHARMACOKINETICS

Absorption: Rapidly and completely absorbed following oral and IM administration.
Distribution: UK.
Metabolism and Excretion: UK.
Half-life: UK.

CONTRAINDICATIONS AND PRECAUTIONS

Contraindicated in: ▪ Hypersensitivity ▪ Children <3 yr ▪ Narrow-angle glaucoma ▪ Tardive dyskinesia.
Use Cautiously in: ▪ Elderly patients (increased risk of adverse reactions) ▪ Pregnancy and lactation (safety not established).

ADVERSE REACTIONS AND SIDE EFFECTS*

CNS: confusion, weakness, hallucinations, headache, sedation, depression, dizziness.
EENT: dry eyes, blurred vision, mydriasis.
CV: tachycardia, arrhythmias, palpitations, hypotension.
GI: constipation, dry mouth, nausea, ileus.
GU: urinary retention, hesitancy.
Misc: decreased sweating.

INTERACTIONS

Drug-Drug: ▪ Additive anticholinergic affects with **drugs sharing anticholinergic properties** such as **antihistamines, phenothiazines, quinidine, disopyramide,** and **tricyclic antidepressants** ▪ Counteracts the cholinergic effects of **bethanecol** ▪ **Antacids** and **antidiarrheals** may decrease absorption.

{} = Available in Canada only.
*Underlines indicate most frequent; **CAPITALS** indicate life-threatening.

ROUTE AND DOSAGE

Parkinsonism

- **PO (Adults):** 0.5–6 mg/day in 1–2 divided doses.

Acute Dystonic Reactions

- **IM, IV (Adults):** 2 mg initially, then 1–2 mg PO bid.

Drug-Induced Extrapyramidal Reactions

- **PO, IM, IV (Adults):** 1–4 mg one 1–2 times daily.

PHARMACODYNAMICS (antidyskinetic activity)

	ONSET	PEAK	DURATION
PO	1–2 hr	several days	24 hr
IM, IV	within mins	UK	24 hr

NURSING IMPLICATIONS

Assessment

- **General Info:** Assess parkinson and extrapyramidal symptoms (akinesia, rigidity, tremors, pill rolling, mask facies, shuffling gait, muscle spasms, twisting motions, and drooling) prior to and throughout course of therapy.
  - Assess bowel function daily. Monitor for constipation, abdominal pain, distention, or the absence of bowel sounds. Report abnormal findings promptly.
  - Monitor intake and output ratios and assess patient for urinary retention (dysuria, distended abdomen, infrequent voiding of small amounts, overflow incontinence).
- Patients with mental illness are at risk of developing exaggerated symptoms of their disorder during early therapy with this medication. Withhold drug and notify physician if significant behavioral changes occur.
- **Parenteral Administration:** Monitor pulse and blood pressure closely and maintain bedrest for 1 hr after administration. Advise patients to make position changes slowly to minimize orthostatic hypotension.

Potential Nursing Diagnoses

- Mobility, impaired physical (indications).
- Injury, high risk for (indications).
- Knowledge deficit related to medication regimen (patient/family teaching).

Implementation

- **PO:** Administer with food or immediately after meals to minimize gastric irritation. May be crushed and administered with food if patient has difficulty swallowing.
- **IM:** Parenteral doses of the drug are only used in acute situations.
- **Direct IV:** IV route is rarely used because onset is same as with IM route.
  - *Rate:* Administer at a rate of 1 mg over 1 min.
- **Syringe Compatibility:** metoclopramide.

Patient/Family Teaching

- Encourage patient to take this drug exactly as directed. Missed doses should be taken as soon as remembered up to 2 hr before the next dose. Drug should be tapered off gradually when discontinuing or a withdrawal reaction may occur (anxiety, tachycardia, insomnia, return of parkinson or extrapyramidal symptoms).
- May cause drowsiness or dizziness. Advise patient to avoid driving or other activities that require alertness until response to the drug is known.
- Instruct patient that frequent rinsing of mouth, good oral hygiene, and sugarless gum or candy may decrease dry mouth. Patient should notify physician if dryness persists (saliva substitutes may be used). Also notify the dentist if dryness interferes with use of dentures.
- Caution patient to make position changes slowly to minimize orthostatic hypotension.
- Instruct patient to notify physician if difficulty with urination, constipation, or abdominal discomfort occurs.
- Advise patient to confer with physician or pharmacist prior to taking

over-the-counter medications, especially cold remedies, or drinking alcoholic beverages.

- Caution patient that this medication decreases perspiration. Overheating may occur during hot weather. Patients should notify physician if they cannot remain indoors in an air-conditioned environment during hot weather.
- Advise patient to avoid taking antacids or antidiarrheals within 1–2 hr of this medication.
- Emphasize the importance of routine follow-up examinations.

Evaluation

Effectiveness of therapy can be demonstrated by: ▪ Decrease in drooling and rigidity and an improvement in gait and balance. Therapeutic effects are usually seen 2–3 days after the initiation of therapy.

BEPRIDIL
(be-pri-dil)
Vascor

CLASSIFICATION(S):
Calcium channel blocker, Antianginal, Coronary vasodilator
Pregnancy Category C

INDICATIONS

▪ Management of effort-induced angina pectoris due to coronary insufficiency in patients who fail to respond to conventional therapy. Has been used with beta blockers or nitrates.

ACTION

▪ Inhibits the transport of calcium into myocardial and vascular smooth muscle cells, resulting in inhibition of excitation-contraction coupling and subsequent contraction. ▪ May decrease SA and AV node conduction. **Therapeutic Effect:** ▪ Coronary vasodilation with subsequent decrease in frequency and severity of attacks of angina pectoris.

PHARMACOKINETICS

Absorption: Well absorbed following oral administration.
Distribution: Crosses the placenta and enters breast milk, remainder of distribution not known.
Metabolism and Excretion: Mostly metabolized by the liver. Inactive metabolites excreted by the kidneys.
Half-life: 42 hr (following cessation of multiple dosing).

CONTRAINDICATIONS AND PRECAUTIONS

Contraindicated in: ▪ Hypersensitivity ▪ Serious ventricular arrhythmias (may be proarrhythmic) ▪ Hypotension ▪ Cardiac insufficiency ▪ Sick sinus syndrome (unless a pacemaker is placed) ▪ 2nd- and 3rd-degree heart block ▪ Congenital or drug-induced prolongation of the QT interval on ECG ▪ Recent (within 3 mon) myocardial infarction.
Use Cautiously in: ▪ Hepatic or renal impairment ▪ Left bundle branch block ▪ Sinus bradycardia (<50 bpm) ▪ Pregnancy, lactation, or children (safety not established).

ADVERSE REACTIONS AND SIDE EFFECTS*

CNS: headache, weakness, dizziness, drowsiness, insomnia, nervousness.
EENT: dry mouth, tinnitus.
Resp: dyspnea, respiratory infection.
CV: CONGESTIVE HEART FAILURE, VENTRICULAR ARRHYTHMIAS, prolonged QT interval, palpitations.
GI: nausea, dyspepsia, anorexia, diarrhea, abdominal pain, constipation.
Hemat: AGRANULOCYTOSIS.
Neuro: tremor, paresthesia.
Misc: flu-like syndrome.

INTERACTIONS

Drug-Drug: ▪ **Antiarrhythmics, antidepressants,** and **cardiac glycosides** may increase the likelihood of ventricular arrhythmias ▪ Increases serum **digoxin** levels.

*Underlines indicate most frequent; **CAPITALS** indicate life-threatening.

ROUTE AND DOSAGE

- **PO (Adults):** 200 mg once daily, may increase after 10 days to 300 mg/day (not to exceed 400 mg/day).

PHARMACODYNAMICS

	ONSET	PEAK	DURATION
PO	8 days*	UK	24 hr

*Onset of steady state antianginal effects with chronic dosing.

NURSING IMPLICATIONS

Assessment

- Assess location, duration, intensity, and precipitating factors of patient's anginal pain.
- Monitor pulse before administering medication. Monitor ECG periodically in patients receiving prolonged therapy.
- Monitor intake and output ratios and daily weight. Assess patient for signs of congestive heart failure (peripheral edema, rales/crackles, dyspnea, weight gain, jugular venous distention).
- Patients receiving cardiac glycosides concurrently with bepridil should have routine serum cardiac glycoside levels and be monitored for signs and symptoms of digitalis glycoside toxicity.
- **Lab Test Considerations:** Monitor WBC periodically in patients receiving long-term therapy.

Potential Nursing Diagnoses

- Cardiac output, decreased (indications).
- Comfort, altered: pain (indications).
- Knowledge deficit related to medication regimen (patient/family teaching).

Implementation

- **PO:** May be administered with meals if gastric irritation becomes a problem.

Patient/Family Teaching

- Advise patient to take medication exactly as prescribed, not to skip or double up on missed doses. Bepridil may need to be discontinued gradually.
- Instruct patients on concurrent nitrate or beta-blocker therapy to continue taking both medications as ordered and using SL nitroglycerin as needed for anginal attacks.
- May cause dizziness. Advise patient to avoid driving or other activities requiring alertness until response to the medication is known.
- Instruct patient to avoid concurrent use of alcohol or over-the-counter medications without consulting physician or pharmacist.
- Advise patient to contact physician if chest pain does not improve or worsens after therapy, or is accompanied by diaphoresis, or shortness of breath, or if severe, persistent headache occurs. Also notify the physician if irregular heart beats, dyspnea, swelling of hands and feet, pronounced dizziness, nausea, or constipation occur.

Evaluation

Effectiveness of therapy can be demonstrated by: ▪ Decrease in frequency and severity of anginal attacks ▫ Decreased need for nitrate therapy ▫ Increase in activity tolerance and sense of well-being.

BETAMETHASONE

(bay-ta-**meth**-a-sone)

Alphatrex, {Betacort}, {Betaderm}, Betameth, Betatrex, Beta-Val, {Betnelan}, {Betnesol}, {Betnovate}, Celestone, Cel-U-Jec, Dermabet, Diprolene, Diprosone, {Ectosone}, {Metaderm}, {Novabetamet}, Prelestone, Selestoject, Valisone, Valnac

CLASSIFICATION(S):
Glucocorticoid—long-acting
Pregnancy Category C (topical), UK (systemic)

{} = Available in Canada only.

INDICATIONS

▪ Used systemically and locally in a wide variety of chronic inflammatory, allergic, hematologic, neoplastic, and autoimmune diseases ▪ Not suitable for alternate-day therapy.

ACTION

▪ Suppresses inflammation and normal immune response. Has numerous intense metabolic effects (see *Adverse Reactions and Side Effects*). Suppresses adrenal function at chronic oral doses of 0.6 mg/day. **Therapeutic Effects:** ▪ Suppression of inflammation and modification of normal immune response.

PHARMACOKINETICS

Absorption: Well absorbed following oral administrations. Sodium phosphate salt is rapidly absorbed following IM administration. Acetate suspension is slowly absorbed. When injected locally, absorption is slow but complete. Systemic absorption also follows topical administration.

Distribution: Crosses the placenta. Small amounts enter breast milk.

Metabolism and Excretion: Mostly metabolized by the liver.

Half-life: 3–5 hr (plasma), 36–54 hr (tissue); adrenal suppression lasts 3.25 days.

CONTRAINDICATIONS AND PRECAUTIONS

Contraindicated in: ▪ Acute untreated infections except for some forms of meningitis ▪ Lactation (avoid chronic use) ▪ Avoid abrupt discontinuation.

Use Cautiously in: ▪ Chronic treatment (leads to adrenal suppression) ▪ Stress (supplemental doses necessary) ▪ Glaucoma ▪ Diabetes mellitus ▪ Pregnancy (safety not established) ▪ Children (chronic treatment results in decreased growth; use of short- or intermediate-acting glucorticoids is recommended) ▪ Use lowest dose for shortest period of time ▪ Some products contain bisulfites and/or tartrazine—use with caution in hypersensitive patients.

ADVERSE REACTIONS AND SIDE EFFECTS*

CNS: headache, restlessness, psychoses, depression, euphoria, personality changes, increased intracranial pressure (children only).

EENT: cataracts, increased intraocular pressure.

CV: hypertension.

GI: nausea, vomiting, anorexia, peptic ulceration, increased appetite.

Derm: impaired wound healing, petechiae, ecchymoses, skin fragility, hirsutism, acne.

Endo: adrenal suppression, hyperglycemia.

F and E: hypokalemia, hypokalemic alkalosis, fluid retention.

Hemat: thromboembolism, thrombophlebitis.

MS: muscle wasting, muscle pain, aseptic necrosis of joints, osteoporosis.

Misc: increased susceptibility to infection, cushingoid appearance (moon face, buffalo hump).

INTERACTIONS

Drug–Drug: ▪ Additive hypokalemia with **diuretics, amphotercin B, mezlocillin,** or **ticarcillin** ▪ Hypokalemia may increase the risk of **cardiac glycoside** toxicity ▪ **Barbiturates, phenytoin,** and **rifampin** increase metabolism and may decrease effectiveness ▪ May increase the need for **insulin** or **hypoglycemic agents.**

ROUTE AND DOSAGE

Note: 0.6 mg betamethasone is equivalent to 20 mg hydrocortisone.

Adrenocortical Insufficiency

- **PO (Children):** 17.5 mcg/kg (500 mcg/m^2) daily in 3 divided doses.
- **IM (Children):** 17.5 mcg/kg (500 mcg/m^2) daily in 3 divided doses every third day; or 5.8–8.75 mcg/kg (166–250 mcg/m^2) daily as a single dose.

*Underlines indicate most frequent; **CAPITALS** indicate life-threatening.

Other Oral Uses

- **PO (Adults):** 0.6 mg–7.2 mg/day as single daily dose or in divided doses.
- **PO (Children):** 62.5–250 mcg/kg (1.875–7.5 mg/m^2) daily in 3–4 divided doses.

Betamethasone Sodium Phosphate

- **IM, IV (Adults):** Up to 9 mg of betamethsone base (12 mg of betamethasone phosphate); given as needed.
- **IM (Children):** 20.8–125 mcg/kg (0.625–3.75 mg/m^2) of the base q 12–24 hr.
- **IA, IL, (Adults):** Up to 9 mg of betamethasone base (12 mg of betamethasone phosphate); given as needed.

Betamethasone Sodium Phosphate/ Betamethasone Acetate Suspension

- **IM (Adults):** 0.5–9 mg/day.
- **IA (Adults):** 1.5–12 mg (dose depends on joint); may be repeated as needed.
- **IL (Adults):** 1.2 mg/m^2 of affected skin (not to exceed 6 mg); may be repeated weekly.

Topical

- **Top (Adults):** Apply 1–3 times daily.
- **Top (Children):** Apply once daily.

PHARMACODYNAMICS (anti-inflammatory activity)

	ONSET	PEAK	DURATION
PO	UK	1–2 hr	3.25 days
IV	rapid	UK	UK
IM (phosphate)	rapid	UK	UK
IM (acetate/ phosphate)	1–3 hr	UK	1 wk
IS, IA	UK	UK	1–2 wk
IL, ST	UK	UK	1 wk
Top	hrs	UK	8–24 hr

NURSING IMPLICATIONS

Assessment

- **General Info:** Assess patient for signs of adrenal insufficiency prior to and periodically throughout therapy.
- □ Monitor intake and output ratios and daily weight. Assess for fluid overload (edema, steady weight gain, rales/crackles, or dyspnea).
- **IA:** Monitor pain, edema, and range of motion of affected joints.
- **Top:** Assess affected skin prior to and daily during therapy. Note degree of inflammation and pruritus.
- **Lab Test Considerations:** *Systemic*—Monitor serum electrolytes and glucose. May cause hyperglycemia, especially in persons with diabetes. May cause hypokalemia.
- □ Guaiac stools. Promptly report presence of guaiac-positive stools.
- □ Periodic adrenal function tests may be ordered to assess degree of hypothalamic-pituitary-adrenal axis suppression in systemic and chronic topical therapy.

Potential Nursing Diagnoses

- Skin integrity, impaired (indications).
- Infection, high risk for (side effects).
- Knowledge deficit related to medication regimen (patient/family teaching).

Implementation

- **General Info:** Suspension of betamethasone sodium phosphate and betamethasone acetate may be combined with 1% or 2% lidocaine without preservatives for injection into joint, tendon, or bursa.
- **PO:** Administer with meals to minimize GI irritation. For daily dose, give in AM to coincide with body's normal secretion of cortisol.
- **Direct IV:** Only betamethasone sodium phosphate may be given IV.
- □ *Rate:* Administer over at least 1 min.
- **Intermittent Infusion:** May be administered as infusion in D5W, 0.9% NaCl, Ringers soln, D5/Ringers soln, or D5/LR.
- **Y-Site Compatibility:** heparin, hydrocortisone sodium succinate, or potassium chloride.
- **Top:** Available as a powder, gel, cream, lotion, ointment, and in aerosol form.
- □ Apply to clean, slightly moist skin. Wear gloves. Do not apply occlusive dressing.

□ Apply aerosol form from a distance of 15 cm for 3 sec.

Patient/Family Teaching

▪ **General Info:** Instruct patient on correct technique of medication administration. Emphasize importance of avoiding the eyes. Advise patient to take medication exactly as directed. Missed doses should be taken as soon as remembered unless almost time for next dose. Do not double doses. Stopping the medication suddenly may result in adrenal insufficiency (anorexia, nausea, weakness, fatigue, hypotension, hypoglycemia). If these signs appear notify physician immediately. This can be life-threatening.

□ This drug causes immunosuppression and may mask symptoms of infection. Instruct patient to avoid persons with known contagious illnesses and to notify physician if infection occurs.

□ Caution patient to avoid vaccinations without first consulting with physician.

□ Instruct patient to notify physician if severe abdominal pain, tarry stools, unusual pain, swelling, weight gain, tiredness, bone pain, bruising, nonhealing sores, visual disturbances, or behavior changes occur.

□ Explain need for continued medical follow-up to assess effectiveness and possible side effects of medication. Physician may order periodic lab tests and eye examinations.

□ Instruct patient to inform physician if symptoms of underlying disease return or worsen.

□ Advise patient to carry identification describing disease process and medication regimen in the event of emergency in which patient cannot relate medical history.

▪ **Long-term Therapy:** Encourage patient to eat a diet high in protein, calcium, and potassium, and low in sodium and carbohydrates (see Appendix K). Alcohol should be avoided during therapy.

Evaluation

Effectiveness of therapy can be demonstrated by: ▪ Decrease in presenting symptoms with minimal systemic side effects.

BETAXOLOL

(be-**tax**-oh-lol)
Betoptic, Kerlone

CLASSIFICATION(S):
Antiglaucoma agent—beta-adrenergic blocker; Beta-adrenergic blocker—selective, Antihypertensive—beta-adrenergic blocker
Pregnancy Category C

INDICATIONS

▪ **PO:** Used alone or in combination with other agents in the treatment of hypertension ▪ **Ophth:** Decreases intraocular pressure in patients with chronic open-angle glaucoma.

ACTION

▪ **PO:** Blocks stimulation of $beta_1$ (myocardial) receptors ▪ **Ophth:** Decreases the production of aqueous humor. **Therapeutic Effect:** ▪ ***PO:*** Decreased blood pressure ▪ ***Ophth:*** Decreased intraocular pressure.

PHARMACOKINETICS

Absorption: Well absorbed following oral administration. Systemic absorption is minimal following ophthalmic administration.
Distribution: Widely distributed when administered systemically.
Metabolism and Excretion: Mostly metabolized by the liver; 20% excreted unchanged by the kidneys following systemic administration.
Half-life: 15–20 hr.

CONTRAINDICATIONS AND PRECAUTIONS

Contraindicated in: ▪ Hypersensitivity to benzalkonium chloride or edetate disodium (ophthalmic preparation only) ▪ Uncompensated congestive heart failure ▪ Pulmonary edema ▪ Cardiogenic shock ▪ Bradycardia ▪ Heart block.

Use Cautiously in: ▪ Cardiac failure ▪ Diabetes mellitus (may block some symptoms of hypoglycemia) ▪ Pulmonary disease including asthma ▪ Thyrotoxicosis ▪ Children, pregnancy, or lactation (safety not established) ▪ Renal impairment (dosage reduction recommended for oral dosage form) ▪ Ophthalmic administration (systemic effects may occur).

ADVERSE REACTIONS AND SIDE EFFECTS*

CNS: Ophth—insomnia, depressive neurosis; PO—dizziness, anxiety, nervousness, nightmares, vivid dreams, tiredness, weakness, confusion.

EENT: Ophth—ocular stinging, tearing, erythema, itching, keratitis, corneal staining, unequal pupil size, photophobia; PO—dry eyes, sore eyes, stuffy nose.

Resp: Ophth and PO—bronchospasm.

CV: PO—bradycardia, CONGESTIVE HEART FAILURE.

GI: PO—diarrhea, nausea, vomiting.

GU: PO—impotence.

Derm: rash.

Hemat: PO—thrombocytopenia.

MS: PO—back pain, joint pain.

Misc: Raynaud's phenomenon.

INTERACTIONS

Drug-Drug: ▪ **PO: General anesthesia, IV phenytoin,** and **verapamil** may cause additive myocardial depression ▪ Additive bradycardia may occur with concurrent use of **cardiac glycosides** ▪ Additive hypotension may occur with other **antihypertensive agents,** acute ingestion of **alcohol,** or **nitrates** ▪ Concurrent use with **amphetamines, cocaine, ephedrine, epinephrine, norepinephrine, phenylephrine,** or **pseudoephedrine** may result in excess alpha-adrenergic stimulation, hypertension and bradycardia ▪ May negate the beneficial $beta_1$ cardiac effects of **dopamine** or **dobutamine** ▪ Concurrent **thyroid** administration may decrease effectiveness ▪ Use with **insulin** may result in prolonged hypoglycemia. ▪ **Ophth:** Additive beta-adrenergic blockade may occur with concurrent **systemic beta-adrenergic blocking agents** ▪ Use cautiously in patients receiving **reserpine** or **adrenergic psychotropic agents**.

ROUTE AND DOSAGE

- **PO (Adults):** 10 mg once daily, may be increased to 20 mg/day after 7–14 days of therapy.
- **Ophth (Adults):** One drop of 0.25% or 0.5% soln twice daily.

PHARMACODYNAMICS

	ONSET	PEAK	DURATION
PO	3–4 hr	7–14 days*	24 hr
Ophth	30 min	2 hr	12 hr

*With multiple dosing.

NURSING IMPLICATIONS

Assessment

- **PO:** Monitor blood pressure and pulse frequently during period of dosage adjustment and periodically throughout therapy. Confer with physician prior to giving drug if pulse is <50 bpm.
- **Ophth:** Intraocular pressure should be monitored during the first mon of therapy and periodically thereafter.

Potential Nursing Diagnoses

- Cardiac output, decreased (indications).
- Knowledge deficit related to medication regimen (patient/family teaching).

Implementation

- **PO:** May be administered concurrently with diuretic therapy.
- **Ophth:** Administer ophthalmic soln by having patient tilt head back and look up, gently depress lower lid with index finger until conjunctival sac is exposed and instill medication. After instillation, maintain gentle pressure on the inner canthus for 1 min to

*Underlines indicate most frequent; CAPITALS indicate life-threatening.

avoid systemic absorption of the drug. Wait at least 5 min before administering other types of eyedrops.
- ▫ When using betaxolol to replace other antiglaucoma agents, continue administration of all medications on the first day of betaxolol therapy. Decrease use of other medications weekly, one at a time, based on patient response.
- ▫ To control intraocular pressure, betaxolol may be used concurrently with muscarinic agonists (pilocarpine, echothiophate, carbachol), beta-agonists (ophthalmic epinephrine, dipivefrin), or systemic carbonic anhydrase inhibitors (acetazolamide).

Patient/Family Teaching

- ▪ **General Info:** Advise patient to take medication exactly as directed. Missed doses should be administered as soon as remembered unless almost time for the next dose; administer next dose at scheduled time.
- ▫ Inform diabetic patients that betaxolol may mask some signs of hypoglycemia.
- ▫ Advise patient to inform physician or dentist of medication regimen prior to treatment or surgery. Gradual withdrawal of betaxolol may be necessary.
- ▫ Instruct patient to notify physician if confusion, depression, sleep disturbance, weakness, wheezing, or dyspnea occur.
- ▫ Emphasize the importance of regular follow-up examinations to monitor progress.
- ▪ **PO:** Teach patient and family how to check blood pressure and pulse. Instruct them to take pulse daily and blood pressure biweekly. Advise patient to hold dose and contact physician if pulse is <50 bpm or blood changes significantly.
- ▫ Reinforce need to continue additional therapies for hypertension (weight loss, restricted sodium intake, stress reduction, regular exercise, moderation of alcohol consumption, cessation of smoking). Betaxolol controls but does not cure hypertension.
- ▫ Caution patient that this medication may cause increased sensitivity to cold.
- ▫ Advise patient to consult physician before taking any over-the-counter drugs, especially cold remedies, concurrently with this medication. Patient should also avoid excessive amounts of coffee, tea, and cola.
- ▫ Advise patient to carry identification describing medication regimen at all times.
- ▪ **Ophth:** Instruct patient in proper technique for instillation of ophthalmic medications. Emphasize the importance of not touching the applicator tip to any surface.
- ▫ Advise patient to wear sunglasses and avoid exposure to bright light to prevent photophobia.

Evaluation

Effectiveness of therapy can be demonstrated by: ▪ Decreased blood pressure ▪ Decreased intraocular pressure.

BETHANECHOL

(be-**than**-e-kole)
Duvoid, Urecholine, Urolax

CLASSIFICATION(S):
Cholinergic—direct-acting
Pregnancy Category C

INDICATIONS

▪ Treatment of postpartum and postoperative nonobstructive urinary retention or urinary retention due to neurogenic bladder.

ACTION

▪ Stimulates cholinergic receptors. Effects include: ▫ Contraction of the urinary bladder ▫ Decreased bladder capacity ▫ Increased frequency of ureteral periostaltic waves ▫ Increased tone and peristalsis in the GI tract ▫ Increased pressure in the lower esophageal sphincter ▫ Increased gastric secretions. **Therapeutic Effect:** ▪ Bladder emptying.

PHARMACOKINETICS

Absorption: Poorly absorbed following oral administration, requiring larger doses by mouth than subcutaneously.
Distribution: Does not cross the blood–brain barrier.
Metabolism and Excretion: UK.
Half-life: UK.

CONTRAINDICATIONS AND PRECAUTIONS

Contraindicated in: ▪ Hypersensitivity ▪ Mechanical obstruction of the GI or GU tract.
Use Cautiously in: ▪ History of asthma ▪ Ulcer disease ▪ Cardiovascular disease ▪ Epilepsy ▪ Hyperthyroidism ▪ Children, pregnancy, and lactation (safety not established) ▪ Sensitivity to cholinergic agents or effects.

ADVERSE REACTIONS AND SIDE EFFECTS*

CNS: malaise, headache.
EENT: lacrimation, miosis.
Resp: bronchospasm.
CV: hypotension, bradycardia, SYNCOPE WITH CARDIAC ARREST, heart block.
GI: abdominal discomfort, diarrhea, nausea, vomiting, salivation.
GU: urgency.
Misc: hypothermia, flushing, sweating.

INTERACTIONS

Drug–Drug: ▪ **Quinidine** and **procainamide** may antagonize cholinergic effects ▪ Additive cholinergic effects with **cholinesterase inhibitors** ▪ Use with **ganglionic blocking agents** may result in severe hypotension ▪ Do not use with **depolarizing neuromuscular blocking agents**.

ROUTE AND DOSAGE

- **PO (Adults):** Initially dose may be determined by administering 5–10 mg hourly until response obtained or total of 50 mg administered. Maintenance dose is 10–50 mg 2–4 times daily (doses up to 50–100 mg 4 times daily have been used).
- **SC (Adults):** Initially dose may be determined by administering 2.5 mg q 15–30 min until response obtained or total of 4 doses administered. Maintenance dose is 2.5–5 mg 3–4 times daily, up to 7.5–10 mg q 4 hr for neurogenic bladder.

PHARMACODYNAMICS (response on bladder muscle)

	ONSET	PEAK	DURATION
PO	30–90	1 hr	6 hr
SC	5–15	15–30 min	2 hr

NURSING IMPLICATIONS

Assessment

- □ Monitor blood pressure, pulse, and respirations before administering and for at least 1 hr following SC administration.
- □ Monitor input and output ratios. Palpate abdomen for bladder distention. Notify physician if drug fails to relieve condition for which it was prescribed. Physician may order catheterization to assess postvoid residual.
- ▪ **Lab Test Considerations:** May cause an increase in serum amylase and lipase, SGOT (AST), and serum bilirubin.
- ▪ **Toxicity and Overdose:** Observe patient for drug toxicity (sweating, flushing, abdominal cramps, nausea, salivation). If overdosage occurs, treatment includes atropine sulfate (specific antidote).

Potential Nursing Diagnoses

- ▪ Urinary elimination, altered (indications).
- ▪ Knowledge deficit related to medication regimen (patient/family teaching).

Implementation

- ▪ **General Info:** A test dose is usually used prior to maintenance.
- □ Oral and SC doses are *not* interchangeable.
- ▪ **PO:** Administer medication on an empty stomach, 1 hr before or 2 hr af-

*Underlines indicate most frequent; CAPITALS indicate life-threatening.

ter meals, to prevent nausea and vomiting.

- **SC:** Parenteral soln is intended only for subcutaneous administration. Do not give IM or IV. Inadvertent IM or IV administration may cause cholinergic overstimulation (circulatory collapse, drop in blood pressure, abdominal cramps, bloody diarrhea, shock, and cardiac arrest).
- □ Do not use if soln is discolored or contains a precipitate.

Patient/Family Teaching

- □ Instruct patient to take medication exactly as directed. Missed doses should be taken as soon as remembered within 1 hr; otherwise, return to regular dosing schedule. Do not double doses.
- □ Caution patient to make position changes slowly to minimize orthostatic hypotension.
- □ Advise patient to report abdominal discomfort, salivation, or flushing to physician.

Evaluation

Effectiveness of therapy can be demonstrated by: ▪ Increase in bladder function and tone ▪ Decrease in abdominal distention.

BIPERIDIN
(by-**per**-i-den)
Akineton

CLASSIFICATION(S):
Antiparkinson agent—anticholinergic
Pregnancy Category C

INDICATIONS

▪ Adjunctive treatment of all forms of Parkinson's disease, including drug-induced extrapyramidal effects and acute dystonic reactions.

ACTION

▪ Blocks cholinergic activity in the CNS, which is partially responsible for the symptoms of Parkinson's disease ▪ Restores the natural balance of neurotransmitters in the CNS. **Therapeutic Effect:** ▪ Reduction of rigidity and tremors.

PHARMACOKINETICS

Absorption: Well absorbed following oral or IM administration.
Distribution: UK.
Metabolism and Excretion: UK.
Half-life: UK.

CONTRAINDICATIONS AND PRECAUTIONS

Contraindicated in: ▪ Hypersensitivity ▪ Narrow-angle glaucoma ▪ Bowel obstruction ▪ Megacolon ▪ Tardive dyskinesia.
Use Cautiously in: ▪ Elderly patients (increased risk of adverse reactions) ▪ Prostatic enlargement ▪ Seizure disorders ▪ Cardiac arrhythmias ▪ Pregnancy and lactation (safety not established).

ADVERSE REACTIONS AND SIDE EFFECTS*

CNS: confusion, weakness, hallucinations, headache, sedation, depression, dizziness.
EENT: dry eyes, blurred vision, mydriasis.
CV: tachycardia, arrhythmias, palpitations, hypotension.
GI: constipation, dry mouth, nausea, ileus.
GU: urinary retention, hesitancy.
Misc: decreased sweating.

INTERACTIONS

Drug-Drug: ▪ Additive anticholinergic affects with **drugs sharing anticholinergic properties** such as **antihistamines, phenothiazines, quinidine, disopyramide,** and **tricyclic antidepressants** ▪ Counteracts the cholinergic effects of **bethanecol** ▪ **Antacids** or **antidiarrheals** may decrease absorption.

ROUTE AND DOSAGE

Parkinsonian Syndrome

▪ **PO (Adults):** 2 mg 3–4 times daily initially (not to exceed 16 mg/day).

*Underlines indicate most frequent; **CAPITALS** indicate life-threatening.

Extrapyramidal Reactions
- **PO (Adults):** 2 mg 1–3 times daily.
- **IM, IV (Adults):** 2 mg, may repeat q 30 min (not to exceed 8 mg in 24 hr).

PHARMACODYNAMICS (relief of parkinsonian symptoms or extrapyramidal reaction)

	ONSET	PEAK	DURATION
PO	UK	UK	UK
IM, IV	UK	UK	UK

NURSING IMPLICATIONS

Assessment
- **General Info:** Assess parkinson and extrapyramidal symptoms (akinesia, rigidity, tremors, pill rolling, mask facies, shuffling gait, muscle spasms, twisting motions, and drooling) prior to and throughout course of therapy.
- Assess bowel function daily. Monitor for constipation, abdominal pain, distention, or the absence of bowel sounds. Report abnormal findings promptly.
- Monitor intake and output ratios and assess patient for urinary retention (dysuria, distended abdomen, infrequent voiding of small amounts, overflow incontinence).
- After parenteral administration, monitor pulse and blood pressure closely and maintain bedrest for 1 hr. Advise patients to make position changes slowly to minimize orthostatic hypotension.

Potential Nursing Diagnoses
- Mobility, impaired physical (indications).
- Infection, high risk for (indications).
- Knowledge deficit related to medication regimen (patient/family teaching).

Implementation
- **PO:** Administer with food or immediately after meals to minimize gastric irritation.
- **IM:** Parenteral dose may be repeated every 30 min if tolerated until symptoms resolve. Limit to 4 doses per day.
- **Direct IV:** Administer each dose over at least 1 min to minimize hypotension and mild bradycardia.

Patient/Family Teaching
- Advise patient to take medication exactly as directed. Missed doses should be taken as soon as remembered up to 2 hr before the next dose. Drug should be tapered off gradually when discontinuing or a withdrawal reaction may occur (anxiety, tachycardia, insomnia, return of parkinson or extrapyramidal symptoms).
- May cause drowsiness, dizziness, or blurred vision. Advise patient to avoid driving or other activities that require alertness until response to the drug is known.
- Advise patient to make position changes slowly to minimize orthostatic hypotension.
- Advise patient that frequent mouth rinses, good oral hygiene, and sugarless gum or candy may decrease dry mouth. Patient should notify physician if dry mouth persists (saliva substitutes may be used). Also notify the dentist if dry mouth interferes with use of dentures.
- Instruct patient/family to notify physician if difficulty with urination, persistent constipation, peristent visual changes, or altered mental status occur.
- Advise patient to confer with physician or pharmacist prior to taking over-the-counter medications, especially cold remedies, or drinking alcoholic beverages.
- Caution patient that this medication decreases perspiration. Overheating may occur during hot weather. Patients should notify physician if they cannot remain indoors in an air-conditioned environment during hot weather.
- Advise patient to avoid antacids or antidiarrheals within 1–2 hr of this medication.
- Emphasize the importance of routine follow-up examinations.

B

Evaluation

Effectiveness of therapy can be demonstrated by: ▪ Decrease in drooling and rigidity in Parkinson's disease ▪ Resolution of drug-induced extrapyramidal reactions.

BISACODYL

(bis-a-**koe**-dill)
{Bisacolax}, Bisco-Lax, Carter's Little Pills, Clysodrast, Dacodyl, Deficol, Dulcolax, {Laxit}, Theralax

CLASSIFICATION(S):
Laxative—stimulant
Pregnancy Category UK

INDICATIONS

▪ Treatment of constipation, particularly when associated with: ▫ Prolonged bed rest ▫ Constipating drugs ▫ Slow transit time ▫ Irritable bowel syndrome ▪ Evacuation of the bowel prior to radiologic studies or surgery ▪ Also useful in patients with spinal cord injury as part of a bowel regimen.

ACTION

▪ Stimulates peristalsis ▪ Alters fluid and electrolyte transport producing fluid accumulation in the colon. **Therapeutic Effect:** ▪ Evacuation of the colon.

PHARMACOKINETICS

Absorption: Minimal absorption following oral administration. Action is local in the colon.
Distribution: Small amounts of metabolites excreted in breast milk.
Metabolism and Excretion: Small amounts absorbed are metabolized by the liver.
Half-life: UK.

CONTRAINDICATIONS AND PRECAUTIONS

Contraindicated in: ▪ Hypersensitivity ▪ Abdominal pain ▪ Obstruction ▪ Nausea or vomiting, especially when associated with fever or other signs of an acute abdomen.
Use Cautiously in: ▪ Severe cardiovascular disease ▪ Anal or rectal fissures ▪ Excess or prolonged use (may result in dependence) ▪ Has been used during pregnancy and lactation.

ADVERSE REACTIONS AND SIDE EFFECTS*

GI: <u>nausea</u>, <u>abdominal cramps</u>, diarrhea, rectal burning.
MS: muscle weakness (chronic use).
F and E: hypokalemia (with chronic use).
Misc: protein losing enteropathy, tetany (with chronic use).

INTERACTIONS

Drug-Drug: ▪ **Antacids** may remove enteric coating of tablets ▪ May decrease the absorption of other **orally administered drugs** because of increased motility and decreased transit time.

ROUTE AND DOSAGE

- **PO (Adults):** 5–15 mg (up to 30 mg).
- **PO (Children >3 yr):** 5–10 mg or 0.3 mg/kg.
- **Rect—Suppository (Adults and Children >2 yr):** 10 mg.
- **Rect—Suppository (Children <2 yr and Infants):** 5 mg.
- **Rect—Enema (Adults):** 1.5–4.5 mg (1–3 pkts)—contains tannex.

PHARMACODYNAMICS (evacuation of bowel)

	ONSET	PEAK	DURATION
PO	6–12 hr	UK	UK
Rect	15–60 min	UK	UK

NURSING IMPLICATIONS

Assessment

- **General Info:** Assess patient for abdominal distention, presence of bowel sounds, and usual pattern of bowel function.

{} = Available in Canada only.
*<u>Underlines</u> indicate most frequent; **CAPITALS** indicate life-threatening.

- Assess color, consistency, and amount of stool produced.

Potential Nursing Diagnoses

- Bowel elimination, altered: constipation (indications).
- Knowledge deficit related to medication regimen (patient/family teaching).

Implementation

- **General Info:** May be administered at bedtime for morning results.
- **PO:** Taking oral doses on an empty stomach will produce more rapid results.
- Do not crush or chew enteric-coated tablets. Take with a full glass of water or juice.
- Do not administer oral doses within 1 hr of milk or antacids; this may lead to premature dissolution of tablet and subsequent gastric or duodenal irritation.
- **Rect:** Suppository or enema can be given at the time a bowel movement is desired. Lubricate suppositories with water or water-soluble lubricant prior to insertion. Encourage patient to retain the suppository or enema 15–30 min before expelling.

Patient/Family Teaching

- Advise patients, other than those with spinal cord injuries, that laxatives should be used only for short-term therapy. Long-term therapy may cause electrolyte imbalance and dependence.
- Advise patient to increase fluid intake to a minimum of 1500–2000 ml/day during therapy to prevent dehydration.
- Encourage patients to utilize other forms of bowel regulation such as increasing bulk in the diet, increasing fluid intake, increasing mobility. Normal bowel habits are individualized and may vary from 3 times/day to 3 times/wk.
- Instruct patients with cardiac disease to avoid straining during bowel movements (Valsalva maneuver).
- Advise patient that bisacodyl should not be used when constipation is accompanied by abdominal pain, fever, nausea, or vomiting.

Evaluation

Effectiveness of therapy can be demonstrated by: ▪ The patient having a soft, formed bowel movement when used for constipation ▪ Evacuation of colon when used before surgery or radiologic studies, or for patients with spinal cord injury.

BISMUTH SUBSALICYLATE

(**bis**-muth sub-sa-**li**-si-late)
Pepto-Bismol

CLASSIFICATION(S):
Antidiarrheal—miscellaneous
Pregnancy Category UK

INDICATIONS

▪ Adjunctive therapy in the treatment of mild to moderate diarrhea ▪ Treatment of nausea, abdominal cramping, heartburn, and indigestion that may accompany diarrheal illnesses. **Unlabeled Use:** ▪ Treatment and prevention of traveler's (enterotoxigenic *Escherchia coli*) diarrhea.

ACTION

▪ Promotes intestinal adsorption of fluids and electrolytes ▪ Decreases synthesis of intestinal prostaglandins. **Therapeutic Effect:** ▪ Relief of diarrhea.

PHARMACOKINETICS

Absorption: Not absorbed.
Distribution: None.
Metabolism and Excretion: Excreted unchanged in the feces.
Half-life: UK.

CONTRAINDICATIONS AND PRECAUTIONS

Contraindicated in: ▪ Elderly patients who may be impacted ▪ Children or teenagers during or after recovery from chickenpox or flu-like illness (contains salicylate) ▪ Aspirin hypersensitivity.
Use Cautiously in: ▪ Infants, elderly or debilitated patients (impaction may oc-

B

cur) ▪ Patients undergoing radiologic examination of the GI tract (bismuth is radiopaque) ▪ Pregnancy or lactation (safety not established) ▪ Diabetes mellitus ▪ Gout.

ADVERSE REACTIONS AND SIDE EFFECTS*

GI: constipation, impaction, gray-black stools.

INTERACTIONS

Drug–Drug: ▪ If taken with **aspirin,** may potentiate signs of salicylate toxicity ▪ May decrease the absorption of **tetracycline** ▪ May alter the effect of **oral anticoagulants.**

ROUTE AND DOSAGE

- **PO (Adults):** 2 tablets or 30 ml; may repeat q 30 min–1 hr, up to 8 doses/24 hr.
- **PO (Children 9–12 yr):** 1 tablet or 15 ml; may repeat q 30 min–1 hr, up to 8 doses/24 hr.
- **PO (Children 6–9 yr):** ⅔ tablet or 10 ml; may repeat q 30 min–1 hr, up to 8 doses/24 hr.
- **PO (Children 3–6 yr):** ⅓ tablet or 5 ml; may repeat q 30 min–1 hr, up to 8 doses/24 hr.
- **PO (Children <3 yr weighing 28 lb or more):** 5 ml; may repeat q 4 hr, up to 6 doses/24 hr.
- **PO (Children <3 yr weighing 14–18 lb):** 2.5 ml; may repeat q 4 hr, up to 6 doses/24 hr.

PHARMACODYNAMICS (relief of diarrhea and other GI symptoms)

	ONSET	PEAK	DURATION
PO	within 24 hr	UK	UK

NURSING IMPLICATIONS

Assessment

- Assess the frequency and consistency of stools, presence of nausea and indigestion, and bowel sounds prior to and throughout course of therapy.
- Assess patient's fluid and electrolyte balance and skin turgor for dehydration if diarrhea is prolonged.

Potential Nursing Diagnoses

- Bowel elimination, altered: diarrhea (indications).
- Bowel elimination, altered: constipation (side effects).
- Knowledge deficit related to medication regimen (patient/family teaching).

Implementation

- **PO:** Shake liquid well before using. Chewable tablets may be chewed well or allowed to dissolve before swallowing.

Patient/Family Teaching

- Instruct patient to take medication exactly as directed.
- Inform patient that medication may temporarily cause stools and tongue to appear gray-black.
- Advise patient taking concurrent aspirin products that bismuth subsalicylate should be discontinued if ringing in the ears occurs.
- Instruct patient to notify physician if diarrhea persists for more than 2 days or if accompanied by a high fever.
- Centers for Disease Control warn against giving salicylates to children or adolescents with varicella (chickenpox) or influenza-ike or viral illnesses because of a possible association with Reye's syndrome.

Evaluation

Effectiveness of therapy may be determined by: ▪ Decrease in diarrhea ▪ Decrease in symptoms of indigestion ▪ Prevention of traveler's diarrhea.

BLEOMYCIN

(blee-oh-**mye**-sin)
Blenoxane

CLASSIFICATION(S):
Antineoplastic—antitumor antibiotic
Pregnancy Category UK

*Underlines indicate most frequent; **CAPITALS** indicate life-threatening.

INDICATIONS

▪ Used alone or in combination with other antineoplastic agents in the treatment of: ▫ Lymphomas ▫ Squamous cell carcinoma ▫ Testicular embryonal cell carcinoma ▫ Choriocarcinoma ▫ Teratocarcinoma. **Unlabeled Use:** ▪ Intrapleural administration to prevent the reaccumulation of malignant effusions.

ACTION

▪ Inhibits DNA and RNA synthesis. **Therapeutic Effect:** ▪ Death of rapidly replicating cells, particularly malignant ones.

PHARMACOKINETICS

Absorption: Not absorbed from the GI tract. Well absorbed from IM and SC sites. Absorption also occurs following intrapleural and intraperitoneal administration.

Distribution: Widely distributed, concentrates mainly in skin, lung, peritoneum, kidneys, and lymphatics.

Metabolism and Excretion: 60–70% excreted unchanged by the kidneys.

Half-life: 2 hr (increased in renal impairment).

CONTRAINDICATIONS AND PRECAUTIONS

Contraindicated in: ▪ Hypersensitivity.

Use Cautiously in: ▪ Renal impairment (dosage reduction required) ▪ Pulmonary impairment ▪ Patients with childbearing potential ▪ Nonmalignant chronic debilitating illness ▪ Elderly patients (increased risk of pulmonary toxicity).

ADVERSE REACTIONS AND SIDE EFFECTS*

CNS: weakness, disorientation, aggressive behavior.

Resp: pneumonitis, **PULMONARY FIBROSIS.**

CV: hypotension, peripheral vasoconstriction.

GI: nausea, vomiting, anorexia, stomatitis.

Derm: mucocutaneous toxicity, urticaria, erythema, hyperpigmentation, alopecia, rashes, vesiculation, alopecia.

Hemat: thrombocytopenia, leukopenia, anemia.

Local: pain at tumor site, phlebitis at IV site.

Metab: weight loss.

Misc: fever, chills, **ANAPHYLACTOID REACTIONS.**

INTERACTIONS

Drug–Drug: ▪ Hematologic toxicity increased with concurrent use of **radiation therapy** and other **antineoplastic agents** ▪ Concurrent use with **cisplatin** decreases elimination of bleomycin and may increase toxicity ▪ Increased risk of pulmonary toxicity with other **antineoplastic agents** or thoracic **radiation**.

ROUTE AND DOSAGE

Note: Lymphoma patients should receive initial test doses of 2 units or less for the first 2 doses.

- **IV, IM, SC (Adults):** 0.25–0.5 units/kg (10–20 units/m^2) weekly or twice weekly initially. If favorable response occurs, lower maintenance doses are employed (1 unit/day or 5 units/wk).
- **Intrapleural (Adults):** 60–120 units instilled into pleural cavity.

PHARMACODYNAMICS (tumor response)

	ONSET	PEAK	DURATION
IV, IM, SC	2–3 wk	UK	UK

NURSING IMPLICATIONS

Assessment

▫ Monitor vital signs prior to and frequently during therapy.

▫ Assess for fever and chills. May occur 2–6 hr after administration and last 4–6 hr. Confer with physician regarding antipyretic therapy.

▫ Monitor for anaphylactic reaction (fever, chills, hypotension, and wheez-

*Underlines indicate most frequent; **CAPITALS** indicate life-threatening.

B

ing). Keep resuscitation equipment and medications on hand. Lymphoma patients are at particular risk.

- Assess respiratory status for dyspnea and rales/crackles. Pulmonary toxicity occurs primarily in elderly patients (age 70 or older) who have received 400 or more units. May occur 4–10 wk after therapy. Physician may order periodic pulmonary function tests and carbon monoxide diffusion capacity for early detection of pulmonary toxicity. Pulmonary toxicity may occur at lower doses in patients also having received other antineoplastics or thoracic radiation.
- Assess nausea, vomiting, and appetite. Weigh weekly. Modify diet as tolerated. Confer with physician regarding an antiemetic prior to administration.
- **Lab Test Considerations:** Monitor CBC prior to and periodically throughout therapy. May cause mild thrombocytopenia and leukopenia (nadir occurs in 2 wk).
- Monitor baseline and periodic renal and hepatic function.

Potential Nursing Diagnoses

- Injury, high risk for (side effects).
- Body image disturbance (side effects).
- Knowledge deficit related to medication regimen (patient/family teaching).

Implementation

- **General Info:** Soln should be prepared in a biologic cabinet. Wear gloves, gown, and mask while handling medication. Discard equipment in specially designated containers (see Appendix I).
- Physician may order lymphoma patients to receive 2 test doses of 2 units initially. Monitor closely for anaphylactic reaction.
- May be administered through thoracostomy tube by physician. Position patient as directed.
- Reconstituted soln is stable for 24 hr at room temperature and 14 days if refrigerated.
- **IM/SC:** Reconstitute vial with 1–5 ml of sterile water for injection, 0.9% NaCl, D5W, or bacteriostatic water for injection. Do not reconstitute with diluents containing benzyl alcohol when used for neonates.
- **Direct IV:** Prepare IV and intra-arterial doses by diluting 15-unit vial with 5 ml of D5W or 0.9% NaCl.
- *Rate:* Administer slowly over 10 min.
- **Intermittent Infusion:** May be further diluted in 50–100 ml of D5W or 0.9% NaCl.
- **Syringe Compatibility:** cisplatin, cyclophosphamide, doxorubicin, droperidol, fluorouracil, furosemide, heparin, leucovorin calcium, methotrexate, metoclopramide, mitomycin, vinblastine, or vincristine.
- **Y-Site Compatibility:** cisplatin, cyclophosphamide, doxorubicin, droperidol, fluorouracil, heparin, leucovorin calcium, methotrexate, metoclopramide, mitomycin, ondansetron, vinblastine, or vincristine.
- **Additive Compatibility:** amikacin, cephapirin, dexamethasone, diphenhydramine, fluorouracil, gentamicin, heparin, hydrocortisone sodium phosphate, phenytoin, streptomycin, tobramycin, vinblastine, or vincristine.
- **Additive Incompatibility:** aminophylline, ascorbic acid injection, cefazolin, cephalothin, diazepam, hydrocortisone sodium succinate, methotrexate, mitomycin, nafcillin, penicillin, or terbutaline.

Patient/Family Teaching

- Instruct patient to notify physician if fever, chills, wheezing, faintness, diaphoresis, shortness of breath, prolonged nausea and vomiting, or mouth sores occur.
- Encourage patient not to smoke as this may worsen pulmonary toxicity.
- Explain to the patient that skin toxicity may manifest itself as skin sensitivity, hyperpigmentation (especially at skin folds and points of skin irritation), and skin rashes and thickening.
- Instruct patient to inspect oral mu-

cosa for erythema and ulceration. If ulceration occurs, advise patient to use sponge brush and rinse mouth with water after eating and drinking. Physician may order viscous lidocaine swishes if pain interferes with eating.

- □ Discuss with patient the possibility of hair loss. Explore coping strategies.
- □ Advise patient of the need for contraception.
- □ Instruct patient not to receive any vaccinations without advice of physician.
- □ Emphasize need for periodic lab tests to monitor for side effects.

EVALUATION

Effectiveness of therapy can be demonstrated by: ▪ Decrease in tumor size without evidence of hypersensitivity or pulmonary toxicity.

BRETYLIUM
(bre-till-ee-yum)
{Bretylate}, Bretylol

CLASSIFICATION(S):
Antiarrhythmic—type III
Pregnancy Category UK

INDICATIONS
▪ Treatment of ventricular tachycardia and prophylaxis against ventricular fibrillation ▪ Treatment of other serious ventricular arrhythmias resistant to lidocaine.

ACTION
▪ Initially releases norepinephrine, then blocks its release. **Therapeutic Effect:** ▪ Suppression of ventricular tachycardia and fibrillation.

PHARMACOKINETICS
Absorption: Well absorbed following IM administration.
Distribution: Reaches high concentration in areas of adrenergic innervation.
Metabolism and Excretion: Eliminated entirely unchanged by the kidneys.
Half-life: 5–10 hr (increased in renal impairment).

CONTRAINDICATIONS AND PRECAUTIONS
Contraindicated in: ▪ No significant contraindications.
Use Cautiously in: ▪ Suspected cardiac glycoside toxicity (increased risk of arrhythmias) ▪ Patients with fixed cardiac output (may produce severe hypotension requiring supportive therapy) ▪ Renal insufficiency (dosage reduction required) ▪ Pregnancy, lactation, and children (safety not established).

ADVERSE REACTIONS AND SIDE EFFECTS*
CNS: syncope, faintness, vertigo, dizziness.
EENT: nasal stuffiness.
CV: postural hypotension, transient hypertension, bradycardia, angina.
GI: nausea, vomiting (rapid IV administration to conscious patients), diarrhea.

INTERACTIONS
Drug-Drug: ▪ Combination with other **antiarrhythmics** may be additive or antagonistic ▪ Avoid using in suspected **cardiac glycoside** toxicity (initial release of norepinephrine may aggravate arrhythmias).

ROUTE AND DOSAGE
Note: See infusion rate table in Appendix D.

Ventricular Fibrillation
- **IV (Adults):** 5 mg/kg bolus over 15–30 sec initially; if no response, increase to 10 mg/kg, repeat as necessary (not to exceed 30 mg/kg/24 hr). For maintenance: dilute and infuse at 1–2 mg/min *or* dilute and infuse 5–10 mg/kg over 10–30 min q 6 hr.

Other Ventricular Arrhythmias
- **IV (Adults):** Dilute and infuse 5–10 mg/kg over 10–30 min q 6–8 hr.

{} = Available in Canada only.
*Underlines indicate most frequent; **CAPITALS** indicate life-threatening.

B

- **IM (Adults):** 5–10 mg/kg, repeat q 1–2 hr if arrhythmia persists, then q 6–8 hr.

Use in Children (Unlabeled)

- **IM (Children):** 2–5 mg/kg as single dose.

PHARMACODYNAMICS (suppression of arrhythmias)

	ONSET	PEAK	DURATION
IM	15 min–1 hr (fibrillation) 20 min–6 hr (VT, PVCs)	UK	6–24 hr
IV	within min (fibrillation) 20 min–6 hr (VT, PVCs)	end of infusion	6–24 hr

NURSING IMPLICATIONS

Assessment

- Patients receiving this medication should be hospitalized in a unit where ECG and blood pressure can be constantly monitored. Assess patient for arrhythmias and changes in blood pressure frequently. A transient increase in arrhythmias and hypertension may occur within 1 hr after initial administration.
- Assess patient frequently for orthostatic hypotension, keep supine until tolerance to hypotension develops. Instruct patient to make position changes slowly, assist with ambulation. If systolic blood pressure <75 mmHg or symptomatic notify physician. Dopamine, dobutamine, or norepinephrine, and volume replacement may be necessary.

Potential Nursing Diagnoses

- Cardiac output, decreased (indications).
- Injury, high risk for (adverse reactions).

Implementation

- **General Info:** Dosage should be reduced gradually and discontinued over 3–5 days with close ECG monitoring. Maintenance with an oral antiarrhythmic may be initiated.
- Available in premixed soln with 5% dextrose.
- **IM:** Do not dilute bretylium for IM injection. Rotate injection sites frequently during IM injection to prevent atrophy and necrosis of muscle tissue caused by repeated injections. May repeat injection at 1–2 hr intervals if arrhythmia persists.
- **Direct IV:** For ventricular fibrillation, give IV undiluted; arrhythmia usually resolves within mins. Repeat in 15–30 min if arrhythmia persists. Do not exceed 30 mg/kg/24 hr. Employ usual resusitative procedures, including CPR and electrical cardioversion, prior to and following injection.
- *Rate:* Administer over 15–30 sec.
- **Intermittent Infusion:** For other ventricular arrhythmias, dilute 500 mg in at least 50 ml of D5W, 0.9% NaCl, D5/0.45% NaCl, D5/0.9% NaCl, D5/LR, ⅙ M sodium lactate, or lactated Ringer's soln for intermittent infusion.
- *Rate:* Administer over 10–30 min. More rapid infusion in the alert patient may cause nausea and vomiting. May repeat after 1–2 hr if necessary. Ventricular tachycardia usually resolves within 20 min.
- **Continuous Infusion:** Bretylium can be diluted in any amount of soln (1 g in 1000 ml equals 1 mg/ml).
- *Rate:* Infuse at 1–2 mg of diluted soln/min. Administer via infusion pump to ensure accurate dosage. (See Appendix D for Infusion Rate Table).
- **Y-Site Compatibility:** amrinone, dobutamine, famotidine, isoproterenol, or ranitidine.
- **Additive Compatibility:** 5% sodium bicarbonate, 20% mannitol, aminophylline, calcium chloride, calcium gluconate, digoxin, dopamine, esmolol, insulin, lidocaine, potassium chloride, quinidine, or verapamil.
- **Additive Incompatibility:** phenytoin sodium.

Patient/Family Teaching

- Instruct patient to make position changes slowly to minimize the effects of drug-induced orthostatic hypotension.

EVALUATION

Clinical response can be demonstrated by: ▪ Suppression of existing ventricular arrhythmias ▪ Prevention of additional arrhythmias.

BROMOCRIPTINE

(broe-moe-**krip**-teen)
Parlodel

CLASSIFICATION(S):
Antiparkinson agent
Pregnancy Category UK

INDICATIONS

▪ Adjunct to levodopa in the treatment of Parkinsonism ▪ Treatment of hyperprolactinemia (amenorrhea/galactorrhea) including associated female infertility ▪ Suppression of lactation ▪ Treatment of acromegaly.

ACTION

▪ Activates dopamine receptors in the CNS ▪ Decreases prolactin secretion. **Therapeutic Effects**: ▪ Relief of rigidity and tremor in Parkinsonism ▪ Restoration of fertility in hyperprolactinemia ▪ Suppression of lactation ▪ Decreased growth hormone in acromegaly.

PHARMACOKINETICS

Absorption: Poorly absorbed (30%) from the GI tract.
Distribution: Distribution not known.
Metabolism and Excretion: Completely metabolized by the liver and excreted mainly in the feces via biliary elimination.
Half-life: Biphasic—initial phase 4–4.5 hr, terminal phase 45–50 hr.

CONTRAINDICATIONS AND PRECAUTIONS

Contraindicated in: ▪ Hypersensitivity to bromocriptine or ergot alkaloids ▪ Children <15 yr.

Use Cautiously in: ▪ Cardiac disease ▪ Mental disturbances ▪ May restore fertility (additional contraception may be required if pregnancy is undesirable) ▪ Pregnancy (safety not established) ▪ Severe liver impairment (dosage reduction required).

ADVERSE REACTIONS AND SIDE EFFECTS*

CNS: headache, <u>dizziness</u>, drowsiness, insomnia, confusion, hallucinations, nightmares.
EENT: burning eyes, visual disturbances, nasal stuffiness.
Resp: pulmonary infiltrates, effusions.
CV: <u>hypotension</u>.
GI: <u>nausea</u>, vomiting, anorexia, abdominal pain, dry mouth, metallic taste.
Derm: urticaria.
MS: leg cramps.
Misc: digital vasospasm (acromegaly only).

INTERACTIONS

Drug-Drug: ▪ Additive hypotension with **antihypertensives** ▪ Additive CNS depression with **antihistamines, alcohol, narcotic analgesics,** and **sedative/hypnotics** ▪ Additive neurologic effects with **levodopa** ▪ Effective on prolactin levels may be antagonized by **phenothiazines, haloperidol, methyldopa, tricyclic antidepressants,** and **reserpine.**

ROUTE AND DOSAGE

Parkinsonism

- **PO (Adults):** 1.25 mg twice daily, increased by 2.5 mg/day in 2–4 wk intervals (usual dose range is 30–90 mg/day in 3 divided doses).

Hyperprolactinemia

- **PO (Adults):** 1.25–2.5 mg/day initially, may be gradually increased up to 30 mg/day.

Postpartum Lactation

- **PO (Adults):** 2.5 mg 2–3 times daily.

Acromegaly

- **PO (Adults):** 1.25–2.5 mg/day for 3 days, increase by 1.25–2.5 mg q 3–7

*<u>Underlines</u> indicate most frequent; **CAPITALS** indicate life-threatening.

days until optimal response is obtained (not to exceed 100 mg/day).

PHARMACODYNAMICS (suppression of tremor in Parkinson's disease)

	ONSET	PEAK	DURATION
PO	30–90 min	1–2 hr	8–12 hr

NURSING IMPLICATIONS

Assessment

- **General Info:** Assess patient for allergy to ergot derivatives.
- ▫ Monitor blood pressure prior to and frequently during drug therapy. Instruct patient to remain supine during and for several hrs after first dose, because severe hypotension may occur. Supervise ambulation and transfer during initial dosing to prevent injury from hypotension.
- **Parkinson's Disease:** Assess symptoms (akinesia, rigidity, tremors, pill rolling, mask facies, shuffling gait, muscle spasms, twisting motions, drooling) prior to and throughout course of therapy.
- **Lactation Suppression:** Assess breasts for firmness, discomfort, and milk production.
- **Lab Test Considerations:** May cause elevated serum BUN, SGOT (ALT), SGPT (AST), CPK, alkaline phosphatase, and uric acid levels. Elevations are usually transient and not clinically significant.

Potential Nursing Diagnoses

- Mobility, impaired physical (indications).
- Injury, high risk for (indications, side effects).
- Knowledge deficit related to medication regimen (patient/family teaching).

Implementation

- **General Info:** This medication is often given concurrently with levodopa or a levodopa-carbidopa combination in the treatment of Parkinson's disease.
- **PO:** Administer with food or milk to minimize gastric distress. Tablets may be crushed if patient has difficulty swallowing.

Patient/Family Teaching

- **General Info:** Instruct patient to take medication exactly as directed. If a dose is missed it should be taken within 4 hr of the scheduled dose or omitted. Do not double doses.
- ▫ May cause drowsiness and dizziness. Caution patients to avoid driving and other activities requiring alertness until response to medication is known.
- ▫ Caution patient to avoid concurrent use of alcohol during the course of therapy.
- ▫ Instruct patient to inform physician if increasing shortness of breath is noted; pulmonary infiltrates and pleural effusions may occur with long-term therapy.
- ▫ Advise women to consult with physician regarding a nonhormonal method of birth control. Women should contact the physician promptly if pregnancy is suspected.
- ▫ Emphasize the importance of regular follow-up examinations to determine effectiveness and monitor side effects.
- **Pituitary Tumors:** Instruct patients taking bromocriptine for pituitary tumors to inform physician immediately if signs of tumor enlargement (blurred vision, sudden headache, severe nausea, and vomiting) occur.
- **Infertility:** Instruct women treated for infertility to obtain daily basal body temperatures to determine when ovulation occurs.
- **Lactation Suppression:** Explain that course of therapy usually lasts 2–3 wk. Mild to moderate breast engorgement may occur after therapy is discontinued.

Evaluation

Effectiveness of therapy can be demonstrated by: ▪ Decrease in tremor, rigidity, and bradykinesia ▫ Improvement in balance and gait in patients with Parkinson's disease ▪ Decreased serum levels of growth hormone in patients with acromegaly ▪ Decreased breast engorgement and galactorrhea ▪ Resumption of normal ovulatory menstrual cycles with restoration of fertility. In patients with amenorrhea and galactorrhea, menses usually resume within 6–8 wk, and galactorrhea subsides within 8–12 wk.

BROMPHENIRAMINE

(brome-fen-**eer**-a-meen)
Brombay, Bromphen, Chlorphed, Codimal-A, Conjec-B, Copene-B, Dehist, Diamine, Dimetane, Histaject Modified, Nasahist B, ND Stat Revised, Oraminic II, Veltane

CLASSIFICATION(S):
Antihistamine
Pregnancy Category B

INDICATIONS

▪ Symptomatic relief of allergic symptoms caused by histamine release; conditions in which it is most useful include nasal allergies and allergic dermatoses ▪ Management of severe allergic or hypersensitivity reactions, including anaphylaxis and transfusion reactions.

ACTION

▪ Blocks the following effects of histamine: ▫ Vasodilation ▫ Increased GI tract secretions ▫ Increased heart rate ▫ Hypotension. **Therapeutic Effect:** ▪ Relief of symptoms associated with histamine excess usually seen in allergic conditions. Does not block the release of histamine.

PHARMACOKINETICS

Absorption: Well absorbed following oral and IM administration.
Distribution: Widely distributed. Minimal amounts excreted in breast milk. Crosses the blood–brain barrier.
Metabolism and Excretion: Extensively metabolized by the liver.
Half-life: 12–35 hr.

CONTRAINDICATIONS AND PRECAUTIONS

Contraindicated in: ▪ Hypersensitivity ▪ Acute attacks of asthma ▪ Lactation (avoid use).
Use Cautiously in: ▪ Narrow-angle glaucoma ▪ Liver disease ▪ Elderly patients (more susceptible to adverse reaction) ▪ Pregnancy (safety not established).

ADVERSE REACTIONS AND SIDE EFFECTS*

CNS: drowsiness, sedation, excitation (in children), dizziness.
CV: hypotension, hypertension, palpitations, arrhythmias.
EENT: blurred vision.
GI: dry mouth, obstruction, constipation.
GU: urinary hesitancy, retention.
Derm: sweating.
Misc: hypersensitivity reaction (IV use).

INTERACTIONS

Drug-Drug: ▪ Additive CNS depression with other **CNS depressants** including **alcohol, narcotics,** and **sedative/hypnotics** ▪ **MAO inhibitors** intensify and prolong the anticholinergic effects of antihistamines.

ROUTE AND DOSAGE

- **PO (Adults):** 4 mg q 4–6 hr daily (not to exceed 24 mg/day), or 8 mg q 8 hr of extended-release form or 12 mg q 12 hr of extended-release form.
- **PO (Children 6–12 yr):** 2 mg q 4–6 hr (not to exceed 12 mg/day) or 8–12 mg of extended-release form q 12 hr.
- **PO (Children 2–6 yr):** 1 mg q 4–6 hr (not to exceed 6 mg/day).
- **SC, IM, IV (Adults):** 5–20 mg q 6–12 hr (not to exceed 40 mg/day).
- **SC, IM, IV (Children):** 0.125 mg/kg or 3.75 mg/m^2 3–4 times daily.

*Underlines indicate most frequent; **CAPITALS** indicate life-threatening.

B

PHARMACODYNAMICS (relief of allergic symptoms)

	ONSET	PEAK	DURATION
PO	15–30 min	1–2 hr	6–8 hr*
SC	20–30 min	UK	8–12 hr
IM	20–30 min	UK	8–12 hr
IV	rapid	UK	8–12 hr

*Duration is longer (8–12 hr) for sustained-release oral preparations.

NURSING IMPLICATIONS

Assessment

- **Allergy:** Assess allergy symptoms (rhinitis, conjunctivitis, hives) prior to and periodically throughout course of therapy.
- □ Assess lung sounds and character of bronchial secretions. Maintain fluid intake of 1500–2000 ml/day to decrease viscosity of secretions.
- **Transfusion Reaction or Anaphylaxis:** Monitor for resolution of symptoms of allergic transfusion reaction or anaphylaxis (urticaria, wheezing, bronchospasm, hypotension). Monitor pulse and blood pressure prior to and throughout therapy.
- **IV:** Observe patient for sweating, hypotension, dizziness, drowsiness, or hypersensitivity reactions when administering medication intravenously. Elderly patients are more susceptible to side effects with this medication.
- **Lab Test Considerations:** May cause false negatives in allergy skin testing. Discontinue antihistamines at least 72 hr before testing.

Potential Nursing Diagnoses

- Airway clearance, ineffective (indications).
- Injury, high risk for (adverse reactions).
- Knowledge deficit related to medication regimen (patient/family teaching).

Implementation

- **General Info:** Available in tablets, elixir, extended-release tablets, and injectable (SC, IM, IV) forms.
- **PO:** Administer oral doses with food or milk to decrease GI irritation. Extended-release tablets should be swallowed whole; do not crush, break, or chew.
- **Direct IV:** May be given IV undiluted, but further dilution of each ml of 10 mg/ml soln with 10 ml of 0.9% NaCl for injection is recommended to reduce side effects.
- □ *Rate:* Administer each single dose slowly over at least 1 min.
- **Intermittent Infusion:** May be further diluted in 0.9% NaCl, D5W, or whole blood for IV infusion. The 100 mg/ml concentration is not recommended for IV use.

Patient/Family Teaching

- □ Instruct patient to take medication exactly as directed; do not double doses.
- □ Commonly causes drowsiness. Caution patient to avoid driving or other activities requiring alertness until response to the medication is known.
- □ Advise patient to avoid taking alcohol or other CNS depressants concurrently with this drug.
- □ Frequent oral rinses, good oral hygiene, and sugarless gum or candy may help relieve dry mouth.
- □ Instruct patient to contact physician if symptoms persist.

Evaluation

Effectiveness of therapy may be determined by: ▪ Decrease in allergic symptoms.

BUMETANIDE

(byoo-**met**-a-nide)
Bumex

CLASSIFICATION(S):
Diuretic—loop
Pregnancy Category C

INDICATIONS

▪ Management of edema secondary to congestive heart failure, hepatic or renal disease. **Unlabeled Use:** Used alone or in combination with antihypertensives in the treatment of hypertension.

ACTION

■ Inhibits the reabsorption of sodium and chloride from the loop of Henle and distal renal tubule ■ Increases renal excretion of water, sodium, chloride, magnesium, hydrogen, and calcium ■ Has renal and peripheral vasodilatory effects ■ Effectiveness persists in impaired renal function. **Therapeutic Effects:** ■ Diuresis and subsequent mobilization of excess fluid (edema, pleural effusions); also lowers blood pressure.

PHARMACOKINETICS

Absorption: Rapidly and completely absorbed following oral or IM administration.

Distribution: Distribution not known.

Metabolism and Excretion: Partially metabolized by the liver. 50% eliminated unchanged by the kidneys. 20% excreted in the feces.

Half-life: 1–1.5 hr.

CONTRAINDICATIONS AND PRECAUTIONS

Contraindicated in: ■ Hypersensitivity ■ Cross-sensitivity with sulfonamides may exist ■ Pregnancy or lactation ■ Anuria or increasing azotemia.

Use Cautiously in: ■ Severe liver disease ■ Electrolyte depletion ■ Diabetes mellitus.

ADVERSE REACTIONS AND SIDE EFFECTS*

CNS: dizziness, headache, encephalopathy.

CV: hypotension.

Derm: rashes.

EENT: hearing loss, tinnitus.

F and E: metabolic alkalosis, hypovolemia, dehydration, hyponatremia, hypokalemia, hypochloremia, hypomagnesemia.

GI: nausea, vomiting, diarrhea, constipation, dry mouth.

GU: frequency.

Metab: hyperglycemia, hyperuricemia.

MS: muscle cramps.

INTERACTIONS

Drug-Drug: ■ Additive hypotension with **antihypertensives**, acute ingestion of **alcohol**, or **nitrates** ■ Additive hypokalemia with other **diuretics, ticarcillin, mezlocillin, piperacillin, amphotericin** B, and **glucocorticoids** ■ Hypokalemia may increase **cardiac glycoside** toxicity ■ Decreases **lithium** excretion, may cause toxicity ■ Increased risk of ototoxicity with **aminoglycosides**.

ROUTE AND DOSAGE

Note: 1 mg bumetanide approx. equivalent to 40 mg furosemide.

- **PO (Adults):** 0.5–2 mg/day (up to 10 mg/day; larger doses may be required in renal insufficiency).
- **IM, IV (Adults):** 0.5–1.0 mg; may give 1–2 more doses q 2–3 hr (not to exceed 10 mg/24 hr).

PHARMACODYNAMICS (onset of diuresis)

	ONSET	PEAK	DURATION
PO	30–60 min	1–2 hr	3–6 hr
IM	40 min	1–2 hr	4–6 hr
IV	within mins	15–45 min	3–6 hr

NURSING IMPLICATIONS

ASSESSMENT

- □ Assess fluid status throughout therapy. Monitor daily weight, intake and output ratios, amount and location of edema, lung sounds, skin turgor, and mucous membranes. Notify physician if thirst, dry mouth, lethargy, weakness, hypotension, or oliguria occur.
- □ Monitor blood pressure and pulse before and during administration.
- □ Assess patients receiving cardiac glycosides for anorexia, nausea, vomiting, muscle cramps, paresthesia, confusion. Notify physician if these symptoms occur.
- □ Assess patient for hearing loss. Audiometry is recommended for patients receiving prolonged therapy. Hearing loss is most common following rapid or high-dose IV administration in pa-

*Underlines indicate most frequent; **CAPITALS** indicate life-threatening.

B

tients with decreased renal function or those taking other ototoxic drugs.
- ▫ Assess for allergy to sulfonamides.
- ▪ **Lab Test Considerations:** Monitor electrolytes, renal and hepatic function, glucose, and uric acid prior to and periodically throughout course of therapy. May cause decreased electrolyte levels (especially potassium). May cause elevated blood glucose, BUN, uric acid, and urinary phosphate levels.

Potential Nursing Diagnoses
- ▪ Fluid volume excess (indications).
- ▪ Fluid volume deficit (side effects).
- ▪ Knowledge deficit related to medication regimen (patient/family teaching).

Implementation
- ▪ **General Info:** Administer medication in the morning to prevent disruption of sleep cycle.
- ▫ Intermittent dose, given on alternate days or for 3–4 days with rest periods of 1–2 days in between, may be used for continued control of edema.
- ▪ **PO:** Administer orally with food or milk to minimize gastric irritation.
- ▪ **Direct IV:** Administer over 1–2 min. May repeat at 2–3 hr intervals, not to exceed 10 mg/day.
- ▪ **Intermittent Infusion:** Dilute in D5W, 0.9% NaCl, or lactated Ringer's soln, and administer through Y-tubing or 3-way stopcock. Use reconstituted soln within 24 hr.
- ▪ **Additive Incompatibility:** dobutamine.

Patient/Family Teaching
- ▪ **General Info:** Instruct patient to take bumetanide exactly as directed. Missed doses should be taken as soon as possible; do not double doses. Advise patients on antihypertensive regimen to continue taking medication, even if feeling better. Bumetanide controls but does not cure hypertension.
- ▫ Caution patient to make position changes slowly to minimize orthostatic hypotension. Caution patient that the use of alcohol, exercise during hot weather, or standing for long periods during therapy may enhance orthostatic hypotension.
- ▫ Instruct patient to consult physician regarding a diet high in potassium (see Appendix K).
- ▫ Advise patient to consult physician or pharmacist before taking over-the-counter medication concurrently with this therapy.
- ▫ Instruct patient to notify physician or dentist of medication regimen prior to treatment or surgery.
- ▫ Advise patient to contact physician immediately if muscle weakness, cramps, nausea, dizziness, numbness, or tingling of extremities occur.
- ▫ Emphasize the importance of routine follow-up examinations.
- ▪ **Hypertension:** Reinforce the need to continue additional therapies for hypertension (weight loss, exercise, restricted sodium intake, stress reduction, regular exercise, moderation of alcohol consumption, cessation of smoking).

Evaluation
Effectiveness of therapy can be demonstrated by: ▪ Decrease in edema ▫ Decrease in abdominal girth ▫ Increase in urinary output ▪ Decrease in blood pressure.

BUPRENORPHINE
(byoo-pre-**nor**-feen)
Buprenex

CLASSIFICATION(S):
Narcotic analgesic—agonist/antagonist
Schedule V
Pregnancy Category C

INDICATIONS
▪ Management of moderate to severe pain.

ACTION
▪ Binds to opiate receptors in the CNS ▪ Alters the perception of and response to painful stimuli, while producing gen-

eralized CNS depression ▪ Has partial antagonist properties that may result in narcotic withdrawal in physically dependent patients. **Therapeutic Effect:** ▪ Decreased severity of pain.

PHARMACOKINETICS

Absorption: Well absorbed from IM sites.
Distribution: Crosses the placenta and enters breast milk.
Metabolism and Excretion: Mostly metabolized by the liver.
Half-life: 2–3 hr.

CONTRAINDICATIONS AND PRECAUTIONS

Contraindicated in: ▪ Hypersensitivity.
Use Cautiously in: ▪ Increased intracranial pressure ▪ Severe renal, hepatic, or pulmonary disease ▪ Hypothyroidism ▪ Adrenal insufficiency ▪ Alcoholism ▪ Elderly or debilitated patients (dosage reduction required) ▪ Undiagnosed abdominal pain ▪ Prostatic hypertrophy ▪ Pregnancy, labor, lactation, or children (safety not established).

ADVERSE REACTIONS AND SIDE EFFECTS*

CNS: <u>sedation</u>, <u>confusion</u>, headache, euphoria, floating feeling, unusual dreams, <u>hallucinations</u>, <u>dysphoria</u>, dizziness.
EENT: miosis (high doses), blurred vision, diplopia.
Resp: respiratory depression.
CV: hypotension, hypertension, palpitations.
GI: <u>nausea</u>, vomiting, constipation, ileus, dry mouth.
GU: urinary retention.
Derm: <u>sweating</u>, clammy feeling.
Misc: <u>sweating</u>, tolerance, physical dependence, psychological dependence.

INTERACTIONS

Drug-Drug: ▪ Use with caution in patients receiving **MAO inhibitors** (increased CNS and respiratory depression and hypotension; decrease buprenorphine dose by 50%, may need to decrease MAO inhibitor dose) ▪ Additive CNS depression with **alcohol, antihistamines, antidepressants,** and **sedative/hypnotics** ▪ May precipitate withdrawal in patients who are **narcotic**-dependent and have not been detoxified ▪ May decrease effectiveness of other **narcotic analgesics**.

ROUTE AND DOSAGE

- **IM, IV (Adults):** 0.3–0.6 mg q 4–6 hr as needed.

PHARMACODYNAMICS (pain relief)

	ONSET	PEAK	DURATION
IM	15 min	60 min	6 hr
IV	rapid	rapid	6 hr

NURSING IMPLICATIONS

Assessment

- □ Assess type, location, and intensity of pain prior to and 15 min following IM and 5 min following IV administration.
- □ Assess blood pressure, pulse, and respirations before and periodically during administration. Buprenorphine 0.3 mg has approximately equal respiratory depression with morphine 10 mg.
- □ While this drug has a low potential for dependence, prolonged use may lead to physical and psychological dependence and tolerance. This should not prevent patient from receiving adequate analgesia. Most patients receiving buprenorphine for medical reasons do not develop psychological dependence. Progressively higher doses may be required to relieve pain with long-term therapy.
- □ Antagonistic properties may induce withdrawal symptoms (vomiting, restlessness, abdominal cramps, increased blood pressure and temperature) in narcotic-dependent patients. Symptoms may occur up to 15 days after discontinuation and persist for 1–2 wk.

*<u>Underlines</u> indicate most frequent; **CAPITALS** indicate life-threatening.

- **Lab Test Considerations:** May cause elevated serum amylase and lipase levels.
- **Toxicity and Overdose:** If overdose occurs, respiratory depression may be partially reversed by naloxone (Narcan), the antidote. Doxapram may also be ordered as a respiratory stimulant.

POTENTIAL NURSING DIAGNOSES
- Comfort, altered: pain (indications).
- Injury, high risk for (side effects).

IMPLEMENTATION
- **General Info:** Explain therapeutic value of medication prior to administration to enhance the analgesic effect.
- □ Regularly administered doses may be more effective than prn administration. Analgesic is more effective if given before pain becomes severe.
- □ Coadministration with non-narcotic analgesics may have additive effects and permit lower narcotic doses.
- **IM:** Administer IM injections deep into well-developed muscle. Rotate sites of injections.
- **Direct IV:** May give IV undiluted. Administer slowly. Rapid administration may cause respiratory depression, hypotension, and cardiac arrest.
- **Syringe Compatibility:** midazolam.
- **Additive Compatibility:** 0.9% NaCl, D5W, D5/0.9% NaCl, lactated Ringer's soln, atropine, diphenhydramine, droperidol, glycopyrrolate, haloperidol, hydroxyzine, promethazine, or scopolamine.
- **Additive Incompatibility:** diazepam or lorazepam.

PATIENT/FAMILY TEACHING
- □ Instruct patient on how and when to ask for prn pain medication.
- □ Medication may cause drowsiness or dizziness. Advise patient to call for assistance when ambulating and to avoid driving or other activities requiring alertness until response to medication is known.
- □ Encourage patient to turn, cough, and deep breathe every 2 hr to prevent atelectasis.
- □ Advise patient that good oral hygiene, frequent mouth rinses, and sugarless gum or candy may decrease dry mouth.
- □ Instruct patient to change positions slowly to minimize orthostatic hypotension.
- □ Advise patient to avoid concurrent use of alcohol or other CNS depressants.

EVALUATION

Effectiveness of therapy can be demonstrated by: ▪ Decrease in severity of pain without a significant alteration in level of consciousness or respiratory status.

BUPROPION
(byoo-**proe**-pee-on)
Wellbutrin

CLASSIFICATION(S):
Antidepressant—miscellaneous
Pregnancy Category B

INDICATIONS
- Treatment of depression, often in conjunction with psychotherapy.

ACTION
- Decreases neuronal reuptake of dopamine in the CNS ▪ Diminished neuronal uptake of serotonin and norepinephrine (less than tricyclic antidepressants). **Therapeutic Effect:** ▪ Diminished depression.

PHARMACOKINETICS
Absorption: Although well absorbed, bioavailability appears to be low due to extensive rapid metabolic clearance by the liver.
Distribution: Distribution not known.
Metabolism and Excretion: Extensively metabolized by the liver. Some conversion to active metabolites.
Half-life: 14 hr (active metabolites may have longer half-lives).

CONTRAINDICATIONS AND PRECAUTIONS

Contraindicated in: ▪ Hypersensitivity ▪ History of seizures, bullemia, and anorexia nervosa ▪ Concurrent MAO inhibitor therapy.

Use Cautiously in: ▪ History of cranial trauma ▪ Renal or hepatic impairment (dosage reduction recommended) ▪ Pregnancy, lactation, or children (safety not established) ▪ Recent history of myocardial infarction ▪ Unstable cardiovascular status

ADVERSE REACTIONS AND SIDE EFFECTS*

CNS: SEIZURES, agitation, insomnia, psychoses, mania, headache.

GI: dry mouth, nausea, vomiting, change in appetite, weight gain, weight loss.

Neuro: tremor.

INTERACTIONS

Drug–Drug: ▪ Increased risk of adverse reactions when used with **levodopa** or **MAO inhibitors** ▪ Increased risk of seizures with **phenothiazines, antidepressants**, cessation of **benzodiazepines,** or cessation of **alcohol**.

ROUTE AND DOSAGE

- **PO (Adults):** 100 mg twice daily (morning and evening) initially; after 3 days may be increased to 100 mg 3 times daily depending on response. If no response after 4 wk of therapy, may increase to a maximum daily dose of 450 mg/day in divided doses. (No single dose to exceed 150 mg, wait at least 6 hr between doses at the 300 mg/day dose, or at least 4 hr between doses at the 450 mg/day dose).

PHARMACODYNAMICS (antidepressant effect)

	ONSET	PEAK	DURATION
PO	up to 4 wk	UK	UK

NURSING IMPLICATIONS

Assessment

- □ Monitor mood changes. Inform physician if patient demonstrates significant increase in anxiety, nervousness, or insomnia.
- □ Assess for suicidal tendencies, especially during early therapy. Restrict amount of drug available to patient.

Potential Nursing Diagnoses

- ▪ Coping, ineffective individual, (indications).
- ▪ Knowledge deficit related to medication regimen (patient/family teaching).

Implementation

- ▪ **PO:** Administer doses in equally spaced time increments throughout day to minimize the risk of seizures.
- □ May be initially administered concurrently with sedatives to minimize agitation. This is not usually required after the first wk of therapy.
- □ Insomnia may be decreased by avoiding bedtime doses.

Patient/Family Teaching

- □ Instruct patient to take bupropion exactly as directed. If a dose is missed, omit dose and return to regular dosing schedule. Do not double doses.
- □ Bupropion may impair judgement or motor and cognitive skills. Caution patient to avoid driving and other activities requiring alertness until response to medication is known.
- □ Advise patient to avoid alcohol during therapy and to consult with physician before taking other medications with bupropion.
- □ Inform patient that frequent mouth rinses, good oral hygiene, and sugarless gum or candy may minimize dry mouth. If dry mouth persists for more than 2 wk consult physician or dentist regarding use of saliva substitute.
- □ Instruct female patients to inform physician if pregnancy is planned or suspected.
- □ Emphasize the importance of follow-up examinations to monitor progress.

*Underlines indicate most frequent; **CAPITALS** indicate life-threatening.

Encourage patient participation in psychotherapy.

EVALUATION

Effectiveness of therapy can be demonstrated by: ▪ Increased sense of well-being ▫ Renewed interest in surroundings. Acute episodes of depression may require several mons of treatment.

BUSPIRONE
(byoo-**spye**-rone)
BuSpar

CLASSIFICATION(S):
Antianxiety agent
Pregnancy Category B

INDICATIONS

▪ Management of anxiety.

ACTION

▪ Binds to serotonin and dopamine receptors in the brain ▪ Increases norepinephrine metabolism in the brain. **Therapeutic Effect:** ▪ Relief of anxiety.

PHARMACOKINETICS

Absorption: Rapidly absorbed.
Distribution: Distribution not known.
Metabolism and Excretion: Extensively metabolized by the liver. 20–40% excreted in feces.
Half-life: 2–3 hr.

CONTRAINDICATIONS AND PRECAUTIONS

Contraindicated in: ▪ Hypersensitivity.
Use Cautiously in: ▪ Patients receiving other antianxiety agents (other agents should be slowly withdrawn to prevent withdrawal or rebound phenomenon) ▪ Severe liver disease ▪ Pregnancy, lactation, and children (safety not established) ▪ Patients receiving other psychoactive drugs.

ADVERSE REACTIONS AND SIDE EFFECTS*

CNS: dizziness, insomnia, nervousness, drowsiness, light-headedness, excitement, headache, personality changes, fatigue, weakness.
EENT: tinnitus, sore throat, blurred vision, nasal congestion, altered taste or smell, conjunctivitis.
Resp: hyperventilation, shortness of breath, chest congestion.
CV: chest pain, palpitations, tachycardia, syncope, hypotension, hypertension.
GI: nausea, dry mouth, diarrhea, constipation, abdominal pain, vomiting.
GU: frequency, hesitancy, dysuria, changes in libido.
Derm: rashes, pruritis, edema, flushing, easy bruising, hair loss, dry skin, blisters.
Endo: irregular menses.
MS: myalgia.
Neuro: paresthesia, numbness, incoordination, tremor.
Misc: sweating, clamminess, fever.

INTERACTIONS

Drug-Drug: ▪ Use with **MAO inhibitors** may result in hypertension ▪ May increase the risk of hepatic effects from **trazadone** ▪ Avoid concurrent use with **alcohol**.

ROUTE AND DOSAGE

▪ **PO (Adults):** 15 mg/day in 3 divided doses, increase by 5 mg/day at 2–3-day intervals, (not to exceed 60 mg/day). Usual dose is 20–30 mg/day.

PHARMACODYNAMICS (relief of anxiety)

	ONSET	PEAK	DURATION
PO	7–14 days	3–4 wk	UK

NURSING IMPLICATIONS

ASSESSMENT

▪ **General Info:** Assess degree and manifestations of anxiety prior to and periodically throughout therapy.

*Underlines indicate most frequent; **CAPITALS** indicate life-threatening.

□ Buspirone does not appear to cause physical or psychological dependence or tolerance. However, patients with a history of drug abuse should be assessed for tolerance or dependence, and the amount of drug available to these patients should be restricted.

Potential Nursing Diagnoses

- Anxiety (indications).
- Injury, high risk for (side effects).
- Knowledge deficit related to medication regimen (patient/family teaching).

Implementation

- **General Info:** Patients changing from other antianxiety agents should receive gradually decreasing doses because buspirone will not prevent withdrawal symptoms.
- **PO:** May be administered with food to minimize gastric irritation. Food slows but does not alter extent of absorption.

Patient/Family Teaching

□ Instruct patient to take buspirone exactly as directed. If a dose is missed, take as soon as remembered if not just before next dose; do not double doses. Do not take more than amount prescribed; 1–2 wk of therapy may be required before antianxiety effect is noticeable.

□ May cause dizziness or drowsiness. Caution patient to avoid driving or other activities requiring alertness until response to the medication is known.

□ Advise patient to avoid concurrent use of alcohol or other CNS depressants with this medication.

□ Advise patient to consult physician or pharmacist before taking over-the-counter medications with this drug.

□ Instruct patient to notify the physician if any chronic abnormal movements occur (dystonia, motor restlessness, involuntary movements of facial or cervical muscles) or if pregnancy is suspected.

□ Emphasize the importance of follow-up examinations to determine effectiveness of this medication.

Evaluation

Effectiveness of therapy can be demonstrated by: ■ Increase in well-being □ Decrease in subjective feelings of anxiety. Buspirone is usually used for short-term therapy (3–4 wk). If prescribed for long-term therapy, efficacy should be periodically assessed.

BUSULFAN

(byoo-**sul**-fan)
Myleran

CLASSIFICATION(S):
Antineoplastic—alkylating agent
Pregnancy Category D

INDICATIONS

■ Treatment of chronic myelogenous leukemia and bone marrow disorders.

ACTION

■ Disrupts nucleic acid function and protein synthesis (cell cycle-phase nonspecific). **Therapeutic Effect:** ■ Death of rapidly growing cells, especially malignant ones.

PHARMACOKINETICS

Absorption: Rapidly absorbed from the GI tract.
Distribution: Distribution not known.
Metabolism and Excretion: Extensively metabolized by the liver.
Half-life: UK.

CONTRAINDICATIONS AND PRECAUTIONS

Contraindicated in: ■ Hypersensitivity ■ Failure to respond to previous courses ■ Pregnancy or lactation.
Use Cautiously in: ■ Patients with childbearing potential ■ Active infections ■ Decreased bone marrow reserve ■ Other chronic debilitating diseases.

B

ADVERSE REACTIONS AND SIDE EFFECTS*

Resp: PULMONARY FIBROSIS.
GI: nausea, vomiting, hepatitis.
Derm: alopecia.
Endo: gynecomastia, gonadal suppression.
Hemat: bone marrow depression.
Metab: hyperuricemia.

INTERACTIONS

Drug-Drug: ▪ Additive bone marrow suppression with other **antineoplastic agents** or **radiation therapy**.

ROUTE AND DOSAGE

- **PO (Adults):** 4–8 mg/day initially; maintenance 2 mg twice weekly—4 mg/day.
- **PO (Children):** 0.06–0.12 mg/kg/day or 1.8–4.6 mg/m^2/day.

PHARMACODYNAMICS (effects on blood counts)

	ONSET	PEAK	DURATION
PO	10–15 days	wks	up to 1 mon*

*Complete recovery may take up to 20 mon.

NURSING IMPLICATIONS

Assessment

- Assess for fever, sore throat, and signs of infection. If these symptoms occur, notify physician immediately.
- Assess for bleeding (bleeding gums, bruising, petechiae; guaiac stools, urine, emesis). Avoid IM injections and rectal temperatures or products containing aspirin. Hold pressure on all venipuncture sites for at least 10 min.
- Monitor intake and output ratios and daily weights. Notify physician if significant changes in totals occur.
- Monitor for symptoms of gout (increased uric acid, joint pain, swelling). Encourage patient to drink at least 2 liters of fluid each day. Allopurinol may be given to decrease uric acid levels. Alkalinization of urine may be ordered to increase excretion of uric acid.
- Anemia may occur. Monitor for increased fatigue, dyspnea, and orthostatic hypotension.
- **Lab Test Considerations:** Monitor CBC and differential prior to and weekly during course of therapy. The nadir of leukopenia occurs within 10–30 days. Recovery usually occurs within 12–20 wk. Notify physician if WBC is <15,000 mm^3 or if a precipitous drop occurs. Institute thrombocytopenia precautions if platelet count is <150,000/mm^3.
- Monitor liver function tests, BUN, serum creatinine, and uric acid prior to and periodically during course of therapy.
- May cause false-positive cytology results of breast, bladder, cervix, and lung tissues.

Potential Nursing Diagnoses

- Body image disturbance (side effects).
- Injury, high risk for (side effects).
- Infection, high risk for (side effects).

Implementation

- **PO:** Administer either 1 hr before or 2 hr after meals.

Patient/Family Teaching

- Instruct patient to take medication exactly as directed, even if nausea and vomiting is a problem. Consult physician if vomiting occurs shortly after dose is taken. If a dose is missed do not take at all; do not double doses.
- Instruct patient to report unusual bleeding. Advise patient of thrombocytopenia precautions (use soft tooth brush, electric razor, and avoid falls). Do not drink alcoholic beverages or take medication containing aspirin, as these may precipitate gastric bleeding.
- Caution patient to avoid crowds and persons with known infections. Physician should be informed immediately if symptoms of infection occur.
- Discuss with patient the possibility of

*Underlines indicate most frequent; **CAPITALS** indicate life-threatening.

hair loss. Explore methods of coping.

- Review with patient the need for contraception during therapy. Women need to use contraception even if amenorrhea occurs.
- Instruct patient not to receive any vaccinations without advice of physician.
- Advise patient to notify physician if unusual bleeding or bruising, or flank, stomach, or joint pain occurs. Advise patients on long-term therapy to notify physician immediately if cough, shortness of breath, and fever occur. Patients should also notify physician if darkening of skin, diarrhea, dizziness, fatigue, anorexia, confusion, or nausea and vomiting become pronounced.

EVALUATION

Effectiveness of therapy can be demonstrated by: ▪ Decrease in leukocyte count to within normal limits ▫ Decreased night sweats ▫ Increase in appetite ▫ Increased sense of well-being. Therapy is resumed when leukocyte count reaches 50,000/mm^3.

BUTALBITAL COMPOUND
(byoo-**tal**-bi-tal)

butalbital, acetaminophen
Bancap, Bucet, Phrenilin, Phrenilin Forte, Sedapap-10, Triaprin

butalbital, acetaminophen, caffeine
Amaphen, Anoquan, Arcet, Butace, Endolor, Esgic, Esgic Plus, Femcet, Fioricet, G-1, Medigesic Plus, Repan, Tencet, Triad, Two-Dyne

butalbital, aspirin
Axotal, Pacaps

butalbital, aspirin, caffeine
B-A-C, Fiorgan PF, Fiorinal, Isollyl Improved, Lanorinal, Lorprn, Marnal, {Tecanl}

CLASSIFICATION(S):
Non-narcotic analgesics with barbiturates
Schedule III
Pregnancy Category D

INDICATIONS

▪ Management of mild to moderate pain.

ACTION

▪ Contains an analgesic (aspirin or acetaminophen) for relief of pain, a barbiturate (butalbital) for its sedative effect, and some contain caffeine, which may be of benefit in vascular headaches. **Therapeutic Effect:** ▪ Decreased severity of pain with some sedation.

PHARMACOKINETICS

Absorption: All components are well absorbed.

Distribution: All components are widely distributed, cross the placenta, and enter breast milk.

Metabolism and Excretion: All components are mostly metabolized by the liver.

Half-life: Aspirin, 2–3 hr (low doses); acetaminophen, 1–4 hr; butalbital, UK.

CONTRAINDICATIONS AND PRECAUTIONS

Contraindicated in: ▪ Hypersensitivity to aspirin, acetaminophen, or butalbital ▪ Cross-sensitivity may exist with other nonsteroidal anti-inflammatory agents or barbiturates ▪ Aspirin should be avoided in patients with bleeding disorders or thrombocytopenia ▪ Acetaminophen should be avoided in patients with severe hepatic or renal disease ▪ Butalbital should not be used in comatose patients or those with pre-existing CNS depression ▪ Uncontrolled severe pain ▪ Pregnancy or lactation ▪ Caffeine should be avoided in patients with severe cardiovascular disease.

Use Cautiously in: ▪ Patients who may be suicidal or who may have been addicted to drugs previously ▪ Elderly patients (dosage reduction required) ▪ Use should be short term only ▪ Children (safety not established).

ADVERSE REACTIONS AND SIDE EFFECTS*

CNS: **caffeine**—nervousness, irritability, insomnia; **butalbital**—drowsiness, lethargy, vertigo, depression, hangover, excitation, delerium.
EENT: **aspirin**—tinnitus, hearing loss.
Resp: **butalbital**—respiratory depression.
CV: **caffeine**—tachycardia, palpitations.
GI: **acetaminophen**—HEPATIC NECROSIS (overdose); **aspirin**—dyspepsia, heartburn, epigastric distress, nausea, vomiting, anorexia, abdominal pain, GI BLEEDING, hepatotoxicity; **caffeine**—heartburn, epigastric distress; **butalbital**—nausea, vomiting, diarrhea, constipation.
Derm: **acetaminophen**—rash, dermatitis.
Hemat: **aspirin**—increased bleeding time, anemia, hemolysis.
Misc: **aspirin**—noncardiogenic pulmonary edema, allergic reactions including ANAPHYLAXIS and LARYNGOSPASM; **butalbital**—hypersensitivity reactions including ANGIOEDEMA and serum sickness, physical dependence, psychological dependence.

INTERACTIONS

Drug-Drug: ▪ *Aspirin*—May potentiate **oral anticoagulants** ▪ May enhance the activity of **penicillins, phenytoin, methotrexate, valproic acid, oral hypoglycemic agents,** and **sulfonamides** ▪ May antagonize the beneficial effects of **uricosuric agents** ▪ May decrease effects of most nonsteroidal anti-inflammatory agents. ▪ **Glucocorticoids** may decrease salicylate levels ▪ **Urinary acidification** may increase salicylate levels. ▪ **Alkalinization** may decrease salicylate levels ▪ May blunt the therapeutic response to **diuretics.** ▪ *Acetaminophen*—Hepatotoxicity may be additive with other **hepatotoxic agents** including **alcohol** ▪ **Phenobarbital** may potentiate hepatotoxicity in overdosage ▪ **Cholestyramine** and **colestipol** may decrease absorption ▪ *Butalbital*—Additive CNS depression with other **CNS depressants,** including **alcohol, antihistamines, antidepressants, narcotic analgesics,** and **sedative/hypnotics** ▪ May increase the liver metabolism and decrease the effectiveness of other drugs including **oral contraceptives, chloramphenicol, acebutolol, propranolol, metoprolol, timolol, doxycycline, glucocorticoids, tricyclic antidepressants, phenothiazines, phenylbutazone,** and **quinidine.** ▪ **MAO inhibitors, primidone,** and **valproic acid** may prevent metabolism and increase the effectiveness of butalbital. ▪ May enhance the hematologic toxicity of **cyclophosphamide.**

ROUTE AND DOSAGE

- **PO (Adults):** 1–2 capsules or tablets every 2–6 hr as needed for pain.

PHARMACODYNAMICS

	ONSET	PEAK	DURATION
PO	15–30 min	1–2 hr	2–6 hr

NURSING IMPLICATIONS

Assessment

- □ Assess type, location, and intensity of pain prior to and 60 min following administration.
- □ Prolonged use may lead to physical and psychological dependence and tolerance. This should not prevent patient from receiving adequate analgesia. Most patients who receive butalbital compound for medical reasons do not develop psychological dependency.
- ▪ **Lab Test Considerations:** Aspirin prolongs bleeding time for 4–7 days and, in large doses, may cause prolonged prothrombin time.
- □ False-negative urine glucose test results with glucose oxidase method (Clinistix, Tes-Tape), and false-posi-

*Underlines indicate most frequent; **CAPITALS** indicate life-threatening.

tive urine glucose test results with copper sulfate method (Clinitest).

POTENTIAL NURSING DIAGNOSES

- Comfort, altered: pain (indications).
- Injury, high risk for (side effects).

IMPLEMENTATION

- **General Info:** Explain therapeutic value of medication prior to administration to enhance the analgesic effect.
  - Regularly administered doses may be more effective than prn administration. Analgesic is more effective if given before pain becomes severe.
  - Medication should be discontinued gradually after long-term use to prevent withdrawal symptoms.
  - Available in combination with aspirin, acetaminophen, and codeine (see Appendix A).
- **PO:** Oral doses may be administered with food or milk to minimize GI irritation.

PATIENT/FAMILY TEACHING

- Instruct patient to take medication exactly as directed. Do not increase dose due to the habit-forming potential of butalbital. If medication appears less effective after a few wks, consult physician.
- Instruct patient on how and when to ask for prn pain medication.
- Medication may cause drowsiness or dizziness. Advise patient to avoid driving and other activities requiring alertness until response to medication is known.
- Caution patient to avoid concurrent use of alcohol or other CNS depressants.
- Tablets containing aspirin that have an acetic (vinegar-like) odor should be discarded.
- Centers for Disease Control warn against giving aspirin to children or adolescents with varicella (chickenpox) or influenza-like or viral illnesses because of a possible association with Reye's syndrome.

EVALUATION

Effectiveness of therapy can be demonstrated by: ▪ Decrease in severity of pain without a significant alteration in level of consciousness.

BUTORPHANOL
(byoo-**tor**-fa-nole)
Stadol

CLASSIFICATION(S):
Narcotic analgesic—agonist/antagonist
Pregnancy Category UK

INDICATIONS

▪ Management of moderate to severe pain ▪ Analgesia during labor ▪ Sedation prior to surgery ▪ Supplement in balanced anesthesia.

ACTION

▪ Binds to opiate receptors in the CNS ▪ Alters the perception of and response to painful stimuli, while producing generalized CNS depression ▪ Has partial antagonist properties that may result in narcotic withdrawal in physically dependent patients. **Therapeutic Effect:** ▪ Decreased severity of pain.

PHARMACOKINETICS

Absorption: Well absorbed from IM sites.

Distribution: Crosses the placenta and enters breast milk.

Metabolism and Excretion: Mostly metabolized by the liver; 11–14% excreted in the feces. Minimal amounts excreted unchanged by the kidneys.

Half-life: 3–4 hr.

CONTRAINDICATIONS AND PRECAUTIONS

Contraindicated in: ▪ Hypersensitivity ▪ Narcotic-dependent patients who have not been detoxified (may precipitate withdrawal).

Use Cautiously in: ▪ Head trauma ▪ Increased intracranial pressure ▪ Severe renal, hepatic, or pulmonary disease ▪ Hypothyroidism ▪ Adrenal insufficiency ▪ Alcoholism ▪ Elderly or debilitated patients (dosage reduction required) ▪ Undiagnosed abdominal pain ▪ Prostatic hypertrophy ▪ Pregnancy, lactation, or children (safety not established, but has been used during labor—may cause respiratory depression in the newborn).

ADVERSE REACTIONS AND SIDE EFFECTS*

CNS: sedation, confusion, headache, euphoria, floating feeling, unusual dreams, hallucinations, dysphoria.
EENT: miosis (high doses), blurred vision, diplopia.
Resp: respiratory depression.
CV: hypotension, hypertension, palpitations.
GI: nausea, vomiting, constipation, ileus, dry mouth.
GU: urinary retention.
Derm: sweating, clammy feeling.
Misc: tolerance, physical dependence, psychological dependence.

INTERACTIONS

Drug-Drug: ▪ Use with extreme caution in patients receiving **MAO inhibitors** (may produce severe, potentially fatal reactions—reduce initial dose of butorphanol to 25% of usual dose) ▪ Additive CNS depression with **alcohol, antihistamines, antidepressants,** and **sedative/hypnotics** ▪ May precipitate withdrawal in patients who are physically dependent on narcotic analgesics and have not been detoxified ▪ May decrease effects of concurrently administered **narcotic analgesics.**

ROUTE AND DOSAGE

- **IM (Adults):** 2 mg q 3–4 hr as needed (range 1–4 mg).
- **IV (Adults):** 0.5–2.0 mg q 3–4 hr as needed (range 0.5–2 mg).

PHARMACODYNAMICS (analgesia)

	ONSET	PEAK	DURATION
IM	1–30 min	30–60 min	3–4 hr
IV	1 min	4–5 min	2–4 hr

NURSING IMPLICATIONS

Assessment

- Assess type, location, and intensity of pain prior to and 30–60 min following IM and 5 min following IV administration.
- Assess blood pressure, pulse, and respirations before and periodically during administration. Butorphanol 2 mg produces approximately equal respiratory depression to morphine 10 mg, but respiratory depression does not increase in severity, only in duration, with increased dosage.
- While this drug has a low potential for dependence, prolonged use may lead to physical and psychological dependence and tolerance. This should not prevent patient from receiving adequate analgesia. Most patients who receive butorphanol for medical reasons do not develop psychological dependence. Progressively higher doses may be required to relieve pain with long-term therapy.
- Antagonistic properties may induce withdrawal symptoms (vomiting, restlessness, abdominal cramps, increased blood pressure and temperature) in narcotic-dependent patients.
- **Lab Test Considerations:** May cause elevated serum amylase and lipase levels.
- **Toxicity and Overdose:** If overdose occurs, respiratory depression may be partially reversed by naloxone (Narcan), the antidote.

Potential Nursing Diagnoses

- Comfort, altered: pain (indications).
- Injury, high risk for (side effects).
- Sensory-perceptual alteration: visual, auditory (side effects).

Implementation

- **General Info:** Explain therapeutic value of medication prior to administration to enhance the analgesic effect.
- Regularly administered doses may be

*Underlines indicate most frequent; **CAPITALS** indicate life-threatening.

more effective than prn administration. Analgesic is more effective if given before pain becomes severe.
- □ Coadministration with non-narcotic analgesics may have additive analgesic effects and permit lower narcotic doses.
- ▪ **IM:** Administer IM injections deep into well-developed muscle. Rotate sites of injections.
- ▪ **Direct IV:** May give IV undiluted.
- □ *Rate:* Administer over 3–5 min.
- □ Rapid administration may cause respiratory depression, hypotension, and cardiac arrest.
- ▪ **Syringe Compatibility:** atropine, chlorpromazine, cimetidine, diphenhydramine, droperidol, fentanyl, hydroxyzine, meperidine, midazolam, morphine, pentazocine, perphenazine, prochlorperazine, promethazine, scopolamine, or thiethylperazine.
- ▪ **Syringe Incompatibility:** dimenhydrinate or pentobarbital.
- ▪ **Y-Site Compatibility:** enalaprilat.

Patient/Family Teaching

- □ Instruct patient on how and when to ask for prn pain medication.
- □ Medication may cause drowsiness or dizziness. Advise patient to call for assistance when ambulating and to avoid driving or other activities requiring alertness until response to the medication is known.
- □ Encourage patient to turn, cough, and breathe deeply every 2 hr to prevent atelectasis.
- □ Instruct patient to change positions slowly to minimize orthostatic hypotension.
- □ Caution patient to avoid concurrent use of alcohol or other CNS depressants with this medication.

Evaluation

Effectiveness of therapy can be demonstrated by: ▪ Decrease in severity of pain without a significant alteration in level of consciousness or respiratory status.

CALCITONIN—salmon

(kal-si-**toe**-nin)
Calcimar, Miacalcin

CALCITONIN—human

Cibacalcin

CLASSIFICATION(S):
Hormone, Electrolyte modifier—hypocalcemic
Pregnancy Category C

INDICATIONS

▪ Treatment of Paget's disease of bone (human and salmon) ▪ Adjunctive therapy for hypercalcemia (salmon only) ▪ Management of postmenopausal osteoporosis (salmon only).

ACTION

▪ Decreases serum calcium by a direct effect on bone, kidney, and GI tract ▪ Promotes renal excretion of calcium. ▪ Salmon source is more potent on a weight basis and has a longer duration of action. **Therapeutic Effects:** ▪ Decreased rate of bone turnover ▪ Lowering of serum calcium.

PHARMACOKINETICS

Absorption: Destroyed in GI tract, necessitating parenteral administration. Completely absorbed from IM and SC sites.

Distribution: Distribution not known. Does not appear to cross the placenta.

Metabolism and Excretion: Rapidly metabolized in kidneys, blood, and tissues.

Half-life: Human, 60 min; salmon, 70–90 min.

CONTRAINDICATIONS AND PRECAUTIONS

Contraindicated in: ▪ Hypersensitivity to salmon protein or gelatin diluent (salmon product) ▪ Pregnancy or lactation (use not recommended).

Use Cautiously in: Children (safety not established).

ADVERSE REACTIONS AND SIDE EFFECTS*

CNS: headaches.
GI: nausea, vomiting, diarrhea, strange taste.
GU: urinary frequency.
Derm: rashes.
Local: injection site reactions.
Misc: allergic reactions including ANAPHYLAXIS (more common with salmon product), swelling, tingling, and tenderness in the hands, facial flushing.

INTERACTIONS

Drug-Drug: ■ None significant.

ROUTE AND DOSAGE

Calcitonin—Salmon

Note: Precede therapy with 1-IU intradermal skin test. 1 IU = 1 MRC unit.

Paget's Disease

- **IM, SC (Adults):** 100 IU/day initially, 50 IU/day or 50–100 IU q 1–3 days maintenance dose.

Hypercalcemia

- **IM, SC (Adults):** initially 4 IU/kg q 12 hr, can increase up to 8 IU/kg q 12 hr.

Osteoporosis

- **IM, SC (Adults):** 100 IU/day.

Calcitonin—Human

Paget's Disease

- **SC (Adults):** 0.25–0.5 mg daily or 2–3 times weekly as single daily dose, up to 1.0 mg/day in 2 divided doses.

PHARMACODYNAMICS (Noted as effects of salmon calcitonin on serum calcium concentrations. Clinical improvement in Paget's disease may take several mons of continuous therapy.)

	ONSET	PEAK	DURATION
IM	15 min	4 hr	8–24
SC	15 min	4 hr	8–24

NURSING IMPLICATIONS

Assessment

- □ Observe patient for signs of hypersensitivity (skin rash, fever, hives, anaphylaxis, serum sickness). Keep epinephrine, antihistamines, and oxygen nearby in the event of a reaction.
- □ Assess patient for signs of hypocalcemic tetany (nervousness, irritability, paresthesia, muscle twitching, tetanic spasms, convulsions) during the first several doses of calcitonin. Parenteral calcium, such as calcium gluconate, should be available in case of this event.
- ■ **Lab Test Considerations:** Serum calcium and alkaline phosphatase should be monitored periodically throughout therapy. These levels should normalize within a few mons of initiation of therapy.
- □ Urine sediment should be monitored for the presence of casts periodically during the course of therapy.

Potential Nursing Diagnoses

- ■ Comfort, altered: pain (indications).
- ■ Injury, high risk for (indications, side effects).
- ■ Knowledge deficit related to medication regimen (patient/family teaching).

Implementation

- ■ **General Info:** Assess for sensitivity to calcitonin-salmon by administering an intradermal test dose on the inner aspect of the forearm prior to initiating therapy. Test dose is prepared in a dilution of 10 IU/ml by withdrawing 0.05 ml in a tuberculin syringe and filling to 1 ml with 0.9% NaCl for injection. Mix well and discard 0.9 ml. Administer 0.1 ml and observe site for 15 min. More than mild erythema or wheal constitutes positive response.
- □ Store soln in refrigerator.
- ■ **IM/SC:** Inspect injection site for the appearance of redness, swelling, or pain. Rotate injection sites. SC is the preferred route. Use IM route if dose exceeds 2 ml in volume. Use multiple sites to minimize inflammatory reaction.

Patient/Family Teaching

- ■ **General Info:** Advise patient to take medication exactly as ordered. If dose

*Underlines indicate most frequent; **CAPITALS** indicate life-threatening.

is missed and medication is scheduled for twice a day, take only if remembered within 2 hr of correct time. If scheduled for daily dose, take only if remembered that day. If scheduled for every other day, take when remembered and restart alternate day schedule. Do not double doses.

- Instruct patient in the proper method of self-injection.
- Advise patient to report signs of hypercalcemic relapse (deep bone or flank pain, renal calculi, anorexia, nausea, vomiting, thirst, lethargy) or allergic response to the physician promptly.
- Reassure patient that flushing and warmth following injection is transient and usually lasts about 1 hr.
- Explain that nausea following injection tends to decrease even with continued therapy.
- Instruct patient to follow low-calcium diet if ordered by physician (see Appendix K). Women with postmenopausal osteoporosis should adhere to diet high in calcium and vitamin D.

▪ **Osteoporosis:** Advise patients receiving calcitonin for the treatment of osteoporosis that exercise has been found to arrest and reverse bone loss. The patient should discuss any exercise limitations with physician before beginning program.

Evaluation

Effectiveness of therapy can be measured by: ▪ Lowered serum calcium levels ▪ Decreased bone pain ▪ Slowed progression of postmenopausal osteoporosis.

CALCITRIOL

(kal-si-**trye**-ole)
1,25 dihydroxycholecalciferol, Calcijex, Rocaltrol, vitamin D_3

CLASSIFICATION(S):
Vitamin—fat-soluble
Pregnancy Category C

INDICATIONS

▪ Management of hypocalcemia in chronic renal failure patients ▪ Treatment of hypoparathyroidism or pseudohypoparathyroidism.

ACTION

▪ Synthetic active form of vitamin D_3 ▪ Promotes the absorption of calcium from the GI tract ▪ Regulates calcium homeostasis in conjunction with parathyroid hormone and calcitonin. **Therapeutic Effect:** ▪ Normalization of serum calcium levels in hypocalcemic chronic renal failure patients receiving dialysis. May also reduce elevated parathyroid hormone levels.

PHARMACOKINETICS

Absorption: Well absorbed following oral administration.
Distribution: Primarily stored in liver. Crosses the placenta.
Metabolism and Excretion: Metabolized by the liver, excreted primarily in bile.
Half-life: 3–8 hr.

CONTRAINDICATIONS AND PRECAUTIONS

Contraindicated in: ▪ Hypercalcemia ▪ Any other evidence of vitamin D toxicity.
Use Cautiously in: ▪ Sarcoidosis ▪ Hyperparathyroidism ▪ Pregnancy, lactation, or children (safety not established).

ADVERSE REACTIONS AND SIDE EFFECTS*

Note: Seen primarily as manifestations of toxicity (hypercalcemia).
CNS: weakness, headache, somnolence.
EENT: photophobia, conjunctivitis, rhinorrhea.
CV: hypertension, arrhythmias.
GI: nausea, vomiting, dry mouth, constipation, metallic taste, polydipsia, anorexia, weight loss.
GU: polyuria, nocturia, decreased libido, albuminuria.

*Underlines indicate most frequent; **CAPITALS** indicate life-threatening.

Derm: pruritus.
F and E: hypercalcemia.
Metab: hyperthermia.
MS: muscle pain, bone pain.

INTERACTIONS

Drug–Drug: ▪ Use with caution in patients receiving **cardiac glycosides, magnesium-containing antacids,** or **thiazide diuretics** ▪ Absorption may be decreased by concurrent administration of **cholestyramine** or **colestipol** ▪ **Glucocorticoids** may antagonize the effects of calcitriol.
Drug–Food: ▪ Ingestion of foods high in **calcium** content (see Appendix K) may lead to hypercalcemia.

ROUTE AND DOSAGE

Hypocalcemia in Chronic Renal Failure Patients

- **PO (Adults):** 0.25 mcg/day or every other day initially, increase by 0.25 mcg/day at 4–8 wk intervals. Usual dose range 0.5–1.0 mcg/day.
- **IV (Adults):** 0.5 mcg (0.01 mcg/kg) 3 times weekly. May be increased by 0.25–0.5 mcg/dose at 2–4 wk intervals. Usual dose is 0.5–3.0 mcg 3 times weekly (0.01–0.05 mcg/kg 3 times weekly).

Hypoparathyroidism or Pseudohypoparathyroidism

- **PO (Adults and Children > 6 yr):** 0.25 mcg/day, may be increased at 2–4 wk intervals (usual range, 0.5–2.0 mcg/day).
- **PO (Children 1–5 yr):** 0.25–0.75 mcg/day (0.04–0.08 mcg/kg/day).

PHARMACODYNAMICS

	ONSET	PEAK	DURATION
PO	2–6 hr	2–6 hr	1–5 days
IV	UK	UK	UK

NURSING IMPLICATIONS

Assessment

- □ Assess patient for bone pain and weakness prior to and throughout course of therapy.
- □ Observe patient carefully for evidence of hypocalcemia (paresthesia, muscle twitching, laryngospasm, colic, cardiac arrhythmias, and Chvostek's or Trousseau's sign). Protect symptomatic patient by raising and padding side rails; keep bed in low position.
- ▪ **Lab Test Considerations:** Serum calcium levels should be drawn weekly during initial therapy.
- □ Monitor BUN, serum creatinine, alkaline phosphatase parathyroid hormone levels, creatine clearance, 24–hr urinary calcium periodically.
- □ Monitor serum phosphorous levels prior to and periodically throughout course of therapy. Serum phosphorous must be controlled prior to initiating calcitriol. Aluminum carbonate or aluminum hydroxide is used for this purpose in dialysis patients.
- □ A fall in alkaline phosphatase levels may signal onset of hypercalcemia. Overdosage is associated with a serum calcium times phosphate (Ca × P) level of greater than 70 and elevated BUN, SGOT (AST), and SGPT (ALT).
- □ May cause false elevated cholesterol levels.
- ▪ **Toxicity and Overdose:** Toxicity is manifested as hypercalcemia, hypercalciuria, and hyperphosphatemia. Assess patient for appearance of nausea, vomiting, anorexia, weakness, constipation, headache, bone pain, and metallic taste. Later symptoms include polyuria, polydipsia, photophobia, rhinorrhea, pruritus, and cardiac arrhythmias. Notify physician immediately if these signs of hypervitaminosis D occur. Treatment usually consists of discontinuation of calcitriol, low calcium diet, and use of low calcium dialysate in dialysis patients.

Potential Nursing Diagnoses

- ▪ Nutrition, altered: less than body requirements (indications).
- ▪ Knowledge deficit related to medication regimen (patient/family teaching).

IMPLEMENTATION

- **PO:** May be administered without regard to meals.

PATIENT/FAMILY TEACHING

- Advise patient to take calcitriol exactly as directed. If dose is missed take as soon as remembered; do not double up on doses.
- Review diet modifications with patient. Foods high in vitamin D include fish livers and oils, and fortified milk, bread, and cereals. Foods high in calcium include dairy products, canned salmon and sardines, broccoli, bok choy, tofu, molasses, and cream soups. Renal patients must still consider renal failure diet in food selection. Physician may order concurrent calcium supplement (see Appendix K).
- Review symptoms of overdosage and instruct patient to report these promptly to physician.

EVALUATION

Effectiveness of therapy can be demonstrated by: ▪ Normalization of serum calcium and parathyroid hormone levels ▪ Decreased bone pain and weakness in patients with renal osteodystrophy.

CALCIUM CARBONATE

(**kal**-see-um **kar**-boh-nate)
BioCal, Calciday, Cal-Sup, Caltrate, Gencalc, Nephro-calci, Oscal, Oysco, Oystca, Rolaids, Suplical, Titrilac, Tums

CLASSIFICATION(S):
Electrolyte—calcium salt
Pregnancy Category C

INDICATIONS

▪ Treatment and prevention of calcium depletion in diseases associated with hypocalcemia including: ▫ Hypoparathyroidism ▫ Achlorhydria ▫ Chronic diarrhea ▫ Pancreatitis ▫ Vitamin D deficiency ▫ Hyperphosphatemia ▪ Adjunct in the prevention of postmenopausal osteoporosis ▪ Has been used as an antacid.

ACTION

▪ Essential for nervous, muscular, and skeletal systems ▪ Maintains cell membrane and capillary permeability ▪ Acts as an activator in the transmission of nerve impulses, contraction of cardiac, skeletal, and smooth muscle ▪ Essential for bone formation and blood coagulation. **Therapeutic Effect:** ▪ Replacement of calcium in deficiency states.

PHARMACOKINETICS

Absorption: Absorption from the GI tract requires vitamin D.
Distribution: Readily enters extracellular fluid. Crosses the placenta and enters breast milk.
Metabolism and Excretion: Excreted mostly in the feces. 20% eliminated by the kidneys.
Half-life: UK.

CONTRAINDICATIONS AND PRECAUTIONS

Contraindicated in: ▪ Hypercalcemia ▪ Renal calculi ▪ Ventricular fibrillation.
Use Cautiously in: ▪ Patients receiving cardiac glycosides ▪ Severe respiratory insufficiency ▪ Renal disease ▪ Cardiac disease.

ADVERSE REACTIONS AND SIDE EFFECTS*

GI: nausea, vomiting, constipation.
GU: hypercalcuria, calculi.
F and E: hypercalcemia.

INTERACTIONS

Drug–Drug: ▪ Hypercalcemia increases the risk of **cardiac glycoside** toxicity ▪ Chronic use with **antacids** in renal insufficiency may lead to milk–alkali syndrome ▪ Ingestion by mouth with **tetracyclines** decreases the absorption of tetracycline.
Drug–Food: ▪ **Cereals, spinach,** or **rhubarb** may decrease the absorption of calcium supplements.

*Underlines indicate most frequent; **CAPITALS** indicate life-threatening.

C

ROUTE AND DOSAGE

Note: Doses are expressed in g or mEq of elemental calcium. Contains 40% calcium by weight or 20 mEq/g.

Prevention of Hypocalcemia, Treatment of Depletion, Osteoporosis

- **PO (Adults):** 1–2 g/day in divided doses 4 times daily.

Supplementation

- **PO (Children):** 45–65 mg/kg/day.

Neonatal Hypocalcemia

- **PO (Infants):** 50–150 mg/kg (not to exceed 1 g).

PHARMACODYNAMICS (effects on serum calcium)

	ONSET	PEAK	DURATION
PO	hrs–days	UK	UK

NURSING IMPLICATIONS

Assessment

- **Calcium Supplement:** Monitor for signs of hypocalcemia (paresthesia, muscle twitching, laryngospasm, colic, cardiac arrhythmias, Chvostek's or Trousseau's sign). Notify physician if these occur.
- **Antacid:** When used as an antacid assess for heartburn, indigestion, abdominal pain. Inspect abdomen; auscultate bowel sounds.
- **Lab Test Considerations:** Monitor serum calcium levels. Used to treat hyperphosphatemia in renal failure patients; monitor phosphate levels.
- **Toxicity and Overdose:** Observe patient for appearance of nausea, vomiting, anorexia, thirst, severe constipation, paralytic ileus, and bradycardia. Contact physician immediately if these signs of hypercalcemia occur.

Potential Nursing Diagnoses

- Nutrition, altered: less than body requirements (indications).
- Injury, high risk for, related to osteoporosis or electrolyte imbalance (indications).
- Knowledge deficit related to medication and dietary regimens (patient/family teaching).

Implementation

- **General Info:** Physician may order concurrent vitamin D therapy for patients receiving calcium carbonate as a calcium supplement.
- **PO:** Administer 1 hr after meals and at bedtime.
  - Chewable tablets should be well chewed before swallowing; follow with a full glass of water.
  - Do not administer concurrently with foods containing large amounts of oxalic acid (spinach, rhubarb), phytic acid (brans, cereals), or phosphorus (milk or dairy products). Administration with milk products may lead to milk-alkali syndrome (nausea, vomiting, confusion, headache).

Patient/Family Teaching

- **General Info:** Instruct patient not to take enteric-coated tablets within 1 hr of calcium carbonate as this will result in premature dissolution of the tablets.
  - Advise patient that calcium carbonate may cause constipation. Review methods of preventing constipation (increasing bulk in diet, increasing fluid intake, increasing mobility). Patient may need to discuss use of laxatives with the physician. Severe constipation may indicate toxicity.
- **Calcium Supplement:** Encourage patients to maintain a diet adequate in vitamin D and calcium.
- **Osteoporosis:** Advise patients that exercise has been found to arrest and reverse bone loss. The patient should discuss any exercise limitations with physician before beginning program.

Evaluation

Effectiveness of therapy can be demonstrated by: ▪ Increase in serum calcium levels ▫ Decrease in the signs and symptoms of hypocalcemia ▪ Resolution of indigestion ▪ Control of hyperphosphatemia in patients with renal failure.

CALCIUM CHLORIDE
(**kal**-see-um **klor**-ide)

CLASSIFICATION(S):
Electrolyte—calcium salt
Pregnancy Category C

INDICATIONS
▪ Treatment and prevention of calcium depletion in diseases associated with hypocalcemia including: ▫ Hypoparathyroidism ▫ Achlorhydria ▫ Chronic diarrhea ▫ Pancreatitis ▫ Vitamin D deficiency ▫ Hyperphosphatemia ▪ Treatment of certain heavy metal poisonings.

ACTION
▪ Essential for nervous, muscular, and skeletal systems ▪ Maintains cell membrane and capillary permeability ▪ Acts as an activator in the transmission of nerve impulses, contraction of cardiac, skeletal, and smooth muscle ▪ Essential for bone formation and blood coagulation. **Therapeutic Effect:** ▪ Replacement of calcium in deficiency states.

PHARMACOKINETICS
Absorption: Absorption from the GI tract requires vitamin D.
Distribution: Readily enters extracellular fluid. Crosses the placenta and enters breast milk.
Metabolism and Excretion: Excreted mostly in the feces. 20% eliminated by the kidneys.
Half-life: UK.

CONTRAINDICATIONS AND PRECAUTIONS
Contraindicated in: ▪ Hypercalcemia ▪ Renal calculi ▪ Ventricular fibrillation.
Use Cautiously in: ▪ Patients receiving cardiac glycosides ▪ Severe respiratory insufficiency ▪ Renal disease ▪ Cardiac disease.

ADVERSE REACTIONS AND SIDE EFFECTS*
CNS: tingling, syncope.
CV: bradycardia, <u>arrhythmias</u>, <u>cardiac arrest</u>.
GI: nausea, vomiting, <u>constipation</u>.
GU: hypercalcemia, calculi.
Local: <u>phlebitis</u> at IV site.

INTERACTIONS
Drug-Drug: ▪ Increases the risk of **cardiac glycoside** toxicity ▪ Chronic use with **antacids** in renal insufficiency may lead to milk-alkali syndrome.

ROUTE AND DOSAGE
Note: Doses are expressed in g or mEq of elemental calcium. Contains 27% calcium by weight or 13.6 mEq/g.

Emergency Treatment of Hypocalcemia
- **IV (Adults):** 7–14 mEq.
- **IV (Children):** 1–7 mEq.
- **IV (Infants):** <1 mEq.

Hypocalcemia Tetany
- **IV (Adults):** 4.5–16 mEq repeat until symptoms are controlled.
- **IV (Children):** 0.5–0.7 mEq/kg 3–4 times daily.
- **IV (Neonates):** 2.4 mEq/kg/day in divided doses.

PHARMACODYNAMICS (effects on serum calcium)

	ONSET	PEAK	DURATION
IV	immediate	immediate	0.5–2 hr

NURSING IMPLICATIONS
Assessment
- ▫ Observe patient carefully for evidence of hypocalcemia (parathesias, muscle twitching, laryngospasm, colic, cardiac arrhythmias, and Chvostek's or Trousseau's sign). Protect symptomatic patients by elevating and padding side rails; keep bed in low position.
- ▫ Monitor blood pressure, pulse, and ECG frequently throughout therapy.

*<u>Underlines</u> indicate most frequent; **CAPITALS** indicate life-threatening.

May cause vasodilation with resulting hypotension, bradycardia, arrhythmias, and cardiac arrest.
- □ Assess IV site for patency. Extravasation may cause cellulitis, necrosis, and sloughing.
- □ Monitor client on cardiac glycosides for signs of toxicity.
- ▪ **Lab Test Considerations:** Monitor electrolytes (especially calcium) prior to and periodically throughout therapy. May cause false decreased serum and urine magnesium levels.
- □ Digitalis levels should be monitored in patients receiving calcium and digitalis glycosides concurrently, as hypercalcemia increases the risk of cardiac toxicity.
- ▪ **Toxicity and Overdose:** Observe patient for appearance of nausea, vomiting, anorexia, thirst, weakness, constipation, paralytic ileus, and bradycardia. Contact physician immediately if these signs of hypercalcemia occur.

Potential Nursing Diagnoses
- ▪ Nutrition, altered: less than body requirements (indications).
- ▪ Knowledge deficit related to medication and dietary regimens (patient/family teaching).

Implementation
- ▪ **General Info:** Do not administer IM or SC.
- □ In arrest situations, the use of calcium chloride is now limited to patients with hyperkalemia, hypocalcemia, and calcium channel blocker toxicity. Physician should specify form of calcium desired. Crash cart may contain both calcium chloride and calcium gluconate—ml doses are not equivalent. Doses should be expressed in mEq.
- □ Available as an intracardiac preparation.
- ▪ **IV:** IV soln should be warmed to body temperature and given through a small-bore needle in a large vein to minimize phlebitis. Do not administer through a scalp vein.
- □ If infiltration occurs, discontinue IV. Confer with physician about local infiltration of 1% procaine HCL or hyaluronidase, or application of heat.
- □ *Rate:* Maximum rate for adults is 0.7–1.5 mEq/min (0.5–1 ml of 10% soln); for children 0.5 ml/min. Rapid administration may cause tingling, sensation of warmth, and a metallic taste. Halt infusion if these symptoms occur and resume infusion at a slower rate when they subside.
- ▪ **Direct IV:** May be administered undiluted by IV push.
- ▪ **Intermittent/Continuous Infusion:** Calcium chloride may be diluted with D5W, D10W, 0.9% NaCl, D5/0.25% NaCl, D5/0.45% NaCl, D5/0.9% NaCl, or D5/LR.
- ▪ **Y-Site Compatibility:** amrinone, dobutamine, epinephrine, esmolol, or morphine.
- ▪ **Y-Site Incompatibility:** sodium bicarbonate.
- ▪ **Additive Compatibility:** amikacin, ascorbic acid, bretyllium, cephapirin, chloramphenicol, dopamine, hydrocortisone, isoproterenol, lidocaine, methicillin, norepinephrine, penicillin, pentobarbitol, phenobarbitol, sodium bicarbonate, or verapamil.
- ▪ **Additive Incompatibility:** amphotericin B, cephalothin, chlorphenarimine, phosphates, sulfates, or tartrates.

Patient/Family Teaching
- □ Instruct patient to remain recumbent for 15–30 min after IV administration.
- □ Encourage patients with chronic hypocalcemia to maintain a diet adequate in vitamin D (fish livers and oils, fortified milk, breads, and cereals) and calcium (milk, leafy green vegetables, sardines, oysters, clams); see Appendix K.

Evaluation
Effectiveness of therapy may be determined by: ▪ Increase in serum calcium levels ▪ Decrease in symptoms of hypocalcemia.

CALCIUM GLUCEPTATE
(**kal**-see-um **gloo**-sep-tate)

CLASSIFICATION(S):
Electrolyte—calcium salt
Pregnancy Category C

INDICATIONS
▪ Treatment and prevention of calcium depletion in diseases associated with hypocalcemia including: ▫ Hypoparathyroidism ▫ Achlorhydria ▫ Chronic diarrhea ▫ Pancreatitis ▫ Vitamin D deficiency ▫ Hyperphosphatemia ▪ Also used to treat certain heavy metal poisonings.

ACTION
▪ Essential for nervous, muscular, and skeletal systems ▪ Maintains cell membrane and capillary permeability ▪ Acts as an activator in the transmission of nerve impulses, contraction of cardiac, skeletal, and smooth muscle ▪ Essential for bone formation and blood coagulation. **Therapeutic Effect:** ▪ Replacement of calcium in deficiency states.

PHARMACOKINETICS
Absorption: Absorption from the GI tract requires vitamin D.
Distribution: Readily enters extracellular fluid. Crosses the placenta and enters breast milk.
Metabolism and Excretion: Excreted mostly in the feces. 20% eliminated by the kidneys.
Half-life: UK.

CONTRAINDICATIONS AND PRECAUTIONS
Contraindicated in: ▪ Hypercalcemia ▪ Renal calculi ▪ Ventricular fibrillation.
Use Cautiously in: ▪ Patients receiving cardiac glycosides ▪ Severe respiratory insufficiency ▪ Renal disease ▪ Cardiac disease.

ADVERSE REACTIONS AND SIDE EFFECTS*
CNS: tingling, syncope.
CV: bradycardia, arrhythmias, cardiac arrest.
GI: nausea, vomiting, constipation.
GU: hypercalcuria, calculi.
Local: phlebitis at IV site.

INTERACTIONS
Drug-Drug: ▪ Increases the risk of **cardiac glycoside** toxicity ▪ Chronic use with **actacids** in renal insufficiency may lead to milk–alkali syndrome.

ROUTE AND DOSAGE
Note: Doses are expressed in g or mEq of elemental calcium. Contains 8.2% calcium by weight or 4.1 mEq/g.

Emergency Treatment of Hypocalcemia.
- **IV (Adults):** 7–14 mEq.
- **IV (Children):** 1–7 mEq.
- **IV (Infants):** $<$1 mEq.

Hypocalcemic Tetany
- **IV (Adults):** 4.5–16 mEq repeat until symptoms are controlled.
- **IV (Children):** 0.5–0.7 mEq/kg 3–4 times daily.
- **IV (Neonates):** 2.4 mEq/kg/day in divided doses.

PHARMACODYNAMICS

	ONSET	PEAK	DURATION
IV	immediate	immediate	0.5–2 hr

NURSING IMPLICATIONS
Assessment
- ▫ Observe patient carefully for evidence of hypocalcemia (paresthesia, muscle twitching, laryngospasm, colic, cardiac arrhythmias, and Chvostek's or Trousseau's sign). Protect symptomatic patients by raising and padding side rails; keep bed in low position.
- ▫ Monitor blood pressure, pulse, and ECG frequently throughout therapy. May cause hypotension, bradycardia, arrhythmias, and cardiac arrest.
- ▫ Assess IV site for patency. Extravasa-

*Underlines indicate most frequent; **CAPITALS** indicate life-threatening.

C

tion may cause cellulitis, necrosis, and sloughing. If extravasation occurs, 1% procaine and hyaluronidase may be infiltrated into the area to decrease venospasm. Local application of heat may be helpful.
- Monitor patients taking cardiac glycosides for signs of digitalis toxicity.
- **Lab Test Considerations:** Monitor electrolytes (especially calcium) and albumin concentrations prior to and periodically throughout therapy. May cause false decrease in serum and urine magnesium levels.
- Digitalis levels should be monitored in patients receiving calcium and cardiac glycosides concurrently, because hypercalcemia increases the risk of digitalis toxicity.
- **Toxicity and Overdose:** Observe patient for appearance of nausea, vomiting, anorexia, thirst, weakness, constipation, paralytic ileus, and bradycardia. Contact physician immediately if these signs of hypercalcemia occur.

Potential Nursing Diagnoses
- Nutrition, altered: less than body requirements (indications).
- Knowledge deficit related to medication and dietary regimens (patient/family teaching).

Implementation
- **General Info:** Milligram doses of calcium chloride, calcium gluconate, and calcium gluceptate are not equal. Doses should be expressed in mEq of calcium.
- **IM:** May be administered IM in emergency situation if venous access not available. For child administer only in thigh. For adult administer only in gluteal region.
- **IV:** IV soln should be warmed to body temperature and given through a small-bore needle in a large vein to minimize phlebitis. Do not administer through a scalp vein.
- *Rate:* Rapid administration may cause tingling, sensation of warmth, and a metallic taste. If these symptoms occur, stop infusion; resume administration at slower rate when symptoms subside.
- **Direct IV:** Administer by direct IV push at a rate not to exceed 2 ml/(1.8 mEq)/min for adults; 0.5 ml/(0.45 mEq)/min for children. In exchange transfusion for neonates, 0.5 ml (0.45 mEq) is given after each 100 ml of citrated blood.
- **Intermittent Infusion:** May be further diluted in D5W, D10W, 0.9% NaCl, 0.45% NaCl, D5/LR, or lactated Ringer's soln. Soln should be clear; do not use if crystals are present.
- **Y-Site Compatibility:** dobutamine, epinephrine, or morphine.
- **Y-Site Incompatibility:** sodium bicarbonate.
- **Additive Compatibility:** ascorbic acid, isoproterenol, lidocaine, norepinephrine, phytonadione, or sodium bicarbonate.
- **Additive Incompatibility:** cefamandole, cefazolin, cephalothin, magnesium sulfate, prednisolone, prochlorperazine, tobramycin, phosphates, sulfates, or tartrates.

Patient/Family Teaching
- Instruct patient to remain recumbent for 15–30 min after IV administration.
- Encourage patients with chronic hypocalcemia to maintain a diet adequate in vitamin D (fish livers and oils, fortified milk, breads, and cereals) and calcium (milk, leafy green vegetables, sardines, oysters, clams); see Appendix K.

Evaluation
Effectiveness of therapy can be demonstrated by: ▪ Increase in serum calcium levels ▫ Decrease in symptoms of hypocalcemia.

CALCIUM GLUCONATE
(**kal**-see-um **gloo**-koh-nate)
Kalcinate

CLASSIFICATION(S):
Electrolyte—calcium salt
Pregnancy Category C

INDICATIONS

■ Treatment and prevention of calcium depletion in diseases associated with hypocalcemia including: □ Hypoparathyroidism □ Achlorhydria □ Chronic diarrhea □ Pancreatitis □ Vitamin D deficiency □ Hyperphosphatemia ■ Adjunct in the prevention of postmenopausal osteoporosis ■ Used to treat certain heavy metal poisonings.

ACTION

■ Essential for nervous, muscular, and skeletal systems ■ Maintains cell membrane and capillary permeability ■ Acts as an activator in the transmission of nerve impulses, contraction of cardiac, skeletal, and smooth muscle ■ Essential for bone formation and blood coagulation. **Therapeutic Effect:** ■ Replacement of calcium in deficiency states.

PHARMACOKINETICS

Absorption: Absorption from the GI tract requires vitamin D.
Distribution: Readily enters extracellular fluid. Crosses the placenta and enters breast milk.
Metabolism and Excretion: Excreted mostly in the feces; 20% eliminated by the kidneys.
Half-life: UK.

CONTRAINDICATIONS AND PRECAUTIONS

Contraindicated in: ■ Hypercalcemia ■ Renal calculi ■ Ventricular fibrillation.
Use Cautiously in: ■ Patients receiving cardiac glycosides ■ Severe respiratory insufficiency ■ Renal disease ■ Cardiac disease.

ADVERSE REACTIONS AND SIDE EFFECTS*

CNS: IV—tingling, syncope.
CV: IV—bradycardia, arrhythmias, cardiac arrest.
GI: nausea, vomiting, constipation, metallic taste.
GU: hypercalcuria, calculi.
Local: phlebitis at IV site.

INTERACTIONS

Drug-Drug: ■ Hypercalcemia increases the risk of **cardiac glycoside** toxicity ■ Chronic use with **antacids** in renal insufficiency may lead to milk-alkali syndrome ■ Ingestion by mouth with **tetracyclines** decreases the absorption of tetracycline.
Drug-Food: ■ **Cereals, spinach,** or **rhubarb** may decrease the absorption of oral calcium supplements.

ROUTE AND DOSAGE

Note: Doses are expressed in g or mEq of elemental calcium. Contains 9% calcium by weight or 4.5 mEq/g.

Prevention of Hypocalcemia, Treatment of Depletion, Osteoporosis

- **PO (Adults):** 1–2 g/day.

Supplementation

- **PO (Children):** 45–65 mg/kg/day.

Neonatal Hypocalcemia

- **PO (Infants):** 50–150 mg/kg (not to exceed 1 g).

Emergency Treatment of Hypocalcemia

- **IV (Adults):** 7–14 mEq.
- **IV (Children):** 1–7 mEq.
- **IV (Infants):** <1 mEq.

Hypocalcemia Tetany

- **IV (Adults):** 4.5–16 mEq; repeat until symptoms are controlled.
- **IV (Children):** 0.5–0.7 mEq/kg 3–4 times daily.
- **IV (Neonates):** 2.4 mEq/kg/day in divided doses.

PHARMACODYNAMICS (effects on serum calcium)

	ONSET	PEAK	DURATION
PO	UK	UK	UK
IV	immediate	immediate	0.5–2 hr

NURSING IMPLICATIONS

Assessment

■ **General Info:** Observe patient carefully for evidence of hypocalcemia

*Underlines indicate most frequent; **CAPITALS** indicate life-threatening.

(paresthesia, muscle twitching, laryngospasm, colic, cardiac arrhythmias, and Chvostek's or Trousseau's sign). Protect symptomatic patients by raising and padding side rails; keep bed in low position.

- Monitor patient on cardiac glycosides for signs of digitalis toxicity.

- **IV:** Monitor blood pressure, pulse, and ECG frequently throughout IV therapy. May cause vasodilation with resulting hypotension, bradycardia, arrhythmias, and cardiac arrest.
- Assess site for patency. Extravasation may cause cellulitis, necrosis, and sloughing.
- **Lab Test Considerations:** Monitor electrolytes (especially calcium) and albumin concentrations prior to and periodically throughout therapy. May cause false decrease in serum and urine magnesium levels.
- Digitalis levels should be monitored in patients receiving calcium and cardiac glycosides concurrently, because hypercalcemia increases the risk of digitalis toxicity.
- **Toxicity and Overdose:** Observe patient for appearance of nausea, vomiting, anorexia, thirst, weakness, constipation, paralytic ileus, and bradycardia. Contact physician immediately if these signs of hypercalcemia occur.

Potential Nursing Diagnoses

- Nutrition, altered: less than body requirements (indications).
- Knowledge deficit related to medication and dietary regimens (patient/family teaching).

Implementation

- **General Info:** Milligram doses of calcium chloride, calcium gluconate, and calcium gluceptate are not equal. Doses should be expressed in mEq of calcium.
- In arrest situations, calcium use is now limited to patients with hyperkalemia, hypocalcemia, and calcium channel blocker toxicity. Physician should specify form of calcium desired. Crash cart may contain both calcium chloride and calcium gluconate—mg doses are not equivalent.
- **PO:** Administer oral calcium 1–1½ hr after meals. Chewable tablets should not be swallowed whole. Chew well before swallowing and follow with a full glass of water.
- Available in combination with vitamins and other minerals.
- **IM/SC:** Avoid SC route.
- **IM:** IM administration of calcium gluconate may be tolerated if IV route is not accessible. Limit use to emergency situations. Do not use IM route in infants and children.
- **IV:** Soln should be warmed to body temperature and given through a small-bore needle in a large vein to minimize phlebitis. Do not use scalp vein. May cause cutaneous burning sensation, peripheral vasodilation, and a drop in blood pressure.
- Soln should be clear; do not use if crystals are present.
- Patients should remain recumbent for 30 min to 1 hr following IV administration.
- **Direct IV:** Administer slowly by direct IV push.
- *Rate:* Maximum administration rate for adults is 1.5–3 ml (0.7–1.5 mEq)/min. Rapid administration may cause tingling, sensation of warmth, and a metallic taste. If these symptoms occur, stop infusion; resume infusion at slower rate when symptoms subside. Administer slowly; high concentrations may cause cardiac arrest.
- **Continuous Infusion:** May be further diluted in 1000 ml of D5W, D10W, D20W, D5/0.9% NaCl, 0.9% NaCl, D5/LR, or lactated Ringer's soln.
- *Rate:* Administer over 12–24 hr.
- **Syringe Incompatibility:** metoclopramide.
- **Y-Site Compatibility:** cefazolin, dobutamine, enalaprilat, epinephrine, heparin with hydrocortisone sodium succinate, labetolol, netilmicin, potassium chloride, or tolazoline.
- **Additive Compatibility:** amikacin,

aminophylline, ascorbic acid, bretylium, cephapirin, chloramphenicol, corticotropin, dimenhydrinate, erythromycin, heparin, hydrocortisone, lidocaine, magnesium sulfate, methicillin, norepinephrine, penicillin G, phenobarbital, potassium chloride, vancomycin, or verapamil.

- **Additive Incompatibility:** amphotericin, cefamandole, cephalothin, cefazolin, clindamycin, dobutamine, or prednisolone.

Patient/Family Teaching

- □ Instruct patient to remain recumbent for 30 min to 1 hr after IV administration.
- □ With physician's order, encourage patient to maintain a diet adequate in vitamin D (fish liver and oils, fortified milk, breads, and cereals) and calcium (milk, leafy green vegetables, sardines, oysters, clams); see Appendix K.
- □ Caution patient not to take oral calcium preparations with cereal, spinach, or rhubarb as these will interfere with calcium absorption.
- □ Advise patients receiving calcium for the treatment of osteoporosis that exercise has been found to arrest and reverse bone loss. The patient should discuss any exercise limitations with physician before beginning program.
- □ Instruct patient to contact physician immediately if signs of hypocalcemia or hypercalcemia occur.
- □ Advise patient that calcium may cause constipation. Review methods of preventing constipation (increasing bulk in diet, increasing fluid intake, increasing mobility). Patient may need to discuss use of laxatives with the physician. Severe constipation may indicate toxicity.

Evaluation

Effectiveness of therapy can be demonstrated by: ▪ Increase in serum calcium levels □ Decrease in the signs and symptoms of hypocalcemia ▪ Control of osteoporotic bone changes.

CALCIUM LACTATE
(**kal**-see-um **lak**-tate)

CLASSIFICATION(S):
Electrolyte—calcium salt
Pregnancy Category C

INDICATIONS

▪ Treatment and prevention of calcium depletion in diseases associated with hypocalcemia including: □ Hypoparathyroidism □ Achlorhydria □ Chronic diarrhea □ Pancreatitis □ Vitamin D deficiency □ Hyperphosphatemia ▪ Adjunct in the prevention of postmenopausal osteoporosis.

ACTION

▪ Essential for nervous, muscular, and skeletal systems. ▪ Maintains cell membrane and capillary permeability ▪ Acts as an activator in the transmission of nerve impulses, contraction of cardiac, skeletal, and smooth muscle ▪ Essential for bone formation and blood coagulation. **Therapeutic Effect:** ▪ Replacement of calcium in deficiency states.

PHARMACOKINETICS

Absorption: Absorption from the GI tract requires vitamin D.
Distribution: Readily enters extracellular fluid. Crosses the placenta and enters breast milk.
Metabolism and Excretion: Excreted mostly in the feces. 20% eliminated by the kidneys.
Half-life: UK.

CONTRAINDICATIONS AND PRECAUTIONS

Contraindicated in: ▪ Hypercalcemia ▪ Renal calculi ▪ Ventricular fibrillation.
Use Cautiously in: ▪ Patients receiving cardiac glycosides ▪ Severe respiratory insufficiency ▪ Renal disease ▪ Cardiac disease.

ADVERSE REACTIONS AND SIDE EFFECTS*

GI: nausea, vomiting, constipation.

*Underlines indicate most frequent; **CAPITALS** indicate life-threatening.

C

GU: hypercalcuria, calculi.
F and E: hypercalcemia.

INTERACTIONS

Drug–Drug: ▪ Hypercalcemia increases the risk of **cardiac glycoside toxicity** ▪ Chronic use with **antacids** in renal insufficiency may lead to milk–alkali syndrome ▪ Ingestion by mouth with **tetracyclines** decreases the absorption of tetracycline.

Drug–Food: ▪ **Cereals, spinach,** or **rhubarb** may decrease the absorption of calcium supplements.

ROUTE AND DOSAGE

Note: Doses are expressed in g or mg of elemental calcium. Contains 13% elemental calcium by weight or 6.5 mEq/g.

Prevention of Hypocalcemia, Treatment of Depletion, Osteoporosis

- **PO (Adults):** 1–2 g/day.

Supplementation

- **PO (Children):** 45–65 mg/kg/day.

Neonatal Hypocalcemia

- **PO (Infants):** 50–150 mg/kg (not to exceed 1 g).

PHARMACODYNAMICS (effects on serum calium levels)

	ONSET	PEAK	DURATION
PO	UK	UK	UK

NURSING IMPLICATIONS

Assessment

- **General Info:** Monitor for signs of hypocalcemia (paresthesia, muscle twitching, laryngospasm, colic, cardiac arrhythmias, and Chvostek's or Trousseau's sign). Notify physician if these occur.
- **Lab Test Considerations:** Monitor sodium, chloride, potassium, magnesium, albumin, and calcium levels prior to and periodically throughout therapy. May cause false decreases in serum and urine magnesium concentrations.
  - ▫ Digitalis levels should be monitored in patients receiving calcium and cardiac glycosides concurrently, because hypercalcemia increases the risk of digitalis toxicity.
- **Toxicity and Overdose:** Observe patient for appearance of nausea, vomiting, anorexia, thirst, severe constipation, paralytic ileus, and bradycardia. Contact physician immediately if these signs of hyperglycemia occur.

Potential Nursing Diagnoses

- Nutrition, altered: less than body requirements (indications).
- Injury, high risk for, related to osteoporosis or electrolyte imbalance (indications).
- Knowledge deficit related to medication regimen (patient/family teaching).

Implementation

- **General Info:** Physician may order concurrent vitamin D therapy for patients receiving calcium supplement.
- **PO:** Administer 1–1½ hr after meals.
  - ▫ Chewable tablets should not be swallowed whole. Chew well before swallowing; follow with a full glass of water.
  - ▫ Administration with milk products may lead to milk–alkali syndrome (nausea, vomiting, confusion, headache).

Patient/Family Teaching

- ▫ With physician's order, encourage patient to maintain a diet adequate in vitamin D (fish livers and oils, fortified milk, breads, and cereals) and calcium (milk, leafy green vegetables, sardines, oysters, clams); see Appendix K.
- ▫ Caution patient not to take oral calcium preparations with cereal, bran, spinach, or rhubarb as these will interfere with calcium absorption.
- ▫ Advise patients receiving calcium for the treatment of osteoporosis that exercise has been found to arrest and reverse bone loss. The patient should discuss any exercise limitations with physician before beginning program.
- ▫ Advise patient to contact physician immediately if signs of hypocalcemia or hypercalcemia occur.

□ Advise patient that calcium may cause constipation. Review methods of preventing constipation (increasing bulk in diet, increasing fluid intake, increasing mobility.) Patient may need to discuss use of laxatives with the physician. Severe constipation may indicate toxicity.

Evaluation

Effectiveness of therapy can be demonstrated by: ▪ Increase in serum calcium levels □ Decrease in the signs and symptoms of hypocalcemia ▪ Control of osteoporotic bone changes.

CAPSAICIN

(cap-**say**-sin)
Axsain (0.075% cream), Zostrix (0.025% cream)

CLASSIFICATION(S):
Analgesic—topical
Pregnancy Category UK

INDICATIONS

▪ 0.025% cream—used in the temporary management of neuralgia following healing of open skin lesions in herpes zoster or pain associated with diabetic neuropathy, rheumatoid arthritis, or osteoarthritis ▪ 0.075% cream—management of neuralgia associated with diabetic neuropathy or postsurgical pain.

ACTION

▪ May deplete and prevent the reaccumulation of a chemical (substance P) responsible for transmitting painful impulses from peripheral sites to the central nervous system. **Therapeutic Effect:** ▪ Relief of discomfort associated with peripheral painful syndromes.

PHARMACOKINETICS

Absorption: Absorption not known.
Distribution: Distribution not known.
Metabolism and Excretion: Metabolism and excretion not known.
Half-life: Half-life not known.

CONTRAINDICATIONS AND PRECAUTIONS

Contraindicated in: ▪ Hypersensitivity ▪ Use near eyes or on open or broken skin.
Use Cautiously in: ▪ Pregnancy, lactation, or children <2 yr (safety not established).

ADVERSE REACTIONS AND SIDE EFFECTS*

Derm: transient burning.
Misc: Hypersensitivity to capsaicin or components in preparations.

INTERACTIONS

Drug-Drug: ▪ None known.

ROUTE AND DOSAGE

▪ **Top:** Apply to affected areas not more than 3–4 times/day.

PHARMACODYNAMICS

	ONSET	PEAK	DURATION
Top	UK	UK	UK

NURSING IMPLICATIONS

Assessment

□ Assess pain intensity and location prior to and periodically throughout therapy.

Potential Nursing Diagnoses

▪ Comfort, altered (indications).
▪ Knowledge deficit related to medication regimen (patient/family teaching).

Implementation

▪ **Top:** Apply to affected area not more than 3–4 times daily. Avoid getting medication into eyes or broken or irritated skin. Do not bandage tightly.

Patient/Family Teaching

□ Instruct patient on the correct method for application of capsaicin. Gloves should be worn during application or hands should be washed immediately after application.
□ Advise patient that transient burning may occur with application, espe-

*Underlines indicate most frequent; **CAPITALS** indicate life-threatening.

cially if applied less than 3–4 times daily.

- Advise patient to discontinue use and notify physician if pain persists longer than 14–28 days or clears up and recurs within a few days or if signs of infection are present.

EVALUATION

Effectiveness of therapy can be demonstrated by: ■ Decrease in discomfort associated with: ▫ Postherpetic neuropathy ▫ Diabetic neuropathy ▫ Rheumatoid arthritis ▫ Osteoarthritis.

CAPTOPRIL

(**kap**-toe-pril)

Capoten

CLASSIFICATION(S):

Antihypertensive—angiotensin converting enzyme (ACE) inhibitor

Pregnancy Category C

INDICATIONS

■ Alone or in combination with other antihypertensives in the management of hypertension ■ Used in combination with other drugs in the treatment of congestive heart failure.

ACTION

■ Prevents the production of angiotensin II, a potent vasoconstrictor that stimulates the production of aldosterone, by blocking its conversion to the active form. Result is systemic vasodilation. **Therapeutic Effects:** ■ Lowering of blood pressure in hypertensive patients ■ Decreased preload and afterload in patients with congestive heart failure.

PHARMACOKINETICS

Absorption: Rapidly absorbed (75%) from the GI tract. Food decreases absorption.

Distribution: Widely distributed but does not cross blood–brain barrier. Crosses the placenta. Small amounts enter breast milk.

Metabolism and Excretion: 50% metabolized by the liver. 50% excreted unchanged by the kidneys.

Half-life: <2 hr.

CONTRAINDICATIONS AND PRECAUTIONS

Contraindicated in: ■ Hypersensitivity ■ Cross-sensitivity with other ACE inhibitors may exist.

Use Cautiously in: ■ Renal impairment (dosage reduction required) ■ Aortic stenosis ■ Cerebrovascular or cardiac insufficiency ■ Pregnancy (may cause fetal malformation; hypotension, oliguria, or hypokalemia may occur in newborns) ■ Lactation, and children (safety not established) ■ Surgery/anesthesia (hypotension may be exaggerated).

Extreme Caution in: Family history of hereditary angioedema.

ADVERSE REACTIONS AND SIDE EFFECTS*

CNS: dizziness.

Resp: cough.

CV: <u>hypotension</u>, tachycardia, angina pectoris.

GI: anorexia, <u>loss of taste perception</u>.

GU: <u>proteinuria</u>, renal failure.

Derm: <u>rashes</u>.

Hemat: **LEUKOPENIA, AGRANULOCYTOSIS.**

Misc: fever.

INTERACTIONS

Drug–Drug: ■ Additive hypotension with other **antihypertensives, phenothiazines,** acute ingestion of **alcohol,** and **vasodilators** ■ Hyperkalemia may result from concurrent use of **potassium supplements** or **potassium-sparing diuretics** ■ Antihypertensive response may be blunted by **nonsteroidal anti-inflammatory agents** ■ Absorption may be decreased by **antacids** ■ Increases levels and may increase risk of **digoxin** or **lithium** toxicity ■ **Probenecid** decreases elimination and increases levels of cap-

*<u>Underlines</u> indicate most frequent; **CAPITALS** indicate life-threatening.

topril ▪ Risk of hypersensitivity reactions increased by concurrent **allopurinol.**

ROUTE AND DOSAGE

Hypertension

- **PO (Adults):** Initial dose 25 mg 2–3 times daily; may increase at 1–2 wk intervals up to 150 mg 3 times daily (usual dose, 50 mg 3 times daily).

Congestive Heart Failure

- **PO (Adults):** 6.25–25 mg 3 times daily (range 12.5–4.50 mg/day).

PHARMACODYNAMICS (effect on blood pressure)*

	ONSET	PEAK	DURATION
PO	15–60 min	60–90 min	6–12 hr

*Full effects may not be noted until several wks of therapy.

NURSING IMPLICATIONS

Assessment

- Monitor blood pressure and pulse frequently during initial dosage adjustment and periodically throughout course of therapy. Notify physician of significant changes.
- Monitor weight and assess patient routinely for resolution of fluid overload (peripheral edema, rales/crackles, dyspnea, weight gain, jugular venous distension) if on concurrent diuretic therapy.
- **Lab Test Considerations:** Periodic assessments of urine protein may be ordered, because proteinuria and nephrotic syndrome may occur with patients on captopril therapy.
- Monitor BUN, creatinine, and electrolyte levels periodically. Serum potassium may be increased and BUN and creatinine transiently increased, while sodium levels may be decreased.
- WBC with differential should be monitored prior to initiation of therapy, every 2 wk for the first 3 mon, and periodically thereafter during the course of therapy.
- May cause false-positive test results for urine acetone.

Potential Nursing Diagnoses

- Cardiac output, decreased (indications, side effects).
- Knowledge deficit related to medication regimen (patient/family teaching).
- Noncompliance (patient/family teaching).

Implementation

- **General Info:** Precipitous drop in blood pressure during first 1–3 hr following first dose may require volume expansion with normal saline, but is not normally considered an indication for stopping therapy.
- Available in combination with hydrochlorothiazide (Capozide); see Appendix A.
- **PO:** Administer 1 hr before or 2 hr after meals, because food reduces absorption by 30–40%. May be crushed if patient has difficulty swallowing. Tablets may have a sulfurous odor.
- An oral soln may be prepared by crushing a 25-mg tablet and dissolving it in 25–100 ml of water. Shake for at least 5 min and administer within 30 min.

Patient/Family Teaching

- Instruct patient to take captopril exactly as directed, even if feeling better. Missed doses should be taken as soon as remembered but not if almost time for next dose. Do not double doses. Medication controls but does not cure hypertension. Warn patients not to discontinue captopril therapy unless directed by the physician.
- Encourage patient to comply with additional interventions for hypertension (weight reduction, discontinuation of smoking, moderation of alcohol consumption, regular exercise, and stress management).
- Instruct patient and family on proper technique for blood pressure monitoring. Advise them to check blood pressure at least weekly and report significant changes to physician.
- Caution patient to avoid salt substitutes or foods containing high levels of potassium or sodium unless di-

rected by physician (see Appendix K).

- Advise patient that captopril may cause an impairment of taste that generally reverses itself within 8–12 wk, even with continued therapy.
- Caution patient to change positions slowly to minimize orthostatic hypotension, particularly after initial dose. Patients should also be advised that exercising in hot weather may increase hypotensive effects.
- Advise patient to consult physician or pharmacist before taking any over-the-counter medications, especially cold remedies. Patients should also avoid excessive amounts of tea, coffee, or cola.
- Captopril may cause dizziness. Caution patient to avoid driving and other activities requiring alertness until response to medication is known.
- Advise patient to inform physician or dentist of medication regimen prior to treatment or surgery.
- Instruct patient to notify physician if rash, sore throat, fever, irregular heart beat, chest pain, swelling of face, eyes, lips, or tongue, or difficulty breathing occurs.
- Emphasize the importance of follow-up examinations to monitor progress.

Evaluation

Effectiveness of therapy can be demonstrated by: ▪ Decrease in blood pressure without appearance of side effects ▪ Decrease in signs and symptoms of congestive heart failure. Several wks may be necessary before full effects of the drug are recognized.

CARBACHOL

(**kar**-ba-kole)
Isopto Carbochol, Miostat

CLASSIFICATION(S):
Ophthalmic—miotic—direct-acting cholinergic
Pregnancy Category UK

INDICATIONS

▪ Induction of miosis during ocular surgery ▪ Treatment of chronic open-angle glaucoma.

ACTION

▪ Directly stimulates cholinergic receptors in the eye, producing miosis and accommodation (contraction of the ciliary muscle) ▪ Increases outflow of aqueous humor. **Therapeutic Effects:** ▪ Miosis ▪ Lowering of intraocular pressure.

PHARMACOKINETICS

Absorption: Minimal absorption may follow intraocular administration.
Distribution: Systemic distribution following intraocular administration not known.
Metabolism and Excretion: Not known following intraocular administration.
Half-life: UK.

CONTRAINDICATIONS AND PRECAUTIONS

Contraindicated in: ▪ Hypersensitivity ▪ Hypersensitivity to benzalkonium chloride or hydroxypropyl methylcellulose ▪ Acute iritis ▪ Certain forms of secondary glaucoma ▪ Inflammatory diseases of the anterior chamber.
Use Cautiously in: ▪ Patients at risk for retinal detachment or retinal tears ▪ Children (safety not established) ▪ Corneal abrasions, following tonometry or trauma (systemic absorption may occur) ▪ Although unlikely to cause systemic problems, use cautiously in patients with: □ Acute heart failure □ Asthma □ Ulcer disease □ Hyperthyroidism □ Urinary tract obstruction □ Parkinson's disease.

ADVERSE REACTIONS AND SIDE EFFECTS*

EENT: transient opacities of the lens, blurred vision, eye ache, eye brow ache, impaired night vision.
CV: bradycardia, hypotension.
Resp: difficulty breathing.

*Underlines indicate most frequent; **CAPITALS** indicate life-threatening.

GI: abdominal cramping.
Derm: flushing, sweating.

INTERACTIONS

Drug–Drug: ▪ May be ineffective when used with **ophthalmic flurbiprofen** ▪ **Local anesthetics** may decrease epithelial barriers and promote systemic absorption.

ROUTE AND DOSAGE

- **Ophth (Adults):** 1–2 drops of 0.75–3% soln q 4–8 hr.
- **Intraocular (Adults):** Instill not more than 0.5 ml of 0.01% soln into anterior chamber.

PHARMACODYNAMICS (miosis)

	ONSET	PEAK	DURATION
Ophth	10–20 min	<4 hr*	4–8 hr*

*Also denotes effects on intraocular pressure.

NURSING IMPLICATIONS

Assessment

- Monitor pulse, blood pressure, and lung sounds. Inform physician if hypotension, bradycardia, or bronchospasm occurs.
- Assess for symptoms of systemic absorption (nausea, vomiting, diarrhea, abdominal cramping, increased urge to urinate, shortness of breath, increased sweating, salivation). Notify physician if these symptoms occur.
- **Toxicity and Overdose:** Systemic effects may be reversed with atropine.

Potential Nursing Diagnoses

- Knowledge deficit related to medication regimen (patient/family teaching).

Implementation

- **General Info:** May be administered via intraocular injection intraoperatively by physician. Vials are for single use only.
- **Ophth:** Administer ophthalmic soln by having patient tilt head back and look up. Gently depress lower lid with index finger until conjunctival sac is exposed and instill medication. After instillation, maintain gentle pressure on the inner canthus for 1 min to avoid systemic absorption of the drug. Wait at least 5 min before administering other types of eyedrops.

Patient/Family Teaching

- Instruct patient in proper technique for instillation of ophthalmic medications. Emphasize the importance of not touching the applicator tip to any surface.
- Advise patient to take exactly as prescribed. A missed dose should be taken as soon as remembered unless almost time for next dose.
- Explain to patient that pupil size will decrease. This may cause blurred vision and eye or brow ache. Night vision will be impaired, so patient should not drive at night.
- Instruct patient to notify physician if visual changes, eye or brow ache, or headache persist or if symptoms of systemic absorption occur.
- Emphasize the importance of regular follow-up examinations to monitor intraocular pressure.

Evaluation

Effectiveness of therapy can be demonstrated by: ▪ Miosis resulting in decreased intraocular pressure.

CARBAMAZEPINE

(kar-ba-**maz**-e-peen)
{Apo-Carbamazepine}, Epitol, {Mazepine}, Tegretol

CLASSIFICATION(S):
Anticonvulsant
Pregnancy Category C

INDICATIONS

▪ Prophylaxis of tonic–clonic, mixed, and complex–partial seizures ▪ Management of pain in trigeminal neuralgia. **Unlabeled Uses:** ▪ Other forms of neurogenic pain ▪ Prophylaxis and treatment of bipolar disorders and other psychiatric illnesses ▪ Management of diabetes insipidus.

C

ACTION

▪ Decreases synaptic transmission in the CNS. **Therapeutic Effects:** ▪ Prevention of seizures ▪ Decreased severity of pain in trigeminal neuralgia.

PHARMACOKINETICS

Absorption: Slowly but completely absorbed from the GI tract. Absorption of suspension results in earlier and higher peak and lower trough levels than tablets.
Distribution: Widely distributed. Crosses the blood–brain barrier. Crosses the placenta and enters breast milk.
Metabolism and Excretion: Extensively metabolized by the liver.
Half-life: 14–30 hr or longer.

CONTRAINDICATIONS AND PRECAUTIONS

Contraindicated in: ▪ Hypersensitivity ▪ Bone marrow depression.
Use Cautiously in: ▪ Cardiac disease ▪ Hepatic disease ▪ Elderly men with prostatic hypertrophy ▪ Increased intraocular pressure ▪ Pregnancy and lactation (safety not established).

ADVERSE REACTIONS AND SIDE EFFECTS*

CNS: vertigo, <u>drowsiness</u>, fatigue, <u>ataxia</u>, psychosis.
EENT: blurred vision, corneal opacities.
Resp: pneumonitis.
CV: congestive heart failure, syncope, hypertension, hypotension.
GI: hepatitis.
GU: hesitancy, urinary retention.
Derm: rashes, urticaria, photosensitivity.
Hemat: APLASTIC ANEMIA, AGRANULOCYTOSIS, THROMBOCYTOPENIA, leukopenia, leukocytosis, eosinophilia.
Misc: fever, chills, lymphadenopathy.

INTERACTIONS

Drug-Drug: ▪ May decrease effectiveness of **glucocorticoids, doxycycline, quinidine, warfarin, oral contraceptives, barbiturates, benzodiazepines,** and other **anticonvulsants** by increasing their metabolism ▪ Concurrent use (within 14 days) of **MAO inhibitors** may result in hyperpyrexia, hypertension, seizures, and death ▪ **Verapamil, diltiazem, propoxyphene,** or **erythromycin** increase carbamazepine levels and may cause toxicity ▪ May increase risk of hepatotoxicity from **isoniazid.**

ROUTE AND DOSAGE

Anticonvulsant

- **PO (Adults):** Start with 200 mg twice daily (tablets) or 100 mg 4 times daily (suspension); increase by 200 mg/day until therapeutic levels are achieved. Range is 800–1200 mg/day in divided doses given q 6–8 hr. Not to exceed 1 g/day in 12–15 yr olds.
- **PO (Children 6–12 yr):** 200 mg/day in 2–4 divided doses increased until therapeutic levels are achieved (Range 400–800 mg/day) not to exceed 1 g/day.

Trigeminal Neuralgia

- **PO (Adults):** 200 mg/day in 2–4 divided doses; increase until pain is relieved. Range 200–1200 mg/day.

Antipsychotic

- **PO (Adults):** 200–400 mg/day in 2–4 divided doses initially; may be gradually increased at weekly intervals (not to exceed 1.6 g/day).

Antidiuretic (Diabetes Insipidus)

- **PO (Adults):** 300–600 mg/day in 3–4 divided doses if used alone; 200–400 mg/day in 3–4 divided doses if used with other agents.

PHARMACODYNAMICS

	ONSET	PEAK	DURATION
PO	2–4 days*	2–12 hr	UK hr

*Onset of anticonvulsant activity; relief of neuritic pain takes 8–72 hr.

NURSING IMPLICATIONS

Assessment

- **Seizures:** Assess location, duration, and characteristics of seizure activity.

*<u>Underlines</u> indicate most frequent; **CAPITALS** indicate life-threatening.

- **Trigeminal Neuralgia:** Assess for facial pain. Ask patient to identify stimuli that may precipitate facial pain (hot or cold foods, bed clothes, touching face).
- **Psychiatric Disorders:** Assess mental status and behavior.
- **Lab Test Considerations:** Monitor CBC, including platelet count, reticulocyte count, and serum iron, weekly during the first 3 mon and monthly thereafter, for evidence of potentially fatal blood cell abnormalities. Medication should be discontinued if bone marrow depression occurs.
  - Liver function tests, urinalysis, and BUN should be routinely performed. May cause elevated SCOT (AST), SGPT (ALT), serum bilirubin, BUN, urine protein, and urine glucose levels.
  - Thyroid function tests and serum calcium concentrations may be decreased.
  - May cause false-negative pregnancy test results with tests that determine human chorionic gonadotropin.
- **Toxicity and Overdose:** Serum blood levels should be routinely monitored throughout course of therapy. Therapeutic levels range from 6–12 mcg/ml.

POTENTIAL NURSING DIAGNOSES

- Injury, high risk for (indications, side effects).
- Comfort, altered: pain (indications).
- Knowledge deficit related to medication regimen (patient/family teaching).

IMPLEMENTATION

- **General Info:** Implement seizure precautions.
- **PO:** Administer medication with food to minimize gastric irritation. Tablets may be crushed if patient has difficulty swallowing. Also available in chewable tablets.

PATIENT/FAMILY TEACHING

- **General Info:** Instruct patient to take carbamazepine around the clock, exactly as directed. If a dose is missed, take as soon as remembered but not just before next dose; do not double doses. Notify physician if more than one dose is missed. Medication should be gradually discontinued to prevent seizures and status epilepticus.
  - May cause dizziness or drowsiness. Advise patients to avoid driving or other activities requiring alertness until response to medication is known.
  - Instruct patients that fever, sore throat, mouth ulcers, easy bruising, petechiae, unusual bleeding, abdominal pain, chills, pale stools, dark urine, or jaundice should be reported to the physician immediately.
  - Advise patient not to take alcohol or other CNS depressants concurrently with this medication.
  - Caution patients to use sunscreen and protective clothing to prevent photosensitivity reactions.
  - Inform patient that frequent mouth rinses, good oral hygiene, and sugarless gum or candy may help reduce dry mouth. Saliva substitute may be used. Consult dentist if dry mouth persists >2 wk.
  - Advise patients to use a nonhormonal form of contraception while taking carbamazepine.
  - Instruct patient to notify physician or dentist of medication regimen prior to treatment or surgery.
  - Emphasize the importance of follow-up lab tests and eye examinations to monitor for side effects.
- **Seizures:** Advise patients to carry identification describing disease and medication regimen at all times.

EVALUATION

Clinical response to therapy can be indicated by: ▪ Absence or reduction of seizure activity ▪ Decrease in trigeminal neuralgia pain. Patients with trigeminal neuralgia should be re-evaluated every 3 mon to determine minimum effective dose ▪ Management of diabetes insipidus ▪ Improvement in affect and mental status in psychiatric patients.

C

CARBENICILLIN
(kar-ben-i-**sill**-in)
Geocillin

CLASSIFICATION(S):
Anti-infective—extended-spectrum penicillin
Pregnancy Category B

INDICATIONS

▪ Treatment of urinary tract infections or prostatitis due to susceptible organisms.

ACTION

▪ Binds to bacterial cell wall membrane, causing cell death. **Therapeutic Effect:** ▪ Bactericidal against susceptible bacteria. Spectrum is broader than other penicillins. **Spectrum:** ▪ Active against: ▫ *Pseudomas aeruginosa* ▫ Escherichia coli ▫ Proteus mirabilis ▫ Proteus vulgaris ▫ Morganella morganii ▫ Pseudomonas ▫ Enterobacter ▫ Enterococci ▪ Also active against some anaerobic bacteria including Bacteroides ▪ Not active against penicillinase-producing staphylococci.

PHARMACOKINETICS

Absorption: Oral form is rapidly but incompletely absorbed. Well absorbed from IM sites.
Distribution: Widely distributed. Enters CSF well only when meninges are inflamed. Crosses the placenta and enters breast milk in low concentrations.
Metabolism and Excretion: Metabolized by plasma and tissues to yield free carbenicillin. 80–99% excreted unchanged by the kidneys.
Half-life: 0.8–1 hr (increased in renal impairment).

CONTRAINDICATIONS AND PRECAUTIONS

Contraindicated in: ▪ Hypersensitivity to penicillins or cephalosporins.
Use Cautiously in: ▪ Renal impairment (dosage reduction required) ▪ Severe liver disease ▪ Pregnancy or lactation (safety not established).

ADVERSE REACTIONS AND SIDE EFFECTS*

GI: nausea, diarrhea.
Derm: rashes, urticaria.
Hemat: blood dyscrasias.
Misc: superinfection, hypersensitivity reactions including ANAPHYLAXIS and serum sickness.

INTERACTIONS

Drug-Drug: ▪ **Probenecid** decreases renal excretion and increases blood levels.

ROUTE AND DOSAGE

▪ **PO (Adults):** 382–764 mg (1–2 tablets) every 6 hr.

PHARMACODYNAMICS (blood levels)

	ONSET	PEAK
PO	30 min	30–120 min

NURSING IMPLICATIONS

Assessment

▫ Assess patient for infection (vital signs; appearance of wound, sputum, urine, and stool; WBC) at beginning and throughout course of therapy.
▫ Obtain a history before initiating therapy to determine previous use and reactions to penicillins or cephalosporins. Persons with a negative history of penicillin sensitivity may still have an allergic response.
▫ Obtain specimens for culture and sensitivity prior to initiating therapy. First dose may be given before receiving results.
▫ Observe patient for signs and symptoms of anaphylaxis (rash, pruritus, laryngeal edema, wheezing). Discontinue the drug and notify the physician immediately if these occur. Keep epinephrine, an antihistamine, and resuscitation equipment close by in the event of an anaphylactic reaction.
▪ **Lab Test Considerations:** Renal and

*Underlines indicate most frequent; **CAPITALS** indicate life-threatening.

hepatic function, CBC, serum potassium, and bleeding times should be evaluated prior to and routinely throughout therapy.
- May cause elevated SGOT (AST) and SGPT (ALT) levels.

POTENTIAL NURSING DIAGNOSES
- Infection, high risk for (indications, side effects).
- Knowledge deficit related to medication regimen (patient/family teaching).
- Noncompliance related to medication regimen (patient/family teaching).

IMPLEMENTATION
- **PO:** Administer around the clock on an empty stomach at least 1 hr before or 2 hr after meals, with a full glass of water.

PATIENT/FAMILY TEACHING
- Instruct patient to take medication around the clock and to finish the drug completely as directed, even if feeling better. Advise patient that sharing of this medication may be dangerous.
- Advise patient to report the signs of superinfection (furry overgrowth on the tongue, vaginal itching or discharge, loose or foul smelling stools) and allergy.
- Instruct the patient to notify the physician if symptoms do not improve.

EVALUATION

Clinical response to therapy may be determined by: ▪ Resolution of the signs and symptoms of infection. Length of time for complete resolution depends on the organism and site of infection.

CARBIDOPA/LEVODOPA
(**kar**-bi-doe-pa/**lee**-voe-doe-pa)
Sinemet, Sinemet CR

CLASSIFICATION(S):
Antiparkinson—decarboxylase inhibitor/dopamine agonist
Pregnancy Category UK

INDICATIONS
▪ Treatment of Parkinson's disease and other forms of parkinsonism. Not useful for drug-induced extrapyramidal reactions.

ACTION
▪ Levodopa is converted to dopamine in the CNS where it serves as a neurotransmitter. Carbidopa prevents peripheral destruction of levodopa so more is available to the CNS. **Therapeutic Effect:** ▪ Relief of tremor and rigidity in parkinsonian syndrome.

PHARMACOKINETICS
Absorption: Both agents are well absorbed following oral administration. CR dosage form is absorbed more slowly.

Distribution: Both agents are widely distributed. Levodopa administered alone enters the CNS in small concentrations. Carbidopa does not cross the blood–brain barrier, but does cross the placenta and enter breast milk.

Metabolism and Excretion: Levodopa is mostly metabolized by the GI tract and liver. 30% of carbidopa is excreted unchanged by the kidneys.

Half-life: Levodopa—1 hr; carbidopa—1–2 hr.

CONTRAINDICATIONS AND PRECAUTIONS
Contraindicated in: ▪ Hypersensitivity ▪ Narrow-angle glaucoma ▪ Patients receiving MAO inhibitors ▪ Malignant melanoma ▪ Undiagnosed skin lesions ▪ Lactation.

Use Cautiously in: ▪ History of cardiac, psychiatric, or ulcer disease ▪ Pregnancy or children <18 yr (safety not established).

ADVERSE REACTIONS AND SIDE EFFECTS*
CNS: <u>involuntary movements</u>, memory loss, anxiety, psychiatric problems, hallucinations, dizziness, drowsiness.
EENT: mydriasis, blurred vision.

*<u>Underlines</u> indicate most frequent; **CAPITALS** indicate life-threatening.

C

CV: hypertension, hypotension.
GI: nausea, vomiting, anorexia, dry mouth, hepatotoxicity.
Derm: melanoma.
Hemat: hemolytic anemia, leukopenia.

INTERACTIONS

Drug–Drug: ▪ Concurrent use with **MAO inhibitors** (within 14 days) may result in hypertensive crisis ▪ **Phenothiazines, haloperidol, papaverine, phenytoin, reserpine,** and large doses of **pyridoxine** may antagonize the beneficial effect of levodopa ▪ Additive hypotension with **methyldopa, quanethidine,** or **tricyclic antidepressants.**
Drug–Food: Ingestion of food containing high amounts of **pyridoxine** may reverse the beneficial effect of levodopa.

ROUTE AND DOSAGE

Note: Carbidopa/Levodopa tablets contain 10/100, 25/100, or 25/250 mg of carbidopa and levodopa, respectively.

Sinemet

- **PO (Adults):** 75/300–150/1500 mg/day in three to four divided doses, can increase up to 200/2000 mg/day.

Sinemet CR

- **PO (Adults):** Usual dose 1 tablet bid at intervals of not less than 6 hr. Doses of 2–8 tablets/day in divided doses at intervals of 4–8 hr while awake have been used. Add 3 days between dosage adjustments.

PHARMACODYNAMICS (antiparkinson effect)

	ONSET	PEAK	DURATION
PO carbidopa	UK	UK	5–24 hr
PO levodopa	10–15 min	UK	5–24 hr or more

NURSING IMPLICATIONS

Assessment

- □ Assess symptoms of Parkinsonism (akinesia, rigidity, tremors, pill rolling, shuffling gait, mask facies, twisting motions, and drooling) prior to and throughout course of therapy.
- □ Assess blood pressure and pulse frequently during period of dose adjustment.
- □ Assess for signs of toxicity (involuntary muscle twitching, facial grimacing, spasmodic eye winking, exaggerated protrusion of tongue, or behavioral changes). Consult physician promptly if these symptoms occur.
- ▪ **Lab Test Considerations:** May cause false-positive Coombs' test, serum and urine uric acid, serum gonadotropin, urine norepinephrine, and urine protein concentrations.
- □ May interfere with results of urine glucose and urine ketone tests. Copper reduction method of testing urine glucose (Clinitest) and dipstick for urine ketones may reveal false-positive results. Glucose oxidase method of testing urine glucose (Tes-Tape) may yield false-negative results.
- □ Patients on long-term therapy should have hepatic and renal function and CBC monitored periodically. May cause elevated BUN, SGOT (AST), SGPT (ALT), bilirubin, alkaline phosphatase, LDH, and serum protein-bound iodine concentrations.

Potential Nursing Diagnoses

- ▪ Mobility, impaired physical (indications).
- ▪ Injury, high risk for (indications).
- ▪ Knowledge deficit related to medication regimen (patient/family teaching).

Implementation

- ▪ **General Info:** In the carbidopa/levodopa combination, the numbers following the drug name represent the mg of each respective drug.
- □ Wait 8 hr after last levodopa dose before switching patient to carbidopa/levodopa. Addition of carbidopa reduces the need for levodopa by 75%. Administering carbidopa shortly after a full dose of levodopa may result in toxicity.
- □ In preoperative patients or patients that are NPO, confer with physician

regarding continuing medication administration.

- **PO:** Administer food shortly after medication to minimize gastric irritation; taking food before or concurrently may retard levodopa's effects.
- ▫ Controlled-release tablets may be administered as whole or half tablets, but should not be crushed or chewed.

Patient/Family Teaching

- ▫ Instruct patient to take this drug exactly as prescribed. If a dose is missed, take as soon as remembered, unless next scheduled dose is within 2 hr; do not double doses.
- ▫ Explain that gastric irritation may be decreased by taking medication with or after meals, but that high-protein meals may impair levodopa's effects. Dividing the daily protein intake between all the meals may help ensure adequate protein intake and drug effectiveness.
- ▫ May cause drowsiness or dizziness. Advise patient to avoid driving or other activities that require alertness until response to the drug is known.
- ▫ Caution patient to make position changes slowly to minimize orthostatic hypotension.
- ▫ Instruct patient that frequent rinsing of mouth, good oral hygiene, and sugarless gum or candy may decrease dry mouth.
- ▫ Caution patient to monitor skin lesions for any changes. Physician should be notified promptly as carbidopa/levodopa may activate a malignant melanoma.
- ▫ Advise patient to confer with physician or pharmacist prior to taking over-the-counter medications, especially cold remedies.
- ▫ Inform patient that harmless darkening of urine or sweat may occur.
- ▫ Advise patient to notify physician if palpitations, urinary retention, involuntary movements, behavioral changes, or severe nausea and vomiting occur.

Evaluation

Effectiveness of therapy can be demonstrated by: ▪ Resolution of parkinsonian signs and symptoms. Therapeutic effects usually become evident after 2 to 3 wk of therapy, but may require up to 6 mon. Patients who take this medication for several yrs may experience a decrease in the effectiveness of this drug. An increased response to the drug may occur after a drug holiday.

CARBOPLATIN

(kar-boe-**pla**-tin)
Paraplatin

CLASSIFICATION(S):
Antineoplastic agent—alkylating agent
Pregnancy Category D

INDICATIONS

▪ Treatment of ovarian carcinoma alone or in combination with cyclophosphamide.

ACTION

▪ Inhibits DNA synthesis by producing cross-linking of parent DNA strands (cell cycle-phase nonspecific). **Therapeutic Effect:** ▪ Death of rapidly replicating cells, particularly malignant cells.

PHARMACOKINETICS

Absorption: Administered IV only, resulting in complete bioavailability.
Distribution: Distribution not known.
Metabolism and Excretion: Excreted mostly by the kidneys.
Half-life: 2.6–5.9 hr (increased in renal impairment).

CONTRAINDICATIONS AND PRECAUTIONS

Contraindicated in: ▪ Hypersensitivity to carboplatin, cisplatin, or mannitol ▪ Pregnancy or lactation.
Use Cautiously in: ▪ Hearing loss ▪ Electrolyte abnormalities ▪ Patients

C

with childbearing potential ▪ Active infections ▪ Diminished bone marrow reserve ▪ Other chronic debilitating illnesses ▪ Renal impairment (dosage reduction recommended).

ADVERSE REACTIONS AND SIDE EFFECTS*

CNS: weakness.
EENT: ototoxicity.
GI: vomiting, nausea, abdominal pain, diarrhea, constipation, hepatitis, stomatitis.
GU: nephrotoxicity, gonadal suppression.
Derm: rash, alopecia.
F and E: hyponatremia, hypocalcemia, hypomagnesemia, hypokalemia.
Hemat: leukopenia, thrombocytopenia, anemia.
Neuro: peripheral neuropathy.
Misc: hypersensitivity reactions including ANAPHYLAXIS.

INTERACTIONS

Drug–Drug: ▪ Additive nephrotoxicity and ototoxicity with other **nephro-** and **ototoxic drugs (aminoglycosides, loop diuretics)** ▪ Additive bone marrow depression with other **bone-marrow-depressing drugs** or **radiation therapy**.

ROUTE AND DOSAGE

- **IV (Adults):** 360 mg/m^2 as a single dose; may be repeated at 4-wk intervals depending on response, or 300 mg/m^2 with cyclophosphamide at 4-wk intervals.

PHARMACODYNAMICS (effects on blood counts)

	ONSET	PEAK	DURATION
IV	UK	21 days	28 days

NURSING IMPLICATIONS

Assessment

- ▫ Assess for nausea and vomiting. Mild to moderately severe nausea and vomiting often occur 6–12 hr after therapy and may persist for 24 hr. Confer with physician about prophylactic use of antiemetics. Adjust diet as tolerated to maintain fluid and electrolyte balance and ensure adequate nutritional intake.
- ▫ Monitor platelet count throughout therapy. Assess for bleeding (bleeding gums, bruising, petechiae; guaiac stools, urine, and emesis). Avoid IM injections and rectal temperatures. Apply pressure to venipuncture sites for 10 min.
- ▫ Assess for fever, chills, sore throat, and signs of infection. Notify physician if these symptoms occur.
- ▫ Anemia may occur. Monitor for increased fatigue, dyspnea, and orthostatic hypotension.
- ▫ Monitor for signs of anaphylaxis (rash, urticaria, pruritus, wheezing, tachycardia, hypotension). Discontinue medication immediately and notify physician if these occur. Epinephrine and resuscitation equipment should be readily available.
- ▪ **Lab Test Considerations:** CBC, differential, and clotting studies should be monitored prior to and routinely throughout course of therapy. The nadir of thrombocytopenia occurs within 14–28 days. Withhold subsequent doses until neutrophil count is >2,000/mm^3 and platelet count is >100,000/mm^3.
- ▫ Monitor renal and hepatic function prior to and periodically throughout course of therapy.

Potential Nursing Diagnoses

- ▪ Infection, high risk for (adverse reactions).
- ▪ Injury, high risk for (side effects).
- ▪ Knowledge deficit related to medication regimen (patient/family teaching).

Implementation

- ▪ **General Info:** Do not use aluminum needles or equipment during preparation or administration, because aluminum reacts with the drug.
- ▫ Soln should be prepared in a biologic

*Underlines indicate most frequent; **CAPITALS** indicate life-threatening.

cabinet. Wear gloves, gown, and mask while handling medication. Discard equipment in specially designated containers (see Appendix I).

- **Intermittent Infusion:** Reconstitute to a concentration of 10 mg/ml with sterile water for injection, D5W, or 0.9% NaCl for injection. May be further diluted in D5W or 0.9% NaCl to a concentration of 0.5 mg/ml. Stable for 8 hr at room temperature.
  - *Rate:* Administered as a bolus over 15–60 min.
- **Y-Site Compatibility:** ondansetron.

Patient/Family Teaching

- Instruct patient to notify physician promptly if fever, sore throat, signs of infection, bleeding gums, bruising, petechiae; blood in stools, urine or emesis; increased fatigue, dyspnea, or orthostatic hypotension occur. Caution patient to avoid crowds and persons with known infections. Instruct patient to use soft toothbrush, electric razor, and to avoid falls. Patients should be cautioned not to drink alcoholic beverages or take medication containing aspirin, because these may precipitate gastric bleeding.
- Instruct patient to promptly report any numbness or tingling in extremities or face, decreased coordination, difficulty with hearing or tinnitus, unusual swelling or weight gain to physician. The risks of ototoxicity, neurotoxicity, and nephrotoxicity are less than with cisplatin.
- Instruct patient not to receive any vaccinations without advice of physician.
- Advise patient of the need for contraception (if patient is not infertile as a result of surgical or radiation therapy).
- Instruct patient to inspect oral mucosa for erythema and ulceration. If ulceration occurs advise patient to notify physician, rinse mouth with water after eating, and use sponge brush. Physician may order viscous lidocaine swishes if mouth pain interferes with eating.
- Discuss with patient the possibility of hair loss. Explore methods of coping.
- Emphasize the need for periodic lab tests to monitor for side effects.

Evaluation

Effectiveness of therapy can be demonstrated by: ▪ Decrease in size or spread of ovarian carcinoma.

CARBOPROST

(**kar**-bo-prost)
Prostin/15M

CLASSIFICATION(S):
Abortifacient—prostaglandin, Oxytocic
Pregnancy Category C

INDICATIONS

▪ Induction of midtrimester abortion ▪ Treatment of postpartum hemorrhage that has not responded to conventional therapy.

ACTION

▪ Causes uterine contractions by directly stimulating the myometrium. Also produces cervical softening and dilation. **Therapeutic Effects:** ▪ Expulsion of fetus ▪ Control of postpartum bleeding.

PHARMACOKINETICS

Absorption: Well absorbed following IM administration.
Distribution: UK.
Metabolism and Excretion: Metabolized by tissue enzymes.
Half-life: UK.

CONTRAINDICATIONS AND PRECAUTIONS

Contraindicated in: ▪ Hypersensitivity ▪ Acute pelvic inflammatory disease ▪ Active pulmonary, renal, or hepatic disease.
Use Cautiously in: ▪ Uterine scarring ▪ Asthma ▪ Hypotension ▪ Hypertension ▪ Cardiac disease ▪ Adrenal disease ▪ Anemia ▪ Jaundice ▪ Diabetes mellitus.

C

ADVERSE REACTIONS AND SIDE EFFECTS*

CNS: headache.
Resp: wheezing.
GI: diarrhea, vomiting, nausea, abdominal pain, cramps.
GU: UTERINE RUPTURE.
Derm: flushing, redness of the face.
Misc: fever, chills, shivering.

INTERACTIONS

Drug-Drug: ▪ Augments the effects of other **oxytocics**.

ROUTE AND DOSAGE

Test Dose

- **IM (Adults):** 0.1 mg.

Abortifacient

- **IM (Adults):** 0.25 mg every 1.5–3.5 hr may be increased to 0.5 mg if doses of 0.25 mg produce inadequate response (not to exceed 2 days of continuous therapy or total dose of 12 mg).

Antihemorrhagic

- **IM (Adults):** 0.25 mg; may be repeated every 15–90 min (total dose not to exceed 2 mg).

PHARMACODYNAMICS (peak noted as mean abortion time)

	ONSET	PEAK	DURATION
IM	UK	16 hr	UK

NURSING IMPLICATIONS

Assessment

- Monitor frequency, duration, and force of contractions and uterine resting tone. Notify physician if contractions absent or last more than 1 min.
- Monitor temperature, pulse, and blood pressure periodically throughout course of therapy. Large dose may cause hypertension. Temperature elevation beginning 1 to 16 hr after initiation of therapy and lasting for several hrs is not unusual.
- Auscultate breath sounds. Wheezing and sensation of chest tightness may indicate hypersensitivity reaction.
- Assess for nausea, vomiting, and diarrhea. Vomiting and diarrhea occur in approximately two thirds of patients. Premedication with antiemetic and antidiarrheal may be ordered.
- Monitor amount and type of vaginal discharge. Notify physician immediately if symptoms of hemorrhage (increased bleeding, hypotension, pallor, tachycardia) occur.

Potential Nursing Diagnoses

- Knowledge deficit related to medication regimen (patient/family teaching).

Implementation

- **General Info:** Avoid contact with skin. Thoroughly wash skin immediately after spillage.
- Premedication with meperidine may be ordered for uterine cramping.
- Store in refrigerator.
- **IM/SC:** Administer deep IM. Dose may be repeated every 1½–3½ hr. Rotate sites.

Patient/Family Teaching

- **General Info:** Explain purpose of vaginal examinations (to assess for trauma to cervix).
- Instruct patient to notify physician immediately if fever and chills, foul-smelling vaginal discharge, lower abdominal pain, or increased bleeding occurs.

Evaluation

Effectiveness of therapy can be demonstrated by: ▪ Complete abortion ▪ Control of postpartum or postabortal hemorrhage.

CARISOPRODOL

(kar-i-soe-**proe**-dole)
Rela, Sodol, Soma, Soprodol, Soridol

CLASSIFICATION(S):
Skeletal muscle relaxant—centrally acting
Pregnancy Category UK

*Underlines indicate most frequent; **CAPITALS** indicate life-threatening.

INDICATIONS

▪ Adjunct to rest and physical therapy in the treatment of muscle spasm associated with acute painful musculoskeletal conditions.

ACTION

▪ Skeletal muscle relaxation, probably due to CNS depression. **Therapeutic Effect:** ▪ Skeletal muscle relaxation.

PHARMACOKINETICS

Absorption: Appears to be well absorbed following oral administration.
Distribution: Crosses the placenta. High concentrations in breast milk.
Metabolism and Excretion: Mostly metabolized by the liver.
Half-life: 8 hr.

CONTRAINDICATIONS AND PRECAUTIONS

Contraindicated in: ▪ Hypersensitivity to carisoprodol or to meprobamate ▪ Porphyria or suspected porphyria.
Use Cautiously in: ▪ Severe liver or kidney disease ▪ Pregnancy, lactation, or children <12 yr (safety not established) ▪ Some products may contain tartrazine; use cautiously in patients with tartrazine sensitivity.

ADVERSE REACTIONS AND SIDE EFFECTS*

CNS: dizziness, drowsiness, ataxia, vertigo, agitation, irritability, headache, depression, syncope, insomnia.
Resp: asthmatic attacks.
CV: tachycardia, hypotension.
GI: nausea, vomiting, hiccups, epigastric distress.
Derm: rashes, flushing.
Hemat: eosinophilia, leukopenia.
Misc: severe idiosyncratic reaction, fever, ANAPHYLACTIC SHOCK.

INTERACTIONS

Drug–Drug: ▪ Additive CNS depression with other **CNS depressants** including **alcohol, antihistamines, narcotic analgesics,** and **sedative/hypnotics**.

ROUTE AND DOSAGE

▪ **PO (Adults):** 350 mg 4 times daily.

PHARMACODYNAMICS (skeletal muscle relaxation)

	ONSET	PEAK	DURATION
PO	30 min	UK	4–6 hr

NURSING IMPLICATIONS

Assessment

□ Assess patient for pain, muscle stiffness, and range of motion prior to and periodically throughout therapy.
□ Observe patient for idiosyncratic symptoms that may appear within mins or hrs of administration during the first dose. Symptoms include extreme weakness, quadriplegia, dizziness, ataxia, dysarthria, visual disturbances, agitation, euphoria, confusion, and disorientation. Usually subsides over several hrs.

Potential Nursing Diagnoses

▪ Comfort, altered: pain (indications).
▪ Mobility, impaired physical (indications).
▪ Injury, high risk for (side effects).

Implementation

▪ **General Info:** Provide safety measures as indicated. Supervise ambulation and transfer of patients.
□ Available in combinations with aspirin and codeine (Soma Compound, Soma Compound with Codeine); see Appendix A.
▪ **PO:** Administer with food to minimize GI irritation. Last dose should be given at bedtime.

Patient/Family Teaching

□ Instruct patient to take medication exactly as directed. Missed doses should be taken within 1 hr; if not, return to regular dosing schedule. Do not double doses.
□ Encourage patient to comply with additional therapies prescribed for muscle spasm (rest, physical therapy, heat, etc).
□ May cause dizziness or drowsiness.

*Underlines indicate most frequent; **CAPITALS** indicate life-threatening.

C

Advise patient to avoid driving or other activities requiring alertness until response to drug is known.
- Instruct patient to make position changes slowly to minimize orthostatic hypotension.
- Advise patient to avoid concurrent use of alcohol and other CNS depressants while taking this medication.
- Instruct patient to notify physician if signs of allergy (rash, hives, swelling of tongue or lips, dyspnea) or idiosyncratic reaction occur.

EVALUATION

Effectiveness of therapy can be demonstrated by: ▪ Decreased musculoskeletal pain and muscle spasticity ▫ Increased range of motion.

CARMUSTINE
(kar-**mus**-teen)
BCNU, BiCNU

CLASSIFICATION(S):
Antineoplastic—alkylating agent
Pregnancy Category D

INDICATIONS

▪ Alone or in combination with other treatment modalities (surgery, radiation) in the treatment of: ▫ Brain tumors ▫ Multiple myeloma ▫ Hodgkin's disease ▫ Other lymphomas.

ACTION

▪ Inhibits DNA and RNA synthesis (cell cycle-phase nonspecific). **Therapeutic Effect:** ▪ Death of rapidly replicating cells, especially malignant ones.

PHARMACOKINETICS

Absorption: Following IV administration absorption is essentially complete.
Distribution: Highly lipid-soluble, readily penetrates CSF. Enters breast milk.
Metabolism and Excretion: Rapidly metabolized. Some metabolites have antineoplastic activity.
Half-life: UK.

CONTRAINDICATIONS AND PRECAUTIONS

Contraindicated in: ▪ Hypersensitivity ▪ Pregnancy or lactation.
Use Cautiously in: ▪ Patients with childbearing potential ▪ Infections ▪ Depressed bone-marrow reserve ▪ Other chronic debilitating illnesses.

ADVERSE REACTIONS AND SIDE EFFECTS*

Resp: pulmonary infiltrates, pulmonary fibrosis.
GI: nausea, vomiting, diarrhea, esophagitis, anorexia, hepatotoxicity.
GU: renal failure.
Derm: alopecia.
Hemat: leukopenia, thrombocytopenia, anemia.
Local: pain at IV site.

INTERACTIONS

Drug-Drug: ▪ Additive bone marrow depression with other **antineoplastics** or **radiation therapy** ▪ **Smoking** increases the risk of pulmonary toxicity.

ROUTE AND DOSAGE

▪ **IV (Adults and Children):** 200 mg/m^2 given as a single dose every 6 wk or 75–100 mg/m^2 daily for 2 days every 6 wk or 40 mg/m^2/day for 5 days q 6 wk.

PHARMACODYNAMICS (noted as effect on platelet counts)

	ONSET	PEAK	DURATION
IV	days	4–5 wk	6 wk

NURSING IMPLICATIONS

ASSESSMENT

- Monitor vital signs prior to and frequently during therapy.
- Assess for fever, chills, sore throat, and signs of infection. Notify physician if these symptoms occur.
- Assess respiratory status for dyspnea

*Underlines indicate most frequent; **CAPITALS** indicate life-threatening.

or cough. Pulmonary toxicity usually occurs after high cumulative doses or several courses of therapy. Notify physician promptly if these symptoms occur.

- Monitor platelet count throughout therapy. Assess for bleeding (bleeding gums, bruising, petechiae; guaiac stools, urine, and emesis). Avoid IM injections, rectal temperatures, and aspirin-containing products. Apply pressure to venipuncture sites for 10 min.
- Anemia may occur. Monitor for increased fatigue, dyspnea, and orthostatic hypotension.
- Monitor IV site closely. Carmustine is an irritant. Instruct patient to notify nurse immediately if discomfort at IV site occurs. Discontinue IV immediately if infiltration occurs. Confer with physician about application of ice to site. May cause hyperpigmentation of skin along vein.
- Monitor intake and output, appetite, and nutritional intake. Assess for nausea and vomiting, which may occur within 2 hr of administration and persist for 6 hr. Administration of an antiemetic prior to and periodically during therapy and adjusting diet as tolerated may help maintain fluid and electrolyte balance and nutritional status.
- **Lab Test Considerations:** Monitor CBC and differential prior to and periodically throughout therapy. The nadir of thrombocytopenia occurs in 4–5 wk; the nadir of leukopenia in 5–6 wk. Withhold dose and notify physician if platelet count is $<100,000/mm^3$ or leukocyte count is $<4000/mm^3$. Anemia is usually mild.
- May cause mild, reversible increase in SGOT (AST), alkaline phosphatase, and bilirubin.
- Monitor renal studies; notify physician if BUN is elevated.

Potential Nursing Diagnoses

- Injury, high risk for (side effects).
- Body image disturbance (side effects).
- Knowledge deficit related to medication regimen (patient/family teaching).

Implementation

- **General Info:** Soln should be prepared in a biologic cabinet. Wear gloves, gown, and mask while handling medication. Discard equipment in designated containers. Contact with skin may cause transient hyperpigmentation (see Appendix I).
- **Intermittent Infusion:** Dilute contents of each 100-mg vial with 3 ml of absolute ethyl alcohol provided as a diluent. Dilute this soln with 27 ml of sterile water for injection. Further dilute with 500 ml of D5W or 0.9% NaCl in a glass container.
- Soln is clear and colorless. Do not use vials that contain an oily film, which is indicative of decomposition. Reconstituted soln is stable for 24 hr when refrigerated and protected from light. Soln contains no preservatives and should not be used as multi-dose vials.
- IV lines may be flushed with 5–10 ml of 0.9% NaCl prior to and following carmustine infusion.
- *Rate:* Administer dose over 1–2 hr. Rapid infusion rate may cause local pain, burning at site, and flushing. Facial flushing may persist for 4 hr.
- **Y-Site Compatibility:** ondansetron
- **Additive Incompatibility:** sodium bicarbonate.

Patient/Family Teaching

- Instruct patient to notify physician if fever, chills, sore throat, signs of infection, bleeding gums, bruising, petechiae, or blood in urine, stool, or emesis occur. Caution patient to avoid crowds and persons with known infections. Instruct patient to use soft toothbrush and electric razor. Patients should be cautioned not to drink alcoholic beverages or take aspirin-containing products.

- Instruct patient to notify physician if shortness of breath or increased cough occurs. Encourage patient not to smoke, because smokers are at greater risk for pulmonary toxicity.
- Instruct patient to inspect oral mucosa for redness and ulceration. If mouth sores occur advise patient to use sponge brush and rinse mouth with water after eating and drinking. Consult physician if pain interferes with eating.
- Discuss with patient the possibility of hair loss. Explore coping strategies.
- Advise patient of the need for contraception.
- Instruct patient not to receive any vaccinations without advice of physician.
- Emphasize need for periodic lab tests to monitor for side effects.

EVALUATION

Effectiveness of therapy can be demonstrated by: ▪ Decrease in size and spread of tumor on improvement in hematologic parameters in nonsolid cancers.

CARTEOLOL

(kar-**tee**-oh-lole)
Cartrol

CLASSIFICATION(S):
Beta-adrenergic blocking agent—nonselective, Antihypertensive—beta-adrenergic blocker
Pregnancy Category C

INDICATIONS

▪ Alone or with other agents in the management of hypertension.

ACTION

▪ Blocks stimulation of $beta_1$ (myocardial) and $beta_2$ (pulmonary, vascular, or uterine) receptor sites ▪ Possesses mild intrinsic sympathomimetic (ISA) activity. **Therapeutic Effects:** ▪ Decreased heart rate and blood pressure.

PHARMACOKINETICS

Absorption: 85% absorbed following oral administration.
Distribution: Distribution not known.
Metabolism and Excretion: Some metabolism by the liver, with conversion to at least one active compound (8-hydroxycarteolol). 50–70% excreted unchanged by the kidneys.
Half-life: Carteolol 6–8 hr, 8-hydroxycarteolol 8–12 hr (both increased in renal impairment).

CONTRAINDICATIONS AND PRECAUTIONS

Contraindicated in: ▪ Uncompensated congestive heart failure ▪ Pulmonary edema ▪ Cardiogenic shock ▪ Bradycardia ▪ Heart block ▪ COPD or asthma.
Use Cautiously in: ▪ Thyrotoxicosis or hypoglycemia (may mask symptoms) ▪ Diabetes mellitus (may mask symptoms of hypoglycemia) ▪ Renal impairment (dosage reduction suggested) ▪ Pregnancy or lactation (may cause apnea, low apgar scores, bradycardia, and hypoglycemia in the newborn) ▪ Children (safety not established).

ADVERSE REACTIONS AND SIDE EFFECTS*

CNS: <u>fatigue</u>, <u>weakness</u>, drowsiness, depression, memory loss, mental change.
EENT: dry eyes, blurred vision, nasal stuffiness.
Resp: bronchospasm, wheezing.
CV: **BRADYCARDIA, CONGESTIVE HEART FAILURE, PULMONARY EDEMA,** hypotension, peripheral vasoconstriction, chest pain.
GI: diarrhea, nausea.
GU: impotence, diminished libido.
Derm: rash, itching.
Endo: hyperglycemia, hypoglycemia.
MS: muscle cramps, back pain.
Neuro: paresthesia.
Misc: Raynaud's phenomenon.

INTERACTIONS

Drug-Drug: ▪ **General anesthesia, IV phenytoin,** and **verapamil** may cause

*<u>Underlines</u> indicate most frequent; **CAPITALS** indicate life-threatening.

additive myocardial depression ▪ Additive bradycardia may occur with concurrent use of **cardiac glycosides** ▪ Additive hypotension may occur with other **antihypertensive agents,** acute ingestion of **alcohol,** or **nitrates** ▪ Concurrent use with **amphetamines, cocaine, ephedrine, epinephrine, norepinephrine, phenylephrine,** or **pseudoephedrine** may result in excess alpha-adrenergic stimulation, hypertension, and bradycardia ▪ May negate the beneficial $beta_1$ cardiac effects of **dopamine** or **dobutamine** ▪ Concurrent **thyroid** administration may decrease effectiveness ▪ Use with **insulin** may result in prolonged hypoglycemia.

ROUTE AND DOSAGE

- **PO (Adults):** 2.5 mg/day as a single dose; may be increased up to 10 mg/day (usual dose 2.5–5.0 mg/day).

PHARMACODYNAMICS

	ONSET	PEAK	DURATION
PO	UK	2–4 wk	UK

NURSING IMPLICATIONS

Assessment

- □ Monitor blood pressure and pulse frequently during dosage adjustment period and periodically throughout therapy. Confer with physician prior to giving drug if pulse is <50 bpm.
- □ Monitor intake and output ratios and daily weight. Assess patient routinely for evidence of fluid overload (peripheral edema, dyspnea, rales/crackles, fatigue, weight gain, jugular venous distension).

Potential Nursing Diagnoses

- Cardiac output, decreased (side effects).
- Knowledge deficit related to medication regimen (patient/family teaching).
- Noncompliance related to medication regimen (patient/family teaching).

Implementation

- **PO:** Administered as a single daily dose. Doses >10 mg do not usually increase effectiveness and may decrease response.

Patient/Family Teaching

- □ Instruct patient to take medication exactly as prescribed, even if feeling well. If a dose is missed, it may be taken as soon as remembered up to 4 hr before next dose. Abrupt withdrawal may result in life-threatening arrhythmias, hypertension, or myocardial ischemia.
- □ Teach patient and family how to check pulse and blood pressure. Instruct them to take pulse daily and blood pressure biweekly. Advise patient to withhold dose and contact physician if pulse is <50 bpm or blood pressure changes significantly.
- □ May occasionally cause drowsiness. Caution patients to avoid driving or other activities that require alertness until response to medication is known.
- □ Reinforce the need to continue additional therapies for hypertension (weight loss, exercise, restricted sodium intake, stress reduction, regular exercise, moderation of alcohol consumption, and cessation of smoking). Carteolol controls but does not cure hypertension.
- □ Caution patient that this medication may cause increased sensitivity to cold.
- □ Advise patient to consult physician or pharmacist before taking any over-the-counter medications, especially cold remedies, concurrently with this medication. Patients on antihypertensive therapy should also avoid excessive amounts of coffee, tea, and cola.
- □ Diabetics should closely monitor blood sugar, especially if weakness, malaise, irritability, or fatigue occur.
- □ Advise patient to notify physician if slow pulse rate, fever, dizziness, lightheadedness, confusion, or depression, skin rash, sore throat, or unusual bleeding or bruising occur.
- □ Instruct patient to inform physician or dentist of medication regimen prior to treatment or surgery.

□ Advise patient to carry identification describing disease process and medication regimen at all times.

EVALUATION

Effectiveness of therapy can be demonstrated by: ▪ Decrease in blood pressure.

CASANTHRANOL
(ka-**san**-thra-nole)

CASCARA
(kas-**kar**-a)

CASCARA SAGRADA
(kas-**kar**-a sa-**grad**-a)

CLASSIFICATION(S):
Laxative—stimulant
Pregnancy Category UK

INDICATIONS

▪ Treatment of constipation. Particularly useful when constipation is secondary to prolonged bed rest or constipating drugs.

ACTION

▪ Stimulates peristalsis ▪ Alters fluid and electrolyte transport, producing fluid accumulation in the colon. **Therapeutic Effect:** ▪ Evacuation of the colon. Cascara is another name for cascara sagrada, which is naturally derived from the bark of the Buckhorn tree. Casanthranol is the active ingredient that has been extracted from cascara.

PHARMACOKINETICS

Absorption: Minimally absorbed. Converted in the colon to active drug.
Distribution: Distribution not known.
Metabolism and Excretion: Small amounts absorbed are metabolized by the liver.
Half-life: Unknown.

CONTRAINDICATIONS AND PRECAUTIONS

Contraindicated in: ▪ Hypersensitivity ▪ Abdominal pain, obstruction, nausea or vomiting, especially when associated with fever or other signs of acute abdomen ▪ Pregnancy or lactation.
Use Cautiously in: ▪ Severe cardiovascular disease ▪ Anal or rectal fissures ▪ Excessive or prolonged use may lead to dependence.

ADVERSE REACTIONS AND SIDE EFFECTS*

GI: nausea, abdominal cramps, diarrhea.
GU: discoloration of urine.
F and E: hypokalemia (with chronic use).

INTERACTIONS

Drug-Drug: ▪ May decrease the absorption of concurrently administered **oral medications** due to increased motility and decreased transit time.

ROUTE AND DOSAGE

Casanthranol
- **PO (Adults):** 30–90 mg once daily.
- **PO (Children 2–11 yr):** 50% of adult dose.
- **PO (Younger Children and Infants):** 25% of adult dose.

Cascara Sagrada
- **PO (Adults):** 300 mg–1 g once daily.
- **PO (Children 2–11 yr):** 50% of adult dose.
- **PO (Younger Children and Infants):** 25% of adult dose.

Cascara Sagrada Extract
- **PO (Adults):** 200–400 mg once daily.
- **PO (Children 2–11 yr):** 50% of adult dose.
- **PO (Younger Children and Infants):** 25% of adult dose.

Cascara Sagrada Fluidextract
- **PO (Adults):** 0.5–1.5 ml once daily.
- **PO (Children 2–11 yr):** 50% of adult dose.
- **PO (Younger Children and Infants):** 25% of adult dose.

Aromatic Cascara Fluidextract
- **PO (Adults):** 2–6 ml once daily.
- **PO (Children 2–11 yr):** 50% of adult dose.

*Underlines indicate most frequent; **CAPITALS** indicate life-threatening.

- **PO (Younger Children and Infants):** 25% of adult dose.

PHARMACODYNAMICS (evacuation of colon)

	ONSET	PEAK	DURATION
PO	6–12 hr	UK	UK

NURSING IMPLICATIONS

Assessment

- ▫ Assess patient for abdominal distention, presence of bowel sounds, and usual pattern of bowel function.
- ▫ Assess color, consistency, and amount of stool produced.

Potential Nursing Diagnoses

- Bowel elimination, altered: constipation (indications).
- Bowel elimination, altered: diarrhea (side effects).
- Knowledge deficit related to medication regimen (patient/family teaching).

Implementation

- **PO:** Administer with full glass of water. Administer at bedtime for evacuation 6–12 hr later. Administer on an empty stomach for more rapid results.
- ▫ Available in tablet, capsule, and liquid forms. Available in combination with milk of magnesia, docusate, and mineral oil (see Appendix A).

Patient/Family Teaching

- ▫ Advise patients that laxatives should be used only for short-term therapy. Long-term therapy may cause electrolyte imbalance and dependence.
- ▫ Encourage patients to utilize other forms of bowel regulation such as increasing bulk in the diet, increasing fluid intake, increasing mobility. Normal bowel habits are individualized and may vary from 3 times/day to 3 times/wk.
- ▫ Inform patients that this medication may cause a change in urine color to a pink, red, violet, or brown color.
- ▫ Instruct patients with cardiac disease to avoid straining during bowel movements (Valsalva maneuver).
- ▫ Advise patients not to use laxatives when abdominal pain, nausea, vomiting, or fever are present.

Evaluation

Effectiveness of therapy can be demonstrated by: ▪ The patient having a soft, formed bowel movement.

CEFACLOR
(sef-a-klor)
Ceclor

CLASSIFICATION(S):
Anti-infective—second generation cephalosporin
Pregnancy Category B

INDICATIONS

▪ Useful in the treatment of the following infections due to susceptible organisms: ▫ Otitis media ▫ Respiratory tract infections ▫ Skin and skin structure infections ▫ Bone and joint infections ▫ Urinary tract and gynecologic infections ▫ Septicemia.

ACTION

▪ Binds to bacterial cell wall membrane, causing cell death. **Therapeutic Effect:** ▪ Bactericidal action against susceptible bacteria. **Spectrum:** ▪ Many gram-positive cocci including: ▫ *Streptococcus pneumoniae* ▫ Group A beta-hemolytic streptococci ▫ Penicillinase-producing staphylococci ▪ Has increased activity against several other important gram-negative pathogens including: ▫ *Haemophilus influenzae* ▫ Acinetobacter ▫ Enterobacter ▫ *Escherichia coli* ▫ *Klebsiella pneumoniae* ▫ *Neisseria gonorrhea* (including penicillinase-producing strains) ▫ Providencia ▫ Proteus ▫ Serratia ▪ Has no activity against: ▫ Methicillin-resistant staphylococci ▫ Enterococcus.

PHARMACOKINETICS

Absorption: Well absorbed following oral administration.
Distribution: Widely distributed. Penetration into CSF is poor. Crosses the

placenta and enters breast milk in low concentrations.
Metabolism and Excretion: Excreted primarily unchanged by the kidneys.
Half-life: 0.6–0.9 hr (increased in renal impairment).

CONTRAINDICATIONS AND PRECAUTIONS

Contraindicated in: ▪ Hypersensitivity to cephalosporins ▪ Serious hypersensitivity to penicillins.
Use Cautiously in: ▪ Renal impairment (dosage reduction required if severe) ▪ Pregnancy and lactation (safety not established, but has been used in obstetrical surgery).

ADVERSE REACTIONS AND SIDE EFFECTS*

GI: nausea, vomiting, cramps, diarrhea, PSEUDOMEMBRANOUS COLITIS.
Derm: rashes, urticaria.
Hemat: blood dyscrasias, hemolytic anemia.
Misc: superinfection, allergic reactions including ANAPHYLAXIS and serum sickness.

INTERACTIONS

Drug–Drug: ▪ **Probenecid** decreases excretion and increases blood levels.

ROUTE AND DOSAGE

Cefaclor

- **PO (Adults):** 250–500 mg q 8 hr.
- **PO (Children >1 mon):** 20–40 mg/kg/day in divided doses q 8 hr.

PHARMACODYNAMICS (blood levels)

	ONSET	PEAK
PO	rapid	30–60 min

NURSING IMPLICATIONS

Assessment

- Assess patient for infection (vital signs; appearance of wound, sputum, urine, and stool; WBC; earache) at beginning and throughout course of therapy.
- Obtain a history before initiating therapy to determine previous use of and reactions to penicillins or cephalosporins. Persons with a negative history of penicillin sensitivity may still have an allergic response.
- Obtain specimens for culture and sensitivity prior to initiating therapy. First dose may be given before receiving results.
- Observe patient for signs and symptoms of anaphylaxis (rash, pruritus, laryngeal edema, wheezing). Discontinue the drug and notify the physician immediately if these occur. Keep epinephrine, an antihistamine, and resuscitation equipment close by in the event of an anaphylactic reaction.
- **Lab Test Considerations:** May cause false-positive results for Coombs' test and urine glucose when tested with copper sulfate method (Clinitest). Use glucose oxidase method (Clinistix or Tes-tape) to test urine glucose.
- May cause elevated BUN, creatinine, SGOT (AST), SGPT (ALT), and alkaline phosphatase levels.

Potential Nursing Diagnoses

- Infection, high risk for (indications, side effects).
- Bowel elimination, altered: diarrhea (adverse reactions).
- Knowledge deficit related to medication regimen (patient/family teaching).

Implementation

- **General Info:** Available in capsules or oral suspension.
- **PO:** Administer around the clock. May be administered without regard to meals. If gastric irritation occurs administer with food. Food slows but does not effect amount absorbed.
- Shake suspension well before administering. Suspension is stable for 14 days if refrigerated.

Patient/Family Teaching

- Instruct patient to take cefaclor around the clock and to finish the drug completely, even if feeling better. Advise patient that sharing of this medication may be dangerous.

*Underlines indicate most frequent; CAPITALS indicate life-threatening.

- ▫ Instruct patients receiving suspension on the correct method for measuring liquid.
- ▫ Advise patient to report the signs of superinfection (furry overgrowth on the tongue, vaginal itching or discharge, loose or foul-smelling stools) and allergy.
- ▫ Instruct patient to notify physician if fever and diarrhea develop, especially if stool contains blood, pus, or mucus. Advise patient not to treat diarrhea without consulting physician or pharmacist.

EVALUATION

Clinical response to therapy can be evaluated by: ▪ Resolution of the signs and symptoms of infection. Length of time for complete resolution depends on the organism and site of infection.

CEFADROXIL
(sef-a-**drox**-ill)
Duricef, Ultracef

CLASSIFICATION(S):
Anti-infective—first generation cephalosporin
Pregnancy Category B

INDICATIONS

▪ Treatment of: ▫ Serious skin and skin structure infections ▫ Urinary tract infections ▫ Bone and joint infections ▫ Septicemia due to susceptible organisms ▫ Group A beta-hemolytic streptococcal pharyngitis.

ACTION

▪ Binds to bacterial cell wall membrane, causing cell death. **Therapeutic Effect:** ▪ Bactericidal action against susceptible bacteria. **Spectrum:** ▪ Active against many gram-positive cocci including: ▫ *Streptococcus pneumoniae* ▫ Group A beta-hemolytic streptococci ▫ Penicillinase-producing staphylococci ▪ Has limited activity against some gram-negative rods: ▫ *Klebsiella pneumoniae* ▫ *Proteus mirabilis* ▫ *Escherichia coli* ▪ Not active against: ▫ Methicillin-resistant staphylococci ▫ *Bacteroides fragilis* ▫ Enterococcus.

PHARMACOKINETICS

Absorption: Well absorbed following oral administration.
Distribution: Widely distributed. Crosses the placenta and enters breast milk in low concentrations. Minimal penetration into CSF.
Metabolism and Excretion: Excreted almost entirely unchanged by the kidneys.
Half-life: Cefadroxil 1.1–2 hr.

CONTRAINDICATIONS AND PRECAUTIONS

Contraindicated in: ▪ Hypersensitivity to cephalosporins ▪ Serious hypersensitivity to penicillins.
Use Cautiously in: ▪ Renal impairment (dosage reduction required) ▪ Pregnancy or lactation (safety not established).

ADVERSE REACTIONS AND SIDE EFFECTS*

GI: nausea, vomiting, cramps, diarrhea, PSEUDOMEMBRANOUS COLITIS.
Derm: rashes, urticaria.
GU: interstitial nephritis.
Hemat: blood dyscrasias, hemolytic anemia.
Misc: superinfection, allergic reactions including ANAPHYLAXIS and serum sickness.

INTERACTIONS

Drug–Drug: ▪ **Probenecid** decreases excretion and increases blood levels.

ROUTE AND DOSAGE

- ▪ **PO (Adults):** 1–2 g/day in one dose or divided dose q 12 hr.
- ▪ **PO (Children):** 15 mg/kg twice daily.

PHARMACODYNAMICS (blood levels)

	ONSET	PEAK
PO	rapid	1.5–2 hr

*Underlines indicate most frequent; CAPITALS indicate life-threatening.

C

NURSING IMPLICATIONS

ASSESSMENT

- ▫ Assess patient for infection (vital signs; appearance of wound, sputum, urine, and stool; WBC) at beginning and throughout course of therapy.
- ▫ Obtain a history before initiating therapy to determine previous use of and reactions to penicillins or cephalosporins. Persons with a negative history of penicillin sensitivity may still have an allergic response.
- ▫ Obtain specimens for culture and sensitivity prior to initiating therapy. First dose may be given before receiving results.
- ▫ Observe patient for signs and symptoms of anaphylaxis (rash, pruritus, laryngeal edema, wheezing). Discontinue the drug and notify the physician immediately if these occur. Keep epinephrine, an antihistamine, and resuscitation equipment close by in the event of an anaphylactic reaction.
- ▪ **Lab Test Considerations:** May cause false-positive results for Coombs' test and urine glucose when tested with copper sulfate method (Clinitest). Use glucose oxidase method (Clinistix or Tes-Tape) to test urine glucose.
- ▫ May cause transient increase in SGOT (AST), SGPT (ALT), and alkaline phosphatase.

POTENTIAL NURSING DIAGNOSES

- ▪ Infection, high risk for (indications, side effects).
- ▪ Knowledge deficit related to medication regimen (patient/family teaching).
- ▪ Noncompliance related to medication regimen (patient/family teaching).

IMPLEMENTATION

- ▪ **General Info:** Available in tablets, capsules, and oral suspension.
- ▪ **PO:** Administer around the clock. May be administered without regard to food or meals. If gastric irritation occurs, administer with food.
- ▫ Shake suspensions well before administering. Suspension is stable for 14 days if refrigerated.

PATIENT/FAMILY TEACHING

- ▫ Instruct patient to take cefadroxil around the clock and to finish the drug completely, even if feeling better. Advise patients that sharing of this medication may be dangerous.
- ▫ Instruct patients receiving suspension on correct method for measuring liquid.
- ▫ Advise patient to report the signs of superinfection (furry overgrowth on the tongue, vaginal itching or discharge, loose or foul-smelling stools) and allergy.
- ▫ Instruct patient to notify physician if fever and diarrhea develop, especially if stool contains blood, mucus, or pus. Advise patient not to treat diarrhea without consulting physician or pharmacist.

EVALUATION

Clinical response to therapy can be evaluated by: ▪ Resolution of the signs and symptoms of infection. Length of time for complete resolution depends on the organism and site of infection.

CEFAMANDOLE

(sef-a-**man**-dole)
Mandol

CLASSIFICATION(S):
Anti-infective—second generation cephalosporin
Pregnancy Category B

INDICATIONS

▪ Treatment of the following infections due to susceptible organisms: ▫ Respiratory tract infections ▫ Skin and skin structure infections ▫ Bone and joint infections ▫ Urinary tract and gynecologic infections ▫ Septicemia ▫ Intra-abdominal and biliary tract infections ▪ Has also been used as a perioperative prophylactic anti-infective.

ACTION

▪ Binds to bacterial cell wall membrane, causing cell death. **Therapeutic Effect:**

▪ Bactericidal action against susceptible bacteria. **Spectrum:** ▪ Many gram-positive cocci including: ▫ *Streptococcus pneumoniae* ▫ Group A beta-hemolytic streptococci ▫ Penicillinase-producing staphylococci ▪ Increased activity against several other important gram-negative pathogens including: ▫ *Haemophilus influenzae* ▫ Acinetobacter ▫ Enterobacter ▫ *Escherichia coli* ▫ *Klebsiella pneumoniae* ▫ *Neisseria gonorrhea* (including penicillinase-producing strains) ▫ Providencia ▫ Proteus ▫ Serratia ▪ Also active against *Bacteroides fragilis* ▪ Has no activity against: ▫ Methicillin-resistant staphylococci ▫ Enterococcus.

PHARMACOKINETICS

Absorption: Well absorbed following IM administration.

Distribution: Widely distributed. Penetration into CSF is poor. Crosses the placenta and enters breast milk in low concentrations.

Metabolism and Excretion: Excreted primarily unchanged by the kidneys.

Half-life: 0.5–1.2 hr (increased in renal impairment).

CONTRAINDICATIONS AND PRECAUTIONS

Contraindicated in: ▪ Hypersensitivity to cephalosporins ▪ Serious hypersensitivity to penicillins.

Use Cautiously in: ▪ Renal impairment (dosage reduction required) ▪ Pregnancy and lactation (safety not established, but has been used in obstetrical surgery).

ADVERSE REACTIONS AND SIDE EFFECTS*

GI: nausea, vomiting, cramps, diarrhea, PSEUDOMEMBRANOUS COLITIS.

Derm: rashes, urticaria.

Hemat: blood dyscrasias, hemolytic anemia, bleeding.

Local: phlebitis at IV site, pain at IM site.

Misc: superinfection, allergic reactions including ANAPHYLAXIS and serum sickness.

INTERACTIONS

Drug-Drug: ▪ **Probenecid** decreases excretion and increases blood levels ▪ If **alcohol** is ingested within 48–72 hr, a disulfiram-like reaction may occur ▪ May increase risk of bleeding with **oral anticoagulants, thrombolytics, nonsteroidal anti-inflammatory agents, plicamycin,** or **valproic acid.**

ROUTE AND DOSAGE

- **IM, IV (Adults):** 500–1000 mg q 4–8 hr.
- **IM, IV (Children >1 mon):** 50–100 mg/kg/day in divided doses q 4–8 hr.

PHARMACODYNAMICS (blood levels)

	ONSET	PEAK
cefamandole IM	rapid	30–120 min
cefamandole IV	rapid	end of infusion

NURSING IMPLICATIONS

Assessment

- **General Info:** Assess patient for infection (vital signs; appearance of wound, sputum, urine, and stool; WBC) at beginning and throughout course of therapy.
  - ▫ Obtain a history before initiating therapy to determine previous use of and reactions to penicillins or cephalosporins. Persons with a negative history of penicillin sensitivity may still have an allergic response.
  - ▫ Obtain specimens for culture and sensitivity prior to initiating therapy. First dose may be given before receiving results.
  - ▫ Observe patient for signs and symptoms of anaphylaxis (rash, pruritus, laryngeal edema, wheezing). Discontinue the drug and notify the physician immediately if these occur. Keep epinephrine, an antihistamine, and resuscitation equipment close by in the event of an anaphylactic reaction.
- **Lab Test Considerations:** Monitor

*Underlines indicate most frequent; CAPITALS indicate life-threatening.

prothrombin time and assess for bleeding (guaiac stools; check for hematuria, bleeding gums, ecchymosis) daily in patients receiving cefamandole, because it may cause hypoprothrombinemia. Elderly or debilitated patients are at increased risk for hypoprothrombinemia. If bleeding occurs, it can be reversed with vitamin K, or prophylactic vitamin K 10 mg/wk may be given.

- May cause transient increase in BUN, creatinine, SGOT (AST), SGPT (ALT), LDH, and alkaline phosphatase.
- May cause false-positive proteinuria, Coombs' test, and urine glucose when tested with copper sulfate method (Clinitest). Use glucose oxidase method (Clinistix or Tes-Tape) to test urine glucose.

Potential Nursing Diagnoses

- Infection, high risk for (indications, side effects).
- Bowel elimination, altered: diarrhea (adverse reactions).
- Knowledge deficit related to medication regimen (patient/family teaching).

Implementation

- **General Info:** Soln ranges in color from light yellow to amber. Do not use if soln is a different color or contains a precipitate.
- Reconstitution causes gas to form. Vial can be vented prior to withdrawal, or use gas to assist in withdrawal of the soln by inverting the vial over the syringe needle, allowing the soln to flow into the needle.
- Powder is difficult to dissolve. Reconstitute by keeping powder at stopper end of vial and adding diluent to other end of vial. Shake vigorously to dissolve.
- **IM:** Reconstitute IM doses with 3 ml of sterile or bacteriostatic water for injection or 0.9% NaCl for injection. Physician may order dilution with 0.5–2.0% lidocaine HCl to minimize injection discomfort. Inject deep into a well-developed muscle mass; massage well.
- **IV:** Change IV sites every 48–72 hr to prevent phlebitis.
- Manufacturer recommends discontinuing other IV solns during IV administration of cephalosporins.
- **Direct IV:** Dilute each g with 10 ml of sterile water for injection, D5W, or 0.9% NaCl.
- *Rate:* Administer slowly over 3–5 min. Monitor for phlebitis.
- **Intermittent Infusion:** Reconstituted soln may be further diluted in 100 ml of 0.9% NaCl, D5W, D10W, D5/0.25% NaCl, D5/0.45% NaCl, D5/0.9% NaCl, or D5/LR. Soln is stable for 24 hr at room temperature and 96 hr if refrigerated.
- *Rate:* Administer over 15–30 min.
- **Continuous Infusion:** May be diluted in up to 1000 ml for continuous infusion.
- **Syringe Compatibility:** heparin.
- **Syringe Incompatibility:** cimetidine, gentamicin, or tobramycin.
- **Y-Site Compatibility:** acyclovir, cyclophosphamide, hydromorphone, magnesium sulfate, meperidine, morphine, or perphenazine.
- **Y-Site Incompatibility:** hetastarch.
- **Additive Compatibility:** fat emulsion, mannitol, clindamycin, metronidazole, or verapamil.
- **Additive Incompatibility:** calcium, cimetidine, gentamicin, lactated Ringer's soln, Ringer's soln, or tobramycin.
- Do not admix with aminoglycosides.

Patient/Family Teaching

- Advise patient to report the signs of superinfection (furry overgrowth on the tongue, vaginal itching or discharge, loose or foul-smelling stools) and allergy.
- Caution patient that concurrent use of alcohol with cefamandole may cause a disulfiram-like reaction (abdominal cramps, nausea, vomiting, hypotension, palpitations, dyspnea, tachycardia, sweating, flushing). Alcohol and medications containing alcohol should be avoided during and for several days after therapy.

□ Instruct patient to notify physician if fever and diarrhea develop, especially if stool contains blood, pus, or mucus. Advise patient not to treat diarrhea without consulting physician or pharmacist.

Evaluation

Clinical response to therapy can be evaluated by: ■ Resolution of the signs and symptoms of infection. Length of time for complete resolution depends on the organism and site of infection.

CEFAZOLIN
(sef-a-zoe-lin)
Ancef, Kefzol, Zolicef

CLASSIFICATION(S):
Anti-infective—first generation cephalosporin
Pregnancy Category B

INDICATIONS

■ Treatment of: □ Serious skin and skin structure infections □ Urinary tract infections □ Bone and joint infections □ Septicemia due to susceptible organisms ■ Has been used to treat intra-abdominal and biliary tract infections and as a perioperative prophylactic anti-infective.

ACTION

■ Binds to bacterial cell wall membrane, causing cell death. **Therapeutic Effect:** ■ Bactericidal action against susceptible bacteria. **Spectrum:** ■ Active against many gram-positive cocci including: □ *Streptococcus pneumoniae* □ Group A beta-hemolytic streptococci □ Penicillinase-producing staphylococci ■ Limited activity against some gram-negative rods including: □ *Klebsiella pneumoniae* □ *Proteus mirabilis* □ *Escherichia coli* ■ Not active against: □ Methicillin-resistant staphylococci □ *Bacteroides fragilis* □ Enterococcus.

PHARMACOKINETICS

Absorption: Well absorbed following IM administration.
Distribution: Widely distributed. Crosses the placenta and enters breast milk in low concentrations. Minimal penetration into CSF.
Metabolism and Excretion: Excreted almost entirely unchanged by the kidneys.
Half-life: 1.2–2.2 hr.

CONTRAINDICATIONS AND PRECAUTIONS

Contraindicated in: ■ Hypersensitivity to cephalosporins ■ Serious hypersensitivity to penicillins.
Use Cautiously in: ■ Renal impairment (dosage reduction required) ■ Patients >50 yr old (increased risk of renal toxicity) ■ Pregnancy or lactation (safety not established).

ADVERSE REACTIONS AND SIDE EFFECTS*

CNS: SEIZURES (high doses).
GI: nausea, vomiting, cramps, diarrhea, PSEUDOMEMBRANOUS COLITIS.
GU: nephrotoxicity.
Derm: rashes, urticaria.
Hemat: blood dyscrasias, hemolytic anemia.
Local: phlebitis at IV site, pain at IM site.
Misc: superinfection, allergic reactions including ANAPHYLAXIS and serum sickness.

INTERACTIONS

Drug-Drug: ■ **Probenecid** decreases excretion and increases blood levels ■ May potentiate nephrotoxicity from other **nephrotoxic agents (aminoglycosides)**.

ROUTE AND DOSAGE

- **IM, IV (Adults):** 0.5–2 g q 6–8 hr.
- **IM, IV (Children and Infants >1 mon):** 25–50 mg/kg/day in divided doses every 6–8 hr.

*Underlines indicate most frequent; **CAPITALS** indicate life-threatening.

C

PHARMACODYNAMICS (blood levels)

	ONSET	PEAK
IM	rapid	1–2 hr
IV	rapid	end of infusion

NURSING IMPLICATIONS

Assessment

- Assess patient for infection (vital signs; appearance of wound, sputum, urine, and stool; WBC) at beginning and throughout course of therapy.
- Obtain a history before initiating therapy to determine previous use of and reactions to penicillins or cephalosporins. Persons with a negative history of penicillin sensitivity may still have an allergic response.
- Obtain specimens for culture and sensitivity prior to initiating therapy. First dose may be given before receiving results.
- Observe patient for signs and symptoms of anaphylaxis (rash, pruritus, laryngeal edema, wheezing). Discontinue the drug and notify the physician immediately if these occur. Keep epinephrine, an antihistamine, and resuscitation equipment close by in the event of an anaphylactic reaction.
- Monitor intake and output ratios and daily weight. Patients with impaired renal function, over the age of 50, or taking other nephrotoxic drugs are at risk for developing nephrotoxicity with high-dose therapy.
- **Lab Test Considerations:** May cause false-positive results for Coombs' test and urine glucose when tested with copper sulfate method (Clinitest). Use glucose oxidase method (Clinistix or Tes-Tape) to test urine glucose.
  - May cause transient elevation in BUN, SGOT (AST), SGPT (ALT), and alkaline phosphatase.

Potential Nursing Diagnoses

- Infection, high risk for (indications, side effects)
- Bowel elimination, altered: diarrhea (adverse reactions).
- Knowledge deficit related to medication regimen (patient/family teaching).

Implementation

- **General Info:** Do not use soln that is cloudy or contains a precipitate.
- **IM:** Reconstitute IM doses with 2 ml of sterile or bacteriostatic water for injection or 0.9% NaCl for injection in the 250-mg or 500-mg vial and 2.5 ml in the 1-g vial for concentrations of 125, 225, or 330 mg/ml, respectively. Inject deep into a well-developed muscle mass, massage well.
- **IV:** Change IV sites every 48–72 hr to prevent phlebitis. Manufacturer recommends discontinuation of other IV solns during IV administration of cephalosporins.
- **Direct IV:** For direct IV administration dilute in 10 ml of sterile water for injection.
  - *Rate:* Administer slowly over 3–5 min. Monitor for phlebitis.
- **Intermittent Infusion:** Reconstituted 500-mg or 1-g soln may be diluted in 50–100 ml of 0.9% NaCl, D5W, D10W, D5/0.25% NaCl, D5/0.45% NaCl, D5/0.9% NaCl, D5/LR, or lactated Ringer's soln. Soln is stable for 24 hr at room temperature and 96 hr if refrigerated.
  - *Rate:* Administer over 30–60 min.
- **Syringe Compatibility:** heparin or vitamin B complex.
- **Syringe Incompatibility:** ascorbic acid injection, cimetidine, or lidocaine.
- **Y-Site Compatibility:** acyclovir, atracurium, calcium gluconate, enalaprilat, cyclophosphamide, esmolol, famotidine, foscarnet, hydromorphone, labetalol, lidocaine, magnesium sulfate, meperidine, morphine, multivitamins, ondansetron, perphenazine, pancuronium, or vecuronium.
- **Additive Compatibility:** aztreonam, clindamycin, metronidazole, or verapamil.
- **Additive Incompatibility:** amikacin, amobarbital, bleomycin, calcium gluceptate, calcium gluconate, colistimethate, erythromycin, kanamycin,

oxytetracycline, pentobarbital, polymyxin B, or tetracycline.

PATIENT/FAMILY TEACHING

- Advise patient to report the signs of superinfection (furry overgrowth on the tongue, vaginal itching or discharge, loose or foul-smelling stools) and allergy.
- Instruct patient to notify physician if fever and diarrhea develop, especially if stool contains blood, mucus, or pus. Advise patient not to treat diarrhea without consulting physician or pharmacist.

EVALUATION

Clinical response to therapy can be evaluated by: ▪ Resolution of the signs and symptoms of infection. Length of time for complete resolution depends on the organism and site of infection.

CEFIXIME

(se-**fix**-eem)
Suprax

CLASSIFICATION(S):
Anti-infective—third generation cephalosporin
Pregnancy Category B

INDICATIONS

▪ Treatment of the following infections due to susceptible organisms: ▫ Uncomplicated urinary tract infections ▫ Otitis media ▫ Bronchitis (acute and exacerbations) ▫ Pharyngitis or tonsillitis.

ACTION

▪ Binds to the bacterial cell wall membrane causing cell death. **Therapeutic Effect:** ▪ Bactericidal action against susceptible bacteria. **Spectrum:** ▪ Spectrum is similar to that of second generation cephalosporins, however, activity against staphylococci is diminished in comparison, while activity against gram-negative pathogens is enhanced, even for organisms resistant to first and second generation agents ▪ Notable for activity against: ▫ *Hemophilus influenzae* (including β-lactamase-producing strains) ▫ *Escherichia coli* ▫ *Branhamella catarrhalis* ▫ *Proteus mirabilis*.

PHARMACOKINETICS

Absorption: 40–50% absorbed following oral administration (suspension produces higher blood levels than tablets).
Distribution: Widely distributed.
Metabolism and Excretion: 50% excreted unchanged by the kidneys, >10% excreted in bile.
Half-life: 180–240 min (increased in renal impairment).

CONTRAINDICATIONS AND PRECAUTIONS

Contraindicated in: ▪ Hypersensitivity to cephalosporins ▪ Serious hypersensitivity to penicillins.
Use Cautiously in: ▪ Renal impairment (dosage reduction recommended) ▪ Pregnancy or lactation (safety not established).

ADVERSE REACTIONS AND SIDE EFFECTS*

CNS: headache, dizziness.
GI: diarrhea, abdominal pain, nausea, dyspepsia, flatulence, PSEUDOMEMBRANOUS COLITIS.
Derm: rashes, urticaria.
Misc: superinfection, allergic reactions including ANAPHYLAXIS, fever.

INTERACTIONS

Drug–Drug: ▪ None significant.

ROUTE AND DOSAGE

- **PO (Adults, Children >12 yr or >50 kg):** 400 mg/day as a single dose or 200 mg q 12 hr.
- **PO (Children):** 8 mg/kg/day as a single dose or in 2 divided doses q 12 hr; when treating otitis media use only suspension.

*Underlines indicate most frequent; **CAPITALS** indicate life-threatening.

C

PHARMACODYNAMICS (blood levels)

	ONSET	PEAK
PO	rapid	2–6 hr

NURSING IMPLICATIONS

Assessment

- ▫ Assess patient for infection (vital signs; appearance of wound, sputum, urine, and stool; WBC; earache) at beginning and throughout course of therapy.
- ▫ Obtain a history before initiating therapy to determine previous use of and reactions to penicillins or cephalosporins. Persons with a negative history of penicillin sensitivity may still have an allergic response.
- ▫ Obtain specimens for culture and sensitivity prior to initiating therapy. First dose may be given before receiving results.
- ▫ Observe patient for signs and symptoms of anaphylaxis (rash, pruritus, laryngeal edema, wheezing). Discontinue the drug and notify the physician immediately if these occur. Keep epinephrine, an antihistamine, and resuscitation equipment close by in the event of an anaphylactic reaction.
- ▪ **Lab Test Considerations:** May cause false positive results for Coombs' test and urine glucose when tested with copper sulfate method (Clinitest). Use glucose oxidase method (Clinistix or Tes-Tape) to test urine glucose.
- ▫ May cause elevated BUN, creatinine, SGOT (AST), SGPT (ALT), and alkaline phosphatase levels.

Potential Nursing Diagnoses

- ▪ Infection, high risk for (indications, side effects).
- ▪ Bowel elimination, altered: diarrhea (adverse reactions).
- ▪ Knowledge deficit related to medication regimen (patient/family teaching).

Implementation

- ▪ **General Info:** Available in tablets or oral suspension.
- ▪ **PO:** Administer around the clock. Shake suspension well before administering.

Patient/Family Teaching

- ▫ Instruct patient to take cefixime around the clock and to finish the drug completely, even if feeling better. Advise patient that sharing of this medication may be dangerous.
- ▫ Instruct patients receiving suspension on the correct method for measuring liquid.
- ▫ Advise patient to report the signs of superinfection (furry overgrowth on the tongue, vaginal itching or discharge, loose or foul-smelling stools) and allergy.
- ▫ Instruct patient to notify physician if fever and diarrhea develop, especially if stool contains blood, pus, or mucus. Advise patient not to treat diarrhea without consulting physician or pharmacist.

Evaluation

Clinical response to therapy can be evaluated by: ▪ Resolution of the signs and symptoms of infection. Length of time for complete resolution depends on the organism and site of infection.

CEFMETAZOLE

(sef-**met**-a-zole)
Zefazone

CLASSIFICATION(S):
Anti-infective—second generation cephalosporin
Pregnancy Category B

INDICATIONS

▪ Treatment of the following infections due to susceptible organisms: ▫ Lower respiratory tract infections ▫ Skin and skin structure infections ▫ Urinary tract and intra-abdominal infections ▫ Has also been used as a perioperative prophylactic anti-infective in patients undergoing: ▫ Cesarian section ▫ Abdominal or vaginal hysterectomy ▫ Cholecystectomy ▫ Colorectal surgery.

ACTION

▪ Binds to bacterial cell wall membrane, causing cell death. **Therapeutic Effect:** ▪ Bactericidal action against susceptible bacteria. **Spectrum:** ▪ Many gram-positive cocci including: ▫ *Streptococcus pneumoniae* ▫ Group A beta-hemolytic streptococci ▫ Penicillinase-producing staphylococci. ▪ In addition has increased activity against several other important gram-negative pathogens including: ▫ *Haemophilus influenzae* ▫ Acinetobacter ▫ Enterobacter ▫ *Escherichia coli* ▫ *Klebsiella sp* ▫ *Neisseria gonorrhea (including penicillinase-producing strains)* ▫ Providencia ▫ Proteus ▫ Serratia ▪ Also active against *Bacteroides fragilis* ▪ Has no activity against: ▫ Methicillin-resistant staphylococci ▫ Enterococcus.

PHARMACOKINETICS

Absorption: Following IV administration absorption is essentially complete.
Distribution: Widely distributed. Penetration into CSF is poor. Crosses the placenta and enters breast milk in low concentrations.
Metabolism and Excretion: 85% excreted unchanged by the kidneys.
Half-life: 0.8–1.8 (increased in renal impairment).

CONTRAINDICATIONS AND PRECAUTIONS

Contraindicated in: ▪ Hypersensitivity to cephalosporins ▪ Serious hypersensitivity to penicillins.
Use Cautiously in: ▪ Renal impairment (dosage reduction required) ▪ Pregnancy, lactation, and children (safety not established, but has been used in obstetrical surgery).

ADVERSE REACTIONS AND SIDE EFFECTS*

GI: nausea, vomiting, cramps, diarrhea, PSEUDOMEMBRANOUS COLITIS.
Derm: rashes, urticaria.
Hemat: blood dyscrasias, hemolytic anemia, bleeding, bruising.
Local: phlebitis at IV site.
Misc: superinfection, allergic reactions including ANAPHYLAXIS and serum sickness.

INTERACTIONS

Drug–Drug: ▪ **Probenecid** decreases excretion and increases blood levels ▪ If **alcohol** is ingested within 48–72 hr a disulfiram-like reaction may occur ▪ May increase risk of bleeding with **anticoagulants, thrombolytics, nonsteroidal anti-inflammatory agents, plicamycin,** or **valproic acid**.

ROUTE AND DOSAGE

▪ **IV (Adults):** 1–2 g q 6–12 hr.

PHARMACODYNAMICS

	ONSET	PEAK
IV	rapid	end of infusion

NURSING IMPLICATIONS

Assessment

- ▫ Assess patient for infection (vital signs; appearance of wound, sputum, urine, and stool; WBC) at beginning and throughout course of therapy.
- ▫ Obtain a history before initiating therapy to determine previous use of and reactions to penicillins or cephalosporins. Persons with a negative history of penicillin sensitivity may still have an allergic response.
- ▫ Obtain specimens for culture and sensitivity prior to initiating therapy. First dose may be given before receiving results.
- ▫ Observe patient for signs and symptoms of anaphylaxis (rash, pruritus, laryngeal edema, wheezing). Discontinue the drug and notify the physician immediately if these occur. Keep epinephrine, an antihistamine, and resuscitation equipment close by in the event of an anaphylactic reaction.
- ▪ **Lab Test Considerations:** Monitor prothrombin time and assess patient for bleeding (guaiac stools; check for hematuria, bleeding gums, ecchymo-

*Underlines indicate most frequent; **CAPITALS** indicate life-threatening.

C

sis) daily in patient receiving cefmetazole as it may cause hypoprothrombinemia. Elderly or debilitated patients are at increased risk for hypoprothrombinemia. If bleeding occurs, it can be reversed with vitamin K, or prophylactic vitamin K 10 mg/wk may be given.

Potential Nursing Diagnoses

- Infection, high risk for (indications, side effects).
- Bowel elimination, altered: diarrhea (adverse reactions).
- Knowledge deficit related to medication regimen (patient/family teaching).

Implementation

- **IV:** Change IV sites every 48–72 hr to prevent phlebitis.
  - Manufacturer recommends discontinuation of other IV solns during IV administration of cephalosporins.
- **Intermittent Infusion:** Reconstitute with sterile water, bacteriostatic water, or 0.9% NaCl for injection. Reconstituted soln may be further diluted to concentrations of 1–20 mg/ml in 0.9% NaCl, D5W, or LR. Soln is stable for 24 hr at room temperature and 7 days if refrigerated.
  - *Rate:* Administer over 30–60 min.

Patient/Family Teaching

- Advise patient to report the signs of superinfection (furry overgrowth on the tongue, vaginal itching or discharge, loose or foul-smelling stools) and allergy.
- Caution patient that concurrent use of alcohol with cefmetazole may cause a disulfiram-like reaction (abdominal cramps, nausea, vomiting, hypotension, palpitations, dyspnea, tachycardia sweating, flushing). Alcohol and medications containing alcohol should be avoided during and for several days after therapy.
- Instruct patient to notify physician if fever and diarrhea develop, especially if stool contains blood, pus, or mucus. Advise patient not to treat diarrhea without consulting physician or pharmacist.

Evaluation

Effectiveness of therapy can be demonstrated by: ▪ Resolution of the signs and symptoms of infection. Length of time for complete resolution depends on the organism and site of infection.

CEFONICID

(se-**fon**-i-sid)
Monocid

CLASSIFICATION(S):
Anti-infective—second generation cephalosporin
Pregnancy Category B

INDICATIONS

▪ Treatment of the following infections due to susceptible organisms: ▫ Respiratory tract infections ▫ Skin and skin structure infections ▫ Bone and joint infections ▫ Urinary tract and gynecologic infections ▫ Septicemia ▪ Has also been used as a perioperative prophylactic anti-infective.

ACTION

▪ Binds to bacterial cell wall membrane, causing cell death. **Therapeutic Effect:** ▪ Bactericidal action against susceptible bacteria. **Spectrum:** ▪ Many gram-positive cocci, including: ▫ *Streptococcus pneumoniae* ▫ Group A beta-hemolytic streptococci ▫ Penicillinase-producing staphylococci ▪ Increased activity against several other important gram-negative pathogens, including: ▫ *Haemophilus influenzae* ▫ Acinetobacter ▫ Enterobacter ▫ *Escherichia coli* ▫ *Klebsiella pneumoniae* ▫ *Neisseria gonorrhea* (including penicillinase-producing strains) ▫ Providencia ▫ Proteus ▫ Serratia ▪ Also active against *Bacteroides fragilis* ▪ Has no activity against: ▫ Methicillin-resistant staphylococci ▫ Enterococcus.

PHARMACOKINETICS

Absorption: Well absorbed following IM administration.
Distribution: Widely distributed. Pen-

etration into CSF is poor. Crosses the placenta and enters breast milk in low concentrations.

Metabolism and Excretion: Excreted primarily unchanged by the kidneys.

Half-life: 4.5 hr (increased in renal impairment).

CONTRAINDICATIONS AND PRECAUTIONS

Contraindicated in: ▪ Hypersensitivity to cephalosporins ▪ Serious hypersensitivity to penicillins.

Use Cautiously in: ▪ Renal impairment (dosage reduction required) ▪ Pregnancy and lactation (safety not established, but has been used in obstetrical surgery).

ADVERSE REACTIONS AND SIDE EFFECTS*

Derm: rashes, urticaria.

GI: nausea, vomiting, cramps, diarrhea, PSEUDOMEMBRANOUS COLITIS.

Hemat: blood dyscrasias, hemolytic anemia.

Local: phlebitis at IV site, pain at IM site.

Misc: superinfection, allergic reactions including ANAPHYLAXIS and serum sickness.

INTERACTIONS

Drug–Drug: ▪ **Probenecid** decreases excretion and increases blood levels.

ROUTE AND DOSAGE

- **IM, IV (Adults):** 0.5–2 g/day—single dose.

PHARMACODYNAMICS (blood levels)

	ONSET	PEAK
IM	rapid	60 min
IV	rapid	end of infusion

NURSING IMPLICATIONS

Assessment

- **General Info:** Assess patient for infection (vital signs; appearance of wound, sputum, urine, and stool; WBC) at beginning and throughout course of therapy.
- □ Obtain a history before initiating therapy to determine previous use of and reactions to penicillins or cephalosporins. Persons with a negative history of penicillin sensitivity may still have an allergic response.
- □ Obtain specimens for culture and sensitivity prior to initiating therapy. First dose may be given before receiving results.
- □ Observe patient for signs and symptoms of anaphylaxis (rash, pruritus, laryngeal edema, wheezing). Discontinue the drug and notify the physician immediately if these occur. Keep epinephrine, an antihistamine, and resuscitation equipment close by in the event of an anaphylactic reaction.
- **Lab Test Considerations:** May cause false-positive results for Coombs' test and urine glucose when tested with the copper sulfate method (Clinitest). Use glucose oxidase method (Clinistix, Tes-Tape) to test urine glucose.
- □ May cause increase in SGOT (AST), SGPT (ALT), LDH, and alkaline phosphatase levels.

Potential Nursing Diagnoses

- Infection, high risk for (indications, side effects).
- Bowel elimination, altered: diarrhea (adverse reactions).
- Knowledge deficit related to medication regimen (patient/family teaching).

Implementation

- **General Info:** Reconstitute IM and IV doses with 2 ml of sterile water for injection to each 500-mg vial and 2.5 ml to each 1-g vial for concentrations of 220 and 325 mg/ml, respectively. Soln may be colorless to light amber.
- **IM:** Administer IM doses deep into a well-developed muscle mass; massage well. When administering 2-g dose, divide in half and inject into 2 large muscle mass sites.
- **IV:** Change IV sites every 48–72 hr to

*Underlines indicate most frequent; CAPITALS indicate life-threatening.

prevent phlebitis. Discontinue other IV solns during IV administration of cephalosporins.
- **Direct IV:** Direct IV administration can be administered slowly over 3–5 min. Monitor for phlebitis.
- **Intermittent Infusion:** Reconstituted soln may be further diluted in 50–100 ml of D5W, D10W, D5/LR, D5/0.25% NaCl, D5/0.45% NaCl, D5/0.9% NaCl, 0.9% NaCl, or Ringer's or lactated Ringer's soln. Stable for 24 hr at room temperature and 72 hr if refrigerated.
  - *Rate:* Administer over 30 min.
- **Y-Site Compatibility:** acyclovir.
- **Additive Compatibility:** clindamycin.
- **Additive Incompatibility:** Do not admix with aminoglycosides.

Patient/Family Teaching

- Advise patient to report the signs of superinfection (furry overgrowth on the tongue, vaginal itching or discharge, loose or foul-smelling stools) and allergy.
- Instruct patient to notify physician if fever and diarrhea develop, especially if stool contains blood, pus, or mucus. Advise patient not to treat diarrhea without consulting physician or pharmacist.

Evaluation

Clinical response to therapy can be evaluated by: ▪ Resolution of the signs and symptoms of infection. Length of time for complete resolution depends on the organism and site of infection.

CEFOPERAZONE
(sef-oh-**per**-a-zone)
Cefobid

CLASSIFICATION(S):
Anti-infective—third generation cephalosporin
Pregnancy Category B

INDICATIONS

▪ Treatment of: ▫ Skin and skin structure infections ▫ Bone and joint infections ▫ Urinary and gynecologic infections ▫ Respiratory tract infections ▫ Intra-abdominal infections ▫ Septicemia.

ACTION

▪ Binds to the bacterial cell wall membrane causing cell death. **Therapeutic Effect:** ▪ Bactericidal action against susceptible bacteria. **Spectrum:** ▪ Activity against staphylococci is diminished in comparison to second generation cephalosporins, while action against gram-negative pathogens is enhanced, even for organisms resistant to first and second generation agents ▪ Notable is increased action against: ▫ Citrobacter ▫ Enterobacter ▫ *Escherichia coli* ▫ *Klebsiella pneumoniae* ▫ Neisseria ▫ Proteus ▫ Providencia ▫ Serratia ▫ *Pseudomonas aeruginosa* ▫ Hemophilus influenzae ▪ Has some activity against anaerobes including *Bacteroides fragilis.*

PHARMACOKINETICS

Absorption: Well absorbed following IM administration.
Distribution: Widely distributed. Crosses the placenta and enters breast milk in low concentrations.
Metabolism and Excretion: Excreted in the bile.
Half-life: 1.6–2 hr.

CONTRAINDICATIONS AND PRECAUTIONS

Contraindicated in: ▪ Hypersensitivity to cephalosporins ▪ Serious hypersensitivity to penicillins.
Use Cautiously in: ▪ Severe hepatic impairment (dosage reduction required) ▪ Pregnancy, lactation, or children <12 yr (safety not established).

ADVERSE REACTIONS AND SIDE EFFECTS*

Derm: rashes, urticaria.
GI: nausea, vomiting, diarrhea, cramps, PSEUDOMEMBRANOUS COLITIS.
Hemat: blood dyscrasias, hemolytic anemia, bleeding.

*Underlines indicate most frequent; CAPITALS indicate life-threatening.

Local: phlebitis at IV site, pain at IM site.
Misc: superinfection, allergic reactions including **ANAPHYLAXIS** and serum sickness.

INTERACTIONS

Drug–Drug: ▪ **Probenecid** decreases excretion and increases serum levels ▪ Ingestion of **alcohol** within 48–72 hr may result in a disulfiram-like reaction ▪ May increase risk of bleeding with **anticoagulants, thrombolytics, nonsteroidal anti-inflammatory agents, plicamycin,** or **valproic acid.**

ROUTE AND DOSAGE

- **IM, IV (Adults):** 2–4 g/day in divided doses q 12 hr (up to 16 g/day).

PHARMACODYNAMICS (blood levels)

	ONSET	PEAK
IM	rapid	1–2 hr
IV	rapid	end of infusion

NURSING IMPLICATIONS

Assessment

- **General Info:** Assess patient for infection (vital signs; appearance of wound, sputum, urine, and stool; WBC) at beginning and throughout course of therapy.
- ▫ Obtain a careful history before initiating therapy to determine previous use of and reactions to penicillins or cephalosporins. Persons with a negative history of penicillin sensitivity may still have an allergic response.
- ▫ Obtain specimens for culture and sensitivity prior to initiating therapy. First dose may be given before receiving results.
- ▫ Observe patient for signs and symptoms of anaphylaxis (rash, pruritus, laryngeal edema, wheezing). Discontinue the drug and notify the physician immediately if these occur. Keep epinephrine, an antihistamine, and resuscitation equipment close by in the event of an anaphylactic reaction.
- **Lab Test Considerations:** Monitor prothrombin time and assess for bleeding (guaiac stools; check for hematuria, bleeding gums, ecchymosis) daily in patients receiving cefoperazone, because it may cause hypoprothrombinemia. Elderly or debilitated patients are at greater risk of hypoprothrombinemia. If bleeding occurs, it can be reversed with vitamin K, or prophylactic vitamin K 10 mg/wk may be given.
- ▫ May cause false-positive results for Coombs' test and urine glucose when tested with copper sulfate method (Clinitest). Use glucose oxidase method (Clinistix or Tes-Tape) to test urine glucose.
- ▫ May cause elevated BUN, creatinine, SGOT (AST), SGPT (ALT), and alkaline phosphatase levels. Peak and trough blood levels should be drawn periodically on patients with hepatic, biliary, or renal dysfunction.

Potential Nursing Diagnoses

- Infection, high risk for (indications, side effects).
- Bowel elimination, altered: diarrhea (adverse reactions).
- Knowledge deficit related to medication regimen (patient/family teaching).

Implementation

- **General Info:** Soln may be colorless to straw-colored.
- **IM:** Reconstitute IM doses with 2.8 ml of sterile or bacteriostatic water for injection to each 1-g vial or 5.4 ml to each 2-g vial. Physician may order additional dilution of 1 ml or 1.8 ml of 2% lidocaine, respectively, to minimize injection discomfort. Allow vial to stand so that foaming may dissipate.
- ▫ Inject deep into a well-developed muscle mass; massage well.
- **IV:** Change IV sites every 48–72 hr to prevent phlebitis.
- ▫ Manufacture recommends discontinuation of other IV solns during IV administration of cephalosporins.
- **Direct IV:** Manufacturer does not recommend direct IV administration.
- **Intermittent Infusion:** For IV admin-

istration reconstitute each g with at least 2.8 ml of sterile or bacteriostatic water for injection or 0.9% NaCl. Do not use preparations containing benzyl alcohol when used for neonates. Shake vigorously and allow to stand following reconstitution for visualization of clarity.

- Each g in soln should be further diluted in 20–40 ml of 0.9% NaCl, D5W, D10W, D5/0.25% NaCl, D5/0.9% NaCl, D5/LR, or lactated Ringer's soln. Soln is stable for 24 hr at room temperature and 5 days if refrigerated.
- *Rate:* Administer intermittent infusions over 15–30 min. Monitor for phlebitis.

- **Continuous Infusion:** For continuous infusion concentration should be 2–25 mg/ml.
- **Syringe Compatibility:** heparin.
- **Y-Site Compatibility:** acyclovir, cyclophosphamide, enalaprilat, esmolol, famotidine, foscarnet, hydromorphone, magnesium sulfate, or morphine.
- **Y-Site Incompatibility:** hetastarch, labetalol, meperidine, ondansetron, perphenazine, or promethazine.
- **Additive Incompatibility:** Do not admix with aminoglycosides.

PATIENT/FAMILY TEACHING

- Advise patient to report the signs of superinfection (furry overgrowth on the tongue, vaginal itching or discharge, loose or foul-smelling stools) and allergy.
- Caution patient that concurrent use of alcohol with cefoperazone may cause a disulfiram-like reaction (abdominal cramps, nausea, vomiting, hypotension, palpitations, dyspnea, tachycardia, sweating, flushing). Alcohol and medications containing alcohol should be avoided during and for several days after therapy.
- Instruct patient to notify physician if fever and diarrhea develop, especially if stool contains blood, pus, or mucus. Advise patient not to treat diarrhea without consulting physician or pharmacist.

EVALUATION

Clinical response to therapy can be evaluated by: ▪ Resolution of the signs and symptoms of infection. Length of time for complete resolution depends on the organism and site of infection.

CEFORANIDE

(se-**for**-i-nide)
Precef

CLASSIFICATION(S):
Anti-infective—second generation cephalosporin
Pregnancy Category B

INDICATIONS

▪ Treatment of the following infections due to susceptible organisms: ▫ Respiratory tract infections ▫ Skin and skin structure infections ▫ Bone and joint infections ▫ Urinary tract and gynecologic infections ▫ Septicemia ▪ Has also been used as a perioperative prophylactic anti-infective.

ACTION

▪ Binds to bacterial cell wall membrane, causing cell death. **Therapeutic Effect:** ▪ Bactericidal action against susceptible bacteria. **Spectrum:** ▪ Many gram-positive cocci including: ▫ *Streptococcus pneumoniae* ▫ Group A beta-hemolytic streptococci ▫ Penicillinase-producing staphylococci ▪ Increased activity against several other important gram-negative pathogens including: ▫ *Haemophilus influenzae* ▫ Acinetobacter ▫ Enterobacter ▫ *Escherichia coli* ▫ *Klebsiella pneumoniae* ▫ *Neisseria gonorrhea* (including penicillinase-producing strains) ▫ Providencia ▫ Proteus ▫ Serratia ▪ Also active against *Bacteroides fragilis* ▪ Has no activity against: ▫ Methicillin-resistant staphylococci ▫ Enterococcus.

PHARMACOKINETICS

Absorption: Well absorbed following IM administration.
Distribution: Widely distributed. Pen-

etration into CSF is poor. Crosses the placenta and enters breast milk in low concentrations.
Metabolism and Excretion: Excreted primarily unchanged by the kidneys.
Half-life: 2.9 hr (increased in renal impairment).

CONTRAINDICATIONS AND PRECAUTIONS

Contraindicated in: ▪ Hypersensitivity to cephalosporins ▪ Serious hypersensitivity to penicillins.
Use Cautiously in: ▪ Renal impairment (dosage reduction required) ▪ Pregnancy and lactation (safety not estabished, but has been used in obstetrical surgery).

ADVERSE REACTIONS AND SIDE EFFECTS*

Derm: rashes, urticaria.
GI: nausea, vomiting, cramps, diarrhea, PSEUDOMEMBRANOUS COLITIS.
Hemat: blood dyscrasias, hemolytic anemia.
Local: phlebitis at IV site, pain at IM site.
Misc: superinfection, allergic reactions including ANAPHYLAXIS and serum sickness.

INTERACTIONS

Drug–Drug: ▪ **Probenecid** decreases excretion and increases blood levels.

ROUTE AND DOSAGE

- **IM, IV (Adults):** 1–2 g/day in divided doses every 12 hr.
- **IM, IV (Children):** 20–40 mg/kg/day in divided doses q 12 hr.

PHARMACODYNAMICS (blood levels)

	ONSET	PEAK
IM	rapid	60 min
IV	rapid	end of infusion

NURSING IMPLICATIONS

Assessment

- □ Assess patient for infection (vital signs; appearance of wound, sputum, urine, and stool; WBC) at beginning and throughout course of therapy.
- □ Obtain a history before initiating therapy to determine previous use of and reactions to penicillins or cephalosporins. Persons with a negative history of penicillin sensitivity may still have an allergic response.
- □ Obtain specimens for culture and sensitivity prior to initiating therapy. First dose may be given before receiving results.
- □ Observe patient for signs and symptoms of anaphylaxis (rash, pruritus, laryngeal edema, wheezing). Discontinue the drug and notify the physician immediatley if these occur. Keep epinephrine, an antihistamine, and resuscitation equipment close by in the event of an anphylactic reaction.
- ▪ **Lab Test Considerations:** May cause false-positive results for Coombs' test.
- □ May cause increase in BUN, creatinine, SGOT (AST), SGPT (ALT), and alkaline phosphatase levels.

Potential Nursing Diagnoses

- ▪ Infection, high risk for (indications, side effects).
- ▪ Bowel elimination, altered: diarrhea (adverse reactions).
- ▪ Knowledge deficit related to medication regimen (patient/family teaching).

Implementation

- ▪ **General Info:** Soln may appear cloudy but will clear upon standing. Color may vary from light yellow to amber.
- ▪ **IM:** Reconstitute IM doses with 1.7 ml of sterile or bacteriostatic water for injection or 0.9% NaCl for injection to each 500-mg vial or 3.2 ml to each 1-g vial. Shake immediately.
- □ Inject deep into a well-developed muscle mass; massage well.
- ▪ **IV:** Change IV sites every 48–72 hr to prevent phlebitis.
- □ Manufacturer recommends discontinuing other IV solns during IV administration of cephalosporins.
- ▪ **Direct IV:** Add 5 ml of sterile or bacteriostatic water or 0.9% NaCl for injec-

*Underlines indicate most frequent; **CAPITALS** indicate life-threatening.

tion to each 500-mg vial or 10 ml to each 1-g vial and shake immediately.

- *Rate:* Administer slowly over 3–5 min. Monitor for phlebitis.
- **Intermittent Infusion:** Reconstituted soln may be further diluted in at least 1 g/10 ml of 0.9% NaCl, D5W, D10W, D5/0.25% NaCl, D5/0.45% NaCl, D5/LR, or lactated Ringer's soln. Stable for 24 hr at room temperature.
- *Rate:* Administer over 30 min.
- **Y-Site Compatibility:** acyclovir, cyclophosphamide, hydromorphone, magnesium sulfate, meperidine, morphine, ondansetron, or perphenazine.
- **Additive Incompatibility:** Do not admix with aminoglycosides.

Patient/Family Teaching

- Advise patient to report the signs of superinfection (furry overgrowth on the tongue, vaginal itching or discharge, loose or foul-smelling stools) and allergy.
- Instruct patient to notify physician if fever and diarrhea develop, especially if stool contains blood, pus, or mucus. Advise patient not to treat diarrhea without consulting physician or pharmacist.

Evaluation

Clinical response to therapy can be evaluated by: ▪ Resolution of the signs and symptoms of infection. Length of time for complete resolution depends on the organism and site of infection.

CEFOTAXIME

(sef-oh-**tax**-eem)

Claforan

CLASSIFICATION(S):

Anti-infective—third generation cephalosporin

Pregnancy Category B

INDICATIONS

▪ Treatment of: ▫ Skin and skin structure infections ▫ Bone and joint infections ▫ Urinary and gynecologic infections ▫ Respiratory tract infections ▫ Intra-abdominal infections ▫ Septicemia and meningitis due to susceptible organisms ▪ Has also been used as a perioperative prophylatic anti-infective.

ACTION

▪ Binds to the bacterial cell wall membrane, causing cell death. **Therapeutic Effect:** ▪ Bactericidal action against susceptible bacteria. **Spectrum:** ▪ Activity against staphylococci is diminished in comparison to second generation cephalosporins, while action against gram-negative pathogens is enhanced, even for organisms resistant to first and second generation agents ▪ Notable is increased action against: ▫ Citrobacter ▫ Enterobacter ▫ *Escherichia coli* ▫ *Klebsiella pneumoniae* ▫ Neisseria ▫ Proteus ▫ Providencia ▫ Serratia ▫ *Pseudomonas aeruginosa* ▫ Hemophilus influenzae ▪ Has some activity against anaerobes including *Bacteroides fragilis.*

PHARMACOKINETICS

Absorption: Well absorbed following IM administration.

Distribution: Widely distributed. Crosses the placenta and enters breast milk in low concentrations. CSF penetration sufficient to treat meningitis.

Metabolism and Excretion: Partly metabolized and partly excreted in the urine.

Half-life: 0.9–1.7 hr.

CONTRAINDICATIONS AND PRECAUTIONS

Contraindicated in: ▪ Hypersensitivity to cephalosporins ▪ Serious hypersensitivity to penicillins.

Use Cautiously in: ▪ Pregnancy or lactation (safety not established) ▪ Renal impairment (dosage reduction required).

ADVERSE REACTIONS AND SIDE EFFECTS*

Derm: rashes, urticaria.

GI: nausea, vomiting, diarrhea,

*Underlines indicate most frequent; **CAPITALS** indicate life-threatening.

cramps, **PSEUDOMEMBRANOUS COLITIS.**
Hemat: blood dyscrasias, hemolytic anemia.
Local: phlebitis at IV site, pain at IM site.
Misc: superinfection, allergic reactions including **ANAPHYLAXIS** and serum sickness.

INTERACTIONS

Drug–Drug: ▪ **Probenecid** decreases excretion and increases serum levels.

ROUTE AND DOSAGE

- **IM, IV (Adults):** 1–2 g q 6–8 hr (up to 12 g/day).
- **IM, IV (Children >1 mon):** 50–180 mg/kg/day in divided doses q 4–6 hr.
- **IV (Infants 1–4 wk):** 50 mg/kg q 8 hr.
- **IV (Infants 0–1 wk):** 50 mg/kg q 12 hr.

PHARMACODYNAMICS (blood levels)

	ONSET	PEAK
IM	rapid	0.5 hr
IV	rapid	end of infusion

NURSING IMPLICATIONS

Assessment

- Assess patient for infection (vital signs; appearance of wound, sputum, urine, and stool; WBC) at beginning and throughout course of therapy.
- Obtain a history before initiating therapy to determine previous use of and reactions to penicillins or cephalosporins. Persons with a negative history of penicillin sensitivity may still have an allergic response.
- Obtain specimens for culture and sensitivity prior to initiating therapy. First dose may be given before receiving results.
- Observe patient for signs and symptoms of anaphylaxis (rash, pruritus, laryngeal edema, wheezing). Discontinue the drug and notify the physician immediatley if these occur. Keep epinephrine, an antihistamine, and resuscitation equipment close by in the event of an anaphylactic reaction.
- **Lab Test Considerations:** May cause false-positive Coombs' test.
- May cause transient increase in BUN, SGOT (AST), SGPT (ALT), LDH, and alkaline phosphatase levels.

Potential Nursing Diagnoses

- Infection, high risk for (indications, side effects).
- Bowel elimination, altered: diarrhea (adverse reactions).
- Knowledge deficit related to medication regimen (patient/family teaching).

Implementation

- **General Info:** Reconstituted soln may range in color from light yellow to amber.
- Change IV sites every 48–72 hr to prevent phlebitis.
- Manufacturer recommends discontinuation of other IV solns during IV administration of cephalosporins.
- **IM:** Reconstitute IM doses with 2, 3, or 5 ml of sterile or bacteriostatic water for injection in the 500-mg, 1-g, and 2-g vials, respectively. Shake well to dissolve.
- Inject deep into well-developed muscle mass, massage well.
- **Direct IV:** Dilute in 10 ml of sterile or bacteriostatic water for injection. Do not use preparations containing benzyl alcohol when used for neonates.
- *Rate:* Administer slowly over 3–5 min. Monitor for phlebitis.
- **Intermittent Infusion:** Reconstituted soln may be further diluted in 50–100 ml of D5W, D10W, lactated Ringer's soln, D5/0.25% NaCl, D5/0.45% NaCl, D5/0.9% NaCl, or 0.9% NaCl. Stable for 24 hr at room temperature and 5 days if refrigerated.
- *Rate:* Administer IV infusion over 30 min.
- **Syringe Compatibility:** heparin.
- **Y-Site Compatibility:** acyclovir, cyclophosphamide, famotidine, hydromorphone, magnesium sulfate, meperidine, morphine, ondansetron, or perphenazine.
- **Y-Site Incompatibility:** hetastarch.

C

- **Additive Compatibility:** clindamycin, metronidazole, or verapamil.
- **Additive Incompatibility:** Do not admix with aminoglycosides.

PATIENT/FAMILY TEACHING

- Advise patient to report the signs of superinfection (furry overgrowth on the tongue, vaginal itching or discharge, loose or foul-smelling stools) and allergy.
- Instruct patient to notify physician if fever and diarrhea develop, especially if stool contains blood, pus, or mucus. Advise patient not to treat diarrhea without consulting physician or pharmacist.

EVALUATION

Clinical response to therapy can be evaluated by: ▪ Resolution of the signs and symptoms of infection. Length of time for complete resolution depends on the organism and site of infection.

CEFOTETAN

(sef-oh-**tee**-tan)
Cefotan

CLASSIFICATION(S):
Anti-infective—second generation cephalosporin
Pregnancy Category B

INDICATIONS

▪ Treatment of the following infections due to susceptible organisms: ▫ Respiratory tract infections ▫ Skin and skin structure infections ▫ Bone and joint infections ▫ Urinary tract and gynecologic infections ▫ Septicemia ▫ Intra-abdominal and biliary tract infections ▪ Has also been used as a perioperative prophylactic anti-infective.

ACTION

▪ Binds to bacterial cell wall membrane, causing cell death. **Therapeutic Effect:** ▪ Bactericidal action against susceptible bacteria. **Spectrum:** ▪ Many gram-positive cocci including: ▫ *Streptococcus pneumoniae* ▫ group A beta-hemolytic streptococci ▫ penicillinase-producing staphylococci ▪ Increased activity against several other important gram-negative pathogens including: ▫ *Haemophilus influenzae* ▫ Acinetobacter ▫ Enterobacter ▫ *Escherichia coli* ▫ *Klebsiella pneumoniae* ▫ *Neisseria gonorrhea* (including penicillinase-producing strains) ▫ Providencia ▫ Proteus ▫ Serratia ▪ Also active against *Bacteroides fragilis* ▪ Has no activity against: ▫ Methicillin-resistant staphylococci ▫ Enterococcus.

PHARMACOKINETICS

Absorption: Well absorbed following IM administration.

Distribution: Widely distributed. Penetration into CSF is poor. Crosses the placenta and enters breast milk in low concentrations.

Metabolism and Excretion: Excreted primarily unchanged by the kidneys.

Half-life: 3–4.6 hr (increased in renal impairment).

CONTRAINDICATIONS AND PRECAUTIONS

Contraindicated in: ▪ Hypersensitivity to cephalosporins ▪ Serious hypersensitivity to penicillins.

Use Cautiously in: ▪ Renal impairment (dosage reduction required) ▪ Pregnancy and lactation (safety not established, but has been used in obstetrical surgery).

ADVERSE REACTIONS AND SIDE EFFECTS*

Derm: rashes, urticaria.

GI: nausea, vomiting, cramps, diarrhea, PSEUDOMEMBRANOUS COLITIS.

Hemat: blood dyscrasias, hemolytic anemia, bleeding.

Local: phlebitis at IV site, pain at IM site.

Misc: superinfection, allergic reactions including ANAPHYLAXIS and serum sickness.

*Underlines indicate most frequent; CAPITALS indicate life-threatening.

INTERACTIONS

Drug–Drug: ▪ **Probenecid** decreases excretion and increases blood levels ▪ If **alcohol** is ingested within 48–72 hr, a disulfiram-like reaction may occur ▪ May increase risk of bleeding with **anticoagulants, thrombolytics, nonsteroidal anti-inflammatory agents, plicamycin,** or **valproic acid**.

ROUTE AND DOSAGE

- **IM, IV (Adults):** 1–6 g/day in divided doses q 12 hr (1–2 g may be given q 24 hr for urinary tract infections).

PHARMACODYNAMICS (blood levels)

	ONSET	PEAK
IM	rapid	1–3 hr
IV	rapid	end of infusion

NURSING IMPLICATIONS

Assessment

- **General Info:** Assess patient for infection (vital signs; appearance of wound, sputum, urine, and stool; WBC) at beginning and throughout course of therapy.
  - Obtain a history before initiating therapy to determine previous use of and reactions to penicillins or cephalosporins. Persons with a negative history of penicillin sensitivity may still have an allergic response.
  - Obtain specimens for culture and sensitivity prior to initiating therapy. First dose may be given before receiving results.
  - Observe patient for signs and symptoms of anaphylaxis (rash, pruritus, laryngeal edema, wheezing). Discontinue the drug and notify the physician immediately if these occur. Keep epinephrine, an antihistamine, and resuscitation equipment close by in the event of an anaphylactic reaction.
- **Lab Test Considerations:** Monitor prothrombin time and assess patient for bleeding (guaiac stools; check for hematuria, bleeding gums, ecchymosis) daily in patients receiving cefotetan as it may cause hypoprothrombinemia. Elderly or debilitated patients are at greater risk of developing hypoprothrombinemia. If bleeding occurs it can be reversed with vitamin K, or prophylactic vitamin K 10 mg/wk can be given.
  - May cause false-positive results for Coombs' test and urine glucose when tested with copper sulfate method (Clinitest). Use glucose oxidase method (Clinistix or Tes-Tape) to test urine glucose.
  - May cause transient elevations in SGOT (AST), SGPT (ALT), LDH, and alkaline phosphatase concentrations.
  - May cause falsely elevated serum and urine creatinine concentrations. Do not draw serum samples within 2 hr of administration.

Potential Nursing Diagnoses

- Infection, high risk for (indications, side effects).
- Bowel elimination, altered: diarrhea (adverse reactions).
- Knowledge deficit related to medication regimen (patient/family teaching).

Implementation

- **General Info:** Reconstituted soln may range from colorless to yellow in color.
- **IM:** Reconstitute IM doses with 2 ml of sterile or bacteriostatic water for injection or 0.9% NaCl for injection for each 1-g vial, and 3 ml for each 2-g vial. Physician may order dilution with 0.5% or 1% lidocaine to minimize injection discomfort.
  - Inject deep into a well-developed muscle mass, massage well.
- **IV:** Change IV sites every 48–72 hr to prevent phlebitis.
  - Manufacturer recommends discontinuation of other IV solns during IV administration of cephalosporins.
- **Direct IV:** Dilute in at least 1 g/10 ml.
  - *Rate:* Administer slowly over 3–5 min. Monitor for phlebitis.
- **Intermittent Infusion:** Dilute further in 50–100 ml of D5W or 0.9% NaCl.

Soln is stable for 24 hr at room temperature and 96 hr if refrigerated.

□ *Rate:* Administer over 30–60 min.

- **Y-Site Compatibility:** famotidine, meperidine, or morphine.
- **Additive Incompatibility:** Do not admix with aminoglycosides.

Patient/Family Teaching

- **General Info:** Advise patient to report the signs of superinfection (furry overgrowth on the tongue, vaginal itching or discharge, loose or foul-smelling stools) and allergy.

□ Caution patient that concurrent use of alcohol with cefotetan may cause a disulfiram-like reaction (abdominal cramps, nausea, vomiting, hypotension, palpitations, dyspnea, tachycardia, sweating, flushing). Alcohol and medications containing alcohol should be avoided during and for several days after therapy.

□ Instruct patient to notify physician if fever and diarrhea develop, especially if stool contains blood, pus, or mucus. Advise patient not to treat diarrhea without consulting physician or pharmacist.

Evaluation

Clinical response to therapy can be evaluated by: ▪ Resolution of the signs and symptoms of infection. Length of time for complete resolution depends on the organism and site of infection.

CEFOXITIN
(se-**fox**-i-tin)
Mefoxin

CLASSIFICATION(S):
Anti-infective—second generation cephalosporin
Pregnancy Category B

INDICATIONS

▪ Treatment of the following infections due to susceptible organisms: □ Respiratory tract infections □ Skin and skin structure infections □ Bone and joint infections □ Urinary tract and gynecologic infections □ Septicemia ▪ Has also been used as a perioperative prophylactic anti-infective.

ACTION

▪ Binds to bacterial cell wall membrane, causing cell death. **Therapeutic Effect:** ▪ Bactericidal action against susceptible bacteria. **Spectrum:** ▪ Many gram-positive cocci including: □ *Streptococcus pneumoniae* □ Group A beta-hemolytic streptococci □ Penicillinase-producing staphylococci ▪ Increased activity against several other important gram-negative pathogens including: □ *Haemophilus influenzae* □ Acinetobacter □ Enterobacter □ *Escherichia coli* □ *Klebsiella pneumoniae* □ *Neisseria gonorrhea* (including penicillinase-producing strains) □ Providencia □ Proteus □ Serratia ▪ Also active against *Bacteroides fragilis* ▪ Has no activity against: □ Methicillin-resistant staphylococci □ Enterococcus.

PHARMACOKINETICS

Absorption: Well absorbed following IM administration.

Distribution: Widely distributed. Penetration into CSF is poor. Crosses the placenta and enters breast milk in low concentrations.

Metabolism and Excretion: Excreted primarily unchanged by the kidneys.

Half-life: 0.7–1.1 hr (increased in renal impairment).

CONTRAINDICATIONS AND PRECAUTIONS

Contraindicated in: ▪ Hypersensitivity to cephalosporins ▪ Serious hypersensitivity to penicillins.

Use Cautiously in: ▪ Renal impairment (dosage reduction required) ▪ Pregnancy and lactation (safety not established, but has been used in obstetrical surgery).

ADVERSE REACTIONS AND SIDE EFFECTS*

Derm: rashes, urticaria.

GI: nausea, vomiting, cramps, diar-

*Underlines indicate most frequent; **CAPITALS** indicate life-threatening.

rhea, PSEUDOMEMBRANOUS COLITIS.
Hemat: blood dyscrasias, hemolytic anemia.
Local: phlebitis at IV site, pain at IM site.
Misc: superinfection, allergic reactions including ANAPHYLAXIS and serum sickness.

INTERACTIONS

Drug–Drug: ▪ **Probenecid** decreases excretion and increases blood levels.

ROUTE AND DOSAGE

- **IM, IV (Adults):** 1–2 g q 6–8 hr (IM injection is painful).
- **IM, IV (Children and Infants >3 mon):** 80–160 mg/kg/day in divided doses q 4–6 hr.

PHARMACODYNAMICS (blood levels)

	ONSET	PEAK
IM	rapid	30 min
IV	rapid	end of infusion

NURSING IMPLICATIONS

Assessment

- Assess patient for infection (vital signs; appearance of wound, sputum, urine, and stool; WBC) at beginning and throughout course of therapy.
- Obtain a history before initiating therapy to determine previous use of and reactions to penicillins or cephalosporins. Persons with a negative history of penicillin sensitivity may still have an allergic response.
- Obtain specimens for culture and sensitivity prior to initiating therapy. First dose may be given before receiving results.
- Observe patient for signs and symptoms of anaphylaxis (rash, pruritus, laryngeal edema, wheezing). Discontinue the drug and notify the physician immediately if these occur. Keep epinephrine, an antihistamine, and resuscitation equipment close by in the event of an anaphylactic reaction.
- **Lab Test Considerations:** May cause false-positive results for Coombs' test and urine glucose when tested with copper sulfate method (Clinitest). Use glucose oxidase method (Clinistix or Tes-Tape) to test urine glucose.
- May cause transient increase in BUN, SGOT (AST), SGPT (ALT), LDH, and alkaline phosphatase levels.
- May cause falsely elevated serum and urine creatinine concentrations. Do not draw serum samples within 2 hr of administration.

Potential Nursing Diagnoses

- Infection, high risk for (indications, side effects).
- Bowel elimination, altered: diarrhea (adverse reactions).
- Knowledge deficit related to medication regimen (patient/family teaching).

Implementation

- **General Info:** Darkened powder does not alter potency.
- **IM:** Reconstitute IM doses with 2 ml of sterile water for injection to each 1-g vial. Physician may order dilution with 0.5% or 1% lidocaine HCl to minimize injection discomfort.
- Inject deep into a well-developed muscle mass, massage well.
- **IV:** Change IV sites every 48–72 hr to prevent phlebitis.
- Manufacturer recommends discontinuing other IV solns during IV administration of cephalosporins.
- **Direct IV:** Dilute with 10 ml of sterile water for injection to each 1-g vial and 20 ml to each 2-g vial. Shake well and allow to stand until soln becomes clear.
- *Rate:* Administer slowly over 3–5 min.
- **Intermittent Infusion:** Dilute further with 50–100 ml of D5W, D10W, D5/0.25% NaCl, D5/0.45% NaCl, D5/0.9% NaCl, 0.9% NaCl, D5/LR, D5/0.02%, sodium bicarbonate, or Ringer's or lactated Ringer's soln. Stable for 24 hr at room temperature and 1 wk if refrigerated.
- *Rate:* Administer infusion over 15–30 min. Monitor for phlebitis.
- **Continuous Infusion:** May be diluted in 500–1000 ml.

- **Syringe Compatibility:** heparin.
- **Y-Site Compatibility:** acyclovir, cyclophasphamide, famotidine, foscarnet, hydromorphone, magnesium sulfate, meperidine, morphine, ondansetron, or perphenazine.
- **Y-Site Incompatibility:** hetastarch.
- **Additive Compatibility:** cimetidine, clindamycin, heparin, insulin, metronidazole, multivitamin infusion, sodium bicarbonate, or verapamil.
- **Additive Incompatibility:** Do not admix with aminoglycosides.

PATIENT/FAMILY TEACHING

- □ Advise patient to report the signs of superinfection (furry overgrowth on the tongue, vaginal itching or discharge, loose or foul-smelling stools) and allergy.
- □ Instruct patient to notify physician if fever and diarrhea develop, especially if stool contains blood, pus, or mucus. Advise patient not to treat diarrhea without consulting physician or pharmacist.

EVALUATION

Clinical response to therapy can be evaluated by: ▪ Resolution of the signs and symptoms of infection. Length of time for complete resolution depends on the organism and site of infection.

CEFTAZIDIME

(sef-**tay**-zi-deem)

Ceptaz, Fortaz, {Magnacef}, Tazicef, Tazidime

CLASSIFICATION(S):
Anti-infective—third generation cephalosporins
Pregnancy Category B

INDICATIONS

▪ Treatment of: □ Skin and skin structure infections □ Bone and joint infections □ Urinary and gynecologic infections □ Respiratory tract infections □ Intra-abdominal infections □ Septicemia and meningitis due to susceptible organisms.

ACTION

▪ Binds to the bacterial cell wall membrane, causing cell death. **Therapeutic Effect:** ▪ Bactericidal action against susceptible bacteria. **Spectrum:** ▪ Activity against staphylococci is diminished in comparison to second generation cephalosporins, while action against gram-negative pathogens is enhanced, even for organisms resistant to first and second generation agents ▪ Notable is increased action against: □ Citrobacter □ Enterobacter □ *Escherichia coli* □ *Klebsiella pneumoniae* □ Neisseria □ Proteus □ Providencia □ Serratia □ *Pseudomonas aeruginosa* □ *Hemophilus influenzae* ▪ Has some activity against anaerobes including *Bacteroides fragilis*.

PHARMACOKINETICS

Absorption: Well absorbed following IM administration.
Distribution: Widely distributed. Crosses the placenta and enters breast milk in low concentrations. CSF penetration sufficient to treat meningitis.
Metabolism and Excretion: >90% excreted unchanged by the kidneys.
Half-life: 1.4–2 hr (increased in renal impairment).

CONTRAINDICATIONS AND PRECAUTIONS

Contraindicated in: ▪ Hypersensitivity to cephalosporins ▪ Serious hypersensitivity to penicillins ▪ Hypersensitivity to L-Arginine (Ceptaz formulation only).
Use Cautiously in: ▪ Renal impairment (dosage reduction required) ▪ Patients >50 yr (increased risk of renal toxicity) ▪ Pregnancy or lactation (safety not established).

ADVERSE REACTIONS AND SIDE EFFECTS*

Derm: rashes, urticaria.
GI: nausea, vomiting, diarrhea,

{} = Available in Canada only.
*Underlines indicate most frequent; **CAPITALS** indicate life-threatening.

cramps, PSEUDOMEMBRANOUS COLITIS.
Hemat: blood dyscrasias, hemolytic anemia.
Local: phlebitis at IV site, pain at IM site.
Misc: superinfection, allergic reactions including ANAPHYLAXIS and serum sickness.

INTERACTIONS

Drug-Drug: ▪ **Probenecid** decreases excretion and increases serum levels.

ROUTE AND DOSAGE

- **IM, IV (Adults):** 1–2 g q 8–12 hr (250–500 mg q 12 hr for urinary tract infections).
- **IM, IV (Children 1 mon–12 yr):** 30–50 mg/kg q 8 hr.
- **IV (Neonates <4 wk):** 30–50 mg/kg q 12 hr.

PHARMACODYNAMICS (blood levels)

	ONSET	PEAK
IM	rapid	1 hr
IV	rapid	end of infusion

NURSING IMPLICATIONS

Assessment

- Assess patient for infection (vital signs; appearance of wound, sputum, urine, and stool; WBC) at beginning and throughout course of therapy.
- Obtain a history before initiating therapy to determine previous use of and reactions to penicillins or cephalosporins. Persons with a negative history of penicillin sensitivity may still have an allergic response.
- Obtain specimens for culture and sensitivity prior to initiating therapy. First dose may be given before receiving results.
- Observe patient for signs and symptoms of anaphylaxis (rash, pruritus, laryngeal edema, wheezing). Discontinue the drug and notify the physician immediately if these occur. Keep epinephrine, an antihistamine, and resuscitation equipment close by in the event of an anaphylactic reaction.
- **Lab Test Considerations:** May cause false-positive results for Coombs' test and urine glucose when tested with copper sulfate method (Clinitest). Use glucose oxidase method (Clinistix or Tes-Tape) to test urine glucose.
- May cause increased BUN, creatinine, SGOT (AST), SGPT (ALT), LDH, and alkaline phosphatase levels.

Potential Nursing Diagnoses

- Infection, high risk for (indications, side effects).
- Bowel elimination, altered: diarrhea (adverse reactions).
- Knowledge deficit related to medication regimen (patient/family teaching).

Implementation

- **General Info:** Dilution causes carbon dioxide to form inside vial resulting in positive pressure; vial may require venting after dissolution to preserve sterility of vial. Not required with L-Arginine formulation (Ceptaz).
- Soln may range from light yellow to amber; darkened soln or powder does not alter potency.
- **IM:** Reconstitute IM doses with 1.5 ml of sterile or bacteriostatic water for injection in each 500-mg vial and 3 ml in each 1 g-vial. Physician may order dilution with 0.5% or 1% lidocaine HCl to minimize injection discomfort.
- Inject deep into a well-developed muscle mass; massage well.
- **IV:** Change IV sites every 48–72 hr to prevent phlebitis.
- Manufacturer recommends discontinuing other IV solns during IV administration of cephalosporins.
- **Direct IV:** Add 5 ml of sterile water for injection to each 500-mg vial or 10 ml to each 1- or 2-g vial. Do not use preparations with benzyl alcohol when used for neonates.
- *Rate:* Administer slowly over 3–5 min.
- **Intermittent Infusion:** Reconstituted soln may be further diluted in at least 1 g/10 ml of 0.9% NaCl, D5W, D10W, D5/0.25% NaCl, D5/0.45% NaCl, D5/0.9% NaCl, or lactated Ringer's

soln. Stable for 18 hr at room temperature and 7 days if refrigerated.

- *Rate:* Administer over 30–60 min. Monitor for phlebitis.
- **Y-Site Compatibility:** acyclovir, ciprofloxacin, enalaprilat, esmolol, foscarnet, labetolol, ondansetron, or zidovudine.
- **Additive Compatibility:** ciprofloxacin, clindamycin, or metronidazole.
- **Additive Incompatibility:** Do not admix with aminoglycosides or sodium bicarbonate.

Patient/Family Teaching

- Advise patient to report the signs of superinfection (furry overgrowth on the tongue, vaginal itching or discharge, loose or foul-smelling stools) and allergy.
- Instruct patient to notify physician if fever and diarrhea develop, especially if stool contains blood, pus, or mucus. Advise patient not to treat diarrhea without consulting physician or pharmacist.

Evaluation

Clinical response to therapy can be evaluated by: ▪ Resolution of the signs and symptoms of infection. Length of time for complete resolution depends on the organism and site of infection.

CEFTIZOXIME

(sef-ti-**zox**-eem)
Cefizox

CLASSIFICATION(S):
Anti-infective—third generation cephalosporin
Pregnancy Category B

INDICATIONS

▪ Treatment of: ▫ Skin and skin structure infections ▫ Bone and joint infections ▫ Urinary and gynecologic infections ▫ Respiratory tract infections ▫ Intra-abdominal infections ▫ Septicemia and meningitis due to susceptible organisms.

ACTION

▪ Binds to the bacterial cell wall membrane, causing cell death. **Therapeutic Effect:** ▪ Bactericidal action against susceptible bacteria. **Spectrum:** ▪ Activity against staphylococci is diminished in comparison to second generation cephalosporins, while action against gram-negative pathogens is enhanced, even for organisms resistant to first and second generation agents ▪ Notable is increased action against: ▫ Citrobacter ▫ Enterobacter ▫ *Escherichia coli* ▫ *Klebsiella pneumoniae* ▫ Neisseria ▫ Proteus ▫ Providencia ▫ Serratia ▫ *Pseudomonas aeruginosa* ▫ Hemophilus influenzae ▪ Has some activity against anaerobes including *Bacteroides fragilis*.

PHARMACOKINETICS

Absorption: Well absorbed following IM administration.
Distribution: Widely distributed. Crosses the placenta and enters breast milk in low concentrations. CSF penetration sufficient to treat meningitis.
Metabolism and Excretion: >90% excreted unchanged by the kidneys.
Half-life: 1.4–1.9 hr.

CONTRAINDICATIONS AND PRECAUTIONS

Contraindicated in: ▪ Hypersensitivity to cephalosporins ▪ Serious hypersensitivity to penicillins.
Use Cautiously in: ▪ Renal impairment (dosage reduction required) ▪ Pregnancy or lactation (safety not established).

ADVERSE REACTIONS AND SIDE EFFECTS*

GI: nausea, vomiting, diarrhea, cramps, PSEUDOMEMBRANOUS COLITIS.
Derm: rashes, urticaria.
Hemat: blood dyscrasias, hemolytic anemia.
Local: phlebitis at IV site, pain at IM site.
Misc: superinfection, allergic reactions

*Underlines indicate most frequent; **CAPITALS** indicate life-threatening.

including ANAPHYLAXIS and serum sickness.

INTERACTIONS

Drug–Drug: ▪ **Probenecid** decreases excretion and increases serum levels.

ROUTE AND DOSAGE

- **IM, IV (Adults):** 1–2 g q 8–12 hr.
- **IM, IV (Children >6 mon):** 50 mg/kg q 6–8 hr.

PHARMACODYNAMICS (blood levels)

	ONSET	PEAK
IM	rapid	0.5–1.5 hr
IV	rapid	end of infusion

NURSING IMPLICATIONS

Assessment

- ▫ Assess patient for infection (vital signs; appearance of wound, sputum, urine, and stool; WBC) at beginning and throughout course of therapy.
- ▫ Obtain a history before initiating therapy to determine previous use of and reactions to penicillins or cephalosporins. Persons with a negative history of penicillin sensitivity may still have an allergic response.
- ▫ Obtain specimens for culture and sensitivity prior to initiating therapy. First dose may be given before receiving results.
- ▫ Observe patient for signs and symptoms of anaphylaxis (rash, pruritus, laryngeal edema, wheezing). Discontinue the drug and notify the physician immediately if these occur. Keep epinephrine, an antihistamine, and resuscitation equipment close by in the event of an anaphylactic reaction.
- ▪ **Lab Test Considerations:** May cause false-positive results for Coombs' test.
- ▫ May cause increased BUN, creatinine, SGOT (AST), SGPT (ALT), and alkaline phosphatase levels.

Potential Nursing Diagnoses

- ▪ Infection, high risk for (indications, side effects).
- ▪ Bowel elimination, altered: diarrhea (adverse reactions).
- ▪ Knowledge deficit related to medication regimen (patient/family teaching).

Implementation

- ▪ **General Info:** Soln varies in color from yellow to amber.
- ▪ **IM:** Reconstitute IM doses with 3 ml of sterile water for injection in each 1-g vial or 6 ml in each 2-g vial for a concentration of 270 mg/ml.
- ▫ Inject deep into a well-developed muscle mass; massage well.
- ▪ **IV:** Change IV sites every 48–72 hr to prevent phlebitis.
- ▫ Manufacturer recommends discontinuing other IV solns during IV administration of cephalosporins.
- ▪ **Direct IV:** For direct IV administration dilute with 10 ml of sterile water for injection in each 1-g vial or 20 ml in each 2-g vial.
- ▫ *Rate:* Administer slowly over 3–5 min.
- ▪ **Intermittent Infusion:** May be further diluted in 50–100 ml of D5W, D10W, 0.9% NaCl, D5/0.25% NaCl, D5/0.45% NaCl, D5/0.9% NaCl, or lactated Ringer's soln. Stable for 8 hr at room temperature and 48 hr if refrigerated.
- ▫ *Rate:* Administer over 30 min. Monitor for phlebitis.
- ▪ **Y-Site Compatibility:** acyclovir, enalaprilat, esmolol, famotidine, foscarnet, hydromorphone, labetalol, meperidine, morphine, or ondansetron.
- ▪ **Additive Compatibility:** clindamycin.
- ▪ **Additive Incompatibility:** Do not admix with aminoglycosides.

Patient/Family Teaching

- ▫ Advise patient to report the signs of superinfection (furry overgrowth on the tongue, vaginal itching or discharge, loose or foul-smelling stools) and allergy.
- ▫ Instruct patient to notify physician if fever and diarrhea develop, especially if stool contains blood, pus, or mucus. Advise patient not to treat diarrhea without consulting physician or pharmacist.

C

EVALUATION

Clinical response to therapy can be evaluated by: ▪ Resolution of the signs and symptoms of infection. Length of time for complete resolution depends on the organism and site of infection.

CEFTRIAXONE
(cef-try-**ax**-one)
Rocephin

CLASSIFICATION(S):
Anti-infective—third generation cephalosporin
Pregnancy Category B

INDICATIONS

▪ Treatment of: ▫ Skin and skin structure infections ▫ Bone and joint infections ▫ Urinary and gynecologic infections ▫ Respiratory tract infections ▫ Intra-abdominal infections ▫ Meningitis due to susceptible organisms ▪ Has also been used as a perioperative prophylactic anti-infective.

ACTION

▪ Binds to the bacterial cell wall membrane, causing cell death. **Therapeutic Effect:** ▪ Bactericidal action against susceptible bacteria. **Spectrum:** ▪ Activity against staphylococci is diminished in comparison to second generation cephalosporins, while action against gram-negative pathogens is enhanced, even for organisms resistant to first and second generation agents ▪ Notable is increased action against: ▫ Citrobacter ▫ Enterobacter ▫ *Escherichia coli* ▫ *Klebsiella pneumoniae* ▫ Neisseria ▫ Proteus ▫ Providencia ▫ Serratia ▫ Hemophilus influenzae ▫ *Pseudomonas aeruginosa* ▪ Has some activity against anaerobes including *Bacteroides fragilis*.

PHARMACOKINETICS

Absorption: Well absorbed following IM administation.

Distribution: Widely distributed. Crosses the placenta and enters breast milk in low concentrations. CSF penetration sufficient to treat meningitis.

Metabolism and Excretion: Partly metabolized and partly excreted in the urine.

Half-life: 5.4–10.9 hr.

CONTRAINDICATIONS AND PRECAUTIONS

Contraindicated in: ▪ Hypersensitivity to cephalosporins ▪ Serious hypersensitivity to penicillins.

Use Cautiously in: ▪ Pregnancy or lactation (safety not established).

ADVERSE REACTIONS AND SIDE EFFECTS*

GI: nausea, vomiting, diarrhea, cramps, PSEUDOMEMBRANOUS COLITIS.

Derm: rashes, urticaria.

Hemat: blood dyscrasias, hemolytic anemia.

Local: phlebitis at IV site, pain at IM site.

Misc: superinfection, allergic reactions including ANAPHYLAXIS and serum sickness.

INTERACTIONS

Drug-Drug: ▪ **Probenecid** decreases excretion and increases serum levels.

ROUTE AND DOSAGE

- **IM, IV (Adults):** 1–2 g/day, single dose or q 12 hr.
- **IM, IV (Children):** 50–75 mg/kg/day in divided doses q 12 hr (100 mg/kg/day for meningitis).

PHARMACODYNAMICS (blood levels)

	ONSET	PEAK
IM	rapid	1–2 hr
IV	rapid	end of infusion

NURSING IMPLICATIONS

ASSESSMENT

▫ Assess patient for infection (vital signs; appearance of wound, sputum,

*Underlines indicate most frequent; CAPITALS indicate life-threatening.

urine, and stool; WBC) at beginning and throughout course of therapy.

- Obtain a history before initiating therapy to determine previous use of and reactions to penicillins or cephalosporins. Persons with a negative history of penicillin sensitivity may still have an allergic response.
- Obtain specimens for culture and sensitivity prior to initiating therapy. First dose may be given before receiving results.
- Observe patient for signs and symptoms of anaphylaxis (rash, pruritus, laryngeal edema, wheezing). Discontinue the drug and notify the physician immediately if these occur. Keep epinephrine, an antihistamine, and resuscitation equipment close by in the event of an anaphylactic reaction.
- **Lab Test Considerations:** May cause increased BUN, creatinine, SGOT (AST), SGPT (ALT), bilirubin, and alkaline phosphatase levels.
- May cause false-positive results for Coombs' test and urine glucose when copper sulfate method is used (Clinitest). Use glucose oxidase method (Clinistix, Tes-Tape) to test urine glucose.

Potential Nursing Diagnoses

- Infection, high risk for (indications, side effects).
- Bowel elimination, altered: diarrhea (adverse reactions).
- Knowledge deficit related to medication regimen (patient/family teaching).

Implementation

- **General Info:** Reconstituted soln may vary in color from light yellow to amber.
- **IM:** Reconstitute IM doses with 0.9 ml of sterile or bacteriostatic water for injection, D5W, or 0.9% NaCl for injection in each 250-mg vial, 1.8 ml in each 500-mg vial, 3.6 ml in each 1-g vial or 7.2 ml in each 2-g vial. Physician may order dilution with 1% lidocaine HCl to minimize injection discomfort.
- Inject deep into a well-developed muscle mass; massage well.
- **IV:** Change IV sites every 48–72 hr to prevent phlebitis.
- Manufacturer recommends discontinuation of other IV solns during IV administration of cephalosporins.
- **Intermittent Infusion:** For intermittent infusion reconstitute each 250-mg vial with 2.4 ml, each 500-mg vial with 4.8 ml, each 1-g vial with 9.6 ml, and each 2-g vial with 19.2 ml sterile water for injection, 0.9% NaCl, or D5W. Do not use preparations containing benzyl alcohol when used for neonates.
- Soln may be diluted further in 50–100 ml of 0.9% NaCl, D5W, D10W, D5/0.45% NaCl, or lactated Ringer's soln. Stable for 3 days at room temperature.
- *Rate:* Administer infusion over 30–60 min. Monitor for phlebitis.
- **Y-Site Compatibility:** acyclovir or zidovudine.
- **Additive Compatibility:** amino acids or sodium bicarbonate.
- **Additive Incompatibility:** Do not admix with aminoglycosides or clindamycin.

Patient/Family Teaching

- Advise patient to report the signs of superinfection (furry overgrowth on the tongue, vaginal itching or discharge, loose or foul-smelling stools) and allergy.
- Instruct patient to notify physician if fever and diarrhea develop, especially if stool contains blood, pus, or mucus. Advise patient not to treat diarrhea without consulting physician or pharmacist.

Evaluation

Clinical response to therapy can be evaluated by: ▪ Resolution of the signs and symptoms of infection. Length of time for complete resolution depends on the organism and site of infection.

C

CEFUROXIME
(se-fyoor-**ox**-eem)
Ceftin, Kefurox, Zinacef

CLASSIFICATION(S):
Anti-infective—second generation cephalosporin
Pregnancy Category B

INDICATIONS

▪ Treatment of the following infections due to susceptible organisms: ▫ Respiratory tract infections ▫ Skin and skin structure infections ▫ Bone and joint infections ▫ Urinary tract and gynecologic infections ▫ Septicemia and meningitis ▪ Oral form to treat pharyngitis, tonsillitis, and otitis ▪ Has been used as a perioperative prophylactic anti-infective.

ACTION

▪ Binds to bacterial cell wall membrane, causing cell death. **Therapeutic Effect:** ▪ Bactericidal action against susceptible bacteria. **Spectrum:** ▪ Many gram-positive cocci including: ▫ *Streptococcus pneumoniae* ▫ Group A beta-hemolytic streptococci ▫ Penicillinase-producing staphylococci ▪ Increased activity against several other important gram-negative pathogens including: ▫ *Haemophilus influenzae* ▫ Acinetobacer ▫ Enterobacter ▫ *Escherichia coli* ▫ *Klebsiella pneumoniae* ▫ *Neisseria gonorrhea* (including penicillinase-producing strains) ▫ Providencia ▫ Proteus ▫ Serratia ▪ Also active against *Bacteroides fragilis* ▪ Has no activity against: ▫ Methicillin-resistant staphylococci ▫ Enterococcus.

PHARMACOKINETICS

Absorption: Well absorbed following IM administration. Oral absorption is enhanced by food (52% with food, 37% fasting).
Distribution: Widely distributed. Penetration into CSF sufficient to treat meningitis. Crosses the placenta and enters breast milk in low concentrations.
Metabolism and Excretion: Excreted primarily unchanged by the kidneys.
Half-life: 1.3 hr (increased in renal impairment).

CONTRAINDICATIONS AND PRECAUTIONS

Contraindicated in: ▪ Hypersensitivity to cephalosporins ▪ Serious hypersensitivity to penicillins.
Use Cautiously in: ▪ Renal impairment (dosage reduction required) ▪ Pregnancy and lactation (safety not established, but has been used in obstetrical surgery).

ADVERSE REACTIONS AND SIDE EFFECTS*

GI: nausea, vomiting, cramps, diarrhea, PSEUDOMEMBRANOUS COLITIS.
Derm: rashes, urticaria.
Hemat: blood dyscrasias, hemolytic anemia.
Local: phlebitis at IV site, pain at IM site.
Misc: superinfection, allergic reactions including ANAPHYLAXIS and serum sickness.

INTERACTIONS

Drug-Drug: ▪ **Probenecid** decreases excretion and increases blood levels.

ROUTE AND DOSAGE

- **PO (Adults and Children >12 yr):** 125–500 mg twice daily.
- **IM, IV (Adults):** 750–1000 mg q 8 hr.
- **PO (Children <12 yr):** 125 mg twice daily (250 mg twice daily for otitis media in children >2 yr).
- **IM, IV (Children and Infants >3 mon):** 50–100 mg/kg/day in divided doses every 6–8 hr (for meningitis: 200–240 mg/kg/day).

PHARMACODYNAMICS (blood levels)

	ONSET	PEAK
PO	rapid	2 hr
IM	rapid	15–60 min
IV	rapid	end of infusion

*Underlines indicate most frequent; **CAPITALS** indicate life-threatening.

NURSING IMPLICATIONS

Assessment

- Assess patient for infection (vital signs; appearance of wound, sputum, urine, and stool; WBC) at beginning and throughout course of therapy.
- Obtain a history before initiating therapy to determine previous use of and reactions to penicillins or cephalosporins. Persons with a negative history of penicillin sensitivity may still have an allergic response.
- Obtain specimens for culture and sensitivity prior to initiating therapy. First dose may be given before receiving results.
- Observe patient for signs and symptoms of anaphylaxis (rash, pruritus, laryngeal edema, wheezing). Discontinue the drug and notify the physician immediately if these occur. Keep epinephrine, an antihistamine, and resuscitation equipment close by in the event of an anaphylactic reaction.
- **Lab Test Considerations:** May cause false-positive results for Coombs' test and urine glucose when tested with copper sulfate method (Clinitest). Use glucose oxidase method (Clinistix or Tes-Tape) to test urine glucose.
- May cause false-negative blood glucose test results with ferricyanide tests. Use glucose enzymatic or hexokinase tests to determine blood glucose concentrations.
- May cause increased SGOT (AST), SGPT (ALT), alkaline phosphatase and bilirubin levels and decreased hemoglobin and hematocrit levels.

Potential Nursing Diagnoses

- Infection, high risk for (indications, side effects).
- Bowel elimination, altered: diarrhea (adverse reactions).
- Knowledge deficit related to medication regimen (patient/family teaching).

Implementation

- **General Info:** Reconstituted soln is light yellow to amber in color. Do not use soln that is cloudy or contains a precipitate.
- **PO:** Tablets may be crushed and mixed with food; however, crushed tablets have a strong, persistent bitter taste. Alternative therapy should be considered for children that cannot swallow tablets.
- **IM:** Reconstitute IM doses with 3.6 ml of sterile water for injection to each 750-mg vial.
- Inject deep into a well-developed muscle mass; massage well.
- **IV:** Change IV sites every 48–72 hr to prevent phlebitis.
- Discontinue other IV solns during IV administration of cephalosporins.
- **Direct IV:** Add 8 ml of sterile water for injection to each 750-mg vial or 16 ml to 1.5-g vial for a concentration of 90 mg/ml.
- *Rate:* Administer slowly over 3–5 min.
- **Intermittent Infusion:** Soln may be further diluted in 100 ml of 0.9% NaCl, D5W, D10W, D5/0.45% NaCl, or D5/0.9% NaCl. Stable for 24 hr at room temperature and 1 wk if refrigerated.
- *Rate:* Administer over 30 min. Monitor for phlebitis.
- **Continuous Infusion:** May also be diluted in 500–1000 ml for continuous infusion.
- **Y-Site Compatibility:** acyclovir, foscarnet, hydromorphone, meperidine, morphine, or perphenazine.
- **Additive Compatibility:** clindamycin or metronidazole.
- **Additive Incompatibility:** Do not admix with aminoglycosides.

Patient/Family Teaching

- Instruct patient to take medication around the clock and to finish drug completely, even if feeling better. Caution patient that sharing of this medication may be dangerous.
- Advise patient to report the signs of superinfection (furry overgrowth on the tongue, vaginal itching or discharge, loose or foul-smelling stools) and allergy.
- Instruct patient to notify physician if fever and diarrhea develop, especially

C

if stool contains blood, pus, or mucus. Advise patient not to treat diarrhea without consulting physician or pharmacist.

EVALUATION

Clinical response to therapy can be evaluated by: ▪ Resolution of the signs and symptoms of infection. Length of time for complete resolution depends on the organism and site of infection.

CEPHALEXIN

(sef-a-**lex**-in)
{Ceporex}, Keflet, Keflex, Keftab, {Novolexin}

CLASSIFICATION(S):
Anti-infective—first generation cephalosporin
Pregnancy Category B

INDICATIONS

▪ Treatment of: ▫ Serious skin and skin structure infections ▫ Urinary tract infections ▫ Bone and joint infections ▫ Septicemia ▫ Respiratory tract infections ▫ Otitis media due to susceptible organisms.

ACTION

▪ Binds to bacterial cell wall membrane, causing cell death. **Therapeutic Effect:** ▪ Bactericidal action against susceptible bacteria. **Spectrum:** ▪ Active against many gram-positive cocci including: ▫ *Streptococcus pneumoniae* ▫ Group A beta-hemolytic streptococci ▫ Penicillinase-producing staphylococci ▪ Active against some gram-negative rods including: ▫ *Klebsiella pneumoniae* ▫ *Proteus mirabilis* ▫ *Escherichia coli* ▪ Not active against: ▫ Methicillin-resistant staphylococci ▫ *Bacteroides fragilis* ▫ Enterococcus.

PHARMACOKINETICS

Absorption: Well absorbed following oral administration.
Distribution: Widely distributed. Crosses the placenta and enters breast milk in low concentrations. Minimal penetration into CSF.
Metabolism and Excretion: Excreted almost entirely unchanged by the kidneys.
Half-life: 0.5–1.2 hr; cephradine, 0.7–2 hr.

CONTRAINDICATIONS AND PRECAUTIONS

Contraindicated in: ▪ Hypersensitivity to cephalosporins ▪ Serious hypersensitivity to penicillins.
Use Cautiously in: ▪ Renal impairment (dosage reduction required) ▪ Patients >50 yr (increased risk of renal toxicity) ▪ Pregnancy or lactation (safety not established).

ADVERSE REACTIONS AND SIDE EFFECTS*

GI: nausea, vomiting, cramps, diarrhea, PSEUDOMEMBRANOUS COLITIS.
GU: nephrotoxicity.
Derm: rashes, urticaria.
Hemat: blood dyscrasias, hemolytic anemia.
Local: phlebitis at IV site, pain at IM site.
Misc: superinfection, allergic reactions including ANAPHYLAXIS and serum sickness.

INTERACTIONS

Drug-Drug: ▪ **Probenecid** decreases excretion and increases blood levels ▪ May potentiate nephrotoxicity from other **nephrotoxic agents (aminoglycosides)**.

ROUTE AND DOSAGE

- **PO (Adults):** 250–500 mg q 6 hr.
- **PO (Children):** 25–50 mg/kg/day in divided doses q 6 hr.

PHARMACODYNAMICS (blood levels)

	ONSET	PEAK
PO	rapid	1 hr

{} = Available in Canada only.
*Underlines indicate most frequent; CAPITALS indicate life-threatening.

NURSING IMPLICATIONS

Assessment

- □ Assess patient for infection (vital signs; appearance of wound, sputum, urine, and stool; WBC) at beginning and throughout course of therapy.
- □ Obtain a history before initiating therapy to determine previous use of and reactions to penicillins or cephalosporins. Persons with a negative history of penicillin sensitivity may still have an allergic response.
- □ Obtain specimens for culture and sensitivity prior to initiating therapy. First dose may be given before receiving results.
- □ Observe patient for signs and symptoms of anaphylaxis (rash, pruritus, laryngeal edema, wheezing). Discontinue the drug and notify the physician immediately if these occur. Keep epinephrine, an antihistamine, and resuscitation equipment close by in the event of an anaphylactic reaction.
- □ Monitor intake and output ratios and daily weight. Patients with impaired renal function, over age 50, or receiving other nephrotoxic drugs are at risk for developing nephrotoxicity with high-dose therapy.
- ■ **Lab Test Considerations:** May cause false-positive results for Coombs' test and urine glucose when tested with copper sulfate method (Clinitest). Use glucose oxidase method (Clinistix or Tes-Tape) to test urine glucose.
- □ May cause elevated SGOT (AST), SGPT (ALT), and alkaline phosphatase levels.

Potential Nursing Diagnoses

- ■ Infection, high risk for (indications, side effects).
- ■ Knowledge deficit related to medication regimen (patient/family teaching).
- ■ Noncompliance related to medication regimen (patient/family teaching).

Implementation

- ■ **PO:** Administer with food or milk to minimize GI irritation. Food slows but does not decrease absorption.
- □ Also available as a suspension. Refrigerate oral suspensions.

Patient/Family Teaching

- □ Instruct patients to finish the medication completely as directed, even if feeling better. Advise patients that sharing of this medication may be dangerous.
- □ Advise patient to report the signs of superinfection (furry overgrowth on the tongue, vaginal itching or discharge, loose or foul-smelling stools) and allergy.
- □ Instruct patient to notify physician if fever and diarrhea develop, especially if stool contains blood, mucus, or pus. Advise patient not to treat diarrhea without consulting physician or pharmacist.

Evaluation

Clinical response to therapy can be evaluated by: ■ Resolution of the signs and symptoms of infection. Length of time for complete resolution depends on the organism and site of infection.

CEPHALOTHIN

(sef-**a**-loe-thin)
{Ceporacin}, {Keflin}, Keflin Neutral, Seffin Neutral

CLASSIFICATION(S):
Anti-infective—first generation cephalosporin.
Pregnancy Category B

INDICATIONS

■ Treatment of: □ Serious skin and skin structure infections □ Urinary tract infections □ Bone and joint infections □ Endocarditis □ Septicemia due to susceptible organisms ■ Has also been used as a perioperative prophylactic anti-infective.

ACTION

■ Binds to bacterial cell wall membrane, causing cell death. **Therapeutic Effect:** ■ Bactericidal action against susceptible bacteria. **Spectrum:** ■ Active against many gram-positive cocci including: □ *Streptococcus pneumoniae* □ Group A beta-hemolytic streptococci □ Penicillinase-producing staphylococci ■ Active against some gram-negative rods including: □ *Klebsiella pneumoniae* □ *Proteus mirabilis* □ *Escherichia coli* ■ Not active against: □ Methicillin-resistant staphylococci □ *Bacteroides fragilis* □ Enterococcus.

PHARMACOKINETICS

Absorption: Well absorbed following IM administration.

Distribution: Widely distributed. Crosses the placenta and enters breast milk in low concentrations. Minimal penetration into CSF.

Metabolism and Excretion: Excreted almost entirely unchanged by the kidneys.

Half-life: 0.5–1 hr.

CONTRAINDICATIONS AND PRECAUTIONS

Contraindicated in: ■ Hypersensitivity to cephalosporins ■ Serious hypersensitivity to penicillins.

Use Cautiously in: ■ Renal impairment (dosage reduction required) ■ Patients >50 yr (increased risk of renal toxicity) ■ Pregnancy or lactation (safety not established).

ADVERSE REACTIONS AND SIDE EFFECTS*

GI: nausea, vomiting, cramps, diarrhea, PSEUDOMEMBRANOUS COLITIS.

GU: nephrotoxicity.

Derm: rashes, urticaria.

Hemat: blood dyscrasias, hemolytic anemia.

Local: phlebitis at IV site, pain at IM site.

Misc: superinfection, allergic reactions including ANAPHYLAXIS and serum sickness.

INTERACTIONS

Drug-Drug: ■ **Probenecid** decreases excretion and increases blood levels ■ May potentiate nephrotoxicity from other **nephrotoxic agents (aminoglycosides)**.

ROUTE AND DOSAGE

- **IM, IV (Adults):** 1–2 g q 4–6 hr.
- **IM, IV (Children):** 80–160 mg/kg/day in divided doses q 6 hr.

PHARMACODYNAMICS (blood levels)

	ONSET	PEAK
IM	rapid	0.5 hr
IV	rapid	end of infusion

NURSING IMPLICATIONS

Assessment

- □ Assess patient for infection (vital signs; appearance of wound, sputum, urine, and stool; WBC) at beginning and throughout course of therapy.
- □ Obtain a history before initiating therapy to determine previous use of and reactions to penicillins or cephalosporins. Persons with a negative history of penicillin sensitivity may still have an allergic response.
- □ Obtain specimens for culture and sensitivity prior to initiating therapy. First dose may be given before receiving results.
- □ Observe patient for signs and symptoms of anaphylaxis (rash, pruritus, laryngeal edema, wheezing). Discontinue the drug and notify the physician immediately if these occur. Keep epinephrine, an antihistamine, and resuscitation equipment close by in the event of an anaphylactic reaction.
- □ Monitor intake and output ratios and daily weight. Patients with impaired renal function, over age 50, or receiving other nephrotoxic drugs are at risk for developing nephrotoxicity with high-dose therapy.
- ■ **Lab Test Considerations:** May cause false-positive results for Coombs' test and urine glucose when tested with copper sulfate method (Clinitest). Use glucose oxidase method (Clinistix or Tes-Tape) to test urine glucose.

*Underlines indicate most frequent; **CAPITALS** indicate life-threatening.

□ May cause increased BUN, SGOT (AST), SGPT (ALT), and alkaline phosphatase levels.

Potential Nursing Diagnoses

- Infection, high risk for (indications, side effects).
- Bowel elimination, altered: diarrhea (adverse reactions).
- Knowledge deficit related to medication regimen (patient/family teaching).

Implementation

- **General Info:** Darkened color of soln does not affect potency. Do not administer soln that is cloudy or contains a precipitate.
- **IM:** Reconstitute IM doses with 4 ml of sterile water for injection to each 1-g vial. May use additional diluent (0.2–0.4 ml) and warm slightly to facilitate dissolution.

□ Inject deep into a well-developed muscle mass; massage well.

- **IV:** Change IV sites every 48–72 hr to prevent phlebitis.

□ Discontinue other IV solns during IV administration of cephalosporins.

□ Hydrocortisone 10–25 mg may be added to infusions containing 4–6 g or more of cephalothin to decrease the incidence of thrombophlebitis.

- **Direct IV:** Dilute in at least 1 g/10 ml of sterile water for injection, D5W, or 0.9% NaCl.

□ *Rate:* Administer slowly over 3–5 min.

- **Intermittent Infusion:** Reconstituted 1-g or 2-g soln may be further diluted in 50 ml of D5W, D10W, D5/0.9% NaCl, D5/LR, lactated Ringer's soln, or 0.9% NaCl. Stable for 24 hr at room temperature and 96 hr if refrigerated.

□ *Rate:* Administer over 15–30 min. Monitor for phlebitis.

- **Continuous Infusion:** May also be diluted in 500–1000 ml for continuous infusion.
- **Syringe Compatibility:** cimetidine.
- **Syringe Incompatibility:** metoclopramide.
- **Y-Site Compatibility:** cyclophosphamide, famotidine, heparin, hydromorphone, magnesium sulfate, meperidine, morphine, multivitamins, perphenazine, or potassium chloride.
- **Additive Compatibility:** ascorbic acid, chloramphenicol, clindamycin, fluorouracil, hydrocortisone sodium succinate, isoproterenol, magnesium sulfate, metaraminol bitartrate, methicillin, methotrexate, potassium chloride, prednisolone sodium phosphate, procaine hydrochloride, or sodium bicarbonate.
- **Additive Incompatibility:** amikacin, aminophylline, amobarbital, bleomycin, calcium chloride, calcium gluceptate, calcium gluconate, colistimethate, diphenydramine, doxorubicin, erythromycin, gentamicin, kanamycin, oxytetracycline, pentobarbital, penicillin G sodium, phenobarbital, polymyxin B, prochlorperazine, or tetracycline. Do not admix with aminoglycosides.

Patient/Family Teaching

□ Advise patient to report the signs of superinfection (furry overgrowth on the tongue, vaginal itching or discharge, loose or foul-smelling stools) and allergy.

□ Instruct patient to notify physician if fever and diarrhea develop, especially if stool contains blood, mucus, or pus. Advise patient not to treat diarrhea without consulting physician or pharmacist.

Evaluation

Clinical response to therapy can be evaluated by: ▪ Resolution of the signs and symptoms of infection. Length of time for complete resolution depends on the organism and site of infection.

CEPHAPIRIN

(sef-a-pye-rin)

Cefadyl

CLASSIFICATION(S):

Anti-infective—first generation cephalosporin

Pregnancy Category B

INDICATIONS

■ Treatment of: □ Serious skin and skin structure infections □ Urinary tract infections □ Bone and joint infections □ Endocarditis □ Septicemia due to susceptible organisms ■ Has also been used as a perioperative prophylactic anti-infective.

ACTION

■ Binds to bacterial cell wall membrane, causing cell death. **Therapeutic Effect:** ■ Bactericidal action against susceptible bacteria. **Spectrum:** ■ Active against many gram-positive cocci including: □ *Streptococcus pneumoniae* □ Group A beta-hemolytic streptococci □ Penicillinase-producing staphylococci ■ Active against some gram-negative rods including: □ *Klebsiella pneumoniae* □ *Proteus mirabilis* □ *Escherichia coli* ■ Not active against: □ Methicillin-resistant staphylococci □ *Bacteroides fragilis* □ Enterococcus.

PHARMACOKINETICS

Absorption: Well absorbed following IM administration.
Distribution: Widely distributed. Crosses the placenta and enters breast milk in low concentrations. Minimal penetration into CSF.
Metabolism and Excretion: Excreted almost entirely unchanged by the kidneys.
Half-life: 0.4–0.8 hr.

CONTRAINDICATIONS AND PRECAUTIONS

Contraindicated in: ■ Hypersensitivity to cephalosporins ■ Serious hypersensitivity to penicillins.
Use Cautiously in: ■ Renal impairment (dosage reduction required) ■ Pregnancy or lactation (safety not established).

ADVERSE REACTIONS AND SIDE EFFECTS*

GI: nausea, vomiting, cramps, diarrhea.
Derm: rashes, urticaria.
Hemat: blood dyscrasias, hemolytic anemia, bleeding.
Local: phlebitis at IV site, pain at IM site.
Misc: superinfection, allergic reactions including ANAPHYLAXIS and serum sickness.

INTERACTIONS

Drug-Drug: ■ **Probenecid** decreases excretion and increases blood levels.

ROUTE AND DOSAGE

- **IM, IV (Adults):** 500–1000 mg q 4–6 hr.
- **IM, IV (Children > 3 mon):** 40–80 mg/kg/day in divided doses every 6 hr.

PHARMACODYNAMICS (blood levels)

	ONSET	PEAK
IM	rapid	0.5
IV	rapid	end of infusion

NURSING IMPLICATIONS

Assessment

□ Assess patient for infection (vital signs; appearance of wound, sputum, urine, and stool; WBC) at beginning and throughout course of therapy.

□ Obtain a history before initiating therapy to determine previous use of and reactions to penicillins or cephalosporins. Persons with a negative history of penicillin sensitivity may still have an allergic response.

□ Obtain specimens for culture and sensitivity prior to initiating therapy. First dose may be given before receiving results.

□ Observe patient for signs and symptoms of anaphylaxis (rash, pruritus, laryngeal edema, wheezing). Discontinue the drug and notify the physician immediately if these occur. Keep epinephrine, an antihistamine, and resuscitation equipment close by in the event of an anaphylactic reaction.

■ **Lab Test Considerations:** May cause false-positive results for Coombs' test

*Underlines indicate most frequent; **CAPITALS** indicate life-threatening.

and urine glucose when tested with copper sulfate method (Clinitest). Use glucose oxidase method (Clinistix or Tes-Tape) to test urine glucose.
- □ May cause transient increase in BUN, SGOT (AST), SGPT (ALT), alkaline phosphatase and bilirubin levels.

POTENTIAL NURSING DIAGNOSES

- ■ Infection, high risk for (indications, side effects).
- ■ Bowel elimination, altered: diarrhea (adverse reactions).
- ■ Knowledge deficit related to medication regimen (patient/family teaching).

IMPLEMENTATION

- ■ **General Info:** Soln color changes do not alter potency.
- ■ **IM:** Reconstitute IM doses with 1 or 2 ml of sterile or bacteriostatic water for injection to each 1- or 2-g vial, respectively.
- □ Inject deep into a well-developed muscle mass; massage well.
- ■ **IV:** Change IV sites every 48–72 hr to prevent phlebitis.
- □ Discontinue other IV solns during IV administration of cephalosporins.
- ■ **Direct IV:** Dilute in 10 ml or more of bacteriostatic water for injection, D5W, or 0.9% NaCl.
- □ *Rate:* Administer slowly over 3–5 min.
- ■ **Intermittent Infusion:** Reconstituted soln may be further diluted in 50–100 ml of 0.9% NaCl, D5W, D10W, D20W, D5/0.25% NaCl, D5/0.45% NaCl, D5/0.9% NaCl, or D5/LR. Stable for 24 hr at room temperature and 10 days if refrigerated.
- □ *Rate:* Administer over 15–20 min. Monitor for phlebitis.
- ■ **Continuous Infusion:** Soln may also be diluted in 500–1000 ml for continuous infusion.
- ■ **Y-Site Compatibility:** acyclovir, cyclophosphamide, famotidine, heparin, hydrocortisone sodium succinate, hydromorphone, magnesium sulfate, meperidine, morphine, multivitamins, perphenazine, or potassium chloride.
- ■ **Additive Compatibility:** bleomycin, calcium chloride, calcium gluconate, chloramphenicol, diphenhydramine, ergonovine maleate, heparin, hydrocortisone sodium phosphate, hydrocortisone sodium succinate, metaraminol bitartrate, oxacillin, penicillin G potassium, pentobarbital, phenobarbital, phytonadione, potassium chloride, sodium bicarbonate, succinylcholine, verapamil, or warfarin.
- ■ **Additive Incompatibility:** amikacin, ascorbic acid, epinephrine, gentamicin, kanamycin, mannitol, norepinephrine, oxytetracycline, phenytoin, tetracycline, or thiopental. Do not admix with aminoglycosides.

PATIENT/FAMILY TEACHING

- □ Advise patient to report the signs of superinfection (furry overgrowth on the tongue, vaginal itching or discharge, loose or foul-smelling stools) and allergy.
- □ Instruct patient to notify physician if fever and diarrhea develop, especially if stool contains blood, mucus, or pus. Advise patient not to treat diarrhea without consulting physician or pharmacist.

EVALUATION

Clinical response to therapy can be evaluated by: ■ Resolution of the signs and symptoms of infection. Length of time for complete resolution depends on the organism and site of infection.

CEPHRADINE

(**sef**-re-deen)
Anspor, Velosef

CLASSIFICATION(S):
Anti-infective—first generation cephalosporin
Pregnancy Category B

INDICATIONS

■ Treatment of: □ Serious skin and skin structure infections □ Urinary tract infections □ Bone and joint infection □ Respiratory tract infections ▫ Otitis media ▫ Septicemia due to susceptible organisms ▪ Has also been used as a perioperative prophylactic anti-infective.

ACTION

▪ Binds to bacterial cell wall membrane, causing cell death. **Therapeutic Effect:** ▪ Bactericidal action against susceptible bacteria. **Spectrum:** ▪ Active against many gram-positive cocci including: ▫ *Streptococcus pneumoniae* ▫ Group A beta-hemolytic streptococci ▫ Penicillinase-producing staphylococci ▪ Active against some gram-negative rods including: ▫ *Klebsiella pneumoniae* ▫ *Proteus mirabilis* ▫ *Escherichia coli* ▪ Not active against: ▫ Methicillin-resistant staphylococci ▫ *Bacteroides fragilis* ▫ Enterococcus.

PHARMACOKINETICS

Absorption: Well absorbed following oral and IM administration.

Distribution: Widely distributed. Crosses the placenta and enters breast milk in low concentrations. Minimal penetration into CSF.

Metabolism and Excretion: Excreted almost entirely unchanged by the kidneys.

Half-life: 0.7–2 hr.

CONTRAINDICATIONS AND PRECAUTIONS

Contraindicated in: ▪ Hypersensitivity to cephalosporins ▪ Serious hypersensitivity to penicillins.

Use Cautiously in: ▪ Renal impairment (dosage reduction required). ▪ Pregnancy or lactation (safety not established).

ADVERSE REACTIONS AND SIDE EFFECTS*

GI: <u>nausea</u>, <u>vomiting</u>, cramps, <u>diarrhea</u>, PSEUDOMEMBRANOUS COLITIS.

Derm: <u>rashes</u>, urticaria.

Hemat: blood dyscrasias, hemolytic anemia.

Local: <u>phlebitis</u> at IV site, <u>pain</u> at IM site.

Misc: superinfection, allergic reactions including ANAPHYLAXIS and serum sickness.

INTERACTIONS

Drug-Drug: ▪ **Probenecid** decreases excretion and increases blood levels.

ROUTE AND DOSAGE

- **PO (Adults):** 250 mg q 6 hr or 500 mg q 12 hr.
- **PO (Children >9 mon):** 25–100 mg/kg/day in divided doses q 6–12 hr.
- **IM, IV (Adults):** 500–1000 mg q 6 hr.
- **IM, IV (Children >1 yr):** 50–100 mg/kg/day in divided doses q 6 hr.

PHARMACODYNAMICS (blood levels)

	ONSET	PEAK
PO, IM	rapid	1–2
IV	rapid	end of infusion

NURSING IMPLICATIONS

Assessment

- ▫ Assess patient for infection (vital signs; appearance of wound, sputum, urine, and stool; WBC) at beginning and throughout course of therapy.
- ▫ Obtain a history before initiating therapy to determine previous use of and reactions to penicillins or cephalosporins. Persons with a negative history of penicillin sensitivity may still have an allergic response.
- ▫ Obtain specimens for culture and sensitivity prior to initiating therapy. First dose may be given before receiving results.
- ▫ Observe patient for signs and symptoms of anaphylaxis (rash, pruritus, laryngeal edema, wheezing). Discontinue the drug and notify the physician immediately if these occur. Keep epinephrine, an antihistamine, and resusitation equipment close by in the event of an anaphylactic reaction.
- ▪ **Lab Test Considerations:** May cause false-positive results for Coombs' test and urine glucose when tested with copper sulfate method (Clinitest).

*<u>Underlines</u> indicate most frequent; **CAPITALS** indicate life-threatening.

Use glucose oxidase method (Clinistix or Tes-Tape) to test urine glucose.
- May cause transient increase in BUN, SGOT (AST), SGPT (ALT), LDH, alkaline phosphatase, and bilirubin levels.

Potential Nursing Diagnoses
- Infection, high risk for (indications, side effects).
- Knowledge deficit related to medication regimen (patient/family teaching).
- Noncompliance related to medication regimen (patient/family teaching).

Implementation
- **General Info:** Reconstituted parenteral doses may vary in color from light straw to yellow. Color changes do not alter potency.
- **PO:** Administer oral doses with food or milk to minimize GI irritation.
- Oral doses are also available as a suspension. Shake well. Refrigerate oral suspensions.
- **IM:** Reconstitute IM doses with 1.2 ml of sterile or bacteriostatic water for injection in each 250-mg vial, 2 ml in each 500-mg vial, 4 ml in each 1-g vial.
- Inject deep into a well-developed muscle mass; massage well.
- **IV:** Change IV sites every 48–72 hr to prevent phlebitis.
- Manufacturer recommends discontinuation of other IV solns during IV administration of cephalosporins.
- **Direct IV:** Add 5 ml of sterile water, D5W, or 0.9% NaCl to each 250- or 500-mg vial, 10 ml of diluent to each 1-g vial, and 20 ml to each 2-g vial.
- *Rate:* Administer slowly over 3–5 min.
- **Intermittent Infusion:** Dilute each g in at least 10 ml of D5W, D10W, 0.9% NaCl, or D5/0.9% NaCl. Stable for 10 hr at room temperature and 48 hr if refrigerated.
- *Rate:* Administer over 30–60 min. Monitor for phlebitis.
- **Additive Incompatibility:** other antibiotics, calcium salts, epinephrine, lidocaine, Ringer's or lactated Ringer's soln, or tetracyclines.

Patient/Family Teaching
- Instruct patients to finish the drug completely as directed, even if feeling better. Advise patients that sharing of this medication may be dangerous.
- Advise patient to report the signs of superinfection (furry overgrowth on the tongue, vaginal itching or discharge, loose or foul-smelling stools) and allergy.
- Instruct patient to notify physician if fever and diarrhea develop, especially if stool contains blood, mucus, or pus. Advise patient not to treat diarrhea without consulting physician or pharmacist.

Evaluation

Clinical response to therapy can be evaluated by: ▪ Resolution of the signs and symptoms of infection. Length of time for complete resolution depends on the organism and site of infection.

CHLORAL HYDRATE
(klor-al-**hye**-drate)
Aquachloral, Noctec, {Novachlor-hydrate}

CLASSIFICATION(S):
Sedative/hypnotic
Schedule IV
Pregnancy Category C

INDICATIONS
▪ Short-term sedative and hypnotic (effectiveness decreases after 2 wk of use) ▪ Sedation or reduction of anxiety preoperatively (anesthetic adjunct) ▪ With analgesics to control pain postoperatively (analgesic adjunct).

ACTION
▪ Converted to trichloroethanol, which is the active drug. Has generalized CNS depressant properties. **Therapeutic Effect:** ▪ Sedation or induction of sleep.

C

PHARMACOKINETICS

Absorption: Well absorbed following oral or rectal administration.

Distribution: Widely distributed. Crosses the placenta and enters breast milk in low concentrations.

Metabolism and Excretion: Converted by liver to trichloroethanol, which is active. Trichloroethanol is, in turn, metabolized by the liver and kidneys to inactive compounds.

Half-life: 8–10 hr (trichloroethanol).

CONTRAINDICATIONS AND PRECAUTIONS

Contraindicated in: ▪ Hypersensitivity ▪ Coma or pre-existing CNS depression ▪ Uncontrolled severe pain ▪ Pregnancy and lactation ▪ Esophagitis, gastritis, or ulcer disease ▪ Proctitis (rectal use).

Use Cautiously in: ▪ Hepatic dysfunction ▪ Severe renal impairment ▪ Patients who may be suicidal or who may have been addicted to drugs previously ▪ Elderly patients (reduce dosage).

ADVERSE REACTIONS AND SIDE EFFECTS*

CNS: excess sedation, hangover, disorientation, headache, irritability, dizziness, incoordination.

Resp: respiratory depression.

Derm: rashes.

GI: nausea, vomiting, diarrhea, flatulence.

Misc: tolerance, psychological dependence, physical dependence.

INTERACTIONS

Drug-Drug: ▪ Additive CNS depression with other **CNS depressants** including **alcohol, antihistamines, antidepressants, sedative/hypnotics,** and **narcotic analgesics** ▪ May potentiate **oral anticoagulants** ▪ When given within 24 hr of IV **furosemide** may cause diaphoresis, changes in blood pressure, and flushing.

ROUTE AND DOSAGE

Anxiety, Sedation

- **PO, Rect (Adults):** 250 mg 3 times daily.
- **PO, Rect (Children):** 25 mg/kg/day in divided doses.

Insomnia

- **PO, Rect (Adults):** 500–1000 mg at bedtime.
- **PO, Rect (Children):** 50 mg/kg.

Preoperative

- **PO (Adults):** 500 mg–1 g 30 min before surgery.

Pre-EEG Sedation

- **PO (Children):** 25–50 mg/kg.

PHARMACODYNAMICS (sedation)

	ONSET	PEAK	DURATION
PO	30 min	UK	4–8 hr
Rect	0.5–1 hr	UK	4–8 hr

NURSING IMPLICATIONS

Assessment

- □ Assess mental status, sleep patterns, and potential for abuse prior to administering this medication. Prolonged use may lead to physical and psychological dependence. Limit amount of drug available to the patient.
- □ Assess alertness at time of peak effect. Notify physician if desired sedation does not occur or if paradoxical reaction occurs.
- ▪ **Lab Test Considerations:** Interferes with copper sulfate urine glucose test results (Clinitest). Test for urine glucose with glucose oxidase method (Ketodiastix or Tes-Tape).
- □ Interferes with tests for urinary 17-hydroxycorticosteroids and urinary catecholamines.

Potential Nursing Diagnoses

- ▪ Sleep pattern disturbance (indications).

*Underlines indicate most frequent; **CAPITALS** indicate life-threatening.

- Anxiety (indications).
- Injury, high risk for (side effects).

IMPLEMENTATION

- **General Info:** Before administering, reduce external stimuli and provide comfort measures to increase effectiveness of medication.
- Protect patient from injury. Place bed side rails up. Assist with ambulation. Remove cigarettes from patients receiving hypnotic dose.
- **PO:** Capsules should be swallowed whole with a full glass of water or juice to minimize gastric irritaton; do not chew. Dilute syrup in ½ glass of water or juice.
- **Rect:** If suppository is too soft for insertion, chill in refrigerator for 30 min or run under cold water before removing foil wrapper.

PATIENT/FAMILY TEACHING

- Instruct patient to take chloral hydrate exactly as directed. Missed doses should be omitted; do not double doses. If used for 2 wk or longer, abrupt withdrawal may result in CNS excitement, tremor, anxiety, hallucinations, and delirium.
- Chloral hydrate causes drowsiness or dizziness. Caution patient to avoid driving or other activities requiring alertness until response to medication is known.
- Caution patient that concurrent alcohol use may create an additive effect that results in tachycardia, vasodilation, flushing, headache, hypotension, and pronounced CNS depression. Alcohol and other CNS depressants should be avoided while taking chloral hydrate.
- Advise patient to discontinue use and notify physician if skin rash, dizziness, irritability, impaired thought processes, headache, or motor incoordination occur.

EVALUATION

Effectiveness of therapy can be demonstrated by: ▪ Sedation ▪ Improvement in sleep pattern.

CHLORAMBUCIL

(klor-**am**-byoo-sill)
Leukeran

CLASSIFICATION(S):
Antineoplastic—alkylating agent
Pregnancy Category D

INDICATIONS

▪ Management of chronic lymphocytic leukemia, malignant lymphoma, and Hodgkin's disease (alone and in combination with other agents).

ACTION

▪ An alkylating agent that interferes with cellular protein synthesis (cell cycle-phase nonspecific). **Therapeutic Effect:** ▪ Death of rapidly replicating cells, particularly malignant cells.

PHARMACOKINETICS

Absorption: Rapidly and completely absorbed from the GI tract.
Distribution: Crosses the placenta.
Metabolism and Excretion: Extensively metabolized by the liver.
Half-life: 1.5 hr.

CONTRAINDICATIONS AND PRECAUTIONS

Contraindicated in: ▪ Hypersensitivity ▪ Previous resistance ▪ Pregnancy or lactation.
Use Cautiously in: Patients with childbearing potential ▪ Infection ▪ Other chronic debilitating diseases.

ADVERSE REACTIONS AND SIDE EFFECTS*

Resp: pulmonary fibrosis.
GI: nausea, vomiting, stomatitis (rare).
GU: decreased sperm count, infertility.
Derm: rash, dermatitis, alopecia (rare).
Hemat: anemia, leukopenia, thrombocytopenia.
Metab: <u>hyperuricemia</u>.
Misc: allergic reactions, risk of second malignancy.

*<u>Underlines</u> indicate most frequent; **CAPITALS** indicate life-threatening.

INTERACTIONS

Drug–Drug: Additive bone marrow depression with other **bone marrow depressants (antineoplastics)** ▪ May decrease antibody response to **live vaccines** and increase the risk of adverse reactions.

ROUTE AND DOSAGE

- **PO (Adults):** 0.1–0.2 mg/kg/day for 3–6 wk, then adjust dose on basis of blood counts—usual maintenance dose is 2 mg/day.
- **PO (Children):** 0.1–0.2 mg/kg/day or 4.5 mg/m²/day.

PHARMACODYNAMICS (effects on white blood cell counts)

	ONSET	PEAK	DURATION
PO	7–14 days	7–14 days	14–28 days

NURSING IMPLICATIONS

Assessment

- ▫ Assess for fever, sore throat, and signs of infection. If these symptoms occur notify physician immediately.
- ▫ Assess for bleeding (bleeding gums, bruising, petechiae; guaiac stools, urine, emesis). Avoid IM injections and rectal temperatures. Hold pressure on all venipuncture sites for at least 10 min.
- ▫ Monitor intake and output ratios and daily weights. Notify physician if significant changes in totals occur.
- ▫ Monitor for symptoms of gout (increased uric acid, joint pain, edema). Encourage patient to drink at least 2 liters of fluid each day. Allopurinol may be given to decrease uric acid levels. Alkalinization of urine may be ordered to increase excretion of uric acid.
- ▫ Anemia may occur. Monitor for increased fatigue, dyspnea, and orthostatic hypotension.
- ▪ **Lab Test Considerations:** Monitor CBC and differential prior to and weekly during course of therapy. Notify physician of significant drops in granulocyte count. Leukopenia usually occurs around the third wk of therapy and persists for 1–2 wk following a short course of therapy. The nadir of leukopenia occurs in 7–14 days after a single high dose, with recovery in 2–3 wk. The neutrophil count may decrease for 10 days after last dose. Monitor platelet count throughout therapy. Thrombocytopenia usually occurs around third wk of therapy and persists for 1–2 wk following a short course of therapy. The nadir of thrombocytopenia occurs in 1–2 wk after a single dose, with recovery in 2–3 wk. Institute thrombocytopenia precautions if platelet count is <150,000/mm.³
- ▫ Monitor liver function tests, BUN, serum creatinine, and uric acid prior to and periodically during course of therapy. May cause elevated SGPT (ALT) and alkaline phosphatase, which may reflect hepatotoxicity.

Potential Nursing Diagnoses

- ▪ Injury, high risk for (side effects).
- ▪ Infection, high risk for (side effects).
- ▪ Knowledge deficit related to medication regimen (patient/family teaching).

Implementation

- ▪ **PO:** Administer oral medication either 1 hr before or 2 hr after meals. Can be compounded into a suspension by pharmacist for patients who have difficulty swallowing.

Patient/Family Teaching

- ▫ Instruct patient to take medication exactly as directed, even if nausea or vomiting is a problem. Consult physician if vomiting occurs shortly after dose is taken. If a dose is missed and the medication is ordered daily, take when remembered that day. If ordered more frequently, take unless almost time for next dose. Do not double doses.
- ▫ Instruct patient to report unusual bleeding. Advise patient of thrombocytopenia precautions (use soft toothbrush, electric razor, and avoid falls; do not drink alcoholic beverages or take medication containing aspirin,

because these may precipitate gastric bleeding).
- ▫ Caution patient to avoid crowds and persons with known infections. Physician should be informed immediately if symptoms of infection occur.
- ▫ Instruct patient to inspect oral mucosa for redness and ulceration. If mouth sores occur, advise patient to use sponge brush and rinse mouth with water after eating and drinking. Consult physician if pain interferes with eating.
- ▫ Advise patients on long-term therapy to notify physician immediately if cough, shortness of breath, and fever occur.
- ▫ Instruct patient to inform physician if nausea and vomiting persist. Physician may order an antiemetic, although these side effects usually last less than 1 day and tend to decrease with continued therapy.
- ▫ Discuss with patient the possibility of hair loss. Explore methods of coping.
- ▫ This drug may cause irreversible gonadal suppression; however, patient should still practice birth control. Instruct patient to inform physician if pregnancy is suspected.
- ▫ Instruct patient not to receive any vaccinations without advice of physician.

EVALUATION

Effectiveness of therapy can be demonstrated by: ▪ Improvement of hematopoietic values in leukemia ▪ Decrease in size and spread of the tumor. Therapeutic effects of this drug are usually seen by the third wk of therapy.

CHLORAMPHENICOL

(klor-am-**fen**-i-kole)
Chloromycetin, {Novochlorocap}, {Pentamycetin}

CLASSIFICATION(S):
Anti-infective—miscellaneous
Pregnancy Category UK

INDICATIONS

▪ **PO, IV:** Management of the following serious infections due to susceptible organisms when less toxic agents cannot be used: ▫ Skin and soft tissue infections ▫ Intra-abdominal infections ▫ CNS infections ▫ Meningitis ▫ Bacteremia ▪ **Top, Otic, Ophth:** Local management of superficial infections due to susceptible organisms.

ACTION

▪ Inhibits protein synthesis in susceptible bacteria at the level of the 50S bacterial ribosome. **Therapeutic Effect:** ▪ Bacteriostatic action in susceptible organisms. **Spectrum:** ▪ Wide variety of gram-positive aerobic organisms including: ▫ *Streptococcus pneumoniae* and other streptococci ▪ Gram-negative pathogens: ▫ *Haemophilus influenzae* ▫ *Neisseria menigitidis* ▫ Salmonella ▫ Shigella ▪ Anaerobes: ▫ *Bacteroides fragilis* ▫ *Bacteroides melaninogenicus* ▪ Other organisms inhibited: ▫ Rickettsia ▫ Chlamydia ▫ Mycoplasma.

PHARMACOKINETICS

Absorption: Well absorbed following oral administration.
Distribution: Widely distributed. Crosses the blood–brain barrier with CSF levels 60% of serum values. Readily crosses the placenta and enters breast milk.
Metabolism and Excretion: Mostly metabolized by the liver. <10% excreted unchanged by the kidneys.
Half-life: 1.5–3.5 hr.

CONTRAINDICATIONS AND PRECAUTIONS

Contraindicated in: ▪ Hypersensitivity ▪ Previous toxic reaction.
Use Cautiously in: ▪ Newborns ▪ Severe liver or renal disease (increased risk of adverse reactions) ▪ Elderly patients (increased risk of adverse reactions) ▪ Discontinue if neuritis develops or blood counts fall ▪ Pregnancy or lactation (safety not established).

ADVERSE REACTIONS AND SIDE EFFECTS*

CNS: depression, confusion, headache.
EENT: optic neuritis, blurred vision.
GI: nausea, vomiting, diarrhea, bitter taste (IV only).
Derm: rashes.
Hemat: bone marrow depression, APLASTIC ANEMIA.
Neuro: peripherial neuritis.
Misc: GRAY SYNDROME in newborns, fever.

INTERACTIONS

Drug–Drug: ▪ Inhibits drug metabolizing ability of the liver and may increase effects of the following drugs: **oral hypoglycemic agents, oral anticoagulants,** and **phenytoin** ▪ **Phenobarbital** or **rifampin** may decrease blood levels of chloramphenicol ▪ May delay the therapeutic response to **vitamin B_{12}** or **folic acid** therapy ▪ Bone marrow depression may be additive with other **bone-marrow-depressing agents (antineoplastics)** ▪ Chronic high-dose **acetaminophen** may prolong half-life and increase toxicity.

ROUTE AND DOSAGE

- **PO, IV (Adults and Children):** 50 mg/kg/day in divided doses q 6 hr.
- **PO, IV (Neonates >7 days):** 25 mg/kg q 12 hr.
- **Ophth (Adults and Children):** 1–2 drops of soln or small amount of ointment q 3–6 hr.
- **Otic (Adults and Children):** 2–3 drops 2–3 times/day.
- **Top (Adults and Children):** 1% cream applied 3–4 times daily.

PHARMACODYNAMICS (blood levels)

	ONSET	PEAK
PO	rapid	1–3 hr
IV	rapid	end of infusion

NURSING IMPLICATIONS

Assessment

- **General Info:** Assess patient for infection (vital signs; wound appearance; sputum, urine, and stool; WBC) at beginning and throughout course of therapy.
- □ This drug should be administered systemically only to hospitalized patients or those under close medical supervision. Diagnosis should be confirmed with cultures prior to administration.
- □ Assess patients daily for signs of bone marrow depression (petechiae, sore throat, fatigue, unusual bleeding, bruising). Patients that have impaired liver or renal function, infants, children, and the elderly are at the greatest risk of developing adverse effects.
- **Premature Infants and Neonates:** Assess for gray syndrome (abdominal distension, drowsiness, low body temperature, cyanosis, hypotension, and respiratory distress).
- **Lab Test Considerations:** CBC and platelet count should be monitored every 2 days throughout therapy. The drug should be stopped if anemia, reticulocytopenia, leukopenia, or thrombocytopenia develops. Notify physician promptly.
- □ May cause false-positive copper sulfate urine glucose tests (Clinitest). Test urine glucose with glucose oxidase method (Ketodiastix or Tes-Tape).
- **Toxicity and Overdose:** Monitor serum levels weekly. Therapeutic levels: peak, 5–20 mcg/ml.

Potential Nursing Diagnoses

- Infection, high risk for (indications, adverse effects).
- Knowledge deficit related to medication regimen (patient/family teaching).

Implementation

- **General Info:** Medication should be administered around the clock.
- **PO:** Give oral doses with a full glass of water 1 hr before or 2 hr after meals. Available as an oral suspension for patients with difficulty swallowing.

*Underlines indicate most frequent; **CAPITALS** indicate life-threatening.

- **Direct IV:** Reconstitute to a 10% soln by adding 10 ml of sterile water for injection or D5W to each 1 g. Do not use preparations containing benzyl alcohol in neonates.
  - *Rate:* Inject slowly over at least 1 min.
- **Intermittent Infusion:** May be further diluted in 50–100 ml of D5W, D10W, D5/0.9% NaCl, D5/0.45% NaCl, D5/0.25% NaCl, D5/LR, 0.45% NaCl, 0.9% NaCl, or lactated Ringer's soln. Soln may form crystals at low temperatures. Shake well to dissolve crystals. Do not administer cloudy solns.
  - *Rate:* Administer over 30–60 min.
- **Syringe Compatibility:** ampicillin, heparin, methicillin, or penicillin G sodium.
- **Syringe Incompatibility:** glycopyrrolate or metoclopramide.
- **Y-Site Compatibility:** acyclovir, cyclophosphamide, enalaprilat, esmolol, foscarnet, hydromorphone, labetalol, magnesium sulfate, meperidine, or morphine, perphenazine.
- **Additive Compatibility:** amikacin, aminophylline, ascorbic acid, calcium chloride, calcium gluconate, cephalothin, cephapirin, colistimethate, corticotropin, cyanocobalamin, dimenhydrinate, dopamine, ephedrine, heparin, hydrocortisone sodium succinate, kanamycin, lidocaine, magnesium sulfate, metaraminol, methicillin, methyldopate, methylprednisolone, metronidazole, nafcillin, oxacillin, oxytocin, penicillin G, pentobarbital, phenylephrine, phytonadione, plasma protein fraction, potassium chloride, promazine, ranitidine, sodium bicarbonate, thiopental, or verapamil.
- **Additive Incompatibility:** chlorpromazine, erythromycin, hydroxyzine, oxytetracycline, phenytoin, polymyxin B, prochlorperazine, promethazine, tetracycline, or vancomycin.
- **Ophth:** See Appendix H for instillation of ophthalmic soln.
  - Ophathalmic preparation is available in combination with hydrocortisone and polymyxin B (see Appendix A).
- **Top:** Cleanse area with soap and water prior to application.

Patient/Family Teaching

- **General Info:** Instruct patient to take medication exactly as directed and to finish prescription, even if feeling better. Missed doses should be taken as soon as remembered if not almost time for next dose. Do not double doses. Caution patient that sharing of this medication may be dangerous.
  - Advise patient to contact physician immediately if signs of unusual bleeding; bruising; fever; sore throat; nausea; vomiting; diarrhea; numbness, tingling, burning pain or weakness in hands or feet, occur. Medication should be discontinued with the onset of these symptoms.
  - Instruct patient to report signs of superinfection (stomatitis, perianal itching, vaginal discharge, fever).
  - Emphasize the importance of follow-up examinations. Bone marrow depression may develop wks to mons after drug therapy has been discontinued.
- **IV:** Reassure patient that bitter taste 15–20 sec following injection is limited to 2–3 min.
- **Ophth:** Inform patient soln may cause blurred vision for a few mins after instillation.

Evaluation

Clinical response to therapy may be determined by: ▪ Resolution of the signs and symptoms of infection. Length of time for complete resolution depends on the organism and site of infection.

CHLORDIAZEPOXIDE

(klor-dye-az-e-**pox**-ide)
{Apo-Chlordiazepoxide}, Libritabs, Lipoxide, Librium, {Medilium}, Mitran, {Novopoxide}, Reposans, Sereen, {Solium}

CLASSIFICATION(S):
Sedative/hypnotic—benzodiazepine
Schedule: IV
Pregnancy Category D

INDICATIONS

▪ Adjunct in the management of anxiety and as a preoperative sedative ▪ Treatment of symptoms of alcohol withdrawal.

ACTION

▪ Acts at many levels of the CNS to produce anxiolytic effect ▪ Depresses the CNS, probably by potentiating gamma aminobutyric acid (GABA), an inhibitory neurotransmitter. **Therapeutic Effects:** ▪ Sedation ▪ Relief of anxiety.

PHARMACOKINETICS

Absorption: Well absorbed from the GI tract. Absorption from IM sites may be slow and unpredictable.
Distribution: Widely distributed. Crosses the blood–brain barrier. Crosses the placenta and enters breast milk.
Metabolism and Excretion: Highly metabolized by the liver. Some products of metabolism are active as CNS depressants.
Half-life: 5–30 hr.

CONTRAINDICATIONS AND PRECAUTIONS

Contraindicated in: ▪ Hypersensitivity ▪ Cross-sensitivity with other benzodiazepines may exist ▪ Comatose patients or those with pre-existing CNS depression ▪ Uncontrolled severe pain ▪ Narrow-angle glaucoma ▪ Pregnancy and lactation.
Use Cautiously in: ▪ Hepatic dysfunction ▪ Severe renal impairment ▪ Patients who may be suicidal or who may have been addicted to drugs previously ▪ Elderly or debilitated patients (dosage reduction required).

ADVERSE REACTIONS AND SIDE EFFECTS*

CNS: dizziness, drowsiness, hangover, paradoxical excitation, headache.
EENT: blurred vision.
GI: nausea, vomiting, diarrhea, constipation.
Derm: rashes.
Local: pain at IM site.
Misc: tolerance, psychological dependence, physical dependence.

INTERACTIONS

Drug-Drug: ▪ **Alcohol, antidepressants, antihistamines,** and **narcotic analgesics**—concurrent use results in additive CNS depression ▪ **Cimetidine, oral contraceptives, disulfiram, fluoxetine, isoniazid, ketoconazole, metoprolol, propoxyphene, propranolol,** or **valproic acid** may decrease the metabolism of chlordiazepoxide, enhancing its actions ▪ May decrease efficacy of **levodopa** ▪ **Rifampin** or **barbiturates** may increase the metabolism and decrease effectiveness of chlordiazepoxide ▪ Sedative effects may be decreased by **theophylline.**

ROUTE AND DOSAGE

Alcohol Withdrawal

- **PO (Adults):** 50–100 mg, repeated until agitation is controlled, up to 300 mg/day.
- **IM, IV (Adults):** 50–100 mg initially; may be repeated in 2–4 hr.

Anxiety

- **PO (Adults):** 5–25 mg 3–4 times daily.
- **PO (Children >6 yr):** 5 mg 2–4 times daily, up to 10 mg 3 times daily.
- **IM, IV (Adults):** 50–100 mg initially, then 25–50 mg 3–4 times daily as required.

Preoperative Sedation

- **PO (Adults):** 5–10 mg 3–4 times daily for 24 hr preop.
- **IM (Adults):** 50–100 mg 1 hr preop.

*Underlines indicate most frequent; **CAPITALS** indicate life-threatening.

PHARMACODYNAMICS (sedation)

	ONSET	PEAK	DURATION
PO	1–2 hr	0.5–4 hr	up to 24 hr
IM	15–30 min	UK	UK
IV	1–5 min	UK	0.25–1 hr

NURSING IMPLICATIONS

Assessment

- **General Info:** Assess patient for anxiety and level of sedation (ataxia, dizziness, slurred speech) periodically throughout course of therapy.
- Monitor blood pressure, heart rate, and respiratory rate frequently when administering parenterally. Contact physician immediately if significant changes occur.
- Prolonged high-dose therapy may lead to psychological or physical dependence. Restrict the amount of drug available to patient.
- **Alcohol Withdrawal:** Assess patient for tremors, agitation, delirium, and hallucinations. Protect patient from injury.
- **Lab Test Considerations:** Patients on prolonged therapy should have CBC and liver function tests evaluated periodically. May cause an increase in serum bilirubin, SGOT (AST), and SGPT (ALT).

Potential Nursing Diagnoses

- Anxiety (indications).
- Injury, high risk for (side effects).
- Knowledge deficit related to medication regimen (patient/family teaching).

Implementation

- **General Info:** Use parenteral soln immediately after reconstitution and discard any unused portion.
- Following parenteral administration have patient remain recumbent, and observe for 3 hr.
- Available in combination with amitriptyline, esterified estrogens, and clinidium bromide (see Appendix A).
- **PO:** Administer after meals or with milk to minimize GI irritation. Tablets may be crushed and taken with food or fluids if patient has difficulty swallowing. Do not open capsules.
- **IM:** Reconstitute with 2 ml of diluent provided by manufacturer only. Do not use soln if opalescent or hazy. Agitate gently to minimize bubbling. Administer slowly, deep into a well-developed muscle mass to minimize pain at injection site. Soln reconstituted with IM diluent should not be given IV.
- **Direct IV:** Reconstitute 100 mg in 5 ml of 0.9% NaCl or sterile water for injection. Do not use IM diluent.
- *Rate:* Administer prescribed dose slowly over at least 1 min. Rapid administration may cause apnea, hypotension, bradycardia, or cardiac arrest.
- **Syringe Incompatibility:** benzquinamide.
- **Y-Site Compatibility:** heparin, hydrocortisone sodium succinate, or potassium chloride.

Patient/Family Teaching

- Instruct patient to take chlordiazepoxide exactly as directed. If medication is less effective after a few wks, check with physician, do not increase dose. Medication should be tapered at the completion of long-term therapy. Sudden cessation of medication may lead to withdrawal (insomnia, irritability, nervousness, tremors).
- May cause drowsiness or dizziness. Caution patient to avoid driving or other activities requiring alertness until response to medication is known.
- Advise patient to avoid the use of alcohol and other CNS depressants concurrently with this medication. Instruct patient to consult physician or pharmacist before taking over-the-counter medications.
- Instruct patient to notify physician if pregnancy is suspected.

Evaluation

Effectiveness of therapy can be demonstrated by: ▪ Decreased sense of anxiety ▫ Increased ability to cope ▪ Decreased tremulousness and more rational ide-

C

ation when used for alcohol withdrawal.

CHLOROQUINE

(klor-oh-kwin)

Aralen

CLASSIFICATION(S):
Antimalarial
Pregnancy Category UK

INDICATIONS

▪ Suppression and prophylaxis of malaria. **Unlabeled Uses:** ▪ Treatment of extraintestinal (hepatic) amebiasis ▪ Treatment of severe rheumatoid arthritis or systemic lupus erythematosus.

ACTION

▪ Inhibits protein synthesis in susceptible organisms by inhibiting DNA and RNA polymerase. **Therapeutic Effects:** ▪ Death of plasmodia responsible for causing malaria ▪ Elimination of amebiasis ▪ Improvement in inflammatory arthritis.

PHARMACOKINETICS

Absorption: Well absorbed following oral administration.
Distribution: Widely distributed; high tissue concentrations achieved. Crosses the placenta, enters breast milk.
Metabolism and Excretion: 30% metabolized by the liver. Metabolite also has antiplasmodial activity. 70% excreted unchanged by the kidneys.
Half-life: 72–120 hr.

CONTRAINDICATIONS AND PRECAUTIONS

Contraindicated in: ▪ Hypersensitivity ▪ Hypersensitivity to other 4-aminoquinolones (hydroxychloroquine) ▪ Visual damage caused by chloroquine or other 4-aminoquinolones ▪ Children (parenteral form).
Use Cautiously in: ▪ Liver disease ▪ Alcoholism ▪ Patients receiving hepatotoxic drugs ▪ Psoriasis ▪ G6-PD deficiency ▪ Bone marrow depression ▪ Pregnancy (although safety not established, has been used).

ADVERSE REACTIONS AND SIDE EFFECTS*

CNS: headache, fatigue, nervousness, anxiety, irritability, personality changes, confusion, SEIZURES, dizziness.
EENT: visual disturbances, keratopathy, retinopathy, ototoxicity.
CV: hypotension, EKG changes.
GI: epigastric discomfort, anorexia, nausea, vomiting, abdominal cramps, diarrhea.
GU: rusty yellow or brown discoloration of urine.
Derm: pigmentary changes, alopecia, pruritus, photosensitivity, skin erruptions, dermatoses.
Hemat: leukopenia, thrombocytopenia, agranulocytosis, APLASTIC ANEMIA.
Neuro: peripheral neuritis, neuromyopathy.

INTERACTIONS

Drug-Drug: ▪ May increase the risk of hepatotoxicity when administered with other **hepatotoxic agents** ▪ **Penicillamine** increases the risk of hematologic toxicity ▪ Increased risk of dermatologic toxicity when given with other **agents having dermatologic toxicity** ▪ May decrease rabies antibody titers when given concurrently with human diplod cell **rabies vaccine** ▪ **Urinary acidifiers** may increase renal excretion and decrease effectiveness.
Drug-Food: ▪ **Foods that acidify urine** (see Appendix K) may increase excretion and decrease effectiveness.

ROUTE AND DOSAGE

Note: Doses expressed as chloroquine base: 1 mg of chloroquine base = 1.67 mg chloroquine phosphate or 1.25 mg chloroquine hydrochloride.

Malaria (Suppression or Chemoprophylaxis)

▪ **PO (Adults):** 300 mg once weekly, starting 1–2 wk prior to entering ma-

*Underlines indicate most frequent; CAPITALS indicate life-threatening.

larious areas and for 6–8 wk afterwards.

- **PO (Children):** 5 mg/kg once weekly, starting 1–2 wk prior to entering malarious areas and for 6–8 wk afterwards (not to exceed 300 mg/day).

Malaria (Uncomplicated Attacks)

- **PO (Adults):** 600 mg initially, then 300 mg at 6 hr, 24 hr, and 48 hr after initial dose (not to exceed 1 g/24 hr).
- **PO (Children):** 10 mg/kg initially, 5 mg/kg at 6 hr, 24 hr, and 48 hr after initial dose (not to exceed 12.5 mg/kg/24 hr).

Malaria (Severe)

- **IM (Adults):** 200 mg q 6 hr.

Extraintestinal Amebiasis

- **PO (Adults):** 600 mg once daily for 2 days, then 300 mg (500 mg phophate) once daily for at least 2–3 wk.
- **PO (Children):** 10 mg/kg once daily for at least 2–3 wk (not to exceed 300 mg/day).

Rheumatoid Arthritis, Systemic Lupus Erythematosus

- **PO (Adults):** 150 mg/day.

PHARMACODYNAMICS (onset of antimalarial activity is rapid, anti-inflammatory activity may take up to 6 mon)

	ONSET	PEAK	DURATION
PO	rapid	1–2 hr	days–wks
IM	rapid	UK	days–wks

NURSING IMPLICATIONS

Assessment

- **General Info:** Determine baseline for future reference that includes current symptoms of disease prior to administration.
- □ Assess deep tendon reflexes periodically to determine muscle weakness. Therapy may be discontinued should this occur.
- **Malaria, Amebiasis, or Lupus Erythematosus:** Assess patient for improvement in signs and symptoms of condition daily throughout course of therapy.
- **Rheumatoid Arthritis:** Assess degree of joint pain and limitation of motion monthly.
- **Lab Test Considerations:** Monitor CBC and platelet count periodically throughout therapy. May cause decreased WBC and platelet counts.

Potential Nursing Diagnoses

- Infection, high risk for (indications).
- Comfort, altered: pain (indications).
- Knowledge deficit related to medication regimen (patient/family teaching).

Implementation

- **General Info:** For malaria prophylaxis, chloroquine therapy should be started 2 wk prior to potential exposures and continued for 6 wk after leaving the area.
- **PO:** Administer with milk or meals to minimize GI distress.
- □ Tablets may be crushed and placed inside empty capsules for patients with difficulty swallowing. Can be compounded into a suspension by pharmacist.
- **IM:** Parenteral administration may cause severe reaction (seizures, respiratory distress, shock, and cardiovascular collapse) or sudden death in children. Avoid if possible.
- □ Avoid intravenous injection; aspirate to ensure needle placement in muscle. Rotate sites. IM dose may be repeated in 6 hr if necessary. Change to oral route as soon as possible.

Patient/Family Teaching

- □ Instruct patient to take medication exactly as directed, and continue full course of therapy, even if feeling better. Missed doses should be taken as soon as remembered, except with regimens requiring doses more than once a day, for which missed doses should be taken within 1 hr or omitted. Do not double doses.
- □ Review methods of minimizing exposure to mosquitos with patients receiving chloroquine prophylactically (use repellant, wear long-sleeved shirt and long trousers, use screen or netting).
- □ Chloroquine may cause dizziness or

C

lightheadedness. Caution patient to avoid driving or other activities requiring alertness until response to medication is known.
- Advise patients to avoid use of alcohol while taking chloroquine.
- Caution patient to keep chloroquine out of the reach of children; fatalities have occurred with ingestion of 3 or 4 tablets.
- Explain need for periodic ophthalmic examinations for patients on prolonged high-dose therapy. Advise patient that the risk of ocular damage may be decreased by the use of dark glasses in bright light. Protective clothing and sunscreen should also be used to reduce risk of dermatoses.
- Inform patient that chloroquine may cause rusty yellow or brown discoloration of the urine.
- Advise patient to notify physician promptly if sore throat, fever, unusual bleeding or bruising, blurred vision, difficulty reading, visual changes, ringing in the ears, difficulty hearing, mental changes, or muscle weakness occur. Most adverse reactions are dose related.

▪ **Rheumatoid Arthritis:** Instruct patient to contact physician if no improvement is noticed within a few days. Treatment may require up to 6 mon for full benefit.

Evaluation

Effectiveness of therapy may be demonstrated by: ▪ Prevention of or improvement in signs and symptoms of malaria ▪ Improvement in signs and symptoms of amebiasis ▪ Management of rheumatoid arthritis ▪ Management of lupus erythematosus.

CHLOROTHIAZIDE

(klor-oh-**thye**-a-zide)
Diachlor, Diurigen, Diuril

CLASSIFICATION(S):
Diuretic—thiazide, Antihypertensive—thiazide
Pregnancy Category UK

INDICATIONS

▪ Alone or in combination with other agents in the management of mild to moderate hypertension ▪ Alone or in combination in the treatment of edema associated with congestive heart failure, the nephrotic syndrome, or pregnancy.

ACTION

▪ Increases excretion of sodium and water ▪ Promotes excretion of chloride, potassium, magnesium, and bicarbonate ▪ May produce arteriolar dilation. **Therapeutic Effects:** ▪ Lowering of blood pressure in hypertensive patients ▪ Diuresis with subsequent mobilization of edema.

PHARMACOKINETICS

Absorption: Incompletely absorbed from the GI tract. Only 50 mg absorbed from doses of 250–500 mg.

Distribution: Distributed into extracellular space. Crosses the placenta and enters breast milk.

Metabolism and Excretion: Excreted mainly unchanged by the kidneys.

Half-life: 1–2 hr.

CONTRAINDICATIONS AND PRECAUTIONS

Contraindicated in: ▪ Hypersensitivity ▪ Cross-sensitivity with other thiazides or sulfonamides may exist ▪ Anuria ▪ Lactation.

Use Cautiously in: ▪ Renal impairment ▪ Severe hepatic impairment ▪ Pregnancy (jaundice or thrombocytopenia have been seen in the newborn).

ADVERSE REACTIONS AND SIDE EFFECTS*

CNS: drowsiness, lethargy, dizziness, weakness.

CV: hypotension.

GI: anorexia, nausea, vomiting, cramping, hepatitis.

Derm: rashes, photosensitivity.

Endo: hyperglycemia.

F and E: <u>hypokalemia</u>, hypochloremic alkalosis, hyponatremia, hypercalce-

*Underlines indicate most frequent; CAPITALS indicate life-threatening.

mia, hypophosphatemia, hypomagnesemia, dehydration, hypovolemia.
Hemat: blood dyscrasias.
Metab: hyperuricemia, hyperlipidemia.
MS: muscle cramps.
Misc: pancreatitis.

INTERACTIONS

Drug–Drug: ▪ Additive hypotension with other **antihypertensives,** acute ingestion of **alcohol,** and **nitrates** ▪ Additive hypokalemia with **glucocorticoids, amphotericin B, mezlocillin, piperacillin,** or **ticarcillin** ▪ Decreases the excretion of **lithium,** may cause toxicity ▪ **Cholestyramine** decreases absorption.
Drug–Food: ▪ **Food** may increase extent of absorption.

ROUTE AND DOSAGE

- **PO, IV (Adults):** 500–2000 mg/day in 1–2 doses.
- **PO, IV (Children >6 mon):** 20 mg/kg/day in 2 divided doses.
- **PO, IV (Children <6 mon):** 30 mg/kg/day in 2 divided doses.

PHARMACODYNAMICS

	ONSET	PEAK	DURATION
PO (diuretic)	1–2 hr	4 hr	6–12 hr
PO (antihypertensive)	3–4 days	7–14 days	7 days
IV (diuretic)	15 min	30 min	2 hr

NURSING IMPLICATIONS

Assessment

- ▫ Monitor blood pressure, intake and output, daily weight and assess feet, legs, and sacral area for edema daily.
- ▫ Assess patient, especially if taking cardiac glycosides, for anorexia, nausea, vomiting, muscle cramps, paresthesia, and confusion. Patients taking cardiac glycosides are at increased risk of digitalis toxicity due to the potassium-depleting effect of the diuretic.
- ▫ Assess patient for allergy to sulfonamides.
- ▪ **Lab Test Considerations:** Monitor electrolytes (especially potassium), blood glucose, BUN, and serum uric acid levels prior to and periodically throughout course of therapy.
- ▫ May cause increase in serum and urine glucose in diabetic patients. May cause an increase in serum bilirubin, calcium, and uric acid, and a decrease in serum magnesium, potassium, and sodium levels.
- ▫ May cause increased serum cholesterol, low-density lipoprotein, and triglyceride concentrations.

Potential Nursing Diagnoses

- ▪ Fluid volume excess (indications).
- ▪ Fluid volume deficit (side effects).
- ▪ Knowledge deficit related to medication regimen (patient/family teaching).

Implementation

- ▪ **General Info:** Administer in the morning to prevent disruption of sleep cycle.
- ▫ Available in tablet, oral suspension, and injectable forms.
- ▫ Also available in combination with reserpine and methyldopa (see Appendix A).
- ▪ **PO:** May give with food or milk to minimize GI irritation. Tablets may be crushed and mixed with fluid for patients with difficulty swallowing.
- ▫ Shake suspension well before administering.
- ▫ Intermittent dose schedule may be used for continued control of edema.
- ▪ **Direct IV:** Dilute each 0.5 g with at least 18 ml of sterile water. May dilute further in D5W, D10W, Ringer's or lactated Ringer's injections, 0.45% NaCl, 0.9% NaCl, or dextrose/saline, dextrose/Ringer's, or dextrose/lactated Ringer's combinations. Soln is stable for 24 hr at room temperature.
- ▫ *Rate:* Administer at a rate of 0.5 g over 5 min. Avoid extravasation.
- ▪ **Additive Compatibility:** cimetidine, lidocaine, nafcillin, or sodium bicarbonate.
- ▪ **Additive Incompatibility:** blood and blood products, amikacin, chlorpromazine, codeine, hydralazine, in-

sulin, levorphanol, methadone, morphine, norepinephrine, polymyxin B, procaine, prochlorperazine, promazine, promethazine, streptomycin, tetracycline, triflupromazine, or vancomycin.

Patient/Family Teaching

- Instruct patient to take this medication at the same time each day. If a dose is missed, take as soon as remembered but not just before next dose is due. Do not double doses. Advise patients using chlorothiazide for hypertension to continue taking the medication even if feeling well. Medication controls but does not cure hypertension.
- Encourage patient to comply with additional interventions for hypertension (weight reduction, low-sodium diet, regular exercise, discontinuation of smoking, moderation of alcohol consumption, and stress management).
- Instruct patient to monitor weight biweekly and notify physician of significant changes. Instruct patients with hypertension in correct technique for monitoring weekly blood pressure.
- Caution patient to make position changes slowly to minimize orthostatic hypotension. This may be potentiated by alcohol.
- Advise patient to use sunscreen (avoid those containing PABA) and protective clothing when in the sun to prevent photosensitivity reactions.
- Instruct patient to follow a diet high in potassium (see Appendix K).
- Advise patient to consult physician or pharmacist before taking over-the-counter medication concurrently with this therapy.
- Advise patient to report muscle weakness, cramps, nausea, or dizziness to the physician.
- Instruct patient to notify physician or dentist of medication regimen prior to treatment or surgery.
- Emphasize the importance of routine follow-up examinations.

Evaluation

Effectiveness of therapy can be demonstrated by: ▪ Increase in urine output ▫ Decrease in edema ▪ Decreased blood pressure.

CHLOROTRIANISENE

(klor-oh-trye-**an**-i-seen)
TACE

CLASSIFICATION(S):
Hormone—estrogen
Pregnancy Category X

INDICATIONS

▪ Moderate to severe vasomotor symptoms of menopause ▪ Atrophic vaginitis ▪ Female hypogonadism ▪ Advanced, metastatic prostate cancer.

ACTION

▪ Promotes growth and development of female sex organs and the maintenance of secondary sex characteristics in women. **Therapeutic Effects:** ▪ Restoration of hormonal balance in various deficiency states ▪ Regression of advanced prostate cancer.

PHARMACOKINETICS

Absorption: Well absorbed following oral administration.
Distribution: Widely distributed. Stored in adipose tissue and then slowly released.
Metabolism and Excretion: Metabolized by the liver to a compound with more estrogenic activity.
Half-life: UK.

CONTRAINDICATIONS AND PRECAUTIONS

Contraindicated in: ▪ Thromboembolic disease ▪ Undiagnosed vaginal bleeding ▪ Pregnancy (use may harm fetus) ▪ Lactation ▪ Hypersensitivity to tartrazine (capsules contain tartrazine-FDC yellow dye #5).
Use Cautiously in: ▪ Cardiovascular disease ▪ Severe hepatic or renal dis-

ease ▪ May increase the risk of endometrial cancer.

ADVERSE REACTIONS AND SIDE EFFECTS*

CNS: headache, dizziness, lethargy, depression.
EENT: worsening of astigmatism or myopia, intolerance to contact lenses.
CV: edema, **THROMBOEMBOLISM**, hypertension, **MYOCARDIAL INFARCTION**.
GI: nausea, vomiting, weight changes, jaundice.
GU: women—breakthrough bleeding, dysmenorrhea, amenorrhea, cervical erosions, vaginal candidiasis, loss of libido; men—testicular atrophy, impotence.
Derm: acne, urticaria, oily skin, hyperpigmentation, photosensitivity.
Endo: hyperglycemia, gynecomastia (men), breast tenderness.
F and E: sodium and water retention, hypercalcemia.
MS: leg cramps.

INTERACTIONS

Drug-Drug: ▪ May alter requirements for **oral anticoagulants, oral hypoglycemic agents**, or **insulin** ▪ **Barbiturates** or **rifampin** may increase metabolism and decrease effectiveness ▪ **Smoking** increases risk of adverse cardiovascular reactions.

ROUTE AND DOSAGE

Vasomotor Symptoms of Menopause
- **PO (Adults):** 12–25 mg/day for 30-day cycle.

Atrophic Vaginitis
- **PO (Adults):** 12–25 mg daily in a 30–60-day cycle.

Female Hypogonadism
- **PO (Adults):** 12–25 mg daily in a 21-day cycle. Progesterone or progestin may be given on last 5 days. New cycle may begin on fifth day of bleeding.

Advanced Prostate Cancer
- **PO (Adult Male):** 12–25 mg/day.

PHARMACODYNAMICS (estrogenic effects)

	ONSET	PEAK	DURATION
PO	hrs–days	days–wks	days–wks

NURSING IMPLICATIONS

Assessment
- **General Info:** Assess blood pressure prior to and periodically throughout therapy.
  - Monitor intake and output ratios and weekly weight. Report significant discrepancies or steady weight gain to physician.
- **Menopause:** Assess frequency and severity of vasomotor symptoms.
- **Lab Test Considerations:** Monitor hepatic function periodically during long-term therapy.
  - May cause increased serum glucose, sodium, triglyceride, phospholipid, prothrombin, clotting factors VII, VIII, IX, and X and cortisol levels. May cause decreased serum folate, pyridoxine, antithrombin III, and pregnanediol excretion concentrations.
  - May cause elevated serum calcium levels in patients with bone metastases.
  - May cause false interpretations of thyroid function tests, false increases in sulfobromophtalein (BSP) and norepinephrine platelet-induced aggregability, and false decreases in metyrapone tests.

Potential Nursing Diagnoses
- Sexual dysfunction (indications).
- Knowledge deficit related to medication regimen (patient/family teaching).

Implementation
- **PO:** Administer oral doses with or immediately after food to reduce nausea.

*Underlines indicate most frequent; **CAPITALS** indicate life-threatening.

C

Patient/Family Teaching

- □ Instruct patient to take medication as directed. Missed doses should be taken as soon as remembered if not just before next dose. Do not double doses.
- □ Explain medication schedule to women on 21-day cycle followed by 7 days of not taking medication. Encourage patient to take medication at the same time each day.
- □ If nausea becomes a problem, advise patient that eating solid food often provides relief.
- □ Advise patient to report signs and symptoms of fluid retention (swelling of ankles and feet, weight gain), thromboembolic disorders (pain, swelling, tenderness in extremities, headache, chest pain, blurred vision), mental depression, hepatic dysfunction (yellowed skin or eyes, pruritus, dark urine, light-colored stools), or abnormal vaginal bleeding to physician.
- □ Instruct patient to stop taking medication and notify physician if pregnancy is suspected.
- □ Caution patient that cigarette smoking during estrogen therapy may cause increased risk of serious side effects, especially for women over 35 yr of age.
- □ Advise patient to notify physicians or dentist of medication regimen prior to treatment or surgery.
- □ Caution patient to use protective clothing and sunscreen to prevent photosensitivity rections.
- □ Emphasize the importance of routine follow-up physical examinations including blood pressure; breast, abdomen, and pelvic examinations; and PAP smears every 6–12 mon.

Evaluation

Effectiveness of therapy can be demonstrated by: ▪ Reduction in menopausal vasomotor symptoms ▪ Arrested spread of advanced prostatic cancer.

CHLORPHENIRAMINE

(klor-fen-**eer**-a-meen)
Aller-Chlor, Chlo-Amine, Chlorate, Chlor-Niramine, Chlor-Pro, Chlor-Trimeton, {Chlor-Tripolon}, Chlorotab, Genallerate, {Nonopheniram}, Teldrin, Pfeiffer's Allergy, Phenetron, Trimegen

CLASSIFICATION(S):
Antihistamine
Pregnancy Category B

INDICATIONS

▪ Symptomatic relief of allergic symptoms caused by histamine release; conditions in which drug is most useful include nasal allergies and allergic dermatoses ▪ Management of severe allergic or hypersensitivity reactions including anaphylaxis and transfusion reactions.

ACTION

▪ Blocks the following effects of histamine: □ Vasodilation □ Increased GI tract secretions □ Increased heart rate □ Hypotension. **Therapeutic Effect:** ▪ Relief of symptoms associated with histamine excess usually seen in allergic conditions. Does not block the release of histamine.

PHARMACOKINETICS

Absorption: Well absorbed following oral and parenteral administration.
Distribution: Widely distributed. Minimal amounts excreted in breast milk. Crosses the blood–brain barrier.
Metabolism and Excretion: Extensively metabolized by the liver.
Half-life: 12–15 hr.

CONTRAINDICATIONS AND PRECAUTIONS

Contraindicated in: ▪ Hypersensitivity ▪ Acute attacks of asthma ▪ Lactation (avoid use).
Use Cautiously in: ▪ Narrow-angle

glaucoma ▪ Liver disease ▪ Elderly patients (more susceptible to adverse reactions) ▪ Pregnancy (safety not established).

ADVERSE REACTIONS AND SIDE EFFECTS*

CNS: drowsiness, sedation, excitation (in children), dizziness.
CV: hypotension, hypertension, palpitations, arrhythmias.
EENT: blurred vision.
GI: dry mouth, obstruction, constipation.
GU: urinary hesitancy, retention.

INTERACTIONS

Drug–Drug: ▪ Additive CNS depression with other **CNS depressants** including **alcohol, narcotic analgesics,** and **sedative/hypnotics** ▪ **MAO inhibitors** intensify and prolong the anticholinergic effects of antihistamines ▪ Additive anticholinergic effects with other **drugs possessing anticholinergic properties** including **antihistamines, antidepressants, atropine, haloperidol, phenothiazines, quinidine,** and **disopyramide.**

ROUTE AND DOSAGE

- **PO (Adults):** 4 mg q 4–6 hr or 8–12 mg of extended-release formulation q 8–12 hr (not to exceed 24 mg/day).
- **PO (Children 6–12 yr):** 2 mg q 4–6 hr or 8 mg of extended-release formulation once daily (not to exceed 12 mg/day).
- **PO (Children 2–6 yr):** 1 mg q 4–6 hr.
- **SC, IM, IV (Adults):** 5–20 mg single dose (not to exceed 40 mg/day).
- **SC (Children):** 0.0875 mg/kg q 6 hr.

PHARMACODYNAMICS (antihistaminic effects)

	ONSET	PEAK	DURATION
PO	15–30 min	1–2 hr	4–12 hr
SC	UK	UK	4–12 hr
IM	UK	UK	4–12 hr
IV	rapid	UK	4–12 hr

NURSING IMPLICATIONS

Assessment

- Assess allergy symptoms (rhinitis, conjunctivitis, hives) prior to and periodically throughout course of therapy.
- Monitor pulse and blood pressure before initiating and throughout IV therapy.
- Assess lung sounds and character of bronchial secretions. Maintain fluid intake of 1500–2000 ml/day to decrease viscosity of secretions.
- **Lab Test Considerations:** May cause false-negative reactions on allergy skin tests; discontinue 4 days prior to testing.

Potential Nursing Diagnoses

- Airway clearance, ineffective (indications).
- Injury, high risk for (adverse reactions).
- Knowledge deficit related to medication regimen (patient/family teaching).

Implementation

- **General Info:** Available in tablets, chewable tablets, extended-release tablets and capsules, syrup, and injectable (SC, IM, IV) forms. Also available in combination with decongestants (see Appendix A).
- **PO:** Administer oral doses with food or milk to decrease GI irritation. Extended-release tablets and capsules should be swallowed whole, do not crush, break, or chew. Chewable tablets should not be swallowed whole; chew well before swallowing.
- **IM/SC:** The 20 mg/ml and 100 mg/ml soln are recommended for IM or SC route only.
- **Direct IV:** May be given undiluted. Use only the 10 mg/ml strength for IV administration.
  - *Rate:* Administer each 10 mg dose over at least 1 min.
- **Additive Compatibility:** standard IV solns or amikacin.
- **Additive Incompatibility:** calcium

*Underlines indicate most frequent; **CAPITALS** indicate life-threatening.

chloride, kanamycin, norepinephrine, or pentobarbital.

Patient/Family Teaching

- Instruct patient to take chlorpheniramine exactly as directed.
- Chlorpheniramine may cause drowsiness. Caution patient to avoid driving or other activities requiring alertness until response to drug is known.
- Caution patient to avoid using alcohol or other CNS depressants concurrently with this drug.
- Advise patient that good oral hygiene, frequent rinsing of mouth with water, and sugarless gum or candy may help relieve dryness of mouth.
- Instruct patient to contact physician if symptoms persist.

Evaluation

Effectiveness of therapy can be demonstrated by: ▪ Decrease in allergic symptoms.

CHLORPROMAZINE

(klor-**proe**-ma-zeen)
{Chlorpromanyl}, {Largactil}, {Novo-Chlorpromazine}, Thorazine, Thor-prom

CLASSIFICATION(S):
Antipsychotic—phenothiazine, Antiemetic—phenothiazine
Pregnancy Category UK

INDICATIONS

▪ Treatment of acute and chronic psychoses, particularly when accompanied by increased psychomotor activity ▪ Management of nausea and vomiting ▪ Control of intractable hiccups ▪ Preoperative sedation.

ACTION

▪ Alters the effects of dopamine in the CNS ▪ Possesses significant anticholinergic and alpha-adrenergic blocking activity. **Therapeutic Effects:** ▪ Diminished signs and symptoms of psychosis ▪ Relief of nausea and vomiting ▪ Control of intractable hiccups ▪ Tetanus ▪ Porhyria.

PHARMACOKINETICS

Absorption: Absorption is variable following oral administration. Well absorbed following IM administration.
Distribution: Widely distributed, high concentrations in the CNS. Crosses the placenta and enters breast milk.
Metabolism and Excretion: Highly metabolized by the liver and GI mucosa. Converted to some compounds with antipsychotic activity.
Half-life: 30 hr.

CONTRAINDICATIONS AND PRECAUTIONS

Contraindicated in: ▪ Hypersensitivity ▪ Hypersensitivity to sulfites (injectable), povidone or benzyl alcohol (spansules) ▪ Cross-sensitivity with other phenothiazines may exist ▪ Narrow-angle glaucoma ▪ Bone marrow depression ▪ Severe liver disease ▪ Severe cardiovascular disease.
Use Cautiously in: ▪ Elderly or debilitated patients (dosage reduction required) ▪ Pregnancy or lactation (safety not established) ▪ Diabetes ▪ Respiratory disease ▪ Prostatic hypertrophy ▪ CNS tumors ▪ Epilepsy ▪ Intestinal obstruction.

ADVERSE REACTIONS AND SIDE EFFECTS*

CNS: sedation, extrapyramidal reactions, tardive dyskinesia.
EENT: dry eyes, blurred vision, lens opacities.
CV: hypotension, tachycardia.
GI: constipation, dry mouth, ileus, anorexia, hepatitis.
GU: urinary retention.
Derm: rashes, photosensitivity, pigment changes.
Endo: galactorrhea.
Hemat: AGRANULOCYTOSIS, leukopenia.
Metab: hyperthermia.
Misc: allergic reactions.

{} = Available in Canada only.
*Underlines indicate most frequent; **CAPITALS** indicate life-threatening.

INTERACTIONS

Drug–Drug: ▪ Additive hypotension with **antihypertensive agents** ▪ Additive CNS depression with other **CNS depressants** including **alcohol, antidepressants, antihistamines, MAO inhibitors, narcotics, sedative/hypnotics,** or **general anesthetics** ▪ **Phenobarbital** may increase metabolism and decrease effectiveness ▪ Concurrent use with **lithium** may produce any of the following—acute encephalopathy, decreased chlorpromazine absorption, increased excretion of lithium, increased risk of extrapyramidal reactions, or masking of the early signs of **lithium** toxicity ▪ **Antacids** or **adsorbent antidiarrheals (kaolin)** may decrease adsorption ▪ Increased risk of agranulocytosis with **antithyroid drugs** ▪ May decrease antiparkinson activity of **levodopa** and **bromocriptine** ▪ Decreases vasopressorresponse to **epinephrine** and **norepinephrine** ▪ Decreases antihypertensive effect of **guanethidine** ▪ Concurrent use with **beta blockers** may result in inhibition of metabolism of one or both drugs producing an increased response ▪ Increased risk or anticholinergic effects with other **agents having anticholinergic properties** including **antihistamines, tricyclic antidepressants, quinidine,** or **disopyramide.**

ROUTE AND DOSAGE

Psychoses

- **PO (Adults):** 10–25 mg 2–4 times daily; increase by 20–50 mg/day every 3–4 days up to 30–800 mg/day in 1–4 divided doses (usual dose is 200 mg/day; 1–2 g/day may be needed in some patients).
- **PO (Children):** 0.55 mg/kg q 4–6 hr.
- **IM (Adults):** 25–50 mg initially, may be repeated in 1 hr, increase to maximum of 400 mg q 4–6 hr if needed (1–2 g/day may be needed in some patients).
- **IM (Children >6 mon):** 0.55 mg/kg or 15 mg/m² q 6–8 hr (not to exceed 40 mg/day in children 6 mon–5 yr, or 75 mg/day in children 5–12 yr except in unmanagable cases).

Nausea and Vomiting

- **PO (Adults):** 10–25 mg q 4–6 hr.
- **PO (Children >6 mon):** 0.55 mg/kg or 15 mg/m² q 6–8 hr.
- **IM (Adults):** 25–50 mg q 3–4 hr.
- **IM (Children):** 0.55 mg/kg or 15 mg/m² q 6–8 hr.
- **Rect (Adults):** 50–100 mg q 6–8 hr.
- **Rect (Children):** 1.1 mg/kg q 6–8 hr.

Nausea and Vomiting During Surgery

- **IM (Adults):** 12.5 mg; may be repeated in 30 min.
- **IM (Children):** 0.275 mg/kg; may be repeated in 30 min.
- **IV (Adults):** 25 mg as a slow infusion at no more than 1 mg/min.
- **IV (Children):** 0.275 mg/kg as a slow infusion at no more than 1 mg every 2 min.

Preoperative Sedation

- **IM (Adults):** 12.5–25 mg 1–2 hr before surgery.
- **IM (Children):** 0.55 mg/kg 1–2 hr before surgery.

Intractable Hiccups

- **PO (Adults):** 25–50 mg 3–4 times daily.
- **IM (Adults):** 25–50 mg 3–4 times daily, if no response to PO.
- **IV (Adults):** 25–50 mg by slow infusion, rate not to exceed 1 mg/min.

PHARMACODYNAMICS (antipsychotic activity, antiemetic activity, sedation)

	ONSET	PEAK	DURATION
PO	30–60 min	UK	4–6 hr
PO–ER	30–60 min	UK	10–12 hr
Rect	1–2 hr	UK	3–4 hr
IM	UK	UK	4–8 hr
IV	rapid	UK	UK

NURSING IMPLICATIONS

Assessment

- **General Info:** Assess patient's mental status (orientation, mood, behavior) prior to and periodically throughout therapy.
- □ Monitor blood pressure (sitting, standing, lying), ECG, pulse, and re-

spiratory rate prior to and frequently during the period of dosage adjustment. May cause Q-wave and T-wave changes in ECG.
- Observe patient carefully when administering medication to ensure medication is actually taken and not hoarded.
- Assess fluid intake and bowel function. Increased bulk and fluids in the diet may help minimize constipation.
- Observe patient carefully for extrapyramidal symptoms (pill-rolling motions, drooling, tremors, rigidity, shuffling gait) and tardive dyskinesia (uncontrolled movements of face, mouth, tongue, or jaw, and involuntary movements of extremities). Notify physician immediately at the onset of these symptoms.
- **Preoperative Sedation:** Assess level of anxiety prior to and following administration.
- **Lab Test Considerations:** CBC, liver function tests, and ocular examinations should be evaluated periodically throughout course of therapy. May cause decreased hematocrit, hemoglobin, leukocytes, granulocytes, platelets. May cause elevated bilirubin, SGOT (AST), SGPT (ALT), and alkaline phosphatase.
- May cause false-positive or false-negative pregnancy tests and false-positive urine bilirubin test results.

Potential Nursing Diagnoses
- Thought processes, altered (indications).
- Knowledge deficit related to medication regimen (patient/family teaching).
- Noncompliance (patient/family teaching).

Implementation
- **General Info:** Available in tablet, sustained-release capsule, syrup, concentrate, suppository, and injectable forms.
- Keep patient recumbent for at least 30 min following parenteral administration to minimize hypotensive effects.
- To prevent contact dermatitis, avoid getting soln on hands.
- Phenothiazines should be discontinued 48 hr before and not resumed for 24 hr following metrizamide myelography, because they lower the seizure threshold.
- **PO:** Administer oral doses with food, milk, or a full glass of water to minimize gastric irritation. Tablets may be crushed. Do not open capsules; swallow whole. Spansules may be opened but contents should not be chewed. Dilute concentrate just prior to administration in 120 ml of coffee, tea, tomato or fruit juice, milk, water, soup, or carbonated beverages.
- **Rect:** If suppository is too soft for insertion, chill in refrigerator for 30 min or run under cold water before removing foil wrapper.
- **IM:** Do not inject SC. Inject slowly into deep, well-developed muscle. May be diluted with 0.9% NaCl or 2% procaine if ordered. Lemon-yellow color does not alter potency of soln. Do not administer soln that is markedly discolored or contains a precipitate.
- **Direct IV:** For IV administration dilute with 0.9% NaCl in a 1 mg/ml concentration.
- *Rate:* Inject slowly at a rate of 1 mg/1–2 min.
- **Continuous Infusion:** May dilute 25–50 mg in 500–1000 ml of D5W, D10W, 0.45% NaCl, 0.9% NaCl, Ringer's or lactated Ringer's injection, dextrose/Ringer's or dextrose/lactated Ringer's combinations for intractable hiccups.
- **Syringe Compatibility:** atropine, butorphanol, diphenhydramine, doxapram, droperidol, fentanyl, glycopyrrolate, hydromorphone, hydroxyzine, meperidine, metoclopramide, midazolam, morphine, pentazocine, perphenazine, prochlorperazine, promazine, promethazine, or scopolamine.
- **Syringe Incompatibility:** cimetidine, dimenhydrinate, heparin, pentobarbital, or thiopental.
- **Y-Site Compatibility:** heparin, hydro-

cortisone sodium succinate, ondansetron, or potassium chloride.

- **Additive Compatibility:** ascorbic acid, ethacrynate, or netilmicin.
- **Additive Incompatibility:** aminophylline, amphotericin B, ampicillin, chloramphenicol, chlorothiazide, methicillin, methohexital, penicillin G, or phenobarbital.

Patient/Family Teaching

- Advise patient to take medication exactly as directed and not to skip doses or double up on missed doses. Abrupt withdrawal may lead to gastritis, nausea, vomiting, dizziness, headache, tachycardia, and insomnia.
- Inform patient of possibility of extrapyramidal symptoms and tardive dyskinesia. Instruct patient to report these symptoms immediately to physician.
- Advise patients to make position changes slowly to minimize orthostatic hypotension.
- Medication may cause drowsiness. Caution patient to avoid driving or other activities requiring alertness until response to the medication is known.
- Caution patient to avoid taking alcohol or other CNS depressants concurrently with this medication.
- Advise patient to use sunscreen and protective clothing when exposed to the sun. Exposed surfaces may develop a temporary pigment change (ranging from yellow-brown to grayish purple). Extremes of temperature (exercise, hot weather, hot baths or showers) should also be avoided, because this drug impairs body temperature regulation.
- Instruct patient to use frequent mouth rinses, good oral hygiene, and sugarless gum or candy to minimize dry mouth. Consult physician or dentist if dry mouth continues for >2 wk.
- Advise patient not to take chlorpromazine within 2 hr of antacids or antidiarrheal medication.
- Inform patient that this medication may turn urine a pink-to-reddish-brown color.
- Advise patient to notify physician or dentist of medication regimen prior to treatment or surgery.
- Instruct patient to notify physician promptly if sore throat, fever, unusual bleeding or bruising, rash, weakness, tremors, visual disturbances, dark-colored urine, or clay-colored stools occur.
- Emphasize the importance of routine follow-up examinations and continued participation in psychotherapy as indicated.

Evaluation

Effectiveness of therapy can be demonstrated by: ▪ Decrease in excitable, paranoic, or withdrawn behavior. Therapeutic effects may not be seen for 7–8 wk ▪ Relief of nausea and vomiting ▪ Relief of hiccups ▪ Preoperative sedation.

CHLORPROPAMIDE

(klor-**proe**-pa-mide)
{Apo-Chlorpropamide}, Diabinese, Glucamide, {Novopropamide}

CLASSIFICATION(S):
Oral hypoglycemic agent—sulfonylurea
Pregnancy Category C

INDICATIONS

▪ Control of blood sugar in adult-onset, noninsulin-dependent diabetes (NIDDM, type II, adult-onset, nonketosis-prone) when dietary therapy fails. Requires some pancreatic function.

ACTION

▪ Lowers blood sugar by stimulating the release of insulin from the pancreas and increasing sensitivity to insulin at receptor sites ▪ May also decrease hepatic glucose production. **Therapeutic Effect:** ▪ Lowering of blood sugar in diabetic (NIDDM) patients.

PHARMACOKINETICS

Absorption: Well absorbed following oral administration.
Distribution: Distribution not known.
Metabolism and Excretion: Metabolized by the liver (up to 80%).
Half-life: 36 hr (range, 25–60 hr).

CONTRAINDICATIONS AND PRECAUTIONS

Contraindicated in: ▪ Hypersensitivity ▪ Cross-sensitivity with sulfonamides may exist ▪ Insulin-dependent diabetics (type I, juvenile-onset, ketosis-prone, brittle) ▪ Severe renal impairment ▪ Severe hepatic impairment ▪ Thyroid or other endocrine disease.
Use Cautiously in: ▪ Severe cardiovascular disease (increased risk of congestive heart failure) ▪ Elderly patients (dosage reduction may be required) ▪ Infection, stress, or changes in diet may alter requirements for control of blood sugar.

ADVERSE REACTIONS AND SIDE EFFECTS*

CNS: headache, weakness.
CV: congestive heart failure.
GI: nausea, vomiting, diarrhea, cramps, hepatitis.
Hemat: APLASTIC ANEMIA, leukopenia, pancytopenia, thrombocytopenia.
Derm: photosensitivity, rashes.
Endo: hypoglycemia, syndrome of inappropriate secretion of antidiuretic hormone.
F and E: hyponatremia.

INTERACTIONS

Drug-Drug: ▪ Ingestion of **alcohol** may result in disulfiram-like reaction ▪ **Alcohol, glucocorticoids, rifampin,** and **thiazides** may decrease effectiveness ▪ **Androgens (testosterone), chloramphenicol, clofibrate, guanethidine, monoamine oxidase inhibitors, phenylbutazone, salicylates,** and **sulfonamides** may increase risk of hypoglycemia ▪ Concurrent **oral anticoagulant** therapy may result in altered response to chlorpropamide (dosage adjustments of both agents may be necessary) ▪ Concurrent **beta blocker** therapy may produce prolonged hypoglycemia and may mask symptoms.

ROUTE AND DOSAGE

- **PO (Adults):** 250–500 mg day in 1–2 divided doses (initial dose in elderly patients should be 100 mg).

PHARMACODYNAMICS (hypoglycemic activity)

	ONSET	PEAK	DURATION
PO	1 hr	3–6 hr	24 hr

NURSING IMPLICATIONS

Assessment

- □ Observe patient for signs and symptoms of hypoglycemic reactions (sweating, hunger, weakness, dizziness, tremor, tachycardia, anxiety). Long duration of action increases the risk of recurrent hypoglycemia. Monitor patients who experience a hypoglycemic episode closely for 3–5 days.
- □ Assess patient for allergy to sulfonamides.
- □ Monitor intake and output ratios and daily weight. Notify physician promptly if peripheral edema, rales/crackles, or a significant discrepancy in totals develops.
- ▪ **Lab Test Considerations:** Monitor serum or urine glucose and ketones daily.
- □ Serum sodium levels, plasma osmolarity, and CBC should be monitored periodically throughout therapy.

Potential Nursing Diagnoses

- ▪ Nutrition, altered: more than body requirements (indications).
- ▪ Knowledge deficit related to medication regimen (patient/family teaching).
- ▪ Noncompliance (patient/family teaching).

Implementation

- ▪ **General Info:** To convert from other oral hypoglycemic agents or insulin

*Underlines indicate most frequent; **CAPITALS** indicate life-threatening.

dosage of less than 40 units/day, change may be made without gradual dosage adjustment. Patients taking insulin of greater than 40 units/day should convert gradually by receiving chlorpropamide and 50% of previous insulin dosage for initial few days. Monitor serum or urine glucose and ketones at least 3 times/day during conversion.

- **PO:** May be administered once in the morning or divided into 2 doses. Administer with meals to ensure best diabetic control and minimize gastric irritation. Do not administer after last meal of the day.
  - Tablets may be crushed and taken with fluids if patient has difficulty swallowing.

PATIENT/FAMILY TEACHING

- Instruct patient to take medication at same time each day. If a dose is missed, take as soon as remembered unless almost time for next dose. Do not take if unable to eat.
- Explain to patient that this medication controls hyperglycemia but does not cure diabetes. Therapy is long term.
- Review signs of hypoglycemia and hyperglycemia with patient. If hypoglycemia occurs, advise patient to take a glass of orange juice or 2–3 tsp of sugar, honey, or corn syrup dissolved in water and notify physician.
- Encourage patient to follow prescribed diet, medication, and exercise regimen to prevent hypoglycemic or hyperglycemia episodes.
- Instruct patient in proper testing of serum glucose or urine glucose and ketones. Stress the importance of double-voided urine specimens for accuracy. These tests should be closely monitored during periods of stress or illness and physician notified if significant changes occur.
- Caution patient to avoid other medications, especially aspirin and alcohol, while on this therapy without consulting physician or pharmacist.
- Concurrent use of alcohol may cause a disulfiram-like reaction (abdominal cramps, nausea, flushing, headaches, and hypoglycemia).
- Caution patient to use sunscreen and protective clothing to prevent photosensitivity reactions.
- Advise patient to inform physician or dentist of medication regimen prior to treatment or surgery.
- Advise patient to carry sugar and identification describing disease process and medication regimen at all times.
- Advise patient to notify physician promptly if unusual weight gain, swelling of ankles, drowsiness, shortness of breath, muscle cramps, weakness, sore throat, rash, or unusual bleeding or bruising occur.
- Emphasize the importance of routine follow-up examinations.

EVALUATION

Effectiveness of therapy can be demonstrated by: ▪ Control of blood glucose levels without the appearance of hypoglycemic or hyperglycemic episodes.

CHLORTHALIDONE

(klor-**thal**-i-doan)
{Apo-Chlorthalidone}, Hygroton, Thalitone, {Novothalidone}, {Uridon}

CLASSIFICATION(S):
Antihypertensive—diuretic, Diuretic—thiazide-like
Pregnancy Category B

INDICATIONS

▪ Alone or in combination with other agents in the management of mild to moderate hypertension ▪ Alone or in combination in the treatment of edema associated with congestive heart failure, the nephrotic syndrome, or pregnancy.

ACTION

▪ Increases excretion of sodium and water ▪ Promotes excretion of chloride, potassium, magnesium, and bicarbonate ▪ May produce arteriolar dilation.
Therapeutic Effects: ▪ Lowering of blood pressure in hypertensive patients ▪ Diuresis with subsequent mobilization of edema.

PHARMACOKINETICS

Absorption: Well absorbed following oral administration.
Distribution: Distributed into extracellular space. Crosses the placenta and enters breast milk.
Metabolism and Excretion: 30–60% excreted unchanged by the kidneys.
Half-life: 54 hr.

CONTRAINDICATIONS AND PRECAUTIONS

Contraindicated in: ▪ Hypersensitivity ▪ Cross-sensitivity with sulfonamides may exist ▪ Anuria ▪ Lactation.
Use Cautiously in: ▪ Renal impairment ▪ Severe hepatic impairment ▪ Pregnancy (jaundice or thrombocytopenia may be seen in the newborn).

ADVERSE REACTIONS AND SIDE EFFECTS*

CNS: drowsiness, lethargy.
CV: hypotension.
GI: anorexia, nausea, vomiting, cramping, hepatitis.
Derm: rashes, photosensitivity.
Endo: hyperglycemia.
F and E: hypokalemia, hypochloremic alkalosis, hyponatremia, hypercalcemia, hypophosphatemia, hypomagnesemia, dehydration, hypovolemia.
Hemat: blood dyscrasias.
Metab: hyperuricemia, hyperlipidemia.
MS: muscle cramps.
Misc: pancreatitis.

INTERACTIONS

Drug–Drug: ▪ Additive hypotension with other **antihypertensives,** acute ingestion of **alcohol,** or **nitrates** ▪ Additive hypokalemia with **glucocorticoids, amphotericin B, mezlocillin, piperacillin,** or **ticarcillin** ▪ Decreases **lithium** excretion, may cause toxicity ▪ **Cholestyramine** decreases absorption.
Drug–Food: ▪ **Food** may increase extent of absorption.

ROUTE AND DOSAGE

- **PO (Adults):** 25–100 mg/day or 100 mg 3 times weekly.
- **PO (Children):** 2 mg/kg 3 times weekly.

PHARMACODYNAMICS (diuretic effect)

	ONSET	PEAK	DURATION
PO	2 hr	2–6 hr	24–72 hr

NURSING IMPLICATIONS

Assessment

- **General Info:** Monitor blood pressure, intake and output, daily weight and assess feet, legs, and sacral area for edema daily.
  - Assess patient, especially if taking cardiac glycosides, for anorexia, nausea, vomiting, muscle cramps, paresthesia, and confusion. Patients taking cardiac glycosides are at increased risk of digitalis toxicity due to the potassium-depleting effect of the diuretic.
  - Assess patient for allergy to sulfonamides.
- **Lab Test Considerations:** Monitor electrolytes (especially potassium), blood glucose, BUN, and serum uric acid levels prior to and periodically throughout course of therapy.
  - May cause increase in serum and urine glucose in diabetic patients. May cause an increase in serum bilirubin, calcium, and uric acid, and a decrease in serum magnesium, potassium, and sodium levels.
  - May cause increased serum cholesterol, low-density lipoprotein, and triglyceride concentrations.

Potential Nursing Diagnoses

- Fluid volume excess (indications).

*Underlines indicate most frequent; **CAPITALS** indicate life-threatening.

- Fluid volume deficit (side effects).
- Knowledge deficit related to medication regimen (patient/family teaching).

IMPLEMENTATION

- **General Info:** Administer in the morning to prevent disruption of sleep cycle.
- □ Available in combination with clonidine, atenolol, and reserpine (see Appendix A).
- **PO:** May give with food or milk to minimize GI irritation. Tablets may be crushed and mixed with fluid to facilitate swallowing.
- □ Intermittent dose schedule may be used for continued control of edema.

PATIENT/FAMILY TEACHING

- □ Instruct patient to take this medication at the same time each day. If a dose is missed, take as soon as remembered, but not just before next dose is due. Do not double doses. Advise patients using chlorthalidone for hypertension to continue taking the medication even if feeling better.
- □ Medication controls but does not cure hypertension.
- □ Encourage patient to comply with additional interventions for hypertension (weight reduction, low-sodium diet, regular exercises, discontinuation of smoking, moderation of alcohol consumption, and stress management).
- □ Instruct patient to monitor weight biweekly and notify physician of significant changes. Instruct patients with hypertension in correct technique for monitoring weekly blood pressure.
- □ Caution patient to make position changes slowly to minimize orthostatic hypotension. This may be potentiated by alcohol.
- □ Advise patient to use sunscreen (avoid those containing PABA) and protective clothing when in the sun to prevent photosensitivity reactions.
- □ Instruct patient to follow a diet high in potassium (see Appendix K).
- □ Advise patient to consult physician or pharmacist before taking over-the-counter medication concurrently with this therapy.
- □ Advise patient to report muscle weakness, cramps, nausea, or dizziness to the physician.
- □ Instruct patient to notify physician or dentist of medication regimen prior to treatment or surgery.
- □ Emphasize the importance of routine follow-up examinations.

EVALUATION

Effectiveness of therapy can be demonstrated by: ▪ Increase in urine output □ Decrease in edema ▪ Decrease in blood pressure.

CHOLESTYRAMINE

(koe-less-**tear**-a-meen)
Cholybar, Questran, Questran Light

CLASSIFICATION(S):
Lipid-lowering agent—bile acid sequestrant
Pregnancy Category UK

INDICATIONS

▪ Adjunct in the management of primary hypercholesterolemia ▪ Relief of pruritis associated with elevated levels of bile acids.

ACTION

▪ Binds bile acids in the GI tract, forming an insoluble complex. Result is increased clearance of cholesterol. **Therapeutic Effect:** ▪ Decreased plasma cholesterol and low-density lipoproteins.

PHARMACOKINETICS

Absorption: Action takes place in the GI tract. No absorption occurs.
Distribution: No distribution.
Metabolism and Excretion: After binding bile acids, insoluble complex is eliminated in the feces.
Half-life: UK.

C

CONTRAINDICATIONS AND PRECAUTIONS

Contraindicated in: ▪ Hypersensitivity ▪ Complete biliary obstruction ▪ Hypersensitivity to propylene glycol (Questran) or aspartame (Questran Light) ▪ Phenylketonuria (Questran Light).

Use Cautiously in: ▪ History of constipation (causes severe constipation) ▪ Other concurrently administered oral medications (may interfere with absorption).

ADVERSE REACTIONS AND SIDE EFFECTS*

EENT: irritation of the tongue.
GI: nausea, vomiting, constipation, impaction, hemorrhoids, flatulence, perianal irritation, steatorrhea, abdominal discomfort.
Derm: rashes, irritation.
F and E: hyperchloremic acidosis.
Hemat: bleeding.
Metab: Vitamin A, D, K deficiency.

INTERACTIONS

Drug–Drug: ▪ Decreases absorption of orally administered **acetaminophen, amiodarone, glucocorticoids, cardiac glycosides, methotrexate, naproxen, phenylbutazone piroxicam, propranolol, thiazide diuretics, thyroid, ursodiol, oral anticoagulants,** and **fat-soluble vitamins (A, D, E and K)** ▪ May increase effect of **oral anticoagulants** due to depletion of vitamin K ▪ May decrease absorption of other **orally administered medications**.

ROUTE AND DOSAGE

▪ **PO (Adults):** 3–4 g 3–4 times daily.

PHARMACODYNAMICS (hypocholesterolemic effects)

ONSET	PEAK	DURATION
24–48 hr	1–3 wk	2–4 wk

NURSING IMPLICATIONS

Assessment

▪ **Hypercholesterolemia:** Obtain a diet history, especially in regard to fat consumption.
▪ **Pruritus:** Assess severity of itching and skin integrity.
▪ **Lab Test Considerations:** Serum cholesterol and triglyceride levels should be evaluated before initiating and periodically throughout course of therapy. Medication should be discontinued if paradoxical increase in cholesterol level occurs.
□ May cause an increase in SGOT (AST), phosphate, chloride, and alkaline phosphatase and a decrease in serum calcium, sodium, and potassium levels.

Potential Nursing Diagnoses

▪ Bowel elimination, altered: constipation (side effects).
▪ Knowledge deficit related to medication regimen (patient/family teaching).
▪ Noncompliance (patient/family teaching).

Implementation

□ Physician may order parenteral or water-miscible forms of fat-soluble vitamins (A, D, K) and folic acid for patients on chronic therapy.
□ Available in powder or bar (Cholybar) form.
▪ **PO:** Administer other medications 1 hr before or 4–6 hr after the administration of this medication.

Patient/Family Teaching

□ Instruct patient to take medication exactly as directed, do not skip doses or double up on missed doses.
□ Instruct patient to take medication before meals. Mix with 4–6 oz of water, milk, fruit juice, or other noncarbonated beverages. Rinse glass with small amount of additional beverage to ensure all medication is taken. May also mix with highly fluid soups, cereals, or pulpy fruits (applesauce, crushed pineapple). Allow powder to sit on fluid and hydrate for 1–2 min prior to mixing. Do not take

*Underlines indicate most frequent; **CAPITALS** indicate life-threatening.

dry. Color variations do not alter stability.

- Advise patient that this medication should be used in conjunction with diet restrictions (fat, cholesterol, carbohydrates, alcohol), exercise, and cessation of smoking.
- Explain that constipation may occur. Increasing fluids and bulk in diet, exercise, stool softeners, and laxatives may be required to minimize the constipating effects. Instruct patient to notify physician if constipation, nausea, flatulence, and heartburn persist or if stools become frothy and foul smelling.
- Advise patient to notify physician if unusual bleeding or bruising, petechiae, or black, tarry stools occur. Treatment with vitamin K may be necessary.

EVALUATION

Effectiveness of therapy can be demonstrated by: ▪ Decrease in serum low-density lipoprotein (LDL) cholesterol levels. Cholesterol levels should begin to decrease in 48 hr but may take 1 yr to stabilize. Therapy is usually discontinued if the clinical response remains poor after 3 mon of therapy ▪ Decrease in severity of pruritus. Relief usually occurs 1–3 wk after therapy is initiated.

CHOLINE MAGNESIUM TRISALICYLATE

(**koe**-leen **mag**-neez-ee-um **try**-sal-i-sil-ate)
Trilisate

CLASSIFICATION(S):
Non-narcotic analgesic, Nonsteroidal anti-inflammatory agent, Antipyretic
Pregnancy Category C

INDICATIONS

▪ Treatment of mild to moderate pain ▪ Management of inflammatory disorders including: ▫ Rheumatoid arthritis ▫ Osteoarthritis ▪ Treatment of fever.

ACTION

▪ Produces analgesia and reduces inflammation by inhibiting the production of prostaglandins ▪ Unlike aspirin, has no effect on platelet function. **Therapeutic Effects:** ▪ Analgesia resulting in reduction of mild to moderate pain ▪ Reduction of inflammation ▪ Reduction of fever.

PHARMACOKINETICS

Absorption: Well absorbed following oral administration.
Distribution: Rapidly and widely distributed. Crosses the placenta and enters breast milk.
Metabolism and Excretion: Extensively metabolized by the liver. Inactive metabolites excreted by the kidneys.
Half-life: 2–3 hr for low doses. For larger doses, half-life may increase up to 15–30 hr due to saturation of liver metabolism.

CONTRAINDICATIONS AND PRECAUTIONS

Contraindicated in: ▪ Hypersensitivity to aspirin or other nonsteroidal anti-inflammatory agents (less cross-sensitivity than aspirin).
Use Cautiously in: ▪ Renal insufficiency (magnesium toxicity may occur) ▪ Severe liver impairment ▪ Pregnancy (may have adverse effects on fetus and mother) ▪ Lactation (safety not established) ▪ Children or adolescents with viral infections (may increase the risk of Reye's Syndrome).

ADVERSE REACTIONS AND SIDE EFFECTS*

EENT: tinnitus, hearing loss.
GI: <u>dyspepsia</u>, <u>heartburn</u>, <u>epigastric distress</u>, <u>nausea</u>, vomiting, anorexia, abdominal pain, **GI BLEEDING**, hepatotoxicity.
Misc: noncardiogenic pulmonary

*<u>Underlines</u> indicate most frequent; **CAPITALS** indicate life-threatening.

edema, allergic reactions including ANAPHYLAXIS or LARYNGEAL EDEMA.

INTERACTIONS

Drug–Drug: ▪ May potentiate **oral anticoagulants, heparin,** or **thrombolytic agents** (effect less than aspirin) ▪ May enhance the activity of **penicillins, phenytoin, methotrexate, valproic acid, oral hypoglycemic agents,** and **sulfonamides.** ▪ May antagonize the beneficial effects of **probenecid** or **sulfinpyrazone** ▪ May decrease effectiveness of concurrently administered **nonsteroidal anti-inflammatory agents** (except ketoprofen) ▪ **Glucocorticoids** may decrease serum salicylate levels ▪ **Urinary acidification** enhances reabsorption and may increase serum salicylate levels ▪ **Alkalinization of the urine** or the ingestion of large amounts of **antacids** promotes excretion and decreases serum salicylate levels ▪ May blunt the therapeutic response to **diuretics** or **antihypertensives** ▪ May increase the risk of bleeding with **cefamandole, cefoperazone, cefotetan, moxalactam, valproic acid,** or **plicamycin** (effect less than aspirin) ▪ Increased risk of gastrointestinal irritation with **nonsteroidal anti-inflammatory agents** (effect less than aspirin) ▪ Increased risk of ototoxicity with **vancomycin.**

Drug–Food: ▪ **Foods capable of acidifying the urine** (see Appendix K) may enhance reabsorption and increase serum salicylate levels.

ROUTE AND DOSAGE

Note: 5 ml of liquid equivalent to 500 mg salicylate or 650 mg of aspirin. Tablet strength expressed in mg of salicylate: 500 mg tablet equivalent to 650 mg of aspirin, 750 mg tablet equivalent to 975 mg of aspirin, 1000 mg tablet equivalent to 1.3 g of aspirin.

- **PO (Adults):** 2–3 g of salicylate/day in 1–3 divided doses.
- **PO (Children >37 kg):** 2.2 g of salicylate/day in 2 divided doses.
- **PO (Children <37 kg):** 50 mg of salicylate/kg/day in 2 divided doses.

PHARMACODYNAMICS (analgesia and fever reduction)*

	ONSET	PEAK	DURATION
PO	5–30 min	1–3 hr	3–6 hr

*Antirheumatic effect may take 2–3 wk of chronic dosing.

NURSING IMPLICATIONS

Assessment

- **General Info:** Patients who have asthma, allergies, and nasal polyps or who are allergic to tartrazine dyes are at an increased risk for developing hypersensitivity reactions.
- **Pain:** Assess pain and limitation of movement; note type, location, and intensity prior to and 1–3 hr following administration.
- **Fever:** Assess fever and note associated signs (diaphoresis, tachycardia, malaise, chills).
- **Toxicity and Overdose:** Observe patient for the onset of tinnitus, hyperventilation, agitation, mental confusion, lethargy, diarrhea, and sweating. If these symptoms appear, withhold medication and notify physician immediately.

Potential Nursing Diagnoses

- Comfort, altered: pain (indications).
- Mobility, impaired physical (indications).
- Knowledge deficit related to medication regimen (patient/family teaching).

Implementation

- **General Info:** Available in tablet and liquid preparations.
- **PO:** Administer after meals or with food or an antacid to minimize gastric irritation. Food slows but will not alter the total amount absorbed.

Patient/Family Teaching

- ▫ Instruct patient to take with a full glass of water and to remain in an upright position for 15–30 min after administration.
- ▫ Advise patient to report tinnitus, unusual bleeding of gums, bruising, or black, tarry stools, or fever lasting longer than three days.

- ▫ Caution patient to avoid concurrent use of alcohol with this medication to minimize possible gastric irritation.
- ▫ Advise patients on long-term therapy to inform physician or dentist of medication regimen prior to surgery.
- ▫ Centers for Disease Control warn against giving salicylates to children or adolescents with varicella (chickenpox), influenza-like or viral illnesses because of a possible association with Reye's syndrome.

EVALUATION

Effectiveness of therapy can be demonstrated by: ▪ Decrease in severity of mild to moderate discomfort ▪ Increased ease of joint movement ▪ Reduction of fever.

CHOLINE SALICYLATE

(**koe**-leen sal-i-sil-ate)

Arthropan

CLASSIFICATION(S):

Non-narcotic analgesic, Nonsteroidal anti-inflammatory agent, Antipyretic

Pregnancy Category UK

INDICATIONS

▪ Treatment of mild to moderate pain ▪ Management of inflammatory disorders including: ▫ Rheumatoid arthritis ▫ Osteoarthritis ▪ Treatment of fever.

ACTION

▪ Produces analgesia and reduces inflammation by inhibiting the production of prostaglandins ▪ Unlike aspirin, has no effect on platelet function. **Therapeutic Effects:** ▪ Analgesia resulting in reduction of mild to moderate pain ▪ Reduction of inflammation ▪ Reduction of fever.

PHARMACOKINETICS

Absorption: Well absorbed following oral administration.

Distribution: Rapidly and widely distributed. Crosses the placenta and enters breast milk.

Metabolism and Excretion: Extensively metabolized by the liver. Inactive metabolites excreted by the kidneys.

Half-life: 2–3 hr for low doses. For larger doses, half-life may increase up to 15–30 hr due to saturation of liver metabolism.

CONTRAINDICATIONS AND PRECAUTIONS

Contraindicated in: ▪ Hypersensitivity to aspirin or other nonsteroidal anti-inflammatory agents (less cross-sensitivity than aspirin).

Use Cautiously in: ▪ Renal insufficiency (magnesium toxicity may occur) ▪ Severe liver impairment ▪ Pregnancy (may have adverse effects on fetus and mother) ▪ Lactation (safety not established) ▪ Children or adolescents with viral infections (may increase the risk of Reye's Syndrome).

ADVERSE REACTIONS AND SIDE EFFECTS*

EENT: tinnitus, hearing loss.

GI: <u>dyspepsia</u>, <u>heartburn</u>, <u>epigastric distress</u>, <u>nausea</u>, vomiting, anorexia, abdominal pain, **GI BLEEDING**, hepatotoxicity.

Misc: noncardiogenic pulmonary edema, allergic reactions including **ANAPHYLAXIS** or **LARYNGEAL EDEMA**.

INTERACTIONS

Drug–Drug: ▪ May potentiate **oral anticoagulants, heparin,** or **thrombolytic agents** (effect less than aspirin) ▪ May enhance the activity of **penicillins, phenytoin, methotrexate, valproic acid, oral hypoglycemic agents,** and **sulfonamides** ▪ May antagonize the beneficial effects of **probenecid** or **sulfinpyrazone** ▪ May decrease effectiveness of concurrently administered **nonsteroidal anti-inflammatory agents** (except ketoprofen) ▪ **Glucocorticoids** may decrease serum salicylate levels ▪ **Urinary acidification** enhances reabsorption and may increase serum salicylate levels ▪ **Alka-**

*<u>Underlines</u> indicate most frequent; **CAPITALS** indicate life-threatening.

C

linization of the urine or the ingestion of large amounts of **antacids** promotes excretion and decreases serum salicylate levels ▪ May blunt the therapeutic response to **diuretics** or **antihypertensives** ▪ May increase the risk of bleeding with **cefamandole, cefoperazone, cefotetan, moxalactam, valproic acid,** or **plicamycin** (effect less than aspirin) ▪ Increased risk of gastrointestinal irritation with **nonsteroidal anti-inflammatory agents** (effect less than aspirin) ▪ Increased risk of ototoxicity with **vancomycin.**

Drug–Food: ▪ **Foods capable of acidifying the urine** (see Appendix K) may enhance reabsorption and increase serum salicylate levels.

ROUTE AND DOSAGE

Note: 5 ml of liquid equivalent to 870 mg salicylate or 650 mg of aspirin.

Analgesic/Antipyretic

- **PO (Adults):** 435–669 mg q 3 hr or 435–870 mg q 4 hr or 870–1338 mg q 6 hr as needed.
- **PO (Children):** 2 g/m^2/day in 4–6 divided doses as needed.
- **PO (Children 11–12 yr):** 435–652.5 mg q 4 hr as needed.
- **PO (Children 9–11 yr):** 435–543.8 mg q 4 hr as needed.
- **PO (Children 6–9 yr):** 435 mg q 4 hr as needed.
- **PO (Children 4–6 yr):** 326.5 mg q 4 hr as needed.
- **PO (Children 2–4 yr):** 217.5 mg q 4 hr as needed.

Anti-Inflammatory

- **PO (Adults):** 4.8–7.2 g/day in divided doses.
- **PO (Children):** 107–133 mg/kg/day in divided doses.

PHARMACODYNAMICS (analgesia and fever reduction)*

	ONSET	PEAK	DURATION
PO	5–30 min	1–3 hr	3–6 hr

*Antirheumatic effect may take 2–3 wk of chronic dosing.

NURSING IMPLICATIONS

Assessment

- **General Info:** Patients who have asthma, allergies, and nasal polyps or who are allergic to tartrazine dyes are at an increased risk for developing hypersensitivity reactions.
- **Pain:** Assess pain and limitation of movement; note type, location, and intensity prior to and 1–3 hr following administration.
- **Fever:** Assess fever and note associated signs (diaphoresis, tachycardia, malaise, chills).
- **Toxicity and Overdose:** Observe patient for the onset of tinnitus, hyperventilation, agitation, mental confusion, lethargy, diarrhea, and sweating. If these symptoms appear, withhold medication and notify physician immediately.

Potential Nursing Diagnoses

- Comfort, altered: pain (indications).
- Mobility, impaired physical (indications).
- Knowledge deficit related to medication regimen (patient/family teaching).

Implementation

- **General Info:** Available only in a liquid preparation.
- **PO:** Administer after meals or with food or an antacid to minimize gastric irritation. Food slows but will not alter the total amount absorbed.

Patient/Family Teaching

- ▫ Instruct patient to take with a full glass of water and to remain in an upright position for 15–30 min after administration.
- ▫ Advise patient to report tinnitus, unusual bleeding of gums, bruising, or black, tarry stools, or fever lasting longer than three days.
- ▫ Caution patient to avoid concurrent use of alcohol with this medication to minimize possible gastric irritation.
- ▫ Advise patients on long-term therapy to inform physician or dentist of medication regimen prior to surgery.
- ▫ Centers for Disease Control warn

against giving salicylates to children or adolescents with varicella (chickenpox), influenza-like or viral illnesses because of a possible association with Reye's syndrome.

Evaluation

Effectiveness of therapy can be demonstrated by: ▪ Decrease in severity of mild to moderate discomfort ▪ Increased ease of joint movement ▪ Reduction of fever.

CIMETIDINE

(sye-**met**-i-deen)
{Apo-Cimetidine}, {Novocimetine}, {Peptol}, Tagamet

CLASSIFICATION(S):
Histamine H_2 Antagonist, Antiulcer
Pregnancy Category B

INDICATIONS

▪ Treatment of active duodenal ulcers and benign gastric ulcers ▪ Prophylaxis of duodenal ulcer ▪ Management of gastroesophageal reflux disease (GERD) ▪ Managment of gastric hypersecretory states (Zollinger–Ellison Syndrome). **Unlabeled Uses:** ▪ Treatment of upper GI bleeding ▪ Prevention of stress ulceration or aspiration pneumonitis.

ACTION

▪ Inhibits the action of histamine at the H_2-receptor site located primarily in gastric parietal cells, resulting in inhibition of gastric acid secretion. **Therapeutic Effects:** ▪ Healing and prevention of ulcers ▪ Decreased symptoms of gastroesophageal reflux ▪ Decreased secretion of gastric acid.

PHARMACOKINETICS

Absorption: Well absorbed following oral and IM administration.
Distribution: Widely distributed. Enters breast milk and probably crosses the placenta.
Metabolism and Excretion: 30% metabolized by the liver. Remainder is eliminated unchanged by the kidneys.
Half-life: 2 hr (increased in renal impairment).

CONTRAINDICATIONS AND PRECAUTIONS

Contraindicated in: ▪ Hypersensitivity.
Use Cautiously in: ▪ Elderly (more susceptible to adverse CNS reactions; dosage reduction recommended) ▪ Renal impairment (more susceptible to adverse CNS reactions; dosage reduction recommended) ▪ Pregnancy or lactation.

ADVERSE REACTIONS AND SIDE EFFECTS*

CNS: <u>confusion</u>, dizziness, headache, drowsiness.
CV: bradycardia.
GI: nausea, diarrhea, constipation, hepatitis.
GU: nephritis, decreased sperm count.
Derm: rashes, exfoliative dermatitis, urticaria.
Endo: gynecomastia.
Hemat: **AGRANULOCYTOSIS, APLASTIC ANEMIA**, neutropenia, thrombocytopenia, anemia.
Local: pain at IM site.
MS: muscle pain.

INTERACTIONS

Drug-Drug: ▪ Cimetidine inhibits drug metabolizing enzymes in the liver; likely to lead to increased blood levels and toxicity of the following—**oral anticoagulants, lidocaine, phenytoin,** and **theophylline** ▪ May have a similar but less predictable effect with **metronidazole, triamterene, metoprolol, mexiletine, flecainide, procainamide, quinidine, quinine, caffeine, some benzodiazepines (diazepam, chlordiazepoxide) succinyl choline, narcotic analgesics, pentoxiphylline, carbamazepine, chloroquine, calcium channel blockers, some sulfonylureas (glybur-**

{} = Available in Canada only.
*<u>Underlines</u> indicate most frequent; **CAPITALS** indicate life-threatening.

ide, glipizide) and **some tricyclic antidepressants** ▪ May potentiate myelosuppressive properties of **carmustine** ▪ **Antacids** may decrease the absorption of cimetidine ▪ Cigarette **smoking** decreases the effectiveness of cimetidine ▪ Cimetidine decreases absorption of **iron salts, indomethacin, ketoconazole,** and **tetracyclines** ▪ May decrease the pharmacologic effects of **tocainide**.

ROUTE AND DOSAGE

Short-Term Treatment of Active Ulcers

- **PO (Adults):** 300 mg 4 times daily or 800 mg at bedtime or 400 mg twice daily for up to 8 wk (not to exceed 2.4 g/day).
- **PO (Children):** 20–40 mg/kg/day in 4 divided doses.
- **IM, IV (Adults):** 300 mg q 6 hr (not to exceed 2.4 g/day).
- **IM, IV (Children):** 5–10 mg/kg q 6–8 g.
- **IV Infusion (Adults):** 900 mg infused over 24 hr; may be preceded by a 150 mg bolus dose.

Duodenal Ulcer Prophylaxis

- **PO (Adults):** 400–800 mg at bedtime.

Gastric Hypersecretory Conditions

- **PO, IM, IV (Adults):** 300–600 mg q 6 hr (up to 12 g/day has been used).

Gastroesophageal Reflux, Upper GI Bleeding

- **PO (Adults):** 300 mg 4 times daily or 600 mg twice daily.

Prophylaxis of Stress Ulcers

- **IV (Adults):** 300 mg q 6 hr (or more as needed to maintain gastric pH >4).

Prophylaxis of Aspiration Pneumonitis

- **IM, IV (Adults):** 300 mg IM 1 hr before anesthesia, then 300 mg IV q 4 h until patient is conscious.

PHARMACODYNAMICS (suppression of gastric acid secretion)

	ONSET	PEAK	DURATION
PO	30 min	45–90 min	4–5 hr
IM, IV	10 min	30 min	4–5 hr

NURSING IMPLICATIONS

Assessment

- Assess patient for epigastric or abdominal pain and frank or occult blood in the stool, emesis, or gastric aspirate.
- Assess elderly and debilitated patients routinely for confusion. Notify physician promptly should this occur.
- **Lab Test Considerations:** CBC with differential should be monitored periodically throughout therapy.
- May cause transient increase in serum transaminase and serum creatinine. Serum prolactin concentration may be increased following IV bolus. May also cause decreased parathyroid concentrations.
- Antagonizes effects of pentagastrin and histamine during gastric acid secretion testing. Avoid administration for 24 hr preceding the test.
- May cause false-negative results in skin tests using allergenic extracts. Cimetidine should be discontinued 24 hr prior to the test.

Potential Nursing Diagnoses

- Comfort, altered: pain (indications).
- Knowledge deficit related to medication regimen (patient/family teaching).

Implementation

- **General Info:** Available in tablet, oral solution, and injectable forms.
- **PO:** Administer medication with meals or immediately afterward and at bedtime to prolong effect. If administering oral doses concurrently with antacids, give at least 1 hr apart.
- Tablets have a characteristic odor.
- **Direct IV:** Dilute each 300 mg in 20 ml of 0.9% NaCl for injection.
- *Rate:* Administer over at least 2 min. Rapid administration may cause hypotension and arrhythmias.
- **Intermittent Infusion:** Dilute each 300 mg in 50 ml of 0.9% NaCl, D5W, D10W, D5/LR, D5/0.9% NaCl, D5/0.45% NaCl, D5/0.25% NaCl, Ringer's or lactated Ringer's soln, or sodium bicarbonate. Diluted soln is

stable for 48 hr at room temperature. Refrigeration may cause cloudiness but will not affect potency. Do not use soln that is discolored or contains precipitate.

- *Rate:* Administer over 15–20 min.
- **Continuous Infusion:** Dilute cimetidine 900 mg in 100–1000 ml of compatible soln (see Intermittent Infusion).
- *Rate:* Usually infused at a rate of 37.5 mg/hr, but should be individualized.
- **Syringe Compatibility:** atropine, butorphanol, cephalothin, diazepam, diphenhydramine, doxapram, droperidol, fentanyl, glycopyrrolate, heparin, hydromorphone, hydroxyzine, lorazepam, meperidine, midazolam, morphine, nafcillin, nalbuphine, penicillin G sodium, pentazocine, perphenizine, prochlorperizine, promazine, promethazine, scopolamine, sodium acetate, NaCl, sodium lactate, or sterile water.
- **Syringe Incompatibility:** cefamandole, cefazolin, chlorpromazine, pentobarbital, or secobarbital.
- **Y-Site Compatibility:** acyclovir, aminophylline, amrinone, atracurium, enalaprilat, esmolol, foscarnet, heparin, hetastarch, labetalol, ondansetron, pancuronium, tolazoline, vecuronium, or zidovudine.
- **Additive Compatibility:** acetazolamide, amikacin, aminophylline, cefoxitin, chlorothiazide, clindamycin, colistimethate, dexamethasone, digoxin, epinephrine, erythromycin, ethacrynate, furosemide, gentamicin, insulin, isoproterenol, lidocaine, lincomycin, metaraminol bitartrate, methylprednisolone, norepinephrine, penicillin G potassium, phytonadione, polymyxin B, potassium chloride, protamine sulfate, quinidine, sodium nitroprusside, tetracycline, verapamil, or vitamin B complex.
- **Additive Incompatibility:** amphotericin B.

Patient/Family Teaching

- **General Info:** Instruct patient to take medication as prescribed for the full course of therapy, even if feeling better. If a dose is missed, it should be taken as soon as remembered but not if almost time for next dose. Do not double doses.
- Inform patient that smoking interferes with the action of cimetidine. Encourage patient to quit smoking or at least not to smoke after last dose of the day.
- Cimetidine may cause drowsiness or dizziness. Caution patient to avoid driving or other activities requiring alertness until response to the drug is known.
- Advise patient to avoid alcohol, products containing aspirin, and foods that may cause an increase in GI irritation.
- Advise patient to report onset of black, tarry stools, fever, sore throat, diarrhea, dizziness, rash, confusion, or hallucinations to the physician promptly.

Evaluation

Effectiveness of therapy can be demonstrated by: ▪ Decrease in abdominal pain or prevention of gastric irritation and bleeding. Healing of duodenal ulcers can be seen by x-rays or endoscopy. Therapy is continued for at least 6 wk in treatment of ulcers ▪ Decreased symptoms of esophageal reflux.

CIPROFLOXACIN

(sip-roe-**flox**-a-sin)
Ciloxan, Cipro

CLASSIFICATION(S):
Anti-infective—fluoroquinolone
Pregnancy Category C

INDICATIONS

▪ **PO, IV:** Treatment of the following infections due to susceptible organisms: ▫ Lower respiratory tract infections ▫ Skin and skin structure infections ▫ Bone and joint infections ▫ Urinary tract infections ▪ **PO:** Infectious diarrhea ▪ **Ophth:** Management of corneal ulcers and conjunctivitis.

C

ACTION

■ Inhibits bacterial DNA synthesis by inhibiting DNA gyrase. **Therapeutic Effect:** ■ Death of susceptible bacteria. **Spectrum:** ■ Broad activity includes many gram-positive pathogens: □ Staphylococci (including *Staphylococcus epidermidis* and methicillin-resistant strains of *Staphylococcus aureus*) □ *Streptococcus pyogenes* □ *Streptococcus pneumoniae* ■ Gram-negative spectrum notable for activity against: □ *E. coli* □ Klebsiella species □ Enterobacter □ Salmonella □ Shigella □ *Proteus vulgaris* □ *Providencia stuartii* □ Providencia retgerii □ *Morganella morganii* □ *Pseudomonas aeruginoa* □ Serratia □ Haemophilus species □ Acinetobacter □ *Neisseria gonorrhea* and *meningitidis* □ *Branhamella catarrhalis* □ Yersinia □ Vibrio □ Brucella □ Campylobacter □ Aeromonas species.

PHARMACOKINETICS

Absorption: Well absorbed (70%) following oral administration.
Distribution: Widely distributed. High tissue concentrations are achieved.
Metabolism and Excretion: 15% metabolized by the liver. 40–50% excreted unchanged by the kidneys.
Half-life: 4 hr (increased in renal disease).

CONTRAINDICATIONS AND PRECAUTIONS

Contraindicated in: ■ Hypersensitivity ■ Cross-sensitivity with other fluoroquinolones may exist ■ Children <18 yr ■ Pregnancy ■ Hypersensitivity to benzalkoniun chloride or EDTA (ophth only).
Use Cautiously in: ■ Underlying CNS pathology ■ Lactation (safety not established) ■ Severe renal impairment (dosage reduction required).

ADVERSE REACTIONS AND SIDE EFFECTS*

CNS: tremors, restlessness, confusion, hallucination, SEIZURES, dizziness.
EENT: Ophth—lid margin crusting, crystals/scales, foreign body sensation, itching, conjuntival hyperemia.
GI: nausea, diarrhea, vomiting, abdominal pain; Ophth—bad taste in mouth.
GU: crystalluria, cylinduria, hematuria.
Derm: rash, photosensitivity.
Local: phlebitis at IV site (especially if infusion time is <30 min).
Misc: allergic reactions including ANAPHYLAXIS.

INTERACTIONS

Drug-Drug: ■ Increases serum **theophylline** levels may lead to toxicity ■ Administration with **antacids, iron salts, sucralfate,** or **zinc sulfate** decrease absorption of ciprofloxacin ■ **Drugs that alkalinize the urine** increase the risk of crystalluria ■ May increase nephrotoxicity of **cyclosporine** ■ **Nitrofurantoin** may decrease effectiveness ■ **Probenecid** increases blood levels ■ May increase the effect of **oral anticoagulants** ■ **Antineoplastics** may decrease ciprofloxacin blood levels.

ROUTE AND DOSAGE

- **IV (Adults):** 200–400 mg q 12 hr (administered as an infusion over 60 min).
- **PO (Adults):** 250–750 mg q 12 hr.
- **Ophth: (Adults):** 1–2 drops q 15–30 min until infection is controlled, then 1–2 drops 4–6 times daily.

PHARMACODYNAMICS (blood levels)

	ONSET	PEAK
PO	rapid	1–2 hr
IV	rapid	end of infusion

NURSING IMPLICATIONS

Assessment

□ Assess patient for infection (vital signs; appearance of wound, sputum, urine, and stool; WBC) at beginning and throughout course of therapy.
□ Obtain specimens for culture and sensitivity prior to initiating therapy.

*Underlines indicate most frequent; **CAPITALS** indicate life-threatening.

First dose may be given before receiving results.

□ Monitor intake and output. Intake should be at least 2000–3000 ml/day to prevent crystalluria.

■ **Lab Test Considerations:** May cause elevated SGOT (AST), SGPT (ALT), alkaline phosphatase, bilirubin, BUN, creatinine, and LDH concentrations.

□ May cause elevated or decreased serum platelets and decreased RBCs and WBCs.

Potential Nursing Diagnoses

■ Infection, high risk for (indications, side effects).

■ Knowledge deficit related to medication regimen (patient/family teaching).

■ Noncompliance related to medication regimen (patient/family teaching).

Implementation

■ **PO:** Administer on an empty stomach, 2 hr after meals. If gastric irritation occurs, may be administered with meals. Food slows and may slightly decrease absorption.

□ If antacids are prescribed concurrently, administer at least 2 hr before or after ciprofloxacin.

■ **Intermittent Infusion:** Dilute ciprofloxacin to a concentration of 1–2 mg/ml with 0.9% NaCl or D5W. Stable for 14 days at refrigerated or room temperature.

□ Temporarily discontinue other solns when administering ciprofloxacin.

□ *Rate:* Administer over 60 min into a large vein to minimize venous irritation.

■ **Ophth:** Administer drops by having patient lie down or tilt head back and look at ceiling. Pull down on lower lid creating a small pocket and instill soln into pocket. Instruct patient to gently close eye. Wait 5 min before instilling other ophthalmic soln.

Patient/Family Teaching

□ Instruct patients to take medication completely as directed, even if feeling better. Advise patients that sharing of this medication may be dangerous.

□ Ciprofloxacin may cause dizziness or lightheadedness. Caution patient to avoid driving or other activities requiring alertness until response to medication is known.

□ Caution patient to use sunscreen and protective clothing to prevent photosensitivity reactions.

□ Advise patient to report signs of superinfection (furry overgrowth on the tongue, vaginal itching or discharge, loose or foul-smelling stools).

□ Instruct the patient to notify physician if symptoms do not improve.

Evaluation

Clinical response to therapy can be evaluated by: ■ Resolution of the signs and symptoms of infection. Length of time for complete resolution depends on the organism and site of infection.

CISPLATIN

(sis-**pla**-tin)
{Abiplatin}, CDDP, Platinol, {Platinol-AQ}

CLASSIFICATION(S):
Antineoplastic—alkylating agent
Pregnancy Category UK

INDICATIONS

■ Alone or in combination (with other antineoplastics, surgery, or radiation) in the management of: □ Metastatic testicular and ovarian carcinoma □ Advanced bladder cancer □ Head and neck cancer □ Cervical cancer □ Lung cancer □ Other tumors.

ACTION

■ Inhibits DNA synthesis by producing cross-linking of parent DNA strands. (cell cycle-phase nonspecific). **Therapeutic Effect:** ■ Death of rapidly replicating cells, particularly malignant cells.

{} = Available in Canada only.

C

PHARMACOKINETICS

Absorption: Following IV administration absorption is essentially complete.
Distribution: Widely distributed. Accumulation continues for mons after administration.
Metabolism and Excretion: Excreted mainly by the kidneys.
Half-life: 30–100 hr.

CONTRAINDICATIONS AND PRECAUTIONS

Contraindicated in: ▪ Hypersensitivity ▪ Pregnancy or lactation.
Use Cautiously in: ▪ Renal disease (dosage modification required) ▪ Hearing loss ▪ Electrolyte abnormalities ▪ Patients with childbearing potential ▪ Active infections ▪ Bone marrow depression ▪ Chronic debilitating illnesses.

ADVERSE REACTIONS AND SIDE EFFECTS*

CNS: SEIZURES.
EENT: ototoxicity, tinnitus.
GI: severe nausea, vomiting, diarrhea, hepatotoxicity.
GU: nephrotoxicity, infertility.
F and E: hypomagnesemia, hypokalemia, hypocalcemia.
Hemat: anemia, leukopenia, thrombocytopenia.
Local: phlebitis at IV site.
Metab: hyperuricemia.
Neuro: peripheral neuropathy.
Misc: anaphylactoid reactions.

INTERACTIONS

Drug-Drug: ▪ Additive nephrotoxicity and ototoxicity with other **nephro-** and **ototoxic drugs (aminoglycosides, loop diuretics)** ▪ Additive bone marrow depression with other **antineoplastic agents** or **radiation therapy**.

ROUTE AND DOSAGE

▪ **IV (Adults):** 20 mg/m^2 daily for 5 days or 50–70 mg/m^2, repeat q 3 wk.

PHARMACODYNAMICS (effects on blood counts)

	ONSET	PEAK	DURATION
IV	UK	18–23 days	39 days

NURSING IMPLICATIONS

Assessment

- Monitor blood pressure, pulse, respiratory rate, and temperature frequently during administration. Notify physician of significant changes.
- Monitor intake and output and specific gravity frequently throughout therapy. Physician should be notified immediately if discrepancies in these totals occur. To reduce the risk of nephrotoxicity, a urinary output of at least 100 ml/hr should be maintained for 4 hr before initiating and for at least 24 hr after administration.
- Encourage patient to drink 2000–3000 ml/day to promote excretion of uric acid. Allopurinol and alkalinization of the urine may be ordered to help prevent uric acid nephropathy.
- Assess patency of IV site frequently during therapy. This medication may cause severe irritation and necrosis of tissue if extravasation occurs.
- Severe and protracted nausea and vomiting may occur as early as 1 hr after therapy and may last for 24 hr. Parenteral antiemetic agents should be administered 30–45 min prior to therapy and routinely around the clock for the next 24 hr as indicated. Monitor amount of emesis and notify physician if emesis exceeds guidelines to prevent dehydration.
- Assess for fever, chills, sore throat, and signs of infection. Notify physician if these symptoms occur.
- Monitor platelet count throughout therapy. Assess for bleeding (bleeding gums, bruising, petechiae; guaiac stools, urine, and emesis). Avoid IM injections and rectal temperatures. Apply pressure to venipuncture sites for 10 min.

*Underlines indicate most frequent; **CAPITALS** indicate life-threatening.

- Anemia may occur. Monitor for increased fatigue, dyspnea, and orthostatic hypotension.
- Monitor for signs of anaphylaxis (facial edema, wheezing, tachycardia, hypotension). Discontinue medication immediately and notify physician if these occur. Epinephrine and resuscitation equipment should be readily available.
- Medication may cause ototoxicity (especially in children) and neurotoxicity. Assess patient frequently for dizziness, tinnitus, hearing loss, loss of coordination, or numbness and tingling of extremities. These symptoms may be irreversible. Notify physician promptly if these occur.
- **Lab Test Considerations:** Monitor CBC prior to and routinely throughout course of therapy. The nadir of leukopenia, thrombocytopenia, and anemia occur within 18–23 days. Withhold further doses until WBC is $>4000/mm^3$ and platelet count is $>100,000/mm^3$.
- Monitor renal and hepatic function prior to and periodically throughout course of therapy. May cause nephrotoxicity (increased BUN and creatinine, and decreased calcium, magnesium, phosphate, and potassium levels). Do not administer additional doses until BUN is <25 mg/100 ml and serum creatinine is <1.5 mg/100 ml. May cause increased uric acid levels. Hepatotoxity may be manifested by increased SGOT (AST), SGPT (ALT), and bilirubin.

Potential Nursing Diagnoses

- Infection, high risk for (adverse reactions).
- Injury, high risk for (side effects).
- Knowledge deficit related to medication regimen (patient/family teaching).

Implementation

- **General Info:** Hydrate patient with at least 1–2 liters of IV fluid 8–12 hr before initiating therapy with cisplatin.
- Do not use aluminum needles or equipment during preparation or administration. Aluminum reacts with the drug, forms a black or brown precipitate, and renders it ineffective.
- Unopened vials of powder must be refrigerated.
- Soln should be prepared in a biologic cabinet. Wear gloves, gown, and mask while handling medication. Discard equipment in specially designated containers (see Appendix I).
- **Intermittent Infusion:** Reconstitute 10-mg vial with 10 ml of sterile water for injection and 50-mg vial with 50 ml. Stable for 2 hr if reconstituted with sterile water, for 72 hr with bacteriostatic water. Do not refrigerate, as crystals will form. Soln should be clear and colorless; discard if turbid or contains precipitates.
- Dilution in 2 liters of 5% dextrose in 0.3% or 0.45% NaCl containing 37.5 g of mannitol is recommended.
- *Rate:* Infuse over 6–8 hr.
- **Continuous Infusion:** Has been administered as continuous infusion over 24 hr to 5 days with resultant decrease in nausea and vomiting.
- **Syringe/Y-Site Compatability:** Compatible in syringe for limited duration and via Y-site injection into a free-flowing IV with bleomycin, cyclophosphamide, doxorubicin, droperidol, fluorouracil, furosemide, heparin, leucovorin calcium, methotrexate, metoclopromide, mitomycin, ondansetron, vinblastine, or vincristine.
- **Additive Compatability:** etoposide, hydroxyzine, magnesium sulfate, mannitol, 0.9% NaCl, or D5/0.9% NaCl.
- **Additive Incompatability:** fluorouracil, metoclopramide, or sodium bicarbonate.

Patient/Family Teaching

- Instruct patient to report pain at injection site immediately.
- Instruct patient to notify physician promptly if fever, sore throat, signs of infection, bleeding gums, bruising, petechiae; blood in stools, urine, or emesis; increased fatigue, dyspnea, or orthostatic hypotension occur.

Caution patient to avoid crowds and persons with known infections. Instruct patient to use soft toothbrush and electric razor, and to avoid falls. Caution patient not to drink alcoholic beverages or take medication containing aspirin, as these may precipitate gastric bleeding.

- Instruct patient to report promptly any numbness or tingling in extremities or face, difficulty with hearing or tinnitus, unusual swelling, or joint pain to physician.
- Instruct patient not to receive any vaccinations without advice of physician.
- Advise patient of the need for contraception although cisplatin may cause infertility.
- Emphasize the need for periodic lab tests to monitor for side effects.

EVALUATION

Effectiveness of therapy may be determined by: ▪ Decrease in size or spread of malignancies ▪ Therapy should not be administered more frequently than every 3–4 wk, and only if lab values are within acceptable parameters and patient is not exhibiting signs of ototoxicity or other serious adverse effects.

CLARITHROMYCIN

(klare-**ith**-row-my-sin)
Biaxin

CLASSIFICATION(S):
Anti-infective—macrolide
Pregnancy Category C

INDICATIONS

▪ Treatment of the following infections due to susceptible organisms: □ Upper respiratory tract infections including streptococcal pharyngitis and sinusitis □ Lower respiratory tract infections including bronchitis and pneumonia.

ACTION

▪ Inhibits protein synthesis at the level of the 50S bacterial ribosome. **Therapeutic Effects:** ▪ Bacteriostatic action against susceptible bacteria. **Spectrum:** ▪ Active against the following gram-positive aerobic bacteria: □ *Staphylococcus aureus* □ *Streptococcus pneumoniae* □ *Streptococcus pyogenes* (group A strep) ▪ Active against these gram-negative aerobic bacteria: □ *Haemophilus influenzae* □ *Moraxella catarrhalis* ▪ Also active against: □ *Mycoplasma* □ *Legionella* ▪ Not active against methicillin-resistant *Staphylococcus aureus*.

PHARMACOKINETICS

Absorption: Rapidly absorbed (50%) following oral administration.

Distribution: Widely distributed to body tissues and fluids. Tissue levels may exceed those in serum.

Metabolism and Excretion: 10–15% conversion by the liver to 14-hydroxyclarithromycin, which has anti-infective activity. 20–30% excreted unchanged in urine.

Half-life: 250-mg dose—3–4 hr; 500-mg dose—5–7 hr.

CONTRAINDICATIONS AND PRECAUTIONS

Contraindicated in: ▪ Hypersensitivity to clarithromycin, erythromycin, or other macrolide anti-infectives.

Use Cautiously in: ▪ Pregnancy (avoid use unless no alternatives available) ▪ Lactation and children <12 yr (safety not established) ▪ Severe liver and/or renal impairment (dosage adjustment may be required).

ADVERSE REACTIONS AND SIDE EFFECTS*

CNS: headache.

GI: diarrhea, nausea, abnormal taste, dyspepsia, abdominal pain/discomfort.

Hemat: leukopenia, elevated prothrombin time.

INTERACTIONS

Drug-Drug: ▪ May increase serum levels and the risk of toxicity from **theo-**

*Underlines indicate most frequent; **CAPITALS** indicate life-threatening.

phylline or **carbamazepine** ▪ May increase the effect of **oral anticoagulants** ▪ May increase serum **digoxin** levels ▪ May increase the effects of **triazolam**.

ROUTE AND DOSAGE

- **PO (Adults):** 250–500 mg bid.

PHARMACODYNAMICS (serum levels)

	ONSET	PEAK
PO	UK	2 hr

NURSING IMPLICATIONS

Assessment

- □ Assess patient for infection (vital signs; appearance of wound, sputum, urine, and stool; WBC) at beginning and throughout course of therapy.
- □ Obtain specimens for culture and sensitivity prior to initiating therapy. First dose may be given before receiving results.
- ▪ **Lab Test Considerations:** May cause increased serum bilirubin, SGOT (AST), SGPT (ALT), LDH, and alkaline phosphatase concentrations.
- □ May rarely cause elevated prothrombin time, BUN, and serum creatinine. May occasionally cause decreased WBC.

Potential Nursing Diagnoses

- ▪ Infection, high risk for (indications, side effects).
- ▪ Knowledge deficit related to medication regimen (patient/family teaching).
- ▪ Noncompliance related to medication regimen (patient/family teaching).

Implementation

- ▪ **PO:** Administer around the clock, without regard to meals. Food slows but does not decrease the extent of absorption.

Patient/Family Teaching

- □ Instruct patients to take medication around the clock and to finish the drug completely as directed, even if feeling better. Missed doses should be taken as soon as possible, with remaining doses evenly spaced throughout day. Advise patients that sharing of this medication may be dangerous.
- □ Advise patient to report the signs of superinfection (black, furry overgrowth on the tongue, vaginal itching or discharge, loose or foul-smelling stools).
- □ Instruct patient to notify the physician if fever and diarrhea develop, especially if stool contains blood, pus, or mucus. Advise patient not to treat diarrhea without consulting physician or pharmacist.
- □ Advise patient to notify physician if pregnancy is planned or suspected.
- □ Instruct the patient to notify the physician if symptoms do not improve.

Evaluation

Clinical response to therapy may be determined by: ▪ Resolution of the signs and symptoms of infection. Length of time for complete resolution depends on the organism and site of infection.

CLEMASTINE
(**klem**-as-teen)
Tavist

CLASSIFICATION(S):
Antihistamine
Pregnancy Category B

INDICATIONS

▪ Relief of allergic symptoms caused by histamine release. Conditions in which it is most useful include allergic urticaria and angioedema.

ACTION

▪ Blocks the following effects of histamine: □ Vasodilation □ Increased GI tract secretions □ Increased heart rate □ Hypotension. **Therapeutic Effect:** ▪ Relief of symptoms associated with histamine excess usually seen in allergic conditions. Does not block the release of histamine.

PHARMACOKINETICS

Absorption: Well absorbed following oral administration.

Distribution: Enters breast milk in high concentrations.

Metabolism and Excretion: Extensively metabolized by the liver.

Half-life: UK.

CONTRAINDICATIONS AND PRECAUTIONS

Contraindicated in: ▪ Hypersensitivity ▪ Acute attacks of asthma ▪ Lactation (avoid use).

Use Cautiously in: ▪ Narrow-angle glaucoma ▪ Liver disease ▪ Elderly patients (more susceptible to adverse reactions) ▪ Pregnancy or children <6 yr (safety not established).

ADVERSE REACTIONS AND SIDE EFFECTS*

CNS: drowsiness, sedation, dizziness, confusion, paradoxical excitation (children).

CV: hypotension, hypertension, palpitations, arrhythmias.

EENT: blurred vision.

GI: dry mouth, obstruction, constipation.

GU: urinary hesitancy, retention.

Derm: sweating.

INTERACTIONS

Drug-Drug: ▪ Additive CNS depression with other **CNS depressants,** including **alcohol, narcotic analgesics,** and **sedative/hypnotics** ▪ **MAO inhibitors** intensify and prolong the anticholinergic effects of antihistamines.

ROUTE AND DOSAGE

Allergic Rhinitis

- **PO (Adults and Children >12 yr):** 1.34 mg bid; may be increased as needed (not to exceed 8.04 mg/day).
- **PO (Children 6–12 yr):** 0.67 mg bid; may be increased to 3.02 mg bid (not to exceed 4.02 mg/day).

Allergic Urticaria and Angioedema

- **PO (Adults and Children >12 yr):** 2.68 mg 1–3 times daily (not to exceed 8.04 mg/day).
- **PO (Children 6–12 yr):** 1.34 mg bid; may be increased (not to exceed 4.02 mg/day).

PHARMACODYNAMICS (antihistaminic effects)

	ONSET	PEAK	DURATION
PO	15–60 min	1–2 hr	12 hr

NURSING IMPLICATIONS

Assessment

- ▫ Assess allergy symptoms (rhinitis, conjunctivitis, hives, urticaria) prior to and periodically throughout course of therapy.
- ▫ Assess lung sounds and character of bronchial secretions. Maintain fluid intake of 1500–2000 ml/day to decrease viscosity of secretions.
- **Lab Test Considerations:** May cause false-negative reactions on allergy skin tests; discontinue 3 days prior to testing.
- **Toxicity and Overdose:** Symptoms of toxicity in children include excitement, hyperreflexia, hallucinations, tremors, ataxia, fever, seizures, fixed dilated pupils, dry mouth, and facial flushing. The dose that causes seizures approximates the lethal dose. Adults are more likely to experience severe drowsiness.

Potential Nursing Diagnoses

- Airway clearance, ineffective (indications).
- Injury, high risk for (adverse reactions).
- Knowledge deficit related to medication regimen (patient/family teaching).

Implementation

- **General Info:** Available in tablet and syrup form.
- **PO:** Administer with food or milk to decrease GI irritation.

*Underlines indicate most frequent; **CAPITALS** indicate life-threatening.

PATIENT/FAMILY TEACHING

- Instruct patient to take medication as directed. Do not take more than recommended amount. Missed doses should be taken as soon as remembered unless almost time for next dose. Do not double dose.
- Clemastine may cause drowsiness. Caution patient to avoid driving or other activities requiring alertness until response to drug is known.
- Caution patient to avoid using alcohol or other CNS depressants concurrently with this drug.
- Advise patient that good oral hygiene, frequent rinsing of mouth with water, and sugarless gum or candy may help relieve dry mouth. Patient should notify dentist if dry mouth persists for >2 wk.
- Elderly patients are at risk for orthostatic hypotension. Advise patient to make position changes slowly.
- Instruct patient to contact physician if symptoms persist or difficulty with urination, changes in vision, confusion, severe dry mouth, nose, and throat, or dizziness occur. Parents should notify physician if their child has difficulty sleeping, becomes unusually excited or irritable, or develops shortness of breath or facial flushing.

EVALUATION

Effectiveness of therapy can be demonstrated by: ▪ Decrease in allergic symptoms.

CLINDAMYCIN

(klin-da-**mye**-sin)
Cleocin, Dalacin C

CLASSIFICATION(S):
Anti-infective—miscellaneous
Pregnancy Category UK

INDICATIONS

▪ **PO, IM, IV:** Treatment of the following serious infections due to susceptible organisms: ▫ Skin and skin structure infections ▫ Respiratory tract infections ▫ Septicemia ▫ Intra-abdominal infections ▫ Gynecologic infections ▫ Osteomyeolitis ▪ Endocarditis prophylaxis ▪ **Top:** Treatment of severe acne.

ACTION

▪ Inhibits protein synthesis in susceptible bacteria at the level of the 50S ribosome. **Therapeutic Effect:** ▪ Bactericidal or bacteriostatic, depending on susceptibility and concentration. **Spectrum:** ▪ Active against most gram-positive aerobic cocci, including: ▫ Staphylococci ▫ *Streptococcus pneumoniae* ▫ Other streptococci, but not enterococcus ▪ Has good activity against many anaerobic bacteria, including *Bacteroides fragilis.*

PHARMACOKINETICS

Absorption: Well absorbed following oral and IM administration. Minimal absorption following topical application.
Distribution: Widely distributed. Does not significantly cross blood–brain barrier. Crosses the placenta and enters breast milk.
Metabolism and Excretion: Mostly metabolized by the liver.
Half-life: 2–3 hr.

CONTRAINDICATIONS AND PRECAUTIONS

Contraindicated in: ▪ Hypersensitivity ▪ Previous pseudomembranous colitis ▪ Severe liver impairment ▪ Diarrhea.
Use Cautiously in: ▪ Pregnancy or lactation (safety not established).

ADVERSE REACTIONS AND SIDE EFFECTS*

CNS: dizziness, vertigo, headache.
CV: hypotension, arrhythmias.
Derm: rashes.
GI: diarrhea, nausea, vomiting, PSEUDOMEMBRANOUS COLITIS, bitter taste (IV only).
Local: phlebitis at IV site.

*Underlines indicate most frequent; **CAPITALS** indicate life-threatening.

C

INTERACTIONS

Drug-Drug: ▪ **Kaolin** may decrease GI absorption ▪ May enhance the neuromuscular blocking action of other **neuromuscular blocking agents** ▪ **Top:** Concurrent use with **irritants, abrasives, or desquamating agents** may result in additive irritation ▪ **Top:** Antagonizes the effects of topical **erythromycin.**

ROUTE AND DOSAGE

- **PO (Adults):** 150–600 mg q 6 hr.
- **PO (Children):** 8–25 mg/kg/day in divided doses q 6–8 hr.
- **IM, IV (Adults):** 300–600 mg q 6–8 hr (up to 4.8 g/day IV has been used, single IM doses of >600 mg are not recommended).
- **IM, IV (Children):** 15–40 mg/kg/day in divided doses q 6–8 hr.
- **IM, IV (Neonates):** 15–20 mg/kg/day in divided doses q 6–8 hr.
- **Top:** 1% soln applied twice daily.

PHARMACODYNAMICS (blood levels)

	ONSET	PEAK
PO	rapid	45 min
IM	rapid	1.3 hr
IV	rapid	end of infusion

NURSING IMPLICATIONS

Assessment

- Assess patient for infection (vital signs; appearance of wound, sputum, urine, and stool; WBC) at beginning and throughout course of therapy.
- Obtain specimens for culture and sensitivity prior to initiating therapy. First dose may be given before receiving results.
- Monitor bowel elimination. Diarrhea, abdominal cramping, fever, and bloody stools should be reported to physician promptly as a sign of drug-induced pseudomembranous colitis. This may begin up to several wks following the cessation of therapy.
- Assess patient for hypersensitivity (skin rash, urticaria).
- **Lab Test Considerations:** Monitor CBC; may cause transient decrease in leukocytes, eosinophils, and platelets.
- May cause elevated alkaline phosphatase, bilirubin, CPK, SGOT (AST), and SGPT (ALT) concentrations.

Potential Nursing Diagnoses

- Infection, high risk for (indications, side effects).
- Bowel elimination, altered: diarrhea (side effects).
- Knowledge deficit related to medication regimen (patient/family teaching).

Implementation

- **PO:** Administer the oral form of the drug with a full glass of water. May be given with meals. Shake liquid preparations well. Do not refrigerate. Stable for 14 days at room temperature.
- **IM:** Do not administer >600 mg in a single IM injection.
- **Intermittent Infusion:** Do not administer as an undiluted IV bolus. Dilute each 300 mg for IV administration with at least 50 ml of D5W, D10W, D5/0.45% NaCl, D5/0.9% NaCl, D5/Ringer's injection, 0.9% NaCl, or lactated Ringer's soln for injection. Stable for 24 hr at room temperature. Crystals may occur if refrigerated but dissolve when warmed to room temperature. Do not administer soln with undissolved crystals.
- *Rate:* Administer each 300 mg over a minimum of 10 min. Do not give more than 1200 mg in a single 1-hr infusion.
- **Continuous Infusion:** May also be initially administered as a single rapid infusion, followed by continuous IV infusion.
- **Syringe Compatibility:** amikacin, aztreonam, gentamicin, or heparin.
- **Syringe Incompatibility:** tobramycin.
- **Y-Site Compatibility:** cyclophosphamide, enalaprilat, esmolol, foscarnet, hydromorphone, labetolol, magnesium sulfate, meperidine, morphine, multivitamins, ondansetron, perphenazine, or zidovudine.
- **Additive Compatibility:** amikacin, aztreonam, cefamandole, cefazolin,

cefonicid, cefoperazone, cefotaxime, cefoxitin, ceftazidime, ceftizoxime, cefuroxime, cephalothin, cimetidine, heparin, hydrocortisone sodium succinate, kanamycin, methylprednisolone, metoclopramide, metronidazole, netilmicin, penicillin G, piperacillin, potassium chloride, sodium bicarbonate, tobramycin, or verapamil.

▪ **Additive Incompatibility:** aminophylline, ceftriaxone, barbiturates, calcium gluconate, magnesium sulfate, phenytoin, or ranitidine.

▪ **Top:** Contact with eyes, mucous membranes, and open cuts should be avoided during topical application. If accidental contact occurs, rinse with copious amounts of cool water.

□ Wash affected areas with warm water and soap, rinse, and pat dry prior to application. Apply to entire affected area.

PATIENT/FAMILY TEACHING

▪ **General Info:** Instruct patient to take medication around the clock and to finish the drug completely as directed, even if feeling better. If a dose is missed, take as soon as remembered. If almost time for next dose, space doses 2–4 hr apart. Advise patient that sharing of this medication may be dangerous.

□ Instruct patient to notify physician immediately if diarrhea, abdominal cramping, fever, or bloody stools occur and not to treat with antidiarrheals without physician's approval.

□ Advise patient to report signs of superinfection (furry overgrowth on the tongue, vaginal or anal itching or discharge).

□ Notify physician if no improvement within a few days.

□ Patients with a history of rheumatic heart disease or valve replacement need to be taught the importance of antimicrobial prophylaxis before invasive medical or dental procedures.

▪ **IV:** Inform patient that bitter taste occurring with IV administration is not significant.

▪ **Top:** Caution patient applying topical clindamycin that soln is flammable (vehicle is isopropyl alcohol). Avoid application while smoking or near heat or flame.

□ Advise patient to notify physician if excessive drying of skin occurs.

□ Advise patient to wait 30 min after washing or shaving area before applying.

EVALUATION

Clinical response to therapy can be evaluated by: ▪ Resolution of the signs and symptoms of infection. Length of time for complete resolution depends on the organism and site of infection ▪ Endocarditis prophylaxis ▪ Improvement in acne vulgaris lesions. Improvement should be seen in 6 wk but may take 8–12 wk for maximum benefit.

CLOFAZIMINE
(kloe-**fa**-zi-meen)
Lamprene

CLASSIFICATION(S):
Anti-infective—miscellaneous
Pregnancy Category C

INDICATIONS

▪ In combination with other agents in the treatment of leprosy (Hansen's disease). **Unlabeled Use:** ▪ In combination with other agents in the treatment of atypical mycobacterial infections (*Mycobacterium avium-intracellulare*) in AIDS patients.

ACTION

▪ Binds to mycobacterial DNA, inhibiting mycobacterial protein synthesis and growth. **Therapeutic Effects:** ▪ Slow bactericidal action against susceptible mycobacteria ▪ Also has anti-inflammatory and immunosuppressive properties.

PHARMACOKINETICS

Absorption: Incompletely absorbed following oral administration. Degree

C

of absorption depends on type of formulation and dose.
Distribution: Distributes to fatty and reticuloendothelial tissue concentrating as crystals. Does not enter CSF. Crosses the placenta and enters breast milk.
Metabolism and Excretion: 35–75% excreted unchanged in the feces. Small amounts eliminated in bile.
Half-life: 8 days (70 days in tissue).

CONTRAINDICATIONS AND PRECAUTIONS

Contraindicated in: ▪ Hypersensitivity.
Use Cautiously in: ▪ Has been used in pregnancy safely (skin discoloration of infants noted) ▪ Lactation (causes skin discoloration of nursing infant) ▪ Children <12 yr (safety not established) ▪ Abdominal pain or diarrhea ▪ Suicidal tendencies.

ADVERSE REACTIONS AND SIDE EFFECTS*

CNS: anxiety, depression, dizziness, drowsiness, fatigue.
EENT: red-brown discoloration of conjunctiva, cornea, and lacrimal fluid, dryness, burning, itching, irritation, lacrimation, visual loss.
GI: SPLENIC INFARCTION, BOWEL OBSTRUCTION, GI BLEEDING, abdominal pain, epigastric pain, diarrhea, nausea, vomiting, anorexia, constipation.
Derm: dry skin, pinkish-brown discoloration of skin, rash, phototoxicity.
Misc: reddish-brown discoloration of sweat, sputum, urine, breast milk, feces, nasal secretions, and semen.

INTERACTIONS

Drug-Drug: ▪ **Dapsone** may negate the anti-inflammatory properties of clofazimine ▪ **Isoniazid** decreases skin concentrations and increases urinary excretion of clofazimine.

ROUTE AND DOSAGE

Leprosy

- **PO (Adults):** 50–100 mg/day (up to 300 mg/day).

Atypical Mycobacterium Infections

- **PO (Adults):** 100 mg q 8 hr.

PHARMACODYNAMICS

	ONSET	PEAK	DURATION
PO	UK	UK	UK

NURSING IMPLICATIONS

Assessment

- **General Info:** Assess patient for mental depression and suicidal tendencies if skin discoloration occurs.
- **Leprosy:** Assess skin lesions periodically throughout treatment.
- **AIDS:** Assess vital signs, lung sounds, and respiratory status in patients with atypical mycobacterial infections.
- **Lab Test Considerations:** May cause increased erythrocyte sedimentation rate (ESR).
- □ May cause elevated serum glucose, albumin, SGOT (AST), and bilirubin concentrations. May cause decreased serum potassium concentrations.

Potential Nursing Diagnoses

- Skin integrity, impaired (indications).
- Body image disturbance (adverse reactions).
- Knowledge deficit related to medication regimen (patient/family teaching).

Implementation

- **PO:** Administer medication with meals or milk.

Patient/Family Teaching

- □ Instruct patient to take clofazimine as directed, at the same time every day; therapy may take yrs. Missed doses should be taken as soon as remembered if not almost time for next dose; do not double doses.
- □ May cause loss of vision, dizziness, or

*Underlines indicate most frequent; **CAPITALS** indicate life-threatening.

drowsiness. Caution patient to avoid driving or other activities requiring alertness until response to medication is known.

- ▫ Inform diabetic patients that clofazimine may cause elevated blood glucose test results.
- ▫ Advise patient to use sunscreen and protective clothing to prevent phototoxicity reactions.
- ▫ Instruct patient to use skin creams, lotions, or oils to treat rough, dry, or scaly skin.
- ▫ Inform patient that a reversible pink or red to brownish-black discoloration of the skin may occur within a few wks of treatment. Several mons or yrs after discontinuing clofazimine may be required for discoloration to disappear completely. May also cause discoloration of feces, lining of eyelids, sputum, sweat, tears, and urine.
- ▫ Instruct patient to notify physician promptly if abdominal pain, diarrhea, nausea or vomiting, jaundice, tarry stools, loss of vision, skin discoloration, or mental depression occurs.
- ▫ Advise patient to notify physician if no improvement is seen within 1–3 mon.

EVALUATION

Effectiveness of therapy may be determined by: ▪ Improvement in skin lesions. Full therapeutic benefits may take up to 6 mon ▪ Resolution of symptoms of atypical mycobacterial infection.

CLOFIBRATE

(kloe-**fye**-brate)

Atromid-S, {Claripe}, {Novofibrate}

CLASSIFICATION(S):
Lipid-lowering agent

Pregnancy Category UK

INDICATIONS

▪ Adjunct to dietary therapy in the management of hyperlipidemias associated with high triglyceride levels. **Unlabeled Use:** ▪ Management of central diabetes insipidus (some pituitary function required).

ACTION

▪ Decreases hepatic synthesis of and accelerates the breakdown of very low-density lipoproteins to low-density lipoproteins. **Therapeutic Effect:** ▪ Lowering of plasma triglycerides and very low-density lipoproteins.

PHARMACOKINETICS

Absorption: Following conversion to active compound in the GI tract, absorption is slow but complete.

Distribution: Distributed into extracellular space. Crosses the placenta.

Metabolism and Excretion: Mostly metabolized by the liver. 10–20% excreted unchanged by the kidneys.

Half-life: 6–25 hr.

CONTRAINDICATIONS AND PRECAUTIONS

Contraindicated in: ▪ Hypersensitivity ▪ Severe hepatic or renal impairment ▪ Primary biliary cirrhosis ▪ Pregnancy, lactation, and children $<$14 yr.

Use Cautiously in: ▪ Renal or hepatic impairment ▪ Discontinue use if flu-like syndrome develops (myalgia, fever).

ADVERSE REACTIONS AND SIDE EFFECTS*

CNS: fatigue, weakness.

CV: arrhythmias, angina.

GI: nausea, vomiting, diarrhea, abdominal discomfort, flatulence, polyphagia, weight gain, gallstones, hepatitis.

GU: decreased libido, renal failure.

Derm: rashes.

Hemat: blood dyscrasias.

MS: myalgia, arthralgia.

INTERACTIONS

Drug–Drug: ▪ Enhances the effect of **oral anticoagulants** ▪ May displace and enhance the effects of other **highly protein-bound drugs,** including **furose-**

{} = Available in Canada only.

*Underlines indicate most frequent; **CAPITALS** indicate life-threatening.

C

mide and **oral hypoglycemic agents** ▪ **Cholestyramine** may slow the absorption of the active compound of clofibrate.

ROUTE AND DOSAGE

Lipid Lowering

- **PO (Adults):** 500 mg 4 times daily.

Diabetes Insipidus

- **PO (Adults):** 6–8 g/day in 2–4 divided doses.

PHARMACODYNAMICS (lipid lowering effect)

	ONSET	PEAK	DURATION
PO	2–5 days	3 wk	2–3 wk

NURSING IMPLICATIONS

Assessment

- **General Info:** Obtain a diet history, especially regarding fat and alcohol consumption.
- □ Monitor weight at baseline and weekly throughout therapy.
- **Lab Test Considerations:** Monitor serum triglyceride and cholesterol levels closely. LDL and VLDL levels should be assessed prior to beginning therapy, every 2 wk during initial therapy, and then monthly. Medication should be discontinued if paradoxical increase in lipid levels occurs.
- □ May cause an increase in CPK and serum amylase levels and a decrease in plasma fibrinogen levels.
- □ Liver function tests should be assessed prior to therapy, monthly for the initial 2 mon, every 2 mon until clinical response occurs, then every 4 mon. Hepatotoxicity may be indicated by an increase in SGOT (AST) and SGPT (ALT).
- □ CBC and electrolytes should be routinely evaluated throughout course of therapy. Notify physician if anemia or leukopenia occurs.

Potential Nursing Diagnoses

- Knowledge deficit related to medication regimen (patient/family teaching).
- Noncompliance (patient/family teaching).

Implementation

- **PO:** Administer medication with food or milk to minimize gastric irritation.

Patient/Family Teaching

- □ Instruct patient to take medication exactly as directed. If a dose is missed take as soon as remembered unless almost time for next dose.
- □ Advise patient that this medication should be used in conjunction with dietary restrictions (fat, cholesterol, carbohydrates, alcohol), exercise, and cessation of smoking.
- □ Instruct patient to notify physician promptly if any of the following symptoms occur: chest pain, dyspnea, irregular heart beat, severe stomach pains with nausea and vomiting, fever, chills, sore throat, hematuria, dysuria, swelling of the lower extremities, or weight gain.
- □ Caution women that this medication may have teratogenic properties. Advise patient to practice contraception while taking this medication and for at least 2 mon following the completion of therapy.

Evaluation

Effectiveness of therapy can be demonstrated by: ▪ Decrease in serum cholesterol levels and triglyceride levels. Improved values are usually seen within 3 wk. If decreased levels are not seen within 3 mon medication is usually discontinued.

CLOMIPHENE

(**kloe**-mi-feen)
Clomid, Serophene

CLASSIFICATION(S):
Hormone—ovulation inducer
Pregnancy Category UK

INDICATIONS

- Induces ovulation in anovulatory women who desire to become pregnant.

Requires intact anterior pituitary, thyroid, and adrenal function. **Unlabeled Use:** ▪ Male infertility caused by oligospermia.

ACTION

▪ Stimulates release of pituitary gonadotropins, follicle-stimulating hormone, and luteinizing hormone, resulting in ovulation and the development of the corpus luteum. **Therapeutic Effect:** ▪ Induction of ovulation.

PHARMACOKINETICS

Absorption: Well absorbed following oral administration.
Distribution: Not known.
Metabolism and Excretion: Apparently metabolized by the liver, with enterohepatic recirculation and biliary elimination. Excreted in feces.
Half-life: 5 days.

CONTRAINDICATIONS AND PRECAUTIONS

Contraindicated in: ▪ Liver disease ▪ Ovarian cysts ▪ Pregnancy.
Use Cautiously in: ▪ Known sensitivity to pituitary gonadotropins ▪ Polycystic ovary syndrome.

ADVERSE REACTIONS AND SIDE EFFECTS*

CNS: nervousness, restlessness, headache, insomnia, lightheadedness, fatigue.
EENT: blurred vision, scotoma, photophobia, visual disturbances.
CV: flushing, <u>hot flashes</u>.
GI: distention, bloating, abdominal pain, nausea, vomiting, increased appetite.
GU: urinary frequency, increased urine volume.
Derm: rashes, urticaria, allergic dermatitis, reversible hair loss.
Endo: <u>ovarian enlargement</u>, <u>cyst formation</u>, breast discomfort, multiple births.
Metab: weight gain.

INTERACTIONS

Drug–Drug: None significant.

ROUTE AND DOSAGE

▪ **PO (Adults):** 50 mg/day for 5 days; if ovulation does not occur a second course of 100 mg/day for 5 days may be given 30 days after the initial course. A maximum of 3 courses may be administered.

PHARMACODYNAMICS (ovulation)

	ONSET	PEAK	DURATION
PO	5–14 days	UK	UK

NURSING IMPLICATIONS

Assessment

□ A pelvic examination to determine ovarian size should be completed prior to course of therapy.
□ An endometrial biopsy is recommended in older patients prior to clomiphene therapy to rule out the presence of endometrial carcinoma.
□ Liver function tests should be performed prior to course of therapy.
▪ **Lab Test Considerations:** Estrogen excretion determinations, histological studies of the luteal phase endometrium, serum progesterone, and urinary excretion of pregnanediol may be used to determine whether ovulation has occurred following a course of clomiphene.
□ May cause increased serum thyroxine and thyroxine-binding globulin levels.

Potential Nursing Diagnoses

▪ Knowledge deficit related to medication regimen (patient/family teaching).

Implementation

▪ **General Info:** Clomiphene therapy is usually begun on the fifth day of the menstrual cycle.

Patient/Family Teaching

□ Instruct patient to take clomiphene exactly as directed at the same time each day. Missed doses should be taken as soon as remembered and the

*<u>Underlines</u> indicate most frequent; **CAPITALS** indicate life-threatening.

dose doubled if not remembered until the time of the next dose. Notify physician if more than 1 dose is missed.
- Advise patient that conception should be attempted with intercourse every other day starting 48 hr prior to ovulation.
- Instruct patient in the correct method for measuring basal body temperature. A record of the daily basal body temperature should be maintained prior to and throughout course of therapy. Emphaszie the importance of compliance with all aspects of therapy.
- Prior to therapy, patient should be informed of the potential for multiple births.
- Medication may cause visual disturbances or dizziness. Caution patient to avoid driving until the response to the medication is known.
- Instruct patient to notify physician immediately if pregnancy is suspected; clomiphene should not be taken during pregnancy.
- Advise patient that ophthalmologic examinations should be performed to evaluate the possibility of ocular toxicity if treatment is continued for more than 1 yr.
- Advise patient to notify physician promptly if bloating, stomach or pelvic pain, blurred vision, jaundice, persistent hot flashes, breast discomfort, headache, or nausea and vomiting occur.
- Emphasize the importance of close monitoring by the physician throughout course of therapy.

EVALUATION

Effectiveness of therapy can be demonstrated by: ▪ Occurrence of ovulation measured by estrogen excretion, biphasic body temperature curve, urinary excretion of pregnanediol at postovulatory levels, and endometrial histologic changes. If conception is not achieved after 3–4 courses of clomiphene, diagnosis should be re-evaluated.

C

CLOMIPRAMINE
(kloe-**mip**-ra-meen)
Anafranil

CLASSIFICATION(S):
Antipsychotic—miscellaneous, Antiobsessive agent
Pregnancy Category UK

INDICATIONS

▪ Management of obsessive-compulsive disorder (OCD).

ACTION

▪ Potentiates the effect of serotonin (antiobsessional effect) and norepinephrine in the CNS. Also has moderate anticholinergic properties. **Therapeutic Effect:** ▪ Diminished obsessive-compulsive behavior.

PHARMACOKINETICS

Absorption: Well absorbed from the GI tract.
Distribution: Widely distributed.
Metabolism and Excretion: Extensively metabolized by the liver. Some conversion to a pharmacologically active metabolite (desmethylclomipramine). Undergoes enterohepatic recirculation and secretion into gastric juices. Appears to enter breast milk.
Half-life: 21–31 hr.

CONTRAINDICATIONS AND PRECAUTIONS

Contraindicated in: ▪ Hypersensitivity ▪ Pregnancy or lactation ▪ Narrow-angle glaucoma ▪ Recent myocardial infarction.
Use Cautiously in: ▪ History of seizures (threshold may be lowered) ▪ Children <10 yr (safety not established) ▪ Elderly patients ▪ Concurrent MAO inhibitor or clonidine use (avoid if possible) ▪ Patients with pre-existing cardiovascular disease ▪ Elderly men with prostatic hypertrophy (may be more susceptible to urinary retention) ▪ Hy-

perthyroidism (increased risk of arrhythmias).

ADVERSE REACTIONS AND SIDE EFFECTS*

CNS: SEIZURES, sedation, drowsiness, lethargy, weakness, aggressive behavior.
EENT: dry eyes, dry mouth, blurred vision, vestibular disorder.
CV: hypotension, ARRHYTHMIAS, ECG changes.
GI: orthostatic constipation, eructation.
GU: urinary retention, male sexual dysfunction.
Derm: photosensitivity, dry skin.
Endo: gynecomastia.
Hemat: anemia.
MS: muscle weakness.
Neuro: extrapyramidal reactions.
Misc: hyperthermia, weight gain.

INTERACTIONS

Drug-Drug: ▪ May cause hypotension and tachycardia when used with **MAO inhibitors** ▪ May prevent the therapeutic response to **antihypertensives** ▪ Use with **clonidine** may result in hypertensive crisis ▪ Additive CNS depression with other **CNS depressants** including **alcohol, antihistamines, narcotic analgesics,** and **sedative/hypnotics** ▪ **Adrenergic** and **anticholinergic** side effects may be additive with other **agents having these properties** ▪ Effects and toxicity may be increased by concurrent **fluoxetine, phenothazines, cimetidine,** or **oral contraceptives** ▪ **Nicotine** (cigarette smoke or nicotine gum) may increase metabolism and decrease effectiveness ▪ Organic brain syndrome may occur with **disulfiram.**

ROUTE AND DOSAGE

- **PO (Adults):** 25 mg/day initially, increased over 2 wk period to 100 mg/day in divided doses. May be further increased over several wks to maximum of 250 mg/day in divided doses. Once stabilizing dose is reached, entire daily dose may be given at bedtime.
- **PO (Children and Adolescents):** 25 mg/day initially, increased over 2 wk period to 3 mg/kg/day or 100 mg/day (whichever is smaller) in divided doses. May be further increased to 3 mg/kg/day or 200 mg/day (whichever is smaller) in divided doses. Once stabilizing dose is reached, entire daily dose may be given at bedtime.

PHARMACODYNAMICS

	ONSET	PEAK	DURATION
PO	1–6 wk	UK	UK

NURSING IMPLICATIONS

Assessment

- □ Monitor mental status and affect. Assess patient for frequency of obsessive-compulsive behaviors. Note degree to which these thoughts and behaviors interfere with daily functioning.
- □ Observe for onset of extrapyramidal side effects (pill-rolling motions, drooling, tremors, rigidity, mask facies, shuffling gait, restlessness, muscle spasms, twisting motions). Notify physician immediately if these symptoms occur. Dosage reduction or discontinuation may be necessary. Physician may order antiparkinson agents to control extrapyramidal effects.

Potential Nursing Diagnosis

- Coping, ineffective individual (obsessive-compulsive behaviors) related to repressed anxiety (indications).
- Injury, high risk for (side effects).
- Knowledge deficit related to medication regimen (patient/family teaching).

Implementation

- **PO:** Administer medication with or immediately following a meal to minimize gastric irritation. After titration of dosage total daily dose may be given at bedtime.

Patient/Family Teaching

- □ Instruct patient to take medication exactly as prescribed. Abrupt discontin-

*Underlines indicate most frequent; **CAPITALS** indicate life-threatening.

uation may cause nausea, headache, and malaise.

- □ May cause drowsiness and blurred vision. Caution patient to avoid driving and other activities requiring alertness until response to drug is known.
- □ Advise patient to avoid alcohol or other CNS depressant drugs during course of therapy and for 3–7 days after cessation of therapy.
- □ Instruct patient to notify physician if dry mouth or constipation persists or if urinary retention or uncontrolled movements or rigidity occur. Sugarless candy or gum may diminish dry mouth, and an increase in fluid intake or bulk may prevent constipation. If these symptoms persist dosage reduction or discontinuation may be necessary.
- □ Advise patient to inform physician if breast enlargement or sexual dysfunction occurs.
- □ Caution patient to use sunscreen and protective clothing to prevent photosensitivity reactions.
- □ Inform patient of need to monitor dietary intake as possible increase in appetite may lead to undesired weight gain.
- □ Advise patient to notify physician or dentist of medication regimen prior to treatment or surgery.
- □ Emphasize the importance of follow-up examinations to monitor effectiveness and side effects.

EVALUATION

Effectiveness of therapy can be demonstrated by: ▪ Diminished obsessive-compulsive behavior.

CLONAZEPAM

(kloe-**na**-ze-pan)
Klonipin, {Rivotril}

CLASSIFICATION(S):
Anticonvulsant—benzodiazepine
Schedule IV
Pregnancy Category UK

INDICATIONS

▪ Prophylaxis of: □ Petit mal □ Petit mal variant □ Akinetic □ Myoclonic seizures.

ACTION

▪ Produces anticonvulsant and sedative effects in the CNS. Mechanism is unknown but is probably similar to that of benzodiazepines (chlordiazepoxide, diazepam). **Therapeutic Effect:** ▪ Prevention of seizures.

PHARMACOKINETICS

Absorption: Well absorbed from the GI tract.
Distribution: Appears to cross the blood–brain barrier and the placenta.
Metabolism and Excretion: Mostly metabolized by the liver.
Half-life: 18–50 hr.

CONTRAINDICATIONS AND PRECAUTIONS

Contraindicated in: ▪ Hypersensitivity to clonazepam or other benzodiazepines ▪ Severe liver disease.
Use Cautiously in: ▪ Narrow-angle glaucoma ▪ Chronic respiratory disease ▪ Pregnancy or lactation (safety not established) ▪ Children (long-term effects on growth and maturation not known) ▪ Do not discontinue abruptly.

ADVERSE REACTIONS AND SIDE EFFECTS*

CNS: <u>drowsiness</u>, <u>ataxia</u>, hypotonia, <u>behavioral changes</u>.
EENT: abnormal eye movements, diplopia, nystagmus.
Resp: increased secretions.
CV: palpitations.
GI: constipation, diarrhea, hepatitis.
GU: dysuria, nocturia, urinary retention.
Hemat: anemia, leukopenia, thrombocytopenia, eosinophilia.
Misc: fever.

INTERACTIONS

Drug-Drug: ▪ **Alcohol, antidepressants, antihistamines,** and **narcotic an-**

{} = Available in Canada only.
*<u>Underlines</u> indicate most frequent; **CAPITALS** indicate life-threatening.

algesics,—concurrent use results in additive CNS depression ▪ **Cimetidine, oral contraceptives, disulfiram, fluoxetine, isoniazid, ketoconazole, metoprolol, propoxyphene, propranolol,** or **valproic acid** may decrease the metabolism of clonazepam, enhancing its actions ▪ May decrease efficacy of **levodopa** ▪ **Rifampin** or **barbiturates** may increase the metabolism and decrease effectiveness of clonazepam ▪ Sedative effects may be decreased by **theophylline** ▪ May increase serum **phenytoin** levels ▪ **Phenytoin** may decrease serum clonazepam levels.

ROUTE AND DOSAGE

- **PO (Adults):** Initial daily dose not to exceed 1.5 mg given in 3 divided doses; may increase by 0.5–1 mg q 3rd day. Total daily maintenance dose not to exceed 20 mg.
- **PO (Children up to 10 yr or 30 kg):** Initial daily dose 0.01–0.03 mg/kg (not to exceed 0.05 mg/kg) given in 2–3 divided doses; increase by no more than 0.5 mg q 3rd day until therapeutic blood levels are reached. Daily dose not to exceed 0.2 mg/kg.

PHARMACODYNAMICS (anticonvulsant activity)

	ONSET	PEAK	DURATION
PO	20–60 min	1–2 hr	6–12 hr

NURSING IMPLICATIONS

Assessment

- ▫ Observe and record intensity, duration, and location of seizure activity.
- ▫ Assess patient for drowsiness, unsteadiness, and clumsiness. These symptoms are dose-related and most severe during initial therapy; may decrease in severity or disappear with continued or long-term therapy.
- ▪ **Lab Test Considerations:** Evaluate liver function, CBC, and platelet counts periodically throughout course of prolonged therapy.
- ▫ May cause decreased RBCs, WBCs, and platelets. May also cause increased SGOT (AST), SGPT (ALT), and alkaline phosphatase.

Potential Nursing Diagnoses

- ▪ Injury, high risk for (indications, side effects).
- ▪ Knowledge deficit related to medication regimen (patient/family teaching).

Implementation

- ▪ **General Info:** Institute seizure precautions for patients on initial therapy or undergoing dosage manipulations.
- ▪ **PO:** Administer with food to minimize gastric irritation. Tablets may be crushed if patient has difficulty swallowing.

Patient/Family Teaching

- ▫ Instruct patient to take medication exactly as directed. Missed doses should be taken within 1 hr or omitted; do not double doses. Abrupt withdrawal of clonazepam may cause status epilepticus, tremors, nausea, vomiting, and abdominal and muscle cramps.
- ▫ Medication may cause drowsiness or dizziness. Advise patient to avoid driving or other activities requiring alertness until response to drug is known.
- ▫ Caution patient to avoid taking alcohol or other CNS depressants concurrently with this medication.
- ▫ Advise patient to notify physician or dentist of medication regimen prior to treatment or surgery.
- ▫ Instruct patient and family to notify physician of unusual tiredness, bleeding, sore throat, fever, clay-colored stools, yellowing of skin, or behavioral changes.
- ▫ Emphasize the importance of follow-up examinations to determine effectiveness of the medication.
- ▫ Patient on anticonvulsant therapy should carry identification describing disease process and medication regimen at all times.

Evaluation

Effectiveness of therapy can be demonstrated by: ▪ Decrease or cessation of seizure activity without undue sedation. Dosage adjustments may be required after several mons of therapy.

CLONIDINE
(**klon**-i-deen)
Catapres, Catapress-TTS, {Dixarit}

CLASSIFICATION(S):
Antihypertensive—centrally acting adrenergic
Pregnancy Category C

INDICATIONS

▪ Alone and in combination with other antihypertensives in the management of mild to moderate hypertension. **Unlabeled Uses:** ▪ Management of narcotic withdrawal, prophylaxis of vascular headaches, treatment of dysmenorrhea, treatment of menopausal syndrome.

ACTION

▪ Stimulates alpha-adrenergic receptors in the CNS. Result is inhibition of cardioacceleration and vasoconstriction center. **Therapeutic Effect:** ▪ Decrease in blood pressure.

PHARMACOKINETICS

Absorption: Well absorbed from the GI tract and through the skin.
Distribution: Widely distributed and crosses the blood–brain barrier. Enters breast milk.
Metabolism and Excretion: Mostly metabolized by the liver. 30% eliminated unchanged by the kidneys.
Half-life: 12–20 hr.

CONTRAINDICATIONS AND PRECAUTIONS

Contraindicated in: ▪ Hypersensitivity.
Use Cautiously in: ▪ Serious cardiac disease ▪ Cerebrovascular disease ▪ Renal insufficiency ▪ Pregnancy, lactation, or children (safety not established) ▪ Elderly patients (dosage reduction may be required) ▪ Do not discontinue abruptly.

ADVERSE REACTIONS AND SIDE EFFECTS*

CNS: drowsiness, nightmares, nervousness, depression.
CV: hypotension, bradycardia, palpitations.
GI: dry mouth, constipation.
GU: impotence.
Derm: rash.
F and E: sodium retention.
Metab: weight gain.
Misc: withdrawal phenomenon.

INTERACTIONS

Drug–Drug: ▪ Additive sedation with **CNS depressants** including **alcohol, antihistamines, narcotic analgesics,** and **sedative/hypnotics** ▪ Additive hypotension with other **antihypertensive agents** and **nitrates** ▪ Additive bradycardia with **myocardial depressants,** including **beta-adrenergic blockers** ▪ **MAO inhibitors, amphetamines,** or **tricyclic antidepressants** may decrease antihypertensive effect ▪ Withdrawal phenomenon may be exaggerated by concurrent **tricyclic antidepressants** or discontinuation of **beta blockers** (discontinue beta blockers several days prior to discontinuing clonidine).

ROUTE AND DOSAGE

Hypertension

- **PO (Adults):** Initial dose 0.1 mg bid. Usual maintenance dose is 0.2–1.2 mg/day in 2–3 divided doses.
- **Top (Adults):** 1–3 mg applied weekly as transdermal delivery system.

Hypertensive Urgency

- **PO (Adults):** 0.1–0.2 mg initially, then 0.05–0.1 mg q h until BP controlled or total of 0.5–0.7 mg given, then start maintenance therapy.

Narcotic Withdrawal

- **PO (Adults):** 0.3–1.2 mg/day, may be decreased by 50%/day for 3 days then

{} = Available in Canada only.
*Underlines indicate most frequent; **CAPITALS** indicate life-threatening.

discontinued or decreased by 0.1–0.2 mg/day.

Vascular Headache Prophylaxis

- **PO (Adults):** 0.025 mg 2–4 times daily (up to 0.15 mg/day in divided doses).

Dysmenorrhea

- **PO (Adults):** 0.025 mg twice daily for 14 days before and during menses.

Menopausal Syndrome

- **PO (Adults):** 0.025–0.075 mg twice daily.

PHARMACODYNAMICS (antihypertensive effect)

	ONSET	PEAK	DURATION
PO	30–60 min	2–4 hr	8 hr
Top	2–3 days	UK	7 days*

*8 hr following removal of patch.

NURSING IMPLICATIONS

Assessment

- **General Info:** Monitor intake and output ratios and daily weight, and assess for edema daily, especially at beginning of therapy.
- **Hypertension:** Monitor blood pressure and pulse frequently during initial dosage adjustment and periodically throughout course of therapy. Notify physician of significant changes.
- **Narcotic Withdrawal:** Monitor patient for signs and symptoms of narcotic withdrawal (tachycardia, fever, runny nose, diarrhea, sweating, nausea, vomiting, irritability, stomach cramps, shivering, unusually large pupils, weakness, difficulty sleeping, gooseflesh).
- **Lab Test Considerations:** May cause transient increase in blood glucose levels.

Potential Nursing Diagnoses

- Injury, high risk for (side effects).
- Knowledge deficit related to medication regimen (patient/family teaching).
- Noncompliance (patient/family teaching).

Implementation

- **General Info:** Available in combination with chlorthalidone (see Appendix A).
- **PO:** Administer last dose of the day at bedtime.
- **Topical:** Transdermal system should be applied once every 7 days. May be applied to any hairless site; avoid cuts or callouses. Absorption is greater when placed on chest or upper arm, and decreased when placed on thigh. Rotate sites. Wash area with soap and water, dry thoroughly before application. Apply firm pressure over patch to ensure contact with skin, especially around edges. Remove old system and discard. System includes a protective adhesive overlay to be applied over medication patch to ensure adhesion should medication patch loosen.

Patient/Family Teaching

- **General Info:** Instruct patient to take clonidine at the same time each day, even if feeling well. Clonidine controls but does not cure hypertension. If a dose is missed, take as soon as remembered. If more than one oral dose in a row is missed, or if transdermal system is late being changed by 3 or more days, consult physician. Oral clonidine should be gradually discontinued over 2–4 days to prevent rebound hypertension.
- □ Encourage patient to comply with additional interventions for hypertension (weight reduction, low-sodium diet, discontinuation of smoking, moderation of alcohol consumption, regular exercise, and stress management). Patient should also avoid excessive amounts of tea, coffee, and cola.
- □ Instruct patient and family on proper technique for blood pressure monitoring. Advise them to check blood pressure at least weekly and report significant changes to physician.
- □ Clonidine may cause drowsiness. Advise patient to avoid driving or other activities requiring alertness until response to medication is known.

- ▫ Caution patient to avoid sudden changes in position to decrease orthostatic hypotension. Use of alcohol, standing for long periods, exercising, and hot weather may increase orthostatic hypotension.
- ▫ If dry mouth occurs, frequent mouth rinses, good oral hygiene, and sugarless gum or candy may decrease effect. If dry mouth continues for more than 2 wk, consult physician or dentist.
- ▫ Caution patient to avoid concurrent use of alcohol or other CNS depressants with this medication.
- ▫ Advise patient to consult physician or pharmacist before taking any cough, cold, or allergy remedies.
- ▫ Advise patient to notify physician or dentist of medication regimen prior to treatment or surgery.
- ▪ **Top:** Instruct patient on proper application of transdermal system. Do not cut or trim unit. Transdermal system can remain in place during bathing or swimming.

Evaluation

Effectiveness of therapy can be demonstrated by: ▪ Decrease in blood pressure ▪ Decrease in the signs and symptoms of narcotic withdrawal ▪ Prevention of vascular headaches ▪ Decrease in dysmenorrhea ▪ Decrease in symptoms of menopausal syndrome.

CLORAZEPATE

(klor-**az**-e-pate)
Cloraze-Caps, {Novoclopate}, Tranxene

CLASSIFICATION(S):
Antianxiety agent, Sedative/hypnotic—benzodiazepine, Anticonvulsant
Schedule IV
Pregnancy Category UK

INDICATIONS

▪ Treatment of anxiety ▪ Management of alcohol withdrawal ▪ Management of simple partial seizures.

ACTION

▪ Acts at many levels in the CNS to produce anxiolytic effect and CNS depression (by stimulating inhibitory GABA receptors) ▪ Produces skeletal muscle relaxation (by inhibiting spinal polysynaptic afferent pathways) ▪ Also has anticonvulsant effect (enhances presynaptic inhibition). **Therapeutic Effects:** ▪ Relief of anxiety ▪ Sedation ▪ Prevention of seizures.

PHARMACOKINETICS

Absorption: Well absorbed from the GI tract.
Distribution: Widely distributed. Crosses the placenta and enters breast milk.
Metabolism and Excretion: Metabolized by the liver. Some conversion to active compounds.
Half-life: 48 hr.

CONTRAINDICATIONS AND PRECAUTIONS

Contraindicated in: ▪ Hypersensitivity ▪ Cross-sensitivity with other benzodiazepines may exist ▪ Pre-existing CNS depression ▪ Severe uncontrolled pain ▪ Narrow-angle glaucoma ▪ Pregnancy or lactation.
Use Cautiously in: ▪ Pre-existing hepatic dysfunction ▪ Patients who may be suicidal or have been addicted to drugs in the past ▪ Elderly or debilitated patients (dosage reduction required) ▪ Severe pulmonary disease.

ADVERSE REACTIONS AND SIDE EFFECTS*

CNS: dizziness, drowsiness, lethargy, hangover, paradoxical excitation, mental depression, headache.
EENT: blurred vision.
Resp: respiratory depression.

{} = Available in Canada only.
*Underlines indicate most frequent; **CAPITALS** indicate life-threatening.

GI: nausea, vomiting, diarrhea, constipation.
Derm: rashes.
Misc: tolerance, psychological dependence, physical dependence.

INTERACTIONS

Drug-Drug: ▪ **Alcohol, antidepressants, antihistamines,** and **narcotic analgesics**—concurrent use results in additive CNS depression ▪ **Cimetidine, oral contraceptives, disulfram, fluoxetine, isoniazid, ketoconazole, metoprolol, propoxyphene, propranolol,** or **valproic acid** may decrease the metabolism of clorazepate, enhancing its actions ▪ May decrease efficacy of **levodopa** ▪ **Rifampin** or **barbiturates** may increase the metabolism and decrease effectiveness of clorazepate ▪ Sedative effects may be decreased by **theophylline.**

ROUTE AND DOSAGE

Anxiety

- **PO (Adults):** 7.5–15 mg 2–4 times daily. May be given in a single dose of up to 22.5 mg at bedtime.

Alcohol Withdrawal

- **PO (Adults):** 30 mg initially, then 15 mg 2–4 times daily on first day, then gradually decreased over subsequent days.

Anticonvulsant

- **PO (Adults):** 7.5 mg 3 times daily; can increase by no more than 7.5 mg/day at weekly intervals (daily dose not to exceed 90 mg).
- **PO (Children 9–12 yr):** 7.5 mg bid; increase dose by no more than 7.5 mg/day at weekly intervals (daily dose not to exceed 60 mg).

PHARMACODYNAMICS (sedation)

	ONSET	PEAK	DURATION
PO	1–2 hr	1–2 hr	up to 24 hr

NURSING IMPLICATIONS

Assessment

- **General Info:** Prolonged high-dose therapy may lead to psychological or physical dependence. Restrict amount of drug available to patient.
- **Anxiety:** Assess degree and manifestations of anxiety prior to and periodically throughout therapy.
- **Alcohol Withdrawal:** Assess patient experiencing alcohol withdrawal for tremors, agitation, delirium, and hallucinations. Protect patient from injury.
- **Seizures:** Observe and record intensity, duration, and location of seizure activity.
- **Lab Test Considerations:** Patients on high-dose therapy should receive routine evaluation of renal, hepatic, and hematologic function. May cause increased serum bilirubin, SGOT (AST), SGPT (ALT), and alkaline phosphatase concentrations.

Potential Nursing Diagnoses

- Anxiety (indications).
- Injury, high risk for (indications, side effects).
- Knowledge deficit related to medication regimen (patient/family teaching).

Implementation

- **General Info:** Available in tablets and sustained-duration capsules. Sustained-duration capsules should not be used for initiation of therapy.
- **PO:** If gastric irritation is a problem, may be administered with food or fluids. Capsule should be swallowed whole; do not open.
- ▫ Avoid administration of antacids within 1 hr of medication, as absorption of clorazepate may be delayed.

Patient/Family Teaching

- **General Info:** Instruct patient to take medication exactly as directed, not to skip or double up on missed doses. Abrupt withdrawal of clorazepate may cause status epilepticus, tremors, nausea, vomiting, and abdominal and muscle cramps.
- ▫ Medication may cause drowsiness or dizziness. Advise patient to avoid driving or other activities requiring alertness until response to drug is known.

- ▫ Caution patient to avoid taking alcohol or other CNS depressants concurrently with this medication.
- ▫ Instruct patient to contact physician immediately if pregnancy is suspected.
- ▫ Advise patient to notify physician or dentist of medication regimen prior to treatment or surgery.
- ▫ Emphasize the importance of follow-up examinations to determine effectiveness of the medication.
- ▪ **Seizures:** Patients on anticonvulsant therapy should carry identification describing disease process and medication regimen at all times.

EVALUATION

Effectiveness of therapy can be demonstrated by: ▪ Increase in sense of well-being ▫ Decrease in subjective feelings of anxiety ▪ Control of acute alcohol withdrawal ▪ Decrease or cessation of seizure activity without undue sedation.

CLOTRIMAZOLE

(kloe-**trim**-a-zole)
{Canesten}, Gyne-Lotrimin, Lotrimin, Mycelex, {Myclo}

CLASSIFICATION(S):
Antifungal—imidazole
Pregnancy Category B

INDICATIONS

▪ Treatment of the following infections due to susceptible fungi: ▫ Orophayngeal candidiasis ▫ Superficial fungal infections ▫ Cutaneous and vulvovaginal candidiasis.

ACTION

▪ Damages fungal cell membrane, allowing leakage of cellular contents. May also alter metabolism in fungal cells. **Therapeutic Effect:** ▪ Fungicidal or fungistatic, depending on the organism and concentration. **Spectrum:** ▪ Active against many fungi, including: ▫ *Candida albicans* ▫ *Tricophyton rubrum* ▫ *Malassezia furfur.*

PHARMACOKINETICS

Absorption: Only small amounts are absorbed from lozenge, topical, or vaginal administration.
Distribution: Distribution not known. Action is primarily local.
Metabolism and Excretion: Action is local. Elimination is not known.
Half-life: UK.

CONTRAINDICATIONS AND PRECAUTIONS

Contraindicated in: ▪ Hypersensitivity ▪ Cross-sensitivity with other imidazole antifungals may exist.
Use Cautiously in: ▪ Safety of lozenges in children <3 yr is not established ▪ Has been used without adverse effects in second and third trimesters of pregnancy.

ADVERSE REACTIONS AND SIDE EFFECTS*

GI: <u>nausea</u>, <u>vomiting</u> (with lozenges only).
GU: Vag—vaginal irritation.
Derm: irritation, pruritus, burning.
Misc: hepatitis.

INTERACTIONS

Drug–Drug: ▪ None significant.

ROUTE AND DOSAGE

- ▪ **PO (Adults and Children >3 yr):** 10 mg lozenge dissolved slowly 5 times daily.
- ▪ **Top (Adults and Children):** 1% cream, lotion, or soln applied bid.
- ▪ **Vag (Adults):** 100-mg vaginal tablet daily for 7 days or 200 mg vaginally for 3 days (nonpregnant women only) or 500 mg-vaginal tablet single dose (uncomplicated infections only) or 5

{} = Available in Canada only.
*Underlines indicate most frequent; **CAPITALS** indicate life-threatening.

g of 1% vaginal cream daily for 7–14 days.

PHARMACODYNAMICS (antifungal action)

	ONSET	PEAK	DURATION
PO	15–30 min	UK	3 hr
Top	upon application	UK	UK
Vag	upon application	UK	up to 72 hr

NURSING IMPLICATIONS

Assessment

- Inspect involved areas of skin prior to and frequently throughout course of therapy. Increased skin irritation may indicate need to discontinue medication.
- **Lab Test Considerations:** The oral form of this medication may cause elevated SGOT (AST), SGPT (ALT), alkaline phosphatase, and serum bilirubin levels.

Potential Nursing Diagnoses

- Oral mucous membranes, altered (indications).
- Skin integrity, impaired (indications).
- Knowledge deficit related to medication regimen (patient/family teaching).

Implementation

- **General Info:** Available as a lozenge, topical cream and soln, and over-the-counter vaginal cream and tablet.
- **PO:** Lozenges should be kept in mouth and allowed to dissolve slowly and completely while swallowing saliva over 15–30 min. Do not chew or swallow lozenge whole.
- **Top:** Consult physician for proper cleansing technique prior to applying medication. Skin cream and solns should be applied sparingly with a gloved hand.
- **Vag:** Vaginal preparations should be used at bedtime for maximum contact with mucous membranes. Applicators are supplied for vaginal administration. Sitz baths and vaginal douches may be ordered concurrently with this therapy.

Patient/Family Teaching

- **General Info:** Instruct patient to take medication as directed, even if feeling better. If a dose is missed take as soon as remembered, if not almost time for next dose. Do not double doses.
- Advise patient to report increased skin irritation or lack of response to therapy to physician.
- **Top:** Instruct patient to change clothing in contact with infected area after each application. Occlusive dressings or bandages are contraindicated unless specifically ordered by physician. Avoid use of other topical lotions or ointments without consulting physician.
- Patients receiving therapy for ringworm (tinea corporis) should be instructed to wear loose, light-weight clothing or footwear, to launder personal articles separately from those of other family members, and to keep skin clean and dry.
- **Vag:** Instruct patient on proper use of vaginal applicator for vaginal creams or tablets. Patient should remain recumbent for at least 30 min following insertion. Advise use of sanitary napkins to prevent staining of clothing or bedding.
- Advise patient to consult physician regarding douching and intercourse during therapy. Vaginal medication may cause minor skin irritation in sexual partner. Advise patient to refrain from sexual contact during therapy or have partner wear a condom.

Evaluation

Effectiveness of therapy can be demonstrated by: ▪ Decrease in skin irritation and discomfort ▫ Resolution of infection. Length of time for complete resolution depends on the organism and site of infection.

C

CLOXACILLIN
(klox-a-**sill**-in)
{Apo-Cloxi}, Cloxapen, {Novocloxin}, {Orbenin}, Tegopen

CLASSIFICATION(S):
Anti-infective—penicillinase-resistant penicillin
Pregnancy Category B

INDICATIONS

▪ Treatment of the following infections due to susceptible strains of streptococci or penicillinase-producing staphylococci: ▫ Respiratory tract infections ▫ Sinusitis ▫ Skin and skin structure infections.

ACTION

▪ Binds to bacterial cell wall, leading to cell death. Resists the action of penicillinase, an enzyme capable of inactivating penicillin. **Therapeutic Effect:** ▪ Bactericidal action against susceptible bacteria. **Spectrum:** ▪ Active against most gram-positive aerobic cocci, but less so than penicillin. ▪ Spectrum is notable for activity against: ▫ Penicillinase-producing strains of *Staphylococcus aureus* ▫ *Staphylococcus epidermidis* ▪ Not active against methicillin-resistant staphylococci.

PHARMACOKINETICS

Absorption: Moderately absorbed (37–60%) following oral administration.
Distribution: Widely distributed. Penetration into CSF is minimal. Crosses the placenta and enters breast milk.
Metabolism and Excretion: Some metabolism by the liver (9–22%) and some renal excretion of unchanged drug (30–45%).
Half-life: 0.5–1.1 hr (increased in severe hepatic and renal dysfunction).

CONTRAINDICATIONS AND PRECAUTIONS

Contraindicated in: ▪ Hypersensitivity to penicillins ▪ Should not be used as initial therapy in serious infections or in patients experiencing nausea or vomiting.
Use Cautiously in: ▪ Severe renal or hepatic impairment (dosage reduction required) ▪ Pregnancy or lactation (safety not established).

ADVERSE REACTIONS AND SIDE EFFECTS*

CNS: SEIZURES (high doses).
GI: nausea, vomiting, diarrhea, hepatitis.
GU: interstitial nephritis.
Derm: rashes, urticaria.
Hemat: blood dyscrasias.
Misc: superinfection, allergic reactions, including ANAPHYLAXIS and serum sickness.

INTERACTIONS

Drug-Drug: ▪ **Probenecid** decreases renal excretion and increases blood levels ▪ May alter the effect of **oral anticoagulants**.
Drug-Food: ▪ **Food** and **acidic juices** decrease absorption.

ROUTE AND DOSAGE

- **PO (Adults and Children >20 kg):** 250–500 mg q 6 hr.
- **PO (Children >1 mon and <20 kg):** 50–100 mg/kg/day in divided doses q 6 hr.

PHARMACODYNAMICS (blood levels)

	ONSET	PEAK
PO	30 min	30–120 min

NURSING IMPLICATIONS

Assessement

▫ Assess patient for infection (vital signs; appearance of wound, sputum, urine, and stool; WBC) at beginning and throughout course of therapy.
▫ Obtain a history before initiating therapy to determine previous use of and reactions to penicillins or cephalosporins. Persons with a negative his-

{} = Available in Canada only.
*Underlines indicate most frequent; CAPITALS indicate life-threatening.

tory of penicillin sensitivity may still have an allergic response.
- □ Obtain specimens for culture and sensitivity prior to initiating therapy. First dose may be given before receiving results.
- □ Observe patient for signs and symptoms of anaphylaxis (rash, pruritus, laryngeal edema, wheezing, abdominal pain). Discontinue the drug and notify the physician immediately if these occur. Keep epinephrine, an antihistamine, and resuscitation equipment close by in the event of an anaphylactic reaction.
- ▪ **Lab Test Considerations:** CBC, BUN, creatinine, urinalysis, and liver function tests should be monitored periodically during therapy.
- □ May cause an increased SGOT (AST) concentrations.

Potential Nursing Diagnoses
- ▪ Infection, high risk for (indications, side effects).
- ▪ Knowledge deficit related to medication regimen (patient/family teaching).
- ▪ Noncompliance related to medication regimen (patient/family teaching).

Implementation
- ▪ **PO:** Administer around the clock on an empty stomach at least 1 hr before or 2 hr after meals. Take with a full glass of water; acidic juices may decrease absorption of penicillins.
- □ Use calibrated measuring device for liquid preparations. Shake well. Soln stable for 14 days if refrigerated.

Patient/Family Teaching
- □ Instruct patient to take medication around the clock and to finish the drug completely as directed by the physician, even if feeling better. Missed doses should be taken as soon as remembered. Advise patient that sharing of this medication may be dangerous.
- □ Advise patient to report signs of superinfection (black, furry overgrowth on the tongue, vaginal itching or discharge, loose or foul-smelling stools) and allergy.
- □ Instruct patient to notify physician if fever and diarrhea develop, especially if stool contains blood, pus, or mucus. Advise patient not to treat diarrhea without consulting physician or pharmacist.
- □ Instruct patient to notify physician if symptoms do not improve.

Evaluation

Clinical response can be evaluated by:
▪ Resolution of the signs and symptoms of infection. Length of time for complete resolution depends on the organism and site of infection.

CLOZAPINE
(**cloz**-a-peen)
Clozaril

CLASSIFICATION(S):
Antipsychotic—miscellaneous
Pregnancy Category B

INDICATIONS
▪ Treatment of schizophrenic patients who are unresponsive to or cannot tolerate standard therapy with other antipsychotic agents.

ACTION
▪ Binds to dopamine receptors in the CNS ▪ Also has anticholinergic and alpha-adrenergic blocking activity ▪ Produces less extrapyramidal reactions and tardive dyskinesia than standard antipsychotic therapy but carries high risk of hematologic abnormalities. **Therapeutic Effect:** ▪ Diminished schizophrenic behavior.

PHARMACOKINETICS
Absorption: Well absorbed following oral administration.
Distribution: Rapid and extensive distribution, crosses blood-brain barrier and placenta. 95% bound to plasma proteins.
Metabolism and Excretion: Mostly

metabolized on first pass through the liver.

Half-life: 8–12 hr.

CONTRAINDICATIONS AND PRECAUTIONS

Contraindicated in: ▪ Hypersensitivity ▪ Bone marrow depression ▪ Lactation ▪ Severe CNS depression or coma.

Use Cautiously in: ▪ Prostatic enlargement (extreme caution) ▪ Narrow-angle glaucoma (extreme caution) ▪ Children <16 yr (safety not established) ▪ Cardiovascular, hepatic, or renal disease ▪ Seizure disorder.

ADVERSE REACTIONS AND SIDE EFFECTS*

CNS: sedation, SEIZURES, dizziness.

EENT: visual disturbances, dry mouth, increased salivation.

CV: hypotension, tachycardia, ECG changes, hypertension.

GI: constipation, nausea, vomiting, abdominal discomfort.

Derm: sweating, rash.

Hemat: AGRANULOCYTOSIS, LEUKOPENIA.

Neuro: extrapyramidal reactions.

Misc: fever, weight gain.

INTERACTIONS

Drug-Drug: ▪ Additive anticholinergic effects with other **agents having anticholinergic properties** including **antihistamines, quinidine, disopyramide,** and **antidepressants** ▪ Additive CNS depression with **alcohol, antidepressants, antihistamines, narcotic analgesics,** or **sedative/hypnotics** ▪ Additive hypotension with **nitrates,** acute ingestion of **alcohol,** or **antihypertensives** ▪ Increased risk of bone marrow suppression with **antineoplastic agents** or **radiation therapy** ▪ Use with **lithium** increases the risk of adverse CNS reactions, including seizures.

ROUTE AND DOSAGE

- **PO (Adults):** 25 mg 1–2 times daily initially, increase by 25–50 mg/day over a period of 2 wk up to target dose of 300–450 mg/day. May increase by up to 100 mg/day once or twice weekly (not to exceed 900 mg/day).

PHARMACODYNAMICS

	ONSET	PEAK	DURATION
PO	UK	wks	4–12 hr

NURSING IMPLICATIONS

Assessment

- Monitor patient's mental status (delusions, hallucinations, and behavior) prior to and periodically throughout therapy.
- Monitor blood pressure (sitting, standing, lying) and pulse rate prior to and frequently during initial dosage titration.
- Observe patient carefully when administering medication to ensure medication is actually taken and not hoarded.
- Monitor patient for onset of extrapyramidal side effects (akathesia—restlessness, dystonia—muscle spasms and twisting motions, or pseudoparkinsonism—mask facies, rigidity, tremors, drooling, shuffling gait, dysphagia). Notify physician if these symptoms occur because reduction in dosage or discontinuation of medication may be necessary. Physician may also order antiparkinson agents (trihexyphenidyl, benztropine) to control these symptoms.
- Although not yet reported for clozapine, monitor for possible tardive dyskinesia (rhythmic movement of mouth, face, and extremities). Notify physician immediately if these symptoms occur as these side effects may be irreversible.
- Monitor frequency and consistency of bowel movements. Increasing bulk and fluids in the diet may help minimize constipation.
- Clozapine lowers the seizure threshold. Institute seizure precautions for patients with history of seizure disorder.

*Underlines indicate most frequent; **CAPITALS** indicate life-threatening.

- Transient fevers may occur, especially during first 3 wk of therapy. Fever is usually self-limiting, but may require discontinuation of medication. Also, monitor for development of neuroleptic malignant syndrome (fever, respiratory distress, tachycardia, convulsions, diaphoresis, hypertension or hypotension, pallor, tiredness). Notify physician immediately if these symptoms occur.

- **Lab Test Considerations:** Monitor WBC and differential count prior to initiation of therapy, and WBC count weekly during therapy and for 4 wk after discontinuation of clozapine. Due to the risk of agranulocytosis, clozapine is only available in a 1 wk supply through the *Clozaril Patient Management System,* which combines WBC testing, patient monitoring, pharmacy, and drug distribution. If WBC is <3000 mm^3 or granulocyte count is <1500 mm^3 withhold clozapine and monitor patient for signs and symptoms of infection.
- **Toxicity and Overdose:** Overdose is treated with activated charcoal and supportive therapy. Monitor patient for several days due to risk of delayed effects.
  - Avoid use of epinephrine and its derivatives when treating hypotension, and quinidine and procainamide when treating arrhythmias.

Potential Nursing Diagnoses

- Violence, high risk for: directed at others related to mistrust and panic (indications).
- Thought processes, altered: related to panic anxiety (indications).
- Injury, high risk for (side effects).

Implementation

- **PO:** Administer capsules with food or milk to decrease gastric irritation.

Patient/Family Teaching

- Instruct patient to take medication exactly as directed. Patients on long-term therapy may need to discontinue gradually over 1–2 wk.
- Inform patient of possibility of extrapyramidal symptoms. Instruct patient to report these symptoms immediately to physician.
- Advise patients to make position changes slowly to minimize orthostatic hypotension.
- May cause seizures and drowsiness. Caution patient to avoid driving or other activities requiring alertness while taking clozapine.
- Caution patient to avoid concurrent use of alcohol, other CNS depressants, and over-the-counter medications without consulting physician.
- Instruct patient to use frequent mouth rinses, good oral hygiene, and sugarless gum or candy to minimize dry mouth.
- Advise patient to notify physician or dentist of medication regimen prior to treatment or surgery.
- Instruct patient to notify physician promptly if sore throat, fever, lethargy, weakness, malaise, or flu-like symptoms occur. Patients should also notify physician if they become or intend to become pregnant.
- Advise patient of need for continued medical follow-up for psychotherapy, eye examinations, and laboratory tests.

Evaluation

Effectiveness of therapy can be demonstrated by: ▪ Decreased psychotic ideation.

CODEINE
(koe-**deen**)
{Paveral}

CLASSIFICATION(S):
Narcotic analgesic—agonist, Antitussive
Schedules II, III, IV, V
Pregnancy Category C

INDICATIONS

▪ Alone and in combination with nonnarcotic analgesics in the management of mild to moderate pain ▪ Antitussive

C

(in smaller doses). **Unlabeled Use:** ▪ Management of diarrhea.

ACTION

▪ Binds to the opiate receptor in the CNS. Alters the perception of and response to painful stimuli, while producing generalized CNS depression. ▪ Decreases cough reflex ▪ Decreases GI motility. **Therapeutic Effects:** ▪ Decreased severity of pain ▪ Suppression of the cough reflex ▪ Decreased diarrhea.

PHARMACOKINETICS

Absorption: 50% absorbed from the GI tract. Completely absorbed from IM sites. Oral and parenteral doses are not equal.
Distribution: Widely distributed. Crosses the placenta and enters breast milk.
Metabolism and Excretion: Mostly metabolized by the liver. 10% converted to morphine. Minimal renal excretion (5–15%) of unchanged drug.
Half-life: 2.5–4 hr.

CONTRAINDICATIONS AND PRECAUTIONS

Contraindicated in: ▪ Hypersensitivity ▪ Pregnancy or lactation (avoid chronic use).
Use Cautiously in: ▪ Head trauma ▪ Increased intracranial pressure ▪ Severe renal, hepatic, or pulmonary disease ▪ Hypothyroidism ▪ Adrenal insufficiency ▪ Alcoholism ▪ Elderly or debilitated patients (dosage reduction required) ▪ Patients with undiagnosed abdominal pain ▪ Prostatic hypertrophy ▪ Has been used during labor; respiratory depression may occur in the newborn.

ADVERSE REACTIONS AND SIDE EFFECTS*

CNS: sedation, confusion, headache, euphoria, floating feeling, unusual dreams, hallucinations, dysphoria: hypotension, bradycardia.
EENT: miosis, diplopia, blurred vision.
Resp: respiratory depression.
GI: nausea, vomiting, constipation.
GU: urinary retention.
Derm: sweating, flushing.
Misc: tolerance, physical dependence, psychological dependence.

INTERACTIONS

Drug-Drug: ▪ Use with caution in patients receiving **MAO inhibitors** (reduce initial dosage to 25% of usual dose) ▪ Additive CNS depression with **alcohol, antidepressants, antihistamines,** and **sedative/hypnotics** ▪ Administration of **partial antagonists (buprenorphine, butorphanol, nalbuphine,** or **pentazocine)** may precipitate narcotic withdrawal in physically dependent patients ▪ **Nalbuphine** or **pentazocine** may decrease alalgesia.

ROUTE AND DOSAGE

Analgesia

- **PO, IM, SC (Adults):** 15–60 mg q 4 hr as needed.
- **PO, IM, SC (Children):** 0.5 mg/kg q 4–6 hr as needed.

Antitussive

- **PO, IM, SC (Adults):** 10–20 mg q 4–6 hr as needed (not to exceed 120 mg/day).
- **PO, IM, SC (Children 6–11 yr):** 5–10 mg q 4–6 hr as needed (not to exceed 60 mg/day).
- **PO, IM, SC (Children 2–5 yr):** 2.5–5 mg q 4–6 hr (not to exceed 30 mg/day).

Antidiarrheal

- **PO (Adults):** 30 mg, may be repeated up to 4 times daily.

PHARMACODYNAMICS (analgesia)

	ONSET	PEAK	DURATION
PO	30–45 min	60–120 min	4 hr
IM	10–30 min	30–60 min	4 hr
SC	10–30 min	UK	4 hr

NURSING IMPLICATIONS

Assessment

- **General Info:** Assess blood pressure, pulse, and respiratory rate before and

*Underlines indicate most frequent; **CAPITALS** indicate life-threatening.

periodically during administration.

- Assess bowel function routinely. Increased intake of fluids and bulk, stool softeners, and laxatives may minimize constipating effects.
- **Pain:** Assess type, location, and intensity of pain prior to and 60 min following administration.
- Prolonged use may lead to physical and psychological dependence and tolerance. This should not prevent patient from receiving adequate analgesia. Most patients who receive codeine for medical reasons do not develop psychological dependency. Potential for dependence is less than that of morphine. Progressively higher doses may be required to relieve pain with long-term therapy.
- **Cough:** Assess cough and lung sounds during antitussive use.
- **Lab Test Considerations:** May cause increased plasma amylase and lipase concentrations.
- **Toxicity and Overdose:** If overdosage occurs, naloxone (Narcan) is the antidote.

POTENTIAL NURSING DIAGNOSES

- Comfort, altered: pain (indications).
- Sensory-perceptual alteration: visual, auditory (side effects).
- Injury, high risk for (side effects).

IMPLEMENTATION

- **General Info:** Explain therapeutic value of medication prior to administration to enhance the analgesic effect.
- Regularly administered doses may be more effective than prn administration. Analgesic is more effective if given before pain becomes severe.
- Coadministration with non-narcotic analgesics may have additive analgesic effects and permit lower doses.
- Medications should be discontinued gradually after long-term use to prevent withdrawal symptoms.
- Available in tablet, various cough syrups and elixirs, and injectable forms. Also available in combination with non-narcotic analgesics (aspirin, acetaminophen; #2 = 15 mg, #3 = 30 mg, #4 = 60 mg codeine). Codeine as an individual drug is a Schedule II substance. In combination with other drugs, tablet form is Schedule III, liquid is Schedule IV, and elixir or cough suppressant is Schedule V.
- **PO:** Oral doses may be administered with food or milk to minimize GI irritation.
- **IM/SC:** Do not administer soln that is more than slightly discolored or contains a precipitate.
- **Syringe Compatibility:** glycopyrrolate or hydroxyzine.

PATIENT/FAMILY TEACHING

- Instruct patient on how and when to ask for prn pain medication.
- Codeine may cause drowsiness or dizziness. Advise patient to call for assistance when ambulating or smoking. Caution ambulatory patient to avoid driving or other activities requiring alertness until response to medication is known.
- Advise patient to make position changes slowly to minimize orthostatic hypotension.
- Caution patient to avoid concurrent use of alcohol or other CNS depressants with this medication.
- Encourage patient to turn, cough, and breathe deeply every 2 hr to prevent atelectasis.

EVALUATION

Effectiveness of therapy can be demonstrated by: ▪ Decrease in severity of pain without a significant alteration in level of consciousness or respiratory status ▪ Suppression of cough ▪ Control of diarrhea.

COLCHICINE

(**kol**-chi-seen)

CLASSIFICATION(S):
Antigout agent
Pregnancy Category C (IV form is Category D)

C

INDICATIONS

▪ Treatment of acute attacks of gouty arthritis (larger doses) ▪ Prevention of recurrences of gout (smaller doses). **Unlabeled Uses:** ▪ Treatment of hepatic cirrhosis and familial Mediterranean fever.

ACTION

▪ Interferes with the functions of white blood cells in initiating and perpetuating the inflammatory response to monosodium urate crystals. **Therapeutic Effects:** ▪ Decreased pain and inflammation in acute attacks of gout ▪ Prevention of recurrent attacks of gout.

PHARMACOKINETICS

Absorption: Absorbed from the GI tract, then re-enters GI tract from biliary secretions, when more absorption may occur.
Distribution: Concentrates in white blood cells.
Metabolism and Excretion: Partially metabolized by the liver. Secreted in bile back into GI tract. Eliminated in the feces. Small amount excreted in the urine.
Half-life: 20 min (plasma), 60 hr (white blood cells).

CONTRAINDICATIONS AND PRECAUTIONS

Contraindicated in: ▪ Hypersensitivity ▪ Pregnancy ▪ Severe renal or GI disease.
Use Cautiously in: ▪ Elderly or debilitated patients (toxicity may be cumulative) ▪ IV dosing (not intended for prolonged use) ▪ Lactation or children (safety not established).

ADVERSE REACTIONS AND SIDE EFFECTS*

GI: nausea, vomiting, abdominal pain, diarrhea.
GU: anuria, hematuria, renal damage.
Derm: alopecia.
Hemat: AGRANULOCYTOSIS, APLASTIC ANEMIA, leukopenia, thrombocytopenia.
Local: phlebitis at IV site.
Neuro: peripheral neuritis.

INTERACTIONS

Drug-Drug: ▪ May cause reversible malabsorption of **vitamin B_{12}**.

ROUTE AND DOSAGE

Acute Gouty Arthritis

- **PO (Adults):** 0.5–1.2 mg, then 0.5–0.6 mg q 1–2 hr or 1–1.2 mg q 2 hr until relief or GI side effects occur (control of acute attack usually requires total cumulative dose of 4–8 mg).
- **IV (Adults):** 1–3 mg initially, then 0.5 mg q 6 hr until response (total daily dose not to exceed 4 mg).

Prophylaxis of Recurrence of Gouty Arthritis

- **PO (Adults):** 0.5–1.2 mg daily.

PHARMACODYNAMICS (anti-inflammatory activity)

	ONSET	PEAK	DURATION
PO	12 hr	24–72 hr	UK
IV	6–12 hr	24–72 hr	UK

NURSING IMPLICATIONS

Assessment

- □ Assess involved joints for pain, mobility, and edema throughout course of therapy. During initiation of therapy, monitor for drug response every 1–2 hr.
- □ Monitor intake and output ratios. Fluids should be encouraged to promote a urinary output of at least 2000 ml/day.
- ▪ **Lab Test Considerations:** In patients receiving prolonged therapy, monitor baseline and periodic CBC; notify physician if a significant decrease in values occurs.
- □ May cause an increase in SGOT (AST) and alkaline phosphatase.
- □ May cause false-positive results for urine hemoglobin.
- □ May interfere with results of urinary 17-hydroxycorticosteroid concentrations.

*Underlines indicate most frequent; **CAPITALS** indicate life-threatening.

- **Toxicity and Overdose:** Assess patient for toxicity (weakness, abdominal discomfort, nausea, vomiting, diarrhea). If these symptoms occur, discontinue medication and notify physician.

POTENTIAL NURSING DIAGNOSES
- Comfort, altered: pain (indications).
- Mobility, impaired physical (indications).
- Knowledge deficit related to medication regimen (patient/family teaching).

IMPLEMENTATION
- **General Info:** Physician may order intermittent therapy with 3 days between courses to decrease risk of toxicity.
- **PO:** Administer oral doses with food to minimize gastric irritation.
- **IV:** Do not administer SC or IM, as tissue damage and necrosis may result. Observe IV site frequently to prevent extravasation. If extravasation occurs confer with physician regarding local application of heat or cold and analgesics.
- **Direct IV:** May administer IV undiluted or dilute with 10–20 ml of 0.9% NaCl without a bacteriostatic agent or sterile water for injection. Do not administer turbid soln.
- □ *Rate:* Administer each dose over 2–5 min.
- **Additive Incompatibility:** Incompatible with dextrose; do not dilute with or inject into tubing containing dextrose.

PATIENT/FAMILY TEACHING
- □ Review medication administration schedule. Emphasize importance of taking medication at correct time: begin or increase dose when first symptoms of attack occur; stop or return to prophylactic dose when attack subsides. If dose is missed, take as soon as remembered unless almost time for next dose. Do not double doses.
- □ Advise patient to follow physician's recommendations regarding weight loss, diet, and alcohol consumption.
- □ Instruct patient to report nausea, vomiting, abdominal pain, diarrhea, unusual bleeding, or bruising, sore throat, fatigue, malaise, or rash to physician promptly. Medication should be withheld if gastric symptoms occur.
- □ Surgery may precipitate an acute attack of gout. Advise patient to confer with physician regarding dose 3 days before surgical or dental procedures.

EVALUATION
Therapeutic effects can be demonstrated by: ■ Decrease in pain and swelling in affected joints within 12 hr □ Relief of symptoms within 24–48 hr ■ Prevention of acute gout attacks.

COLESTIPOL
(koe-**less**-ti-pole)
Colestid

CLASSIFICATION(S):
Lipid-lowering agent—bile acid sequestrant
Pregnancy Category UK

INDICATIONS
■ Adjunct in the management of primary hypercholesterolemia ■ Relief of pruritis associated with elevated levels of bile acids.

ACTION
■ Binds bile acids in the GI tract forming an insoluble complex. Result is increased clearance of cholesterol. **Therapeutic Effect:** ■ Decreased plasma cholesterol and low-density lipoproteins.

PHARMACOKINETICS
Absorption: Action takes place in the GI tract. No absorption occurs.
Distribution: No distribution.
Metabolism and Excretion: After binding bile acids, insoluble complex is eliminated in the feces.
Half-life: UK.

C

CONTRAINDICATIONS AND PRECAUTIONS

Contraindicated in: ▪ Hypersensitivity ▪ Complete biliary obstruction.
Use Cautiously in: ▪ Constipation (causes severe constipation).

ADVERSE REACTIONS AND SIDE EFFECTS*

EENT: irritation of the tongue.
GI: nausea, vomiting, constipation, impaction, hemorrhoids, flatulence, perianal irritation, steatorrhea, abdominal discomfort.
Derm: rashes, irritation.
F and E: hyperchloremic acidosis.
Hemat: bleeding.
Metab: Vitamin A, D, K deficiency.

INTERACTIONS

Drug–Drug: ▪ May decrease absorption of orally administered **acetaminophen, amiodarone, glucocorticoids, cardiac glycosides, methotrexate, naproxen, phenylbutazone, piroxicam, propranolol, thiazide diuretics, thyroid, chenodrol, ursodiol, oral anticoagulants,** and **fat-soluble vitamins (A, D, E, and K)** ▪ May increase effect of **oral anticoagulants** due to depletion of vitamin K ▪ May decrease absorption of other **orally administered medications.**

ROUTE AND DOSAGE

- **PO (Adults):** 4 g qid (not to exceed 32 g/day).
- **PO (Children >6 yr):** 80 mg/kg 3 times daily.

PHARMACODYNAMICS (hypocholesterolemic effects)

	ONSET	PEAK	DURATION
PO	24–48 hr	1 mon	1 mon

NURSING IMPLICATIONS

Assessment

- □ Obtain a diet history, especially in regard to fat consumption.
- ▪ **Lab Test Considerations:** Serum cholesterol and triglyceride levels should be evaluated before initiating and periodically throughout course of therapy. Medication should be discontinued if paradoxical increase in cholesterol level occurs.
- □ May cause an increase in SGOT (AST), phosphate, chloride, and alkaline phosphatase and a decrease in serum calcium, sodium, and potassium levels.

Potential Nursing Diagnoses

- ▪ Bowel elimination, altered: constipation (side effects).
- ▪ Knowledge deficit related to medication regimen (patient/family teaching).
- ▪ Noncompliance (patient/family teaching).

Implementation

- ▪ **General Info:** Physician may order parenteral or water-miscible forms of fat-soluble vitamins (A, D, K,) and folic acid for patients on chronic therapy.
- ▪ **PO:** Administer other medications 1 hr before or 4–6 hr after the administration of this medication.

Patient/Family Teaching

- □ Instruct patient to take medication exactly as directed; do not skip doses or double up on missed doses.
- □ Instruct patient to take medication before meals. Colestipol can be mixed with water, juice, or carbonated beverages, slowly stirred in a large glass. Rinse glass with small amount of additional beverage to ensure that all medication is taken. May also mix with highly fluid soups, cereals, or pulpy fruits (applesauce, crushed pineapple). Allow powder to sit on fluid and hydrate for 1–2 min prior to mixing. Do not take dry. Color variations do not alter stability.
- □ Advise patient that this medication should be used in conjunction with diet restrictions (fat, cholesterol, carbohydrates, alcohol), exercise, and cessation of smoking.
- □ Explain that constipation may occur.

*Underlines indicate most frequent; **CAPITALS** indicate life-threatening.

Increasing fluids and bulk in diet, exercise, stool softeners, and laxatives may be required to minimize the constipating effects. Instruct patient to notify physician if constipation, nausea, flatulence, and heartburn persist or if stools become frothy and foul-smelling.

- □ Advise patient to notify physician if unusual bleeding or bruising, petechiae, or tarry, black stools occur. Treatment with vitamin K may be necessary.

EVALUATION

Effectiveness of therapy can be demonstrated by: ▪ Decrease in serum cholesterol levels. Cholesterol levels should begin to decrease in 48 hr but may take 1 yr to stabilize. Therapy is usually discontinued if the clinical response remains poor after 3 mon of therapy.

COLFOSCERIL PALMITATE

(koll-**foss**-er-ill **pal**-mi-tate)
dipalmitoylphosphatidylcholine, DPPC, Exosurf Neonatal

CLASSIFICATION(S):
Pulmonary surfactant
Pregnancy Category UK

INDICATIONS

▪ Treatment and prophylaxis of respiratory distress syndrome (RDS, hyaline membrane disease) in premature infants.

ACTION

▪ Replaces endogenous pulmonary surfactant in premature infants, allowing normal surface activity in alveoli. Cetyl alcohol in formulation spreads colfosceril on air-fluid surface whereas Tyloxapal, a surfactant, disperses colfosceril and cetyl alcohol. **Therapeutic Effects:** ▪ Decreased incidence, mortality, and complications from RDS in premature infants.

PHARMACOKINETICS

Absorption: Administered directly to site of action. Systemic absorption not known.
Distribution: Rapidly distributes to lung tissue.
Metabolism and Excretion: Enters surfactant pathways where recycling and reutilization occur.
Half-life: UK.

CONTRAINDICATIONS AND PRECAUTIONS

Contraindications in: ▪ No known contraindications.
Use Cautiously in: ▪ No known cautions.

ADVERSE REACTIONS AND SIDE EFFECTS*

Resp: pulmonary hemorrhage, apnea
CV: <u>bradycardia</u>, hypotension, vasoconstriction.
Misc: increased risk of sepsis following treatment.

INTERACTIONS

Drug–Drug: ▪ None known.

ROUTE AND DOSAGE

Prophylactic Treatment

- ▪ **Intratracheal (Premature Infants):** 5 ml/kg given as 2 half-doses of 2.5 ml/kg as soon as possible after birth, give 2 more doses 12 and 24 hr later.

Rescue Treatment

- ▪ **Intratracheal (Premature Infants):** 5 ml/kg given as 2 half-doses of 2.5 ml/kg as soon as diagnosis of RDS is made, give a second dose 12 hr later.

PHARMACODYNAMICS

	ONSET	PEAK	DURATION
Intratracheal	rapid	UK	12 hr

NURSING IMPLICATIONS

ASSESSMENT

- □ Monitor ECG, heart rate, color, chest expansion, facial expression, transcutaneous oxygen saturation, and endo-

*<u>Underlines</u> indicate most frequent; **CAPITALS** indicate life-threatening.

C

tracheal tube patency continuously during dosing. Continuous bedside monitoring should continue for at least 30 min following dosing.

- **Lab Test Considerations:** Monitor arterial blood gases frequently to prevent hyperoxia or hypocarbia.
- **Toxicity and Overdose:** If chest expansion improves substantially after dosing, reduce peak inspiratory ventilator pressures immediately to prevent lung overdistension and fatal pulmonary leak.
  - If infant becomes pink and transcutaneous oxygen saturation is in excess of 95%, reduce FiO_2 in small but repeated steps immediately to prevent hyperoxia.
  - If arterial or transcutaneous CO_2 measurements are less than 30 mmHg, ventilator rate should be reduced immediately to prevent hypocarbia.

Potential Nursing Diagnoses

- Impaired gas exchange (indications).

Implementation

- **General Info:** Only trained medical personnel with experience in airway and clinical management of unstable neonates should perform colfosceril instillation.
  - Suction the infant endotracheally prior to instillation. Check position of endotracheal tube prior to instillation. Do not suction for 2 hr following instillation unless clinically necessary.
  - If reflux occurs after instillation, stop drug administration and increase the peak inspiratory pressure on the ventilator by 4–5 cm H_2O until the endotracheal tube clears.
  - If transcutaneous oxygen saturation drops more than 20% during instillation, stop administration and increase peak inspiratory pressure on the ventilator by 4–5 cm H_2O and increase the FiO_2 for 1–2 min, if necessary.
- **Inhaln:** Reconstitute *only* with diluent provided (preservative-free sterile water for injection). Fill a 10- or 12-ml syringe with 8 ml of diluent using an 18- or 19-gauge needle. Allow the vacuum in the vial to draw the sterile water into the vial. Aspirate as much of the 8 ml as possible out of the vial and into the syringe while maintaining the vacuum, then suddenly release the syringe plunger. Repeat process 3–4 times to ensure mixing of contents. If vacuum is not present, do not use the vial.
  - Draw the entire dose from below the froth line in the vial. Reconstituted drug is a milky white suspension. If suspension separates, gently shake or swirl to resuspend. Do not use if persistent large flakes or particles are present.
  - Instillation is accomplished through a special endotracheal tube adaptor.
  - *Rate:* Instill each half-dose slowly over 1–2 min in small bursts timed with inspiration. After the first 2.5 ml/kg half-dose is administered in the midline position, turn the infant's head and torso 45° to the right and continue mechanical ventilation for 30 sec. Once returned to the midline position, instill the second 2.5 ml/kg half-dose over 1–2 min and turn the infant's head and torso to the left for 30 sec while continuing mechanical ventilation. Then return infant to midline.

Patient/Family Teaching

- Explain purpose of medication to parents.

Evaluation

Effectiveness of therapy may be determined by: ▪ Prevention of RDS ▪ Improvement in lung compliance ▫ Improved oxygenation ▫ Normalization of arterial blood gases.

COLISTIN

(koe-**lis**-tin)
Coly-mycin S, Polymyxin E

COLISTIMETHATE

(koe-lis-ti-**meth**-ate)
Coly-mycin M

CLASSIFICATION(S):
Anti-infective—polymyxin
Pregnancy Category UK

INDICATIONS

Colistimethate: ▪ Treatment of the following infections due to susceptible organisms: ▫ Serious gram-negative infections (only where less toxic agents are contraindicated) ▫ Urinary tract infections due to resistant strains of *Psuedomonas aeruginosa*. **Colistin:** ▪ Treatment of gastroenteritis in infants and children due to enteropathogenic strains of *Escherichia coli* or *Shigella* (other agents or treatments usually preferred).

ACTION

▪ Binds to bacterial cell wall, allowing leakage of intracellular contents. **Therapeutic Effect:** ▪ Bactericidal action against susceptible organisms. **Spectrum:** ▪ Most gram-negative pathogens, including: ▫ *E. coli* ▫ *Shigella* ▪ Not active against *Proteus* species.

PHARMACOKINETICS

Absorption: Minimal absorption may follow oral administration.
Distribution: Widely distributed following parenteral administration. Does not enter CSF. Crosses the placenta and enters breast milk.
Metabolism and Excretion: Colistimethate is hydrolyzed to colistin. Remainder of metabolic fate not known.
Half-life: 1.5–8 hr (increased in renal impairment).

CONTRAINDICATIONS AND PRECAUTIONS

Contraindicated in: ▪ Hypersensitivity.
Use Cautiously in: ▪ Impaired renal function (dosage adjustment of parenteral forms necessary).

ADVERSE REACTIONS AND SIDE EFFECTS*

Note: Occur only at higher-than-recommended doses.

CNS: neurotoxicity.
GU: nephrotoxicity.

INTERACTIONS

Drug-Drug: ▪ Increased neuromuscular blockade with **neuromuscular blocking agents** ▪ Additive nephrotoxicity or neurotoxicity with **nephrotoxic** or **neurotoxic agents**.

ROUTE AND DOSAGE

- **PO (Children):** 5–15 mg/kg/day in 3 divided doses.
- **IM, IV (Adults and Children):** 2.5–5 mg/kg/day in 2–4 divided doses (dosage reduction required in renal impairment).

PHARMACODYNAMICS (blood levels)

	ONSET	PEAK
IM	UK	2 hr
IV	rapid	end of infusion

NURSING IMPLICATIONS

Assessment

- **General Info:** Assess patient for infection (vital signs, tympanic membrane, earache, urine, stool, and WBC) at beginning and throughout course of therapy.
  ▫ Obtain specimens for culture and sensitivity prior to initiating therapy. First dose may be given before receiving results.
- **Diarrhea:** Assess hydration status (intake and output, weight, skin turgor, moistness of mucous membranes). Notify physician promptly if dehydration present.
- **Lab Test Considerations:** May cause nephrotoxicity; monitor BUN and serum creatinine.

Potential Nursing Diagnoses

- Infection, high risk for (indications, side effects).
- Fluid volume deficit (indications).
- Knowledge deficit related to medication regimen (patient/family teaching).

*Underlines indicate most frequent; **CAPITALS** indicate life-threatening.

C

Implementation

- **General Info:** Available in combination with neomycin and hydrocortisone (see Appendix A).
- **PO:** Shake suspension well before measuring dose. Stable for 2 wk when refrigerated.
- **IM/IV:** Reconstitute the 150-mg vial with 2 ml of sterile water for injection. Swirl gently to avoid frothing.
- **Direct IV:** Administer initial dose (½ daily dose) via direct IV slowly over 3–5 min.
- **Continous Infusion:** Second dose (remaining ½ of daily dose) may be diluted in D5W, D5/0.25% NaCl, D5/0.45% NaCl, or D5/0.9% NaCl.
  - *Rate:* Administer second dose 1–2 hr after initial dose slowly at a rate of 5–6 mg/hr.
- **Syringe Compatibility:** ampicillin, methicillin, or penicillin G sodium.
- **Additive Compatibility:** amikacin, ascorbic acid, chloramphenicol, cimetidine, diphenhydramine, heparin, methicillin, oxytetracycline, penicillin G potassium and sodium, phenobarbital, polymyxin B, or tetracycline.
- **Additive Incompatibility:** cefazolin, cephalothin, erythromycin, hydrocortisone sodium succinate, or kanamycin.

Patient/Family Teaching

- **General Info:** Instruct patient to administer medication around the clock and to finish the drug completely as directed, even if feeling better. Advise patient that sharing of this medication may be dangerous.
  - Advise patient to report signs of superinfection (furry overgrowth on the tongue, vaginal itching or discharge, loose, foul-smelling stools) and allergy.
  - Instruct patient to notify physician if symptoms do not improve.
- **Diarrhea:** Emphasize importance of accurately measuring oral dose with provided calibrated device. Review methods of preventing spread of diarrhea (good handwashing, preparation of food, etc.). Discuss risk and symptoms of dehydration, review dietary restrictions.

Evaluation

Clinical response to therapy can be evaluated by: ▪ Resolution of the signs and symptoms of infection.

CONTRACEPTIVES, HORMONAL

MONOPHASIC ORAL CONTRACEPTIVES

mestranol/norethindrone
(**mes**-tre-nole)/(nor-eth-**in**-drone)
Genora 1/50, Nelova 1/50M, Norethin 1/50M, Norinyl 1 + 50, Ortho-Novum 1/50

ethinyl estradiol/norethindrone
(**eth**-in-il ess-tra-**dye**-ole/(nor-eth-**in**-drone)
Brevicon, Genora 0.5/35, Genora 1/35, Loestrin 21 1.5/30, Loestrin 21 1/20, Modicon, N.E.E. 1/35, Nelova 0.5/35E, Nelova 1/35E, Norcept-E 1/35, Norethin 1/35E, Norinyl 1 + 35, Ortho-Novum 1/35, Ovcon 35, Ovcon-50, Norlestrin 1/50, Norlestrin 2.5/50

ethinyl estradiol/ethynodiol
(**eth**-in-il ess-tra-**dye**-ole/e-thye-noe-**dye**-ole)
Demulen, Demulen 1/35

ethinyl estradiol/norgestrel
(**eth**-in-il ess-tra-**dye**-ole/nor-**jess**-trel)
Lo-Ovral, Ovral

ethinyl estradiol/levonorgestrel
(**eth**-in-il ess-tra-**dye**-ole/lee-voe-nor-**jess**-trel)
Levlen, Nordette

BIPHASIC ORAL CONTRACEPTIVES

ethinyl estradiol/norethindrone
Nelova 10/11, Ortho Novum 10/11

TRIPHASIC ORAL CONTRACEPTIVES

ethinyl estradiol/norethindrone
Tri-Norinyl, Ortho Novum 7/7/7

ethinyl estradiol/norgestrel
Tri-Levlen, Triphasil

PROGESTIN-ONLY ORAL CONTRACEPTIVES
norethindrone
Micronor, Nor-Q.D.
norgestrel
Ovrette

CONTRACEPTIVE IMPLANT
levonorgestrel
Norplant

CLASSIFICATION(S):
Hormones—estrogens, progestins, contraceptives
Pregnancy Category X

INDICATIONS

▪ Prevention of pregnancy.

ACTION

▪ **Monophasic Oral Contraceptives:** Provide a fixed dosage of estrogen/progestin over a 21-day cycle. Ovulation is inhibited by suppression of follicle-stimulating hormone (FSH) and luteinizing hormone (LH). May alter cervical mucus and the endometrial environment, preventing penetration by sperm and implantation of the egg ▪ **Biphasic Oral Contraceptives:** Ovulation is inhibited by suppression of follicle-stimulating hormone (FSH) and luteinizing hormone (LH). May alter cervical mucus and the endometrial environment, preventing penetration by sperm and implantation of the egg. In addition, smaller dose of progestin in phase 1 allows for proliferation of endometrium. Larger amount in phase 2 allows for adequate secretory development ▪ **Triphasic Oral Contraceptives:** Ovulation is inhibited by suppression of follicle-stimulating hormone (FSH) and luteinizing hormone (LH). May alter cervical mucus and the endometrial environment, preventing penetration by sperm and implantation of the egg. Varying doses of estrogen/progestin may more closely mimic natural hormonal fluctuations ▪ **Progestin-Only Contraceptives and Contraceptive Implant:** Mechanism not clearly known. May alter cervical mucus and the endometrial environment, preventing penetration by sperm and implantation of the egg. Ovulation may also be suppressed.
Therapeutic Effect: ▪ Prevention of pregnancy.

PHARMACOKINETICS

Absorption: Well absorbed following oral administration.
Distribution: UK.
Metabolism and Excretion: Mostly metabolized by the liver.
Half-life: UK.

CONTRAINDICATIONS AND PRECAUTIONS

Contraindicated in: ▪ History of thromboembolic disorders, cardiovascular disease, cerebrovascular disease, liver tumors, or gallbladder disease ▪ Lactation (avoid use).
Use Cautiously in: ▪ Surgical procedures (discontinue 2–4 wk prior to surgery) ▪ History of cigarette smoking or age >30–35 yr (increased risk of cardiovascular or thromboembolic phenomenon ▪ Presence of other cardiovascular risk factors (obesity, hyperglycemia, elevated lipids, hypertension) ▪ History of diabetes mellitus, bleeding disorders, or headaches.

ADVERSE REACTIONS AND SIDE EFFECTS*

CNS: migraine headache, depression.
EENT: contact lens intolerance, retinal thrombosis, optic neuritis.
CV: PULMONARY EMBOLISM, CORONARY THROMBOSIS, CEREBRAL HEMORRHAGE, CEREBRAL THROMBOSIS, thrombophlebitis, thromboembolic phenomenon, Raynaud's disease, hypertension, edema.
GI: nausea, vomiting, abdominal cramps, bloating, gallbladder disease, cholestatic jaundice, liver tumors.
GU: breakthrough bleeding, spotting, dysmenorrhea, amenorrhea.
Derm: melasma, rash.

*Underlines indicate most frequent; **CAPITALS** indicate life-threatening.

Endo: hyperglycemia.
Misc: weight change.

INTERACTIONS

Drug–Drug: ▪ Oral contraceptive efficacy may be decreased by **penicillins, chloramphenicol, dihydroergotamine, mineral oil, oral neomycin, sulfonamides, barbiturates (except butalbital), chronic alcohol use, carbamazepine, glucocorticoids (systemic), griseofulvin, phenylbutazone, phenytoin, primidone, rifampin,** or **tetracyclines** ▪ May increase the risk of toxicity from **tricyclic antidepressants** ▪ Increased risk of hepatic toxicity with **dantrolene** (estrogen only) ▪ **Carbamazepine** or **phenytoin** may decrease the efficacy of contraceptive implants ▪ **Cigarette smoking** increases the risk of thromboembolic phenomenon (estrogen only) ▪ May interfere with the effectiveness of **bromocriptine** ▪ May alter the effects of **warfarin** (increase or decrease).

ROUTE AND DOSAGE

Monophasic Oral Contraceptives

- **PO (Adults):** On 21-day regimen, take first tablet on first Sunday after menses begin (take on Sunday if menses begin on Sunday) for 21 days, then skip seven days, then begin again. Regimen may also be started on first day of menses, continued for 21 days, then skip 7 days and begin again. Some regimens contain 7 placebo tablets, so that one tablet is taken every day for 28 days.

Biphasic Oral Contraceptives

- **PO (Adults):** Given in 2 phases. First phase is 10 days of smaller amount of progestin. Second phase is larger amount of progestin. Amount of estrogen remains constant for same length of time (total of 21 days), then skip 7 days, then begin again. Some regimens contain 7 placebo tablets for 28-day regimen.

Triphasic Oral Contraceptives

- **PO (Adults):** Progestin amount varies throughout a 21-day cycle. Estrogen component stays the same or may vary. Some regimens contain 7 placebo tablets for 28-day regimen.

Progestin Only Oral Contraceptives

- **PO (Adults):** Start on first day of menses. Taken daily and continuously.

Contraceptive Implant

- **Subdermal (Adults):** 6 capsules implanted subdermally during first 7 days of menses.

PHARMACODYNAMICS (prevention of pregnancy)

	ONSET	PEAK	DURATION
PO	1 mon	1 mon	1 mon*
Implant	1 mon	1 mon	5 yr

*Only during mon of taking contraceptive.

NURSING IMPLICATIONS

Assessment

- □ Assess blood pressure prior to and periodically throughout therapy.
- ▪ **Lab Test Considerations:** Monitor hepatic function periodically throughout therapy.
- □ *Estrogens-only*—May cause increased serum glucose, sodium, triglyceride, high-density lipoproteins (HDL), phospholipid, cortisol, prothrombin, and Factors VII, VIII, IX, and X levels. May cause decreased serum folate, pyridoxine, and antithrombin III levels.
- □ May cause false interpretations of thyroid function tests, false increases in norepinephrine platelet-induced aggregability, and false decreases in metyrapone tests.
- □ *Progestins-only*—May cause increased serum alkaline phosphatase, low-density lipoproteins (LDL), and urinary nitrogen concentrations. May cause decreased amino acids and high-density lipoprotein (HDL) concentrations.
- □ *Estrogens and Progestins*—May cause decreased pregnanediol excretion concentrations. May cause increased serum proteins.

Potential Nursing Diagnoses

- Knowledge deficit related to medication regimen (patient/family teaching).

Implementation

- **PO:** Oral doses may be administered with or immediately after food to reduce nausea.
- **Levonorgestrel Implant:** Six-capsule implant is inserted subdermally in midportion of upper arm about 8–10 cm above the elbow crease.

Patient/Family Teaching

- Instruct patient to take oral medication as directed at the same time each day. Pills should be taken in proper sequence and kept in the original container.
- *If single daily dose is missed:* take as soon as remembered; if not until next day, take 2 tablets and continue on regular dosing schedule. *If 2 days in a row are missed:* take 2 tablets a day for the next 2 days and continue on regular dosing schedule, using a second method of birth control for the remaining cycle. *If 3 days in a row are missed:* discontinue medication and use another form of birth control until period begins or pregnancy is ruled out; then begin a new cycle of tablets. *For 28-day dosing schedule:* if schedule is followed for first 21 days and one dose is missed of the last 7 tablets, it is important to take first tablet of next month's cycle on the regularly scheduled day.
- Advise patient of the need to use another form of contraception for the first 3 wk when beginning to use oral contraceptives.
- Advise patient that a second method of birth control should also be used during each cycle in which any of the following are used: *Oral Contraceptives*—alcohol (chronic use), barbiturates (except butalbital), carbamazepine, chloramphenicol, dihydroergotamine, glucocorticoids (systemic), griseofulvin, mineral oil, oral neomycin, penicillins, rifampin, sulfonamides, or tetracyclines. *Levonorgestrel Implant*—carbamazepine or phenytoin.
- Explain dosage schedule and maintenance routine. Discontinuing medication suddenly may cause withdrawal bleeding.
- If nausea becomes a problem, advise patient that eating solid food often provides relief.
- Advise patient to report signs and symptoms of fluid retention (swelling of ankles and feet, weight gain), thromboembolic disorders (pain, swelling, tenderness in extremities, headache, chest pain, blurred vision), mental depression, or hepatic dysfunction (yellowed skin or eyes, pruritus, dark urine, light colored stools), or abnormal vaginal bleeding to physician.
- Instruct patient to stop taking medication and notify physician if pregnancy is suspected.
- Caution patient that cigarette smoking during estrogen therapy may cause increased risk of serious side effects, especially for women over age 35.
- Caution patients to use sunscreen and protective clothing to prevent increased pigmentation.
- Advise patient to notify physicians or dentist of medication regimen prior to treatment or surgery.
- Emphasize the importance of routine follow-up physical examinations including blood pressure; breast, abdomen, and pelvic examinations; and PAP smears every 6–12 mon.

Evaluation

Effectiveness of therapy can be demonstrated by: ▪ Prevention of pregnancy.

CORTICOTROPIN

(kor-ti-koe-**troe**-pin)

ACTH, Acthar, Cortrophin-Zinc, H.P. Acthar Gel

CLASSIFICATION(S):
Hormone-adrenocorticotrophic
Pregnancy Category C

INDICATIONS

■ Diagnosis of adrenocortical disorders ■ Used as an anti-inflammatory or immunosuppressant when conventional glucorticoid therapy has failed. **Unlabeled Use:** ■ Myasthenia gravis.

ACTION

■ Normally produced by the pituitary, stimulates the adrenal gland to produce both glucocorticoids (hydrocortisone) and mineralocorticoids (sodium retention). Action requires intact adrenal responsiveness ■ Actions resemble those in glucorticoid administration and include suppression of the normal immune response and inflammation ■ Additional numerous intense metabolic effects ■ Potent mineralocorticoid (soduim retention) ■ Suppresses adrenal function with chronic use. **Therapeutic Effect:** ■ Production of adrenal steroids following administration.

PHARMACOKINETICS

Absorption: ACTH is rapidly absorbed from IM and SC sites. Repository forms or zinc hydroxide are more slowly absorbed from IM and SC sites.
Distribution: Removed from plasma to many tissues. Does not cross the placenta.
Metabolism and Excretion: Metabolic fate not known.
Half-life: 15 min (plasma).

CONTRAINDICATIONS AND PRECAUTIONS

Contraindicated in: ■ Hypersensitivity to pork proteins ■ Serious infections, except for septic shock or tuberculous meningitis.
Use Cautiously in: ■ Children (chronic use may lead to growth suppression) ■ Chronic treatment may result in adrenal suppression ■ Do not discontinue abrupty ■ Additional doses may be needed during stress (infections, surgery) ■ Use lowest possible dose for shortest period of time ■ Pregnancy or lactation (safety not established).

ADVERSE REACTIONS AND SIDE EFFECTS* (with chronic use)

CNS: psychoses, depression, euphoria.
EENT: cataracts, increased intraocular pressure.
CV: edema, hypertension, congestive heart failure, thromboembolism.
GI: nausea, vomiting, increased appetite, weight gain, peptic ulceration.
Derm: petechiae, ecchymoses, fragility, decreased wound healing, hirsutism, acne.
Endo: menstrual irregularities, hyperglycemia, decreased growth in children, ADRENAL SUPPRESSION.
F and E: hypokalemia, sodium retention, metabolic alkalosis, hypocalcemia.
Local: atrophy at IM sites (repository dosage forms).
MS: weakness, myopathy, aseptic necrosis of joints, osteoporosis.
Misc: increases susceptibility to infections, pancreatitis, Cushingoid appearance (moon face, buffalo hump).

INTERACTIONS

Drug-Drug: ■ Additive hypokalemia with **amphotericin B, mezlocillin, piperacillin, ticarcillin,** or **diuretics** ■ Hypokalemia may increase the risk of **cardiac glycoside** toxicity ■ May increase requirements for **insulin** or **oral hypoglycemic agents** ■ **Phenytoin, phenobarbital,** and **rifampin** stimulate metabolism, may decrease effectiveness ■ **Oral contraceptives** may block metabolism.

ROUTE AND DOSAGE

Anti-Inflammatory/Immunosuppressant

- **IM, SC (Adults):** 20 units qid (up to 120 units/day for multiple sclerosis) or 40–80 units q 24–48 hr of repository gelatin form or 40 units q 12–24 hr of zinc hydroxide form (zinc hydroxide form for IM use only).
- **IM, SC (Children):** 1.6 units/kg/day or 50 units/m^2/day in 3–4 divided doses or 0.8 units/kg/day or 25 units/m^2/day

*Underlines indicate most frequent; **CAPITALS** indicate life-threatening.

of repository form in 1–2 divided doses.

Myasthenia Gravis

- **IV (Adults):** 100 mg of corticotropin injection infused over 8 hr daily for 10 days, repeated after a 5–10-day rest period.

Diagnosis of Adrenal Disorders

- **IV (Adults):** 10–25 units infused over 8 hr.
- **IM (Adults):** 25 units.

PHARMACODYNAMICS (effects on plasma cortisol levels)

	ONSET	PEAK	DURATION
IM (zinc hydroxide)	UK	7–24 hr	31–48 hr
IM (gelatin repository)	UK	3–12 hr	10–25 hr
IV	UK	1 hr	UK

NURSING IMPLICATIONS

Assessment

- In patients with a history of allergic reactions, monitor for hypersensitivity response (wheezing, rash or hives, bradycardia, irritability seizures, nausea, and vomiting). These reactions are more likely to occur with SC route or prolonged therapy. Patients allergic to porcine proteins should receive intradermal test dose prior to therapeutic or diagnostic dose.
- Monitor intake and output ratios and daily weights. Observe patient for peripheral edema, steady weight gain, rales/crackles, or dyspnea. Notify physician should these occur.
- **Lab Test Considerations:** When used to diagnose adrenal insufficiency, plasma cortisol concentrations, and urine 17-ketosteroids and 17-hydroxyketosteroids will be measured prior to and after administration of corticotropin. Therapeutic response is a rise in the plasma and urine steroid concentrations.
- Patients on prolonged courses of therapy should routinely have hematologic values, serum electrolytes, serum and urine glucose evaluated. May decrease WBC counts. May cause hyperglycemia, especially in persons with diabetes. May decrease serum potassium and calcium and increase serum sodium concentrations.
- Guaiac stools. Promptly report presence of guaiac-positive stools.
- May increase serum cholesterol and lipid values. May decrease serum protein-bound iodine and thyroxine concentrations.
- Suppresses reactions to allergy skin tests.

Potential Nursing Diagnoses

- Infection, high risk for (side effects).
- Knowledge deficit related to medication regimen (patient/family teaching).

Implementation

- **General Info:** Reconstitute 25-unit vial with 1 ml of sterile water or 0.9% NaCl for injection. Reconstitute 40-unit vial with 2 ml. Stable for 24 hr at room temperature, 7 days if refrigerated.
- **IM/SC:** Shake suspension well before drawing up dose.
- Refrigerate repository form. Warm to room temperature before administering. Use 22-gauge needle. Administer deep IM; massage well. Rotate sites. Inform patient that injection is painful.
- **IV:** Do not administer repository or zinc hydroxide form IV. Ensure that label on vial states it is for IV use.
- **Direct IV:** Administer over 2 min.
- **Intermittent Infusion:** Dilute 10–25 units in 500 ml of D5W, D5/0.9% NaCl, 0.9% NaCl, or lactated Ringer's soln.
- *Rate:* Infuse over 8 hr. May also be ordered as 40 units to be infused over 12–48 hr.
- **Additive Compatibility:** calcium gluconate, chloramphenicol, cytarabine (for 8 hr), dimenhydrinate, erythromycin gluceptate, heparin, hydrocortisone sodium succinate, methicillin, norepinephrine, oxytetracycline, penicillin G potassium, potassium chloride, tetracycline, or vancomycin.

- **Additive Incompatibility:** aminophylline or sodium bicarbonate.

PATIENT/FAMILY TEACHING

- **General Info:** This drug causes immunosuppression and may mask symptoms of infection. Instruct patient to avoid people with known contagious illness and to report possible infections immediately.
  - Review side effects with patient. Instruct patient to inform physician promptly if severe abdominal pain or tarry stools occur. Patient should also report unusual swelling, weight gain, tiredness, bone pain, bruising, nonhealing sores, visual disturbances, or behavior changes.
  - Encourage patients on long-term therapy to eat a diet high in protein, calcium, and potassium and low in sodium and carbohydrates (see Appendix K).
  - Instruct patient to inform physician if symptoms of underlying disease return or worsen.
  - Caution patient to avoid vaccinations without consulting physician.
- **Diagnostic Aid:** Explain purpose of corticotropin and need for lab tests.

EVALUATION

Effectiveness of therapy can be demonstrated by: ▪ Differentiation of primary from secondary adrenocortical insufficiency ▪ Decrease in presenting symptoms ▪ Induction of remission in multiple sclerosis.

CORTISONE

(**kor**-ti-sone)
Cortone

CLASSIFICATION(S):
Glucocorticoid—short-acting
Pregnancy Category C

INDICATIONS

▪ Management of adrenocortical insufficiency. Use in other situations is limited due to mineralocorticoid activity.

ACTION

▪ Suppresses the normal immune response and inflammation ▪ Additional numerous intense metabolic effects ▪ Potent mineralocorticoid (sodium retention) ▪ Suppresses adrenal function with chronic use at doses >20 mg/day. **Therapeutic Effect:** ▪ Replacement of cortisol in adrenal insufficiency.

PHARMACOKINETICS

Absorption: Absorption from the GI tract, but large amounts are rapidly inactivated. Converted to hydrocortisone following absorption. Slowly absorbed from IM sites.
Distribution: Widely distributed. Crosses the placenta and probably enters breast milk.
Metabolism and Excretion: Converted by the liver to hydrocortisone.
Half-life: 30 min.

CONTRAINDICATIONS AND PRECAUTIONS

Contraindications in: ▪ Serious infections.
Use Cautiously in: ▪ Children (chronic use may lead to growth suppression) ▪ Chronic treatment with doses >20 mg/day may also result in adrenal suppression ▪ Stress, including surgery or infection (additional doses may be required in patients receiving chronic therapy) ▪ Pregnancy or lactation (safety not established).

ADVERSE REACTIONS AND SIDE EFFECTS*

CNS: psychoses, depression, euphoria.
EENT: cataracts, increased intraocular pressure.
CV: edema, hypertension, congestive heart failure, thromboembolism.
GI: nausea, vomiting, increased appetite, weight gain, peptic ulceration.
Derm: petechiae, ecchymoses, fragility, decreased wound healing, hirsutism, acne.
Endo: menstrual irregularities, hyper-

*Underlines indicate most frequent; **CAPITALS** indicate life-threatening.

glycemia, decreased growth in children, ADRENAL SUPPRESSION.
F and E: hypokalemia, sodium retention, metabolic alkalosis, hypocalcemia.
Local: atrophy at IM sites (repository dosage forms).
MS: weakness, myopathy, aseptic necrosis of joints, osteoporosis.
Misc: increases susceptibility to infections, pancreatitis, Cushingoid appearance (moon face, buffalo hump).

INTERACTIONS

Drug-Drug: ▪ Additive hypokalemia with **amphotericin B, mezlocillin, piperacillin, ticarcillin,** or **diuretics** ▪ Hypokalemia may increase the risk of **cardiac glycoside** toxicity ▪ May increase requirements for **insulin** or **oral hypoglycemic agents** ▪ **Phenytoin, phenobarbital,** and **rifampin** stimulate metabolism, may decrease effectiveness ▪ **Oral contraceptives** may block metabolism.

ROUTE AND DOSAGE

- **PO, IM (Adults):** 25–300 mg/day.

PHARMACODYNAMICS (peak = blood levels; duration = duration of adrenal suppression or anti-inflammatory activity)

	ONSET	PEAK	DURATION
PO	rapid	2 hr	1.25–1.5 days
IM	slow	20–48 hr	1.25–1.5 days

NURSING IMPLICATIONS

Assessment

- Assess patient for signs of adrenal insufficiency (hypotension, weight loss, weakness, nausea, vomiting, anorexia, lethargy confusion, restlessness) prior to and periodically throughout course of therapy.
- Monitor intake and output ratios and daily weights. Observe patient for peripheral edema, steady weight gain, rales/crackles, or dyspnea. Notify physician should these occur.
- Children should also have periodic evaluations of growth.

- **Lab Test Considerations:** Patients on prolonged courses of therapy should routinely have hematologic values, serum electrolytes, serum and urine glucose evaluated. May decrease WBC counts. May cause hyperglycemia, especially in persons with diabetes. May decrease serum potassium and calcium and increase serum sodium concentrations.
  - Promptly report presence of guaiac-positive stools.
  - May increase serum cholesterol and lipid values. May decrease serum protein-bound iodine and thyroxine concentrations.
  - Suppresses reactions to allergy skin tests.
  - Periodic adrenal function tests may be ordered to assess degree of hypothalamic-pituitary-adrenal axis suppression.

Potential Nursing Diagnoses

- Infection, high risk for (side effects).
- Knowledge deficit related to medication regimen (patient/family teaching).

Implementation

- **General Info:** If dose is ordered daily or every other day, administer in the morning to coincide with the body's normal secretion of cortisol.
- **PO:** Administer with meals to minimize gastric irritation.
- **IM/SC:** Shake suspension well before drawing up. IM doses should not be administered when rapid effect is desirable. Do not dilute with other soln or admix. Do not administer this preparation IV.

Patient/Family Teaching

- Instruct patient to take medication exactly as directed; do not skip or double up on missed doses. Stopping the medication suddenly may result in adrenal insufficiency (anorexia, nausea, fatigue, weakness, hypotension, dyspnea, and hypoglycemia). If these signs appear notify physician immediately. This can be life-threatening.

- Encourage patients on long-term therapy to eat a diet high in protein, calcium, and potassium and low in sodium and carbohydrates (see Appendix K).
- This drug causes immunosuppression and may mask symptoms of infection. Instruct patient to avoid people with known contagious illnesses and to report possible infections immediately.
- Review side effects with patient. Instruct patient to inform physician promptly if severe abdominal pain or tarry stools occur. Patient should also report unusual swelling, weight gain, tiredness, bone pain, bruising, nonhealing sores, visual disturbances, or behavior changes.
- Advise patient to notify physician or dentist of medication regimen prior to treatment or surgery.
- Instruct patient to inform physician if symptoms of underlying disease return or worsen.
- Advise patient to carry identification in the event of an emergency in which patient cannot relate medical history.
- Caution patient to avoid vaccinations without consulting physician.
- Emphasize the importance of follow-up examinations to monitor progress and side effects.

Evaluation

Effectiveness of therapy can be demonstrated by: ▪ Decrease in presenting symptoms with minimal drug-related side effects.

COSYNTROPIN

(**koe**-sin-troe-pin)
Cortrosyn, Synacthen, Tetracosactrin

CLASSIFICATION(S):
Hormone—adrenocorticotrophic
Pregnancy Category C

INDICATIONS

▪ Diagnosis of adrenocortical disorders.

ACTION

▪ A synthetic form of corticotropin (ACTH); stimulates the adrenal gland to produce both glucocorticoids (hydrocortisone) and mineralocorticoids (aldosterone). Action requires intact adrenal responsiveness ▪ Actions resemble those of glucocorticoid administration and include suppression of the normal immune response and inflammation ▪ Additional numerous intense metabolic effects ▪ Potent mineralocorticoid (sodium retention). **Therapeutic Effect:** ▪ Production of adrenal steroids following administration.

PHARMACOKINETICS

Absorption: ACTH is rapidly absorbed. Repository forms (gelatin or zinc hydroxide) are more slowly absorbed.

Distribution: Removed from plasma to many tissues. Does not cross the placenta.

Metabolism and Excretion: Metabolic fate not known.

Half-life: 15 min (plasma).

CONTRAINDICATIONS AND PRECAUTIONS

Contraindicated in: ▪ Hypersensitivity ▪ Serious infections.

Use Cautiously in: ▪ Pregnancy or lactation (safety not established).

ADVERSE REACTIONS AND SIDE EFFECTS*

Misc: hypersensitivity reactions, including ANAPHYLAXIS.

INTERACTIONS

Drug-Drug: ▪ **Estrogens** may block metabolism ▪ **Glucocorticoids** will alter the results of testing.

ROUTE AND DOSAGE

- **IM, IV (Adults):** 0.25 mg; determine plasma cortisol prior to and 30 min after administration.
- **IM, IV (Children <2 yr):** 0.125 mg; determine plasma cortisol prior to and 30 min after administration.

*Underlines indicate most frequent; **CAPITALS** indicate life-threatening.

PHARMACODYNAMICS (effects on plasma cortisol levels)

	ONSET	PEAK	DURATION
IM, IV	UK	45–60 min	UK

NURSING IMPLICATIONS

Assessment

- □ In patients with a history of allergic reactions, monitor for hypersensitivity response (wheezing, rash or hives, bradycardia, irritability seizures, nausea,and vomiting). Cosyntropin is less likely than ACTH to cause such a response.
- ■ **Lab Test Considerations:** Plasma cortisol concentrations will be measured prior to and 30 or 60 min after administration of cosyntropin. Therapeutic response is a rise in the plasma cortisol of at least 7 mcg/100 ml above baseline or a final concentration of at least 18 mcg/100 ml. Administration of glucocorticoids on the day of the test will interfere with test results by causing elevated baseline plasma cortisol concentrations.

Potential Nursing Diagnoses

- ■ Knowledge deficit related to medication regimen (patient/family teaching).

Implementation

- ■ **General Info:** May be administered SC, IM, direct IV, and by IV infusion.
- □ Reconstitute 250-mcg vial with 1 ml of 0.9% NaCl for injection.
- □ Stable for 24 hr at room temperature, 21 days if refrigerated.
- ■ **Direct IV:** Administer over 2 min.
- ■ **Intermittent Infusion:** May be further diluted in D5W or 0.9% NaCl. Stable for 12 hr at room temperature.
- □ *Rate:* Infuse at a rate of 40 mcg/hr over 6 hr.

Patient/Family Teaching

- □ Explain purpose of cosyntropin and need for lab tests.

Evaluation

Effectiveness of therapy can be demonstrated by: ■ Differentiation of primary from secondary adrenocortical insufficiency.

CO-TRIMOXAZOLE

(koe-tyre-**mox**-a-zole)
{Apo-Sulfatrim}, Bactrim, {Novo-trime}, {Protrin}, {Roubac}, Septra, Sulfomethaprim, Sulmeprim, trimethoprim/sulfamethoxazole, SMX/TMP, TMP/SMX, Uroplus

CLASSIFICATION(S):
Anti-infective—sulfonamide
Pregnancy Category C

INDICATIONS

■ Treatment of the following infections due to susceptible organisms: □ Bronchitis □ *Shigella* enteritis □ Otitis media □ *Pneumocyctis carinii* pneumonia □ Urinary tract infections ■ Treatment of traveler's diarrhea. **Unlabeled Uses:** ■ Biliary tract infections, osteomyelitis, burn and wound infections, clamydial infections, endocarditis, gonorrhea, intra-abdominal infections, nocardiosis, rheumatic fever prophylaxis, sinusitis, erradication of meningococcal carriers, and prophylaxis of urinary tract infections.

ACTION

■ Combination inhibits the metabolism of folic acid in bacteria at two different points. **Therapeutic Effect:** ■ Bactericidal action against susceptible bacteria. **Spectrum:** ■ Active against many strains of gram-positive aerobic pathogens, including: □ *Streptococcus pneumoniae* □ *Staphylococcus aureus* □ Group A beta-hemolytic streptococci □ Nocardia □ Enterococcus ■ Has activity against many aerobic gram-negative pathogens, such as: □ *Acinetobacter* □ *Enterobacter* □ *Klebsiella pneumoniae* □ *Escherichia coli* □ *Proteus mirabilis* □ *Shigella* □ *Salmonella* ■ Good activity against: □ *Hemophilus influenzae* (including ampicillin-resistant strains)

▪ *Pneumocystis carinii,* a protozoa, is also susceptible ▪ Not active against *Pseudomonas aeruginosa.*

PHARMACOKINETICS

Absorption: Well absorbed from the GI tract.
Distribution: Widely distributed. Crosses the blood-brain barrier and placenta and enters breast milk.
Half-life: trimethoprim 8–11 hr, sulfamethoxazole 7–12 hr.

CONTRAINDICATIONS AND PRECAUTIONS

Contraindicated in: ▪ Hypersensitivity to sulfonamides or trimethoprim ▪ Megaloblastic anemia secondary to folate deficiency ▪ Pregnancy, lactation, or children <2 mon ▪ Severe renal impairment.
Use Cautiously in: ▪ Impaired hepatic or renal function (dosage reduction required) ▪ AIDS (increased incidence of adverse reactions).

ADVERSE REACTIONS AND SIDE EFFECTS*

CNS: headache, insomnia, fatigue, depression, hallucinations.
GI: nausea, vomiting, stomatitis, diarrhea, HEPATICONECROSIS.
GU: crystalluria.
Derm: rashes, TOXIC EPIDERMAL NECROLYSIS, photosensitivity.
Hemat: APLASTIC ANEMIA, AGRANULOCYTOSIS, leukopenia, thrombocytopenia, megaloblastic anemia, hemolytic anemia.
Local: phlebitis at IV site.
Misc: allergic reactions, including STEVENS-JOHNSON SYNDROME, ERYTHEMA MULTIFORME, fever.

INTERACTIONS

Drug-Drug: ▪ May increase half-life, decrease clearance, and exaggerate folic acid deficiency caused by **phenytoin** ▪ May enhance the effects of **oral hypoglycemic agents** and **oral anticoagulants** ▪ May increase the toxicity of **methotrexate** ▪ Increases the risk of thrombocytopenia from **thiazide diuretics** (elderly patients) ▪ Decreases efficacy of **cyclosporine** and increases risk of nephrotoxicity.

ROUTE AND DOSAGE

Note: TMP = trimethoprim, SMX = sulfamethoxazole.

Chronic Bronchitis

- **PO (Adults):** 160 mg TMP/800 mg SMX q 12 hr.

Otitis Media

- **PO (Children >2 mon):** 7.5–8 mg/kg TMP/40 mg/kg SMX daily in divided doses q 12 hr.

Pneumocyctis carinii Pneumonia

- **PO, IV (Adults and Children):** 5 mg/kg TMP/25 mg SMX q 6 hr.

Urinary Tract Infections, Shigellosis

- **PO (Adults):** 160 mg TMP/800 mg SMX q 12 hr.
- **PO (Children):** 7.5–8 mg/kg TMP/37.5–40 mg/kg SMX daily in divided doses q 12 hr.

Severe Urinary Tract Infections, Shigellosis

- **IV (Children):** 8–10 mg/kg TMP/40–50 mg/kg SMX daily in divided doses q 6–12 hr.

PHARMACODYNAMICS (blood levels)

	ONSET	PEAK
PO	rapid	2–4 hr
IV	rapid	end of infusion

NURSING IMPLICATIONS

Assessment

- ▫ Assess patient for infection (vital signs; appearance of wound, sputum, urine, and stool; WBC) at beginning and throughout course of therapy.
- ▫ Obtain specimens for culture and sensitivity prior to initiating therapy. First dose may be given before receiving results.
- ▫ Assess patient for allergy to sulfonamides.
- ▫ Monitor intake and output ratios. Fluid intake should be sufficient to

*Underlines indicate most frequent; **CAPITALS** indicate life-threatening.

maintain a urine output of at least 1200–1500 ml daily to prevent crystalluria and stone formation.

- **Lab Test Considerations:** Monitor CBC and urinalysis periodically throughout therapy.
- □ May produce elevated serum bilirubin, creatinine, and alkaline phosphatase.

Potential Nursing Diagnoses

- Infection, high risk for (indications, side effects).
- Knowledge deficit related to medication regimen (patient/family teaching).
- Noncompliance related to medication regimen (patient/family teaching).

Implementation

- **General Info:** Available in a double-strength (DS) tablet. Single-strength tablet (SS) contains trimethoprim 80 mg/sulfamethoxazole 400 mg. Double-strength tablet (DS) contains trimethoprim 160 mg/sulfamethoxazole 800 mg.
- □ Do not administer medication IM.
- **PO:** Administer around the clock on an empty stomach at least 1 hr before or 2 hr after meals, with a full glass of water. Use calibrated measuring device for liquid preparations.
- **Intermittent Infusion:** Dilute each 5-ml ampule with 125 ml of D5W. May reduce diluent to 75 ml if fluid restriction required. Do not use if soln is cloudy or contains a precipitate. Do not mix with other medications or soln. Soln is stable for 6 hr in standard dilution and 2 hr in fluid-restricted dilution at room temperature. Do not refrigerate.
- □ *Rate:* Infuse over 60–90 min. Do not administer rapidly or by bolus injection.
- **Syringe Compatibility:** heparin.
- **Y-Site Compatibility:** acyclovir, atracurium, cyclophosphamide, enalaprilat, esmolol, hydromorphone, labetolol, magnesium sulfate, meperidine, morphine, pancuronium, perphenazine, vecuronium, or zidovudine.
- **Y-Site Incompatibility:** foscarnet.
- **Additive Compatibility:** D5/0.45% NaCl or 0.45% NaCl.
- **Additive Incompatibility:** verapamil.

Patient/Family Teaching

- □ Instruct patient to take medication around the clock and to finish the drug completely as directed, even if feeling better. If a dose is missed, it should be taken as soon as remembered. Advise patient that sharing of this medication may be dangerous.
- □ Caution patient to use sunscreen and protective clothing to prevent photosensitivity reactions.
- □ Advise patient to notify physician if skin rash, sore throat, fever, mouth sores, or unusual bleeding or bruising occurs.
- □ Instruct patient to notify physician if symptoms do not improve within a few days.

Evaluation

Clinical response to therapy can be evaluated by: ▪ Resolution of the signs and symptoms of infection. Length of time for complete resolution depends on the organism and site of infection.

CROMOLYN

(**kroe**-moe-lin)
cromoglycate, {Fivent}, Intal, Gastrochrom, {Nalcrom}, Nasalcrom, Opticrom, {Rynocrom}, {Vistacrom}

CLASSIFICATION(S):
Antihistamine—mast cell stabilizer
Pregnancy Category B

INDICATIONS

▪ **PO:** Treatment of mastocytosis ▪ **Inhaln, Ophth, Nasal:** Adjunct in the prophylaxis of allergic disorders including rhinitis, conjunctivitis, and asthma ▪ Inhalation product has also been used in the prevention of exercise-induced bronchospasm.

C

ACTION

▪ Prevents the release of histamine and slow reacting substance of anaphylaxis (SRS-A) from sensitized mast cells. **Therapeutic Effects:** ▪ Decreased symptoms of mastocytosis (diarrhea, flushing, headache, vomiting, urticaria, abdominal pain, nausea, itching) ▪ Decreased frequency and intensity of allergic reactions including rhinitis, conjunctivitis, and asthma.

PHARMACOKINETICS

Absorption: Poorly absorbed following all routes of administration; action is local. Small amounts may reach systemic circulation after inhalation, even less from other routes.
Distribution: Because only small amounts are absorbed, distribution is not known. Does not cross biologic membranes well.
Metabolism and Excretion: Small amounts absorbed are excreted unchanged in bile and urine.
Half-life: 80 min.

CONTRAINDICATIONS AND PRECAUTIONS

Contraindicated in: ▪ Hypersensitivity ▪ Acute attacks of asthma.
Use Cautiously in: ▪ Pregnancy and lactation (safety not established) ▪ Children <2 yr (oral use reserved for severe mastocytosis) ▪ Will not relieve and may worsen acute attacks of bronchospasm (inhaln).

ADVERSE REACTIONS AND SIDE EFFECTS*

CNS: All routes—headache; PO—irritability, trouble sleeping.
EENT: Nasal—nasal irritation, sneezing; Ophth:—ocular burning, stinging unpleasant taste.
GI: PO—diarrhea, abdominal pain.
Resp: Inhaln—irritation of the throat and trachea, cough, bronchospasm.
Derm: All routes—rash, erythema, urticaria.
MS: PO—myalgia.
Misc: allergic reactions, including ANAPHYLAXIS or worsening of conditions being treated.

INTERACTIONS

Drug-Drug: None significant.

ROUTE AND DOSAGE

- **PO (Adults):** 200 mg 4 times daily.
- **PO (Children 2–12 yr):** 100 mg 4 times daily.
- **PO (Children <2 yr):** 20 mg/kg/day in 4 divided doses, dose may be increased up to 30 mg/kg/day.
- **Inhaln (Adults and Children >5 yr):** 20 mg 4 times daily as nebulizer soln or 2 sprays (800 mcg/spray) as aerosol. For prevention of bronchospasm use 2 sprays 10–15 min prior to exposure to known precipitating situation.
- **Nasal (Adults and Children >6 yr):** 1 spray (5.2 mg) each nostril 3–4 times daily (up to 6 times daily).
- **Ophth (Adults and Children >4 yr):** 1–2 drops (1.6 mg/drop) each eye 4–6 times daily.

PHARMACODYNAMICS (effects on diminishing symptoms)

	ONSET	PEAK	DURATION
PO	UK	2–3 wk	UK
Inhaln	< 1 wk	2–4 wk	UK
Nasal	< 1 wk	2–4 wk	UK
Ophth	<1 wk	2–4 wk	UK

NURSING IMPLICATIONS

Assessment

- **PO:** Assess patient for signs of mastocytosis (diarrhea, flushing, headaches, vomiting, urticaria, abdominal pain, nausea, and itching) prior to and periodically throughout therapy.
- **Inhaln:** Pulmonary function testing should be evaluated prior to initiating therapy in asthmatics.
- □ Assess lung sounds and respiratory function prior to and periodically throughout therapy.
- **Ophth:** Assess eye for redness, tearing, and irritation.
- **Nasal Spray:** Assess for symptoms of rhinitis (stuffiness, rhinorrhea).

*Underlines indicate most frequent; CAPITALS indicate life-threatening.

Potential Nursing Diagnoses

- Airway clearance, ineffective (indications).
- Knowledge deficit related to medication regimen (patient/family teaching).

Implementation

- **General Info:** Available in oral capsules, inhalation aerosol, nasal spray, soln for nebulization, and ophthalmic soln.
  - Reduction in dosage of other asthma medications may be possible after 2–4 wk of therapy.
- **PO:** Administer at regular intervals 30 min before meals and at bedtime. Dose may be reduced once therapeutic response is achieved.
  - To prepare, open capsule(s) and pour into a glass half full of hot water. Stir until completely dissolved and soln is clear. Add an equal quantity of cold water while stirring. Do not mix with fruit juice, milk, or foods. Patient should drink all of the liquid.
- **Inhaln:** Medication should be used prophylactically, not for use during acute asthma attacks or status asthmaticus.
  - Pretreatment with bronchodilator may be required to increase delivery of inhalation product.
- **Ophth:** Instruct patient to lie down or tilt head back and look at ceiling. Pull down on lower lid creating a small pocket and instill soln into pocket. Instruct patient to gently close eye. Wait 5 min before instilling any other ophthalmic soln.

Patient/Family Teaching

- **General Info:** Medication must be used routinely. If a dose is missed, take as soon as remembered and space other doses at regular intervals, do not double doses. Do not discontinue therapy without consulting physician or exacerbation of symptoms may occur.
  - If cromolyn is prescribed before contact with known allergen or exercise, explain that it should be administered 10–15 min, and no earlier than 60 min, in advance.
- **PO:** Emphasize the importance of taking at least 30 min before meals; not mixing with fruit juice, milk, or food; and drinking all of the liquid to prevent relapse.
- **Metered-Dose Aerosol Inhaler:** Instruct patient in the proper use of the metered-dose inhaler. Shake well, exhale, close lips firmly around mouth piece, administer during second half of inhalation and hold breath as long as possible after treatment to ensure deep instillation of medication. Do not take more than 2 inhalations at one time; allow 1–2 min between inhalations. Wash inhalation assembly at least daily in warm running water.
  - Advise patient that gargling and rinsing the mouth after each dose helps to decrease dryness of mouth, throat irritation, and hoarseness.
  - Caution patient to notify physician if asthmatic symptoms recur.
- **Ophth:** Instruct patient on correct technique for instillation of eye drops. Advise patient to notify physician if eye irritation increases; a mild, transient burning immediately following administration is not unusual.
- **Nasal Spray:** Instruct patient to clear nasal passages prior to and to inhale through nose during administration.

Evaluation

Therapeutic effects, observable within 2–4 wk after beginning therapy, are demonstrated by: ▪ Decrease in symptoms of mastocytosis ▪ Reduction in symptoms of asthma ▪ Decrease in the symptoms of conjunctivitis ▪ Decrease in the symptoms of rhinitis.

CYANOCOBALAMIN

(sye-an-oh-koe-**bal**-a-min)
{Anacobin}, {Bedoz}, Berubigen, Betalin 12, {Cyanabin}, Redisol, {Rubion}, Rubramin PC, vitamin B_{12}

C

CLASSIFICATION(S):
Vitamin—water-soluble,
Antianemic
Pregnancy Category C

INDICATIONS

▪ Treatment and prevention of vitamin B_{12} deficiency ▪ Treatment of pernicious anemia.

ACTION

▪ A necessary coenzyme for many metabolic processes, including fat and carbohydrate metabolism and protein synthesis ▪ Required for the formation of red blood cells. **Therapeutic Effects:** ▪ Correction of manifestations of pernicious anemia (megaloblastic indeces, GI lesions, and neurologic damage) ▪ Prevention of vitamin B_{12} deficiency.

PHARMACOKINETICS

Absorption: Absorption from the GI tract requires intrinsic factor and calcium. Well absorbed following IM and SC administration.
Distribution: Stored in the liver. Crosses the placenta and enters breast milk.
Metabolism and Excretion: Excess amounts are eliminated unchanged in the urine.
Half-life: 6 days (400 days in liver).

CONTRAINDICATIONS AND PRECAUTIONS

Contraindicated in: ▪ Hypersensivity ▪ Hereditary optic nerve atrophy ▪ Avoid using benzyl alcohol containing preparations in premature infants (associated with fatal "gasping syndrome").
Use Cautiously in: ▪ Cardiac disease ▪ Uremia, folic acid deficiency, concurrent infection, iron deficiency (response to B_{12} will be impaired).

ADVERSE REACTIONS AND SIDE EFFECTS*

CV: peripheral vascular thrombosis.
GI: diarrhea.
Derm: itching, swelling of the body, urticaria.
F and E: hypokalemia.
Local: pain at IM site.
Misc: hypersensitivity reactions including **ANAPHYLAXIS**.

INTERACTIONS

Drug-Drug: Chloramphenicol and **antineoplastic agents** may decrease the hematologic response to vitamin B_{12} ▪ **Aminoglycosides, colchicine, extended-release potassium supplements, anticonvulsants, cimetidine,** excess intake of **alcohol** or **vitamin C** may decrease oral absorption of vitamin B_{12}.

ROUTE AND DOSAGE

Vitamin B_{12} Deficiency

- **IM, SC (Adults):** 30 mcg/day for 5–10 days (up to 1000 mcg has been used), then 100–200 mcg/mon.
- **IM, SC (Children):** 1–5 mg, given as single doses of 100 mcg over at least 2 wk, then 60 mcg/mon.

Dietary Supplementation

- **PO (Adults and Children):** 1–25 mcg/day (up to 100 mcg has been used).

PHARMACODYNAMICS (reticulocytosis)

	ONSET	PEAK	DURATION
PO	UK	UK	UK
IM, SC	UK	3–10 days	UK

NURSING IMPLICATIONS

Assessment

- Assess patient for signs of vitamin B_{12} deficiency (pallor, neuropathy, psychosis, red inflamed tongue) prior to and periodically throughout therapy.
- **Lab Test Considerations:** Monitor plasma folic acid levels, reticulocyte count, and plasma vitamin B_{12} levels prior to and between the fifth and seventh day of therapy with vitamin B_{12}. Patients receiving vitamin B_{12} for megaloblastic anemia should have serum potassium level evaluated for hypokalemia during the first 48 hr of treatment.

*Underlines indicate most frequent; **CAPITALS** indicate life-threatening.

POTENTIAL NURSING DIAGNOSES
- Nutrition, altered: less than body requirements (indications).
- Activity intolerance (indications).
- Knowledge deficit related to medication regimen (patient/family teaching).

IMPLEMENTATION
- **General Info:** Usually administered in combination with other vitamins, as solitary vitamin B deficiencies are rare.
- □ Administration of vitamin B_{12} by the oral route is useful only for nutritional deficiencies. Patients with small bowel disease, malabsorption syndrome, or gastric or ileal resections require parenteral administration.
- **PO:** Administer with meals to increase absorption.
- □ May be mixed with fruit juices. Administer immediately after mixing, as ascorbic acid alters stability.
- **IV:** IV route is not recommended, however cyanocobalamin may be admixed in TPN soln.
- **Y-Site Compatibility:** heparin, hydrocortisone sodium succinate, or potassium chloride.
- **Additive Compatibility:** dextrose/Ringer's or lactated Ringer's combinations, dextrose/saline combinations, D5W, D10W, 0.45% NaCl, 0.9% NaCl, Ringer's or lactated Ringer's soln, ascorbic acid, chloramphenicol, or metaraminol bitartrate.

PATIENT/FAMILY TEACHING
- □ Encourage patients to comply with diet recommendations of physician. Explain that the best source of vitamins is a well-balanced diet with foods from the 4 basic food groups.
- □ Foods high in vitamin B_{12} include meats, seafood, egg yolk, and fermented cheeses; little lost with ordinary cooking.
- □ Patients self-medicating with vitamin supplements should be cautioned not to exceed RDA (see Appendix L). The effectiveness of megadoses for treatment of various medical conditions is unproven and may cause side effects.
- □ Inform patients of the lifelong need for vitamin B_{12} replacement following gastrectomy or ileal resection.
- □ Emphasize the importance of follow-up examinations to evaluate progress.

EVALUATION
Effectiveness of therapy can be demonstrated by: ▪ Resolution of the symptoms of vitamin B_{12} deficiency ▪ Increase in reticulocyte count.

CYCLIZINE
(sye-kli-zeen)
Marezine, {Marzine}

CLASSIFICATION(S):
Antiemetic—antihistamine
Pregnancy Category B

INDICATIONS
▪ Prevention and treatment of dizziness, nausea, and vomiting associated with motion sickness. **Unlabeled Use:** ▪ Postoperative vomiting.

ACTION
▪ Central anticholinergic effects result in decreased vestibular and labyrinthine function ▪ Also has antihistaminic properties and may depress the chemoreceptive trigger zone in the medulla. **Therapeutic Effects:** ▪ Decreased dizziness, nausea, and vomiting.

PHARMACOKINETICS
Absorption: Absorption following oral administration not known.
Distribution: Distributed throughout most tissues.
Metabolism and Excretion: Probably metabolized by the liver.
Half-life: UK.

CONTRAINDICATIONS AND PRECAUTIONS
Contraindicated in: ▪ Hypersensitivity ▪ Children (IM use).

{} = Available in Canada only.

C

Use Cautiously in: ▪ Elderly patients and children (increased risk of adverse reactions) ▪ Prostatic enlargement ▪ Glaucoma ▪ GI obstruction.

ADVERSE REACTIONS AND SIDE EFFECTS*

CNS: drowsiness, dizziness, nervousness, restlessness, insomnia.
EENT: blurred vision, dry eyes, nasal dryness.
CV: hypotension (IM use), tachycardia.
GI: dry mouth, anorexia, upset stomach.
GU: urinary retention, urinary frequency.
Derm: rash.
Misc: hypersensitivity reactions, including ANAPHYLAXIS.

INTERACTIONS

Drug–Drug: ▪ Additive CNS depression with other **CNS depressants,** including **alcohol, antihistamines, antidepressants, narcotic analgesics,** and **sedative/hypnotics** ▪ Additive anticholinergic effects (dry mouth, dry eyes, blurred vision, constipation) with other **agents having anticholinergic properties,** including **antihistamines, antidepressants, quinidine,** and **disopyramide.**

ROUTE AND DOSAGE

Motion Sickness

- **PO (Adults):** 50 mg 30 min prior to travel, may repeat in 4–6 hr as needed.
- **PO (Children 6–12 yr):** 25 mg 30 min prior to travel, may repeat in 4–6 hr as needed, or 1 mg/kg or 33 mg/m^2 3 times daily (not to exceed 75 mg/day).
- **IM (Adults):** 50 mg q 4–6 h.
- **IM (Children 6–12 yr):** 1 mg/kg or 33 mg/m^2 3 times daily (unlabeled).

Postoperative Vomiting (Unlabeled Use)

- **IM (Adults):** 50 mg 15–30 min before end of surgery, may be repeated 3 times daily for first few postoperative days.
- **IM (Children 6–12 yr):** 25 mg 15–30 min before end of surgery, may be repeated 3 times daily for first few postoperative days.
- **IM (Children <6 yr):** 12.5 mg 15–30 min before end of surgery, may be repeated 3 times daily for first few postoperative days.

PHARMACODYNAMICS

	ONSET	PEAK	DURATION
PO	30–60 min	UK	4–6 hr
IM	30–60 min	UK	4–6 hr

NURSING IMPLICATIONS

Assessment

- □ Assess nausea, vomiting, bowel sounds, and abdominal pain prior to and following administration. Monitor hydration status and intake and output. Patients with severe nausea and vomiting may require IV fluids in addition to antiemetics.
- ▪ **Lab Test Considerations:** May alter results of skin tests using allergens. Discontinue use of cyclizine 72 hr prior to test.

Potential Nursing Diagnoses

- ▪ Fluid volume deficit (indications).
- ▪ Nutrition, altered: less than body requirements (indications).
- ▪ Injury, high risk for (side effects).

Implementation

- ▪ **PO:** Administer with food, water, or milk to minimize GI irritation.
- ▪ **IM:** May be administered prophylactically at least 15–30 min prior to emergence from anesthesia.
- ▪ **Syringe Compatibility:** atropine, codeine, hydromorphone, meperidine, morphine, pyridoxine, ranitidine, scopolamine, streptomycin, or tetracycline.

Patient/Family Teaching

- □ Instruct patient to take cyclizine 30 min before travel.
- □ Advise patient and family to use general measures to decrease nausea (be-

*Underlines indicate most frequent; CAPITALS indicate life-threatening.

gin with sips of liquids, small nongreasy meals, provide oral hygiene, remove noxious stimuli from environment).

- □ Cyclizine may cause drowsiness. Caution patient to avoid driving or other activities requiring alertness until reponse to medication is known.
- □ Inform patient that this drug may cause dry mouth. Frequent oral rinses, good oral hygiene, and sugarless gum or candy may minimize this effect.
- □ Caution patient to avoid concurrent use of alcohol or other CNS depressants with this medication.

EVALUATION

Effectiveness of therapy can be demonstrated by: ▪ Prevention and treatment of motion sickness ▪ Prevention and treatment of postoperative nausea and vomiting.

CYCLOBENZAPRINE

(sye-kloe-**ben**-za-preen)
Flexeril

CLASSIFICATION(S):
Skeletal muscle relaxant—centrally acting
Pregnancy Category B

INDICATIONS

▪ In combination with other treatment modalities (physical therapy, bed rest) in the management of acute painful musculoskeletal conditions associated with muscle spasm.

ACTION

▪ Reduces tonic somatic muscle activity at the level of the brainstem. Structually similar to tricyclic antidrepressants. **Therapeutic Effect:** ▪ Reduction in muscle spasm and hyperactivity without loss of function.

PHARMACOKINETICS

Absorption: Well absorbed from the GI tract.
Distribution: Distribution not known.
Metabolism and Excretion: Mostly metabolized by the liver.
Half-life: 1–3 days.

CONTRAINDICATIONS AND PRECAUTIONS

Contraindicated in: ▪ Hypersensitivity ▪ Should not be used within 14 days of MAO inhibitor therapy ▪ Immediate period after myocardial infarction ▪ Severe or symptomatic cardiovascular disease ▪ Cardiac conduction disturbances ▪ Hyperthyroidism.
Use Cautiously in: ▪ Cardiovascular disease ▪ Pregnancy, lactation, and children (safety not established) ▪ Therapy should be limited to 2–3 wk.

ADVERSE REACTIONS AND SIDE EFFECTS*

CNS: <u>drowsiness</u>, <u>dizziness</u>, fatigue, headache, nervousness, confusion.
EENT: <u>dry mouth</u>, blurred vision.
CV: arrhythmias.
GI: constipation, unpleasant taste, dyspepsia, nausea.
GU: urinary retention.

INTERACTIONS

Drug-Drug: ▪ Additive CNS depression with other **CNS depressants,** including **alcohol, antihistamines, narcotic analgesics,** and **sedative/hypnotics** ▪ Additive anticholinergic effects with other **drugs possessing anticholinergic properties,** including **antihistamines, antidepressants, atropine, haloperidol,** and **phenothiazines** ▪ Avoid use within 14 days of **MAO inhibitor** therapy (hyperpyretic crisis, convulsions, and death may occur) ▪ May blunt the response to **guanadrel** or **guanethidine.**

ROUTE AND DOSAGE

▪ **PO (Adults):** 10 mg 3 times daily (range 20–40 mg/day, not to exceed 60 mg/day).

*<u>Underlines</u> indicate most frequent; **CAPITALS** indicate life-threatening.

PHARMACODYNAMICS (skeletal muscle relaxation)

	ONSET	PEAK*	DURATION
PO	1 hr	4–6 hr	12–24 hr

*Full effects may not occur for 1–2 wk.

NURSING IMPLICATIONS

Assessment

- Assess patient for pain, muscle stiffness, and range of motion prior to and periodically throughout therapy.

Potential Nursing Diagnoses

- Comfort, altered: pain (indications).
- Mobility, impaired physical (indications).
- Injury, high risk for (side effects).

Implementation

- **PO:** May be administered with meals to minimize gastric irritation.

Patient/Family Teaching

- Instruct patient to take medication exactly as directed; do not take more than the prescribed amount. Missed doses should be taken within 1 hr of time ordered, otherwise return to normal dosage schedule. Do not double doses.
- Medication may cause drowsiness, dizziness, and blurred vision. Caution patient to avoid driving or other activities requiring alertness until response to drug is known.
- Advise patient to avoid concurrent use of alcohol or other CNS depressants with this medication.
- If constipation becomes a problem, advise patient that increasing fluid intake and bulk in diet, and stool softeners may alleviate this condition.
- Advise patient to notify physician if symptoms of urinary retention (distended abdomen, feeling of fullness, overflow incontinence, voiding small amounts) occur.
- Inform patient that good oral hygiene, frequent mouth rinses, and sugarless gum or candy may help relieve dry mouth.

Evaluation

Effectiveness of therapy can be demonstrated by: ■ Relief of muscular spasm in acute skeletal muscle conditions. Effects may not be evident for 1–2 wk.

CYCLOPENTOLATE

(sye-kloe-**pen**-toe-late)
Ak-pentolate, Cyclogyl, 1-Pentolate, Pentolair

CLASSIFICATION(S):
Ophthalmic—mydriatic, Anticholinergic
Pregnancy Category UK

INDICATIONS

■ Used to produce mydriasis and cycloplegia and thereby allow ophthalmic examination.

ACTION

■ Blocks the response to acetylcholine in the eye, resulting in mydriasis and cycloplegia. **Therapeutic Effects:** ■ Mydriasis and cycloplegia.

PHARMACOKINETICS

Absorption: Small amounts may be systemically absorbed.
Distribution: Distribution not known.
Metabolism and Excretion: Not known.
Half-life: Not known.

CONTRAINDICATIONS AND PRECAUTIONS

Contraindicated in: ■ Hypersensitivity ■ Angle-closure glaucoma.
Use Cautiously in: ■ Children (increased risk of psychotic reactions).

ADVERSE REACTIONS AND SIDE EFFECTS*

CNS: psychotic reaction (children).
EENT: burning sensation, increased intraocular pressure, hypersensitivity reaction.

*Underlines indicate most frequent; **CAPITALS** indicate life-threatening.

INTERACTIONS

Drug–Drug: None significant.

ROUTE AND DOSAGE

- **Ophth (Adults):** 1 drop of 1–2% soln, followed by a second drop in 5 min, 40–50 min prior to procedure.
- **Ophth (Children):** 1 drop of 0.5–2% soln, followed by a second drop in 5 min, 40–50 min prior to procedure.

PHARMACODYNAMICS

	ONSET	PEAK	DURATION
Ophth (mydriasis)	rapid	15–60 min	24 hr (up to several days)
Ophth (cycloplegia)	rapid	25–75 min	6–24 hr

NURSING IMPLICATIONS

Assessment

- **General Info:** Assess for symptoms of systemic absorption (tachycardia, flushed face, dry mouth, drowsiness, or confusion). Notify physician if these symptoms occur.
- **Children:** Assess for psychotic response (ataxia, incoherent speech, disorientation, hallucinations, restlessness, tachycardia). Notify physician immediately if these symptoms occur.

Potential Nursing Diagnoses

- Sensory-perceptual alteration: visual (side effects).
- Knowledge deficit related to medication regimen (patient/family teaching).

Implementation

- **Ophth:** Available in three concentrations: 0.5%, 1%, and 2%.
  - □ Have patient tilt head back and look up, gently depress lower lid with index finger until conjunctival sac is exposed, and instill 1 drop. After instillation, maintain gentle pressure on inner canthus for 1 min to avoid systemic absorption of the drug. Wait at least 5 min before instilling second drop or other types of eyedrops.

Patient/Family Teaching

- □ Prior to instillation of drops, warn patient that burning sensation may occur (especially with 1% and 2% soln).
- □ Advise patient that ophthalmic preparations may temporarily impair ability to judge distances. Dark glasses may be needed to protect eyes from bright light.

Evaluation

Effectivenesss of therapy can be demonstrated by: ▪ Mydriasis and cycloplegia in preparation for ophthalmic examination.

CYCLOPHOSPHAMIDE

(sye-kloe-**foss**-fa-mide)
Cytoxan, Neosar, {Procytox}

CLASSIFICATION(S):
Antineoplastic—alkylating agent, Immunosuppressant
Pregnancy Category C

INDICATIONS

▪ Alone or with other modalities (other chemotherapeutic agents, radiation therapy, surgery) in the management of: □ Hodgkin's disease □ Malignant lymphomas □ Multiple myeloma □ Leukemias □ Mycosis fungoides □ Neuroblastoma □ Ovarian carcinoma □ Breast carcinoma, and a variety of other tumors ▪ Treatment of minimal change nephrotic syndrome in children. **Unlabeled Uses:** ▪ Used as an immunosuppressant in the treatment of severe active rheumatoid arthritis or Wegener's granulomatosis.

ACTION

▪ Interferes with DNA replication and RNA transcription, ultimately disrupting protein synthesis (cell cycle-phase nonspecific). **Therapeutic Effects:** ▪ Death of rapidly replicating cells, particularly malignant ones ▪ Also has immunosuppressant action in smaller doses.

C

PHARMACOKINETICS

Absorption: Inactive parent drug is well absorbed from the GI tract. Converted to active drug by the liver.
Distribution: Widely distributed. Limited penetration of the blood-brain barrier. Crosses the placenta and enters breast milk.
Metabolism and Excretion: Converted to active drug by the liver. 30% eliminated unchanged by the kidneys.
Half-life: 4–6.5 hr.

CONTRAINDICATIONS AND PRECAUTIONS

Contraindicated in: ▪ Hypersensitivity ▪ Pregnancy or lactation.
Use Cautiously in: ▪ Patients with childbearing potential ▪ Active infections ▪ Decreased bone marrow ▪ Other chronic debilitating illnesses.

ADVERSE REACTIONS AND SIDE EFFECTS*

CV: MYOCARDIAL FIBROSIS, hypotension.
Resp: pulmonary fibrosis.
GI: anorexia, nausea, vomiting.
GU: hemorrhagic cystitis, hematuria.
Derm: alopecia.
Endo: syndrome of inappropriate secretion of antidiuretic hormone (SIADH), gonadal suppression.
Hemat: anemia, thrombocytopenia, leukopenia.
Metab: hyperuricemia.
Misc: secondary neoplasms.

INTERACTIONS

Drug–Drug: ▪ **Phenobarbital** or **rifampin** may increase the toxicity of cyclophosphamide ▪ Concurrent **allopurinol** may exaggerate bone marrow depression ▪ May prolong neuromuscular blockade from **succinylcholine** ▪ Cardiotoxicity may be additive with **other cardiotoxic agents (doxorubicin)** ▪ Additive bone marrow depression with other **antineoplastics** or **radiation therapy** ▪ May potentiate the effects of **oral anticoagulants** ▪ May decrease antibody response to **live virus vaccines** and increase the risk of adverse reactions.

ROUTE AND DOSAGE

Induction

- **IV (Adults):** 40–50 mg/kg (1.5–1.8 g/m^2) in divided doses over 2–5 days (up to 100 mg/kg has been used).
- **IV (Children):** 2–8 mg/kg/day (60–250 mg/m^2).
- **PO (Adults):** 1–5 mg/kg/day.
- **PO (Children):** 2–8 mg/kg/day (60–250 mg/m^2).

Maintenance

- **IV (Adults):** 10–15 mg/kg (350–550 mg/m^2) every 7–10 days or 3–5 mg/kg twice weekly (110–185 mg/m^2).
- **PO (Adults):** 1–5 mg/kg/day.
- **PO (Children):** 2–5 mg/kg (50–150 mg/m^2) twice weekly.

PHARMACODYNAMICS (effects on blood counts)

	ONSET	PEAK	DURATION
PO	7 days	10–14 days	21 days
IV	7 days	10–14 days	21 days

NURSING IMPLICATIONS

ASSESSMENT

- ▫ Monitor blood pressure, pulse, respiratory rate, and temperature frequently during administration. Notify physician of significant changes.
- ▫ Monitor urinary output frequently throughout therapy. To reduce the risk of hemorrhagic cystitis, fluid intake should be at least 3000 ml/day for adults and 1000–2000 ml/day for children.
- ▫ Assess for fever, chills, sore throat, and signs of infection. Notify physician if these symptoms occur.
- ▫ Monitor platelet count throughout therapy. Assess for bleeding (bleeding gums, bruising, petechiae; guaiac stools, urine, and emesis). Avoid IM injections and rectal temperatures.

*Underlines indicate most frequent; **CAPITALS** indicate life-threatening.

Apply pressure to venipuncture sites for 10 min.

- Assess nausea, vomiting, and appetite. Weigh weekly. Antiemetics may be given 30 min prior to administration of medication to minimize GI effects. Anorexia and weight loss can be minimized by feeding frequent light meals.
- Encourage patient to drink 2000–3000 ml/day to promote excretion of uric acid. Alkalinization of the urine may be ordered to help prevent uric acid nephropathy.
- Anemia may occur. Monitor for increased fatigue, dyspnea, and orthostatic hypotension.
- Assess cardiac and respiratory status for dyspnea, rales/crackles, weight gain, edema. Pulmonary toxicity may occur after prolonged therapy. Cardiotoxicity may occur early in therapy and is characterized by symptoms of congestive heart failure.

- **Lab Test Considerations:** Monitor CBC and differential prior to and periodically throughout course of therapy. The nadir of leukopenia occurs in 7–12 days (recovery in 17–21 days). Leukocytes should be maintained between 2500–4000/mm^3. May also cause thrombocytopenia (nadir 10–15 days) and rarely causes anemia.
  - Monitor BUN, creatinine, and uric acid prior to and frequently during course of therapy to detect nephrotoxicity.
  - Monitor SGPT (ALT), SGOT (AST), LDH, and serum bilirubin prior to and frequently during course of therapy to detect hepatotoxicity.
  - Urinalysis should be evaluated before initiating therapy and frequently during course of therapy to detect hematuria or change in specific gravity indicative of SIADH.
  - May suppress positive reactions to skin tests for candida, mumps, trichophyton, and tuberculin PPD. May also produce false-positive results in PAP smears.

Potential Nursing Diagnoses

- Infection, high risk for (side effects).
- Body image disturbance (side effects).
- Knowledge deficit related to medication regimen (patient/family teaching).

Implementation

- **PO:** Administer medication on an empty stomach. If severe gastric irritation develops, medication may be given with food.
  - Oral preparations can be formed by diluting powder for injection in aromatic elixir to a concentration of 1–5 mg of cyclophosphamide/ml. Reconstituted preparations should be refrigerated and used within 2 wk.
- **IV:** Soln for IV administration should be prepared in a biologic cabinet. Wear gloves, gown, and mask while handling IV medication. Discard IV equipment in specially designated containers (see Appendix I).
  - Prepare IV soln by diluting each 100 mg with 5 ml of sterile water or bacteriostatic water for injection containing parabens. Shake soln gently and allow to stand until clear. Use soln prepared without bacteriostatic water within 6 hr. Soln prepared with bacteriostatic water is stable for 24 hr at room temperature, 6 days if refrigerated.
- **Direct IV:** Administer reconstituted soln directly at a rate of 100 mg over 1 min.
- **Intermittent Infusion:** May be further diluted in up to 250 ml of D5W, 0.9% NaCl, D5/0.9% NaCl, 0.45% NaCl, lactated Ringer's soln, or dextrose/Ringer's soln.
- **Syringe Compatibility:** bleomycin, cisplatin, doxapram, doxorubicin, droperidol, fentanyl, fluorouracil, furosemide, heparin, leucovorin calcium, methotrexate, metoclopramide, mitomycin, vinblastine, or vincristine.
- **Y-Site Compatibility:** Compatible via Y-site injection into port of free-flowing IV with amikacin, ampicillin,

C

bleomycin, cefamandole, cefazolin, cefoperazone, ceforanide, cefotaxime, cefoxitin, cefuroxime, cephalothin, cephapirin, chloramphenicol, cisplatin, clindamycin, co-trimoxazole, doxorubicin, doxycycline, droperidol, erythromycin, fluorouracil, furosemide, gentamicin, heparin, kanamycin, leucovorin calcium, methotrexate, metoclopramide, metronidazole, mezlocillin, minocycline, mitomycin, moxalactam, nafcillin, ondanestron, oxacillin, penicillin G potassium, piperacillin, tetracycline, ticarcillin, tobramycin, vancomycin, vinblastine, or vincristine.

Patient/Family Teaching

- Instruct patient to take dose in early morning. Emphasize need for adequate fluid intake for 72 hr after therapy. Patient should void frequently to decrease bladder irritation from metabolites excreted by the kidneys. Physician should be notified immediately if hematuria is noted. If a dose is missed physician should be contacted.
- Instruct patient to notify physician promptly if fever, sore throat, signs of infection, bleeding gums, bruising, petechiae, blood in urine, stool, or emesis or unusual swelling, joint pain, shortness of breath, or confusion occurs. Caution patient to avoid crowds and persons with known infections. Instruct patient to use soft toothbrush and electric razor and to avoid falls. Patient should also be cautioned not to drink alcoholic beverages or to take products containing aspirin, as these may precipitate GI hemorrhage.
- Advise patient that this medication may cause sterility and menstrual irregularities or cessation of menses. This drug is also teratogenic, and contraceptive measures should continue for at least 4 mon after completion of therapy.
- Discuss with patient the possibility of hair loss. Explore methods of coping. May also cause darkening of skin and fingernails.
- Instruct patient not to receive any vaccinations without advice of physician.

Evaluation

Effectiveness of therapy can be demonstrated by: ▪ Decrease in size or spread of malignant tumors ▪ Improvement of hematologic status in patients with leukemia. Maintenance therapy is instituted if leukocyte count remains between 2500–4000/mm^3 and patient does not demonstrate serious side effects.

CYCLOSPORINE

(**sye**-kloe-spor-een)
Ciclosporin, Cyclosporin A, Sandimmune

CLASSIFICATION(S):
Immunosuppressant
Pregnancy Category C

INDICATIONS

▪ Used with glucocorticoids to prevent rejection in renal, cardiac, and hepatic transplantation. **Unlabeled Use:** ▪ Prevention of rejection in heart-lung, pancreatic, and bone marrow transplantation.

ACTION

▪ Inhibits normal immune responses (cellular and humoral) by inhibiting interleukin-2, a factor necessary for initiation of T-cell activity. **Therapeutic Effect:** ▪ Prevention of rejection reactions.

PHARMACOKINETICS

Absorption: Erratically absorbed (range 10–60%) after oral administration, with significant first-pass metabolism by the liver.

Distribution: Widely distributed, mainly into extracellular fluid and blood cells. Crosses the placenta and enters breast milk.

Metabolism and Excretion: Extensively metabolized by the liver, excreted in bile, small amounts (6%) excreted unchanged by the kidneys.

Half-life: 19–27 hr.

CONTRAINDICATIONS AND PRECAUTIONS

Contraindicated in: ▪ Hypersensitivity to cyclosporine or polyoxethylated castor oil (vehicle for IV form) ▪ Should not be given to pregnant or lactating women unless benefits outweigh risks ▪ Disulfiram therapy (IV and oral liquid dosage forms contain alcohol).

Use Cautiously in: ▪ Severe hepatic impairment (dosage reduction recommended) ▪ Renal impairment ▪ Active infection.

ADVERSE REACTIONS AND SIDE EFFECTS*

CNS: tremor, SEIZURES, headache, flushing, confusion, psychiatric problems.

CV: hypertension.

Derm: hirsutism, gingival hyperplasia, acne.

GI: nausea, vomiting, diarrhea, anorexia, abdominal discomfort.

GU: nephrotoxicity.

F and E: hypomagnesemia, hyperkalemia.

Hemat: leukopenia, anemia, thrombocytopenia.

Metab: hyperuricemia, hyperlipidemia.

Neuro: paresthesia, hyperesthesia.

Misc: hepatotoxicity, infections, hypersensitivity reactions, hyperlipidemia.

INTERACTIONS

Drug-Drug: ▪ Increased risk of nephrotoxicity with **amphotericin B, aminoglycosides, fluoroquinolones, erythromycin, ketoconazole, NSAIDs, melphelan,** or **sulfonamides** ▪ Blood levels and risk of toxicity of cyclosporine are increased by **anabolic steroids, oral contraceptives, erythromycin, cimetidine, fluconazole, ketoconazole, miconazole,** and **calcium channel blockers** ▪ Additive immunosuppression with other **immunosuppressants (cyclophosphamide, azathioprine, glucocorticoids)** or **verapamil** ▪ **Barbiturates, phenytoin, rifampin, carbamazepine,** or **sulfonamides** may decrease the effect of cyclosporine ▪ Additive hyperkalemia may occur with **potassium-sparing diuretics, potassium supplements,** or **ACE inhibitors** ▪ Increases serum levels and the risk of toxicity from **digoxin** (decrease digoxin dose by 50%) ▪ Prolongs the action of **neuromuscular blocking agents** ▪ Increased risk of seizures with **imipenem/cilastatin** ▪ May decrease antibody response to **live virus vaccines** and increase the risk of adverse reactions.

ROUTE AND DOSAGE

Note: Many regimens used.

- **PO (Adults and Children):** 15 mg/kg/day (first dose before transplant) for 1–2 wk, taper by 5% weekly to maintenance dose of 5–10 mg/kg/day.
- **IV (Adults and Children):** 5–6 mg/kg/day (1/3 PO dose) initially, change to PO as soon as possible.

PHARMACODYNAMICS (blood levels)

	ONSET	PEAK	DURATION
PO	UK	3.5 hr	UK
IV	UK	end of infusion	UK

NURSING IMPLICATIONS

Assessment

- **General Info:** Assess for symptoms of organ rejection throughout therapy.
- ▫ Monitor intake and output ratios, daily weight, and blood pressure throughout therapy. Notify physician of significant changes.
- **IV:** Monitor patient for signs and symptoms of hypersensitivity (wheezing, dyspnea, flushing of face or neck). Oxygen, epinephrine, and equipment for treatment of anaphylaxis should be available with each IV dose.
- **Lab Test Considerations:** Serum cyclosporine levels should be evaluated periodically during therapy. Dosage may be adjusted daily, in response to levels, during initiation of therapy. Trough levels of 250–800 ng/ml (blood) or 50–300 ng/ml

*Underlines indicate most frequent; **CAPITALS** indicate life-threatening.

(plasma) 24 hr after a dose is given have been shown to minimize side effects and rejection events.

- Nephrotoxicity may occur; monitor BUN and serum creatinine periodically. Notify physician if significant increases occur. May also cause decreased serum magnesium levels.
- May cause hepatotoxicity; monitor for elevated SGOT (AST), SGPT (ALT), alkaline phoshatase, amylase, and bilirubin.
- May cause increased serum potassium and uric acid levels.
- Serum lipid levels may be elevated.

Potential Nursing Diagnoses

- Infection, high risk for (side effects).
- Knowledge deficit related to medication regimen (patient/family teaching).

Implementation

- **General Info:** Given with other immunosuppresive agents. Protect transplant patients from staff and visitors who may carry infection. Maintain protective isolation as indicated.
- **PO:** Draw up oral soln in the pipette provided with the medication. Mix oral soln with milk, chocolate milk, or orange juice, preferably at room temperature. Stir well and drink at once. Use a glass container and rinse with more diluent to ensure that total dose is taken. Administer oral doses with meals. Wipe pipette dry; do not wash after use.
- **Intermittent Infusion:** Dilute each 1 ml (50 mg) of IV concentrate immediately before use with 20–100 ml of D5W or 0.9% NaCl for injection. Soln is stable for 24 hr in D5W. In 0.9% NaCl it is stable for 6 hr in a polyvinylchloride container and 12 hr in a glass container at room temperature.
  - *Rate:* Recommended rate of infusion is slowly, over 2–6 hr via infusion pump.
- **Continuous Infusion:** May be administered as a continuous infusion over 24 hr.

Patient/Family Teaching

- Instruct patient to take medication at the same time each day, as directed. Do not skip doses or double up on missed doses. Take a missed dose as soon as remembered within 12 hr. Do not discontinue medication without physician's advice.
- Reinforce the need for lifelong therapy to prevent transplant rejection. Review symptoms of rejection for transplanted organ and stress need to notify physician immediately if they occur.
- Advise patient of common side effects (nephrotoxicity, increased blood pressure, hand tremors, increased facial hair, gingival hyperplasia).
- Teach patient the correct method for monitoring blood pressure at home. Instruct patient to notify physician of significant changes in blood pressure or if hematuria, frequency, cloudy urine, or decreased urine output occur.
- Instruct patient on proper oral hygiene. Meticulous oral hygiene and regular dental care will help decrease gingival inflammation and hyperplasia.
- Instruct patient to consult with physician or pharmacist before taking any over-the-counter medications or receiving any vaccinations while taking this medication.
- Advise patient to notify physician if pregnancy is planned or suspected.
- Emphasize the importance of follow-up examinations and lab tests.

Evaluation

Effectiveness of therapy may be determined by: ▪ Prevention of rejection of transplanted tissues.

CYPROHEPTADINE

(si-proe-**hep**-ta-deen)
Periactin

CLASSIFICATION(S):
Antihistamine
Pregnancy Category B

INDICATIONS

■ Relief of allergic symptoms caused by histamine release. Most useful in conditions such as: □ Nasal allergies □ Allergic dermatoses □ Cold urticaria. **Unlabeled Uses:** ■ Has been used to stimulate appetite ■ Suppression of vascular headaches.

ACTION

■ Blocks the following effects of histamine: □ Vasodilation □ Increased GI tract secretions □ Increased heart rate □ Hypotension ■ Also blocks the effects of serotonin which may result in increased appetite and decreased vascular headaches. **Therapeutic Effects:** ■ Relief of symptoms associated with histamine excess usually seen in allergic conditions, including cold urticaria ■ Stimulation of appetite.

PHARMACOKINETICS

Absorption: Apparently well absorbed after oral dosing.
Distribution: Distribution not known.
Metabolism and Excretion: Almost completely metabolized by the liver.
Half-life: UK.

CONTRAINDICATIONS AND PRECAUTIONS

Contraindicated in: ■ Hypersensitivity ■ Acute attacks of asthma ■ Lactation.
Use Cautiously in: ■ Elderly (more susceptible to adverse reactions) ■ Pregnancy (safety not established) ■ Narrow-angle glaucoma ■ Liver disease.

ADVERSE REACTIONS AND SIDE EFFECTS*

CNS: drowsiness, sedation, excitation (in children).
CV: hypotension, palpitations, arrhythmias.
EENT: blurred vision.
GI: dry mouth, constipation.
GU: urinary hesitancy, retention.
Derm: rashes, photosensitivity.

INTERACTIONS

Drug-Drug: ■ Additive CNS depression with other **CNS depressants,** including **alcohol, narcotic analgesics,** and **sedative/hypnotics** ■ **MAO inhibitors** may intensify and prolong the anticholinergic effects of antihistamines.

ROUTE AND DOSAGE

- **PO (Adults):** 12–20 mg/day q 8 hr (not to exceed 0.5 mg/kg/day).
- **PO (Children 7–14 yr):** 4 mg q 8–12 hr (not to exceed 16 mg/day).
- **PO (Children 2–6 yr):** 2 mg q 8–12 hr (not to exceed 12 mg/day).

PHARMACODYNAMICS (antihistaminic effects)

	ONSET	PEAK	DURATION
PO	15–60 min	1–2 hr	8 hr

NURSING IMPLICATIONS

Assessment

- **Allergy:** Assess symptoms (rhinitis, conjunctivitis, hives) prior to and periodically throughout course of therapy.
- □ Assess lung sounds and respiratory function prior to and periodically throughout course of therapy. Medication may cause thickening of bronchial secretions. Maintain fluid intake of 1500–2000 ml/day to decrease viscosity of secretions.
- **Appetite Stimulant:** Monitor food intake and weight routinely.
- **Lab Test Considerations:** May cause false-negative reactions on allergy skin tests; discontinue 72 hr prior to testing.
- □ Increased serum amylase and prolactin concentrations may occur when cyproheptadine is administered with a thyrotropin-releasing hormone.

Potential Nursing Diagnoses

- Airway clearance, ineffective (indications).
- Injury, high risk for (side effects).
- Knowledge deficit related to medica-

*Underlines indicate most frequent; **CAPITALS** indicate life-threatening.

tion regimen (patient/family teaching).

Implementation

- **PO:** Administer with food, water, or milk to minimize gastric irritation.
- Available as a syrup for patients with difficulty swallowing.

Patient/Family Teaching

- Instruct patient to take cyproheptadine exactly as directed. Missed dose should be taken as soon as remembered. Do not double doses. Syrup should be accurately measured using calibrated medication cup or measuring device.
- Medication may cause drowsiness. Advise patient to avoid driving or other activities requiring alertness until response to the drug is known.
- Advise patient to use sunscreen and protective clothing to prevent a photosensitivity reaction.
- Caution patient to avoid concurrent use of alcohol and other CNS depressants.
- Advise patient that frequent mouth rinses, good oral hygiene, and sugarless gum or candy may decrease dryness of mouth. Patient should notify dentist if dry mouth persists for >2 wk.

Evaluation

Effectiveness of therapy can be demonstrated by: ▪ Alleviation of allergic symptoms ▫ Alleviation of cold urticaria ▪ Improvement of appetite.

CYTARABINE

(sye-**tare**-a-been)

Ara-C, cytosine arabinoside, Cytosar-U, {Cytosar}, Tarabine PFS

CLASSIFICATION(S):

Antineoplastic—antimetabolite

Pregnancy Category C

INDICATIONS

▪ **IV:** Used mainly in combination chemotherapeutic regimens for the treatment of leukemias and non-Hodgkin's lymphomas ▪ **IT:** Treatment of meningeal leukemia.

ACTION

▪ Inhibits DNA synthesis by inhibiting DNA polymerase (cell cycle-S phase specific). **Therapeutic Effect:** ▪ Death of rapidly replicating cells, particularly malignant ones.

PHARMACOKINETICS

Absorption: Absorption occurs from SC sites, but blood levels are less than with IV administration.

Distribution: Widely distributed. Crosses the blood-brain barrier, but not in sufficient quantities. Crosses the placenta.

Metabolism and Excretion: Metabolized mostly by the liver; small amounts (<10%) excreted unchanged by the kidneys.

Half-life: 1–3 hr.

CONTRAINDICATIONS AND PRECAUTIONS

Contraindicated in: ▪ Hypersensitivity ▪ Pregnancy or lactation.

Use Cautiously in: ▪ Patients with childbearing potential ▪ Active infections ▪ Decreased bone marrow reserve ▪ Other chronic debilitating illnesses.

ADVERSE REACTIONS AND SIDE EFFECTS*

CNS: headache, CNS dysfunction (high dose).

EENT: high dose—hemorrhagic conjunctivitis, corneal toxicity.

Resp: high dose—pulmonary edema.

GI: nausea, vomiting, hepatitis; high dose—severe GI ulceration, hepatotoxicity, stomatitis.

Derm: rash, alopecia.

Endo: gonadal suppression.

Hemat: bone marrow depression.

{} = Available in Canada only.

*Underlines indicate most frequent; **CAPITALS** indicate life-threatening.

Metab: hyperuricemia.
Misc: fever.

INTERACTIONS

Drug–Drug: Additive bone marrow depression with other **antineoplastics** or **radiation therapy** ▪ Increased risk of cardiomyopathy when used in high-dose regimens with **cyclophosphamide** ▪ May decrease antibody response to **live virus vaccines** and increase the risk of adverse reactions.

ROUTE AND DOSAGE

- **IV (Adults and Children):** 100–200 mg/m^2/day or 3 mg/kg/day as a continuous infusion over 24 hr or divided doses by rapid injection for 5–10 days; course may be repeated in 2 wk. High-dose regimen—2–3 g/m^2 over 1–3 hr every 12 hr for 2–6 days.
- **SC (Adults and Children):** Maintenance dose—1 mg/kg q 1–4 wk.
- **IT (Adults):** 30 mg/m^2 once every 4 days until CSF is normal, followed by an additional dose (range 5–75 mg/m^2 given every 1–4 days for 4 days).

PHARMACODYNAMICS (effects on white blood cell counts)

	ONSET	PEAK	DURATION
SC—1st phase	24 hr	7–9 days	12 days
SC—2nd phase	15–24 days	15–24 days	25–34 days
IV—1st phase	24 hr	7–9 days	12 days
IV—2nd phase	15–24 days	15–24 days	25–34 days

NURSING IMPLICATIONS

Assessment

- Assess for fever, sore throat, and signs of infection. If these symptoms occur notify physician immediately.
- Assess for bleeding (bleeding gums, bruising, petechiae; guaiac stools, urine, emesis). Avoid IM injections and rectal temperatures. Hold pressure on all venipuncture sites for at least 10 min.
- Monitor intake and output ratios and daily weights. Notify physician if significant changes in totals occur.
- Monitor for symptoms of gout (increased uric acid, joint pain, edema). Encourage patient to drink at least 2 liters of fluid each day. Allopurinol may be given to decrease uric acid levels. Alkalinization of urine may be ordered to increase excretion of uric acid.
- Assess nutritional status. Nausea and vomiting may occur within 1 hr of administration of medication, especially if IV dose is administered rapidly. Administering an antiemetic prior to and periodically throughout therapy and adjusting diet as tolerated may help maintain fluid and electrolyte balance and nutritional status.
- Anemia may occur. Monitor for increased fatigue, dyspnea, and orthostatic hypotension.

▪ **Lab Test Considerations:** Monitor CBC and differential prior to and frequently throughout therapy. Leukocyte counts begins to drop within 24 hr of administration. The initial nadir occurs in 7–9 days. After a small rise in the count the second, deeper nadir occurs 15–24 days after administration. Leukocyte and thrombocyte counts usually begin to rise 10 days after the nadirs. Therapy is usually withdrawn if leukocyte count is $<$1000/mm^3 or platelet count is $<$50,000/mm^3. Frequent bone marrow examinations are also indicated.

- Renal (BUN and creatinine) and hepatic function (SGPT [ALT], SGOT [AST], bilirubin, and LDH) should be monitored prior to and routinely throughout course of therapy.
- May cause increase uric acid concentrations.

Potential Nursing Diagnoses

- Infection, high risk for (adverse reactions).
- Injury, high risk for (side effects).
- Knowledge deficit related to medication regimen (patient/family teaching).

Implementation

- **General Info:** Soln should be prepared in a biologic cabinet. Wear gloves, gown, and mask while handling IV medication. Discard IV equipment in specially designated containers (see Appendix I).
- May be given SC, direct IV, intermittent IV, continuous IV, or IT.
- **SC/IV:** Reconstitute 100-mg vials with 5 ml of bacteriostatic water for injection with benzyl alcohol 0.9%. Reconstitute 500-mg vials with 10 ml. Reconstituted soln is stable for 48 hr. Do not administer a cloudy soln.
- **Direct IV:** Administer each 100 mg direct IV push over 1–3 min.
- **Intermittent Infusion:** May be further diluted in 100 ml of 0.9% NaCl or D5W.
- *Rate:* Infuse over 30 min.
- **Continuous Infusion:** Rate and concentration for IV infusion are ordered individually by physician.
- **Syringe Compatibility:** metoclopramide.
- **Y-Site Compatibility:** ondansetron
- **Additive Compatibility:** corticotropin, hydroxyzine, lincomycin, methotrexate, potassium chloride, prednisolone sodium phosphate, sodium bicarbonate, or vincristine. May also be diluted in D10W, D5/0.9% NaCl, Ringer's soln, lactated Ringer's soln, or D5/LR.
- **Additive Incompatibility:** fluorouracil, heparin, regular insulin, nafcillin, oxacillin, or penicillin G sodium.
- **IT:** Reconstitute with preservative-free 0.9% NaCl or other suitable diluent. Use immediately to prevent bacterial contamination.

Patient/Family Teaching

- Caution patient to avoid crowds and persons with known infections. Physician should be informed immediately if symptoms of infection occur.
- Instruct patient to report unusual bleeding. Advise patient of thrombocytopenia precautions (use soft toothbrush and electric razor; avoid falls; do not drink alcoholic beverages or take medication containing aspirin, as these may precipitate gastric bleeding).
- Instruct patient to inspect oral mucosa for redness and ulceration. If mouth sores occur advise patient to use sponge brush and rinse mouth with water after eating and drinking. Consult physician if pain interferes with eating.
- Advise patient that this medication may have teratogenic effects. Contraception should be practiced during therapy and for at least 4 mon after therapy is concluded.
- Instruct patient not to receive any vaccinations without advice of physician.
- Emphasize the need for periodic lab tests to monitor for side effects.

Evaluation

Effectiveness of therapy can be demonstrated by: ▪ Improvement of hematopoietic values in leukemias ▪ Decrease in size and spread of the tumor in non-Hodgkin's lymphomas. Therapy is continued every 2 wk until patient is in complete remission or thrombocyte count or leukocyte count falls below acceptable levels.

CYTOMEGALOVIRUS IMMUNE GLOBULIN

(site-oh-**meg**-a-loe-vye-rus)

CMVIG

CLASSIFICATION(S):
Vaccine—immune globulin
Pregnancy Category UK

INDICATIONS

- Suppression of cytomegalovirus (CMV) disease in CMV-negative recipients of transplanted CMV-positive kidneys.

ACTION

- Consists of IgG antibodies capable of providing passive immunity against CMV disease. **Therapeutic Effect:**

- Prevention of serious sequelae of CMV disease in renal transplant patients.

PHARMACOKINETICS

Absorption: Administered IV only, resulting in complete bioavailability.
Distribution: Distribution not known.
Metabolism and Excretion: UK
Half-life: UK

CONTRAINDICATIONS AND PRECAUTIONS

Contraindicated in: ▪ Hypersensitivity to immune globulins or albumin ▪ Selective IgA deficiency.
Use Cautiously in: ▪ Pregnancy or lactation (safety not established).

ADVERSE REACTIONS AND SIDE EFFECTS*

CV: hypotension.
Resp: wheezing.
GI: vomiting, nausea.
Derm: flushing.
MS: muscle cramps, back pain.
Misc: chills, fever, allergic reactions including ANAPHYLAXIS.

INTERACTIONS

Drug-Drug: ▪ May interfere with the normal immune response to some **live virus vaccines** including **measles, mumps,** and **rubella virus vaccine** (do not administer within 3 mon of immune globulin).

ROUTE AND DOSAGE

- **IV (Adults):** 150 mg/kg within 72 hr of transplantation, followed by 100 mg/kg after 2, 4, 6, and 8 wk, then 50 mg/kg at 12 and 16 wk.

PHARMACODYNAMICS

	ONSET	PEAK	DURATION
IV	rapid	UK	UK

NURSING IMPLICATIONS

Assessment

- Monitor vital signs prior to, during, and following infusion, and before any increases in infusion rate.
- Monitor patient for adverse reactions throughout therapy. If patient develops minor side effects (nausea, vomiting, muscle cramps, back pain, fever, flushing, chills) slow infusion rate or stop infusion temporarily. If hypotension or anaphylaxis occurs, stop infusion and administer treatment (epinephrine and diphenhydramine).

Potential Nursing Diagnoses

- Infection, high risk for (indications)
- Knowledge deficit related to medication regimen (patient/family teaching).

Implementation

- **General Info:** Reconstitute with 50 ml of sterile water for injection with a double-ended needle or large syringe. To avoid foaming, do not shake vial. If using a double-ended needle, insert into water first as powder is supplied in an evacuated vial and water will transfer by suction. After water is transferred release residual vacuum to speed dissolution. Rotate gently to wet undissolved powder. Allow 30 min for powder to dissolve. Soln should be clear, colorless, and free of particulate matter.
- **Intermittent Infusion:** Infusion should be started within 6 hr and completed within 12 hr of reconstitution.
- Administer via infusion pump through a separate IV line. If not possible, soln may be piggy-backed in an IV line containing 0.9% NaCl, D5W, D10W, D20W, or combinations of dextrose and saline, but do not dilute to more than 1:2. Do not use filters.
- *Rate:* Administer initial dose at 15 mg/kg/hr for first 30 min. If no adverse reactions occur, rate may be increased to 30 mg/kg/hr; if no adverse reactions occur in subsequent 30 min, rate may be increased to 60 mg/kg/hr. Do not exceed 75 ml/hr volume or 60 mg/kg/hr rate. Monitor patient closely during rate changes. May cause pain at injection site.
- During subsequent doses, rate may be

*Underlines indicate most frequent; **CAPITALS** indicate life-threatening.

increased in same increments every 15 min if no adverse reactions occur, until 60 mg/kg/hr maximum is reached.

Patient/Family Teaching

- Instruct patient to notify physician if any adverse reactions occur.
- May cause drowsiness. Caution patient to avoid driving or other activities requiring alertness after receiving medication until response to medication is known.

Evaluation

Effectiveness of therapy can be demonstrated by: ▪ Prevention of serious sequelae of CMV disease, including blindness, in renal transplant patients.

DACARBAZINE
(da-**kar**-ba-zeen)
DTIC-Dome, {DTIC}

CLASSIFICATION(S):
Antineoplastic—alkylating agent
Pregnancy Category C

INDICATIONS

▪ Used alone in the treatment of metastatic malignant melanoma ▪ Used in combination with other antineoplastic agents in the treatment of advanced Hodgkin's disease. **Unlabeled Use:** ▪ Treatment of metastatic sarcomas.

ACTION

▪ Disrupts DNA and RNA synthesis (cell cycle-phase nonspecific). **Therapeutic Effect:** ▪ Death of rapidly growing tissue cells, especially malignant cells.

PHARMACOKINETICS

Absorption: Poorly absorbed following oral administration. Must be given IV.
Distribution: Large volume of distribution; appears to concentrate in liver. Some penetration of CNS.
Metabolism and Excretion: 50% metabolized by the liver, 50% excreted unchanged by the kidneys.
Half-life: 5 hr (increased in renal disease).

CONTRAINDICATIONS AND PRECAUTIONS

Contraindicated in: ▪ Hypersensitivity ▪ Pregnancy or lactation.
Use Cautiously in: ▪ Patients with childbearing potential ▪ Active infections ▪ Decreased bone marrow reserve ▪ Other chronic debilitating diseases ▪ Children (safety not established) ▪ Renal disease.

ADVERSE REACTIONS AND SIDE EFFECTS*

GI: nausea, vomiting, anorexia, diarrhea, hepatic vein thrombosis, HEPATIC NECROSIS.
Derm: alopecia, photosensitivity, facial flushing.
Endo: gonadal suppression.
Hemat: bone marrow depression.
Local: pain at IV site, phlebitis at IV site, tissue necrosis.
MS: mylagia.
Neuro: facial paresthesia.
Misc: facial flushing, flu-like syndrome, malaise, fever, ANAPHYLAXIS.

INTERACTIONS

Drug-Drug: ▪ Additive bone marrow depression with other **antineoplastic agents** or **radiation therapy** ▪ Additive hepatotoxicity with other **hepatotoxic drugs** ▪ **Phenytoin** or **phenobarbital** may increase metabolism and decrease effectiveness ▪ May decrease antibody response to **live virus vaccines** and increase the risk of adverse reactions.

ROUTE AND DOSAGE

Malignant Melanoma

- **IV (Adults):** 2–4.5 mg/kg/day for 10 days repeated every 4 wk or 250 mg/m^2/day for 5 days repeated every 3 wk.

Hodgkin's Disease

- **IV (Adults):** 150 mg/m^2/day for 5 days

{} = Available in Canada only.
*Underlines indicate most frequent; CAPITALS indicate life-threatening.

in combination with other agents given every 4 wk or 375 mg/m² given on the first day with other agents and repeated every 15 days.

PHARMACODYNAMICS (effects on blood counts)

	ONSET	PEAK	DURATION
IV—WBC	16–20 days	21–25 days	3–5 days
IV—platelets	UK	16 days	3–5 days

NURSING IMPLICATIONS

Assessment

- Monitor vital signs prior to and frequently during therapy.
- Assess for fever, chills, sore throat, and signs of infection. Notify physician if these symptoms occur.
- Monitor platelet count throughout therapy. Assess for bleeding (bleeding gums, bruising, petechiae; guaiac stools, urine, and emesis). Avoid IM injections and rectal temperatures. Apply pressure to venipuncture sites for 10 min.
- Monitor IV site closely. Dacarbazine is an irritant. Instruct patient to notify nurse immediately if discomfort at IV site occurs. Discontinue IV immediately if infiltration occurs. Confer with physician regarding application of ice to site.
- Monitor intake and output, appetite, and nutritional intake. Assess for nausea and vomiting, which may be severe and last 1–12 hr. Administration of an antiemetic prior to and periodically during therapy and adjusting diet as tolerated may help maintain fluid and electrolyte balance and nutritional status. Nausea usually decreases on subsequent doses.
- **Lab Test Considerations:** Monitor CBC and differential prior to and periodically throughout therapy. The nadir of thrombocytopenia occurs in 16 days. The nadir of leukopenia occurs in 3–4 wk. Recovery begins in 5 days. Withhold dose and notify physician if platelet count is <100,000/mm³ or leukocyte count is <4000/mm³.
- Monitor for increased SGOT (AST), SGPT (ALT), uric acid, and BUN.

Potential Nursing Diagnoses

- Infection, high risk for (side effects).
- Injury, high risk for (side effects).
- Knowledge deficit related to medication regimen (patient/family teaching).

Implementation

- **General Info:** Reconstitute each 100-mg vial with 9.9 ml of sterile water and each 200-mg vial with 19.7 ml to yield a concentration of 10 mg/ml. Soln is colorless or clear yellow. Do not use soln that has turned pink. Soln is stable for 8 hr at room temperature and for 72 hr if refrigerated.
- Soln should be prepared in a biologic cabinet. Wear gloves, gown, and mask while handling medication. Discard equipment in designated containers (see Appendix I).
- **Direct IV:** Administer over 1 min.
- **Intermittent Infusion:** Further dilute with 250 ml of D5W or 0.9% NaCl. Stable for 24 hr if refrigerated or 8 hr at room temperature.
- *Rate:* Administer over 15–30 min.
- **Y-Site Compatibility:** ondansetron.
- **Additive Compatibility:** bleomycin, carmustine, cyclophosphamide, cytarabine, dactinomycin, doxorubicin, fluorouracil, mercaptopurine, methotrexate, or vinblastine.
- **Additive Incompatibility:** hydrocortisone sodium succinate.

Patient/Family Teaching

- Instruct patient to notify physician if fever, chills, sore throat, signs of infection, bleeding gums, bruising, petechiae; or blood in urine, stool, or emesis occurs. Caution patient to avoid crowds and persons with known infections. Instruct patient to use soft toothbrush and electric razor. Patients should be cautioned not to drink alcoholic beverages or take products containing aspirin.
- May occasionally cause photosensitivity. Instruct patient to avoid sun-

light or wear protective clothing and use sunscreen for 2 days after therapy.

- Instruct patient to inform physician if flu-like syndrome occurs. Symptoms include fever, myalgia, and general malaise. May occur after several courses of therapy. Usually occurs 1 wk after administration. May persist for 1–3 wk. Physician may order acetaminophen for relief of symptoms.
- Discuss with patient the possibility of hair loss. Explore coping strategies.
- Advise patient of the need for contraception.
- Instruct patient not to receive any vaccinations without advice of physician.

Evaluation

Effectiveness of therapy and be demonstrated by: ▪ Decrease in size and spread of malignant melanoma or Hodgkin's lymphoma.

DACTINOMYCIN

(dak-ti-noe-**mye**-sin)
Actinomycin D, Cosmegen

CLASSIFICATION(S):
Antineoplastic—antibiotic
Pregnancy Category C

INDICATIONS

▪ Used alone and in combination with other treatment modalities (other antineoplastic agents, radiation therapy, or surgery) in the management of: ▫ Wilms' tumor ▫ Rhabdomyosarcoma ▫ Ewing sarcoma ▫ Trophoblastic neoplasms ▫ Testicular carcinoma ▫ Other malignancies.

ACTION

▪ Inhibits RNA synthesis by forming a complex with DNA (cell cycle-phase nonspecific). **Therapeutic Effects:** ▪ Death of rapidly replicating cells, particularly malignant ones ▪ Also has immunosuppressive properties.

PHARMACOKINETICS

Absorption: Administered IV only.
Distribution: Widely distributed, but does not cross the blood-brain barrier. Crosses the placenta.
Metabolism and Excretion: Excreted in bile and subsequently in the feces as unchanged drug (50%); small amounts (10%) excreted unchanged by the kidneys.
Half-life: 36 hr.

CONTRAINDICATIONS AND PRECAUTIONS

Contraindicated in: ▪ Hypersensitivity ▪ Pregnant or lactating women.
Use Cautiously in: ▪ Patients with childbearing potential ▪ Active infections ▪ Decreased bone marrow reserve ▪ Other chronic debilitating illnesses.

ADVERSE REACTIONS AND SIDE EFFECTS*

CNS: lethargy.
GI: <u>nausea</u>, <u>vomiting</u>, <u>stomatitis</u>, ulceration.
Derm: <u>alopecia</u>, rashes.
Endo: gonadal suppression.
Hemat: <u>anemia</u>, <u>leukopenia</u>, <u>thrombocytopenia</u>.
Local: <u>phlebitis</u> at IV site.
Misc: fever.

INTERACTIONS

Drug-Drug: ▪ Additive bone marrow depression with other **antineoplastics** or **radiation therapy** ▪ May decrease antibody response to **live virus vaccines** and increase risk of adverse reactions.

ROUTE AND DOSAGE

- **IV (Adults):** 500 mcg/day for 5 days, repeat q 2–4 wk.
- **IV (Children >6 mon):** 15 mcg/kg daily for 5 days, repeat q 2–4 wk.

PHARMACODYNAMICS (effects on blood counts)

	ONSET	PEAK	DURATION
IV	7 days	14 days	21–28 days

*<u>Underlines</u> indicate most frequent; **CAPITALS** indicate life-threatening.

NURSING IMPLICATIONS

Assessment

- Monitor vital signs prior to and frequently during therapy.
- Assess for fever, chills, sore throat, and signs of infection. Notify physician if these symptoms occur.
- Monitor platelet count throughout therapy. Assess for bleeding (bleeding gums, bruising, petechiae; guaiac stools, urine, and emesis). Avoid IM injections and rectal temperatures. Apply pressure to venipuncture sites for 10 min.
- Assess IV site frequently for inflammation or infiltration. Patient should notify nurse if pain or irritation at injection site occurs. If extravasation occurs infusion must be stopped and restarted in another vein to avoid damage to SC tissue. Notify physician immediately. Standard treatments include local injections of steroids and application of ice compresses.
- Monitor intake and output, appetite, and nutritional intake. Assess for nausea and vomiting, which usually begins a few hrs after administration and persists for up to 20 hr. Administration of an antiemetic prior to and periodically during therapy and adjusting diet as tolerated may help maintain fluid and electrolyte balance and nutritional status. IV fluids and allopurinol may be given to decrease uric acid levels in patients unable to maintain satisfactory oral intake.
- **Lab Test Considerations:** May cause increased uric acid levels.
- Monitor CBC and differential prior to and periodically throughout therapy. Platelets and leukocyte counts begin to drop 7–10 days after beginning therapy. The nadirs of thrombocytopenia and leukopenia occur in 3 wk. Recovery occurs 3 wk later.
- Monitor for hepatotoxicity (increased SGOT [AST], SGPT [ALT], LDH, and serum bilirubin).

Potential Nursing Diagnoses

- Infection, high risk for (adverse reactions).
- Oral mucous membranes, altered (side effects).
- Knowledge deficit related to medication regimen (patient/family teaching).

Implementation

- **General Info:** Avoid contact with skin. If spillage occurs, irrigate skin with copious amount of water for 15 min. If splashed into eye, irrigate with water and consult ophthalmologist.
- Soln for IV administration should be prepared in a biologic cabinet. Wear gloves, gown, and mask while handling IV medication. Discard IV equipment in specially designated containers (see Appendix I).
- **IV:** Reconstitute each 0.5 mg vial with 1.1 ml of sterile water for injection without preservatives. Soln color is gold. Discard any unused soln.
- **Direct IV:** Change needle between reconstitution and direct IV administration.
- *Rate:* May be injected into Y-site or 3-way stopcock of free-flowing infusions of 0.9% NaCl or D5W at a rate of 500 mcg/min.
- **Intermittent Infusion:** May be further diluted in 50 ml of 0.9% NaCl or D5W.
- *Rate:* Infuse over 10–15 min.

Patient/Family Teaching

- Instruct patient to notify physician if fever, chills, sore throat, signs of infection, bleeding gums, bruising, petechiae, blood in urine, stool, or emesis occurs. Caution patient to avoid crowds and persons with known infections. Instruct patient to use soft toothbrush and electric razor. Patients should be cautioned not to drink alcoholic beverages or take products containing aspirin.
- Instruct patient to inspect oral mucosa for erythema and ulceration. If ulceration occurs advise patient to use sponge brush and rinse mouth

with water after eating and drinking. Physician may order viscous lidocaine swishes if mouth pain interferes with eating.
- ☐ Inform patient that this medication may cause irreversible gonadal suppression. Advise patient that this medication may have teratogenic effects. Contraception should be practiced during therapy and for at least 4 mon after therapy is concluded.
- ☐ Discuss with patient the possibility of hair loss, which usually occurs 7–10 days after administration of dactinomycin. Explore coping strategies.
- ☐ Instruct patient not to receive any vaccinations without advice of physician.
- ☐ Emphasize the need for periodic lab tests to monitor for side effects.

Evaluation

Effectiveness of therapy can be demonstrated by: ▪ Decrease in size or spread of malignancy.

DANAZOL
(**da**-na-zole)
Danocrine, {Cyclomen}

CLASSIFICATION(S):
Hormone—androgen
Pregnancy Category UK

INDICATIONS

▪ Treatment of moderate endometriosis unresponsive to more conventional therapy ▪ Palliative therapy of fibrocystic breast disease ▪ Prophylaxis of hereditary angioedema. **Unlabeled Uses:** ▪ Precocious puberty, gynecomastia, menorrhagia, idiopathic immune thrombocytopenia, lupus-associated thrombocytopenia, and autoimmune hemolytic anemia.

ACTION

▪ Inhibits pituitary output of gonadotropins, resulting in suppression of ovarian function. Has weak androgenic-anabolic activity. **Therapeutic Effects:** ▪ Atrophy of ectopic endometrial tissue in endometriosis ▪ Decreased pain and nodularity in fibrocystic breast disease ▪ Correction of biochemical abnormalities in hereditary angioedema.

PHARMACOKINETICS

Absorption: Absorbed from the GI tract.
Distribution: Distribution not known.
Metabolism and Excretion: Metabolized by the liver.
Half-life: 4.5 hr.

CONTRAINDICATIONS AND PRECAUTIONS

Contraindicated in: ▪ Hypersensitivity ▪ Male patients with breast or prostate cancer ▪ Hypercalcemia ▪ Severe hepatic, renal, or cardiac disease ▪ Pregnancy or lactation.
Use Cautiously in: ▪ Previous history of liver disease ▪ Coronary artery disease ▪ Prepubertal males.

ADVERSE REACTIONS AND SIDE EFFECTS*

CNS: emotional lability.
CV: edema.
Derm: hirsutism, acne, oiliness.
EENT: deepening of voice.
Endo: decreased breast size (females), anovulation, amenorrhea, decreased libido.
GU: testicular atrophy, clitoral enlargement, amenorrhea.
Metab: weight gain.
Misc: hepatitis (cholestatic jaundice).

INTERACTIONS

Drug-Drug: ▪ May potentiate **oral anticoagulants, oral hypoglycemic agents, insulin,** or **glucocorticoids** ▪ May increase **cyclosporine** levels and risk of toxicity.

ROUTE AND DOSAGE

Endometriosis

▪ **PO (Adults):** 200–800 mg/day in 2 di-

{} = Available in Canada only.

*Underlines indicate most frequent; **CAPITALS** indicate life-threatening.

vided doses for 3–6 mon (up to 9 mon).

Fibrocystic Breast Disease

- **PO (Adults):** 100–400 mg/day in 2 divided doses for 2–6 mon.

Hereditary Angioedema

- **PO (Adults):** 400–600 mg/day in 2–3 divided doses.

PHARMACODYNAMICS

	ONSET	PEAK	DURATION
PO (endometriosis)	UK	6–8 wk	60–90 days
PO (fibrocystic disease)	1 mon	2–6 mon	1 yr
PO (angioedema)	UK	1–3 mon	UK

NURSING IMPLICATIONS

Assessment

- **Endometriosis:** Assess patient for endometrial pain prior to and periodically throughout therapy.
- **Fibrocystic Breast Disease:** Assess patient for breast pain, tenderness, and nodules prior to and monthly throughout therapy.
- **Hereditary Angioedema:** Monitor patient for edematous attacks throughout therapy, especially during dosage adjustments.
- **Lab Test Considerations:** Liver function tests should be monitored periodically throughout therapy.
  - Semen count and volume, viscosity, and motility determinations are recommended every 3–4 mon during treatment for hereditary angioedema, especially in adolescents.
  - May alter results of glucose tolerance or thyroid function tests.

Potential Nursing Diagnoses

- Sexual dysfunction (side effects).
- Body image disturbance (side effects).
- Knowledge deficit related to medication regimen (patient/family teaching).

Implementation

- **General Info:** In patients with endometriosis or fibrocystic breast disease therapy should be started during menstruation or preceded by a pregnancy test. Advise patient to notify physician immediately if pregnancy is suspected.
- **PO:** Medication may be administered with meals to minimize GI irritation.

Patient/Family Teaching

- **General Info:** Instruct patient to take medication exactly as prescribed. Missed doses should be taken as soon as remembered, if not almost time for next dose; do not double doses.
  - Advise patient to use a form of contraception other than oral contraceptives during therapy. Inform patient that amenorrhea is expected with higher doses. Instruct patient to notify physician if regular menstruation does not occur within 60–90 days after discontinuation of therapy.
  - Advise patient to notify physician if masculinizing effects occur (abnormal growth of facial hair or other body hair, deepening of the voice).
  - Emphasize the importance of routine visits to physician to check progress during therapy.
- **Fibrocystic Breast Disease:** Teach patient the correct technique for monthly breast self-examination. Instruct patient to report increase in size of nodules to physician promptly.

Evaluation

Effectiveness of therapy can be demonstrated by: ▪ Decrease in symptoms of endometriosis. Therapy for endometriosis usually requires 3–6 mon and may extend to 9 mon to decrease symptoms ▪ Relief of pain and tenderness in fibrocystic breast disease, which is usually relieved by the first mon and eliminated in 2–3 mon. Elimination of nodularity usually requires 4–6 mon ▪ Resolutions of signs and symptoms of hereditary angioedema. Initial response in hereditary angioedema may require

D

1–3 mon of therapy; efforts should be made to decrease dosage at 1–3-mon intervals.

DANTROLENE
(**dan**-troe-leen)
Dantrium

CLASSIFICATION(S):
Skeletal muscle relaxant—direct acting
Pregnancy Category C (IV use)

INDICATIONS

▪ **PO:** Treatment of spasticity associated with: ▫ Spinal cord injury ▫ Stroke ▫ Cerebral palsy ▫ Multiple sclerosis ▪ **PO:** Prophylaxis of malignant hyperthermia ▪ **IV:** Emergency treatment of malignant hyperthermia.

ACTION

▪ Acts directly on skeletal muscle causing relaxation by decreasing calcium release from sarcoplasmic reticulum in muscle cells ▪ Prevents intense catabolic process associated with malignant hyperthermia. **Therapeutic Effects:** ▪ Reduction of muscle spasticity ▪ Prevention of malignant hyperthermia.

PHARMACOKINETICS

Absorption: 35% absorbed after oral administration.
Distribution: Distribution not known.
Metabolism and Excretion: Almost entirely metabolized by the liver.
Half-life: 8.7 hr.

CONTRAINDICATIONS AND PRECAUTIONS

Contraindicated in: ▪ No contraindications to IV form in treatment of hyperthermia ▪ Pregnancy and lactation ▪ In situations where spasticity is used to maintain posture or balance.
Use Cautiously in: ▪ Cardiac, pulmonary, or previous liver disease.

ADVERSE REACTIONS AND SIDE EFFECTS*

CNS: muscle weakness, drowsiness, dizziness, malaise, headache, confusion, nervousness, insomnia, lightheadedness.
EENT: excessive lacrimation, visual disturbances.
Resp: pleural effusions.
CV: tachycardia, changes in blood pressure.
GI: diarrhea, anorexia, vomiting, cramps, dysphagia, **HEPATITIS**.
GU: frequency, incontinence, nocturia, dysuria, crytalluria, impotence.
Derm: pruritis, urticaria, photosensitivity, sweating.
Hemat: eosinophilia.
MS: myalgia.
Misc: drooling, chills, fever.

INTERACTIONS

Drug-Drug: ▪ Additive CNS depression with **CNS depressants,** including **alcohol, antihistamines, narcotic analgesics, sedative/hypnotics,** and **parenteral magnesium sulfate** ▪ Increased risk of hepatotoxicity with other **hepatotoxic agents**.

ROUTE AND DOSAGE

Spasticity

- **PO (Adults):** 25 mg/day initially, increase to 25 mg 2–4 times daily, then by increments of 25 mg up to 100 mg 2–4 times daily if needed—dosage increments may be made q 4–7 days (not to exceed 400 mg/day).
- **PO (Children >5 yr):** 0.5 mg/kg twice daily; increase to 0.5 mg/kg 3–4 times daily, then by increments of 0.5 mg/kg up to 3 mg/kg 2–4 times daily (not to exceed 100 mg 4 times daily).

Hyperthermic Crisis

- **IV (Adults and Children):** 1 mg/kg; may repeat dose up to cumulative dose of 10 mg/kg, followed by 1–3 days of PO therapy (4–8 mg/kg/day in 4 divided doses).

*Underlines indicate most frequent; **CAPITALS** indicate life-threatening.

Hyperthermia Prevention

- **PO (Adults and Children):** 4–8 mg/kg/day in 3–4 divided doses for 1–2 days prior to procedure, last dose 3–4 hr preop.

PHARMACODYNAMICS (effects on spasticity)

	ONSET	PEAK	DURATION
PO	1 wk	UK	6–12 hr
IV	rapid	rapid	UK

NURSING IMPLICATIONS

Assessment

- **General Info:** Assess bowel function periodically. Persistent diarrhea may warrant discontinuation of therapy.
- **Muscle Spasticity:** Assess neuromuscular status and muscle spasticity before initiating therapy and periodically during its course to determine response to therapy.
- **Malignant Hyperthermia:** Assess previous anesthesia history of all surgical patients. Also assess for family history of reactions to anesthesia (malignant hyperthermia or perioperative death).
  - Monitor ECG, vital signs, electrolytes, and urine output continuously when administering IV for malignant hyperthermia.
- **Lab Test Considerations:** Hepatic and renal function and CBC should be evaluated prior to and periodically during therapy in patients receiving prolonged therapy. Liver function abnormalities may require discontinuation of therapy.

Potential Nursing Diagnoses

- Mobility, impaired physical (indication).
- Comfort, altered: pain (indications).
- Injury, high risk for (side effects).

Implementation

- **PO:** If gastric irritation becomes a problem, may be administered with food. Oral suspensions may be made by opening capsules and adding them to fruit juices or other liquid. Drink immediately after mixing.
- **Direct IV:** Reconstitute each 20 mg with 60 ml of sterile water for injection without a bacteriostatic agent for a concentration of 333 mcg/ml. Shake until soln is clear. Soln must be used within 6 hr. Protect diluted soln from direct light.
  - *Rate:* Administer each single dose by rapid continuous IV push through Y tubing or 3-way stopcock. Follow immediately with subsequent doses as indicated. Medication is very irritating to tissues; observe infusion site frequently to avoid extravasation.

Patient/Family Teaching

- **General Info:** Advise patient not to take more medication than the amount prescribed, to minimize risk of hepatotoxicity and other side effects. If a dose is missed, do not take unless remembered within 1 hr. Do not double doses.
  - May cause dizziness, drowsiness, lightheadedness, visual disturbances, and muscle weakness. Advise patient to avoid driving and other activities requiring alertness until response to drug is known.
  - Caution patient to use sunscreen and protective clothing to prevent photosensitivity reactions.
  - Advise patient to avoid taking alcohol or other CNS depressants concurrently with this medication.
  - Instruct patient to notify physician if nausea, vomiting, abdominal discomfort, yellow eyes, dark urine, or clay-colored stools occur.
  - Emphasize the importance of follow-up examinations to check progress in long-term therapy and blood tests to monitor for side effects.
- **Malignant Hyperthermia:** Patients with malignant hyperthemia should carry identification describing disease process at all times.

Evaluation

Effectiveness of therapy can be demonstrated by: ▪ Relief of muscle spasm in musculoskeletal conditions. One week or more may be required to see improvement; if there is no observed improvement in 45 days the medication is usually discontinued ▪ Prevention or decrease in temperature and skeletal rigidity in malignant hyperthermia.

DAPIPRAZOLE
(da-**pip**-ra-zole)
Rev-Eyes

CLASSIFICATION(S):
Ophthalmic—alpha-adrenergic blocker
Pregnancy Category B

INDICATIONS
▪ Reversal of mydriasis produced by phenylephrine or tropicamide.

ACTION
▪ Blocks alpha-adrenergic receptors in dilator muscle of the iris producing miosis. **Therapeutic Effect:** ▪ Restoration of pupillary function following ophthalmic examination.

PHARMACOKINETICS
Absorption: Not known.
Distribution: Not known.
Metabolism and Excretion: Not known.
Half-life: Not known.

CONTRAINDICATIONS AND PRECAUTIONS
Contraindicated in: ▪ Hypersensitivity to dapiprazole or other components (hydroxypropyl methylcellulose, edetate sodium, sodium phosphate dibasic and monobasic, benzalkonium chloride) ▪ Acute iritis or other situations where pupillary constriction should be avoided.
Use Cautiously in: ▪ Pregnancy, lactation, or children (safety not established).

ADVERSE REACTIONS AND SIDE EFFECTS*
CNS: headache.
EENT: conjunctival injection, ocular burning, ptosis, lid erythema, lid edema, chemosis, itching, punctate keratitis, cornela edema, browache, photophobia, dry eyes, blurred vision, tearing.

INTERACTIONS
Drug-Drug: ▪ None significant.

ROUTE AND DOSAGE
- **Ophth (Adults):** 2 drops to conjunctiva, followed by 2 more drops 5 min later in each eye (should not be used more than once a wk).

PHARMACODYNAMICS

	ONSET	PEAK	DURATION
Ophth	rapid (within min)	UK	UK

NURSING IMPLICATIONS
ASSESSMENT
□ Assess pupil size prior to and following administration.

POTENTIAL NURSING DIAGNOSES
- Sensory-perceptual alteration: visual (indications).
- Injury, high risk for (indications).
- Knowledge deficit related to medication regimen (patient/family teaching).

IMPLEMENTATION
- **General Info:** To prepare soln, tear off seals and remove rubber plugs from drug and diluent. Pour diluent into drug vial and shake for several mins to ensure mixing. Stable at room temperature for 21 days. Discard soln that is not clear and colorless.
- **Ophth:** Have patient lie down or tilt head back and look at ceiling. Pull down on lower lid creating a small pocket and instill soln into pocket. Instruct patient to gently close eye. Do

*Underlines indicate most frequent; **CAPITALS** indicate life-threatening.

not touch the dropper tip to the eye lid or any surface.
- Do not use more frequently than once per wk.

Patient/Family Teaching
- Explain the purpose of the medication to patient. Instruct patient to report adverse reactions to physician.

Evaluation

Effectiveness of therapy can be demonstrated by: ▪ Restoration of pupillary function following ophthalmic examination.

DAUNORUBICIN
(daw-noe-**roo**-bi-sin)
Daunomycin, Rubidomycin, Cerubidine

CLASSIFICATION(S):
Antineoplastic—antibiotic
Pregnancy Category D

INDICATIONS

▪ Used in combination with other antineoplastic agents in the treatment of leukemias.

ACTION

▪ Forms a complex with DNA, which subsequently inhibits DNA and RNA synthesis (cell cycle-phase nonspecific). **Therapeutic Effect:** ▪ Death of rapidly replicating cells, particularly malignant ones. Also has immunosuppressive properties.

PHARMACOKINETICS

Absorption: Administered IV only, resulting in complete bioavailability.
Distribution: Widely distributed. Crosses the placenta.
Metabolism and Excretion: Extensively metabolized by the liver. Converted partially to a compound that also has antineoplastic activity. 40% eliminated by biliary excretion.
Half-life: 18.5 hr.

CONTRAINDICATIONS AND PRECAUTIONS

Contraindicated in: ▪ Hypersensitivity ▪ Underlying congestive heart failure ▪ Cardiac arrhythmias ▪ Pregnant or lactating women.
Use Cautiously in: ▪ Patients with childbearing potential ▪ Active infections ▪ Decreased bone marrow reserve ▪ Other chronic debilitating illnesses ▪ May reactivate skin lesions produced by previous radiation therapy ▪ Hepatic or renal impairment (dosage reduction recommended).

ADVERSE REACTIONS AND SIDE EFFECTS*

CV: CONGESTIVE HEART FAILURE, arrhythmias.
GI: nausea, vomiting, stomatitis, esophagitis.
GU: red urine.
Derm: alopecia.
Endo: gonadal suppression.
Hemat: bone marrow depression.
Local: phlebitis at IV site.
Metab: hyperuricemia.
Misc: fever, chills.

INTERACTIONS

Drug-Drug: ▪ Additive myelosuppression with other **antineoplastic agents** ▪ **Cyclophosphamide** increases the risk of cardiotoxicity ▪ May decrease antibody response to **live virus vaccines** and increase risk of adverse reactions.

ROUTE AND DOSAGE

- **IV (Adults):** 30–60 mg/m^2/day for 3–5 days, repeated q 3–4 wk. Total cumulative dose in adults should not exceed 400–600 mg/m^2
- **IV (Children):** 25–45 mg/m^2.

PHARMACODYNAMICS (effects on blood counts)

	ONSET	PEAK	DURATION
IV	7–10 days	10–14 days	21 days

*Underlines indicate most frequent; **CAPITALS** indicate life-threatening.

D

NURSING IMPLICATIONS

Assessment

- Monitor vital signs prior to and frequently during therapy.
- Assess for fever, chills, sore throat, and signs of infection. Notify physician if these symptoms occur.
- Monitor platelet count throughout therapy. Assess for bleeding (bleeding gums, bruising, petechiae, guaiac stools, urine, and emesis). Avoid IM injections and rectal temperatures. Apply pressure to venipuncture sites for 10 min.
- Assess IV site frequently for inflammation or infiltration. Patient should notify nurse if pain or irritation at injection site occurs. If extravasation occurs infusion must be stopped and restarted in another vein to avoid damage to SC tissue. Notify physician immediately. Standard treatments include local injections of steroids and application of ice compresses.
- Monitor intake and output, appetite, and nutritional intake. Assess for nausea and vomiting, which although mild, may persist for 24–48 hr. Administration of an antiemetic prior to and periodically during therapy and adjusting diet as tolerated may help maintain fluid and electrolyte balance and nutritional status. Encourage fluid intake of 2000–3000 ml/day. Physician may also order allopurinol and alkalinization of the urine to help prevent urate stone formation.
- Assess patient for evidence of congestive heart failure (peripheral edema, dyspnea, rales/crackles, weight gain, jugular venous distension); usually cumulative dose-related. Chest x-ray, echocardiography, and ECGs may be ordered prior to and periodically throughout therapy. A 30% decrease in QRS voltage and decrease in systolic ejection fraction are early signs of cardiomyopathy.
- **Lab Test Considerations:** Monitor CBC and differential prior to and periodically throughout therapy. The leukocyte count nadir occurs 10–14 days after administration. Recovery usually occurs within 21 days after administration of daunorubicin.
- Monitor SGOT (AST), SGPT (ALT), LDH, and serum bilirubin. May cause transiently elevated serum phosphatase, bilirubin, and SGOT (AST) concentrations.
- Monitor uric acid levels.

Potential Nursing Diagnoses

- Infection, high risk for (adverse reactions).
- Cardiac output, decreased (side effects).
- Knowledge deficit related to medication regimen (patient/family teaching).

Implementation

- **General Info:** Soln for IV administrations should be prepared in a biologic cabinet. Wear gloves, gown, and mask while handling IV medication. Discard IV equipment in specially designated containers (see Appendix I).
- **IV:** Reconstitute each 20 mg with 4 ml of sterile water for injection. Reconstituted medication is stable for 24 hr at room temperature, 48 hr if refrigerated. Protect from sunlight.
- Do not use aluminum needles when reconstituting or injecting daunorubicin, as aluminum darkens the soln.
- **Direct IV:** Further dilute in 10–15 ml of 0.9% NaCl. Administer direct IV push through Y-site or 3-way stopcock into free-flowing infusion of 0.9% NaCl or D5W.
- *Rate:* Administer over at least 3–5 min. Rapid administration rate may cause facial flushing or erythema along the vein.
- **Intermittent Infusion:** May be further diluted in 50 ml of D5W, 0.9% NaCl, or lactated Ringer's soln and infused over 10–15 min. May also be diluted in 100 ml and infused over 30–45 min.
- **Y-Site Compatibility:** ondansetron.
- **Additive Incompatibility:** dexamethasone or heparin. Manufacturer does

not recommend admixing daunorubicin.

PATIENT/FAMILY TEACHING

- Instruct patient to notify physician if fever, chills, sore throat, signs of infection, bleeding gums, bruising, petechiae, blood in urine, stool, or emesis occurs. Caution patient to avoid crowds and persons with known infections. Instruct patient to use soft toothbrush and electric razor. Patient should be cautioned not to drink alcoholic beverages or take products containing aspirin.
- Instruct patient to inspect oral mucosa for erythema and ulceration. If ulceration occurs advise patient to use sponge brush and rinse mouth with water after eating and drinking. Consult physician if mouth pain interferes with eating. Period of highest risk is 3–7 days after administration of dose.
- Instruct patient to notify physician immediately if irregular heartbeat, shortness of breath, or swelling of lower extremities occurs.
- Discuss with patient possibility of hair loss. Explore methods of coping. Regrowth of hair usually begins within 5 wk after discontinuing therapy.
- Inform patient that medication may turn urine reddish color for 1–2 days following administration.
- Inform patient that this medication may cause irreversible gonadal suppresssion. Advise patient that this medication may have teratogenic effects. Contraception should be practiced during therapy and for at least 4 mon after therapy is concluded.
- Instruct patient not to receive any vaccinations without advice of physician.
- Emphasize the need for periodic lab tests to monitor for side effects.

EVALUATION

Effectiveness of therapy can be demonstrated by: ▪ Improvement of hematologic status. Courses of therapy are usually administered no more frequently than every 21 days, to allow for bone marrow recovery.

DEFEROXAMINE

(dee-fer-**ox**-a-men)
Desferal

CLASSIFICATION(S):
Antidote—heavy metal antagonist
Pregnancy Category C

INDICATIONS

▪ Management of acute toxic iron ingestion ▪ Management of secondary iron overload syndromes associated with multiple transfusion therapy.

ACTION

▪ Chelates unbound iron, forming a water-soluble complex (ferrioxamine) in plasma that is easily excreted by the kidneys. **Therapeutic Effect:** ▪ Removal of excess iron. Also chelates aluminum.

PHARMACOKINETICS

Absorption: Poorly absorbed following oral administration. Well absorbed following IM administration and SC administration.

Distribution: Appears to be widely distributed.

Metabolism and Excretion: Metabolized by tissues and plasma enzymes. Unchanged drug and chelated form excreted by the kidneys. 33% of iron removed is eliminated in the feces via the biliary excretion.

Half-life: 1 hr.

CONTRAINDICATIONS AND PRECAUTIONS

Contraindicated in: ▪ Avoid use during pregnancy or in women who may become pregnant ▪ Severe renal disease ▪ Anuria.

Use Cautiously in: ▪ Safe use in children <3 yr not established.

D

ADVERSE REACTIONS AND SIDE EFFECTS*

CV: tachycardia.
EENT: cataracts, blurred vision, ototoxicity.
GI: abdominal pain, diarrhea.
GU: red urine.
Local: pain at injection site, induration at injection site.
MS: leg cramps.
Misc: flushing, erythema, urticaria, hypotension, shock following rapid IV administration, allergic reactions, fever.

INTERACTIONS

Drug-Drug: ▪ **Ascorbic acid** may increase the effectiveness of deferoxamine but may also increase cardiac iron toxicity.

ROUTE AND DOSAGE

Note: IV infusions are to be given slowly, rate not to exceed 15 mg/kg/hr; IM route is preferred in acute intoxication unless accompanied by shock.

Acute Iron Intoxication

- **IM, IV (Adults):** 1 g initially, then 500 mg q 4 hr for 2 more doses. Additional doses of 500 mg given at 4–12-hr intervals may be required, not to exceed 6 g/day.
- **IM, IV (Children):** 1 g initially, then 500 mg q 4 hr for 2 more doses. Additional doses of 500 mg given at 4–12-hr intervals may be required, not to exceed 6 g/day or 20 mg/kg (600 mg/m^2) initially followed by 10 mg/kg (300 mg/m^2) q 4 hr for 2 more doses. Additional doses of 10 mg/kg (300 mg/m^2) may be given at 4–12-hr intervals, not to exceed 6 g/day.

Chronic Iron Overload

- **IM (Adults and Children):** 0.5–1 g/day.
- **IV (Adults and Children):** In addition to above IM dosage for chronic iron overload, 2-g doses may be given by slow IV infusion at the time each unit of blood is transfused (not in same line).
- **SC (Adults and Children):** 1–2 g/day (20–40 mg/kg/day) by continuous SC infusion given over 8–24 hr.

PHARMACODYNAMICS (effects on hematologic parameters)

	ONSET	PEAK	DURATION
IV	rapid	UK	UK
IM	UK	UK	UK
SC	UK	UK	UK

NURSING IMPLICATIONS

Assessment

- ▫ In acute poisoning, assess time, amount, and type of iron preparation ingested.
- ▫ Monitor signs of iron toxicity: early acute (abdominal pain, bloody diarrhea, emesis), late acute (decreased level of consciousness, shock, metabolic acidosis).
- ▫ Monitor vital signs closely, especially during IV administration. Notify physician if hypotension, erythema, urticaria, or signs of allergic reaction occur. Keep epinephrine, an antihistamine, and resuscitation equipment close by in the event of an anaphylactic reaction.
- ▫ May cause ocular or ototoxicity. Inform physician if decreased visual acuity or hearing loss occurs.
- ▫ Monitor intake and output and urine color. Inform physician if patient is anuric. Chelated iron is excreted primarily by the kidneys; urine may turn red.
- ▪ **Lab Test Considerations:** Monitor serum iron, iron binding capacity, transferrin levels, and urinary iron excretion prior to and periodically throughout course of therapy.
- ▫ Monitor liver function studies to assess damage from iron poisoning.

Potential Nursing Diagnosis

- ▪ Injury, high risk for: poisoning (patient/family teaching).
- ▪ Knowledge deficit related to medication regimen (patient/family teaching).

*Underlines indicate most frequent; **CAPITALS** indicate life-threatening.

Implementation

- **General Info:** Reconstitute contents of each vial with 2 ml of sterile water for injection. Soln is stable for 1 wk after reconstitution if protected from light.
- □ Used in conjunction with induction of emesis or gastric aspiration and lavage with sodium bicarbonate, and supportive measures for shock and metabolic acidosis in acute poisoning.
- **IM:** IM is the preferred route for acute poisoning. Administer deep IM and massage well. Rotate sites. IM administration may cause transient severe pain.
- **SC:** SC route is used to treat chronically elevated iron levels.
- □ Therapy is administered into abdominal subcutaneous tissue via infusion pump for 8–24 hr per treatment.
- **IV:** IV route is reserved for severe life-threatening poisoning. Reconstitute, then further dilute in D5W, 0.9% NaCl, or lactated Ringer's soln.
- □ *Rate:* Maximum infusion rate is 15 mg/kg/hr. Rapid infusion rate may cause hypotension, erythema, urticaria, wheezing, convulsions, tachycardia, or shock.
- □ May be administered at the same time as blood transfusion in persons with chronically elevated serum iron levels. Use separate site for administration.

Patient/Family Teaching

- □ Reinforce need to keep iron preparations, all medications, and hazardous substances out of the reach of children.
- □ Reassure patient that red coloration of urine is expected and reflects excretion of excess iron.
- □ Advise patient not to take vitamin C preparations without consulting physician, as tissue toxicity may increase.
- □ Encourage patients requiring chronic therapy to keep follow-up appointments for lab tests. Physician may also order eye and hearing examinations every 3 mon.

Evaluation

Effectiveness of therapy can be demonstrated by: ▪ Return of serum iron concentrations to a normal level (50–150 mcg/100 ml).

DEMECARIUM

(dem-e-**kare**-ee-um)
Humorsol

CLASSIFICATION(S):
Ophthalmic—cholinergic, Antiglaucoma
Pregnancy Category C

INDICATIONS

▪ Treatment of open-angle and other chronic glaucomas that have not responded to more conventional therapy ▪ Diagnosis and treatment of accommodative esotropia (abnormal alignment of the eyes) when not accompanied by amblyopia (decreased vision) and anisometropia (unequal refractive ability).

ACTION

▪ Long-lasting inhibition of the enzyme cholinesterase, resulting in accumulation and prolonged effects of acetylcholine. **Therapeutic Effects:** ▪ Contraction of iris sphincter muscle causing miosis ▪ Ciliary muscle constriction resulting in increased accommodation ▪ Decreased resistance to aqueous humor outflow, resulting in decreased intraocular pressure.

PHARMACOKINETICS

Absorption: Rapidly penetrates the cornea. Systemic absorption follows ophthalmic administration.
Distribution: Not known.
Metabolism and Excretion: Metabolized slowly in tissues and fluids by cholinesterases.
Half-life: UK.

CONTRAINDICATIONS AND PRECAUTIONS

Contraindicated in: ▪ Hypersensitivity ▪ Risk or history of retinal detachment

D

■ Acute ocular inflammation ■ Posterior synechiae (adhesion between the iris and the lens).

Use Cautiously in: ■ Corneal abrasion ■ Asthma ■ Hypertension ■ Hyperthyroidism ■ Cardiovascular disease ■ Epilepsy ■ Parkinsonism ■ Bradycardia ■ Ulcer disease ■ Urinary tract obstruction ■ Hypotension ■ GI obstruction.

ADVERSE REACTIONS AND SIDE EFFECTS*

CV: bradycardia, hypotension.

EENT: accommodative spasm, myopia, blurred vision, poor night vision, retinal detachment, stinging, burning, lacrimation, eye ache, brow ache, conjuntival conjestion, lacrimal duct stenosis, eyelid twitching, iris cysts (children), anterior chamber hyperemia, nasal congestion.

Resp: bronchospasm.

GI: nausea, vomiting, diarrhea, abdominal pain, cramps, excessive salivation.

GU: urinary frequency.

Derm: sweating, pallor, cyanosis.

MS: muscle weakness.

Neuro: paresthesia.

INTERACTIONS

Drug–Drug: ■ Additive intraocular pressure-lowering effects with ophthalmic administration of **epinephrine, beta-adrenergic blockers (timolol, metipranolol, levobunolol, betaxolol)**, and systemic **carbonic anhydrase inhibitors** ■ **Physostigmine, cyclopentolate,** local or systemic **glucocorticoids,** systemic **anticholinergics, antihistamines, meperidine, sympathomimetics,** and **tricyclic antidepressants** may decrease the effects of demecarium ■ Increases the duration of action of **ester-type local anesthetics (benzocaine, butacaine, tetracaine)** ■ Decreases the metabolism of and enhances the activity of **cocaine** ■ May enhance neuromuscular blockade from **succinylcholine** ■ Additive cholinergic toxicity with **cholinesterase inhibitors,** including **carbamate** and **organophosphate insecticides** ■ **Clofibrate** potentiates miosis ■ May potentiate the action of **general anesthetics,** including **cyclopropane** and **halothane**.

ROUTE AND DOSAGE

Glaucoma

- **Ophth (Adults and Children):** 1 drop of 0.125% soln twice daily (range 1–2 drops of 0.125–0.25% soln twice daily–twice weekly).

Accommodative Esotropia

- **Ophth (Adults and Children):** 1 drop of 0.125–0.25% soln once daily for 2–3 wk, then 1 drop every 2 days for 3–4 wk, then 1 drop every 2–4 days.

Diagnosis of Accommodative Esotropia

- **Ophth (Adults and Children):** 1 drop of 0.125–0.25% soln once daily for 2 wk, then 1 drop every 2 days for 2–3 wk.

PHARMACODYNAMICS

	ONSET	PEAK	DURATION
Ophth (miosis)	15–60 min	2–4 hr	3–10 days (up to 3–4 wk)
Ophth (intraocular pressure)	UK	24 hr	9 days or more

NURSING IMPLICATIONS

Assessment

- □ Assess for symptoms of systemic absorption (bradycardia, hypotension, dyspnea, increased salivation, sweating, nausea, vomiting, or diarrhea). Notify physician if these symptoms occur.
- **Toxicity and Overdose:** Toxicity is manifested as systemic side effects. Atropine is the antidote.

Potential Nursing Diagnoses

- Sensory-perceptual alteration: visual (side effect).
- Knowledge deficit related to medication regimen (patient/family teaching).

*Underlines indicate most frequent; **CAPITALS** indicate life-threatening.

Implementation

- **Ophth:** Available in two concentrations, 0.125% and 0.25%. Carefully check percentage on label prior to administration.
- □ Have patient tilt head back and look up, gently depress lower lid with index finger until conjunctival sac is exposed, and instill 1 drop. After instillation, maintain gentle pressure on inner canthus for 1 min to avoid systemic absorption of the drug. Wait at least 5 min before instilling other types of eyedrops.

Patient/Family Teaching

- □ Instruct patient on correct method of instillation of eyedrops. Instruct patient to take as ordered and not to discontinue without physician's approval. A missed dose should be taken as soon as remembered unless almost time for next dose. If not ordered daily, take when remembered, then resume correct spacing of demecarium.
- □ Caution patient that night vision may be impaired. Advise patient not to drive at night until response to medication is known. To prevent injury at night, patient should use a night light and keep environment uncluttered.
- □ Advise patient of the need for regular eye examinations to monitor intraocular pressure.
- □ Review symptoms of systemic absorption and instruct patient to notify physician should these symptoms occur. Patient also should inform physician if persistent vision changes, eye irritation, or persistent brow ache occur.
- □ Instruct patient to avoid use of pesticides with carbamate and organophosphate bases during therapy.
- □ Advise patient to inform physician or dentist of medication regimen prior to surgery as interaction with anesthetic agents may occur.

Evaluation

Effectiveness of therapy can be demonstrated by: ▪ Miosis with subsequent decrease in intraocular pressure.

DEMECLOCYCLINE

(dem-e-kloe-**sye**-kleen)
Declomycin

CLASSIFICATION(S):
Anti-infective—tetracycline
Pregnancy Category UK

INDICATIONS

▪ Treatment of various infections due to unusual organisms, including: □ *Mycoplasma* □ *Chlamydia* □ *Rickettsia* ▪ Treatment of gonorrhea and syphillis in penicillin-allergic patients ▪ Adjunctive treatment of severe acne and inclusion conjunctivitis and prevention of exacerbations of chronic bronchitis. **Unlabeled Use:** ▪ Management of chronic syndrome of inappropriate secretion of antidiuretic hormone (SIADH).

ACTION

▪ Inhibits bacterial protein synthesis at the level of the 30S ribosome. **Therapeutic Effect:** ▪ Bacteriostatic action against susceptible bacteria. **Spectrum:** ▪ Some gram-positive pathogens: □ *Bacillus anthracis* □ *Clostridium perfringens* □ *Clostridium tetani* □ *Listeria monocytogenes* □ *Nocardia* □ Propionibacterium acnes □ *Actinomyces isrealii* ▪ Some gram-negative pathogens: □ *Haemophilus influenzae* □ *Legionella pneumophila* □ *Yersinia entercolitica* □ *Yersinia pestis* □ *Neisseria gonorrhea* □ *Neisseria meningitidis*. ▪ Also active against several unusual pathogens, including: □ *Mycoplasma* □ *Chlamydia* □ *Rickettsia*.

PHARMACOKINETICS

Absorption: Well absorbed (60–80%) following oral administration.
Distribution: Widely distributed throughout body fluids. Concentrates in bone, liver, spleen, tumors, and teeth.
Metabolism and Excretion: Some biliary secretion, 40% excreted unchanged by the kidneys.

Half-life: 10–17 hr (increased in renal impairment).

CONTRAINDICATIONS AND PRECAUTIONS

Contraindicated in: ▪ Hypersensitivity ▪ Pregnancy (permanent staining of teeth in child) ▪ Lactation and children <8 yr.

Use Cautiously in: ▪ Cachectic or debilitated patients ▪ Liver disease ▪ Renal disease ▪ Nephrogenic diabetes insipidus.

ADVERSE REACTIONS AND SIDE EFFECTS*

GI: nausea, vomiting, diarrhea, pancreatitis, esophagitis.

Derm: rashes, photosensitivity, urticaria.

Endo: nephrogenic diabetes insipidus (increased thirst, increased urination, weakness, fatigue).

Hemat: blood dyscrasias.

Misc: superinfection, hypersensitivity reactions.

INTERACTIONS

Drug-Drug: ▪ May enhance the effect of **oral anticoagulants** ▪ May decrease the effectiveness of **oral contraceptives** ▪ **Calcium, iron,** and **magnesium** form insoluble compounds (chelates) and decrease absorption of demeclocycline ▪ Decreases antidiuretic effect of **desmopressin.**

Drug-Food: ▪ **Calcium** in foods or dairy products decreases absorption by forming insoluble compounds (chelates) ▪ **Food** decreases absorption of demeclocycline.

ROUTE AND DOSAGE

Anti-infective

- **PO (Adults):** 150 mg q 6 hr or 300 mg q 12 hr (up to 2.4 g/day).

SIADH

- **PO (Adults):** 600–1200 mg/day in 3–4 divided doses.

PHARMACODYNAMICS

	ONSET	PEAK	DURATION
PO (anti-infective)	UK	3–4 hr	
PO (SIADH)	5 days	UK	2–6 days

NURSING IMPLICATIONS

Assessment

- **General Info:** Assess patient for infection (vital signs; appearance of wound, sputum, urine, and stool; WBC) at beginning and throughout course of therapy.
  - ▫ Obtain specimens for culture and sensitivity prior to initiating therapy. First dose may be given before receiving results.
- **SIADH:** Monitor intake and output ratios and assess edema in patients treated for syndrome of inappropriate antidiuretic hormone.
- **Lab Test Considerations:** Renal, hepatic, and hematopoietic functions should be monitored periodically during long-term therapy.
  - ▫ May cause SGOT (AST), SGPT (ALT), serum alkaline phosphatase, bilirubin, and amylase concentrations. May interfere with urine glucose testing with copper sulfate method (Clinitest); use glucose oxidase reagent (Tes-Tape, Ketodiastix).

Potential Nursing Diagnoses

- Infections, high risk for (indications, side effects).
- Knowledge deficit related to medication regimen (patient/family teaching).
- Noncompliance related to medication regimen (patient/family teaching).

Implementation

- **General Info:** May cause yellow-brown discoloration and softening of teeth and bones if administered prenatally or during early childhood. Not recommended for children under 8 yr of age or during pregnancy or lactation.
- **PO:** Administer around the clock. May be taken with food if GI irritation oc-

*Underlines indicate most frequent; **CAPITALS** indicate life-threatening.

curs. Take with a full glass of liquid and at least 1 hr before going to bed to avoid esophageal irritation. Do not administer within 1–3 hr of other medications.

- Avoid administration of milk, calcium, antacids, magnesium-containing medications, or iron supplements within 1–3 hr of oral demeclocycline.

Patient/Family Teaching

- Instruct patient to take medication around the clock and to finish the drug completely as directed, even if feeling well. Advise patient that sharing of this medication may be dangerous.
- Advise patient to avoid taking milk or other dairy products concurrently with this medication.
- Caution patient to use sunscreen and protective clothing to prevent phototoxicity reactions.
- Advise patient to report signs of superinfection (black, furry overgrowth on the tongue, vaginal itching or discharge, loose or foul-smelling stools). Skin rash, pruritus, and urticaria should also be reported.
- Instruct patient to notify physician if symptoms do not improve.
- Caution patient to discard outdated or decomposed products, as they may be toxic.

Evaluation

Clinical response can be evaluated by: ▪ Resolution of the signs and symptoms of infection. Length of time for complete resolution depends on the organism and site of infection ▪ Resolution of the signs and symptoms of SIADH.

DESLANOSIDE

(des-**lan**-oh-side)
Cedilanid, {Cedilanid-D}

CLASSIFICATION(S):
Cardiac glycoside, Inotropic agent, Antiarrhythmic
Pregnancy Category C

INDICATIONS

▪ Alone or in combination with other agents (diuretics, vasodilators) in the initial treatment of congestive heart failure ▪ Used to slow the ventricular rate in tachyarrhythmias, such as atrial fibrillation and atrial flutter ▪ Used to terminate paroxysmal atrial tachycardia.

ACTION

▪ Increases the force of myocardial contraction ▪ Prolongs refractory period of the AV node ▪ Decreases conduction through the SA and AV node. **Therapeutic Effects:** ▪ Increased cardiac output ▪ Slowing of the heart rate.

PHARMACOKINETICS

Absorption: Well absorbed from IM sites.

Distribution: Widely distributed. Crosses the placenta and enters breast milk.

Metabolism and Excretion: Excreted almost entirely unchanged by the kidneys.

Half-life: 33–36 hr (increased in renal impairment).

CONTRAINDICATIONS AND PRECAUTIONS

Contraindicated in: ▪ Hypersensitivity ▪ Uncontrolled ventricular arrhythmias ▪ AV block ▪ Idiopathic hypertrophic subaortic stenosis ▪ Constrictive pericarditis.

Use Cautiously in: Electrolyte abnormalities (hypokalemia, hypercalcemia, and hypomagnesemia may predispose to cardiac glycoside toxicity) ▪ Pregnancy and lactation (safety has not been established) ▪ Children (safety not established; unlabeled) ▪ Elderly patients (particularly sensitive to toxic effects) ▪ Myocardial infarction ▪ Renal impairment (dosage reduction required) ▪ Hypothyroidism.

D

ADVERSE REACTIONS AND SIDE EFFECTS*

CNS: fatigue, weakness, headache, blurred vision, yellow vision.
CV: ARRHYTHMIAS, bradycardia, ECG changes.
GI: nausea, vomiting, anorexia, diarrhea, abdominal pain.
Endo: gynecomastia.
Hemat: thrombocytopenia.
Local: irritation at IV site, pain at IM site.

INTERACTIONS

Drug-Drug: ▪ **Thiazide** and **loop diuretics, mezlocillin, piperacillin, ticarcillin, amphotericin B,** and **glucocorticoids,** which cause hypokalemia, may increase the risk of toxicity ▪ Additive bradycardia may occur with **beta-adrenergic blocking agents** and other **antiarrhythmic agents (quinidine, disopyramide)** ▪ **Thyroid hormone** may decrease effects of cardiac glycosides.

ROUTE AND DOSAGE

Note: Used to initiate therapy or provide loading doses only, IV route preferred.

- **IV (Adults):** Loading dose—1.6 mg or 0.8 mg initially, then repeated in 4 hr (not to exceed 2 mg in 24 hr).
- **IM (Adults):** 2 doses of 0.8 mg given at separate sites (not to exceed 2 mg in 24 hr).
- **IM, IV (Children >3 yr):** Loading dose—22.5 mcg/kg in 2–3 divided doses given at 3–4-hr intervals (in emergency can be given as single dose).
- **IM, IV (Children 2 wk–3 yr):** Loading dose—25 mcg/kg in 2–3 divided doses given at 3–4-hr intervals (in emergency can give as single dose).
- **IM, IV (Premature and Full-Term Neonates or Children with Reduced Renal Function or Myocarditis):** Loading dose—22 mcg/kg in 2–3 divided doses given at 3–4-hr intervals (in emergency can give as single dose).

PHARMACODYNAMICS (cardiac effects)

	ONSET	PEAK	DURATION
IM	UK	UK	UK
IV	10–30 min	1–3 hr	2–5 days

NURSING IMPLICATIONS

Assessment

- Monitor apical pulse for 1 full min prior to administering. Withhold dose and notify physician if pulse rate is <60 bpm in an adult, <70 bpm in a child, or <90 bpm in an infant. Also notify physician promptly of any significant changes in rate, rhythm, or quality of pulse.
- Blood pressure should be monitored periodically in patients receiving IV deslanoside.
- Monitor ECG throughout IV administration. Notify physician if bradycardia or new arrhythmias occur. Observe IV site for redness or infiltration; extravasation can lead to tissue irritation and sloughing.
- Serum electrolyte levels, especially potassium, magnesium, and calcium, renal and hepatic functions, and ECGs should be evaluated periodically during course of therapy. Notify physician prior to giving dose if patient is hypokalemic. Hypokalemia, hypomagnesemia, or hypercalcemia may make patient more susceptible to digitalis toxicity.
- Monitor intake and output ratios and daily weights. Assess for peripheral edema and auscultate lungs for rales at least every 8 hr.
- Before administering initial loading dose, determine if patient has taken any digitalis preparations in the preceding 2–3 wk.
- **Toxicity and Overdose:** Observe patient for signs and symptoms of toxicity. In adults and older children the first signs of toxicity usually include abdominal pain, anorexia, nausea, vomiting, visual disturbances, bradycardia, and other arrhythmias. In in-

*Underlines indicate most frequent; **CAPITALS** indicate life-threatening.

fants and small children the first symptoms of overdose are usually cardiac arrhythmias. If these appear, withhold drug and notify physician immediately.
- If signs of toxicity occur and are not severe, discontinuation of deslanoside may be all that is required.
- If hypokalemia is present and renal function is adequate, potassium salts may be administered. Do not administer if hyperkalemia or heart block exists.
- Correction of arrhythmias due to digitalis toxicity may be attempted with lidocaine, procainamide, quinidine, propranolol, and phenytoin. Temporary ventricular pacing may be useful in advanced heart block.

Potential Nursing Diagnoses
- Cardiac output, decreased (indications).
- Knowledge deficit related to medication regimen (patient/family teaching).

Implementation
- **General Info:** To achieve a therapeutic maintenance level dose an orally effective cardiac glycoside should be administered within 12 hr of deslanoside.
- **IM:** Do not administer more than 0.8 mg in each site. Inject deep into gluteal muscle and massage well.
- **Direct IV:** IV doses may be given undiluted or diluted in 10 ml of 0.9% NaCl.
- *Rate;* Administer through Y-site injection or 3-way stopcock at a rate of each single dose over a minimum of 5 min.
- **Y-Site Compatibility:** heparin, hydrocortisone sodium succinate, or potassium chloride.

Patient/Family Teaching
- Review signs and symptoms of digitalis toxicity with patient and family. Advise patient to notify physician immediately if these symptoms or those of congestive heart failure occur. Inform patients that these symptoms may be mistaken for those of colds or flu.
- Caution patient to avoid concurrent use of over-the-counter medications without consulting the physician.
- Advise patient to notify physician or dentist of this medication regimen prior to treatment.
- Patients taking cardiac glycosides should carry identification describing disease process and medication regimen at all times.
- Emphasize the importance of routine follow-up examinations to determine effectiveness and to monitor for toxicity.

Evaluation
Effectiveness of therapy can be demonstrated by: ▪ Decrease in severity of congestive heart failure and peripheral edema ▫ Increase in cardiac output ▪ Decrease in ventricular response in tachyarrhythmias ▪ Termination of paroxysmal atrial tachycardia.

DESMOPRESSIN
(des-moe-**press**-in)
Concentraid, DDAVP, Stimate

CLASSIFICATION(S):
Hormone—antidiuretic
Pregnancy Category B

INDICATIONS
▪ **Intranasal:** Management of primary nocturnal enuresis unresponsive to other treatment modalities ▪ **Intranasal, SC, IV:** Treatment of diabetes insipidus caused by a deficiency of vasopressin ▪ **SC, IV:** Control bleeding in certain types of hemophilia and von Willebrand's disease ▪ **Intranasal:** Concentraid product only used for testing of renal concentrating ability.

ACTION
▪ An analogue of naturally occurring vasopressin (antidiuretic hormone). Primary action is enhanced reabsorption of water in the kidneys. **Therapeu-**

D

tic Effects: ▪ Prevention of nocturnal enuresis ▪ Maintenance of appropriate body water content in diabetes insipidus ▪ Control of bleeding in certain types of hemophilia or von Willebrand's disease.

PHARMACOKINETICS

Absorption: Some absorption (10–20%) from nasal mucosa.
Distribution: Distribution not fully known. Enters breast milk.
Metabolism and Excretion: Metabolism and excretion not known.
Half-life: 75 min.

CONTRAINDICATIONS AND PRECAUTIONS

Contraindicated in: ▪ Hypersensitivity ▪ Hypersensitivity to chlorobutanol ▪ Patients with type 11B or platelet-type (pseudo) von Willebrand's disease.
Use Cautiously in: ▪ Angina pectoris ▪ Hypertension ▪ Pregnancy or lactation (safety not established).

ADVERSE REACTIONS AND SIDE EFFECTS*

CNS: headache, drowsiness, listlessness.
EENT: rhinitis, nasal congestion.
Resp: dyspnea.
CV: hypertension, hypotension, and tachycardia (large IV doses only).
GI: nausea, mild abdominal cramps.
GU: vulval pain.
Derm: flushing.
F and E: water intoxication and hyponatremia.
Local: phlebitis at IV site.

INTERACTIONS

Drug–Drug: ▪ **Chlorpropamide, clofibrate,** or **carbamazepine** may enhance the antidiuretic response to desmopressin ▪ **Demeclocycline, lithium,** or **norepinephrine** may diminish the antidiuretic response to desmopressin.

ROUTE AND DOSAGE

Primary Nocturnal Enuresis

- **Intranasal (Children ≥6 yr):** 20 mcg (10 mcg in each nostril) at bedtime (range 10–40 mcg).

Diabetes Insipidus

- **Intranasal (Adults):** 5–40 mcg (0.05–0.4 ml of 0.01% soln) as single dose or in divided doses 1–3 times daily.
- **Intranasal (Children 3 mon–12 yr):** 5–30 mcg (0.05–0.3 ml of 0.01% soln) as a single dose or in divided doses 2 times daily.
- **SC, IV (Adults):** 2–4 mcg/day in 2 divided doses.

Hemophilia A and Type I von Willebrand's Disease

- **IV (Adults and Children >3 mon):** 0.3 mcg/kg by slow infusion 30 min preop.

Renal Concentrating Test

- **Intranasal (Adults):** 40 mcg (20 mcg in each nostril—contents of 2 pipets).
- **Intranasal (Children 1–12 yr):** 20 mcg (1 pipet).

PHARMACODYNAMICS (intranasal = antidiuretic effect; IV = effect on factor VIII activity)

	ONSET	PEAK	DURATION
Intranasal	1 hr	1–5 hr	8–20 hr
IV	within min	15–30 min	3 hr (4–24 hr in mild hemophilia A)

NURSING IMPLICATIONS

Assessment

- **Nocturnal Enuresis:** Monitor frequency of enuresis throughout therapy.
- **Diabetes Insipidus:** Monitor urine osmolality and urine volume frequently to determine effects of medication. Assess patient for symptoms of dehydration (excessive thirst, dry skin and mucous membranes, tachycardia, poor skin turgor). Weigh patient daily and assess for edema.
- **Hemophilia:** When used in hemophilia A and von Willebrand's disease, monitor plasma factor VIII concentrations and bleeding time. Assess patient for signs of bleeding.

*Underlines indicate most frequent; **CAPITALS** indicate life-threatening.

Monitor ristocetin cofactor and Willebrand factor when used for von Willebrand's disease.

- □ Monitor blood pressure and pulse during IV infusion.
- □ Monitor intake and output and adjust fluid intake (especially in children and elderly) to avoid overhydration in patients receiving desmopressin for hemophilia.
- ■ **Toxicity and Overdose:** Signs and symptoms of water intoxication include confusion, drowsiness, headache, weight gain, difficulty urinating, seizures, and coma.
- □ Treatment of overdose includes decreasing dosage and, if symptoms are severe, administration of furosemide.

POTENTIAL NURSING DIAGNOSES

- ■ Fluid volume deficit (indications).
- ■ Fluid volume excess (adverse reactions).
- ■ Knowledge deficit related to medication regimen (patient/family teaching).

IMPLEMENTATION

- ■ **General Info:** IV desmopressin has 10 times the antidiuretic effect of intranasal desmopressin.
- ■ **Diabetes Insipidus:** Parenteral dose for antidiuretic effect is administered direct IV or SC.
- ■ **Hemophilia:** Parenteral for antihemorrhage is administered via IV infusion.
- ■ **Direct IV:** Administer each dose over 1 min for diabetes insipidus.
- ■ **Intermittent Infusion:** Dilute each dose in 50 ml of 0.9% NaCl.
- □ *Rate:* Infuse slowly over 15–30 min for hemophilia.

PATIENT/FAMILY TEACHING

- ■ **General Info:** Advise patient to notify physician if drowsiness, listlessness, headache, dyspnea, heartburn, nausea, abdominal cramps, vulval pain, or severe nasal congestion or irritation occurs.
- □ Caution patient to avoid concurrent use of alcohol with this medication.
- ■ **Diabetes Insipidus:** Instruct patient on intranasal administration. Medication is supplied with a flexible calibrated catheter (rhinyle). Draw soln into rhinyle. Insert one end of tube into nostril, blow on the other end to deposit soln deep into nasal cavity. An air-filled syringe may be attached to the plastic catheter for children, infants, or obtunded patients. Tube should be rinsed under water after each use.
- □ If a dose is missed, instruct patient to take it as soon as remembered, not using if it is almost time for the next dose. Do not double doses.
- □ Advise patient that rhinitis or upper respiratory infection may decrease effectiveness of this therapy. If increased urine output occurs patient should contact physician for dosage adjustment.
- □ Patients with diabetes insipidus should carry identification describing disease process and medication regimen at all times.

EVALUATION

Effectiveness of therapy can be demonstrated by: ■ Decreased frequency of nocturnal enuresis ■ Decrease in urine volume □ Relief of polydipsia □ Increased urine osmolality ■ Control of bleeding in hemophilia.

DEXAMETHASONE

(dex-a-**meth**-a-sone)

Ak-Dex, Dalalone, Decadrol, Decadron, Decaject, Decameth, {Deronil}, Dexacen, Dexasone, Dexon, Hexadrol, Mymethasone, Oradexon, Solurex

CLASSIFICATION(S):

Glucocorticoid—long-acting, Anti-inflammatory agent

Pregnancy Category UK

D

INDICATIONS

■ Used systemically and locally in a wide variety of disorders including: □ Chronic inflammatory disorders □ Allergies □ Hematologic diseases □ Neoplasms □ Autoimmune problems □ Management of cerebral edema and septic shock □ Diagnostic agent in adrenal disorders. **Unlabeled Use:** ■ Short-term administration to high-risk mothers before delivery to prevent respiratory distress syndrome in the newborn.

ACTION

■ Suppresses inflammation and the normal immune response. Has numerous intense metabolic effects ■ Suppresses adrenal function at chronic doses of 0.75 mg/day. Practically devoid of mineralocorticoid (sodium-retaining) activity. **Therapeutic Effects:** ■ Suppression of inflammation and modification of the normal immune response.

PHARMACOKINETICS

Absorption: Well absorbed following oral and IM administration. Chronic high-dose topical application may also lead to systemic absorption. IM acetate salt is long-acting.
Distribution: Widely distributed. Crosses the placenta and probably enters breast milk.
Metabolism and Excretion: Mostly metabolized by the liver; small amounts excreted unchanged by the kidneys.
Half-life: 110–210 min; Adrenal suppression lasts 2.75 days.

CONTRAINDICATIONS AND PRECAUTIONS

Contraindicated in: ■ Active untreated infections (except for certain forms of meningitis) ■ Avoid chronic use during lactation ■ Bisulfite, paraben, or alcohol hypersensitivity—some products contain bisulfites, parabens, or alcohol.
Use Cautiously in: ■ Chronic treatment (will lead to adrenal suppression) ■ Should never be abruptly discontinued ■ Supplemental doses may be needed during stress (surgery, infection) ■ Pregnancy (safety not established) ■ Children (chronic use will result in decreased growth) ■ Use lowest possible dose for shortest period of time.

ADVERSE REACTIONS AND SIDE EFFECTS*

CNS: headache, restlessness, psychoses, depression, euphoria, personality changes, increased intracranial pressure (children only).
EENT: cataracts, increased intraocular pressure.
CV: hypertension.
GI: nausea, vomiting, anorexia, peptic ulceration.
Derm: decreased wound healing, petechiae, ecchymoses, fragility, hirsutism, acne.
Endo: adrenal suppression, hyperglycemia.
F and E: hypokalemia, hypokalemic alkalosis, fluid retention (long-term high doses).
Hemat: thromboembolism, thrombophlebitis.
Metab: weight loss, weight gain.
MS: muscle wasting, muscle pain, aseptic necrosis of joints, osteoporosis.
Misc: increased susceptibility to infection, cushingoid appearance (moon face, buffalo hump).

INTERACTIONS

Drug-Drug: ■ Additive hypokalemia with **diuretics, amphotericin B, mezlocillin, piperacillin,** or **ticarcillin** ■ Hypokalemia may increase the risk of **cardiac glycoside** toxicity ■ May increase requirement for **insulin** or **hypoglycemic agents**.

ROUTE AND DOSAGE

Note: 0.75 mg dexamethasone is equivalent to approximately 20 mg hydrocortisone.

*Underlines indicate most frequent; **CAPITALS** indicate life-threatening.

Adrenal Insufficiency

- **PO (Children):** 23.3 mcg (0.0233 mg)/kg or 670 mcg (0.67 mg)/m^2/day in 3 divided doses.

Anti-Inflammatory and Most Other Uses (Note: doses are usually determined by response.)

- **PO (Adults):** 0.5–9 mg daily in single or 3–4 divided doses.
- **PO (Children):** 83.3–333.3 mcg/kg (0.0833–0.3333 mg/kg) or 2.5–10 mg/m^2/day in 3–4 divided doses.
- **IM, IV (Adults):** 0.5–24 mg/day (phosphate).
- **IM (Adults):** 8–16 mg/day (acetate).
- **Intra-Articular (Adults):** 4–16 mg (acetate) single dose, may be repeated q 1–3 wk.
- **Top (Adults):** 0.1% cream, 0.1% gel, or 0.01% or 0.04% spray 3–4 times daily.
- **Top (Children):** 0.1% cream, 0.1% gel, or 0.01% or 0.04% spray 1–2 times daily.
- **Inhaln (Adults):** (100 mcg/spray) 3 sprays 2–4 times daily (up to 12 sprays/day).
- **Inhaln (Children):** (100 mcg/spray) 2 sprays 2–4 times daily.
- **Ophth (Adults and Children):** 1–2 drops of 0.1% soln or susp q 1 hr during the day and q 2 hr at night or 1.25–2.5 cm of 0.05% oint 3–4 times daily initially, then 1–2 times daily, or use soln during day and ointment at night.
- **Nasal (Adults):** 2 sprays in each nostril 2–3 times daily (200 mcg/spray, not to exceed 1200 mcg/day).
- **Nasal (Children 6–12 yr):** 1–2 sprays in each nostril bid (200 mcg/spray, not to exceed 800 mcg/day).

Cerebral Edema

- **IM, IV (Adults):** 10 mg initially, 4–6 mg q 6 hr (phosphate), may be decreased to 2 mg q 8–12 hr, then change to PO.
- **PO (Adults):** 2 mg q 8–12 hr.

Dexamethasone Suppression Test

- **PO (Adults):** 1 mg at 11 p.m. or 0.5 mg q 6 hr for 48 hr.

PHARMACODYNAMICS (peak = peak blood levels; duration = duration of adrenal suppression or anti-inflammatory activity)

	ONSET	PEAK	DURATION
PO	UK	1–2 hr	2.75 days
IM (phosphate)	rapid	UK	2.75 days
IV (phosphate)	rapid	UK	2.75 days
IM (acetate)	UK	8 hr	6 days
IA (acetate)	UK	UK	1–3 wk

NURSING IMPLICATIONS

Assessment

- **General Info:** This drug is indicated for many conditions. Assess involved systems prior to and periodically throughout course of therapy.
  - Monitor intake and output ratios and daily weights. Observe patient for the appearance of peripheral edema, steady weight gain, rales/crackles, or dyspnea. Notify physician should these occur.
  - Children should have periodic evaluations of growth.
- **Cerebral Edema:** Assess patient for changes in level of consciousness and headache throughout therapy.
- **Intra-articular:** Monitor pain, edema, and range of motion of affected joints.
- **Top:** Assess affected skin prior to and daily during therapy. Note degree of inflammation and pruritis.
- **Inhaln:** Monitor respiratory status and lung sounds.
- **Lab Test Considerations:** Monitor serum electrolytes and glucose. May cause hyperglycemia, especially in persons with diabetes. May cause hypokalemia.
  - Promptly report presence of guaiac-positive stools.
  - Periodic adrenal function tests may be ordered to assess degree of hypothalamic-pituitary-adrenal axis suppression in systemic and chronic topical therapy.

D

- **Dexamethasone Suppression Test:** To diagnose Cushing's syndrome: obtain baseline cortisol level; administer dexamethasone at 11 p.m. and obtain cortisol levels at 8 a.m. the next day. Normal response is a decreased cortisol level.
- □ Alternative method: Obtain baseline 24-hr urine for 17-hydroxycorticosteroid (OHCS) concentrations, then begin 48-hr administration of dexamethasone. Second 24-hr urine for 17-OHCS is obtained after 24 hr of dexamethasone.

Potential Nursing Diagnoses

- Infection, high risk for (side effects).
- Knowledge deficit related to medication regimen (patient/family teaching).

Implementation

- **General Info:** If dose is ordered daily, administer in the morning to coincide with the body's normal secretion of cortisol.
- □ Available in oral, topical, otic, nasal, ophthalmic, inhalation, and injectable forms. Injectable forms are for IM, IV, intra-articular, and intralesional administration.
- **PO:** Administer with meals to minimize gastric irritation.
- **Direct IV:** May be given undiluted over 1 min. Do not administer suspension IV.
- **Intermittent IV:** May be added to D5W or 0.9% NaCl soln. Administer infusions at prescribed rate. Diluted soln should be used within 24 hr.

Dexamethasone sodium phosphate

- **Syringe Compatibility:** metoclopramide or ranitadine.
- **Syringe Incompatibility:** doxapram or glycopyrrolate.
- **Y-Site Compatibility:** acyclovir, famotidine, foscarnet, heparin, hydrocortisone, potassium, ondansetron, or zidovudine.
- **Additive Compatibility:** aminophylline, bleomycin, cimetidine, lidocaine, nafcillin, netilmicin, prochlorperazine, or verapamil.
- **Additive Incompatibility:** daunorubicin, doxorubicin, metaraminol, or vancomycin.
- **Top:** Apply to clean, slightly moist skin. Wear gloves.
- □ Apply occulsive dressing only with physician's order. Apply aerosol form from a distance of 15 cm for 1–2 sec.
- **Inhaln:** Allow at least 1 min between inhalations of aerosol medication.
- **Ophth:** Have patient tilt head back and look up, gently depress lower lid with index finger until conjunctival sac is exposed, and instill medication. Wait at least 5 min before instilling other types of eyedrops.

Patient/Family Teaching

- **General Info:** Instruct patient to take medication exactly as directed, not to skip doses or double up on missed doses. Stopping the medication suddenly may result in adrenal insufficiency (anorexia, nausea, fatigue, weakness, hypotension, dyspnea, and hypoglycemia). If these signs appear notify physician immediately. This can be life-threatening.
- □ Instruct patient on correct technique of medication administration. Emphasize importance of avoiding the eyes unless ophthalmic form is specified.
- □ Encourage patient on long-term therapy to eat diet high in protein, calcium, and potassium and low in sodium and carbohydrates (see Appendix K for foods included).
- □ This drug causes immunosuppression and may mask symptoms of infection. Instruct patient to avoid people with known contagious illnesses and to report possible infections immediately.
- □ Review side effects with patient. Instruct patient to inform physician promptly if severe abdominal pain or tarry stools occur. Patient should also report unusual swelling, weight gain, tiredness, bone pain, bruising, nonhealing sores, visual disturbances, or behavior changes.
- □ Instruct patient to inform physician if symptoms of underlying disease return or worsen.

- ▫ Advise patient to carry identification describing medication regimen in the event of an emergency in which patient cannot relate medical history.
- ▫ Caution patient to avoid vaccinations without consulting physician.
- ▫ Explain need for continued medical follow-up to assess effectiveness and possible side effects of medication. Physician may order periodic lab tests and eye examinations.
- ▫ Emphasize the importance of follow-up examinations to monitor progress and side effects.
- ▪ **Inhaln:** Advise patients using inhalation glucocorticoids and bronchodilator to use bronchodilator first and to allow 5 min to elapse before administering the glucocorticoid, unless otherwise directed by physician.
- ▫ Instruct patient in the proper use of the metered-dose inhaler. Shake well, exhale, close lips firmly around mouthpiece, administer during second half of inhalation, and hold breath as long as possible after treatment to ensure deep instillation of medication. Do not take more than 2 inhalations at one time; allow 1–2 min between inhalations. Wash inhalation assembly at least daily in warm running water.

EVALUATION

Effectiveness of therapy can be demonstrated by: ▪ Suppression of the inflammatory and immune responses in autoimmune disorders and allergic reactions ▪ Decrease in intracranial pressure.

DEXTROAMPHETAMINE

(dex-troe-am-**fet**-a-meen)
Dexampex, Dexedrine, Ferndex, Oxydess II, Spancap #1

CLASSIFICATION(S):
CNS Stimulant
Schedule II
Pregnancy Category C

INDICATIONS

▪ Treatment of narcolepsy ▪ Adjunct in the management of attention deficit disorder (ADD).

ACTION

▪ Produces CNS stimulation by releasing norepinephrine from nerve endings. Pharmacologic effects: ▫ CNS and respiratory stimulation ▫ Vasoconstriction ▫ Mydriasis (pupillary dilation) ▫ Contraction of the urinary bladder sphincter. **Therapeutic Effects:** ▪ Increased motor activity and mental alertness and decreased fatigue in narcoleptic patients ▪ Increased attention span in attention deficit disorder.

PHARMACOKINETICS

Absorption: Well absorbed following oral administration.
Distribution: Widely distributed throughout body tissues with high concentrations in the brain and CSF. Crosses the placenta and enters breast milk. Potentially embryotoxic.
Metabolism and Excretion: Some metabolism by the liver. Urinary excretion is pH-dependent. Alkaline urine promotes reabsorption and prolongs action.
Half-life: 10–12 hr (6.8 hr in children).

CONTRAINDICATIONS AND PRECAUTIONS

Contraindicated in: ▪ Pregnancy or lactation ▪ Hyperexcitable states, including hyperthyroidism ▪ Psychotic personalities ▪ Suicidal or homicidal tendencies ▪ Chemical dependence ▪ Glaucoma.
Use Cautiously in: ▪ Cardiovascular disease ▪ Hypertension ▪ Diabetes mellitus ▪ Elderly or debilitated patients ▪ Continual use (may result in psychological dependence or physical addiction).

ADVERSE REACTIONS AND SIDE EFFECTS*

CNS: restlessness, tremor, hyperactiv-

*Underlines indicate most frequent; **CAPITALS** indicate life-threatening.

ity, insomnia, irritability, dizziness, headache.
CV: tachycardia, palpitations, hypertension, hypotension.
GI: nausea, vomiting, anorexia, dry mouth, cramps, diarrhea, constipation, metallic taste.
GU: impotence, increased libido.
Derm: urticaria.
Misc: psychological dependence, physical dependence.

INTERACTIONS

Drug–Drug: ▪ Additive adrenergic effects with other **adrenergic agents** ▪ Use with **monoamine oxidase inhibitors** can result in hypertensive crisis ▪ Alkalinizing the urine (**sodium bicarbonate, acetazolamide**) decreases excretion, prolongs effect ▪ Acidification of urine (**ammonium chloride,** large doses of **ascorbic acid**) decreases effect ▪ **Phenothiazines** may decrease effect of dextroamphetamine ▪ May antagonize the response to **antihypertensives** ▪ Increased risk of cardiovascular side effects with **beta blockers** or **tricyclic antidepressants**.

ROUTE AND DOSAGE

Attention Deficit Disorder

- **PO (Children >6 yr):** 5–10 mg/day in 1–2 doses, increase by 5 mg at weekly intervals.
- **PO (Children 3–5 yr):** 2.5 mg/day, increase by 2.5 mg at weekly intervals.

Narcolepsy

- **PO (Adults):** 5–60 mg/day in divided doses.
- **PO (Children >12 yr):** 10 mg/day, increase by 10 mg at weekly intervals.
- **PO (Children 6–12 yr):** 5 mg/day, increase by 5 mg/day at weekly intervals.

PHARMACODYNAMICS (CNS stimulation)

	ONSET	PEAK	DURATION
PO	1–2 hr	UK	2–10 hr

NURSING IMPLICATIONS

Assessment

- **General Info:** Monitor blood pressure, pulse, and respiration before administering and periodically throughout course of therapy.
- □ May produce a false sense of euphoria and well-being. Provide frequent rest periods and observe patient for rebound depression after the effects of the medication have worn off.
- □ Has high dependence and abuse potential. Tolerance to medication occurs rapidly; do not increase dose.
- **Attention Deficit Disorders:** Assess attention span, impulse control, and interactions with others in children.
- **Narcolepsy:** Observe and document frequency of episodes.

Potential Nursing Diagnoses

- Thought processes, altered (side effects).
- Knowledge deficit related to medication regimen (patient/family teaching).

Implementation

- **General Info:** Therapy should utilize the lowest effective dose.
- □ Available in tablets, capsules, and elixir preparations.
- **PO:** Extended-release capsules should be swallowed whole; do not break, crush, or chew.

Patient/Family Teaching

- **General Info:** Instruct patient to take medication at least 6 hr before bedtime to avoid sleep disturbances. Missed doses should be taken as soon as remembered up to 6 hr before bedtime. Do not double doses. Instruct patient not to alter dosage without consulting physician. Abrupt cessation with high doses may cause extreme fatigue and mental depression.
- □ Inform patient that the effects of drug-induced dry mouth can be minimized by rinsing frequently with water or chewing sugarless gum or candies.
- □ Advise patient to avoid the intake of large amounts of caffeine.

- Medication may impair judgment. Advise patients to use caution when driving or during other activities requiring alertness.
- Advise patient to notify physician if nervousness, restlessness, insomnia, dizziness, anorexia, or dry mouth becomes severe.
- Inform patient that physician may order periodic holiday from the drug to assess progress and decrease dependence.

EVALUATION

Effectiveness of therapy can be demonstrated by: ▪ Decreased incidence of narcolepsy ▪ Improved attention span and social interactions.

DEXTROMETHORPHAN

(dex-troe-meth-**or**-fan)
{Balminil DM}, Benylin DM, {Broncho-Grippol-DM}, Cremacoat 1, Delsym, DM Cough, {DM Syrup}, Hold, {Koffex}, {Neo-DM}, Pertussin 8-Hour Cough Formula, {Robidex}, Romilar, St. Joseph for Children, {Sedatuss}, Sucrets Cough Control Formula

CLASSIFICATION(S):
Antitussive
Pregnancy Category UK

INDICATIONS

▪ Symptomatic relief of coughs caused by minor viral upper respiratory tract infections or inhaled irritants ▪ Most effective for chronic nonproductive cough ▪ A common ingredient in nonprescription cough and cold preparations.

ACTION

▪ Suppresses the cough reflex by a direct effect on the cough center in the medulla. Related to narcotics structurally but has no analgesic properties. **Therapeutic Effect:** ▪ Relief of irritating nonproductive cough.

PHARMACOKINETICS

Absorption: Rapidly absorbed from the GI tract.
Distribution: Distribution not known. Probably crosses the placenta and enters breast milk.
Metabolism and Excretion: Probably metabolized by the liver.
Half-life: UK.

CONTRAINDICATIONS AND PRECAUTIONS

Contraindicated in: ▪ Hypersensitivity ▪ Patients taking monoamine oxidase inhibitors ▪ Should not be used for chronic productive coughs.
Use Cautiously in: ▪ Cough that lasts more than 1 wk or is accompanied by fever, rash, or headache—physician should be consulted ▪ Pregnancy, lactation, or children <2 yr (safety not established).

ADVERSE REACTIONS AND SIDE EFFECTS*

CNS: high dose—dizziness, sedation.
GI: nausea.

INTERACTIONS

Drug–Drug: ▪ Use with **MAO inhibitors** may result in excitation, hypotension, and hyperpyrexia. ▪ Additive CNS depression with **antihistamines, alcohol, antidepressants, sedative/hypnotics,** or **narcotic analgesics**.

ROUTE AND DOSAGE

- **PO (Adults):** 10–20 mg q 4 hr or 30 mg q 6–8 hr or 60 mg of extended-release preparation bid (not to exceed 120 mg/day).
- **PO (Children 6–11 yr):** 5–10 mg q 4 hr or 15 mg q 6–8 hr or 30 mg of extended-release preparation bid.
- **PO (Children 2–5 yr):** 2.5–5 mg q 4 hr or 7.5 mg q 6–8 hr or 15 mg of extended-release preparation bid.

{} = Available in Canada only.

*Underlines indicate most frequent; **CAPITALS** indicate life-threatening.

PHARMACODYNAMICS (cough suppression)

	ONSET	PEAK	DURATION
PO	15–30 min	UK	3–6 hr

NURSING IMPLICATIONS

Assessment

- **General Info:** Assess frequency and nature of cough, lung sounds, and amount and type of sputum produced. Unless contraindicated, maintain fluid intake of 1500–2000 ml to decrease viscosity of bronchial secretions.

Potential Nursing Diagnoses

- Airway clearance, ineffective (indications).
- Knowledge deficit related to medication regimen (patient/family teaching).

Implementation

- **General Info:** Available in many over-the-counter combination products. Forms include chewable tablets, lozenges, syrups, and suspensions.
  - Available in combination with other products (see Appendix A).
- **PO:** Do not give fluids immediately after administering to prevent dilution of vehicle. Shake oral suspension well before administration. Chewable tablets should be chewed well and not swallowed whole.

Patient/Family Teaching

- Instruct patient to cough effectively: sit upright and take several deep breaths before attempting to cough.
- Advise patient to minimize cough by avoiding irritants, such as cigarette smoke, fumes, and dust. Humidification of environmental air, frequent sips of water, and sugarless hard candy may also decrease the frequency of dry, irritating cough.
- Caution patient to avoid taking alcohol or other CNS depressants concurrently with this medication.
- May occasionally cause dizziness or drowsiness. Caution patient to avoid driving or other activities requiring alertness until response to the medication is known.
- Advise patient that any cough lasting over 1 wk or accompanied by fever, chest pain, persistent headache, or skin rash warrants medical attention.

Evaluation

Effectiveness of therapy can be demonstrated by: ■ Decrease in frequency and intensity of cough without eliminating patient's cough reflex.

DEXTROSE

Glucose, Insta-glucose

CLASSIFICATION(S):
Caloric agent—carbohydrate
Pregnancy Category C

INDICATIONS

■ Lower-concentration (2.5–11.5%) injection is used to provide hydration and calories ■ Higher concentrations (up to 70%) are used IV to treat hyperglycemia and in combination with amino acids to provide calories for parenteral nutrition ■ Oral forms are used to correct hypoglycemia in conscious patients.

ACTION

■ Provides calories. **Therapeutic Effects:** ■ Provision of calories ■ Prevention and treatment of hypoglycemia.

PHARMACOKINETICS

Absorption: Well absorbed following oral administration.

Distribution: Widely distributed and rapidly utilized.

Metabolism and Excretion: Metabolized to carbon dioxide and water. When renal threshold is exceeded, dextrose is excreted unchanged by the kidneys.

Half-life: UK.

CONTRAINDICATIONS AND PRECAUTIONS

Contraindicated in: ■ Allergy to corn or corn products ■ Hypertonic soln (>5%) should not be given to patients with CNS bleeding or anuria or who are at risk of dehydration.

Use Cautiously in: ▪ Known diabetic patients (frequent lab assessment necessary to quantitate appropriate doses) ▪ Chronic alcoholics (administration requires initial pretreatment with thiamine).

ADVERSE REACTIONS AND SIDE EFFECTS*

Endo: inappropriate insulin secretion (long-term use).

F and E: hypokalemia, hypophosphatemia, hypomagnesemia, fluid overload.

Local: local pain and irritation at IV site (hypertonic soln).

Metab: hyperglycemia, glycosuria.

INTERACTIONS

Drug-Drug: ▪ Will alter requirements for **insulin** or **oral hypoglycemic agents** in diabetic patients.

ROUTE AND DOSAGE

Hydration (as 5% soln)

- **IV (Adults and Children):** 0.5–0.8 g/kg/hr.

Hypoglycemia

- **PO (Conscious Adults and Children):** 10–20 g, may repeat in 10–20 min.
- **IV (Adults):** 20–50 ml of 50% soln infused slowly (3 ml/min).
- **IV (Infants and Neonates):** 2 ml/kg of 10–15% soln infused slowly.

PHARMACODYNAMICS (effects on blood sugar in diabetic patients)

	ONSET	PEAK	DURATION
PO	rapid	rapid	brief
IV	rapid	rapid	brief

NURSING IMPLICATIONS

Assessment

- ▫ Assess the hydration status of patients receiving IV dextrose. Monitor intake and output and electrolyte concentrations. Assess patient for dehydration or edema.
- ▫ Assess nutritional status, function of gastrointestinal tract, and caloric needs of patient.
- ▫ Diabetics and patients receiving hypertonic dextrose soln (>5%) should have serum glucose monitored regularly.
- ▫ Monitor IV site frequently for phlebitis and infection.
- ▪ **Lab Test Considerations:** May cause an elevated serum glucose.

Potential Nursing Diagnoses

- ▪ Fluid volume deficit (indications).
- ▪ Nutrition, altered: less than body requirements (indications).
- ▪ Fluid volume excess (adverse reactions).

Implementation

- ▪ **General Info:** Dextrose soln alone does not contain enough calories to sustain an individual for a prolonged period. Dextrose contains 3.4 kcal/g. D5W contains 170 cal/liter and D10W contains 340 cal/liter.
- ▫ Available parenterally in combination with alcohol, dextran, hetastarch, NaCl, potassium, and electrolyte soln.
- ▪ **PO:** Concentrated dextrose gels and chewable tablets may be used in the treatment of hypoglycemia in conscious patients. The dose should be repeated if symptoms persist and serum glucose has not increased by at least 20 mg/100 ml within 20 min.
- ▪ **IV:** Hypertonic dextrose soln (>5%) should be administered IV into a central vein. For emergency treatment of hypoglycemia administer slowly into a large peripheral vein to prevent phlebitis or sclerosis of the vein. Assess IV site frequently. Rapid infusions may cause hyperglycemia or fluid shifts. When hypertonic soln is discontinued, taper soln and administer D5W or D10W to prevent rebound hypoglycemia.
- ▫ Patients requiring prolonged infusions of dextrose should have electrolytes added to the dextrose soln to prevent water intoxication and main-

*Underlines indicate most frequent; **CAPITALS** indicate life-threatening.

D

tain fluid and electrolyte balance.
- **Additive Incompatibility:** warfarin or whole blood.

Patient/Family Teaching
- Explain the purpose of dextrose administration to patient.
- Instruct diabetic patient on the correct method for self-blood glucose monitoring.
- Advise patient on when and how to administer dextrose products for hypoglycemia.

Evaluation
Effectiveness of therapy can be demonstrated by: ▪ Correction and maintenance of adequate hydration status and normal serum glucose levels ▪ Maintenance of adequate caloric intake.

DEZOCINE
(**dez**-oh-seen)
Dalgan

CLASSIFICATION(S):
Narcotic analgesic—agonist/antagonist
Pregnancy Category C

INDICATIONS
- Management of moderate to severe pain.

ACTION
▪ Binds to opiate receptors in the CNS ▪ Alters the perception of and the response to painful stimuli, while causing generalized CNS depression ▪ Has partial antagonist properties, which may result in narcotic withdrawal in physically dependent patients. **Therapeutic Effect:** ▪ Relief of moderate to severe pain.

PHARMACOKINETICS
Absorption: Rapidly and completely absorbed following IM administration.
Distribution: Distribution not known.
Metabolism and Excretion: Mostly metabolized by the liver. <1% excreted unchanged by the kidneys.
Half-life: 2.4 hr (range 1.2–7.4 hr).

CONTRAINDICATIONS AND PRECAUTIONS
Contraindicated in: ▪ Hypersensitivity to dezocine or bisulfites.
Use Cautiously in: ▪ Head trauma ▪ Increased intracranial pressure ▪ Severe renal, hepatic, or pulmonary disease (dosage reduction recommended) ▪ Undiagnosed abdominal pain ▪ Geriatric patients (initial dosage reduction recommended) ▪ Pregnancy, labor, lactation, or children <18 yr (safety not established).

ADVERSE REACTIONS AND SIDE EFFECTS*
CNS: drowsiness, anxiety, confusion, crying, dizziness, lightheadedness, slurred speech.
EENT: miosis, blurred vision, double vision.
CV: orthostatic hypotension.
Resp: respiratory depression.
GI: nausea, vomiting, abdominal pain, constipation, dry mouth.
GU: urinary frequency, hesitancy, retention.
Derm: flushing or redness of skin.
Misc: tolerance, physical dependence, psychological dependence.

INTERACTIONS
Drug-Drug: ▪ Use with caution in patients receiving **MAO inhibitors** (may result in unpredictable reactions) ▪ Additive CNS depression with **alcohol, antihistamines,** and **sedative/hypnotics** ▪ May precipitate withdrawal in patients who are dependent on **narcotic analgesic agonists** and have not been detoxified ▪ May diminish the analgesic effects of other **narcotic analgesics**.

ROUTE AND DOSAGE
- **IM (Adults):** 10 mg (range: 5–20 mg) every 3–6 hr as needed.
- **IV (Adults):** 5 mg initially (range: 2.5–10 mg) every 2–4 hr as needed.

*Underlines indicate most frequent; **CAPITALS** indicate life-threatening.

PHARMACODYNAMICS

	ONSET	PEAK	DURATION
IM	within 30 min	1–2 hr	3–6 hr
IV	within 15 min	UK	2–4 hr

NURSING IMPLICATIONS

Assessment

- Assess type, location, and intensity of pain prior to and 60 min following IM and 30 min following IV administration.
- Assess blood pressure, pulse, and respirations before and periodically during administration. Dezocine does produce respiratory depression, but this does not markedly increase with increased doses.
- While this drug has a low potential for dependence, prolonged use may lead to physical and psychological dependence and tolerance. This should not prevent patient from receiving adequate analgesia. Most patients who receive dezocine for medical reasons do not develop psychological dependence. Progressively higher doses may be required to relieve pain with long-term therapy.
- Assess prior analgesic history. Antagonistic properties may induce withdrawal symptoms (vomiting, restlessness, abdominal cramps, and increased blood pressure and temperature) in narcotic-dependent patients.
- **Toxicity and Overdose:** If overdose occurs, respiratory depression may be partially reversed by naloxone (Narcan), the antidote.

Potential Nursing Diagnoses

- Comfort, altered: pain (indications).
- Injury, high risk for (side effects).
- Sensory-perceptual alteration: visual, auditory (side effects).

Implementation

- **General Info:** Explain therapeutic value of medication prior to administration to enhance the analgesic effect.
- Regularly administered doses may be more effective than prn administration. Analgesic is more effective if given before pain becomes severe.
- Coadministration with non-narcotic analgesics may have additive effects and permit lower narcotic doses.
- **IM:** Administer IM injections deep into well-developed muscle. Rotate sites of injections. Avoid SC injections.
- **Direct IV:** May give IV undiluted.
- *Rate:* Administer slowly, each 5 mg over 3–5 min.

Patient/Family Teaching

- Instruct patient on how and when to ask for prn pain medication.
- Dezocine may cause drowsiness or dizziness. Advise patient to call for assistance when ambulating and to avoid driving or other activities requiring alertness until response to the medication is known.
- Caution patient to make position changes slowly to minimize orthostatic hypotension.
- Advise patient that frequent mouth rinses, good oral hygiene, and sugarless gum or candy may decrease dry mouth.
- Encourage patient to turn, cough, and breathe deeply every 2 hr to prevent atelectasis.
- Advise patient to avoid concurrent use of alcohol or other CNS depressants with this medication.

Evaluation

Effectiveness of therapy can be demonstrated by: ▪ Decrease in severity of pain without a significant alteration in level of consciousness or respiratory status.

DIAZEPAM

(dye-**az**-e-pam)
{Apo-Diazepam}, {Diazemuls}, {E-Pam}, {Meval}, {Novodipam}, Q-Pam, {Rival}, Stress-Pam, Valium, Valrelease, Vasepam, {Vivol}, Zetran

CLASSIFICATION(S):
Sedative/hypnotic—benzodiazepine, Anticonvulsant—benzodiazepine, Skeletal muscle relaxant—centrally acting
Schedule IV
Pregnancy Category D

INDICATIONS

▪ Management of anxiety ▪ Preoperative sedation ▪ Light anesthesia ▪ Amnesia ▪ Treatment of status epilepticus ▪ Skeletal muscle relaxant ▪ Management of the symptoms of alcohol withdrawal.

ACTION

▪ Depresses the CNS, probably by potentiating gamma-aminobutyric acid (GABA), an inhibitory neurotransmitter ▪ Produces skeletal muscle relaxation by inhibiting spinal polysynaptic afferent pathways ▪ Has anticonvulsant properties due to enhanced presynaptic inhibition. **Therapeutic Effects:** ▪ Relief of anxiety ▪ Sedation ▪ Amnesia ▪ Skeletal muscle relaxation ▪ Cessation of seizure activity.

PHARMACOKINETICS

Absorption: Rapidly absorbed from the GI tract. Absorption from IM sites may be slow and unpredictable.
Distribution: Widely distributed. Crosses the blood-brain barrier. Crosses the placenta and enters breast milk.
Metabolism and Excretion: Highly metabolized by the liver. Some products of metabolism are active as CNS depressants.
Half-life: 20–70 hr.

CONTRAINDICATIONS AND PRECAUTIONS

Contraindicated in: ▪ Hypersensitivity ▪ Cross-sensitivity with other benzodiazepines may exist ▪ Comatose patients ▪ Pre-existing CNS depression ▪ Uncontrolled severe pain ▪ Narrow-angle glaucoma ▪ Pregnancy or lactation.
Use Cautiously in: ▪ Hepatic dysfunction ▪ Severe renal impairment ▪ Patients who may be suicidal or who may have been addicted to drugs previously ▪ Elderly or debilitated patients (dosage reduction required).

ADVERSE REACTIONS AND SIDE EFFECTS*

CNS: <u>dizziness</u>, <u>drowsiness</u>, <u>lethargy</u>, hangover, paradoxical excitation, mental depression, headache.
CV: hypotension (IV only).
Derm: rashes.
EENT: blurred vision.
GI: nausea, vomiting, diarrhea, constipation.
Local: venous thrombosis, phlebitis (IV).
Resp: respiratory depression.
Misc: tolerance, psychological dependence, physical dependence.

INTERACTIONS

Drug-Drug: ▪ **Alcohol, antidepressants, antihistamines,** and **narcotic analgesics**—concurrent use results in additive CNS depression ▪ **Cimetidine, oral contraceptives, disulfiram, fluoxetine, isoniazid, ketoconazole, metoprolol, propoxyphene, propranolol,** or **valproic acid** may decrease the metabolism of diazepam, enhancing its actions ▪ May decrease the efficacy of **levodopa** ▪ **Rifampin** or **barbiturates** may increase the metabolism and decrease effectiveness of diazepam ▪ Sedative effects may be decreased by **theophylline.**

ROUTE AND DOSAGE

Antianxiety, Anticonvulsant

- **PO (Adults):** 2–10 mg 2–4 times daily (15–30 mg of extended-release form once daily).
- **PO (Children >6 mon):** 1–2.5 mg 3–4 times daily.
- **IM, IV (Adults):** 2–10 mg, may repeat in 3–4 hr if needed.

*<u>Underlines</u> indicate most frequent; **CAPITALS** indicate life-threatening.

Precardioversion
- **IV (Adults):** 5–15 mg 5–10 min pre-cardioversion.

Pre-Endoscopy
- **IV (Adults):** up to 20 mg
- **IM (Adults):** 5–10 mg 30 min pre-endoscopy.

Status Epilepticus
- **IV (Adults):** 5–10 mg, followed by up to total of 30 mg in 1 hr, may repeat in 2–4 hr (IM route may be used if IV route unavailable).
- **IM, IV (Children >5 yr):** 1 mg q 2–5 min total of 10 mg, repeat q 2–4 hr.
- **IM, IV (Children 30 days–5 yr):** 0.2–0.5 mg q 2–5 min to maximum of 5 mg.

Skeletal Muscle Relaxation
- **PO (Adults):** 2–10 mg 2–4 times daily (15–30 mg of extended-release form once daily).
- **IM, IV (Adults):** 5–10 mg, may repeat in 2–4 hr.

Tetanic Muscle Spasms
- **IM, IV (Children >5 yr):** 5–10 mg q 3–4 hr as needed.
- **IM, IV (Infants >30 days):** 1–2 mg q 3–4 hr as needed.

Alcohol Withdrawal
- **PO (Adults):** 10 mg 3–4 times in 1st 24 hr, decrease to 5 mg 3–4 times daily.
- **IM, IV (Adults):** 10 mg initially, then 5–10 mg in 3–4 hr as needed.

PHARMACODYNAMICS (sedation)

	ONSET	PEAK	DURATION
PO	30–60 min	1–2 hr	up to 24 hr
IM	within 20 min	0.5–1.5 hr	UK
IV	1–5 min	15–30 min	15–60 min*

*In status epilepticus anticonvulsant duration is 15–20 min.

NURSING IMPLICATIONS

Assessment
- **General Info:** Monitor blood pressure, pulse, and respiratory rate prior to and periodically throughout therapy and frequently during IV therapy.
- □ Assess IV site frequently during administration, as diazepam may cause phlebitis and venous thrombosis.
- □ Prolonged high-dose therapy may lead to psychological or physical dependence. Restrict amount of drug available to patient. Observe depressed patients closely for suicidal tendencies.
- **Anxiety:** Assess degree of anxiety and level of sedation (ataxia, dizziness, slurred speech) prior to and periodically throughout therapy.
- **Seizures:** Observe and record intensity, duration, and location of seizure activity. The initial dose of diazepam offers seizure control for 15–20 min after administration. Institute seizure precautions.
- **Muscle Spasms:** Assess muscle spasm, associated pain, and limitation of movement prior to and throughout course of therapy.
- **Alcohol Withdrawal:** Assess patient experiencing alcohol withdrawal for tremors, agitation, delirium, and hallucinations. Protect patient from injury.
- **Lab Test Considerations:** Hepatic and renal function, and CBC should be evaluated periodically throughout course of prolonged therapy.

Potential Nursing Diagnoses
- Anxiety (indications).
- Mobility, impaired physical (indications).
- Injury, high risk for (side effects).

Implementation
- **General Info:** Available in tablet, extended-release capsule, oral soln, and injectable forms.
- □ Patient should be kept on bedrest and observed for at least 3 hr following parenteral administration.
- **PO:** Administer with food to minimize gastric irritation. Tablets may be crushed and taken with food or water if patient has difficulty swallowing. Swallow extended-release capsules whole; do not crush, break, or chew.
- **IM:** IM injections are painful and erratically absorbed. If IM route is used,

inject deeply into deltoid muscle for maximum absorption.

- **IV:** Resuscitation equipment should be available when diazepam is administered IV.
- **Direct IV:** For IV administration do not dilute or mix with any other drug. If direct IV push is not feasible, administer IV push into tubing as close to insertion site as possible. Continuous infusion is not recommended because of precipitation in IV fluids and absorption of diazepam into infusion bags and tubing. Injection may cause burning and venous irritation; avoid small veins.
  - *Rate:* Administer slowly at a rate of 5 mg over at least 1 min. Infants and children should receive total dose over a minimum of 3–5 min. Rapid injection may cause apnea, hypotension, bradycardia, or cardiac arrest.
- **Syringe Compatibility:** cimetidine.
- **Syringe Incompatibility:** benzquinamide, buprenorphine, doxapram, glycopyrrolate, heparin, or nalbuphine.
- **Y-Site Compatibility:** dobutamine, nafcillin, or quinidine gluconate.
- **Y-Site Incompatibility:** atracurium, heparin, foscarnet, pancuronium, potassium chloride, or vecuronium.
- **Additive Compatibility:** netilmicin or verapamil.
- **Additive Incompatibility:** bleomycin, dobutamine, doxorubicin, or fluorouracil.

PATIENT/FAMILY TEACHING

- **General Info:** Instruct patient to take medication exactly as directed; not to take more than prescribed, or to increase dose if less effective after a few wks without checking with physician. Abrupt withdrawal of diazepam may cause insomnia, unusual irritability or nervousness, and seizures. Advise patient that sharing of this medication may be dangerous.
  - Medication may cause drowsiness, clumsiness, or unsteadiness. Advise patient to avoid driving or other activities requiring alertness until response to drug is known.
  - Caution patient to avoid taking alcohol or other CNS depressants concurrently with this medication.
  - Advise patient to notify physician if pregnancy is suspected or planned.
  - Emphasize the importance of follow-up examinations to determine effectiveness of the medication.
- **Seizures:** Patients on anticonvulsant therapy should carry identification describing disease process and medication regimen at all times.

EVALUATION

Effectiveness of therapy can be demonstrated by: ▪ Decrease in anxiety level. Full therapeutic antianxiety effects occur after 1–2 wk of therapy ▪ Control of seizures ▪ Decrease in muscle spasms ▪ Decreased tremulousness and more rational ideation when used for alcohol withdrawal. Tolerance to medication effects may occur within 4 wk and may require dosage adjustments.

DIAZOXIDE
(dye-az-**ox**-ide)
Hyperstat, Proglycem

CLASSIFICATION(S):
Antihypertensive—vasodilator, Hyperglycemic
Pregnancy Category C (PO)

INDICATIONS

▪ **IV:** Emergency treatment of malignant hypertension ▪ **PO:** Treatment of hypoglycemia associated with hyperinsulinism or other causes.

ACTION

▪ Directly relaxes vascular smooth muscle in peripheral arterioles. Produces reflex tachycardia and increased cardiac output ▪ Inhibits insulin release from the pancreas and decreases peripheral utilization of glucose. **Therapeutic Ef-**

fects: ▪ Lowering of blood pressure ▪ Increased blood glucose.

PHARMACOKINETICS

Absorption: Well absorbed following oral administration.
Distribution: Crosses the blood-brain barrier and placenta.
Metabolism and Excretion: 50% metabolized by the liver. 50% excreted unchanged by the kidneys.
Half-life: 21–45 hr.

CONTRAINDICATIONS AND PRECAUTIONS

Contraindicated in: ▪ Hypersensitivity.
Use Cautiously in: ▪ Diabetics (hyperglycemia accompanies use) ▪ Pregnancy and lactation (safety not established—may inhibit labor) ▪ Cardiovascular disease ▪ Uremia.

ADVERSE REACTIONS AND SIDE EFFECTS*

CV: edema, tachycardia, angina, arrhythmias, hypotension, flushing, congestive heart failure.
Derm: hirsutism.
Endo: hyperglycemia.
F and E: sodium and water retention.
Local: phlebitis at IV site.

INTERACTIONS

Drug-Drug: ▪ Concurrent **diuretic** therapy may potentiate hyperglycemic, hyperuricemic, and hypotensive effects ▪ May increase the metabolism and decrease the effectiveness of **phenytoin** ▪ **Phenytoin, corticosteroids,** and **estrogen/progesterone** may increase hyperglycemia.

ROUTE AND DOSAGE

Hypertension

- **IV (Adults and Children):** 1–3 mg/kg every 5–15 min.

Hypoglycemia

- **PO (Adults and Children):** 3–8 mg/kg/day given in divided doses every 8–12 hr.
- **PO (Infants and Newborns):** 8–15 mg/kg/day in divided doses every 8–12 hr.

PHARMACODYNAMICS

	ONSET	PEAK	DURATION
PO (blood sugar)	1 hr	8–12 hr	8 hr
IV (blood pressure)	immediate	5 min	3–12 hr

NURSING IMPLICATIONS

Assessment

- **General Info:** Assess for allergy to sulfonamide drugs.
- □ Assess patient routinely for signs and symptoms of congestive heart failure (peripheral edema, dyspnea, rales/crackles, fatigue, weight gain, jugular venous distension). Notify physician if these occur.
- **Hypertension:** Monitor blood pressure and pulse every 5 min until stable and then hourly. Report significant changes to physician immediately.
- **Hypoglycemia:** Assess patient for signs of hyperglycemia (drowsiness, fruity breath, increased urination, unusual thirst). Monitor blood glucose on diabetic patients requiring frequent doses.
- **Lab Test Considerations:** May cause increased serum glucose, BUN, alkaline phosphatase, SGOT (AST), sodium and uric acid levels.
- □ Monitor blood glucose in diabetic patients requiring frequent parenteral doses.
- □ May cause decreased creatinine clearance, hematocrit, and hemoglobin.
- **Toxicity and Overdose:** If severe hypotension occurs, treatment includes Trendelenburg position, volume infusion, and sympathomimetics (norepinephrine).
- □ Patients who develop marked hyperglycemia must be monitored for 7 days while blood glucose concentrations stabilize.

*Underlines indicate most frequent; **CAPITALS** indicate life-threatening.

D

Potential Nursing Diagnoses

- Cardiac output, decreased (side effects).
- Knowledge deficit related to medication regimen (patient/family teaching).

Implementation

- **General Info:** Loop diuretics are commonly given concurrently with this medication to prevent sodium and water retention.
  - Oral and injectable soln must be protected from light. Do not administer darkened soln.
  - Available in capsules and oral suspension for hyperglycemia and injectable form for hypertension.
- **PO:** Shake oral suspension well before use.
- **Direct IV:** Do not administer SC or IM. Injection may cause warmth and pain along injected vein. Monitor IV site closely; extravasation causes cellulitis and pain. Cold packs may be applied if extravasation occurs.
  - *Rate:* Administer undiluted over 30 sec or less only into a peripheral vein to prevent cardiac arrhythmias. May be repeated every 5–15 min as indicated.
  - Have patient remain recumbent for at least 1 hr following IV administration. Take blood pressure standing prior to ambulation.
- **Syringe Compatibility:** heparin.
- **Y-Site Incompatibility:** hydralazine or propranolol.

Patient/Family Teaching

- **Hypoglycemia:** Instruct patient to take medication as directed, at the same time each day.
  - Encourage patient to follow prescribed diet, medication, and exercise regimen to prevent hypoglycemic or hyperglycemic episodes.
  - Review signs of hypoglycemia and hyperglycemia with patient.
  - Advise patient not to switch from capsule to oral suspension form without consulting physician, as oral suspension produces higher blood concentrations.
- **Hypertension:** Instruct patient to make position changes slowly to minimize orthostatic hypotension.
  - Caution patient to avoid taking other medications, especially over-the-counter cold medicine, without consulting physician or pharmacist.
  - Emphasize the importance of routine follow-up examinations, especially during the first few wks of therapy.

Evaluation

Effectiveness of therapy can be demonstrated by: ■ Decrease in blood pressure without the appearance of side effects. This drug is utilized in short-term treatment of hypertension. Oral antihypertensives should be introduced as soon as the hypertensive crisis is controlled ■ Management of hypoglycemia and return to normal serum glucose concentrations. If diazoxide is not effective within 2–3 wk, therapy should be reevaluated.

DIBUCAINE
(dye-byoo-kane)
Nupercainal

CLASSIFICATION(S):
Anesthetic—local
Pregnancy Category C

INDICATIONS

■ Relief of pruritus or pain associated with minor skin disorders including: □ Burns □ Abrasions □ Bruises □ Hemorrhoids □ Other forms of skin irritation.

ACTION

■ Inhibits initiation and conduction of sensory nerve impulses. **Therapeutic Effect:** ■ Local anesthesia with subsequent relief of pain and/or pruritus.

PHARMACOKINETICS

Absorption: Poorly absorbed through intact skin; absorption increases with surface area and abrasions.
Distribution: Distribution not known.

Metabolism and Excretion: Small amounts that may be absorbed are primarily metabolized by the liver.
Half-life: UK.

CONTRAINDICATIONS AND PRECAUTIONS

Contraindicated in: ▪ Hypersensitivity to lidocaine or other amide-type local anesthetics ▪ Hypersensitivity to any components of preparations including stabilizers, colorants, or bases ▪ Active, untreated infection of affected area ▪ Not to be used in the eye.
Use Cautiously in: ▪ Large or severely abraded areas of skin or mucous membrane ▪ Prolonged use (not recommended) ▪ Elderly patients, debilitated patients, and children (use smaller doses) ▪ Children <2 yr (safety not established).

ADVERSE REACTIONS AND SIDE EFFECTS*

Derm: contact dermatitis, urticaria, edema, burning, stinging, tenderness, irritation.
Misc: allergic reactions, including ANAPHYLAXIS.

INTERACTIONS

Drug-Drug: ▪ None signficant.

ROUTE AND DOSAGE

- **Top (Adults):** Apply 0.5% cream or 1% ointment as needed (not to exceed 30 g in 24 hr).
- **Top (Children):** Apply 0.5% cream or 1% ointment as needed (not to exceed 7.5 g in cream or 15 g in ointment in 24 hr).

PHARMACODYNAMICS (anesthetic effect following application to skin)

	ONSET	PEAK	DURATION
Top	up to 15 min	15 min	2–4 hr

NURSING IMPLICATIONS

Assessment

- Assess type, location, and intensity of pain prior to and a few min after administration of dibucaine.
- Assess integrity of involved skin or hemorrhoids prior to and periodically throughout course of therapy. Notify physician if signs of infection or irritation develop.

Potential Nursing Diagnoses

- Comfort, altered: pain (indications).
- Knowledge deficit related to medication regimen (patient/family teaching).

Implementation

- **General Info:** Available as ointment, cream, or suppository.
- **Top:** Apply ointment lightly to affected areas. A light dressing may be applied over the site.
- Apply cream liberally, then gently rub in.
- **Hemorrhoids:** Administer using applicator provided by the manufacturer. Attach applicator to tube and squeeze until small amount of ointment comes through holes in applicator. After administration of internal dose, a small amount of ointment may be applied to anus using a gloved finger.

Patient/Family Teaching

- **General Info:** Instruct patient on correct application technique. Emphasize need to avoid the eyes and not to apply medication to large areas of denuded skin.
- Advise patient to discontinue use if erythema or irritation at site of administration occurs or if the symptoms worsen or persist for more than 7 days.
- **Hemorrhoids:** Instruct patient to notify physician if rectal bleeding occurs.

Evaluation

Effectiveness of therapy can be demonstrated by: ▪ Temporary relief of discomfort associated with minor irritations of skin ▪ Relief of pain and itching associated with hemorrhoids.

*Underlines indicate most frequent; CAPITALS indicate life-threatening.

D

DICLOFENAC

(dye-**kloe**-fen-ak)
Voltaren

CLASSIFICATION(S):
Nonsteroidal anti-inflammatory agent
Pregnancy Category B

INDICATIONS

▪ **PO:** Management of inflammatory disorders including: ▫ Rheumatoid arthritis ▫ Osteoarthritis ▫ Ankylosing spondylitis ▪ **Ophth:** Management of inflammation following cataract extraction.

ACTION

▪ Inhibits prostaglandin synthesis. **Therapeutic Effects:** ▪ Suppression of pain and inflammation.

PHARMACOKINETICS

Absorption: Well absorbed following oral administration. Tablets are delayed-release dosage form. Absorbtion also occurs following ophthalmic administration.
Distribution: Crosses the placenta and enters breast milk.
Metabolism and Excretion: At least 50% metabolized on first pass through the liver.
Half-life: 1.2–2 hr.

CONTRAINDICATIONS AND PRECAUTIONS

Contraindicated in: ▪ Hypersensitivity ▪ Cross-sensitivity may exist with other nonsteroidal anti-inflammatory agents, including aspirin ▪ Active GI bleeding or ulcer disease ▪ Patients who wear soft contact lenses (ophthalmic product only).
Use Cautiously in: ▪ Severe cardiovascular, renal, or hepatic disease ▪ Past history of ulcer disease ▪ Pregnancy, lactation, and children (safety not established) ▪ Elderly patients (dosage reduction recommended; may be more susceptible to adverse reactions) ▪ History of bleeding tendency.

ADVERSE REACTIONS AND SIDE EFFECTS*

Note: Listed as occurring with oral use of dicofenac, except for **EENT**.

CV: hypertension, drowsiness, dizziness, headache.
EENT: Ophth—stinging, anterior chamber reactions, ocular allergy.
GI: abdominal pain, dyspepsia, heartburn, diarrhea, GI BLEEDING, elevated liver enzymes.
GU: frequency, dysuria, hematuria, nephritis, proteinuria, acute renal failure.
Derm: rashes, eczema, photosensitivity.
F and E: edema.
Hemat: prolonged bleeding time.
Misc: allergic reactions, including ANAPHYLAXIS.

INTERACTIONS (Listed as occurring with oral use of dicofenac)

Drug-Drug: ▪ Concurrent use with **aspirin** may decrease effectiveness ▪ Additive adverse GI effects with **aspirin**, other **nonsteroidal anti-inflammatory agents, potassium supplements, glucocorticoids,** or **alcohol** ▪ Chronic use with **acetaminophen** may increase the risk of adverse renal reactions ▪ May decrease the effectiveness of **diuretics, antihypertensive** therapy, **insulin,** or **hypoglycemic agents.** ▪ Increases serum **digoxin** levels (dosage adjustment may be necessary) ▪ May increase serum **lithium** levels and increase the risk of toxicity ▪ Increases the risk of toxicity from **methotrexate** ▪ **Probenecid** increases risk of toxicity from diclofenac ▪ Increased risk of bleeding with **cefamandole, cefotetan, cefoperazone, moxalactam** or **plicamycin, thrombolytic agents,** or **anticoagulants** ▪ Increased risk of adverse hematologic reactions with **antineoplastic agents** or **radiation therapy**.

*Underlines indicate most frequent; **CAPITALS** indicate life-threatening.

ROUTE AND DOSAGE

Rheumatoid Arthritis

- **PO (Adults):** 150–200 mg/day in 2–4 divided doses initially; when response is obtained, decrease dosage to minimum amount required to control symptoms (range 75–100 mg/day in 3 divided doses).

Osteoarthritis

- **PO (Adults):** 100–150 mg/day in 2–3 divided doses initially; when response is obtained, decrease dosage to minimum amount required to control symptoms.

Ankylosing Spondylitis

- **PO (Adults):** 100–125 mg/day in 4–5 divided doses initially; when response is obtained, decrease dosage to minimum amount required to control symptoms.

Postcataract Surgery

- **Ophth (Adults):** 1 drop of 0.1% soln 4 times daily for 2 wk starting 24 hr after procedure.

PHARMACODYNAMICS (anti-inflammatory effects)

	ONSET	PEAK	DURATION
PO	few days–1 wk	2 wk or more	UK
Ophth	rapid	UK	UK

NURSING IMPLICATIONS

Assessment

- **PO:** Assess arthritic pain (note type, location, intensity) and limitation of movement prior to and 30–60 min following administration.
- □ Patients who have asthma, aspirin-induced allergy, and nasal polyps are at increased risk for developing hypersensitivity reactions.
- **Ophth:** Assess patient for eye inflammation throughout therapy.

Potential Nursing Diagnoses

- Comfort, altered: pain (indications).
- Mobility, impaired physical (indications).
- Knowledge deficit related to medication regimen (patient/family teaching).

Implementation

- **PO:** Administer after meals or with food to minimize gastric irritation. Do not crush or chew extended-release tablets.
- **Ophth:** Administer by having patient lie down or tilt head back and look at ceiling. Gently depress lower lid with index finger until conjunctival sac is exposed, and instill 1 drop. Wait at least 5 min before instilling other types of eye drops.

Patient/Family Teaching

- **PO:** Instruct patient to take diclofenac with a full glass of water and to remain in an upright position for 15–30 min after administration.
- □ Caution patient to avoid concurrent use of alcohol or aspirin with this medication.
- □ May cause drowsiness or dizziness. Caution patient to avoid driving or other activities requiring alertness until response to medication is known.
- □ Advise patient to consult physician if rash, itching, visual disturbances, tinnitus, weight gain, edema, black stools, or perisitent headache occurs.
- **Ophth:** Instruct patient on correct technique for instillation of drops.
- □ Inform patient that concurrent use of hydrogel soft contact lenses may cause ocular irritation.

Evaluation

Effectiveness of therapy can be demonstrated by: ▪ Decrease in severity of mild to moderate discomfort □ Increased ease of joint movement. Patients who do not respond to one nonsteroidal anti-inflammatory agent may respond to another ▪ Decrease in ocular irritation following cataract surgery.

DICLOXACILLIN

(dye-**klox**-a-sill-in)
Dicloxacil, Dycill, Dynapen, Pathocil

D

CLASSIFICATION(S):
Anti-infective—penicillinase-resistant penicillin
Pregnancy Category B

INDICATIONS

▪ Treatment of the following infections due to susceptible strains of streptococci or penicillinase-producing staphylococci: ▫ Respiratory tract infections ▫ Sinusitis ▫ Skin and skin structure infections.

ACTION

▪ Binds to bacterial cell wall, leading to cell death. Resists the action of penicillinase, an enzyme capable of inactivating penicillin. **Therapeutic Effect:** ▪ Bactericidal action against susceptible bacteria. **Spectrum:** ▪ Active against most gram-positive aerobic cocci, but less so than penicillin. Spectrum is notable for activity against penicillinase-producing strains of: ▫ *Staphylococcus aureus* ▫ *Staphylococcus epidermidis* ▪ Not active against methicillin-resistant staphylococci.

PHARMACOKINETICS

Absorption: Rapidly but incompletely (35–76%) absorbed from the GI tract.
Distribution: Widely distributed. Penetration into CSF is minimal. Crosses the placenta and enters breast milk.
Metabolism and Excretion: Some metabolism by the liver (6–10%) and some renal excretion of unchanged drug (60%). Small amounts eliminated in the feces via the bile.
Half-life: 0.5–1 hr (increased in severe hepatic and renal dysfunction).

CONTRAINDICATIONS AND PRECAUTIONS

Contraindicated in: ▪ Hypersensitivity ▪ Should not be used as initial therapy in serious infections or in patients experiencing nausea or vomiting.
Use Cautiously in: ▪ Severe renal or hepatic impairment (dosage reduction required) ▪ Pregnancy or lactation (safety not established).

ADVERSE REACTIONS AND SIDE EFFECTS*

CNS: SEIZURES (high doses).
GI: nausea, vomiting, diarrhea, hepatitis.
GU: interstitial nephritis.
Derm: rashes, urticaria.
Hemat: blood dyscrasias.
Misc: superinfection, allergic reactions, including ANAPHYLAXIS and serum sickness.

INTERACTIONS

Drug-Drug: ▪ **Probenecid** decreases renal excretion and increases blood levels ▪ May alter the effect of **oral anticoagulants.**
Drug-Food: ▪ **Food** or **acidic beverages** decreases absorption.

ROUTE AND DOSAGE

- **PO (Adults and Children >40 kg):** 125–250 mg q 6 hr (up to 6 g/day).
- **PO (Children >1 mon and <40 kg):** 12.5–25 mg/kg/day in divided doses q 6 hr.

PHARMACODYNAMICS (blood levels)

	ONSET	PEAK
PO	30 min	0.5–2 hr

NURSING IMPLICATIONS

Assessment

▫ Assess patient for infection (vital signs; appearance of wound, sputum, urine, and stool; WBC) at beginning and throughout course of therapy.
▫ Obtain a history before initiating therapy to determine previous use of and reactions to penicillins or cephalosporins. Persons with a negative history of penicillin sensitivity may still have an allergic response.
▫ Obtain specimens for culture and sensitivity prior to initiating therapy. First dose may be given before receiving results.

*Underlines indicate most frequent; **CAPITALS** indicate life-threatening.

□ Observe patient for signs and symptoms of anaphylaxis (rash, pruritus, laryngeal edema, wheezing, abdominal pain). Discontinue drug and notify physician immediately if these occur. Keep epinephrine, an antihistamine, and resuscitation equipment close by in the event of an anaphylactic reaction.

■ **Lab Test Considerations:** CBC, BUN, creatinine, urinalysis, and liver function tests should be monitored periodically during therapy. May cause an increased SGOT (AST) concentrations.

Potential Nursing Diagnoses

■ Infection, high risk for (indications, side effects).
■ Knowledge deficit related to medications regimen (patient/family teaching).
■ Noncompliance related to medication regimen (patient/family teaching).

Implementation

■ **PO:** Administer around the clock on an empty stomach at least 1 hr before or 2 hr after meals. Take with a full glass of water; acidic juices may decrease absorption of penicillins.
□ Use calibrated measuring device for liquid preparations. Shake well. Soln is stable for 14 days if refrigerated.

Patient/Family Teaching

□ Instruct patient to take medication around the clock and to finish the drug completely as directed, even if feeling better. Missed doses should be taken as soon as remembered. Advise patient that sharing of this medication may be dangerous.
□ Advise patient to report signs of superinfection (black, furry overgrowth on the tongue, vaginal itching or discharge, loose or foul-smelling stools) and allergy.
□ Instruct patient to notify physician if fever and diarrhea develop, especially if stool contains blood, pus, or mucus. Advise patient not to treat diarrhea without consulting physician or pharmacist.
□ Instruct patient to notify physician if symptoms do not improve.

Evaluation

Clinical response to therapy can be evaluated by: ■ Resolution of the signs and symptoms of infection. Length of time for complete resolution depends on the organism and site of infection.

DIDANOSINE

(dye-**dan**-oh-seen)
ddI, dideoxyinosine, Videx

CLASSIFICATION(S):
Antiviral
Pregnancy Category B

INDICATIONS

■ Treatment of symptomatic human immunodeficiency virus (HIV) infection (acquired immunodeficiency syndrome [AIDS] in patients who are unable to tolerate zidovudine (AZT) ■ Treatment of advanced AIDS-related complex (ARC) in patients who are unable to tolerate zidovudine (AZT).

ACTION

■ Inhibits viral replication by interfering with viral RNA-directed DNA polymerase (reverse transcriptase). Must be converted intracellulary by the phosphorylation process to its active form. **Therapeutic Effects:** ■ Virustatic action against susceptible viruses ■ Increase in CD4 cell counts that may result in slowed progression and decreased incidence of opportunistic infections in HIV-infected patients. **Spectrum:** ■ Active against retroviruses, including the human immunodeficiency virus.

PHARMACOKINETICS

Absorption: Rapidly degrades at gastric pH. Buffers in formulation neutralize gastric acid and allow for maximal absorption (33–37%).
Distribution: CSF levels are 21% of plasma levels in adults.

D

Metabolism and Excretion: 55% eliminated by the kidneys (urinary excretion appears to be less in children).
Half-life: 1.6 hr (0.8 hr in children).

CONTRAINDICATIONS AND PRECAUTIONS

Contraindicated in: ▪ Hypersensitivity ▪ Lactation ▪ Phenylketonuria (tablets contain phenylalanine).
Use Cautiously in: ▪ History of gout ▪ Patients on sodium-restricted diets (tablets contain 264.5 mg sodium) ▪ Renal impairment (dosage modification required) ▪ History of seizures.

ADVERSE REACTIONS AND SIDE EFFECTS*

CNS: headache, weakness, insomnia, pain, dizziness, SEIZURES, lethargy.
EENT: rhinitis, ear pain, photophobia, epistaxis.
Resp: cough, asthma.
CV: hypertension, edema, vasodilation, arrhythmias.
GI: PANCREATITIS, diarrhea, nausea, vomiting, (more common with buffered powder for oral soln), abdominal pain, dry mouth, anorexia, weight loss, constipation, stomatitis, liver function abnormalities, LIVER FAILURE.
GU: urinary frequency.
Derm: rash, alopecia, ecchymoses.
Metab: hyperlipidemia.
Hemat: leukopenia, granulocytopenia, anemia, bleeding.
MS: myalgia, arthritis.
Neuro: peripheral neuropathy, poor coordination.
Misc: chills, fever.

INTERACTIONS

Drug-Drug: ▪ Presence of buffers will decrease absorption of **ketoconazole, dapsone, tetracyclines, fluoroquinolones** (wait 2 hr before administering didanosine) ▪ Increased risk of peripheral neuropathy with other **drugs causing peripheral neuropathy** ▪ Increased risk of pancreatitis increased with other **drugs causing pancreatitis.**
Drug-Food: ▪ Administration of didanosine with **food** decreases absorption by 50%.

ROUTE AND DOSAGE

- **PO (Adults ≥75 kg):** 300 mg q 12 hr as tablets or 375 mg q 12 hr as buffered powder. Use two tablets to give each dose.
- **PO (Adults 50–74 kg):** 200 mg q 12 hr as tablets or 250 mg q 12 hr as buffered powder. Use two tablets to give each dose.
- **PO (Adults 35–49 kg):** 125 mg q 12 hr as tablets or 167 mg q 12 hr as buffered powder. Use two tablets to give each dose.
- **PO (Children >6 mon):** 200 mg/m^2/day given q 12 hr as didanosine pediatric powder. Use two tablets to give each dose, unless child is <1 yr.

PHARMACODYNAMICS (antiviral plasma levels)

	ONSET	PEAK
PO	UK	UK

NURSING IMPLICATIONS

Assessment

- ▫ Monitor patient for symptoms of AIDS or AIDS-related complex prior to and throughout course of therapy.
- ▫ Monitor patient for peripheral neuropathy (distal numbness, tingling, or pain in feet or hands) throughout therapy. Dose may need to be decreased.
- ▫ Monitor patient for symptoms of pancreatitis (abdominal pain, nausea, vomiting, increased amylase concentrations). May require discontinuation of therapy. Pancreatitis may be fatal.
- **Lab Test Considerations:** Monitor CBC and hepatic function throughout therapy. May cause leukopenia, granulocytopenia, thrombocytopenia, and anemia. May cause elevated SGOT (AST), SGPT (ALT), alkaline phosphatase, bilirubin, uric acid, and amylase concentrations.

*Underlines indicate most frequent; **CAPITALS** indicate life-threatening.

Potential Nursing Diagnoses
- Infection, high risk for (indications, side effects).
- Injury, high risk for (side effects).
- Knowledge deficit related to medication regimen (patient/family teaching).

Implementation
- **General Info:** If diarrhea develops in patients taking buffered powder for oral soln, chewable/dispersible buffered tablets may cause less diarrhea.
  - If soln or powder spills or leaks, a wet mop or damp sponge should be used for cleaning to avoid generation of dust. Clean surface with soap and water as needed.
- **PO:** Administer every 12 hr on an empty stomach, 1 hr before or 2 hr after meals. Food may decrease the absorption of didanosine by 50%. Do not administer ketoconazole, dapsone, tetracyclines, or fluoroquinolones within 2 hr of didanosine.
  - Tablets should be chewed thoroughly, manually crushed or dispersed in at least 1 oz of water prior to administration. To disperse, add one or two tablets to at least 1 oz of water and stir until a uniform dispersion forms. Dispersion should be taken immediately.
  - Buffered powder for oral soln should be mixed in at least 4 oz of water; do not mix with fruit juice or other acid-containing liquid. Stir 2–3 min until the powder dissolves completely. Soln should be taken immediately.
  - Soln for pediatric use is mixed by pharmacist and is stable for 30 days if refrigerated. Shake admixture immediately before administering.

Patient/Family Teaching
- Instruct patient on the importance of taking didanosine exactly as directed, even if feeling better. Caution patient not to share or trade this medication with others.
- May cause dizziness. Caution patient to avoid driving or other activities requiring alertness until response to medication is known.
- Advise patient to consult physician or pharmacist before taking other medications concurrently with didanosine.
- Caution patient to avoid crowds and persons with known infections.
- Advise patient to notify physician immediately if numbness or tingling of the hands or feet, stomach pain, nausea, or vomiting occur.
- Caution patient to avoid sexual contact, to use a condom to prevent transmission of the AIDS virus, and not to share needles with anyone.
- Children should have dilated retinal examinations every 6 mon during therapy.
- Emphasize the importance of regular examinations to monitor for side effects.

Evaluation
Effectiveness of therapy may be determined by: ■ Decrease in the symptoms of AIDS or AIDS-related complex infections.

DIENESTROL
(dye-en-**ess**-trole)
DV, Estraguard, Ortho Dienestrol

CLASSIFICATION(S):
Hormone—estrogen
Pregnancy Category X

INDICATIONS
- Symptomatic management of atrophic vaginitis in postmenopausal women.

ACTION
- Estrogens promote the growth and development of female sex organs and the maintenance of secondary sex characteristics in women. Metabolic effects include: □ Reduced blood cholesterol □ Protein synthesis □ Sodium and water retention. **Therapeutic Effect:** ■ Restoration of integrity of the vaginal mucosa in postmenopausal women.

PHARMACOKINETICS
Absorption: Readily absorbed through skin and mucous membranes.

D

Distribution: Amounts absorbed are widely distributed.
Metabolism and Excretion: Amounts absorbed are metabolized by the liver.
Half-life: UK.

CONTRAINDICATIONS AND PRECAUTIONS

Contraindicated in: ▪ Thromboembolic disease ▪ Undiagnosed vaginal bleeding ▪ Pregnancy (use may result in harm to the fetus) ▪ Lactation.
Use Cautiously in: ▪ Patients with serious cardiac, hepatic, or renal disease ▪ May increase the risk of endometrial carcinoma.

ADVERSE REACTIONS AND SIDE EFFECTS*

CNS: headache, dizziness, depression.
CV: edema, hypertension.
GI: nausea, vomiting, abdominal cramps, bloating, jaundice.
GU: breakthrough bleeding, dysmenorrhea, vaginal candidiasis, cystitis.
Derm: pigmentation, rashes.
Endo: hyperglycemia.
F and E: hypercalcemia, sodium and water retention.
Hemat: thromboembolism.
Misc: breast tenderness, enlargement, change in libido.

INTERACTIONS

Drug-Drug: ▪ May alter requirements for **oral anticoagulants, oral hypoglycemic agents,** or **insulin.**

ROUTE AND DOSAGE

Note: 1 applicator = 6 g containing 0.6 mg dienestrol.

- **Vag (Adults):** 1–2 applicator/day for 2 wk, then ½ dose for 2 wk. Maintenance dose of 1 applicator 1–3 times/wk for 3 wk of every month.

PHARMACODYNAMICS (symptomatic relief of atrophic vaginitis)*

	ONSET	PEAK	DURATION
Vag	days	UK	UK

*Response is highly variable.

NURSING IMPLICATIONS

Assessment

- □ Blood pressure should be monitored periodically throughout therapy.
- □ Monitor intake and output ratios and weekly weight. Report significant discrepancies or steady weight gain to physician.
- ▪ **Lab Test Considerations:** May cause increased serum glucose and triglycerides and may alter prothrombin levels.

Potential Nursing Diagnoses

- ▪ Sexual dysfunction (indications).
- ▪ Knowledge deficit related to medication regimen (patient/family teaching).

Implementation

- ▪ **Vag:** Manufacturer provides applicator with cream.

Patient/Family Teaching

- □ Instruct patient in the correct use of vaginal applicator. Patient should remain recumbent for at least 30 min after administration. May use sanitary napkin to protect clothing, but do not use tampons.
- □ Explain dosage schedule and maintenance routine. Discontinuing medication suddenly may cause withdrawal bleeding.
- □ Advise patient to report signs and symptoms of fluid retention (swelling of ankles and feet, weight gain), thromboembolic disorders (pain, swelling, tenderness in extremities, headache, chest pain, blurred vision), mental depression, unusual vaginal bleeding, or hepatic dysfunction (yellowed skin or eyes, pruritus, dark urine, light-colored stools) to physician.
- □ Instruct patient to stop taking medication and notify physician if pregnancy is suspected.
- □ Caution patient that cigarette smoking during estrogen therapy may cause increased risk of serious side effects, especially for women over age 35.

- Emphasize the importance of routine follow-up physical examinations, including blood pressure; breast, abdomen, and pelvic examinations; and PAP smears every 6–12 mon.

EVALUATION

Effectiveness of therapy can be demonstrated by: ▪ Decrease in vaginal and vulval itching, inflammation, and dryness.

DIETHYLSTILBESTROL

(dye-eth-il-stil-**bess**-trole)
DES, {Honvol}, Stilphostrol

CLASSIFICATION(S):
Hormone—estrogen, antineoplastic—hormone
Pregnancy Category X

INDICATIONS

▪ Management of severe vasomotor symptoms of menopause ▪ Replacement of estrogen in female hypogonadism or castration ▪ Prophylaxis of postmenopausal osteoporosis ▪ Palliatively in advanced, inoperable metastatic prostate carcinoma and postmenopausal breast carcinoma.

ACTION

▪ Promotes the growth and development of female sex organs and the maintenance of secondary sex characteristics in women ▪ Metabolic effects include reduced blood cholesterol, protein synthesis, and sodium and water retention.
Therapeutic Effects: ▪ Replacement of estrogen effect lost due to a number of causes, decreased tumor spread in androgen-sensitive tumors.

PHARMACOKINETICS

Absorption: Well absorbed from the GI tract.
Distribution: Widely distributed. Crosses the placenta and probably enters breast milk.
Metabolism and Excretion: Metabolized by the liver.
Half-life: UK.

CONTRAINDICATIONS AND PRECAUTIONS

Contraindicated in: ▪ Thromboembolic disease ▪ Undiagnosed vaginal bleeding ▪ Pregnancy (use may result in harm to the fetus) ▪ Lactation.
Use Cautiously in: ▪ Underlying cardiovascular disease ▪ Severe hepatic or renal disease ▪ May increase the risk of endometrial carcinoma.

ADVERSE REACTIONS AND SIDE EFFECTS*

CNS: headache, dizziness, lethargy.
CV: edema, THROMBOEMBOLISM, hypertension, MYOCARDIAL INFARCTION.
EENT: worsening of myopia or astigmatism, intolerance to contact lenses.
GI: nausea, vomiting, anorexia, increased appetite, weight changes, jaundice.
GU: females—breakthrough bleeding, dysmenorrhea, amenorrhea, cervical erosions, vaginal candidiasis, loss of libido; males—testicular atrophy, impotence.
Derm: acne, urticaria, oily skin, pigmentation, photosensitivity.
Endo: hyperglycemia, gynecomastia, (males).
F and E: sodium and water retention, hypercalcemia.
MS: leg cramps.
Misc: breast tenderness.

INTERACTIONS

Drug-Drug: ▪ May alter requirement for **oral anticoagulants, oral hypoglycemic agents,** or **insulin** ▪ **Barbiturates** or **rifampin** may decrease effectiveness.

ROUTE AND DOSAGE

Hypogonadism, Ovarian Failure
- **PO (Adults):** 0.2–0.5 mg/day.

Menopausal Symptoms
- **PO (Adults):** 0.1–2 mg/day for 3 wk, 1 wk off.

{} = Available in Canada only.
*Underlines indicate most frequent; **CAPITALS** indicate life-threatening.

D

Postmenopausal Breast Carcinoma
- **PO (Adults):** 15 mg/day.

Prostate Carcinoma
- **PO (Adults):** 1–3 mg/day of diethylstilbestrol or 50–200 mg 3 times daily as diethylstilbestrol diphosphate (stilphostrol).
- **IV (Adults):** 500 mg as an infusion/day, may be increased to 1 g/day initially until response is obtained (5 or more days), then 250–500 mg 1–2 times weekly.

Postcoital Contraception
- **PO (Adults):** 25 mg bid for 5 days.

PHARMACODYNAMICS (estrogen replacement effect)

	ONSET	PEAK	DURATION
PO	rapid*	UK	UK

*Onset of response for carcinomas may take 4–8 wk.

NURSING IMPLICATIONS

Assessment
- Assess blood pressure prior to and periodically throughout therapy.
- Monitor intake and output ratios and weekly weight. Report significant discrepancies or steady weight gain to physician.
- **Lab Test Considerations:** May cause increased serum glucose, sodium, triglyceride, phospholipid, cortisol, prolactin, prothrombin, and factors VII, VIII, IX, and X levels. May decrease serum folate, pyridoxine, antithrombin III, and pregnanediol excretion concentrations.
- May alter thyroid hormone assays.
- May cause hypercalcemia in patients with metastatic bone lesions.

Potential Nursing Diagnoses
- Sexual dysfunction (indications).
- Knowledge deficit related to medication regimen (patient/family teaching).

Implementation
- **PO:** Administer oral doses with or immediately after food to reduce nausea.
- Do not crush or chew enteric-coated tablets.
- **IV:** Dilute soln in 250–500 ml of D5W or 0.9% NaCl.
- *Rate:* Infuse at a rate of 1–2 ml/min for the first 10–15 min. If infusion is tolerated, adjust the rate so that the entire dose has infused within 1 hr.

Patient/Family Teaching
- Instruct patient to take oral medication as prescribed. If a dose is missed, take as soon as remembered as long as it is not just before next dose. Do not double doses.
- If nausea becomes a problem, advise patient that eating solid food often provides relief.
- Advise patient to report signs and symptoms of fluid retention (swelling of ankles and feet, weight gain), thromboembolic disorders (pain, swelling, tenderness in extremities, headache, chest pain, blurred vision), mental depression, or hepatic dysfunction (yellowed skin or eyes, pruritus, dark urine, light-colored stools) to physician.
- Instruct patient to stop taking medication and notify physician if pregnancy is suspected. Caution patient of the increase in cervical and vaginal carcinoma in female offspring and in testicular tumors in male offspring if this drug is taken during pregnancy.
- Caution patient that cigarette smoking during estrogen therapy may cause increased risk of serious side effects, especially for women over age 35.
- Advise patient to notify physician or dentist of medication regimen prior to treatment or surgery.
- Diethylstilbestrol may occasionally cause a photosensitivity reaction. Caution patient to use sunscreen and protective clothing.
- Emphasize the importance of routine follow-up physical examinations including blood pressure; breast, abdomen, and pelvic examinations; and PAP smears every 6–12 mon.

Evaluation
Effectiveness of therapy can be demonstrated by: ■ Resolution of menopausal

vasomotor symptoms ▫ Decreased vaginal and vulval itching, inflammation, or dryness associated with menopause ▪ Normalization of estrogen levels in female castration or hypogonadism ▪ Control of the spread of advanced metastatic breast or prostatic cancer.

DIFENOXIN/ATROPINE
(dye-fen-**ox**-in/**a**-troe-peen)
Motofen

CLASSIFICATION(S):
Antidiarrheal
Pregnancy Category C

INDICATIONS
▪ Adjunctive therapy in the treatment of diarrhea.

ACTION
▪ Inhibits excess GI motility ▪ Structurally related to narcotic analgesics but has no analgesic properties. **Therapeutic Effect:** ▪ Decreased GI motility with subsequent decrease in diarrhea.

PHARMACOKINETICS
Absorption: Well absorbed from the GI tract.
Distribution: Distribution not known. Probably enters breast milk.
Metabolism and Excretion: Mostly metabolized by the liver to inactive compounds.
Half-life: UK.

CONTRAINDICATIONS AND PRECAUTIONS
Contraindicated in: ▪ Hypersensitivity ▪ Severe liver disease ▪ Infectious diarrhea (due to *E. Coli, Salmonella,* or *Shigella*) ▪ Diarrhea associated with Pseudomembranous colitis ▪ Dehydrated patients ▪ Narrow-angle glaucoma ▪ Children <2 yr.
Use Cautiously in: ▪ Patients physically dependent on narcotic analgesics ▪ Inflammatory bowel disease ▪ Prostatic hypertrophy ▪ Pregnancy, lactation, and children <12 yr (safety not established).

ADVERSE REACTIONS AND SIDE EFFECTS*
CNS: dizziness, lightheadedness, drowsiness, headache, tiredness, nervousness, insomnia, confusion.
EENT: blurred vision, burning eyes.
GI: nausea, vomiting, constipation, dry mouth, epigastric distress.

INTERACTIONS
Drug–Drug: ▪ Additive CNS depression with other CNS **depressants,** including **alcohol, antihistamines, narcotic analgesics,** and **sedative/hypnotics** ▪ Additive anticholinergic properties with other drugs having **anticholinergic** properties, including **tricyclic antidepressants, quinidine,** and **disopyramide** ▪ Use with **MAO inhibitors** may result in hypertensive crisis.

ROUTE AND DOSAGE
Note: Doses given are in terms of difenoxin—each tablet contains 1 mg difenoxin with 0.025 mg of atropine.

- **PO (Adults):** 2 tablets initially then 1 tablet after each loose stool or every 3–4 hr as needed (not to exceed 8 tablets/day).

PHARMACODYNAMICS (antidiarrheal action)

	ONSET	PEAK	DURATION
PO	45–60 min	2 hr	3–4 hr

NURSING IMPLICATIONS
Assessment
▫ Assess frequency and consistency of stools and bowel sounds prior to and throughout course of therapy.
▫ Assess patient's fluid and electrolyte balance and skin turgor for dehydration.
- **Lab Test Considerations:** Liver function tests should be evaluated periodically during prolonged therapy.

*Underlines indicate most frequent; **CAPITALS** indicate life-threatening.

D

Potential Nursing Diagnoses

- Bowel elimination, altered: diarrhea (indications).
- Bowel elimination, altered: constipation (side effects).
- Knowledge deficit related to medication regimen (patient/family teaching).

Implementation

- **General Info:** Risk of dependence increases with high-dose, long-term use. Atropine has been added to discourage abuse.
- **PO:** May be administered with food if GI irritation occurs.

Patient/Family Teaching

- Instruct patient to take medication exactly as directed. Do not take more than the prescribed amount, due to the habit-forming potential.
- Medication may cause drowsiness. Advise patient to avoid driving or other activities requiring alertness until response to drug is known.
- Advise patient that frequent mouth rinses, good oral hygiene, and sugarless gum or candy may relieve dry mouth.
- Caution patient to avoid using alcohol and other CNS depressants concurrently with this medication.
- Instruct patient to notify physician if diarrhea persists or if fever or palpitations occur.

Evaluation

Effectiveness of therapy can be demonstrated by: ▪ Decrease in diarrhea. Treatment should be continued for 24–36 hr before it is considered ineffective in acute diarrhea.

DIFLUNISAL

(dye-**floo**-ni-sal)
Dolobid

CLASSIFICATION(S):
Non-narcotic analgesic—nonsteroidal anti-inflammatory agent, Anti-inflammatory agent
Pregnancy Category C

INDICATIONS

▪ Management of inflammatory disorders including: ▫ Rheumatoid arthritis ▫ Osteoarthritis ▪ Analgesic in the treatment of mild to moderate pain.

ACTION

▪ Inhibits prostaglandin synthesis. **Therapeutic Effects:** ▪ Suppression of pain and inflammation.

PHARMACOKINETICS

Absorption: Well absorbed from the GI tract.
Distribution: Crosses the placenta and enters breast milk.
Metabolism and Excretion: Metabolized by the liver.
Half-life: 8–12 hr.

CONTRAINDICATIONS AND PRECAUTIONS

Contraindicated in: ▪ Hypersensitivity ▪ Cross-sensitivity may exist with other NSAIAs, including aspirin ▪ Active GI bleeding or ulcer disease.
Use Cautiously in: ▪ Severe cardiovascular, renal, or hepatic disease ▪ History of ulcer disease ▪ Pregnancy, lactation, or children (safety not established).

ADVERSE REACTIONS AND SIDE EFFECTS*

CNS: headache, drowsiness, psychic disturbances, dizziness.
EENT: blurred vision, tinnitus, rhinitis.
CV: edema, changes in blood pressure, arrhythmias.
GI: nausea, vomiting, diarrhea, constipation, GI bleeding, discomfort.
GU: renal failure.
Derm: rashes.
Hemat: blood dyscrasias, prolonged bleeding time.
MS: muscle aches.
Misc: allergic reactions, including ANAPHYLAXIS, chills.

INTERACTIONS

Drug-Drug: ▪ Concurrent use with **aspirin** may decrease effectiveness ▪ Additive adverse GI effects with **aspi-**

*Underlines indicate most frequent; **CAPITALS** indicate life-threatening.

rin, other **nonsteroidal anti-inflammatory agents, potassium supplements, glucocorticoids,** or **alcohol** ▪ Chronic use with **acetaminophen** may increase the risk of adverse renal reactions ▪ May decrease the effectiveness of **diuretics, antihypertensive** therapy, **insulin,** or **oral hypoglycemic agents** ▪ May increase serum **lithium** levels and increase the risk of toxicity ▪ Increases the risk of toxicity from **methotrexate** ▪ **Probenecid** increases risk of toxicity from diflunisal ▪ Increased risk of bleeding with **cefamandole, cefotetan, cefoperazone, moxalactam** or **plicamycin, thrombolytic agents,** or **anticoagulants** ▪ Increased risk of adverse hematologic reactions with **antineoplastic agents** or **radiation therapy.**

ROUTE AND DOSAGE

Pain

- **PO (Adults):** 500–1000 mg initally, then 250–500 mg q 8–12 hr.

Inflammatory Conditions

- **PO (Adults):** 500–1000 mg/day in 2 divided doses.

PHARMACODYNAMICS

	ONSET	PEAK	DURATION
PO (analagesic)	60 min	2–3 hr	8–12 hr
PO (anti-inflammatory)	few days–1 wk	2 wk	UK

NURSING IMPLICATIONS

Assessment

- **General Info:** Patients who have asthma, aspirin-induced allergy, and nasal polyps are at increased risk for developing hypersensitivity reactions.
- **Arthritis:** Assess pain and range of motion prior to and 1–2 hr following administration.
- **Pain:** Assess pain (type, location, and intensity) prior to and 1–2 hr following administration.
- **Lab Test Considerations:** BUN, serum creatinine, CBC, and liver function tests should be evaluated periodically in patients receiving prolonged course of therapy.
  - □ Serum potassium, creatinine, SGOT (AST), SGPT (ALT), and LDH may show increased levels. Serum uric acid levels may be decreased.
  - □ May cause minimally prolonged bleeding time, which may persist for less than 1 day following discontinuation of therapy.

Potential Nursing Diagnoses

- Comfort, altered: pain (indications).
- Mobility, impaired physical (indications).
- Knowledge deficit related to medication regimen (patient/family teaching).

Implementation

- **General Info:** Coadministration with narcotic analgesics may have additive analgesic effects and may permit lower narcotic doses.
- **PO:** For rapid initial effect, administer 30 min before or 2 hr after meals. May be administered with food, milk, or antacids to decrease GI irritation. Food slows but does not reduce the extent of absorption. Capsules should be swallowed whole; do not crush or chew.

Patient/Family Teaching

- □ Advise patient to take this medication with a full glass of water and to remain in an upright position for 15–30 min after administration.
- □ Instruct patient to take medication exactly as prescribed. If a dose is missed, it should be taken as soon as remembered but not if almost time for the next dose. Do not double doses.
- □ This medication may cause drowsiness or dizziness. Advise patient to avoid driving or other activities requiring alertness until response to the medication is known.
- □ Caution patient to avoid concurrent use of alcohol, aspirin, acetaminophen, or other over-the-counter medications without consulting physician or pharmacist.
- □ Instruct patient to notify physician if rash, itching, chills, rhinitis, fever,

D

muscle aches, visual disturbances, weight gain, edema, black stools, or persistent headache occur.

EVALUATION

Effectiveness of therapy can be demonstrated by: ▪ Decrease in severity of moderate pain ▪ Improved joint mobility. Partial arthritic relief is usually seen within 1–2 wk with maximum effectiveness seen in several wks. Patients who do not respond to one nonsteroidal anti-inflammatory agent may respond to another.

DIGITOXIN

(di-ji-**tox**-in)
Crystodigin

CLASSIFICATION(S):
Cardiac glycoside, Inotropic agent, Antiarrhythmic
Pregnancy Category C

INDICATIONS

▪ Alone or in combination with other agents (diuretics, vasodilators) in the treatment of congestive heart failure ▪ Used to slow the ventricular rate in tachyarrhythmias, such as atrial fibrillation and atrial flutter ▪ Used to terminate paroxysmal atrial tachycardia.

ACTION

▪ Increases the force of myocardial contraction ▪ Prolongs refractory period of the AV node ▪ Decreases conduction through the SA and AV node. **Therapeutic Effects:** ▪ Increased cardiac output (positive inotropic effect) and slowing of the heart rate (negative chronotropic effect).

PHARMACOKINETICS

Absorption: Completely absorbed following oral administration.
Distribution: Widely distributed.
Metabolism and Excretion: Primarily metabolized by the liver. Some metabolites have cardiac activity.
Half-life: 5–7 days.

CONTRAINDICATIONS AND PRECAUTIONS

Contraindicated in: ▪ Hypersensitivity ▪ Uncontrolled ventricular arrhythmias ▪ AV block ▪ Idiopathic hypertrophic subaortic stenosis ▪ Constrictive pericarditis.

Use Cautiously in: ▪ Electrolyte abnormalities (hypokalemia, hypercalcemia, and hypomagnesemia may predispose to cardiac glycoside toxicity) ▪ Pregnancy and lactation (safety has not been established) ▪ Elderly (particularly sensitive to toxic effects) ▪ Myocardial infarction.

ADVERSE REACTIONS AND SIDE EFFECTS*

CNS: <u>fatigue</u>, weakness, headache.
EENT: blurred vision, yellow vision.
CV: ARRHYTHMIAS, <u>bradycardia</u>, ECG changes.
Endo: gynecomastia.
GI: <u>nausea</u>, <u>vomiting</u>, <u>anorexia</u>, diarrhea.
Hemat: thrombocytopenia.

INTERACTIONS

Drug-Drug: ▪ **Thiazide diuretics, mezlocillin, piperacillin, ticarcillin, amphotericin B,** and **glucocorticoids,** which cause hypokalemia, may increase the risk of toxicity ▪ Use with **quinidine, verapamil,** or **diltiazem** increases serum levels of digitoxin ▪ Additive bradycardia may occur with **beta-adrenergic blocking agents** and other **antiarrhythmic agents (quinidine, disopyramide)** ▪ Absorption is decreased by concurrent **antacids, kaolin-pectin, cholestyramine,** or **colestipol** ▪ Concurrent use with **phenobarbital, phenytoin,** or **rifampin** may result in decreased effectiveness of digitoxin ▪ Use with **succinylcholine** may increase cardiac irritability.

ROUTE AND DOSAGE

▪ **PO (Adults and Children >12 yr):** 1.2–1.6-mg (digitalizing dose) initially given in divided doses over 24

*<u>Underlines</u> indicate most frequent; **CAPITALS** indicate life-threatening.

hr, followed by 150 mcg daily (0.15 mg) daily (range 50–300 mcg).

PHARMACODYNAMICS (antiarrhythmic or inotropic effects, provided that a loading dose has been given)

	ONSET	PEAK	DURATION
PO	30 min–2 hr	4–12 hr	2–3 wk

NURSING IMPLICATIONS

Assessment

- Monitor apical pulse for 1 full min prior to administering. Withhold dose and notify physician if pulse rate is <60 bpm. Also notify physician promptly of any significant changes in rate, rhythm, or quality of pulse.
- Monitor intake and output ratios and daily weights. Assess for peripheral edema and auscultate lungs for rales/crackles throughout course of therapy.
- Before administering initial loading dose, determine if patient has taken any digitalis preparations in the preceding 2–3 wk, to prevent toxicity.
- Monitor ECG periodically throughout therapy.
- **Lab Test Considerations:** Serum electrolyte levels, especially potassium, magnesium, and calcium, and renal and hepatic functions should be evaluated periodically during course of therapy. Notify physician prior to giving dose if patient is hypokalemic. Hypokalemia, hypomagnesemia, or hypercalcemia may make the patient more susceptible to digitalis toxicity.
- **Toxicity and Overdose:** Therapeutic serum digitoxin levels range from 20 to 35 ng/ml. Serum digitoxin levels may be drawn 4–10 hr after a dose, although levels are usually drawn immediately prior to the next dose.
- Observe patient for signs and symptoms of toxicity (anorexia, nausea, vomiting, abdominal pain, visual disturbances, headache, confusion, unusually slow or irregular pulse). If these appear, withhold drug and notify physician immediately.
- If signs of life-threatening digitoxin toxicity occur, potassium, phenytoin, and digoxin immune Fab (Digibind) may be used for treatment.

Potential Nursing Diagnoses

- Cardiac output, decreased (indications).
- Knowledge deficit related to medication regimen (patient/family teaching).

Implementation

- **General Info:** For rapid digitalization the initial dose is higher than the maintenance dose. One fourth to one half the total digitalizing dose may be given initially. The remainder of the dose will be given in one-quarter increments in 4–8-hr intervals.
- **PO:** Oral preparations can be administered without regard to meals. Tablets can be crushed and administered with food or fluids if patient has difficulty swallowing.

Patient/Family Teaching

- Instruct patient to take medication exactly as prescribed, at the same time each day. If a dose is missed, take within 12 hr. Do not double doses. Consult physician if doses for 2 or more days are missed.
- Teach patient to take own pulse and to contact physician before taking medication if pulse rate is < 60 or > 100.
- Review signs and symptoms of digitalis toxicity with patient and family. Advise patient to notify physician immediately if symptoms of toxicity or congestive heart failure occur. Inform patient that these symptoms may be mistaken for those of colds and flu.
- Instruct patient to keep digitoxin tablets in their original container and not to mix in pill boxes with other medications, as they may look similar and be mistaken for other medications.
- Advise patient that sharing of this medication can be dangerous.
- Caution patient to avoid concurrent

D

use of over-the-counter medications, especially antacids and cold preparations, without consulting physician.
- Advise patient to notify physician or dentist of this medication regimen prior to treatment.
- Advise patient to carry identification describing condition and medication regimen at all times.
- Emphasize the importance of routine follow-up examinations to determine effectiveness and to monitor for toxicity.

EVALUATION
Effectiveness of therapy can be demonstrated by: ■ Decrease in severity of congestive heart failure □ Increase in cardiac output ■ Decrease in ventricular response in atrial tachyarrhythmias ■ Resolution of paroxysmal atrial tachycardia.

DIGOXIN
(di-**jox**-in)
Lanoxicaps, Lanoxin, {Novodigoxin}

CLASSIFICATION(S):
Cardiac glycoside, Inotropic agent, Antiarrhythmic
Pregnancy Category C

INDICATIONS

■ Alone or in combination with other agents (diuretics, vasodilators) in the treatment of congestive heart failure ■ Used to slow the ventricular rate in tachyarrhythmias, such as atrial fibrillation and atrial flutter ■ Used to terminate paroxysmal atrial tachycardia.

ACTION

■ Increases the force of myocardial contraction ■ Prolongs refractory period of the AV node ■ Decreases conduction through the SA and AV node. **Therapeutic Effects:** ■ Increased cardiac output and slowing of the heart rate.

PHARMACOKINETICS

Absorption: 60–85% absorbed following oral administration of tablets. 75–80% absorbed following administration of elixir. Absorption from liquid-filled capsules is 90–100%. 80% absorbed from IM sites, but this route is not recommended due to extreme pain and irritation.
Distribution: Widely distributed. Crosses the placenta and enters breast milk.
Metabolism and Excretion: Excreted almost entirely unchanged by the kidneys.
Half-life: 34–44 hr (increased in renal impairment).

CONTRAINDICATIONS AND PRECAUTIONS

Contraindicated in: ■ Hypersensitivity ■ Uncontrolled ventricular arrhythmias ■ AV block ■ Idiopathic hypertrophic subaortic stenosis ■ Constrictive pericarditis.
Use Cautiously in: ■ Electrolyte abnormalities (hypokalemia, hypercalcemia, and hypomagnesemia may predispose to cardiac glycoside toxicity) ■ Pregnancy and lactation (although safety has not been established, digoxin has been used during pregnancy without adverse effects on the fetus) ■ Elderly patients (particularly sensitive to toxic effects) ■ Myocardial infarction ■ Renal impairment (dosage reduction required).

ADVERSE REACTIONS AND SIDE EFFECTS*

CNS: fatigue, weakness, headache, blurred vision, yellow vision.
CV: ARRHYTHMIAS, bradycardia, ECG changes.
GI: nausea, vomiting, anorexia, diarrhea.
Endo: gynecomastia.
Hemat: thrombocytopenia.

{} = Available in Canada only.
*Underlines indicate most frequent; **CAPITALS** indicate life-threatening.

INTERACTIONS

Drug–Drug: ▪ **Thiazide** and **loop diuretics, mezlocillin, piperacillin, ticarcillin, amphotericin B,** and **glucocorticoids** which cause hypokalemia may increase the risk of toxicity ▪ **Quinidine, cyclosporine, amiodarone, verapamil, diltiazem, propofenone,** and **diflunisal** increase serum levels of digoxin and may lead to toxicity (dosage reduction recommended) ▪ **Spironolactone** increases digoxin half-life (reduced dosage or increased dosing interval may be required) ▪ Additive bradycardia may occur with **beta-adrenergic blocking agents** and other **antiarrhythmic agents (quinidine, disopyramide)** ▪ Absorption is decreased by concurrent **antacids, kaolin-pectin, cholestyramine,** or **colestipol** ▪ **Thyroid hormones** may decrease therapeutic effects.

Drug–Food: Concurrent ingestion of a **high-fiber meal** may decrease the absorption of digoxin.

ROUTE AND DOSAGE

Note: For rapid effect, a larger initial loading or "digitalizing" dose should be administered in several divided doses over 12–24 hr. Maintenance doses must be determined by renal function. All dosing must be evaluated by individual response. In general, doses required for atrial arrhythmias are higher than those for inotropic effect. Digoxin 0.25 mg tablets = 0.2 mg liquid-filled capsules.

Oral Digoxin Tablets or Elixir

- **PO (Adults):** 8–12 mcg/kg (6–10 mcg/kg in renal impairment, 10–15 mcg/kg for atrial arrhythmias). Give half of this initially, remainder at 4–8 hr intervals based on response. Maintenance dose: 15–25% of loading dose. Usual adult oral dose 0.1–0.25 mg/day.
- **PO (Children >10 yr):** 10–15 mcg/kg. Give half of this initially, remainder at 6–8 hr intervals based on response. Maintenance dose: 25–35% of loading dose.
- **PO (Children 2–5 yr):** 30–40 mcg/kg initially in several divided doses given every 6–8 hr. Maintenance dose: 25–35% of loading dose given as a single daily dose.
- **PO (Children 1–24 mon):** 35–60 mcg/kg initially in several divided doses given every 6–8 hr. Maintenance dose: 25–35% of loading dose given as a single daily dose.
- **PO (Neonates <1 mon):** 25–35 mcg/kg initially in several divided doses given every 6–8 hr. Maintenance dose: 25–35% of loading dose given as a single daily dose.

Digoxin Liquid-Filled Capsules

- **PO (Adults and Children >10 yr):** 8–12 mcg/kg initially in several divided doses given every 6–8 hr. Maintenance dose: 15–35% of initial dose given as a single daily dose or 2 divided doses (if dose >300 mcg give as 2 divided doses).
- **PO (Children 5–10 yr):** 15–30 mcg/kg initially in several divided doses given every 6–8 hr. Maintenance dose: 25–35% of initial dose given in 2–3 divided doses/day.
- **PO (Children 2–5 yr):** 25–35% mcg/kg initially in several divided doses given every 6–8 hr. Maintenance dose: 25–35% of initial dose given in 2–3 divided doses/day.

IV Digoxin

- **IV (Adults and Children >10 yr):** 8–12 mcg/kg initially in several divided doses given every 4–8 hr (every 6–8 hr in children). Maintenance dose: 25–35% of initial dose given as a single daily dose.
- **IV (Children 5–10 yr):** 15–30 mcg/kg initially in several divided doses given every 6–8 hr. Maintenance dose: 25–35% of initial dose given in 2–3 divided doses/day.
- **IV (Children 2–5 yr):** 25–35 mcg/kg initially in several divided doses given every 6–8 hr. Maintenance dose: 25–35% of initial dose given in 2–3 divided doses/day.
- **IV (Children 1–24 mon):** 30–50 mcg/kg initially in several divided doses given every 6–8 hr. Mainte-

D

nance dose: 25–35% of initial dose given in 2–3 divided doses/day.

- **IV (Neonates):** 20–30 mcg/kg initially in several divided doses given every 6–8 hr. Maintenance dose: 25–35% of initial dose given in 2 divided doses/day.

PHARMACODYNAMICS (antiarrhythmic or inotropic effects, provided that a loading dose has been given. Duration listed is that for normal renal function; in impaired renal function, duration will be longer.)

	ONSET	PEAK	DURATION
PO	0.5–2 hr	6–8 hr	2–4 days
IM	30 min	4–6 hr	2–4 days
IV	5–30 min	1–5 hr	2–4 days

NURSING IMPLICATIONS

Assessment

- ▫ Monitor apical pulse for 1 full min prior to administering. Withhold dose and notify physician if pulse rate is <60 bpm in an adult or <70 bpm in a child, or <90 bpm in an infant. Also notify physician promptly of any significant changes in rate, rhythm, or quality of pulse.
- ▫ Blood pressure should be monitored periodically in patients receiving IV digoxin.
- ▫ Monitor ECG throughout IV administration and periodically throughout therapy. Notify physician if bradycardia or new arrhythmias occur. Observe IV site for redness or infiltration; extravasation can lead to tissue irritation and sloughing.
- ▫ Monitor intake and output ratios and daily weights. Assess for peripheral edema and auscultate lungs for rales/crackles at least every 8 hr.
- ▫ Before administering initial loading dose, determine if patient has taken any digitalis preparations in the preceding 2–3 wk.
- **Lab Test Considerations:** Serum electrolyte levels, especially potassium, magnesium, and calcium, renal, and hepatic functions should be evaluated periodically during course of therapy. Notify physician prior to giving dose if patient is hypokalemic. Hypokalemia, hypomagnesemia, or hypercalcemia may make the patient more susceptible to digitalis toxicity.
- **Toxicity and Overdose:** Therapeutic serum digoxin levels range from 0.5 to 2 ng/ml. Serum digoxin levels may be drawn 4–10 hr after a dose is administered, although they are usually drawn immediately prior to the next dose.
- ▫ Observe patient for signs and symptoms of toxicity. In adults and older children the first signs of toxicity usually include abdominal pain, anorexia, nausea, vomiting, visual disturbances, bradycardia, and other arrhythmias. In infants and small children the first symptoms of overdose are usually cardiac arrhythmias. If these appear, withhold drug and notify physician immediately.
- ▫ If signs of toxicity occur and are not severe, discontinuation of digoxin may be all that is required.
- ▫ If hypokalemia is present and renal function is adequate, potassium salts may be administered. Do not administer if hyperkalemia or heart block exists.
- ▫ Correction of arrhythmias due to digitalis toxicity may be attempted with lidocaine, procainamide, quinidine, propranolol, or phenytoin. Temporary ventricular pacing may be useful in advanced heart block.
- ▫ Treatment of life-threatening arrhythmias may include administration of digoxin immune Fab (Digibind), which binds to the digoxin molecule in the blood and is excreted by the kidneys.

Potential Nursing Diagnoses

- Cardiac output, decreased (indications).
- Knowledge deficit related to medication regimen (patient/family teaching).

Implementation

- **General Info:** Available in tablet, fluid-filled soft capsule, elixir, and injectable forms.
  - For rapid digitalization the initial dose is higher than the maintenance dose. One fourth to one half of the total digitalizing dose is given initially. The remainder of the dose will be administered in one-quarter increments at 4–6-hr intervals.
  - When changing from parenteral to oral dosage forms, dosage adjustments may be necessary because of pharmacokinetic variations in percent of digoxin absorbed, except when changing from parenteral to liquid-filled soft capsules.
- **PO:** Oral preparations can be administered without regard to meals. Tablets can be crushed and administered with food or fluids if patient has difficulty swallowing. Use calibrated measuring device for liquid preparations. Do not alternate between dosage forms; bioavailability of capsules is not equal to that of the tablets or elixir.
- **IM:** If physician orders IM route, administer deep into gluteal muscle and massage well to reduce painful local reactions. Do not administer more than 2 ml of digoxin in each IM site. IM administration is not generally recommended.
- **Direct IV:** IV doses may be given undiluted or each 1 ml may be diluted in 4 ml of sterile water, 0.9% NaCl, D5W, or lactated Ringer's soln for injection. Less diluent will cause precipitation. Use diluted soln immediately. Do not use soln that is discolored or contains precipitate. Mixing with other drugs in the same container or simultaneous administration in the same IV line is not recommended.
  - *Rate:* Administer each dose through Y-site injection or 3-way stopcock over a minimum of 5 min.
- **Syringe Compatibility:** heparin.
- **Y-Site Compatibility:** famotidine, heparin with hydrocortisone sodium succinate, or potassium chloride.
- **Additive Compatibility:** bretylium, cimetidine, lidocaine, or verapamil.
- **Additive Incompatibility:** dobutamine.

Patient/Family Teaching

- Instruct patient to take medication exactly as prescribed, at the same time each day. Missed doses should be taken within 12 hr of scheduled dose or not taken at all. Do not double doses. Consult physician if doses for 2 or more days are missed. Do not discontinue medication without consulting physician.
- Teach patient to take pulse and to contact physician before taking medication if pulse rate is <60 or >100.
- Review signs and symptoms of digitalis toxicity with patient and family. Advise patient to notify physician immediately if these or symptoms of congestive heart failure occur. Inform patient that these symptoms may be mistaken for those of colds or flu.
- Instruct patient to keep digoxin tablets in their original container and not to mix in pill boxes with other medications, as they may look similar and may be mistaken for other medications. Advise patient that sharing of this medication can be dangerous.
- Caution patient to avoid concurrent use of over-the-counter medications without consulting physician. Advise patient to avoid taking antacids or antidiarrheals within 2 hr of digoxin.
- Advise patient to notify physician or dentist of this medication regimen prior to treatment.
- Patients taking digoxin should carry identification describing disease process and medication regimen at all times.
- Emphasize the importance of routine follow-up examinations to determine effectiveness and to monitor for toxicity.

Evaluation

Effectiveness of therapy can be demonstrated by: ▪ Decrease in severity of congestive heart failure ▪ Increase in cardiac output ▪ Decrease in ventricular

D

response in tachyarrhythmias ▪ Termination of paroxysmal atrial tachycardia.

DIGOXIN IMMUNE FAB

(di-**jox**-in im-**myoon** FAB)
Digibind

CLASSIFICATION(S):
Antidote—for digoxin, digitoxin
Pregnancy Category C

INDICATIONS

▪ Management of serious life-threatening overdosage with digoxin or digitoxin.

ACTION

▪ An antibody produced in sheep that binds antigenically to unbound digoxin or digitoxin in serum. **Therapeutic Effect:** ▪ Binding and subsequent removal of digoxin or digitoxin, preventing toxic effects in overdose.

PHARMACOKINETICS

Absorption: Administered IV only, resulting in complete bioavailability.
Distribution: Widely distributed throughout extracellular space.
Metabolism and Excretion: Excreted by the kidneys as the bound complex (digoxin immune Fab plus digoxin or digitoxin).
Half-life: 14–20 hr.

CONTRAINDICATIONS AND PRECAUTIONS

Contraindicated in: ▪ No known contraindications.
Use Cautiously in: ▪ Known hypersensitivity to sheep proteins or products ▪ Children, pregnancy, or lactation (safety not established).

ADVERSE REACTIONS AND SIDE EFFECTS*

CV: re-emergence of atrial fibrillation, re-emergence of congestive heart failure.
F and E: HYPOKALEMIA.

INTERACTIONS

Drug-Drug: ▪ Prevents response to digoxin or digitoxin.

ROUTE AND DOSAGE

When Estimated Digoxin or Digitoxin Dose is *Not* Known

▪ **IV (Adults and Children):** 800 mg.

When Digoxin or Digitoxin Dose is Known

Calculate total dose or body load (TBL) in mg of digoxin or digitoxin. If digoxin was ingested orally as tablets or elixir multiply by 0.8.

▪ **IV (Adults and Children):** Total body load (TBL) × 66.7 = dose of digoxin immune Fab (mg).

Skin Test

▪ **Intradermal (Adults):** 10 mcg (0.1 ml of a 1:100 dilution of 10 mg/ml soln).

PHARMACODYNAMICS (reversal of arrhythmias and hyperkalemia; reversal of inotropic effect may take several hrs)

	ONSET	PEAK	DURATION
IV	30 min (variable)	UK	2–6 hr

NURSING IMPLICATIONS

Assessment

- ▫ Monitor ECG, pulse, blood pressure, and body temperature prior to and throughout treatment. Patients with atrial fibrillation may develop a rapid ventricular response as a result of decreased digoxin or digitoxin levels.
- ▫ Assess patient for increase in signs of congestive heart failure (peripheral edema, dyspnea, rales/crackles, weight gain).
- ▪ **Lab Test Considerations:** Monitor serum digoxin or digitoxin levels prior to administration.
- ▫ Monitor serum potassium levels frequently during treatment. Prior to treatment hyperkalemia usually coexists with toxicity. Levels may decrease rapidly; hypokalemia should be treated promptly.

*Underlines indicate most frequent; **CAPITALS** indicate life-threatening.

□ Free serum digoxin or digitoxin levels fall rapidly following administration. Total body concentrations rise suddenly after administration but are bound to the Fab molecule and are inactive. Total body concentrations will decrease to undetectable levels within several days. Serum digoxin or digitoxin levels are not valid for 5–7 days following administration.

POTENTIAL NURSING DIAGNOSES

■ Knowledge deficit related to medication regimen (patient/family teaching).

IMPLEMENTATION

■ **General Info:** Patients with a high risk for allergy to digoxin immune Fab or sheep proteins should have skin testing for allergy prior to administration. Prepare skin test soln by diluting 0.1 ml of the reconstituted soln (10 mg/ml) in 9.9 ml of 0.9% NaCl to produce a 10 ml soln (100 mcg/ml). Testing may be administered by intradermal injection or scratch test. For intradermal use, inject 0.1 ml intradermally. For scratch test place 1 drop of soln on the skin and make a ¼-in scratch through the drop with a sterile needle. Following either method, inspect for urticarial wheal surrounded by erythema after 20 min. If a positive skin test occurs, use of digoxin immune Fab should be avoided unless absolutely necessary.

□ Cardiopulmonary resuscitation equipment and medications should be available during administration.

□ Delay redigitalization for several days until the elimination of digoxin immune Fab from the body is complete.

■ **Intermittent Infusion:** Reconstitute each 40 mg for IV administration in 4 ml of sterile water and mix gently. Soln will contain a concentration of 10 mg/ml. May be further diluted with 0.9% NaCl for IV infusion. Reconstituted soln should be used immediately but is stable for 4 hr if refrigerated.

□ In infants and small children, monitor for fluid overload. For small doses a reconsituted 40-mg vial can be diluted with 36 ml of 0.9% NaCl for a concentration of 1 mg/ml. Administer with a tuberculin syringe.

□ *Rate:* Administer reconstituted soln by IV infusion through a 0.22-micron membrane filter over 30 min. If cardiac arrest is imminent, rapid direct IV injection may be used.

PATIENT/FAMILY TEACHING

□ Explain the procedure and purpose of the treatment to the patient.

EVALUATION

Effectiveness of therapy can be demonstrated by: ■ Resolution of signs and symptoms of digoxin or digitoxin toxicity □ Decreased digoxin or digitoxin level without major side effects.

DIHYDROTACHYSTEROL

(dye-hye-droh-tak-**iss**-ter-ole)
DHT, Hytakerol, vitamin D analogue

CLASSIFICATION(S):
Vitamin—fat-soluble
Pregnancy Category C

INDICATIONS

■ Treatment of hypophosphatemia ■ Treatment of hypocalcemia ■ Prevention and treatment of rickets ■ Prevention and treatment of vitamin D deficiency ■ Prevention and treatment of postoperative and idiopathic tetany. **Unlabeled Use:** ■ Renal osteodystrophy.

ACTION

■ Promotes the absorption of calcium and phosphorous ■ Regulates calcium homeostasis in conjunction with parathyroid hormone and calcitonin. **Therapeutic Effect:** ■ Treatment and prevention of deficiency states, particularly bone manifestations.

PHARMACOKINETICS

Absorption: Well absorbed in an inactive form.

Distribution: Stored in the liver and other fatty tissues.
Metabolism and Excretion: Converted to active form by sunlight and the liver. Metabolized and excreted by the kidneys.
Half-life: UK.

CONTRAINDICATIONS AND PRECAUTIONS

Contraindicated in: ▪ Hypersensitivity ▪ Hypercalcemia ▪ Vitamin D toxicity ▪ Lactation (large doses).
Use Cautiously in: ▪ Patients receiving cardiac glycosides ▪ Pregnancy (larger doses; safety not established).

ADVERSE REACTIONS AND SIDE EFFECTS*

▪ Do not occur at dose within the range of daily requirements.

INTERACTIONS

Drug-Drug: ▪ **Cholestyramine, colestipol,** or **mineral oil** decrease absorption of vitamin D analogues ▪ Use with **thiazide diuretics** in patients with hypoparathyroidism may result in hypercalcemia ▪ **Glucocorticoids** decrease the effectiveness of vitamin D analogues ▪ Use with **cardiac glycosides** increases the risk of arrhythmias ▪ Vitamin D requirements are increased by **phenytoin** and other **hydantoin anticonvulsants, sucralfate, barbiturates,** and **primidone.**

ROUTE AND DOSAGE

Hypocalcemic Tetany

- **PO (Adults):** 0.2–2.5 mg for 3 days, then 0.2–1 mg daily.

Hypoparathyroidism or Pseudohypoparathyroidism

- **PO (Adults):** 0.75–2.5 mg/day initially for several days, then 0.2–1 mg/day (up to 1.5 mg/day).
- **PO (Children):** 1–5 mg/day for 4 days initially, then one fourth of the initial dose, then maintenance dose of 0.5–1.5 mg/day.

Renal Osteodystrophy

- **PO (Adults):** 0.1–0.25 mg/day initially, then 0.2–1 mg/day.

PHARMACODYNAMICS (effects on serum calcium)

	ONSET	PEAK	DURATION
PO	several hrs	1–2 wk	2 wk

NURSING IMPLICATIONS

Assessment

- □ Observe patient for evidence of hypocalcemia (paresthesia, muscle twitching, laryngospasm, colic, cardiac arrhythmias, and Chvostek's or Trousseau's sign). Protect symptomatic patient by raising and padding side rails; keep bed in low position.
- □ Assess patient for bone pain and weakness prior to and throughout course of therapy.
- ▪ **Lab Test Considerations:** Serum calcium levels should be drawn weekly during initial therapy. Monitor BUN, serum creatinine, alkaline phosphatase parathyroid hormone levels, creatinine clearance, and 24-hr urinary calcium periodically. Monitor serum phosphorous levels prior to and periodically throughout course of therapy.
- ▪ **Toxicity and Overdose:** Toxicity is manifested as hypercalcemia. Assess for nausea, vomiting, anorexia, weakness, constipation, headache, bone pain, and metallic taste. Later symptoms include polyuria, polydipsia, photophobia, rhinorrhea, pruritis, and cardiac arrhythmias.
- □ Treatment includes discontinuing dihydrotachysterol, instituting a low-calcium diet, and administering a laxative. IV hydration and loop diuretics may be ordered to increase urinary excretion of calcium. Hemodialysis may also be used.

Potential Nursing Diagnoses

- ▪ Nutrition, altered: less than body requirements (indications).

*Underlines indicate most frequent; CAPITALS indicate life-threatening.

- Knowledge deficit related to medication regimen (patient/family teaching).

Implementation

- **PO:** May be administered without regard to meals. Measure soln accurately with calibrated dropper provided by manufacturer.

Patient/Family Teaching

- Advise patient to take as directed. If dose is missed take as soon as remembered; do not double up on doses.
- Encourage patient to comply with diet recommendations of physician. Explain that the best source of vitamins is a well-balanced diet with foods from the 4 basic food groups. Foods high in vitamin D include fish livers and oils, fortified milk, bread, and cereals.
- Foods high in calcium include dairy products, canned salmon and sardines, broccoli, bok choy, tofu, molasses, and cream soups (see Appendix K). Renal patients must still consider renal failure diet in food selection. Physician may order concurrent calcium supplement.
- Review symptoms of overdosage and instruct patient to report these promptly to physician.
- Emphasize the importance of follow-up examinations to evaluate progress.

Evaluation

Effectiveness of therapy can be demonstrated by: ■ Normalization of serum calcium levels in hypocalcemic tetany and hypoparathyroidism.

DILTIAZEM

(dil-**tye**-a-zem)

{Apo-Diltiaz}, Cardizem, Cardizem SR

CLASSIFICATION(S):

Calcium channel blocker, Antianginal, Coronary vasodilator

Pregnancy Category C

INDICATIONS

■ Management of angina pectoris due to coronary insufficiency or vasospasm (Prinzmetal's angina) ■ Alone or in combination with other agents in the management of hypertension (SR product only).

ACTION

■ Inhibits the transport of calcium into myocardial and vascular smooth muscle cells, resulting in inhibition of excitation-contraction coupling and subsequent contraction ■ May decrease SA and AV node conduction. **Therapeutic Effect:** ■ Coronary vasodilation and subsequent decrease in frequency and severity of attacks of angina pectoris.

PHARMACOKINETICS

Absorption: Well absorbed after oral administration, but large amounts are rapidly metabolized.

Distribution: Distribution not known.

Metabolism and Excretion: Mostly metabolized by the liver.

Half-life: 3.5–9 hr.

CONTRAINDICATIONS AND PRECAUTIONS

Contraindicated in: ■ Hypersensitivity ■ Sick sinus syndrome (without a pacemaker) ■ 2nd- and 3rd-degree heart block ■ Severe hypotension.

Use Cautiously in: ■ Severe hepatic disease (dosage reduction may be required) ■ Congestive heart failure ■ Pregnancy, lactation, or children (safety not established).

ADVERSE REACTIONS AND SIDE EFFECTS*

CNS: dizziness, headache, tremors, mood changes, fatigue, drowsiness.

CV: arrhythmias, edema, hypotension, syncope, palpitations, congestive heart failure, 2nd- and 3rd-degree heart block.

GI: anorexia, constipation, nausea, abdominal discomfort, hepatitis, gingival hyperplasia.

Derm: rash, petechiae, photosensitivity.

INTERACTIONS

Drug–Drug: ▪ May increase serum **digoxin** levels ▪ Increased risk of bradycardia, conduction defects, or congestive heart failure when used with **beta-adrenergic blockers, digoxin,** or **disopyramide** ▪ **Phenytoin** and **phenobarbital** may hasten metabolism and decrease effectiveness ▪ **Cimetidine** and **propranolol** may slow metabolism and lead to toxicity ▪ May decrease metabolism and increase risk of toxicity from **cyclosporine** or **carbamazepine** ▪ Additive hypotension with other **antihypertensives,** acute ingestion of **alcohol,** or **nitrates.**

ROUTE AND DOSAGE

- **PO (Adults):** 30–120 mg 3–4 times daily or 60–120 mg twice daily as SR capsules (up to 360 mg/day).

PHARMACODYNAMICS (cardiovascular effects)

	ONSET	PEAK	DURATION
PO	30 min	2–3 hr	6–8 hr
PO-SR	UK	UK	12 hr

NURSING IMPLICATIONS

Assessment

- **General Info:** Monitor blood pressure and pulse before and periodically during therapy.
  - Monitor intake and output ratios and daily weight. Assess patient for signs of congestive heart failure (peripheral edema, rales/crackles, dyspnea, weight gain).
  - Patients receiving cardiac glycosides concurrently with diltiazem should have routine serum digoxin levels and be monitored for signs and symptoms of digitalis toxicity.
  - Monitor ECG frequently during dosage titration and periodically in patients receiving long-term therapy. May cause prolonged PR interval.
- **Angina:** Assess location, duration, intensity, and precipitating factors of patient's anginal pain.
- **Lab Test Considerations:** Monitor renal and hepatic functions periodically during long-term therapy. May cause increase in hepatic enzymes after several days of therapy, which return to normal upon discontinuation of therapy.
  - Total serum calcium concentrations are not affected by calcium channel blockers.

Potential Nursing Diagnoses

- Cardiac output, decreased (indications).
- Comfort, altered: pain (indications).
- Knowledge deficit related to medication regimen (patient/family teaching).

Implementation

- **PO:** May be administered with meals if gastric irritation becomes a problem. Crush and mix with food or fluids for patients having difficulty swallowing. Do not open, crush, or chew sustained-release capsules.

Patient/Family Teaching

- **General Info:** Advise patient to take medication exactly as directed, not to skip or double up on missed doses. Consult physician prior to discontinuation of therapy; gradual discontinuation may be necessary.
  - Instruct patient to take pulse prior to taking diltiazem. Patients should hold medication and consult physician if pulse is $<$50 bpm.
  - Caution patients to make position changes slowly to minimize orthostatic hypotension.
  - Medication may cause dizziness. Advise patient to avoid driving or other activities requiring alertness until response to medication is known.
  - Instruct patient to avoid concurrent use of alcohol or over-the-counter medications without consulting physician or pharmacist.
  - Diltiazem may occasionally cause gingival hyperplasia. Advise patient to maintain good oral hygiene and have regular dental examinations and cleaning to prevent gingival tenderness, bleeding, and enlargement.

- ▫ Caution patient to wear protective clothing and use sunscreen to prevent photosensitivity reactions.
- ▪ **Angina:** Advise patient to contact physician if chest pain does not improve or worsens after therapy, or if it is accompanied by diaphoresis or shortness of breath.
- ▫ Caution patient to discuss exercise restrictions with physician prior to exertion.
- ▫ Advise patient that nitroglycerin SL may be used concurrently as directed for acute anginal attacks.
- ▪ **Hypertension:** Encourage patient to comply with additional methods for controlling hypertension (weight reduction, low-sodium diet, discontinuation of smoking, moderation of alcohol consumption, regular exercise, stress management). Diltiazem controls but does not cure hypotension.
- ▫ Instruct patient and family in proper technique for monitoring blood pressure. Advise patient to take blood pressure weekly and to report significant changes to physician.

EVALUATION

Effectiveness of therapy can be demonstrated by: ▪ Decrease in frequency and severity of anginal attacks ▫ Decreased need for nitrate therapy ▫ Increase in activity tolerance and sense of well-being ▪ Decrease in blood pressure.

DIMENHYDRINATE

(dye-men-**hye**-dri-nate)
{Apo-Dimenhydrinate}, Calm X, Diante, Dimentabs, Dommanate, Dramamine, Dramanate, Dramilin, Dramocen, Dramoject, Dymenate, {Gravol}, Hydrate, Marmine, Motion Aid, {Nauseatol}, {Novodimenate}, {PMS-Dimenhydrinate}, Reidamine, {Travamine}, Triptone, Wehamine

CLASSIFICATION(S):
Antihistamine, Antiemetic
Pregnancy Category B

INDICATIONS

▪ Treatment and prevention of nausea, vomiting, dizziness, and vertigo accompanying motion sickness.

ACTION

▪ Inhibits vestibular stimulation ▪ Has significant CNS depressant, anticholinergic, antihistaminic, and antiemetic properties. **Therapeutic Effect:** ▪ Decreased vestibular stimulation, which may prevent motion sickness.

PHARMACOKINETICS

Absorption: Well absorbed following oral or IM administration.
Distribution: Distribution not known. Probably crosses the placenta and enters breast milk.
Metabolism and Excretion: Metabolized by the liver.
Half-life: UK.

CONTRAINDICATIONS AND PRECAUTIONS

Contraindicated in: ▪ Hypersensitivity.
Use Cautiously in: ▪ Narrow-angle glaucoma ▪ Seizure disorders ▪ Prostatic hypertrophy.

ADVERSE REACTIONS AND SIDE EFFECTS*

CNS: drowsiness, paradoxical excitation (children), dizziness, headache.
EENT: blurred vision, tinnitus.
CV: palpitations, hypotension.
GI: dry mouth, anorexia, constipation, diarrhea.
GU: frequency, dysuria.
Local: pain at IM site.

INTERACTIONS

Drug–Drug: ▪ Additive CNS depression with other **antihistamines, alcohol, narcotic analgesics,** and **sedative/hypnotics** ▪ May mask signs or symptoms of ototoxicity in patients receiving **ototoxic drugs (aminoglycosides, ethacrynic acid)** ▪ Additive anticholinergic properties with **tricyclic antide-**

{} = Available in Canada only.
*Underlines indicate most frequent; **CAPITALS** indicate life-threatening.

D

pressants, quinidine, or **disopyramide** ▪ **MAO inhibitors** intensify and prolong the anticholinergic effects of antihistamines.

ROUTE AND DOSAGE

- **PO, IM, IV (Adults):** 50–100 mg q 4–6 hr.
- **PO (Children 6–12 yr):** 25–50 mg q 6–8 hr (not to exceed 150 mg/day).
- **PO (Children 2–5 yr):** 12.5–25 mg q 6–8 hr (not to exceed 75 mg/day).
- **IM (Children):** 1.25 mg/kg q 6 hr.

PHARMACODYNAMICS (antimotion sickness, antiemetic activity)

	ONSET	PEAK	DURATION
PO	15–60 min	1–2 hr	3–6 hr
IM	20–30 min	1–2 hr	3–6 hr
IV	rapid	UK	3–6 hr

NURSING IMPLICATIONS

Assessment

- □ Assess nausea, vomiting, bowel sounds, and abdominal pain prior to and after the administration of this drug. Dimenhydrinate may mask the signs of an acute abdomen.
- □ Monitor intake and output, including emesis. Assess patient for signs of dehydration (excessive thirst, dry skin and mucous membranes, tachycardia, increased urine specific gravity, poor skin turgor).
- ▪ **Lab Test Considerations:** Will cause false-negative allergy skin tests; discontinue 72 hr prior to testing.

Potential Nursing Diagnoses

- ▪ Fluid volume deficit, potential (indications).
- ▪ Nutrition, altered: less than body requirements (indications).
- ▪ Injury, high risk for (side effects).

Implementation

- ▪ **General Info:** When used for prophylaxis of motion sickness, administer at least 30 min and preferably 1–2 hr before exposure to conditions that may precipitate motion sickness.
- ▪ **PO:** Use calibrated measuring device when administering liquid dose.
- ▪ **IM:** Administer into well-developed muscle; massage well.
- ▪ **Direct IV:** Dilute 50 mg in 10 ml of 0.9% NaCl for injection.
- □ *Rate:* Inject over 2 min.
- ▪ **Syringe Compatibility:** atropine, diphenhydramine, droperidol, fentanyl, heparin, meperidine, metoclopramide, morphine, pentazocine, perphenazine, ranitidine, or scopolamine. Mix immediately before use.
- ▪ **Syringe Incompatibility:** butorphanol, chlorpromazine, glycopyrrolate, hydroxyzine, midazolam, pentobarbital, prochlorperazine, promazine, promethazine, or thiopental.
- ▪ **Y-Site Compatibility:** acyclovir.
- ▪ **Y-Site Incompatibility:** aminophylline, heparin, hydrocortisone sodium succinate, hydroxyzine, phenobarbital, phenytoin, prednisolone, prochlorperazine, promazine, or promethazine.
- ▪ **Additive Compatibility:** D5W, 0.45% NaCl, 0.9% NaCl, Ringer's soln, lactated Ringer's soln, dextrose/saline combinations, or dextrose/Ringer's combinations. Also compatible with amikacin, calcium gluconate, chloramphenicol, corticotropin, erythromycin, heparin, hydroxyzine, methicillin, norepinephrine, oxytetracycline, penicillin G potassium, pentobarbital, phenobarbital, potassium chloride, prochlorperazine, or vancomycin.
- ▪ **Additive Incompatibility:** tetracycline or thiopental.

Patient/Family Teaching

- □ Medication may cause drowsiness and sedation. Advise patient to avoid driving or other activities requiring alertness until response to the drug is known.
- □ Inform patient that this medication may cause dry mouth. Frequent oral rinses, good oral hygiene, and sugarless gum or candy may minimize this effect.
- □ Caution patient to avoid alcohol and other CNS depressants concurrently with this medication.

EVALUATION

Effectiveness of therapy can be demonstrated by: ▪ Prevention or decreased severity of nausea and vomiting.

DIMERCAPROL
(dye-mer-**cap**-role)
British anti-lewisite, BAL in Oil, dimercaptopropanol

CLASSIFICATION(S):
Antidote—heavy metal antagonist
Pregnancy Category C

INDICATIONS

▪ Treatment of acute: ▫ Mercury ▫ Gold ▫ Arsenic poisoning ▪ Adjunct (with edetate calcium disodium) in the treatment of severe lead poisoning accompanied by encephalopathy.

ACTION

▪ Binds up heavy metals in a reversible complex so that they cannot bind to tissues and cause organ damage. **Therapeutic Effect:** ▪ Prevention of organ damage from mercury, gold, arsenic, or lead poisoning.

PHARMACOKINETICS

Absorption: Well absorbed following IM administration.
Distribution: Widely distributed with high concentrations in liver and kidneys. Also penetrates brain.
Metabolism and Excretion: 50% excreted as complex with heavy metal by kidneys and in bile. 50% rapidly metabolized by the liver.
Half-life: UK (metabolism and excretion are complete within 6–24 hr).

CONTRAINDICATIONS AND PRECAUTIONS

Contraindicated in: ▪ Hypersensitivity ▪ Hypersensitivity to peanut products (vehicle is peanut oil) ▪ Impaired liver function (except postarsenical jaundice).

Use Cautiously in: ▪ Renal impairment (dosage reduction required) ▪ Hypertension ▪ Pregnancy or lactation (safety not established).

ADVERSE REACTIONS AND SIDE EFFECTS*

CNS: SEIZURES, coma, stupor, anxiety, nervousness, restlessness, weakness.
EENT: blepheral spasm, lacrimation, rhinorrhea.
Resp: unpleasant breath odor.
CV: increased blood pressure.
GI nausea, vomiting, pain in teeth, abdominal pain.
GU: nephrotoxicity.
Derm: sweating.
Hemat: hemolysis (in G6-PD-deficient patients), transient leukopenia (children).
Local: pain at IM site, sterile abscesses at IM sites.
MS: muscle ache, muscle spasm, painful extremities.
Misc: feeling of constriction in throat, chest, or hands; burning sensation in lips, mouth, throat, eyes, or penis; fever (children).

INTERACTIONS

Drug-Drug: ▪ Forms a toxic complex with **iron** ▪ Nephrotoxicity decreased by **agents that alkalinize the urine.**
Drug-Food: ▪ Nephrotoxicity decreased by **foods that alkalinize the urine.**

ROUTE AND DOSAGE

Acute Gold or Arsenic Poisoning

▪ **IM (Adults and Children):** 3 mg/kg q 4 hr for first 2 days, then qid on third day, then bid for 10 days or until recovery is complete.

Severe Gold Dermatitis

▪ **IM (Adults and Children):** 2.5 mg/kg q 4 hr for first 2 days, then bid for 1 wk.

Gold-Induced Thrombocytopenia

▪ **IM (Adults and Children):** 100 mg bid for 15 days.

*Underlines indicate most frequent; **CAPITALS** indicate life-threatening.

Adjunct in Severe Lead Poisoning
- **IM (Adults and Children):** 4 mg/kg (75–83 mg/m^2) q 4 hr for 5 days at same time as edetate calcium disodium.
- **IM (Children):** Alternate regimen—300 mg/m^2/day in divided doses q 4 hr with concurrent edetate calcium disodium for 5 days. If blood lead level decreases to 50 mcg/dl after 3 days, dimercaprol (but not edetate calcium disodium) may be discontinued.

PHARMACODYNAMICS (blood levels of heavy metals)

	ONSET	PEAK	DURATION
IM	UK	UK	4 hr

NURSING IMPLICATIONS

Assessment
- Determine time and amount of ingestion of heavy metal (arsenic, lead, mercury) or time and amount of administration of gold.
- Assess patient for symptoms of toxicity from ingested substance.
- Monitor blood pressure and pulse throughout therapy. Systolic blood pressure may rise and tachycardia may occur 15–30 min after administration. Blood pressure usually returns to normal within 2 hr.
- Monitor intake and output and notify physician if significant discrepancies occur or if urine output decreases. Physician may order alkalinization of urine to prevent nephrotoxicity.
- Monitor temperature throughout therapy. May cause fever in children after second or third dose, which persists until discontinuation of therapy.
- **Lab Test Considerations:** May cause decreased values of I^{131} thyroid uptake if test is performed during or immediately following dimercaprol therapy.

Potential Nursing Diagnoses
- Poisoning, high risk for (indications).
- Home maintenance management, impaired (indications).
- Knowledge deficit related to ingestion and medication regimen (patient/family teaching).

Implementation
- **General Info:** Dimercaprol is most effective when administered within 1–2 hr after ingestion.
- Administration of ephedrine or an antihistamine may prevent or treat histamine-like side effects.
- Commonly used concurrently with edetate calcium disodium when used to treat lead poisoning.
- Contact of the soln with the skin may cause dermatitis. Wash hands immediately.
- **IM:** Administer only deep IM. Injection is painful and may cause sterile abscess.
- Soln is yellow and viscous, with a pungent odor. May be turbid and contain sediment. This does not indicate deterioration of soln.
- If administered concurrently with edetate calcium disodium, use different sites for injections.

Patient/Family Teaching
- Explain purpose of therapy to patient or parents.
- Inform patient that injection is painful and may cause an unpleasant garlic-like breath odor.
- Instruct patient to notify physician if headache, burning of lips, sweating, or tearing occurs.

Evaluation
Effectiveness of therapy can be demonstrated by: ▪ Resolution of the symptoms of arsenic, lead, mercury, or gold toxicity.

DINOPROSTONE
(dye-noe-**prost**-one)
Prostin E_2

CLASSIFICATION(S):
Abortifacient—prostaglandin, Oxytocic
Pregnancy Category UK

INDICATIONS

▪ Induction of midtrimester abortion ▪ Management of missed abortion up to 28 wk ▪ Management of nonmetastatic gestational trophoblastic disease (benign hydatidiform mole). **Unlabeled Use:** ▪ Induction of labor or cervical ripening prior to induction of labor.

ACTION

▪ Causes uterine contractions by directly stimulating the myometrium ▪ Causes cervical softening and dilation. **Therapeutic Effect:** ▪ Expulsion of fetus.

PHARMACOKINETICS

Absorption: Systemic absorption not known.
Distribution: Distribution not known.
Metabolism and Excretion: Metabolized by enzymes in lung, kidneys, spleen, and liver tissue.
Half-life: UK.

CONTRAINDICATIONS AND PRECAUTIONS

Contraindicated in: ▪ Hypersensitivity ▪ Acute pelvic inflammatory disease ▪ Ruptured membranes.
Use Cautiously in: ▪ Uterine scarring ▪ Asthma ▪ Hypotension ▪ Cardiac disease ▪ Adrenal disorders ▪ Anemia ▪ Jaundice ▪ Diabetes mellitus ▪ Epilepsy ▪ Glaucoma ▪ Pulmonary, renal, or hepatic disease.

ADVERSE REACTIONS AND SIDE EFFECTS*

CNS: headache, drowsiness, syncope.
Resp: coughing, dyspnea, wheezing.
CV: hypotension, hypertension.
GI: nausea, vomiting, diarrhea.
GU: uterine rupture, urinary tract infection, vaginal/uterine pain.
Misc: chills, fever, allergic reactions, including ANAPHYLAXIS.

INTERACTIONS

Drug-Drug: ▪ Augments the effects of other **oxytocics**.

ROUTE AND DOSAGE

Abortifacient

▪ **Vag (Adults):** 20 mg, repeat q 3–5 hr until results (not to exceed total dose of 240 mg).

Induction of Labor/Cervical Ripening (Unlabeled Use)

▪ **Vag (Adults):** 0.2–5 mg as suppository or gel prepared by pharmacist (usual dose required: 2–5 mg).

PHARMACODYNAMICS (abortion time)

	ONSET	PEAK	DURATION
Vag	10 min	12–24 hr	2–3 hr

NURSING IMPLICATIONS

Assessment

▫ Monitor frequency, duration, and force of contractions and uterine resting tone.
▫ Monitor temperature, pulse, and blood pressure periodically throughout course of therapy. Dinoprostone-induced fever (elevation >1.1°C or 2°F) usually occurs within 15–45 min following insertion of suppository. This returns to normal 2–6 hr after discontinuation or removal of suppository from vagina.
▫ Auscultate breath sounds. Wheezing and sensation of chest tightness may indicate hypersensitivity reaction.
▫ Assess for nausea, vomiting, and diarrhea. Vomiting occurs in about 67% of patients and diarrhea in about 40% of patients. Premedication with antiemetic and an antidiarrheal may be ordered.
▫ Monitor amount and type of vaginal discharge. Notify physician immediately if symptoms of hemorrhage (increased bleeding, hypotension, pallor, tachycardia) occur.

Potential Nursing Diagnoses

▪ Knowledge deficit related to medication regimen (patient/family teaching).

*Underlines indicate most frequent; **CAPITALS** indicate life-threatening.

Implementation

- **Vag:** Warm the suppository to room temperature just prior to use. Can be made into a gel by pharmacist.
  - Wear gloves when handling unwrapped suppository to prevent absorption through skin.
  - Patient should remain supine for 10 min following insertion of suppository, then she may be ambulatory.

Patient/Family Teaching

- Explain purpose of vaginal examinations (to assess for trauma to cervix).
- Instruct patient to notify physician immediately if fever and chills, foul-smelling vaginal discharge, lower abdominal pain, or increased bleeding occurs.
- Provide emotional support throughout therapy.

Evaluation

Effectiveness of therapy can be demonstrated by: ▪ Complete abortion. Continuous administration for more than 2 days is not usually recommended.

DIPHENHYDRAMINE

(dye-fen-**hye**-dra-meen)
{Allerdryl}, AllerMax, Bena-D, Benadryl, Benahist, Ben-Allergin, Benaphen, Benoject, Benylin, Bydramine, Compoz, Diahist, Dihydrex, Di-phen, Diphenacen, Diphenadryl, Dormarex 2, Fenylhist, Fynex, Hydramine, Hydril, Hyrexin, {Insomnal}, Nervine Nighttime Sleep-Aid, Nordryl, Nytol with DPH, Sleep-Eze 3, Sominex, Tusstat, Twilite, Valdrene, Wehydryl

CLASSIFICATION(S):
Antihistamine, Antitussive
Pregnancy Category B

INDICATIONS

▪ Symptomatic relief of allergic symptoms caused by histamine release including: ▫ Anaphylaxis ▫ Nasal allergies ▫ Allergic dermatoses ▪ Parkinson's disease and dystonic reactions from medications ▪ Mild night-time sedation ▪ Prevention of motion sickness ▪ Antitussive.

ACTION

▪ Blocks the following effects of histamine: ▫ Vasodilation ▫ Increased GI tract secretions ▫ Increased heart rate ▫ Hypotension ▪ Has significant CNS depressant and anticholinergic properties. **Therapeutic Effects:** ▪ Relief of symptoms associated with histamine excess usually seen in allergic conditions ▪ Relief of acute dystonic reactions ▪ Prevention of motion sickness ▪ Suppression of cough.

PHARMACOKINETICS

Absorption: Well absorbed following oral and IM administration. Minimal systemic absorption may follow topical administration.
Distribution: Widely distributed. Crosses the placenta and enters breast milk.
Metabolism and Excretion: Metabolized by the liver (95%).
Half-life: 2.4–7 hr.

CONTRAINDICATIONS AND PRECAUTIONS

Contraindicated in: ▪ Hypersensitivity ▪ Acute attacks of asthma ▪ Lactation.
Use Cautiously in: ▪ Elderly patients (more susceptible to adverse drug reactions; dosage reduction recommended) ▪ Severe liver disease ▪ Narrow-angle glaucoma ▪ Seizure disorders ▪ Prostatic hypertrophy ▪ Pregnancy (safety not established).

ADVERSE REACTIONS AND SIDE EFFECTS*

CNS: drowsiness, paradoxical excitation (children), dizziness, headache.
EENT: blurred vision, tinnitus.
CV: palpitations, hypotension.
GI: dry mouth, anorexia, constipation, diarrhea.

{} = Available in Canada only.
*Underlines indicate most frequent; **CAPITALS** indicate life-threatening.

GU: frequency, dysuria, urinary retention.
Derm: photosensitivity.
Local: pain at IM site.

INTERACTIONS

Drug–Drug: ▪ Additive CNS depression with other **antihistamines, alcohol, narcotic analgesics,** and **sedative/hypnotics** ▪ Additive anticholinergic properties with **tricyclic antidepressants, quinidine,** or **disopyramide** ▪ **MAO inhibitors** intensify and prolong the anticholinergic effects of antihistamines.

ROUTE AND DOSAGE

- **PO (Adults):** 25–50 mg q 4–6 hr.
- **PO (Children >9.1 kg):** 12.5–25 mg q 4–6 hr.
- **PO (Children <9.1 kg):** 6.25–12.5 mg q 4–6 hr.
- **IM, IV (Adults):** 10–50-mg single dose (may need up to 100 mg, not to exceed 400 mg/day).
- **IM, IV (Children):** 5 mg/kg/day or 150 mg/m^2 in divided doses q 6–8 hr (not to exceed 300 mg/day).
- **Top (Adults and Children >2 yr):** 1–2% cream, lotion, or soln 3–4 times daily.

PHARMACODYNAMICS (antihistaminic effects)

	ONSET	PEAK	DURATION
PO	15–60 min	1–4 hr	4–8 hr
IM	20–30 min	1–4 hr	4–8 hr
IV	rapid	UK	4–8 hr

NURSING IMPLICATIONS

Assessment

- **General Info:** Diphenhydramine has multiple uses. Determine why the medication was ordered and assess symptoms that apply to the individual patient.
- **Prevention and Treatment of Anaphylaxis:** Assess for urticaria and for patency of airway.
- **Allergic Rhinitis:** Assess degree of nasal stuffiness, rhinorrhea, and sneezing.
- **Parkinsonism and Extrapyramidal Reactions:** Assess movement disorder prior to and following administration.
- **Insomnia:** Assess sleep patterns.
- **Motion Sickness and Nausea Associated with Chemotherapy:** Assess nausea, vomiting, bowel sounds, and abdominal pain.
- **Cough Suppressant:** Assess frequency and nature of cough, lung sounds, and amount and type of sputum produced. Unless contraindicated, maintain fluid intake of 1500–2000 ml daily to decrease viscosity of bronchial secretions.
- **Pruritis:** Assess degree of itching and skin rash and inflammation.
- **Lab Test Considerations:** Diphenhydramine may decrease skin response to allergy tests. Discontinue 4 days prior to skin testing.

Potential Nursing Diagnoses

- Sleep pattern disturbance (indications).
- Fluid volume deficit, potential (indications).
- Injury, high risk for (side effects).

Implementation

- **General Info:** When used for insomnia, administer 20 min before bedtime and schedule nursing activities to minimize interruption of sleep.
  - When used for prophylaxis of motion sickness administer at least 30 min and preferably 1–2 hr before exposure to conditions that may precipitate motion sickness.
- **PO:** Administer with meals or milk to minimize GI irritation. Capsule may be emptied and contents taken with water or food.
- **IM:** Administer into well-developed muscle. Avoid SC injections.
- **Direct IV:** May give undiluted. May be further diluted in 0.9% NaCl, 0.45% NaCl, D5W, D10W, D5/0.9% NaCl, D5/0.45% NaCl, D5/0.25% NaCl, Ringer's soln, lactated Ringer's soln, and dextrose/Ringer's combinations.
  - *Rate:* Inject each 25 mg over at least 1 min.
- **Syringe Compatibility:** atropine, butorphanol, chlorpromazine, cimeti-

dine, dimenhydrinate, droperidol, fentanyl, glycopyrrolate, hydromorphone, hydroxyzine, meperidine, metoclopramide, midazolam, morphine, nalbuphine, pentazocine, perphenazine, prochlorperazine, promazine, promethazine, ranitidine, or scopolamine. Compatible only for brief periods; prepare immediately before injection.

- **Syringe Incompatibility:** pentobarbital, phenobarbital, phenytoin, or thiopental.
- **Y-Site Compatibility:** acyclovir, heparin, hydrocortisone, ondansetron, or potassium chloride.
- **Y-Site Incompatibility:** foscarnet.
- **Additive Compatibility:** amikacin, aminophylline, ascorbic acid, bleomycin, cephapirin, colistimethate, erythromycin, lidocaine, methicillin, methyldopate, naficillin, netilimicin, penicillin G, polymixin B, or tetracycline.
- **Additive Incompatibility:** amobarbital, amphotericin B, cephalothin, hydrocortisone, phenobarbital, phenytoin, or thiopental.

Patient/Family Teaching

- **General Info:** Instruct patient to take medication exactly as directed; do not exceed recommended amount.
- □ May cause drowsiness and sedation. Advise patient to avoid driving or other activities requiring alertness until response to drug is known.
- □ Inform patient that this drug may cause dry mouth. Frequent oral rinses, good oral hygiene, and sugarless gum or candy may minimize this effect. Notify dentist if dry mouth persists for more than 2 wk.
- □ Advise patient to use sunscreen and protective clothing to prevent photosensitivity reactions.
- □ Caution patient to avoid use of alcohol and other CNS depressants concurrently with this medication.
- □ Advise patients taking diphenhydramine in OTC preparations to notify the physician if symptoms worsen or persist for more than 7 days.
- **Top:** Instruct patient to cleanse affected skin prior to application, to avoid application to raw or blistered skin, and to discontinue use and contact physician if irritation occurs.

Evaluation

Effectiveness of therapy can be demonstrated by: ▪ Prevention of or decreased urticaria in anaphylaxis or other allergic reactions ▪ Decreased dyskinesia in parkinsonism and extrapyramidal reactions ▪ Sedation when used as a sedative/hypnotic ▪ Prevention of or decreased nausea and vomiting caused by motion sickness ▪ Decrease in frequency and intensity of cough without eliminating cough reflex.

DIPHENOXYLATE/ATROPINE

(dye-fen-**ox**-i-late/**a**-troe-peen)
Diphenatol, Lofene, Logen, Lomanate, Lomotil, Lonox, Lo-Trol, Low-Quel, Nor-mil

CLASSIFICATION(S):
Antidiarrheal
Schedule V
Pregnancy Category C

INDICATIONS

▪ Adjunctive therapy in the treatment of diarrhea.

ACTION

▪ Inhibits excess GI motility ▪ Structurally related to narcotic analgesics but has no analgesic properties ▪ Atropine added to discourage abuse. **Therapeutic Effect:** ▪ Decreased GI motility with subsequent decrease in diarrhea.

PHARMACOKINETICS

Absorption: Diphenoxylate is well absorbed from the GI tract.
Distribution: Distribution not known. Diphenoxylate enters breast milk.
Metabolism and Excretion: Diphenoxylate is mostly metabolized by the liver, with some conversion to an active antidiarrheal compound (difenoxin).

Minimal excretion in the urine.
Half-life: 2.5 hr (diphenoxylate).

CONTRAINDICATIONS AND PRECAUTIONS

Contraindicated in: ▪ Hypersensitivity ▪ Severe liver disease ▪ Infectious diarrhea (due to *E. Coli, Salmonella, or Shigella*) ▪ Diarrhea associated with pseudomembranous colitis ▪ Dehydrated patients ▪ Narrow-angle glaucoma ▪ Children <2 yr.
Use Cautiously in: ▪ Patients physically dependent on narcotic analgesics ▪ Inflammatory bowel disease ▪ Prostatic hypertrophy ▪ Pregnancy and lactation (safety not established).

ADVERSE REACTIONS AND SIDE EFFECTS*

CNS: drowsiness, dizziness.
EENT: blurred vision, dry eyes.
CV: tachycardia.
GI: constipation, ileus, dry mouth.
GU: urinary retention.
Derm: flushing.

INTERACTIONS

Drug-Drug: ▪ Additive CNS depression with other **CNS depressants,** including **alcohol, antihistamines, narcotic analgesics,** and **sedative/hypnotics** ▪ Additive anticholinergic properties with other **drugs having anticholinergic properties,** including **tricyclic antidepressants** and **disopyramide** ▪ Use with **MAO inhibitors** may result in hypertensive crisis.

ROUTE AND DOSAGE

Note: Do not exceed recommended doses. Doses given are in terms of diphenoxylate: each tablet contains 2.5 mg diphenoxylate with 0.025 mg of atropine, each 5 ml of liquid contains 2.5 mg diphenoxylate with 0.025 mg of atropine.

- **PO (Adults):** 2.5–5 mg 2–4 times daily (not to exceed 20 mg/day).
- **PO (Children 8–12 yr):** 2 mg 5 times daily (not to exceed 10 mg/day).
- **PO (Children 5–8 yr):** 2 mg 4 times daily (not to exceed 8 mg/day).
- **PO (Children 2–5 yr):** 2 mg 3 times daily (not to exceed 6 mg/day).

PHARMACODYNAMICS (antidiarrheal action)

	ONSET	PEAK	DURATION
PO	45–60 min	2 hr	3–4 hr

NURSING IMPLICATIONS

Assessment

- Assess the frequency and consistency of stools, and bowel sounds prior to and throughout course of therapy.
- Assess patient's fluid and electrolyte balance and skin turgor for dehydration.
- **Lab Test Considerations:** Liver function tests should be evaluated periodically during prolonged therapy.
- May cause increased serum amylase concentrations.

Potential Nursing Diagnoses

- Bowel elimination, altered: diarrhea (indications).
- Bowel elimination, altered: constipation (side effects).
- Knowledge deficit related to medication regimen (patient/family teaching).

Implementation

- **General Info:** Risk of dependence increases with high-dose, long-term use. Atropine has been added to discourage abuse.
- **PO:** May be administered with food if GI irritation occurs. Tablets may be crushed and administered with patient's fluid of choice. Use calibrated measuring device for liquid preparations.

Patient/Family Teaching

- Instruct patient to take medication exactly as directed. Do not take more than the prescribed amount because of the habit-forming potential and risk of overdose in children.
- Medication may cause drowsiness.

*Underlines indicate most frequent; **CAPITALS** indicate life-threatening.

Advise patient to avoid driving or other activities requiring alertness until response to drug is known.
- Advise patient that frequent mouth rinses, good oral hygiene, and sugarless gum or candy may relieve dry mouth.
- Caution patient to avoid alcohol and other CNS depressants concurrently with this medication.
- Instruct patient to notify physician if diarrhea persists or if fever, abdominal pain, or palpitations occur.

Evaluation

Effectiveness of therapy can be demonstrated by: ▪ Decrease in diarrhea. Treatment should be continued for 24–36 hr before it is considered ineffective in treatment of acute diarrhea.

DIPIVEFRIN

(dye-**pi**-ve-frin)
Propine

CLASSIFICATION(S):
Ophthalmic—antiglaucoma
Pregnancy Category B

INDICATIONS

▪ Treatment of open-angle glaucoma.

ACTION

▪ Converted by enzymes in the eye to epinephrine, which decreases intraocular pressure by decreasing production of aqueous humor and increasing aqueous outflow. **Therapeutic Effect:** ▪ Lowering of intraocular pressure.

PHARMACOKINETICS

Absorption: Systemic absorption not known.
Distribution: Highly lipid-soluble, penetrates anterior chamber.
Metabolism and Excretion: Converted to epinephrine in the anterior chamber then metabolized by tissue enzymes.
Half-life: UK.

CONTRAINDICATIONS AND PRECAUTIONS

Contraindicated in: ▪ Hypersensitivity ▪ Hypersensitivity to sulfites ▪ Narrow-angle glaucoma.
Use Cautiously in: ▪ Aphakia (lack of lens)—increased risk of macular edema ▪ Pregnancy, lactation, or children (safety not established).

ADVERSE REACTIONS AND SIDE EFFECTS*

EENT: adrenochrome deposits in conjunctiva and cornea, burning, stinging, irritation, photophobia, macular edema (in aphakic patients), mydriasis.
CV: hypertension, tachycardia, arrhythmias.

INTERACTIONS

Drug-Drug: ▪ Increased risk of arrhythmias with **hydrocarbon inhalation anesthetics** or **cardiac glycosides** ▪ Increased risk of arrhythmias, tachycardia, or hypertension with **tricyclic antidepressants** or **maprotiline** ▪ Increased risk of changes in heart rate or blood pressure with **beta-adrenergic blocking agents** ▪ Additive sympathomimetic effects with other **adrenergic (sympathomimetic) agents.**

ROUTE AND DOSAGE

▪ **Ophth (Adults):** 1 drop of 0.1% q 12 hr.

PHARMACODYNAMICS (effects on intraocular pressure)

	ONSET	PEAK	DURATION
Ophth	30 min	1 hr	12 hr

NURSING IMPLICATIONS

Assessment

- Assess for symptoms of systemic absorption (increased pulse and blood pressure and arrhythmias).

Potential Nursing Diagnoses

▪ Knowledge deficit related to medication regimen (patient/family teaching).

*Underlines indicate most frequent; **CAPITALS** indicate life-threatening.

IMPLEMENTATION

- **General Info:** If miotic agent is ordered concurrently, administer miotic first.
  - *If dipivefrin is the sole antiglaucoma agent:* To switch from epinephine, just administer dipivefrin when next epinephrine dose is due.
  - *To switch from other anitglaucoma agents:* continue other drug for the first day of dipivefrin therapy.
- **Ophth:** Administer ophthalmic soln by having patient tilt head back and look up. Gently depress lower lid with index finger until conjunctival sac is exposed and instill medication. After instillation, maintain gentle pressure on the inner canthus for 1 min to avoid systemic absorption of the drug. Wait at least 5 min before administering other types of eyedrops.

PATIENT/FAMILY TEACHING

- Instruct in proper technique for instillation of ophthalmic medications. Emphasize the importance of not touching the applicator tip to any surface.
- Advise patient to take exactly as prescribed. A missed dose should be taken as soon as remembered unless almost time for next dose.
- Instruct patient to notify physician if eye irritation or visual changes persist. Temporary stinging is not significant.
- Emphasize the importance of regular follow-up examinations to monitor intraocular pressure.

EVALUATION

Effectiveness of therapy can be demonstrated by: ▪ Decreased intraocular pressure.

DIPYRIDAMOLE

(dye-peer-**id**-a-mole)
{Apo-Dipyridamole}, Persantin, Persantine

CLASSIFICATION(S):
Antiplatelet agent, Diagnostic agent—coronary vasodilator
Pregnancy Category B

INDICATIONS

▪ **PO:** Used in combination with anticoagulants (warfarin) to prevent thromboembolism in patients with prosthetic heart valves ▪ **PO:** Used in combination with other antiplatelet agents (aspirin) to maintain patency after surgical grafting procedures, including coronary artery bypass ▪ **IV:** Used as a diagnostic agent in lieu of exercise during thallium myocardial perfusion imaging.

ACTION

▪ **PO:** Decreases platelet aggregation by inhibiting the enzyme phosphodiesterase ▪ **IV:** Produces coronary vasodilation by inhibiting adenosine uptake. **Therapeutic Effects:** ▪ *PO:* Inhibition of platelet aggregation and subsequent thromboembolic events ▪ *IV:* In diagnostic thallium imaging dilates normal coronary arteries, reducing flow to vessels that are narrowed and causing abnormal thallium distribution.

PHARMACOKINETICS

Absorption: Moderately absorbed (30–60%) after oral administration.
Distribution: Widely distributed. Crosses the placenta. Enters breast milk.
Metabolism and Excretion: Metabolized by the liver, excreted in the bile.
Half-life: 10 hr.

CONTRAINDICATIONS AND PRECAUTIONS

Contraindicated in: ▪ Hypersensitivity.
Use Cautiously in: ▪ Hypotensive patients ▪ Patients with platelet defects ▪ Pregnancy (although safety not established, has been used without harm during pregnancy) ▪ Lactation or children <12 yr (safety not established).

D

ADVERSE REACTIONS AND SIDE EFFECTS*

CNS: headache, dizziness, weakness, syncope; IV only—transient cerebral ischemia.

CV: flushing, hypotension; IV only—MYOCARDIAL INFARCTION, arrhythmias.

Resp: IV only—bronchospasm.

GI: GI upset, nausea, vomiting, diarrhea.

Derm: rash.

INTERACTIONS

Drug-Drug: ▪ Additive effects with **aspirin** on platelet aggregation ▪ Risk of bleeding may be increased when used with **anticoagulants, thrombolytics, nonsteroidal anti-inflammatory agents,** or **sulfinpyrazone** ▪ Increased risk of hypotension with **alcohol** ▪ **Theophylline** may negate the effects of dipyridamole during diagnostic thallium imaging.

ROUTE AND DOSAGE

- **PO (Adults):** 100–400 mg/day in 2–4 divided doses.
- **IV (Adults):** 0.57 mg/kg (0.142 mg/kg/min for 4 min).

PHARMACODYNAMICS (PO = antiplatelet activity, IV = coronary vasodilation)

	ONSET	PEAK	DURATION
PO	UK	UK	UK
IV	UK	6.5 min*	30 min

*From start of infusion.

NURSING IMPLICATIONS

Assessment

- **PO:** Monitor blood pressure and pulse before instituting therapy and regularly during period of dosage adjustment.
- **IV:** Monitor vital signs during and for 10–15 min following infusion. Obtain ECG in at least one lead. If severe chest pain or bronchospasm occurs, administer IV aminophylline 50–250 mg at a rate of 50–100 mg over 30–60 sec. If hypotension is severe, place patient in a supine position with head tilting down. If chest pain is unrelieved with aminophylline 250 mg, administer nitroglycerin SL. If chest pain is still unrelieved, treat as myocardial infarction.
- **Lab Test Considerations:** Bleeding time should be monitored periodically throughout course of therapy.

Potential Nursing Diagnoses

- Cardiac output, decreased (indications).
- Comfort, altered: pain (indications).
- Knowledge deficit related to medication regimen (patient/family teaching).

Implementation

- **PO:** Administer with a full glass of water at least 1 hr before or 2 hr after meals for faster absorption. If GI irritation occurs, may be administered with or immediately after meals. Tablets may be crushed and mixed with food if patient has difficulty swallowing. Pharmacist may make a suspension.
- **Intermittent Infusion:** Dilute in at least a 1:2 ration of 0.45% NaCl, 0.9% NaCl, or D5W for a total volume of 20–50 ml. Undiluted dipyridamole may cause venous irritation.
  - *Rate:* Infuse dose over 4 min.

Patient/Family Teaching

- **PO:** Instruct patient to take medication at evenly spaced intervals as prescribed. If a dose is missed, take as soon as remembered unless the next scheduled dose is within 4 hr. Do not double doses. Benefit of medication may not be apparent to patient; encourage patient to continue taking medication as directed.
  - Caution patient to make position changes slowly to minimize orthostatic hypotension.
  - Advise patient to avoid the use of alcohol, as it may potentiate the hypotensive effects. Tobacco products should also be avoided because nicotine causes vasoconstriction.

*Underlines indicate most frequent; **CAPITALS** indicate life-threatening.

- Advise patient to consult physician or pharmacist before taking over-the-counter medications concurrently with this medication.
- Instruct patient to notify physician if unusual bleeding or bruising occurs.
- **IV:** Instruct patient to notify physician immediately if dyspnea or chest pain occur.

Evaluation

Effectiveness of therapy can be demonstrated by: ▪ Prevention of postoperative thromboembolic complications associated with prosthetic heart valves ▪ Maintenance of patency after surgical graft procedures ▪ Coronary vasodilation in thallium myocardial perfusion imaging.

DISOPYRAMIDE

(dye-soe-**peer**-a-mide)

Norpace, Norpace CR, {Rythmodan}, {Rythmodan-LA}

CLASSIFICATION(S):

Antiarrhythmic—class I

Pregnancy Category C

INDICATIONS

▪ Suppression and prevention of unifocal and multifocal PVCs, paired PVCs, and ventricular tachycardia. **Unlabeled Use:** ▪ Treatment and prevention of supraventricular tachyarrhythmias.

ACTION

▪ Decreases myocardial excitability and conduction velocity ▪ May depress myocardial contractility ▪ Also has anticholinergic properties ▪ Little effect on heart rate, but has a direct negative inotropic effect. **Therapeutic Effect:** ▪ Suppression of ventricular arrhythmias.

PHARMACOKINETICS

Absorption: Well absorbed from the GI tract.

Distribution: Widely distributed throughout extracellular fluid. Enters breast milk.

Metabolism and Excretion: Metabolized by the liver. 10% excreted unchanged in the feces, 50% excreted unchanged by the kidneys.

Half-life: 8–18 hr (increased in hepatic or renal impairment).

CONTRAINDICATIONS AND PRECAUTIONS

Contraindicated in: ▪ Hypersensitivity ▪ Cardiogenic shock ▪ 2nd degree and 3rd degree heart block ▪ Sick sinus syndrome (without a pacemaker).

Use Cautiously in: ▪ Cardiomyopathy ▪ Possible cardiac decompensation (dosage reduction recommended) ▪ Hepatic or renal insufficiency (dosage reduction recommended) ▪ Elderly men with prostatic enlargement ▪ Myasthenia gravis ▪ Glaucoma ▪ Pregnancy or lactation (safety not established).

ADVERSE REACTIONS AND SIDE EFFECTS*

CNS: blurred vision, dizziness, headache, fatigue.

CV: CONGESTIVE HEART FAILURE, edema, dyspnea, AV block, hypotension.

EENT: dry eyes, dry throat.

GI: dry mouth, constipation, nausea, abdominal pain, flatulence.

GU: urinary hesitancy, retention.

Endo: hypoglycemia.

Misc: impaired temperature regulation.

INTERACTIONS

Drug-Drug: ▪ May potentiate anticoagulant effect of **warfarin** ▪ **Rifampin, phenobarbital,** and **phenytoin** may decrease blood levels and effectiveness ▪ **Cimetidine** may decrease metabolism and increase blood levels ▪ May have additive toxic cardiac effects when used with other **antiarrhythmics** (prolonged conduction and decreased cardiac output), especially **verapamil**—avoid us-

{} = Available in Canada only.

*Underlines indicate most frequent; **CAPITALS** indicate life-threatening.

ing disopyramide for 48 hr before or 24 hr after ▪ Anticholinergic side effects may be additive with other **drugs having anticholinergic properties** including **antihistamines** and **tricyclic antidepressants** ▪ Increased risk of arrhythmias with **pimozide**.

ROUTE AND DOSAGE

- **PO (Adults >50 kg):** 150 mg q 6 hr (as regular capsules) or 300 mg q 12 hr as CR dosage form (up to 800 mg/day).
- **PO (Adults <50 kg):** 400 mg/day—100 mg q 6 hr (as regular capsules) or 200 mg q 12 hr as CR dosage form (up to 800 mg/day).
- **PO (Children 12–18 yr):** 6–15 mg/kg daily, in divided doses q 6 hr.
- **PO (Children 4–12 yr):** 10–15 mg/kg daily in divided doses q 6 hr.
- **PO (Children 1–4 yr):** 10–20 mg/kg daily in divided doses q 6 hr.
- **PO (Children <1 yr):** 10–30 mg/kg daily in divided doses q 6 hr.

PHARMACODYNAMICS (antiarrhythmic effects)

	ONSET	PEAK	DURATION
PO	0.5–3.5 hr	2.5 hr	1.5–8.5 hr
PO-CR	0.5–3.5 hr	4.9 hr	12 hr

NURSING IMPLICATIONS

Assessment

- Monitor blood pressure, pulse, and ECG prior to and routinely throughout therapy. Check pulse prior to administering medication; withhold and notify physician if <60 or >120 bpm, or if changes in rhythm occur.
- Monitor intake and output ratios and daily weight; assess for edema and urinary retention daily.
- Assess patient for signs of congestive heart failure (peripheral edema, rales/crackles, dyspnea, weight gain, jugular venous distention). Notify physician if these occur.
- **Lab Test Considerations:** Renal and hepatic functions and serum potassium levels should be evaluated periodically throughout course of therapy.
  - May cause elevated serum BUN, cholesterol, and triglyceride concentrations.
  - May cause decreased blood glucose concentrations.

Potential Nursing Diagnoses

- Cardiac output, decreased (indications).
- Oral mucous membranes, altered: (side effects).
- Knowledge deficit related to medication regimen (patient/family teaching).

Implementation

- **General Info:** When changing from quinidine sulfate or procainamide to disopyramide, regular maintenance dose of disopyramide may be given 6–12 hr after last dose of quinidine sulfate or 3–6 hr after last dose of procainamide.
  - Extended-release form is indicated for maintenance therapy only. When changing from regular dosage form to extended-release forms, give the first dose of extended-release form 6 hr after the last regular dose.
- **PO:** Administer medication on an empty stomach, 1 hr before or 2 hr after meals. Controlled-release capsules (CR) must be swallowed whole; do not break open, crush, or chew.
  - Pharmacist may prepare a suspension with 100 mg capsules and cherry syrup.

Patient/Family Teaching

- Advise patient to take medication around the clock, exactly as directed. Do not discontinue medication without consulting physician. If a dose is missed, take as soon as remembered unless within 4 hr of next dose. Do not double doses.
- Medication may cause dizziness. Caution patients to avoid driving or other activities requiring alertness until response to medication is known.
- Instruct patient to make position changes slowly to minimize orthostatic hypotension.

- □ Advise patient that frequent mouth rinses, good oral hygiene, and sugarless gum or candy may help relieve dry mouth.
- □ Caution patient to avoid extremes of temperature, as this medication may cause impairment of body temperature regulation. Patient should use sunscreen and protective clothing to prevent photosensitivity reactions.
- □ Advise patient to consult physician or pharmacist prior to taking over-the-counter medications or alcohol concurrently with this medication.
- □ If constipation becomes a problem, advise patient that increasing bulk and fluids in the diet and exercise may minimize the constipating effects.
- □ Instruct patient to notify physician if dry mouth, difficult urination, constipation, or blurred vision persist.

EVALUATION

Effectiveness of therapy can be demonstrated by: ▪ Suppression of PVCs and ventricular tachycardia ▪ Prevention of further arrhythmias.

DISULFIRAM

(dye-**sul**-fi-ram)
Antabuse

CLASSIFICATION(S):
Alcohol abuse deterrent
Pregnancy Category UK

INDICATIONS

▪ Management of alcohol dependence ▪ Discourages further abuse of alcohol in programs combining support and psychotherapy.

ACTION

▪ Inhibits the enzyme aldehyde dehydrogenase, resulting in accumulation of toxic concentrations of acetaldehyde following ingestion of alcohol. **Therapeutic Effect:** ▪ Production of uncomfortable hypersensitivity reaction following alcohol ingestion (disulfiram reaction or acetaldehyde syndrome).

PHARMACOKINETICS

Absorption: Rapidly absorbed following oral administration, but effect is delayed.
Distribution: Initially distributes to fat.
Metabolism and Excretion: Metabolized by the liver. 5–20% excreted unchanged in feces.
Half-life: UK. Up to 20% remains in the body for 7 days.

CONTRAINDICATIONS AND PRECAUTIONS

Contraindicated in: ▪ Previous allergic reactions to disulfiram or rubber contact dermatitis (thiuram derivatives) ▪ Alcohol intoxication ▪ Cardiovascular disease ▪ Psychoses.
Use Cautiously in: ▪ Diabetes mellitus ▪ Hypothyroidism ▪ Seizures or abnormal EEG ▪ Cerebral hemorrhage ▪ Nephritis ▪ History of liver disease ▪ History of drug dependence ▪ Pregnancy, lactation, or children (safety not established).

ADVERSE REACTIONS AND SIDE EFFECTS*

CNS: drowsiness, fatigue, impotence, headache, vertigo, insomnia, abnormal gait, slurred speech, disorientation, confusion, personality changes, seizures, delirium, psychoses, bizarre behavior.
EENT: optic neuritis.
GU: impotence.
Derm: acneform rash, allergic dermatitis.
Hemat: blood dyscrasias.
Neuro: peripheral neuropathy, polyneuritis.
Misc: ingestion or application of alcohol results in disulfiram reaction (see Drug–Drug Interactions).

INTERACTIONS

Drug–Drug: ▪ Concurrent use with **alcohol** in any form (cough and cold prep-

*Underlines indicate most frequent; **CAPITALS** indicate life-threatening.

arations, skin liniments, aftershaves) will produce the disulfiram reaction ▪ Disulfiram increases blood levels and the risk of toxicity of **phenytoin, isoniazid, metronidazole, diazepam, chlordiazepoxide,** and **paraldehyde.**
Drug–Food: ▪ Concurrent use with any food containing **alcohol** will result in disulfiram reaction.

ROUTE AND DOSAGE

- **PO (Adults):** 500 mg/day for 1–2 wk, then 250 mg/day (range 125–500 mg/day).

PHARMACODYNAMICS (ability to produce disulfiram reaction following exposure to alcohol)

	ONSET	PEAK	DURATION
PO	5–10 min (3–12 hr)*	UK	1–2 wk

*Onset of reaction is 5–10 min following alcohol ingestion during chronic dosing. After initial dose, reaction may be delayed up to 12 hr.

NURSING IMPLICATIONS

Assessment

- □ Assess patient for use of alcohol in any form within the 12 hr prior to administration of disulfiram. Patients should be free of alcohol intake for at least 12 hr prior to initiation of therapy.
- ▪ **Lab Test Considerations:** Monitor CBC periodically and SMA-12 levels every 6 mon throughout therapy.
- □ Doses of 500 mg/day may cause an increase in serum cholesterol concentrations.
- □ Monitor hepatic function tests prior to and at periodic intervals during therapy. May cause elevated SGOT (AST) and SGPT (ALT) levels.

Potential Nursing Diagnoses

- ▪ Coping, ineffective individual (indications).
- ▪ Knowledge deficit related to medication regimen (patient/family teaching).

Implementation

- ▪ **General Info:** Disulfiram should *never* be administered without the patient's knowledge.
- □ Check alcohol content of other medications patient is taking prior to administration. Do not administer within 12 hr of alcohol-containing preparations.
- □ The alcohol-disulfiram test is considered unnecessary by most clinicians and may be associated with increased drug toxicity. Explicit descriptions of the reaction following ingestion of alcohol are considered sufficient to deter the patient from ingesting alcohol during treatment. If the test is considered necessary, it should be performed under careful medical supervision with adequate facilities, including oxygen, in the event of a severe reaction. This test should not be performed on patients over 50 yr. The test consists of administering 15 ml of 100-proof alcohol after 1–2 wk of disulfiram therapy. The dose may be repeated once but should not exceed 30 ml of alcohol. Discontinue alcohol at the first sign of symptoms.
- ▪ **PO:** Tablets may be crushed and mixed with beverages.

Patient/Family Teaching

- □ Inform patient of the nature of the medication, the disulfiram-alcohol reaction, and its consequences. Instruct patient in the importance of compliance with disulfiram therapy. Alcohol in all forms, including beer, wine, liquor, vinegars, cough mixtures, sauces, aftershave lotions, liniments, and colognes, should be avoided. Advise patient that alcohol intake within 12 hr prior to or 14 days following administration may cause the disulfiram-alcohol reaction (blurred vision, chest pain, confusion, dizziness or fainting, fast or pounding heartbeat, flushing or redness of face, nausea, vomiting, dyspnea, unusual sweating, severe weakness, seizures, myocardial infarction, unconsciousness, death). Effects of this reaction may last 30 min to several hrs.

- □ Advise patient to check all medications for alcohol content.
- □ Medication may cause drowsiness. Caution patient to avoid driving or other activities requiring alertness until response to drug is known.
- □ Caution patient to avoid taking CNS depressants during disulfiram therapy.
- □ Instruct patient to carry identification describing medication regimen at all times. Physician should be notified if visual changes or rash occur.
- □ Emphasize the importance of follow-up visits to the physician to monitor progress in long-term therapy and participation in alcohol-abuse therapy.

EVALUATION

Effectiveness of therapy can be demonstrated by: ▪ Maintenance of sobriety in the treatment of chronic alcoholism or avoidance of alcohol intake.

DOBUTAMINE

(doe-**byoo**-ta-meen)
Dobutrex

CLASSIFICATION(S):
Inotropic agent
Pregnancy Category UK

INDICATIONS

▪ Short-term management of heart failure due to depressed contractility from organic heart disease or surgical procedures.

ACTION

▪ Stimulates $beta_1$ (myocardial) adrenergic receptors with relatively minor effect on heart rate or peripheral blood vessels. **Therapeutic Effect:** ▪ Increased cardiac output without significantly increasing heart rate.

PHARMACOKINETICS

Absorption: Administered by IV infusion only, resulting in complete bioavailability.
Distribution: Distribution not known.
Metabolism and Excretion: Metabolized by the liver and other tissues.
Half-life: 2 min.

CONTRAINDICATIONS AND PRECAUTIONS

Contraindicated in: ▪ Hypersensitivity ▪ Hypersensitivity to bisulfites (contains bisulfite) ▪ Idiopathic hypertropic subaortic stenosis.
Use Cautiously in: ▪ Myocardial infarction ▪ Atrial fibrillation (pretreatment with cardiac glycosides recommended) ▪ Pregnancy, lactation, and children (safety not established).

ADVERSE REACTIONS AND SIDE EFFECTS*

CNS: headache.
Resp: shortness of breath.
CV: <u>tachycardia</u>, <u>hypertension</u>, <u>premature ventricular contractions</u>, angina pectoris.
GI: nausea, vomiting.
Misc: nonanginal chest pain.

INTERACTIONS

Drug-Drug: ▪ Use with **nitroprusside** may have a synergistic effect on increasing cardiac output ▪ **Beta-adrenergic blocking agents** may negate the effect of dobutamine ▪ Increased risk of arrhythmias or hypertension with some **anesthetics (cyclopropane, halothane), MAO inhibitors, oxytocics,** or **tricyclic antidepressants**.

ROUTE AND DOSAGE

Note: See infusion rate chart in Appendix D.

- ▪ **IV (Adults):** 2.5–10 mcg/kg/min infusion (up to 40 mcg/kg/min).

PHARMACODYNAMICS (inotropic effects)

	ONSET	PEAK	DURATION
IV	1–2 min	10 min	brief (min)

*<u>Underlines</u> indicate most frequent; **CAPITALS** indicate life-threatening.

D

NURSING IMPLICATIONS

Assessment

- □ Monitor blood pressure, heart rate, ECG, pulmonary capillary wedge pressure (PCWP), cardiac output, central venous pressure (CVP), and urinary output continuously during the administration of this medication.
- □ An increase in systolic blood pressure of 10–20 mmHg and an increase in heart rate of 5–15 bpm occurs in most patients. Observe patient closely for extreme increases in blood pressure, heart rate, or ectopy. This may indicate a need for dosage reduction. Notify physician.
- □ Diabetic patients may require an increase in insulin. Monitor blood glucose levels closely.
- ■ **Toxicity and Overdose:** If overdose occurs, reduction or discontinuation of therapy is the only treatment necessary due to the short duration of dobutamine.

Potential Nursing Diagnoses

- ■ Cardiac output, decreased (indications).
- ■ Tissue perfusion, altered: (indications).

Implementation

- ■ **General Info:** Hypovolemia should be corrected with volume expanders prior to initiating dobutamine therapy.
- ■ **IV:** Reconstitute 250-mg vial with 10 ml of sterile water or D5W for injection. If not completely dissolved, add another 10 ml of diluent. Dilute in at least 50 ml of D5W, 0.9% NaCl, sodium lactate, 0.45% NaCl, D5/0.45% NaCl, D5/0.9% NaCl, D5/LR, or lactated Ringer's soln. Standard concentrations range from 250 mcg/ml to 1000 mcg/ml. Concentrations should not exceed 5 mg of dobutamine per ml. Slight pink color of soln does not alter potency. Soln is stable for 24 hr at room temperature.
- ■ **Continuous Infusion:** Administer via infusion pump. Rate of administration is titrated according to patient response (heart rate, presence of ectopic activity, blood pressure, urine output, CVP, PCWP, cardiac output); see Appendix D.
- ■ **Syringe Compatibility:** heparin or ranitidine.
- ■ **Y-Site Compatibility:** amrinone, atracurium, bretylium, calcium chloride, calcium gluconate, diazepam, dopamine, enalaprilat, famotidine, insulin, lidocaine, magnesium sulfate, nitroglycerin, pancuronium, potassium chloride, ranitidine, sodium nitroprusside, streptokinase, tolazoline, vecuronium, verapamil, or zidovudine.
- ■ **Y-Site Incompatibility:** acyclovir, alteplase, aminophylline, foscarnet, or phytonadione.
- ■ **Additive Compatibility:** atropine, dopamine, epinephrine, hydralazine, isoproterenol, lidocaine, meperidine, metaraminol bitartrate, morphine, nitroglycerin, norepinephrine, phentolamine, phenylephrine, procainamide, propranolol, or ranitidine.
- ■ **Additive Incompatibility:** acyclovir, aminophylline, bumetanide, calcium gluconate, diazepam, digoxin, furosemide, insulin, magnesium sulfate, phenytoin, potassium phosphate, or sodium bicarbonate.

Patient/Family Teaching

- □ Explain to patient the rationale for instituting this medication and the need for frequent monitoring.
- □ Instruct patient to notify nurse immediately of pain or discomfort at the site of administration.

Evaluation

Effectiveness of therapy can be demonstrated by: ■ Increase in cardiac output □ Improved hemodynamic parameters □ Increased urine output.

DOCUSATE

(**dok**-yoo-sate)

DOCUSATE CALCIUM

Pro-Cal-Sof, Surfak

DOCUSATE POTASSIUM

Dialose, Diocto-K, Kasof

DOCUSATE SODIUM

Afko-Lube, Colace, Dioeze, Diocto, Diosuccin, Diosul, Disonate, DiSosul, Doss, DOSS, Doxinate, DSS, Duosol, Laxinate 100, Modane Soft, Pro-Sof, Regulax SS, {Regulex}, Regutol, Stulex

CLASSIFICATION(S):
Laxative—stool softener
Pregnancy Category C

INDICATIONS

▪ **PO:** Prevention of constipation (in patients who should avoid straining, such as after myocardial infarction or rectal surgery) ▪ **Rectal:** Used by enema to soften fecal impaction.

ACTION

▪ Promotes incorporation of water into stool, resulting in softer fecal mass ▪ May also promote electrolyte and water secretion into the colon. **Therapeutic Effect:** ▪ Softening and passage of stool.

PHARMACOKINETICS

Absorption: Small amounts may be absorbed from the small intestine after oral administration. Absorption from the rectum is not known.
Distribution: Distribution not known.
Metabolism and Excretion: Amounts absorbed after oral administration are eliminated in bile.
Half-life: UK.

CONTRAINDICATIONS AND PRECAUTIONS

Contraindicated in: ▪ Hypersensitivity ▪ Abdominal pain, nausea, or vomiting especially when associated with fever or other signs of an acute abdomen.
Use Cautiously in: ▪ Excessive or prolonged use may lead to dependence ▪ Has been used during pregnancy and lactation ▪ Should not be used if prompt results are desired.

ADVERSE REACTIONS AND SIDE EFFECTS*

EENT: throat irritation.
GI: mild cramps.
Derm: rashes.

INTERACTIONS

Drug-Drug: None significant.

ROUTE AND DOSAGE

Docusate Calcium

- **PO (Adults):** 240 mg once daily.
- **PO (Children ≥6 yr and Adults With Minimal Requirements):** 50–150 mg once daily.

Docusate Potassium

- **PO (Adults):** 100–300 mg once daily.
- **PO (Children ≥6 yr):** 100 mg once daily at bedtime.

Docusate Sodium

- **PO (Adults and Older Children):** 50–500 mg once daily.
- **PO (Children 6–12 yr):** 40–120 mg once daily.
- **PO (Children 3–6 yr):** 20–60 mg once daily.
- **PO (Children <3 yr):** 10–40 mg.
- **Rect—Enema (Adults):** 50–100 mg or 3.9 g capsule containing 283 mg docusate sodium, soft soap, and glycerin).

PHARMACODYNAMICS (softening of stool)

	ONSET	PEAK	DURATION
PO	1–3 days	UK	UK
Rectal	min–hr	UK	UK

NURSING IMPLICATIONS

Assessment

- ☐ Assess patient for abdominal distention, presence of bowel sounds, and usual pattern of bowel function.
- ☐ Assess color, consistency, and amount of stool produced.

Potential Nursing Diagnoses

- Bowel elimination, altered: constipation (indications).

{} = Available in Canada only.
*Underlines indicate most frequent; **CAPITALS** indicate life-threatening.

D

- Knowledge deficit related to medication regimen (patient/family teaching).

IMPLEMENTATION

- **General Info:** Available in combination with other products (see Appendix A).
  - This medication does not stimulate intestinal peristalsis.
- **PO:** Administer with a full glass of water or juice. May be administered on an empty stomach for more rapid results.
  - Oral soln may be diluted in milk or fruit juice to decrease bitter taste.

PATIENT/FAMILY TEACHING

- Advise patients that laxatives should be used only for short-term therapy. Long-term therapy may cause electrolyte imbalance and dependence.
- Encourage patients to use other forms of bowel regulation, such as increasing bulk in the diet, increasing fluid intake, increasing mobility. Normal bowel habits are variable and may vary from 3 times/day to 3 times/wk.
- Instruct patients with cardiac disease to avoid straining during bowel movements (Valsalva maneuver).
- Advise patient not to use laxatives when abdominal pain, nausea, vomiting, or fever is present.

EVALUATION

Effectiveness of therapy can be demonstrated by: ▪ A soft, formed bowel movement, usually within 24–48 hr. May require 3–5 days of therapy for results.

DOPAMINE

(dope-a-meen)

Intropin, {Revimine}

CLASSIFICATION(S):
Vasopressor, Inotropic agent
Pregnancy Category C

INDICATIONS

▪ Adjunct to standard measures to improve: ▫ Blood pressure ▫ Cardiac output ▫ Urine output in treatment of shock unresponsive to fluid replacement.

ACTION

▪ Small doses (0.5–2 mcg/kg/min) stimulate dopaminergic receptors, producing renal vasodilation ▪ Larger doses (2–10 mcg/kg/min) stimulate dopaminergic and $beta_1$-adrenergic receptors, producing cardiac stimulation and renal vasodilation ▪ Doses greater than 10 mcg/kg/min stimulate alpha-adrenergic receptors and may cause renal vasoconstriction. **Therapeutic Effects:** ▪ Increased cardiac output, increased blood pressure, and improved renal blood flow.

PHARMACOKINETICS

Absorption: Administered IV only, resulting in complete bioavailability.

Distribution: Widely distributed after IV administration, but does not cross the blood-brain barrier.

Metabolism and Excretion: Metabolized in liver, kidneys, and plasma.

Half-life: 2 min.

CONTRAINDICATIONS AND PRECAUTIONS

Contraindicated in: ▪ Tachyarrhythmias ▪ Pheochromocytoma.

Use Cautiously in: ▪ Occlusive vascular diseases ▪ Pregnancy, lactation, and children (safety not established).

ADVERSE REACTIONS AND SIDE EFFECTS*

CNS: headache.
EENT: mydriasis (high dose).
Resp: dyspnea.
CV: arrhythmias, hypotension, palpitations, angina, ECG change, vasoconstriction.
GI: nausea, vomiting.
Derm: piloerection.
Local: irritation at IV site.

INTERACTIONS

Drug-Drug: ▪ Use with **MAO inhibitors** or **ergot alkaloids (ergotamine)** re-

{} = Available in Canada only.
*Underlines indicate most frequent; CAPITALS indicate life-threatening.

sults in severe hypertension ▪ Use with **IV phenytoin** may cause hypotension and bradycardia ▪ Use with **general anesthetics** may result in arrhythmias ▪ **Beta-adrenergic blockers** may antagonize cardiac effects.

ROUTE AND DOSAGE

Note: See infusion rate table in Appendix D.

- **IV (Adults):** 1–5 mcg/kg/min initially, increase at 10–30 min intervals up to 50 mcg/kg/min, titrate by hemodynamic and renal response.

PHARMACODYNAMICS (hemodynamic effects)

	ONSET	PEAK	DURATION
IV	5 min	rapid	<10 min

NURSING IMPLICATIONS

Assessment

- ▫ Monitor blood pressure, pulse, respiration, ECG, and hemodynamic parameters every 5–15 min during and after administration. Notify physician if significant changes in vital signs or arrhythmias occur. Consult physician for parameters for pulse, blood pressure, or ECG changes for adjusting dosage or discontinuing medication.
- ▫ Monitor urine output frequently throughout administration. Notify physician promptly if urine output decreases.
- ▫ Palpate peripheral pulses and assess appearance of extremities routinely throughout dopamine administration. Notify physician if quality of pulse deteriorates or if extremities become cold or mottled.
- ▫ If hypotension occurs, administration rate should be increased. If hypotension continues, more potent vasoconstrictors (norepinephrine) may be administered.
- ▪ **Toxicity and Overdose:** If excessive hypertension occurs, rate of infusion should be decreased or temporarily discontinued until blood pressure is decreased. Although additional measures are usually not necessary due to short duration of dopamine, phentolamine may be administered if hypertension continues.

Potential Nursing Diagnoses

- ▪ Cardiac output, decreased (indications).
- ▪ Tissue perfusion, altered: (indications).

Implementation

- ▪ **General Info:** Hypovolemia should be corrected prior to administration of dopamine.
- ▫ Administer into a large vein, and assess administration site frequently. Extravasation may cause severe irritation, necrosis, and sloughing of tissue. If extravasation occurs, affected area should be infiltrated with 10–15 ml of 0.9% NaCl containing 5–10 mg of phentolamine.
- ▪ **Continuous Infusion:** Dilute 200–400 mg in 250–500 ml of 0.9% NaCl, D5W, D5/LR, D5/0.45% NaCl, D5/0.9% NaCl, or in lactated Ringer's soln for IV infusion. Concentrations commonly used are 800 mcg/ml or 0.8 mg/ml (200 mg/250 ml) and 1.6 mg/ml (400 mg/250 ml). Dilute immediately prior to administration. Yellow or brown discoloration indicates decomposition. Discard soln that is cloudy, discolored, or contains a precipitate. Soln is stable for 24 hr.
- ▫ *Rate:* Administer at a rate of 1–5 mcg/kg/min, and increase by 1–4 mcg/kg/min at 10–30 min intervals until desired dosage is obtained. Infusion must be administered via infusion pump to ensure precise amount delivered. Rate of administration is titrated according to patient response (blood pressure, heart rate, urine flow, peripheral perfusion, presence of ectopic activity, cardiac output); see Appendix D.
- ▪ **Syringe Compatibility:** doxapram, heparin, or ranitidine.
- ▪ **Y-Site Compatibility:** amrinone, atracurium, dobutamine, enalaprilat, esmolol, famotidine, foscarnet, heparin,

hydrocortisone sodium succinate, labetalol, lidocaine, nitroglycerin, pancuronium, potassium chloride, ranitidine, sodium nitroprusside, streptokinase, tolazoline, vecuronium, or verapamil.

- **Y-Site Incompatibility:** acyclovir or alteplase.
- **Additive Compatibility:** aminophylline, bretylium, calcium chloride, chloramphenicol, dobutamine, heparin, hydrocortisone sodium succinate, kanamycin, lidocaine, methylprednisolone, nitroglycerin, oxacillin, potassium chloride, ranitidine, tetracycline, or verapamil.
- **Additive Incompatibility:** acyclovir, amphotericin B, ampicillin, cephalothin, or penicillin G potassium. Dopamine is inactivated (soln turns pink to violet) in alkaline soln, including sodium bicarbonate.

PATIENT/FAMILY TEACHING

- □ Advise patient to inform nurse immediately if chest pain, dyspnea, numbness, tingling, or burning of extremities occurs.
- □ Instruct patient to inform nurse immediately of pain or discomfort at the site of administration.

EVALUATION

Effectiveness of therapy can be demonstrated by: ▪ Increase in blood pressure □ Increase in peripheral circulation □ Increase in urine output.

DOXACURIUM

(dox-a-**cure**-ee-yum)
Nuromax

CLASSIFICATION(S):
Neuromuscular blocking agent—nondepolarizing
Pregnancy Category C

INDICATIONS

▪ Induction of skeletal muscle paralysis and facilitation of intubation after induction of anesthesia in surgical procedures.

ACTION

▪ Prevents neuromuscular transmission by blocking the effect of acetylcholine at the myoneural junction. Has no analgesic or anxioytic properties. **Therapeutic Effect:** ▪ Skeletal muscle paralysis.

PHARMACOKINETICS

Absorption: Administered IV only, resulting in complete bioavailability.
Distribution: Distribution not known.
Metabolism and Excretion: Excreted primarily unchanged in urine and bile.
Half-life: 90–120 min (increased in kidney transplant patients).

CONTRAINDICATIONS AND PRECAUTIONS

Contraindicated in: ▪ Hypersensitivity to doxacurium or benzyl alcohol ▪ Newborn infants (benzyl alcohol may produce fatal reactions).

Use Cautiously in: ▪ Pregnancy, lactation, or children <2 yr (safety not established) ▪ Elderly patients (slower onset of neuromuscular blockade) ▪ Electrolyte or acid base abnormalities (unpredictable response) ▪ Burn patients (may have resistance) ▪ Neuromuscular diseases (exaggerated response).

ADVERSE REACTIONS AND SIDE EFFECTS*

Note: Almost all adverse reactions to doxacurium are extensions of pharmacologic effects.

Resp: APNEA, respiratory insufficiency.
CV: hypotension.
Derm: flushing.
MS: muscle weakness.

INTERACTIONS

Drug-Drug: ▪ **Carbamazepine** and **phenytoin** decrease duration of block and increase time of onset ▪ Intensity and duration of paralysis may be prolonged by **aminoglycoside antibiotics, polymyxin B, colistin, clindamycin,**

*Underlines indicate most frequent; **CAPITALS** indicate life-threatening.

lidocaine, quinidine, procainamide, beta-adrenergic blocking agents, potassium-losing diuretics, and **magnesium** ▪ **Isoflurane, enflurane, halothane,** or **succinylcholine** potentiate effects (decrease doxacurium dosage).

ROUTE AND DOSAGE

- **IV (Adults):** 0.05 mg/kg (may need up to 0.08 mg/kg for prolonged effect) initially, followed 60–100 min later by 0.005–0.01 mg/kg, repeated as required.
- **IV (Children):** 0.03–0.05 mg/kg initially, maintenance doses may be required more frequently than in adults.

PHARMACODYNAMICS

	ONSET	PEAK	DURATION
IV*	5 min	UK	100 min

*For a 0.05 mg/kg dose in an adult.

NURSING IMPLICATIONS

Assessment

- Assess respiratory status continuously throughout doxacurium therapy. Atracurium should be used only by individuals experienced in endotracheal intubation and equipment for this procedure should be readily available.
- Neuromuscular response to atracurium should be monitored with a peripheral nerve stimulator. Paralysis is initially selective and usually occurs sequentially in the following muscles: levator muscles of eyelids, muscles of mastication, limb muscles, abdominal muscles, muscles of the glottis, intercostal muscles and the diaphragm. Recovery of muscle function usually occurs in reverse order.
- Observe the patient for residual muscle weakness and respiratory distress during the recovery period.
- **Toxicity and Overdose:** If overdose occurs use peripheral nerve stimulator to determine the degree of neuromuscular blockade. Maintain airway patency and ventilation until recovery of normal respirations occur.
- Administration of anticholinesterase agents (neostigmine, pyridostigmine) may be used to antagonize the action of doxacurium once the patient has demonstrated some spontaneous recovery from neuromuscular block. Atropine is usually administered prior to or concurrently with anticholinesterase agents to counteract the muscarinic effects.
- Administration of fluids and vasopressors may be necessary to treat severe hypotension or shock.

Potential Nursing Diagnoses

- Breathing pattern, ineffective (indications).
- Communication, impaired: verbal (side effects).
- Fear (side effects).

Implementation

- **General Info:** Dose is titrated to patient response.
- Doxacurium has no effect on consciousness or the pain threshold. Adequate anesthesia should *always* be used when doxacurium is used as an adjunct to surgical procedures.
- Store at room temperature.
- **Direct IV:** Administer initial IV dose as a bolus over 1 min. Maintenance dose is usually required 60 min following initial dose of 0.025 mg/kg or 100 min following initial dose of 0.05 mg/kg. May be diluted further in D5W or 0.9% NaCl. Use diluted doxacurium within 8 hr. Discard unused diluted doxacurium after 8 hr.
- *Rate:* Administer every 30–45 min.
- **Y-Site Compatibility:** D5/0.9% NaCl, LR, D5/LR, alfentanil, fentanyl, or sufentanil.
- **Additive Incompatibility:** Incompatible with most barbiturates or sodium bicarbonate; do not administer in the same syringe or through the same needle during infusion.

Patient/Family Teaching

- Explain all procedures to patient receiving doxacurium therapy without anesthesia, as consciousness is not affected by atracurium alone.
- Reassure patient that communication

D

abilities will return as the medication wears off.

Evaluation

Effectiveness of therapy can be demonstrated by: ▪ Adequate suppression of the twitch response when tested with peripheral nerve stimulation and subsequent muscle paralysis.

DOXAPRAM
(**dox**-a-pram)
Dopram

CLASSIFICATION(S):
Respiratory and cerebral stimulant
Pregnancy Category B

INDICATIONS

▪ Used in carefully selected short-term situations with other supportive measures to treat postoperative CNS and respiratory depression due to CNS depressants ▪ Short-term postoperative stimulation of deep breathing with other supportive measures ▪ Prevention of acute hypercapnea during administration of oxygen to patients with acute respiratory insufficiency due to COPD (short-term only—less than 2 hr).

ACTION

▪ In low doses, stimulates breathing by activating carotid receptors ▪ Larger doses directly stimulate the respiratory center in medulla as well as produce generalized CNS stimulation. **Therapeutic Effect:** ▪ Transient increase in tidal volume, small increase in respiratory rate. Oxygenation is not increased.

PHARMACOKINETICS

Absorption: Administered IV only, results in complete bioavailability.
Distribution: Distribution in humans not known.
Metabolism and Excretion: Rapidly metabolized. Metabolites mostly excreted by the kidneys.
Half-life: 2.4–4 hr.

CONTRAINDICATIONS AND PRECAUTIONS

Contraindicated in: ▪ Hypersensitivity ▪ Patients on ventilators ▪ Head trauma ▪ Seizures ▪ Flail chest ▪ Pulmonary embolism ▪ Pneumothorax ▪ Pulmonary fibrosis ▪ Acute asthma ▪ Extreme dyspnea ▪ Cardiovascular or cerebrovascular disease ▪ Newborns (contains benzyl alcohol).
Use Cautiously in: ▪ Patients with a history of asthma or arrhythmias ▪ Increased intracranial pressure ▪ Hyperthyroidism ▪ Pheochromocytoma ▪ Serious uncorrected metabolic disorders ▪ Pregnancy, lactation, or children <12 (safety not established) ▪ Should not be used routinely as a respiratory stimulant.

ADVERSE REACTIONS AND SIDE EFFECTS*

CNS: SEIZURES†, headache, dizziness, apprehension, disorientation.
EENT: miosis, sneezing, gagging.
Resp: dyspnea†, bronchospasm, laryngospasm, coughing, rebound hypoventilation.
CV: elevated blood pressure†, tachycardia†, arrhythmias†, hypotension, chest pain, changes in heart rate, T-wave inversion.
GI: nausea, vomiting, diarrhea, desire to defecate.
GU: perineal or genital burning sensation, urinary retention, spontaneous voiding.
Derm: flushing, sweating, pruritus.
Hemat: hemolysis.
Local: irritation at IV site.
Metab: hyperpyrexia.
MS: skeletal muscle hyperactivity†, muscle spasticity†, involuntary movement†.
Neuro: paresthesia, positive bilateral Babinski's sign, generalized clonus.

INTERACTIONS

Drug-Drug: ▪ Pressor effects may be increased by concurrent use of **sympa-**

†Early signs of toxicity.
*Underlines indicate most frequent; **CAPITALS** indicate life-threatening.

thomimetic amines or **MAO inhibitors** ▪ May mask effects of **skeletal muscle relaxants**.

ROUTE AND DOSAGE

Respiratory Depression Following Anesthesia

- **IV (Adults):** 0.5–1 mg/kg (not to exceed 1.5 mg/kg) initially, may repeat every 5 min to a total of 2 mg/kg or as an infusion at 5 mg/min until response is obtained, then decrease infusion rate to 1–3 mg/min (total dose by infusion method should not exceed 4 mg/kg).

Drug-Induced CNS Depression

- **IV (Adults):** 2 doses of 1–2 mg/kg may be repeated at 5 min intervals. Can repeat in 1–2 hr until spontaneous breathing or total of 3 g given. If response occurs in 1–2 hr, can infuse at rate of 1–3 mg/min for up to 2 hr. Total dose not to exceed 3 g/24 hr.

Acute Hypercapnea

- **IV (Adults):** 1–2 mg/min (up to 3 mg/min).

PHARMACODYNAMICS (increases in minute volume)

	ONSET	PEAK	DURATION
IV	20–40 sec	1–2 min	5–12 min

NURSING IMPLICATIONS

Assessment

- □ Because of narrow margin of safety and indications for use, patient must be monitored constantly when receiving doxapram and for 1 hr after medication is discontinued and patient is fully alert.
- □ Monitor respiratory status (rate, rhythm, and depth of respirations) and ABGs. Ensure that patient has patent airway and is adequately oxygenated. Relapse of respiratory depression may occur if CNS depressant has long duration of action. To encourage maximal chest expansion and to prevent aspiration, position patient on side; elevate head of bed.
- □ Monitor neurologic status (level of consciousness and deep tendon reflexes). Notify physician if reflexes become hyperactive or if spasticity occurs.
- □ Monitor vital signs, ECG, and hemodynamic parameters. May cause tachycardia, hypertension, increased cardiac output, increased pulmonary artery pressure. Notify physician if there is significant change in hemodynamic parameters, arrhythmias, or chest pain. Patients with COPD may be at increased risk for arrhythmias because of hypoxia.
- □ Obtain baseline weight to ensure correct dosage.
- □ Inspect infusion site. May cause thrombophlebitis (erythema, swelling, and pain or skin irritation).
- ▪ **Lab Test Considerations:** Monitor ABGs prior to and every 30 min during therapy. Notify physician immediately if ABGs deteriorate. Physician may order cessation of drug, intubation, and mechanical ventilation.
- □ Monitor hemoglobin, hematocrit, erythrocyte, and leukocyte count. Rapid infusion may cause hemolysis.
- □ May cause elevated BUN and proteinuria.
- ▪ **Toxicity and Overdose:** Toxicity is manifested by severe hypertension, tachycardia, and hyperactive reflexes or seizures. Infusion should be stopped immediately. Seizures may be controlled with diazepam or a short-acting barbiturate. Resuscitative equipment should be available at all times.

Potential Nursing Diagnoses

- Breathing pattern, ineffective (indications).
- Knowledge deficit related to medication regimen (patient/family teaching).

Implementation

- **General Info:** Maximum dose is 4 mg/kg or 3 g total.
- **Direct IV:** Administer by direct IV injection over 5 min.
- **IV Infusion:** Dilute 250 mg in 250 ml of D5W, D10W, or 0.9% NaCl to yield

a concentration of 1 mg/ml. Dilute 400 mg (20-mg vial) in 180 ml of IV fluid to yield a 2 mg/ml concentration. Dosages vary with patient's condition. Infusion is limited to 2 hr. Administer via infusion pump to ensure accurate dosage.

- **Syringe Compatibility:** amikacin, bumetanide, chlorpromazine, cimetidine, cisplatin, cyclophosphamide, deslanoside, dopamine, doxycycline, epinephrine, hydroxyzine, imipramine, isoniazid, lincomycin, methotrexate, netilmicin, phytonadione, pyridoxine, terbutaline, thiamine, tobramycin, or vincristine.
- **Syringe Incompatibility:** aminophylline, ascorbic acid, cefoperazone, cefotaxime, cefotetan, cefuroxime, dexamethasone, diazepam, digoxin, dobutamine, folic acid, furosemide, hydrocortisone, ketamine, methylprednisolone, minocycline, thiopental, or ticarcillin.
- **Additive Incompatibility:** aminophylline, sodium bicarbonate, or thiopental.

Patient/Family Teaching

- ☐ Instruct patient to notify nurse immediately if shortness of breath worsens.

Evaluation

Effectiveness of therapy can be demonstrated by: ▪ Reversal of respiratory and nervous system depression associated with CNS depressants ▪ Postoperative respiratory depression not associated with skeletal muscle relaxants ▪ Prevention of acute respiratory insufficiency in patients with COPD. Doxapram is not used often because of its narrow margin of safety.

DOXAZOSIN

(**dox**-a-zoe-sin)
Cardura

CLASSIFICATION(S):
Antihypertensive—peripherally acting antiadrenergic
Pregnancy Category B

INDICATIONS

▪ Treatment of hypertension, alone or in combination with other agents.

ACTION

▪ Dilates both arteries and veins by blocking postsynaptic $alpha_1$-adrenergic receptors. **Therapeutic Effect:** ▪ Lowering of blood pressure.

PHARMACOKINETICS

Absorption: Well absorbed following oral administration.
Distribution: Distribution not known. Appears to enter breast milk. 98% bound to plasma proteins.
Metabolism and Excretion: Extensively metabolized by the liver.
Half-life: 22 hr.

CONTRAINDICATIONS AND PRECAUTIONS

Contraindicated in: ▪ Hypersensitivity.
Use Cautiously in: ▪ Pregnancy, lactation, or children (safety not established) ▪ Hepatic dysfunction.

ADVERSE REACTIONS AND SIDE EFFECTS*

CNS: dizziness, headache, depression, somnolence, nervousness, weakness, fatigue.
EENT: epistaxis, blurred vision, abnormal vision, conjunctivitis, vertigo.
Resp: dyspnea.
CV: first dose orthostatic hypotension, palpitations, arrhythmias, chest pain, edema.
GI: nausea, vomiting, dry mouth, diarrhea, constipation, abdominal discomfort, flatulence.
GU: decreased libido, sexual dysfunction.
Derm: flushing, rash.
MS: arthritis, arthralgia, myalgia, gout.

INTERACTIONS

Drug-Drug: ▪ Additive hypotension with acute ingestion of **alcohol,** other **antihypertensive agents,** or **nitrates** ▪ **Nonsteroidal anti-inflammatory**

*Underlines indicate most frequent; **CAPITALS** indicate life-threatening.

agents may decrease antihypertensive effects.

ROUTE AND DOSAGE

- **PO (Adults):** 1 mg once daily, may be increased to 2–16 mg/day, incidence of postural hypotension greatly increased at doses >4 mg/day.

PHARMACODYNAMICS

	ONSET	PEAK	DURATION
PO	UK	2–6 hr	24 hr

NURSING IMPLICATIONS

Assessment

- Monitor blood pressure and pulse frequently between 2–6 hr after a dose during initial dosage adjustment and with each increase in dose, and periodically throughout course of therapy. Notify physician of significant changes.
- Assess patient for first dose orthostatic hypotension and syncope. Incidence may be dose related. Observe patient closely during this period and take precautions to prevent injury.
- Monitor intake and output ratios and daily weight, and assess for edema daily, especially at beginning of therapy. Notify physician of weight gain or edema.
- **Lab Test Considerations:** May cause elevated serum sodium levels.

Potential Nursing Diagnoses

- Injury, high risk for (side effects).
- Knowledge deficit related to medication regimen (patient/family teaching).
- Noncompliance (patient/family teaching).

Implementation

- May be administered concurrently with a diuretic or other antihypertensive.

Patient/Family Teaching

- Emphasize the importance of continuing to take this medication, even if feeling well. Instruct patient to take medication at the same time each day. If a dose is missed, take as soon as remembered unless almost time for next dose. Do not double doses.
- Encourage patient to comply with additional interventions for hypertension (weight reduction, low sodium diet, discontinuation of smoking, moderation of alcohol consumption, regular exercise, and stress management).
- Instruct patient and family on proper technique for blood pressure monitoring. Advise them to check blood pressure at least weekly and report significant changes to physician.
- Doxazosin may cause drowsiness or dizziness. Advise patient to avoid driving or other activities requiring alertness until response to medication is known.
- Caution patient to avoid sudden changes in position to decrease orthostatic hypotension.
- Advise patient to consult physician or pharmacist before taking any cough, cold, or allergy remedies. Patients should also avoid excessive amounts of coffee, tea, or cola.
- Emphasize the importance of follow-up visits to determine effectiveness of therapy.

Evaluation

Effectiveness of therapy can be measured by: ▪ Decrease in blood pressure without appearance of side effects.

DOXEPIN

(**dox**-e-pin)
Adapin, Sinequan, {Triadapin}

CLASSIFICATION(S):
Antidepressant—tricyclic
Pregnancy Category C

INDICATIONS

- Used in conjunction with psychotherapy in the management of various forms

{} = Available in Canada only.

of endogenous depression ▪ Also been used in the treatment of anxiety. **Unlabeled Use:** ▪ Management of chronic pain syndromes.

ACTION

▪ Prevents the re-uptake of norepinephrine and serotonin by presynaptic neurons; resultant accumulation of neurotransmitters potentiates their activity ▪ Also possesses significant anticholinergic properties. **Therapeutic Effects:** ▪ Relief of depression ▪ Decreased anxiety.

PHARMACOKINETICS

Absorption: Well absorbed from the GI tract, although much is metabolized on first pass through the liver.

Distribution: Widely distributed. Enters breast milk. Probably crosses the placenta.

Metabolism and Excretion: Metabolized by the liver. Some conversion to active antidepressant compound. May re-enter gastric juice via secretion from enterohepatic circulation, where more absorption may occur.

Half-life: 8–25 hr.

CONTRAINDICATIONS AND PRECAUTIONS

Contraindicated in: ▪ Hypersensitivity ▪ Narrow-angle glaucoma ▪ Pregnancy or lactation ▪ Period immediately after myocardial infarction.

Use Cautiously in: ▪ Elderly patients ▪ Pre-existing cardiovascular disease (increased risk of adverse reactions) ▪ Prostatic enlargement (more susceptible to urinary retention) ▪ Seizures ▪ Anticholinergic side effects (may require dosage modification or drug discontinuation) ▪ Dosage requires slow titration, therapeutic response may take up to 6 wk.

ADVERSE REACTIONS AND SIDE EFFECTS*

CNS: drowsiness, sedation, lethargy, fatigue, confusion, agitation, hallucinations.

EENT: blurred vision, increased intraocular pressure.

CV: hypotension, ECG abnormalities, arrhythmias.

GI: dry mouth, constipation, paralytic ileus, hepatitis, nausea, increased appetite.

GU: urinary retention.

Derm: rashes, photosensitivity.

Hemat: blood dyscrasias.

Misc: hypersensitivity reactions.

INTERACTIONS

Drug–Drug: ▪ May cause hypotension, tachycardia, and potentially fatal reactions when used with **MAO inhibitors** (avoid concurrent use—discontinue 2 wk prior to doxepin) ▪ May prevent the therapeutic response to most **antihypertensives** ▪ May cuase severe hypertension when used with **clonidine** (avoid concurrent use) ▪ Additive CNS depression with other **CNS depressants** including **alcohol, antihistamines, narcotic analgesics,** and **sedative/hypnotics** ▪ **Adrenergic** and **anticholinergic** side effects may be additive with other agents having these properties ▪ **Cimetidine, fluoxetine, phenothiazines,** or **oral contraceptives** increase levels and may cause toxicity ▪ May produce organic brain syndrome with **disulfiram** ▪ **Smoking** may increase metabolism and decrease effectiveness.

ROUTE AND DOSAGE

- **PO (Adults):** 10–150 mg/day single bedtime dose or 2–3 divided doses, increase gradually (up to 300 mg/day, single dose should not exceed 150 mg).

PHARMACODYNAMICS (antidepressant activity)

	ONSET	PEAK	DURATION
PO	2–3wk	up to 6 wk	days–wks

NURSING IMPLICATIONS

Assessment

- **General Info:** Monitor blood pressure

*Underlines indicate most frequent; **CAPITALS** indicate life-threatening.

and pulse rate prior to and during initial therapy.

- **Depression:** Assess mental status frequently. Confusion, agitation, and hallucinations may occur during initiation of therapy and may require dosage reduction. Monitor mood changes. Assess for suicidal tendencies, especially during early therapy. Restrict amount of drug available to patient.
- **Pain:** Assess the type, location, and severity of pain prior to and periodically throughout therapy.
- **Lab Test Considerations:** Assess leukocyte and differential blood counts, hepatic function, and serum glucose periodically. May cause elevated serum bilirubin and alkaline phosphatase levels. May cause bone marrow depression. Serum glucose may be increased or decreased.

Potential Nursing Diagnoses

- Coping, ineffective individual (indications).
- Injury, high risk for (side effects).
- Knowledge deficit related to medication regimen (patient/family teaching).

Implementation

- May be given as a single dose at bedtime to minimize sedation during the day. Dose increases should be made at bedtime because of sedation. Dose titration is a slow process; may take wks to mons.
- **PO:** Administer medication with or immediately following a meal to minimize gastric irritation. Capsules may be opened and mixed with foods or fluids if patient has difficulty swallowing.
- Oral concentrates must be diluted in at least 120 ml of water, milk, or juice. Do not mix with carbonated beverages or grape juice. Use calibrated measuring device to ensure accurate amount.

Patient/Family Teaching

- Instruct patient to take medication exactly as prescribed. Do not skip or double up on missed doses. Inform patient that at least 2 wk are needed before drug effects may be noticed. Abrupt discontinuation may cause nausea, headache, and malaise.
- Doxepin may cause drowsiness and blurred vision. Caution patient to avoid driving and other activities requiring alertness until response to the medication is known.
- Orthostatic hypotension, sedation, and confusion are common during early therapy, especially in the elderly. Protect patient from falls and advise patient to make position changes slowly.
- Advise patient to avoid alcohol or other CNS depressant drugs during and for at least 3–7 days after therapy has been discontinued.
- Advise patient to notify physician if urinary retention occurs or if dry mouth or constipation persists. Frequent rinses, good oral hygiene, and sugarless hard candy or gum may diminish dry mouth. An increase in fluid intake, fiber, and exercise may prevent constipation. If these symptoms persist, dosage reduction or discontinuation may be necessary.
- Caution patient to use sunscreen and protective clothing to prevent photosensitivity reactions.
- Inform patient of need to monitor dietary intake. Increase in appetite is possible and may lead to undesired weight gain.
- Advise patient to notify physician or dentist of medication regimen prior to treatment or surgery.
- Therapy for depression is usually prolonged. Emphasize the importance of follow-up examinations to monitor effectiveness and side effects.

Evaluation

Effectiveness of therapy can be demonstrated by: ▪ Increased sense of well-being ▫ Renewed interest in surroundings ▫ Increased appetite ▫ Improved energy level ▫ Improved sleep ▪ Decrease in anxiety ▪ Decrease in chronic pain. Patients may require 2–6 wk of therapy before full therapeutic effects of medication are evident.

DOXORUBICIN

(dox-oh-**roo**-bi-sin)
Adriamycin PFS, Adriamycin RDF

CLASSIFICATION(S):
Antineoplastic—antibiotic
Pregnancy Category UK

INDICATIONS

▪ Alone and in combination with other treatment modalities (surgery, radiation therapy) in the treatment of various solid tumors including: ▫ Breast ▫ Ovarian ▫ Bladder ▫ Bronchogenic carcinoma ▪ Also useful in malignant lymphomas and leukemias.

ACTION

▪ Inhibits DNA and RNA synthesis by forming a complex with DNA; (action is cell cycle-S phase specific) ▪ Also has immunosuppressive properties. **Therapeutic Effect:** ▪ Death of rapidly replicating cells, particularly malignant ones.

PHARMACOKINETICS

Absorption: Administered IV only, resulting in complete bioavailability.
Distribution: Widely distributed. Does not cross the blood-brain barrier.
Metabolism and Excretion: Mostly metabolized by the liver. Converted by liver to compound, which also has antineoplastic activity. Excreted predominantly in the bile, 50% as unchanged drug. Less than 5% eliminated unchanged in the urine.
Half-life: 16.7 hr.

CONTRAINDICATIONS AND PRECAUTIONS

Contraindicated in: ▪ Hypersensitivity ▪ Pregnancy or lactation.
Use Cautiously in: ▪ Previous congestive heart failure or arrhythmias ▪ Patients with childbearing potential ▪ Infections ▪ Depressed bone marrow reserve ▪ Other chronic debilitating illnesses ▪ Liver impairment (dosage reduction required).

ADVERSE REACTIONS AND SIDE EFFECTS*

CV: CARDIOMYOPATHY, ECG changes.
Derm: alopecia.
Endo: gonadal suppression.
GI: stomatitis, esophagitis, nausea, vomiting, diarrhea.
GU: red urine.
Hemat: anemia, leukopenia, thrombocytopenia.
Local: phlebitis at IV site, tissue necrosis.
Metab: hyperuricemia.
Misc: hypersensitivity reactions.

INTERACTIONS

Drug-Drug: ▪ Additive bone marrow depression with other **antineoplastics** or **radiation therapy** ▪ May aggravate skin reactions at previous **radiation therapy** sites ▪ May increase risk of hemorrhagic cystitis from **cyclophosphamide** or hepatitis from **mercaptopurine** ▪ Cardiac toxicity may be enhanced by **radiation therapy** or **cyclophosphamide** ▪ May decrease antibody response to **live virus vaccines** and increase the risk of adverse reactions.

ROUTE AND DOSAGE

▪ **IV (Adults):** 60–75 mg/m^2 daily repeat q 21 days or 30 mg/m^2 daily for 3 days, repeat q 4 wk. Total cumulative dose should not exceed 550 mg/m^2 without monitoring of cardiac function.

PHARMACODYNAMICS (effect on blood counts)

	ONSET	PEAK	DURATION
IV	10 days	14 days	21–24 days

NURSING IMPLICATIONS

Assessment

▫ Monitor blood pressure, pulse, respiratory rate, and temperature frequently during administration. Notify

*Underlines indicate most frequent; **CAPITALS** indicate life-threatening.

physician of significant changes.

- ▫ Assess for fever, chills, sore throat, and signs of infection. Notify physician if these symptoms occur.
- ▫ Monitor platelet count throughout therapy. Assess for bleeding (bleeding gums, bruising, petechiae, guaiac stools, urine, and emesis). Avoid IM injections and rectal temperatures. Apply pressure to venipuncture sites for 10 min.
- ▫ Anemia may occur. Monitor for increased fatigue, dyspnea, and orthostatic hypotension.
- ▫ Monitor intake and output ratios, and inform physician if significant discrepancies occur. Encourage fluid intake of 2000–3000 ml/day. Physician may also order allopurinol and alkalinization of the urine to decrease serum uric acid levels and to help prevent urate stone formation.
- ▫ Severe and protracted nausea and vomiting may occur as early as 1 hr after therapy and may last 24 hr. Parenteral antiemetic agents should be administered 30–45 min prior to therapy and routinely around the clock for the next 24 hr as indicated. Monitor amount of emesis and notify physician if emesis exceeds guidelines to prevent dehydration.
- ▫ Monitor for development of signs of myocardial toxicity, which may be either acute and transient (ST segment depression, flattened T wave, sinus tachycardia, and extrasystoles) or of late onset and characterized by congestive heart failure (peripheral edema, dyspnea, rales/crackles, weight gain). Chest x-ray, echocardiography, ECG's and radionuclide angiography may be ordered prior to and periodically throughout therapy.
- ▫ Assess injection site frequently for redness, irritation, or inflammation. Medication may infiltrate painlessly. If extravasation occurs, infusion must be stopped and restarted elsewhere to avoid damage to SC tissue. Standard treatments include leaving original needle in place, injecting the area with corticosteroids, and applying ice compresses.
- ▫ Monitor CBC and differential prior to and periodically throughout therapy. The leukocyte count nadir occurs 10–14 days after administration and recovery usually occurs by the twenty-first day. Thrombocytopenia and anemia may also occur.
- ▫ Monitor renal (BUN and creatinine) and hepatic (SGOT [AST], SGPT [ALT], LDH, and serum bilirubin) function prior to and periodically throughout course of therapy. May cause increased serum and urine uric acid concentrations.

Potential Nursing Diagnoses

- ▪ Infection, high risk for (adverse reactions).
- ▪ Nutrition, altered: less than body requirements (adverse reactions).
- ▪ Knowledge deficit related to medication regimen (patient/family teaching).

Implementation

- ▪ **General Info:** Soln should be prepared in a biologic cabinet. Wear gloves, gown, and mask while handling medication. Discard IV equipment in specially designated containers (see Appendix I).
- ▫ Aluminum needles may be used to administer doxorubicin but should not be used during storage, as prolonged contact results in discoloration of soln and formation of a dark precipitate.
- ▪ **Direct IV:** Dilute each 10 mg with 5 ml of 0.9% NaCl (nonbacteriostatic) for injection. Shake to dissolve completely. Do not add to IV soln. Reconstituted medication is stable for 24 hr at room temperature and 48 hr if refrigerated. Protect from sunlight. Manufacturer does not recommend admixture.
- ▫ *Rate:* Administer each dose over 3–5 minutes through Y-site or 3-way stopcock of a free-flowing infusion of 0.9% NaCl or D5W. Facial flushing and erythema along vein involved fre-

quently occur when administration is too rapid.

- **Syringe Compatibility:** bleomycin, cisplatin, cyclophosphamide, droperidol, fluorouracil, leucovorin calcium, methotrexate, metoclopromide, mitomycin, or vincristine.
- **Syringe Incompatibility:** furosemide or heparin.
- **Y-site Compatibility:** bleomycin, cisplatin, cyclophosphamide, droperidol, fluorouracil, leucovorin calcium, methotrexate, metoclopromide, mitomycin, ondansetron, vinblastine, or vincristine.
- **Y-Site Incompatibility:** furosemide or heparin.
- **Additive Incompatibility:** aminophylline, cephalothin, dexamethasone, diazepam, fluorouracil, or hydrocortisone.

PATIENT/FAMILY TEACHING

- □ Instruct patient to notify physician promptly if fever; sore throat; signs of infection; bleeding gums; bruising; petechiae; blood in stools, urine, or emesis; increased fatigue; dyspnea; or orthostatic hypotension occur. Caution patient to avoid crowds and persons with known infections. Instruct patient to use soft toothbrush and electric razor and to avoid falls. Patients should be cautioned not to drink alcoholic beverages or take medication containing aspirin, as these may precipitate gastric bleeding.
- □ Instruct patient to report pain at injection site immediately.
- □ Instruct patient to inspect oral mucosa for erythema and ulceration. If ulceration occurs advise patient to use sponge brush, rinse mouth with water after eating and drinking, and confer with physician about viscous lidocaine swishes if mouth pain interferes with eating. The risk of developing stomatitis is greatest 5–10 days after a dose; the usual duration is 3–7 days.
- □ Advise patient that this medication may have teratogenic effects. Contraception should be practiced during and for at least 4 mon after therapy is concluded. Inform patient before initiating therapy that this medication may cause irreversible gonadal suppression.
- □ Instruct patient to notify physician immediately if irregular heartbeat, shortness of breath, or swelling of lower extremities occurs.
- □ Discuss the possibility of hair loss with patient. Explore methods of coping. Regrowth usually occurs 2–3 mon after discontinuation of therapy.
- □ Instruct patient not to receive any vaccinations without advice of physician.
- □ Inform patient that medication may cause urine to appear red for 1–2 days.
- □ Instruct patient to notify physician if skin irritation occurs at site of previous radiation therapy.
- □ Emphasize the need for periodic lab tests to monitor for side effects.

EVALUATION

Effectiveness of therapy can be demonstrated by: ▪ Decrease in size or spread of malignancies in solid tumors ▪ Improvement of hematologic status in leukemias.

DOXYCYCLINE

(dox-i-**sye**-kleen)
{Apo-Doxy}, Doryx, Doxy, Doxy-Caps, Doxychel, Monodox, Vibramycin, Vibra-Tabs, Vovox

CLASSIFICATION(S):
Anti-infective—tetracycline
Pregnancy Category UK

INDICATIONS

▪ Used most commonly in the treatment of infections due to unusual organisms including: □ *Mycoplasma* □ *Chlamydia* □ *Rickettsia* ▪ Also useful in the treatment of gonorrhea and syphilis in penicillin-allergic patients. **Unlabeled Uses:** ▪ Treatment of "traveler's diarrhea" ▪ Prevention of exacerbations of chronic bronchitis.

ACTION

▪ Inhibits bacterial protein synthesis at the level of the 30S ribosome. **Therapeutic Effect:** ▪ Bacteriostatic action against susceptible bacteria. **Spectrum:** ▪ Some gram-positive pathogens: ▫ *Bacillus anthracis* ▫ *Clostridium perfringens* ▫ *Clostridium tetani* ▫ *Listeria monocytogenes* ▫ *Nocardia* ▫ *Propionbacterium acnes* ▫ *Actinomyces isrealii* ▪ Some gram-negative pathogens: ▫ *Haemophilus influenzae* ▫ *Legionella pneumophila* ▫ *Versinia entercolitica* ▫ *Versinia pestis* ▫ *Neisseria gonorrhea* ▫ *Neisseria meningtidis* ▪ Also active against several unusual pathogens, including: ▫ *Mycoplasma* ▫ *Chlamydia* ▫ *Rickettsia.*

PHARMACOKINETICS

Absorption: Well absorbed from the GI tract.
Distribution: Widely distributed, some penetration into CSF. Crosses the placenta and enters breast milk.
Metabolism and Excretion: 20–40% excreted unchanged by the urine. Some inactivation in the intestine and some enterohepatic circulation with excretion in bile and feces.
Half-life: 14–17 hr (increased in severe renal impairment).

CONTRAINDICATIONS AND PRECAUTIONS

Contraindicated in: ▪ Hypersensitivity ▪ Children <8 yr (permanent staining of teeth) ▪ Pregnancy or lactation.
Use Cautiously in: ▪ Cachectic or debilitated patients ▪ Hepatic or renal disease.

ADVERSE REACTIONS AND SIDE EFFECTS*

GI: <u>nausea</u>, <u>vomiting</u>, <u>diarrhea</u>, pancreatitis, esophagitis, hepatotoxicity.
Hemat: blood dyscrasias.
Derm: rashes, photosensitivity.
Local: phlebitis at IV site.
Misc: superinfection, hypersensitivity reactions.

INTERACTIONS

Drug-Drug: ▪ May enhance the effect of **oral anticoagulants** ▪ **Barbiturates, phenytoin,** or **carbamazepine** may decrease the activity of doxycycline ▪ May decrease the effectiveness of **oral contraceptives** ▪ **Calcium, iron,** or **magnesium** form chelates and decrease absorption (effect is less with doxycycline than with other tetracyclines).
Drug-Food: ▪ **Calcium** in foods or dairy products decreases absorption by forming an insoluble chelate (effect is less with doxycycline than with other tetracyclines).

ROUTE AND DOSAGE

- **PO (Adults):** 100 mg q 12–24 hr.
- **PO (Children over 8 yr):** 2.2–4.4 mg/kg/day given in divided doses q 12–24 hr.
- **IV (Adults):** 100–200 mg q 24 hr.
- **IV (Children over 8 yr):** 2.2–4.4 mg/kg/day given in divided doses q 12–24 hr.

PHARMACODYNAMICS (blood levels)

	ONSET	PEAK
PO	1–2 hr	1.5–4 hr
IV	rapid	end of infusion

NURSING IMPLICATIONS

Assessment

- ▫ Assess patient for infection (vital signs; appearance of wound, sputum, urine, and stool; WBC) at beginning and throughout course of therapy.
- ▫ Obtain specimens for culture and sensitivity prior to initiating therapy. First dose may be given before receiving results.
- ▫ Assess IV site frequently; may cause thrombophlebitis.
- ▪ **Lab Test Considerations:** Renal, hepatic, and hematopoietic functions

*<u>Underlines</u> indicate most frequent; **CAPITALS** indicate life-threatening.

should be monitored periodically during long-term therapy.
- May cause increased SGOT (AST), SGPT (ALT), serum alkaline phosphatase, bilirubin, and amylase concentrations. May interfere with urine glucose testing with copper sulfate method (Clinitest); use glucose oxidase reagent (Tes-Tape, Ketodiastix).

POTENTIAL NURSING DIAGNOSES
- Infection, high risk for (indications, side effects).
- Knowledge deficit related to medication regimen (patient/family teaching).
- Noncompliance related to medication regimen (patient/family teaching).

IMPLEMENTATION
- **General Info:** May cause yellow-brown discoloration and softening of teeth and bones if administered prenatally or during early childhood. Not recommended for children under 8 yr or during pregnancy or lactation.
- Available in tablets, capsules, delayed-release capsules, oral suspension, and injectable forms.
- **PO:** Administer the oral form of the drug around the clock. May be taken with food. Take with a full glass of liquid and at least 1 hr before going to bed to avoid esophageal ulceration. Use calibrated measuring for liquid preparations. Shake liquid preparations well. Do not administer within 1–3 hr of other medications.
- Avoid administration of calcium, antacids, magnesium-containing medications, or iron supplements within 1–3 hr of oral doxycycline.
- **SC/IM:** Do not administer SC or IM.
- **Intermittent Infusion:** Dilute each 100 mg with 10 ml of sterile water or 0.9% NaCl for injection. Dilute further in 100–1000 ml of 0.9% NaCl, D5W, D5/LR, Ringer's, or lactated Ringer's soln. Soln is stable for 12 hr at room temperature and 72 hr if refrigerated. If diluted with D5/LR or lactated Ringer's soln, administer within 6 hr. Protect soln from direct sunlight. Concentrations of less than 1 mcg/ml or greater than 1 mg/ml are not recommended.
- *Rate:* Administer over a minimum of 1–4 hr. Avoid rapid administration. Avoid extravasation.
- **Y-Site Compatibility:** acyclovir, cyclophosphamide, hydromorphone, magnesium sulfate, meperidine, morphine, ondansetron, or perphenazine.
- **Additive Compatibility:** ranitidine.

PATIENT/FAMILY TEACHING
- Instruct patient to take medication around the clock and to finish the drug completely as directed, even if feeling better. Advise patient that sharing of this medication may be dangerous.
- Caution patient to use sunscreen and protective clothing to prevent photosensitivity reactions.
- Advise patient to report the signs of superinfection (black, furry overgrowth on the tongue, vaginal itching or discharge, loose or foul-smelling stools). Skin rash, pruritus, and urticaria should also be reported.
- Instruct patient to notify physician if symptoms do not improve.
- Caution patient to discard outdated or decomposed products, as they may be toxic.

EVALUATION
Clinical response to therapy can be evaluated by: ■ Resolution of the signs and symptoms of infection. Length of time for complete resolution depends on the organism and site of infection.

DRONABINOL
(droe-**nab**-i-nol)
delta-9-tetrahydrocannabinol, THC, Marinol

CLASSIFICATION(S):
Antiemetic—cannabinoid
Schedule II
Pregnancy Category B

INDICATIONS

■ Prevention of serious nausea and vomiting from cancer chemotherapy when other more conventional agents have failed.

ACTION

■ Active ingredient in marijuana ■ Has a wide variety of CNS effects, including inhibition of the vomiting control mechanism in the medulla oblongata. **Therapeutic Effects:** ■ Suppression of nausea and vomiting.

PHARMACOKINETICS

Absorption: Extensively metabolized following absorption resulting in poor bioavailability (10–20%).
Distribution: Enters breast milk in high concentrations. Highly lipid-soluble. Persists in tissues for prolonged period of time.
Metabolism and Excretion: Extensively metabolized. 50% excreted via biliary elimination. At least 1 metabolite is psychoactive.
Half-life: 25–36 hr.

CONTRAINDICATIONS AND PRECAUTIONS

Contraindicated in: ■ Hypersensitivity to dronabinol, marijuana, or sesame oil ■ Nausea and vomiting due to any other causes ■ Should be used only in supervised patients ■ Lactation.
Use Cautiously in: ■ Patients who have abused drugs or been drug-dependent in the past ■ Chronic use may lead to withdrawal syndrome on discontinuation ■ Pregnancy (do not use unless clearly indicated) ■ Safety in children <18 not established.

ADVERSE REACTIONS AND SIDE EFFECTS*

CNS: drowsiness, heightened awareness, dizziness, concentration difficulty, perceptual difficulty, coordination impairment, headache, irritability, depression, weakness, hallucinations, memory loss, ataxia, paranoia, disorientation, tinnitus, nightmares, speech difficulty, impaired judgement.
EENT: dry mouth, visual distortion.
CV: tachycardia, syncope.
GI: diarrhea.
Derm: facial flushing, perspiring.
MS: muscular pain.
Neuro: paresthesia.
Misc: physical dependence, psychological dependence (high doses or prolonged therapy).

INTERACTIONS

Drug-Drug: ■ Additive CNS depression with **alcohol, antihistamines, narcotic analgesics,** and **sedative/hypnotics.**

ROUTE AND DOSAGE

■ **PO (Adults):** 5 mg/m^2 1–3 hr prior to chemotherapy; may repeat every 2–4 hr after chemotherapy to a total of 4–6 doses/day. If initial dose is ineffective and no significant adverse reactions have occurred, dosage may be increased by 2.5 mg/m^2 to a maximum of 15 mg/m^2.

PHARMACODYNAMICS (antiemetic effect)

	ONSET	PEAK	DURATION
PO	UK	2 hr	6 hr

NURSING IMPLICATIONS

Assessment

- Assess nausea, vomiting, bowel sounds, and abdominal pain prior to and following the administration of this drug.
- Monitor hydration status and intake and output. Patients with severe nausea and vomiting may require IV fluids in addition to antiemetics.
- Monitor blood pressure and heart rate periodically throughout therapy.
- Patients on dronabinol therapy should be monitored closely for side effects because the effects of dronabinol vary with each patient.

*Underlines indicate most frequent; **CAPITALS** indicate life-threatening.

Potential Nursing Diagnoses
- Fluid volume deficit, potential (indications).
- Nutrition, altered: less than body requirements (indications).
- Injury, high risk for (side effects).

Implementation
- **PO:** This drug may be administered prophylactically 1–3 hr prior to chemotherapy and repeated every 2–4 hr after chemotherapy up to 4–6 doses daily.
- Dronabinol capsules should be refrigerated but not frozen.
- Physical or psychological dependence may occur with high doses or prolonged therapy, causing a withdrawal syndrome (irritability, restlessness, insomnia, hot flashes, sweating, rhinorrhea, loose stools, hiccups, anorexia) when discontinued. This is unlikely to occur with therapeutic doses and short-term use of dronabinol.

Patient/Family Teaching
- Instruct patient to take dronabinol exactly as directed. Take missed doses as soon as remembered but not if almost time for next dose; do not double doses. Signs of overdose (mood changes, confusion, hallucinations, depression, nervousness, fast or pounding heartbeat) may occur with increased doses.
- Advise patient to call for assistance when ambulating, as this drug may cause dizziness, drowsiness, and impaired judgment and coordination. Avoid driving or other activities requiring alertness until response to the drug is known.
- Instruct patient to make position changes slowly to minimize orthostatic hypotension.
- Caution patient to avoid taking alcohol or other CNS depressants during dronabinol therapy.
- Advise patient and family to use general measures to decrease nausea (begin with sips of liquids and small nongreasy meals, provide oral hygiene, remove noxious stimuli from environment).

Evaluation

Effectiveness of therapy can be demonstrated by: ▪ Prevention of and decrease in nausea and vomiting associated with chemotherapy.

DROPERIDOL
(droe-**per**-i-dole)
Inapsine

CLASSIFICATION(S):
Tranquilizer—butyrophenone, Antiemetic—butyrophenone
Pregnancy Category C

INDICATIONS
▪ Used to produce tranquilization and as an adjunct to general and regional anesthesia ▪ Also useful in decreasing postoperative or postprocedure nausea and vomiting ▪ May be used in combination with fentanyl (see **Droperidol/Fentanyl**).

ACTION
▪ Similar to haloperidol, alters the action of dopamine in the CNS. **Therapeutic Effects:** ▪ Tranquilization ▪ Suppression of nausea and vomiting in selected situations.

PHARMACOKINETICS
Absorption: Well absorbed following IM administration.
Distribution: Appears to cross the blood-brain barrier and placenta.
Metabolism and Excretion: Mainly metabolized by the liver. Only 10% excreted unchanged by the kidneys.
Half-life: UK.

CONTRAINDICATIONS AND PRECAUTIONS
Contraindicated in: ▪ Hypersensitivity ▪ Known intolerance ▪ Narrow-angle glaucoma ▪ Bone marrow depression ▪ CNS depression ▪ Severe liver or cardiac disease.

Use Cautiously in: ▪ Elderly or debilitated patients ▪ Severely ill patients ▪ Diabetics ▪ Respiratory insufficiency ▪ Prostatic hypertrophy ▪ CNS tumors ▪ Intestinal obstruction ▪ Cardiac disease ▪ Seizures (may lower seizure threshold) ▪ Severe liver disease ▪ Pregnancy, lactation, and children <2 yr (although safety not established, droperidol has been used during cesarean section without respiratory depression in the newborn).

ADVERSE REACTIONS AND SIDE EFFECTS*

CNS: excessive sedation, extrapyramidal reactions, tardive dyskinesia, restlessness, confusion, hyperactivity, dizziness, nightmares, mental depression, hallucinations, SEIZURES, anxiety, abnormal EEG.
EENT: dry eyes, blurred vision.
Resp: bronchospasm, laryngospasm.
CV: hypotension, tachycardia.
GI: dry mouth, constipation.
Misc: chills, shivering, facial sweating.

INTERACTIONS

Drug-Drug: ▪ Additive hypotension with **antihypertensives** or **nitrates** ▪ Additive CNS depression with other **CNS depressants,** including **alcohol, antihistamines, antidepressants, narcotic analgesics,** and other **sedatives**.

ROUTE AND DOSAGE

Premedication

- **IM, IV (Adults):** 2.5–10 mg 30–60 min prior to induction of anesthesia. Additional doses of 1.25–2.5 mg may be needed.
- **IM, IV (Children 2–12 yr):** 0.088–0.165 mg/kg.

Adjunct Before Induction of General Anesthesia (IV route preferred)

- **IM, IV (Adults):** 0.22–0.275 mg/kg with anesthetic or analgesic. Additional doses of 1.25–2.5 mg may be needed.
- **IM, IV (Children 2–12 yr):** 0.088–0.165 mg/kg.

Adjunct for Maintenance of General Anesthesia

- **IV (Adults):** 1.25–2.5 mg.

Used without General Anesthesia During Diagnostic Procedures

- **IM (Adults):** 2.5–10 mg 30–60 min prior to procedure. Additional IV doses of 1.25–5 mg may be needed.

Adjunct in Regional Anesthesia

- **IM, IV (Adults):** 2.5–5 mg.

PHARMACODYNAMICS (sedation)

	ONSET	PEAK	DURATION*
IM	3–10 min	30 min	2–4 hr
IV	3–10 min	30 min	2–4 hr

*Listed as duration of tranquilization; alterations in consciousness may last up to 12 hr.

NURSING IMPLICATIONS

Assessment

- **General Info:** Monitor blood pressure and heart rate frequently throughout course of therapy. Notify physician of significant changes immediately. Hypotension may be treated with parenteral fluids if hypovolemia is a causal factor. Vasopressors (norepinephrine, phenylephrine) may be needed. Avoid use of epinephrine, as droperidol reverses its pressor effects and may cause paradoxical hypotension.
- □ Assess patient for level of sedation following administration.
- □ Observe patient for extrapyramidal symptoms (dystonia, oculogyric crisis, extended neck, flexed arms, tremor, restlessness, hyperactivity, anxiety) throughout therapy. Notify physician should these occur. An anticholinergic, antiparkinsonian agent may be used to treat these symptoms.
- **Nausea and Vomiting:** Assess nausea, vomiting, bowel sounds, and abdominal pain prior to and following administration.

Potential Nursing Diagnoses

- Injury, high risk for (side effects).
- Knowledge deficit related to medication regimen (patient/family teaching).

*Underlines indicate most frequent; **CAPITALS** indicate life-threatening.

Implementation

- **General Info:** Available in combination with fentanyl (Innovar); see Appendix A.
- **IM/IV:** May be administered IM or IV.
- **Direct IV:** Administer each dose slowly over at least 1 min.
- **Intermittent Infusion:** May be added to 250 ml of D5W, 0.9% NaCl, or lactated Ringer's soln and administered by slow IV infusion.
- **Syringe Compatibility:** atropine, bleomycin, butorphanol, chlorpromazine, cimetidine, cisplatin, cyclophosphamide, dimenhydrinate, diphenhydramine, doxorubicin, fentanyl, glycopyrrolate, hydroxyzine, meperidine, metoclopramide, midazolam, mitomycin, morphine, nalbuphine, pentazocine, perphenazine, prochlorperazine, promazine, promethazine, scopolamine, vinblastine, or vincristine.
- **Syringe Incompatibility:** fluorouracil, furosemide, heparin, leucovorin calcium, methotrexate, or pentobarbital.
- **Y-Site Compatibility:** bleomycin, buprenorphine, cisplatin, cyclophosphamide, doxorubicin, hydrocortisone sodium succinate, metoclopramide, mitomycin, ondansetron, potassium chloride, vinblastine, or vincristine.
- **Y-Site Incompatibility:** fluorouracil, foscarnet, furosemide, leucovorin calcium, methotrexate, or nafcillin.
- **Additive Incompatibility:** barbiturates.

Patient/Family Teaching

- □ Caution patient to make position changes slowly to minimize orthostatic hypotension.
- □ Medication causes drowsiness. Advise patient to call for assistance during ambulation and transfer.

Evaluation

Effectiveness of therapy can be demonstrated by: ▪ General quiescence and reduced motor activity ▪ Decreased nausea and vomiting.

D

DROPERIDOL/FENTANYL

(droe-**per**-i-dole/**fen**-ta-nil)
Innovar

CLASSIFICATION(S):
Combination butyrophenone (droperidol) plus narcotic analgesic (fentanyl)
Schedule II
Pregnancy Category C

INDICATIONS

▪ Used to produce tranquilization and analgesia during diagnostic or surgical procedures ▪ Adjunct in various types of anesthesia.

ACTION

▪ *Droperidol* alters the action of dopamine in the CNS ▪ *Fentanyl* is a narcotic analgesic that binds to opiate receptors in the CNS, altering the response to and perception of pain. **Therapeutic Effect of Combination:** ▪ Neuroleptanalgesia (quiescence, decreased motor activity, and analgesia without loss of consciousness).

PHARMACOKINETICS

Distribution: Droperidol appears to cross the blood-brain barrier and placenta.

Metabolism and Excretion: Both droperidol and fentanyl are mainly metabolized by the liver with small amounts (10–20%) excreted unchanged by the kidneys.

Half-life: UK for both drugs.

CONTRAINDICATIONS AND PRECAUTIONS

Contraindicated in: ▪ Hypersensitivity ▪ Known intolerance ▪ Narrow-angle glaucoma ▪ Bone marrow depression ▪ CNS depression ▪ Severe liver or cardiac disease.

Use Cautiously in: ▪ Elderly or debilitated patients ▪ Severely ill patients ▪ Diabetics ▪ Patients with severe pulmonary or hepatic disease ▪ Prostatic hypertrophy ▪ CNS tumors ▪ Increased intracranial pressure ▪ Head trauma ▪ Intestinal obstruction ▪ Undiagnosed abdominal pain ▪ Adrenal insufficiency ▪ Hypothyroidism ▪ Alcoholism ▪ Cardiac disease ▪ Seizures (may lower seizure threshold) ▪ Pregnancy, lactation, and children <2 yr (safety not established).

ADVERSE REACTIONS AND SIDE EFFECTS*

CNS: excessive sedation, extrapyramidal reactions, tardive dyskinesia, restlessness, confusion, hyperactivity, dizziness, nightmares, mental depression, hallucinations, euphoria, floating feeling, dysphoria.
EENT: dry eyes, blurred vision, miosis, diplopia.
Resp: bronchospasm, laryngospasm, apnea, respiratory depression.
CV: hypotension, tachycardia, bradycardia.
GI: dry mouth, constipation, nausea, vomiting.
GU: urinary retention.
Derm: sweating, flushing.
MS: skeletal and thoracic muscle rigidity.
Misc: chills, shivering, facial sweating.

INTERACTIONS

Drug-Drug: ▪ Additive hypotension with **antihypertensives** or **nitrates** ▪ Additive CNS depression with other **CNS depressants,** including **alcohol, antihistamines, antidepressants,** and other **sedative/hypnotics** or **narcotic analgesics** (decrease dose of narcotics if given within 8 hr of droperidol/fentanyl) ▪ Avoid using in patients who have received **MAO inhibitors** within 14 days.

ROUTE AND DOSAGE

Note: Each ml contains 2.5 mg droperidol and 0.05 mg fentanyl. Because droperidol is much longer acting than fentanyl, additional doses of fentanyl alone may be given to prevent accumulation of droperidol.

Premedication

- **IM (Adults):** 0.5–2 ml 45–60 min prior to surgery.
- **IM (Children):** 0.25 ml/20 lb body weight 45–60 min prior to surgery.

Adjunct to General Anesthesia

- **IV (Adults):** 1 ml/20–25 lb body weight administered in small increments or as an infusion until somnolence occurs. Additional fentanyl used to maintain analgesia. In prolonged procedures, additional doses of 0.5–1 ml of droperidol/fentanyl **IV** may be required if lightening of tranquilization and analgesia occurs.
- **IV (Children) >2 yr):** 0.5 ml/20 lb body weight administered in small increments or as an infusion until somnolence occurs. Additional fentanyl may be used to maintain analgesia.

Used without a General Anesthetic in Diagnostic Procedures

- **IM (Adults):** 0.5–2 ml 45–60 min prior to procedure. Additional fentanyl used to maintain analgesia. In prolonged procedures, additional doses of 0.5–1 ml of droperidol/fentanyl **IV** may be required if lightening of tranquilization and analgesia occurs.

Adjunct to Regional Anesthesia

- **IM, IV (Adults):** 1–2 ml.

PHARMACODYNAMICS (noted as tranquilizing effects of droperidol, analgesic effects of fentanyl)

	ONSET	PEAK	DURATION*
IM droperidol	3–10 min	30 min	up to 12 hr
IM fentanyl	7–15 min	20–30 min	1–2 hr
IV droperidol	3–10 min	30 min	up to 12 hr
IV fentanyl	1–2 min	3–5 min	0.5–1 hr

*Listed as duration of tranquilization; alterations in consciousness may last up to 12 hr. Effects on respiratory depression outlast analgesic effects.

*Underlines indicate most frequent; **CAPITALS** indicate life-threatening.

D

NURSING IMPLICATIONS

Assessment

□ May cause pronounced respiratory depression. Monitor respiratory rate, ECG, and blood pressure frequently throughout course of therapy. Notify physician of significant changes immediately. Hypotension may be treated with parenteral fluids if hypovolemia is a causal factor. Vasopressors (norepinephrine, phenylephrine) may be needed. Avoid use of epinephrine, as droperidol reverses its pressor effects and may cause paradoxical hypotension.

□ Doses of narcotic analgesics administered following administration of droperidol/fentanyl should be decreased to ¼ to ⅓ the normal dose for 8 hr following the administration of droperidol/fentanyl.

□ Observe patient for extrapyramidal symptoms (dystonia, oculogyric crisis, extended neck, flexed arms, tremor, restlessness, hyperactivity, anxiety) throughout therapy. Notify physician should these occur. An anticholinergic antiparkinsonian agent may be used to treat these symptoms.

- **Lab Test Considerations:** May cause elevated serum amylase and lipase concentrations.
- **Toxicity and Overdose:** Naloxone (Narcan) may reverse respiratory depression. Dose may need to be repeated, as fentanyl has a longer duration than naloxone.

□ Bradycardia may be treated with atropine.

Potential Nursing Diagnoses

- Comfort, altered: pain (indications).
- Injury, high risk for (side effects).

Implementation

- **Direct IV:** Direct IV injection should be administered slowly over at least 1 min.
- **Intermittent Infusion:** Droperidol/fentanyl 10 ml may be added to 250 ml of D5W and infused until the onset of somnolence as an adjunct to general anesthesia.
- **Syringe Compatibility:** benzquinamide or glycopyrrolate.
- **Syringe Incompatibility:** heparin.
- **Y-Site Compatibility:** hydrocortisone sodium succinate, or potassium chloride.
- **Y-Site Incompatibility:** nafcillin.
- **Additive Incompatibility:** barbiturates.

Patient/Family Teaching

□ Caution patient to make position changes slowly to minimize orthostatic hypotension.

□ Medication causes drowsiness. Advise patient to call for assistance during ambulation and transfer and to avoid driving or other activities requiring alertness for 24 hr after last dose.

Evaluation

Effectiveness of therapy can be demonstrated by: ▪ General quiescence, reduced motor activity, and pronounced analgesia.

DYPHYLLINE

(**dye**-fi-lin)

Asminyl, Dilor, Dyflex, Dylline, Dy-Phyl-Lin, Lufyllin, Neothylline, {Protophylline}

CLASSIFICATION(S):
Bronchodilator—phosphodiesterase inhibitor
Pregnancy Category C

INDICATIONS

▪ Bronchodilator in reversible airway obstruction due to asthma or COPD.

ACTION

▪ Inhibits phosphodiesterase, producing increases in tissue concentrations of cyclic adenosine monophosphate (cAMP). Increased levels of cAMP result in: □ Bronchodilation □ CNS stimulation □ Positive inotropic and chronotropic effects □ Diuresis □ Gastric acid secretion. Dyphylline is a chemical derivative of theophylline. **Therapeutic Effect:** ▪ Bronchodilation.

PHARMACOKINETICS

Absorption: Well absorbed (75%) following oral administration.
Distribution: Achieves high concentrations in breast milk.
Metabolism and Excretion: 85% excreted unchanged by the kidneys.
Half-life: 1.8–2.1 hr (increased in renal impairment).

CONTRAINDICATIONS AND PRECAUTIONS

Contraindicated in: ▪ Hypersensitivity ▪ Some products contain benzyl alcohol and/or bisulfites—avoid use in patients with hypersensitivities to these compounds ▪ Lactation ▪ Uncontrolled arrhythmias ▪ Hyperthyroidism
Use Cautiously in: ▪ Pregnancy or children (safety not established) ▪ Severe cardiovascular disease ▪ Peptic ulcer disease.

ADVERSE REACTIONS AND SIDE EFFECTS*

CNS: <u>nervousness</u>, <u>anxiety</u>, headache, insomnia, SEIZURES.
Resp: tachypnea.
CV: <u>tachycardia</u>, palpitations, arrhythmias, angina pectoris.
GI: <u>nausea</u>, <u>vomiting</u>, anorexia, cramps.
GU: albuminuria, hematuria, diuresis.
Neuro: tremor.
Misc: hyperglycemia, syndrome of inappropriate secretion of antidiuretic hormone (SIADH).

INTERACTIONS

Drug-Drug: ▪ Additive CV and CNS side effects with **adrenergic (sympathomimetic) agents** ▪ Additive bronchodilation with other **bronchodilators** ▪ **Probenecid** decreases renal excretion and increases blood levels ▪ **Beta-adrenergic blockers** may decrease therapeutic effects of dyphylline.

ROUTE AND DOSAGE

Acute Bronchospasm

- **PO (Adults):** 500 mg.

Chronic Therapy

- **PO (Adults):** 15 mg/kg q 6 hr.
- **IM (Adults):** 250—500 mg q 6 hr.

PHARMACODYNAMICS (bronchodilation)

	ONSET	PEAK	DURATION
PO	UK	1 hr	6 hr

NURSING IMPLICATIONS

Assessment

- Assess blood pressure, pulse, respiration, and lung sounds before administering medication and throughout therapy.
- Patients with a history of cardiovascular problems should be monitored for ECG changes.
- Monitor intake and output ratios for an increase in diuresis.
- **Lab Test Considerations:** Standard theophylline assays do not measure dyphylline concentrations.

Potential Nursing Diagnoses

- Airway clearance, ineffective (indications).
- Activity intolerance (indications).
- Knowledge deficit related to medication regimen (patient/family teaching).

Implementation

- **General Info:** Administer around the clock to maintain therapeutic plasma levels.
- Determine if patient has had another form of theophylline prior to administering initial dose.
- **PO:** Administer 1 hr before or 2 hr after meals for rapid absorption. May be administered after meals to minimize GI irritation. Food slows but does not reduce the extent of absorption. Measure dose of liquid forms, using calibrated medication cup.
- **IM:** Do not use if precipitate is pres-

*<u>Underlines</u> indicate most frequent; **CAPITALS** indicate life-threatening.

ent. May be caused by exposure to cold.
- Inject slowly; avoid IV administration.

Patient/Family Teaching
- Emphasize the importance of taking only the prescribed dose at the prescribed time intervals. Missed doses should be taken as soon as remembered or omitted if close to next dose.
- Encourage patient to drink adequate liquids (2000 ml/day minimum) to decrease the viscosity of the airway secretions.
- Advise patient to avoid over-the-counter cough, cold, or breathing preparations without consulting physician or pharmacist. These medications may increase side effects and cause arrhythmias.
- Advise patient to minimize intake of xanthine-containing foods or beverages (colas, coffee, chocolate).
- Encourage patients not to smoke, as smoking may irritate respiratory tract.
- Advise patient to contact physician promptly if the usual dose of medication fails to produce the desired results, symptoms worsen after treatment, or toxic effects (anorexia, nausea, vomiting, restlessness, insomnia, tachycardia, arrhythmias, seizures) occur.

Evaluation
Effectiveness of therapy can be demonstrated by: ▪ Increased ease in breathing and clearing of lung fields on auscultation.

ECHOTHIOPHATE IODIDE
(ek-oh-**thye**-oh-fate)
Ecostigmine iodide, Echothiophate, Phospholine Iodide

CLASSIFICATION(S):
Ophthalmic—cholinergic, Antiglaucoma
Pregnancy Category C

INDICATIONS
▪ Treatment of open-angle and other chronic glaucomas that have not responded to more conventional therapy ▪ Diagnosis and treatment of accommodative esotropia (abnormal alignment of the eyes) when not accompanied by amblyopia (decreased vision) and anisometropia (unequal refractive ability).

ACTION
▪ Long-lasting inhibition of the enzyme cholinesterase, resulting in accumulation and prolonged effects of acetylcholine. **Therapeutic Effects:** ▪ Produces contraction of iris sphincter muscle, causing miosis, ciliary muscle constriction resulting in increased accommodation and decreased resistance to aqueous humor outflow ▪ Decreased intraocular pressure.

PHARMACOKINETICS
Absorption: Rapidly penetrates the cornea. Extensive systemic absorption follows ophthalmic administration.
Distribution: Distribution not known.
Metabolism and Excretion: Metabolized slowly in tissues and fluids by cholinesterases.
Half-life: UK.

CONTRAINDICATIONS AND PRECAUTIONS
Contraindicated in: ▪ Hypersensitivity ▪ Risk or history of retinal detachment ▪ Acute ocular inflammation ▪ Posterior synechiae.
Use Cautiously in: ▪ Corneal abrasion ▪ Asthma ▪ Hypertension ▪ Hyperthyroidism ▪ Cardiovascular disease ▪ Epilepsy ▪ Parkinsonism ▪ Bradycardia ▪ Ulcer disease ▪ Urinary tract obstruction ▪ Hypotension ▪ GI obstruction.

ADVERSE REACTIONS AND SIDE EFFECTS*
EENT: accommodative spasm, myopia, blurred vision, poor night vision, retinal detachment, stinging, burning, lacrimation, eye ache, brow ache, conjunctival congestion, lacrimal duct stenosis, eye-

*Underlines indicate most frequent; **CAPITALS** indicate life-threatening.

lid twitching, iris cysts (children), anterior chamber hyperemia, nasal congestion.
Resp: bronchospasm.
GI: nausea, vomiting, diarrhea, abdominal pain, cramps, excessive salivation.
GU: urinary frequency.
Derm: sweating, pallor, cyanosis.
MS: muscle weakness.
Neuro: paresthesia.

INTERACTIONS

Drug–Drug: ▪ Additive intraocular pressure lowering effects with ophthalmic administration of **epinephrine, beta-adrenergic blockers,** and systemic **carbonic anhydrase inhibitors** ▪ **Physostigmine, cyclopentolate,** local or systemic **glucocorticoids,** systemic **anticholinergics, antihistamines, meperidine, sympathomimetics,** and **tricyclic antidepressants** may decrease the effects of ecothiophate ▪ Increases the duration of action of **ester-type local anesthetics (benzocaine, butacaine, tetracaine)** ▪ Decreases the metabolism of and enhances the activity of **cocaine** ▪ May enhance neuromuscular blockade from **succinylcholine** ▪ Additive toxicity with **cholinesterase inhibitors** ▪ **Clofibrate** potentiates miosis.

ROUTE AND DOSAGE

Glaucoma

- **Ophth (Adults):** 1 drop of 0.03–0.25% soln 1–2 times daily.

Accommodative Esoptropia

- **Ophth (Adults):** 1 drop of 0.03–0.125% soln 1 time daily or qid.

Diagnostic Aid (Accommodative Esoptropia)

- **Ophth (Adults):** 1 drop of 0.125% soln once daily at bedtime for 2–3 wk.

PHARMACODYNAMICS

	ONSET	PEAK	DURATION
Ophth (miosis)	10–30 min	30 min	7–28 days
Ophth (intraocular pressure)	4–8 hr	within 24 hr	up to 28 days

NURSING IMPLICATIONS

Assessment

- □ Monitor patient for changes in vision, eye irritation, and persistent headache.
- □ Monitor patient for signs of systemic side effects (sweating, increased salivation, nausea, vomiting, diarrhea, and respiratory distress). Notify physician if these signs occur.
- ▪ **Toxicity and Overdose:** Toxicity is manifested as systemic side effects. Atropine is the antidote.

Potential Nursing Diagnoses

- ▪ Sensory-perceptual alteration: visual (indications, side effects).
- ▪ Knowledge deficit related to medication regimen (patient/family teaching).

Implementation

- ▪ **Ophth:** Available in several concentrations. Carefully check percentage on label prior to administration.

Patient/Family Teaching

- □ Instruct patient to take as directed and not to discontinue without physician's approval. Lifelong therapy may be required. A missed dose of eyedrops should be taken as soon as remembered unless almost time for next dose.
- □ Instruct patient on correct method of application of drops. Wash hands. Lie down or tilt head back and look at ceiling. Pull down on lower lid, creating a small pocket. Place prescribed number of drops in pocket. Apply pressure to the inner canthus for 1–2 min to confine effects to the eye. Wait 5 min before applying other prescribed eyedrops.
- □ Explain to patient that pupil constriction and temporary stinging and blurring of vision are expected. Physician should be notified if blurred vision and brow ache persist.
- □ Caution patient that night vision may be impaired. Advise patient not to drive at night until response to medication is known. To prevent injury at night, patient should use a night light

and keep environment uncluttered.
- Advise patient to notify physician or dentist of medication regimen prior to treatment or surgery.
- Advise patient of the need for regular eye examinations to monitor intraocular pressure and visual fields.

EVALUATION

Effectiveness of therapy can be demonstrated by: ▪ Control of elevated intraocular pressure ▪ Diagnosis and treatment of convergent strabismus. Diagnosis is based upon straightening of eyes after 2–3 wk of receiving 1 drop at bedtime. Although therapy may continue for up to 5 yr, usually surgical correction is considered if strabismus does not resolve after 1–2 yr of therapy or recurs after drug withdrawal.

ECONAZOLE
(ee-**kon**-a-zole)
Spectazole

CLASSIFICATION(S):
Antifungal—topical
Pregnancy Category C

INDICATIONS

▪ Treatment of a variety of superficial fungal infections, including: ▫ Tinea pedis ▫ Tinea cruris ▫ Tinea corporis ▫ Tinea versicolor ▫ Cutaneous candidiasis.

ACTION

▪ Damages fungal cell membrane allowing leakage of cellular contents ▪ May also alter metabolism in fungal cells. **Therapeutic Effect:** ▪ Fungicidal or fungistatic depending on the organism and concentration. **Spectrum:** ▪ Active against many fungi including: ▫ *Candida albicans* ▫ *Tricophyton rubrum* ▫ *T. mentagrophytes* ▫ *T. tonsurans* ▫ *Pityrosporum orbiculare.*

PHARMACOKINETICS

Absorption: Minimal systemic absorption follows topical application.
Distribution: Achieves good concentration in stratum corneum, epidermis, and dermis.
Metabolism and Excretion: Metabolism and excretion not known. <1% excreted in urine and feces.
Half-life: UK.

CONTRAINDICATIONS AND PRECAUTIONS

Contraindicated in: ▪ Hypersensitivity to econazole or components of base ▪ First trimester of pregnancy.
Use Cautiously in: ▪ Second and third trimester of pregnancy (use only if clearly needed) ▪ Lactation ▪ Severe hepatic dysfunction.

ADVERSE REACTIONS AND SIDE EFFECTS*

Derm: burning, itching, stinging, erythema.

INTERACTIONS

Drug–Drug: ▪ None significant.

ROUTE AND DOSAGE

Tinea Pedis, Tinea Cruris, Tinea Corporis, Tinea Versicolor
- **Top (Adults and Children):** Apply 1% cream once daily.

Cutaneous Candidiasis
- **Top (Adults and Children):** Apply 1% cream twice daily.

PHARMACODYNAMICS

	ONSET	PEAK	DURATION
Top	2 wk–1 mon	UK	UK

NURSING IMPLICATIONS

ASSESSMENT
- Assess patient for infection prior to and throughout course of therapy.

POTENTIAL NURSING DIAGNOSES
- Infection, high risk for (indications).
- Skin integrity, impaired (indications).
- Knowledge deficit related to medication regimen (patient/family teaching).

*Underlines indicate most frequent; **CAPITALS** indicate life-threatening.

IMPLEMENTATION
- **Top:** Cleanse affected skin with soap and water and dry thoroughly. Apply sufficient amount to cover affected area and rub in gently. Avoid contact with eyes. Do not use occlusive dressings unless directed by physician.

PATIENT/FAMILY TEACHING
- **Top:** Instruct patient to apply topical econazole exactly as directed. Missed doses should be applied as soon as remembered, unless almost time for next dose.
- □ Advise patients with athlete's foot to wear well-fitting, ventilated shoes and to change socks and shoes at least once a day.
- □ Advise patient to consult physician if no improvement is seen in 4 wk or if burning, stinging, redness, or itching occur.

EVALUATION
Effectiveness of therapy can be demonstrated by: ▪ Resolution of the signs and symptoms of infection. May require 2 wk to 1 mon to prevent recurrence.

EDETATE CALCIUM DISODIUM
(**ee**-de-tate **kal**-see-yum dye-**sode**-ee-yum)
Calcium disodium edathamil, Calcium disodium edetate, Calcium Disodium Versenate, Calcium edetate, Calcium EDTA, Sodium calcium edetate

CLASSIFICATION(S):
Antidote—lead chelator
Pregnancy Category UK

INDICATIONS
▪ Management of acute and chronic lead poisoning, including encephalopathy and nephropathy.

ACTION
▪ Removes toxic amounts of lead or other divalent or trivalent cations by their displacement of calcium in edetate calcium disodium. Result is a soluble complex that is excreted by the kidneys. **Therapeutic Effect:** ▪ Removal of toxic amounts of lead from the blood and other tissues.

PHARMACOKINETICS
Absorption: Well absorbed following IM administration.
Distribution: Distributed to extracellular fluid. Does not cross the blood-brain barrier.
Metabolism and Excretion: Rapidly excreted by the kidneys as unchanged drug or lead complex.
Half-life: IM—20–60 min; IV—1.5 hr.

CONTRAINDICATIONS AND PRECAUTIONS
Contraindicated in: ▪ Anuria.
Use Cautiously in: ▪ Underlying renal disease (dosage reduction required if serum creatinine >2 mg/dl) ▪ Cardiac arrhythmias ▪ Pregnancy or lactation (safety not established) ▪ Lead encephalopathy (should be used with concurrent dimercaprol).

ADVERSE REACTIONS AND SIDE EFFECTS*
CNS: headache, malaise, fatigue.
EENT: sneezing, lacrimation, nasal, congestion.
CV: ECG changes (inverted T waves), hypotension.
GI: nausea, vomiting.
GU: <u>nephrotoxicity</u>, glycosuria.
F and E: hypercalcemia.
Local: <u>pain</u> at IM site, phlebitis at IV site.
MS: mylagia, arthralgia, leg cramps.
Neuro: numbness, tingling.
Misc: excessive thirst, fever, chills, histamine-like reaction.

*<u>Underlines</u> indicate most frequent; **CAPITALS** indicate life-threatening.

E

INTERACTIONS

Drug–Drug: ▪ May increase the risk of **cardiac glycoside** toxicity ▪ **Glucocorticoids** increase nephrotoxicity ▪ Decreases the duration of action of **zinc insulin** preparations.

ROUTE AND DOSAGE

Diagnosis of Lead Poisoning
(Calcium EDTA mobilization test)

- **IM, IV (Adults):** 500 mg/m² (not to exceed 1 g).
- **IV (Children):** 500 mg/m².
- **IM (Children):** 500 mg/m² single dose or 500 mg/m² q 12 hr for 2 doses or single dose of 50 mg/kg (not to exceed 1 g).

Lead Poisoning without Encephalopathy

- **IM (Adults):** 1–1.5 g/m²/day given as 2 divided doses for 3–5 days (if given with dimercaprol divide daily dose and give at 4–hr intervals, not to exceed 2 courses; wait at least 2–4 days and preferably 2–3 wk between courses).
- **IM (Children):** 1–1.5 g/m²/day given as 2–3 divided doses for 3–5 days (if given with dimercaprol divide daily dose and give at 4–hr intervals; wait at least 2–4 days and preferably 2–3 wk between courses).
- **IV (Adults):** 1–1.5 g/m²/day for 3–5 days (not to exceed 2 courses; wait at least 2–4 days and preferably 2–3 wk between courses).
- **IV (Children):** 1–1.5 g/m²/day given as 2 divided doses for 3–5 days (if given with dimercaprol divide daily dose and give at 4–hr intervals; wait at least 2–4 days and preferably 2–3 wk between courses).

Lead Poisoning with Encephalopathy

- **IM (Adults and Children):** Start treatment with dimercaprol, then after 4 hr administer dimercaprol and edetate calcium disodium 250 mg/m² q 4 hr for 5 days.
- **IV (Adults and Children):** Start treatment with dimercaprol, then after 4 hr start constant infusion of edetate calcium disodium 1.5 g/m²/day for 5 days.

PHARMACODYNAMICS (urinary lead excretion)

	ONSET	PEAK	DURATION
IM	UK	UK	UK
IV	1 hr	24–48 hr	UK

NURSING IMPLICATIONS

Assessment

- ☐ Assess patient and family members for evidence of lead poisoning prior to and periodically throughout course of therapy. Acute lead poisoning is characterized by a metallic taste, colicky abdominal pain, vomiting, diarrhea, oliguria, and coma. Symptoms of chronic poisoning vary with severity and include anorexia, a blue-black line along the gums, intermittent vomiting, paresthesia, encephalopathy, seizures, and coma.
- ☐ Monitor strict intake and output and daily weight. Notify physician of any discrepancies. If patient is anuric, edetate calcium disodium should be held until urine flow is established by IV hydration.
- ☐ Monitor neurologic status closely (level of consciousness, pupil response, movement). Notify physician immediately of any changes. Infuse slowly; rapid infusion rate may increase intracranial pressure. Physician may also order fluid restriction to prevent increased intracranial pressure.
- ☐ Monitor vital signs and ECG frequently. Notify physician if hypotension or T wave inversion occur. Physician should also be notified if fever, chills, malaise, or nasal congestion occur. This histamine-like response reaction usually resolves in 48 hr.
- ▪ **Lab Test Considerations:** Monitor serum and urine lead levels prior to and periodically throughout therapy. Wait at least 1 hr after infusing edetate calcium disodium before drawing serum lead level.

- □ Monitor urinalysis daily and serum creatinine, BUN, alkaline phosphatase, calcium, and phosphorous levels. Both lead and edetate calcium disodium are nephrotoxic. Notify physician if hematuria, proteinuria, or large renal epithelial cells are present.
- □ May cause an increase in urine glucose.

POTENTIAL NURSING DIAGNOSES

- ▪ Injury, high risk for: poisoning (indications, patient/family teaching).
- ▪ Home maintenance management, impaired (indications).
- ▪ Knowledge deficit related to medication and dietary regimens (patient/family teaching).

IMPLEMENTATION

- ▪ **General Info:** Administer IM or IV; oral administration may increase absorption of lead.
- □ Patients with serum lead levels of 100 mcg/dl or more, or those with lead encephalopathy may also be treated with dimercaprol (BAL). Administer these medications at separate sites.
- ▪ **IM:** IM is the preferred route for children and patients with lead encephalopathy. Procaine hydrochloride 1% (1 ml procaine to 1 ml edetate calcium disodium ratio, for a final concentration of 0.5% procaine) is usually ordered to minimize pain at the injection site. Administer deep IM into well-developed muscle; massage well. Rotate sites.
- ▪ **Intermittent Infusion:** Dilute 5 ml ampule with 250–500 ml of D5W or 0.9% NaCl to yield a final concentration of 2–4 mg/ml.
- □ *Rate:* Administer over 1 hr in asymptomatic adults and over 2 hr in symptomatic patients. Use infusion pump to control rate accurately.
- ▪ **Continuous Infusion:** May also be administered as a single daily infusion over 8–24 hr.
- ▪ **Additive Compatibility:** netilmicin.
- ▪ **Additive Incompatibility:** D10W, lactated Ringer's soln, amphotericin B, or hydralazine.

PATIENT/FAMILY TEACHING

- □ Discuss need for follow-up appointments to monitor lead levels. Additional treatments may be necessary.
- □ Consult public health department regarding potential sources of lead poisoning in the home, workplace, and recreational areas.

EVALUATION

Effectiveness of therapy can be demonstrated by: ▪ Decrease in symptoms of lead poisoning □ Decrease in serum lead levels to below 50 mcg/dl, although the normal upper limit is 29 mcg/dl.

EDROPHONIUM

(ed-roe-**fone**-ee-yum)
Enlon, Reversol, Tensilon

CLASSIFICATION(S):
Cholinergic—anticholinesterase
Pregnancy Category C

INDICATIONS

▪ Diagnosis of myasthenia gravis ▪ Assessment of adequacy of anticholinesterase therapy in myasthenia gravis ▪ Differentiating myasthenic from cholinergic crisis ▪ Reversal of nondepolarizing neuromuscular blockers. **Unlabeled Use:** ▪ Termination of paroxysmal atrial tachycardia.

ACTION

▪ Inhibits the breakdown of acetylcholine so that it accumulates and has a prolonged effect. Effects include miosis, increased intestinal and skeletal muscule tone, bronchial and ureteral constriction, bradycardia, increased salivation, lacrimation, and sweating. **Therapeutic Effects:** ▪ Improved but short-lived cranial muscular function in patients with myasthenia gravis, reversal of nondepolarizing neuromuscular blockers, and suppression of certain arrhythmias.

PHARMACOKINETICS

Absorption: Absorption following IM and SC administration not known.

Distribution: Distribution not known.
Metabolism and Excretion: Metabolic fate not known.
Half-life: UK.

CONTRAINDICATIONS AND PRECAUTIONS

Contraindicated in: ▪ Hypersensitivity ▪ Mechanical obstruction of the GI or GU tract ▪ Pregnancy (may cause uterine irritability after IV administation near term; newborns may display muscle weakness) ▪ Lactation.
Use Cautiously in: ▪ History of asthma ▪ Ulcer disease ▪ Cardiovascular disease ▪ Epilepsy ▪ Hyperthyroidism ▪ Because some patients may be extremely sensitive to the effects of anticholinesterases, atropine should be available in case of excessive dosage.

ADVERSE REACTIONS AND SIDE EFFECTS*

CNS: dizziness, weakness, SEIZURES.
EENT: miosis, lacrimation.
Resp: excess secretions, bronchospasm.
CV: bradycardia, hypotension.
GI: abdominal cramps, nausea, vomiting, diarrhea, excess salivation.
Derm: rashes, sweating.
MS: fasciculation.

INTERACTIONS

Drug-Drug: ▪ Action may be antagonized by **drugs possessing anticholinergic properties,** including **antihistamines, antidepressants, atropine, haloperidol, phenothiazines, quinidine,** and **disopyramide** ▪ Prolongs action of **depolarizing muscle-relaxing agents (succinylcholine, decamethonium)** ▪ May lead to excessive bradycardia in patients receiving **cardiac glycosides.**

ROUTE AND DOSAGE

Diagnosis of Myasthenia Gravis

- **IV (Adults):** 2 mg, if no response administer 8 more mg; may repeat test in 30 min. If cholinergic response occurs, administer atropine 0.4–0.5 mg IV.
- **IV (Children >34 kg):** 2 mg, if no response may administer 1 mg q 30–45 sec to a total of 10 mg. If cholinergic response occurs, administer atropine IV.
- **IV (Children <34 kg):** 1 mg, if no response may administer 1 mg q 30–45 sec to a total of 5 mg. If cholinergic response occurs, administer atropine IV.
- **IV (Infants):** 0.5 mg.
- **IM (Adults):** 10 mg. If cholinergic response occurs, may repeat 2 mg dose in 30 min to rule out false positive reaction.
- **IM (Children <34 kg):** 2 mg.
- **IM (Children >34 kg):** 5 mg.

Assessment of Anticholinesterase Therapy

- **IV (Adults):** 1–2 mg 1 hr after oral anticholinesterase dose.

Differentiation of Cholinergic from Myasthenic Crisis

- **IV (Adults):** 1 mg, may give additional 1 mg 1 min later.

Reversal of Nondepolarizing Neuromuscular Blocking Agents

- **IV (Adults):** 10 mg, may repeat q 5–10 min (not to exceed 40 mg).

Termination of PAT

- **IV (Adults):** 5–10 mg.

Slow Tachyarrhythmias

- **IV (Adults):** 2 mg test dose, then 2 mg q min to a total of 10 mg. May continue therapy with infusion of 0.25–2 mg/min.

PHARMACODYNAMICS (cholinergic activity)

	ONSET	PEAK	DURATION
IM	2–10 min	UK	5–30 min
IV	30–60 sec	UK	5–10 min

NURSING IMPLICATIONS

Assessment

- **General Info:** Assess neuromuscular status (ptosis, diplopia, vital capac-

*Underlines indicate most frequent; **CAPITALS** indicate life-threatening.

ity, ability to swallow, extremity strength) prior to and immediately after administration of medication.

□ To differentiate myasthenic from cholinergic crisis, assess for increased weakness, diaphoresis, increased saliva and bronchial secretions, dyspnea, nausea, vomiting, diarrhea, and bradycardia. If these symptoms occur, patient is in cholinergic crisis. If strength improves, patient is in a myasthenic crisis.

- **Supraventricular Tachycardia:** Monitor pulse, blood pressure, and ECG prior to and throughout administration.
- **Toxicity and Overdose:** Atropine may be used for treatment of cholinergic symptoms. Oxygen and resuscitation equipment should be available.

Potential Nursing Diagnoses

- Breathing pattern, ineffective (indications).
- Knowledge deficit related to medication regimen (patient/family teaching).

Implementation

- **General Info:** For myasthenia gravis patients diagnostic IV dose and dose to differentiate myasthenic from cholinergic crisis is administered by a physician.
- **IV:** IV doses are administered undiluted with a tuberculin syringe.
- **Y-Site Compatibility:** heparin, hydrocortisone, or potassium chloride.

Patient/Family Teaching

□ Inform patient that the effects of this medication last up to 30 min.

Evaluation

Effectiveness of medication can be demonstrated by: ▪ Relief of myasthenic symptoms ▪ Differentiation of myasthenic from cholinergic crisis ▪ Reversal of paralysis after anesthesia ▪ Resolution of supraventricular tachycardia.

ENALAPRIL
(e-**nal**-a-pril)
Vasotec

ENALAPRILAT
(e-**nal**-a-pril-at)
Vasotec

CLASSIFICATION(S):
Antihypertensive—angiotensin converting enzyme (ACE) inhibitor
Pregnancy Category C

INDICATIONS

▪ Alone or in combination with other antihypertensives in the management of hypertension ▪ Used in combination with other drugs in the treatment of congestive heart failure.

ACTION

▪ Prevents the production of angiotensin II, a potent vasoconstrictor that stimulates the production of aldosterone, by blocking its conversion to the active form. Result is systemic vasodilation. **Therapeutic Effects:** ▪ Lowering of blood pressure in hypertensive patients ▪ Decreased preload and afterload in patients with congestive heart failure.

PHARMACOKINETICS

Absorption: Well absorbed following oral administration.

Distribution: Minimal crossing of the blood-brain barrier. Rest of distribution not known.

Metabolism and Excretion: Following absorption, enalapril is converted to enalaprilat, the active metabolite. 60% excreted by the kidneys (40% as enalaprilat, 20% as enalapril).

Half-life: Enalaprilat—11 hr (increased in renal impairment).

CONTRAINDICATIONS AND PRECAUTIONS

Contraindicated in: ▪ Hypersensitivity ▪ Cross-sensitivity with other ACE inhibitors may exist.

Use Cautiously in: ▪ Renal impairment (dosage reduction required) ▪ Pregnancy, lactation, and children (safety not established) ▪ Hypotension

E

may be exaggerated during surgery/anesthesia ▪ Aortic stenosis ▪ Cerebrovascular disease ▪ Cardiac insufficiency.

Extreme Caution in: ▪ Patients with a family history of hereditary angioedema.

ADVERSE REACTIONS AND SIDE EFFECTS*

CNS: headache, dizziness, fatigue.

Resp: cough.

CV: hypotension, tachycardia, angina pectoris.

GI: anorexia, diarrhea, nausea, impaired taste.

GU: impotence.

Derm: rashes.

F and E: hyperkalemia.

Misc: fever, ANGIOEDEMA with laryngospasm.

INTERACTIONS

Drug–Drug: ▪ Additive hypotension with other **antihypertensives,** acute ingestion of **alcohol,** and **vasodilators** ▪ Hyperkalemia may result with concurrent **potassium therapy** or **potassium-sparing diuretics** ▪ Antihypertensive response may be blunted by **nonsteroidal anti-inflammatory agents** ▪ Renal side effects may be exaggerated by concurrent **penicillamine** therapy.

Drug–Food: ▪ Hyperkalemia may result from a **high-potassium diet**.

ROUTE AND DOSAGE

Hypertension

- **PO (Adults):** Initial dose—2.5 mg, then 5 mg/day, increased as required by blood pressure response (usual range 10–40 mg/day in 1–2 divided doses).

Congestive Heart Failure

- **PO (Adults):** Initial dose—2.5 mg, increased as required by clinical response (usual range 5–20 mg/day in 1–2 divided doses).
- **IV (Adults):** 0.625–1.25 mg q 6 hr.

PHARMACODYNAMICS (effect on blood pressure)

	ONSET	PEAK	DURATION
PO	1 hr	4–6 hr	24 hr
IV	15 min	1–4 hr	6 hr

NURSING IMPLICATIONS

Assessment

- □ Monitor blood pressure and pulse frequently during initial dosage adjustment and periodically throughout course of therapy. Notify physician of significant changes.
- □ Monitor weight and assess patient routinely for resolution of fluid overload (peripheral edema, rales/crackles, dyspnea, weight gain, jugular venous distension).
- ▪ **Lab Test Considerations:** Monitor BUN, creatinine, and electrolyte levels periodically. Serum potassium may be increased and BUN and creatinine transiently increased, while sodium levels may be decreased.

Potential Nursing Diagnoses

- ▪ Cardiac output, decreased (indications, side effects).
- ▪ Knowledge deficit related to medication regimen (patient/family teaching).
- ▪ Noncompliance (patient/family teaching).

Implementation

- ▪ **PO:** Precipitous drop in blood pressure during first 1–3 hr following first dose may require volume expansion with normal saline but is not normally considered an indication for stopping therapy. Monitor closely for at least 1 hr after blood pressure has stabilized.
- □ Available in combination with hydrochlorothiazide (Vaseretic); see Appendix A.
- ▪ **Direct IV:** May be administered undiluted over 5 min or diluted in 50 ml of D5W, 0.9% NaCl, D5/0.9% NaCl, or D5/LR. Diluted soln is stable for 24 hr.

*Underlines indicate most frequent; **CAPITALS** indicate life-threatening.

Patient/Family Teaching

- Instruct patient to take enalapril exactly as directed, even if feeling well. Missed doses should be taken as soon as remembered but not if almost time for next dose. Do not double doses. Medication controls but does not cure hypertension. Caution patient not to discontinue enalapril therapy unless directed by physician.
- Encourage patient to comply with additional interventions for hypertension (weight reduction, discontinuation of smoking, moderation of alcohol consumption, regular exercise, and stress management).
- Instruct patient and family on proper technique for blood pressure monitoring. Advise them to check blood pressure at least weekly and report significant changes to physician.
- Caution patient to avoid salt substitutes or foods containing high levels of potassium or sodium, unless directed by physician (see Appendix K).
- Advise patient that enalapril may cause an impairment of taste that generally reverses itself within 8–12 wk, even with continued therapy.
- Caution patient to change positions slowly to minimize orthostatic hypotension, particularly after initial dose. Also advise patient that exercise or hot weather may increase hypotensive effects.
- Advise patient to consult physician or pharmacist before taking any over-the-counter medications, especially cold remedies. Patient should also avoid excessive amounts of tea, coffee, or cola.
- Enalapril may cause dizziness. Caution patient to avoid driving and other activities requiring alertness until response to medication is known.
- Advise patient to inform physician or dentist of medication regimen prior to treatment or surgery.
- Instruct patient to notify physician if rash, mouth sores, sore throat, fever, swelling of hands or feet, irregular heartbeat, chest pain, dry cough, swelling of face, eyes, lips, or tongue, or difficulty breathing occurs.
- Emphasize the importance of follow-up examinations to monitor progress.

Evaluation

Effectiveness of therapy can be demonstrated by: ▪ Decrease in blood pressure without appearance of side effects ▪ Decrease in signs and symptoms of congestive heart failure. Several wks may be necessary before full effects of the drug are recognized.

EPHEDRINE

(e-**fed**-drin)

Efed-II, Efedron nasal jelly, Vatronol Nose Drops

CLASSIFICATION(S):

Bronchodilator—alpha- and beta-adrenergic agonist, Nasal decongestant, Vasopressor

Pregnancy Category C

INDICATIONS

▪ Used as a bronchodilator in the management of reversible airway obstruction due to asthma or COPD ▪ Relief of nasal congestion in viral upper respiratory tract infections or allergic rhinitis ▪ Management of orthostatic hypotension ▪ Management of acute hypotension associated with overdosage of antihypertensive agents ▪ As a CNS stimulant in the management of mental depression or narcolepsy.

ACTION

▪ An alpha- and beta-adrenergic agonist. Beta-adrenergic agonist effects result in accumulation of cyclic AMP at beta-adrenergic receptors, producing bronchodilation, CNS and cardiac stimulation, diuresis, and gastric acid secretion. Primary alpha-adrenergic effect is peripheral vasoconstriction. **Therapeutic Effects:** ▪ Bronchodilation ▪ Vasoconstriction with decreased congestion ▪ Restoration of blood pressure ▪ CNS stimulation.

E

PHARMACOKINETICS

Absorption: Well absorbed following oral, IM, or SC administration.

Distribution: Probably crosses the placenta and enters breast milk.

Metabolism and Excretion: Small amounts slowly metabolized by the liver. Mostly excreted unchanged by the kidneys.

Half-life: 3–6 hr (depends on urine pH).

CONTRAINDICATIONS AND PRECAUTIONS

Contraindicated in: ▪ Hypersensitivity ▪ Known intolerance ▪ Angle-closure glaucoma ▪ Cyclopropane or halothane anesthesia ▪ Thyrotoxicosis ▪ Diabetes mellitus ▪ Pregnancy ▪ Hypertension ▪ Severe cardiovascular disease.

Use Cautiously in: ▪ Cardiovascular disease ▪ Lactation ▪ Prostatic hypertrophy.

ADVERSE REACTIONS AND SIDE EFFECTS*

CNS: CNS stimulation, nervousness, anxiety paranoid state (long-term use), dizziness, lightheadedness, vertigo.

EENT: rebound congestion (nasal use), local irritation.

Resp: breathing difficulties.

CV: angina pectoris, palpitations, tachycardia, ARRHYTHMIAS.

GU: urinary retention, decreased urine output.

Misc: rapid development of tolerance (tachyphylaxis), diaphoresis.

INTERACTIONS

Drug-Drug: **Cyclopropane, cardiac glycosides,** or **halothane** increases risk of arrhythmias ▪ Additive effects with other **adrenergic (sympathomimetic) agents** ▪ Use with **MAO inhibitors** may result in hypertensive crisis ▪ Pressor response may be reduced by **reserpine, methyldopa,** or **furosemide** ▪ **Theophylline** increases the risk of adverse effects ▪ Reflex bradycardia and pressor effects are decreased by **atropine** ▪ **Acidifying the urine (ammonium chloride)** decreases half-life ▪ **Alkalinizing the urine (sodium bicarbonate)** increases the half-life.

ROUTE AND DOSAGE

Bronchodilator, Nasal Decongestant

- **PO (Adults):** 25–50 mg q 3–4 hr as needed or 15–60 mg or sustained-release preparation every 8–12 hr.
- **PO (Children):** 2–3 mg/kg/day or 100 $mg/m^2/day$ in 4–6 divided doses.
- **IV, IM, SC (Adults):** 12.5–25 mg.
- **Top (Adults and Children >6 yr):** Instill 0.5–1% soln directly to nasal mucosa or on a nasal pack q 4 hr or small amount of 0.6% jelly in each nostril (not to be used more frequently than q 4 hr or more than 3–4 days).

Vasopressor

- **IV (Adults):** 10–25 mg as a slow injection; additional doses may be given in 5–10 min (not to exceed 150 mg/24 hr).
- **SC, IM (Adults):** 25–50 mg (range 10–50 mg), may be followed by second **IM** dose of 50 mg or an **IV** dose of 25 mg (not to exceed 150 mg/24 hr).
- **IV, SC (Children):** 3 mg/kg/day or 100 $mg/m^2/day$ in 4–6 divided doses.

Orthostatic Hypotension

- **PO (Adults):** 25 mg 1–4 times daily.
- **PO (Children):** 3 mg/kg/day in 4–6 divided doses.

CNS Stimulant

- **PO (Adults):** 25–50 mg q 3–4 hr as needed or 15–60 mg or sustained-release preparation every 8–12 hr.
- **PO (Children):** 3 mg/kg/day or 100 $mg/m^2/day$ in 4–6 divided doses.

PHARMACODYNAMICS (PO, SC, IM = bronchodilation, IV = pressor response, Top = nasal decongestion)

	ONSET	PEAK	DURATION
PO	15–60 min	UK	3–5 hr
PO-SR	UK	UK	12 hr
SC	UK	UK	1 hr
IM	10–20 min	UK	1 hr
IV	UK	UK	1 hr
Top	UK	UK	6 hr

*Underlines indicate most frequent; **CAPITALS** indicate life-threatening.

NURSING IMPLICATIONS

Assessment

- **Bronchodilator:** Assess lung sounds, pulse, and blood pressure before administration and during peak of medication.
- **Vasopressor:** Monitor blood pressure, pulse, ECG, and respiratory rate frequently during IV administration.
- **Nasal Decongestant:** Assess patient for nasal and sinus congestion prior to and periodically during therapy.
- **CNS Stimulant:** Assess sleep patterns and mental status of patients treated for narcolepsy or mental depression.

Potential Nursing Diagnoses

- Tissue perfusion, altered (indications).
- Airway clearance, ineffective (indications).
- Knowledge deficit related to medication regimen (patient/family teaching).

Implementation

- **General Info:** Available in tablets, capsules, syrup, and injectable forms. Also available in combination with other drugs (see Appendix A).
  - Tolerance to ephedrine may develop with prolonged or excessive use. Effectiveness may be restored by discontinuing for a few days and then readministering.
- **PO:** Administer last dose each day a few hrs before bedtime to minimize insomnia.
- **IV:** Use only clear soln. Discard any unused soln.
- **Direct IV:** Inject undiluted through Y-site or 3-way stopcock.
  - *Rate:* Administer slowly, each 10 mg over at least 1 min.
- **Additive Compatibility:** D5W, D10W, 0.45% NaCl, 0.9% NaCl, Ringer's and lactated Ringer's soln, dextrose/saline combinations, dextrose/Ringer's or lactated Ringer's combinations, chloramphenicol, lidocaine, metaraminol, nafcillin, penicillin G potassium, or tetracycline.
- **Additive Incompatibility:** hydrocortisone sodium succinate, pentobarbital, phenobarbital, or secobarbital.

Patient/Family Teaching

- Instruct patient to take ephedrine exactly as directed. If on a scheduled dosing regimen, take a missed dose as soon as remembered, spacing remaining doses at regular intervals. Do not double doses. Caution patient not to exceed recommended dose.
- Instruct patient to contact physician immediately if shortness of breath is not relieved by medication or is accompanied by diaphoresis, dizziness, palpitations, or chest pain.
- Advise patient to consult physician or pharmacist before taking any over-the-counter medications or alcoholic beverages concurrently with this therapy.

Evaluation

Effectiveness of therapy can be demonstrated by: ■ Prevention or relief of bronchospasm ■ Increase in blood pressure, when used as a vasopressor ■ Decrease in sinus and nasal congestion ■ Improvement in mental status and increase in alertness, when used as a CNS stimulant.

EPINEPHRINE (inhalation)
(ep-i-**nef**-rin)
Adrenalin, AsthmaHaler, Bronkaid, Dysne-Inhal, Medihaler-Epi, Primatene

RACEMIC EPINEPHRINE (inhalation)
AsthmaNefrin, microNEFRIN, S-2 Inhalant, Vaponefrin

EPINEPHRINE (parenteral)
EpiPen, EpiPen Jr

EPINEPHRINE (parenteral suspension)
Sus-Phrine

EPINEPHRINE (ophthalmic)

EPINEPHRINE OPHTH SOLN
Epifrin, Glaucon

EPINEPHRINE BITARTRATE
Epitrate

EPINEPHRYL BORATE
Epinal, Eppy/N

CLASSIFICATION(S):
Bronchodilator, Cardiac stimulant, Ophthalmic—adrenergic, Antiglaucoma
Pregnancy Category C

INDICATIONS

■ **IV, SC, Inhaln:** Bronchodilator in the symptomatic treatment of asthma and other forms of reversible airway disease, which may occur in association with chronic bronchitis and emphysema ■ **IV, SC:** Treatment of anaphylaxis ■ **IV, Intracardiac:** Cardiac arrest ■ **Ophth:** Treatment of open-angle glaucoma ■ **Local:** As an adjunct in the localization of anesthesia.

ACTION

■ $Beta_1$- and $beta_2$-adrenergic agonist, which produces an accumulation of cyclic adenosine monophosphate (cAMP). Increased levels of cAMP at beta-adrenergic receptors produce bronchodilation, CNS and cardiac stimulation, diuresis, and gastric acid secretion ■ When injected locally, stimulates alpha-adrenergic receptors in blood vessels of the skin, producing vasoconstriction. **Therapeutic Effects:** ■ Bronchodilation ■ Cardiac stimulation ■ Vasoconstriction ■ The following ophthalmic effects: □ Decreased formation of aqueous humor □ Increased aqueous outflow □ Conjunctival vasoconstriction □ Mydriasis ■ Localization of anesthetics.

PHARMACOKINETICS

Absorption: Absorbed but rapidly metabolized following oral administration. Systemic absorption may follow ophthalmic administration or large and repeated inhalation doses.
Distribution: Does not cross the blood-brain barrier. Crosses the placenta and enters breast milk.
Metabolism and Excretion: Action is rapidly terminated by metabolism and uptake by nerve endings.
Half-life: UK.

CONTRAINDICATIONS AND PRECAUTIONS

Contraindicated in: ■ Hypersensitivity to sympathomimetics ■ May contain bisulfites—avoid use in patients with bisulfite hypersensitivity.
Use Cautiously in: ■ Elderly (more susceptible to adverse reactions—dosage reduction may be required) ■ Pregnancy and lactation (safety not established) ■ Cardiovascular disease ■ Arrhythmias ■ Hypertension ■ Hyperthyroidism ■ Glaucoma (except for ophthalmic use in open-angle glaucoma) ■ Diabetes mellitus (may increase the need for insulin or oral hypoglycemic agents) ■ Excessive use of inhaler may lead to tolerance, paradoxical bronchospasm, systemic absorption, and side effects.

ADVERSE REACTIONS AND SIDE EFFECTS*

CNS: <u>nervousness</u>, <u>restlessness</u>, <u>insomnia</u>, <u>tremor</u>, <u>headache</u>.
CV: hypertension, <u>arrhythmias</u>, angina.
Endo: hyperglycemia.
GI: nausea, vomiting.
GU: urinary retention, hesitancy.

INTERACTIONS

Drug-Drug: ■ Additive effect with other **adrenergic (sympathomimetic) agents,** including **decongestants** ■ Use with **MAO inhibitors** may lead to hypertensive crisis ■ Increased risk of arrhythmias with **general anesthetics** or **cardiac glycosides** ■ **Beta-adrenergic blockers** may block therapeutic response (however, **ophthalmic beta blockers** may be used with **ophthalmic epinephrine**, resulting in additive lowering of intraocular pressure).

ROUTE AND DOSAGE

Note: See infusion rate table in Appendix D.

*<u>Underlines</u> indicate most frequent; **CAPITALS** indicate life-threatening.

Epinephrine Solution—Parenteral Bronchodilator

- **SC (Adults):** 0.2–0.5 mg q 20 min–4 hr (up to 1 mg/dose).
- **SC (Children):** 0.01 mg/kg repeat q 15 min for 2 doses, then q 4 hr as needed (not to exceed 0.5 mg/dose).

Anaphylactic Reactions

- **IM, SC (Adults):** 0.2–0.5 mg, may repeat q 10–15 min (up to 1 mg/dose).
- **SC (Children):** 0.01 mg/kg repeat q 15 min for 2 doses, then q 4 hr as needed (not to exceed 0.5 mg/dose).

Vasopressor, Anaphylactic Shock

- **IM, SC (Adults):** 0.5 mg, may be followed by IV administration.
- **IV (Adults):** 0.1–0.25 mg, may repeat q 5–15 min or followed by infusion at 0.001 mg/min (1 mcg/min); may be increased to a maximum of 0.004 mg/min (4 mcg/min).
- **IM, IV (Children):** 0.3 mg, may repeat q 15 min for 3–4 doses.

Cardiac Arrest

- **IV, Intracardiac, Endotracheal (Adults):** 0.1–1 mg, repeat q 5 min as needed.
- **IV, Intracardiac, Endotracheal (Children):** 5–10 mcg/kg q 5 min, may be followed by IV infusion at an initial rate of 0.1 mcg/kg/min, not to exceed 1.5 mcg/kg/min.

Epinephrine Suspension—Parenteral Bronchodilator

- **SC (Adults):** 0.5 mg (0.5 ml) of suspension initially, then 0.5–1.5 mg (0.5–1.5 ml) no more often than q 6 hr as needed.
- **SC (Children):** 25 mcg/kg (0.025 mg/kg) of suspension no more often than q 6 hr as needed.

Epinephrine Inhalation

- **Inhaln (Adults and Children):** 1–2 inhalations of 1:100 or 2.25% racepinephrine (0.2 mg/dose).

Epinephrine Ophthalmic

- **Ophth (Adults):** 1 drop of 0.25–2% **epinephrine ophth soln** to conjunctiva 1–2 times daily or 1 drop of 1–2% **epinephrine bitartrate ophth soln** up to 2 times daily or 1 drop of 0.5–2% **epinephryl borate ophth soln** 1–2 times daily.

PHARMACODYNAMICS (SC, IM, IV, Inhaln = bronchodilation, Ophth = lowering of intraocular pressure)

	ONSET	PEAK	DURATION
SC	5–10 min	20 min	20–30 min*
IM	5–10 min	20 min	20–30 min
IV	rapid	20 min	20–30 min
Inhaln	3–5 min	20 min	1–3 hr
Ophth	within 1 hr	4–8 hr	24 hr

*Epinephrine suspension has a duration of 6–12 hr.

NURSING IMPLICATIONS

Assessment

- **IV:** Monitor blood pressure, pulse, and respiratory rate prior to and every 5 min during IV administration. Patients receiving IV epinephrine should have continuous ECG monitoring.
- **Bronchodilator:** Assess lung sounds before and after treatment. Note amount, color, and character of sputum produced, and notify physician of abnormal findings.
  - Observe patient closely for symptoms of relief. If no relief occurs within 20 min of treatment, or if symptoms worsen, notify physician immediately.
  - Observe patient for drug tolerance and rebound bronchospasm. Patients requiring more than 3 inhalation treatments in 24 hr should be under close supervision. If minimal or no relief is seen after 3–5 inhalation treatments within 6–12 hr, further treatment with aerosol alone is not recommended.
- **Lab Test Considerations:** May cause an increase in blood glucose and serum lactic acid concentrations.

Potential Nursing Diagnoses

- Airway clearance, ineffective (indications).
- Cardiac output, decreased (indications).
- Knowledge deficit related to medica-

tion regimen (patient/family teaching).

Implementation

- **General Info:** Medication should be administered promptly at the onset of bronchospasm.
  - Check dose, concentration, and route of administration carefully prior to administration. Fatalities have occurred from medication errors. Use a tuberculin syringe for SC injection to ensure that correct amount of medication is administered. Suspension is for SC use *only*.
  - Do not use soln that is pinkish or brownish or one that contains a precipitate.
  - Administer injection of sterile epinephrine suspension promptly after drawing into syringe, to prevent settling of the suspension.
  - For anaphylactic shock, volume replacement should be administered concurrently with epinephrine. Antihistamines and glucocorticoids may be used in conjunction with epinephrine.
- **SC/IM:** Medication can cause irritation of tissue. Rotate injection sites to prevent tissue necrosis. Massage injection sites well after administration to enhance absorption and to decrease local vasoconstriction. Avoid IM administration in gluteal muscle. Shake suspension well before administering; inject promptly to prevent settling.
- **IV:** For IV administration each 1 mg (1 ml) of 1:1000 soln must be diluted in at least 10 ml of 0.9% NaCl for injection to prepare a 1:10,000 soln. Discard any soln not used within 24 hr of preparation.
- **Direct IV:** Administer each 1 mg over at least 1 min; more rapid administration may be used during cardiac resuscitation.
- **Continuous Infusion:** For maintenance, soln may be further diluted in 500 ml of D5W, D10W, 0.9% NaCl, D5/LR, D5/Ringer's soln, dextrose/saline combinations, or Ringer's or lactated Ringer's soln. Administer through Y-site or 3–way stopcock via infusion pump to ensure accurate dosage.
- **Syringe Compatibility:** doxapram or heparin.
- **Y-Site Compatibility:** amrinone, atracurium, calcium chloride, calcium gluconate, famotidine, heparin, hydrocortisone sodium succinate, pancuronium, potassium chloride, phytonadione, or vecuronium.
- **Additive Compatibility:** amikacin, cimetidine, dobutamine, metaraminol, or verapamil.
- **Additive Incompatibility:** aminophylline, cephapirin, sodium bicarbonate, or warfarin.
- **Inhaln:** When using epinephrine inhalation soln, 10 drops of 1% base soln should be placed in the reservoir of the nebulizer.
  - The 2.25% inhalation soln of racepinephrine must be diluted for use in the combination nebulizer/respirator.
  - Allow 1–2 min to elapse between inhalations of epinephrine inhalation soln, ephinephrine inhalation aerosol, or epinephrine bitartrate inhalation aerosol to make certain the second inhalation is necessary.
  - When epinephrine is used concurrently with glucocorticoid or ipratropium inhalations, administer bronchodilator first and other medications 5 min apart to prevent toxicity from inhaled fluorocarbon propellants.
- **Endotracheal:** Epinephrine can be injected directly into the bronchial tree via the endotracheal tube if the patient has been intubated. Use the same dose as for IV injection.
- **Ophth:** See Appendix H for administration of ophthalmic soln.

Patient/Family Teaching

- **General Info:** Advise patient taking epinephrine for asthma, bronchitis, emphysema, or other obstructive pulmonary diseases to contact physician immediately if there is no response to the usual dose of epinephrine or if angina develops. This may signify worsening of condition and requires evaluation of therapy.

- **Inhaln:** Instruct patient to rinse mouth after each inhalation to prevent dryness.
- Advise patient to consult physician or pharmacist prior to taking any over-the-counter medications concurrently with epinephrine.
- Advise patient to report bronchial irritation, restlessness, or insomnia to physician promptly. A decrease in medication dosage may be necessary.
- **Auto-injector:** Instruct patients using auto-injector for anaphylactic reactions to remove gray safety cap, placing black tip on thigh at right angle to leg. Press hard into thigh until auto-injector functions, hold in place several sec, remove, and discard properly. Massage injected area for 10 sec.

EVALUATION

Effectiveness of therapy can be demonstrated by: ▪ Decrease in wheezing and respiratory distress ▪ Reversal of signs and symptoms of anaphylaxis ▪ Increase in cardiac rate and output, when used in cardiac resuscitation ▪ Decrease in intraocular pressure ▪ Localization of local anesthetic.

EPOETIN ALFA

(ee-**poe**-e-tin **al**-fa)
Epogen, EPO, erythropoietin, Procrit

CLASSIFICATION(S):
Hormone—erythropoietin, recombinant
Pregnancy Category C

INDICATIONS

▪ Treatment of anemia associated with chronic renal failure ▪ Management of anemia secondary to zidovudine (AZT) therapy in HIV-infected patients.

ACTION

▪ Stimulates erythropoiesis (production of red blood cells). **Therapeutic Effects:** ▪ Maintains and may elevate red blood cell counts, decreasing the need for transfusions.

PHARMACOKINETICS

Absorption: Well absorbed following SC administration.
Distribution: Distribution not known.
Metabolism and Excretion: Metabolism and excretion not known.
Half-life: 4–13 hr.

CONTRAINDICATIONS AND PRECAUTIONS

Contraindicated in: ▪ Hypersensitivity to albumin or mammalian cell-derived products ▪ Uncontrolled hypertension.
Use Cautiously in: ▪ History of seizures ▪ Pregnancy, lactation, or children (safety not established).

ADVERSE REACTIONS AND SIDE EFFECTS*

CNS: SEIZURES, headache.
CV: thrombotic events (hemodialysis patients), <u>hypertension</u>.
Derm: transient rashes.
Endo: resumption of menses, restored fertility.

INTERACTIONS

Drug-Drug: ▪ May increase the requirement for **heparin** anticoagulation during hemodialysis.

ROUTE AND DOSAGE

Anemia of Chronic Renal Failure

- **SC, IV (Adults):** 50–100 units/kg 3 times weekly initially, then adjust dosage by changes of 25 units/kg/dose to maintain target range of Hct of 30–33% (not to exceed 36%). Usual maintenance dose 25 units/kg 3 times weekly.

Anemia Secondary to Zidovudine (AZT) Therapy

- **IV, SC (Adults):** 100 units/kg 3 times weekly for 8 wk, if inadequate response, may increase by 50–100

*<u>Underlines</u> indicate most frequent; **CAPITALS** indicate life-threatening.

units/kg every 4–8 wk, up to 300 units/kg 3 times weekly (if Hct >40%, stop therapy until it drops to 36%, then decrease dose by 25% and resume therapy).

PHARMACODYNAMICS (increase in RBCs)

	ONSET*	PEAK	DURATION
IV, SC	10 days	2–6 wks	UK

*Increase in reticulocytes.

NURSING IMPLICATIONS

Assessment

- Monitor blood pressure prior to and throughout course of therapy. Inform physician if severe hypertension is present or if blood pressure begins to increase. Uncontrolled hypertension is a contraindication for epoetin alfa therapy. Additional antihypertensive therapy may be required during initiation of therapy.
- Monitor response for symptoms of anemia (fatigue, dyspnea, pallor).
- Monitor dialysis shunts (thrill and bruit) and status of artificial kidney during hemodialysis. Heparin dose may need to be increased to prevent clotting. Patients with underlying vascular disease should be monitored for impaired circulation.
- **Lab Test Considerations:** Hematocrit should be monitored prior to and twice weekly during initial therapy, and regularly after target range (30–33%) has been reached and maintenance dose is determined. Other hemopoietic parameters (hemoglobin, reticulocyte count, and RBC count) also should be monitored prior to and periodically throughout therapy. Reticulocyte count usually begins to rise 10 days after initiation of therapy. Hemoglobin, hematocrit, and RBC levels begin to increase after 2–6 wk of therapy. Notify physician if hematocrit increases more than 4 points in a 2-wk period, as this increases the likelihood of a hypertensive reaction and seizures. If hematocrit exceeds 36%, dose should be withheld until hematocrit is 33%. Dose should be reduced by 25 units/kg upon resumption.
- Serum ferritin, transferrin, and iron levels should also be monitored to assess need for concurrent iron therapy.
- Monitor renal function studies and electrolytes closely, as resulting increased sense of well-being may lead to decreased compliance with other therapies for renal failure. Increases in BUN, creatinine, uric acid, phosphorous, and potassium may occur.
- May cause increase in WBCs and platelets. May decrease bleeding times.

Potential Nursing Diagnoses

- Activity intolerance (indications).
- Knowledge deficit related to medication and dietary regimen (patient/family teaching).
- Noncompliance (patient/family teaching).

Implementation

- **General Info:** Transfusions are still required for severe symptomatic anemia, as several wks are required before therapeutic response occurs.
- Institute seizure precautions in patients who experience greater than 4 point increase in hematocrit in a 2-wk period or exhibit any change in neurologic status. Risk of seizures is greatest during the first 90 days of therapy.
- Do not shake vial, as inactivation of medication may occur. Discard vial immediately after withdrawing dose.
- **SC:** This route is often used for patients not requiring dialysis.
- **IV:** May be administered as direct injection or bolus via venous line at end of dialysis session.

Patient/Family Teaching

- Stress importance of compliance with dietary restrictions, medications, and dialysis. Foods high in iron and low in potassium include liver, pork, veal, beef, mustard and turnip greens, peas, eggs, broccoli, kale, blackberries, strawberries, apple juice, watermelon, oatmeal, and enriched bread. Epoetin alfa will result in increased sense of well-being, but it does not cure underlying renal disease.

- Explain rationale for concurrent iron therapy (increased red blood cell production requires iron).
- Discuss possible return of menses and fertility in females of childbearing age. Patient should discuss contraceptive options with physician.
- Discuss ways of preventing self-injury in patients at risk for seizures. Driving and activities requiring continuous alertness should be avoided.

EVALUATION

Clinical response is indicated by: ▪ Increase in hematocrit to 30–33% and subsequent improvement in symptoms of anemia in patients with chronic renal failure ▪ Increase in hematocrit to >40% in anemia secondary to zidovudine therapy.

ERGOCALCIFEROL

(er-goe-kal-**sif**-e-role)
Calciferol, Deltalin, Drisdol, {Ostoforte}, {Radiostol}, vitamin D_2

CLASSIFICATION(S):
Vitamin—fat-soluble
Pregnancy Category C

INDICATIONS

▪ Prophylaxis and treatment of vitamin D deficiency ▪ Treatment of hypophosphatemia or hypocalcemia ▪ Treatment of osteodystrophy ▪ Treatment of rickets. **Unlabeled Uses:** ▪ Renal osteodystrophy ▪ Treatment and prophylaxis of postoperative and idiopathic tetany.

ACTION

▪ Promotes the absorption of calcium and phosphorous ▪ Regulates calcium homeostasis in conjunction with parathyroid hormone and calcitonin. **Therapeutic Effects:** ▪ Treatment and prevention of deficiency states, particularly bone manifestations.

PHARMACOKINETICS

Absorption: Well absorbed in an inactive form.
Distribution: Stored in the liver and other fatty tissues.
Metabolism and Excretion: Converted to active form by sunlight and the liver. Metabolized and excreted by the kidney.
Half-life: UK.

CONTRAINDICATIONS AND PRECAUTIONS

Contraindicated in: ▪ Hypersensitivity ▪ Hypercalcemia ▪ Vitamin D toxicity ▪ Lactation (large doses).
Use Cautiously in: ▪ Patients receiving cardiac glycosides ▪ Pregnancy (larger doses; safety not established).

ADVERSE REACTIONS AND SIDE EFFECTS*

▪ Do not occur at doses within the range of daily requirements.

INTERACTIONS

Drug-Drug: ▪ **Cholestyramine, colestipol,** or **mineral oil** decreases absorption of vitamin D analogs ▪ Use with **thiazide diuretics** in patients with hypoparathyroidism may result in hypercalcemia ▪ **Glucocorticoids** decrease the effectiveness of vitamin D analogs ▪ Use with **cardiac glycosides** increases the risk of arrhythmias ▪ Vitamin D requirements are increased by **phenytoin** and other **hydantoin anticonvulsants, sucralfate, barbiturates,** and **primidone**.

ROUTE AND DOSAGE

Vitamin D Deficiency

- **PO (Adults and Children):** 1000–2000 units/day initially, then 400 units/day maintenance.

Vitamin D-Resistant Rickets

- **PO (Adults):** 12,000–500,000 units/day.

{} = Available in Canada only.
*Underlines indicate most frequent; **CAPITALS** indicate life-threatening.

Vitamin D-Dependent Rickets
- **PO (Adults):** 10,000–60,000 units/day (up to 500,000 units/day).
- **PO (Children):** 3000–10,000 units/day, up to 50,000 units/day.

Familial Hypophosphatemia
- **PO (Adults):** 50,000–100,000 units/day.

Hypoparathyroidism
- **PO (Adults):** 50,000–150,000 units/day.
- **PO (Children):** 50,000–200,000 units/day.

Renal Osteodystrophy
- **PO (Adults):** 10,000–300,000 units/day.
- **PO (Children):** 4000–40,000 units/day.

PHARMACODYNAMICS (effects on serum calcium levels)

	ONSET	PEAK	DURATION
PO	12–24 hr*	UK	up to 6 mon*

*Therapeutic effect may take 10–14 days.

NURSING IMPLICATIONS

Assessment
- **General Info:** Assess for symptoms of vitamin deficiency prior to and periodically throughout therapy.
  - Observe patient for evidence of hypocalcemia (paresthesias, muscle twitching, laryngospasm, colic, cardiac arrhythmias, and Chvostek's or Trousseau's sign). Protect symptomatic patient by raising and padding side rails; keep bed in low position.
- **Children:** Monitor height and weight; growth arrest may occur in prolonged high-dose therapy.
- **Ricketts/Osteomalacia:** Assess patient for bone pain and weakness prior to and throughout course of therapy.
- **Lab Test Considerations:** Monitor serum phosphorous levels prior to and periodically throughout course of therapy. Serum phosphorous must be controlled prior to initiating therapy. Aluminum carbonate or aluminum hydroxide is used for this purpose in dialysis patients.
  - Serum calcium levels should be drawn weekly during initial therapy. Monitor BUN, serum creatinine, alkaline phosphatase, parathyroid hormone levels, creatine clearance, and 24–hr urinary calcium periodically. A fall in alkaline phosphatase levels may signal onset of hypercalcemia.
- **Toxicity and Overdose:** Toxicity is manifested as hypercalcemia. Assess for nausea, vomiting, anorexia, weakness, constipation, headache, bone pain, and metallic taste. Later symptoms include polyuria, polydipsia, photophobia, rhinorrhea, pruritis, and cardiac arrhythmias. Treatment includes discontinuing ergocalciferol and instituting a low-calcium diet. IV hydration, loop diuretics, and urinary acidification may be ordered to increase urinary excretion of calcium. Dialysis may also be used.

Potential Nursing Diagnoses
- Nutrition, altered: less than body requirements (indications).
- Knowledge deficit related to medication regimen (patient/family teaching).

Implementation
- **General Info:** Because solitary vitamin deficiencies are rare, combinations are commonly administered.
- **PO:** May be administered without regard to meals. Measure soln accurately with calibrated dropper provided by manufacturer. May be mixed with juice, cereal, or food.
- **IM:** Injection is oil-based; avoid IV administration.

Patient/Family Teaching
- Advise patient to take as directed. If dose is missed, take as soon as remembered; do not double up on doses.
- Encourage patients to comply with diet recommendations of physician. Explain that the best source of vita-

mins is a well-balanced diet with foods from the 4 basic food groups.

- Foods high in vitamin D include fish livers and oils, and fortified milk, bread, and cereals. Foods high in calcium include dairy products, canned salmon and sardines, broccoli, bok choy, tofu, molasses, and cream soups (see Appendix K). Renal patients must still consider renal failure diet in food selection. Physician may order concurrent calcium supplement.
- Patients self-medicating with vitamin supplements should be cautioned not to exceed RDA (see Appendix L). The effectiveness of megadoses for treatment of various medical conditions is unproven and may cause side effects.
- Review symptoms of overdosage and instruct patient to report these promptly to physician.
- Emphasize the importance of follow-up examinations to evaluate progress.

EVALUATION

Effectiveness of therapy can be demonstrated by: ▪ Decrease in the symptoms of vitamin D deficiency ▪ Normalization of serum calcium levels in hypoparathyroidism ▪ Improvement in symptoms of vitamin D-resistant rickets.

ERGONOVINE

(er-goe-**noe**-veen)
Ergometrine, Ergotrate

CLASSIFICATION(S):
Oxytocic
Pregnancy Category UK

INDICATIONS

▪ Prevention and treatment of postpartum or postabortion hemorrhage caused by uterine atony or involution. **Unlabeled Use:** ▪ As a diagnostic agent to provoke coronary artery spasm.

ACTION

▪ Directly stimulates uterine and vascular smooth muscle. **Therapeutic Effect:** ▪ Uterine contraction.

PHARMACOKINETICS

Absorption: Well absorbed following oral or IM administration.
Distribution: Distribution not known.
Metabolism and Excretion: UK. Probably metabolized by the liver.
Half-life: UK.

CONTRAINDICATIONS AND PRECAUTIONS

Contraindicated in: ▪ Hypersensitivity ▪ Avoid chronic use ▪ Should not be used to induce labor.
Use Cautiously in: ▪ Hypertensive or eclamptic patients (increased susceptibility to hypertensive and arrhythmogenic side effects) ▪ Severe hepatic or renal disease ▪ Sepsis ▪ Third stage of labor.

ADVERSE REACTIONS AND SIDE EFFECTS*

CNS: dizziness, headache.
CV: palpitations, chest pain, hypertension, arrhythmias.
Derm: sweating.
EENT: tinnitus.
GI: nausea, vomiting.
Resp: dyspnea.
Misc: allergic reactions.

INTERACTIONS

Drug–Drug: ▪ Excessive vasoconstriction may result when used with other **vasopressors**, such as **dopamine** or **nicotine**.

ROUTE AND DOSAGE

Oxytocic

- **PO (Adults):** 0.2–0.4 mg q 6–12 hr for 2–7 days.
- **IM, IV (Adults):** 0.2 mg q 2–4 hr for up to 5 doses; then change to PO.

*Underlines indicate most frequent; **CAPITALS** indicate life-threatening.

E

Provocative Agent for Coronary Artery Spasm
- **IV (Adults):** 0.1–0.4 mg.

PHARMACODYNAMICS (uterine contractions)

	ONSET	PEAK	DURATION
PO	5–15 min	UK	3 hr or longer
IM	2–5 min	UK	3 hr or longer
IV	immediate	UK	45 min

NURSING IMPLICATIONS

Assessment
- Monitor blood pressure, pulse, and respirations every 15–30 min until transfer to the postpartum unit, then every 1–2 hr. Inform physician if hypertension, chest pain, arrhythmias, headache, or change in neurologic status occurs.
- Monitor amount and type of vaginal discharge. Notify physician immediately if symptoms of hemorrhage (increased bleeding, hypotension, pallor, tachycardia) occur.
- Palpate uterine fundus, note position and consistency. Notify physician if fundus fails to contract in response to ergonovine. Assess patient for severe cramping; physician may reduce the dose.
- Assess for signs of ergotism (cold, numb fingers and toes, nausea, vomiting, diarrhea, headache, muscle pain, weakness).
- If patient fails to respond to ergonovine, check serum calcium level. Correction of hypocalcemia may restore responsiveness.
- **Lab Test Considerations:** May cause decreased serum prolactin level, which inhibits synthesis of breast milk.
- **Toxicity and Overdose:** Toxicity, initially manifested as ergotism, may cause seizures and gangrene. Seizures are treated with anticonvulsants. Vasodilators and heparin may be ordered to improve circulation to extremities. Amputation is required for gangrene.

Potential Nursing Diagnoses
- Tissue perfusion, altered (indications).
- Injury, high risk for (side effects).
- Knowledge deficit related to medication regimen (patient/family teaching).

Implementation
- **General Info:** Do not administer soln that is discolored or contains a precipitate.
- **PO:** Administration is usually limited to 48 hr postpartum, by which time the danger of hemorrhage from uterine atony has passed.
- **IM:** The preferred route is IM. Firm uterine contractions are produced within a few mins. Dose may need to be repeated every 2–4 hr for full therapeutic effect.
- **Direct IV:** The IV route is reserved for severe uterine bleeding. Dilute with 5 ml of 0.9 % NaCl.
  - *Rate:* Administer slow IV push over at least 1 min through Y-site injection of an IV of D5W or 0.9% NaCl.
- **Additive Compatibility:** amikacin, cephapirin, or sodium bicarbonate.

Patient/Family Teaching
- Review symptoms of toxicity with patient. Instruct her to report occurrence of these immediately.
- Inform patient that uterine cramping demonstrates effectiveness of therapy.
- Explain need for pad count to determine degree of bleeding. Instruct patient to report immediately an increase in degree of bleeding or passage of clots.
- Instruct patient to report breastfeeding difficulties.
- Caution patient not to smoke while receiving ergonovine, as nicotine is also a vasoconstrictor.

Evaluation
Effectiveness of therapy is demonstrated by: ▪ Prevention or cessation of uterine hemorrhage after delivery or abortion.

ERGOTAMINE
(er-**got**-a-meen)
Ergomar, Ergostat, {Gynergen}, Medihaler-Ergotamine

CLASSIFICATION(S):
Alpha-adrenergic blocking agent
Pregnancy Category X

INDICATIONS
▪ Treatment and prevention of vascular headaches including: ▫ Migraine and cluster headaches.

ACTION
▪ In therapeutic doses, produces vasoconstriction of dilated blood vessels by stimulating alpha-adrenergic receptors ▪ Larger doses may produce alpha-adrenergic blockade and vasodilation ▪ Also has antiserotonin activity. **Therapeutic Effect:** ▪ Constriction of dilated carotid artery bed with resolution of vascular headache.

PHARMACOKINETICS
Absorption: Rapidly and reliably absorbed following inhalation. Unpredictably absorbed (60%) from the GI tract. Oral absorption may be enhanced by caffeine. Sublingual absorption is poor.
Distribution: Crosses the blood-brain barrier and enters breast milk.
Metabolism and Excretion: Highly metabolized (90%) by the liver.
Half-life: 2 phases: first phase—2.7 hr; second phase—21 hr.

CONTRAINDICATIONS AND PRECAUTIONS
Contraindicated in: ▪ Serious infections ▪ Peripheral vascular disease ▪ Cardiovascular disease ▪ Hypertension ▪ Severe renal or liver disease ▪ Malnutrition ▪ Pregnancy ▪ Lactation.
Use Cautiously in: ▪ Illnesses associated with peripheral vascular pathology, such as diabetes mellitus ▪ Children (safety not established).

ADVERSE REACTIONS AND SIDE EFFECTS*
CV: sinus tachycardia, sinus bradycardia, intermittent claudication, arterial spasm, angina pectoris, **MYOCARDIAL INFARCTION**.
GI: nausea, vomiting, abdominal pain, diarrhea, polydypsia.
MS: muscle pain, extremity stiffness, stiff neck, stiff shoulders.
Neuro: leg weakness, numbness or tingling in fingers or toes.
Misc: fatigue.

INTERACTIONS
Drug-Drug: ▪ Concurrent use with **propranolol, oral contraceptives, vasoconstrictors, troleandomycin,** or heavy cigarette **smoking** may increase the risk of peripheral vasoconstriction ▪ When used concurrently with prophylactic **methysergide** (another ergot alkaloid), dosage of ergotamine should be decreased by 50%.

ROUTE AND DOSAGE
- **PO, SL (Adults):** 2 mg initially, then 1–2 mg q 30 min until attack subsides or a total of 6 mg has been given. Daily dose should not exceed 6 mg or 10 mg weekly. 1–2 mg PO at bedtime daily for 10–14 days has been used to terminate series of cluster headaches.
- **PO, SL (Older Children and Adolescents):** 1 mg followed by 1 mg after 30 min if necessary.
- **Inhaln (Adults):** 1 inhalation (360 mcg), may be repeated at 5-min intervals until attack subsides, not to exceed 6 inhalations in 24 hr or 15 inhalations weekly.

PHARMACODYNAMICS (relief of headache)

	ONSET	PEAK	DURATION
PO	1–2 hr (variable)	UK	UK
SL	UK	UK	UK
Inhaln	UK	UK	UK

{} = Available in Canada only.
*Underlines indicate most frequent; **CAPITALS** indicate life-threatening.

E

NURSING IMPLICATIONS

Assessment

- Assess frequency, location, duration, and characteristics (pain, nausea, vomiting, visual disturbances) of chronic headaches. During acute attack assess type, location, and intensity of pain prior to and 60 min after administration.
- Monitor blood pressure and peripheral pulses periodically during therapy. Inform physician if significant hypertension occurs.
- Assess for signs of ergotism (cold, numb fingers and toes, nausea, vomiting, headache, muscle pain, weakness).
- Assess for nausea and vomiting. Ergotamine stimulates the chemoreceptor trigger zone. Physician may order a phenothiazine as an antiemetic.
- **Toxicity and Overdose:** Toxicity is manifested by severe ergotism (chest pain, abdominal pain, persistent paresthesia in the extremities) and gangrene. Vasodilators, dextran, or heparin may be ordered to improve circulation.

Potential Nursing Diagnoses

- Comfort, altered: pain, acute (indications).
- Injury, high risk for (side effects).
- Knowledge deficit related to medication regimen (patient/family teaching).

Implementation

- **General Info:** Administer as soon as patient reports prodromal symptoms or headache.
- Available in oral, sublingual, and inhalation forms.
- **SL:** Allow tablet to dissolve under tongue. Do not allow patient to eat, drink, or smoke while tablet is dissolving.
- **Metered-Dose Inhaler:** Available as an inhalation via metered-dose inhaler. Wait 5 min between sprays.

Patient/Family Teaching

- **General Info:** Instruct patient to take ergotamine at the first sign of an impending headache and not to exceed the maximum dose prescribed by the physician.
- Encourage patient to rest in a quiet, dark room after taking ergotamine.
- Review symptoms of toxicity. Instruct patient to report these to physician promptly.
- Caution patient not to smoke and to avoid exposure to cold, as these vasoconstrictors may further impair peripheral circulation.
- Advise patient to avoid alcohol, as it may precipitate vascular headaches.
- Instruct female patients to inform physician if they plan or suspect pregnancy. Ergotamine should not be taken during pregnancy.
- **Metered-dose Inhaler:** Instruct patient in the proper use of the metered-dose inhaler. Shake well, exhale, close lips firmly around mouthpiece, administer during second half of inhalation, and hold breath as long as possible after treatment to ensure deep instillation of medication.

Evaluation

Effectiveness of therapy can be demonstrated by: ▪ Prevention or relief of pain from vascular headaches.

ERYTHROMYCIN

(eh-rith-roe-**mye**-sin)

erythromycin base
E-base, E-mycin, Eryc, Eryc-Sprinkle, Ery-tab, {Erythromid}, Ilotycin, {Novorythro}, PCE Dispersatabs, Robimycin

erythromycin estolate
Ilosone, {Novorythro}

erythromycin ethylsuccinate
E.E.S., EryPed

erythromycin gluceptate
Ilotycin

erythromycin lactobionate
Erythrocin
erthromycin stearate
Eramycin, Wyamycin S
erythromycin (ophthalmic)
Ilotycin
erythromycin (topical)
Akne-Mycin, Erycette, Erygel, Erymax, ETS, Mythromycin, Staticin, T-stat

CLASSIFICATION(S):
Anti-infective—macrolide
Pregnancy Category B

INDICATIONS

▪ **PO, IV:** Treatment of the following infections due to susceptible organisms: ▫ Upper and lower respiratory tract infections ▫ Otitis media (with sulfonamides) ▫ Skin and skin structure infections ▫ Pertussis ▫ Diphtheria ▫ Erythrasma ▫ Intestinal amebiasis ▫ Pelvic inflammatory disease ▫ Nongonococcal urethritis ▫ Syphilis ▫ Legionnaire's disease ▫ Rheumatic fever ▪ **Top:** Treatment of acne ▪ **Ophth:** ▪ Treatment of superficial ocular infections ▪ Useful in situations in which penicillin is the most appropriate drug but cannot be used because of previous hypersensitivity reactions, including: ▫ Streptococcal infections ▫ Treatment of syphilis or gonorrhea ▫ Endocarditis prophylaxis.

ACTION

▪ Suppresses protein synthesis at the level of the 50S bacterial ribosome. **Therapeutic Effect:** ▪ Bacteriostatic action against susceptible bacteria. **Spectrum:** ▪ Active against many gram-positive cocci, including: ▫ Streptococci ▫ Staphylococci ▪ Gram-positive bacilli, including: ▫ *Clostridium* ▫ *Corynebacterium* ▪ Several gram-negative pathogens, notably: ▫ *Neisseria* ▫ *Haemophilus influenzae* ▫ *Legionella pneumophila* ▪ *Mycoplasma* and *Chlamydia* are also usually susceptible.

PHARMACOKINETICS

Absorption: Well absorbed from the duodenum following oral administration. Minimal absorption may follow topical or ophthalmic use.
Distribution: Widely distributed. Minimal penetration into CSF. Crosses the placenta and enters breast milk.
Metabolism and Excretion: Partially metabolized by the liver, excreted mainly unchanged in the bile. Small amounts excreted unchanged in the urine.
Half-life: 1.4–2 hr.

CONTRAINDICATIONS AND PRECAUTIONS

Contraindicated in: ▪ Hypersensitivity ▪ Hepatic dysfunction (estolate salt) ▪ Pregnancy (estolate salt).
Use Cautiously in: ▪ Liver disease ▪ Salts other than the estolate may be used in pregnancy to treat *Chlamydia* infections or syphilis ▪ Tartrazine sensitivity (some products contain tartrazine—FDC yellow dye #5).

ADVERSE REACTIONS AND SIDE EFFECTS*

GI: nausea, vomiting, diarrhea, abdominal pain, cramping, hepatitis.
EENT: ototoxicity.
Derm: rashes.
Local: phlebitis at IV site.
Misc: allergic reactions, superinfection.

INTERACTIONS

Drug-Drug: ▪ Increases activity and may increase the risk of toxicity from **alfentanil, bromocriptine, theophylline, carbamazepine, cyclosporine, disopyramide, ergot alkaloids, triazolam, oral anticoagulants,** or **methylprednisolone** ▪ May increase serum **digoxin** levels in a small percentage of patients ▪ **Top:**

*Underlines indicate most frequent; **CAPITALS** indicate life-threatening.

Concurrent use with **irritants, abrasives,** or **desquamating agents** may result in increased irritation ▪ **Top: Topical clindamycin** may antagonize beneficial effects.

ROUTE AND DOSAGE

Note: 250 mg of erythromycin base, estolate, or stearate = 400 mg of erythromycin ethylsuccinate.

- **PO (Adults):** Base, estolate, stearate—250–500 mg q 6–8 hr, ethylsuccinate—400–800 mg q 6–8 hr.
- **PO (Children):** 30–50 mg/kg/day in divided doses q 6 hr (up to 100 mg/kg/day).
- **IV (Adults):** Gluceptate and lactobionate only—1–4 g/day in divided doses q 6 hr, or as a continuous infusion.
- **IV (Children):** Gluceptate and lactobionate only—15–20 mg/kg/day in divided doses q 6 hr or as a continuous infusion.
- **Top (Adults and Children >12 yr):** 2% ointment, gel, or soln bid.
- **Ophth (Adults):** 0.5% ointment to conjunctiva 1 or more times daily.

PHARMACODYNAMICS (blood levels)

	ONSET	PEAK
PO	1 hr	1–4 hr
IV	rapid	end of infusion

NURSING IMPLICATIONS

Assessment

- Assess patient for infection (vital signs; appearance of wound, sputum, urine, and stool; WBC) at beginning and throughout course of therapy.
- Obtain specimens for culture and sensitivity prior to initiating therapy. First dose may be given before receiving results.
- **Lab Test Considerations:** Liver function tests should be performed periodically on patients receiving high-dose, long-term therapy.
- May cause increased serum bilirubin, SGOT (AST), SGPT (ALT), and alkaline phosphatase concentrations.
- May cause false elevations of urinary catecholamines.

Potential Nursing Diagnoses

- Infection, high risk for (indications, side effects).
- Knowledge deficit related to medication regimen (patient/family teaching).
- Noncompliance related to medication regimen (patient/family teaching).

Implementation

- **General Info:** Available in tablets, enteric-coated tablets, capsules, suspension, injectable forms, topical gel and soln, and ophthalmic ointment.
- **PO:** Administer around the clock on an empty stomach, at least 1 hr before or 2 hr after meals. May be taken with food if GI irritation occurs. Should not be taken with fruit juices. Take each dose with a full glass of water.
- Use calibrated measuring device for liquid preparations. Shake well before using.
- Chewable tablets should be crushed or chewed and not swallowed whole.
- Do not open, crush, or chew delayed-release capsules or tablets; swallow whole. Enteric-coated tablets may be administered regardless of meals.
- **IV:** Add 10 ml of sterile water for injection without preservatives to 250- or 500-mg vials and 20 ml to 1-g vial. Soln is stable for 7 days after reconstitution if refrigerated.
- **Intermittent Infusion:** Dilute further in 100–250 ml of 0.9% NaCl or D5W.
- *Rate:* Administer slowly over 20–60 min to avoid phlebitis. Assess for pain along vein; slow rate if pain occurs; apply ice and notify physician if unable to relieve pain.
- **Continuous Infusion:** May also be administered as an infusion in a dilution of 1 g/liter of 0.9% NaCl, D5W, or lactated Ringer's soln over 4 hr.

ERYTHROMYCIN GLUCEPTATE

- **Syringe Incompatibility:** heparin.
- **Y-Site Incompatibility:** chloramphenicol, heparin, phenobarbital, or phenytoin.

- **Additive Compatibility:** calcium gluconate, corticotropin, dimenhydrinate, heparin, hydrocortisone sodium succinate, methicillin, penicillin G potassium, potassium chloride, or sodium bicarbonate.
- **Additive Incompatibility:** aminophylline, oxytetracycline, pentobarbital, secobarbital, streptomycin, or tetracycline.

ERTHROMYCIN LACTOBIONATE

- **Syringe Compatibility:** methicillin.
- **Syringe Incompatibility:** ampicillin or heparin.
- **Y-Site Compatibility:** acyclovir, cyclophosphamide, enalaprilat, esmolol, famotidine, foscarnet, hydromorphone, labetalol, magnesium sulfate, meperidine, morphine, multivitamins, or zidovudine.
- **Additive Compatibility:** aminophylline, ampicillin, cimetidine, diphenhydramine, hydrocortisone sodium succinate, lidocaine, methicillin, penicillin G potassium, penicillin G sodium, pentobarbital, polymyxin B, potassium chloride, prednisolone, prochlorperazine, promazine, sodium bicarbonate, sodium iodide, or verapamil.
- **Additive Incompatibility:** cephalothin, colistimethate, heparin, metaraminol, metoclopramide, or tetracycline.
- **Ophth:** See Appendix H for administration of ophthalmic preparations.
- **Top:** Cleanse area prior to application. Wear gloves during application.

PATIENT/FAMILY TEACHING

- □ Instruct patient to take medication around the clock and to finish the drug completely as directed, even if feeling better. Missed doses should be taken as soon as remembered, with remaining doses evenly spaced throughout day. Advise patient that sharing of this medication may be dangerous.
- □ May cause nausea, vomiting, diarrhea, or stomach cramps; notify physician if these effects persist or if severe abdominal pain, yellow discoloration of the skin or eyes, darkened urine, pale stool, or unusual tiredness develops.
- □ Advise patient to report signs of superinfection (black, furry overgrowth on the tongue, vaginal itching or discharge, loose or foul-smelling stools).
- □ Instruct patient to notify the physician if symptoms do not improve.
- □ Patients with a history of rheumatic heart disease or valve replacement need to be taught the importance of using antimicrobial endocarditis prophylaxis before invasive medical or dental procedures.

EVALUATION

Clinical response can be determined by: ▪ Resolution of the signs and symptoms of infection. Length of time for complete resolution depends on the organism and site of infection ▪ Improvement of acne lesions ▪ Endocarditis prophylaxis.

ESMOLOL

(**ez**-moe-lole)
Brevibloc

CLASSIFICATION(S):
Beta-adrenergic blocker—selective, Antiarrhythmic—type II
Pregnancy Category C

INDICATIONS

▪ Short-term management of supraventricular tachyarrhythmias. **Unlabeled Use:** ▪ Lowering of blood pressure during surgical procedures.

ACTION

▪ Blocks stimulation of $beta_1$ (myocardial) receptor sites, with less effect on $beta_2$ (pulmonary and vascular) receptor sites. Results in decreased heart rate, decreased contractility, lowering of blood pressure, and decreased AV conduction. **Therapeutic Effect:** ▪ Slowing of the ventricular response in supraventricular tachyarrhythmias.

PHARMACOKINETICS

Absorption: Administered by IV route, resulting in complete bioavailability.
Distribution: Rapidly and widely distributed.
Metabolism and Excretion: Metabolized by enzymes in red blood cells and the liver.
Half-life: 9 min.

CONTRAINDICATIONS AND PRECAUTIONS

Contraindicated in: ▪ Uncompensated congestive heart failure ▪ Pulmonary edema ▪ Cardiogenic shock ▪ Bradycardia ▪ 2nd- or 3rd-degree heart block.
Use Cautiously in: ▪ Thyrotoxicosis ▪ Hypoglycemia (symptoms may be masked) ▪ Pregnancy, lactation, or children <18 yr (safety not established).

ADVERSE REACTIONS AND SIDE EFFECTS*

CNS: dizziness, headache, confusion, agitation, somnolence, weakness.
EENT: visual disturbances.
Resp: bronchospasm, wheezing.
CV: hypotension, chest pain, pulmonary edema, PVCs, ECG changes, bradycardia.
GI: nausea, vomiting, constipation, abdominal pain, dyspepsia.
GU: urinary retention.
Derm: rash.
Local: phlebitis at IV site.
Misc: peripheral ischemia, fever, chills.

INTERACTIONS

Drug-Drug: ▪ **General anesthesia, IV phenytoin,** and **verapamil** may cause additive myocardial depression ▪ Additive bradycardia may occur with **cardiac glycosides** ▪ Additive hypotension may occur with other **antihypertensive agents,** acute ingestion of **alcohol,** or **nitrates** ▪ Concurrent use with **amphetamines, cocaine, ephedrine, epinephrine, norepinephrine, phenylephrine,** or **pseudoephedrine** may result in excess alpha-adrenergic stimulation, hypertension, and bradycardia ▪ May negate the beneficial $beta_1$ cardiac effects of **dopamine** or **dobutamine** ▪ Concurrent **thyroid** administration may decrease effectiveness ▪ Use with **insulin** may result in prolonged hypoglycemia ▪ May prolong the effects of **succinylcholine** ▪ Concurrent use with **morphine** may increase activity of esmolol.

ROUTE AND DOSAGE

Note: See infusion rate table in Appendix D.

- **IV (Adults):** 500-mcg/kg loading dose over 1 min initially, followed by 50-mcg/kg/min infusion for 4 min; if no response within 5 min, give second loading dose of 500 mcg/kg over 1 min and increase infusion to 100 mcg kg/min for 4 min. If no response, repeat loading dose of 500 mcg/kg over 1 min and increase infusion rate by 50 mcg/kg/min increments (not to exceed 200 mcg/kg/min). As therapeutic end point is achieved, eliminate loading doses and decrease dosage increments to 25 mcg/kg/min.

PHARMACODYNAMICS (cardiovascular effects)

	ONSET	PEAK	DURATION
IV	min	UK	1–20 min

NURSING IMPLICATIONS

Assessment

- ▫ Monitor blood pressure, heart rate, and ECG frequently throughout course of therapy. The risk of hypotension is greatest within the first 30 min of initiating esmolol infusion.
- ▫ Assess infusion site frequently throughout therapy. Concentrations of greater than 10 mg/ml may cause redness, swelling, skin discoloration, and burning at the injection site. Do not use butterfly needles for administration. If venous irritation occurs,

*Underlines indicate most frequent; **CAPITALS** indicate life-threatening.

stop the infusion and resume at another site.

- Monitor intake and output ratios and daily weight. Assess patient for signs and symptoms of congestive heart failure (peripheral edema, dyspnea, rales/crackles, weight gain, jugular venous distension).
- **Lab Test Considerations:** Monitor blood sugar closely in diabetic patients, because esmolol may mask signs and symptoms of hypoglycemia and may potentiate insulin-induced hypoglycemia.
- **Toxicity and Overdose:** Monitor patient for signs of overdose (bradycardia, severe dizziness or fainting, severe drowsiness, dyspnea, bluish fingernails or palms, seizures). Notify physician immediately if these signs occur.
- Treatment of esmolol overdose is symptomatic and supportive. Due to the short action of esmolol, discontinuation of therapy may relieve acute toxicity.
- Symptomatic bradycardia may be treated with atropine, isoproterenol, dobutamine, epinephrine, or a transvenous pacemaker.
- Premature ventricular contractions may be treated with lidocaine or phenytoin. Avoid the use of quinidine, procainamide, or disopyramide, as they may further depress myocardial function.
- Congestive heart failure may be treated with oxygen, cardiac glycosides, and/or diuretics.
- Hypotension may be treated with Trendelenberg position and IV fluids unless contraindicated. Vasopressors (epinephrine, norepinephrine, dopamine, dobutamine) may also be used. Hypotension does not respond to beta$_2$ agonists.
- Glucagon has been used to treat bradycardia and hypotension.
- A beta$_2$-adrenergic agonist (isoproterenol) and/or theophylline may be used to treat bronchospasm.

Potential Nursing Diagnoses

- Cardiac output, decreased (indications).
- Injury, high risk for (side effects).
- Knowledge deficit related to medication regimen (patient/family teaching).

Implementation

- **General Info:** To convert to other antiarrhythmic agents following esmolol administration, administer the first dose of the antiarrhythmic agent and decrease the esmolol dose by 50% after 30 min. If an adequate response is maintained for 1 hr following the second dose of the antiarrhythmic agent, discontinue the esmolol.
- **IV:** Esmolol must be diluted and administered via IV infusion. To dilute for infusion, remove 20 ml from a 500-ml bottle of D5W, D5/LR, D5/0.45% NaCl, D5/0.9% NaCl, 0.45% NaCl, 0.9% NaCl, or lactated Ringer's soln. Add 5 g of esmolol to the bottle, for a concentration of 10 mg/ml. Soln is stable for 24 hr at room temperature.
- *Rate:* The loading dose of esmolol is administered over 1 min, followed by a maintenance dose via IV infusion over 5 min. If the response is not adequate, the procedure is repeated every 5 min with an increase in the maintenance dose. Titration of dose is based on desired heart rate or undesired decrease in blood pressure. The maintenance dose should not be >200 mcg/kg/min and can be administered for up to 48 hr. Esmolol infusions should not be abruptly discontinued; eliminate loading doses and decrease dosage by 25 mcg/kg/min (see Appendix D).
- **Y-Site Compatibility:** amikacin, aminophylline, ampicillin, atracurium, butorphanol, calcium chloride, cefazolin, cefoperazone, ceftazidime, ceftizoxime, chloramphenicol, cimetidine, clindamycin, co-trimoxazole, dopamine, enalaprilat, erythromycin lactobionate, famotidine, fentanyl, gentamicin, heparin, hydrocortisone

sodium succinate, magnesium sulfate, methyldopate, metronidazole, morphine sulfate, nafcillin, pancuronium, penicillin G potassium, phenytoin, piperacillin, polymyxin B, potassium chloride, potassium phosphate, ranitidine, sodium acetate, streptomycin, tobramycin, vancomycin, or vecuronium.

- **Y-Site Compatibility:** furosemide.
- **Additive Compatibility:** aminophylline, bretylium, or heparin.
- **Additive Incompatibility:** diazepam, procainamide, sodium bicarbonate, or thiopental.

Patient/Family Teaching

- ☐ Caution patient to make position changes slowly to minimize orthostatic hypotension.
- ☐ May cause drowsiness and dizziness. Caution patient to call for assistance during ambulation or transfer.

Evaluation

Effectiveness of therapy can be demonstrated by: ▪ Decrease in or control of supraventricular tachyarrythmias without the appearance of detrimental side effects.

ESTAZOLAM

(ess-**taz**-oh-lam)
ProSom

CLASSIFICATION(S):
Sedative/hypnotic—benzodiazepine
Schedule IV
Pregnancy Category X

INDICATIONS

▪ Short-term management of insomnia.

ACTION

▪ Depresses the CNS, probably by potentiating gamma-aminobutyric acid (GABA), an inhibitory neurotransmitter. **Therapeutic Effect:** ▪ Relief of insomnia.

PHARMACOKINETICS

Absorption: Well absorbed following oral administration.
Distribution: Highly lipid-soluble. Crosses the blood-brain barrier and placenta. Enters breast milk.
Metabolism and Excretion: Mostly metabolized by the liver. Metabolites do not have CNS depressant activity.
Half-life: 10–24 hr.

CONTRAINDICATIONS AND PRECAUTIONS

Contraindicated in: ▪ Hypersensitivity ▪ Cross-sensitivity with other benzodiazepines may exist ▪ Pre-existing CNS depression ▪ Severe uncontrolled pain ▪ Narrow-angle glaucoma ▪ Pregnancy or lactation.
Use Cautiously in: ▪ Hepatic dysfunction, elderly, very small or debilitated patients (dosage reduction may be necessary) ▪ Patients who are suicidal or who may have been addicted to drugs previously.

ADVERSE REACTIONS AND SIDE EFFECTS*

CNS: <u>somnolence</u>, <u>weakness</u>, hypokinesia, hangover, abnormal thinking, anxiety, agitation, amnesia, apathy, hostility, seizures, sleep disorders, stupor, twitch.
EENT: ear pain, eye irritation, photophobia.
Resp: RESPIRATORY DEPRESSION, cold symptoms, pharyngitis, asthma, dyspnea, sinusitus, rhinitus.
GI: dyspepsia, changes in appetite, flatulence, gastritis, abdominal pain.
GU: urinary frequency, urinary hesitancy, menstrual cramps, vaginal discharge, vaginal itching.
Derm: urticaria.
MS: lower extremity pain, back pain, stiffness, neck pain, myalgia, muscle spasm, arthritis.
Misc: allergic reactions, chills, thirst, psychological dependence, physical dependence.

*<u>Underlines</u> indicate most frequent; **CAPITALS** indicate life-threatening.

INTERACTIONS

Drug–Drug: ▪ Additive CNS depression with **alcohol, antihistamines, antidepressants, MAO inhibitors,** other **sedative/hypnotics,** or **narcotic analgesics** ▪ **Cimetidine** or **oral contraceptives** may decrease metabolism and increase effects of estazolam ▪ May decrease efficacy of **levodopa** ▪ **Rifampin** or **cigarette smoking** increase metabolism and decrease effectiveness.

ROUTE AND DOSAGE

- **PO (Adults):** 1 mg at bedtime (range 0.5–2 mg).

PHARMACODYNAMICS (hypnotic activity)

	ONSET	PEAK*	DURATION
PO	15–30 min	2 hr	6–8 hr

*Plasma level.

NURSING IMPLICATIONS

Assessment

- Assess sleep patterns prior to and periodically throughout course of therapy.
- Prolonged therapy may lead to psychological or physical dependence. Restrict amount of drug available topatient, especially if patient is depressed, suicidal, or has a history of addiction.
- **Lab Test Considerations:** Monitor CBC, urinalysis, and serum chemistries periodically during prolonged therapy.

Potential Nursing Diagnoses

- Sleep pattern disturbance (indications).
- Injury, high risk for (side effects).
- Knowledge deficit related to medication regimen (patient/family teaching).

Implementation

- **General Info:** Supervise ambulation and transfer of patients following administration. Remove cigarettes. Side rails should be raised and call bell within reach at all times.

Patient/Family Teaching

- Advise patient to take medication exactly as directed. Discuss the importance of preparing environment for sleep (dark room, quiet, avoidance of nicotine and caffeine). Gradual discontinuation may be required following prolonged therapy. May cause disturbed sleep for the first 2 nights following discontinuation of estazolam.
- Medication may cause daytime drowsiness. Caution patient to avoid driving and other activities requiring alertness until response to medication is known.
- Caution patients to avoid taking alcohol or other CNS depressants concurrently with this medication.
- Instruct patient to contact physician immediately if pregnancy is planned or suspected.

Evaluation

Effectiveness of therapy can be demonstrated by: ▪ Improvement in sleep pattern.

ESTRADIOL
(ess-tra-**dye**-ole)
Estrace

ESTRADIOL CYPIONATE
Depanate, Depestro, dep Gynogen, Depo-Estradiol, Depogen, Dura-Estrin, E-Cypionate, Estralonate P.A., Estra-L, Estro-Cyp, Estrofem, Estroject-LA, Estronol-LA, Hormogen Depot

ESTRADIOL VALERATE
Delestrogen, Dioval, Duragen, Estradiol L.A., Estra-L, Estraval, Estravel-P.A., Feminate, {Femogex}, Gynogen L.A., L.A.E., Menaval,Valergen

ESTRADIOL TRANSDERMAL SYSTEM
Estrace, Estraderm TTS

CLASSIFICATION(S):
Hormone—estrogen
Pregnancy Category X

E

INDICATIONS

▪ **PO, IM, Transdermal:** Treatment of moderate to severe vasomotor symptoms of menopause and of various estrogen-deficiency states including: ▫ Female hypogonadism ▫ Female castration ▫ Primary ovarian failure ▪ **PO:** Inoperable metastatic postmenopausal breast or prostate carcinoma ▪ **Transdermal:** Treatment and prevention of postmenopausal osteoporosis.

ACTION

▪ Estrogens promote the growth and development of female sex organs and the maintenance of secondary sex characteristics in women ▪ Metabolic effects include reduced blood cholesterol, protein synthesis, and sodium and water retention. **Therapeutic Effects:** ▪ Restoration of hormonal balance in various deficiency states ▪ Treatment of hormone-sensitive tumors.

PHARMACOKINETICS

Absorption: Well absorbed following oral administration. Readily absorbed through skin and mucous membranes.
Distribution: Widely distributed. Crosses the placenta and enters breast milk.
Metabolism and Excretion: Mostly metabolized by the liver and other tissues. Enterohepatic recirculation occurs, and more absorption may occur from the GI tract.
Half-life: UK.

CONTRAINDICATIONS AND PRECAUTIONS

Contraindicated in: ▪ Thromboembolic disease ▪ Undiagnosed vaginal bleeding ▪ Pregnancy (may result in harm to the fetus) ▪ Lactation.
Use Cautiously in: ▪ Underlying cardiovascular disease ▪ Severe hepatic or renal disease ▪ May increase the risk of endometrial carcinoma.

ADVERSE REACTIONS AND SIDE EFFECTS*

CNS: headache, dizziness, lethargy.
EENT: worsening of myopia or astigmatism, intolerance to contact lenses.
CV: edema, thromboembolism, hypertension, myocardial infarction.
GI: nausea, vomiting, anorexia, increased appetite, weight changes, jaundice.
GU: females—breakthrough bleeding, dysmenorrhea, amenorrhea, cervical erosions, vaginal candidiasis, loss of libido; males—testicular atrophy, impotence.
Derm: acne, urticaria, oily skin, pigmentation.
Endo: hyperglycemia, gynecomastia (males).
F and E: sodium and water retention, hypercalcemia.
MS: leg cramps.
Misc: breast tenderness.

INTERACTIONS

Drug-Drug: ▪ May alter requirement for **oral anticoagulants, oral hypoglycemic agents,** or **insulin** ▪ **Barbiturates** or **rifampin** may decrease effectiveness.

ROUTE AND DOSAGE

Vasomotor Symptoms of Menopause, Atrophic Vaginitis, Female Hypogonadism, Ovarian Failure

- **PO (Adults):** 1–2 mg/day for 21 days, then off for 7 days, then repeat cycle.
- **IM (Adults):** 1–5 mg q 3–4 wk (estradiol cypionate) or 10–20 mg (estradiol valerate) q 4 wk.
- **Transdermal: (Adults):** 50- or 100-mcg transdermal patch applied twice weekly for 3 wk, then off for 1 wk, then repeat cycle.
- **Vag (Adults):** 2–4 g cream (0.2–0.4 mg estradiol) daily for 1–2 wk, then decrease to 1–2 g (0.1–0.2 mg estradiol) for 1–2 wk, then maintenance dose of 1 g (0.1 mg estradiol) 1–3 times weekly for 3 wk, then off for 1

*Underlines indicate most frequent; **CAPITALS** indicate life-threatening.

wk, then repeat cycle once vaginal mucosa has been restored.

Postmenopausal Breast Carcinoma

- **PO (Adults):** 10 mg 3 times daily for at least 3 mon.

Prostate Carcinoma

- **PO (Adults):** 1–2 mg 3 times daily.
- **IM (Adults):** 30 mg q 1–2 wk (estradiol valerate).

PHARMACODYNAMICS (estrogenic effects)

	ONSET	PEAK	DURATION
PO	UK	UK	UK
IM	UK	UK	UK
Top	UK	UK	UK

NURSING IMPLICATIONS

Assessment

- Assess blood pressure prior to and periodically throughout therapy.
- Monitor intake and output ratios and weekly weight. Report significant discrepancies or steady weight gain to physician.
- **Lab Test Considerations:** Monitor heptic function prior to and periodically throughout therapy.
- May cause increased serum glucose, sodium, triglyceride, phospholipid, cortisol, prolactin, prothrombin and factors VII, VIII, IX, and X levels. May decrease serum folate, pyridoxine, antithrombin III, and pregnanediol excretion concentrations.
- May alter thyroid hormone assays.
- May cause hypercalcemia in patients with metastatic bone lesions.

Potential Nursing Diagnoses

- Sexual dysfunction (indications).
- Knowledge deficit related to medication regimen (patient/family teaching).

Implementation

- **PO:** Administer with or immediately after food to reduce nausea.
- **Vag:** Manufacturer provides applicator with cream. Dosage is marked on the applicator.
- **Transdermal:** When switching from PO, begin transdermal therapy 1 wk after the last dose or when symptoms reappear.
- **IM:** Injection has oil base. Roll syringe to ensure even dispersion. Administer deep IM. Avoid IV administration.

Patient/Family Teaching

- **General Info:** Instruct patient to take medication as prescribed. If a dose is missed, take as soon as remembered as long as it is not just before next dose. Do not double doses.
- If nausea becomes a problem, advise patient that eating solid food often provides relief.
- Advise patient to report signs and symptoms of fluid retention (swelling of ankles and feet, weight gain), thromboembolic disorders (pain, swelling, tenderness in extremities, headache, chest pain, blurred vision), mental depression, or hepatic dysfunction (yellowed skin or eyes, pruritus, dark urine, light-colored stools) to physician.
- Instruct patient to stop taking medication and notify physician if pregnancy is suspected.
- Advise patient to notify physician or dentist of medication regimen prior to treatment or surgery.
- Explain dosage schedule and maintenance routine. Discontinuing medication suddenly may cause withdrawal bleeding.
- Caution patient that cigarette smoking during estrogen therapy may cause increased risk of serious side effects, especially for women over age 35.
- Caution patient to use sunscreen and protective clothing to prevent increased pigmentation.
- Advise patient treated for osteoporosis that exercise has been found to arrest and reverse bone loss. The patient should discuss any exercise limitations with physician before beginning program.
- Emphasize the importance of routine follow-up physical examinations,

including blood presssure; breast, abdomen, and pelvic examinations; and PAP smears, every 6–12 mon.

- **Vag:** Instruct patient in the correct use of applicator. Patient should remain recumbent for at least 30 min after administration. May use sanitary napkin to protect clothing, but do not use tampon.
- **Transdermal Patch:** Instruct patient to wash and dry hands first. Apply disk to intact skin on hairless portion of abdomen. Press disk for 10 sec to ensure contact with skin (especially around edges). Avoid areas where clothing may rub disk loose. Change site with each administration to prevent skin irritation. Do not reuse site for 1 wk. Disk may be reapplied if it falls off.

EVALUATION

Effectiveness of therapy can be demonstrated by: ▪ Resolution of menopausal vasomotor symptoms ▪ Decreased vaginal and vulval itching, inflammation, or dryness associated with menopause ▪ Normalization of estrogen levels in female castration or hypogonadism ▪ Control of the spread of advanced metastatic breast or prostate cancer.

ESTRAMUSTINE

(ess-tra-**muss**-teen)
Emcyt

CLASSIFICATION(S):
Antineoplastic agent–hormone/alkylating agent
Pregnancy Category UK

INDICATIONS

▪ Palliative treatment of advanced metastatic prostate cancer.

ACTION

▪ Consists of combination of mechlorethamine, an alkylating agent, and estradiol, an estrogenic compound. Antineoplastic activity may be due to either component or the combination ▪ Also decreases serum testosterone levels. **Therapeutic Effect:** ▪ Decreased spread of prostate cancer.

PHARMACOKINETICS

Absorption: Well absorbed (75%) following oral administration. During absorption, converted to estromustine and then to estrogenic compounds and mechlorethamine.

Distribution: Presence of estrogen enhances delivery to tissues with estrogen receptors. Concentrates in prostatic tissue.

Metabolism and Excretion: Eliminated primarily by biliary and fecal excretion. Small amounts excreted by kidneys.

Half-life: 20 hr.

CONTRAINDICATIONS AND PRECAUTIONS

Contraindicated in: ▪ Thromboembolism, recent stroke, or myocardial infarction ▪ Cross-sensitivity or tolerance to estradiol or mechlorethamine may exist.

Use Cautiously in: ▪ History of thromboembolic disorders ▪ Hypercalcemia ▪ Peptic ulcer ▪ Active infection including recent chickenpox or herpes zoster ▪ Renal or hepatic impairment ▪ Gallbladder disease ▪ Cardiovascular disease ▪ Cerebrovascular disease ▪ Migraine headaches ▪ Metabolic bone disease ▪ Epilepsy ▪ Asthma ▪ Bone marrow depression ▪ Patients with childbearing potential.

ADVERSE REACTIONS AND SIDE EFFECTS*

CNS: insomnia.

CV: edema, thromboembolism, hypertension.

GI: nausea, diarrhea, vomiting.

Endo: gynecomastia, decreased libido, gonadal suppression (azoospermia), hyperglycemia.

Derm: rashes.

F and E: sodium and water retention.

*Underlines indicate most frequent; **CAPITALS** indicate life-threatening.

Hemat: anemia, leukopenia, thrombocytopenia.
Misc: allergic reactions, fever.

INTERACTIONS

Drug–Drug: ▪ **Cigarette smoking** increases the risk of adverse vascular effects ▪ **Calcium supplements** form an insoluble complex with estramustine that cannot be absorbed ▪ Increases effects and risk of toxicity with **glucocorticoids** (dosage reduction may be necessary) ▪ May decrease appropriate immune response to **live virus vaccines** and increase risk of adverse reactions.
Drug–Food: ▪ **Calcium** in dairy foods or supplements forms an insoluble complex with estramustine that cannot be absorbed.

ROUTE AND DOSAGE

▪ **PO (Adults):** 600 mg/m^2/day in 3 divided doses or 14 mg/kg/day (range 10–16 mg/kg) in3–4 divided doses.

PHARMACODYNAMICS (noted as effect on tumor spread)

	ONSET	PEAK	DURATION
PO	30–90 days	UK	6 wk*

*Persistence of hematologic effects.

NURSING IMPLICATIONS

Assessment

□ Monitor blood pressure periodically throughout therapy.
□ Monitor intake and output ratios and weekly weight. Report significant discrepancies or steady weight gain to physician.
□ Monitor blood glucose closely in diabetic patients. May decrease glucose tolerance.
▪ **Lab Test Considerations:** Monitor hematologic and hepatic functions periodically throughout therapy. May cause leukopenia and thrombocytopenia. May also cause elevated LDH, SGOT (AST), and bilirubin levels.

Potential Nursing Diagnoses

▪ Knowledge deficit related to medication regimen (patient/family teaching).

Implementation

▪ **PO:** Administer with water 1 hr before or 2 hr after meals. Milk, milk products, and calcium-rich foods or calcium-containing antacids impair the absorption of estramustine and must not be taken simultaneously.

Patient/Family Teaching

□ Instruct patient to take estramustine exactly as directed.
□ Instruct patient to store capsules in the refrigerator, but may be kept at room temperature for 24–48 hr without losing potency.
□ Advise patient of the need for contraception throughout therapy.
□ Advise patient to report signs and symptoms of fluid retention (swelling of ankles and feet, weight gain) and thromboembolic disorders (pain, swelling, tenderness in extremities, headache, chest pain, blurred vision) to physician.

Evaluation

Effectiveness of therapy may be demonstrated by: ▪ Decrease in spread of prostate cancer. May require 30–90 days to determine maximum effects of therapy.

ESTROGENS, CONJUGATED

(ess-troe-jenz)
{C.E.S.}, conjugated estrogens, {Conjugated Estrogens C.S.D.}, Premarin

CLASSIFICATION(S):
Hormone—estrogen
Pregnancy Category X

INDICATIONS

▪ **PO:** Treatment of moderate to severe vasomotor symptoms of menopause and in various estrogen-deficiency states, including: □ Female hypogonadism □ Female castration □ Primary ovarian failure ■ **PO:** Adjunctive therapy of postmenopausal osteoporosis ■ **PO:** Adjunctive therapy of advanced inoperable metastatic breast and prostatic carcinoma ■ **IM, IV:** Uterine bleeding due to hormonal imbalance ■ **Vag:** Management of atrophic vaginitis.

ACTION

■ Estrogens promote the growth and development of female sex organs and the maintenance of secondary sex characteristics in women ■ Metabolic effects include reduced blood cholesterol, protein synthesis, and sodium and water retention. **Therapeutic Effects:** ■ Restoration of hormonal balance in various deficiency states and treatment of hormone-sensitive tumors.

PHARMACOKINETICS

Absorption: Well absorbed following oral administration. Readily absorbed through skin and mucous membranes.

Distribution: Widely distributed. Crosses the placenta and enters breast milk.

Metabolism and Excretion: Mostly metabolized by the liver and other tissues. Enterohepatic recirculation occurs, and more absorption may occur from the GI tract.

Half-life: UK.

CONTRAINDICATIONS AND PRECAUTIONS

Contraindicated in: ■ Thromboembolic disease ■ Undiagnosed vaginal bleeding ■ Pregnancy (may result in harm to the fetus) ■ Lactation.

Use Cautiously in: ■ Underlying cardiovascular disease ■ Severe hepatic or renal disease ■ May increase the risk of endometrial carcinoma.

ADVERSE REACTIONS AND SIDE EFFECTS*

CNS: headache, dizziness, lethargy, mental depression.

EENT: worsening of myopia or astigmatism, intolerance to contact lenses.

CV: edema, thromboembolism, hypertension, myocardial infarction.

GI: nausea, vomiting, anorexia, increased appetite, weight changes, jaundice.

GU: females—breakthrough bleeding, dysmenorrhea, amenorrhea, cervical erosions, vaginal candidiasis, loss of libido; males—testicular atrophy, impotence.

Derm: acne, urticaria, oily skin, pigmentation.

Endo: hyperglycemia, gynecomastia (males).

F and E: sodium and water retention, hypercalcemia.

MS: leg cramps.

Misc: breast tenderness.

INTERACTIONS

Drug-Drug: ■ May alter requirement for **oral anticoagulants, oral hypoglycemic agents,** or **insulin** ■ **Barbiturates** or **rifampin** may decrease effectiveness ■ **Cigarette smoking** increases the risk of adverse cardiovascular reactions.

ROUTE AND DOSAGE

Female Castration, Primary Ovarian Failure

■ **PO (Adults):** 1.25 mg/day for 21 days, off 7 days, then repeat.

Hypogonadism, Ovarian Failure

■ **PO (Adults):** 2.5–7.5 mg/day for 20 days, off 10 days; repeat until menses occur.

Inoperable Breast Carcinoma—Males and Postmenopausal Females

■ **PO (Adults):** 10 mg tid.

Inoperable Prostate Carcinoma

■ **PO (Adults):** 1.25–2.5 mg tid.

Menopausal Symptoms

■ **PO (Adults):** 0.3–1.25 mg/day for 21 days, off 7 days, then repeat.

Osteoporosis

■ **PO (Adults):** 0.625 mg/day for 21 days, off 7 days, then repeat.

Uterine Bleeding

■ **IM, IV (Adults):** 25 mg, may repeat in 6–12 hr if necessary.

*Underlines indicate most frequent; **CAPITALS** indicate life-threatening.

Atrophic Vaginitis

- **Vag (Adults):** 2–4 g of 0.0625% cream daily for 21 days, off for 7 days, then repeat.

PHARMACODYNAMICS (estrogenic effects)*

	ONSET	PEAK	DURATION
PO	rapid	UK	UK
IM	delayed	UK	UK
IV	rapid	UK	UK

*Tumor response may take several wks.

NURSING IMPLICATIONS

Assessment

- **General Info:** Assess blood pressure prior to and periodically throughout therapy.
- Monitor intake and output ratios and weekly weight. Report significant discrepancies or steady weight gain to physician.
- **Menopause:** Assess frequency and severity of vasomotor symptoms.
- **Lab Test Considerations:** Monitor hepatic function periodically during long-term therapy.
- May cause increased serum glucose, sodium, triglyceride, phospholipid, cortisol, prolactin, prothrombin and factors VII, VIII, IX, and X levels. May decrease serum folate, pyridoxine, antithrombin III, and pregnanediol excretion concentrations.
- May cause hypercalcemia in patients with metastatic bone lesions.
- May cause false interpretations of thyroid function tests, false increases in sulfobromophthalein (BSP) and norepinephrine platelet-induced aggregability, and false decreases in metyrapone tests.

Potential Nursing Diagnoses

- Sexual dysfunction (indications).
- Knowledge deficit related to medication regimen (patient/family teaching).

Implementation

- **PO:** Administer with or immediately after food to reduce nausea.
- **Vag:** Manufacturer provides applicator with cream. Dosage is marked on the applicator. Wash applicator with mild soap and warm water after each use.
- **IM:** To reconstitute, withdraw at least 5 ml of air from dry container and then slowly introduce the sterile diluent against the container side. Gently agitate container to dissolve; do not shake vigorously. Soln is stable for 60 days if refrigerated. Do not use if precipitate is present or if soln is darkened.
- **Direct IV:** Reconstitute as for IM. Inject into distal port tubing of free-flowing IV of 0.9% NaCl, D5W, or lactated Ringer's soln.
- *Rate:* Administer slowly (no faster than 5 mg/min) to prevent flushing.
- **Y-Site Compatibility:** heparin or potassium chloride.
- **Additive Incompatibility:** ascorbic acid or acidic solns.

Patient/Family Teaching

- **General Info:** Instruct patient to take oral medication as directed. If a dose is missed, take as soon as remembered, but not just before next dose. Do not double doses.
- Explain dosage schedule and maintenance routine. Discontinuing medication suddenly may cause withdrawal bleeding. Bleeding is anticipated on the wk conjugated estrogens are withheld.
- If nausea becomes a problem, advise patient that eating solid food often provides relief.
- Advise patient to report signs and symptoms of fluid retention (swelling of ankles and feet, weight gain), thromboembolic disorders (pain, swelling, tenderness in extremities; headache; chest pain; blurred vision), mental depression, hepatic dysfunction (yellowed skin or eyes, pruritus, dark urine, light-colored stools), or abnormal vaginal bleeding to physician.
- Instruct patient to stop taking medication and notify physician if pregnancy is suspected.
- Caution patient that cigarette smoking during estrogen therapy may

cause increased risk of serious side effects, especially for women over age 35.
- ▫ Caution patients to use sunscreen and protective clothing to prevent increased pigmentation.
- ▫ Advise patient to notify physician or dentist of medication regimen prior to treatment or surgery.
- ▫ Advise patient treated for osteoporosis that exercise has been found to arrest and reverse bone loss. The patient should discuss any exercise limitations with physician before beginning program.
- ▫ Emphasize the importance of routine follow-up physical examinations, including blood pressure; breast, abdomen, and pelvic examinations; and PAP smears, every 6–12 mon. Physician will evaluate possibility of discontinuing medication every 3–6 mon.
- ▪ **Vag:** Instruct patient in the correct use of applicator. Patient should remain recumbent for at least 30 min after administration. May use sanitary napkin to protect clothing, but do not use tampon. If a dose is missed, do not use the missed dose, but return to regular dosing schedule.

EVALUATION

Effectiveness of therapy can be demonstrated by: ▪ Resolution of menopausal vasomotor symptoms ▫ Decreased vaginal and vulval itching, inflammation, or dryness associated with menopause ▪ Normalization of estrogen levels in female castration, or hypogonadism ▪ Control of the spread of advanced metastatic breast or prostate cancer ▪ Prevention of osteoporosis.

ESTROPIPATE

(ess-troe-**pi**-pate)

Ogen, Piperazine estrone sulfate

CLASSIFICATION(S):

Hormone—estrogen

Pregnancy Category X

INDICATIONS

▪ **Vag:** Management of atrophic vaginitis ▪ **PO:** Treatment of vasomotor symptoms of menopause ▪ **PO:** Treatment of various estrogen-deficiency states, including: ▫ Female hypogonadism ▫ Female castration ▫ Primary ovarian failure ▪ Adjunctive therapy of postmenopausal osteoporosis.

ACTION

▪ Estrogens promote the growth and development of female sex organs and the maintenance of secondary sex characteristics in women ▪ Metabolic effects include reduced blood cholesterol, protein synthesis, and sodium and water retention. **Therapeutic Effect:** ▪ Restoration of hormonal balance in various deficiency states.

PHARMACOKINETICS

Absorption: Well absorbed following oral administration. Readily absorbed through skin and mucous membranes.

Distribution: Widely distributed. Crosses the placenta and enters breast milk.

Metabolism and Excretion: Mostly metabolized by the liver and other tissues. Enterohepatic recirculation occurs, and more absorption may occur from the GI tract.

Half-life: UK.

CONTRAINDICATIONS AND PRECAUTIONS

Contraindicated in: ▪ Thromboembolic disease ▪ Undiagnosed vaginal bleeding ▪ Pregnancy (may result in harm to the fetus) ▪ Lactation.

Use Cautiously in: ▪ Underlying cardiovascular disease ▪ Severe hepatic or renal disease ▪ May increase the risk of endometrial carcinoma.

ADVERSE REACTIONS AND SIDE EFFECTS*

CNS: headache, dizziness, lethargy.

EENT: worsening of myopia or astigmatism, intolerance to contact lenses.

*Underlines indicate most frequent; **CAPITALS** indicate life-threatening.

CV: edema, thromboembolism, hypertension, myocardial infarction.
GI: nausea, vomiting, anorexia, increased appetite, weight changes, jaundice.
GU: females—breakthrough bleeding, dysmenorrhea, amenorrhea, cervical erosions, vaginal candidiasis, loss of libido; males—testicular atrophy, impotence.
Derm: acne, urticaria, oily skin, pigmentation.
Endo: hyperglycemia, gynecomastia (males).
F and E: sodium and water retention, hypercalcemia.
MS: leg cramps.
Misc: breast tenderness.

INTERACTIONS

Drug-Drug: ▪ May alter requirement for **oral anticoagulants, oral hypoglycemic agents,** or **insulin** ▪ **Barbiturates** or **rifampin** may decrease effectiveness ▪ **Cigarette smoking** increases the risk of adverse cardiovascular reactions.

ROUTE AND DOSAGE

Vasomotor Symptoms of Menopause, Atrophic Vaginitis, Osteoporosis

- **PO (Adults):** 0.75–6 mg/day for 21 days, off for 7 days, then repeat cycle.
- **Vag (Adults):** 2–4 g of 0.15% cream daily for 3 wk, then off for 1 wk, then repeat cycle.

Female Hypogonadism, Ovarian Failure

- **PO (Adults):** 1.25–7.5 mg/day for 21 days, off for 8–10 days, then repeat cycle.

PHARMACODYNAMICS (estrogenic effects)

	ONSET	PEAK	DURATION
PO	UK	UK	UK

NURSING IMPLICATIONS

Assessment

- **General Info:** Assess blood pressure prior to and periodically throughout therapy.
- □ Monitor intake and output ratios and weekly weight. Report significant discrepancies or steady weight gain to physician.
- **Menopause:** Assess frequency and severity of vasomotor symptoms.
- **Lab Test Considerations:** Monitor hepatic function periodically during long-term therapy.
- □ May cause increased serum glucose, sodium, triglyceride, phospholipid, cortisol, prolactin, prothrombin and factors VII, VIII, IX, and X levels. May decrease serum folate, pyridoxine, antithrombin III, and pregnanediol excretion concentrations.
- □ May cause hypercalcemia in patients with metastatic bone lesions.
- □ May cause hypercalcemia in patients with metastatic bone lesions.
- □ May cause false interpretations of thyroid function tests, false increases in sulfobromophthalein (BSP) and norepinephrine platelet-induced aggregability, and false decreases in metyrapone tests.

Potential Nursing Diagnoses

- Sexual dysfunction (indications).
- Knowledge deficit related to medication regimen (patient/family teaching).

Implementation

- **PO:** Administer PO doses with or immediately after food to reduce nausea.
- **Vag:** Manufacturer provides applicator with cream. Dosage is marked on the applicator. Wash applicator with mild soap and warm water after each use.

Patient/Family Teaching

- **General Info:** Instruct patient to take oral medication as directed. If a dose is missed, take as soon as remembered as long as it is not just before next dose. Do not double doses.
- □ Explain medication schedule to women on 21-day cycle followed by 7 days of not taking medication. Encourage patient to take medication at the same time each day.

- ▫ If nausea becomes a problem, advise patient that eating solid food often provides relief.
- ▫ Advise patient to report signs and symptoms of fluid retention (swelling of ankles and feet, weight gain), thromboembolic disorders (pain, swelling, tenderness in extremities; headache; chest pain; blurred vision), mental depression, hepatic dysfunction (yellowed skin or eyes, pruritus, dark urine, light-colored stools), or abnormal vaginal bleeding to physician.
- ▫ Instruct patient to stop taking medication and notify physician if pregnancy is suspected.
- ▫ Caution patient that cigarette smoking during estrogen therapy may cause increased risk of serious side effects, especially for women over age 35.
- ▫ Caution patient to use sunscreen and protective clothing to prevent increased pigmentation.
- ▫ Advise patient to notify physician or dentist of medication regimen prior to treatment or surgery.
- ▫ Advise patient treated for osteoporosis that exercise has been found to arrest and reverse bone loss. The patient should discuss any exercise limitations with physician before beginning program.
- ▫ Emphasize the importance of routine follow-up physical examinations, including blood pressure; breast, abdomen, and pelvic examinations; and PAP smears, every 6–12 mon. Physician will evaluate possibility of discontinuing medication every 3–6 mon.
- ■ **Vag:** Instruct patient in the correct use of applicator. Patient should remain recumbent for at least 30 min after administration. May use sanitary napkin to protect clothing, but do not use tampon. If a dose is missed, do not use the missed dose, but return to regular dosing schedule.

EVALUATION

Effectiveness of therapy can be demonstrated by: ■ Resolution of menopausal vasomotor symptoms ▫ Decreased vaginal and vulval itching, inflammation, or dryness associated with menopause ■ Normalization of estrogen levels in female castration, or hypogonadism ■ Prevention of osteoporosis.

E

ETHAMBUTOL

(e-**tham**-byoo-tole)
{Etibi}, Myambutol

CLASSIFICATION(S):
Antitubercular
Pregnancy Category UK

INDICATIONS

■ Used in combination with at least one other drug in the treatment of active tuberculosis or other mycobacterial diseases.

ACTION

■ Inhibits the growth of mycobacteria. **Therapeutic Effect:** ■ Tuberculostatic effect against susceptible organisms.

PHARMACOKINETICS

Absorption: Rapidly and well (80%) absorbed from the GI tract.
Distribution: Widely distributed into many body tissues and fluids. Crosses the blood-brain barrier, but only in small amounts. Crosses the placenta and enters breast milk.
Metabolism and Excretion: 50% metabolized by the liver, 50% eliminated unchanged by the kidneys.
Half-life: 3.3 hr (increased in renal or hepatic impairment).

CONTRAINDICATIONS AND PRECAUTIONS

Contraindicated in: ■ Hypersensitivity ■ Optic neuritis.
Use Cautiously in: ■ Renal and severe hepatic impairment (dosage reduction

required) ▪ Children <13 yr (safety not established) ▪ Pregnancy (although safety not established, ethambutol has been used with isoniazid to treat tuberculosis in pregnant women without adverse effects on the fetus) ▪ Lactation.

ADVERSE REACTIONS AND SIDE EFFECTS*

CNS: headache, malaise, dizziness, confusion, hallucinations.
EENT: optic neuritis.
GI: nausea, vomiting, anorexia, abdominal pain, hepatitis.
Metab: hyperuricemia.
MS: joint pain.
Neuro: peripheral neuritis.
Misc: fever, anaphylactoid reactions.

INTERACTIONS

Drug-Drug: ▪ Neurotoxicity may be additive with other **neurotoxic agents**.

ROUTE AND DOSAGE

Initial Treatment of Tuberculosis

- **PO (Adults and Children >13 yr):** 15 mg/kg/day or 50 mg/kg 2–3 times weekly.

Retreatment of Tuberculosis

- **PO (Adults and Children >13 yr):** 25 mg/kg/day for 60 days, then 15 mg/kg/day.

Tuberculous Meningitis or Atypical Mycobacterial Infections

- **PO (Adults and Children >13 yr):** 15–25 mg/kg/day.

PHARMACODYNAMICS (blood levels)

	ONSET	PEAK
PO	rapid	2–4 hr

NURSING IMPLICATIONS

Assessment

- ▫ Specimens for culture and sensitivity should be obtained prior to initiating therapy.
- ▫ Assessments of visual function should be done frequently during course of therapy. Advise patient to report blurring of vision, constriction of visual fields, or changes in color perception immediately. Visual impairment, if not identified early, may lead to permanent sight impairment.
- ▪ **Lab Test Considerations:** Renal and hepatic functions, CBC, and uric acid levels should be monitored routinely throughout therapy.

Potential Nursing Diagnoses

- ▪ Infection, high risk for (indications).
- ▪ Sensory-perceptual alteration (side effect).
- ▪ Knowledge deficit related to medication regimen (patient/family teaching).

Implementation

- ▪ **General Info:** Ethambutol is given as a single daily dose and should be taken at the same time each day. Some regimens require dosing 2–3 times/wk.
- ▪ **PO:** Administer with food or milk to minimize GI irritation.

Patient/Family Teaching

- ▫ Instruct patient to take medication exactly as prescribed by physician. Do not skip or double up on missed doses. A full course of therapy may take mons to yrs. Do not discontinue without consulting physician, even though symptoms may disappear.
- ▫ Advise patient to notify physician if pregnancy is suspected.
- ▫ Instruct patient to notify physician if no improvement is seen in 2–3 wk. Physician should also be notified if unexpected weight gain or decreased urine output occurs.
- ▫ Emphasize the importance of routine examinations to evaluate progress and ophthalmic examinations if signs of optic neuritis occur.

Evaluation

Effectiveness of therapy can be demonstrated by: ▪ Resolution of clinical symptoms of tuberculosis ▫ Decrease in acid-fast bacteria in sputum samples ▫ Improvement in chest x-rays. Therapy for tuberculosis is usually continued for at least 1–2 yr.

*Underlines indicate most frequent; **CAPITALS** indicate life-threatening.

E

ETHCHLORVYNOL
(eth-klor-vi-nole)
Placidyl

CLASSIFICATION(S):
Sedative/hypnotic—miscellaneous
Schedule IV
Pregnancy Category C

INDICATIONS

▪ Short-term (<1 wk) management of insomnia ▪ Sedation.

ACTION

▪ Acts as a CNS depressant—mechanism not known, appears to act similar to barbiturates. **Therapeutic Effects:** ▪ Sedation ▪ Induction of sleep.

PHARMACOKINETICS

Absorption: Rapidly absorbed following oral administration.
Distribution: Widely distributed, concentrates in adipose tissue. Crosses the blood-brain barrier and the placenta.
Metabolism and Excretion: 90% metabolized by the liver.
Half-life: 10–20 hr.

CONTRAINDICATIONS AND PRECAUTIONS

Contraindicated in: ▪ Hypersensitivity.
Use Cautiously in: ▪ Elderly patients (dosage reduction may be necessary) ▪ History of drug dependence ▪ Hepatic or renal impairment (dosage reduction may be required) ▪ Uncontrolled pain ▪ Depression ▪ Pregnancy, lactation, or children (safety not established) ▪ Some products contain tartrazine (FDC yellow dye #5); use cautiously in patients with tartrazine sensitivity.

ADVERSE REACTIONS AND SIDE EFFECTS*

CNS: dizziness, facial numbness, giddiness, ataxia, paradoxical reaction (insomnia, nervousness, excitement), hangover, syncope, hysteria, prolonged hypnosis.
EENT: blurred vision.
CV: hypotension.
GI: vomiting, GI gastric upset, aftertaste, cholestatic jaundice.
Derm: rash, hives.
Hemat: thrombocytopenia.
MS: muscular weakness.
Misc: hypersensitivity reactions, psychological dependence, physical dependence.

INTERACTIONS

Drug-Drug: ▪ Additive CNS depression with other **CNS depressants,** including **alcohol, antihistamines, antidepressants,** other **sedative/hypnotics, MAO inhibitors,** or **narcotic analgesics** ▪ Transient delerium with **amitriptyline** ▪ May alter the response to **oral anticoagulants**.

ROUTE AND DOSAGE

Hypnotic

▪ **PO (Adults):** 500 mg–1 g at bedtime, may give an additional 200 mg if awakening occurs.

Sedative

▪ **PO (Adults):** 200 mg 2–3 times daily.

PHARMACODYNAMICS (induction of sleep)

	ONSET	PEAK	DURATION
PO	15 min–1 hr	UK	5 hr

NURSING IMPLICATIONS

Assessment

▫ Assess sleep patterns and potential for abuse prior to administering this medication. Prolonged use may lead to physical and psychological dependence. Limit amount of drug available to the patient. Not recommended for use longer than 1 wk.
▫ Assess alertness at time of peak effect. Notify physician if desired sedation does not occur or if paradoxical reaction occurs.

*Underlines indicate most frequent; **CAPITALS** indicate life-threatening.

Potential Nursing Diagnoses
- Sleep pattern disturbance (indications).
- Injury, high risk for (side effects).

Implementation
- **General Info:** Before administering, reduce external stimuli and provide comfort measures to increase effectiveness of medication.
  - Protect patient from injury. Place bed side rails up. Assist with ambulation. Remove cigarettes from patient receiving hypnotic dose.
- **PO:** Capsules should be taken with food or milk to minimize dizziness and ataxia.
  - A single 200-mg dose supplement may be ordered for patients who awaken after the original bedtime dose of 500 mg or 750 mg.

Patient/Family Teaching
- Instruct patient to take ethchlorvynol exactly as directed. Missed doses should be omitted; do not double doses. If used for 2 wk or longer, abrupt withdrawal may result in convulsions, hallucinations, muscle twitching, nausea, vomiting, irritability, sweating, trembling, insomnia, and weakness.
- Ethchlorvynol may cause daytime drowsiness or dizziness. Caution patient to avoid driving or other activities requiring alertness until response to medication is known.
- Caution patient to avoid concurrent use of alcohol or other CNS depressants while taking this medication.

Evaluation
Effectiveness of therapy can be demonstrated by: ■ Improvement in sleep pattern ■ Sedation.

ETHOSUXIMIDE
(eth-oh-**sux**-i-mide)
Zarontin

CLASSIFICATION(S):
Anticonvulsant
Pregnancy Category UK

INDICATIONS
■ Management of absence seizures (petit mal). **Unlabeled Use:** ■ Management of myoclonic (partial) seizures.

ACTION
■ Elevates the seizure threshold ■ Suppresses abnormal wave and spike activity associated with absence (petit mal) seizures. **Therapeutic Effect:** ■ Prevention of absence (petit mal) seizures.

PHARMACOKINETICS
Absorption: Rapidly and completely absorbed from the GI tract following oral administration.
Distribution: Freely distributed throughout body water.
Metabolism and Excretion: Mostly metabolized by the liver. 10% excreted unchanged by the kidneys.
Half-life: 60 hr (adults); 30 hr (children).

CONTRAINDICATIONS AND PRECAUTIONS
Contraindicated in: ■ Hypersensitivity.
Use Cautiously in: ■ Hepatic or renal disease ■ Pregnancy or lactation (safety not established) ■ Do not discontinue abruptly.

ADVERSE REACTIONS AND SIDE EFFECTS*
CNS: drowsiness, headaches, euphoria, irritability, hyperactivity, psychiatric disturbances, dizziness, ataxia, increased frequency of grand mal SEIZURES.
Derm: urticaria, rashes, hirsutism.
EENT: blurred vision.
GI: anorexia, gastric upset, nausea, vomiting, cramping, weight loss, diarrhea, hiccups.
GU: vaginal bleeding, pink or brown discoloration of urine.
Hemat: APLASTIC ANEMIA, AGRANULOCYTOSIS, leukopenia, eosinophilia.

*Underlines indicate most frequent; **CAPITALS** indicate life-threatening.

Misc: allergic reactions, including STEVENS-JOHNSON SYNDROME.

INTERACTIONS

Drug–Drug: ▪ Seizure threshold may be lowered by **phenothiazines, antidepressants,** or **MAO inhibitors** ▪ Additive CNS depression with other **CNS depressants,** including **alcohol, antihistamines, antidepressants, narcotic analgesics,** and **sedative/hypnotics** ▪ **Phenytoin** may increase metabolism and decrease effectiveness.

ROUTE AND DOSAGE

- **PO (Adults and Children >6 yr):** 250 mg bid initially, may increase by 250 mg/day q 4–7 days up to 1.5 g/day given in divided doses bid (usual maintenance dose 20 mg/kg/day).
- **PO (Children 3–6 yr):** 250 mg/day as a single dose.

PHARMACODYNAMICS (anticonvulsant activity)

	ONSET	PEAK	DURATION
PO	hr–days	days	days

NURSING IMPLICATIONS

Assessment

- Assess location, duration, and characteristics of seizure activity.
- Assess patient's mood, behavioral patterns, and facial expressions. Patients with a history of psychiatric disorders have an increased risk of developing behavioral changes. These symptoms may necessitate withdrawal of the medication.
- **Lab Test Considerations:** CBC, hepatic function tests, and urinalysis should be monitored routinely throughout the course of prolonged therapy.
- May cause false-positive results of direct Coombs' test.
- **Toxicity and Overdose:** Therapeutic serum ethosuximide levels range from 40–100 mcg/ml.

Potential Nursing Diagnoses

- Injury, high risk for (indications, side effects).
- Knowledge deficit related to medication regimen (patient/family teaching).

Implementation

- **PO:** Available in capsules and liquid preparations. Measure liquid preparations with calibrated measuring device.
- Administer with food or fluids to minimize GI irritation.

Patient/Family Teaching

- Instruct patient to take medication exactly as prescribed by physician. If a dose is missed, take as soon as remembered within 4 hr, then continue on dosage schedule. Do not double doses. Do not discontinue medication without advice of physician. Sudden withdrawal may precipitate seizures.
- Medication may cause dizziness, drowsiness, or blurred vision. Caution patient to avoid driving or other activities requiring alertness until response to medication is known. Do not resume driving until physician gives clearance based on control of seizure disorder.
- Inform patient that medication may turn urine pink or brown.
- Advise patient to avoid alcohol while taking this medication.
- Advise patient to consult physician or pharmacist before taking any over-the-counter medications concurrently with this drug.
- Instruct patient to notify physician if skin rash, sore throat, fever, unusual bleeding or bruising, swollen glands, or pregnancy occurs.
- Advise patient to carry identification describing disease process and medication regimen at all times.
- Emphasize the importance of follow-up examinations to monitor progress and side effects.

Evaluation

Effectiveness of therapy can be demonstrated by: ▪ Decrease or cessation of seizure activity without excessive sedation.

ETIDRONATE
(eh-tih-**droe**-nate)
Didronel, EHDP

CLASSIFICATION(S):
Electrolyte modifier—hypocalcemic
Pregnancy Category B (oral), C (IV)

INDICATIONS

▪ Treatment of Paget's disease of bone ▪ Treatment and prophylaxis of heterotopic calcification associated with total hip replacement or spinal cord injury ▪ Used with other agents (saline diuresis) in the management of hypercalcemia associated with malignancies.

ACTION

▪ Blocks the growth of calcium hydroxyapatite crystals by binding to calcium phosphate. **Therapeutic Effects:** ▪ Decreased bone resorption and turnover.

PHARMACOKINETICS

Absorption: Absorption is generally poor following oral administration (low doses 1%, large doses up to 6%).
Distribution: Half of the absorbed dose is bound to hydroxyapatite crystals in areas of increased osteogenesis.
Metabolism and Excretion: Unabsorbed drug is eliminated in the feces. 50% of the absorbed dose is excreted unchanged by the kidneys.
Half-life: 5–7 hr.

CONTRAINDICATIONS AND PRECAUTIONS

Contraindicated in: ▪ Hypersensitivity ▪ Severe renal impairment (serum creatinine >5 mg/dl) ▪ Hypercalcemia due to hyperparathyroidism.
Use Cautiously in: ▪ Long bone fractures ▪ Congestive heart failure ▪ Hypocalcemia ▪ Hypovitaminosis D ▪ Moderate renal impairment (serum creatinine 2.5–4.9 mg/dl) ▪ Pregnancy, lactation, or children (safety not established).

ADVERSE REACTIONS AND SIDE EFFECTS*

GI: diarrhea, nausea; IV—loss of taste, metallic taste.
GU: nephrotoxicity.
Derm: rash.
MS: bone pain, bone tenderness, microfractures.

INTERACTIONS

Drug-Drug: ▪ **Antacids** or **mineral supplements** or **buffers** (as in didanosine) containing **calcium, aluminum, iron,** or **magnesium** may decrease the absorption of etidronate ▪ Hypocalcemic effect may be additive with **calcitonin.**
Drug-Food: ▪ Foods containing large amounts of **calcium, aluminum, iron,** or **magnesium** may decrease the absorption of etidronate.

ROUTE AND DOSAGE

Paget's Disease

- **PO (Adults):** 5 mg/kg/day single dose for up to 6 mon or 6–20 mg/kg/day for not more than 3 mon.

Heterotopic Ossification, Hip Replacement

- **PO (Adults):** 20 mg/kg/day for 1 mon prior to and 3 mon following surgery.

Heterotopic Ossification, Spinal Cord Injury

- **PO (Adults):** 20 mg/kg/day for 2 wk, then decreased to 10 mg/kg/day for 10 wk.

Hypercalcemia

- **IV (Adults):** 7.5 mg/kg/day for 3 days.

*Underlines indicate most frequent; **CAPITALS** indicate life-threatening.

PHARMACODYNAMICS

	ONSET	PEAK	DURATION
PO (Paget's disease)	1 mon*	UK	1 yr
PO (heterotopic calcification)	UK	UK	several mons
IV (hypercalcemia)	24 hr†	3 days	11 days

*As measured by decreased urinary hydroxyproline.
†As measured by decreased urinary calcium excretion.

NURSING IMPLICATIONS

Assessment

- **General Info:** Assess patient for bone pain, weakness, or loss of function prior to and throughout course of therapy. Bone pain may persist or increase in patients with Paget's disease; it usually subsides days to mons after therapy is discontinued. Confer with physician regarding analgesic to control pain.
- **Heterotopic Ossification:** Monitor for inflammation and pain at the site and loss of function if ossification occurs near a joint.
- **Hypercalcemia:** Monitor symptoms of hypercalcemia (nausea, vomiting, anorexia, weakness, constipation, thirst, and cardiac arrhythmias).
  - Observe patient carefully for evidence of hypocalcemia (paresthesia, muscle twitching, laryngospasm, colic, cardiac arrhythmias, and Chvostek's or Trousseau's sign). Protect symptomatic patients by elevating and padding side rails; keep bed in low position. Risk of hypocalcemia is greatest after 3 days of continuous IV therapy.
- **Lab Test Considerations:** Etidronate interferes with bone uptake of Technetium^{99} in diagnostic scans.
  - *Paget's Disease:* Decreased urinary excretion of hydroxyproline and serum alkaline phosphatase are often the first clinical signs of effectiveness. These values are monitored every 3 mon. Treatment is restarted when levels return to 75% of pretreatment values. Serum phosphate levels are also monitored prior to and 4 wk after beginning therapy. Dosage may be reduced if serum phosphate is elevated without corresponding decrease in urinary excretion of hydroxyproline or serum alkaline phosphatase.
  - *Hypercalcemia:* Monitor serum calcium and albumin levels to determine effectiveness of therapy.
  - Monitor BUN and creatine prior to and periodically throughout course of therapy. Stable or reversible increases in BUN and creatinine may occur in patients with hypercalcemia.

Potential Nursing Diagnoses

- Comfort, altered: pain (indications, side effects).
- Injury, high risk for (indications).
- Knowledge deficit related to medication regimen (patient/family teaching).

Implementation

- **Hypercalcemia:** Used as adjunctive treatment after IV hydration and loop diuretics have restored urine output.
- **PO:** Administer on empty stomach, as food decreases absorption.
- **Intermittent Infusion:** Dilute in at least 250 ml of 0.9% NaCl. Soln is stable for 48 hr.
  - *Rate:* Infuse over at least 2 hr.

Patient/Family Teaching

- Advise patient to take as directed. If dose is missed, take as soon as remembered unless almost time for next dose. Do not double up on doses. Dose should not be taken within 2 hr of eating (especially products high in calcium) or taking vitamins or antacids, as absorption will be impaired.
- Instruct patient to notify physician if diarrhea occurs. Physician may divide the dose throughout the day to control diarrhea.
- Encourage patients to comply with physician's diet recommendations. Diet should contain adequate amounts of calcium and vitamin D.
- Foods high in vitamin D include fish livers and oils, and fortified milk, bread, and cereals. Foods high in cal-

cium include dairy products, canned salmon and sardines, broccoli, bok choy, tofu, molasses, and cream soups (see Appendix K).

- Explain to patient receiving IV dose that metallic taste is not uncommon and usually disappears in a few hrs.
- Advise patient to report signs of hypercalcemic relapse (bone pain, anorexia, nausea, vomiting, thirst, lethargy) to physician promptly.
- Emphasize need for keeping follow-up appointments to monitor progress, even after medication is discontinued, in order to detect relapse.

EVALUATION

Effectiveness of therapy can be demonstrated by: ▪ Lowered serum calcium levels ▪ Decreased bone pain and fractures in Paget's disease ▪ Prevention or treatment of heterotopic ossification. Normal serum calcium levels are usually attained in 2–8 days in hypercalcemia associated with boney metastasis. Therapy may be repeated once after 1 wk.

ETODOLAC

(ee-toe-**doe**-lak)
Lodine

CLASSIFICATION(S):
Nonsteroidal anti-inflammatory agent, Non-narcotic analgesic
Pregnancy Category C

INDICATIONS

▪ Management of osteoarthritis ▪ Used as an analgesic in the treatment of mild to moderate pain.

ACTION

▪ Inhibits prostaglandin synthesis. **Therapeutic Effects:** ▪ Suppression of inflammation and pain.

PHARMACOKINETICS

Absorption: Well absorbed following oral administration.

Distribution: Highly bound to plasma proteins. Remainder of distribution not known.

Metabolism and Excretion: Not known.

Half-life: UK

CONTRAINDICATIONS AND PRECAUTIONS

Contraindicated in: ▪ Hypersensitivity ▪ Active GI bleeding or ulcer disease ▪ Cross-sensitivity may exist with other nonsteroidal anti-inflammatory agents, including aspirin.

Use Cautiously in: ▪ Severe cardiovascular, renal, or hepatic disease ▪ History of ulcer disease ▪ Pregnancy, lactation, or children (safety not established).

ADVERSE REACTIONS AND SIDE EFFECTS*

CNS: weakness, malaise, dizziness, depression, nervousness, somnolence, insomnia, syncope.

EENT: blurred vision, tinnitus, photophobia.

Resp: asthma.

CV: fluid retention, edema, hypertension, congestive heart failure, palpitations.

GI: dyspepsia, abdominal pain, diarrhea, flatulence, nausea, constipation, gastritis, GI BLEEDING, melena, vomiting, thirst, dry mouth, drug-induced hepatitis, stomatitis.

GU: renal failure, dysuria, urinary frequency.

Derm: pruritus, rashes, flushing, ecchymoses, hyperpigmentation, sweating.

Hemat: anemia, prolonged bleeding time, thrombocytopenia.

Misc: chills, fever, allergic reactions including ANAPHYLAXIS, ANGIOEDEMA, STEVENS JOHNSON SYNDROME.

INTERACTIONS

Drug-Drug: ▪ Concurrent use with **aspirin** may decrease effectiveness ▪ Additive adverse GI effects with **aspirin,** other **nonsteroidal anti-inflammatory**

*Underlines indicate most frequent; **CAPITALS** indicate life-threatening.

agents, potassium supplements, glucocorticoids, or **alcohol** ▪ Chronic use with **acetaminophen** may increase the risk of adverse renal reactions ▪ May decrease the effectiveness of **diuretics** or **antihypertensive** therapy ▪ May increase serum **lithium** levels and increase the risk of toxicity ▪ Increases the risk of toxicity from **methotrexate** ▪ Increased risk of bleeding with **cefamandole, cefotetan, cefoperazone, moxalactam** or **plicamycin, thrombolytic agents,** or **anticoagulants** ▪ Increased risk of adverse hematologic reactions with **antineoplastic agents** or **radiation therapy.**

ROUTE AND DOSAGE

Osteoarthritis

- **PO (Adults):** 600–1200 mg/day in divided doses given q 6–8 hr initially, followed by adjustment to maintenance dose of 200–1200 mg/day in divided doses given 2–4 times daily (200 mg 3–4 times daily, 300 mg 2–4 times daily, or 400 mg 2–4 times daily; not to exceed 1200 mg/day or 20 mg/kg in patients ≤60 kg).

Analgesia

- **PO (Adults):** 200–400 mg q 6–8 hr (not to exceed 1200 mg/day or 20 mg/kg in patients ≤60 kg).

PHARMACODYNAMICS (analgesic effect)

	ONSET	PEAK	DURATION
PO	0.5 hr	UK	4–12 hr

NURSING IMPLICATIONS

Assessment

- **General Info:** Patients who have asthma, aspirin-induced allergy, and nasal polyps are at increased risk for developing hypersensitivity reactions. Monitor for rhinitis, asthma, and urticaria.
- **Osteoarthritis:** Assess pain and range of movement prior to and 1–2 hr following administration.
- **Pain:** Assess location, duration, and intensity of the pain prior to and 60 min following administration.

Potential Nursing Diagnoses

- Comfort, altered: pain (indications).
- Mobility, impaired physical (indications).
- Knowledge deficit related to medication regimen (patient/family teaching).

Implementation

- **General Info:** Coadministration with narcotic analgesics may have additive analgesic effects and may permit lower narcotic doses.
- **PO:** For rapid initial effect, administer 30 min before or 2 hr after meals. May be administered with food, milk, or antacids to decrease GI irritation. Food slows but does not reduce the extent of absorption.

Patient/Family Teaching

- □ Advise patients to take this medication with a full glass of water and to remain in an upright position for 15–30 min after administration.
- □ Instruct patient to take medication exactly as prescribed. If a dose is missed, take as soon as remembered but not if almost time for next dose. Do not double doses.
- □ This medication may occasionally cause drowsiness or dizziness. Advise patient to avoid driving or other activities requiring alertness until response to the medication is known.
- □ Caution patient to avoid the concurrent use of alcohol, aspirin, acetaminophen, or other over-the-counter medications without consultation with physician or pharmacist.
- □ Instruct patient to notify physician if rash, itching, chills, fever, visual disturbances, tinnitus, weight gain, edema, black stools, persistent or severe diarrhea, or persistent headache occur.
- □ Advise patient to inform physician or dentist of medication regimen prior to treatment or surgery.

Evaluation

Effectiveness of therapy can be demonstrated by: ▪ Decreased severity of pain ▪ Improved joint mobility. Patients who do not respond to one nonsteroidal anti-inflammatory agent may respond to another.

ETOPOSIDE
(e-**toe**-poe-side)
EPEG, VP-16, VP-213, VePesid

CLASSIFICATION(S):
Antineoplastic—podophyllotoxin derivative
Pregnancy Category D

INDICATIONS
▪ Alone and in combination with other treatment modalities (other antineoplastic agents, radiation therapy, surgery) in the management of refractory testicular neoplasms and small cell carcinoma of the lung. **Unlabeled Uses:** ▪ Lymphomas and some leukemias.

ACTION
▪ Damages DNA prior to mitosis (cycle-dependent and phase-specific). **Therapeutic Effect:** ▪ Death of rapidly replicating cells, particularly malignant ones.

PHARMACOKINETICS
Absorption: Variably absorbed following oral administration.
Distribution: Rapidly distributed, does not appear to enter the CSF significantly but does appear to cross the placenta. Enters breast milk.
Metabolism and Excretion: Some metabolism by the liver, 45% excreted unchanged by the kidneys.
Half-life: 7 hr (range 3–12 hr).

CONTRAINDICATIONS AND PRECAUTIONS
Contraindicated in: ▪ Hypersensitivity ▪ Pregnancy ▪ Lactation.
Use Cautiously in: ▪ Patients with childbearing potential ▪ Active infections ▪ Decreased bone marrow reserve ▪ Other chronic debilitating illnesses.

ADVERSE REACTIONS AND SIDE EFFECTS*
CNS: somnolence, fatigue, headache, vertigo.
Resp: bronchospasm, pulmonary edema.
CV: hypotension (IV), myocardial infarction, congestive heart failure.
GI: nausea, vomiting.
Hemat: leukopenia, thrombocytopenia.
Local: phlebitis at IV site.
Derm: alopecia.
Endo: gonadal suppression.
MS: muscle cramps.
Neuro: peripheral neuropathy.
Misc: allergic reactions, including ANAPHYLAXIS, fever.

INTERACTIONS
Drug-Drug: ▪ Additive bone marrow depression with other **antineoplastics** or **radiation therapy** ▪ May impair normal immune response to **live virus vaccines** and increase the risk of adverse reactions.

ROUTE AND DOSAGE
Note: Infuse over 30–60 min.

Testicular Neoplasms
- **IV (Adults):** 50–100 mg/m^2 daily for 3–5 days, repeat every 3–4 wk, or 100 mg/m^2 on days 1, 3, and 5 every 3–4 wk for 3–4 courses of therapy.

Small Cell Carcinoma of the Lung
- **PO (Adults):** 70–100 mg/m^2 (rounded to the nearest 50 mg)/day for 5 days, repeated every 3–4 wk.
- **IV (Adults):** 35 mg/m^2 daily for 4 days up to 50 mg/m^2 daily for 5 days every 3–4 wk.

PHARMACODYNAMICS (noted as effects on blood counts)

	ONSET	PEAK	DURATION
PO	7–14 days	9–16 days	20 days
IV	7–14 days	9–16 days	20 days

NURSING IMPLICATIONS
Assessment
- ▫ Monitor blood pressure prior to and every 15 min during infusion. If hypo-

*Underlines indicate most frequent; **CAPITALS** indicate life-threatening.

tension occurs, stop infusion and notify physician. After stabilizing blood pressure with IV fluids and supportive measures, infusion may be resumed at slower rate.

- Monitor for hypersensitivity reaction (fever, chills, pruritus, urticaria, bronchospasm, tachycardia, hypotension). If these occur, stop infusion and notify physician. Keep epinephrine, an antihistamine, and resuscitative equipment close by in the event of an anaphylactic reaction.
- Assess for fever, chills, sore throat, and signs of infection. Notify physician if these symptoms occur.
- Assess for bleeding (bleeding gums, bruising, petechiae; guaiac stools, urine, and emesis). Avoid IM injections and rectal temperatures. Apply pressure to venipuncture sites for 10 min.
- Monitor intake and output, appetite, and nutritional intake. Etoposide causes nausea and vomiting in 30% of patients. Confer with physician regarding prophylactic use of an antiemetic.
- Adjust diet as tolerated to help maintain fluid and electrolyte balance and nutritional status.
- **Lab Test Considerations:** Monitor CBC and differential prior to and periodically throughout therapy. The nadir of leukopenia occurs in 7–14 days. Notify physician if leukocyte count is $<1000/mm^3$. The nadir of thrombocytopenia occurs in 9–16 days. Notify physician if the platelet count is $<75{,}000/mm^3$. Recovery of leukopenia and thrombocytopenia occurs in 20 days.
- Monitor liver function studies (SGOT [AST], SGPT [ALT], LDH, bilirubin) and renal function studies (BUN, creatinine) prior to and periodically throughout therapy to detect hepatotoxicity and nephrotoxicity.
- May cause increased uric acid. Monitor levels periodically during therapy.

Potential Nursing Diagnoses

- Injury, high risk for (side effects).
- Infection, high risk for (side effects).
- Knowledge deficit related to medication regimen (patient/family teaching).

Implementation

- **General Info:** Avoid contact with skin. Use Luer-Lok tubing to prevent accidental leakage. If contact with skin occurs, immediately wash skin with soap and water.
- Soln should be prepared in a biologic cabinet. Wear gloves, gown, and mask while handling medication. Discard equipment in designated containers (see Appendix I).
- **PO:** Capsules should be refrigerated.
- **Intermittent Infusion:** Dilute 5-ml vial with 250–500 ml of D5W or 0.9% NaCl for a concentration of 0.4–0.2 mg/ml. The 0.2-mg/ml soln is stable for 96 hr. The 0.4-mg/ml soln is stable for 48 hr. Concentrations >0.4 mg/ml are not recommended, as crystallization is likely. Discard soln if crystals present.
- *Rate:* Infuse slowly over 30–60 min.
- **Y-Site Compatibility:** ondansetron.
- **Additive Compatibility:** cisplatin.

Patient/Family Teaching

- Instruct patient to take etoposide exactly as directed, even if nausea or vomiting occurs. If vomiting occurs shortly after dose is taken, consult physician. If a dose is missed, do not take at all.
- Advise patient to notify physician if fever, chills, sore throat, signs of infection, bleeding gums, bruising, petechiae, or blood in urine, stool, or emesis occurs. Caution patient to avoid crowds and persons with known infections. Instruct patient to use soft toothbrush and electric razor. Patient should be cautioned not to drink alcoholic beverages or take aspirin-containing products.
- Instruct patient to notify physician if abdominal pain, yellow skin, weakness, paresthesia, or gait disturbances occur.
- Instruct patient to inspect oral mucosa for redness and ulceration. If

mouth sores occur, advise patient to use sponge brush and rinse mouth with water after eating and drinking. Physician may order viscous lidocaine swishes if pain interferes with eating.

- Discuss with patient the possibility of hair loss. Explore coping strategies.
- Advise patient of the need for contraception.
- Instruct patient not to receive any vaccinations without advice of physician.
- Emphasize the need for periodic lab tests to monitor for side effects.

Evaluation

Effectiveness of therapy can be demonstrated by: ▪ Decrease in size or spread of malignancies in solid tumors ▪ Improvement of hematologic status in leukemias.

ETRETINATE
(e-**tret**-i-nate)
Tegison

CLASSIFICATION(S):
Antipsoriatic—retinoid
Pregnancy Category X

INDICATIONS

▪ Alone or as adjunct therapy in the management of severe recalcitrant psoriasis resistant to more conventional methods of treatment (topical tars, psoralens, UVB light, or methotrexate).

ACTION

▪ Structurally resembles vitamin A, though mechanism of action is not known. **Therapeutic Effect:** ▪ Improvement in psoriatic lesions.

PHARMACOKINETICS

Absorption: Inactive form is well absorbed following oral administration.
Distribution: Concentrates in dermal tissues and liver; stored in adipose tissue. Crosses the placenta.
Metabolism and Excretion: Highly metabolized by the liver, mostly on first pass through, where conversion to an active metabolite occurs.
Half-life: 120 days.

CONTRAINDICATIONS AND PRECAUTIONS

Contraindicated in: ▪ Hypersensitivity to retinoids ▪ Pregnancy ▪ Lactation ▪ Patients who are trying to conceive, who use unreliable methods of contraception, or who are planning to become pregnant in the future.
Use Cautiously in: ▪ Patients with a history of liver disease ▪ Children (safety not established).

ADVERSE REACTIONS AND SIDE EFFECTS*

CNS: fatigue, headache, fever, dizziness, pseudotumor cerebrii, anxiety, depression, abnormal thinking.
EENT: dry nose, chapped lips, sore throat, nose bleeds, cheilitis, sore tongue, rhinorrhea, eye irritation, eye pain, decreased visual acuity, abnormal lacrimation, visual defects, otitis, hearing changes, photophobia.
Resp: dyspnea, coughing, increased sputum, pharyngitis.
CV: thrombotic events, edema, arrhythmias, chest pain, syncope.
GI: dry mouth, gingival bleeding, abdominal pain, appetite changes, nausea, hepatitis, constipation, weight loss, abnormal taste, melana, mouth ulcers, flatulence.
GU: proteinuria, hemoglobinuria, WBCs in urine, polyuria, urinary retention, atropic vaginitis.
Derm: hair loss, peeling of skin, itching, redness, skin fragility, photosensitivity, abnormal fingernails, clamminess, granuloma, skin odor, increased pore size, sensory impairment, atropy, fissures, impaired healing, herpes simplex, hirsutism, infections, ulceration.
Endo: irregular menses.
F and E: abnormal calcium, abnormal potassium, abnormal phosphorus, ab-

*Underlines indicate most frequent; **CAPITALS** indicate life-threatening.

E

normal CO_2, abnormal sodium, abnormal chloride.
Metab: hyperglycemia, hypoglycemia, hypertriglyceridemia, hypercholesterolemia, elevated HDL.
MS: hyperostosis, bone and joint pain, myalgia, gout, hyperkinesia, hypotonia.
Misc: increased risk of neoplasm.

INTERACTIONS

Drug–Drug: ▪ Electrolyte abnormalities may increase the risk of **cardiac glycoside** toxicity ▪ Additive toxicity with **vitamin A** ▪ Increased risk of pseudotumor cerebrii with **tetracycline** ▪ Use with **alcohol** has an additive effect on increasing serum triglycerides ▪ Additive risk of hepatotoxicity with other **hepatotoxic agents** ▪ Additive risk of photosensitivity with other **photosensitizing agents** ▪ **Top:** Concurrent use with **irritants, abrasives,** or **desquamating agents** may result in additive irritation.
Drug–Food: ▪ Absorption is enhanced by concurrent administration of **high-fat foods** or **milk**.

ROUTE AND DOSAGE

- **PO (Adults):** 0.75–1 mg/kg/day initially in divided doses for 8–16 wk, then lower to maintenance dose of 0.5–0.75 mg/kg/day. Erythrodermic psoriasis may respond to lower doses.

PHARMACODYNAMICS (improvement in skin lesions)

	ONSET	PEAK	DURATION
PO	wks	wks–mons	yrs

NURSING IMPLICATIONS

Assessment

- □ Assess skin prior to and periodically during therapy. Transient worsening of psoriasis may occur at initiation of therapy.
- ▪ **Lab Test Considerations:** Monitor liver function (SGOT [AST], SGPT [ALT], and LDH) every 1–2 wk during the first 1–3 mon of therapy and every 1–3 mon for the rest of the course of therapy. Inform physician if these values become elevated; therapy may be discontinued.
- □ Monitor blood lipids (cholesterol, HDL, triglycerides) every 1–2 wk in the beginning of therapy and periodically thereafter. Inform physician of increased cholesterol and triglyceride levels or decrease in HDL.
- □ Obtain periodic CBC, urinalysis, and serum electrolytes. Etretinate may alter (increase or decrease) hematocrit, hemoglobin, platelets, and WBC. May cause proteinuria, hematuria, glucose, and acetone in the urine. May increase or decrease sodium, potassium, calcium, and phosphate levels. May cause increased BUN and creatinine.

Potential Nursing Diagnoses

- ▪ Body image disturbance (indications).
- ▪ Knowledge deficit related to medication regimen (patient/family teaching).

Implementation

- ▪ **PO:** Absorption is enhanced by taking with milk or fatty foods.

Patient/Family Teaching

- □ Instruct patient to take etretinate exactly as directed. If a dose is missed, take as soon as remembered with milk or fatty food; do not take if almost time for next dose. Do not double doses. Inform patient that condition may appear to worsen during initial therapy.
- □ Caution patient not to take vitamin A supplements while taking etretinate. Hypervitaminosis A may result. Excessive alcohol and excessive ingestion of foods high in fat should be avoided to reduce the risk of hypertriglyceridemia and cardiovascular problems.
- □ May cause dizziness or blurred vision. Caution patient to avoid driving or other activities requiring alertness until response to the medication is

known. May impair night vision. Driving after dark should be avoided.

- □ Inform patient that dry skin and chapped lips will occur. Applying lubricant to lips will help cheilitis. Physician should be notified if these symptoms become bothersome.
- □ Advise patient that oral rinses, sugarless gum or candy, or frequent oral hygiene may help relieve dry mouth.
- □ With patient who wears contact lenses, discuss possibility of excessively dry eyes. Patient may need to wear glasses during course of therapy.
- □ Advise female patients to practice contraception throughout therapy. This drug is contraindicated during pregnancy. Physician may order pregnancy test 2 wk prior to initiation of therapy and start therapy on day 2 or 3 of the menstrual cycle. Teratogenic effects may persist for yrs. Patient should discuss this with the physician before attempting pregnancy.
- □ Caution patient not to donate blood while taking etretinate. After discontinuation, patient should have physician's approval prior to donating blood to prevent the possibility of a pregnant patient receiving the blood.
- □ Caution patient to minimize exposure to sunlight and to avoid sunlamps to prevent photosensitivity reactions.
- □ Instruct patient to report bone or joint pain, eye irritation, visual changes, abdominal pain, yellow skin, or unusual bruising.
- □ Inform patient of need for medical follow-up. Physician may order periodic ophthalmic examinations and bone x-rays.

Evaluation

Effectiveness of therapy can be demonstrated by: ▪ Improvement or resolution of skin lesions in psoriasis. Therapy may take 2–3 mon before full effects are seen. Therapy is discontinued in 1 mon if no effect is seen, when lesions resolve, or after 4–9 mon. Relapse may occur after discontinuation of therapy.

FACTOR IX COMPLEX

Konyne-HT, Profilnine Heat-Treated, Proplex SX-T, Proplex T

CLASSIFICATION(S):
Hemostatic, Blood derivative
Pregnancy Category C

INDICATIONS

▪ Treatment of active or impending bleeding due to factor IX deficiency (hemophilia B, Christmas disease) ▪ Treatment of bleeding in patients with factor VIII inhibitors ▪ Prevention and treatment of bleeding in patients with factor VII deficiency ▪ Rapid reversal of the effect of oral anticoagulants in emergency situations.

ACTION

▪ Contains blood coagulation factors II, VII, IX, and X (Proplex SX-T has less factor VII). **Therapeutic Effects:** ▪ Replacement of deficient factor IX in hemophilia B ▪ Restoration of hemostasis.

PHARMACOKINETICS

Absorption: Administered IV only, resulting in complete bioavailability.
Distribution: Distribution not known.
Metabolism and Excretion: Rapidly cleared from plasma by utilization in clotting process.
Half-life: Factor IX—24–32 hr; factor VII—3–6 hr.

CONTRAINDICATIONS AND PRECAUTIONS

Contraindicated in: ▪ Factor VII deficiency (except Proplex T) ▪ Intravascular coagulation or fibrinolysis associated with liver disease.
Use Cautiously in: ▪ Postoperative period (increased risk of thrombosis) ▪ Blood groups A, B, or AB.

ADVERSE REACTIONS AND SIDE EFFECTS*

CNS: headache, somnolence, lethargy.
CV: changes in heart rate, changes in blood pressure.

*Underlines indicate most frequent; **CAPITALS** indicate life-threatening.

F

GI: nausea, vomiting.
Derm: flushing, urticaria.
Hemat: thrombosis, disseminated intravascular coagulation.
Neuro: tingling.
Misc: fever, chills, risk of transmission of viral hepatitis, risk of transmission of HIV virus, hypersensitivity reactions.

INTERACTIONS

Drug–Drug: ▪ Use with **aminocaproic acid** may increase the risk of thrombosis.

ROUTE AND DOSAGE

Note: The following formula may be used: Dose (units) = 1 units/kg × body weight (kg) × desired increase (% normal in factor IX activity).

Treatment of Bleeding in Patients with Hemophilia B

▪ **IV (Adults and Children):** Amount necessary to establish 25% of normal factor IX activity or 60–75 units/kg initially, followed by 10–20 units/kg/day for 1 wk.

Prophylaxis of Bleeding in Patients with Hemophilia B

▪ **IV (Adults and Children):** 10–20 units/kg 1–2 times weekly.

Treatment of Bleeding in Patients with Hemophilia A and Inhibitors of Factor VIII

▪ **IV (Adults and Children):** 75 units/kg, repeat dose 12 hr later.

Reversal of Oral Anticoagulant Activity

▪ **IV (Adults and Children):** 15 units/kg.

Factor VII Deficiency

▪ **IV (Adults and Children):** 0.5 units/kg × body weight (kg) × desired increase (% of normal). Repeat every 4–6 hr as needed.

PHARMACODYNAMICS (hemostasis)

	ONSET	PEAK	DURATION
IV	immediate	UK	1–2 days

NURSING IMPLICATIONS

Assessment

- ▫ Monitor blood pressure, pulse, and respirations frequently.
- ▫ Obtain history of current trauma; estimate amount of blood loss.
- ▫ Monitor for renewed or increased bleeding every 15–30 min. Immobilize and apply ice to affected joints.
- ▫ Monitor intake and output ratios; note color of urine. Notify physician if significant discrepancy occurs or urine becomes red or orange. Patients with type A, B, and AB blood are particularly at risk for hemolytic reaction.
- ▫ If hypersensitivity reaction (fever, chills, tingling, headache, urticaria, changes in blood pressure or pulse, nausea and vomiting, lethargy) occur, slow infusion and notify physician.
- ▫ Monitor coagulation studies before, during, and after therapy to assess effectiveness of therapy.

Potential Nursing Diagnoses

- ▪ Tissue perfusion, altered: (indications).
- ▪ Injury, high risk for (indications).
- ▪ Knowledge deficit related to medication regimen (patient/family teaching).

Implementation

- ▪ **General Info:** Dosage varies with degree of clotting factor deficit, desired level of clotting factors, and weight.
- ▫ Obtain type and cross-match of blood in case a transfusion is necessary.
- ▫ To control bleeding after major trauma or surgery, factor IX levels should be maintained at 25% of normal for at least 1 wk. At 50% or greater of normal there is a risk of a thromboembolic reaction or disseminated intravascular coagulopathy.
- ▫ Physician may order hepatitis B vaccine prior to therapy to prevent hepatitis.
- ▫ Inform all personnel of patient's bleeding tendency, to prevent further trauma. Apply pressure to all venipuncture sites for at least 5 min; avoid all IM injections.

■ **Direct IV:** Refrigerate concentrate until just prior to reconstitution. Warm diluent (sterile water for injection) to room temperature before reconstituting. Use plastic syringe for preparation and administration. Use the filter needle provided by the manufacturer as an air vent to the vial when reconstituting. After adding diluent rotate vial gently until completely dissolved. Do not refrigerate after reconstitution. Begin administration within 3 hr. Reconstituted soln is stable for 12 hr at room temperature.

□ *Rate:* Administer IV no faster than 3 ml/min (100 units/min). Do not admix. Temporarily stop infusion and resume at slower rate if facial flushing or tingling occurs.

PATIENT/FAMILY TEACHING

□ Instruct patient to notify nurse immediately if bleeding recurs.

□ Advise patient to carry identification describing disease process at all times.

□ Caution patient to avoid aspirin-containing products, as they may further impair clotting.

□ Review with patient methods of preventing bleeding (use of soft toothbrush, avoid IM and SC injections, avoid potentially traumatic activities).

□ Advise patient that the risk of hepatitis or AIDS transmission may be diminished by the use of heat-treated preparations. Current screening programs and vaccination with hepatitis B vaccine should help decrease the risk.

□ Reinforce need for patients with hemophilia to receive close medical supervision. Physician may order factor IX therapy 2–3 times per week for prophylaxis against spontaneous bleeding.

EVALUATION

Effectiveness of therapy can be demonstrated by: ■ Prevention of spontaneous bleeding or cessation of bleeding in patients with factor IX deficiency (hemophilia B, Christmas disease), factor VIII inhibitors, factor VII deficiency, or anticoagulant overdose.

FAMOTIDINE
(fa-**moe**-ti-deen)
Pepcid

CLASSIFICATION(S):
Histamine H_2 receptor antagonist, Antiulcer
Pregnancy Category B

INDICATIONS

■ Short-term and maintenance treatment of active duodenal ulcers ■ Management of gastric hypersecretory states (Zollinger-Ellison syndrome) ■ Short-term treatment of benign gastric ulcers.

ACTION

■ Inhibits the action of histamine at the H_2 receptor site located primarily in gastric parietal cells, thereby inhibiting gastric acid secretion. **Therapeutic Effect:** ■ Healing and prevention of ulcers.

PHARMACOKINETICS

Absorption: 40–45% absorbed following oral administration.
Distribution: Distribution not known. Probably does not cross the placenta or enter CSF.
Metabolism and Excretion: Up to 65–70% eliminated unchanged by the kidneys. 30–35% metabolized by the liver.
Half-life: 2.5–3.5 hr (increased in renal impairment).

CONTRAINDICATIONS AND PRECAUTIONS

Contraindicated in: ■ Hypersensitivity ■ Hypersensitivity to benzyl alcohol (IV only).
Use Cautiously in: ■ Renal impairment (dosage reduction recommended) ■ Pregnancy, lactation, or children (safety not established).

F

ADVERSE REACTIONS AND SIDE EFFECTS*

CNS: dizziness, headache, drowsiness.
EENT: swelling of eyelids, tinnitus.
Resp: bronchospasm.
CV: palpitations, bradycardia, hypotension (IV).
GI: diarrhea, nausea, constipation, dry mouth.
GU: decreased sexual desire.
Derm: facial edema, loss of hair, rash.
MS: joint pain, muscle pain.
Misc: fever.

INTERACTIONS

Drug–Drug: ▪ **Antacids** may slightly decrease the absorption of famotidine ▪ Decreases the absorption of **ketoconazole**.

ROUTE AND DOSAGE

Duodenal Ulcers

- **PO (Adults):** 40 mg at bedtime or 20 mg bid initially for 2–8 wk, followed by maintenance therapy of 20 mg daily at bedtime.
- **IV (Adults):** 20 mg q 12 hr.

Gastric Hypersecretory Conditions

- **PO (Adults):** 20 mg q 6 hr (range 20–160 mg q 6 hr, not to exceed 800 mg/day).
- **IV (Adults):** 20 mg q 6 hr, higher doses may be necessary.

Benign Gastric Ulcer

- **PO (Adults):** 40 mg once daily at bedtime.

PHARMACODYNAMICS (inhibition of gastric acid secretion)

	ONSET	PEAK	DURATION
PO	within 1 hr	1–4 hr	6–12 hr
IV	within 1 hr	0.5–3 hr	8–15 hr

NURSING IMPLICATIONS

Assessment

- □ Assess patient routinely for epigastric or abdominal pain and frank or occult blood in the stool, emesis, or gastric aspirate.
- ▪ **Lab Test Considerations:** CBC with differential should be monitored periodically throughout therapy.
- □ Antagonizes effects of pentagastrin and histamine during gastric acid secretion tests. Avoid administration during the 24 hr preceding the test.
- □ May cause false-negative results in skin tests using allergen extracts. Famotidine should be discontinued prior to the test.

Potential Nursing Diagnoses

- ▪ Comfort, altered: pain (indications).
- ▪ Knowledge deficit related to medication regimen (patient/family teaching).

Implementation

- ▪ **General Info:** Available in tablets, oral suspension, and injectable forms.
- ▪ **PO:** May be administered with food or liquids. Antacids may be administered concurrently for relief of gastric pain.
- □ Shake oral suspension prior to administration. Discard unused suspension after 30 days.
- ▪ **Direct IV:** Dilute 2 ml (10 mg/ml soln) in 5 or 10 ml of 0.9% NaCl for injection.
- □ *Rate:* Administer over at least 2 min. Rapid administration may cause hypotension.
- ▪ **Intermittent Infusion:** Dilute each 20 mg in 100 ml of 0.9% NaCl, D5W, D10W, lactated Ringer's soln, or sodium bicarbonate. Diluted soln is stable for 48 hr at room temperature. Do not use soln that is discolored or contains a precipitate.
- □ *Rate:* Administer over 15–30 min.
- ▪ **Y-Site Compatibility:** aminophylline, ampicillin, ampicillin/sulbactam, amrinone, atropine, bretylium, calcium gluconate, cefazolin, cefoperazone, cefotaxime, cefotetan, cefoxitin, ceftazidime, ceftizoxime, cefuroxime, cephalothin, cephapirin, dexamethasone, dextran 40, digoxin, dobut-

*Underlines indicate most frequent; **CAPITALS** indicate life-threatening.

amine, dopamine, enalaprilat, epinephrine, erythromycin lactobionate, esmolol, folic acid, furosemide, gentamicin, heparin, hydrocortisone sodium succinate, imipenem/cilastatin, insulin, isoproterenol, labetalol, lidocaine, magnesium sulfate, methylprednisolone, metoclopramide, mezlocillin, midazolam, morphine, nafcillin, nitroglycerin, norepinephrine, ondansetron, oxacillin, perphenazine, phenylephrine, phenytoin, phytonadione, piperacillin, potassium chloride, potassium phosphate, procainamide, sodium bicarbonate, sodium nitroprusside, theophylline, thiamine, ticarcillin, or verapamil.

Patient/Family Teaching

- Instruct patient to take medication as prescribed for the full course of therapy, even if feeling better. If a dose is missed it should be taken as soon as remembered, but not if almost time for next dose. Do not double doses.
- Inform patient that smoking interferes with the action of famotidine. Encourage patient to quit smoking or at least not to smoke after last dose of the day.
- Famotidine may cause drowsiness or dizziness. Caution patient to avoid driving or other activities requiring alertness until response to the drug is known.
- Advise patient to avoid alcohol, products containing aspirin, and foods that may cause an increase in GI irritation.
- Inform patient that increased fluid and fiber intake and exercise may minimize constipation.
- Advise patient to report onset of black, tarry stools; fever; diarrhea; dizziness; or rash to the physician promptly.

Evaluation

Effectiveness of therapy can be demonstrated by: ▪ Decrease in abdominal pain ▫ Prevention of gastric irritation and bleeding. Healing of duodenal ulcers can be seen by x-rays or endoscopy.

FAT EMULSION
(fat ee-**mul**-shun)
Intralipid, Lipsyn, NutriLipid, Soyacal, Travamulsion

CLASSIFICATION(S):
Caloric agent—nonprotein source
Pregnancy Category B—Soyacal, C—Other products

INDICATIONS

▪ Provision of nonprotein calories to patients whose total caloric needs cannot be met by carbohydrate (glucose) alone, usually as part of parenteral nutrition ▪ Treatment and prevention of essential fatty acid deficiency in patients receiving long-term parenteral nutrition.

ACTION

▪ Acts as a nonprotein calorie source. **Therapeutic Effect:** ▪ Provision of essential fatty acids and nonprotein calories.

PHARMACOKINETICS

Absorption: Administered IV only, resulting in complete bioavailability.
Distribution: Distributes into intravascular space.
Metabolism and Excretion: Cleared by conversion to triglycerides, then to free fatty acids and glycerol by lipoprotein lipase. Free fatty acids are transported to tissues where they may be oxidized as an energy source or re-stored as triglycerides.
Half-life: UK.

CONTRAINDICATIONS AND PRECAUTIONS

Contraindicated in: ▪ Hyperlipidemias ▪ Lipoid nephrosis ▪ Pancreatitis accompanied by lipemia ▪ Hypersensitivity to egg products (emulsifier is egg yolk phospholipid).
Use Cautiously in: ▪ Thromboembolic disorders ▪ Severe liver or pulmonary disease ▪ Anemia or bleeding disorders ▪ Patients who are at risk for fat embolism ▪ Preterm infants.

F

ADVERSE REACTIONS AND SIDE EFFECTS*

CV: chest pain.
GI: vomiting, hepatomegaly,† splenomegaly.†
Derm: jaundice.†
Local: phlebitis at IV site.
Misc: fever, chills, shivering, overloading syndrome,† infection, hypersensitivity reactions.

INTERACTIONS

Drug–Drug: ▪ None significant.

ROUTE AND DOSAGE

Note: Fat calories should not make up more than 60% of total calories.

Total Parenteral Nutrition

- **IV (Adults):** 10% emulsion—1 ml/min for initial 15–30 min, then increase to 83–125 ml/hr, not to exceed 500 ml on first day. Dosage may be increased on second day. Not to exceed 3 g/kg/day. 20% emulsion—0.5 ml for initial 15–30 min, then increase to 62.5 ml/hr, not to exceed 250 ml of Liposyn or Soyacal or 500 ml of Intralipid or Travamulsion. Dosage may be increased on second day. Not to exceed 3 g/kg/day.
- **IV (Children):** 10% emulsion—0.1 ml/min for initial 10–15 min, then increase to 1 g/kg over 4 hr; rate should not exceed 100 ml/hr. 20% emulsion—0.05 ml/min for initial 10–15 min, then increase to 1 g/kg over 4 hr, rate should not exceed 50 ml/hr. Total should not exceed 4 g/kg/day.

Essential Fatty Acid Deficiency

- **IV (Adults and Children):** Provide 8–10% of caloric intake as fat.

PHARMACODYNAMICS

	ONSET	PEAK	DURATION
IV	UK	UK	UK

NURSING IMPLICATIONS

Assessment

- ▫ Monitor weight every other day in adults and daily in infants and children receiving fat emulsion to assist in meeting caloric requirements.
- ▫ Assess patient for allergy to eggs prior to initiation of therapy. Acute hypersensitivity reaction with pruritic urticaria may occur in patients allergic to eggs.
- **Lab Test Considerations:** Monitor triglyceride and fatty acid levels routinely to determine patient's capacity to eliminate infused fat from the circulation.
- ▫ Monitor hemoglobin, hematocrit, liver function, blood coagulation, and platelet count (especially in neonates). Notify physician promptly for abnormalities. Therapy may be discontinued.
- **Toxicity and Overdose:** If signs of overloading syndrome (focal seizures, fever, leukocytosis, splenomegaly, shock) or elevated triglyceride or free fatty acid levels occur, infusion should be stopped and the patient re-evaluated prior to reinstituting therapy.

Potential Nursing Diagnoses

- Nutrition, altered: less than body requirements (indications).
- Knowledge deficit related to medication regimen (patient/family teaching).

Implementation

- **General Info:** Fat emulsion should comprise no more than 60% of patient's total caloric intake. The remaining 40% should be comprised of carbohydrates and amino acids.
- ▫ Fat emulsion may be administered via peripheral or central venous catheter. Administer via infusion pump to ensure accurate rate. Monitor peripheral sites for phlebitis.
- ▫ Fat emulsion may be admixed ("3-in-1") or administered simultaneously

†Seen only with long-term use.
*Underlines indicate most frequent; **CAPITALS** indicate life-threatening.

with amino acid and dextrose soln. Infuse fat emulsion via Y-site near the infusion site. Due to the lower specific gravity, the fat emulsion soln must be hung higher than the amino acid and dextrose soln to prevent the fat emulsion from backing up into the amino acid and dextrose line.

- □ Do not use filters during administration.
- □ Use tubing provided by the manufacturer. Change IV tubing after each dose of fat emulsion.
- □ Although compatibility studies have been done, manufacturer recommends that fat emulsion not be admixed or piggybacked with any other medication.
- □ Do not use soln in which the emulsion has separated or appears oily.
- □ Discard all unused portions.
- ▪ **Intermittent Infusion:** For adults the initial infusion rate should be 1 ml/min for the 10% soln and 0.5 ml/min for the 20% soln for the first 15–30 min. If no adverse reactions occur, the rate may be increased to infuse 500 ml over 4–6 hr for the 10% soln and 250 ml over 4–6 hr or 500 ml over 8 hr for the 20% soln. Daily dose should not exceed 3 g/kg.
- □ No more than 500 ml of the 10% soln should be infused the first day. Dose may be increased on subsequent days.
- □ No more than 250 ml of the 20% soln of Soyacal or 500 ml of the 20% soln of Intralipid should be infused the first day. Dose may be increased the following day.
- □ For children the initial infusion rate should be 0.1 ml/min of the 10% soln and 0.05 ml/min for the 20% soln for the first 10–15 min. If no adverse reactions occur, the rate may be increased to 1 g/kg over 4 hr. Do not exceed a rate of 100 ml/hr for the 10% soln or 50 ml/hr for the 20% soln. Daily dose should not exceed 4 g/kg.
- ▪ **Y-Site Compatibility:** ampicillin, cefamandole, cefazolin, cefoxitin, cephapirin, clindamycin, digoxin, dopamine, erythromycin lactobionate, furosemide, gentamicin, isoproterenol, lidocaine, kanamycin, norepinephrine, oxacillin, penicillin G potassium, ticarcillin, or tobramycin.
- ▪ **Y-Site Incompatibility:** amikacin or tetracycline.
- ▪ **Additive Compatibility:** □ INTRALIPID with FreAmine II 8.5%, FreAmine III 8.5%, Travasol without electrolytes 8.5% and 10%, or Dextrose Injection 10% and 70%.

PATIENT/FAMILY TEACHING

- □ Explain the purpose of fat emulsion to the patient prior to administration.

EVALUATION

Effectiveness of therapy may be determined by: ▪ Weight gain □ Maintenance of normal serum triglyceride and fatty acid levels.

FELODIPINE

(fell-**oh**-di-peen)
Plendil

CLASSIFICATION(S):
Calcium channel blocker, Antihypertensive—calcium channel blocker
Pregnancy Category C

INDICATIONS

▪ Alone or with other agents in the management of hypertension.

ACTION

▪ Inhibits the transport of calcium into myocardial and vascular smooth muscle cells, resulting in inhibition of excitation-contraction coupling and subsequent contraction. Result is systemic vasodilation. **Therapeutic Effect:** ▪ Reduction of blood pressure in hypertensive patients.

PHARMACOKINETICS

Absorption: Although well absorbed following oral administration, extensive metabolism leads to decreased bioavailability (20%).
Distribution: Distribution not known.

Metabolism and Excretion: Extensively metabolized. <0.5% excreted unchanged in urine.
Half-life: 11–16 hr.

CONTRAINDICATIONS AND PRECAUTIONS

Contraindicated in: ▪ Hypersensitivity.
Use Cautiously in: ▪ Hypotensive patients ▪ Congestive heart failure or compromised left ventricular function (especially in combination with beta-blocker therapy) ▪ Patients >65 yr with impaired liver function (dosage reduction may be required) ▪ Pregnancy, lactation, or children (safety not established) ▪ Cardiac conduction defects.

ADVERSE REACTIONS AND SIDE EFFECTS*

CNS: headache, dizziness, weakness, syncope, anxiety, insomnia, psychiatric disturbances.
EENT: nasal congestion, pharyngitis, epistaxis.
Resp: cough, dyspnea, wheezing.
CV: peripheral edema, MYOCARDIAL INFARCTION, hypotension, chest pain, AV block, tachycardia.
GI: nausea, diarrhea, constipation, vomiting, dry mouth, flatulence, gingival hyperplasia.
GU: sexual difficulties.
Derm: flushing, rash, pruritus.
Hemat: anemia.
MS: muscle cramps, back pain.
Neuro: paresthesia.

INTERACTIONS

Drug-Drug: ▪ Additive hypotension with other **antihypertensives, nitrates,** or acute ingestion of **alcohol** ▪ **Cimetidine** or **ranitidine** decrease metabolism and may increase the effects of felodipine ▪ Combination with **beta blockers** may result in myocardial depression.

ROUTE AND DOSAGE

▪ **PO (Adults):** 5 mg once daily initially. May increase at 2 wk intervals. Usual daily dose is 5–10 mg (not to exceed 20 mg/day).

PHARMACODYNAMICS (antihypertensive effect)

	ONSET	PEAK	DURATION
PO	120–300 min	UK	up to 24 hr

NURSING IMPLICATIONS

Assessment

- ▫ Monitor blood pressure and pulse prior to and periodically throughout therapy. Monitor ECG periodically in patients receiving prolonged therapy.
- ▫ Monitor intake and output ratios and daily weight. Assess patient for signs of congestive heart failure (peripheral edema, rales/crackles, dyspnea, weight gain, jugular venous distention).
- ▪ **Lab Test Considerations:** Monitor hepatic function periodically in patients receiving long-term therapy. May cause elevated liver function tests.

Potential Nursing Diagnoses

- ▪ Cardiac output, decreased (indications).
- ▪ Knowledge deficit related to medication regimen (patient/family teaching).

Implementation

- ▪ **PO:** Administer once daily. Tablets should be swallowed whole; do not crush or chew.

Patient/Family Teaching

- ▫ Advise patient to take medication exactly as directed, not to skip or double up on missed doses. Felodipine may need to be discontinued gradually.
- ▫ Caution patients to make position changes slowly to minimize orthostatic hypotension.
- ▫ Felodipine may cause dizziness. Advise patient to avoid driving or other activities requiring alertness until response to the medication is known.
- ▫ Instruct patient to avoid concurrent use of alcohol or over-the-counter

*Underlines indicate most frequent; **CAPITALS** indicate life-threatening.

medications without consulting physician or pharmacist.
- □ Advise patient to notify the physician if irregular heart beats, dyspnea, swelling of hands and feet, pronounced dizziness, nausea, constipation or hypotension occur.

EVALUATION

Effectiveness of therapy can be demonstrated by: ▪ Decrease in blood pressure.

FENOPROFEN
(fen-oh-**proe**-fen)
Nalfon

CLASSIFICATION(S):
Nonsteroidal anti-inflammatory agent, Non-narcotic analgesic
Pregnancy Category B

INDICATIONS

▪ Management of inflammatory disorders, including: □ Rheumatoid arthritis □ Osteoarthritis ▪ Analgesic in the treatment of mild to moderate pain, including dysmenorrhea.

ACTION

▪ Inhibits prostaglandin synthesis. **Therapeutic Effects:** ▪ Suppression of pain and inflammation.

PHARMACOKINETICS

Absorption: Well absorbed from the GI tract.

Distribution: Does not cross the placenta. Enters breast milk in low concentrations.

Metabolism and Excretion: Mostly metabolized by the liver. Small amounts (2–5%) excreted unchanged by the kidneys.

Half-life: 3 hr.

CONTRAINDICATIONS AND PRECAUTIONS

Contraindicated in: ▪ Hypersensitivity ▪ Cross-sensitivity may exist with other NSAIAs, including aspirin ▪ Active GI bleeding or ulcer disease.

Use Cautiously in: ▪ Severe cardiovascular, renal, or hepatic disease ▪ Patients with a history of ulcer disease ▪ Pregnancy, lactation, or children (safety not established).

ADVERSE REACTIONS AND SIDE EFFECTS*

CNS: <u>headache</u>, <u>drowsiness</u>, psychic disturbances, dizziness.

EENT: blurred vision, tinnitus.

CV: edema, arrhythmias.

GI: <u>nausea</u>, <u>dyspepsia</u>, <u>vomiting</u>, <u>constipation</u>, **GI BLEEDING**, discomfort, **HEPATITIS**.

GU: renal failure, hematuria, cystitis.

Derm: rashes.

Hemat: blood dyscrasias, prolonged bleeding time.

Misc: allergic reactions, including **ANAPHYLAXIS**.

INTERACTIONS

Drug-Drug: ▪ Concurrent use with **aspirin** or **antacids** may decrease effectiveness ▪ Additive adverse GI effects with **aspirin,** other **nonsteroidal anti-inflammatory agents, potassium supplements, glucocorticoids,** or **alcohol** ▪ Chronic use with **acetaminophen** may increase the risk of adverse renal reactions ▪ May increase the risk of hypoglycemia with **insulin** or **oral hypoglycemic agents** ▪ May decrease the effectiveness of **diuretics** or **antihypertensive** therapy ▪ May increase serum **lithium** levels and increase the risk of toxicity ▪ Increases the risk of toxicity from **methotrexate** ▪ Increased risk of bleeding with **cefamandole, cefotetan, cefoperazone, moxalactam** or **plicamycin, heparin, thrombolytic agents,** or **oral anticoagulants** ▪ Increased risk of adverse hematologic reactions with **antineoplastic agents** or **radiation therapy** ▪ **Phenobarbital** may increase metabolism and decrease effectiveness of fenoprofen.

*<u>Underlines</u> indicate most frequent; **CAPITALS** indicate life-threatening.

F

ROUTE AND DOSAGE

Pain

- **PO (Adults):** 200 mg q 4–6 hr.

Inflammatory Conditions

- **PO (Adults):** 300–600 mg 3–4 times daily (not to exceed 3.2 g/day).

PHARMACODYNAMICS

	ONSET	PEAK	DURATION
PO (analgesic activity)	15–30 min	1–2 hr	4–6 hr
PO (anti-inflammatory activity)	several days	2–3 wk	UK

NURSING IMPLICATIONS

Assessment

- **General Info:** Patients who have asthma, aspirin-induced allergy, and nasal polyps are at increased risk for developing hypersensitivity reactions. Monitor for rhinitis, asthma, and urticaria.
- **Arthritis:** Assess pain and range of movement prior to and 1–2 hr following administration.
- **Pain:** Assess pain (type, location, and intensity) prior to and 1–2 hr following administration.
- **Lab Test Considerations:** BUN, serum creatinine, CBC, and liver function tests should be evaluated periodically in patients receiving prolonged course of therapy.
  - Serum potassium, alkaline phosphatase, LDH, SGOT (AST), and SGPT (ALT) may show increased levels. Bleeding time may also be prolonged.

Potential Nursing Diagnoses

- Comfort, altered: pain (indications).
- Mobility, impaired physical (indications).
- Knowledge deficit related to medication regimen (patient/family teaching).

Implementation

- **General Info:** Coadministration with narcotic analgesics may have additive analgesic effects and may permit lower narcotic doses.
- **PO:** For rapid initial effect, administer 30 min before or 2 hr after meals.
- **Dysmenorrhea:** Administer as soon as possible after the onset of menses. Prophylactic use has not been proven effective.

Patient/Family Teaching

- Advise patient to take this medication with a full glass of water and to remain in an upright position for 15–30 min after administration.
- Instruct patient to take medication exactly as prescribed. If a dose is missed, take as soon as remembered, but not if almost time for next dose. Do not double doses.
- May cause drowsiness or dizziness. Advise patient to avoid driving or other activities requiring alertness until response to the medication is known.
- Caution patient to avoid the concurrent use of alcohol, aspirin, acetaminophen, or other over-the-counter medications without consulting physician or pharmacist.
- Instruct patient to notify physician if rash, itching, chills, fever, muscle aches, visual disturbances, tinnitus, weight gain, edema, black stools, or persistent headache occur.
- Advise patient to inform physician or dentist of medication regimen prior to treatment or surgery.

Evaluation

Effectiveness of therapy can be demonstrated by: ▪ Decrease in severity of mild to moderate pain ▪ Improved joint mobility. Partial arthritic relief is usually seen within a few days, but maximum effects may require 2–3 wk of continuous therapy. Patients who do not respond to one nonsteroidal anti-inflammatory agent may respond to another.

FENTANYL (Parenteral)

(fen-ta-nil)

Sublimaze

CLASSIFICATION(S):
Narcotic analgesic—agonist
Schedule II
Pregnancy Category C

INDICATIONS

▪ Management of: ▫ Perioperative pain ▫ Intraoperative pain ▫ Postoperative pain ▪ Treatment and prevention of perioperative tachypnea and emergence delirium ▪ Supplement to general or regional analgesia—combination with droperidol produces neuroleptanalgesia (quiescence, decreased motor activity, and analgesia without loss of consciousness).

ACTION

▪ Binds to opiate receptors in the CNS, altering the response to and perception of pain ▪ Produces CNS depression. **Therapeutic Effect:** ▪ Relief of moderate to severe pain.

PHARMACOKINETICS

Absorption: Well absorbed following IM administration.
Distribution: Distribution not known.
Metabolism and Excretion: Mostly metabolized by the liver. 10–25% excreted unchanged by the kidneys.
Half-life: 3.6 hr (increased after cardiopulmonary bypass and in elderly patients).

CONTRAINDICATIONS AND PRECAUTIONS

Contraindicated in: ▪ Hypersensitivity ▪ Known intolerance.
Use Cautiously in: ▪ Elderly or debilitated patients ▪ Severely ill patients ▪ Diabetics ▪ Patients with severe pulmonary or hepatic disease ▪ CNS tumors ▪ Increased intracranial pressure ▪ Head trauma ▪ Adrenal insufficiency ▪ Undiagnosed abdominal pain ▪ Hypothyroidism ▪ Alcoholism ▪ Cardiac disease, particularly arrhythmias ▪ Pregnancy, lactation, and children <2 yr (safety not established).

ADVERSE REACTIONS AND SIDE EFFECTS*

CNS: euphoria, floating feeling, dysphoria, hallucinations, depression, excessive sedation.
Resp: respiratory depression, APNEA, laryngospasm, bronchoconstriction.
CV: bradycardia.
GI: constipation, nausea, vomiting.
MS: skeletal and thoracic muscle rigidity.

INTERACTIONS

Drug-Drug: ▪ Avoid use in patients who have received **MAO inhibitors** within the previous 14 days (may produce unpredictable, potentially fatal reactions) ▪ Additive CNS and respiratory depression with other **CNS depressants**, including **alcohol, antihistamines, antidepressants,** and other **sedative/hypnotics** ▪ Increased risk of hypotension with **benzodiazepines**.

ROUTE AND DOSAGE

Preoperative Use

▪ **IM (Adults):** 50–100 mcg 30–60 min before surgery.

Adjunct to General Anesthesia

▪ **IV (Adults):** Low dose—2 mcg/kg. Moderate dose—2–20 mcg/kg, additional doses of 25–100 mcg may be given as necessary. High dose—20–50 mcg/kg; additional doses ranging from 25 mcg to 50% of original dose may be repeated as necessary.

Adjunct to Regional Anesthesia

▪ **IM, IV (Adults):** 50–100 mcg.

To Provide General Anesthesia

▪ **IV (Adults):** 50–100 mcg/kg (up to 150 mcg/kg) with oxygen and a skeletal muscle relaxant.
▪ **IV (Children 2–12 yr):** 2–3 mcg/kg.

PHARMACODYNAMICS (analgesia; respiratory depression may last longer than analgesia)

	ONSET	PEAK	DURATION
IM	7–15 min	20–30 min	1–2 hr
IV	1–2 min	3–5 min	0.5–1 hr

*Underlines indicate most frequent; **CAPITALS** indicate life-threatening.

F

NURSING IMPLICATIONS

Assessment

- **General Info:** Monitor respiratory rate and blood pressure frequently throughout course of therapy. Notify physician of significant changes immediately. The respiratory depressant effects of fentanyl last longer than the analgesic effects. Subsequent narcotic doses should be reduced by ¼ to ⅓ of the usually recommended dose. Monitor closely.
- □ Assess type, location, and intensity of pain prior to and 10 min following IM administration or 1–2 min following IV administration when fentanyl is used to treat pain.
- **Lab Test Considerations:** May cause elevated serum amylase and lipase concentrations.
- **Toxicity and Overdose:** If overdose occurs, naloxone (Narcan) is the antidote.

Potential Nursing Diagnoses

- Comfort, altered: pain (indications).
- Breathing pattern, ineffective (adverse reactions).
- Injury, high risk for (side effects).

Implementation

- **General Info:** Benzodiazepines may be administered prior to administration of fentanyl to reduce the induction dose requirements and decrease the time to loss of consciousness. This combination may also increase the risk of hypotension.
- □ Narcotic antagonist, oxygen, and resuscitative equipment should be readily available during the administration of fentanyl.
- □ Available in combination with droperidol (Innovar); see Appendix A.
- **Direct IV:** Administer slowly over at least 1–2 min. Slow IV administration may reduce the incidence or severity of muscle rigidity, bradycardia, or hypotension.
- **Intermittent Infusion:** Fentanyl may also be diluted with D5W, 0.9% NaCl, D5/LR, or lactated Ringer's soln for infusion and administered until the onset of somnolence as an adjunct to general anesthesia.
- **Syringe Compatibility:** atropine, butorphanol, chlorpromazine, cimetidine, dimenhydrinate, diphenhydramine, droperidol, heparin, hydromorphone, hydroxyzine, meperidine, metoclopramide, midazolam, morphine, pentazocine, perphenazine, prochlorperazine edisylate, promazine, promethazine, ranitidine, or scopolamine.
- **Syringe Incompatibility:** pentobarbital.
- **Y-Site Compatibility:** atracurium, enalaprilat, esmolol, heparin, hydrocortisone sodium succinate, labetalol, nafcillin, pancuronium, potassium chloride, or vecuronium.
- **Additive Incompatibility:** methohexital, pentobarbital, or thiopental.

Patient/Family Teaching

- □ Caution patient to make position changes slowly to minimize orthostatic hypotension.
- □ Medication causes dizziness and drowsiness. Advise patient to call for assistance during ambulation and transfer, and to avoid driving or other activities requiring alertness for 24 hr after administration of fentanyl during outpatient surgery.
- □ Instruct patient to avoid alcohol or other CNS depressants for 24 hr after administration of fentanyl for outpatient surgery.

Evaluation

Effectiveness of therapy can be demonstrated by: ▪ General quiescence □ Reduced motor activity ▪ Pronounced analgesia.

FENTANYL TRANSDERMAL

(**fen**-ta-nil)
Duragesic

CLASSIFICATION(S):
Narcotic analgesic—agonist
Schedule II
Pregnancy Category C

INDICATIONS

▪ Management of chronic pain in patients already receiving narcotic analgesic therapy.

ACTION

▪ Binds to opiate receptors in the CNS, altering the response to and perception of pain. **Therapeutic Effect:** ▪ Decrease in severity of chronic pain.

PHARMACOKINETICS

Absorption: Well absorbed (92% of dose) through skin surface under transdermal patch, creating a depot in the upper skin layers. Release from transdermal system into systemic circulation increases gradually to a constant rate providing continuous delivery for 72 hr.
Distribution: Crosses the placenta and enters breast milk.
Metabolism and Excretion: Mostly metabolized by the liver. 10–25% excreted unchanged by the kidneys.
Half-life: 17 hr following removal of patch (due to continued release from deposition of drug in skin layers).

CONTRAINDICATIONS AND PRECAUTIONS

Contraindicated in: ▪ Hypersensitivity to fentanyl or adhesives ▪ Known intolerance ▪ Acute pain (onset not rapid enough) ▪ Alcohol intolerance (small amounts of alcohol released into skin).
Use Cautiously in: ▪ Elderly or debilitated patients (dosage reduction suggested) ▪ Severely ill patients ▪ Diabetics ▪ Patients with severe pulmonary or hepatic disease ▪ CNS tumors ▪ Increased intracranial pressure ▪ Head trauma ▪ Adrenal insufficiency ▪ Undiagnosed abdominal pain ▪ Hypothyroidism ▪ Alcoholism ▪ Cardiac disease, particularly bradyarrhythmias ▪ Pregnancy, lactation, or children <2 yr (safety not established) ▪ Fever (increases release of fentanyl from delivery system) ▪ **Nalbuphine** or **pentazocine** may decrease analgesia.

ADVERSE REACTIONS AND SIDE EFFECTS*

CNS: drowsiness, confusion, weakness, dizziness, restlessness.
Resp: respiratory depression, APNEA, laryngospasm, bronchoconstriction.
CV: bradycardia.
GI: constipation, dry mouth, nausea, vomiting, anorexia.
Derm: sweating, erythema.
Local: application site reactions.
MS: skeletal and thoracic muscle rigidity.
Misc: physical dependence, psychological dependence.

INTERACTIONS

Drug-Drug: ▪ Avoid use in patients who have received **MAO inhibitors** within the previous 14 days (may produce unpredictable, potentially fatal reactions) ▪ Additive CNS and respiratory depression with other **CNS depressants** including **alcohol, antihistamines, antidepressants,** and other **sedative/hypnotics** ▪ **Disulfiram, moxalactam, cefoperazone, cefotetan,** or **cefamandole** may produce adverse reactions due to release of small amounts of alcohol from transdermal system.

ROUTE AND DOSAGE

▪ **Transdermal (Adults):** 25 mcg/hr initially, may be increased until adequate pain relief is achieved (25–300 mcg/hr) Patch is worn for 72 hr. Additional narcotic analgesics may be required during dose titration.

PHARMACODYNAMICS

	ONSET	PEAK	DURATION
TD	6 hr*	12–24 hr	72 hr†

*Achievement of blood levels associated with analgesia; maximal response and dose titration may take up to 6 days.
†While patch is worn.

NURSING IMPLICATIONS

Assessment

□ Assess type, location, and intensity of pain prior to and 24 hr after applica-

*Underlines indicate most frequent; CAPITALS indicate life-threatening.

tion and periodically throughout therapy. Pain should be monitored frequently during initiation of therapy as should dosage changes to assess need for supplementary analgesics.
- Assess blood pressure, pulse, and respiratory rate before and periodically during administration.
- Prolonged use may lead to physical and psychological dependence and tolerance. This should not prevent patient from receiving adequate analgesia. Most patients who receive narcotic analgesics for medical reasons do not develop psychological dependency.
- Progressively higher doses may be required to relieve pain with long-term therapy. It may take up to 6 days after increasing doses to reach equilibrium, so patients should wear higher dose through 2 applications before increasing dose again.
- Assess bowel function routinely. Increased intake of fluids and bulk, stool softeners, and laxatives may minimize constipating effects.
- **Lab Test Considerations:** May increase plasma amylase and lipase levels.
- **Toxicity and Overdose:** If overdosage occurs, naloxone (Narcan) is the antidote. Monitor patient closely, dose may need to be repeated or may need to be administered as an infusion because of long duration of action despite removal of patch.

Potential Nursing Diagnoses
- Comfort, altered: pain (indications).
- Sensory-perceptual alteration: visual, auditory (side effects).
- Injury, high risk for (side effects).
- Knowledge deficit related to medication regimen (patient/family teaching).

Implementation
- **General Info:** Explain therapeutic value of medication prior to administration to enhance the analgesic effect.
- Supplemental doses of short-acting narcotic analgesics should be used to manage pain until relief is obtained with the transdermal system. Patients may continue to require supplemental narcotics for breakthrough pain. If >100 mcg/hr is required, use multiple systems.
- Dosage is titrated based on the patient's report of pain until adequate analgesia is attained. Dosage is determined by calculating the previous 24 hr analgesic requirement and converting to equianalgesic morphine dose using Appendix B. The conversion ratio from morphine to transdermal fentanyl is conservative; 50% of patients may require a dose increase after initial application. Increase after 3 days based on required daily doses of supplemental analgesics. Increases should be based on ratio of 90 mg/24 hr of oral morphine to 25 mcg/hr increase in transdermal fentanyl dose. Patients requiring >300 mcg/hr may need other methods of narcotic analgesic administration.
- Coadministration with non-narcotic analgesics may have additive analgesic effects and permit lower doses.
- To convert to another narcotic analgesic, remove transdermal fentanyl system and begin treatment with half the equianalgesic dose of the new analgesic in 12–18 hr.
- Medication should be discontinued gradually after long–term use to prevent withdrawal symptoms.
- **Transdermal:** Apply system to upper torso on a flat, nonirritated, and nonirradiated site. If skin preparation is necessary, use clear water and clip, do not shave, hair. Allow skin to dry completely before application. Apply immediately after removing from package and press firmly in place with palm of hand for 10–20 sec, especially around the edges, to make sure contact is complete. For continued use, remove used system and fold so that adhesive edges are together. Flush system down toilet immediately upon removal. Apply new system to a different site. Discard un-

used systems by removing from pouch and flushing down the toilet.

Patient/Family Teaching

- Instruct patient how and when to ask for prn pain medication.
- Instruct patient in correct method for application and disposal of transdermal system.
- Medication may cause drowsiness or dizziness. Caution patient to call for assistance when ambulating or smoking and to avoid driving or other activities requiring alertness until response to medication is known.
- Advise patient to make position changes slowly to minimize dizziness.
- Caution patient to avoid concurrent use of alcohol or other CNS depressants with this medication.
- Encourage patient to turn, cough, and breathe deeply every 2 hr to prevent atelectasis.

Evaluation

Effectiveness of therapy can be demonstrated by: ▪ Decrease in severity of pain without a significant alteration in level of consciousness, respiratory status, or blood pressure.

FERROUS FUMARATE

(**fer**-us **fyoo**-ma-rate)
Femiron, Feostat, Fumasorb, Fumerin, Hemocyte, Ircon, {Neo-Fer}, {Novofumar}, {Palafer}, Palmiron, Span-FF

CLASSIFICATION(S):
Antianemic, Iron supplement
Pregnancy Category UK

INDICATIONS

▪ Prevention and treatment of iron-deficiency anemias.

ACTION

▪ An essential mineral found in hemoglobin, myoglobin, and a number of enzymes ▪ Allows oxygen transport from lungs to tissues via hemoglobin. **Therapeutic Effects:** ▪ Correction of iron-deficiency states ▪ Iron supplementation.

PHARMACOKINETICS

Absorption: 5–10% of dietary iron is absorbed. In deficiency states this may increase up to 30%. Therapeutically administered iron may be 60% absorbed. Absorbed by active and passive transport processes.
Distribution: Crosses the placenta.
Metabolism and Excretion: Mostly recycled, small daily losses occurring through desquamation, sweat, urine, and bile.
Half-life: UK.

CONTRAINDICATIONS AND PRECAUTIONS

Contraindicated in: ▪ Primary hemochromatosis ▪ Hemolytic anemias ▪ Some products contain tartrazine (FDC yellow dye #5)—use cautiously in patients with tartrazine sensitivity.
Use Cautiously in: ▪ Peptic ulcer ▪ Ulcerative colitis or regional enteritis (condition may be aggravated) ▪ Indiscriminate chronic use (may lead to iron overload).

ADVERSE REACTIONS AND SIDE EFFECTS*

GI: <u>constipation</u>, <u>diarrhea</u>, <u>nausea</u>, <u>dark stools</u>, <u>epigastric pain</u>, gastric bleeding.
Misc: staining of teeth (liquid preparations).

INTERACTIONS

Drug-Drug: ▪ **Tetracycline** and **antacids** inhibit the absorption of iron by forming insoluble compounds ▪ **Tetracycline** absorption is also decreased by concurrent iron administration ▪ Iron decreases the absorption of **fluoroquinolones** or **penicillamine** ▪ **Chloramphenicol** and **vitamin E** may impair the hematologic response to iron therapy

{} = Available in Canada only.
*<u>Underlines</u> indicate most frequent; **CAPITALS** indicate life-threatening.

- **Vitamin C** may slightly increase the absorption of iron.

Drug–Food: ■ Iron absorption is decreased by ⅓–½ by concurrent administration of food.

ROUTE AND DOSAGE

Note: Ferrous fumarate = 33% elemental iron.

Dosage Expressed in mg Ferrous Fumarate

Ferrous fumarate—prophylactic

- **PO (Adults):** 200 mg/day.
- **PO (Children):** 3 mg/kg/day.

Ferrous fumarate—therapeutic

- **PO (Adults):** 200 mg 3–4 times daily.
- **PO (Children):** 3–6 mg/kg tid.

Dosage Expressed in mg Elemental Iron

- **PO (Adults):** 50–100 mg tid.
- **PO (Children):** 4–6 mg/kg/day in 3 divided doses.
- **PO (Infants):** 1–2 mg/kg/day.
- **PO (Pregnant Women):** 30–60 mg/day.

PHARMACODYNAMICS (effects on erythropoiesis)

	ONSET	PEAK	DURATION
PO	4 days	7–10 days	2–4 mon

NURSING IMPLICATIONS

Assessment

- □ Assess patient's nutritional status and dietary history to determine possible cause of anemia and need for patient teaching.
- □ Assess bowel function for constipation or diarrhea. Notify physician and use appropriate nursing measures should these occur.
- **Lab Test Considerations:** Hemoglobin, hematocrit, and reticulocyte values should be monitored prior to therapy and every 3 wk for the first 2 mon of therapy and periodically thereafter. Serum ferritin and iron levels may also be monitored to assess effectiveness of therapy.
- □ Occult blood in stools may be obscured by black coloration of iron in stool. Guaiac test results may be occasionally false-positive. Benzidine test results are not affected by iron preparations.
- **Toxicity and Overdose:** Early symptoms of overdose include stomach pain, fever, nausea, vomiting (may contain blood), and diarrhea. Late symptoms include bluish lips, fingernails, and palms; drowsiness; weakness; tachycardia; seizures; metabolic acidosis; hepatic injury; and cardiovascular collapse. The patient may appear to recover prior to the onset of late symptoms. Therefore, hospitalization continues for 24 hr after patient becomes asymptomatic to monitor for delayed onset of shock or GI bleeding. Late complications of overdose include intestinal obstruction, pyloric stenosis, and gastric scarring.
- □ Treatment includes inducing emesis with syrup of ipecac. If patient is comatose or seizing, gastric lavage with sodium bicarbonate is performed. Deferoxamine is the antidote. Additional supportive treatments to maintain fluid and electrolyte balance and correction of metabolic acidosis are also indicated.

Potential Nursing Diagnoses

- Activity intolerance (indications).
- Knowledge deficit related to medication and dietary regimen (patient/family teaching).

Implementation

- **General Info:** Available in combination with many vitamins and minerals (see Appendix A). Also available in combination with docusate sodium to reduce constipating effects.
- **PO:** Oral preparations are most effectively absorbed if administered 1 hr before or 2 hr after meals. If gastric irritation occurs, administer with meals. Tablets and capsules should be taken with a full glass of water or juice. Do not open, crush, or chew extended-release capsules. Chewable tablet should be chewed well before swallowing; do not swallow whole.
- □ Shake oral suspension prior to

administration. Liquid preparations may stain teeth. Dilute well and administer with a straw or place drops at back of throat.
- Avoid using antacids, coffee, tea, dairy products, eggs, or whole grain breads within 1 hr before and 2 hr after administration of ferrous salts.

Patient/Family Teaching
- Encourage patient to comply with medication regimen. If a dose is missed, take as soon as remembered within 12 hr, otherwise return to regular dosing schedule; do not double doses.
- Advise patient that stools may become dark green or black and that this change is harmless.
- Instruct patient to follow a diet high in iron (organ meat, leafy green vegetables, dried beans and peas, dried fruit, cereals); see Appendix K.
- Discuss with parents the risk of children overdosing on iron. Medication should be stored in the original child-proof container and kept out of reach of children. Do not refer to vitamins as candy. Medical help should be sought immediately if overdose is suspected, as death may occur. Parents should have syrup of ipecac at home and call pediatrician, emergency department, or poison control center for instructions before administering.

Evaluation

Clinical response to therapy is indicated by: ▪ Increase in hemoglobin, which may reach normal parameters after 1–2 mon of therapy. May require 3–6 mon for normalization of body iron stores.

FERROUS GLUCONATE

(**fer**-us gloo-koe-nate)
{Apo-Ferrous Gluconate}, Fergon, Ferralet, {Novoferrogluc}, Simron

CLASSIFICATION(S):
Antianemic, Iron supplement
Pregnancy Category UK

INDICATIONS

▪ Prevention and treatment of iron-deficiency anemias.

ACTION

▪ An essential mineral found in hemoglobin, myoglobin, and a number of enzymes ▪ Allows oxygen transport from lungs to tissues via hemoglobin. **Therapeutic Effects:** ▪ Correction of iron-deficiency states ▪ Iron supplementation.

PHARMACOKINETICS

Absorption: 5–10% of dietary iron is absorbed. In deficiency states this may increase up to 30%. Therapeutically administered iron may be 60% absorbed. Absorbed by active and passive transport processes.
Distribution: Crosses the placenta.
Metabolism and Excretion: Mostly recycled; small daily losses occurring through desquamation, sweat, urine, and bile.
Half-life: UK.

CONTRAINDICATIONS AND PRECAUTIONS

Contraindicated in: ▪ Primary hemochromatosis ▪ Hemolytic anemias ▪ Some products contain tartrazine (FDC yellow dye #5)—use cautiously in patients with tartrazine sensitivity.
Use Cautiously in: ▪ Peptic ulcer ▪ Ulcerative colitis or regional enteritis (condition may be aggravated) ▪ Indiscriminate chronic use (may lead to iron overload).

ADVERSE REACTIONS AND SIDE EFFECTS*

GI: <u>constipation</u>, <u>diarrhea</u>, <u>nausea</u>, <u>dark stools</u>, <u>epigastric pain</u>, gastric bleeding.

{} = Available in Canada only.
*<u>Underlines</u> indicate most frequent; **CAPITALS** indicate life-threatening.

F

Misc: staining of teeth (liquid preparations).

INTERACTIONS

Drug-Drug: ▪ **Tetracycline** and **antacids** inhibit the absorption of iron by forming insoluble compounds ▪ **Tetracycline** absorption is also decreased by concurrent iron administration ▪ Iron decreases the absorption of **fluoroquinolones** or **penicillamine** ▪ **Chloramphenicol** and **vitamin E** may impair the hematologic response to iron therapy ▪ **Vitamin C** may slightly increase the absorption of iron.

Drug-Food: ▪ Iron absorption is decreased by ⅓–½ by concurrent administration of food.

ROUTE AND DOSAGE

Note: Ferrous gluconate = 11.6% elemental iron.

Dosage Expressed in mg Ferrous Gluconate

Ferrous gluconate—prophylactic

- **PO (Adults):** 325 mg/day.
- **PO (Children >2 yr):** 8 mg/kg/day.

Ferrous gluconate—therapeutic

- **PO (Adults):** 325–650 mg qid.
- **PO (Children: >2 yr):** 16 mg/kg tid.

Dosage Expressed in mg Elemental Iron

- **PO (Adults):** 50–100 mg tid.
- **PO (Children):** 4–6 mg/kg/day in 3 divided doses.
- **PO (Infants):** 1–2 mg/kg/day.
- **PO (Pregnant Women):** 30–60 mg/day.

PHARMACODYNAMICS (effects on erythropoiesis)

	ONSET	PEAK	DURATION
PO	4 days	7–10 days	2–4 mon

NURSING IMPLICATIONS

Assessment

- Assess patient's nutritional status and dietary history to determine possible cause of anemia and need for patient teaching.
- Assess bowel function for constipation or diarrhea. Notify physician and use appropriate nursing measures should these occur.
- **Lab Test Considerations:** Hemoglobin, hematocrit, and reticulocyte values should be monitored prior to and every 3 wk during the first 2 mon of therapy and periodically thereafter. Serum ferritin and iron levels may also be monitored to assess effectiveness of therapy.
- Occult blood in stools may be obscured by black coloration of iron in stool. Guaiac test results may occasionally be false-positive. Benzidine test results are not affected by iron preparations.
- **Toxicity and Overdose:** Early symptoms of overdose include stomach pain, fever, nausea, vomiting (may contain blood), and diarrhea. Late symptoms include bluish lips, fingernails, and palms; drowsiness; weakness; tachycardia; seizures; metabolic acidosis; hepatic injury; and cardiovascular collapse. The patient may appear to recover prior to the onset of late symptoms. Therefore, hospitalization continues for 24 hr after patient becomes asymptomatic, to monitor for delayed onset of shock or GI bleeding. Late complications of overdose include intestinal obstruction, pyloric stenosis, and gastric scarring.
- Treatment includes inducing emesis with syrup of ipecac. If patient is comatose or seizing, gastric lavage with sodium bicarbonate is performed. Deferoxamine is the antidote. Additional supportive treatments to maintain fluid and electrolyte balance and correction of metabolic acidosis are also indicated.

Potential Nursing Diagnoses

- Activity intolerance (indications).
- Knowledge deficit related to medication and dietary regimen (patient teaching).

Implementation

- **General Info:** Available in combination with many vitamins and minerals (see Appendix A).

- **PO:** Oral preparations are most effectively absorbed if administered 1 hr before or 2 hr after meals. If gastric irritation occurs, administer with meals. Tablets and capsules should be taken with a full glass of water or juice.
- □ Liquid preparations may stain teeth. Dilute well and administer with a straw, or place drops at back of throat.
- □ Avoid using antacids, coffee, tea, dairy products, eggs, or whole grain breads within 1 hr before and 2 hr after administration of ferrous salts.

Patient/Family Teaching

- □ Encourage patient to comply with medication regimen. If a dose is missed, take as soon as remembered within 12 hr, otherwise return to regular dosing schedule; do not double doses.
- □ Advise patient that stools may become dark green or black and that this change is harmless.
- □ Instruct patient to follow a diet high in iron (organ meat, leafy green vegetables, dried beans and peas, dried fruit, cereals); see Appendix K.
- □ Discuss with parents the risk of children overdosing on iron. Medication should be stored in the original childproof container and kept out of the reach of children. Do not refer to vitamins as candy. Medical help should be sought immediately if overdose is suspected, as death may occur. Parents should have syrup of ipecac at home and call pediatrician, emergency department, or poison control center for instructions before administering.

Evaluation

Clinical response to therapy is indicated by: ▪ Increase in hemoglobin, which may reach normal parameters after 1–2 mon of therapy. May require 3–6 mon for normalization of body iron stores.

FERROUS SULFATE

(fer-us sul-fate)

{Apo-Ferrous Sulfate}, Feosol, Fer-in-Sol, Fer-Iron, {Fero-Grad}, Fero-Gradumet, $FeSO_4$, Ferralyn, Ferra-TD, Mol-Iron, {Novoferrosulfa}, {PMS Ferrous Sulfate}, Slow Fe

CLASSIFICATION(S):

Antianemic, Iron supplement

Pregnancy Category UK

INDICATIONS

▪ Prevention and treatment of iron-deficiency anemias.

ACTION

▪ An essential mineral found in hemoglobin, myoglobin, and a number of enzymes ▪ Allows oxygen transport from lungs to tissues via hemoglobin. **Therapeutic Effects:** ▪ Correction of iron-deficiency states ▪ Iron supplementation.

PHARMACOKINETICS

Absorption: 5–10% of dietary iron is absorbed. In deficiency states this may increase up to 30%. Therapeutically administered iron may be 60% absorbed. Absorbed by active and passive transport processes.

Distribution: Crosses the placenta.

Metabolism and Excretion: Mostly recycled; small daily losses occurring through desquamation, sweat, urine, and bile.

Half-life: UK.

CONTRAINDICATIONS AND PRECAUTIONS

Contraindicated in: ▪ Primary hemochromatosis ▪ Hemolytic anemias ▪ Some products contain tartrazine (FDC yellow dye #5)—use cautiously in patients with tartrazine sensitivity.

Use Cautiously in: ▪ Peptic ulcer ▪ Ulcerative colitis or regional enteritis (condition may be aggravated) ▪ Indiscriminate chronic use (may lead to iron overload).

ADVERSE REACTIONS AND SIDE EFFECTS*

GI: constipation, diarrhea, nausea, dark stools, epigastric pain, gastric bleeding.
Misc: staining of teeth (liquid preparations).

INTERACTIONS

Drug–Drug: ▪ **Tetracycline** and **antacids** inhibit the absorption of iron by forming insoluble compounds ▪ **Tetracycline** absorption is also decreased by concurrent iron administration ▪ Iron decreases the absorption of **fluoroquinolones** or **penicillamine** ▪ **Chloramphenicol** and **vitamin E** may impair the hematologic response to iron therapy ▪ **Vitamin C** may slightly increase the absorption of iron.
Drug–Food: ▪ Iron absorption is decreased by ⅓–½ by concurrent administration of food.

ROUTE AND DOSAGE

Note: Ferrous sulfate = 20–30% elemental iron.

Dosage Expressed in mg Ferrous Sulfate

Ferrous sulfate—prophylactic
- **PO (Adults):** 300–325 mg/day.
- **PO (Children):** 5 mg/kg/day.

Ferrous sulfate—therapeutic
- **PO (Adults):** 300 mg 2–4 times daily.
- **PO (Children):** 10 mg/kg tid.

Dosage Expressed in mg Elemental Iron

- **PO (Adults):** 50–100 mg 3 tid.
- **PO (Children):** 4–6 mg/kg/day in 3 divided doses.
- **PO (Infants):** 1–2 mg/kg/day.
- **PO (Pregnant Women):** 30–60 mg/day.

PHARMACODYNAMICS (effects on erythropoiesis)

	ONSET	PEAK	DURATION
PO	4 days	7–10 days	2–4 mon

NURSING IMPLICATIONS

Assessment

- ▫ Assess patient's nutritional status and dietary history to determine possible cause of anemia and need for patient teaching.
- ▫ Assess bowel function for constipation or diarrhea. Notify physician and use appropriate nursing measures should these occur.
- ▪ **Lab Test Considerations:** Hemoglobin, hematocrit, and reticulocyte values should be monitored prior to and every 3 wk during the first 2 mon of therapy, and periodically thereafter. Serum ferritin and iron levels may also be monitored to assess effectiveness of therapy.
- ▫ Occult blood in stools may be obscured by black coloration of iron in stool. Guaiac test results may occasionally be false-positive. Benzidine test results are not affected by iron preparations.
- ▪ **Toxicity and Overdose:** Early symptoms of overdose include stomach pain, fever, nausea, vomiting (may contain blood), and diarrhea. Late symptoms include bluish lips, fingernails, and palms; drowsiness; weakness; tachycardia; seizures; metabolic acidosis; hepatic injury; and cardiovascular collapse. The patient may appear to recover prior to the onset of the late symptoms. Therefore, hospitalization continues for 24 hr after patient becomes asymptomatic to monitor for delayed onset of shock or GI bleeding. Late complications of overdose include intestinal obstruction, pyloric stenosis, and gastric scarring.
- ▫ Treatment includes inducing emesis with syrup of ipecac. If patient is comatose or seizing, gastric lavage with sodium bicarbonate is performed. Deferoxamine is the antidote. Additional supportive treatments to maintain fluid and electrolyte balance and correction of metabolic acidosis are also indicated.

*Underlines indicate most frequent; **CAPITALS** indicate life-threatening.

Potential Nursing Diagnoses
- Activity intolerance (indications).
- Knowledge deficit related to medication and dietary regimen (patient/family teaching).

Implementation
- **General Info:** Available in combination with many vitamins and minerals (see Appendix A). Also available in combination with magnesium hydroxide and aluminum hydroxide to minimize GI irritation.
- **PO:** Oral preparations are most effectively absorbed if administered 1 hr before or 2 hr after meals. If gastric irritation occurs, administer with meals. Tablets and capsules should be taken with a full glass of water or juice. Do not crush or chew enteric-coated tablets and do not open capsules.
  - Liquid preparations may stain teeth. Dilute well and administer with a straw or place drops at back of throat. Feosol elixir should be diluted in water only. Fer-in-Sol liquid or syrup may be diluted in water or fruit juice.
  - Avoid using antacids, coffee, tea, dairy products, eggs, or whole grain breads within 1 hr before and 2 hr after administration of ferrous salts.

Patient/Family Teaching
- Encourage patient to comply with medication regimen. If a dose is missed, take as soon as remembered within 12 hr, otherwise return to regular dosing schedule. Do not double doses.
- Advise patient that stools may become dark green or black and that this change is harmless.
- Instruct patient to follow a diet high in iron (organ meat, leafy green vegetables, dried beans and peas, dried fruit, cereals); see Appendix K.
- Discuss with parents the risk of children overdosing on iron. Medication should be stored in the original childproof container and kept out of reach of children. Do not refer to vitamins as candy. Medical help should be sought immediately if overdose is suspected, as death may occur. Parents should have syrup of ipecac at home and call pediatrician, emergency department, or poison control center for instructions before administering.

Evaluation

Clinical response to therapy is indicated by: ▪ Increase in hemoglobin, which may reach normal parameters after 1–2 mon of therapy. May require 3–6 mon for normalization of body iron stores.

FIBRINOLYSIN AND DESOXYRIBONUCLEASE
(fye-brin-oh-**lye**-sin/dez-ox-ee-rye-boe-**nuke**-lee-ase)
Elase

CLASSIFICATION(S):
Topical—enzyme
Pregnancy Category UK

INDICATIONS

▪ Used as a topical debriding agent in the management of surgical wounds and other lesions including: ▫ Burns ▫ Ulcers ▫ Vaginitis ▫ Cervicitis ▪ As a debriding irrigant in: ▫ Infected wounds ▫ Sinus tracts ▫ Fistulae ▫ Lesions (with concurrent systemic anti-infective therapy).

ACTION

▪ Fibrinolysin breaks down fibrin in clots and fibrinous exudates ▪ Desoxyribonuclease degrades proteins present in devitalized tissues found in areas of purulent exudate. **Therapeutic Effect:** ▪ Removal of necrotic material (fibrin, purulent exudates), which may result in improved healing and response to other treatment modalities.

PHARMACOKINETICS

Absorption: Negligible systemic absorption.
Distribution: Distribution not known.

Metabolism and Excretion: Metabolism and excretion not known.
Half-life: UK (no activity left after 24 hr).

CONTRAINDICATIONS AND PRECAUTIONS

Contraindicated in: ▪ Hypersensitivity ▪ Hypersensitivity to bovine products or mercury compounds (contains thimerisol).
Use Cautiously in: ▪ Presence of infection (systemic anti-infectives may be required).

ADVERSE REACTIONS AND SIDE EFFECTS*

Local: hyperemia (large doses only).
Misc: hypersensitivity reactions, including ANAPHYLAXIS.

INTERACTIONS

Drug-Drug: ▪ None significant.

ROUTE AND DOSAGE

- **Top (Adults and Children):** Pack wound with gauze strips soaked in freshly prepared soln (wet to dry method) q 6–8 hr for 2–4 days or instill and irrigate with soln q 6–10 hr.
- **Vag (Adults):** 5 ml of ointment deep into vagina at bedtime nightly for 5 nights or instill 10 ml of soln into vagina, wait 2–3 min, and insert cotton tampon; follow next day with instillation of ointment.

PHARMACODYNAMICS (granulation tissue forms)

	ONSET	PEAK	DURATION
Top	2–4 days	UK	UK

NURSING IMPLICATIONS

Assessment

- **General Info:** Assess wound dimensions, depth, exudate, and tissue characteristics prior to and periodically throughout course of therapy.
- □ Monitor skin surrounding wound. Notify physician if severe irritation and inflammation occur.
- □ Assess for pain associated with dressing changes. Confer with physician regarding analgesics for premedication prior to dressing changes.
- **Vag:** Assess for irritation, bleeding, or discharge.

Potential Nursing Diagnoses

- Tissue integrity, altered (indications).
- Knowledge deficit related to medication regimen (patient/family teaching).

Implementation

- **Top Oint:** Flush wound with water, saline irrigation, or hydrogen peroxide. Pat dry. Apply thin layer of ointment to wound and cover with nonadherent dressing. Change at least daily.
- **Top Soln:** Prepare soln by mixing 1 vial of powder with 10–50 ml of 0.9% NaCl. Soln is stable for 24 hr.
- □ Saturate gauze in soln and apply as wet to dry dressing every 6–8 hr. May be used to irrigate infected cavities or tracts (abscesses, empyemas, subcutaneous hematomas, or fistulae). Drain and replace soln every 6–10 hr to ensure enzyme activity and remove debrided tissue and exudate. Blood-tinged drainage may indicate growth of healthy tissue.
- □ In severe cases, 10 ml should be instilled vaginally by physician. Tampon is then inserted 1–2 min later and kept in place until the next day.
- **Vag Oint:** Administer 5 ml with applicator. Do not use tampons.

Patient/Family Teaching

- **Vag:** Instruct patient in the correct use of applicator. Patient should remain recumbent for at least 30 min after administration. May use sanitary napkin to protect clothing, but do not use tampon. Emphasize importance of follow-up appointment to evaluate Effectiveness of treatment.

*Underlines indicate most frequent; **CAPITALS** indicate life-threatening.

Evaluation

Effectiveness of therapy can be demonstrated by: ▪ Debridement of necrotic tissue ▫ Formulation of granulation tissue ▪ Resolution of symptoms of vaginitis and cervicitis.

FILGRASTIM

(fill-**grass**-stim)
Neupogen, G-CSF, granulocyte-colony stimulating factor

CLASSIFICATION(S):
Colony stimulating factor
Pregnancy Category C

INDICATIONS

▪ Prevention of febrile neutropenia and associated infection in patients who have received bone-marrow-depressing antineoplastic agents for the treatment of nonmyeloid malignancies.

ACTION

▪ A glycoprotein that binds to and stimulates immature neutrophils to divide and differentiate. Also activates mature neutrophils. **Therapeutic Effect:** ▪ Decreased incidence of infection in patients who received bone-marrow-depressing antineoplastic agents.

PHARMACOKINETICS

Absorption: Well absorbed following subcutaneous administration.
Distribution: Distribution not known.
Metabolism and Excretion: Metabolism and excretion not known.
Half-life: UK.

CONTRAINDICATIONS AND PRECAUTIONS

Contraindicated in: ▪ Hypersensitivity to *E. Coli*-derived proteins.
Use Cautiously in: ▪ Pregnancy, lactation, or children (safety not established) ▪ Malignancy with myeloid characteristics ▪ Pre-existing cardiac disease.

ADVERSE REACTIONS AND SIDE EFFECTS*

Resp: respiratory distress syndrome.
CV: hypotension, myocardial, infarction, arrhythmias.
MS: medullary bone pain.

INTERACTIONS

Drug–Drug: ▪ Simultaneous use with **antineoplastic agents** may have adverse effects on rapidly proliferating neutrophils—avoid use for 24 hr before and 24 hr following chemotherapy.

ROUTE AND DOSAGE

▪ **IV, SC (Adults):** 5 mcg/kg/day as a single injection daily for up to 2 wk, until absolute neutrophil count reaches 10,000 mm^3 following expected nadir of chemotherapy-induced neutropenia. Dosage may be increased by 5 mcg/kg during each cycle of chemotherapy depending on severity of nadir.

PHARMACODYNAMICS

	ONSET	PEAK	DURATION
IV, SC	UK	UK	4 days

NURSING IMPLICATIONS

Assessment

▫ Monitor heart rate, blood pressure, and respiratory status prior to and periodically during therapy.

▫ Assess bone pain throughout therapy. Pain is usually mild to moderate and controllable with nonnarcotic analgesics.

▪ **Lab Test Considerations:** Obtain a CBC and platelet count prior to chemotherapy and twice weekly during therapy to avoid leukocytosis. Monitor absolute neutrophil count (ANC). A transient rise is seen 1–2 days after initiation of therapy, but therapy should not be discontinued until ANC $>10,000/mm^3$.

▫ May cause transient increases in uric acid, LDH, and alkaline phosphatase concentrations.

*Underlines indicate most frequent; **CAPITALS** indicate life-threatening.

F

Potential Nursing Diagnoses
- Infection, high risk for (indications).
- Comfort, altered: pain (side effects).
- Knowledge deficit related to medication regimen (patient/family teaching).

Implementation
- □ Administer no earlier than 24 hr following cytotoxic chemotherapy and not during the 24 hr before administration of chemotherapy.
- □ Refrigerate, do not freeze. Do not shake. May warm to room temperature for up to 6 hr prior to injection. Discard if left at room temperature for >6 hr. Vial is for one time use only.
- **SC:** If dose requires >1 ml of soln, may be divided into two injection sites.

Patient/Family Teaching
- □ Instruct patient on correct technique and proper disposal for home administration. Caution patient not to reuse needle, vial, or syringe. Provide patient with a puncture-proof container for needle and syringe disposal.

Evaluation
Effectiveness of therapy can be demonstrated by: ■ Decreased incidence of infection in patients who receive bone-marrow-depressing antineoplastic agents.

FLECAINIDE
(**flek**-a-nide)
Tambocor

CLASSIFICATION(S):
Antiarrhythmic—class IC
Pregnancy Category C

INDICATIONS
■ Treatment of life-threatening ventricular arrhythmias, including ventricular tachycardia ■ Treatment of supraventricular tachyarrythmias.

ACTION
■ Slows conduction in cardiac tissue by altering transport of ions across cell membranes. **Therapeutic Effect:** ■ Suppression of arrhythmias.

PHARMACOKINETICS
Absorption: Well absorbed from the GI tract following oral administration.
Distribution: Widely distributed.
Metabolism and Excretion: Mostly metabolized by the liver. 30% excreted unchanged by the kidneys.
Half-life: 11–14 hr.

CONTRAINDICATIONS AND PRECAUTIONS
Contraindicated in: ■ Hypersensitivity ■ Cardiogenic shock.
Use Cautiously in: ■ Congestive heart failure (dosage reduction may be required) ■ Pre-existing sinus node dysfunction or 2nd- or 3rd-degree heart block (without a pacemaker) ■ Renal impairment (dosage reduction may be required) ■ Pregnancy, lactation, or children (safety not established).

ADVERSE REACTIONS AND SIDE EFFECTS*
CNS: dizziness, nervousness, headache, fatigue, tremor.
EENT: blurred vision, visual disturbances, diplopia.
Resp: dyspnea, bronchospasm.
CV: ARRHYTHMIAS, congestive heart failure, palpitations, chest pain, edema, ECG changes.
GI: nausea, dyspepsia, vomiting, anorexia.
GU: impotence, urinary retention, polyuria.
Derm: rashes, increased sweating.
MS: myalgia, arthralgia.
Neuro: perioral numbness and paresthesia.
Misc: malaise, fever, swelling of tongue and lips.

INTERACTIONS
Drug-Drug: ■ Additive cardiac effects with other **antiarrhythmics,** including

*Underlines indicate most frequent; **CAPITALS** indicate life-threatening.

calcium channel blockers ▪ **Disopyramide** or **verapamil** may have additive myocardial depressant effects ▪ Increases serum **digoxin** levels by a small amount (15–25%) ▪ Concurrent **beta-adrenergic blocker** therapy may result in increased levels of beta-adrenergic blocker and flecainide ▪ **Alkalinizing agents** promote reabsorption, increase blood levels, and may cause toxicity ▪ **Acidifying agents** increase renal elimination and may decrease effectiveness of flecainide (if urine pH <5) ▪ **Amiodarone** increases flecainide levels and may result in toxicity (flecainide dosage reduction recommended).

Drug–Food: ▪ **Foods that increase urine pH** to >7 result in increased blood levels (strict **vegetarian diet**). ▪ **Foods or beverages that decrease urine pH** to <5 increase renal elimination and may decrease effectiveness of flecainide **(acidic juices)**.

ROUTE AND DOSAGE

- **PO (Adults):** 50–100 mg q 12 hr initially, increased by 50 mg bid until response is obtained or maximum total daily dose of 400 mg is reached.

PHARMACODYNAMICS (antiarrhythmic effects)

	ONSET	PEAK	DURATION
PO	days	days–wks	12 hr

NURSING IMPLICATIONS

Assessment

- □ Monitor ECG or Holter monitor prior to and periodically throughout therapy. May cause QRS widening, PR prolongation, and QT prolongation.
- □ Monitor blood pressure and pulse periodically throughout course of therapy.
- □ Monitor intake and output ratios and daily weight. Assess patient for signs of congestive heart failure (peripheral edema, rales/crackles, dyspnea, weight gain, jugular venous distension).
- ▪ **Lab Test Considerations:** Renal, pulmonary, and hepatic functions and CBC should be evaluated periodically on patients receiving long-term therapy.
- □ May cause elevations in serum alkaline phosphatase during prolonged therapy.
- ▪ **Toxicity and Overdose:** Therapeutic blood levels range from 0.2 to 1.0 mcg/ml.

Potential Nursing Diagnoses

- ▪ Cardiac output, decreased (indications).
- ▪ Knowledge deficit related to medication regimen (patient/family teaching).

Implementation

- ▪ **General Info:** Previous antiarrhythmic therapy (except lidocaine) should be withdrawn 2–4 half-lives before starting flecainide.
- □ Dosage adjustments should be at least 4 days apart due to the long half-life of flecainide.
- ▪ **PO:** May be administered with meals if GI irritation becomes a problem.

Patient/Family Teaching

- □ Instruct patient to take medication around the clock exactly as directed, even if feeling better. Missed doses should be taken as soon as remembered if within 6 hr; omit if remembered later. Gradual dosage reduction may be necessary.
- □ Medication may cause dizziness or visual disturbances. Caution patient to avoid driving and other activities requiring alertness until response to medication is known.
- □ Advise patient to notify physician or dentist of medication regimen prior to treatment or surgery.
- □ Instruct patient to notify physician if chest pain, shortness of breath, or diaphoresis occurs.
- □ Advise patient to carry identification describing disease process and medication regimen at all times.
- □ Emphasize the importance of follow-up examinations to monitor progress.

Evaluation

Effectiveness of therapy can be demonstrated by: ▪ Decrease in frequency of life-threatening ventricular arrhythmias ▪ Decrease in supraventricular tachyarrhythmias.

FLOXURIDINE

(flox-**yoor**-i-deen)
FUDR

CLASSIFICATION(S):
Antineoplastic—antimetabolite
Pregnancy Category UK

INDICATIONS

▪ Treatment of hepatic and gastrointestinal carcinoma. **Unlabeled Uses:** ▪ Carcinoma of: ▫ Breast ▫ Ovary ▫ Cervix ▫ Bladder ▫ Kidney.

ACTION

▪ Inhibits DNA and RNA synthesis by preventing thymidine production (cell cycle-S phase specific). **Therapeutic Effect:** ▪ Death of rapidly replicating cells, particularly malignant ones.

PHARMACOKINETICS

Absorption: Administered intra-arterially only, resulting in direct delivery to tumor sites. Rapidly converted to floxuridine monophosphate (an active metabolite) and fluorouracil.
Distribution: Distributes mostly to tumor site as a result of elective intra-arterial administration.
Metabolism and Excretion: Fluorouracil undergoes cellular inactivation and metabolism by the liver. 60–80% excreted by the lungs as respiratory CO_2. Small amounts of fluorouracil (<10–15%) excreted unchanged by the kidneys.
Half-life: Fluorouracil—20 hr.

CONTRAINDICATIONS AND PRECAUTIONS

Contraindicated in: ▪ Hypersensitivity ▪ Pregnancy or lactation.
Use Cautiously in: ▪ Patients with childbearing potential ▪ Infections ▪ Depressed bone marrow reserve ▪ Other chronic debilitating illnesses.

ADVERSE REACTIONS AND SIDE EFFECTS*

CNS: acute cerebellar dysfunction.
GI: nausea, vomiting, stomatitis, diarrhea.
Derm: alopecia, maculopapular rash, nail loss, melanosis of nails, photo-toxicity.
Endo: gonadal suppression.
Hemat: anemia, leukopenia, thrombocytopenia.
Misc: fever.

INTERACTIONS

Drug-Drug: ▪ Additive bone marrow depression with other **bone marrow depressants** (other **antineoplastics** and **radiation therapy**) ▪ May decrease antibody response to **live virus vaccines** and increase risk of adverse reactions.

ROUTE AND DOSAGE

▪ **Intra-Arterial (Adults):** 0.1–0.6 mg/kg/day as a continuous infusion.

PHARMACODYNAMICS (effects on blood counts)

	ONSET	PEAK	DURATION
Intra-arterial	1–9 days	9–21 days	30 days

NURSING IMPLICATIONS

Assessment

▫ Monitor vital signs prior to and frequently during therapy.
▫ Assess mucous membranes, number and consistency of stools, and frequency of vomiting. Assess for fever, chills, sore throat, and signs of infection. Assess for bleeding (bleeding gums, bruising, petechiae; guaiac stools, urine, and emesis). Avoid IM injections and rectal temperatures. Apply pressure to venipuncture sites for 10 min. Notify physician if symptoms of toxicity (stomatitis or esophagopharyngitis, uncontrollable vomit-

*Underlines indicate most frequent; **CAPITALS** indicate life-threatening.

ing, diarrhea, GI bleeding, leukocyte count <3500/mm³, platelet count <100,000/mm³, hemorrhage from any site, or erythema at catheter insertion site) occur, as drug will need to be discontinued.

- Monitor intake and output, appetite, and nutritional intake. Adjusting diet as tolerated may help maintain fluid and electrolyte balance and nutritional status.
- Assess for abdominal pain, cramping, anorexia, or jaundice with hepatic artery infusion. These symptoms may indicate hepatotoxicity. Heartburn or black tarry stools may indicate dislodgement of catheter.
- Monitor site of intra-arterial infusion for bleeding, localized skin reaction, or impaired circulation, which may indicate catheter displacement.
- **Lab Test Considerations:** Hepatic, renal, and hematologic functions should be monitored prior to and periodically throughout therapy. Notify physician immediately if WBC <3500/mm³ or platelets <100,000/mm³. These are criteria for discontinuation of the medication. Increased serum alkaline phosphatase, SGOT (AST), SGPT (ALT), LDH, and bilirubin may indicate drug-induced hepatotoxicity or biliary sclerosis.
- Interferes with BSP, prothrombin, sedimentation rate assays.

Potential Nursing Diagnoses

- Infection, high risk for (side effects).
- Nutrition, altered: less than body requirements (side effects).
- Knowledge deficit related to medication regimen (patient/family teaching).

Implementation

- **General Info:** Soln should be prepared in a biologic cabinet. Wear gloves, gown, and mask while handling medication. Discard equipment in specially designated containers (see Appendix I).
- **Intra-arterial Infusion Pump:** Reconstitute 5-ml vial with 5 ml of sterile water for injection, to yield concentration of 100 mg/ml. Further dilute in D5W or 0.9% NaC1 to volume required by arterial infusion pump. Stable for 2 wk if refrigerated.
- **Additive Compatibility:** heparin.

Patient/Family Teaching

- Instruct patient to notify physician if fever, chills, sore throat, signs of infection, bleeding gums, bruising, petechiae, blood in urine or stool, jaundice, abdominal pain, local irritation at the site of arterial cannulization, or emesis occurs. Caution patient to avoid crowds and persons with known infections. Instruct patient to use soft toothbrush and electric razor. Patient should be cautioned not to drink alcoholic beverages or take aspirin-containing products.
- Advise patient to rinse mouth with clear water after eating and drinking and to avoid flossing to minimize stomatitis. Physician may order viscous lidocaine if mouth pain interferes with eating.
- Discuss with patient the possibility of hair loss. Explore methods of coping.
- Caution patient to use sunscreen and protective clothing to prevent phototoxicity reactions.
- Instruct patient not to receive any vaccinations without advice of physician.
- Emphasize the importance of routine follow-up lab tests to monitor progress and to check for side effects.
- Review with patient the need for contraception during therapy.

Evaluation

Effectiveness of therapy can be demonstrated by: ■ Tumor size regression.

FLUCONAZOLE

(floo-**kon**-a-zole)
Diflucan

CLASSIFICATION(S):
Antifungal
Pregnancy Category C

F

INDICATIONS

■ Treatment of fungal infections due to susceptible organisms, including: □ Oropharyngeal or esophageal candidiasis □ Serious systemic candidal infections □ Urinary tract infections □ Peritonitis □ Cryptococcal meningitis.

ACTION

■ Inhibits synthesis of fungal sterols, a necessary component of the cell wall. **Therapeutic Effects:** ■ Fungistatic action against susceptible organisms ■ May be fungicidal in higher concentrations. **Spectrum:** ■ Cryptococcus neoforms ■ Candida sp.

PHARMACOKINETICS

Absorption: Well absorbed following oral administration.

Distribution: Widely distributed, good penetration into cerebrospinal fluid, eye, and peritoneum.

Metabolism and Excretion: >80% excreted unchanged by the kidneys. <10% metabolized by the liver.

Half-life: 30 hr (increased in renal impairment).

CONTRAINDICATIONS AND PRECAUTIONS

Contraindicated in: ■ Hypersensitivity to fluconazole or other azole antifungals.

Use Cautiously in: ■ Renal impairment (dosage reduction required) ■ Underlying liver disease ■ Pregnancy, lactation, or children (safety not established).

ADVERSE REACTIONS AND SIDE EFFECTS*

Note: Incidence of adverse reactions is increased in AIDS patients.

CNS: headache.

GI: nausea, vomiting, abdominal discomfort, diarrhea, HEPATOTOXICITY.

Derm: exfoliative skin disorders including STEVENS-JOHNSON SYNDROME.

INTERACTIONS

Drug–Drug: ■ Increases the activity of **warfarin** ■ **Rifampin** decreases blood levels ■ Increases the hypoglycemic effects of **tolbutamide, glyburide,** or **glipizide** ■ Increases blood levels of **cyclosporine** and **phenytoin**.

ROUTE AND DOSAGE

Cryptococcal Meningitis

■ **PO, IV (Adults):** Treatment—400 mg once daily until favorable clinical response, then 200–400 mg once daily for at least 10–12 wk following clearing of cerebrospinal fluid, change to oral therapy as soon as possible. Suppressive therapy—200 mg once daily.

Oropharyngeal Candidiasis

■ **PO, IV (Adults):** 200 mg initially, then 100 mg daily for at least 2 wk.

Esophageal Candidiasis

■ **PO, IV (Adults):** 200 mg initially, then 100 mg once daily for at least 3 wk or 2 wk following symptomatic improvement (up to 400 mg/day has been used).

Systemic Candidiasis

■ **PO, IV (Adults):** 400 mg initially, then 200 mg once daily for 4 wk or at least 2 wk following symptomatic improvement.

PHARMACODYNAMICS (blood levels)

	ONSET	PEAK
PO	UK	1–2 hr
IV	rapid	end of infusion

NURSING IMPLICATIONS

Assessment

□ Assess infected area and monitor cerebrospinal fluid cultures prior to an periodically throughout therapy.

□ Specimens for culture should be taken prior to instituting therapy. Therapy may be started before results are obtained.

■ **Lab Test Considerations:** BUN and serum creatinine should be moni-

*Underlines indicate most frequent; **CAPITALS** indicate life-threatening.

tored prior to and periodically during therapy as patients with renal dysfunction will require dosage adjustment.

- □ Liver function tests should be monitored prior to an periodically throughout course of therapy. May cause increased SGOT (ALT), SGPT (AST), serum alkaline phosphate, and bilirubin concentrations.

Potential Nursing Diagnoses

- ▪ Infection, high risk for (indications).
- ▪ Knowledge deficit related to medication regimen (patient/family teaching).

Implementation

- ▪ **General Info:** Since bioavailability is similar, oral and IV doses are equal.
- ▪ **Intermittent Infusion:** Available in 200 mg/100 ml or 400 mg/200 ml soln. Open overwrap immediately before infusion. Inner bag may have slight opacity that will diminish gradually. Do not administer soln that is cloudy or has a precipitate. Check for leaks by squeezing inner bag. If found, discard container as unsterile.
- □ Do not set tubing as part of a series of connections as this may cause air embolism. Do not admix with other medications.
- □ *Rate:* Infuse at a maximum rate of 200 mg/hr.

Patient/Family Teaching

- □ Instruct patient to take medication exactly as directed, even if feeling better. Doses should be taken at the same time each day. If a dose is missed, take as soon as remembered, but not if almost time for next dose. Do not double doses.
- □ Instruct patient to notify physician if abdominal pain, fever, or diarrhea become pronounced or if signs and symptoms of liver dysfunction (unusual fatigue, anorexia, nausea, vomiting, jaundice, dark urine, or pale stools) occur.

Evaluation

Effectiveness of therapy can be demonstrated by: ▪ Resolution of clinical and laboratory indications of fungal infections. Full course of therapy may require wks or mons of treatment following resolution of symptoms.

FLUCYTOSINE

(floo-**sye**-toe-seen)
Ancobon, {Ancotil}, 5-FC

CLASSIFICATION(S):
Antifungal
Pregnancy Category C

INDICATIONS

▪ Used in the treatment of serious fungal infections including: □ Endocarditis □ Meningitis □ Septicemia □ Urinary tract infections □ Pulmonary infections.

ACTION

▪ Following penetration into fungi, converted to fluorouracil, which interferes with fungal DNA and RNA synthesis ▪ Synergistic action with amphotericin B against some fungi. **Therapeutic Effect:** ▪ Fungicidal action against susceptible organisms. **Spectrum:** ▪ Active against only a small number of fungi, mainly □ *Candida* □ *Cryptococcus*.

PHARMACOKINETICS

Absorption: Well absorbed from the GI tract following oral administration.

Distribution: Widely distributed. Crosses the blood-brain barrier. Crosses the placenta.

Metabolism and Excretion: 80–90% excreted unchanged by the kidneys.

Half-life: 2.5–8 hr (increased in renal impairment).

CONTRAINDICATIONS AND PRECAUTIONS

Contraindicated in: ▪ Hypersensitivity ▪ Pregnancy or lactation.

Use Cautiously in: ▪ Renal impairment (dosage reduction required) ▪ Bone marrow depression (especially

F

following radiation therapy or antineoplastic drugs).

ADVERSE REACTIONS AND SIDE EFFECTS*

CNS: dizziness, lightheadedness, drowsiness, confusion.
GI: nausea, vomiting, diarrhea, bloating.
Hemat: leukopenia, anemia, pancytopenia, thrombocytopenia.

INTERACTIONS

Drug-Drug: ▪ Additive bone marrow depression with other bone marrow depressant drugs, including **antineoplastic agents** and **radiation therapy** ▪ **Amphotericin B** may increase toxicity of flucytosine but may also increase antifungal activity ▪ **Cytarabine** may decrease antifungal activity.

ROUTE AND DOSAGE

- **PO (Adults and Children >50 kg):** 50–200 mg/kg/day in divided doses q 6 hr.
- **PO (Children <50 kg):** 1.5–4.5 g/m^2/day in divided doses q 6 hr.

PHARMACODYNAMICS (antifungal blood levels)

	ONSET	PEAK
PO	rapid	4–6 hr

NURSING IMPLICATIONS

Assessment

- Assess patient for signs and symptoms of systemic fungal infection prior to and periodically throughout therapy.
- Obtain specimens for culture and sensitivity prior to initiating therapy. First dose may be given before receiving results.
- **Lab Test Considerations:** Renal, hepatic, and hematologic functions should be monitored prior to and periodically throughout course of therapy.

Potential Nursing Diagnoses

- Infection, high risk for (indications).
- Fluid volume deficit, potential (adverse reactions).
- Knowledge deficit related to medication regimen (patient/family teaching).

Implementation

- **PO:** To reduce nausea and vomiting, administer capsules a few at a time over 15 min.

Patient/Family Teaching

- Advise patient to take medication exactly as directed, even if feeling better. Missed doses should be taken as soon as remembered, if not almost time for next dose; do not double doses.
- May cause dizziness, lightheadedness, or drowsiness. Caution patient to avoid driving and other activities requiring alertness until response to medication is known.
- Instruct patient to notify physician promptly if rash, fever, sore throat, diarrhea, unusual bleeding or bruising, unusual tiredness, or weakness occur.
- Emphasize the importance of follow-up examinations to determine effectiveness of treatment.

Evaluation

Effectiveness of therapy can be demonstrated by: ▪ Resolution of the signs and symptoms of fungal infection. Duration of therapy is generally 4–6 wk but may continue for several mons.

FLUDARABINE

(floo-**dar**-a-been)
Fludara

CLASSIFICATION(S):
Antineoplastic—antimetabolite
Pregnancy Category D

*Underlines indicate most frequent; **CAPITALS** indicate life-threatening.

INDICATIONS

▪ Treatment of B-cell chronic lymphocytic leukemia unresponsive to standard therapy. **Unlabeled Use:** ▪ Treatment of non-Hodgkin's lymphoma.

ACTION

▪ Converted intracellularly to an active phosphorylated metabolite that inhibits DNA synthesis. **Therapeutic Effect:** ▪ Death of rapidly replicating cells, particularly malignant ones.

PHARMACOKINETICS

Absorption: Administered IV only, resulting in complete bioavailability.
Distribution: Distribution not known.
Metabolism and Excretion: Following administration, rapidly converted to an active metabolite, which when phosphorylated intracellularly exerts antineoplastic activity. 23% of initial active metabolite excreted unchanged by the kidneys.
Half-life: 10 hr (for initial active metabolite).

CONTRAINDICATIONS AND PRECAUTIONS

Contraindicated in: ▪ Hypersensitivity to fludarabine, mannitol, or sodium hydroxide ▪ Pregnancy or lactation.
Use Cautiously in: ▪ Renal impairment (dosage reduction may be necessary) ▪ Patients with childbearing potential ▪ Bone marrow depression ▪ Chronic debilitating illness ▪ Children (safety not established).

ADVERSE REACTIONS AND SIDE EFFECTS*

CNS: NEUROTOXICITY, malaise, fatigue, weakness, agitation, confusion, visual disturbances, coma.
Resp: pulmonary hypersensitivity, cough, dyspnea.
CV: edema.
GI: nausea, vomiting, anorexia, diarrhea, GI bleeding, stomatitis.
Derm: rashes.
Endo: gonadal suppression.
Hemat: anemia, leukopenia, thrombocytopenia.
MS: myalgia.
Neuro: peripheral neuropathy.
Misc: tumor lysis syndrome.

INTERACTIONS

Drug-Drug: ▪ Additive bone marrow suppression with other **antineoplastic agents** or **radiation therapy** ▪ May decrease antibody response to **live virus vaccines** and increase the risk of adverse reactions.

ROUTE AND DOSAGE

▪ **IV (Adults):** 25 mg/m^2 daily for 5 days, repeat course every 28 days.

PHARMACODYNAMICS (effects on blood counts)

	ONSET	PEAK	DURATION
IV	UK	13–16 days	UK

NURSING IMPLICATIONS

Assessment

- ▫ Assess patient for visual changes, weakness, confusion, and changes in level of consciousness throughout and for 60 days following therapy as neurologic effects resulting in blindness, coma, and death have been reported.
- ▫ Assess for fever, sore throat, and signs of infection. If these symptoms occur notify physician immediately.
- ▫ Assess for bleeding (bleeding gums, bruising, petechiae, guaiac stools, urine, emesis). Avoid IM injections and rectal temperatures. Hold pressure on all venipuncture sites for at least 10 min.
- ▫ Monitor respiratory status, intake and output ratios, and daily weights. Notify physician if significant changes occur.
- ▫ Assess nutritional status. Administering an antiemetic prior to and periodically throughout therapy and adjusting diet as tolerated may help

*Underlines indicate most frequent; **CAPITALS** indicate life-threatening.

F

maintain fluid and electrolyte balance and nutritional status.

- Anemia may occur. Monitor for increased fatigue, dyspnea, and orthostatic hypotension.
- May cause tumor lysis syndrome resulting in hyperuricemia, hyperphosphatemia, hypocalcemia, metabolic acidosis, hyperkalemia, hematuria, urate crystalluria, and renal failure. Monitor for flank pain and hematuria.
- **Lab Test Considerations:** Monitor CBC, differential, and platelet counts prior to and frequently throughout therapy. The nadir for granulocytes occurs in 13 days (range 3–25 days) and for platelets in 16 days (range 2–32 days) after administration.

POTENTIAL NURSING DIAGNOSES

- Infection, high risk for (adverse reactions).
- Injury, high risk for (side effects).
- Knowledge deficit related to medication regimen (patient/family teaching).

IMPLEMENTATION

- **General Info:** Soln should be prepared in a biologic cabinet. Wear gloves, gown, and mask while handling IV medication. Discard IV equipment in specially designated containers (see Appendix I).
- **IV:** Reconstitute with 2 ml of sterile water for injection; solid cake should dissolve in <15 sec. Reconstituted soln is stable for 8 hr.
- **Intermittent Infusion:** Dilute further in 100–125 ml of 0.9% NaCl or D5W.
- *Rate:* Infuse over 30 min.

PATIENT/FAMILY TEACHING

- Caution patient to avoid crowds and persons with known infections. Physician should be informed immediately if symptoms of infection occur.
- Instruct patient to report unusual bleeding. Advise patient of thrombocytopenia precautions (use soft toothbrush, electric razor, and avoid falls.) Do not drink alcoholic beverages or take medication containing aspirin, as these may precipitate gastric bleeding.
- Instruct patient to inspect oral mucosa for redness and ulceration. If mouth sores occur advise patient to use sponge brush and rinse mouth with water after eating and drinking. Consult physician if pain interferes with eating.
- Advise patient that this medication may have teratogenic effects. Contraception should be practiced during therapy and for at least 4 mon after therapy is concluded.
- Instruct patient not to receive any vaccinations without advice of physician.
- Emphasize the need for periodic lab tests to monitor for side effects.

EVALUATION

Effectiveness of therapy can be demonstrated by: ▪ Improvement of hematopoietic values in leukemias ▪ Decrease in size and spread of the tumor in non-Hodgkin's lymphomas. The 5-day course of therapy is continued every 28 days until patient is in complete remission, or neurotoxicity occurs.

FLUDROCORTISONE

(floo-droe-**kor**-ti-sone)
Florinef

CLASSIFICATION(S):
Mineralocorticoid
Pregnancy Category UK

INDICATIONS

▪ Management of sodium loss and hypotension associated with adrenocortical insufficiency in conjunction with hydrocortisone or cortisone ▪ Management of sodium loss due to congenital adrenogenital syndrome (congenital adrenal hyperplasia).

ACTION

▪ Causes sodium reabsorption, hydrogen and potassium excretion, and water retention by its effects on the distal renal tubule. **Therapeutic Effects:** ▪ Maintenance of sodium balance and blood pressure in patients with adrenocortical insufficiency.

PHARMACOKINETICS

Absorption: Well absorbed following oral administration.
Distribution: Appears to be widely distributed; probably enters breast milk.
Metabolism and Excretion: Mostly metabolized by the liver.
Half-life: 3.5 hr.

CONTRAINDICATIONS AND PRECAUTIONS

Contraindicated in: ▪ Hypersensitivity.
Use Cautiously in: ▪ Congestive heart failure ▪ Addison's disease (patients may have exaggerated response) ▪ Pregnancy, lactation, or children (safety not established).

ADVERSE REACTIONS AND SIDE EFFECTS*

CNS: headaches, dizziness.
CV: edema, congestive heart failure, hypertension, arrhythmias.
GI: nausea, anorexia.
Endo: weight gain, adrenal suppression.
F and E: hypokalemia, hypokalemic alkalosis.
MS: arthralgia, tendon contractures, muscular weakness.
Neuro: ascending paralysis.
Misc: hypersensitivity reactions.

INTERACTIONS

Drug–Drug: ▪ Use with **diuretics, mezlocillin, piperacillin,** or **amphotericin B** may result in exaggerated hypokalemia ▪ Hypokalemia may increase the risk of **cardiac glycoside** toxicity ▪ May produce prolonged neuromuscular blockade following the use of **nondepolarizing neuromuscular blocking agents** ▪ **Phenobarbital** or **rifampin** may increase the metabolism and may decrease the effectiveness of fludrocortisone.
Drug–Food: ▪ Ingestion of large amounts of **salt** or **sodium-containing foods** may cause excessive sodium retention and potassium loss.

ROUTE AND DOSAGE

- **PO (Adults):** 0.1 mg/day (range 0.1 mg 3 times weekly–0.2 mg daily). Doses as small as 0.05 mg daily may be required by some patients. Use with 10–37.5 mg cortisone daily or 10–30 mg hydrocortisone daily.

PHARMACODYNAMICS (mineralocorticoid activity)

	ONSET	PEAK	DURATION
PO	UK	UK	1–2 days

NURSING IMPLICATIONS

Assessment

- ▫ Monitor blood pressure periodically throughout course of therapy. Inform physician of significant changes. Hypotension may indicate insufficient dosage.
- ▫ Monitor for fluid retention (weigh daily, assess for edema, and auscultate lungs for rales/crackles).
- **Lab Test Considerations:** Monitor serum electrolytes periodically throughout therapy. Fludrocortisone causes decreased serum potassium levels.

Potential Nursing Diagnoses

- Fluid volume deficit (indications).
- Fluid volume excess (side effects).
- Knowledge deficit related to medication regimen (patient/family teaching).

Implementation

- **PO:** Tablets are scored and may be broken if dosage adjustment is necessary.

Patient/Family Teaching

- ▫ Instruct patient to take medication exactly as directed. If a dose is missed, take as soon as remembered but not just before next dose is due. Explain that lifelong therapy is necessary and that abrupt discontinuation may lead to Addisonian crisis. Patient should keep an adequate supply available at all times.

*Underlines indicate most frequent; **CAPITALS** indicate life-threatening.

F

- Advise patient to follow dietary modification prescribed by physician. Instruct patient to follow a diet high in potassium (see Appendix K). Amount of sodium allowed in diet varies with pathophysiology.
- Instruct patient to inform physician if weight gain or edema, muscle weakness, cramps, nausea, anorexia, or dizziness occurs.
- Advise patient to carry identification describing disease process and medication regimen at all times.

EVALUATION

Effectiveness of therapy can be demonstrated by: ▪ Normalization of fluid and electrolyte balance without the development of hypokalemia or hypertension.

FLUNISOLIDE

(floo-**nis**-oh-lide)

Aerobid, Nasalide, {Rhinalar}

CLASSIFICATION(S):

Glucocorticoid–long-acting, Anti-inflammatory

Pregnancy Category C

INDICATIONS

▪ **Inhaln:** Anti-inflammatory and immunosuppressant in the treatment of chronic steroid-dependent asthma. May decrease requirement for or avoid use of systemic glucocorticoids ▪ **Intranasal:** Used in the management of allergic rhinitis and other chronic nasal inflammatory conditions, including nasal polyps.

ACTION

▪ Potent, locally acting anti-inflammatory and immune modifier. **Therapeutic Effects:** ▪ Decrease in symptoms of chronic asthma and allergic rhinitis.

PHARMACOKINETICS

Absorption: Action following inhalant is mostly local. Additional drug may be swallowed, but systemic bioavailability is minimal at recommended doses. Readily absorbed following nasal inhalant.

Distribution: Distribution not known.

Metabolism and Excretion: Mostly metabolized by the liver.

Half-life: 1–2 hr.

CONTRAINDICATIONS AND PRECAUTIONS

Contraindicated in: ▪ Hypersensitivity ▪ Hypersensitivity to fluorocarbon propellants (inhaler only) ▪ Acute attacks of asthma or allergic rhinitis.

Use Cautiously in: ▪ Nasal ulcers (intranasal form) ▪ Untreated bacterial, viral, or fungal infections ▪ Chronic treatment at higher-than-recommended doses may lead to adrenal suppression ▪ Systemic glucocorticoid therapy should not be abruptly discontinued when inhalation or intranasal therapy is started ▪ Pregnancy, lactation, or children <6 yr (safety not established).

ADVERSE REACTIONS AND SIDE EFFECTS*

CNS: headache, dizziness.

EENT: Nasal—nasal burning, nasal irritation, nasal bleeding, sneezing attacks; Inhaln—oropharyngeal fungal infections.

Resp: Inhaln—wheezing, bronchospasm.

GI: Nasal—nausea, vomiting, abdominal bloating.

Misc: ADRENAL SUPPRESSION at greater than recommended doses.

INTERACTIONS

Drug-Drug: ▪ None significant at recommended doses.

ROUTE AND DOSAGE

Note: Inhaler provides 250 mcg flunisolide/spray; nasal spray provides 25 mcg/spray.

- **Inhaln (Adults):** 2 sprays bid (not to exceed 4 sprays bid).

{} = Available in Canada only.

*Underlines indicate most frequent; **CAPITALS** indicate life-threatening.

- **Inhaln (Children 4–15 yr):** 2 sprays bid (not to exceed 2 sprays bid).
- **Nasal (Adults):** 2 sprays in each nostril bid, may be increased to 3 sprays in each nostril bid (not to exceed 8 sprays in each nostril daily). Attempts should be made to decrease dose to lowest amount required to control symptoms.
- **Nasal (Children 6–14 yr):** 1 spray in each nostril tid, or 2 sprays in each nostril bid (not to exceed 4 sprays in each nostril daily). Attempts should be made to decrease dose to lowest amount required to control symptoms.

PHARMACODYNAMICS

	ONSET	PEAK	DURATION
Inhaln	UK	1–4 wk	UK
Nasal	2–3 days	2–3 wk	UK

NURSING IMPLICATIONS

Assessment

- **General Info:** Assess patients changing from systemic glucocorticoids to flunisolide for signs of adrenal insufficiency (anorexia, nausea, weakness, fatigue, hypotension, hypoglycemia) during initial therapy. If these signs appear, notify physician immediately. This can be life-threatening.
- **Asthma:** Assess breathing pattern and lung sounds periodically throughout therapy. Alternative therapy is indicated for relief of an acute asthmatic attack.
- **Rhinitis:** Monitor degree of nasal stuffiness, amount and color of nasal discharge, and frequency of sneezing.
- **Lab Test Considerations:** Periodic adrenal function tests may be ordered in chronic therapy to assess degree of hypothalamic-pituitary-adrenal (HPA) axis suppression.

Potential Nursing Diagnoses

- Airway clearance, ineffective (indications).
- Infection, high risk for (side effects).
- Knowledge deficit related to medication regimen (patient/family teaching).

Implementation

- **General Info:** Available as nasal spray or in metered-dose inhaler.
- **Nasal Spray:** Patient also using topical decongestant should be given decongestant 5–15 min before flunisolide. Instruct patient to blow nose gently, if unable to breathe freely through nasal passages, in advance of medication administration.
- **Inhaln:** Patients also using inhalation bronchodilators should be given bronchodilator 5 min before administering flunisolide.
- □ Allow at least 1-2 min between inhalations of aerosol medication.

Patient/Family Teaching

- **General Info:** Advise patient to take medication exactly as directed. If a dose is missed, take as soon as remembered unless almost time for next dose.
- □ Advise patient to carry identification in the event of an emergency in which patient cannot relate medical history.
- □ Caution patient to avoid smoking, known allergens, and other respiratory irritants.
- **Metered-dose Inhaler:** Caution patient not to exceed recommended dose. Maximum dosage for adults is 4 per day.
- □ Instruct patient in proper use of metered-dose inhaler. Shake well, exhale, close lips firmly around mouthpiece, administer during second half of inhalation, and hold breath as long as possible after treatment to ensure deep instillation of medication. Do not take more than 2 inhalations at one time; allow 1–2 min between inhalations. Wash inhalation assembly at least daily in warm running water.
- □ Advise patient to rinse mouth and gargle with water after each dose of inhaler to minimize throat irritation and *Candida* infection.
- □ Explain need for continued medical follow-up to assess effectiveness and

F

possible side effects of medication. Physician may order periodic pulmonary function tests.

- Instruct patient to inform physician if symptoms of asthma attack or oral infection occur.

- **Nasal Spray:** Caution patient not to exceed maximal daily dose of 8 sprays per nostril for adults or 4 sprays for children <14 yr.
  - Instruct patient in correct technique for administering nasal spray. Press gently with finger to occlude one naris. Insert tip of applicator into other nostril and spray while gently inhaling. Warn patient that temporary nasal stinging may occur.
  - Instruct patient to notify physician if symptoms do not improve within 1 mon or if nasal discharge becomes purulent.

Evaluation

Effectiveness of therapy can be demonstrated by: ▪ Prevention of bronchospasm in asthma ▪ Resolution of nasal stuffiness, discharge, and sneezing in seasonal or perennial rhinitis.

FLUOROMETHALONE

(flure-oh-**meth**-oh-lone)
Fluor-Op, FML Fotre, FML Liquifilm, FML S.O.P.

CLASSIFICATION(S):
Ophthalmic—anti-inflammatory
Pregnancy Category C

INDICATIONS

▪ Inflammatory and allergic conditions of the ▫ Conjunctiva ▫ Cornea ▫ Anterior segment of the globe.

ACTION

▪ Potent locally acting anti-inflammatory and immune modifier. **Therapeutic Effects:** ▪ Local suppression of inflammation and immune responses, including relief of discomfort and itching.

PHARMACOKINETICS

Absorption: Systemic absorption may occur with prolonged use of large doses, especially in children.
Distribution: Following ophthalmic administration, distributes into aqueous humor, cornea, iris, choroid, ciliary body, and retina.
Metabolism and Excretion: UK.
Half-life: UK.

CONTRAINDICATIONS AND PRECAUTIONS

Contraindicated in: ▪ Ocular fungal infections ▪ Acute superficial herpes keratitis ▪ Ocular tuberculosis ▪ Degenerative ocular disorders ▪ Acute viral disease (infectious stage) ▪ Hypersensitivity to vehicle or preservatives (phenylmercuric acetate, benzalkonium chloride).
Use Cautiously in: ▪ Cataracts ▪ Diabetes mellitus ▪ Glaucoma (may increase intraocular pressure) ▪ Children <2 yr (safety not established) ▪ Corneal or scleral thinning (may increase risk of perforation).

ADVERSE REACTIONS AND SIDE EFFECTS*

CNS: headache.
EENT: burning, stinging, watering of eyes, eye pain, seeing halos around objects, drooping of eyelids, unusually large pupils, blurred vision.
Endo: adrenal suppression (chronic use of large doses).

INTERACTIONS

Drug-Drug: ▪ **Cyloplegic** and **mydriatic agents,** including **atropine,** may result in additive increase in intraocular pressure ▪ May decrease the efficacy of **antiglaucoma agents.**

ROUTE AND DOSAGE

- **Ophth (Adults):** Thin strip of 0.1% oint 1–3 times daily or 1–2 drops of 0.15% or 0.25% susp 2–4 times daily (may use 1–2 drops q 1 hr initially, decreasing dose as inflammation decreases).

*Underlines indicate most frequent; **CAPITALS** indicate life-threatening.

PHARMACODYNAMICS (anti-inflammatory activity)

	ONSET	PEAK	DURATION
Ophth	min–hr	hr–days	1–12 hr

NURSING IMPLICATIONS

Assessment

- Monitor patient for changes in vision, eye irritation, or persistent headache. Notify physician if signs of infection develop.

Potential Nursing Diagnoses

- Infection, high risk for (side effects).
- Sensory-perceptual alteration: visual (indications).
- Knowledge deficit related to medication regimen (patient/family teaching).

Implementation

- **General Info:** Drops are available in 2 concentrations. Carefully check percentage on label prior to administration.
- **Ophth Drops:** Shake suspension prior to administration. Have patient tilt head back and look up, gently depress lower lid with index finger until conjunctival sac is exposed, and instill medication. Wait at least 5 min before instilling other types of eyedrops.
- **Ophth Oint:** Apply ½-in ribbon of ointment to lower conjunctival sac. Instruct patient to close eye gently and roll eyeball around in all directions. Close cap tightly after use.

Patient/Family Teaching

- **General Info:** Instruct patient on correct technique of medication administration. Medication should be taken exactly as directed. If a dose is missed, take as soon as remembered unless almost time for next dose.
- Instruct patient on correct method of application of drops or ointment. Do not touch cap or tip of container to eye, fingers, or any surface.
- Advise patient to notify physician if improvement is not seen in 5–7 days or if condition worsens.
- Instruct patient to discuss with physician use of contact lens while receiving fluorometholone. Contact lenses may increase risk of eye infections; physician usually recommends use of glasses throughout therapy.
- Instruct patient to notify physician if persistent blurred vision, persistent eye irritation, eye or brow ache, halos around lights, or eyelid drooping occur.
- Advise patient of the need for regular eye examinations to monitor intraocular pressure and visual status.
- **Oint:** Advise patient that vision will be blurred. Advise patient to avoid driving or other activities requiring visual acuity while vision is impaired.

Evaluation

Effectiveness of therapy can be demonstrated by: ▪ Suppression of ocular inflammation.

FLUOROURACIL

(flure-oh-**yoor**-a-sill)
Adrucil, Efudex, Fluoroplex, 5-FU

CLASSIFICATION(S):
Antineoplastic—antimetabolite
Pregnancy Category UK

INDICATIONS

▪ Used alone and in combination with other modalities (surgery, radiation therapy, other antineoplastic agents) in the treatment of: ▫ Colon ▫ Breast ▫ Rectal ▫ Gastric ▫ Pancreatic carcinoma ▪ Used topically in the management of multiple actinic (solar) keratoses.

ACTION

▪ Inhibits DNA and RNA synthesis by preventing thymidine production (cell cycle-S phase specific). **Therapeutic Effect:** ▪ Death of rapidly replicating cells, particularly malignant ones.

PHARMACOKINETICS

Absorption: Minimal absorption (5–10%) following topical application.

F

Distribution: Widely distributed. Concentrates and persists in tumors.
Metabolism and Excretion: Converted to floxuridine monophosphate (an active metabolite). Undergoes cellular inactivation and metabolism by the liver. 60–80% excreted by lungs as respiratory CO_2. Small amounts (<10–15%) excreted unchanged by the kidneys.
Half-life: 20 hr.

CONTRAINDICATIONS AND PRECAUTIONS

Contraindicated in: ▪ Hypersensitivity ▪ Pregnancy or lactation.
Use Cautiously in: ▪ Patients with childbearing potential ▪ Infections ▪ Depressed bone marrow reserve ▪ Other chronic debilitating illnesses.

ADVERSE REACTIONS AND SIDE EFFECTS*

CNS: acute cerebellar dysfunction.
GI: nausea, vomiting, stomatitis, diarrhea.
Derm: alopecia, maculopapular rash, nail loss, melanosis of nails, phototoxicity.
Endo: gonadal suppression.
Hemat: anemia, leukopenia, thrombocytopenia.
Local: thrombophlebitis.
Misc: fever.

INTERACTIONS

Drug–Drug: ▪ Additive bone marrow depression with other **bone marrow depressants** (other **antineoplastics** and **radiation therapy**) ▪ May decrease antibody response to **live virus vaccines** and increase risk of adverse reactions.

ROUTE AND DOSAGE

Note: Doses may vary greatly, depending on tumor, patient condition, and protocol use.

- **IV (Adults):** 12 mg/kg/day for days 1–4, then 6 mg/kg on days 6, 8, 10, and 12; can be repeated 30 days after last dose as maintenance or as weekly maintenance dose of 10–15 mg/kg, not to exceed 1 g/wk (no single daily dose should exceed 800 mg). **Poor-risk patients:** 6 mg/kg/day on days 1–3, 3 mg/kg/day on days 5, 7, 9 (not to exceed 400 mg/dose).
- **Top (Adults):** 1% or 2% soln or cream bid to lesion on head or neck, 5% soln or cream bid to other areas.

PHARMACODYNAMICS (IV = effects on blood counts, Top = dermatologic effects)

	ONSET	PEAK	DURATION
IV	1–9 days	9–21 days (nadir)	30 days
Top	2–3 days	2–6 wk	1–2 mon

NURSING IMPLICATIONS

Assessment

- **General Info:** Monitor vital signs prior to and frequently during therapy.
- Assess mucous membranes, number and consistency of stools, and frequency of vomiting. Assess for fever, chills, sore throat, and signs of infection. Assess for bleeding (bleeding gums, bruising, petechiae; guaiac stools, urine, and emesis). Avoid IM injections and rectal temperatures. Apply pressure to venipuncture sites for 10 min. Notify physician if symptoms of toxicity (stomatitis or esophagopharyngitis, uncontrollable vomiting, diarrhea, GI bleeding, leukocyte count <3500/mm^3, platelet count <100,000/mm^3, or hemorrhage from any site) occur, as drug will need to be discontinued.
- Assess IV site frequently for inflammation or infiltration. Patient should notify nurse if pain or irritation at injection site occurs. May cause thrombophlebitis. If extravasation occurs, infusion must be stopped and restarted in another vein to avoid damage to SC tissue. Notify physician immediately. Standard treatment includes application of ice compresses.
- Monitor intake and output, appetite, and nutritional intake. GI effects usually occur on fourth day of therapy.

*Underlines indicate most frequent; CAPITALS indicate life-threatening.

Adjusting diet as tolerated may help maintain fluid and electrolyte balance and nutritional status.

- Monitor patient for cerebellar dysfunction (weakness, ataxia, dizziness). This may persist after discontinuation of therapy.
- **Top:** Inspect involved skin prior to and throughout course of therapy.
- **Lab Test Considerations:** May cause a decrease in plasma albumin.
- Hepatic, renal, and hematologic functions should be monitored prior to and periodically throughout therapy. CBC should be monitored daily during IV therapy. Notify physician immediately if WBC $<3500/mm^3$ or platelets $<100,000/mm^3$. These are criteria for discontinuation of the medication. Leukopenia usually occurs in 9–14 days, nadir in 21–25 days, with recovery by day 30. May also cause thrombocytopenia (nadir 7–17 days).

Potential Nursing Diagnoses

- Infection, high risk for (side effects).
- Nutrition, altered: less than body requirements (side effects).
- Knowledge deficit related to medication regimen (patient/family teaching).

Implementation

- **General Info:** Soln for IV administration should be prepared in a biologic cabinet. Wear gloves, gown, and mask while handling IV medication. Discard IV equipment in specially designated containers (see Appendix I).
- The number 5 in 5-fluorouracil is part of the drug name and does not refer to the dosage.
- **Direct IV:** Rapid IV push administration (over 1–2 min) is most effective, but there is a more rapid onset of toxicity.
- **Intermittent Infusion:** May be diluted with D5W or 0.9% Nacl.
- Use plastic IV tubing and IV bags to maintain greater stability of medication. Soln is stable for 24 hr at room temperature; do not refrigerate. Manufacturer does not recommend admixing. Discard highly discolored or cloudy soln. If crystals form, dissolve by warming soln to 140°F, shaking vigorously, and cooling to body temperature.
- *Rate:* Onset of toxicity is greatly delayed by administering an infusion over 2–8 hr.
- **Syringe Compatibility:** bleomycin, cisplatin, cyclophosphamide, doxorubicin, furosemide, heparin, leucovorin, methotrexate, metoclopramide, mitomycin, vinblastine, or vincristine. Mix immediately before use.
- **Syringe Incompatibility:** droperidol.
- **Y-Site Compatibility:** bleomycin, cisplatin, cyclophosphamide, doxorubicin, furosemide, heparin, leucovorin, methotrexate, metoclopramide, mitomycin, vinblastine, or vincristine. Mix immediately before use.
- **Y-Site Incompatibility:** droperidol.
- **Additive Compatibility:** D5/LR, bleomycin, cephalothin, prednisolone, or vincristine.
- **Additive Incompatibility:** cisplatin, cytarabine, diazepam, or doxorubicin.
- **Top:** Consult physician before administering topical preparations, to determine what skin preparation regimen should be followed. Tight occlusive dressings are not advised because of irritation to surrounding healthy tissue. A loose gauze dressing for cosmetic purposes is usually preferred. Wear gloves when applying medication. Do not use metallic applicator.

Patient/Family Teaching

- **General Info:** Instruct patient to notify physician if fever, chills, sore throat, signs of infection, bleeding gums, bruising, petechiae, blood in urine or stool, or emesis occurs. Caution patient to avoid crowds and persons with known infections. Instruct patient to use soft toothbrush and electric razor. Patients should be cautioned not to drink alcoholic beverages or take aspirin-containing products.

- Advise patient to rinse mouth with clear water after eating and drinking and to avoid flossing to minimize stomatitis.
- Discuss with patient the possibility of hair loss. Explore methods of coping.
- Caution patient to use sunscreen and protective clothing to prevent phototoxicity reactions.
- Instruct patient not to receive any vaccinations without advice of physician.
- Emphasize the importance of routine follow-up lab tests to monitor progress and to check for side effects.
- Review with patient the need for contraception during therapy.
- **Top:** Instruct patient in correct application of soln or cream. Emphasize importance of avoiding the eyes; caution should also be used when applying medication near mouth and nose. If patient uses clean finger to self-administer, emphasize importance of washing hands thoroughly after application. Explain that erythema, scaling, and blistering with pruritus and burning sensation are expected. Therapy is discontinued when erosion, ulceration, and necrosis occur in 2–6 wk (10–12 wk for basal cell carcinomas). Skin heals 4–8 wk later.

Evaluation

Effectiveness of therapy can be demonstrated by: ▪ Tumor size regression ▪ Removal of solar keratoses or superficial basal cell skin cancers.

FLUOXETINE

(floo-**ox**-uh-teen)
Prozac

CLASSIFICATION(S):
Antidepressant
Pregnancy Category B

INDICATIONS

▪ Treatment of various forms of depression, often in conjunction with psychotherapy.

ACTION

▪ Inhibits the upake of serotonin in the CNS. **Therapeutic Effect:** ▪ Antidepressant action.

PHARMACOKINETICS

Absorption: Well absorbed following oral administration.
Distribution: Crosses the blood-brain barrier well.
Metabolism and Excretion: Converted by the liver to norfluoxetine, another antidepressant compound; fluoxetine and norfluoxetine are mostly metabolized by the liver. 12% excreted by kidneys as unchanged fluoxetine, 7% as unchanged norfluoxetine.
Half-life: 1–3 days (norfluoxetine 5–7 days).

CONTRAINDICATIONS AND PRECAUTIONS

Contraindicated in: ▪ Hypersensitivity.
Use Cautiously in: ▪ Severe hepatic or renal impairment (dosage adjustment may be necessary) ▪ Pregnancy, lactation, or children (safety not established) ▪ History of seizures ▪ Debilitated patients (increased risk of seizures) ▪ Diabetes mellitus ▪ Eating disorders (anorexia, bulimia).

ADVERSE REACTIONS AND SIDE EFFECTS*

CNS: SEIZURES, anxiety, nervousness, insomnia, headache, drowsiness, tremor, dizziness, fatigue, mania, hypomania, weakness, abnormal dreams.
EENT: visual disturbances, stuffy nose.
CV: palpitations, chest pain.
Endo: dysmenorrhea.
GI: anorexia, weight loss, nausea, diarrhea, dry mouth, dyspepsia, constipation, abdominal pain, abnormal taste, vomiting.
GU: urinary frequency.
Derm: rashes, excessive sweating, pruritus, flushing.
MS: back pain, arthralgia, myalgia.
Neuro: trembling.

*Underlines indicate most frequent; **CAPITALS** indicate life-threatening.

Resp: cough.
Misc: flu-like syndrome, fever, hot flashes, sexual dysfunction, sensitivity reaction.

INTERACTIONS

Drug–Drug: ▪ Additive CNS depression with **alcohol, antihistamines,** other **antidepressants, narcotic analgesics,** or **sedative/hypnotics** ▪ May prolong the effect of **diazepam** ▪ Discontinue use of **MAO inhibitors** for 14 days prior to fluoxetine therapy; combined therapy may result in confusion, agitation, seizures, hypertension, hyperpyrexia. Fluoxetine should be discontinued for at least 5 wk before therapy is initiated ▪ Increased risk of side effects and adverse reactions with other **antidepressants** or **phenothiazines** ▪ May increase effectiveness/risk of toxicity of **digitoxin, lithium,** or **oral anticoagulants.**

ROUTE AND DOSAGE

- **PO (Adults):** 20 mg/day in the morning. May increase by 20 mg/day; doses greater than 20 mg/day should be given in 2 divided doses, 1 in the morning and 1 at noon (not to exceed 80 mg/day).

PHARMACODYNAMICS (antidepressant effect)

	ONSET	PEAK	DURATION
PO	1 to 4 wk	UK	2 wk

NURSING IMPLICATIONS

Assessment

- ▫ Monitor mood changes. Inform physician if patient demonstrates significant increase in anxiety, nervousness, or insomnia.
- ▫ Assess for suicidal tendencies, especially during early therapy. Restrict amount of drug available to patient.
- ▫ Monitor appetite and nutritional intake. Weigh weekly. Notify physician of continued weight loss. Adjust diet as tolerated to support nutritional status.
- ▫ Assess patient for possible sensitivity reaction (urticaria, fever, arthralgia, edema, carpal tunnel syndrome, rash, lymphadenopathy, respiratory distress) and notify physician if present; these symptoms usually resolve by stopping fluoxetine but may require administration of antihistamines or glucocorticoids.
- ▪ **Lab Test Considerations:** Monitor CBC and differential periodically during course of therapy. Notify physician if leukopenia, anemia, thrombocytopenia, or increased bleeding time occurs.
- ▫ Proteinuria and mild increase in SGOT (AST) may occur during sensitivity reactions.

Potential Nursing Diagnoses

- ▪ Coping, ineffective individual (indications).
- ▪ Injury, high risk for (side effects).
- ▪ Knowledge deficit related to medication regimen (patient/family teaching).

Implementation

- ▪ **PO:** Administer as a single dose in the morning. Some patients may require increased amounts, in divided doses.

Patient/Family Teaching

- ▫ Instruct patient to take fluoxetine exactly as directed. If a dose is missed, omit dose and return to regular dosing schedule. Do not double doses.
- ▫ May cause drowsiness, dizziness, impaired judgment, and blurred vision. Caution patient to avoid driving and other activities requiring alertness until response to the drug is known.
- ▫ Advise patient to avoid alcohol or other CNS depressant drugs during therapy and to consult with physician before taking other medications with fluoxetine.
- ▫ Inform patient that frequent mouth rinses, good oral hygiene, and sugarless gum or candy may minimize dry mouth. If dry mouth persists for more than 2 wk, consult physician or dentist regarding use of saliva substitute.
- ▫ Instruct female patient to inform physician if pregnancy is planned or suspected.

F

□ Advise patient to notify physician if symptoms of sensitivity reaction occur. Patient should also inform physician if headache, nausea, anorexia, anxiety, or insomnia persist.
□ Emphasize the importance of follow-up examinations to monitor progress. Encourage patient participation in psychotherapy.

EVALUATION

Effectiveness of therapy can be demonstrated by: ▪ Increased sense of well-being □ Renewed interest in surroundings. May require 1–4 wk of therapy to obtain antidepressant effects.

FLUPHENAZINE
(floo-**fen**-a-zeen)
{Apo-Fluphenazine}, {Modicate}, {Moditen}, Permitil, Prolixin

CLASSIFICATION(S):
Antipsychotic—phenothiazine
Pregnancy Category UK

INDICATIONS

▪ Treatment of acute and chronic psychoses.

ACTION

▪ Alters the effects of dopamine in the CNS ▪ Possesses anticholinergic and alpha-adrenergic blocking activity. **Therapeutic Effect:** ▪ Diminished signs and symptoms of psychoses.

PHARMACOKINETICS

Absorption: Well absorbed following oral and IM administration. Decanoate and enanthate salts in sesame oil have delayed onset and prolonged action due to delayed release from oil vehicle and subsequent delayed release from fatty tissues.

Distribution: Widely distributed. Crosses the blood-brain barrier. Crosses the placenta and enters breast milk.

Metabolism and Excretion: Highly metabolized by the liver, undergoes enterohepatic recirculation.

Half-life: Fluphenazine hydrochloride—4.7–15.3 hr; fluphenazine enanthate—3.7 days; fluphenazine decanoate—6.8–9.6 days.

CONTRAINDICATIONS AND PRECAUTIONS

Contraindicated in: ▪ Hypersensitivity ▪ Cross-sensitivity with other phenothiazines may exist ▪ Narrow-angle glaucoma ▪ Bone marrow depression ▪ Severe liver or cardiovascular disease ▪ Hypersensitivity to sesame oil (decanoate and enanthate salts).

Use Cautiously in: ▪ Elderly or debilitated patients (dosage reduction may be necessary) ▪ Pregnancy or lactation (safety not established) ▪ Diabetes mellitus ▪ Respiratory disease ▪ Prostatic hypertrophy ▪ CNS tumors ▪ Epilepsy ▪ Intestinal obstruction.

ADVERSE REACTIONS AND SIDE EFFECTS*

CNS: sedation, <u>extrapyramidal reactions</u>, tardive dyskinesia.

EENT: dry eyes, blurred vision, lens opacities.

CV: hypotension, tachycardia.

GI: constipation, dry mouth, ileus, anorexia, hepatitis.

GU: urinary retention.

Derm: rashes, <u>photosensitivity</u>, pigment changes.

Endo: galactorrhea.

Hemat: AGRANULOCYTOSIS, leukopenia.

Misc: allergic reactions, hyperthermia.

INTERACTIONS

Drug-Drug: ▪ Additive hypotension with **antihypertensive agents** ▪ Additive CNS depression with other **CNS depressants,** including **alcohol, antidepres-**

{} = Available in Canada only.
*<u>Underlines</u> indicate most frequent; **CAPITALS** indicate life-threatening.

sants, antihistamines, MAO inhibitors, narcotic analgesics, sedative/hypnotics, or general anesthetics ▪ Phenobarbital may increase metabolism and decrease effectiveness ▪ Concurrent use with **lithium** may produce any of the following—acute encephalopathy, decreased chlorpromazine absorption, increased excretion of lithium, increased risk of extrapyramidal reactions, or masking of the early signs of lithium toxicity ▪ **Antacids** or **adsorbent antidiarrheals (kaolin)** may decrease absorption ▪ Increased risk of agranulocytosis with **antithyroid drugs** ▪ May decrease antiparkinson activity of **levodopa** and **bromocriptine** ▪ Decreases vasopressor response to **epinephrine** and **norepinephrine** ▪ Decreases antihypertensive effect of **guanethidine** ▪ Concurrent use with **beta blockers** may result in inhibition of metabolism of one or both drugs producing an increased response ▪ Increased risk of anticholinergic effects with other **agents having anticholinergic properties,** including **antihistamines, tricyclic antidepressants, disopyramide,** or **quinidine.**

ROUTE AND DOSAGE

Fluphenazine Hydrochloride

- **PO (Adults):** 0.5–10 mg/day in divided doses q 6–8 hr initially, maintenance dose 1–5 mg/day.
- **IM (Adults):** ⅓–½ of PO dose.

Fluphenazine Enanthate

- **IM, SC (Adults):** 25 mg q 2 wk.

Fluphenazine Decanoate

- **IM, SC (Adults):** 12.5–25 mg initially, then q 4–6 wk as needed.

PHARMACODYNAMICS (antipsychotic activity)

	ONSET	PEAK	DURATION
PO hydrochloride	1 hr	UK	6–8 hr
IM hydrochloride	1 hr	1.5–2 hr	6–8 hr
IM enanthate	24–72 hr	UK	2 wk
IM decanoate	24–72 hr	UK	1–6 wk

NURSING IMPLICATIONS

Assessment

- □ Assess patient's mental status (orientation, mood, behavior) prior to and periodically throughout therapy.
- □ Monitor blood pressure (sitting, standing, lying), pulse, and respiratory rate prior to and frequently during the period of dosage adjustment.
- □ Observe patient carefully when administering oral medication to ensure medication is actually taken and not hoarded.
- □ Assess fluid intake and bowel function. Increased bulk and fluids in the diet help minimize the constipating effects of this medication.
- □ Observe patient carefully for extrapyramidal symptoms (pill-rolling motions, drooling, tremors, rigidity, shuffling gait), tardive dyskinesia (uncontrolled movements of face, mouth, tongue, or jaw and involuntary movements of extremities) and neuroleptic malignant syndrome (fever, respiratory distress, tachycardia, convulsions, diaphoresis, hypertension or hypotension, pallor, tiredness). Notify physician immediately at the onset of these symptoms.
- ▪ **Lab Test Considerations:** Monitor liver function tests, urine bilirubin, and bile for evidence of hepatic toxicity periodically throughout course of therapy. Urine bilirubin may be falsely elevated.
- □ May cause false-positive and false-negative pregnancy tests.
- □ May cause blood dyscrasias; monitor CBC periodically throughout course of therapy.

Potential Nursing Diagnoses

- Thought processes, altered (indications).
- Knowledge deficit related to medication regimen (patient/family teaching).
- Noncompliance (patient/family teaching).

Implementation

- **General Info:** Available in tablet, elixir, concentrate, injection, and long-acting injectable forms. Slight yellow to amber color does not alter potency.

- □ To prevent contact dermatitis avoid getting liquid preparations on hands and wash hands thoroughly if spillage occurs.
- □ Injectable forms must be drawn up with a dry syringe and dry 21-gauge needle to prevent clouding of the soln.
- ▪ **PO:** Dilute concentrate just prior to administration in 120–240 ml of water, milk, carbonated beverage, soup, or tomato or fruit juice. Do not mix with beverages containing caffeine (cola, coffee); tannics (tea); or pectinates (apple juice).
- ▪ **SC:** Fluphenazine decanoate and fluphenazine enanthate are dissolved in sesame oil for long duration of action. They may be administered SC or IM.
- ▪ **IM:** IM dose is usually ⅓ to ½ of oral dose. Because fluphenazine hydrochloride has a shorter duration of action, it is used initially to determine the patient's response to the drug and to treat the acutely agitated patient.
- □ Administer deep IM using a dry syringe and 21-gauge needle into dorsal gluteal site. Instruct patient to remain recumbent for 30 min to prevent hypotension.

Patient/Family Teaching

- □ Advise patient to take medication exactly as directed and not to skip doses or double up on missed doses. Abrupt withdrawal may lead to gastritis, nausea, vomiting, dizziness, headache, tachycardia, and insomnia.
- □ Inform patient of possibility of extrapyramidal symptoms and tardive dyskinesia. Caution patient to report these symptoms immediately to physician.
- □ Advise patient to make position changes slowly to minimize orthostatic hypotension.
- □ Medication may cause drowsiness. Caution patient to avoid driving or other activities requiring alertness until response to medication is known.
- □ Caution patient to avoid taking alcohol or other CNS depressants concurrently with this medication.
- □ Advise patient to use sunscreen and protective clothing when exposed to the sun. Exposed surfaces may develop a blue-grey pigmentation, which may fade following discontinuation of the medication. Extremes of temperature should also be avoided, as this drug impairs body temperature regulation.
- □ Advise patient that good oral hygiene, frequent rinsing of mouth with water, and sugarless gum or candy may help relieve dry mouth. Physician or dentist should be notified if dry mouth persists beyond 2 wk.
- □ Inform patient that this medication may turn urine pink to reddish-brown.
- □ Instruct patient to notify physician promptly if sore throat, fever, unusual bleeding or bruising, skin rashes, weakness, tremors, visual disturbances, dark-colored urine, or clay-colored stools are noted.
- □ Advise patient to notify physician or dentist of medication regimen prior to treatment or surgery.
- □ Emphasize the importance of routine follow-up examinations, including ocular examinations, with long-term therapy and continued participation in psychotherapy.

Evaluation

Effectiveness of therapy can be demonstrated by: ▪ Decrease in excitable, paranoic, or withdrawn behavior.

FLURAZEPAM

(flur-**az**-e-pam)

{Apo-flurazepam}, Dalmane, Durapam, {Novoflupam}, {Somnol}, {Som-Pam}

{} = Available in Canada only.

CLASSIFICATION(S):
Sedative/hypnotic—benzodiazepine
Schedule IV
Pregnancy Category UK

INDICATIONS

- Short-term management of insomnia (<4 wk).

ACTION

- Depresses the CNS, probably by potentiating gamma-aminobutyric acid (GABA), an inhibitory neurotransmitter. **Therapeutic Effect:** ▪ Relief of insomnia.

PHARMACOKINETICS

Absorption: Well absorbed following oral administration.
Distribution: Widely distributed, crosses blood-brain barrier. Probably crosses the placenta and enters breast milk. Accumulation of drug occurs with chronic dosing.
Metabolism and Excretion: Metabolized by the liver. Some metabolites have hypnotic activity.
Half-life: 2.3 hr (half-life of active metabolite may be 30–200 hr).

CONTRAINDICATIONS AND PRECAUTIONS

Contraindicated in: ▪ Hypersensitivity ▪ Cross-sensitivity with other benzodiazepines may exist ▪ Pre-existing CNS depression ▪ Severe uncontrolled pain ▪ Narrow-angle glaucoma ▪ Pregnancy or lactation.
Use Cautiously in: ▪ Hepatic dysfunction (dosage reduction may be necessary) ▪ Patients who may be suicidal or have been addicted to drugs previously ▪ Elderly or debilitated patients (dosage reduction may be necessary).

ADVERSE REACTIONS AND SIDE EFFECTS*

CNS: dizziness, daytime drowsiness, lethargy, hangover, paradoxical excitation, confusion, mental depression, headache.
Derm: rashes.
EENT: blurred vision.
GI: nausea, vomiting, diarrhea, constipation.
Misc: tolerance, psychological dependence, physical dependence.

INTERACTIONS

Drug-Drug: ▪ Concurrent use with **alcohol, antidepressants, antihistamines,** and **narcotic analgesics** may result in additive CNS depression ▪ **Cimetidine, oral contraceptives, disulfiram, fluoxetine, isoniazid, ketoconazole, metoprolol, propoxyphene, propranolol,** or **valproic acid** may decrease the metabolism of flurazepam, enhancing its actions ▪ May decrease efficacy of **levodopa** ▪ **Rifampin** or **barbiturates** may increase the metabolism and decrease effectiveness of flurazepam ▪ Sedative effects may be decreased by **theophylline.**

ROUTE AND DOSAGE

- **PO (Adults):** 15–30 mg at bedtime.

PHARMACODYNAMICS (hypnotic activity)

	ONSET	PEAK	DURATION
PO	15–45 min	0.5–1 hr	7–8 hr

NURSING IMPLICATIONS

Assessment

- Assess sleep patterns prior to and periodically throughout course of therapy.
- Prolonged therapy may lead to psychological or physical dependence. Restrict amount of drug available to patient, especially if patient is depressed, suicidal, or has a history of addiction.

Potential Nursing Diagnoses

- Sleep pattern disturbance (indications).
- Injury, high risk for (side effects).
- Knowledge deficit related to medica-

*Underlines indicate most frequent; **CAPITALS** indicate life-threatening.

F

tion regimen (patient/family teaching).

Implementation

- **General Info:** Supervise ambulation and transfer of patients following administration. Remove cigarettes. Side rails should be raised and call bell within reach at all times.
- **PO:** Capsules may be opened and mixed with food or fluids for patients having difficulty swallowing.

Patient/Family Teaching

- Advise patient to take medication exactly as directed. Discuss the importance of preparing environment for sleep (dark room, quiet, avoidance of nicotine and caffeine).
- Medication may cause daytime drowsiness. Caution patient to avoid driving and other activities requiring alertness until response to medication is known.
- Caution patient to avoid taking alcohol or other CNS depressants concurrently with this medication.
- Instruct patient to contact physician immediately if pregnancy is suspected.

Evaluation

Effectiveness of therapy can be demonstrated by: ▪ Improvement in sleep patterns. Maximum hypnotic properties are apparent 2–3 nights after initiating therapy and may last 1–2 nights after therapy is discontinued.

FLURBIPROFEN
(flure-**bi**-proe-fen)
Ansaid, {Froben}, Ocufen

CLASSIFICATION(S):
Nonsteroidal anti-inflammatory agent.
Pregnancy Category C (Ophth)

INDICATIONS

▪ **PO:** Management of inflammatory disorders including: □ Rheumatoid arthritis □ Osteoarthritis ▪ **Ophth:** Used to inhibit intra-operative miosis ▪ **Ophth:** Ocular anti-inflammatory.

ACTION

▪ Inhibits prostaglandin synthesis, resulting in reduced inflammation and pain when administered orally. Inhibition of prostaglandin synthesis in the eye relaxes the iris sphincter. **Therapeutic Effects:** ▪ ***PO:*** Suppression of pain and inflammation ▪ ***Ophth:*** Miosis.

PHARMACOKINETICS

Absorption: Well absorbed following oral administration. Following ophth administration, penetration of the cornea results in systemic absorption.
Distribution: Systemic distribution following oral administration.
Metabolism and Excretion: Mostly metabolized by the liver. 20–25% excreted unchanged by the kidneys.
Half-life: 3–6 hr.

CONTRAINDICATIONS AND PRECAUTIONS

Contraindicated in: ▪ Hypersensitivity ▪ Cross-sensitivity may exist with other nonsteroidal anti-inflammatory agents, including aspirin ▪ Active GI bleeding or ulcer disease ▪ Herpes simplex keratitis (ophth form only).
Use Cautiously in: ▪ Severe cardiovascular, renal, or hepatic disease ▪ History of ulcer disease ▪ Diabetes mellitus ▪ Bleeding disorders ▪ Pregnancy, lactation, or children (safety not established).

ADVERSE REACTIONS AND SIDE EFFECTS*

CNS: PO—mental depression, headache, drowsiness, psychic disturbances, dizziness, insomnia.
EENT: PO—blurred vision, corneal opacities, tinnitus; Ophth—burning, stinging, itching.
CV: PO—edema, changes in blood pressure, palpitations.

{} = Available in Canada only.
*Underlines indicate most frequent; **CAPITALS** indicate life-threatening.

GI: PO—nausea, abdominal pain, heartburn, bloated feeling, diarrhea, constipation, hepatitis, **GASTRIC BLEEDING**, stomatitis.
GU: PO—incontinence.
Derm: PO—rashes, increased sweating.
Hemat: PO—blood dyscrasias, prolonged bleeding time.
MS: PO—myalgia.
Misc: PO—allergic reactions, including **ANAPHYLAXIS** and **STEVENS-JOHNSON SYNDROME**, chills, fever.

INTERACTIONS

Note: For oral flurbiprofen, unless indicated.

Drug-Drug: ▪ Concurrent use with **aspirin** may decrease effectiveness ▪ Additive adverse GI effects with **aspirin,** other **nonsteroidal anti-inflammatory agents, potassium supplements, glucocorticoids,** or **alcohol** ▪ Chronic use with **acetaminophen** may increase the risk of adverse renal reactions ▪ May decrease the effectiveness of **diuretics** or **antihypertensive** therapy ▪ Increases the risk of toxicity from **methotrexate** ▪ **Probenecid** increases risk of toxicity from diclofenac ▪ Increased risk of bleeding with **cefamandole, cefotetan, cefoperazone, moxalactam** or **plicamycin, heparin, thrombolytic agents,** or **oral anticoagulants** ▪ Increased risk of adverse hematologic reactions with **antineoplastic agents** or **radiation therapy** ▪ Increased risk of nephrotoxicity with other **nephrotoxic agents** ▪ Ophthalmic **acetylcholine** or **carbachol** are not effective when administered after ophthalmic flurbiprofen ▪ Ophthalmic flurbiprofen decreases the intraocular pressure-lowering effect of ophthalmic **epinephrine.**

ROUTE AND DOSAGE

- **PO (Adults):** 200–300 mg daily in 2–4 divided doses (not to exceed 300 mg/day).
- **Ophth (Adults):** 1 drop of 0.03% soln every 30 min beginning 2 hr prior to surgery (total of 4 drops).

PHARMACODYNAMICS

	ONSET	PEAK	DURATION
PO (anti-inflammatory)	few days–1 wk	1–2 wk	UK
Ophth (miosis)	UK	UK	UK

NURSING IMPLICATIONS

Assessment

- **General Info:** Patients who have asthma, aspirin-induced allergy, and nasal polyps are at increased risk for developing hypersensitivity reactions. Monitor for rhinitis, asthma, and urticaria.
- **Arthritis:** Assess pain and range of movement prior to and 1–2 hr following administration.
- **Lab Test Considerations:** May cause prolonged bleeding time.

Potential Nursing Diagnoses

- Comfort, altered: pain (indications).
- Mobility, impaired physical (indications).
- Knowledge deficit related to medication regimen (patient/family teaching).

Implementation

- **PO:** For rapid initial effect, administer 30 min before or 2 hr after meals.
- **Ophth:** Instill 1 drop every 30 min beginning 2 hr prior to surgery, for a total of 4 drops. See Appendix H for administration of ophthalmic soln.

Patient/Family Teaching

- **Arthritis:** Advise patient to take this medication with a full glass of water and to remain in an upright position for 15–30 min after administration.
- ▫ Instruct patient to take medication exactly as prescribed. If a dose is missed, take as soon as remembered, but not if almost time for next dose. Do not double doses.
- ▫ This medication may cause drowsiness or dizziness. Advise patient to avoid driving or other activities requiring alertness until response to medication is known.

- □ Caution patient to avoid the concurrent use of alcohol, aspirin, acetaminophen, or other over-the-counter medications without consulting physician or pharmacist.
- □ Instruct patient to notify physician if rash, itching, chills, fever, muscle aches, visual disturbances, tinnitus, weight gain, edema, black stools, or persistent headache occur.
- □ Advise patient to inform physician or dentist of medication regimen prior to treatment or surgery.

Evaluation

Effectiveness of therapy can be demonstrated by: ▪ Decreased pain □ Improved joint mobility. Patients who do not respond to one nonsteroidal antiinflammatory agent may respond to another. ▪ Inhibition of intraoperative miosis.

FLUTAMIDE
(**floo**-ta-mide)
Eulexin

CLASSIFICATION(S):
Antineoplastic—hormone
Pregnancy Category D

INDICATIONS

▪ Treatment of metastatic prostate carcinoma in conjunction with gonadotropin-releasing hormone analogs (leuprolide).

ACTION

▪ Antagonizes the effects of androgen (testosterone) at the cellular level. **Therapeutic Effect:** ▪ Decreased growth of prostate carcinoma, an androgen-sensitive tumor.

PHARMACOKINETICS

Absorption: Well absorbed following oral administration.
Distribution: Distribution not known.
Metabolism and Excretion: Mostly metabolized by the liver. Some converted to another anti-androgenic compound.
Half-life: UK.

CONTRAINDICATIONS AND PRECAUTIONS

Contraindicated in: ▪ Hypersensitivity.
Use Cautiously in: ▪ Severe cardiovascular disease ▪ Requires concurrent luteinizing hormone releasing hormone (LHRH) agonist therapy.

ADVERSE REACTIONS AND SIDE EFFECTS*

Note: Side effects primarily due to LHRH antagonist.
CNS: drowsiness, confusion, anxiety, nervousness, depression.
CV: edema, hypertension.
GI: diarrhea, nausea, vomiting, other gastric disturbances, hepatitis.
GU: loss of libido, impotence.
Derm: rash, photosensitivity.
Endo: gynecomastia.
Misc: hot flashes.

INTERACTIONS

Drug-Drug: ▪ Acts synergistically with **gonadotropin-releasing hormone analogs (leuprolide).**

ROUTE AND DOSAGE

▪ **PO (Adults):** 250 mg q 8 hr.

PHARMACODYNAMICS

	ONSET	PEAK	DURATION
PO	UK	UK	UK

NURSING IMPLICATIONS

Assessment

- □ Monitor for diarrhea, nausea, and vomiting. Adjust diet as tolerated. Notify physician if these symptoms become severe.
- ▪ **Lab Test Considerations:** May cause elevated SGOT (AST), SGPT (ALT), bilirubin, and creatinine values.

Potential Nursing Diagnoses

- ▪ Sexual dysfunction (indications and side effects).

*Underlines indicate most frequent; **CAPITALS** indicate life-threatening.

- Knowledge deficit related to medication regimen (patient/family teaching).

Implementation

- **General Info:** Used in combination with LHRH agonist, such as leuprolide.

Patient/Family Teaching

- ▫ Explain that flutamide must be taken in conjunction with leuprolide.
- ▫ Warn patient that side effects such as hot flashes, loss of sex drive, impotence, and breast enlargement may be caused by the LHRH agonist. The primary side effect of flutamide alone is diarrhea, but the combination of drugs is necessary to achieve the therapeutic effect.

Evaluation

Effectiveness of therapy can be demonstrated by ▪ Decrease in the spread of prostate cancer.

FOLIC ACID

(**foe**-lik **a**-sid)

{Apo-Folic}, Folate, Folvite, {Novofolacid}, vitamin B_9

CLASSIFICATION(S):

Vitamin—water-soluble, Antianemic

Pregnancy Category UK

INDICATIONS

▪ Used in the treatment of megaloblastic and macrocytic anemias ▪ Given during pregnancy to promote normal fetal development.

ACTION

▪ Required for protein synthesis and red blood cell function. Stimulates the production of red blood cells, white blood cells, and platelets. Necessary for normal fetal development. **Therapeutic Effect:** ▪ Restoration and maintenance of normal hematopoiesis.

PHARMACOKINETICS

Absorption: Well absorbed from the GI tract and IM and SC sites.

Distribution: Half of all stores are in the liver. Enters breast milk. Crosses the placenta.

Metabolism and Excretion: Converted by the liver to its active metabolite, dihydrofolate reductase.

Half-life: Excess amounts are excreted unchanged by the kidneys.

CONTRAINDICATIONS AND PRECAUTIONS

Contraindicated in: ▪ Uncorrected pernicious anemia (neurologic damage will progress despite correction of hematologic abnormalities) ▪ Preparations containing benzyl alcohol should not be used in newborns.

Use Cautiously in: ▪ Undiagnosed anemias.

ADVERSE REACTIONS AND SIDE EFFECTS*

Derm: rashes.

Misc: fever.

INTERACTIONS

Drug-Drug: ▪ **Sulfomanides, methotrexate,** and **triamterene** prevent the activation of folic acid ▪ Absorption of folic acid is decreased by **sulfasalazine** ▪ Folic acid requirements are increased by **estrogens, phenytoin,** or **glucocorticoids.**

ROUTE AND DOSAGE

Anemia

- **PO, IM, IV, SC (Adults and Children):** 0.25–1.0 mg/day.

Pregnancy

- **PO, IM, IV, SC (Adults):** 1.0 mg/day.

Dietary Supplement

- **PO, IM, IV, SC (Adults and Children):** 0.1 mg/day.

{} = Available in Canada only.

*Underlines indicate most frequent; **CAPITALS** indicate life-threatening.

PHARMACODYNAMICS (increase in reticulocyte count)

	ONSET	PEAK	DURATION
PO, IM, SC, IV	3–5 days	5–10 days	UK

NURSING IMPLICATIONS

Assessment

- Assess patient for signs of megaloblastic anemia (fatigue, weakness, dyspnea) prior to and periodically throughout therapy.
- **Lab Test Considerations:** Monitor plasma folic acid levels, hemoglobin, hematocrit, and reticulocyte count prior to and periodically during course of therapy.
- May cause decrease in serum concentrations of vitamin B_{12} when given in high continuous doses.

Potential Nursing Diagnoses

- Nutrition, altered: less than body requirements (indications).
- Activity intolerance (indications).
- Knowledge deficit related to medication regimen (patient/family teaching).

Implementation

- **General Info:** Because of infrequency of solitary vitamin deficiencies, combinations are commonly administered (see Appendix A).
- May be given SC, deep IM, or IV when PO route is not feasible.
- **IV:** Soln ranges from yellow to orange-yellow in color.
- **Direct IV:** Administer at a rate of 5 mg over at least 1 min.
- **Continuous Infusion:** May be added to hyperalimentation soln.
- **Y-Site Compatibility:** famotidine.
- **Additive Compatibility:** D20W.
- **Additive Incompatibility:** D50W or calcium gluconate.

Patient/Family Teaching

- Encourage patient to comply with physician's diet recommendations. Explain that the best source of vitamins is a well-balanced diet with foods from the 4 basic food groups. If physician is trying to diagnose folic acid deficiency without concealing pernicious anemia, a diet low in vitamin B_{12} and folate will be ordered.
- Foods high in folic acid include vegetables, fruits, and organ meats; heat destroys folic acid in foods.
- Patients self-medicating with vitamin supplements should be cautioned not to exceed RDA (see Appendix L). The effectiveness of megadoses for treatment of various medical conditions is unproven and may cause side effects.
- Explain that folic acid may make urine more intensely yellow.
- Instruct patient to notify physician if rash occurs, which may indicate hypersensitivity.
- Emphasize the importance of follow-up examinations to evaluate progress.

Evaluation

Effectiveness of therapy may be demonstrated by: ▪ Reticulocytosis 2–5 days after beginning therapy ▫ Resolution of symptoms of megaloblastic anemia.

FOSCARNET
(foss-**kar**-net)
Foscavir

CLASSIFICATION(S):
Antiviral
Pregnancy Category C

INDICATIONS

- Treatment of cytomegalovirus (CMV) retinitis in patients with the acquired immunodeficiency syndrome (AIDS).

ACTION

- Prevents viral replication by inhibiting viral DNA-polymerase and reverse transcriptase. **Therapeutic Effect:** ▪ Virastatic action against susceptible viruses including CMV.

PHARMACOKINETICS

Absorption: Following IV administration absorption is essentially complete. **Distribution:** Variable penetration into

CSF. May concentrate in and be slowly released from bone. Remainder of distribution not known.
Metabolism and Excretion: 80–90% excreted unchanged in urine.
Half-life: 3 hr (in patients with normal renal function). A longer half-life of 90 hr may reflect release of drug from bone.

CONTRAINDICATIONS AND PRECAUTIONS

Contraindicated in: ▪ Hypersensitivity.
Use Cautiously in: ▪ Renal impairment (dosage reduction required) ▪ Pregnancy, lactation, or children (safety not established) ▪ History of seizures.

ADVERSE REACTIONS AND SIDE EFFECTS*

CNS: SIEZURES, headache, fatigue, weakness, malaise, dizziness, depression, confusion, anxiety.
EENT: vision abnormalities, eye pain, conjunctivitis.
Resp: coughing, dyspnea.
CV: edema, chest pain, palpitations, ECG abnormalities.
GI: nausea, vomiting, diarrhea, anorexia, abdominal pain, constipation, dyspepsia, abnormal taste sensation.
GU: renal failure, albuminuria, dysuria, polyuria, urinary retention, nocturia.
Derm: rash, increased sweating, pruritus, skin ulceration.
F and E: hypocalcemia, hypomagnesemia, hypokalemia, hypophosphatemia, hyperphosphatemia.
Hemat: anemia, granulocytopenia, leukopenia.
Local: pain or inflammation at injection site.
MS: involuntary muscle contraction, back pain, arthralgia, myalgia.
Neuro: paresthesia, hypoesthesia, neuropathy, tremor, ataxia.
Misc: fever, chills, flu-like syndrome, lymphoma, sarcoma.

INTERACTIONS

Drug-Drug: ▪ Concurrent use with patenteral **pentamidine** may result in severe, life-threatening hypocalcemia.

ROUTE AND DOSAGE

- **IV (Adults):** 60 mg/kg q 8 hr for 2–3 wk initially, then 90–120 mg/kg/day as a single dose. Dosage reduction required for any degree of renal impairment.

PHARMACODYNAMICS

	ONSET	PEAK
IV	rapid	end of infusion

NURSING IMPLICATIONS

Assessment

- □ Diagnosis of CMV retinitis should be determined by ophthalmoscopy prior to treatment with foscarnet.
- □ Culture for CMV (urine, blood, throat) may be taken prior to administration. However, a negative CMV culture does not rule out CMV retinitis.
- ▪ **Lab Test Considerations:** Monitor serum creatinine prior to and 2–3 times weekly during induction therapy and at least every 1–2 wk during maintenance therapy. Monitor 24-hr creatinine clearance prior to and periodically throughout therapy. If creatinine clearance drops below 0.4 ml/min/kg foscarnet may need to be discontinued.
- □ Monitor serum calcium, magnesium, potassium, and phosphorous prior to and 2–3 times weekly during induction therapy and at least every 1–2 wk during maintenance therapy.
- □ May cause anemia, granulocytopenia, leukopenia, and thrombocytopenia.
- □ May cause elevated SGOT (AST) and SGPT (ALT) levels and abnormal A-G ratios.

Potential Nursing Diagnoses

- ▪ Infection, high risk for (indications).
- ▪ Knowledge deficit related to medication regimen (patient/family teaching).

*Underlines indicate most frequent; **CAPITALS** indicate life-threatening.

F

IMPLEMENTATION

- **General Info:** Patient should be adequately hydrated prior to and throughout infusion to prevent renal toxicity.
- **Intermittent Infusion:** May be administered via central line in standard 24 mg/ml soln undiluted. If administered via peripheral line, *must* be diluted to 12 mg/ml concentration with D5W or 0.9% NaCl to prevent vein irritation. Do not administer soln that is discolored or contains particulate matter. Use diluted soln within 24 hr.
- □ Do not administer concurrently with other solns in IV catheter except D5W or 0.9% NaCl; precipitate will develop.
- □ Dose is based on patient weight; excess soln may be discarded from bottle prior to administration to prevent overdosage.
- □ Patients who experience progression of CMV retinitis during maintenance therapy may be retreated with induction therapy followed by maintenance therapy.
- □ *Rate:* Induction treatment is infused over 1 hr every 8 hr for 2–3 wk depending on clinical response.
- □ Maintenance treatment is infused over 2 hr.
- □ Infuse soln via infusion pump to ensure accurate infusion rate.
- **Y-Site Incompatibility:** acyclovir, amphotericin B, calcium, co-trimoxazole, diazepam, digoxin, gancyclovir, lactated Ringers soln, leucovorin, midazolam, pentamidine, phenytoin, prochlorperazine, or vancomycin.

PATIENT/FAMILY TEACHING

- □ Inform patient that foscarnet is not a cure for CMV retinitis. Progression of retinitis may continue in immunocompromised patients during and following therapy. Advise patients to have regular ophthalmologic examinations.
- □ Advise patient to notify nurse or physician immediately if perioral tingling or numbness in the extremities or paresthesia occur during or after infusion. If these signs of electrolyte imbalance occur during administration, stop infusion and consult physician. Lab samples for serum electrolyte concentrations should be obtained immediately.
- □ Emphasize the importance of frequent follow-up examinations to monitor renal function and electrolytes.

EVALUATION

Effectiveness of therapy can be demonstrated by: ▪ Resolution of the symptoms of CMV retinitis in patients with AIDS.

FOSINOPRIL

(foss-**in**-o-pril)
Monopril

CLASSIFICATION(S):
Antihypertensive—angiotensin converting enzyme (ACE) inhibitor
Pregnancy Category D

INDICATIONS

▪ Alone or in combination with thiazide diuretics in the management of hypertension.

ACTION

▪ Prevents the production of angiotensin II, a potent vasoconstrictor that stimulates the production of aldosterone, by blocking its conversion to the active form. Result is systemic vasodilation. **Therapeutic Effect:** ▪ Lowering of blood pressure in hypertensive patients.

PHARMACOKINETICS

Absorption: 36% absorbed following oral administration.
Distribution: Crosses the placenta and enters breast milk.
Metabolism and Excretion: Converted to fosinoprilat, the active form, of which 50% excreted in feces, 50% excreted in urine as metabolites. Minimal amounts excreted unchanged.
Half-life: 12 hr (fosinoprilat).

CONTRAINDICATIONS AND PRECAUTIONS

Contraindicated in: ▪ Hypersensitivity ▪ Cross-sensitivity with other ACE inhibitors may exist.

Use Cautiously in: ▪ Hereditary angioedema (extreme caution) ▪ Hypovolemia, hyponatremia, elderly patients (dosage reduction required) ▪ Renal disease ▪ Aortic stenosis ▪ Cerebrovascular or cardiac insufficiency ▪ Pregnancy (may cause fetal hypotension, oliguria, renal failure, skull hypoplasia, other fetal abnormalities, and death) ▪ Lactation or children (safety not established) ▪ Surgery/anesthesia (hypotension may be exaggerated).

Extreme Caution in: ▪ Family history of hereditary angioedema.

ADVERSE REACTIONS AND SIDE EFFECTS*

CNS: headache, dizziness, fatigue.
EENT: ANGIOEDEMA.
Resp: cough.
CV: orthostatic hypotension.
GI: nausea, diarrhea, vomiting.
Misc: allergic reactions.

INTERACTIONS

Drug-Drug: ▪ Additive or possibly excessive hypotension with other **antihypertensives, diuretics, nitrates, phenothiazines,** and acute ingestion of **alcohol** ▪ Hyperkalemia may result with concurrent **potassium supplements** or **potassium-sparing diuretics** ▪ Antihypertensive response may be blunted by **nonsteroidal anti-inflammatory agents** ▪ May increase serum **digoxin** levels ▪ Increases blood levels and risk of toxicity from **lithium** ▪ Increased risk of hypersensitivity reactions with **allopurinol**.

ROUTE AND DOSAGE

- **PO (Adults):** 10 mg once daily initially, may be increased as required. Usual range 20–40 mg/day. Doses as high as 80 mg have been used.

PHARMACODYNAMICS (antihypertensive effect)

	ONSET	PEAK	DURATION
PO	1 hr	2–6 hr	24 hr

NURSING IMPLICATIONS

Assessment

- Monitor blood pressure and pulse frequently during initial dosage adjustment and periodically throughout course of therapy. Notify physician of significant changes.
- **Lab Test Considerations:** Monitor BUN, creatinine, and electrolyte levels periodically. Serum potassium may be increased, and BUN and creatine transiently increased while sodium levels may be decreased.

Potential Nursing Diagnoses

- Cardiac output, decreased (indications, side effects).
- Knowledge deficit related to medication regimen (patient/family teaching).
- Noncompliance (patient/family teaching).

Implementation

- **PO:** Precipitous drop in blood pressure following first dose may occur. Discontinuing diuretic therapy 2–3 days prior to initiation of fosinopril may decrease risk of hypotension. Resume diuretics if blood pressure is not controlled with fosinopril.

Patient/Family Teaching

- Instruct patient to take fosinopril exactly as directed, even if feeling better. Missed doses should be taken as soon as remembered but not if almost time for next dose. Do not double doses. Medication controls but does not cure hypertension. Caution patients not to discontinue fosinopril therapy unless directed by the physician.
- Encourage patient to comply with additional interventions for hypertension (weight reduction, discontinuation of smoking, moderation of

*Underlines indicate most frequent; **CAPITALS** indicate life-threatening.

F

alcohol consumption, regular exercise, and stress management). Fosinopril controls but does not cure hypertension.

- Instruct patient and family on proper technique for blood pressure monitoring. Advise them to check blood pressure at least weekly and report significant changes to physician.
- Caution patient to avoid salt substitutes or foods containing high levels of potassium or sodium unless directed by physician (see Appendix K).
- Caution patient to change positions slowly to minimize orthostatic hypotension, particularly after initial dose. Patients should also be advised that exercising or hot weather may increase hypotensive effects.
- Advise patient to consult physician or pharmacist before taking any over-the-counter medications, especially cold remedies. Patients should also avoid excessive amounts of tea, coffee, or cola. May cause dizziness. Caution patient to avoid driving and other activities requiring alertness until response to medication is known.
- Advise patient to inform physician or dentist of medication regimen prior to treatment or surgery.
- Instruct patient to notify physician if rash, mouth sores, sore throat, fever, swelling of hands or feet, irregular heart beat, chest pain, dry cough, swelling of face, eyes, lips, or tongue, or difficulty breathing occurs or if taste impairment persists.
- Emphasize the importance of follow-up examinations to monitor progress.

EVALUATION

Effectiveness of therapy can be demonstrated by: ▪ Decrease in blood pressure without appearance of side effects.

FUROSEMIDE

(fur-**oh**-se-mide)
{Apo-Furosemide}, {Furoside}, Lasix, Myrosemide, {Novosemide}, {Uritol}

CLASSIFICATION(S):
Diuretic—loop diuretic
Pregnancy Category C

INDICATIONS

▪ Management of: ▫ Edema secondary to congestive heart failure ▫ Hepatic or renal disease ▪ Used alone or in combination with antihypertensives in the treatment of hypertension ▪ Management of hypercalcemia of malignancy.

ACTION

▪ Inhibits the reabsorption of sodium and chloride from the loop of Henle and distal renal tubule ▪ Increases renal excretion of water, sodium, chloride, magnesium, hydrogen, and calcium ▪ May have renal and peripheral vasodilatory effects ▪ Effectiveness persists in impaired renal function. **Therapeutic Effects:** ▪ Diuresis and subsequent mobilization of excess fluid (edema, pleural effusions) ▪ Lowers blood pressure.

PHARMACOKINETICS

Absorption: Absorbed from the GI tract (60–75%) following oral administration. Also absorbed from IM sites.
Distribution: Distribution not known. Crosses the placenta and enters breast milk.
Metabolism and Excretion: Some is metabolized by the liver (30–40%). Some nonhepatic metabolism and some renal excretion as unchanged drug.
Half-life: 30–60 min (increased in renal impairment and neonates, markedly increased in hepatic impairment).

CONTRAINDICATIONS AND PRECAUTIONS

Contraindicated in: ▪ Hypersensitivity ▪ Cross-sensitivity with thiazides and sulfonamides may exist ▪ Pregnancy or lactation.
Use Cautiously in: ▪ Severe liver disease ▪ Electrolyte depletion ▪ Diabetes mellitus ▪ Anuria or increasing azotemia.

ADVERSE REACTIONS AND SIDE EFFECTS*

CNS: dizziness, headache, encephalopathy.
EENT: hearing loss, tinnitus.
CV: hypotension.
GI: nausea, vomiting, diarrhea, constipation.
GU: frequency.
Derm: rashes, photosensitivity.
Endo: hyperglycemia.
F and E: metabolic alkalosis, hypovolemia, dehydration, hyponatremia, hypokalemia, hypochloremia, hypomagnesemia.
Hemat: blood dyscrasias.
Metab: hyperuricemia.
MS: muscle cramps.
Misc: increased BUN.

INTERACTIONS

Drug–Drug: ▪ Additive hypotension with **antihypertensives** or **nitrates** ▪ Additive hypokalemia with other **diuretics, mezlocillin, piperacillin, amphotericin B,** and **glucocorticoids** ▪ Hypokalemia may increase **cardiac glycoside** toxicity ▪ Decreases **lithium** excretion, may cause toxicity ▪ Increased risk of ototoxicity with **aminoglycosides** ▪ May increase the effectiveness of **oral anticoagulants.**

ROUTE AND DOSAGE

- **PO, IM, IV (Adults):** 20–80 mg/day (up to 600 mg may be necessary).
- **PO, IM, IV (Children):** 1–2 mg/kg/day (up to 6 mg/kg/day).

PHARMACODYNAMICS (diuretic effect)

	ONSET	PEAK	DURATION
PO	30–60 min	1–2 hr	6–8 hr
IM	10–30 min	UK	4–8 hr
IV	5 min	30 min	2 hr

NURSING IMPLICATIONS

Assessment

- □ Assess fluid status throughout therapy. Monitor daily weight, intake and output ratios, amount and location of edema, lung sounds, skin turgor, and mucous membranes. Notify physician if thirst, dry mouth, lethargy, weakness, hypotension, or oliguria occur.
- □ Monitor blood pressure and pulse before and during administration.
- □ Assess patients receiving cardiac glycosides for anorexia, nausea, vomiting, muscle cramps, paresthesia, confusion. Notify physician if these symptoms occur.
- □ Assess patient for tinnitus and hearing loss. Audiometry is recommended for patients receiving prolonged therapy. Hearing loss is most common following rapid or high-dose IV administration in patients with decreased renal function or those taking other ototoxic drugs.
- □ Assess for allergy to sulfonamides.
- ▪ **Lab Test Considerations:** Monitor electrolytes, renal and hepatic function, glucose, and uric acid prior to and periodically throughout course of therapy. May cause decreased electrolyte levels (especially potassium). May cause elevated blood glucose, BUN, and uric acid levels.

Potential Nursing Diagnoses

- ▪ Fluid volume excess (indications).
- ▪ Fluid volume deficit (side effects).
- ▪ Knowledge deficit related to medication regimen (patient/family teaching).

Implementation

- ▪ **General Info:** Administer medication in the morning to prevent disruption of sleep cycle.
- □ Do not administer discolored soln or tablets.
- ▪ **PO:** Administer with food or milk to minimize gastric irritation. Tablets may be crushed if patient has difficulty swallowing.
- □ Available in oral soln.
- ▪ **IV:** Do not use soln that is yellow.
- ▪ **Direct IV:** Administer each 20 mg slowly over 1–2 min.
- ▪ **Intermittent Infusion:** Dilute large doses in D5W, D10W, D20W, D5/

*Underlines indicate most frequent; **CAPITALS** indicate life-threatening.

0.9% NaCl, D5/LR, 0.9% NaCl, 3% NaCl, 1/6 M sodium lactate, or lactated Ringer's soln. Use reconstituted soln within 24 hr.

- *Rate:* Administer through Y-tubing or 3-way stopcock at a rate not to exceed 4 mg/min in adults to prevent ototoxicity. Use an infusion pump to ensure accurate dosage.
- **Syringe Compatibility:** bleomycin, cisplatin, cyclophosphamide, fluorouracil, heparin, leucovorin calcium, methotrexate, mitomycin, vinblastine, or vincristine.
- **Syringe Incompatibility:** doxapram, doxorubicin, droperidol, metoclopramide, or milrinone.
- **Y-Site Compatibility:** amikacin, bleomycin, cisplatin, cyclophosphamide, famotidine, fluorouracil, foscarnet, heparin, hydrocortisone sodium succinate, kanamycin, leucovorin calcium, methotrexate, mitomycin, potassium chloride, tobramycin, or tolazoline.
- **Y-Site Incompatibility:** doxorubicin, droperidol, esmolol, gentamicin, hydralazine, metoclopramide, ondansetron, quinidine gluconate, vinblastine, or vincristine.
- **Additive Compatibility:** amikacin, cimetidine, kanamycin, nitroglycerin, tobramycin, or verapamil.
- **Additive Incompatibility:** dobutamine, gentamicin, or netilmicin.

Patient/Family Teaching

- **General Info:** Instruct patient to take furosemide exactly as directed. Missed doses should be taken as soon as remembered; do not double doses.
- Caution patient to make position changes slowly to minimize orthostatic hypotension. Caution patient that the use of alcohol, exercise during hot weather, or standing for long periods during therapy may enhance orthostatic hypotension.
- Instruct patient to consult physician regarding a diet high in potassium (see Appendix K).
- Caution patient to use sunscreen and protective clothing to prevent photosensitivity reactions.
- Advise patient to consult physician or pharmacist before taking over-the-counter medication concurrently with this therapy.
- Instruct patient to notify physician or dentist of medication regimen prior to treatment or surgery.
- Advise patient to contact physician immediately if muscle weakness, cramps, nausea, dizziness, numbness or tingling of extremities occur.
- Emphasize the importance of routine follow-up examinations.
- **Hypertension:** Advise patients on antihypertensive regimen to continue taking medication even if feeling better. Furosemide controls but does not cure hypertension.
- Reinforce the need to continue additional therapies for hypertension (weight loss, exercise, restricted sodium intake, stress reduction, regular exercise, moderation of alcohol consumption, cessation of smoking).

Evaluation

Effectiveness of therapy can be demonstrated by: ▪ Increase in urinary output ▫ Decrease in edema ▪ Decrease in blood pressure ▪ Decrease in serum calcium when used to manage hypercalcemia.

GALLAMINE

(**gal**-a-meen)
Flaxedil

CLASSIFICATION(S):
Neuromuscular blocking agent—nondepolarizing
Pregnancy Category C

INDICATIONS

- Production of skeletal muscle paralysis after induction of anesthesia.

ACTION

- Prevents neuromuscular transmission by blocking the effect of acetylcholine at the myoneural junction. **Therapeutic Effect:** ▪ Skeletal muscle paralysis.

PHARMACOKINETICS

Absorption: Following IV administration absorption is essentially complete.
Distribution: Distributes into extracellular space. Crosses the placenta.
Metabolism and Excretion: Excreted almost entirely unchanged by the kidneys.
Half-life: 2.5 hr.

CONTRAINDICATIONS AND PRECAUTIONS

Contraindicated in: ▪ Hypersensitivity ▪ Hypersensitivity to iodides.
Use Cautiously in: ▪ History of pulmonary disease ▪ Renal or liver impairment ▪ Elderly or debilitated patients ▪ Electrolyte disturbances ▪ Fractures or muscular spasm ▪ Children weighing <5 kg.
Extreme Caution in: Myasthenia gravis or myasthenic syndrome.

ADVERSE REACTIONS AND SIDE EFFECTS*

CV: tachycardia, hypertension.
Resp: wheezing, increased bronchial secretions.
Derm: skin flush, erythema, pruritus, urticaria.
Misc: allergic reactions, including ANAPHYLAXIS.

INTERACTIONS

Drug-Drug: ▪ Intensity and duration of paralysis may be prolonged by pretreatment with **succinylcholine, general anesthesia,** (dosage reduction may be necessary) **aminoglycoside antibiotics, polymyxin B, colistin, clindamycin, lidocaine, quinidine, procainamide, beta-adrenergic blocking agents, potassium-losing diuretics,** and **magnesium** ▪ Additive respiratory depression with **narcotic analgesics.**

ROUTE AND DOSAGE

- **IV (Adults and Children):** 1 mg/kg (not to exceed 100 mg/dose), then 0.5–1 mg/kg may be given 30–40 min later if needed during prolonged procedures.
- **IV (Neonates < 1 mon):** 0.25–0.75 mg/kg; additional doses of 0.1–0.5 mg/kg may be given.

PHARMACODYNAMICS (muscle relaxation)

	ONSET	PEAK	DURATION
IV	1–2 min	3–5 min	15–30 min

NURSING IMPLICATIONS

Assessment

- □ Assess respiratory status continuously throughout gallamine therapy. Gallamine should be used only by individuals experienced in endotracheal intubation; equipment for this procedure should be readily available.
- □ Neuromuscular response to gallamine should be monitored with a peripheral nerve stimulator intraoperatively. Paralysis is initially selective and usually occurs sequentially in the following muscles: levator muscles of eyelids, muscles of mastication, limb muscles, abdominal muscles, muscles of the glottis, intercostal muscles, and the diaphragm. Recovery of muscle function usually occurs in reverse order.
- □ Monitor heart rate and ECG throughout therapy. Tachycardia caused by gallamine occurs after doses of 500 mcg/kg. This reaches a maximum within 3 min and then declines gradually.
- □ Observe the patient for residual muscle weakness and respiratory distress during the recovery period.
- ▪ **Toxicity and Overdose:** If overdose occurs, use peripheral nerve stimulator to determine the degree of neuromuscular blockade. Maintain airway patency and ventilation until recovery of normal respirations occur.
- □ Administration of anticholinesterase agents (edrophonium, neostigmine, pyridostigmine) may be used to an-

*Underlines indicate most frequent; **CAPITALS** indicate life-threatening.

G

tagonize the action of gallamine. Atropine is usually administered prior to or concurrently with anticholinesterase agents to counteract the muscarinic effects.
- Administration of fluids and vasopressors may be necessary to treat severe hypotension or shock.

Potential Nursing Diagnoses
- Breathing pattern, ineffective (indications).
- Communication, impaired: verbal (side effects).
- Fear (patient/family teaching).

Implementation
- **General Info:** Dose is titrated to patient response.
- Gallamine has no effect on consciousness or the pain threshold. Adequate anesthesia should *always* be used when gallamine is used as an adjunct to surgical procedures.
- Should be refrigerated during storage.
- **Direct IV:** Administer each single dose undiluted as a bolus over 30–60 sec.
- **Syringe Incompatibility:** barbiturates or meperidine.

Patient/Family Teaching
- Explain all procedures to patient receiving gallamine therapy without anesthesia, as consciousness is not affected by gallamine alone.
- Reassure patient that communication abilities will return as the medication wears off.

Evaluation

Effectiveness of therapy can be demonstrated by: ▪ Adequate suppression of the twitch response when tested with peripheral nerve stimulation and subsequent muscle paralysis.

GALLIUM NITRATE
(**gal**-ee-yum **nye**-trate)
Ganite

CLASSIFICATION(S):
Electrolyte modifier—hypocalcemic agent
Pregnancy Category C

INDICATIONS
- Management of cancer-related hypercalcemia.

ACTION
- Inhibits calcium resorption from bone. **Therapeutic Effect:** ▪ Lowering of serum calcium levels.

PHARMACOKINETICS
Absorption: Administered IV only, resulting in complete bioavailability.
Distribution: Distribution not known.
Metabolism and Excretion: Mostly excreted unchanged by the kidneys.
Half-life: UK.

CONTRAINDICATIONS AND PRECAUTIONS
Contraindicated in: ▪ Severe renal impairment (creatinine $>$2.5 mg%).
Use Cautiously in: ▪ Renal impairment ▪ Pregnancy, lactation, or children (safety not established).

ADVERSE REACTIONS AND SIDE EFFECTS*
EENT: hearing loss, optic neuritis, visual impairment.
F and E: hypocalcemia, hypophosphatemia.
GU: renal toxicity.

INTERACTIONS
Drug-Drug: ▪ Increased risk of nephrotoxicity with other **nephrotoxic agents,** including **amphotericin B** and **aminoglycosides.**

ROUTE AND DOSAGE
- **IV (Adults):** 100–200 mg/m^2 daily for 5 days.

*Underlines indicate most frequent; **CAPITALS** indicate life-threatening.

PHARMACODYNAMICS (effect on serum calcium)

	ONSET	PEAK	DURATION
IV	within 24 hr	5 days	7.5 days

NURSING IMPLICATIONS

Assessment

- □ Monitor symptoms of hypercalcemia (nausea, vomiting, anorexia, lethargy, fatigue, weakness, constipation, thirst, dehydration, impaired mental status, and cardiac arrhythmias).
- □ Observe patient carefully for evidence of hypocalcemia (paresthesia, muscle twitching, laryngospasm, colic, cardiac arrhythmias, and Chvostek's or Trousseau's sign). Protect symptomatic patients by elevating and padding side rails; keep bed in low position. If hypocalcemia occurs, stop gallium nitrate therapy. Temporary calcium therapy may be needed.
- □ It patient requires other nephrotoxic drugs discontinue gallium nitrate and continue hydration for several days following administration of potentially nephrotoxic drug. Monitor serum creatinine and urine output during and after this period.
- ▪ **Lab Test Considerations:** Monitor BUN and serum creatine prior to and frequently throughout course of therapy. Gallium nitrate therapy should be discontinued if serum creatinine is >2.5 mg/dl.
- □ Monitor serum calcium daily and serum phosphate levels twice weekly to determine effectiveness of therapy. Oral phosphate therapy may be needed for hypophosphatemia. May also cause decreased serum bicarbonate concentrations.

Potential Nursing Diagnoses

- ▪ Injury, high risk for (indications).
- ▪ Urinary elimination, alteration in patterns (adverse reactions).

Implementation

- ▪ **General Info:** Gallium nitrate should be instituted after adequate hydration with IV saline has been established. Saline promotes the renal excretion of calcium. Diuretics may also be used following correction of hypovolemia. Adequate hydration and urine output should be maintained at 2000 mg/day throughout therapy.
- ▪ **Continuous Infusion:** Dilute daily dose in 1000 ml of 0.9% NaCl or D5W. Soln is stable for 48 hr at room temperature and 7 days if refrigerated.
- □ *Rate:* Infuse over 24 hr.

Patient/Family Teaching

- □ Encourage patient to comply with physician's diet recommendations. Diet should contain adequate amounts of calcium and vitamin D.
- □ Foods high in vitamin D include fish livers and oils, and fortified milk, bread, and cereals. Foods high in calcium include dairy products, canned salmon and sardines, broccoli, bok choy, tofu, molasses, and cream soups (see Appendix K).
- □ Emphasize need for keeping follow-up appointments to monitor progress, even after medication is discontinued, in order to detect relapse.

Evaluation

Effectiveness of therapy can be demonstrated by: ▪ Lowered serum calcium levels in patients with cancer-related hypercalcemia.

GANCICLOVIR

(gan-**sye**-kloe-vir)
Cytovene, DHPG

CLASSIFICATION(S):
Antiviral
Pregnancy Category C

INDICATIONS

▪ Treatment of cytomegalovirus (CMV) retinitis in immunocompromised patients, including HIV-infected patients.

ACTION

▪ CMV virus converts ganciclovir to its active form (ganciclovir phosphate) inside host cell, where it inhibits viral DNA polymerase. **Therapeutic Effect:**

G

▪ Antiviral effect directed preferentially against CMV-infected cells.

PHARMACOKINETICS

Absorption: Administered IV only, resulting in complete bioavailability.
Distribution: Enters the CSF. Remainder of distribution not known.
Metabolism and Excretion: 90% excreted unchanged by the kidneys.
Half-life: 2.9 hr (increased in renal impairment).

CONTRAINDICATIONS AND PRECAUTIONS

Contraindicated in: ▪ Hypersensitivity to ganciclovir or acyclovir.
Use Cautiously in: ▪ Renal impairment (dosage reduction required) ▪ Pregnancy, lactation, or children (safety not established) ▪ Elderly patients (dosage reduction recommended) ▪ Bone marrow depression ▪ Immunosuppression.

ADVERSE REACTIONS AND SIDE EFFECTS*

CNS: malaise, abnormal dreams, confusion, dizziness, headache, coma, nervousness, headache, drowsiness.
EENT: retinal detachment.
Resp: dyspnea.
CV: arrhythmias, hypertension, hypotension, edema.
GI: nausea, vomiting, gastric bleeding, abdominal pain, increased liver enzymes.
GU: hematuria, gonadal suppression.
Derm: rash, alopecia, pruritus, urticaria.
Endo: hypoglycemia.
Hemat: neutropenia, thrombocytopenia, anemia, eosinophilia.
Local: pain, phlebitis at IV site.
Neuro: tremor, ataxia.
Misc: fever.

INTERACTIONS

Drug-Drug: ▪ Increased risk of bone marrow depression with **antineoplastic agents, radiation therapy,** or **zidovudine** ▪ Toxicity may be increased by **probenecid** ▪ Increased risk of seizures with **imepenem/cilastatin.**

ROUTE AND DOSAGE

▪ **IV (Adults):** 5 mg/kg q 12 hr for 14–21 days initially, then 5 mg/kg/day or 6 mg/kg for 5 days of each wk. If progression occurs, increase to twice daily regimen.

PHARMACODYNAMICS (blood levels)

	ONSET	PEAK
IV	rapid	end of infusion

NURSING IMPLICATIONS

Assessment

□ Diagnosis of CMV retinitis should be determined by ophthalmoscopy prior to treatment with ganciclovir.
□ Culture for CMV (urine, blood, throat) may be taken prior to administration. However, a negative CMV culture does not rule out CMV retinitis.
▪ **Lab Test Considerations:** Monitor neutrophil and platelet count at least every 2 days during bid therapy and weekly thereafter. Granulocytopenia usually occurs during the first 2 wk of treatment but may occur anytime during therapy. Do not administer if neutrophil count $<500/mm^3$ or platelet count $<25,000/mm^3$. Recovery begins within 3–7 days of discontinuation of therapy.
□ Monitor serum creatinine at least once every 2 wk throughout therapy.

Potential Nursing Diagnoses

▪ Infection, high risk for (indications, patient/family teaching).
▪ Knowledge deficit related to medication regimen (patient/family teaching).

Implementation

▪ **General Info:** Soln should be prepared in a biologic cabinet. Wear gloves, gown, and mask while handling medication. Discard IV equip-

*Underlines indicate most frequent; **CAPITALS** indicate life-threatening.

ment in specially designated containers (see Appendix I).

- ▫ Do not administer SC or IM, as severe tissue irritation may result.
- ▪ **IV:** Observe infusion site for phlebitis. Rotate infusion site to prevent phlebitis.
- ▪ **Intermittent Infusion:** Reconstitute 500 mg with 10 ml of sterile water for injection for a concentration of 50 mg/ml. Do not reconstitute with bacteriostatic water with parabens; precipitation will occur. Shake well to dissolve completely. Discard vial if particulate matter or discoloration occurs. Reconstituted soln is stable for 12 hr at room temperature; do not refrigerate.
- ▫ Dilute in 100 ml of D5W, 0.9% NaCl, Ringer's or lactated Ringer's soln for a concentration not to exceed 10 mg/ml. Once diluted for infusion, soln should be used within 24 hr.
- ▫ Refrigerate but do not freeze.
- ▫ *Rate:* Administer slowly, via infusion pump, over 1 hr. Rapid administration may increase toxicity.
- ▪ **Y-Site Incompatibility:** foscarnet or ondansetron.

Patient/Family Teaching

- ▫ Inform patient that ganciclovir is not a cure for CMV retinitis. Progression of retinitis may continue in immunocompromised patients during and following therapy. Advise patients to have regular ophthalmic examinations.
- ▫ Advise patient that ganciclovir may have teratogenic effects. A nonhormonal method of contraception should be used during and for at least 90 days following therapy.
- ▫ Emphasize the importance of frequent follow-up examinations to monitor blood counts.

Evaluation

Effectiveness of therapy can be demonstrated by: ▪ Resolution of the symptoms of CMV retinitis in immunocompromised patients.

GEMFIBROZIL
(gem-**fi**-broe-zil)
Lopid

CLASSIFICATION(S):
Lipid-lowering agent
Pregnancy Category B

INDICATIONS

▪ Adjunct to dietary therapy in the management of hyperlipidemias associated with high triglyceride levels.

ACTION

▪ Inhibits peripheral lipolysis ▪ Decreases triglyceride (very low-density lipoprotein [VLDL]) production by the liver ▪ Decreases production of the triglyceride carrier protein ▪ Increases high-density lipoproteins (HDL). **Therapeutic Effects:** ▪ Decreased plasma triglycerides and increased HDL.

PHARMACOKINETICS

Absorption: Well absorbed following oral administration.
Distribution: Distribution not known.
Metabolism and Excretion: Some metabolism by the liver, 70% excreted by the kidneys (mostly unchanged) 6% excreted in feces.
Half-life: 1.3–1.5 hr.

CONTRAINDICATIONS AND PRECAUTIONS

Contraindicated in: ▪ Hypersensitivity ▪ Primary biliary cirrhosis.
Use Cautiously in: ▪ Gallbladder disease ▪ Liver disease ▪ Severe renal impairment ▪ Pregnancy, lactation, or children (safety not established).

ADVERSE REACTIONS AND SIDE EFFECTS*

CNS: headache, dizziness.
EENT: blurred vision.
GI: abdominal pain, epigastric pain, heartburn, gallstones, diarrhea, nausea, vomiting, flatulence.
Derm: rashes, urticaria, alopecia.

*Underlines indicate most frequent; **CAPITALS** indicate life-threatening.

G

Hemat: leukopenia, anemia.
MS: myositis.

INTERACTIONS

Drug–Drug: ▪ May increase the effect of **oral anticoagulants** ▪ **Thiazide diuretics, methyldopa,** or **estrogens** may decrease the response to gemfibrozil.

ROUTE AND DOSAGE

- **PO (Adults):** 1.2 g/day in 2 divided doses 30 min before breakfast and dinner (range 900 mg–1.5 g).

PHARMACODYNAMICS (triglyceride—VLDL lowering effect)

	ONSET	PEAK	DURATION
PO	2–5 days	4 wk	several mons

NURSING IMPLICATIONS

Assessment

- ▫ Obtain patient's diet history, especially regarding fat and alcohol consumption.
- ▪ **Lab Test Considerations:** Serum triglyceride and cholesterol levels should be monitored closely. LDL and VLDL levels should be assessed prior to and periodically throughout therapy. Medication should be discontinued if paradoxic increase in lipid levels occurs.
- ▫ Liver function tests should be assessed prior to and periodically throughout therapy. May cause an increase in alkaline phosphatase, CPK, LDH, SGOT (AST), and SGPT (ALT).
- ▫ CBC and electrolytes should be evaluated every 3–6 mon and then yearly throughout course of therapy. May cause mild decrease in hemoglobin, hematocrit, and leukocyte counts. May cause a decrease in serum potassium concentrations.
- ▫ May cause slight increase in serum glucose.

Potential Nursing Diagnoses

- ▪ Knowledge deficit related to medication regimen (patient/family teaching).
- ▪ Noncompliance (patient/family teaching).

Implementation

- ▪ **PO:** Administer 30 min before breakfast or dinner.

Patient/Family Teaching

- ▫ Instruct patient to take medication exactly as directed, not to skip doses or double up on missed doses. If a dose is missed, take as soon as remembered unless almost time for next dose.
- ▫ Advise patient that this medication should be used in conjunction with dietary restrictions (fat, cholesterol, carbohydrates, alcohol), exercise, and cessation of smoking.
- ▫ Instruct patient to notify physician promptly if any of the following symptoms occur: severe stomach pains with nausea and vomiting, fever, chills, sore throat. Physician should also be notified if rash, diarrhea, muscle cramping, general abdominal discomfort, or persistent flatulence occurs.

Evaluation

Effectiveness of therapy can be demonstrated by: ▪ Decrease in serum triglyceride and cholesterol levels and improved high-density lipoprotein (HDL) to total cholesterol ratios. If response is not seen within 3 mon, medication is usually discontinued.

GENTAMICIN

(jen-ta-**mye**-sin)
{Alcomicin}, {Cidomycin}, Garamycin, Genoptic, Gentacidin, Gentafair, {Gentamytrex}, G-Myticin

CLASSIFICATION(S):
Anti-infective—aminoglycoside
Pregnancy Category C

{} = Available in Canada only.

INDICATIONS

■ **IM, IV:** Treatment of gram-negative bacillary infections and infections due to staphylococci when penicillins or other less toxic drugs are contraindicated. Especially useful in the following serious gram-negative bacillary infections due to susceptible organisms: □ Bone infections □ CNS infections (intrathecal administration required) □ Respiratory tract infections □ Skin and soft tissue infections □ Abdominal infections □ Complicated urinary tract infections □ Endocarditis □ Septicemia ■ **IM, IV:** Part of a regimen for endocarditis prophylaxis in certain patient populations ■ **Top, Ophth:** Treatment of localized infections due to susceptible organisms.

ACTION

■ Inhibits protein synthesis in bacteria at the level of the 30S ribosome. **Therapeutic Effect:** ■ Bactericidal action against susceptible bacteria. **Spectrum:** ■ *Pseudomonas aeruginosa* ■ *Klebsiella pneumoniae* ■ *Escherichia coli* ■ *Serratia* ■ *Acenitobacter* ■ In the treatment of enterococcal infections, synergy with a penicillin is required.

PHARMACOKINETICS

Absorption: Well absorbed after IM administration. Minimal systemic absorption following topical, intrathecal, or intraventricular administration.

Distribution: Widely distributed in extracellular fluids following IM or IV administration. Crosses the placenta. Poor penetration into CSF.

Metabolism and Excretion: Excretion is mainly renal (>90%). Dosage adjustments are required for any decrease in renal function. Minimal amounts metabolized by the liver.

Half-life: 2–3 hr (increased in renal impairment).

CONTRAINDICATIONS AND PRECAUTIONS

Contraindicated in: ■ Hypersensitivity ■ Cross-sensitivity with other aminoglycosides may exist.

Use Cautiously in: ■ Renal impairment of any kind (dosage adjustments required) ■ Pregnancy and lactation (safety not established) ■ Neuromuscular diseases, such as myasthenia gravis.

ADVERSE REACTIONS AND SIDE EFFECTS*

EENT: <u>ototoxicity</u> (vestibular and cochlear).

GU: <u>nephrotoxicity</u>.

Neuro: enhanced neuromuscular blockade.

Misc: hypersensitivity reactions, superinfection.

INTERACTIONS

Drug–Drug: ■ Inactivated by **penicillins** when coadministered to patients with renal insufficiency ■ Possible respiratory paralysis after inhalation **anesthetics (ether, cyclopropane, halothane,** or **nitrous oxide)** or **neuromuscular blockers (atracurium, tubocurarine, gallamine, succinylcholine, decamethonium)** ■ Additive possibility of neuromuscular blockade with other **aminoglycoside antibiotics** ■ Increased incidence of ototoxicity with **loop diuretics (ethacrynic acid, furosemide)** ■ Incidence of nephrotoxicity may be increased with other potentially **nephrotoxic drugs (cisplatin)**.

ROUTE AND DOSAGE

Note: All doses after initial loading dose should be determined by renal function/blood levels.

- **IM, IV (Adults):** 3–5 mg/kg/day in divided doses q 8 hr.
- **IM, IV (Children):** 6–7.5 mg/kg/day in divided doses q 8 hr.
- **IM, IV (Infants and Neonates):** 7.5 mg/kg/day in divided doses q 8 hr.
- **IM, IV (Premature Infants, Neonates <1 wk):** 2.5 mg/kg q 12 hr.
- **Top (Adults and Children):** 0.1%

*<u>Underlines</u> indicate most frequent; **CAPITALS** indicate life-threatening.

G

cream or ointment, apply to cleansed area 3–4 times daily.

- **Ophth (Adults and Children):** 0.3% soln—1–2 drops q 2–4 hr or 0.3% ointment 2–3 times daily.
- **Intrathecal or Intraventricular (Adults):** 4–8 mg/day as a single dose.
- **Intrathecal or Intraventricular (Children and Infants >3 mon):** 1–2 mg/day as a single dose.

PHARMACODYNAMICS (blood levels)

	ONSET	PEAK
IM	rapid	30–90 min
IV	rapid	end of infusion

NURSING IMPLICATIONS

Assessment

- Assess patient for infection (vital signs; appearance of wound, sputum, urine, and stool; WBC) at beginning and throughout course of therapy.
- Obtain specimens for culture and sensitivity prior to initiating therapy. First dose may be given before receiving results.
- Evaluate eighth cranial nerve function by audiometry prior to and throughout course of therapy. Hearing loss is usually in the high-frequency range. Prompt recognition and intervention is essential in preventing permanent damage. Also monitor for vestibular dysfunction (vertigo, ataxia, nausea, vomiting). Eighth cranial nerve dysfunction is associated with persistently elevated peak gentamicin levels.
- Monitor intake and output and daily weight to assess hydration status and renal function.
- Assess patient for signs of superinfections (fever, upper respiratory infection, vaginal itching or discharge, increasing malaise, diarrhea). Report to physician.
- **Lab Test Considerations:** Monitor renal function by urinalysis, specific gravity, BUN, creatinine, and creatinine clearance prior to and throughout therapy.
- May cause increased SGOT (AST), SGPT (ALT), LDH, bilirubin, and serum alkaline phosphatase levels.
- May cause decreased serum calcium, magnesium, sodium, and potassium levels.
- **Toxicity and Overdose:** Blood levels should be monitored periodically during therapy. Timing of blood levels is important in interpreting results. Draw blood for peak levels 30–60 min after IM injection and immediately after IV infusion is completed. Trough levels should be drawn just prior to next dose. Acceptable peak level is 4–12 mcg/ml; trough level should not exceed 2 mcg/ml.

Potential Nursing Diagnoses

- Infection, high risk for (indications).
- Sensory-perceptual alteration: auditory (side effects).

Implementation

- **General Info:** Keep patient well hydrated (1500–2000 ml/day) during therapy.
- Do not use soln that is discolored or that contains a precipitate.
- **IM:** IM administration should be deep into a well-developed muscle.
- **Intermittent Infusion:** Dilute each dose of gentamicin in 50–200 ml of D5W, 0.9% NaCl, or Ringer's soln to provide a concentration not to exceed 1 mg/ml (0.1%). Also available in commercially mixed piggyback injections.
- *Rate:* Infuse slowly over 30–60 min. Flush IV linc with D5W or 0.9% NaCl following administration.
- Manufacturer recommends administering separately; do not admix. Give aminoglycosides and penicillins at least 1 hr apart to prevent inactivation.
- **Syringe Compatibility:** clindamycin, methicillin, or penicillin G sodium.
- **Syringe Incompatibility:** ampicillin, cefamandole, clindamycin, or heparin.
- **Y-Site Compatibility:** acyclovir, atracurium, cyclophosphamide, enalaprilat, esmolol, famotidine, foscarnet, la-

betalol, hydromorphone, magnesium sulfate, meperidine, morphine, multivitamins, ondansetron, pancuronium, perphenazine, tolazoline, vecuronium, or zidovudine.

- **Y-Site Incompatibility:** furosemide, heparin, or hetastrach.
- **Additive Compatibility:** aztreonam, bleomycin, cefoxitin, cimetidine, clindamycin, methicillin, metronidazole, penicillin G sodium, ranitidine, or verapamil.
- **Additive Incompatibility:** amphotericin B, ampicillin, cefamandole, cephalothin, cephapirin, clindamycin, furosemide, heparin, nafcillin, or ticarcillin.
- **Ophth:** See Appendix H for administration of ophthalmic preparations.
- **Top:** Cleanse skin prior to application. Wear gloves during application.

Patient/Family Teaching

- **General Info:** Instruct patient to report signs of hypersensitivity, tinnitus, vertigo, or hearing loss.
- Patients with a history of rheumatic heart disease or valve replacement should be taught the importance of using antimicrobial prophylaxis before invasive medical or dental procedures.
- **Top:** Instruct patient on correct technique for application.

Evaluation

Clinical response to therapy can be evaluated by: ▪ Resolution of the signs and symptoms of infection. Length of time for complete resolution depends on the organism and site of infection ▪ Endocarditis prophylaxis.

GLIPIZIDE
(**glip**-i-zide)
Glucotrol

CLASSIFICATION(S):
Oral hypoglycemic agent—sulfonylurea
Pregnancy Category C

INDICATIONS

▪ Control of blood sugar in adult-onset, noninsulin-dependent diabetes (NIDDM, type II, adult-onset, nonketosis-prone) when dietary therapy fails. Requires some pancreatic function.

ACTION

▪ Lowers blood sugar by stimulating the release of insulin from the pancreas and increasing sensitivity to insulin at receptor sites ▪ May also decrease hepatic glucose production. **Therapeutic Effect:** ▪ Lowering of blood sugar in diabetic patients.

PHARMACOKINETICS

Absorption: Well absorbed following oral administration.
Distribution: Distribution not known.
Metabolism and Excretion: Almost completely metabolized by the liver.
Half-life: 2.1–2.6 hr.

CONTRAINDICATIONS AND PRECAUTIONS

Contraindicated in: ▪ Hypersensitivity ▪ Cross-sensitivity with sulfonamides or thiazides may exist ▪ Insulin-dependent diabetics (type I, juvenile-onset, ketosis-prone, brittle) ▪ Severe renal impairment ▪ Severe hepatic impairment ▪ Thyroid or other endocrine disease ▪ Pregnancy or lactation.
Use Cautiously in: ▪ Severe cardiovascular disease (increased risk of congestive heart failure) ▪ Severe liver disease (dosage reduction may be required) ▪ Elderly, debilitated, or malnourished patients (dosage reduction may be required) ▪ Infection, stress, or changes in diet may alter requirements for control of blood sugar.

ADVERSE REACTIONS AND SIDE EFFECTS*

CNS: dizziness, drowsiness, headache.
GI: <u>nausea</u>, <u>vomiting</u>, diarrhea, cramps, hepatitis.
Derm: rashes, photosensitivity.
Endo: <u>hypoglycemia</u>.
Hemat: blood dyscrasias, including

*<u>Underlines</u> indicate most frequent; **CAPITALS** indicate life-threatening.

APLASTIC ANEMIA, AGRANULOCYTOSIS, hemolytic anemia.

INTERACTIONS

Drug–Drug: ▪ Ingestion of **alcohol** may result in disulfiram-like reaction ▪ **Alcohol, glucocorticoids, rifampin,** and **thiazides** may decrease effectiveness ▪ **Androgens (testosterone), chloramphenicol, clofibrate, monoamine oxidase inhibitors, phenylbutazone, salicylates, sulfonamides, NSAIDs,** and **oral anticoagulants** may increase effectiveness and cause hypoglycemia ▪ Concurrent **oral anticoagulant** therapy may result in altered response to glipizide—dosage adjustments of both agents may be necessary ▪ Concurrent **beta-adreneric blocker** therapy may produce prolonged hypoglycemia and may mask symptoms.

ROUTE AND DOSAGE

▪ **PO (Adults):** 2.5–40 mg/day (usually 5–25 mg/day). Doses >15–20 mg/day should be divided and given bid.

PHARMACODYNAMICS (hypoglycemic activity)

	ONSET	PEAK	DURATION
PO	15–30 min	1–2 hr	up to 24 hr

NURSING IMPLICATIONS

Assessment

□ Observe patient for signs and symptoms of hypoglycemic reactions (sweating, hunger, weakness, dizziness, tremor, tachycardia, anxiety). Long duration of action increases the risk of recurrent hypoglycemia. Monitor patients who experience a hypoglycemic episode closely for 1–2 days.

□ Assess patient for allergy to sulfonamides.

▪ **Lab Test Considerations:** Serum glucose and glycosylated hemoglobin should be monitored periodically throughout therapy to evaluate effectiveness of treatment.

□ May cause increase in SGOT (AST), LDH, BUN, and serum creatinine.

□ CBC should be monitored periodically throughout therapy. Notify physician promptly if decrease in blood counts occur.

▪ **Toxicity and Overdose:** Overdose is manifested by symptoms of hypoglycemia. Mild hypoglycemia may be treated with administration of oral glucose. Severe hypoglycemia should be treated with IV D50W followed by continuous IV infusion of more dilute dextrose soln at a rate sufficient to keep serum glucose at approximately 100 mg/dl.

Potential Nursing Diagnoses

▪ Nutrition, altered: more than body requirements (indications).

▪ Knowledge deficit related to medication regimen (patient/family teaching).

▪ Noncompliance (patient/family teaching).

Implementation

▪ **General Info:** May be administered once in the morning or divided into 2 doses.

□ Patients stabilized on a diabetic regimen who are exposed to stress, fever, trauma, infection, or surgery may require administration of insulin.

□ To convert from insulin dosage of less than 20 units/day, change may be made without gradual dosage adjustment. Patients taking >20 units/day should convert gradually, receiving glipizide and 50% of previous insulin dose for 1 day, with gradual dosage adjustment of glipizide as needed. Monitor serum or urine glucose and ketones at least 3 times/day during conversion.

▪ **PO:** Administer 30 min before meals to ensure best diabetic control.

□ Tablets may be crushed and taken with fluids if patient has difficulty swallowing.

Patient/Family Teaching

□ Instruct patient to take medication at same time each day. If a dose is missed, take as soon as remembered unless almost time for next dose. Do not take if unable to eat.

□ Explain to patient that this medication controls hyperglycemia but does not cure diabetes. Therapy is long-term.

- Review signs of hypoglycemia and hyperglycemia with patient. If hypoglycemia occurs, advise patient to take a glass of orange juice or sugar, honey, or corn syrup dissolved in water and notify physician.
- Encourage patient to follow prescribed diet, medication, and exercise regimen to prevent hypoglycemic or hyperglycemic episodes.
- Instruct patient in proper testing of blood or urine for glucose and ketones. Stress the importance of double-voided specimens for accuracy. These tests should be closely monitored during periods of stress or illness and physician notified if significant changes occur. During conversion from insulin to oral antidiabetic agents, patients should check glucose levels at least 3 times/day and report results to physician as directed.
- Glipizide may occasionally cause dizziness or drowsiness. Caution patient to avoid driving or other activities requiring alertness until response to medication is known.
- Caution patient to avoid other medications, especially those containing aspirin, and alcohol while on this therapy without consulting physician or pharmacist.
- Advise patient that concurrent use of alcohol may cause a disulfiram-like reaction (abdominal cramps, nausea, flushing, headaches, and hypoglycemia).
- This medication should not be used during pregnancy. Counsel female patient to use a form of contraception other than oral contraceptives and to notify physician promptly if pregnancy is suspected.
- Caution patient to use sunscreen and protective clothing to prevent photosensitivity reactions.
- Advise patient to inform physician or dentist of medication regimen prior to treatment or surgery.
- Advise patient to carry a form of sugar (sugar packets, candy) and identification describing disease and medication regimen at all times.
- Emphasize the importance of routine follow-up with physician.

EVALUATION

Effectiveness of therapy can be demonstrated by: ■ Control of blood glucose levels without the appearance of hypoglycemic or hyperglycemic episodes.

GLUCAGON
(**gloo**-ka-gon)

CLASSIFICATION(S):
Hormone
Pregnancy Category B

INDICATIONS

■ Acute management of severe hypoglycemia when administration of glucose is not feasible ■ Used to terminate insulin shock therapy in psychiatric patients ■ Used to facilitate radiographic examination of the GI tract.

ACTION

■ Stimulates hepatic production of glucose from glycogen stores (glycogenolysis) ■ Relaxes the musculature of the GI tract ■ Has positive inotropic and chronotropic effects. **Therapeutic Effects:** ■ Increase in blood sugar ■ Relaxation of GI musculature, facilitating radiographic examination.

PHARMACOKINETICS

Absorption: Well absorbed following IM and SC administration.
Distribution: Distribution not known.
Metabolism and Excretion: Extensively metabolized by the liver and kidneys.
Half-life: 3–10 min.

CONTRAINDICATIONS AND PRECAUTIONS

Contraindicated in: ■ Hypersensitivity to beef or pork protein ■ Diluent contains glycerin and phenol—avoid use

G

in patients with hypersensitivities to these ingredients.

Use Cautiously in: ▪ History of insulinoma or pheochromocytoma.

ADVERSE REACTIONS AND SIDE EFFECTS*

GI: nausea, vomiting.
Misc: hypersensitivity reactions.

INTERACTIONS

Drug–Drug: ▪ Large doses may enhance the effect of **oral anticoagulants** ▪ Negates the response to **insulin** or **oral hypoglycemic** agents ▪ Hyperglycemic effect is intensified and prolonged by **epinephrine**.

ROUTE AND DOSAGE

Note: 1 USP unit = 1 mg.

Hypoglycemia, Terminating Insulin Shock

- **IV, IM, SC (Adults):** 0.5–1 unit; if no response, may repeat in 5–20 min for 1–2 more doses.
- **IV, IM, SC (Children):** 0.025 unit/kg; if no response, may repeat in 5–20 min for 1–2 more doses.

Radiographic Examination of the GI Tract

- **IM (Adults):** 1–2 units.
- **IV (Adults):** 0.25–2 units.

PHARMACODYNAMICS

	ONSET	PEAK	DURATION
IV, SC (hyperglycemic action)	5–20 min	30 min	1–2 hr
IV (effect on GI musculature)	1 min	UK	9–25 min
IM (effect on GI musculature)	4–10 min	UK	12–32 min

NURSING IMPLICATIONS

Assessment

- Assess patient for signs of hypoglycemia (sweating, hunger, weakness, headache, dizziness, tremor, irritability, tachycardia, anxiety) prior to and periodically during course of therapy.
- Assess neurologic status throughout course of therapy. Institute safety precautions to protect patient from injury caused by seizures, falling, or aspiration.
- Assess nutritional status. Patients who lack liver glycogen stores (as in starvation, chronic hypoglycemia, and adrenal insufficiency) will require administration of glucose instead of glucagon.
- Assess for nausea and vomiting after administration of dose. Protect patients with depressed level of consciousness from aspiration by positioning on side; ensure that a suction unit is available. Notify physician if vomiting occurs; patient will require parenteral glucose to prevent recurrent hypoglycemia.
- Monitor serum glucose levels to determine effectiveness of therapy. Use of bedside fingerstick blood glucose determination methods is recommended for rapid results. Follow-up lab results may be ordered to validate fingerstick values, but do not delay treatment while awaiting lab results as this could result in neurologic injury or death.

Potential Nursing Diagnoses

- Injury, high risk for (indications).
- Knowledge deficit related to medication regimen (patient/family teaching).
- Noncompliance (patient/family teaching).

Implementation

- **General Info:** May be given SC, IM, or IV. Reconstitute with diluent supplied in kit by manufacturer. Inspect soln prior to use; use only clear, water-like soln. Soln is stable for 48 hr if refrigerated, 24 hr at room temperature.
- Administer supplemental carbohydrates IV or orally to facilitate increase of serum glucose levels.
- **IV:** Reconstitute with diluent supplied in kit by manufacturer. With

*Underlines indicate most frequent; **CAPITALS** indicate life-threatening.

doses >2 units (2 mg), use sterile water for injection instead of diluent supplied by manufacturer. Use immediately after reconstituting. Final concentration should not exceed 1 unit (1 mg/ml).

- **Direct IV:** Administer at a rate not exceeding 1 unit (1 mg) per min. May be administered through IV line containing D5W.
- May be given at the same time as a bolus of dextrose.
- **Additive Incompatibility:** 0.9% NaCl, potassium chloride, or calcium chloride.

Patient/Family Teaching

- Teach patient and family signs and symptoms of hypoglycemia. Instruct patient to take oral glucose as soon as symptoms of hypoglycemia occur—glucagon is reserved for episodes when patient is unable to swallow due to decreased level of consciousness.
- Instruct family on correct technique to prepare, draw up, and administer injection. Physician must be contacted immediately after each dose for orders regarding further therapy or adjustment of insulin dose or diet.
- Advise family that patient should receive oral glucose when alertness returns.
- Instruct family to position patient on side until fully alert. Explain that glucagon may cause nausea and vomiting. Aspiration may occur if patient vomits while lying on back.
- Instruct patient to check expiration date monthly and to replace outdated medication immediately.
- Review hypoglycemic medication regimen, diet, and exercise programs.
- Patients with diabetes mellitus should carry a source of sugar (such as a packet of sugar or candy) and identification describing disease process and treatment regimen at all times.

Evaluation

Effectiveness of therapy can be demonstrated by: ▪ Increase of serum glucose to normal levels with improved level of consciousness ▪ Smooth muscle relaxation of the stomach, duodenum, and small and large intestine in patients undergoing radiologic examination of the GI tract.

GLUTETHIMIDE

(gloo-**teth**-i-mide)
Doriden, Doriglute

CLASSIFICATION(S):
Sedative/hypnotic—miscellaneous
Schedule II
Pregnancy Category C

INDICATIONS

▪ Short-term (3–7 days) management of insomnia.

ACTION

▪ Produces generalized CNS depression similar to barbiturates ▪ Has anticholinergic properties. **Therapeutic Effect:** ▪ Relief of insomnia.

PHARMACOKINETICS

Absorption: Unpredictably absorbed from the GI tract.
Distribution: Widely distributed, concentrates in adipose tissue. Crosses the placenta well; enters breast milk in small amounts.
Metabolism and Excretion: Highly (>95%) metabolized by the liver.
Half-life: 10–12 hr.

CONTRAINDICATIONS AND PRECAUTIONS

Contraindicated in: ▪ Hypersensitivity ▪ Poorly controlled pain ▪ Porphyria ▪ Severe renal disease ▪ Patients who may have been addicted to drugs previously.
Use Cautiously in: ▪ Prostatic hypertrophy ▪ Ulcer disease ▪ GI obstruction ▪ Bladder neck obstruction ▪ Glaucoma ▪ Cardiac arrhythmias ▪ Pregnancy, lac-

tation, or children <12 yr (safety not established) ▪ Elderly patients (dosage reduction recommended).

ADVERSE REACTIONS AND SIDE EFFECTS*

CNS: hangover, paradoxical excitation, headache, vertigo.
EENT: blurred vision.
GI: gastric irritation, nausea, hiccups, dry mouth, diarrhea, hepatitis.
Hemat: blood dyscrasias, porphyria.
Derm: rashes, exfoliative dermatitis.
Neuro: peripheral neuropathy.
Misc: hypersensitivity reactions, psychological dependence, physical dependence.

INTERACTIONS

Drug-Drug: ▪ Additive CNS depression with other **CNS depressants,** including **alcohol, sedative/hypnotics, narcotic analgesics, tricyclic antidepressants,** and **antihistamines** ▪ Additive anticholinergic effects with **tricyclic antidepressants** ▪ May increase the metabolism and decrease the effectiveness of **oral anticoagulants**.

ROUTE AND DOSAGE

- **PO (Adults):** 250–500 mg at bedtime (not to exceed 1 g/day).

PHARMACODYNAMICS (hypnotic effect)

	ONSET	PEAK	DURATION
PO	30 min	UK	4–8 hr

NURSING IMPLICATIONS

Assessment

- Assess mental status, sleep patterns, and potential for abuse prior to administering this medication. Prolonged use of greater than 1 wk may lead to decreased effectiveness and physical and psychological dependence. Limit amount of drug available to the patient.
- Assess alertness at time of peak effect. Notify physician if desired sedation does not occur or if paradoxical reaction occurs.
- Assess patient for pain. Medicate as needed. Untreated pain decreases sedative effects.

Potential Nursing Diagnoses

- Sleep pattern disturbance (indications).
- Injury, high risk for (side effects).

Implementation

- **General Info:** Before administering, reduce external stimuli and provide comfort measures to increase effectiveness of medication. Administer at least 4 hr before usual time of awakening to minimize daytime drowsiness.
- Protect patient from injury. Place bed side rails up. Assist with ambulation. Remove cigarettes from patients with hypnotic dose.
- Available in capsule or tablet.
- **PO:** Capsules should be swallowed whole with a full glass of water.

Patient/Family Teaching

- Instruct patient to take glutethimide exactly as directed. Do not take more than the amount prescribed because of the habit-forming potential. Not recommended for use longer than 1 wk. If used for 2 wk or longer, effectiveness may decrease and abrupt withdrawal may result in convulsions, tachycardia, hallucinations, increased dreaming, muscle cramps, nausea, or vomiting.
- May cause daytime drowsiness or dizziness. Advise patient to avoid driving or other activities requiring alertness until response to this medication is known.
- Caution patient to avoid concurrent use of alcohol or other CNS depressants.
- Advise patient to discontinue use and notify physician if skin rash occurs.

Evaluation

Effectiveness of therapy can be demonstrated by: ▪ Relief of insomnia.

*Underlines indicate most frequent; **CAPITALS** indicate life-threatening.

GLYBURIDE
(glye-byoo-ride)
Diabeta, {Euglucon}, Glybenclamide, Micronase

CLASSIFICATION(S):
Oral hypoglycemic agent—sulfonylurea
Pregnancy Category B

INDICATIONS

▪ Control of blood sugar in adult-onset, noninsulin-dependent diabetes (NIDDM, type II, adult-onset, nonketosis-prone) when dietary therapy fails. Requires some pancreatic function.

ACTION

▪ Lowers blood sugar by stimulating the release of insulin from the pancreas and increasing sensitivity to insulin at receptor sites ▪ May also decrease hepatic glucose production. **Therapeutic Effect:** ▪ Lowering of blood sugar in diabetic patients.

PHARMACOKINETICS

Absorption: Well absorbed following oral administration.
Distribution: Reaches high concentrations in bile. Crosses the placenta.
Metabolism and Excretion: Almost completely metabolized by the liver.
Half-life: 10 hr.

CONTRAINDICATIONS AND PRECAUTIONS

Contraindicated in: ▪ Hypersensitivity ▪ Cross-sensitivity with thiazides and sulfonylureas may exist ▪ Insulin-dependent diabetics (type I, juvenile-onset, ketosis-prone, brittle) ▪ Severe renal impairment ▪ Severe hepatic impairment ▪ Thyroid or other endocrine disease ▪ Pregnancy or lactation.
Use Cautiously in: ▪ Severe cardiovascular disease (increased risk of congestive heart failure) ▪ Severe liver disease (dosage reduction may be required) ▪ Elderly, debilitated, or malnourished patients (dosage reduction may be required) ▪ Infection, stress, or changes in diet may alter requirements for control of blood sugar.

ADVERSE REACTIONS AND SIDE EFFECTS*

CNS: dizziness, drowsiness, headache.
GI: <u>nausea</u>, <u>vomiting</u>, diarrhea, cramps, hepatitis.
Derm: rashes, photosensitivity.
Endo: <u>hypoglycemia</u>.
Hemat: blood dyscrasias, including APLASTIC ANEMIA, AGRANULOCYTOSIS, hemolytic anemia.

INTERACTIONS

Drug-Drug: ▪ Ingestion of **alcohol** may result in disulfiram-like reaction ▪ **Alcohol, glucocorticoids, rifampin,** and **thiazides** may decrease effectiveness ▪ **Androgens (testosterone), chloramphenicol, clofibrate, monoamine oxidase inhibitors, phenylbutazone, salicylates, sulfonamides, NSAIDs,** and **oral anticoagulants** may increase effectiveness and cause hypoglycemia ▪ Concurrent **oral anticoagulant** therapy may result in altered response to glyburide—dosage adjustments of both agents may be necessary ▪ Concurrent **beta-adrenergic blocker** therapy may produce prolonged hypoglycemia and may mask symptoms.

ROUTE AND DOSAGE

▪ **PO (Adults):** 1.25–20 mg (usual dose 2.5–10 mg/day), single dose. Doses >10 mg/day should be divided and given bid.

PHARMACODYNAMICS (hypoglycemic activity)

	ONSET	PEAK	DURATION
PO	45–60 min	1.5–3 hr	24 hr

NURSING IMPLICATIONS

ASSESSMENT

□ Observe patient for signs and symptoms of hypoglycemic reactions

{} = Available in Canada only.
*<u>Underlines</u> indicate most frequent; **CAPITALS** indicate life-threatening.

(sweating, hunger, weakness, dizziness, tremor, tachycardia, anxiety). Long duration of action increases the risk of recurrent hypoglycemia. Monitor patients who experience a hypoglycemic episode closely for 1–2 days.

- Assess patient for allergy to sulfonamides.
- **Lab Test Considerations:** Serum glucose and glycosylated hemoglobin should be monitored periodically throughout therapy to evaluate effectiveness of treatment.
- CBC should be monitored periodically throughout therapy. Notify physician promptly if decrease in blood counts occurs.
- **Toxicity and Overdose:** Overdose is manifested by symptoms of hypoglycemia. Mild hypoglycemia may be treated with administration of oral glucose. Severe hypoglycemia should be treated with IV D50W followed by continuous IV infusion of more dilute dextrose soln at a rate sufficient to keep serum glucose at approximately 100 mg/dl.

Potential Nursing Diagnoses

- Nutrition, altered: more than body requirements (indications).
- Knowledge deficit related to medication regimen (patient/family teaching).
- Noncompliance (patient/family teaching).

Implementation

- **General Info:** May be administered once in the morning or divided into 2 doses.
- Patients stabilized on a diabetic regimen who are exposed to stress, fever, trauma, infection, or surgery may require administration of insulin.
- To convert from insulin dosage of $<$40 units/day, change may be made without gradual dosage adjustment. Patients taking $>$40 units/day should convert gradually by receiving glyburide and 50% of previous insulin dose for 1 day, with gradual dosage adjustment of glyburide as needed. Monitor serum or urine glucose and ketones at least 3 times/day during conversion.
- **PO:** Administer with meals.
- Tablets may be crushed and taken with fluids if patient has difficulty swallowing.

Patient/Family Teaching

- Instruct patient to take medication at same time each day. If a dose is missed, take as soon as remembered unless almost time for next dose. Do not take if unable to eat.
- Explain to patient that this medication controls hyperglycemia but does not cure diabetes. Therapy is long-term.
- Review with patient signs of hypoglycemia and hyperglycemia. If hypoglycemia occurs, advise patient to take a glass of orange juice or sugar, honey, or corn syrup dissolved in water and notify physician.
- Encourage patient to follow prescribed diet, medication, and exercise regimen to prevent hypoglycemic or hyperglycemic episodes.
- Instruct patient in proper testing of blood or urine for glucose and ketones. Stress the importance of double-voided specimens for accuracy. These tests should be closely monitored during periods of stress or illness and physician notified if significant changes occur. During conversion from insulin to oral antidiabetic agents, patients should check glucose levels at least 3 times/day and report results to physician as directed.
- Glyburide may occasionally cause dizziness or drowsiness. Caution patient to avoid driving or other activities requiring alertness until response to medication is known.
- Caution patient to avoid taking other medications, especially those containing aspirin, and alcohol while on this therapy without consulting physician or pharmacist.
- Advise patient that concurrent use of alcohol may cause a disulfiram-like

reaction (abdominal cramps, nausea, flushing, headaches, and hypoglycemia).

- This medication should not be used during pregnancy. Counsel female patient to use a form of contraception other than oral contraceptives and to notify physician promptly if pregnancy is suspected.
- Caution patient to use sunscreen and protective clothing to prevent photosensitivity reactions.
- Advise patient to carry a form of sugar (sugar packets, candy) and identification describing disease and medication regimen at all times.
- Emphasize the importance of routine follow-up with physician.

EVALUATION

Effectiveness of therapy can be demonstrated by: ▪ Control of blood glucose levels without the appearance of hypoglycemic or hyperglycemic episodes.

GLYCERIN

(gli-ser-in)

Baby-lax, Glyrol, Ophthalgan, Osmoglyn, Sani-Supp

CLASSIFICATION(S):
Laxative—osmotic, Diuretic—osmotic, Antiglaucoma agent
Pregnancy Category C

INDICATIONS

▪ **Rect:** Treatment of constipation ▪ **PO:** Short-term reduction of intraocular pressure ▪ **Ophth:** Management of edema of the superficial layers of the cornea. **Unlabeled Use:** ▪ ***PO:*** Reduction of elevated intracranial pressure.

ACTION

▪ Draws water into the lumen of the colon ▪ Osmotically draws water from extravascular spaces, including the eye, into intravascular compartment. **Therapeutic Effects:** ▪ Relief of constipation ▪ Reduction of intraocular and intracranial pressure ▪ Reduced swelling of superficial layers of the cornea.

PHARMACOKINETICS

Absorption: Not significantly absorbed from colonic mucosa. Well absorbed following oral administration.
Distribution: Remains in the intravascular space.
Metabolism and Excretion: 80% metabolized by the liver, 10–20% metabolized by the kidneys.
Half-life: 30–45 min.

CONTRAINDICATIONS AND PRECAUTIONS

Contraindicated in: ▪ Hypersensitivity ▪ Hypersensitivity to ingredients in preparations (ophth soln contains chlorobutanol).
Use Cautiously in: ▪ Cardiovascular disease ▪ Mental confusion ▪ Severe dehydration ▪ Diabetes mellitus ▪ Hypervolemia ▪ Renal disease ▪ Elderly patients (increased risk of dehydration).

ADVERSE REACTIONS AND SIDE EFFECTS*

CNS: confusion, headache, **SEIZURES**.
GI: nausea, vomiting, diarrhea.
F and E: dehydration.
Misc: thirst.

INTERACTIONS

Drug-Drug: ▪ **Diuretics** increase the intraocular pressure-lowering effects of glycerin.

ROUTE AND DOSAGE

Laxative

- **Rect (Adults and Children >6 yr):** 2–3 g as a suppository or 5–15 ml as an enema.
- **Rect (Children <6 yr):** 1–1.7 g as a suppository or 2–5 ml as an enema.

Reduction of Intraocular Pressure

- **PO (Adults):** 1–1.5 g/kg as a single dose, may be followed by 500 mg/kg q 6 hr.
- **PO (Children):** 1–1.5 g/kg as a single

*Underlines indicate most frequent; **CAPITALS** indicate life-threatening.

dose, may be followed by 500 mg/kg 4–8 hr later.

Management of Superficial Edema of the Cornea

- **Ophth (Adults):** 1–2 drops every 3–4 hr.

PHARMACODYNAMICS

	ONSET	PEAK	DURATION
Rect (laxative effect)	UK	15–30 min	UK
PO (reduction of intraocular pressure)	10–30 min	30 min–2 hr	4–8 hr
Ophth (reduced corneal swelling)	UK	UK	3–4 hr

NURSING IMPLICATIONS

Assessment

- **Laxative:** Assess patient for abdominal distension, presence of bowel sounds, and normal pattern of bowel function.
  - Assess color, consistency, and amount of stool produced.
- **Lab Test Considerations:** May cause slightly elevated serum and urine glucose concentrations.

Potential Nursing Diagnoses

- Bowel elimination, altered: constipation (indications).
- Knowledge deficit related to medication regimen (patient/family teaching).

Implementation

- **PO:** Soln is clear, colorless, and syrupy, with a sweet taste.
  - Administer 50% glycerin soln with 0.9% NaCl flavored with lemon, lime, or orange juice or commercially prepared 50% or 75% flavored soln to improve taste and to minimize nausea and vomiting. Pour over cracked ice and sip through a straw.
  - Have patient lie down during and after administration to prevent headache from cerebral dehydration.
  - When used to decrease intraocular pressure, do not give the patient hypotonic fluids following administration, as these will cancel the osmotic effect of glycerin.
- **Rect:** Glycerin suppositories or enema usually cause evacuation of the colon in 15–30 min.
- **Ophth:** Do not administer soln that is cloudy or discolored or that contains crystals or a precipitate.
  - Ophthalmic soln may cause pain and eye irritation. Topical local anesthetic should be instilled shortly before administration of glycerin ophthalmic soln.
  - See Appendix H for administration of ophthalmic soln.

Patient/Family Teaching

- **General Info:** Instruct patient to take glycerin as directed.
- **Laxative:** Advise patient that laxatives should be used only for short-term therapy. Long-term therapy may cause electrolyte imbalance and dependence.
  - Caution patients not to use laxatives when abdominal pain, nausea, vomiting, or fever are present.

Evaluation

Effectiveness of therapy can be demonstrated by: ▪ Soft, formed bowel movement ▪ Reduction of intraocular pressure ▪ Reduction of corneal edema.

GLYCOPYRROLATE

(glye-koe-**pye**-roe-late)
Robinul, Robinul-Forte

CLASSIFICATION(S):
Anticholinergic—antimuscarinic
Pregnancy Category B

INDICATIONS

▪ Used as a preoperative medication to inhibit salivation and excessive respiratory secretions ▪ Used to reverse some of the secretory and vagal actions of cholinesterase inhibitors used to treat nondepolarizing neuromuscular blockade (cholinergic adjunct) ▪ Adjunct in the management of peptic ulcer disease.

ACTION

▪ Inhibits the action of acetylcholine at postganglionic sites located in smooth muscle, secretory glands, and the CNS (antimuscarinic activity) ▪ Low doses decrease sweating, salivation, and respiratory secretions ▪ Intermediate doses result in increased heart rate ▪ GI and GU tract motility are decreased at larger doses. **Therapeutic Effects:** ▪ Decreased GI and respiratory secretions.

PHARMACOKINETICS

Absorption: Incompletely absorbed following oral administration. Well absorbed following IM administration.
Distribution: Distribution not fully known. Does not significantly cross the blood-brain barrier or eye. Crosses the placenta.
Metabolism and Excretion: Eliminated primarily unchanged in the feces, via biliary excretion.
Half-life: 1.7 hr (0.6–4.6 hr).

CONTRAINDICATIONS AND PRECAUTIONS

Contraindicated in: ▪ Hypersensitivity ▪ Narrow-angle glaucoma ▪ Acute hemorrhage ▪ Tachycardia secondary to cardiac insufficiency or thyrotoxicosis.
Use Cautiously in: ▪ Elderly and the very young (increased susceptibility to adverse reactions) ▪ Patients who may have intra-abdominal infections ▪ Prostatic hypertrophy ▪ Chronic renal, hepatic, pulmonary, or cardiac disease ▪ Pregnancy and lactation (safety not established).

ADVERSE REACTIONS AND SIDE EFFECTS*

CNS: drowsiness, confusion.
EENT: dry eyes, blurred vision, mydriasis, cycloplegia.
CV: palpitations, tachycardia, orthostatic hypotension.
GI: dry mouth, constipation.
GU: urinary hesitancy, retention.

INTERACTIONS

Drug-Drug: ▪ Additive anticholinergic effects with other **anticholinergic compounds,** including **antihistamines, tricyclic antidepressants, quinidine,** and **disopyramide** ▪ May alter the absorption of **other orally administered drugs** by slowing motility of the GI tract ▪ **Antacids** or **adsorbent antidiarrheals** decrease the absorption of anticholinergics ▪ May increase GI mucosal lesions in patients taking **oral potassium chloride tablets.**

ROUTE AND DOSAGE

Control of Secretions During Surgery

- **IM (Adults and Children >2 yr):** 0.1 mg (4.4 mcg/kg) 30–60 min preop (not to exceed 0.1 mg).
- **IM (Children <2 yr):** 4.4–8.8 mcg/kg 30–60 min preop.

Cholinergic Adjunct

- **IV (Adults and Children):** 200 mcg for each 1 mg of neostigmine or 5 mg of pyridostigmine given at the same time.

Peptic Ulcer

- **PO (Adults):** 1–2 mg 2–3 times daily.
- **IM, IV (Adults):** 100–200 mcg q 4 hr 3–4 times daily.

PHARMACODYNAMICS (anticholinergic effects)

	ONSET	PEAK	DURATION
PO	UK	UK	8–12 hr
IM	15–30 min	30–45 min	2–7 hr
IV	1 min	UK	2–7 hr

NURSING IMPLICATIONS

Assessment

- ▫ Assess heart rate, blood pressure, and respiratory rate prior to and periodically during parenteral therapy.
- ▫ Monitor intake and output ratios in elderly or surgical patients, as glycopyrrolate may cause urinary retention.

*Underlines indicate most frequent; CAPITALS indicate life-threatening.

Instruct patient to void prior to administration.

- □ Assess patient routinely for abdominal distention and auscultate for bowel sounds. If constipation becomes a problem, increasing fluids and adding bulk to the diet may help alleviate the constipating effects of the drug.
- □ Periodic intraocular pressure determinations should be made on patients receiving long-term therapy.
- ▪ **Lab Test Considerations:** Antagonizes effects of pentagastrin and histamine during the gastric acid secretion test. Avoid administration for 24 hr preceding the test.
- □ May cause decreased uric acid levels in patients with gout or hyperuricemia.
- ▪ **Toxicity and Overdose:** If overdosage occurs, neostigmine is the antidote.

Potential Nursing Diagnoses

- ▪ Oral mucous membranes, altered (side effects).
- ▪ Bowel elimination, altered: constipation (side effects).
- ▪ Knowledge deficit related to medication regimen (patient/family teaching).

Implementation

- ▪ **General Info:** Do not administer cloudy or discolored soln.
- ▪ **PO:** Administer 30–60 min before meals to maximize absorption.
- □ Do not administer within 1 hr of antacids or antidiarrheal medications.
- ▪ **IM:** May be administered undiluted or mixed and administered with D5W, D10W, or 0.9% NaCl.
- ▪ **Direct IV:** May be given undiluted through Y-site injection or 3-way stopcock.
- □ *Rate:* Administer at a rate of 0.2 mg over 1–2 min.
- ▪ **Syringe Compatibility:** atropine, benzquinamide, chlorpromazine, cimetidine, codeine, diphenhydramine, droperidol, droperidol/fentanyl, hydromorphone, hydroxyzine, levorphanol, lidocaine, meperidine, midazolam, morphine, nalbuphine, neostigmine, oxymorphone, procaine, prochlorperazine, promazine, promethazine, propiomazine, pyridostigmine, ranitidine, scopolamine, triflupromazine, or trimethobenzamide.
- ▪ **Syringe Incompatibility:** chloramphenicol, dexamethasone, diazepam, dimenhydrinate, methohexital, pentazocine, pentobarbital, secobarbital, sodium bicarbonate, or thiopental.
- ▪ **Additive Compatibility:** D5/0.45% NaCl, D5W, 0.9% NaCl, or Ringer's soln. Administer immediately after admixing.
- ▪ **Additive Incompatibility:** methylprednisolone sodium succinate.

Patient/Family Teaching

- □ Instruct patient to take glycopyrrolate exactly as directed and not to take more than the prescribed amount. Missed doses should be taken as soon as remembered if not just before next dose.
- □ Medication may cause drowsiness and blurred vision. Caution patient to avoid driving or other activities requiring alertness until response to the medication is known.
- □ Inform patient that frequent oral rinses, sugarless gum or candy, and good oral hygiene may help relieve dry mouth. Consult physician or dentist regarding use of saliva substitute if dry mouth persists for more than 2 wk.
- □ Advise patient receiving glycopyrrolate to make position changes slowly to minimize the effects of drug-induced orthostatic hypotension.
- □ Caution patient to avoid extremes of temperature. This medication decreases the ability to sweat and may increase the risk of heat stroke.
- □ Advise patient to notify physician immediately if eye pain or increased sensitivity to light occurs. Emphasize the importance of routine eye examinations throughout therapy.
- □ Advise patient to consult physician or pharmacist prior to taking any over-the-counter medications concurrently with this therapy.

Evaluation

Effectiveness of therapy can be demonstrated by: ▪ Mouth dryness preoperatively ▪ Reversal of cholinergic medications ▪ Decrease in GI motility and pain in patients with peptic ulcer disease.

GOLD SODIUM THIOMALATE

(gold **so**-dee-um thye-oh-**mah**-late)

Aurothiomalate, Myochrisine

CLASSIFICATION(S):
Anti-inflammatory agent
Pregnancy Category C

INDICATIONS

▪ Treatment of progressive rheumatoid arthritis resistant to conventional therapy.

ACTION

▪ Inhibits the inflammatory process ▪ Modifies the immune response (immunomodulating properties). **Therapeutic Effects:** ▪ Relief of pain and inflammation and slowing of the disease process in rheumatoid arthritis.

PHARMACOKINETICS

Absorption: Rapidly absorbed following IM administration.

Distribution: Widely distributed, appears to concentrate in arthritic joints more than uninvolved joints. Enters breast milk.

Metabolism and Excretion: 60–90% slowly excreted by the kidneys (up to 15 mon). 10–40% excreted in the feces.

Half-life: Gold—26 days in blood, 40–128 days in tissue.

CONTRAINDICATIONS AND PRECAUTIONS

Contraindicated in: ▪ Hypersensitivity ▪ Severe hepatic or renal dysfunction ▪ Previous heavy metal toxicity ▪ History of colitis or exfoliative dermatitis ▪ Uncontrolled diabetes mellitus ▪ Tuberculosis ▪ Congestive heart failure ▪ Systemic lupus erythematosus ▪ Recent radiation therapy ▪ Pregnancy or lactation ▪ Debilitated patients.

Use Cautiously in: ▪ History of blood dyscrasias ▪ Hypertension ▪ Rashes ▪ Discontinue at first sign of toxicity, skin rash, proteinuria, or stomatitis.

ADVERSE REACTIONS AND SIDE EFFECTS*

CNS: dizziness, syncope, headache, neuropathy.

EENT: corneal gold deposition, corneal ulcerations.

Resp: pneumonitis.

CV: bradycardia.

GI: metallic taste, difficulty swallowing, stomatitis, nausea, vomiting, diarrhea, abdominal pain, cramping, anorexia, dyspepsia, flatulence, hepatitis.

GU: proteinuria, nephrotoxicity.

Derm: rash, dermatitis, pruritus, photosensitivity reactions.

Hemat: thrombocytopenia, **APLASTIC ANEMIA, AGRANULOCYTOSIS,** leukopenia, eosinophilia.

Misc: allergic reactions, including **ANAPHYLAXIS,** angioneurotic edema, nitritoid reactions.

INTERACTIONS

Drug-Drug: ▪ Bone marrow toxicity may be additive with other **agents capable of bone marrow depression (antineoplastics, radiation therapy)** ▪ Increased risk of renal and hematologic toxicity with **penicillamine** ▪ Increased risk of dermatitis, hepatotoxicity, or renal toxicity with **agents causing similar toxicities**.

ROUTE AND DOSAGE

- **IM (Adults):** 10 mg test dose, then 25 mg first week, then 50 mg weekly for 14–20 doses; if improvement, then 50 mg q 2 wk for 4 doses, then q 3 wk for 4 doses, then monthly as maintenance dose.

*Underlines indicate most frequent; **CAPITALS** indicate life-threatening.

- **IM (Children):** 10 mg initially, then 1 mg/kg/wk or 2.5–5 mg once weekly for 2 wk, then 1 mg/kg/wk. When desired response is obtained, increase dosing interval to every 3–4 wk.

PHARMACODYNAMICS (anti-inflammatory activity)

	ONSET	PEAK	DURATION
IM	6–8 wk	UK	mons

NURSING IMPLICATIONS

Assessment

- Assess patient's range of motion and degree of swelling and pain in affected joints prior to and periodically throughout therapy. Injections may be followed by joint pain for 1–2 days.
- **Lab Test Considerations:** Monitor renal, hepatic, and hematologic function and urinalysis prior to and monthly throughout therapy. Notify physician immediately if WBC $<4000/mm^3$, eosinophils $>5\%$, granulocytes $<1500/mm^3$, or platelets $<100,000/mm^3$. These values may indicate a hypersensitivity reaction and should improve upon discontinuation. Proteinuria or hematuria may necessitate discontinuation of therapy.
- May interfere with serum protein-bound iodine determinations during and for several wks following discontinuation of therapy.
- **Toxicity and Overdose:** If signs of overdose occur, glucocorticoids are usually used to reverse effects. A chelating agent, dimercaprol (BAL), may be given to enhance gold excretion when glucocorticoids are ineffective.

Potential Nursing Diagnoses

- Mobility, impaired physical (indications).
- Bowel elimination, altered: diarrhea (adverse effects).
- Knowledge deficit related to medication regimen (patient/family teaching).

Implementation

- **General Info:** Concurrent therapy with salicylates or other nonsteroidal anti-inflammatory agents or glucocorticoids is usually necessary, especially during the first few mons of gold therapy.
- Never administer IV.
- **IM:** Using an 18-gauge, 1½-in needle, inject deep into gluteal muscle. Soln is pale yellow; do not use soln that has darkened or contains a precipitate.
- Instruct patient to remain recumbent for 15 min after injection. Monitor for nitritoid (dizziness, flushing, fainting, diaphoresis, dyspnea, bradycardia, swelling of face, lips, or eyelids, thickening of tongue) or allergic reaction.

Patient/Family Teaching

- Patient should continue physical therapy and obtain adequate rest. Explain that joint damage will not be reversed; the goal is to slow or stop disease process.
- Emphasize the importance of good oral hygiene to reduce the incidence of stomatitis.
- Caution patient to use sunscreen and protective clothing to prevent photosensitivity reactions.
- Instruct patient to report symptoms of leukopenia (fever, sore throat, signs of infection) or thrombocytopenia (bleeding gums; bruising; petechiae; blood in stools, urine, or emesis) immediately to physician.
- Discuss the need for contraception while receiving this medication. Advise patient to notify physician promptly if pregnancy is suspected.
- Instruct patient to notify physician immediately if symptoms of gold toxicity (pruritus, skin rash, metallic taste in mouth, stomatitis, diarrhea) occur. Diarrhea may be resolved by decreasing the dose.
- Emphasize the importance of regular visits to physician to monitor progress and to evaluate blood and urine tests for side effects.

EVALUATION

Effectiveness of therapy can be demonstrated by: ▪ Decrease in swelling, pain, and stiffness of joints ▫ Increase in mobility. Continuous therapy for 3–6 mon may be required before therapeutic effects are seen.

GONADOTROPIN, CHORIONIC

(goe-**nad**-oh-troe-pin, kor-ee-**on**-ik)
{Antuitrin}, A.P.L., CG, Chorex, Follutein, Glucor, Gonic, HCG, Pregnyl, Profasi

CLASSIFICATION(S):
Hormone—gonadotropin
Pregnancy Category C

INDICATIONS

▪ Treatment of: ▫ Cryptorchidism ▫ Male infertility (secondary to hypogonadism) ▫ Female infertility (to induce ovulation in patients who do not respond to clomiphene) ▪ To induce ovulation in patients undergoing *in vitro* fertilization. **Unlabeled Uses:** ▪ Diagnosis of male hypogonadism ▪ Treatment of corpus luteum dysfunction.

ACTION

▪ Has action similar to that of luteinizing hormone—causes ovulation ▪ Stimulates androgen production by the testes. **Therapeutic Effects:** ▪ Promotion of androgen production by the testes and subsequent descent ▪ Induction of ovulation.

PHARMACOKINETICS

Absorption: Destroyed in the GI tract, necessitating IM administration.
Distribution: Distributed primarily to the ovaries in females and to the testes in males.
Metabolism and Excretion: 10–12% excreted in urine in first 24 hr.
Half-life: 23 hr.

CONTRAINDICATIONS AND PRECAUTIONS

Contraindicated in: ▪ Previous hypersensitivity reactions ▪ Precocious puberty ▪ Carcinoma of the prostate or other androgen-sensitive tumor.
Use Cautiously in: ▪ Asthma ▪ History of seizures ▪ Migraine headaches ▪ Renal disease ▪ Cardiac disease.

ADVERSE REACTIONS AND SIDE EFFECTS*

CNS: headache, irritability, restlessness, depression, fatigue.
CV: edema, fluid retention, ascites (with menotropins), pleural effusion (with menotropins), thromboembolism (with menotropins).
Endo: gynecomastia (males), precocius puberty (prepubertal males), ovarian enlargement (with menotropins), rupture of ovarian cyst (with menotropins).
Local: pain at IM site.
Misc: multiple births (with menotropins).

INTERACTIONS

Drug-Drug: ▪ None significant.

ROUTE AND DOSAGE

Hypogonadism

- **IM (Adults):** 1000–4000 units 2–3 times/wk.

Induction of Ovulation

- **IM (Adults):** 5000–10,000 units 1 day after last dose of menotropins or urofollitropin or 7 days following clomiphene.

Prepubertal Cryptorchidism

- **IM (Children):** 1000–5000 units 2–3 times/wk (not to exceed 8 wk of treatment). Other regimens with doses as small as 500 units are used.

PHARMACODYNAMICS (ovulation)

	ONSET	PEAK	DURATION
IM	UK	18 hr	UK

{} = Available in Canada only.
*Underlines indicate most frequent; **CAPITALS** indicate life-threatening.

NURSING IMPLICATIONS

Assessment

- **General Info:** Assess blood pressure prior to and periodically throughout therapy.
- Monitor intake and output ratios and weekly weight. Report significant discrepancies or steady weight gain to physician.
- **Cryptorchidism:** Monitor for development of precocious puberty (acne, sudden increase in height, secondary sex characteristics—pubic, axillary, or facial hair, voice changes, penile growth. Notify physician; therapy should be discontinued.
- **Anovulatory Infertility:** An ultrasound examination should be conducted prior to therapy to determine number of follicles and degree of development. A pelvic examination to determine ovarian size should be completed prior to course of therapy and daily for 2 wk after chorionic gonadotropin injection. Cervical mucus should be monitored to determine whether ovulation has occurred.
- **Lab Test Considerations:** May cause false results in pregnancy testing. May cause false elevations in tests of urinary steroid excretion.
- **Female Infertility:** Estrogen excretion or serum estrogen level should be monitored prior to administration of chorionic gonadotropin. Levels should be assessed daily beginning 1 wk after course of menotropins.
- **Male Infertility:** Sperm count and motility should be evaluated prior to and after course of therapy.

Potential Nursing Diagnoses

- Sexual dysfunction (indications).
- Body image disturbance (indications).
- Knowledge deficit related to medication regimen (patient/family teaching).

Implementation

- **General Info:** Female infertility—chorionic gonadotropin is usually administered 1 day following a course of human menotropins.
- **IM:** Reconstitute powder with 10-ml vial of normal saline for injection provided by manufacturer. Withdraw sterile air from vial that contains powder, inject air into diluent vial, withdraw same volume of diluent, and inject into vial containing powder. Shake gently until powder fully dissolved. Stable for 90 days when refrigerated.

Patient/Family Teaching

- **General Info:** Advise patient to report signs and symptoms of fluid retention (swelling of ankles and feet, weight gain), thromboembolic disorders (pain, swelling, tenderness in extremities, headache, chest pain, blurred vision), and abdominal or pelvic pain or bloating to physician.
- **Cryptorchidism:** Review symptoms of precocious puberty with parents; instruct them to notify physician immediately if these symptoms occur.
- **Female Infertility:** Instruct patient in the correct method for measuring basal body temperature. A record of the daily basal body temperature should be maintained prior to and throughout course of therapy.
- Reinforce physician's instructions regarding timing of sexual intercourse (usually daily beginning 1 day after administration of chorionic gonadotropin).
- Emphasize the importance of close monitoring by physician throughout course of therapy.
- Inform patient prior to therapy of the potential for multiple births.
- Instruct patient to notify physician immediately if pregnancy is suspected (menses do not occur when expected and basal body temperature is biphasic).

Evaluation

Effectiveness of therapy can be demonstrated by: ▪ Testicular descent in boys (age 4–9) with cryptorchidism ▪ Ovulation 18 hr after therapy in women with anovulatory cycles, with subsequent pregnancy ▪ Increase in spermatogenesis. Therapy may be discontinued in boys with cryptorchidism if testicular descent is progressing poorly after 8 wk of therapy or in infertile woman if ovulation does not occur after 3–6 menstrual cycles.

GOSERELIN
(**goe**-se-rel-lin)
Zoladex
CLASSIFICATION(S):
Antineoplastic—hormone
Pregnancy Category X

INDICATIONS
▪ Treatment (palliative) of prostate cancer in patients who will not tolerate orchiectomy or estrogen therapy.

ACTION
▪ Acts as a synthetic form of leuteinizing hormone releasing hormone (LHRH, GnRH). Inhibits the production of gonadotropins by the pituitary gland. Initially, levels of luteinizing hormone (LH), follicle stimulating hormone (FSH), and testosterone increase. Continued administration leads to decreased production, particularly of testosterone. **Therapeutic Effect:** ▪ Decreased spread of cancer of the prostate.

PHARMACOKINETICS
Absorption: Well absorbed from SC implant. Absorption is slower in first 8 days, then is faster and continuous for remainder of 28-day dosing cycle.
Distribution: Distribution not known.
Metabolism and Excretion: Metabolism and excretion not known.
Half-life: 4.2 hr.

CONTRAINDICATIONS AND PRECAUTIONS
Contraindicated in: ▪ Hypersensitivity ▪ Pregnancy.
Use Cautiously in: ▪ Lactation or children <18 yrs (safety not established).

ADVERSE REACTIONS AND SIDE EFFECTS*
CNS: weakness, anxiety, depression, dizziness, headache, insomnia, fatigue.
Resp: dyspnea.
CV: chest pain, palitations, hypertension, MYOCARDIAL INFARCTION, CEREBROVASCULAR ACCIDENT.
GI: constipation, diarrhea, anorexia, nausea, vomiting, ulcer.
GU: renal insufficiency, urinary obstruction.
Derm: rashes.
Endo: decreased libido, impotence, breast tenderness, breast swelling, infertility.
F and E: peripheral edema.
Hemat: anemia.
Metab: hyperglycemia, gout.
MS: increased bone pain, arthralgia.
Misc: hot flashes, chills, fever, weight gain.

INTERACTIONS
Drug-Drug: ▪ None significant.

ROUTE AND DOSAGE
- **SC (Adults):** 3.6 mg every 28 days (as an implant).

PHARMACODYNAMICS decrease in serum testosterone levels)

	ONSET	PEAK	DURATION
SC	UK	2–4 wk	UK

NURSING IMPLICATIONS
ASSESSMENT
- Monitor patients with vertebral metastases for increased back pain and decreased sensory/motor function.
- Monitor intake and output ratios and assess for bladder distention in patients with urinary tract obstruction during initiation of therapy.
- Initially increases then decreases luteinizing hormone (LH), follicle stimulating hormone (FSH). This leads to castration levels of testosterone in males 2–4 wk after initial increase in concentrations.

*Underlines indicate most frequent; **CAPITALS** indicate life-threatening.

G

Potential Nursing Diagnoses
- Sexual dysfunction (indications, side effects).
- Knowledge deficit related to medication regimen (patient/family teaching).

Implementation
- **SC:** Implant is inserted in upper SC tissue of abdominal wall every 28 days.

Patient/Family Teaching
- Advise patient that bone pain may increase at initiation of therapy. This will resolve with time. Patient should discuss use of analgesics to control pain with physician.
- Advise patient that medication may cause hot flashes. Notify physician if these become bothersome.
- Instruct patient to notify physician promptly if difficulty urinating occurs.

Evaluation
Effectiveness of therapy can be demonstrated by: ▪ Decrease in the spread of prostate cancer.

GRISEOFULVIN
(gris-ee-oh-**ful**-vin)
Fulvicin P/G, Fulvicin-U/F, Grifulvin V, Grisactin, Grisactin Ultra, {Grisovin-FP}, Gris-PEG

CLASSIFICATION(S):
Antifungal
Pregnancy Category UK

INDICATIONS
▪ Treatment of various Tinea (ringworm) infections, including: ▫ *Tinea barbae* ▫ *Tinea capitis* ▫ *Tinea corporis* ▫ *Tinea cruris* ▫ *Tinea pedis* ▫ *Tinea unguium,* caused by one or a combination of susceptible ▫ *Trichophyton* ▫ *Microsporum* ▫ *Epidermatophyton* ▪ Not to be used for superficial infections that may respond to topical antifungals.

ACTION
▪ Inhibits mitosis of fungal cells. Deposits in precursor cells of hair, skin, and nails, making them resistant to fungal invasion. **Therapeutic Effect:** ▪ New cells that are resistant to invasion by fungi.

PHARMACOKINETICS
Absorption: Microsize (Grisactin, Grisovin-FP, Grifulvin V, Fulvicin-U/F, Grifulvin V) preparations are variably (25–70%) absorbed following oral administration. Ultramicrosize products (Fulvicin P/G, Grisactin Ultra, Gris-PEG) are almost completely absorbed.
Distribution: Mostly deposited in keratin layer of skin. Also found in liver, fat, and skeletal muscle.
Metabolism and Excretion: Metabolized by the liver, some excreted in feces and perspiration.
Half-life: 9–24 hr.

CONTRAINDICATIONS AND PRECAUTIONS
Contraindicated in: ▪ Hypersensitivity ▪ Severe liver disease or porphyria.
Use Cautiously in: ▪ Pregnancy or lactation (safety not established) ▪ Possible cross-sensitivity with penicillin.

ADVERSE REACTIONS AND SIDE EFFECTS*
CNS: <u>headache</u>, dizziness.
EENT: hearing loss.
GI: epigastric distress, nausea, vomiting, extreme thirst, flatulence, diarrhea.
Derm: photosensitivity, rashes.
Hemat: leukopenia.
Misc: hypersensitivity reactions, including serum sickness, lupus-like syndrome.

INTERACTIONS
Drug-Drug: ▪ Tachycardia, flushing, and increased CNS depression may result if taken concurrently with **alcohol** ▪ **Phenobarbital** decreases blood levels and may decrease effectiveness ▪ May decrease the effectiveness of **oral anti-**

{} = Available in Canada only.
*<u>Underlines</u> indicate most frequent; **CAPITALS** indicate life-threatening.

coagulants ▪ May decrease the effectiveness of **oral contraceptive agents.**

ROUTE AND DOSAGE

Microsize

- **PO (Adults):** 500–1000 mg/day, single or divided doses.
- **PO (Children):** 10 mg/kg/day, single or divided doses.

Ultramicrosize

- **PO (Adults):** 330–375 mg/day (up to 660–750 mg/day), single or divided doses.
- **PO (Children >2 yr):** 7.3 mg/kg/day, single or divided doses.

PHARMACODYNAMICS (antifungal activity)

	ONSET	PEAK	DURATION
PO	4 hr	24 hr	2 days

NURSING IMPLICATIONS

Assessment

- □ Assess skin at site of fungal infection routinely throughout course of therapy.
- □ Assess patient for allergy to penicillin; potential cross-sensitivity exists.
- ▪ **Lab Test Considerations:** Hematologic, hepatic, and renal functions should be monitored periodically throughout treatment.

Potential Nursing Diagnoses

- Skin integrity, impaired: actual (indications).
- Infection, high risk for (indications, side effects).
- Knowledge deficit related to medication regimen (patient/family teaching).

Implementation

- ▪ **General Info:** Concurrent use of a topical agent is usually required.
- □ Ultramicrosize griseofulvin 250 mg provides serum concentration equal to that of microsize griseofulvin 500 mg.
- □ Available in tablet and oral suspension.
- ▪ **PO:** Administer with or after meals, preferably meals with high fat content, to minimize GI irritation and increase absorption.

Patient/Family Teaching

- □ Instruct patient to complete full course of therapy; several wks of therapy may be necessary. If a dose is missed, take as soon as remembered, but do not take if almost time for next dose.
- □ Instruct patient on hygiene to control sources of infection or reinfection.
- □ Griseofulvin may cause dizziness. Caution patient to avoid driving or other activities requiring alertness until response to medication is known.
- □ Advise patient to wear sunscreen and protective clothing to prevent photosensitivity reaction.
- □ Caution patient not to drink alcohol while taking this medication.
- □ Advise patient to use a nonhormonal form of contraception and to notify physician if pregnancy is planned or suspected.
- □ Advise patient to notify physician if rash, sore throat, fever, diarrhea, or soreness of mouth or tongue occurs.
- □ Emphasize importance of follow-up examinations to monitor progress of therapy.

Evaluation

Effectiveness of therapy can be demonstrated by: ▪ Resolution of signs and symptoms of fungal infection. To prevent relapse, treatment may take wks to mons.

GUAIFENESIN

(gwye-**fen**-e-sin)

Anti-tuss, {Balminil Expectorant}, Baytussin, Breonesin, Colrex Expectorant, Cremacoat 2, 2/G, Gee-Gee, GG-Cen, Glyate, glyceryl guaiacolate, Glycotuss,

{} = Available in Canada only.

G

glytuss, Guiatuss, Halotussin, Humibid L.A., Hytuss, Hytuss-2X, Malotuss, {Neo-Spec}, Notussin, {Resyl}, Robitussin

CLASSIFICATION(S):
Expectorant
Pregnancy Category C

INDICATIONS

▪ Symptomatic management of coughs associated with viral upper respiratory tract infections.

ACTION

▪ Reduces the viscosity of tenacious secretions by increasing respiratory tract fluid. **Therapeutic Effect:** ▪ Easier mobilization and subsequent expectoration of mucus.

PHARMACOKINETICS

Absorption: Well absorbed after oral administration.
Distribution: Distribution not known.
Metabolism and Excretion: Metabolism or excretion not known.
Half-life: UK.

CONTRAINDICATIONS AND PRECAUTIONS

Contraindicated in: ▪ Hypersensitivity.
Use Cautiously in: ▪ Cough lasting >1 wk or accompanied by fever, rash, or headache (if self-medicating, physician should be consulted) ▪ Pregnancy—although safety has not been established, guaifenesin has been used without adverse effects ▪ Patients receiving disulfiram (liquid products may contain alcohol) ▪ Diabetics (products may contain sugar).

ADVERSE REACTIONS AND SIDE EFFECTS*

CNS: drowsiness.
GI: nausea, vomiting, diarrhea, stomach pain.

INTERACTIONS

Drug-Drug: ▪ None significant.

ROUTE AND DOSAGE

- **PO (Adults):** 200–400 mg q 4 hr (not to exceed 2400 mg/day).
- **PO (Children 6–11 yr):** 100–200 mg q 4 hr (not to exceed 1200 mg/day).
- **PO (Children 2–5 yr):** 50–100 mg q 4 hr (not to exceed 600 mg/day).

PHARMACODYNAMICS (expectorant action)

	ONSET	PEAK	DURATION
PO	30 min	UK	4–6 hr

NURSING IMPLICATIONS

Assessment

□ Assess lung sounds, frequency and type of cough, and character of bronchial secretions periodically throughout therapy. Maintain fluid intake of 1500–2000 ml/day to decrease viscosity secretions.

Potential Nursing Diagnoses

- Airway clearance, ineffective (indications).
- Knowledge deficit related to medication regimen (patient/family teaching).

Implementation

- **General Info:** Available in tablets, capsules, and syrups. Also available in combination form in several over-the-counter preparations (see Appendix A).
- **PO:** Do not give fluids immediately after administering liquid preparations, to prevent dilution of the vehicle.

□ Capsules should be swallowed whole; do not open or chew.

Patient/Family Teaching

□ Instruct patient to cough effectively. Patient should sit upright and take several deep breaths before attempting to cough.

*Underlines indicate most frequent; **CAPITALS** indicate life-threatening.

- Inform patient that drug may occasionally cause drowsiness. Avoid driving or other activities requiring alertness until response to drug is known.
- Advise patient to limit talking, stop smoking, maintain moisture in environmental air, and take some sugarless gum or hard candy to help alleviate the discomfort caused by a chronic nonproductive cough.
- Instruct patient to contact physician if cough persists longer than 1 wk or is accompanied by fever or chest pain.

EVALUATION

Effectiveness of therapy can be demonstrated by: ▪ Decreased frequency of a dry, nonproductive cough. Thick, viscous secretions are thinned, which allows easier expectoration.

GUANABENZ

(**gwahn**-a-benz)
Wytensin

CLASSIFICATION(S):
Antihypertensive—centrally acting alpha-adrenergic agonist
Pregnancy Category C

INDICATIONS

▪ Used alone and in combination with other antihypertensives in the management of hypertension. **Unlabeled Use:** ▪ In combination with naltrexone in the management of opiate withdrawal.

ACTION

▪ Stimulates CNS alpha-adrenergic receptors, resulting in decreased sympathetic outflow. Result is decreased peripheral resistance, a slight decrease in heart rate, and no change in cardiac output. **Therapeutic Effect:** ▪ Lowering of blood pressure.

PHARMACOKINETICS

Absorption: 70–80% absorbed following oral administration.
Distribution: Appears to be widely distributed.
Metabolism and Excretion: >95% metabolized by the liver.
Half-life: 4–14 hr.

CONTRAINDICATIONS AND PRECAUTIONS

Contraindicated in: ▪ Hypersensitivity.
Use Cautiously in: ▪ Serious cardiac, cerebrovascular disease, renal or hepatic insufficiency ▪ Elderly patients (more prone to adverse reactions) ▪ Pregnancy, lactation, or children <12 yr (safety not established) ▪ Do not withdraw abruptly.

ADVERSE REACTIONS AND SIDE EFFECTS*

CNS: drowsiness, dizziness, weakness, headache, irritability, nervousness.
EENT: nasal congestion, blurred vision, dry eyes, miosis.
Resp: dyspnea.
CV: chest pain, bradycardia, edema, arrhythmias, palpitations, hypotension.
GI: dry mouth, nausea, abdominal pain, diarrhea, vomiting, anorexia, constipation, change in taste.
GU: frequency, impotence.
Derm: rashes, pruritus, sweating.
Endo: gynecomastia.
MS: painful extremities, backache.
Misc: withdrawal phenomenon.

INTERACTIONS

Drug-Drug: ▪ Additive sedation with **CNS depressants**, including **alcohol, antihistamines, narcotic analgesics,** and **sedative/hypnotics** ▪ **Tricyclic antidepressants** and **nonsteroidal anti-inflammatory agents** may decrease antihypertensive effects ▪ **MAO inhibitors** decrease effectiveness ▪ Additive hypotension with other **antihypertensives, nitrates,** and acute ingestion of **alcohol**.

ROUTE AND DOSAGE

▪ **PO (Adults):** 4 mg bid; may increase

*Underlines indicate most frequent; **CAPITALS** indicate life-threatening.

q 1–2 wk in 4–8 mg increments (range 8–32 mg/day).

PHARMACODYNAMICS (antihypertensive effect)

	ONSET	PEAK	DURATION
PO	1 hr	2–7 hr	6–12 hr

NURSING IMPLICATIONS

Assessment

- Monitor blood pressure (lying and standing) and pulse frequently during initial dosage adjustment and periodically throughout course of therapy. Notify physician of significant changes.
- Monitor intake and output ratios and daily weight; assess for edema daily.
- **Lab Test Considerations:** With chronic use, may decrease serum cholesterol and triglyceride levels.

Potential Nursing Diagnoses

- Injury, high risk for (side effects).
- Knowledge deficit related to medication regimen (patient/family teaching).
- Noncompliance (patient/family teaching).

Implementation

- **PO:** Administer last dose at bedtime to minimize daytime sedation.
- May be used in conjunction with a thiazide diuretic in patients who fail to respond to diet, exercise, and initial antihypertensive drug therapy.

Patient/Family Teaching

- Emphasize the importance of continuing to take this medication, as directed, even if feeling well. Medication controls but does not cure hypertension. Instruct patient to take medication at the same time each day. If a dose is missed, take as soon as remembered; do not double doses. Instruct patient to inform physician if more than 1 consecutive dose is missed. Do not discontinue abruptly; may cause sympathetic overstimulation (nervousness, anxiety, rebound hypertension).
- Encourage patient to comply with additional interventions for hypertension (weight reduction, low-sodium diet, discontinuation of smoking, moderation of alcohol consumption, regular exercise, and stress management).
- Instruct patient and family on proper technique for blood pressure monitoring. Advise them to check blood pressure at least weekly and report significant changes to physician.
- Patients should also weigh themselves twice weekly and assess feet and ankles for fluid retention.
- Guanabenz may cause drowsiness or dizziness. Caution patient to avoid driving or other activities requiring alertness until response to the medication is known.
- Advise patient to consult physician or pharmacist before taking any cough, cold, or allergy remedies. Patients should also avoid excessive amounts of coffee, tea, and cola.
- Frequent mouth rinses, good oral hygiene, and sugarless gum or candy may minimize dry mouth. If dry mouth persists for more than 2 wk consult dentist regarding use of saliva substitute.
- Advise women of childbearing age to use contraception and notify the physician if pregnancy is suspected or planned.
- Instruct patient to notify physician or dentist of medication regimen prior to treatment or surgery.
- Advise patient to notify physician if frequent dizziness or weakness, irritability or nervousness, slow heart rate, pinpoint pupils, unusual tiredness, or persistent dry mouth occur.
- Emphasize the importance of follow-up examinations to evaluate effectiveness of medication.

Evaluation

Effectiveness of therapy can be demonstrated by: ▪ Decrease in blood pressure without appearance of excessive side effects.

GUANADREL
(**gwahn**-a-drel)
Hylorel

CLASSIFICATION(S):
Antihypertensive—peripherally acting antiadrenergic
Pregnancy Category B

INDICATIONS
■ Treatment of moderate to severe hypertension, usually in combination with at least one other agent, most commonly a diuretic.

ACTION
■ Prevents the release of norepinephrine from adrenergic nerve endings and the adrenal medulla in response to sympathetic (adrenergic) stimulation ■ Depletes norepinephrine from nerve endings. Result is decreased sympathetically mediated vasoconstriction. **Therapeutic Effect:** ■ Lowering of blood pressure.

PHARMACOKINETICS
Absorption: Well absorbed following oral administration.
Distribution: Widely distributed. CNS penetration is minimal.
Metabolism and Excretion: 50% metabolized by the liver, 50% excreted unchanged by the kidneys.
Half-life: 10–12 hr.

CONTRAINDICATIONS AND PRECAUTIONS
Contraindicated in: ■ Hypersensitivity ■ Congestive heart failure ■ Pheochromocytoma ■ Lactation.
Use Cautiously in: ■ Asthma ■ Cardiovascular or cerebrovascular insufficiency ■ Peptic ulcer disease ■ Pregnancy, lactation, or children <18 yr (safety not established) ■ Elderly patients and patients with renal failure (dosage reduction may be required) ■ Discontinue 2–3 days prior to surgical procedures if possible.

ADVERSE REACTIONS AND SIDE EFFECTS*
CNS: drowsiness, fatigue, confusion, headaches, sleep disturbances, dizziness, fainting, depression, anxiety.
EENT: nasal stuffiness, chest pain, palpitations, visual disturbances.
Resp: cough, shortness of breath.
CV: orthostatic hypotension, edema, palpitations.
GI: diarrhea, gas pain, indigestion, constipation, dry mouth, anorexia, nausea, abdominal pain.
GU: ejaculation disturbances, impotence, nocturia, frequency.
MS: leg cramps, aching limbs.
Neuro: paresthesia.

INTERACTIONS
Drug-Drug: ■ Additive hypotension with other **antihypertensives, levodopa, nitrates,** or acute ingestion of **alcohol** ■ **Tricyclic antidepressants, phenothiazines, MAO inhibitors,** or **ephedrine** may block the antihypertensive effect of guanadrel ■ May potentiate the pressor and mydriatic effects of **norepinephrine, amphetamines,** or **phenylephrine** ■ Rapid withdrawal of concurrent **tricyclic antidepressant** therapy will potentiate the hypotensive response.

ROUTE AND DOSAGE
- **PO (Adults):** 5 mg bid, may increase weekly by 10–40 mg/day. Usual daily dose is 20–75 mg given in 2 divided doses, up to 400–600 mg/day.

PHARMACODYNAMICS (antihypertensive effect following single dose)

	ONSET	PEAK	DURATION
PO	2 hr	4–6 hr	9 hr

NURSING IMPLICATIONS
Assessment
□ Monitor blood pressure (lying and standing) and pulse prior to administration, frequently during initial dos-

*Underlines indicate most frequent; **CAPITALS** indicate life-threatening.

age adjustment, and periodically throughout course of therapy. Notify physician of significant changes.
- Monitor intake and output ratios and daily weight; assess for edema daily, especially at beginning of therapy.
- Monitor frequency and consistency of stools. Notify physician if excessive diarrhea occurs.

Potential Nursing Diagnoses

- Injury, high risk for (side effects).
- Knowledge deficit related to medication regimen (patient/family teaching).
- Noncompliance (patient/family teaching).

Implementation

- **General Info:** Dosage adjustments should not be made unless there is no decrease in blood pressure when taken supine and after standing for 10 min.
- May be administered concurrently with diuretics to minimize tolerance and fluid retention.

Patient/Family Teaching

- Emphasize the importance of continuing to take this medication as directed, even if feeling well. Medication controls but does not cure hypertension. Instruct patient to take medication at the same time each day. If a dose is missed, take as soon as remembered; do not double doses.
- Encourage patient to comply with additional interventions for hypertension (weight reduction, low-sodium diet, discontinuation of smoking, moderation of alcohol consumption, regular exercise, and stress management).
- Instruct patient and family on proper technique for blood pressure monitoring. Advise them to check blood pressure at least weekly and report significant changes to physician.
- Patients should weigh themselves twice weekly and assess feet and ankles for fluid retention.
- Inform patient that severity of side effects is usually reduced after the initial 8 wk of therapy.
- Guanadrel may cause drowsiness or dizziness. Advise patient to avoid driving or other activities requiring alertness until response to the medication is known.
- Caution patient to avoid sudden changes in position, especially upon arising in the morning, to minimize orthostatic hypotension. Alcohol and other CNS depressants, standing for long periods, hot showers, and exercising in hot weather should be avoided because of enhanced orthostatic effects.
- Advise patient to consult physician or pharmacist before taking any cough, cold, or allergy remedies. Patient should also avoid excessive amounts of tea, coffee, and cola.
- Instruct patient to notify physician or dentist of medication regimen prior to any surgery.
- Advise patient to notify physician if severe diarrhea, frequent dizziness or fainting, fever, or swelling of feet or lower legs occurs.
- Emphasize the importance of follow-up examinations to evaluate effectiveness of medication.

Evaluation

Effectiveness of therapy can be demonstrated by: ▪ Decrease in blood pressure without appearance of excessive side effects.

GUANETHIDINE

(gwahn-**eth**-i-deen)
{Apo-Guanethidine}, Ismelin

CLASSIFICATION(S):
Antihypertensive—peripherally acting antiadrenergic
Pregnancy Category UK

INDICATIONS

- Treatment of moderate to severe hypertension, usually in combination with at least one other agent, usually a diuretic.

ACTION

▪ Prevents the release of norepinephrine from (adrenergic) nerve endings in response to sympathetic stimulation ▪ Depletes norepinephrine from nerve endings. Result is decreased sympathetically mediated vasoconstriction.
Therapeutic Effect: ▪ Gradual and prolonged fall in blood pressure.

PHARMACOKINETICS

Absorption: Incompletely absorbed (3–50%) from the GI tract following oral administration.
Distribution: Widely distributed to storage sites, including adrenergic neurons. Minimal amounts enter breast milk. Does not appreciably cross the blood-brain barrier.
Metabolism and Excretion: Partially metabolized by the liver.
Half-life: 5 days.

CONTRAINDICATIONS AND PRECAUTIONS

Contraindicated in: ▪ Hypersensitivity ▪ Congestive heart failure ▪ Pheochromocytoma.
Use Cautiously in: ▪ Asthma ▪ Cardiovascular or cerebrovascular insufficiency ▪ Peptic ulcer disease ▪ Pregnancy, lactation, or children (safety not established) ▪ Discontinue 3–4 wk prior to surgical procedures if possible ▪ Impaired renal function (dosage reduction required).

ADVERSE REACTIONS AND SIDE EFFECTS*

CNS: drowsiness, fatigue, confusion, headaches, sleep disturbances, dizziness, fainting, depression, anxiety.
EENT: nasal stuffiness, chest pain, palpitations, visual disturbances.
Resp: cough, shortness of breath.
CV: orthostatic hypotension, edema, palpitations.
GI: diarrhea, gas pain, indigestion, constipation, dry mouth, anorexia, nausea, abdominal pain.
GU: ejaculation disturbances, impotence, nocturia, urinary frequency.
MS: leg cramps, aching limbs.

INTERACTIONS

Drug-Drug: ▪ Additive hypotension with other **antihypertensives,** acute ingestion of **alcohol, levodopa, nitrates,** or **alcohol** ▪ Additive bradycardia with **reserpine** or **cardiac glycosides** ▪ **Tricyclic antidepressants, phenothiazines, MAO inhibitors, nonsteroidal anti-inflammatory agents,** and **oral contraceptives** may block antihypertensive action of guanethidine ▪ May potentiate the pressor and mydriatic effects of **norepinephrine, amphetamines, phenylephrine,** and **metaraminol.**

ROUTE AND DOSAGE

- **PO (Adults):** Initial dose—10 mg/day, increase at 7–21 day intervals to desired maintenance dosage of 25–50 mg/day as single dose (maximum dose 300 mg/day). In hospitalized patients a more rapid loading regimen may be used as follows: day 1—50 mg at 8 a.m., 75 mg at 2 p.m., 25 mg at 8 p.m.; day 2—50 mg at 8 a.m., 75 mg at 2 p.m., 75 mg at 8 p.m.; day 3—100 mg at 8 a.m., 2 p.m., and 8 p.m. Regimen is stopped when desired standing BP is obtained. Starting the next day maintenance therapy is started with 1/5–1/7 of the total loading dose given as a single daily dose.

PHARMACODYNAMICS (antihypertensive effect; more rapid effect is achieved with loading regimen)

	ONSET	PEAK	DURATION
PO	1–3 wk	1–3 wk	1–3 wk

NURSING IMPLICATIONS

Assessment

- □ Monitor blood pressure (lying and standing) and pulse frequently dur-

*Underlines indicate most frequent; **CAPITALS** indicate life-threatening.

ing initial dosage adjustment and periodically throughout course of therapy. Notify physician of significant changes.

- Monitor intake and output ratios and daily weight and assess for edema daily, especially at beginning of therapy.
- Monitor frequency and consistency of stools. Notify physician if excessive diarrhea occurs.
- **Lab Test Considerations:** Renal function should be evaluated periodically during prolonged therapy.

Potential Nursing Diagnoses

- Injury, high risk for (side effects).
- Knowledge deficit related to medication regimen (patient/family teaching).
- Noncompliance (patient/family teaching).

Implementation

- **General Info:** Dosage adjustments should not be made unless there is no decrease in blood pressure when taken supine and after standing for 10 min.
- Usually administered concurrently with diuretics to minimize tolerance and fluid retention.
- Available in combination with hydrochlorothiazide (Esimil); see Appendix A.
- **PO:** Tablet may be crushed prior to administration and taken with fluid of patient's choice for patients with difficulty swallowing.

Patient/Family Teaching

- Emphasize the importance of continuing to take this medication, even if feeling well. Instruct patient to take medication at the same time each day. If a dose is missed, take as soon as remembered; do not double doses. If 2 doses in a row are missed, consult physician. Guanethidine controls but does not cure hypertension. Do not discontinue medication without consulting physician.
- Encourage patient to comply with additional interventions for hypertension (weight reduction, low-sodium diet, discontinuation of smoking, moderation of alcohol consumption, regular exercise, and stress management).
- Instruct patient and family on proper technique for blood pressure monitoring. Advise them to check blood pressure at least weekly and report significant changes to physician.
- Patients should weigh themselves twice weekly and assess feet and ankles for fluid retention.
- Guanethidine may occasionally cause drowsiness. Advise patient to avoid driving or other activities requiring alertness until response to medication is known.
- Caution patient to avoid sudden changes in position to minimize orthostatic hypotension, especially upon arising in the morning. Alcohol or other CNS depressants, standing for long periods, hot showers, and exercising in hot weather should be avoided because of enhanced orthostatic effects.
- If dry mouth occurs, frequent mouth rinses, good oral hygiene, and sugarless gum or candy may decrease effect. If dry mouth persists for more than 2 wk consult dentist regarding use of saliva substitute.
- Advise patient to consult physician or pharmacist before taking any cough, cold, or allergy remedies. Patient should also avoid excessive amounts of tea, coffee, and cola.
- Instruct patient to notify physician or dentist of medication regimen prior to treatment or surgery.
- Advise patient to notify physician if severe diarrhea, frequent dizziness, or fainting occur.
- Emphasize the importance of follow-up examinations to evaluate effectiveness of medication.

Evaluation

Effectiveness of therapy can be demonstrated by: ▪ Decrease in blood pressure without excessive side effects.

GUANFACINE
(**gwahn**-fa-seen)
Tenex

CLASSIFICATION(S):
Antihypertensive—centrally acting alpha-andrenergic agonist
Pregnancy Category B

INDICATIONS

▪ Used with thiazide-type diuretics in the management of hypertension.

ACTION

▪ Stimulates CNS alpha-adrenergic receptors, resulting in decreased sympathetic outflow. Overall result is decrease in peripheral resistance, a slight decrease in heart rate, and no change in cardiac output. **Therapeutic Effect:** ▪ Lowering of blood pressure.

PHARMACOKINETICS

Absorption: Well absorbed (80%) following oral administration.
Distribution: Appears to be widely distributed.
Metabolism and Excretion: 50% metabolized by the liver, 50% excreted unchanged by the kidneys.
Half-life: 17 hr.

CONTRAINDICATIONS AND PRECAUTIONS

Contraindicated in: ▪ Hypersensitivity.
Use Cautiously in: ▪ Severe coronary artery disease or recent myocardial infarction ▪ Cerebrovascular disease ▪ Severe renal or liver disease ▪ Pregnancy, lactation, or children <12 yr (safety not established).

ADVERSE REACTIONS AND SIDE EFFECTS*

CNS: drowsiness, weakness, fatigue, dizziness, headache, insomnia, depression.
EENT: tinnitus.
Resp: dyspnea.
CV: bradycardia, palpitations, chest pain.
GI: dry mouth, constipation, abdominal pain, nausea.
GU: impotence.

INTERACTIONS

Drug-Drug: ▪ Additive hypotension with other **antihypertensive agents, nitrates,** and acute ingestion of **alcohol** ▪ Additive CNS depression may occur with other **CNS depressants,** including **alcohol, antihistamines, narcotic analgesics, tricyclic antidepressants,** and **sedative/hypnotics.**

ROUTE AND DOSAGE

▪ **PO (Adults):** 1 mg daily given at bedtime, may be increased if necessary at 3–4-wk intervals up to 3 mg/day.

PHARMACODYNAMICS (antihypertensive effect)

	ONSET	PEAK	DURATION
PO (single dose)	UK	8–12 hr	24 hr
PO (multiple doses)	within 1 wk	1–3 mon	UK

NURSING IMPLICATIONS

Assessment

□ Monitor blood pressure (lying and standing) and pulse frequently during initial dosage adjustment and periodically throughout course of therapy. Notify physician of significant changes.
▪ **Lab Test Considerations:** May cause temporary, clinically insignificant increase in plasma growth hormone levels.
□ May cause decrease in urinary catecholamines and vanillylmandelic acid levels.

Potential Nursing Diagnoses

▪ Injury, high risk for (side effects).
▪ Knowledge deficit related to medication regimen (patient/family teaching).

*Underlines indicate most frequent; **CAPITALS** indicate life-threatening.

H

- Noncompliance (patient/family teaching).

Implementation

- **General Info:** Administer daily dose at bedtime to minimize daytime sedation.
- May be used in conjunction with a thiazide diuretic.

Patient/Family Teaching

- Emphasize the importance of continuing to take medication as directed, even if feeling well. Medication controls but does not cure hypertension. Instruct patient to take medication at the same time each day. If a dose is missed, take as soon as remembered; do not double doses. If 2 or more doses are missed, consult physician. Do not discontinue abruptly; may cause sympathetic overstimulation (nervousness, anxiety, rebound hypertension). These effects may occur 2–7 days after discontinuation, although rebound hypertension is rare and more likely to occur with high doses.
- Encourage patient to comply with additional interventions for hypertension (weight reduction, low-sodium diet, discontinuation of smoking, moderation of alcohol consumption, regular exercise, and stress management).
- Instruct patient and family on proper technique for blood pressure monitoring. Advise them to check blood pressure at least weekly and to report significant changes to physician.
- Guanfacine may cause drowsiness or dizziness. Advise patient to avoid driving or other activities requiring alertness until response to the medication is known.
- Caution patient to avoid alcohol and over-the-counter medications without consulting physician or pharmacist.
- Advise patient to notify physician if dry mouth or constipation persists. Frequent mouth rinses, good oral hygiene, and sugarless gum or candy may minimize dry mouth. Increase in fluid and fiber intake and exercise may decrease constipation.
- Instruct patient to notify physician or dentist of medication regimen prior to treatment or surgery.
- Advise patient to notify physician if dizziness, prolonged drowsiness, fatigue, weakness, depression, headache, sexual dysfunction, or sleep pattern disturbance occur.
- Emphasize the importance of follow-up examinations to evaluate effectiveness of medication.

Evaluation

Effectiveness of therapy can be demonstrated by: ▪ Decrease in blood pressure without excessive side effects.

HALAZEPAM
(hal-**az**-e-pam)
Paxipam

CLASSIFICATION(S):
Sedative/hypnotic—benzodiazepine
Schedule IV
Pregnancy Category D

INDICATIONS

- Adjunct in the management of anxiety.

ACTION

- Depresses the CNS, probably by potentiating gamma-aminobutyric acid (GABA), an inhibitory neurotransmitter. **Therapeutic Effect:** ▪ Relief of anxiety.

PHARMACOKINETICS

Absorption: Well absorbed following oral administration.

Distribution: Widely distributed. Crosses the placenta and enters breast milk.

Metabolism and Excretion: Mostly metabolized by the liver (some conversion to desmethyldiazepam, an active sedative compound). $<1\%$ excreted unchanged by the kidneys.

Half-life: 2 g (desmethyldiazepam 30–100 hr).

CONTRAINDICATIONS AND PRECAUTIONS

Contraindicated in: ▪ Hypersensitivity ▪ Cross-sensitivity with other benzodiazepines may exist ▪ Comatose patients ▪ Pre-existing CNS depression ▪ Uncontrolled severe pain ▪ Narrow-angle glaucoma ▪ Pregnancy or lactation.
Use Cautiously in: ▪ Hepatic dysfunction ▪ Severe renal impairment ▪ Patients who may be suicidal or who may have been addicted to drugs previously ▪ Elderly or debilitated patients (dosage reduction required).

ADVERSE REACTIONS AND SIDE EFFECTS*

CNS: dizziness, drowsiness, lethargy, hangover, paradoxical excitation, mental depression, headache.
EENT: blurred vision.
Resp: respiratory depression.
GI: nausea, vomiting, diarrhea, constipation, dry mouth.
Derm: rashes.
Misc: tolerance, psychological dependence, physical dependence.

INTERACTIONS

Drug–Drug: ▪ Additive CNS depression with other **CNS depressants,** including **alcohol, antihistamines, antidepressants, narcotic analgesics,** and other **sedative/hypnotics** ▪ **Cimetidine, oral contraceptives, disulfiram, fluoxetine, isoniazid, ketoconazole, metoprolol, propoxyphene, propranolol,** or **valproic acid** may decrease metabolism and increase CNS depression ▪ May decrease the efficacy of **levodopa** ▪ **Rifampin** or **barbiturates** may increase metabolism and decrease effectiveness.

ROUTE AND DOSAGE

- **PO (Adults):** 20–40 mg 3–4 times daily.

PHARMACODYNAMICS (antianxiety effect)

	ONSET	PEAK	DURATION
PO	UK	UK	UK

NURSING IMPLICATIONS

Assessment

- Assess degree and manifestations of anxiety and mental status prior to and periodically throughout therapy.
- Assess patient for drowsiness, lightheadedness, and dizziness. These symptoms usually disappear as therapy progresses. Dosage should be reduced if these symptoms persist.
- Prolonged high-dose therapy may lead to psychological or physical dependence. Restrict the amount of drug available to patient.

Potential Nursing Diagnoses

- Anxiety (indications).
- Injury, high risk for (side effects).
- Knowledge deficit related to medication regimen (patient/family teaching).

Implementation

- **PO:** Tablets may be crushed and taken with food or fluids if patient has difficulty swallowing.

Patient/Family Teaching

- Instruct patient to take medication exactly as prescribed; do not skip or double up on missed doses. If a dose is missed, it can be taken within 1 hr, otherwise skip the dose and return to the regular schedule. If medication is less effective after a few wks, check with physician; do not increase dose. Abrupt withdrawal of halazepam may cause sweating, vomiting, muscle cramps, tremors, and convulsions.
- Halazepam may cause drowsiness or dizziness. Caution patient to avoid driving and other activities requiring alertness until response to the medication is known.
- Advise patient to avoid the use of alcohol or other CNS depressants con-

*Underlines indicate most frequent; **CAPITALS** indicate life-threatening.

H

currently with this medication. Instruct patient to consult physician or pharmacist before taking over-the-counter medications concurrently with this medication.
□ Inform patient that frequent mouth rinses, good oral hygiene, and sugarless gum or candy may minimize dry mouth.

EVALUATION

Effectiveness of therapy can be demonstrated by: ▪ Decreased sense of anxiety □ Increased ability to cope. Treatment with this medication should not continue without periodic re-evaluation of the patient's need for the drug.

HALOPERIDOL

(ha-loe-**per**-i-dole)
{Apo-Haloperidol}, Haldol, {Haldol L.A.}, Halperon, {Novoperidol}, {Peridol}

CLASSIFICATION(S):
Anti-Psychotic—butyrophenone
Pregnancy Category C (decanoate salt only, others UK)

INDICATIONS

▪ Treatment of acute and chronic psychoses ▪ Used to control Tourette's disorder and severe behavioral problems in children.

ACTION

▪ Alters the effects of dopamine in the CNS ▪ Also has anticholinergic and alpha-adrenergic blocking activity. **Therapeutic Effect:** ▪ Diminished signs and symptoms of psychoses.

PHARMACOKINETICS

Absorption: Well absorbed following oral and IM administration.
Distribution: Distribution not fully known. High concentrations in the liver. Crosses the placenta. Enters breast milk.
Metabolism and Excretion: Mostly metabolized by the liver.
Half-life: 21–24 hr.

CONTRAINDICATIONS AND PRECAUTIONS

Contraindicated in: ▪ Hypersensitivity ▪ Narrow-angle glaucoma ▪ Bone marrow depression ▪ CNS depression ▪ Severe liver disease ▪ Severe cardiovascular disease.
Use Cautiously in: ▪ Elderly or debilitated patients (dosage reduction required) ▪ Pregnancy and lactation (safety not established) ▪ Cardiac disease ▪ Severely ill patients and diabetics ▪ Respiratory insufficiency ▪ Prostatic hypertrophy ▪ CNS tumors ▪ Intestinal obstruction ▪ History of seizures.

ADVERSE REACTIONS AND SIDE EFFECTS*

CNS: sedation, extrapyramidal reactions, tardive dyskinesia, restlessness, confusion, seizures.
EENT: dry eyes, blurred vision.
Resp: respiratory depression.
CV: hypotension, tachycardia.
GI: constipation, ileus, anorexia, dry mouth, hepatitis.
GU: urinary retention.
Derm: rashes, photosensitivity, diaphoresis.
Endo: galactorrhea.
Hemat: anemia, leukopenia.
Metab: hyperpyrexia.
Misc: hypersensitivity reactions.

INTERACTIONS

Drug-Drug: ▪ Additive hypotension with **antihypertensives, nitrates,** or acute ingestion of **alcohol** ▪ Additive anticholinergic effects with **drugs having anticholinergic properties,** including **antihistamines, antidepressants, atropine, phenothiazines, quinidine,** and **disopyramide** ▪ Additive CNS depression with other **CNS depressants,** including **alcohol, antihistamines, narcotic analgesics,** and **sedative/hypnot-**

{} = Available in Canada only.
*Underlines indicate most frequent; **CAPITALS** indicate life-threatening.

ics ▪ Concurrent use with **epinephrine** may result in severe hypotension and tachycardia ▪ May decrease therapeutic effects of **levodopa** ▪ Acute encephalopathic syndrome may occur when used with **lithium** ▪ Dementia may occur with **methyldopa**.

ROUTE AND DOSAGE

Haloperidol

- **PO (Adults):** 0.5–5 mg 2–3 times daily (daily doses up to 100 mg/day may be required in some patients).
- **IM (Adults):** 2–5 mg q 4–8 hr as needed.
- **PO (Children 3–12 yr or 15–40 kg):** 0.05–0.15 mg/kg/day in 2–3 divided doses.

Haloperidol Decanoate

- **IM (Adults):** 10–15 times the previous daily PO dose, but not to exceed 100 mg initially, given monthly (not to exceed 300 mg/mon).

PHARMACODYNAMICS (antipsychotic activity)

	ONSET	PEAK	DURATION
PO	2 hr	2–6 hr	8–12 hr
IM	20–30 min	30–45 min	4–8 hr*
IM (decanoate)	3–9 days	UK	1 mon

*Effect may persist for several days.

NURSING IMPLICATIONS

Assessment

- Assess patient's mental status (orientation, mood, behavior) prior to and periodically throughout therapy.
- Monitor blood pressure (sitting, standing, lying) and pulse prior to and frequently during the period of dosage adjustment.
- Observe patient carefully when administering medication, to ensure that medication is actually taken and not hoarded.
- Monitor intake and output ratios and daily weight. Assess patient for signs and symptoms of dehydration (decreased thirst, lethargy, hemoconcentration).
- Assess fluid intake and bowel function. Increased bulk and fluids in the diet help minimize the constipating effects of this medication.
- Observe patient carefully for extrapyramidal symptoms (pill-rolling motions, drooling, tremors, rigidity, shuffling gait), tardive dyskinesia (uncontrolled movements of face, mouth, tongue, or jaw and involuntary movements of extremities), and neuroleptic malignant syndrome (pale skin, hyperthermia, skeletal muscle rigidity, autonomic dysfunction, altered consciousness, leukocytosis, elevated liver function tests, elevated CPK). Notify physician immediately at the onset of these symptoms.
- **Lab Test Considerations:** CBC and liver function tests should be evaluated periodically throughout course of therapy.

Potential Nursing Diagnoses

- Thought processes, altered (indications).
- Knowledge deficit related to medication regimen (patient/family teaching).

Implementation

- **General Info:** Available in tablet, concentrate, and injectable forms.
- **PO:** Administer with food or full glass of water or milk to minimize GI irritation.
- Use calibrated measuring device for accurate dosage. Do not dilute concentrate with coffee or tea; may cause precipitation. Should be given undiluted, but if necessary may dilute in at least 60 ml of liquid.
- **IM:** Inject slowly using 2-in, 21-gauge needle into well-developed muscle. Do not exceed 3 ml per injection site. Slight yellow color does not indicate altered potency. Keep patient recumbent for at least 30 min following injection to minimize hypotensive effects.
- **Syringe Incompatibility:** heparin.
- **Y-Site Compatibility:** ondansetron.
- **Y-Site Incompatibility:** foscarnet.

Patient/Family Teaching

- Advise patient to take medication exactly as directed. Missed doses should be taken as soon as remembered, with remaining doses evenly spaced throughout the day. May require several wks to obtain desired effects. Do not increase dose or discontinue medication without consulting physician. Abrupt withdrawal may cause dizziness, nausea, vomiting, GI upset, trembling, or uncontrolled movements of mouth, tongue, or jaw.
- Inform patient of possibility of extrapyramidal symptoms and tardive dyskinesia. Caution patient to report these symptoms immediately to physician.
- Advise patient to make position changes slowly to minimize orthostatic hypotension.
- Medication may cause drowsiness. Caution patient to avoid driving or other activities requiring alertness until response to medication is known.
- Caution patient to avoid taking alcohol or other CNS depressants concurrently with this medication.
- Advise patient to use sunscreen and protective clothing when exposed to the sun to prevent photosensitivity reactions. Extremes of temperature should also be avoided, as this drug impairs body temperature regulation.
- Instruct patient to use frequent mouth rinses, good oral hygiene, and sugarless gum or candy to minimize dry mouth.
- Instruct patient to notify physician promptly if weakness, tremors, visual disturbances, dark-colored urine or clay-colored stools, sore throat, or fever is noted.
- Emphasize the importance of routine follow-up examinations.

Evaluation

Effectiveness of therapy can be demonstrated by: ▪ Decrease in hallucinations, insomnia, agitation, hostility, and delusions ▪ Decreased tics and vocalization in Tourette's syndrome. If no therapeutic effects are seen in 2–4 wk, dosage may be increased.

H

HEPARIN
(**hep**-a-rin)
{Calcilean}, Calciparine, {Hepalean}, Lipo-hepin, Liquaemin

HEPARIN LOCK FLUSH
Hep-Lock, Hep-Lock U/P

CLASSIFICATION(S):
Anticoagulant
Pregnancy Category C

INDICATIONS

▪ Prophylaxis and treatment of various thromboembolic disorders including: ▫ Venous thromboembolism ▫ Pulmonary emboli ▫ Atrial fibrillation with embolization ▫ Acute and chronic consumptive coagulopathies ▫ Peripheral arterial thromboembolism ▪ Used in very low doses (10–100 units) to maintain patency of IV catheters ("heparin flush").

ACTION

▪ Potentiates the effects of antithrombin III ▪ In low doses prevents the conversion of prothrombin to thrombin ▪ Higher doses neutralize thrombin, preventing the conversion of fibrinogen to fibrin. **Therapeutic Effects:** ▪ Prevention of thrombus formation ▪ Prevention of extension of existing thrombi.

PHARMACOKINETICS

Absorption: Destroyed by enzymes in the GI tract, necessitating parenteral administration. Well absorbed following SC administration.
Distribution: Does not cross the placenta or enter breast milk.
Metabolism and Excretion: Appears to be removed by the reticuloendothelial system (lymph nodes, spleen).

Half-life: 1–2 hr (increases with increasing dosage).

CONTRAINDICATIONS AND PRECAUTIONS

Contraindicated in: ▪ Hypersensitivity ▪ Hypersensitivity to pig or beef proteins (some products are derived from pig intestinal mucosa, others from beef lung) ▪ Uncontrolled bleeding ▪ Open wounds ▪ Severe liver or kidney disease ▪ Products containing benzyl alcohol should not be used in premature infants.

Use Cautiously in: ▪ Untreated hypertension ▪ Ulcer disease ▪ Spinal cord or brain injury ▪ Malignancy ▪ May be used during pregnancy, but use with caution during the last trimester and in the immediate postpartum period.

ADVERSE REACTIONS AND SIDE EFFECTS*

GI: hepatitis.
Hemat: BLEEDING, thrombocytopenia.
Derm: rashes, urticaria.
Misc: hypersensitivity, fever.

INTERACTIONS

Drug–Drug: ▪ Risk of bleeding may be increased by concurrent use of **drugs that affect platelet function,** including **aspirin, nonsteroidal anti-inflammatory agents, dipyridamole,** and **dextran** ▪ Risk of bleeding may be increased by concurrent use of **drugs that cause hypoprothrombinemia,** including **quinidine, cefamandole, cefmetazole, cefoperazone, cefotetan, moxalaxtam,** and **plicamycin** ▪ Concurrent use of **thrombolytic agents** increases the risk of bleeding ▪ Heparin affects the prothrombin time used in assessing the response to **warfarin** ▪ **Probenecid** increases the intensity and duration of the action of heparin.

ROUTE AND DOSAGE

Note: See infusion rate table in Appendix D.

Therapeutic Anticoagulation

Dosage depends on results of PTT.

- **Intermittent IV Bolus (Adults):** 10,000 units, followed by 5000–10,000 units q 4–6 hr.
- **Intermittent IV Bolus (Children):** 100 units/kg, followed by 50–100 units/kg q 4 hr.
- **IV Infusion (Adults):** 5000 units (35–70 units/kg), followed by 20,000–40,000 units infused over 24 hr (approx. 1000 units/hr).
- **IV Infusion (Children):** 50 units/kg followed by 100 units/kg/4 hr or 20,000 units/m^2/24 hr.
- **SC (Adults):** 5000 units IV followed by 8000–10,000 units q 8 hr, or 15,000–20,000 units q 12 hr.

Prophylaxis of Thromboembolic Events

- **SC (Adults):** 5000 units q 8–12 hr (may be started 2 hr prior to surgery).

Heparin Flush

- **IV (Adults and Children):** 10–100 units.

PHARMACODYNAMICS (anticoagulant effect)

	ONSET	PEAK	DURATION
SC	20–60 min	2 hr	8–12 hr
IV	immediate	5–10 min	2–6 hr

NURSING IMPLICATIONS

Assessment

- **General Info:** Assess patient for signs of bleeding and hemorrhage (bleeding gums, nose bleed, unusual bruising, black tarry stools, hematuria, fall in hematocrit or blood pressure, guaiac-positive stools). Notify physician if these occur.
- ▫ Assess patient for evidence of additional or increased thrombosis. Symptoms will depend on area of involvement.
- ▫ Monitor patient for hypersensitivity reactions (chills, fever, urticaria). Report signs to physician.
- **SC:** Observe injection sites for hematomas or ecchymosis or inflammation.

*Underlines indicate most frequent; CAPITALS indicate life-threatening.

- **Lab Test Considerations:** Activated partial thromboplastin time (aPTT) and hematocrit should be monitored prior to and periodically throughout course of therapy. When intermittent IV therapy is used, draw aPTT levels 30 min before next dose. During continuous administration, blood for aPTT levels can be drawn 1.5–2 hr after initiation of heparin therapy.
  - Monitor platelet count every 2–3 days throughout course of therapy. May cause mild thrombocytopenia, which appears on fourth day and resolves despite continued heparin therapy. Thrombocytopenia, which necessitates discontinuing medication, may develop on eighth day of therapy. Patients who have received a previous course of heparin may be at higher risk for severe thrombocytopenia for several months after the initial course.
  - May cause prolonged PT levels, false elevations of serum thyroxine, T_3 resin, sulfobromopthalein (BSP), and false-negative ^{125}I fibrinogen uptake tests. May cause decreased serum triglyceride and cholesterol levels and increased plasma free fatty acid concentrations. May also cause elevated SGOT (AST) and SGPT (ALT) levels.
- **Toxicity and Overdose:** Protamine sulfate is the antidote. However, because of the short half-life of heparin, overdosage can often be treated by withdrawing the drug.

Potential Nursing Diagnoses

- Tissue perfusion, altered (indications).
- Injury, potential for (side effects).
- Knowledge deficit related to medication regimen (patient/family teaching).

Implementation

- **General Info:** Inform all personnel caring for patient of anticoagulant therapy. Venipunctures and injection sites require application of pressure to prevent bleeding or hematoma formation. IM injections of other medications should be avoided, as hematomas may develop.
  - In patients requiring long-term anticoagulation, oral anticoagulant therapy should be instituted 4–5 days prior to discontinuing heparin therapy.
- **SC:** Administer deep into SC tissue with a small-gauge (25–27), ⅜–⅝-in needle. Check dosage for accuracy with another licensed nurse prior to administration. Inject into lower abdomen (preferred site); do not aspirate or massage. Rotate sites frequently. Do not administer IM, because of the danger of hematoma formation.
- **Direct IV:** Loading dose usually precedes continuous infusion.
  - *Rate:* May be given undiluted over at least 1 min.
- **Intermittent/Continuous Infusion:** Dilute in prescribed amount of 0.9% NaCl, D5W, or Ringer's soln for injection and give as a continuous or intermittent infusion. Ensure adequate mixing of heparin in soln. Manufacturer does not recommend piggybacking other medications into IV line while heparin is running or admixing heparin soln.
  - *Rate:* Infusion may be administered over 4–24 hr. Use an infusion pump to ensure accuracy.
- **Heparin Lock:** To prevent clot formation in intermittent infusion (heparin lock) sets, inject dilute heparin soln of 10–100 units/0.5–1 ml after each medication injection or every 8–12 hr. To prevent incompatibility of heparin with medication, flush heparin lock set with sterile water or 0.9% NaCl for injection before and after medication is administered.
- **Syringe Compatibility:** aminophylline, amphotericin, ampicillin, atropine, bleomycin, cefamandole, cefazolin, cefoperazone, cefotaxime, cefoxitin, chloramphenicol, cimetidine, cisplatin, clindamycin, co-trimoxazole, cyclophosphamide, diazoxide, digoxin, dimenhydrinate, dobuta-

mine, dopamine, epinephrine, fentanyl, fluorouracil, furosemide, leucovorin, lidocaine, lincomycin, methotrexate, metoclopramide, mezlocillin, mitomycin, moxalactam, nafcillin, naloxone, neostigmine, norepinephrine, oxytetracycline, pancuronium, penicillin G, phenobarbital, piperacillin, nitroprusside, succinylcholine, tetracycline, verapamil, or vincristine.

- **Syringe Incompatibility:** amikacin, chlorpromazine, diazepam, doxorubicin, droperidol, erythromycin, droperidol/fentanyl, gentamicin, haloperidol, kanamycin, meperidine, methicillin, methotrimeprazine, netilmicin, pentazocine, promethazine, streptomycin, tobramycin, triflupromazine, vancomycin, or vinblastine.
- **Y-Site Compatibility:** acyclovir, aminophylline, ampicillin, atracurium, atropine, betamethasone, bleomycin, calcium gluconate, cephalothin, cephapirin, chlordiazepoxide, chlorpromazine, cimetidine, cisplatin, cyancobalamin, cyclophosphamide, deslanoside, dexamethasone, digoxin, dopamine, edrophonium, enalaprilat, epinephrine, esmolol, conjugated estrogens, ethacrynate, famotidine, fentanyl, fluorouracil, foscarnet, furosemide, hydralazine, hydrocortisone, insulin, isoproterenol, kanamycin, labetalol, leucovorin, lidocaine, magnesium sulfate, menadiol sodium, meperidine, methicillin, methotrexate, methoxamine, methylergonovine, metoclopramide, minocycline, mitomycin, morphine, neostigmine, norepinephrine, ondansetron, oxacillin, oxytocin, pancuronium, penicillin G potassium, pentazocine, phytonadione, prednisolone, procainamide, propranolol, pyridostigmine, ranitidine, scopolamine, sodium bicarbonate, streptokinase, succinylcholine, trimethophan camsylate, vecuronium, verapamil, vinblastine, or vincristine.
- **Y-Site Incompatibility:** alteplase, diazepam, dimenhydrinate, doxorubicin, ergotamine tartrate, erythromycin, gentamicin, haloperidol, hydroxyzine, kanamycin, methotrimeprazine, phenytoin, prochlorperazine, promazine, promethazine, tetracycline, tobramycin, triflupromazine, or vancomycin.
- **Additive Compatibility:** aminophylline, amphotericin, ascorbic acid, bleomycin, calcium gluconate, cephalothin, cephapirin, chloramphenicol, clindamycin, colistimethate, dimenhydrinate, dopamine, erythromycin gluceptate, esmolol, isoproterenol, lidocaine, methicillin, methyldopate, methylprednisolone, nafcillin, norepinephrine, potassium chloride, prednisolone, promazine, ranitidine, sodium bicarbonate, or verapamil. Also compatible with TPN solns or fat emulsion.
- **Additive Incompatibility:** amikacin, codeine, cytarabine, daunorubicin, erythromycin lactobionate, gentamicin, hyaluronidase, kanamycin, levorphanol, meperidine, methadone, morphine, polymyxin B, promethazine, streptomycin, or vancomycin.

Patient/Family Teaching

- □ Caution patient to avoid IM injections and activities leading to injury and to use a soft toothbrush and electric razor during heparin therapy.
- □ Advise patient to report any symptoms of unusual bleeding or bruising to physician immediately.
- □ Instruct patient not to take aspirin, medications containing aspirin, or ibuprofen while on heparin therapy.
- □ Advise patient to inform physician and dentist of medication regimen prior to treatment or surgery.
- □ Patients on anticoagulant therapy should carry an identification card with this information at all times.

Evaluation

Clinical response to therapy is indicated by: ▪ Prolonged PTT of 1.5–2.5 times the control, without signs of hemorrhage ▪ Prevention of thromboembolism ▪ Patency of IV catheters.

HEPATITIS B IMMUNE GLOBULIN

(hep-a-**tite**-iss B i-**myoon** **glo**-byoo-lin)
H-BIG, Hep-B-Gammagee, HyperHep

CLASSIFICATION(S):
Serum—immune globulin
Pregnancy Category UK

INDICATIONS

■ Prevents hepatitis B infection in patients who are known to have been exposed, including neonates born to HBsAg-positive women, by providing passive immunity.

ACTION

■ An immune gamma-globulin fraction containing high titers of antibodies to the hepatitis B surface antigen. Confers passive immunity to hepatitis B infection. **Therapeutic Effect:** ■ Prevention of hepatitis B infection.

PHARMACOKINETICS

Absorption: Slowly absorbed following IM administration.
Distribution: Distribution not known. Probably crosses the placenta.
Metabolism and Excretion: Metabolism and excretion not known.
Half-life: 21 days.

CONTRAINDICATIONS AND PRECAUTIONS

Contraindicated in: ■ Hypersensitivity to immune globulins, glycine, or thimerisol.
Use Cautiously in: ■ Thrombocytopenia ■ IgA deficiency ■ Lactation ■ Has been used during pregnancy.

ADVERSE REACTIONS AND SIDE EFFECTS*

CNS: faintness, dizziness, weakness, malaise.
Derm: rashes, urticaria, pruritus.
MS: joint pain.
Local: pain, swelling, tenderness, erythema at IM site.
Misc: allergic reactions, including angioedema and ANAPHYLACTIC SHOCK.

INTERACTIONS

Drug-Drug: ■ May interfere with the immune response to **live vaccines.**

ROUTE AND DOSAGE

- **IM (Adults):** 0.06 ml/kg (usual dose 3–5 ml).
- **IM (Neonates):** 0.5 ml.

PHARMACODYNAMICS (development of anti-HBs antibodies)

	ONSET	PEAK	DURATION
IM	1–6 days	3–11 days	2–6 mon

NURSING IMPLICATIONS

Assessment

- □ For passive immunity, determine the date of exposure to infection. Hepatitis B immune globulin should be administered preferably within 24 hr but not later than 7 days of exposure to hepatitis B.
- □ Assess patient for signs of anaphylaxis (hypotension, flushing, chest tightness, wheezing, fever, dizziness, nausea, vomiting, diaphoresis) following administration. Epinephrine and antihistamines should be available for treatment of anaphylactic reactions.

Potential Nursing Diagnoses

- ■ Infection, high risk for (indications).
- ■ Knowledge deficit related to medication regimen (patient/family teaching).

Implementation

- ■ **General Info:** Soln for injection is clear, slightly amber, and viscous. Soln should be refrigerated.
- □ If administered with hepatitis B virus vaccine, do not administer via same syringe or into same injection site.
- ■ **IM:** Administer hepatitis B immune globulin (HBIG) in adults and chil-

*Underlines indicate most frequent; **CAPITALS** indicate life-threatening.

dren into the deltoid muscle or anterolateral thigh. The gluteal site should be used only in adults with injections of large volumes or when large volumes are divided into multiple doses.
- Do not administer IV.

PATIENT/FAMILY TEACHING
- Explain to patient the use and purpose of hepatitis B immune globulin therapy.
- Advise patient to report symptoms of anaphylaxis immediately.
- Inform patient that pain, tenderness, swelling, and erythema at the injection site may occur following IM injections.

EVALUATION

Effectiveness of immune globulin therapy can be demonstrated by: ▪ Prevention of hepatitis B infection in exposed patients by providing passive immunity.

HETASTARCH
HES, Hespan, Hydroxyethyl starch

CLASSIFICATION(S):
Volume expander
Pregnancy Category UK

INDICATIONS
▪ Adjunct in the early management of shock or impending shock due to: □ Burns □ Hemorrhage □ Surgery □ Sepsis □ Trauma when fluid replacement and plasma volume expansion are needed.

ACTION
▪ A synthetic molecule that acts as a colloidal osmotic agent similar to albumin. **Therapeutic Effect:** ▪ Plasma volume expansion.

PHARMACOKINETICS
Absorption: Administered IV only, resulting in complete bioavailability.
Distribution: Not known.
Metabolism and Excretion: Molecules with a molecular weight of 50,000 or less are excreted unchanged by the kidneys. Larger molecules are slowly degraded before excretion.
Half-life: 90% has half-life of 17 days, remaining 10% has half-life of 48 days.

CONTRAINDICATIONS AND PRECAUTIONS
Contraindicated in: ▪ Hypersensitivity ▪ Severe bleeding disorders ▪ Congestive heart failure ▪ Pulmonary edema ▪ Oliguric or anuric renal failure ▪ Early pregnancy.
Use Cautiously in: ▪ Thrombocytopenia ▪ Elderly patients ▪ Lactation or children (safety not established).

ADVERSE REACTIONS AND SIDE EFFECTS*
CNS: headache.
CV: pulmonary edema, congestive heart failure.
GI: vomiting.
Hemat: decreased platelet function, decreased hematocrit.
Derm: pruritus, urticaria.
F and E: fluid overload, peripheral edema of the lower extremities.
MS: mylagia.
Misc: hypersensitivity reactions, including ANAPHYLACTOID REACTIONS, chills, fever, parotid and submaxillary gland enlargement.

INTERACTIONS
Drug-Drug: ▪ No known interactions.

ROUTE AND DOSAGE
- **IV (Adults):** 30–60 g (500–1000 ml of 6% soln), may be repeated, not to exceed 90 g (1500 ml/day). In acute hemorrhagic shock, up to 20 ml/kg/hr may be used.

PHARMACODYNAMICS (volume expansion)

	ONSET	PEAK	DURATION
IV	rapid	end of infusion	24 hr or longer

*Underlines indicate most frequent; **CAPITALS** indicate life-threatening.

H

NURSING IMPLICATIONS

ASSESSMENT

- Monitor vital signs, CVP, cardiac output, pulmonary capillary wedge pressure, and urinary output prior to and frequently throughout therapy. Assess patient for signs of vascular overload (elevated CVP, rales/crackles, dyspnea, hypertension, jugular venous distention) during and following administration.
- If fever, wheezing, flu-like symptoms, urticaria, periorbital edema, or submaxillary and parotid gland enlargement occur, stop infusion and notify physician immediately. Antihistamines, epinephrine, corticosteroids, and airway management may be required to suppress this response.
- Assess surgical patients for increased bleeding following administration caused by interference with platelet function and clotting factors.
- **Lab Test Considerations:** Monitor CBC with differential, hemoglobin, hematocrit, platelet count, prothrombin time, partial thromboplastin time, and clotting time throughout course of therapy. Large volumes of hetastarch may cause hemodilution; do not allow hematocrit to drop below 30% by volume. May cause increased erythrocyte sedimentation rate; prolonged bleeding time; and prolonged prothrombin, partial thromboplastin, and clotting times.
- May cause elevated indirect serum bilirubin and amylase concentrations.

POTENTIAL NURSING DIAGNOSES

- Tissue perfusion, altered (indications).
- Fluid volume deficit, actual (indications).
- Fluid volume excess (side effects).

IMPLEMENTATION

- **General Info:** Available in a 6% soln diluted with 0.9% NaCl. Soln should be clear pale yellow to amber; do not administer soln that is cloudy or that contains a precipitate. Store at room temperature. Discard unused soln.
- There is no danger of serum hepatitis or AIDS from hetastarch. Crossmatching is not required.
- **Continuous Infusion:** Administer hetastarch undiluted by IV infusion.
- *Rate:* Rate of administration is determined by blood volume, indication, and patient response.
- In acute hemorrhagic shock hetastarch may be administered up to 1.2 g/kg (20 ml/kg) per hr. Slower rates are generally used with burns and septic shock.

PATIENT/FAMILY TEACHING

- Explain to patient the rationale for use of this soln.
- Instruct patient to notify physician or nurse if dyspnsea, itching, or flu-like symptoms occur.

EVALUATION

Effectiveness of therapy can be demonstrated by: ▪ Increase in blood pressure, blood volume, and urinary output when used to treat shock and burns.

HOMATROPINE

(hoe-**ma**-troe-peen)
AK-Homatropine, Homapin, I-Homatrin, Isopto-Homatropine, {Minims Homatropine}

CLASSIFICATION(S):
Ophthalmic—mydriatic, Anticholinergic—antimuscarinic, Antispasmodic
Pregnancy Category C (Ophth)

INDICATIONS

▪ **Ophth:** Production of mydriasis and cycloplegia in order to allow ophthalmic examination ▪ **Ophth:** Treatment of uveitis ▪ **PO:** Adjunct therapy (with antacids or histamine H_2 receptor antagonists) in the management of peptic ulcer disease.

ACTION

▪ Inhibits the action of acetylcholine at postganglionic sites located in smooth muscle, secretory glands, and the CNS (antimuscarinic activity) ▪ Low doses decrease sweating, salivation, and respiratory secretions ▪ Intermediate doses result in mydriasis (pupillary dilation), cycloplegia (loss of visual accommodation), and increased heart rate ▪ GI and GU tract motility are decreased at larger doses. **Therapeutic Effects:** ▪ ***Ophth:*** Mydriasis and cycloplegia ▪ ***PO:*** Decreased GI secretions.

PHARMACOKINETICS

Absorption: Unreliably absorbed following oral administration (10–25%).
Distribution: Minimal penetration of CNS and eye following oral administration.
Metabolism and Excretion: UK.
Half-life: UK.

CONTRAINDICATIONS AND PRECAUTIONS

Contraindicated in: ▪ Hypersensitivity ▪ Narrow-angle glaucoma ▪ Acute hemorrhage ▪ Tachycardia due to cardiac insufficiency ▪ Thyrotoxicosis.
Use Cautiously in: ▪ Elderly patients (increased risk of adverse reactions) ▪ Children (increased risk of adverse reactions) ▪ Suspicion of intra-abdominal infection ▪ Prostatic hypertrophy ▪ Chronic renal, hepatic, or pulmonary disease ▪ Pregnancy or lactation (safety not established).

ADVERSE REACTIONS AND SIDE EFFECTS*

CNS: drowsiness, confusion, dizziness.
EENT: dry eyes, blurred vision, mydriasis, cycloplegia, increased sensitivity to light.
CV: palpitations, tachycardia, hypotension.
GI: dry mouth.
GU: urinary hesitancy, retention.
Misc: decreased sweating.

INTERACTIONS

Drug-Drug: ▪ Additive anticholinergic effects with **antihistamines, antidepressants, quinidine,** and **disopyramide** ▪ Anticholinergics may alter the absorption of **other orally administered drugs** by slowing motility of the GI tract. **Antacids** or **adsorbent antidiarrheals** decrease the absorption of anticholinergics ▪ May increase GI mucosa lesions in patients taking **wax-matrix potassium chloride** preparations ▪ Concurrent use of ophthalmic homatropine may decrease the antiglaucoma effects of **ophthalmic pilocarpine, carbochol,** or **cholinesterase inhibitors.**

ROUTE AND DOSAGE

Note: Patients with heavily pigmented irides may require larger doses.

Cycloplegic Refraction

- **Ophth (Adults):** 1 drop of 2% or 5% soln to conjunctiva, may repeat q 5–10 min for 2–5 doses prior to refraction.
- **Ophth (Children):** 1 drop of 2% soln to conjunctiva, may repeat q 10 min for 3–5 doses prior to refraction.

Uveitis

- **Ophth (Adults):** 1 drop of 2% or 5% soln to conjunctiva 2–3 times daily up to q 3–4 hr.
- **Ophth (Children):** 1 drop of 2% soln to conjunctiva 2–3 times daily.

Peptic Ulcer Adjunct Therapy

- **PO (Adults):** 5–10 mg 3–4 times daily.

PHARMACODYNAMICS (PO = GI effects, ophth = mydriasis and cycloplegia)

	ONSET	PEAK	DURATION
Ophth (mydriasis)	40–60 min	UK	1–3 days
Ophth (cycloplegia)	30–60 min	UK	1–3 days
PO	UK	UK	UK

*Underlines indicate most frequent; **CAPITALS** indicate life-threatening.

H

NURSING IMPLICATIONS

Assessment

- **Ophth:** Assess for symptoms of systemic absorption (tachycardia, flushed face, dry mouth, drowsiness, or confusion). Notify physician if these symptoms occur.
- **Toxicity and Overdose:** If overdose occurs, physostigmine IV is the antidote.

Potential Nursing Diagnoses

- Sensory-perceptual alteration: visual (side effect).
- Knowledge deficit related to medication regimen (patient/family teaching).

Implementation

- **Ophth:** Available in two concentrations (2% and 5%).
- □ Have patient tilt head back and look up, gently depress lower lid with index finger until conjunctival sac is exposed, and instill 1 drop. After instillation, maintain gentle pressure on inner canthus for 1 min to avoid systemic absorption of the drug. Wait at least 5 min before instilling other types of eyedrops.

Patient/Family Teaching

- □ Instruct patient on how to instill eyedrops. Emphasize need to avoid touching applicator tip. If a dose is missed, it should be applied as soon as remembered unless almost time for the next dose. Do not double up on missed doses.
- □ Advise patient that medication may temporarily blur vision and impair ability to judge distances. Driving and other activities that require visual acuity should be avoided until vision clears. Dark glasses may be needed to protect eyes from bright light.
- □ Instruct patient to notify physician if eye irritation, blurred vision, or increased sensitivity to light persists more than 3 days. Periodic ophthalmic examinations to monitor intraocular pressure may be ordered for patients receiving homatropine on a regular basis for uveitis.

Evaluation

Effectiveness of therapy can be demonstrated by: ▪ Mydriasis and cycloplegia. ▪ Management of peptic ulcer disease.

HYDRALAZINE

(hyr-**dral**-a-zeen)
Alazine, Apresoline, Dralzine, {Novo-Hylazin}, Rolzine

CLASSIFICATION(S):
Antihypertensive—vasodilator
Pregnancy Category C

INDICATIONS

▪ In combination with a diuretic in the management of moderate to severe hypertension ▪ Treatment of congestive heart failure unresponsive to conventional therapy with cardiac glycosides and diuretics.

ACTION

▪ Direct-acting peripheral arteriolar vasodilator. **Therapeutic Effects:** ▪ Lowering of blood pressure in hypertensive patients and decreased afterload in patients with congestive heart failure.

PHARMACOKINETICS

Absorption: Rapidly absorbed following oral administration. Well absorbed from IM sites.
Distribution: Widely distributed. Crosses the placenta. Enters breast milk in minimal concentrations.
Metabolism and Excretion: Mostly metabolized by the GI mucosa and liver.
Half-life: 2–8 hr.

CONTRAINDICATIONS AND PRECAUTIONS

Contraindicated in: ▪ Hypersensitivity ▪ Some products contain tartrazine (FDC yellow dye #5)—avoid use in patients with tartrazine hypersensitivity.
Use Cautiously in: ▪ Cardiovascular or cerebrovascular disease ▪ Severe renal

and hepatic disease ▪ Pregnancy, lactation, or children (safety not established).

ADVERSE REACTIONS AND SIDE EFFECTS*

CNS: headache, peripheral neuropathy, dizziness, drowsiness.
CV: tachycardia, angina, arrhythmias, orthostatic hypotension, edema.
GI: nausea, vomiting, diarrhea.
Derm: rashes.
F and E: sodium retention.
MS: arthritis, arthralgias.
Neuro: peripheral neuropathy.
Misc: drug-induced lupus syndrome.

INTERACTIONS

Drug-Drug: ▪ Additive hypotension with other **antihypertensive agents,** acute ingestion of **alcohol,** or **nitrates** ▪ **MAO inhibitors** may exaggerate hypotension ▪ May reduce the pressor response to **epinephrine** ▪ **Nonsteroidal anti-inflammatory agents** may decrease antihypertensive response ▪ **Beta-adrenergic blockers** decrease tachycardia from hydralazine (therapy may be combined for this reason).

ROUTE AND DOSAGE

- **PO (Adults):** 40–400 mg/day in 4 divided doses.
- **PO (Children):** 0.75 mg/kg/day (25 mg/m^2) in 4 divided doses; may increase gradually to 7.5 mg/kg/day in 4 divided doses (unlabeled).
- **IM, IV (Adults):** 20–40 mg repeated q 4–6 hr as needed.
- **IM, IV (Children):** 1.7–3.5 mg/kg/day or 50–100 mg/m^2/day in 4–6 divided doses (unlabeled).

PHARMACODYNAMICS (antihypertensive effect)

	ONSET	PEAK	DURATION
PO	20–30 min	2 hr	6–12 hr
IM	10–30 min	1 hr	4–6 hr
IV	5–20 min	10–80 min	4–6 hr

NURSING IMPLICATIONS

Assessment

- Monitor blood pressure and pulse frequently during initial dosage adjustment and periodically throughout course of therapy. Notify physician of significant changes.
- **Lab Test Considerations:** CBC, electrolytes, LE cell prep, and antinuclear antibody (ANA) titer should be monitored prior to and periodically during prolonged therapy.
- May cause a positive direct Coombs' test.

Potential Nursing Diagnoses

- Tissue perfusion, altered (indications).
- Knowledge deficit related to medication regimen (patient/family teaching).
- Noncompliance (patient/family teaching).

Implementation

- **General Info:** IM or IV route should be used only when drug cannot be given orally.
- May be administered concurrently with diuretics or beta-adrenergic blocking agents to permit lower doses and minimize side effects.
- Available in combination with hydrochlorothiazide (see Appendix A).
- **PO:** Administer with meals consistently to enhance absorption.
- Pharmacist may prepare oral soln from hydralazine injection for patients with difficulty swallowing.
- **Direct IV:** Inject undiluted through Y-tubing or 3-way stopcock.
- Use soln as quickly as possible after drawing through needle into syringe. Hydralazine changes color after contact with a metal filter.
- *Rate:* Administer at a rate of 10 mg over at least 1 min. Monitor blood pressure and pulse frequently after injection.
- **Y-Site Compatibility:** heparin, hydrocortisone sodium succinate, potassium chloride, or verapamil.

*Underlines indicate most frequent; **CAPITALS** indicate life-threatening.

- **Y-Site Incompatibility:** aminophylline, ampicillin, diazoxide, or furosemide.
- **Additive Compatibility:** dextrose/saline combinations, dextrose/Ringer's soln combinations, D5/LR, D5W, D10W, D10/LR, 0.45% NaCl, 0.9% NaCl, Ringer's or lactated Ringer's soln, or dobutamine.
- **Additive Incompatibility:** aminophylline, ampicillin, chlorothiazide, edetate calcium disodium, ethacrynate sodium, hydrocortisone sodium succinate, methohexital, nitroglycerin, phenobarbital, or verapamil.

Patient/Family Teaching

- Emphasize the importance of continuing to take this medication, even if feeling well. Instruct patient to take medication at the same time each day; last dose of the day should be taken at bedtime. If a dose is missed, take as soon as remembered; do not double doses. If more than 2 doses in a row are missed, consult physician. Must be discontinued gradually to avoid sudden increase in blood pressure. Hydralazine controls but does not cure hypertension.
- Encourage patient to comply with additional interventions for hypertension (weight reduction, low-sodium diet, discontinuation of smoking, moderation of alcohol intake, regular exercise, and stress management). Instruct patient and family on proper technique for blood pressure monitoring. Advise them to check blood pressure at least weekly and report significant changes to physician.
- Patients should weigh themselves twice weekly and assess feet and ankles for fluid retention.
- Hydralazine may occasionally cause drowsiness. Advise patient to avoid driving or other activities requiring alertness until response to medication is known.
- Caution patient to avoid sudden changes in position to minimize orthostatic hypotension.
- Advise patient to consult physician or pharmacist before taking any cough, cold, or allergy remedies. Patient should also avoid excessive amounts of tea, coffee, and cola.
- Instruct patient to notify physician or dentist of medication prior to treatment or surgery.
- Advise patient to notify physician immediately if general tiredness, fever, muscle or joint aching, chest pain, skin rash, sore throat or numbness, tingling, pain, or weakness of hands and feet occur. Vitamin B_6 (pyridoxine) may be used to treat peripheral neuritis.
- Emphasize the importance of follow-up examinations to evaluate effectiveness of medication.

Evaluation

Effectiveness of therapy can be demonstrated by: ▪ Decrease in blood pressure without appearance of side effects.

HYDROCHLOROTHIAZIDE

(hye-droe-klor-oh-**thye**-a-zide)
{Apo-Hydro}, {Duiclor H}, Esidrex, HCTZ, HydroDIURIL, Mictrin, {Natrimax}, {Neo-Codema}, {Novohydrazide}, Oretic, Thiuretic, {Urozide}

CLASSIFICATION(S):
Diuretic—thiazide, Antihypertensive—thiazide diuretic
Pregnancy Category B

INDICATIONS

▪ Used alone or in combination with other agents in the management of mild to moderate hypertension ▪ Used alone or in combination in the treatment of edema associated with: ▫ Congestive heart failure ▫ Nephrotic syndrome ▫ Pregnancy.

ACTION

▪ Increases excretion of sodium and water by inhibiting sodium reabsorption in the distal tubule ▪ Promotes excretion of chloride, potassium, magnesium, and bicarbonate ▪ May produce arteriolar dilation. **Therapeutic Effects:** ▪ Lowering of blood pressure in hypertensive patients and diuresis with subsequent mobilization of edema.

PHARMACOKINETICS

Absorption: Variably absorbed from the GI tract following oral administration.
Distribution: Distributed into extracellular space. Crosses the placenta and enters breast milk.
Metabolism and Excretion: Excreted mainly unchanged by the kidneys.
Half-life: 6–15 hr.

CONTRAINDICATION AND PRECAUTIONS

Contraindicated in: ▪ Hypersensitivity ▪ Cross-sensitivity with other thiazides or sulfonamides may exist ▪ Anuria ▪ Lactation.
Use Cautiously in: ▪ Renal or severe hepatic impairment ▪ Pregnancy (jaundice or thrombocytopenia may be seen in the newborn.)

ADVERSE REACTIONS AND SIDE EFFECTS*

CNS: drowsiness, lethargy, dizziness, weakness.
CV: hypotension.
Derm: rashes, photosensitivity.
Endo: hyperglycemia.
F and E: <u>hypokalemia</u>, hypochloremic alkalosis, hyponatremia, hypercalcemia, hypophosphatemia, hypomagnesemia, dehydration, hypovolemia.
GI: anorexia, nausea, vomiting, cramping, hepatitis.
Hemat: blood dyscrasias.
Metab: <u>hyperuricemia</u>, elevated lipids.
MS: muscle cramps.
Misc: pancreatitis.

INTERACTIONS

Drug–Drug: ▪ Additive hypotension with other **antihypertensive agents,** acute ingestion of **alcohol,** or **nitrates** ▪ Additive hypokalemia with **glucocorticoids, amphotericin B, mezlocillin, piperacillin,** or **ticarcillin** ▪ Hypokalemia increases the risk of **cardiac glycoside** toxicity ▪ Decreases the excretion of **lithium** and may cause toxicity ▪ **Cholestyramine** or **colestipol** decreases absorption.
Drug–Food: ▪ **Food** may increase extent of absorption.

ROUTE AND DOSAGE

- **PO (Adults):** 25–100 mg/day in 1–2 doses.
- **PO (Children >6 mon):** 2.2 mg/kg/day in 2 divided doses.
- **PO (Children <6 mon):** up to 3.3 mg/kg/day in 2 divided doses.

PHARMACODYNAMICS

	ONSET	PEAK	DURATION
PO (diuretic)	2 hr	3–6 hr	6–12 hr
PO (antihypertensive)	3–4 days	7–14 days	7 days

NURSING IMPLICATIONS

Assessment

- ▫ Monitor blood pressure, intake and output, and daily weight; assess feet, legs, and sacral area for edema daily.
- ▫ Assess patient for anorexia, nausea, vomiting, muscle cramps, paresthesia, and confusion, especially if patient is taking cardiac glycosides. Patients on cardiac glycosides are at increased risk of digitalis toxicity because of the potassium-depleting effect of the diuretic.
- ▫ Assess patient for allergy to sulfonamides.
- ▪ **Lab Test Considerations:** Monitor electrolytes (especially potassium), blood glucose, BUN, and serum uric acid levels prior to and periodically throughout course of therapy.
- ▫ May cause increase in serum and urine glucose in diabetic patients.
- ▫ May cause an increase in serum bilirubin, calcium, and uric acid and a

*<u>Underlines</u> indicate most frequent; **CAPITALS** indicate life-threatening.

decrease in serum magnesium, potassium, and sodium levels.
- □ May cause increased serum cholesterol, low-density lipoprotein, and triglyceride concentrations.

Potential Nursing Diagnoses
- ■ Fluid volume excess (indications).
- ■ Fluid volume deficit (side effects).
- ■ Knowledge deficit related to medication regimen (patient/family teaching).

Implementation
- ■ **General Info:** Administer in the morning to prevent disruption of sleep cycle.
- □ Available as a tablet, oral soln (10 mg/ml), and concentrated oral soln (100 mg/ml).
- □ Available in combination with antihypertensives and potassium-sparing diuretics (see Appendix A).
- ■ **PO:** May give with food or milk to minimize GI irritation. Tablets may be crushed and mixed with fluid for patients with difficulty swallowing.
- □ Intermittent dose schedule may be used for continued control of edema.

Patient/Family Teaching
- □ Instruct patient to take this medication at the same time each day. If a dose is missed, take as soon as remembered but not just before next dose is due. Do not double doses. Advise patients using hydrochlorothiazide for hypertension to continue taking the medication even if feeling well. Medication controls but does not cure hypertension.
- □ Encourage patient to comply with additional interventions for hypertension (weight reduction, low-sodium diet, regular exercise, discontinuation of smoking, moderation of alcohol consumption, and stress management).
- □ Instruct patient to monitor weight biweekly and to notify physician of significant changes. Instruct patients with hypertension in correct technique for monitoring weekly blood pressure.
- □ Caution patient to make position changes slowly to minimize orthostatic hypotension. This may be potentiated by alcohol.
- □ Advise patient to use sunscreen (avoid those containing PABA) and protective clothing when in the sun to prevent photosensitivity reactions.
- □ Instruct patient to follow a diet high in potassium (see Appendix K).
- □ Advise patient to consult physician or pharmacist before taking over-the-counter medication concurrently with this therapy.
- □ Advise patient to report muscle weakness, cramps, nausea, or dizziness to the physician.
- □ Instruct patient to notify physician or dentist of medication regimen prior to treatment or surgery.
- □ Emphasize the importance of routine follow-up examinations.

Evaluation

Effectiveness of therapy can be demonstrated by: ■ Decrease in blood pressure ■ Increase in urine output □ Decrease in edema.

HYDROCODONE

(hye-droe-**koe**-done)
Hycodan, (U.S. formulation contains homatropine)

CLASSIFICATION(S):
Narcotic analgesic—agonist (combination), Antitussive (combination)
Schedule III
Pregnancy Category C

INDICATIONS

■ Alone and in combination with nonnarcotic analgesics in the management of moderate to severe pain ■ Antitussive (usually in combination products with decongestants).

ACTION

■ Binds to opiate receptors in the CNS. Alters the perception of and response to painful stimuli while producing generalized CNS depression. **Therapeutic Effects:** ▪ Decrease in severity of moderate pain ▪ Suppression of the cough reflex.

PHARMACOKINETICS

Absorption: Well absorbed following oral administration.
Distribution: Distribution not known.
Metabolism and Excretion: Mostly metabolized by the liver.
Half-life: 3.8 hr.

CONTRAINDICATIONS AND PRECAUTIONS

Contraindicated in: ▪ Hypersensitivity ▪ Pregnancy or lactation (avoid chronic use) ▪ Products may contain tartrazine, sulfites, or alcohol; avoid use in hypersensitive patients.
Use Cautiously in: ▪ Head trauma ▪ Increased intracranial pressure ▪ Severe renal, hepatic, or pulmonary disease ▪ Hypothyroidism ▪ Adrenal insufficiency ▪ Alcoholism ▪ Elderly or debilitated patients (dosage reduction required) ▪ Patients with undiagnosed abdominal pain ▪ Prostatic hypertrophy ▪ Pregnancy and lactation (safety not established).

ADVERSE REACTIONS AND SIDE EFFECTS*

CNS: sedation, confusion, headache, euphoria, floating feeling, unusual dreams, hallucinations, dysphoria.
CV: hypotension, bradycardia.
EENT: miosis, diplopia, blurred vision.
Resp: respiratory depression.
GI: nausea, vomiting, constipation.
GU: urinary retention.
Derm: sweating, flushing.
Misc: tolerance, physical dependence, psychological dependence.

INTERACTIONS

Drug–Drug: ▪ Use with extreme caution in patients receiving **MAO inhibitors** (may produce severe, unpredictable reactions—reduce initial dose of hydrocodone to 25% of usual dose) ▪ Additive CNS depression with **alcohol, antihistamines,** and **sedative/hypnotics** ▪ Administration of **partial-antagonist narcotic analgesics** may precipitate withdrawal in narcotic dependent patients ▪ **Nalbuphine** or **pentazocine** may decrease analgesia.

ROUTE AND DOSAGE

Analgesic

- **PO (Adults):** 5–10 mg q 4–6 hr as needed.
- **PO (Children):** 0.15 mg/kg q 6 hr as needed.

Antitussive

- **PO (Adults):** 5–10 mg q 4–6 hr as needed (not to exceed 15 mg/dose) or 10 mg q 12 hr as long-acting preparation.
- **PO (Children):** 0.6 mg/kg/day (20 mg/m²/day) in 3–4 divided doses (not to exceed 10 mg/single dose in children >12 yr; 5 mg/single dose in children 2–12 yr or 1.25 mg/single dose in children <2 yr) or 5 mg q 12 hr as extended-release preparation in children 6–12 yr (not to exceed 10 mg/day).

PHARMACODYNAMICS

	ONSET	PEAK	DURATION
PO (analgesic)	10–30 min	30–60 min	4–6 hr
PO (antitussive)	UK	UK	4–6 hr

NURSING IMPLICATIONS

Assessment

- ▫ Assess blood pressure, pulse, and respiratory rate before and periodically during administration.
- ▫ Assess bowel function routinely. Increased intake of fluids and bulk, stool softeners, and laxatives may minimize constipating effects.
- ▪ **Pain:** Assess type, location, and intensity of pain prior to and 60 min following administration.
- ▫ Prolonged use may lead to physical and psychological dependence and tolerance. This should not prevent

*Underlines indicate most frequent; **CAPITALS** indicate life-threatening.

patient from receiving adequate analgesia. Most patients who receive hydrocodone for medical reasons do not develop psychological dependency. Potential for dependence is less than that of morphine. Progressively higher doses may be required to relieve pain with long-term therapy.

- **Cough:** Assess cough, sputum, and lung sounds during antitussive use.
- **Lab Test Considerations:** May increase plasma amylase and lipase levels.
- **Toxicity and Overdose:** If overdosage occurs, naloxone (Narcan) is the antidote.

POTENTIAL NURSING DIAGNOSES

- Comfort, altered: pain (indications).
- Sensory-perceptual alteration: visual, auditory (side effects).
- Injury, high risk for (side effects).

IMPLEMENTATION

- **General Info:** Explain therapeutic value of medication prior to administration to enhance the analgesic effect.
  - Regularly administered doses may be more effective than prn administration. Analgesic is more effective if given before pain becomes severe.
  - Medication should be discontinued gradually after long-term use to prevent withdrawal symptoms.
  - Available only in combination with other drugs. Available in various cough syrups, elixirs, resins, and suspensions. Usually in combination with non-narcotic analgesics (aspirin, acetaminophen); see Appendix A.
- **PO:** May be administered with food or milk to minimize GI irritation.

PATIENT/FAMILY TEACHING

- Instruct patient on how and when to ask for pain medication prn.
- Medication may cause drowsiness or dizziness. Advise patient to call for assistance when ambulating or smoking. Caution patient to avoid driving or other activities requiring alertness until response to the medication is known.
- Advise patient to make position changes slowly to minimize orthostatic hypotension.
- Caution patient to avoid concurrent use of alcohol or other CNS depressants with this medication.
- Encourage patient to turn, cough, and breathe deeply every 2 hr to prevent atelectasis.

EVALUATION

Effectiveness of therapy can be demonstrated by: ▪ Decrease in severity of pain without a significant alteration in level of consciousness or respiratory status ▪ Suppression of nonproductive cough.

HYDROCORTISONE

(hye-droe-**kor**-ti-sone)
A-hydroCort, Biosone, Cortef, Cortenema, Cortifoam, Cortisol, {Hycort}, Hydrocortone, Solu-Cortef

CLASSIFICATION(S):
Glucocorticoid—short-acting
Pregnancy Category UK

INDICATIONS

▪ Management of adrenocortical insufficiency ▪ Short-term management of a variety of inflammatory and allergic conditions, including asthma and ulcerative colitis ▪ Chronic use is limited due to mineralocorticoid activity ▪ Not suitable for alternate-day therapy.

ACTION

▪ Replaces cortisol in deficiency states ▪ Suppresses the normal immune response and inflammation ▪ Has additional profound and varied metabolic effects ▪ Potent mineralocorticoid (sodium retention) ▪ Suppresses adrenal function with chronic use at doses >20 mg/day. **Therapeutic Effects:** ▪ Replaces cortisol in deficiency states ▪ Suppression of inflammation.

PHARMACOKINETICS

Absorption: Well absorbed following oral administration. Phosphate and succinate salts are rapidly absorbed following IM administration. The acetate salt provides slower absorption and a longer duration of action. Some systemic absorption may occur with chronic use of topical preparations.
Distribution: Widely distributed. Crosses the placenta and probably enters breast milk.
Metabolism and Excretion: Metabolized by the liver.
Half-life: 80–120 min.

CONTRAINDICATIONS AND PRECAUTIONS

Contraindicated in: ▪ Serious infections—except for some forms of meningitis ▪ Do not administer live vaccines to patients receiving more than 20 mg/day.
Use Cautiously in: ▪ Children (chronic use may lead to growth suppression) ▪ Chronic treatment with doses greater than 20 mg/day (results in adrenal suppression) ▪ Do not discontinue abruptly ▪ Periods of stress (infections, surgery) may need additional doses ▪ May mask signs of infection ▪ Use lowest possible dose for shortest period of time ▪ Pregnancy or lactation (safety not established).

ADVERSE REACTIONS AND SIDE EFFECTS*

CNS: psychoses, depression, euphoria.
EENT: cataracts, increased intraocular pressure.
CV: edema, hypertension, congestive heart failure, thromboembolism.
GI: nausea, vomiting, increased appetite, weight gain, GI bleeding, peptic ulceration.
Derm: petechiae, ecchymoses, fragility, decreased wound healing, hirsutism, acne.
Endo: menstrual irregularities, hyperglycemia, decreased growth in children, adrenal suppression.
F and E: hypokalemia, sodium retention, metabolic alkalosis, hypocalcemia.
Local: atrophy at IM sites (sustained-release dosage forms).
MS: weakness, myopathy, aseptic necrosis of joints, osteoporosis.
Misc: increases susceptibility to infections, pancreatitis, cushingoid appearance (moon face, buffalo hump).

INTERACTIONS

Drug-Drug: ▪ Additive hypokalemia with **amphotericin B, mezlocillin, piperacillin, ticarcillin,** or **diuretics** ▪ Hypokalemia may increase the risk of **cardiac glycoside** toxicity ▪ May increase requirements for **insulin** or **oral hypoglycemic agents** ▪ **Phenytoin, phenobarbital,** and **rifampin** stimulate metabolism; may decrease effectiveness ▪ **Oral contraceptives** may block metabolism ▪ May decrease antibody response to **live virus vaccines** and increase the risk of adverse reactions.

ROUTE AND DOSAGE

- **PO (Adults):** 10–320 mg/day in 2–4 divided doses.
- **IM, IV (Adults):** 100–500 mg q 2–10 hr (succinate); 15–240 mg (phosphate) q 12 hr (range 100–8000 mg/day).
- **Intra-Articular (Adults):** 5–75 mg (acetate).
- **Rect (Adults):** 10–100 mg 1–2 times daily as enema, suppository, or foam.
- **Top (Adults and Children):** 0.1–2.5% ointment, cream; apply 1–4 times daily; also available as spray or lotion; apply 3–4 times daily.

PHARMACODYNAMICS (anti-inflammatory activity)

	ONSET	PEAK	DURATION
PO	6 hr	UK	1.25–1.5 days
IM	rapid	UK	1.25–1.5 days
IV	rapid	UK	1.25–1.5 days

*Underlines indicate most frequent; **CAPITALS** indicate life-threatening.

H

NURSING IMPLICATIONS

Assessment

- **General Info:** This drug is indicated for many conditions. Assess involved systems prior to and periodically throughout course of therapy.
- □ Assess patient for signs of adrenal insufficiency (hypotension, weight loss, weakness, nausea, vomiting, anorexia, lethargy, confusion, restlessness) prior to and periodically throughout course of therapy.
- □ Monitor intake and output ratios and daily weights. Observe patient for the appearance of peripheral edema, steady weight gain, rales/crackles, or dyspnea. Notify physician if these occur.
- □ Children should also have periodic evaluations of growth.
- **Intra-articular:** Monitor pain, edema, and range of motion of affected joints.
- **Top:** Assess affected skin prior to and daily during therapy. Note degree of inflammation and pruritus.
- **Lab Test Considerations:** Patients on prolonged courses of therapy should routinely have hematologic values, serum electrolytes, and serum and urine glucose evaluated. May cause decreased WBC counts. May cause hyperglycemia, especially in persons with diabetes. May decrease serum potassium and calcium and increase serum sodium concentrations.
- □ Promptly report presence of guaiac-positive stools.
- □ May increase serum cholesterol and lipid values. May decrease serum protein–bound iodine and thyroxine concentrations.
- □ Suppresses reactions to allergy skin tests.
- □ Periodic adrenal function tests may be ordered to assess degree of hypothalamic-pituitary-adrenal (HPA) axis suppression.

Potential Nursing Diagnoses

- Infection, high risk for (side effects).
- Knowledge deficit related to medication regimen (patient/family teaching).

Implementation

- **General Info:** Available in many forms: tablet; oral suspension; ophthalmic ointment; otic soln and suspension in combination with antibiotics (Cortisporin); topical cream, ointment, spray, gel, foam, soln; rectal enema, foam, ointment, suppository; and parenterally for SC, IM, IV injection, infusion, and direct injection into joints and soft tissue lesions.
- □ If dose is ordered daily, administer in the morning to coincide with the body's normal secretion of cortisol.
- **PO:** Administer with meals to minimize gastric irritation.
- **Direct IV:** Reconstitute with provided soln (i.e., Mix-O-Vials) or 2 ml of bacteriostatic water or saline for injection.
- □ *Rate:* Administer each 100 mg over at least 30 sec. Doses 500 mg and larger should be infused over at least 10 min.
- **Intermittent IV:** May be added to 50–1000 ml of D5W, 0.9% NaCl, or D5/0.9% NaCl. Administer infusions at prescribed rate. Diluted soln should be used within 24 hr.
- **Syringe Compatibility:** □ HYDROCORTISONE SODIUM PHOSPHATE with metoclopramide.
- □ HYDROCORTISONE SODIUM SUCCINATE with metoclopramide or thiopental.
- **Y-Site Compatibility:** □ HYDROCORTISONE SODIUM PHOSPHATE with ondansetron.
- □ HYDROCORTISONE SODIUM SUCCINATE with acyclovir, aminophylline, ampicillin, amrinone, atracurium, atropine, betamethasone, calcium gluconate, cephalothin, cephapirin, chlordiazepoxide, chlorpromazine, cyanocobalamin, deslanoside, dexamethasone, digoxin, diphenhydramine, dopamine, droperidol, edrophonium, enalaprilat, epinephrine, esmolol, conjugated estrogens, ethacrynate, fentanyl, fentanyl/droperidol, fluorouracil, furosemide, hydralazine, insulin, isoproterenol, kanamycin, lidocaine, magnesium

sulfate, menadiol, methicillin, methoxamine, methylergonovine, minocycline, morphine, neostigmine, norepinephrine, ondansetron, oxacillin, oxytocin, pancuronium, penicillin G potassium, pentazocine, phytonadione, prednisolone, procainamide, prochlorperazine, propranolol, pyridostigmine, scopolamine, sodium bicarbonate, succinylcholine, trimethobenzamide, trimethaphan camsylate, or vecuronium.

- **Y-Site Incompatibility:** ▫ HYDROCORTISONE SODIUM SUCCINATE with diazepam, ergotamine tartrate, or phenytoin.
- **Additive Compatibility:** ▫ HYDROCORTISON SODIUM PHOSPHATE with amikacin, amphotericin B, bleomycin, dacarbazine, heparin, cephapirin, metaraminol, sodium bicarbonate, or verapamil.

▫ HYDROCORTISONE SODIUM SUCCINATE with amikacin, aminophylline, amphotericin, calcium chloride, calcium gluconate, cephalothin, cephapirin, chloramphenicol, clindamycin, corticotropin, daunorubicin, dopamine, erythromycin, lidocaine, magnesium sulfate, metronidazole, netilmicin, norepinephrine, penicillin G, piperacillin, polymyxin B, potassium chloride, procaine, sodium bicarbonate, thiopental, vancomycin, or verapamil.

- **Additive Incompatibility:** ▫ HYDROCORTISONE SODIUM SUCCINATE with bleomycin, colistimethate, dimenhydrinate, diphenhydramine, doxorubicin, ephedrine, hydralazine, nafcillin, pentobarbital, phenobarbital, prochlorperazine, promazine, promethazine, secobarbital, or tetracycline.
- **Top:** Apply in a thin layer to clean, slightly moist skin. Gloves should be worn. Apply occlusive dressing only with physician's order. Apply aerosol form from a distance of 15 cm for 1–2 sec.
- **Rect:** Applicator is provided by manufacturer. Do not insert aerosol container into rectum. Instructions are provided for correct usage of applicator. Clean applicator after each use.

Patient/Family Teaching

- ▫ Instruct patient on correct technique of administration for prescribed form. Patient should take medication exactly as directed and not skip doses or double up on missed doses. Stopping the medication suddenly may result in adrenal insufficiency (anorexia, nausea, fatigue, weakness, hypotension, dyspnea, and hypoglycemia). If these signs appear, notify physician immediately. This can be life-threatening.
- ▫ Encourage patients on long-term therapy to eat a diet high in protein, calcium, and potassium and low in sodium and carbohydrates (see Appendix K for foods included).
- ▫ This drug causes immunosuppression and may mask symptoms of infection. Instruct patient to avoid people with known contagious illnesses and to report possible infections.
- ▫ Review side effects with patient. Instruct patient to inform physician promptly if severe abdominal pain or tarry stools occur. Patient should also report unusual swelling, weight gain, tiredness, bone pain, bruising, nonhealing sores, visual disturbances, or behavior changes.
- ▫ Instruct patient to inform physician if symptoms of underlying disease return or worsen.
- ▫ Advise patient to carry identification in the event of an emergency in which patient cannot relate medical history.
- ▫ Advise parents not to administer topical preparations to a child <2 yr unless directed by physician.
- ▫ Caution patient to avoid vaccinations without consulting physician.
- ▫ Emphasize the importance of follow-up examinations to monitor progress and side effects.

Evaluation

Effectiveness of therapy can be demonstrated by: ▪ Suppression of the inflammatory and immune responses in autoimmune disorders and allergic reactions.

HYDROMORPHONE
(hye-droe-**mor**-fone)
dihydromorphinone, Dilaudid, Dilaudid-HP

CLASSIFICATION(S):
Narcotic analgesic—agonist, Antitussive
Schedule II
Pregnancy Category C

INDICATIONS
▪ Used alone and in combination with non-narcotic analgesics (acetaminophen or aspirin) in the management of moderate to severe pain ▪ Used as an antitussive in lower doses.

ACTION
▪ Binds to opiate receptors in the CNS ▪ Alters the perception of and response to painful stimuli while producing generalized CNS depression. **Therapeutic Effects:** ▪ Decrease in moderate to severe pain ▪ Suppression of cough.

PHARMACOKINETICS
Absorption: Well absorbed following oral, Rect, SC, and IM administration.
Distribution: Widely distributed. Crosses the placenta and enters breast milk.
Metabolism and Excretion: Mostly metabolized by the liver.
Half-life: 2–4 hr.

CONTRAINDICATIONS AND PRECAUTIONS
Contraindicated in: ▪ Hypersensitivity ▪ Avoid chronic use during pregnancy or lactation.
Use Cautiously in: ▪ Head trauma ▪ Increased intracranial pressure ▪ Severe renal, hepatic, or pulmonary disease ▪ Hypothyroidism ▪ Adrenal insufficiency ▪ Alcoholism ▪ Elderly or debilitated patients (dosage reduction recommended) ▪ Undiagnosed abdominal pain ▪ Prostatic hypertrophy.

ADVERSE REACTIONS AND SIDE EFFECTS*
CNS: sedation, confusion, headache, euphoria, floating feeling, unusual dreams, hallucinations, dysphoria, dizziness.
EENT: miosis, diplopia, blurred vision.
Resp: respiratory depression.
CV: hypotension, bradycardia.
GI: nausea, vomiting, constipation.
GU: urinary retention.
Derm: sweating, flushing.
Misc: tolerance, physical dependence, psychological dependence.

INTERACTIONS
Drug-Drug: ▪ Use with extreme caution in patients receiving **MAO inhibitors** (may produce severe, unpredictable reactions—reduce initial dose of hydromorphone to 25% of usual dose) ▪ Additive CNS depression with **alcohol, antidepressants, antihistamines,** and **sedative/hypnotics** ▪ Administration of **partial-antagonist narcotic analgesics** may precipitate narcotic withdrawal in physically dependent patients ▪ **Nalbuphine** or **pentazocine** may decrease analgesia.

ROUTE AND DOSAGE
Analgesic
- **PO (Adults):** 2 mg q 3–6 hr as needed; may be increased to 4 mg q 4–6 hr.
- **IM, SC (Adult):** 1–2 mg q 3–6 hr as needed; may be increased to 3–4 mg q 4–6 hr.
- **IV (Adults):** 0.5–1 mg q 3 hr as needed.
- **Rect (Adults):** 3 mg q 4–8 hr as needed.

Antitussive
- **PO (Adults):** 1 mg q 3–4 hr.
- **PO (Children 6–12 yr):** 0.5 mg q 3–4 hr.

*Underlines indicate most frequent; **CAPITALS** indicate life-threatening.

PHARMACODYNAMICS (analgesic effect)

	ONSET	PEAK	DURATION
PO	15–30 min	30–90 min	4–5 hr
SC	15–30 min	30–90 min	4–5 hr
IM	15–30 min	30–90 min	4–5 hr
IV	10–15 min	15–30 min	2–3 hr
Rect	15–30 min	30–90 min	4–5 hr

NURSING IMPLICATIONS

Assessment

- **General Info:** Assess blood pressure, pulse, and respiratory rate before and periodically during administration.
- □ Assess bowel function routinely. Increased intake of fluids and bulk, stool softeners, and laxatives may minimize constipating effects.
- **Pain:** Assess type, location, and intensity of pain prior to and 30 min following administration.
- □ Prolonged use may lead to physical and psychological dependence and tolerance. This should not prevent patient from receiving adequate analgesia. Most patients who receive hydromorphone for medical reasons do not develop psychological dependence. Progressively higher doses may be required to relieve pain with long-term therapy.
- **Cough:** Assess cough and lung sounds during antitussive use.
- **Lab Test Considerations:** May increase plasma amylase and lipase concentrations.
- **Toxicity and Overdose:** If overdosage occurs, naloxone (Narcan) is the antidote. Monitor patient closely; dose may need to be repeated or naloxone infusion administered.

Potential Nursing Diagnoses

- Comfort, altered: pain (indications).
- Sensory-perceptual alteration: visual, auditory (side effects).
- Injury, high risk for (side effects).

Implementation

- **General Info:** Explain therapeutic value of medication prior to administration to enhance the analgesic effect.
- □ Regularly administered doses may be more effective than prn administration. Analgesic is more effective if given before pain becomes severe.
- □ Coadministration with non-narcotic analgesics may have additive analgesic effects and permit lower narcotic doses.
- □ Medication should be discontinued gradually after long-term use to prevent withdrawal symptoms.
- □ Available in tablet, suppository, injectable, and high-potency injectable (10 mg/ml) forms. Also available as an antitussive cough syrup.
- **PO:** May be administered with food or milk to minimize GI irritation.
- **Direct IV:** Dilute with at least 5 ml of sterile water or 0.9% NaCl for injection.
- □ *Rate:* Administer slowly, at a rate not to exceed 2 mg over 3–5 min. Rapid administration may lead to increased respiratory depression, hypotension, and circulatory collapse. Do not use IV without antidote available.
- **Syringe Compatibility:** atropine, chlorpromazine, cimetidine, diphenhydramine, fentanyl, glycopyrrolate, hydroxyzine, midazolam, pentazocine, pentobarbital, promethazine, ranitidine, scopolamine, thiethylperazine, or trimethobenzamide.
- **Y-Site Compatibility:** acyclovir, amikacin, ampicillin, cefamandole, cefazolin, cefoperazone, ceforanide, cefotaxime, cefoxitin, ceftizoxime, cefuroxime, cephalothin, cephapirin, chloramphenicol, clindamycin, co-trimoxazole, doxycycline, erythromycin lactobionate, gentamicin, kanamycin, metronidazole, mezlocillin, moxalactam, nafcillin, ondansetron, oxacillin, penicillin G potassium, piperacillin, ticarcillin, tobramycin, or vancomycin.
- **Y-Site Incompatibility:** minocycline or tetracycline.
- **Additive/Solution Compatibility:** D5W, D5/0.45% NaCl, D5/0.9% NaCl, D5/LR, D5/Ringer's soln, 0.45% NaCl, 0.9% NaCl, Ringer's and lactated Ringer's soln, or verapamil.

H

■ **Additive Incompatibility:** sodium bicarbonate or thiopental.

Patient/Family Teaching

- Instruct patient on how and when to ask for prn pain medication.
- Medication may cause drowsiness or dizziness. Advise patient to call for assistance when ambulating or smoking. Caution patient to avoid driving or other activities requiring alertness until response to medication is known.
- Advise patient to make position changes slowly to minimize orthostatic hypotension.
- Instruct patient to avoid concurrent use of alcohol or other CNS depressants.
- Encourage patient to turn, cough, and breathe deeply every 2 hr to prevent atelectasis.

Evaluation

Effectiveness of therapy can be demonstrated by: ■ Decrease in severity of pain without a significant alteration in level of consciousness or respiratory status ■ Suppression of cough.

HYDROXYCHLOROQUINE

(hye-drox-ee-**klor**-oh-kwin)
Plaquenil

CLASSIFICATION(S):
Antimalarial, Antiarthritic
Pregnancy Category UK

INDICATIONS

■ Suppression and chemoprophylaxis of malaria ■ Treatment of severe rheumatoid arthritis and systemic lupus erythematosus.

ACTION

■ Inhibits protein synthesis in susceptible organisms by inhibiting DNA and RNA polymerase. **Therapeutic Effects:** ■ Death of plasmodia responsible for causing malaria ■ Also has anti-inflammatory properties.

PHARMACOKINETICS

Absorption: Appears to be well absorbed following oral administration.
Distribution: Appears to be widely distributed; high tissue concentrations achieved (especially liver). Probably enters breast milk.
Metabolism and Excretion: Partially metabolized by the liver, partially excreted unchanged by the kidneys.
Half-life: 72–120 hr.

CONTRAINDICATIONS AND PRECAUTIONS

Contraindicated in: ■ Hypersensitivity to hydroxychloroquine or chloroquine ■ Patients with visual damage caused by hydroxychloroquine or chloroquine.
Use Cautiously in: ■ Patients receiving other hepatotoxic drugs ■ Patients with liver disease ■ Alcoholism ■ G6-PD deficiency ■ Psoriasis ■ Bone marrow depression.

ADVERSE REACTIONS AND SIDE EFFECTS*

CNS: headache, fatigue, nervousness, anxiety, apathy, irritability, agitation, aggressiveness, confusion, personality changes, psychoses, SEIZURES.
EENT: visual disturbances, keratopathy, retinopathy, ototoxicity, tinnitus.
CV: hypotension, ECG changes.
GI: epigastric discomfort, anorexia, nausea, vomiting, abdominal cramps, diarrhea.
Derm: dermatoses.
Hemat: leukopenia, thrombocytopenia, AGRANULOCYTOSIS, APLASTIC ANEMIA.
Neuro: peripheral neuritis, neuromyopathy.

INTERACTIONS

Drug-Drug: ■ May increase the risk of hepatotoxicity when administered with **hepatotoxic drugs** ■ May increase the risk of hematologic toxicity when administered with **penicillamine** ■ May increase risk of dermatitis when admin-

*Underlines indicate most frequent; **CAPITALS** indicate life-threatening.

istered with other **agents having dermatologic toxicity** ▪ May decrease serum titers of rabies antibody when given concurrently with **human diploid-cell rabies vaccine** ▪ **Urinary acidifiers** may increase renal excretion ▪ May increase serum levels of **digoxin**.

ROUTE AND DOSAGE

Note: Doses expressed as mg of hydroxychloroquine base: 155 mg of hydroxychloroquine base = 200 mg hydroxychloroquine sulfate.

Malaria (Suppression or Chemoprophylaxis)

- **PO (Adults):** 310 mg once weekly; start 1–2 wk prior to entering malarious area; continue for 6–8 wk after leaving area.
- **PO (Children):** 5 mg/kg once weekly; start 1–2 wk prior to entering malarious area; continue for 6–8 wk after leaving area.

Malaria (Uncomplicated Attacks)

- **PO (Adults):** 620 mg initially, then 310 mg 6–8 hr, 24–26 hr, and 48 hr after initial dose or a single 620 mg dose.
- **PO (Children):** 10 mg/kg initially, then 5 mg/kg at 6 hr, 24 hr, and 48 hr after initial dose.

Rheumatoid Arthritis

- **PO (Adults):** 310–465 mg/day initially; may increase after 5–10 days until optimal effect, then decrease dose by 50% to maintenance dose of 155–310 mg.

Systemic Lupus Erythematosus

- **PO (Adults):** 310 mg (400 mg sulfate) 1–2 times daily for several wks–mons. Usual maintenance dose is 155–310 mg.

PHARMACODYNAMICS (blood levels)

	ONSET	PEAK	DURATION
PO	rapid	1–2 hr	days–wk

NURSING IMPLICATIONS

Assessment

- **General Info:** Assess deep tendon reflexes periodically to determine muscle weakness. Therapy may be discontinued should this occur.
- □ Patients on prolonged high-dose therapy should have eye examinations prior to and every 3 mon during therapy to detect retinal damage.
- **Malaria or Lupus Erythematosus:** Assess patient for improvement in signs and symptoms of condition daily throughout course of therapy.
- **Rheumatoid Arthritis:** Assess patient monthly for pain, swelling, and range of motion.
- **Lab Test Considerations:** Monitor CBC and platelet count periodically throughout therapy. May cause decreased RBC, WBC, and platelet counts.

Implementation

- **PO:** Administer with milk or meals to minimize GI distress. Tablets may be crushed and placed inside empty capsules for patients with difficulty swallowing. Contents of capsules may also be mixed with a teaspoonful of jam, jelly, or jello prior to administration.
- **Malaria Prophylaxis:** Hydroxychloroquine therapy should be started 2 wk prior to potential exposure and continued for 6 wk after leaving the area.

Patient/Family Teaching

- □ Instruct patient to take medication exactly as directed and continue full course of therapy even if feeling better. Missed doses should be taken as soon as remembered except with regimens requiring doses more than once a day, for which missed doses should be taken within 1 hr or omitted. Do not double doses.
- □ Review methods of minimizing exposure to mosquitos with patients receiving hydroxychloroquine prophylactically (use repellant, wear long-sleeved shirt and long trousers, use screen or netting).
- □ Hydroxychloroquine may cause dizziness or lightheadedness. Caution patient to avoid driving or other activities requiring alertness until response to medication is known.

H

- Advise patients to avoid use of alcohol while taking hydroxychloroquine.
- Caution patient to keep hydroxychloroquine out of reach of children; fatalities have occurred with ingestion of 3 or 4 tablets.
- Advise patient that the risk of ocular damage may be decreased by the use of dark glasses in bright light. Protective clothing and sunscreen should also be used to reduce risk of dermatoses.
- Advise patient to notify physician promptly if sore throat, fever, unusual bleeding or bruising, blurred vision, visual changes, ringing in the ears, difficulty hearing, or muscle weakness occurs.
- Instruct patient to contact physician if no improvement is noticed within a few days. Treatment for rheumatoid arthritis may require up to 6 mon for full benefit.

Evaluation

Effectiveness of therapy may be demonstrated by: ▪ Prevention or resolution of malaria ▪ Improvement in signs and symptoms of rheumatoid arthritis ▪ Improvement in symptoms of lupus erythematosus.

HYDROXYCOBALAMIN

(hye-drox-e-koe-**bal**-a-min)
{Acti-B_{12}}, alphaRedisol, Alphamin, Codroxomin, Droxomin, Hydrobexan, Hydrocobex, LA-12, Hydro-Crysti-12, vitamin B_{12}

CLASSIFICATION(S):
Vitamin—water-soluble, Antianemic
Pregnancy Category C

INDICATIONS

▪ Treatment and prevention of vitamin B_{12} deficiency ▪ Treatment of pernicious anemia ▪ Used diagnostically as part of the Schilling test.

ACTION

▪ A necessary coenzyme for many metabolic processes, including fat and carbohydrate metabolism and protein synthesis ▪ Required for the formation of red blood cells. **Therapeutic Effects:** ▪ Correction of manifestations of pernicious anemia (megaloblastic indices, GI lesions, and neurologic damage) ▪ Prevention of vitamin B_{12} deficiency.

PHARMACOKINETICS

Absorption: Absorption from the GI tract requires intrinsic factor and calcium. Well absorbed following IM and SC administration.

Distribution: Stored in the liver. Crosses the placenta and enters breast milk.

Metabolism and Excretion: Excess amounts are eliminated unchanged in the urine.

Half-life: 6 days (400 days in liver).

CONTRAINDICATIONS AND PRECAUTIONS

Contraindicated in: ▪ Hypersensitivity ▪ Hereditary optic nerve atrophy ▪ Avoid using benzyl alcohol–containing preparations in premature infants (associated with fatal "gasping syndrome").

Use Cautiously in: ▪ Cardiac disease ▪ Uremia, folic acid deficiency, concurrent infection, iron deficiency (response to B_{12} will be impaired).

ADVERSE REACTIONS AND SIDE EFFECTS*

CV: peripheral vascular thrombosis.

GI: diarrhea.

Derm: itching, swelling of the body, urticaria.

F and E: hypokalemia.

Local: pain at IM site.

Misc: hypersensitivity reactions, including ANAPHYLAXIS.

INTERACTIONS

Drug-Drug: ▪ **Chloramphenicol** and **antineoplastic agents** may decrease the hematologic response to vitamin

{} = Available in Canada only.
*Underlines indicate most frequent; CAPITALS indicate life-threatening.

B_{12} ▪ **Aminoglycosides, colchicine, extended-release potassium supplements, anticonvulsants, cimetidine,** excess intake of **alcohol,** or **vitamin C** may decrease oral absorption of vitamin B_{12}.

ROUTE AND DOSAGE

Vitamin B_{12} Deficiency

- **IM, SC (Adults):** 30–50 mcg/day (up to 100 mcg/day) for 5–10 days, then 100–200 mcg/mon.
- **IM, SC (Children):** 30–50 mcg/day for 1–2 wk to a total of 1–5 mg, then 60–100 mcg/mon.

PHARMACODYNAMICS (reticulocytosis)

	ONSET	PEAK	DURATION
IM, SC	UK	3–10 days	UK

NURSING IMPLICATIONS

Assessment

- Assess patient for signs of vitamin B_{12} deficiency (pallor, neuropathy, psychosis, red inflamed tongue) prior to and periodically throughout therapy.
- **Lab Test Considerations:** Monitor plasma folic acid levels, reticulocyte count, and plasma vitamin B_{12} levels prior to and between the third and tenth days of therapy.
- Patients receiving vitamin B_{12} for megaloblastic anemia should have the serum potassium level evaluated for hypokalemia during the first 48 hr of treatment.

Potential Nursing Diagnoses

- Nutrition, altered: less than body requirements (indications).
- Activity intolerance (indications).
- Knowledge deficit related to medication regimen (patient/family teaching).

Implementation

- **General Info:** Usually administered in combination with other vitamins, as solitary vitamin B deficiencies are rare.

Patient/Family Teaching

- Encourage patients to comply with diet recommendations of physician. Explain that the best source of vitamins is a well-balanced diet with foods from the 4 basic food groups.
- Foods high in vitamin B_{12} include meats, seafood, egg yolk, and fermented cheeses; little lost with ordinary cooking.
- Inform patients of the lifelong need for vitamin B_{12} replacement following gastrectomy or ileal resection.
- Emphasize the importance of follow-up examinations to evaluate progress.

Evaluation

Effectiveness of therapy may be demonstrated by: ▪ Prevention or resolution of the symptoms of vitamin B_{12} deficiency ▫ Increase in reticulocyte count.

HYDROXYPROGESTERONE

(hye-drox-ee-pro-**jess**-te-rone)
Dalalutin, Duralutin, Gesterol LA, Hy-Gestrone, Hylutin, Hyprogest, Hyproval PA, Pro-Depo, Prodrox

CLASSIFICATION(S):
Hormone—progestin
Pregnancy Category D

INDICATIONS

▪ Treatment of amenorrhea and functional uterine bleeding associated with hormonal imbalance ▪ Production of secretory endometrium and desquamation ▪ Diagnostic agent for endogenous estrogen production ▪ Treatment of uterine carcinoma.

ACTION

▪ A synthetic analog of progesterone ▪ Produces secretory changes in the endometrium ▪ Increases basal temperature ▪ Produces changes in the vaginal epithelium ▪ Relaxes uterine smooth muscle ▪ Stimulates mammary alveolar growth ▪ Inhibits pituitary function

▪ Produces withdrawal bleeding (requires estrogen). **Therapeutic Effects:** ▪ Restoration of normal hormonal balance ▪ Decreased tumor growth.

PHARMACOKINETICS

Absorption: Systemic absorption follows IM administration.
Distribution: Distribution not known.
Metabolism and Excretion: Metabolism and excretion, not known.
Half-life: UK.

CONTRAINDICATIONS AND PRECAUTIONS

Contraindicated in: ▪ Hypersensitivity ▪ Hypersensitivity to castor oil or benzyl alcohol ▪ Pregnancy, lactation, or children ▪ Thromboembolic disorders ▪ Undiagnosed vaginal bleeding ▪ Missed abortion ▪ Severe liver disease ▪ Breast carcinoma.
Use Cautiously in: ▪ Cardiac disease ▪ Renal dysfunction ▪ Asthma ▪ Seizures ▪ Migraine headaches ▪ Diabetes mellitus.

ADVERSE REACTIONS AND SIDE EFFECTS*

CNS: depression, cerebral thrombosis.
Resp: coughing, dyspnea.
CV: thrombophlebitis, PULMONARY EMBOLISM, edema.
GI: cholestatic jaundice.
GU: breakthrough bleeding, amenorrhea, cervical changes.
Derm: rashes, increased pigmentation.
Misc: weight changes, allergic reactions.

INTERACTIONS

Drug-Drug: ▪ Interferes with the effects of **bromocriptine** (causes amenorrhea or galactorrhea).

ROUTE AND DOSAGE

Amenorrhea and Uterine Bleeding

- **IM (Adults):** 375 mg q 4 wk. May be followed by cyclic therapy consisting of 20 mg estradiol valerate on day 1, then 250 mg of hydroxyprogesterone with 5 mg estradiol valerate are given on day 15, repeated at 4-wk intervals.

Production of Secretory Endometrium

- **IM (Adults):** 125–250 mg on 10th day of cycle, repeat q 7 days.

Uterine Carcinoma

- **IM (Adults):** 1 g/1–7 times/wk.

PHARMACODYNAMICS (hormonal effects)

	ONSET	PEAK	DURATION
IM	UK	UK	7–14 days

NURSING IMPLICATIONS

Assessment

- Blood pressure should be monitored periodically throughout therapy.
- Monitor intake and output ratios and weekly weight. Report significant discrepancies or steady weight gain to physician.
- Monitor pattern and amount of vaginal bleeding (pad count).
- **Lab Test Considerations:** Monitor hepatic function prior to and periodically throughout therapy.
- May cause increased serum glucose and alkaline phosphatase levels. May decrease pregnandiol excretion concentrations.
- May alter thyroid hormone assays.

Potential Nursing Diagnoses

- Sexual dysfunction (indications).
- Knowledge deficit related to medication regimen (patient/family teaching).

Implementation

- **IM:** Administer deep IM. Use dry needle and syringe to prevent clouding of soln.

Patient/Family Teaching

- **General Info:** Advise patient to report signs and symptoms of fluid retention (swelling of ankles and feet, weight gain), thromboembolic disorders (pain, swelling, tenderness in extremities, headache, chest pain, blurred

*Underlines indicate most frequent; **CAPITALS** indicate life-threatening.

vision), mental depression, or hepatic dysfunction (yellowed skin or eyes, pruritus, dark urine, light-colored stools) to physician.
- ▫ Instruct patient to notify physician if change in vaginal bleeding pattern or spotting occurs.
- ▫ Instruct patient to stop taking medication and notify physician if pregnancy is suspected.
- ▫ Caution patient to use sunscreen and protective clothing to prevent increased pigmentation.
- ▫ Advise patient to notify physician or dentist of medication regimen prior to treatment or surgery.
- ▫ Emphasize the importance of routine follow-up physical examinations, including blood pressure; breast, abdomen, and pelvic examinations; and PAP smears.
- ▪ **Amenorrhea or Functional Uterine Bleeding:** Explain 28-day cyclic dosage schedule. Cyclic therapy begins after 4 days of desquamation from initial dose or 21 days after injection if bleeding did not occur. Explain that several mons of estrogen therapy may be required before menstruation occurs.

EVALUATION

Effectiveness of therapy can be demonstrated by: ▪ Development of normal cyclic menses ▪ Control of the spread of advanced metastatic uterine cancer.

HYDROXYUREA

(hye-drox-ee-yoo-**ree**-ah)
Hydrea

CLASSIFICATION(S):
Antineoplastic—antimetabolite
Pregnancy Category UK

INDICATIONS

▪ Treatment of head and neck carcinoma ▪ Treatment of ovarian carcinoma ▪ Treatment of resistant chronic myelogenous leukemia ▪ Treatment of melanoma.

ACTION

▪ Interferes with DNA synthesis (cell cycle-S phase specific). **Therapeutic Effect:** ▪ Death of rapidly replicating cells, particularly malignant ones.

PHARMACOKINETICS

Absorption: Well absorbed following oral administration.
Distribution: Crosses the blood-brain barrier.
Metabolism and Excretion: 50% excreted unchanged by the kidneys, 50% metabolized by the liver and eliminated as respiratory CO_2.
Half-life: 3–4 hr.

CONTRAINDICATIONS AND PRECAUTIONS

Contraindicated in: ▪ Hypersensitivity ▪ Pregnancy or lactation.
Use Cautiously in: ▪ Patients with childbearing potential ▪ Active infections ▪ Decreased bone marrow reserve ▪ Other chronic debilitating illness.

ADVERSE REACTIONS AND SIDE EFFECTS*

CNS: drowsiness (large doses).
GI: stomatitis, anorexia, nausea, vomiting, diarrhea, constipation, hepatitis.
GU: dysuria, renal tubular dysfunction, gonadal suppression.
Derm: rashes, erythema, pruritus, alopecia.
Hemat: leukopenia, thrombocytopenia, anemia.
Metab: hyperuricemia.
Misc: fever, chills, malaise.

INTERACTIONS

Drug-Drug: ▪ Additive bone marrow depression with **agents that depress bone marrow,** including **radiation therapy**.

*Underlines indicate most frequent; **CAPITALS** indicate life-threatening.

ROUTE AND DOSAGE

Head and Neck Cancer, Ovarian Cancer, Malignant Melanoma

- **PO (Adults):** 60–80 mg/kg as a single daily dose q third day or 20–30 mg/kg/day.

Resistant Chronic Myelogenous Leukemia

- **PO (Adults):** 20–30 mg/kg/day as a single dose.

PHARMACODYNAMICS (effects on blood counts)

	ONSET	PEAK	DURATION
PO	7 days	10 days	21 days

NURSING IMPLICATIONS

Assessment

- □ Assess for fever, sore throat, and signs of infection. If these symptoms occur, notify physician immediately.
- □ Anemia may occur. Monitor for increased fatigue, dyspnea, and orthostatic hypotension.
- □ Assess for bleeding (bleeding gums; bruising; petechiae; guaiac stools, urine, and emesis). Avoid IM injections and rectal temperatures. Hold pressure on all venipuncture sites for at least 10 min.
- □ Monitor intake and output, appetite, and nutritional intake. Adjust diet as tolerated to maintain nutritional status.
- **Lab Test Considerations:** Monitor CBC and differential prior to and weekly during course of therapy. The onset of leukopenia occurs within 10 days of beginning therapy. Recovery usually occurs within 30 days. Notify physician if WBC <2500 mm^3 or if a precipitous drop occurs. Institute thrombocytopenia precautions if platelet count $<100,000$/mm^3. May cause temporary increase in mean corpuscular volume (MCV).
- □ Monitor renal (BUN, creatinine, and uric acid) and liver function tests (SGOT [AST], SGPT [ALT], bilirubin and LDH) prior to and periodically during course of therapy. May cause increased BUN, creatinine, and uric acid concentrations.

Potential Nursing Diagnoses

- Injury, high risk for (side effects).
- Infection, high risk for (side effects).
- Knowledge deficit related to medication regimen (patient/family teaching).

Implementation

- **PO:** Capsules may be opened and contents mixed into a glass of water and taken immediately if patient has difficulty swallowing. Some inert powder may float on the surface.

Patient/Family Teaching

- **General Info:** Instruct patient to take medication exactly as directed, even if nausea, vomiting, or diarrhea is a problem. Consult physician if vomiting occurs shortly after dose is taken. If a dose is missed, do not take at all; do not double doses.
- □ Instruct patient to notify physician if fever, chills, sore throat, signs of infection, bleeding gums, bruising, petechiae, or blood in urine, stool, or emesis occurs. Caution patient to avoid crowds and persons with known infections. Instruct patient to use soft toothbrush and electric razor. Patients should be cautioned not to drink alcoholic beverages or take aspirin-containing products.
- □ Instruct patient to inspect oral mucosa for erythema and ulceration. If ulceration occurs, advise patient to use sponge brush and rinse mouth with water after eating and drinking. Consult physician if mouth pain interferes with eating.
- □ Discuss possibility of drowsiness with patients receiving large doses. Advise patient to avoid driving or other activities until response to drug is known.
- □ Review with patient the need for contraception during therapy. Women need to use contraception even if amenorrhea occurs.
- □ Instruct patient not to receive any vaccinations without advice of physician.

- Discuss need for lab tests and follow-up visits to monitor progress and detect side effects.
- **Leukemia:** Encourage fluid intake of 2000–3000 ml/day. Physician may also order allopurinol and alkalinization of the urine to help prevent urate stone formation.

EVALUATION

Effectiveness of therapy can be demonstrated by: ▪ Decrease in size and spread of tumors ▪ Improved hematologic values in leukemia. Therapy is held if leukocytes are less than 2500/mm^3 or platelets less than 100,000/mm^3 and resumed when these values begin to return to normal limits, usually within 3 days.

HYDROXYZINE
(hye-**drox**-i-zeen)
Anxanil, {Apo-Hydroxyzine}, Atarax, Atozine, Durrax, E-Vista, Hydroxacen, Hy-Pam, Hyzine-50, {Multipax}, {Novohydroxyzin}, Quiess, Vamate, Vistaject-25, Vistaject-50, Vistaquel 50, Vistaril, Vistazine 50

CLASSIFICATION(S):
Sedative/hypnotic, Antihistamine
Pregnancy Category UK

INDICATIONS

▪ Treatment of anxiety ▪ Preoperative sedation ▪ Antiemetic ▪ Antipruritic ▪ Management of alcohol and drug withdrawal. Often combined with narcotic analgesics.

ACTION

▪ Acts as a CNS depressant at the subcortical level of the CNS ▪ Has anticholinergic, antihistaminic, and antiemetic properties. **Therapeutic Effects:** ▪ Sedation ▪ Relief of anxiety ▪ Relief of nausea and vomiting ▪ Relieves allergic symptoms associated with release of histamine, including pruritus.

PHARMACOKINETICS

Absorption: Well absorbed following oral or IM administration.
Distribution: Distribution not known.
Metabolism and Excretion: Completely metabolized by the liver. Eliminated in the feces via biliary excretion.
Half-life: 3 hr.

CONTRAINDICATIONS AND PRECAUTIONS

Contraindicated in: ▪ Hypersensitivity ▪ Pregnancy.
Use Cautiously in: ▪ Severe hepatic dysfunction ▪ Elderly patients (dosage reduction recommended) ▪ Has been used during labor ▪ Lactation (safety not established).

ADVERSE REACTIONS AND SIDE EFFECTS*

CNS: excess sedation, drowsiness, dizziness, ataxia, weakness, headache, paradoxical agitation.
Resp: wheezing.
GI: dry mouth, bitter taste, nausea, constipation.
GU: urinary retention.
Derm: flushing.
Local: pain at IM site, abscesses at IM sites.
Misc: chest tightness.

INTERACTIONS

Drug-Drug: ▪ Additive CNS depression with other **CNS depressants,** including **alcohol, antidepressants, antihistamines, narcotic analgesics,** and **sedative/hypnotics** ▪ Additive anticholinergic effects with other **drugs possessing anticholinergic properties,** including **antihistamines, antidepressants, atropine, haloperidol, phenothiazines, quinidine,** and **disopyramide.**

ROUTE AND DOSAGE

Anxiety

- **PO (Adults):** 50–100 mg 4 times daily (not to exceed 150–200 mg/day).
- **PO (Children >6 yr):** 50–100 mg/day in 3–4 divided doses.

{} = Available in Canada only.
*Underlines indicate most frequent; **CAPITALS** indicate life-threatening.

- **PO (Children <6 yr):** 50 mg/day in 3–4 divided doses.

Preoperative Sedation

- **PO (Adults):** 50–100 mg.
- **PO (Children):** 0.6 mg/kg.
- **IM (Adults):** 25–100 mg.
- **IM (Children):** 1.1 mg/kg.

Antiemetic

- **IM (Adults):** 25–100 mg.
- **IM (Children):** 1.1 mg/kg.

Antipruritic

- **PO (Adults):** 25 mg 3–4 times daily (not to exceed 150–200 mg/day).
- **PO (Children >6 yr):** 50–100 mg/day in 3–4 divided doses.
- **PO (Children <6 yr):** 50 mg/day in 3–4 divided doses.

Alcohol Withdrawal

- **IM (Adults):** 50–100 mg may repeat q 4–6 hr (not to exceed 150–200 mg/day).

PHARMACODYNAMICS (antihistaminic, sedative, antiemetic effects)

	ONSET	PEAK	DURATION
PO	15–30 min	2–4 hr	4–6 hr
IM	15–30 min	2–4 hr	4–6 hr

NURSING IMPLICATIONS

Assessment

- **General Info:** Assess patient for profound sedation and provide safety precautions as indicated (side rails up, bed in low position, call bell within reach, supervision of ambulation and transfer).
- **Anxiety:** Assess mental status, mood, and behavior.
- **Nausea and Vomiting:** Assess degree of nausea and frequency and amount of emesis.
- **Pruritus:** Assess degree of itching and character of involved skin.
- **Lab Test Considerations:** May cause false-negative skin tests using allergen extracts. Discontinue hydroxyzine at least 72 hr prior to test.

Potential Nursing Diagnoses

- Anxiety (indications).
- Skin integrity, impaired: actual (indications).
- Injury, high risk for (side effects).

Implementation

- **General Info:** Available in tablet, capsule, syrup, suspension, and injectable forms.
- **PO:** Tablets may be crushed and capsules opened and administered with food or fluids for patients having difficulty swallowing.
  - Shake suspension well before administration.
- **IM:** Administer IM deep into well-developed muscle, preferably with Z-track technique. Do not use deltoid site. Significant tissue damage, necrosis, and sloughing may result from SC or intra-arterial injections. Hemolysis may result from IV injections. Rotate injection sites frequently.
- **Syringe Compatibility:** atropine, benzquinamide, butorphanol, chlorpromazine, cimetidine, codeine, diphenhydramine, doxapram, droperidol, fentanyl, glycopyrrolate, hydromorphone, lidocaine, meperidine, methotrimeprazine, metoclopramide, midazolam, morphine, nalbuphine, oxymorphone, pentazocine, procaine, prochlorperazine, promazine, promethazine, ranitidine, or scopolamine.
- **Syringe Incompatibility:** aminophylline, chloramphenicol, dimenhydrinate, heparin, penicillin G potassium, pentobarbital, phenobarbital, or phenytoin.

Patient/Family Teaching

- Instruct patient to take medication exactly as directed. Missed doses should be taken as soon as remembered unless almost time for next dose; do not double doses.
- Medication may cause drowsiness or dizziness. Caution patient to avoid driving or other activities requiring alertness until response to medication is known.
- Advise patient to avoid concurrent use of alcohol or other CNS depressants with this medication.

- ▫ Inform patient that frequent mouth rinses, good oral hygiene, and sugarless gum or candy may help decrease dry mouth. If dry mouth persists for more than 2 wk, consult dentist regarding saliva substitute.

EVALUATION

Effectiveness of therapy can be demonstrated by: ▪ Decrease in anxiety ▪ Relief of nausea and vomiting ▪ Relief of pruritus ▪ Sedation when used as a sedative/hypnotic.

IBUPROFEN

(eye-byoo-**proe**-fen)

Advil, {Amersol}, {Apo-Ibuprofen}, Cap-profen, Haltran, Ibuprin, Ifen, Medipren, Midol 200, Motrin, {Novoprofen}, Nuprin, Pamprin-IB, Pedia Profen, Rufin, Tab-Profen, Trendar

CLASSIFICATION(S):
Nonsteroidal anti-inflammatory agent, Antipyretic
Pregnancy Category UK

INDICATIONS

▪ Management of inflammatory disorders including: ▫ Rheumatoid arthritis ▫ Osteoarthritis ▪ Used as an analgesic in the treatment of mild to moderate pain or dysmenorrhea ▪ Lowering of fever.

ACTION

▪ Inhibits prostaglandin synthesis. **Therapeutic Effects:** ▪ Suppression of pain and inflammation ▪ Reduction of fever.

PHARMACOKINETICS

Absorption: Well absorbed from the GI tract.

Distribution: Distribution not known. Probably crosses the placenta. Does not appear to enter breast milk.

Metabolism and Excretion: Mostly metabolized by the liver. Small amounts (10%) excreted unchanged by the kidneys.

Half-life: 2–4 hr.

CONTRAINDICATIONS AND PRECAUTIONS

Contraindicated in: ▪ Hypersensitivity ▪ Cross-sensitivity may exist with other nonsteroidal anti-inflammatory agents, including aspirin ▪ Active GI bleeding or ulcer disease.

Use Cautiously in: ▪ Severe cardiovascular, renal, or hepatic disease ▪ History of ulcer disease ▪ Pregnancy, lactation, or children (safety not established).

ADVERSE REACTIONS AND SIDE EFFECTS*

CNS: headache, drowsiness, psychic disturbances, dizziness.

EENT: blurred vision, tinnitus, amblyopia.

CV: edema, arrhythmias.

GI: nausea, dyspepsia, vomiting, constipation, GI BLEEDING, discomfort, HEPATITIS.

GU: renal failure, hematuria, cystitis.

Derm: rashes.

Hemat: blood dyscrasias, prolonged bleeding time.

Misc: allergic reactions, including ANAPHYLAXIS.

INTERACTIONS

Drug-Drug: ▪ Concurrent use with **aspirin** may decrease effectiveness ▪ Additive adverse GI side effects with **aspirin,** other **nonsteroidal anti-inflammatory agents, potassium supplements, glucocorticoids,** or **alcohol** ▪ Chronic use with **acetaminophen** may increase the risk of adverse renal reactions ▪ May decrease the effectiveness of **diuretics** or **antihypertensive** therapy ▪ May increase the hypoglycemic effects of **insulin** or **oral hypoglycemic agents** ▪ Increases serum **digoxin** levels (dosage adjustment may be necessary) ▪ May increase serum **lithium** levels and increase the risk of toxicity ▪ Increases the

{} = Available in Canada only.
*Underlines indicate most frequent; **CAPITALS** indicate life-threatening.

I

risk of toxicity from **methotrexate** ▪ **Probenecid** increases risk of toxicity from ibuprofen ▪ Increased risk of bleeding with **cefamandole, cefotetan, cefoperazone, moxalactam** or **plicamycin, thrombolytic agents,** or **anticoagulants** ▪ Increased risk of adverse hematologic reactions with **antineoplastic agents** or **radiation therapy.**

ROUTE AND DOSAGE

Analgesia

- **PO (Adults):** 200–400 mg q 4–6 hr (not to exceed 3200 mg/day).

Antipyretic

- **PO (Children 6 mon–12 yr):** 5 mg/kg for temperature <102.5°F or 10 mg/kg for temperature >102.5°F (not to exceed 40 mg/kg/day).

Inflammatory Disorders

- **PO (Adults):** 300–800 mg 3–4 times daily (not to exceed 3200 mg/day).

PHARMACODYNAMICS

	ONSET	PEAK	DURATION
PO (analgesic)	30 min	1–2 hr	4–6 hr
PO (anti-inflammatory)	7 days	1–2 wk	UK

NURSING IMPLICATIONS

Assessment

- **General Info:** Patients who have asthma, aspirin-induced allergy, and nasal polyps are at increased risk for developing hypersensitivity reactions. Assess for rhinitis, asthma, and urticaria.
- **Arthritis:** Assess pain and range of motion prior to and 1–2 hr following administration.
- **Pain:** Assess pain (note type, location, and intensity) prior to and 1–2 hr following administration.
- **Fever:** Monitor temperature; note signs associated with fever (diaphoresis, tachycardia, malaise).
- **Lab Test Considerations:** BUN, serum creatinine, CBC, and liver function tests should be evaluated periodically in patients receiving prolonged courses of therapy.
  - ▫ Serum potassium, BUN, serum creatinine, SGOT (AST), and SGPT (ALT) tests may show increased levels. Blood glucose, hemoglobin, and hematocrit concentrations and creatinine clearance may be decreased.
  - ▫ May cause prolonged bleeding time, which may persist for 2 days following discontinuation of therapy.

Potential Nursing Diagnoses

- Comfort, altered: pain (indications).
- Mobility, impaired physical (indications).
- Knowledge deficit related to medication regimen (patient/family teaching).

Implementation

- **General Info:** Coadministration with narcotic analgesics may have additive analgesic effects and may permit lower narcotic doses.
- **PO:** For rapid initial effect, administer 30 min before or 2 hr after meals. May be administered with food, milk, or antacids to decrease GI irritation. Food slows but does not reduce the extent of absorption. Tablets may be crushed and mixed with fluids or food. 800 mg tablet can be dissolved in water.
- **Dysmenorrhea:** Administer as soon as possible after the onset of menses. Prophylactic treatment has not been shown to be effective.

Patient/Family Teaching

- ▫ Advise patients to take this medication with a full glass of water and to remain in an upright position for 15–30 min after administration.
- ▫ Instruct patient to take medication exactly as prescribed. If dose is missed, it should be taken as soon as remembered but not if almost time for next dose. Do not double doses.
- ▫ This medication may cause drowsiness or dizziness. Advise patient to avoid driving or other activities requiring alertness until response to medication is known.
- ▫ Caution patient to avoid the concurrent use of alcohol, aspirin, acetaminophen, or other over-the-counter med-

ications without consultation with physician or pharmacist.
- Advise patient to inform physician or dentist of medication regimen prior to treatment or surgery.
- Instruct patients not to take the over-the-counter ibuprofen preparations for more than 10 days for pain or 3 days for fever and to consult physician if symptoms persist or worsen.
- Instruct patient to notify physician if rash, itching, chills, fever, muscle aches, visual disturbances, weight gain, edema, black stools, or persistent headache occurs.

Evaluation

Effectiveness of therapy can be demonstrated by: ▪ Improved joint mobility. Partial arthritic relief is usually seen within 7 days, but maximum effectiveness may require 1–2 wk of continuous therapy ▪ Decrease in severity of moderate pain ▪ Reduction in fever. Patients who do not respond to one nonsteroidal anti-inflammatory agent may respond to another.

IDARUBICIN

(eye-da-**roo**-bi-sin)
Idamycin

CLASSIFICATION(S):
Antineoplastic agent—anthracycline
Pregnancy Category D

INDICATIONS

▪ As part of combination chemotherapy in the treatment of acute myelogenous leukemia in adults.

ACTION

▪ Inhibits nucleic acid synthesis. **Therapeutic Effect:** ▪ Death of rapidly replicating cells, particularly malignant ones.

PHARMACOKINETICS

Absorption: IV administration results in complete bioavailability.
Distribution: Rapidly distributed with extensive tissue binding. High degree of cellular uptake.
Metabolism and Excretion: Extensive enterohepatic metabolism. One metabolite is active (idarubicinol). Primarily eliminated via biliary excretion.
Half-life: 22 hr (range 4–46 hr).

CONTRAINDICATIONS AND PRECAUTIONS

Contraindicated in: ▪ Pregnancy or lactation.
Use Cautiously in: ▪ Children (safety not established) ▪ Patients with child-bearing potential ▪ Active infection ▪ Decreased bone marrow reserve ▪ Other chronic debilitating illnesses ▪ Hepatic impairment (dosage reduction may be required; avoid if bilirubin ≥5 mg/dl) ▪ Renal impairment ▪ Pre-existing cardiac disease ▪ Previous daunorubicin or doxorubicin therapy.

ADVERSE REACTIONS AND SIDE EFFECTS*

CNS: headache, mental status changes.
Resp: pulmonary toxicity, pulmonary allergic reactions.
CV: CARDIOTOXICITY, CONGESTIVE HEART FAILURE, ARRHYTHMIAS.
GI: nausea, vomiting, abdominal cramps, diarrhea, mucositis.
Derm: alopecia, rashes.
Endo: gonadal suppression.
Hemat: anemia, leukopenia, thrombocytopenia, BLEEDING.
Local: phlebitis at IV site.
Metab: hyperuricemia.
Neuro: peripheral neuropathy.
Misc: fever.

INTERACTIONS

Drug-Drug: ▪ Additive myelosuppression with other **antineoplastic agents** or **radiation therapy** ▪ May decrease antibody response to and increase risk of adverse reactions from **live virus vaccines**.

*Underlines indicate most frequent; **CAPITALS** indicate life-threatening.

I

ROUTE AND DOSAGE

- **IV (Adults):** 12 mg/m^2 daily for 3 days in combination with cytarabine.

PHARMACODYNAMICS (effects on blood counts)

	ONSET	PEAK	DURATION
IV	UK	UK	UK

NURSING IMPLICATIONS

Assessment

- ▫ Monitor blood pressure, pulse, respiratory rate, and temperature frequently during administration. Notify physician of significant changes.
- ▫ Assess for fever, chills, sore throat, and signs of infection. Notify physician if these symptoms occur.
- ▫ Monitor platelet count throughout therapy. Assess for bleeding (bleeding gums, bruising, petechiae; guaiac stools, urine, and emesis). Avoid IM injections and rectal temperatures. Apply pressure to venipuncture sites for 10 min.
- ▫ Anemia may occur. Monitor for increased fatigue, dyspnea, and orthostatic hypotension.
- ▫ Monitor intake and output ratios and inform physician if significant discrepancies occur. Encourage fluid intake of 2000–3000 ml/day. Physician may also order allopurinol and alkalinization of the urine to decrease serum uric acid levels and to help prevent urate stone formation.
- ▫ Severe and protracted nausea and vomiting may occur as early as 1 hr after therapy and may last 24 hr. Parenteral antiemetic agents should be administered 30–45 min prior to therapy and routinely around the clock for the next 24 hr as indicated. Monitor amount of emesis and notify physician if emesis exceeds guidelines to prevent dehydration.
- ▫ Monitor for development of signs of myocardial toxicity manifested by life-threatening arrhythmias, cardiomyopathy, and congestive heart failure (peripheral edema, dyspnea, rales/crackles, weight gain).
- ▫ Assess injection site frequently for redness, irritation, or inflammation. Medication may infiltrate painlessly. If extravasation occurs infusion must be stopped and restarted elsewhere to avoid damage to SC tissue. Treatment of extravasation includes intermittent ice packs (apply for 30 min immediately and 30 min qid for 3 days). If pain, erythema, or vesication occur plastic surgery may be warranted.
- **Lab Test Considerations:** Monitor CBC, differential, and renal and hepatic function prior to and frequently throughout therapy. May cause hyperuricemia.

Potential Nursing Diagnosis

- Infection, high risk for (adverse reactions).
- Nutrition; altered: less than body requirements (adverse reactions).
- Knowledge deficit related to medication regimen (patient/family teaching).

Implementation

- **General Info:** Soln should be prepared in a biologic cabinet. Wear gloves, gown, and mask while handling medication. Discard IV equipment in specially designated containers (see Appendix I).
- ▫ See cytarabine monograph for specific information on administration of cytarabine with idarubicin.
- **Direct IV:** Reconstitute 5-mg and 10-mg vials with 5 ml and 10 ml, respectively, of 0.9% NaCl (nonbacteriostatic) for injection for a concentration of 1 mg/ml. Vial contents are under pressure, use care when inserting needle. Do not add to IV soln.
- ▫ Reconstituted medication is stable for 72 hr at room temperature and 7 days if refrigerated. Manufacturer does not recommend admixture.
- ▫ *Rate:* Administer each dose slowly over 10–15 min through Y-site or 3-

way stopcock of a free-flowing infusion of 0.9% NaCl or D5W. Tubing may be attached to a butterfly needle and injected into a large vein.
- **Syringe Incompatibility:** heparin.

Patient/Family Teaching

- Instruct patient to notify physician promptly if fever, sore throat, signs of infection, bleeding gums, bruising, petechiae; or blood in stools, urine, or emesis; increased fatigue, dyspnea, or orthostatic hypotension occur. Caution patient to avoid crowds and persons with known infections. Instruct patient to use soft toothbrush, electric razor, and to avoid falls. Patients should be cautioned not to drink alcoholic beverages or take medication containing aspirin as these may precipitate gastric bleeding.
- Instruct patient to report pain at injection site immediately.
- Instruct patient to inspect oral mucosa for erythema and ulceration. If ulceration occurs advise patient to use sponge brush, rinse mouth with water after eating and drinking, and confer with physician about viscous lidocaine swishes if mouth pain interferes with eating. Further courses of idarubicin should be withheld until recovery from mucositis and subsequent doses should be decreased by 25%.
- Advise patient that this medication may have teratogenic effects. Contraception should be practiced during and for at least 4 mon after therapy is concluded.
- Instruct patient to notify physician immediately if irregular heart beat, shortness of breath or swelling of lower extremities occur.
- Discuss the possibility of hair loss with patient. Explore methods of coping.
- Instruct patient not to receive any vaccinations without advice of physician.
- Emphasize the need for periodic lab tests to monitor for side effects.

Evaluation

Effectiveness of therapy can be demonstrated by: ▪ Improvement of hematologic status in leukemias.

IDOXURIDINE
(eye-dox-**yoor**-i-deen)
Herplex, Stoxil

CLASSIFICATION(S):
Ophthalmic—antiviral
Pregnancy Category UK

INDICATIONS

▪ Treatment of herpes simplex keratitis.

ACTION

▪ Inhibits the incorporation of thymidine into viral DNA, resulting in inhibition of viral DNA synthesis. **Therapeutic Effect:** ▪ Antiviral effect against susceptible viruses.

PHARMACOKINETICS

Absorption: Minimal systemic absorption following ophthalmic instillation.
Distribution: Distribution not known.
Metabolism and Excretion: Rapidly destroyed by enzymes in tissues and fluids.
Half-life: UK.

CONTRAINDICATIONS AND PRECAUTIONS

Contraindicated in: ▪ Hypersensitivity ▪ Hypersensitivity to iodine ▪ Hypersensitivity to thimerisol, benzalkonium chloride, or edetate disodium (soln only) ▪ Lactation ▪ Deep ulceration of stromal layers of cornea.
Use Cautiously in: ▪ Pregnancy (safety not established).

ADVERSE REACTIONS AND SIDE EFFECTS*

EENT: visual haze (ointment), irritation, pain, inflammation, pruritus, conjunctivitis, edema of the eyelid, edema of the cornea, photophobia, punctate defects in corneal epithelium.

*Underlines indicate most frequent; **CAPITALS** indicate life-threatening.

INTERACTIONS

Drug–Drug: ▪ Avoid concurrent use with **boric acid** (increased irritation) ▪ Ophthalmic **glucocorticoids** (increased spread of infection).

ROUTE AND DOSAGE

- **Ophth (Adults and Children):** 1 drop of 0.1% soln q 1 hr during day and q 2 hr at night, or 1 drop q 1 min for 5 min every 4 hr, or instill 0.5% ointment 5 times daily (q 4 hr), with last application at bedtime.

PHARMACODYNAMICS (antiviral effects)

	ONSET	PEAK	DURATION
Ophth	5–8 days	UK	UK

NURSING IMPLICATIONS

Assessment

- Assess eye lesions daily prior to and throughout therapy.

Potential Nursing Diagnoses

- Infection, high risk for (indications).
- Knowledge deficit related to medication regimen (patient/family teaching).

Implementation

- **Ophth Soln:** Instill soln by having patient lie down or tilt head back and look at ceiling. Pull down on lower lid, creating a small pocket, and instill soln in pocket. Gently close eye. Wait 5 min before instilling other ophthalmic medications. Refrigerate soln.
- **Ophth Oint:** Prior to instillation, hold tube in hand for several mins until warm. Squeeze a small amount of ointment (1 cm) inside lower lid. Close eye gently and roll eyeball around in all directions with eye closed. Wait 10 min before instilling other ophthalmic medications.

Patient/Family Teaching

- Instruct patient in the correct technique for instillation of ophthalmic medications. Emphasize the importance of not touching the cap or tip of tube to eye, fingers, or any other surface.
- Instruct patient to instill medication exactly as directed, even if feeling better or if procedure is inconvenient. Herpetic keratitis may recur if idoxuridine is discontinued before microscopic staining with fluorescein has cleared. Missed doses should be instilled as soon as remembered, unless almost time for next dose. Do not use more frequently or for longer than directed.
- Idoxuridine ointment may temporarily cause blurred vision. Caution patient not to drive until vision has cleared.
- Advise patient to wear sunglasses and to avoid prolonged exposure to bright light to prevent photophobic reactions.
- Burning on instillation or failure to respond to treatment may suggest deterioration of soln. Notify physician if this occurs.
- Advise patient to consult physician if there is no improvement after 1 wk of therapy.
- Emphasize the importance of follow-up examinations to determine progress.

Evaluation

Effectiveness of therapy can be demonstrated by: ▪ Resolution of eye lesions in herpetic keratitis.

IFOSFAMIDE

(eye-foss-fam-ide)
Ifex

CLASSIFICATION(S):
Antineoplastic agent—alkylating agent
Pregnancy Category D

INDICATIONS

▪ In combination with other agents in the treatment of germ cell testicular carcinoma ▪ Used in combination with mesna, which prevents ifosfamide-induced hemorrhagic cystitis.

ACTION

▪ Following conversion to active compounds, interferes with DNA replication and RNA transcription, ultimately disrupting protein synthesis (cell cycle-phase nonspecific). **Therapeutic Effect:** ▪ Death of rapidly replicating cells, particularly malignant ones.

PHARMACOKINETICS

Absorption: Administered IV only, inactive prior to conversion to metabolites.
Distribution: Excreted in breast milk.
Metabolism and Excretion: Metabolized by the liver to active antineoplastic compounds.
Half-life: 15 hr.

CONTRAINDICATIONS AND PRECAUTIONS

Contraindicated in: ▪ Hypersensitivity ▪ Pregnancy, lactation, or children.
Use Cautiously in: ▪ Patients with childbearing potential ▪ Active infections ▪ Decreased bone marrow reserve ▪ Other chronic debilitating illness ▪ Impaired renal function.

ADVERSE REACTIONS AND SIDE EFFECTS*

CNS: CNS toxicity (somnolence, confusion, hallucinations, coma), dizziness, disorientation, cranial nerve dysfunction.
CV: cardiotoxicity.
GI: nausea, vomiting, anorexia, diarrhea, constipation, liver dysfunction.
GU: hemorrhagic cystitis, renal toxicity, dysuria, gonadal suppression.
Derm: alopecia.
Hemat: leukopenia, thrombocytopenia, anemia.
Local: phlebitis.
Misc: allergic reactions.

INTERACTIONS

Drug-Drug: ▪ Additive myelosuppression with other **antineoplastic agents** or **radiation therapy** ▪ May decrease antibody response to and increase risk of adverse reactions from **live virus vaccines.**

ROUTE AND DOSAGE

▪ **IV (Adults):** 1.2 g/m^2/day for 5 days, coadminister with mesna. May repeat cycle q 3 wk.

PHARMACODYNAMICS (effects on blood counts)

	ONSET	PEAK	DURATION
IV	UK	UK	UK

NURSING IMPLICATIONS

Assessment

▪ **General Info:** Monitor blood pressure, pulse, respiratory rate, and temperature frequently during administration. Notify physician of significant changes.
□ Monitor urinary output frequently throughout therapy. Notify physician if hematuria occurs. To reduce the risk of hemorrhagic cystitis, fluid intake should be at least 3000 ml/day for adults and 1000–2000 ml/day for children. Mesna is given concurrently to prevent hemorrhagic cystitis.
□ Monitor neurologic status. Inform physician if lethargy, confusion, or hallucinations occur.
□ Assess nausea, vomiting, and appetite. Weigh weekly. Confer with physician about premedication with an antiemetic to minimize GI effects. Adjust diet as tolerated.
□ Assess for fever, chills, sore throat, and signs of infection. Notify physician if these symptoms occur.
□ Monitor platelet count throughout therapy. Assess for bleeding (bleeding gums, bruising, petechiae; guaiac stools, urine, and emesis). Avoid IM injections and rectal temperatures. Apply pressure to venipuncture sites for 10 min.
▪ **Lab Test Considerations:** Monitor CBC and differential prior to and periodically throughout course of therapy. Withhold dose and notify physi-

*Underlines indicate most frequent; **CAPITALS** indicate life-threatening.

cian if WBC $<2,000/\text{mm}^3$ or platelets $<50,000/\text{mm}^3$.

- ▫ Urinalysis should be evaluated before each dose. Withhold dose and notify physician if urinalysis shows >10 RBCs per high power field.
- ▫ May cause elevation in liver enzymes and serum bilirubin.

Potential Nursing Diagnoses

- ▪ Infection, high risk for (side effects).
- ▪ Body image disturbance (side effects).
- ▪ Knowledge deficit related to medication regimen (patient/family teaching).

Implementation

- ▪ **General Info:** Soln for IV administration should be prepared in a biologic cabinet. Wear gloves, gown, and mask while handling IV medication. Discard IV equipment in specially designated containers (see Appendix I).
- ▪ **IV:** Prepare soln by diluting each 1-g vial with 20 ml of sterile water or bacteriostatic water for injection containing parabens. Use soln prepared without bacteriostatic water within 6 hr. Soln prepared with bacteriostatic water is stable for 1 wk at 30°C or 6 wk at 5°C.
- ▪ **Intermittent Infusion:** May be further diluted to a concentration of 0.6 to 20 mg/ml in D5W, 0.9% NaCl, lactated Ringer's soln, or sterile water for injection
- ▫ *Rate:* Administer over 30 min.
- ▪ **Syringe Compatibility:** mesna.
- ▪ **Y-Site Compatibility:** ondansetron.
- ▪ **Additive Compatibility:** mesna.

Patient/Family Teaching

- ▫ Emphasize need for adequate fluid intake throughout course of therapy. Patient should void frequently to decrease bladder irritation from metabolites excreted by the kidneys. Physician should be notified immediately if hematuria is noted.
- ▫ Instruct patient to notify physician promptly if fever, sore throat, signs of infection, bleeding gums, bruising, petechiae, or blood in urine, stool, or emesis, or confusion occurs.
- ▫ Caution patient to avoid crowds and persons with known infections. Instruct patient to use soft toothbrush, electric razor, and to avoid falls. Patients should also be cautioned not to drink alcoholic beverages or to take aspirin-containing products, as these may precipitate GI hemorrhage.
- ▫ Review with patient the need for contraception during therapy.
- ▫ Discuss with patient the possibility of hair loss. Explore methods of coping.
- ▫ Instruct patient not to receive any vaccinations without advice of physician.

Evaluation

Effectiveness of therapy can be demonstrated by: ▪ Decrease in size or spread of malignant germ cell testicular carcinoma.

IMIPENEM/CILASTATIN

(i-me-**pen**-em/sye-la-**stat**-in)
Primaxin

CLASSIFICATION(S):
Anti-infective—miscellaneous penicillin
Pregnancy Category C

INDICATIONS

▪ Treatment of the following serious infections due to susceptible organisms: ▫ Lower respiratory tract infections ▫ Urinary tract infections ▫ Abdominal infections ▫ Gynecologic infections ▫ Skin and skin structure infections ▫ Bone and joint infections ▫ Bacteremia ▫ Endocarditis ▫ Polymicrobic infections.

ACTION

▪ Binds to bacterial cell wall, resulting in cell death ▪ Combination with cilastatin prevents renal inactivation of imipenem, resulting in high urinary concentrations ▪ Resists the actions of many enzymes that degrade most other penicillins and pencillinlike anti-infectives. **Therapeutic Effect:** ▪ Bactericidal action against susceptible bacteria. **Spectrum:** ▪ Spectrum is broad ▪ Active against most gram-positive aerobic cocci: ▫ *Streptococcus pneumoniae* ▫ Group A beta-hemolytic streptococci ▫ Enterococcus ▫ Staphylococus aureus ▪ Active against many gram-negative bacillary organisms: ▫ *Escherichia coli* ▫ *Klebsiella* ▫ *Acinetobacter* ▫ *Proteus* ▫ *Serratia* ▫ *Pseudomonas aeruginosa* ▪ Also displays activity against: ▫ *Salmonella* ▫ *Shigella* ▫ *Neisseria gonorrhoeae* ▫ Numerous anaerobes.

PHARMACOKINETICS

Absorption: Administered IV only, resulting in complete bioavailability.
Distribution: Widely distributed. Crosses the placenta. Enters breast milk.
Metabolism and Excretion: 70% excreted unchanged by the kidneys.
Half-life: 1 hr (prolonged in renal impairment).

CONTRAINDICATIONS AND PRECAUTIONS

Contraindicated in: ▪ Hypersensitivity ▪ Cross-sensitivity may exist with penicillins and cephalosporins.
Use Cautiously in: ▪ Previous history of multiple hypersensitivity reactions ▪ Seizure disorders ▪ Renal impairment (dosage reduction required) ▪ Pregnancy, lactation, or children (safety not established).

ADVERSE REACTIONS AND SIDE EFFECTS*

CNS: SEIZURES, dizziness, somnolence.
CV: hypotension.
GI: <u>nausea</u>, <u>diarrhea</u>, <u>vomiting</u>.
Derm: <u>rash</u>, pruritus, urticaria, sweating.
Hemat: eosinophilia.
Local: <u>phlebitis at IV site</u>.
Misc: allergic reaction, including ANAPHYLAXIS, fever, superinfection.

INTERACTIONS

Drug-Drug: ▪ May antagonize the action of **penicillins** and **cephalosporins** ▪ Do not admix with **aminoglycosides** (inactivation may occur) ▪ **Probenecid** decreases renal excretion and increases blood levels ▪ Increased risk of seizures with **ganciclovir** (avoid concurrent use).

ROUTE AND DOSAGE

- **IV (Adults):** 250–500 mg q 6 hr.
- **IM (Adults):** 500–750 mg q 12 hr.

PHARMACODYNAMICS (blood levels)

	ONSET	PEAK
IV	rapid	end of infusion

NURSING IMPLICATIONS

Assessment

▫ Assess patient for infection (vital signs; appearance of wound, sputum, urine, and stool; WBC) at beginning and throughout course of therapy.
▫ Obtain a history before initiating therapy to determine previous use of and reactions to penicillins. Persons with a negative history of penicillin sensitivity may still have an allergic response.
▫ Obtain specimens for culture and sensitivity prior to initiating therapy. First dose may be given before receiving results.
▫ Observe patient for signs and symptoms of anaphylaxis (rash, pruritus, laryngeal edema, wheezing). Discontinue the drug and notify the physician immediately if these occur. Have epinephrine, an antihistamine, and resuscitative equipment close by in the event of an anaphylactic reaction.
▪ **Lab Test Considerations:** BUN, SGOT (AST), SGPT (ALT), LDH, serum alkaline phosphatase, bilirubin, and creatinine may be transiently increased.
▫ Hemoglobin and hematocrit concentrations may be decreased.

*<u>Underlines</u> indicate most frequent; **CAPITALS** indicate life-threatening.

□ May cause positive direct Coombs' test.

Potential Nursing Diagnoses

- Infection, high risk for (indications, side effects).
- Knowledge deficit related to medication regimen (patient/family teaching).

Implementation

- **IM:** Reconstitute 500-mg vial with 2 ml and 750-mg vial with 3 ml of lidocaine without epinephrine. Shake well to form a suspension. Withdraw and inject entire contents of the vial IM.
- **IV:** Reconstitute each 250- or 500-mg vial with 10 ml of compatible diluent and shake well. Transfer the resulting suspension to not less than 100 ml of compatible diluent. Add an additional 10 ml to each previously reconstituted vial and shake well to ensure all medication is used. Transfer the remaining contents of the vial to the infusion container. Do not administer suspension by direct injection.

□ Reconstitute 120 ml infusion bottles with 100 ml of a compatible diluent. Shake well until clear.

□ *Compatible diluents* include 0.9% NaCl, D5W, D10W, D5/0.2% sodium bicarbonate, D5/0.9% NaCl, D5/0.45% NaCl, D5/0.225% NaCl, or mannitol 2.5%, 5%, or 10%. Soln may range from clear to yellow in color. Do not administer cloudy soln. Soln is stable for 4 hr at room temperature and 24 hr if refrigerated.

- **Intermittent Infusion:** Administer each 250- or 500-mg dose over 20–30 min and each 1-g dose over 40–60 min. Administer over 15–20 min for pediatric patients. Do not administer direct IV. Do not admix with other antibiotics.

□ Rapid infusion may cause nausea, vomiting, hypotension, dizziness, or sweating. If these symptoms develop, slow infusion. Discontinuation of medication may be necessary.

- **Y-Site Compatibility:** acyclovir, famotidine, foscarnet, ondansetron, or zidovudine.

Patient/Family Teaching

□ Advise patient to report the signs of superinfection (black, furry overgrowth on the tongue, vaginal itching or discharge, loose or foul-smelling stools) and allergy.

Evaluation

Clinical response can be evaluated by:
- Resolution of the signs and symptoms of infection. Length of time for complete resolution depends on the organism and site of infection.

IMIPRAMINE

(im-**ip**-ra-meen)
{Apo-Imipramine}, {Impril}, Janimine, {Nono-Pramine}, SK-Pramine, Tipramine, Tofranil, Tofranil PM

CLASSIFICATION(S):
Antidepressant—tricyclic
Pregnancy Category C

INDICATIONS

- Treatment of various forms of depression, often in conjunction with psychotherapy ■ Management of enuresis in children. **Unlabeled Uses:** ■ Adjunct in the management of chronic pain, migraine prophylaxis, and cluster headache.

ACTION

- Potentiates the effect of serotonin and norepinephrine ■ Has significant anticholinergic properties. **Therapeutic Effect:** ■ Antidepressant action that develops slowly over several wks.

PHARMACOKINETICS

Absorption: Well absorbed from the GI tract.
Distribution: Widely distributed. Appears to cross the placenta and enter breast milk.
Metabolism and Excretion: Extensi-

viely metabolized by the liver, much of it on its first pass through the liver. Some is converted to active compounds. Undergoes enterohepatic recirculation and secretion into gastric juices.
Half-life: 8–16 hr.

CONTRAINDICATIONS AND PRECAUTIONS

Contraindicated in: ▪ Hypersensitivity ▪ Cross-sensitivity with other antidepressants may exist ▪ Narrow-angle glaucoma ▪ Pregnancy and lactation ▪ Hypersensitivity to tartrazine, parabens, sulfites, propylene glycol, or povidone (in some preparations).
Use Cautiously in: ▪ Elderly patients (more susceptible to adverse reaction) ▪ Pre-existing cardiovascular disease ▪ Elderly men with prostatic hypertrophy (more susceptible to urinary retention) ▪ Seizures or history of seizure disorder.

ADVERSE REACTIONS AND SIDE EFFECTS*

CNS: drowsiness, sedation, lethargy, fatigue, confusion, agitation, hallucinations, insomnia.
CV: hypotension, ECG changes, ARRHYTHMIAS.
Derm: photosensitivity.
EENT: dry mouth, dry eyes, blurred vision.
Endo: gynecomastia.
GI: constipation, paralytic ileus, nausea.
GU: urinary retention.
Hemat: blood dyscrasias.

INTERACTIONS

Drug-Drug: ▪ May cause hypotension and tachycardia when used with **MAO inhibitors** (avoid concurrent use—discontinue 2 wk prior to impramine) ▪ May prevent therapeutic response to most **antihypertensives** ▪ May cause severe hypertension when used with **clonidine** (avoid concurrent use) ▪ Additive CNS depression with other **CNS depressants,** including **alcohol, antihistamines, narcotics,** and **sedative/hypnotics** ▪ **Adrenergic** and **anticholinergic** side effects may be additive with other agents having these properties ▪ **Cimetidine, fluoxetine, phenothiazines,** or **oral contraceptives** increase levels and may cause toxicity ▪ May produce organic brain syndrome with **disulfiram** ▪ **Smoking** may increase metabolism and decrease effectiveness.

ROUTE AND DOSAGE

Antidepressant

- **PO, IM (Adults):** 25–50 mg 3–4 times daily (not to exceed 300 mg/day); total daily dose may be given at bedtime.

Enuresis

- **PO (Children >6 yr):** 25 mg once daily 1 hr before bedtime; increase if necessary by 25 mg at weekly intervals to 50 mg in children <12 yr, up to 75 mg in children >12 yr.

PHARMACODYNAMICS (antidepressant effect)

	ONSET	PEAK	DURATION
PO	hr	2–6 wk	wk
IM	hr	2–6 wk	wk

NURSING IMPLICATIONS

Assessment

- **General Info:** Monitor blood pressure and pulse rate prior to and during initial therapy.
- Monitor baseline and periodic ECGs in elderly or patients with heart disease and before increasing dosage with children treated for enuresis. May cause prolonged PR and QT intervals and may flatten T waves.
- **Depression:** Assess mental status frequently. Confusion, agitation, and hallucinations may occur during initiation of therapy and may require dosage reduction. Monitor mood changes. Assess for suicidal tendencies, especially during early therapy. Restrict amount of drug available to patient.
- **Pain:** Assess location, duration, and

*Underlines indicate most frequent; CAPITALS indicate life-threatening.

severity of pain periodically throughout therapy.

- **Lab Test Considerations:** Assess leukocyte and differential blood counts and renal and hepatic functions prior to and periodically during prolonged or high-dose therapy.
- □ Serum levels may be monitored in patients who fail to respond to usual therapeutic dose. Therapeutic plasma concentration range is 200–350 ng/ml.
- □ May cause alterations in blood glucose levels.
- **Toxicity and Overdose:** Symptoms of acute overdose include disturbed concentration, confusion, restlessness, agitation, convulsions, drowsiness, mydriasis, arrhythmias, fever, hallucinations, vomiting, and dyspnea.
- □ Treatment of overdose includes gastric lavage, activated charcoal, and a stimulant cathartic. Maintain respiratory and cardiac function (monitor ECG for at least 5 days) and temperature. Medications may include digoxin for congestive heart failure, antiarrhythmics, anticonvulsants, and physostigmine to help reverse anticholinergic effects.

Potential Nursing Diagnoses

- Coping, ineffective individual (indications).
- Anxiety (indications).
- Knowledge deficit related to medication regimen (patient/family teaching).

Implementation

- **General Info:** May be given as a single dose at bedtime to minimize sedation during the day.
- **PO:** Administer medication with or immediately following a meal to minimize gastric irritation.
- **IM:** May be slightly yellow or red in color. Crystals may develop if soln is cool; place ampule under warm running water for 1 min to dissolve.

Patient/Family Teaching

- **General Info:** Instruct patient to take medication exactly as directed. Do not skip or double up on missed doses. Inform patient that at least 2 wk are needed before drug effects may be noticed. Abrupt discontinuation may cause nausea, headache, and malaise.
- □ May cause drowsiness and blurred vision. Caution patient to avoid driving and other activities requiring alertness until response to drug is known.
- □ Instruct patient to notify physician if visual changes occur. Inform patient that physician may order periodic glaucoma testing during long-term therapy.
- □ Caution patient to make position changes slowly to minimize orthostatic hypotension.
- □ Advise patient to avoid alcohol or other CNS depressant drugs during therapy and for at least 3–7 days after therapy has been discontinued.
- □ Instruct patient to notify physician if urinary retention or uncontrolled movements occur or if dry mouth or constipation persists. Sugarless candy or gum may diminish dry mouth, and an increase in fluid intake or bulk may prevent constipation.
- □ Caution patient to use sunscreen and protective clothing to prevent photosensitivity reactions.
- □ Inform patient of need to monitor dietary intake, as possible increase in appetite may lead to undesired weight gain.
- □ Advise patient to notify physician or dentist of medication regimen prior to treatment or surgery.
- □ Therapy for depression is usually prolonged. Emphasize the importance of follow-up examinations to evaluate progress.
- **Children:** Inform parents that the side effects most likely to occur include nervousness, insomnia, unusual tiredness, and mild nausea and vomiting. Notify physician if these symptoms become pronounced.
- □ Advise parents to keep medication out of reach of children to prevent inadvertent overdose.

Evaluation

Effectiveness of therapy can be demonstrated by: ▪ Increased sense of well-being ▫ Renewed interest in surroundings ▫ Increased appetite ▫ Improved energy level ▫ Improved sleep ▪ Control of bedwetting in children >6 yr ▪ Prevention and management of chronic neurogenic pain. Patients may require 2–6 wk of therapy before full therapeutic effects of medication are noticeable.

IMMUNE GLOBULIN
(im-**myoon glo**-byoo-lin)
gamma globulin, IG, ISG, immune serum globulin

IMMUNE GLOBULIN IM
IGIM, Gamastan, Gammar

IMMUNE GLOBULIN IV
Gamimune N, Gammagard, Sandoglobulin, Venoglobulin-I

CLASSIFICATION(S):
Serum—immune globulin
Pregnancy Category UK

INDICATIONS

▪ **IM:** Provides passive immunity to a variety of infections including: ▫ Hepatitis A ▫ Hepatitis B ▫ Measles (rubeola) when immune sera are unavailable or there is insufficient time for active immunization to take place ▪ **IV:** Useful in patients with immunodeficiency syndromes who are unable to produce IgG-type antibodies ▪ **IV:** Treatment of idiopathic thrombocytopenic purpura.

ACTION

▪ A human serum fraction containing gamma globulin antibodies (IgG). **Therapeutic Effect:** ▪ Provision of passive immunity against many infections.

PHARMACOKINETICS

Absorption: Well absorbed following IM administration.

Distribution: Rapidly and evenly distributed.

Metabolism and Excretion: Removed by redistribution, tissue binding, and catabolism.

Half-life: 21–24 days.

CONTRAINDICATIONS AND PRECAUTIONS

Contraindicated in: ▪ Hypersensitivity to immune globulins or additives (maltose, thimerisol, glycine, polyethylene glycol, albumin) ▪ Selective IgA deficiency.

Use Cautiously in: ▪ IM form should be used cautiously in patients with thrombocytopenia ▪ Gamimune N product should be used cautiously in patients with acid-base disorders ▪ Agammaglobulinemia or hypogammaglobulinemia (increased risk of hypotension and anaphylaxis following rapid IV administration) ▪ Has been used during pregnancy, though safety is not established.

ADVERSE REACTIONS AND SIDE EFFECTS*

CNS: faintness, lightheadedness, headache, malaise.

Resp: dyspnea, wheezing.

CV: chest pain.

GI: nausea.

GU: diuresis (if maltose in preparation), nephrotic syndrome.

Derm: urticaria, cyanosis.

Local: <u>pain</u>, <u>tenderness</u>, <u>muscle stiffness at IM site</u>, local inflammation, urticaria at site, phlebitis.

MS: hip pain, back pain. arthralgia.

Misc: allergic reactions, including **ANAPHYLAXIS**, angioedema, fever, chills, sweating.

INTERACTIONS

Drug-Drug: ▪ May interfere with the normal immune response to some **live vaccines,** including **measles, mumps,** and **rubella virus vaccine** (do not administer within 3 mon of immune globulin).

*<u>Underlines</u> indicate most frequent; **CAPITALS** indicate life-threatening.

ROUTE AND DOSAGE

Pre-Exposure and Postexposure Hepatitis A Prophylaxis

- **IM (Adults and Children):** 0.02 ml/kg (for pre-exposure prophylaxis, higher doses—0.05–0.06 ml/kg q 4–6 mon are used if exposure will last >3 mon).

Postexposure Hepatitis B Prophylaxis (HBIG Unavailable)

- **IM (Adults and Children):** 0.06 ml/kg.

Postexposure Measles Prophylaxis

- **IM (Adults and Children):** 0.25 ml/kg (0.5 ml/kg if immunosuppressed).

Immunodeficiency Syndrome

- **IM (Adults and Children):** 1.2 ml/kg initially, then 0.6 ml/kg q 2–4 wk (single dose should not exceed 30–50 ml in adults or 20–30 ml in infants and small children).
- **IV (Adults and Children):** Gamimune N—100–200 mg/kg (2–4 ml/kg) monthly, may be increased to 400 mg/kg (8 ml/kg) or given more frequently.
- **IV (Adults and Children):** Gammagard—200–400 mg/kg monthly.
- **IV (Adults and Children):** Sandoglobulin—200 mg/kg monthly, may be increased to 300 mg/kg monthly or given more frequently.
- **IV (Adults and Children):** Venoglobulin-I—200 mg/kg/mon, may be increased to 300–400 mg/kg/mon or given more frequently if antibody response is inadequate.

Idiopopathic Thrombocytopenic Purpura

- **IV (Adults and Children):** Gamimune N or Sandoglobulin—400 mg/kg daily for 5 days.
- **IV (Adults and Children):** Gammagard—1 g/kg single dose; up to 3 doses may be given on alternate days.

PHARMACODYNAMICS (antibody levels)

	ONSET	PEAK	DURATION
IM	UK	2 days	UK
IV	immediate	UK	UK

NURSING IMPLICATIONS

Assessment

- For passive immunity, determine the date of exposure to infection. Immune globulin should be administered within 2 wk of exposure to hepatitis A, within 6 days after exposure to measles, and within 7 days after exposure to hepatitis B.
- Monitor vital signs continuously during infusion of immune globulin IV and assess patient for signs of anaphylaxis (hypotension, flushing, chest tightness, wheezing, fever, dizziness, nausea, vomiting, diaphoresis) for 1 hr following initiation of infusion. Epinephrine and antihistamines should be available for treatment of anaphylactic reactions.
- Patients receiving repeated injections of immune globulin IM should be monitored for sensitization (fever, chills, sweating).
- Monitor platelet counts in patients being treated for idiopathic thrombocytopenic purpura.

Potential Nursing Diagnoses

- Infection, high risk for (indications).
- Knowledge deficit related to medication regimen (patient/family teaching).

Implementation

- **IM:** Administer immune globulin IM (IGIM) in adults and children into the deltoid muscle or anterolateral thigh. Volumes greater than 10 ml should be divided into several injections to minimize local pain. Avoid IM administration of doses exceeding 20 ml. Use of the gluteal site should be reserved only for volumes >3 ml or when large volumes are divided into multiple injections to prevent damage to the sciatic nerve. Do not administer SC, intradermally, or IV. Soln of IGIM should be transparent or opalescent and may be colorless or brownish in color.
- **Intermittent Infusion:** Immune globulin IV (IGIV) should be administered by IV infusion using separate tubing.

Do not mix with other drugs or solns. If adverse reactions occur during infusion, decrease the rate of infusion or stop the infusion until the adverse reactions subside. The infusion may then be resumed at a rate of tolerance for the individual. Do not use turbid soln. Do not administer IGIV SC or IM.

- *Gamimune N* should be diluted with D5W and infused at a rate of 0.01–0.02 ml/kg/min for 30 min. If no adverse reactions occur, the infusion rate may be gradually increased to a maximum of 0.08 ml/kg/hr. Solns of Gamimune N should be refrigerated but not frozen. Discard soln that has been frozen.
- *Gammagard* should be reconstituted with sterile water for injection for a soln containing 50 mg protein per ml. Warm the powder and sterile water for injection to room temperature prior to reconstitution and use the transfer device provided by the manufacturer for preparation. Administer soln as soon as possible within 2 hr of reconstitution. Infuse via the administration set containing an integral airway and 15 micron filter provided by the manufacturer. Infuse at a rate of 0.5 ml/kg/hr initially. If no adverse reactions occur, the rate of infusion may be increased gradually to a maximum of 4 ml/kg/hr.
- *Sandoglobulin* should be reconstituted with the 0.9% NaCl provided by the manufacturer for a soln containing 30 or 60 mg of protein per ml. For patients with agammaglobulinemia or hypogammaglobulinemia, use a soln containing 30 mg/ml for the initial dose. Infuse at an initial rate of 0.5–1 ml/min. After 15–30 min, the rate may be increased to 1.5–2.5 ml/min, and subsequent infusions may be given at a rate of 2–2.5 ml/min. When infusing the soln containing 60 mg/ml, the initial rate should be 1–1.5 ml/min and increased to a maximum of 2.5 ml/min after 15–30 minutes. Solns of Sandoglobulin should be stored at room temperature.

PATIENT/FAMILY TEACHING

- Explain the use and purpose of immune globulin therapy to the patient.
- Advise patient to report symptoms of anaphylaxis immediately.
- Inform patients that pain, tenderness, and muscle stiffness at the injection site may occur following IM injections of immune globulin. These may persist for several hrs following administration.

EVALUATION

Effectiveness of therapy can be demonstrated by: ▪ Prevention of certain infectious diseases by provision of passive immunity in patients exposed to the infections or patients with immunodeficiency diseases ▪ Increased platelet counts in patients with idiopathic thrombocytopenic purpura.

INDAPAMIDE

(in-**dap**-a-mide)
{Lozide}, Lozol

CLASSIFICATION(S):
Diuretic—sulfonamide, Antihypertensive—diuretic
Pregnancy Category B

INDICATIONS

▪ Used alone or in combination with other agents in the management of mild to moderate hypertension. **Unlabeled Use:** ▪ Used alone or in combination with other agents in the treatment of edema associated with congestive heart failure and other causes.

ACTION

▪ Increases excretion of sodium and water by inhibiting sodium reabsorption in the distal tubule ▪ Promotes excretion of chloride, potassium, magnesium, and bicarbonate ▪ May produce arteriolar dilation. **Therapeutic Effects:**

■ Lowering of blood pressure in hypertensive patients and diuresis with subsequent mobilization of edema.

PHARMACOKINETICS

Absorption: Well absorbed from the GI tract following oral administration.
Distribution: Widely distributed.
Metabolism and Excretion: Mostly metabolized by the liver. Small amounts (7%) excreted unchanged by the kidneys.
Half-life: 14–18 hr.

CONTRAINDICATIONS AND PRECAUTIONS

Contraindicated in: ■ Hypersensitivity ■ Cross-sensitivity with sulfonamides may exist ■ Anuria ■ Lactation.
Use Cautiously in: ■ Renal or severe hepatic impairment ■ Pregnancy or children (safety not established).

ADVERSE REACTIONS AND SIDE EFFECTS*

CNS: drowsiness, lethargy, dizziness.
CV: hypotension, arrhythmias.
GI: anorexia, nausea, vomiting, cramping.
Derm: rashes, photosensitivity.
Endo: hyperglycemia.
F and E: hypokalemia, hypochloremic alkalosis, hyponatremia, dehydration, hypovolemia.
Metab: hyperuricemia.
MS: muscle cramps.

INTERACTIONS

Drug-Drug: ■ Additive hypotension with other **antihypertensives, nitrates,** or acute ingestion of **alcohol** ■ Additive hypokalemia with **glucocorticoids, amphotericin B, mezlocillin, piperacillin,** or **ticarcillin** ■ Decreases the excretion of **lithium**; may cause toxicity ■ Hypokalemia may increase risk of **cardiac glycoside toxicity**.

ROUTE AND DOSAGE

- **PO (Adults):** 2.5–5 mg single daily dose.

PHARMACODYNAMICS (antihypertensive effect)

	ONSET	PEAK	DURATION
PO (single dose)	UK	24 hr	UK
PO (multiple dose)	1–2 wk	8–12 wk	up to 8 wk

NURSING IMPLICATIONS

Assessment

- Monitor blood pressure, intake and output, and daily weight and assess feet, legs, and sacral area for edema daily.
- Assess patient, especially if taking cardiac glycosides, for anorexia, nausea, vomiting, muscle cramps, paresthesia, and confusion. Notify physician if these signs of electrolyte imbalance occur. Patients taking cardiac glycosides have an increased risk of digitalis toxicity due to the potassium-depleting effect of the diuretic.
- Assess patient for allergy to sulfonamides.
- **Lab Test Considerations:** Monitor electrolytes (especially potassium), blood glucose, BUN, and serum creatinine and uric acid levels prior to and periodically throughout course of therapy. May cause decreased potassium, sodium, and chloride concentrations. May increase serum glucose; diabetic patients may require increased oral hypoglycemic or insulin dosage. Increases uric acid level an average of 1.0 mg/100 ml; may precipitate an episode of gout.

Potential Nursing Diagnoses

- Fluid volume excess (indications).
- Fluid volume deficit (side effects).
- Knowledge deficit related to medication regimen (patient/family teaching).

Implementation

- **General Info:** Administer in the morning to prevent disruption of sleep cycle.

*Underlines indicate most frequent; **CAPITALS** indicate life-threatening.

- Intermittent dose given on alternate days for 3–4 days with rest periods of 1–2 days may be used for continued control of edema.
- **PO:** May be given with food or milk to minimize GI irritation.

Patient/Family Teaching

- **General Info:** Instruct patient to take this medication at the same time each day. If a dose is missed, take as soon as remembered, but not just before next dose is due. Do not double doses. Advise patients using indapamide for hypertension to continue taking the medication even if feeling better.
  - Caution patient to make position changes slowly to minimize orthostatic hypotension. This may be potentiated by alcohol.
  - Advise patient to use sunscreen (avoid those containing PABA) and protective clothing when in the sun to prevent photosensitivity reactions.
  - Instruct patient to follow a diet high in potassium (see Appendix K).
  - Advise patient to report muscle weakness, cramps, nausea, or dizziness to physician.
  - Advise patient to consult physician or pharmacist before taking over-the-counter medication concurrently with this therapy.
  - Emphasize the importance of routine follow-up examinations.
- **Hypertension:** Instruct patient and family on proper technique of blood pressure monitoring. Advise them to check blood pressure at least weekly and to report significant changes to physician.
  - Encourage patient to comply with additional interventions for hypertension (weight reduction, low-sodium diet, regular exercise, discontinuation of smoking, moderation of alcohol consumption, and stress management). Indapamide helps control but does not cure hypertension.

Evaluation

Effectiveness of therapy can be demonstrated by: ▪ Control of hypertension ▪ Decrease in edema secondary to congestive heart failure.

INDOMETHACIN

(in-doe-meth-a-sin)
{Apo-Indomethacin}, Indameth, {Indocid}, Indocin, Indocin I.V., {Indocin PDA}, Indocin SR, {Novomethacin}

CLASSIFICATION(S):
Nonsteroidal anti-inflammatory agent
Pregnancy Category UK

INDICATIONS

▪ **PO, Rect:** Management of inflammatory disorders including: ▫ Rheumatoid arthritis ▫ Gouty arthritis ▫ Osteoarthritis ▪ **IV:** Alternative to surgery in the management of patent ductus arteriosus in premature neonates.

ACTION

▪ Inhibits prostaglandin synthesis. **Therapeutic Effects:** ▪ Suppression of pain and inflammation. Therapeutic effect of IV form is closure of patent ductus arteriosus.

PHARMACOKINETICS

Absorption: Well absorbed from the GI tract.
Distribution: Crosses the blood-brain barrier and the placenta. Enters breast milk.
Metabolism and Excretion: Mostly metabolized by the liver.
Half-life: 2.6–11 hr (prolonged in neonates—up to 60 hr, average range 12–21 hr).

CONTRAINDICATIONS AND PRECAUTIONS

Contraindicated in: ▪ Hypersensitivity ▪ Hypersensitivity to ingredients (suspensions may contain alcohol, parabens, or propylene glycol) ▪ Cross-sensitivity may exist with other nonsteroidal anti-inflammatory agents, including aspirin ▪ Active GI bleeding ▪ Ulcer disease ▪ Proctitis or a recent history of rectal bleeding.

Use Cautiously in: ▪ Severe cardiovascular, renal, or hepatic disease ▪ History of ulcer disease ▪ Pregnancy or lactation (safety not established) ▪ Children <14 yr.

ADVERSE REACTIONS AND SIDE EFFECTS*

CNS: headache, drowsiness, psychic disturbances, dizziness.

CV: edema, arrhythmias.

Derm: rashes.

EENT: blurred vision, tinnitus.

F and E: hyperkalemia.

GI: PO—nausea, dyspepsia, vomiting, constipation, GI BLEEDING, discomfort, HEPATITIS; Rect—rectal irritation, tenesmus.

GU: renal failure, hematuria, cystitis.

Hemat: blood dyscrasias, prolonged bleeding time.

Local: phlebitis at IV site (IV only).

Misc: allergic reactions, including ANAPHYLAXIS.

INTERACTIONS

Drug-Drug: ▪ Concurrent use with **aspirin** may decrease effectiveness ▪ Additive adverse GI effects with **aspirin,** other **nonsteroidal anti-inflammatory agents, potassium supplements, glucocorticoids,** or **alcohol** ▪ Chronic use with **acetaminophen** may increase the risk of adverse renal reactions ▪ May decrease the effectiveness of **diuretics** or **antihypertensive** therapy ▪ May increase hypoglycemia from **insulin** or **oral hypoglycemia agents** ▪ May increase serum levels and risk of toxicity from **lithium, zidovudine, digoxin,** or **aminoglycosides** (dosage adjustment may be necessary) ▪ Increases the risk of toxicity from **methotrexate** ▪ **Probenecid** increases risk of toxicity from indomethacin ▪ Increased risk of bleeding with **cefamandole, cefotetan, cefoperazone, moxalactam** or **plicamycin, thrombolytic agents,** or **anticoagulants** ▪ Increased risk of adverse hematologic reactions with **antineoplastic agents** or **radiation therapy**.

ROUTE AND DOSAGE

Anti-Inflammatory/Analgesic

- **PO, Rect (Adults):** 25–50 mg 2–3 times daily or 75 mg extended-release capsule once or twice daily (not to exceed 200 mg or 150 mg of SR/day).
- **PO (Children 2–14 yr):** 2–4 mg/kg/day in 2–4 divided doses (not to exceed 150–200 mg/day); unlabeled use.

Closure of Patent Ductus Arteriosus

- **IV (Neonates):** 0.2 mg/kg initially, then 2 subsequent doses at 12–24-hr intervals of 0.1 mg/kg if age <48 hr at time of inital dose, 0.2 mg/kg if 2–7 days at time of initial dose, 0.25 mg/kg if >7 days at time of initial dose.

PHARMACODYNAMICS

	ONSET	PEAK	DURATION
PO (analgesic)	30 min	0.5–2 hr	4–6 hr
PO—ER (analgesic)	30 min	UK	4–6 hr
PO (anti-inflammatory)	up to 7 days	1–2 wk	UK
PO—ER (anti-inflammatory)	up to 7 days	1–2 wk	UK
IV (closure of PDA)	up to 48 hr	UK	UK

NURSING IMPLICATIONS

Assessment

- **General Info:** Patients who have asthma, aspirin-induced allergy, and nasal polyps are at increased risk for developing hypersensitivity reactions. Monitor for rhinitis, asthma, and urticaria.

*Underlines indicate most frequent; **CAPITALS** indicate life-threatening.

- **Arthritis:** Assess limitation of movement and pain—note type, location, and intensity prior to and 1–2 hr following administration.
- **Patent Ductus Arteriosus:** Monitor respiratory status and heart sounds routinely throughout therapy.
- □ Monitor intake and output. Fluid restriction is usually instituted throughout therapy.
- **Lab Test Considerations:** BUN, serum creatinine, CBC, serum potassium levels, and liver function tests should be evaluated periodically in patients receiving prolonged courses of therapy.
- □ Serum potassium, BUN, serum creatinine, SGOT (ALT), and SGPT (AST) tests may show increased levels. Blood glucose concentrations may be altered.
- □ Urine glucose and urine protein concentrations may be increased. May cause decreased creatinine clearance; serum sodium concentrations; urine chloride, potassium, and sodium concentrations; urine osmolality; and urine volume.
- □ Leukocyte and platelet count may be decreased. Bleeding time may be prolonged for 1 day after discontinuation.

Potential Nursing Diagnoses

- Comfort, altered: pain (indications).
- Mobility, impaired physical (indications).
- Knowledge deficit related to medication regimen (patient/family teaching).

Implementation

- **PO:** Administer after meals or with food or administer antacids to decrease GI irritation.
- □ Shake suspension prior to administration. Do not mix with antacid or any other liquid.
- **Direct IV:** Reconstitute with 1 or 2 ml of preservative-free 0.9% NaCl or preservative-free sterile water for a concentration of 0.1 mg/ml or 0.05 mg/ml, respectively. Reconstitute immediately prior to use and discard any unused soln. Do not dilute further or admix.
- □ *Rate:* Administer over 5–10 sec. Avoid extravasation, as soln is irritating to tissues.
- **Rect:** Encourage patient to retain suppository for 1 hr following administration.

Patient/Family Teaching

- **General Info:** Advise patient to take this medication with a full glass of water and to remain in an upright position for 15–30 min after administration.
- □ Instruct patient to take medication exactly as directed. Missed doses should be taken as soon as remembered if not almost time for next dose. Do not double doses.
- □ May cause drowsiness or dizziness. Advise patient to avoid driving or other activities requiring alertness until response to medication is known.
- □ Caution patient to avoid the concurrent use of alcohol, aspirin, acetaminophen, or other over-the-counter medications without consulting physician or pharmacist.
- □ Instruct patient to notify physician if rash, itching, chills, fever, muscle aches, visual disturbances, weight gain, edema, abdominal pain, black stools, or persistent headache occur.
- □ Advise patient to inform physician or dentist of medication regimen prior to treatment or surgery.
- **Patent Ductus Arteriosus:** Explain to parents the purpose of medication and the need for frequent monitoring.

Evaluation

Effectiveness of therapy can be demonstrated by: ▪ Decrease in severity of moderate pain □ Improved joint mobility. Partial arthritic relief is usually seen within 2 wk, but maximum effectiveness may require up to 1 mon of continuous therapy ▪ Successful closure of patent ductus arteriosus.

I

INSULIN
(in-su-lin)

Rapid-acting Insulins
regular (Actrapid, Humulin R, Humulin BR, Ilentin I, Iletin II, Novolin R, Velosulin)
prompt zinc suspension (Semilente, Semilente Iletin, Semitard)

Intermediate-acting Insulins
isophane suspension (Humulin N, Iletin II, Insultard NPH, Lentard, Novolin N, NPH, NPH Purified)
zinc suspension (Humulin L, Lente, Lente Iletin, Monotard, Novolin L)

Long-acting Insulins
protamine zinc suspension (PZI)
extended zinc suspension (Humulin U, Ultralente, Ultralente Iletin, Ultratard)

Insulin Mixture
regular plus NPH (Humulin 70/30, Mixtard 70/30, Novolin 70/30)

CLASSIFICATION(S):
Hormone—insulin
Pregnancy Category UK

INDICATIONS
▪ Treatment of insulin-dependent diabetes mellitus (IDDM, type I) ▪ Management of noninsulin-dependent diabetes mellitus (NIDDM, type II) unresponsive to treatment with diet and/or oral hypoglycemic agents.

ACTION
▪ Lowers blood glucose by increasing transport into cells and promoting the conversion of glucose to glycogen ▪ Promotes the conversion of amino acids to proteins in muscle and stimulates triglyceride formation ▪ Inhibits the release of free fatty acids ▪ Sources include beef, pork, beef/pork combinations, semisynthetic, and human insulin prepared by recombinant DNA technology. **Therapeutic Effect:** ▪ Control of blood sugar in diabetic patients.

PHARMACOKINETICS
Absorption: Rapidly absorbed from SC administration sites. Absorption rate is determined by type of insulin, injection site, volume of injectate, and other factors.
Distribution: Widely distributed.
Metabolism and Excretion: Metabolized by liver, kidney, and muscle.
Half-life: 9 min (prolonged in diabetics).

CONTRAINDICATIONS AND PRECAUTIONS
Contraindicated in: ▪ Allergy or hypersensitivity to a particular type of insulin, preservatives, or other additives.
Use Cautiously in: ▪ Stress, pregnancy, and infection (temporarily increase insulin requirements).

ADVERSE REACTIONS AND SIDE EFFECTS*
Derm: urticaria.
Endo: HYPOGLYCEMIA, rebound hyperglycemia (Somogyi effect).
Local: lipodystrophy, lipohypertrophy, itching, swelling, redness.
Misc: allergic reactions, including ANAPHYLAXIS.

INTERACTIONS
Drug-Drug: ▪ **Beta-adrenergic blocking agents** may block some of the signs and symptoms of hypoglycemia ▪ **Thiazide diuretics,** acute ingestion of **alcohol, glucocorticoids, thyroid preparations, estrogens, smoking,** and **rifampin** may increase insulin requirements ▪ **Anabolic steroids (testosterone), clofibrate, guanethidine, tricyclic antidepressants, MAO inhibitors, salicylates, phenylbutazone,** and **oral anticoagulants** may decrease insulin requirements.

ROUTE AND DOSAGE
Note: Depends on blood sugar, response, and many other factors.

Ketoacidosis—Regular Insulin Only
▪ **IV, SC (Adults):** 25–150 units ini-

*Underlines indicate most frequent; **CAPITALS** indicate life-threatening.

tially, then additional doses q 1 hr based on blood sugar until stable, then change to SC dosing q 6 hr or 50–100 units IV initially plus 50–100 units SC, then additional SC q 2–6 hr, or 0.33 units/kg bolus, or smaller boluses of 5–10 units followed by 0.1 units/kg/hr infusion.

- **IV, SC (Children):** 0.5–1 units/kg divided into 2 doses ½ IV, ½ SC, followed by 0.5–1 units/kg IV q 1–2 hr or 0.1 units/kg IV bolus, then 0.1 units/kg/hr infusion.
- **IM (Adults):** 0.22 units/kg followed by 5 units/hr.
- **IM (Children):** 0.25 units/kg followed by 0.1 units/kg/hr.

Maintenance Therapy

- **SC (Adults and Children):** 0.5 units/kg/day.
- **SC (Adolescents During Growth Spurts):** 0.8–1.2 units/kg/day.

PHARMACODYNAMICS (hypoglycemic effect)

	ONSET	PEAK	DURATION
regular IV	10–30 min	15–30 min	30–60 min
regular SC	0.5–1 hr	2–4 hr	5–7 hr
Semilente SC	1–3 hr	2–8 hr	12–16 hr
NPH SC	1–4 hr	6–12 hr	18–28 hr
Lente SC	1–3 hr	8–12 hr	18–28 hr
PZI SC	4–6 hr	14–24 hr	36 hr
Ultralente SC	4–6 hr	18–24 hr	36 hr

NURSING IMPLICATIONS

Assessment

- Assess patient for signs and symptoms of hypoglycemia (anxiety, chills, cold sweats, confusion, cool pale skin, difficulty in concentration, drowsiness, excessive hunger, headache, irritability, nausea, nervousness, rapid pulse, shakiness, unusual tiredness or weakness) and hyperglycemia (drowsiness, flushed dry skin, fruit-like breath odor, frequent urination, loss of appetite, tiredness, unusual thirst) periodically throughout therapy.
- Monitor body weight periodically. Changes in weight may necessitate changes in insulin dosage.
- **Lab Test Considerations:** May cause decreased serum inorganic phosphate, magnesium, and potassium levels.
- Monitor blood glucose or urine glucose and ketones every 6 hr throughout course of therapy, more frequently in ketoacidosis and times of stress. Glycosylated hemoglobin may also be monitored to determine effectiveness of therapy.
- **Toxicity and Overdose:** Overdose is manifested by symptoms of hypoglycemia. Mild hypoglycemia may be treated by ingestion of oral glucose. Severe hypoglycemia is a life-threatening emergency; treatment consists of IV glucose, glucagon, or epinephrine.

Potential Nursing Diagnoses

- Knowledge deficit related to medication regimen (patient/family teaching).
- Noncompliance (patient/family teaching).

Implementation

- **General Info:** Available in different types and strengths and from different species. Check type, species source, dose, and expiration date with another licensed nurse. Do not interchange insulins without physician's order.
- Use *only* insulin syringes to draw up dose. The unit markings on the insulin syringe must match the insulin's units/ml. Special syringes for doses <50 units are available. Prior to withdrawing dose, rotate vial between palms to ensure uniform soln; do not shake.
- When mixing insulins, draw regular insulin into syringe first to avoid contamination of regular insulin vial.
- Insulin should be stored in a cool place but does not need to be refrigerated.
- **IV:** Regular insulin is the ONLY insulin that can be administered IV. Do

not use if cloudy, discolored, or unusually viscous.

- Regular insulin U500 is not intended for IV route.
- **Direct IV:** May be administered IV undiluted directly into vein or through Y-site injection or 3-way stopcock.
- *Rate:* Administer each 50 units over 1 min.
- **Continuous Infusion:** May be diluted in commonly used IV solns as an infusion; however, insulin potency may be reduced by at least 20–80% by the plastic or glass container or tubing before reaching the venous system.
- *Rate:* When administered as an infusion, rate should be ordered by physician, and infusion should be placed on an IV pump for accurate administration.
- Rate of administration should be decreased when serum glucose level reaches 250 mg/100 ml.
- **Syringe Compatibility:** metoclopramide.
- **Y-Site Compatibility:** dobutamine, famotidine, heparin with hydrocortisone sodium succinate, meperidine, morphine, pentobarbital, potassium chloride, or sodium bicarbonate.
- **Additive Compatibility:** bretylium, cimetidine, lidocaine, oxytetracycline, or verapamil. May be added to TPN soln.
- **Additive Incompatibility:** aminophylline, amobarbital, chlorothiazide, cytarabine, dobutamine, methylprednisolone, pentobarbital, phenobarbital, phenytoin, secobarbital, sodium bicarbonate, or thiopental.

Patient/Family Teaching

- Instruct patient on proper technique for administration. Include type of insulin, equipment (syringe, cartridge pens, alcohol swabs), storage, and where to discard syringes. Discuss the importance of not changing brands of insulin or syringes, selection and rotation of injection sites, and compliance with therapeutic regimen.
- Demonstrate technique for mixing insulins by drawing up regular insulin first and rolling intermediate-acting insulin vial between palms to mix, rather than shaking (may cause inaccurate dose).
- Explain to patient that this medication controls hyperglycemia but does not cure diabetes. Therapy is long-term.
- Instruct patient in proper testing of serum glucose or urine glucose and ketones. Stress the importance of double-voided specimens for accuracy. These tests should be closely monitored during periods of stress or illness and physician notified if significant changes occur.
- Emphasize the importance of compliance with diabetic diet and exchange system for meals and regular exercise as directed by physician.
- Advise patient to consult physician or pharmacist prior to using alcohol or other medications concurrently with insulin.
- Advise patient to notify physician or dentist of medication regimen prior to treatment or surgery.
- Advise patient to notify physician if nausea, vomiting, or fever develops, if unable to eat regular diet, or if blood sugar levels are not controlled.
- Instruct patient on signs and symptoms of hypoglycemia and hyperglycemia and what to do if they occur.
- Patients with diabetes mellitus should carry a source of sugar (candy, sugar packets) and identification describing their disease and treatment regimen at all times.

Evaluation

Effectiveness of therapy can be demonstrated by: ▪ Control of blood glucose levels without the appearance of hypoglycemic or hyperglycemic episodes.

INTERFERON ALFA-2a

(in-ter-**feer**-on)

IFLrA, rIFN-A, Roferon-A

CLASSIFICATION(S):
Antineoplastic—miscellaneous
Pregnancy Category C

INDICATIONS

▪ Treatment of hairy cell leukemia ▪ Treatment of AIDS-associated Kaposi's sarcoma. **Unlabeled Use:** ▪ Variety of other tumors.

ACTION

▪ A protein produced by recombinant DNA techniques that modulates the immune response and has an antiproliferative action against tumor cells ▪ Antiviral activity. **Therapeutic Effects:** ▪ Antineoplastic and antiproliferative activity.

PHARMACOKINETICS

Absorption: Not absorbed orally. Well absorbed (>80%) following IM and SC administration.
Distribution: Distribution not known.
Metabolism and Excretion: Filtered by the kidneys and subsequently degraded in the renal tubule.
Half-life: 3.7–8.5 hr.

CONTRAINDICATIONS AND PRECAUTIONS

Contraindicated in: ▪ Hypersensitivity to interferon alpha-2a, human serum albumin, or phenol ▪ Pregnancy.
Use Cautiously in: ▪ Severe cardiovascular, renal, or hepatic disease ▪ Active infections ▪ Decreased bone marrow reserve ▪ Previous or concurrent radiation therapy ▪ Other debilitating illnesses ▪ Patients with childbearing potential ▪ Lactation and children <18 yr (safety not established).

ADVERSE REACTIONS AND SIDE EFFECTS*

Note: Most reactions are dose-dependent.

CNS: fatigue, depression, decreased mental status, sleep disturbances, SEIZURES, nervousness, confusion, gait disturbances, coordination difficulties, speech difficulties.
EENT: conjunctivitis.
Resp: bronchospasm.
CV: hypotension, edema, hypertension, chest pain, arrhythmias, palpitations.
GI: nausea, anorexia, diarrhea, vomiting, abdominal fullness, hypermotility, hepatitis, dry mouth, altered taste.
GU: impotence, gonadal suppression.
Derm: rash, pruritus, alopecia, sweating, dry skin.
Hemat: anemia, leukopenia, thrombocytopenia.
MS: myalgia.
Neuro: paresthesia, numbness, peripheral neuropathy.
Misc: flu-like syndrome, fever, chills, weight loss.

INTERACTIONS

Drug-Drug: ▪ Additive myelosuppression with other **antineoplastic agents** or **radiation therapy** ▪ May decrease metabolism and increase blood levels and toxicity of **aminophylline**.

ROUTE AND DOSAGE

Hairy Cell Leukemia

▪ **IM, SC (Adults):** 3 million IU/day for 16–24 wk. If severe adverse reactions occur, reduce dosage by 50%. Maintenance dose 3 million IU 3 times weekly.

Kaposi's Sarcoma

▪ **IM, SC (Adults):** 36 million IU/day for 10–12 wks or 3 million IU/day for 3 days, then 9 million IU/day for next 3 days, then 18 million IU/day for next 3 days, then 36 million IU/day for next 3 days for rest of 10–12 wk course. If severe adverse reactions occur, reduce dosage by 50%. Maintenance dose 36 million IU 3 times weekly.

*Underlines indicate most frequent; **CAPITALS** indicate life-threatening.

PHARMACODYNAMICS

	ONSET	PEAK	DURATION
IM, SC (effects on blood counts)	UK	17–19 days	several wks
IM, SC (clinical response)	1–3 mon	UK	UK

NURSING IMPLICATIONS

Assessment

- **General Info:** Monitor vital signs prior to and periodically throughout course of therapy. Hypotension may occur up to 2 days after therapy.
  - Assess patient for development of flu-like syndrome (fever, chills, myalgia, headache). Symptoms often appear suddenly 3–6 hr after therapy. Symptoms tend to decrease, even with continued therapy. Confer with physician regarding acetaminophen for control of these symptoms.
  - Monitor cardiac status, especially in patients with underlying cardiac disease or advanced malignancy. Assess heart sounds and chest pain, auscultate lung sounds for rales/crackles, and assess for edema. Physician may order periodic ECGs.
  - Assess for fever, sore throat, and signs of infection. Notify physician if these symptoms occur.
  - Assess for bleeding (bleeding gums; bruising; petechiae; guaiac stools, urine, and emesis). Avoid other IM injections and rectal temperatures. Hold pressure on venipuncture sites for at least 10 min.
  - May cause nausea and vomiting. Confer with physician regarding prophylactic use of an antiemetic. Monitor intake and output, daily weight, and appetite. Adjust diet as tolerated for anorexia. Encourage fluid intake of at least 2 liters/day.
  - Monitor neurologic status throughout course of therapy. Notify physician if confusion, decreased coordination, dizziness, gait disturbances, paresthesia, difficulty with speech, or psychological disturbances occur.
- **Kaposi's Sarcoma:** Monitor number, size, and character of lesions prior to and throughout therapy.
- **Lab Test Considerations:** Monitor CBC and differential prior to and periodically throughout course of therapy. May cause leukopenia, neutropenia, thrombocytopenia, and decreased hemoglobin and hematocrit. The nadir of leukopenia occurs in 22–38 days and the nadir of thrombocytopenia in 17–19 days. Recovery of leukopenia and thrombocytopenia occur a few wks after withdrawal of interferon alfa-2a.
  - Monitor liver function tests (SGOT [AST], SGPT [ALT], LDH, bilirubin) and renal function tests (BUN, creatinine, urinalysis) prior to and periodically throughout therapy.
  - May cause increased uric acid; monitor levels periodically during therapy.

Potential Nursing Diagnoses

- Injury, high risk for (side effects).
- Infection, high risk for (side effects).
- Knowledge deficit related to medication regimen (patient/family teaching).

Implementation

- **General Info:** Soln should be prepared in a biologic cabinet. Wear gloves, gown, and mask while handling medication. Discard equipment in specially designated containers (see Appendix I).
- **SC/IM:** SC route is preferred for patients with a platelet count $<50{,}000/mm^3$.
  - Interferon alfa-2a is available in soln or as a powder requiring reconstitution. Reconstitute the 18-million-IU vial with 3 ml of diluent provided. Refrigerate after reconstitution and use within 30 days.

Patient/Family Teaching

- Advise patient to take medication exactly as directed. If a dose is missed, omit dose and return to the regular schedule. The patient should notify the physician if more than 1 dose is missed.

- Instruct patient and family on preparation and correct technique for administration of injection. Explain to patient that brands should not be switched without physician's approval, as this may result in a change of dosage.
- Discuss possibility of flu-like reaction 3–6 hr after dose. Physician may recommend that patient take acetaminophen prior to injection and every 3–4 hr afterward as needed to control symptoms.
- Review side effects with patient. Physician may temporarily discontinue interferon or decrease dose by 50% if serious side effects occur.
- Advise patient to notify physician if fever, chills, sore throat, signs of infection, bleeding gums, bruising, petechiae, or blood in urine, stool, or emesis occurs. Caution patient to avoid crowds and persons with known infections. Instruct patient to use soft toothbrush, avoid flossing, and use electric razor. Caution patient not to drink alcoholic beverages or take aspirin-containing products. Caution patient against use of CNS depressants concurrently with this medication.
- Discuss with patient the possibility of hair loss. Explore coping strategies.
- Explain to patient that fertility may be impaired and that contraception is needed throughout course of treatment to prevent potential harm to the fetus.
- Instruct patient not to receive any vaccinations without advice of physician.
- Emphasize need for periodic lab tests to monitor for side effects.

EVALUATION

Effectiveness of therapy can be demonstrated by: ▪ Normalized blood parameters (hemoglobin, neutrophils, platelets, monocytes, and bone marrow and peripheral hairy cells) in hairy cell leukemia ▪ Decrease in the size and number of lesions in Kaposi's sarcoma. Six mons of therapy may be required before full response is seen. Therapy is discontinued when there is no further clinical improvement and parameters have stabilized for 3 mon.

INTERFERON ALFA-2b

(in-ter-**feer**-on)

a-2-interferon, IFN-alpf-2, Intron A, rIFN-a2

CLASSIFICATION(S):
Antineoplastic—miscellaneous
Pregnancy Category C

INDICATIONS

▪ Treatment of hairy cell leukemia ▪ Treatment of AIDS-associated Kaposi's sarcoma ▪ Treatment of condylomata acuminata (intralesional) ▪ Treatment of chronic hepatitis non-A, non-B/C.

ACTION

▪ A protein produced by recombinant DNA techniques that modulates the immune response and has an antiproliferative action against tumor cells ▪ Antiviral activity. **Therapeutic Effects:** ▪ Antineoplastic and antiproliferative activity ▪ Improvement in liver function in patients with chronic hepatitis non-A, non-B/C.

PHARMACOKINETICS

Absorption: Not absorbed orally. Well absorbed (>80%) following IM and SC administration.
Distribution: Distribution not known.
Metabolism and Excretion: Filtered by the kidneys and subsequently degraded in the renal tubule.
Half-life: 2–3 hr.

CONTRAINDICATIONS AND PRECAUTIONS

Contraindicated in: ▪ Hypersensitivity to interferon alfa-2b, human serum albumin ▪ Pregnancy.
Use Cautiously in: ▪ Severe cardiovascular, renal, or hepatic disease ▪ Active infections ▪ Decreased bone marrow re-

serve ▪ Previous or concurrent radiation therapy ▪ Other debilitating illnesses ▪ Patients with childbearing potential ▪ Lactation and children <18 yr (safety not established).

ADVERSE REACTIONS AND SIDE EFFECTS*

CNS: fatigue, depression, decreased mental status, sleep, seizures, disturbances, nervousness, gait disturbances, coordination difficulties, speech difficulties.
EENT: conjunctivitis.
Resp: bronchospasm.
CV: hypotension, edema, hypertension, chest pain, arrhythmias, palpitations.
GI: nausea, anorexia, diarrhea, vomiting, abdominal fullness, hypermotility, hepatitis, dry mouth, altered taste.
GU: impotence, gonadal suppression.
Derm: rash, pruritus, alopecia, sweating.
Hemat: anemia, leukopenia, thrombocytopenia.
MS: myalgia.
Neuro: paresthesia, numbness.
Misc: flu-like syndrome, fever, chills, weight loss.

INTERACTIONS

Drug-Drug: ▪ Additive myelosuppression with other **antineoplastic agents** or **radiation therapy** ▪ May decrease metabolism and increase blood levels and toxicity of **aminophylline** ▪ Increases the risk of neutropenia associated with **zidovudine** therapy.

ROUTE AND DOSAGE

Hairy Cell Leukemia

- **IM, SC (Adults):** 2 million IU/m^2 3 times weekly. If severe adverse reactions occur, reduce dosage by 50%.

Kaposi's Sarcoma

- **IM, SC (Adults):** 30 million IU/m^2 3 times weekly.

Condylomata Acuminata

- **Intralesional (Adults):** 1 million IU/lesion 3 times weekly for 3 wk, treat only 5 lesions per course.

PHARMACODYNAMICS (IM, SC-CR = clinical response, IM, SC-BC = effects on platelet counts, IM, SC-LFT = effects on liver function in patients with hepatitis. Intralesional = regression of lesions)

	ONSET	PEAK	DURATION
IM, SC-CR	1–3 mon	UK	UK
IM, SC-BC	UK	3–5 days	3–5 days
IM, SC-LFT	2 wk	UK	UK
Intralesional	UK	4–8 wk	UK

NURSING IMPLICATIONS

Assessment

- **General Info:** Monitor vital signs prior to and periodically throughout course of therapy. Hypotension may occur up to 2 days after therapy.
- Assess patient for development of flu-like syndrome (fever, chills, myalgia, headache). Symptoms often appear suddenly 3–6 hr after therapy. Symptoms tend to decrease, even with continued therapy. Confer with physician regarding acetaminophen for control of these symptoms.
- Monitor cardiac status, especially in patients with underlying cardiac disease or advanced malignancy. Assess heart sounds and chest pain, auscultate lung sounds for rales/crackles, and assess for edema. Physician may order periodic ECGs.
- Assess for fever, sore throat, and signs of infection. Notify physician if these symptoms occur.
- Assess for bleeding (bleeding gums; bruising; petechiae; guaiac stools, urine, and emesis). Avoid other IM injections and rectal temperatures. Hold pressure on venipuncture sites for at least 10 min.
- May cause nausea and vomiting. Confer with physician regarding prophylactic use of an antiemetic. Monitor intake and output, daily weight, and appetite. Adjust diet as tolerated for anorexia. Encourage fluid intake of at least 2 liters/day.

*Underlines indicate most frequent; **CAPITALS** indicate life-threatening.

- Monitor neurologic status throughout course of therapy. Notify physician if confusion, decreased coordination, dizziness, gait disturbances, paresthesia, difficulty with speech, or psychologic disturbances occur.
- **Kaposi's Sarcoma:** Monitor number, size, and character of lesions prior to and throughout therapy.
- **Lab Test Considerations:** Monitor CBC and differential prior to and periodically throughout course of therapy. May cause leukopenia, neutropenia, thrombocytopenia, and decreased hemoglobin and hematocrit. The nadirs of leukopenia and thrombocytopenia occur in 3–5 days, with recovery 3–5 days after withdrawal of interferon alfa-2b.
- Monitor liver function tests (SGOT [AST], SGPT [ALT], LDH, bilirubin) and renal function tests (BUN, creatinine, urinalysis) prior to and periodically throughout therapy.
- May cause increased uric acid; monitor levels periodically during therapy.
- **Intralesional Route:** Monitor CBC and liver function tests. May cause mild to moderate leukopenia and elevated SGOT (AST).

Potential Nursing Diagnoses

- Injury, high risk for (side effects).
- Infection, high risk for (side effects).
- Knowledge deficit related to medication regimen (patient/family teaching).

Implementation

- **General Info:** Soln should be prepared in a biologic cabinet. Wear gloves, gown, and mask while handling medication. Discard equipment in specially designated containers (see Appendix I).
- Interferon alfa-2b is available in 3-, 5-, and 25-million-IU vials for SC/IM use and 10-million-IU vials for SC/IM and intralesional use.
- **SC/IM:** SC route is preferred for patients with a platelet count <50,000/mm^3.
- Reconstitute 3- and 5-million-IU vials with 1 ml, 10-million-IU dose with 2 ml, and 25-million-IU vial with 5 ml of diluent provided by manufacturer (bacteriostatic water for injection). Agitate gently. Soln may be colorless to light yellow. Refrigerate after reconstitution. Stable for 1 mon.
- **Intralesional:** Reconstitute 10-million-IU vial with 1 ml of bacteriostatic water for injection. Use a TB syringe with 25–30-gauge needle to administer. Each 0.1-ml dose is injected into the center of the base of the wart using the intradermal injection approach. As many as 5 lesions can be treated at one time.

Patient/Family Teaching

- Advise patient to take medication exactly as directed. If a dose is missed, skip the next dose and return to the regular schedule. The patient should notify the physician if more than 1 dose is missed.
- Instruct patient and family on preparation and correct technique for administration of injection. Explain to patient that brands should not be switched without physician's approval, as this may result in a change of dosage.
- Discuss possibility of flu-like reaction 3–6 hr after dose. Physician may recommend that patient take acetaminophen prior to injection and every 3–4 hr afterward as needed to control symptoms.
- Review side effects with patient. Physician may temporarily discontinue interferon or decrease dose by 50% if serious side effects occur.
- Advise patient to notify physician if fever, chills, sore throat, signs of infection, bleeding gums, bruising, petechiae, or blood in urine, stool, or emesis occurs. Caution patient to avoid crowds and persons with known infections. Instruct patient to use soft toothbrush, avoid flossing, and use electric razor. Caution patient not to drink alcoholic beverages or take aspirin-containing products. Caution patient against use of CNS

depressants concurrently with this medication.

- Discuss with patient the possibility of hair loss. Explore coping strategies.
- Explain to patient that fertility may be impaired and that contraception is needed throughout course of treatment to prevent potential harm to the fetus.
- Instruct patient not to receive any vaccinations without advice of physician.
- Emphasize need for periodic lab tests to monitor for side effects.

Evaluation

Effectiveness of therapy can be demonstrated by: ▪ Normalized blood parameters (hemoglobin, neutrophils, platelets, monocytes, and bone marrow and peripheral hairy cells) in hairy cell leukemia. Six mons or more of therapy may be required before full response is seen ▪ Decrease in the size and number of lesions in Kaposi's sarcoma ▪ Disappearance of or decrease in size and number of genital warts. Condylomata acuminata usually respond in 4–8 wk. The course of therapy may need to be extended to 16 wk; a second course may be required if genital warts persist and laboratory values remain in acceptable limits.

INTERFERON ALFA-N3 (human leukocyte derived)

(in-ter-**feer**-on)

Alferon N

CLASSIFICATION(S):

Antineoplastic—miscellaneous

Pregnancy Category C

INDICATIONS

▪ Treatment of condylomata acuminata (venereal or genital warts) in patients >18 yr who have not responded to conventional therapy (podophyllin resin, surgery, laser, or crotherapy). Condylomata acuminata is considered to be of viral origin (human papilloma virus). **Unlabeled Uses:** ▪ Bladder tumors, some lymphomas, other viral infections.

ACTION

▪ A protein derived from human leukocytes that upon binding to cellular membranes initiates responses capable of inhibiting viral replication and suppressing cellular proliferation ▪ Also enhances phagocytosis, augments cytotoxic action of lymphocytes, and increases antigen expression. **Therapeutic Effect:** ▪ Resolution of warts in condylmata acuminata.

PHARMACOKINETICS

Absorption: Small amounts probably enter systemic circulation following intralesion injection.

Distribution: Distribution not known.

Metabolism and Excretion: Metabolism and excretion not known.

Half-life: UK.

CONTRAINDICATIONS AND PRECAUTIONS

Contraindicated in: ▪ Hypersensitivity to human interferon alfa, phenol, or albumin ▪ Previous anaphylactic reaction to mouse immunoglobulin.

Use Cautiously in: ▪ Severe cardiovascular or pulmonary disease ▪ Diabetes mellitus with ketacidosis ▪ Coagulation disorders ▪ Bone marrow depression ▪ History of seizure disorder ▪ Other chronic debilitating illnesses ▪ Pregnancy, lactation, or children (safety not established).

ADVERSE REACTIONS AND SIDE EFFECTS*

CNS: <u>malaise</u>, <u>fatigue</u>, <u>headache</u>, insomnia, <u>dizziness</u>, depression.

EENT: sinus drainage.

GI: nausea, vomiting, dyspepsia, diarrhea.

Derm: sweating, generalized pruritus.

MS: <u>myalgia</u>, back pain, arthralgia.

*<u>Underlines</u> indicate most frequent; **CAPITALS** indicate life-threatening.

Misc: flu-like syndrome, fever, chills, vasovagal reactions.

INTERACTIONS

Drug–Drug: ▪ None significant.

ROUTE AND DOSAGE

- **Intralesional (Adults):** 0.05 ml (250,000 IU)/wart twice weekly for up to 8 wk (not to exceed 0.5 ml (2.5 million IU) total/treatment session.

PHARMACODYNAMICS (resolution of warts)

	ONSET	PEAK	DURATION
Intra-lesional	several wks	8 wk–3 mon	UK

NURSING IMPLICATIONS

Assessment

- ▫ Assess number, size, and location of condylomata prior to and periodically throughout therapy.
- ▫ Assess patient for signs and symptoms of flu-like syndrome (fever, myalgia, headache). May be treated with acetaminophen and may decrease with repeated dosing.
- ▪ **Lab Test Considerations:** May cause decrease in white blood count.

Potential Nursing Diagnoses

- ▪ Skin integrity, impaired (indications).
- ▪ Knowledge deficit related to medication regimen (patient/family teaching).

Implementation

- ▪ **General Info:** Administered via intralesional injection at the base of each wart using a 30-gauge needle.
- ▫ Types of interferon are not interchangeable. They differ in manufacturing process and strength of interferon.

Patient/Family Teaching

- ▫ Instruct patient to notify physician if signs of hypersensitivity (hives, urticaria, chest tightness, wheezing, hypotension, anaphylaxis) occur.

Evaluation

Effectiveness of therapy can be demonstrated by: ▪ Resolution of genital warts refractory to other treatments. Therapy is continued for 8 wk but may take up to 3 mon for complete resolution. Therapy is not administered within 3 mon of the initial 8 wk course unless warts enlarge or reappear.

INTERFERON GAMMA 1B
(in-ter-**feer**-on)
Actimmune

CLASSIFICATION(S):
Immune modifier
Pregnancy Category C

INDICATIONS

▪ Diminished severity and frequency of infectious complications of chronic granulomatous disease.

ACTION

▪ A protein produced by recombinant DNA technology that is capable of activating phagocytes, enhancing their ability to kill pathogens, including: ▫ *Staphylococcus aureus* ▫ *Toxoplasma gondii* ▫ *Leishmania donovani* ▫ *Listeria monocytognes* ▫ *Myobacterium avium intracellulare*. **Therapeutic Effects:** ▪ Decreased incidence and severity of infection in patients with chronic granulomatous disease.

PHARMACOKINETICS

Absorption: Slowly absorbed following SC administration.
Distribution: Distribution not known.
Metabolism and Excretion: Metabolism and excretion not known.
Half-life: 5.9 hr.

CONTRAINDICATIONS AND PRECAUTIONS

Contraindicated in: ▪ Hypersensitivity to interferon gamma, *E. coli*-derived products, mannitol, or polysorbate.
Use Cautiously in: ▪ Pregnancy, lacta-

tion, or children <1 yr (safety not established) ■ Cardiovascular disease ■ Bone marrow depression.

ADVERSE REACTIONS AND SIDE EFFECTS*

CNS: headache, decreased mental status, dizziness.
GI: nausea, vomiting, abdominal pain.
Derm: rash.
Hemat: neutropenia, thrombocytopenia.
Local: edema or tenderness at injection site.
MS: myalgia, arthralgia, back pain.
Neuro: gait disturbances.
Misc: fever, chills.

INTERACTIONS

Drug–Drug: ■ May have additive bone marrow depressing effects with **antineoplastic agents** or **radiation therapy**.

ROUTE AND DOSAGE

Body Surface Area >0.5 m^2

- **SC (Adults):** 50 mcg/m^2 (1.5 million units/m^2) 3 times weekly.

Body Surface Area <0.5 m^2

- **SC (Adults and Children <1 yr):** 1.5 mcg/kg 3 times weekly.

PHARMACODYNAMICS (blood levels)

	ONSET	PEAK	DURATION
SC	UK	4 hr	UK

NURSING IMPLICATIONS

Assessment

- Assess patient for signs and symptoms of infection prior to and throughout therapy. Flu-like syndrome (fever, headache, chills, myalgia, fatigue) is a frequent side effect that may decrease in severity as treatment continues. Side effects may be minimized by administering at bedtime. Headache and fever may be treated with acetaminophen. If adverse reactions are severe, dose may be reduced by 50% or discontinued.
- **Lab Test Considerations:** Monitor CBC with differential, platelet count, blood chemistries including liver and kidney function, and urinalysis prior to and every 3 mon throughout therapy.

Potential Nursing Diagnoses

- Infection, high risk for (indications).
- Knowledge deficit related to medication regimen (patient/family teaching).

Implementation

- **General Info:** Vial must be refrigerated; do not freeze. If left at room temperature for more than 12 hr, discard vial. Vials do not contain a preservative and are for single use only. Do not shake.
- **SC:** Administer in the right or left arm or anterior thigh.

Patient/Family Teaching

- Instruct patient or family on proper technique for administering injection. Provide a puncture-proof container for disposal of needles.
- Advise patient of the need for contraception throughout therapy.

Evaluation

Effectiveness of therapy can be demonstrated by: ■ Decrease in frequency and severity of infections in patients with chronic granulomatous disease.

IPECAC SYRUP
(ip-e-kak)

CLASSIFICATION(S):
Emetic
Pregnancy Category C

INDICATIONS

■ Used to induce vomiting in the early management of overdose or poisoning of noncaustic substances in conscious patients.

*Underlines indicate most frequent; **CAPITALS** indicate life-threatening.

ACTION

▪ Stimulates the chemoreceptor trigger zone in the CNS and irritates the gastric mucosa. **Therapeutic Effect:** ▪ Induction of emesis in overdose situations.

PHARMACOKINETICS

Absorption: Absorption is minimal.
Distribution: Distribution not known.
Metabolism and Excretion: Metabolism and excretion not known.
Half-life: UK.

CONTRAINDICATIONS AND PRECAUTIONS

Contraindicated in: ▪ Semicomatose, inebriated, unconscious, or seizing patients ▪ Shock ▪ Patients who may not have a gag reflex ▪ Ingestion of caustic substances.
Use Cautiously in: ▪ Pregnancy, lactation, or children <6 mon (safety not established) ▪ Do not confuse syrup with fluidextract, which is 14 times more concentrated.

ADVERSE REACTIONS AND SIDE EFFECTS*

CNS: sedation.
CV: <u>arrhythmias</u>, MYOCARDITIS (if drug is absorbed or overdosage ingested).
GI: diarrhea.

INTERACTIONS

Drug-Drug: ▪ Should not be given concurrently with **antiemetics** or **activated charcoal** (may reduce emetic efficacy).
Drug-Food: ▪ Concurrent administration with **milk** decreases effectiveness ▪ Avoid concurrent use of **carbonated beverages** (causes abdominal distention).

ROUTE AND DOSAGE

- **PO (Adults):** 15 ml followed by 100–200 ml of water.
- **PO (Children ≥1 yr):** 15 ml, followed by 100–200 ml of water.
- **PO (Children <1 yr):** 5–10 ml, followed by 100–200 ml of water. Dose may be repeated after 20 min if necessary.

PHARMACODYNAMICS (onset of emesis)

	ONSET	PEAK	DURATION
PO	20–30 min	UK	20–25 min

NURSING IMPLICATIONS

Assessment

□ A history is essential in determining treatment and antidotes for accidental poisoning. Do not induce vomiting if patient has ingested petroleum distillates, volatile oils, or caustic substances.

□ Assess level of consciousness prior to administration. Do not administer ipecac if patient is unconscious, semiconscious, or convulsing.

Potential Nursing Diagnoses

- Injury, high risk for (indications).
- Knowledge deficit related to medication regimen (patient/family teaching).

Implementation

▪ **General Info:** Check label carefully before administering medication. Do not confuse ipecac syrup with ipecac fluidextract, which is 14 times more concentrated than the syrup.

□ If vomiting does not occur within 30 min, dose may be repeated. If vomiting does not occur within 20 min after second dose, gastric lavage must be performed to recover the medication.

□ Administer activated charcoal only after vomiting has been induced and completed.

▪ **PO:** Administer syrup followed immediately by adequate amounts of water (1–2 glasses for adults and ½–1 glass for children).

□ Do not administer concurrently with milk, as it decreases the effectiveness of ipecac, or carbonated beverages, as they cause stomach distention.

Patient/Family Teaching

□ Advise parents with children >1 yr to keep a small amount of ipecac syrup on hand for emergency use. If child ingests a dangerous substance, the

*<u>Underlines</u> indicate most frequent; **CAPITALS** indicate life-threatening.

parents should contact a poison control center, physician, or emergency department for advice before administering this medication.

- □ Caution parents to avoid inducing emesis if child swallowed caustic substances, volatile oils, or petroleum distillates or if child is unconscious, semiconscious, or convulsing.
- □ Advise parents that the drug has a 1-yr shelf life and therefore needs to be replaced yearly. Advise parents to check expiration date of product before purchasing.

Evaluation

Effectiveness of therapy can be demonstrated by: ▪ Emesis within 30 min of administration.

IPRATROPIUM

(i-pra-**troe**-pee-um)
Atrovent

CLASSIFICATION(S):
Bronchodilator—anticholinergic
Pregnancy Category B

INDICATIONS

▪ Bronchodilator in maintenance therapy of reversible airway obstruction due to asthma or COPD.

ACTION

▪ Inhibits cholinergic receptors in bronchial smooth muscle, resulting in decreased concentrations of cyclic guanosine monophosphate (cGMP). Decreased levels of cGMP produce local bronchodilation. **Therapeutic Effect:** ▪ Bronchodilation without systemic anticholinergic properties.

PHARMACOKINETICS

Absorption: Minimal systemic absorption.
Distribution: Does not appear to cross the blood-brain barrier.
Metabolism and Excretion: Small amounts absorbed are metabolized by the liver.
Half-life: 2 hr.

CONTRAINDICATIONS AND PRECAUTIONS

Contraindicated in: ▪ Hypersensitivity to ipratropium, atropine, belladonna alkaloids, or fluorocarbons ▪ Avoid use during acute bronchospasm.
Use Cautiously in: ▪ Patients with bladder neck obstruction, prostatic hypertrophy, glaucoma, or urinary retention.

ADVERSE REACTIONS AND SIDE EFFECTS*

CNS: nervousness, dizziness, headache.
EENT: blurred vision, sore throat.
Resp: cough, bronchospasm.
CV: palpitations.
GI: nausea, GI irritation.
Derm: rash.

INTERACTIONS

Drug–Drug: ▪ Potential additive fluorocarbon toxicity when used with other **inhalation bronchodilators having a fluorocarbon propellant**.

ROUTE AND DOSAGE

Note: Each inhalation contains 18 mcg ipratropium.

- ▪ **Inhaln (Adults):** 1–2 inhaln 3–4 times daily (not to exceed 12 inhaln/24 hr).

PHARMACODYNAMICS (bronchodilation)

	ONSET	PEAK	DURATION
Inhaln	5–15 min	1–2 hr	3–4 hr (up to 6 hr)

NURSING IMPLICATIONS

Assessment

- □ Assess respiratory status (rate, breath sounds, degree of dyspnea, pulse) before administration and at peak of medication. Confer with physician about alternative medication if severe

*Underlines indicate most frequent; **CAPITALS** indicate life-threatening.

bronchospasm is present, as onset of action is too slow for patients in acute distress. If paradoxical bronchospasm (wheezing) occurs, withhold medication and notify physician immediately.

- □ Assess for allergy to atropine and belladonna alkaloids; patients with these allergies may also be sensitive to ipratropium.

Potential Nursing Diagnoses

- ▪ Airway clearance, ineffective (indications).
- ▪ Activity intolerance (indications).
- ▪ Knowledge deficit related to medication regimen (patient/family teaching).

Implementation

- ▪ **Inhaln:** Shake metered-dose inhaler well. Instruct patient to exhale and close lips firmly around mouthpiece. Administer dose during second half of inhalation and have patient hold breath as long as possible to ensure deep inhalation of medication. If more than 1 inhalation is required, wait at least 1 min between inhalations and wait at least 5 min between inhalations of ipratropium and other inhalation medications. Wash mouthpiece at least daily in warm running water.
- □ When ipratropium is administered concurrently with other inhalation medications, administer ipratropium first.

Patient/Family Teaching

- □ Instruct patient on proper use of inhaler. Instruct patient to take medication as directed. If a dose is missed, take as soon as remembered unless almost time for the next dose. Do not double doses.
- □ Caution patient not to exceed 12 doses within 24 hr. Patient should notify physician if symptoms do not improve within 30 min after administration of medication or if condition worsens.
- □ Explain need for pulmonary function tests prior to and periodically throughout therapy to determine effectiveness of medication.
- □ Caution patient to avoid spraying medication in eyes; may cause blurring of vision or irritation.
- □ Advise patient that rinsing mouth after using inhaler, good oral hygiene, and sugarless gum or candy may minimize dry mouth. Physician should be notified if stomatitis occurs or if dry mouth persists for more than 2 wk.
- □ Advise patient to inform physician if cough, nervousness, headache, dizziness, nausea, or GI distress occurs.

Evaluation

Effectiveness of therapy can be demonstrated by: ▪ Decreased dyspnea □ Improved breath sounds.

IRON DEXTRAN

(**eye**-ern **dex**-tran)
Dextraron, Feronim, Hematran, Hydextran, Imferon, Irodex, Norferan

CLASSIFICATION(S):
Antianemic, Iron supplement
Pregnancy Category C

INDICATIONS

▪ Treatment and prevention of iron-deficiency anemia in patients who are unable to tolerate oral iron preparations.

ACTION

▪ Enters the bloodstream and organs of the reticuloendothelial system (liver, spleen, bone marrow), where iron is separated from the dextran complex and becomes part of the body's iron stores. **Therapeutic Effect:** ▪ Prevention and treatment of iron deficiency.

PHARMACOKINETICS

Absorption: Well absorbed following IM administration.
Distribution: Remains in the body for

many mons. Crosses the placenta and enters breast milk.
Metabolism and Excretion: Lost slowly from the body through desquamation or blood loss.
Half-life: 6 hr.

CONTRAINDICATIONS AND PRECAUTIONS

Contraindicated in: ▪ Hypersensitivity ▪ All other types of anemias.
Use Cautiously in: ▪ Autoimmune disorders and arthritis (more susceptible to allergic reactions).

ADVERSE REACTIONS AND SIDE EFFECTS*

CNS: headache, dizziness, SEIZURES, syncope.
EENT: bad taste.
CV: hypotension, tachycardia.
GI: nausea, vomiting.
Derm: urticaria, flushing.
Local: pain at IM site, staining at IM site, phlebitis at IV site.
MS: arthralgia.
Misc: allergic reactions, including ANAPHYLAXIS, fever, lymphadenopathy.

INTERACTIONS

Drug-Drug: ▪ **Chloramphenicol** and **vitamin E** may impare the normal hematologic response to parenteral iron.

ROUTE AND DOSAGE

Note: Each ml contains 50 mg of elemental iron. Administer a test dose of 25 mg IM or IV 1 hr prior to first dose. Total dosage is calculated by degree of iron deficiency or blood loss.

- **IM (Adults >50 kg):** not to exceed 250 mg/day.
- **IM (Children 9–50 kg):** not to exceed 100 mg/day.
- **IM (Children 4.5–9 kg):** not to exceed 50 mg/day.
- **IM (Children <4.5 kg):** Not to exceed 25 mg/day.
- **IV (Adults):** 100 mg/day as a bolus or dilute total dose and infuse over 1–6 hr.

PHARMACODYNAMICS (effects on reticulocyte counts)

	ONSET	PEAK	DURATION
IV	4 days	1–2 wk	wk–mons
IM	4 days	1–2 wk	wk–mons

NURSING IMPLICATIONS

Assessment

- □ Assess patient's nutritional status and dietary history to determine possible cause of anemia and need for patient teaching.
- □ Monitor blood pressure and heart rate frequently following IV administration until stable. Rapid infusion rate may cause hypotension and flushing.
- □ Assess patient for signs and symptoms of anaphylaxis (rash, pruritus, laryngeal edema, wheezing). Notify physician immediately if these occur. Keep epinephrine and resuscitation equipment close by in the event of an anaphylactic reaction.
- □ Monitor hemoglobin, hematocrit, reticulocyte values, transferrin, ferritin, total iron-binding capacity, and plasma iron concentrations periodically throughout therapy. Serum ferritin levels peak in 7–9 days and return to normal in 3 wk. Serum iron determinations may be inaccurate for 1–2 wk after therapy with large doses, therefore hemoglobin and hematocrit are used to gauge initial response.
- ▪ **Lab Test Considerations:** May impart a brownish hue to serum when blood drawn within 4 hr of administration. May cause false increase in serum bilirubin and false decrease in serum calcium values. Prolonged PTT may be calculated when blood sample is anticoagulated with citrate dextrose soln; use sodium citrate instead.

Potential Nursing Diagnoses

- ▪ Activity intolerance (indications).
- ▪ Knowledge deficit related to medication and dietary regimen (patient/family teaching).

*Underlines indicate most frequent; **CAPITALS** indicate life-threatening.

Implementation

- **General Info:** Oral iron preparations should be discontinued prior to parenteral administration.
  - The 2-ml and 5-ml ampules may be used for IM or IV administration; the 10-ml multi-dose vials may be used only for IM administration.
  - Prior to initial IM or IV dose, a test dose of 25 mg should be given by the same route as the dose is to be given, to determine reaction. The IV test dose should be administered over 5 min. The IM dose should be administered in same injection site and by same technique as the therapeutic dose. The remaining portion may be administered after 1 hr, if no adverse symptoms have occurred.
- **IM:** Inject deeply via Z-track technique into upper outer quadrant of buttock, never into arm or other exposed areas. Use a 2–3 in, 19-gauge or 20-gauge needle. Change needles between withdrawal from container and injection to minimize staining of subcutaneous tissues. Stains are usually permanent.
- **Direct IV:** Give undiluted at a rate of 50 mg over at least 1 min.
- **Intermittent Infusion:** Dilute dose in 200–1000 ml of 0.9% NaCl. Discontinue other IV solns during infusion. Flush line with 10 ml of 0.9% NaCl at completion of the infusion. Do not dilute in D5W, as increased pain and phlebitis may occur.
  - *Rate:* Infuse over 1–6 hr.
  - Following IV administration, patient should remain recumbent for at least 30 min to prevent orthostatic hypotension.

Patient/Family Teaching

- Delayed reaction may occur 1–2 days after administration and last 3–4 days if IV route used, 3–7 days with IM route. Instruct patient to contact physician if fever, chills, malaise, muscle and joint aches, nausea, vomiting, dizziness, and backache occur.
- Instruct patient to follow a diet high in iron (organ meat, leafy green vegetables, dried beans and peas, dried fruit, cereals).

Evaluation

Clinical response can be determined by: ▪ Increase in hemoglobin, hematocrit, and plasma iron levels. The diagnosis of iron-deficiency anemia should be reconfirmed if hemoglobin has not increased by 1 g/100 ml in 2 wk.

ISONIAZID

(eye-soe-**nye**-a-zid)
INH, {Isotamine}, Laniazid, Nydrazid, {PMS Isoniazid}

CLASSIFICATION(S):
Antitubercular
Pregnancy Category UK

INDICATIONS

▪ Used as a first-line antitubercular in combination with other agents in the treatment of active disease ▪ Prevention of tuberculosis in patients exposed to active disease.

ACTION

▪ Inhibits mycobacterial cell wall synthesis and interferes with metabolism. **Therapeutic Effect:** ▪ Bacteriostatic or bactericidal action against susceptible mycobacteria.

PHARMACOKINETICS

Absorption: Well absorbed following oral and IM administration.
Distribution: Widely distributed to many body tissues and fluids. Readily crosses the blood-brain barrier. Crosses the placenta and enters breast milk in concentrations equal to plasma.
Metabolism and Excretion: 50% metabolized by the liver at rates that vary

widely among individuals. Remainder is excreted unchanged by the kidneys.
Half-life: 1–4 hr.

CONTRAINDICATIONS AND PRECAUTIONS

Contraindicated in: ▪ Hypersensitivity ▪ Acute liver disease ▪ Previous hepatitis from isoniazid.
Use Cautiously in: ▪ History of liver damage or chronic alcohol ingestion ▪ Pregnancy and lactation (although safety is not established, isoniazid has been used with ethambutol to treat tuberculosis in pregnant women without harm to the fetus) ▪ Severe renal impairment (dosage reduction may be necessary).

ADVERSE REACTIONS AND SIDE EFFECTS*

CNS: peripheral neuropathy, seizures, psychosis.
EENT: visual disturbances.
GI: nausea, vomiting, **HEPATITIS**.
Derm: rashes.
Endo: gynecomastia.
Hemat: blood dyscrasias.
Misc: fever.

INTERACTIONS

Drug-Drug: ▪ Additive CNS toxicity with other antituberculars ▪ **BCG vaccine** may not be effective during isoniazid therapy ▪ Isoniazid inhibits the metabolism of **phenytoin** ▪ **Aluminum-containing antacids** may decrease absorption ▪ Psychotic reactions and coordination difficulties may result with **disulfiram** ▪ Concurrent administration of **pyridoxine** may prevent neuropathy.
Drug-Food: ▪ Severe reactions may occur with ingestion of foods containing high concentrations of **tyramine** (see Appendix K).

ROUTE AND DOSAGE

- **PO, IM (Adults):** 5–10 mg/kg/day (usually 300 mg) or 15 mg/kg 2–3 times weekly.
- **PO, IM (Children):** 10–20 mg/kg/day or 20–40 mg/kg twice weekly.

PHARMACODYNAMICS (blood levels)

	ONSET	PEAK
PO	rapid	1–2 hr
IM	rapid	1–2 hr

NURSING IMPLICATIONS

Assessment

- □ Mycobacterial studies and susceptibility tests should be performed prior to and periodically throughout therapy to detect possible resistance.
- ▪ **Lab Test Considerations:** May cause false-positive test results for copper sulfate urine glucose tests (Clinitest). Diabetic patients should test urine glucose with enzymatic tests (Ketodiastix, Clinistix, Tes-Tape).
- □ Hepatic function should be evaluated prior to and monthly throughout course of therapy. Increased SGOT (AST), SGPT (ALT), and serum bilirubin may indicate drug-induced hepatitis. Patients >50 yr are at highest risk. The risk is lower in children; therefore liver function tests are usually ordered less frequently for children.
- ▪ **Toxicity and Overdose:** If isoniazid overdosage occurs, treatment with pyridoxine (vitamin B_6) is instituted.

Potential Nursing Diagnoses

- Infection, high risk for (indications).
- Knowledge deficit related to medication regimen (patient/family teaching).
- Noncompliance (patient/family teaching).

Implementation

- ▪ **General Info:** Available in tablet, syrup, and injectable forms.
- □ Also available in combination with rifampin (Rifamate); see Appendix A.
- ▪ **PO:** Administer medication on an empty stomach, at least 1 hr before or

*Underlines indicate most frequent; **CAPITALS** indicate life-threatening.

2 hr after meals. If GI irritation becomes a problem, may be administered with food, although food decreases absorption of isoniazid. Antacids may also be taken 1 hr prior to administration.
- **IM:** Medication may cause discomfort at injection site. Massage site after administration and rotate injection sites.

PATIENT/FAMILY TEACHING
- Advise patient to take medication exactly as directed, not to skip doses or double up on missed doses. Emphasize the importance of continuing therapy even after symptoms have subsided.
- Advise patient to notify physician promptly if signs and symptoms of hepatitis (yellow eyes and skin, nausea, vomiting, anorexia, dark urine, unusual tiredness, or weakness) or peripheral neuritis (numbness, tingling, paresthesia) occur. Pyridoxine may be used concurrently to prevent neuropathy. Any changes in visual acuity, eye pain, or blurred vision should also be reported to the physician immediately.
- Caution patient to avoid the use of alcohol during this therapy, as this may increase the risk of hepatotoxicity. Ingestion of Swiss or Cheshire cheeses, fish (tuna, skipjack, and Sardinella), and possibly tyramine-containing foods (see Appendix K) should also be avoided, as they may result in redness or itching of the skin, hot feeling, rapid or pounding heart beat, sweating, chills, cold clammy feeling, headache, or lightheadedness.
- Emphasize the importance of regular follow-up physical and ophthalmologic examinations to monitor progress and to check for side effects.

EVALUATION

Effectiveness of therapy can be demonstrated by: ▪ Resolution of signs and symptoms of tuberculosis ▫ Negative sputum cultures.

ISOPROTERENOL

(eye-soe-proe-**ter**-e-nole)
Aerolone, Isuprel, Medihaler-Iso, Vapo-Iso

CLASSIFICATION(S):
Bronchodilator—beta-adrenergic agonist, Antiarrhythmic, Inotropic agent
Pregnancy Category UK

INDICATIONS

▪ **Inhaln:** Used as a bronchodilator in reversible airway obstruction due to asthma or COPD ▪ **IV, SL, Rect:** Management of ventricular arrhythmias due to AV nodal block ▪ **IV:** Treatment of shock associated with decreased cardiac output and vasoconstriction.

ACTION

▪ A beta-adrenergic agonist that results in the accumulation of cyclic adenosine monophosphate (cAMP) ▪ Results of increased levels of cAMP at beta-adrenergic receptors include bronchodilation, CNS and cardiac stimulation, diuresis, and gastric acid secretion ▪ Stimulates both $beta_1$ (myocardial) and $beta_2$ (pulmonary) receptors. **Therapeutic Effects:** ▪ Bronchodilation ▪ Increased heart rate ▪ Increased cardiac output.

PHARMACOKINETICS

Absorption: Rapidly absorbed following oral inhalation and from parenteral sites. Orally administered isoproterenol is rapidly metabolized. Sublingual and rectal absorption is erratic and unreliable.
Distribution: Distribution not known.
Metabolism and Excretion: If swallowed, metabolized in the GI tract. Following other routes of administration, drug is metabolized by the lung, liver, and other tissues. 50% excreted unchanged by the kidneys following IV administration.
Half-life: UK.

CONTRAINDICATIONS AND PRECAUTIONS

Contraindicated in: ▪ Hypersensitivity to adrenergic amines or any ingredients in preparations (fluorocarbons in inhalers, bisulfites in injection and SL tablets).

Use Cautiously in: ▪ Elderly patients (more susceptible to adverse reactions; may require dosage reduction) ▪ Lactation (safety not established) ▪ Cardiac disease ▪ Hypertension ▪ Hyperthyroidism ▪ Diabetes ▪ Glaucoma ▪ Pregnancy (near term).

ADVERSE REACTIONS AND SIDE EFFECTS*

CNS: nervousness, restlessness, insomnia, tremor, headache.
Resp: paradoxical bronchospasm (with excessive use).
CV: hypertension, arrhythmias, angina.
GI: nausea, vomiting.
Endo: hyperglycemia.

INTERACTIONS

Drug-Drug: ▪ Additive adrenergic effects with other **adrenergic (sympathomimetic) agents** ▪ Use with **MAO inhibitors** may lead to hypertensive crisis ▪ **Beta-adrenergic blockers** may block therapeutic effect ▪ Arrhythmias may be increased with **cyclopropane** or **halothane-type anesthesia**.

ROUTE AND DOSAGE

Bronchodilation (80–130 mcg/metered-dose spray)

- **Inhaln (Adults and Children):** *Metered-dose inhaler* (120–130 mcg/spray)—1–2 inhalations 4–6 times daily. *Nebulization*—6–12 inhalations of 0.025% nebulized soln repeated q 15 min for 3 treatments up to 8 times/day. *IPPB* (Adults): 2 ml of 0.125% soln or 2.5 ml of 0.1% soln up to 5 times/day. *IPPB* (Children): 2 ml of 0.0625% soln or 2.5 ml of 0.05% soln 5 times/day.
- **SL (Adults):** 10–20 mg (not to exceed 60 mg/day, not to be administered more than 3 times daily or more often than q 3–4 hr).
- **SL (Children):** 5–10 mg (not to exceed 30 mg/day, not to be administered more than 3 times daily or more often than q 3–4 hr).
- **IV (Adults):** For bronchodilation during anesthesia—0.01–0.02 mg.

Cardiac Standstill and Arrhythmias

See infusion rate table in Appendix D

- **IV Bolus (Adults):** 0.01–0.06 mg.
- **IV Infusion (Adults):** 5 mcg/min (range 2–20 mcg/min).
- **IV Bolus (Children):** 0.005–0.03 mg.
- **IV Infusion (Children):** 2.5 mcg/min or 0.1–1 mcg/kg/min.
- **SL (Adults):** 10–30 mg 4–6 times daily or 10 mg initially, followed by 5–50 mg as needed.
- **Rect (Adults):** 5 mg followed by 1–15 mg as needed.

Shock

See infusion rate table in Appendix D

- **IV Infusion (Adults):** 0.5–5 mcg/min.

PHARMACODYNAMICS (Inhaln = bronchodilation, IV = cardiovascular effects)

	ONSET	PEAK	DURATION
Inhaln	rapid	UK	1 hr
IV	rapid	UK	min
SL	UK	UK	2 hr
Rect	UK	UK	2–4 hr

NURSING IMPLICATIONS

ASSESSMENT

- **General Info:** Assess blood pressure, pulse, respiratory pattern, lung sounds, arterial blood gases, and character of secretions frequently during course of therapy. ECG, hemodynamic parameters, and urine output should be monitored continuously during IV administration.
- ▫ Monitor for chest pain, arrhythmias, heart rate >110 bpm, and hypertension. Consult physician for parameters of pulse, blood pressure, and ECG changes for adjusting dosage or discontinuing medication.

*Underlines indicate most frequent; **CAPITALS** indicate life-threatening.

- **Bronchospasm:** Observe patient for appearance of drug tolerance and rebound bronchospasm. Patients requiring more than 3 aerosol treatments within 24 hr should be under close supervision. If minimal or no relief is seen after 3–5 aerosol treatments within 6–12 hr, further treatment with aerosol alone is not recommended.
- **Shock:** Assess volume status. Hypovolemia should be corrected prior to administering isoproterenol IV.
- **Lab Test Considerations:** May cause decreased serum potassium concentrations.

Potential Nursing Diagnoses

- Airway clearance, ineffective (indications).
- Cardiac output, altered: decreased (indications).
- Knowledge deficit related to medication regimen (patient/family teaching).

Implementation

- **General Info:** In treatment of heart block, SL tablet may be administered rectally.
- **Direct IV:** May be administered by diluting 0.2 mg (1 ml) of a 1:5000 soln with 10 ml of 0.9% NaCl for injection, to make a 1:50,000 soln. Do not use if soln is pinkish to brownish or contains a precipitate.
  - *Rate:* Administer each 1 ml of 1:50,000 soln (0.02 mg) over 1 min.
- **Continuous Infusion:** Prepare by adding 2 mg (10 ml) of a 1:5000 soln to 500 ml of D5W, D10W, 0.9% NaCl, 0.45% NaCl, dextrose/saline combinations, dextrose/Ringer's or lactated Ringer's combinations, Ringer's or lactated Ringer's soln for a 1:250,000 soln (4 mcg = 1 ml).
  - *Rate:* Administer at a rate of 1 ml/min, adjusting according to patient response and parameters for blood pressure, hemodynamic values, and urine output specified by physician. Administer via infusion pump to ensure delivery of precise amounts of medication.
- **Syringe Compatibility:** ranitidine.
- **Y-Site Compatibility:** amrinone, atracurium, bretyllium, famotidine, heparin, hydrocortisone sodium succinate, pancuronium, potassium chloride, or vecuronium.
- **Additive Compatibility:** calcium chloride, calcium gluceptate, cephalothin, cimetidine, dobutamine, heparin, magnesium sulfate, multivitamins, netilmicin, oxytetracycline, potassium chloride, succinylcholine, tetracycline, or verapamil.
- **Additive Incompatibility:** aminophylline, barbiturates, lidocaine, or sodium bicarbonate.
- **Inhaln:** For aerosol administration, dilute ordered dose in sterile water or 0.45% or 0.9% NaCl. Administer aerosol medications over 15–20 min.

Patient/Family Teaching

- **General Info:** Instruct patient to take medication exactly as prescribed. Taking more often than prescribed may lead to tolerance or paradoxical bronchospasm.
- **SL:** Instruct patient to hold SL tablet under tongue until completely dissolved. Do not chew or swallow. Encourage patient to rinse mouth frequently between doses and to practice good oral hygiene.
- **Inhaln:** Review correct administration technique (aerosolization, IPPB, metered-dose inhaler) with patient. For administration with metered-dose inhaler, instruct patient to shake inhaler well, clear airways before taking medication, exhale deeply before placing inhaler in mouth, close lips tightly around mouthpiece, inhale deeply while administering medication, and hold breath for several secs after receiving dose. Wait 1–5 min before administering next dose. Mouthpiece should be washed after each use. Medication should be discarded if pinkish to brownish or if it contains a precipitate.
  - Patients taking inhalation glucocorticoids concurrently with isoproterenol should be advised to take isoprotere-

nol first and to allow 15 min to elapse between using the 2 aerosols, unless directed by physician.

- Inform patient that medication may tinge sputum pink or red.
- Advise patient to maintain an adequate fluid intake (2000–3000 ml/day) to help liquify tenacious secretions.
- Advise patient to consult physician if respiratory symptoms are not relieved or worsen after treatment. Patient should also inform physician if chest pain, headache, severe dizziness, palpitations, nervousness, or weakness occurs.

EVALUATION

Effectiveness of therapy can be demonstrated by: ▪ Decrease in bronchoconstriction and bronchospasm ▫ Increase in ease of breathing ▪ Increase in heart rate ▪ Increase in cardiac output.

ISOSORBIDE DINITRATE

(eye-soe-**sor**-bide dye-**nye**-trate)
{Apo-ISDN}, {Cedocard-SR}, {Coronex}, Dilatrate-SR, ISDN, Iso-Bid, Isonate, Isorbid, Isordil, Isotrate, {Novosorbide}, Sorbitrate, Sorbitrate SA

CLASSIFICATION(S):
Vasodilator—nitrate
Pregnancy Category C

INDICATIONS

▪ Acute treatment of anginal attacks ▪ Long-term prophylactic management of angina pectoris ▪ Treatment of chronic congestive heart failure.

ACTION

▪ Produces vasodilation (venous greater than arterial) ▪ Decreases left ventricular end-diastolic pressure and left ventricular end-diastolic volume (preload). Net effect is reduced myocardial oxygen consumption ▪ Increases coronary blood flow by dilating coronary arteries and improving collateral flow to ischemic regions. **Therapeutic Effects:** ▪ Relief of anginal attacks and increased cardiac output.

PHARMACOKINETICS

Absorption: Well absorbed following oral and SL administration.
Distribution: Distribution not known.
Metabolism and Excretion: Mostly metabolized by the liver.
Half-life: 50 min.

CONTRAINDICATIONS AND PRECAUTIONS

Contraindicated in: ▪ Hypersensitivity ▪ Severe anemia.
Use Cautiously in: ▪ Head trauma or cerebral hemorrhage ▪ Pregnancy (may compromise maternal/fetal circulation) ▪ Children or lactation (safety not established).

ADVERSE REACTIONS AND SIDE EFFECTS*

CNS: <u>headache</u>, apprehension, weakness, <u>dizziness</u>.
CV: <u>hypotension</u>, <u>tachycardia</u>, syncope.
GI: nausea, vomiting, abdominal pain.
Misc: flushing, tolerance, cross-tolerance.

INTERACTIONS

Drug–Drug: ▪ Additive hypotension with **antihypertensives,** acute ingestion of **alcohol, beta-adrenergic blocking agents, calcium channel blockers,** and **phenothiazines.**

ROUTE AND DOSAGE

Acute Attack of Angina Pectoris

- **SL, Chew, Intrabuccal (Adults):** 2.5–10 mg, may be repeated q 5–10 min for 3 doses in 15–30 min (inital dose of chewable tablet should not exceed 5 mg).

Prophylaxis of Angina Pectoris

- **SL, Chew, Intrabuccal (Adults):** 2.5–10 mg, may be repeated q 2–3 hr (ini-

{} = Available in Canada only.
*<u>Underlines</u> indicate most frequent; **CAPITALS** indicate life-threatening.

tial dose of chewable tablet should not exceed 5 mg).

- **PO (Adults):** 2.5–30 mg qid or 20 mg q 6–12 hr of extended-release form or 80 mg q 12 hr as extended-release form.

PHARMACODYNAMICS (cardiovascular effects)

	ONSET	PEAK	DURATION
SL, Chew	2–5 min	UK	1–2 hr
PO	15–40 min	UK	4 hr
PO-ER	30 min	UK	up to 12 hr

NURSING IMPLICATIONS

Assessment

- Assess location, duration, intensity, and precipitating factors of anginal pain.
- Monitor blood pressure and pulse routinely during period of dosage adjustment.

Potential Nursing Diagnoses

- Tissue perfusion, altered (indications).
- Activity intolerance (indications).
- Knowledge deficit related to medication regimen (patient/family teaching).

Implementation

- **PO:** Administer 1 hr before or 2 hr after meals with a full glass of water for faster absorption.
- Chewable tablets should be chewed well before swallowing and held in mouth for 2 min. Do not swallow whole.
- Extended-release tablets and capsules should be swallowed whole. Do not crush, break, or chew.
- **SL:** SL tablets should be held under tongue until dissolved.
- Avoid eating, drinking, or smoking until tablet is dissolved. Replace tablet if inadvertently swallowed.

Patient/Family Teaching

- Instruct patient to take medication exactly as directed, even if feeling better. If a dose is missed, take as soon as remembered unless next dose is scheduled within 2 hr (6 hr with extended-release preparations). Do not double doses. Do not discontinue abruptly.
- When used for acute anginal attacks, advise patient to sit down and use medication at first sign of attack. Relief usually occurs within 5 min. Dose may be repeated if pain is not relieved in 5–10 min; call physician or go to nearest emergency room if angina pain is not relieved by 3 tablets in 15 min. Only SL and chewable tablets should be used for anginal attacks.
- Caution patient to make position changes slowly to minimize orthostatic hypotension.
- Advise patient to avoid concurrent use of alcohol with this medication. Patients should also consult physician or pharmacist before taking over-the-counter medications while taking isosorbide dinitrate.
- Inform patient that headache is a common side effect that should decrease with continuing therapy. Aspirin or acetaminophen may be ordered to treat headache. Notify physician if headache is persistent or severe.
- Advise patient to notify physician if dry mouth or blurred vision occurs or if undigested extended-release tablets appear in stool.

Evaluation

Effectiveness of therapy can be demonstrated by: ▪ Decrease in frequency and severity of anginal attacks ▫ Increase in activity tolerance.

ISOTRETINOIN

(eye-soe-**tret**-i-noyn)
Accutane, {Accutane Roche}

CLASSIFICATION(S):
Antiacne agent
Pregnancy Category X

INDICATIONS

- Management of cystic acne resistant to more conventional therapy, including topical therapy and systemic antibiotics.

ACTION

▪ A metabolite of vitamin A (retinol); reduces sebaceous gland size and differentiation. **Therapeutic Effects:** ▪ Diminution and resolution of severe acne. May also prevent abnormal keratinization.

PHARMACOKINETICS

Absorption: 23–25% absorbed following oral administration.
Distribution: Appears to be widely distributed. Probably crosses the placenta.
Metabolism and Excretion: Mostly metabolized by the liver.
Half-life: 10–20 hr.

CONTRAINDICATIONS AND PRECAUTIONS

Contraindicated in: ▪ Hypersensitivity to retinoids or parabens ▪ Pregnant patients ▪ Women of childbearing age who may become or intend to become pregnant ▪ Lactation ▪ Patients planning to donate blood.
Use Cautiously in: ▪ Pre-existing hypertriglyceridemia ▪ Diabetes mellitus ▪ Alcoholics ▪ Obese patients ▪ Inflammatory bowel disease.

ADVERSE REACTIONS AND SIDE EFFECTS*

CNS: pseudotumor cerebrii.
EENT: epistaxis, conjunctivitis, dry eyes, cornea opacities, blurred vision, decreased night vision.
CV: edema.
GI: cheilitis, dry mouth, anorexia, nausea, vomiting, abdominal pain, increased appetite, hepatitis.
Derm: pruritus, thinning of hair, palmar desquamation, skin infections, photosensitivity.
Hemat: decreased hemoglobin, decreased hematocrit.
Metab: hypertriglyceridemia, hypercholesterolemia, decreased high-density lipoproteins, hyperglycemia, hyperuricemia.
MS: bone pain, arthralgia, hyperostosis.
Misc: thirst.

INTERACTIONS

Drug–Drug: ▪ Additive toxicity with **vitamin A** and **related compounds** ▪ Increased risk of pseudotumor cerebreii with **tetracycline** or **minocycline** ▪ Concurrent use with **alcohol** increases hypertriglyceridemia ▪ Drying effects increased by concurrent use of **benzoyl peroxide, sulfur, tretinoin,** and **other topical agents.**
Drug–Food: ▪ Excessive ingestion of **foods high in vitamin A content** may result in additive toxicity.

ROUTE AND DOSAGE

▪ **PO (Adults):** 0.5–1 mg/kg/day (up to 2 mg/kg/day) in 2 divided doses for 15–20 wk. Once discontinued, if relapse occurs, therapy may be reinstituted after an 8-wk rest period.

PHARMACODYNAMICS (diminution of acne)

	ONSET	PEAK	DURATION
PO	UK	up to 8 wk	UK

NURSING IMPLICATIONS

Assessment

- □ Assess skin prior to and periodically during therapy. Transient worsening of acne may occur at initiation of therapy. Note number and severity of cysts, degree of skin dryness, erythema, and itching.
- □ Assess for allergy to parabens, as capsules contain parabens as a preservative.
- ▪ **Lab Test Consideration:** Monitor liver function (SGOT [AST], SGPT [ALT], and LDH) prior to therapy, after 1 mon of therapy, and periodically thereafter. Inform physician if these values become elevated; therapy may need to be discontinued.
- □ Monitor blood lipids (cholesterol, high-density lipoproteins, triglycer-

*Underlines indicate most frequent; **CAPITALS** indicate life-threatening.

ides) prior to beginning therapy, after 1 mon, and periodically thereafter. Inform physician of increase in cholesterol and triglyceride levels or decrease in high-density lipoproteins.

- □ Obtain baseline and periodic CBC, urinalysis, and SMA-12. May cause increased blood glucose, CPK, platelet counts, and sedimentation rate. May decrease RBC and WBC parameters. May cause proteinuria, red and white blood cells in urine, and elevated uric acid.

Potential Nursing Diagnoses

- Skin integrity, impaired (indications, side effects).
- Body image disturbance (indications).
- Knowledge deficit related to medication regimen (patient/family teaching).

Implementation

- **PO:** Daily dose is administered in 2 divided doses.

Patient/Family Teaching

- □ Instruct patient to take isotretinoin exactly as directed. Do not take more than the amount prescribed. If a dose is missed, take as soon as remembered if not almost time for next dose. Do not double doses.
- □ Explain to patient that a temporary worsening of acne may occur at beginning of therapy.
- □ Instruct female patients to use contraception 1 mon before therapy, throughout therapy, and for at least 1 mon after discontinuation of drug. This drug is contraindicated during pregnancy and may cause birth defects. Physician may order pregnancy test 2 wk prior to initiation of therapy. Patient should discontinue medication and inform physician immediately if pregnancy is suspected. Recommended consent form prepared by manufacturer stresses fetal risk. Parents of minors should also read and sign form.
- □ May cause sudden decrease in night vision. Caution patient to avoid driving at night until response to the medication is known.
- □ Advise patient to consult with physician before using other acne preparations while taking isotretinoin. Soaps, cosmetics, and shaving lotion may also worsen dry skin.
- □ Inform patient that dry skin and chapped lips will occur. Lubricant to lips may help cheilitis.
- □ Instruct patient that oral rinses, good oral hygiene, and sugarless gum or candy may help minimize dry mouth. Notify physician if dry mouth persists for more than 2 wk.
- □ Discuss possibility of excessively dry eyes with patients who wear contact lenses. Patient should contact physician about eye lubricant. Patient may need to switch to glasses during course of therapy and for up to 2 wk following discontinuation.
- □ Advise patient to avoid alcoholic beverages while taking isotretinoin, as this may further increase triglyceride levels.
- □ Caution patient to use sunscreen and protective clothing to prevent photosensitivity reactions. Physician should be consulted about sunscreen, as some sunscreens may worsen acne.
- □ Instruct patient not to take vitamin A supplements and to avoid excessive ingestion of foods high in vitamin A (liver, fish liver oils, egg yolks, yellow-orange fruits and vegetables, dark green leafy vegetables, whole milk, vitamin A-fortified skim milk, butter, margarine) while taking isotretinoin; this may result in hypervitaminosis.
- □ Advise patient not to donate blood while receiving this medication. After discontinuing isotretinoin, wait at least 1 mon before donating blood to prevent the possibility of a pregnant patient receiving the blood.
- □ Instruct patient to report burning of eyes, visual changes, rash, abdominal pain, diarrhea, headache, nausea, and vomiting to physician.

- Inform patient of need for medical follow-up. Physician may order periodic lab tests.

EVALUATION

Effectiveness of therapy can be demonstrated by: ▪ Decrease in the number and severity of cysts in severe acne. Therapy may take 4–5 mon before full effects are seen. Therapy is discontinued when the number of cysts is reduced by 70% or after 5 mon. Improvement may occur after discontinuation of therapy; therefore, a delay of at least 8 wk is recommended before a second course of therapy is considered.

ISRADIPINE

(is-**ra**-di-peen)
DynaCirc

CLASSIFICATION(S):
Calcium channel blocker, Antihypertensive—calcium channel blocker
Pregnancy Category C

INDICATIONS

▪ Management of hypertension, alone or in combination with thiazide-type diuretics.

ACTION

▪ Inhibits the transport of calcium into vascular smooth muscle cells, resulting in the inhibition of excitation-contraction coupling and subsequent contraction. Net result is vasodilation. **Therapeutic Effect:** ▪ Lowering of blood pressure.

PHARMACOKINETICS

Absorption: Well absorbed following oral administration, but large amounts are rapidly metabolized resulting in decreased bioavailability.
Distribution: Distribution not known. 95% bound to plasma proteins.
Metabolism and Excretion: Mostly metabolized by the liver.
Half-life: 8 hr.

CONTRAINDICATIONS AND PRECAUTIONS

Contraindicated in: ▪ Hypersensitivity ▪ Sick sinus syndrome, 2nd- or 3rd-degree heart block (without a pacemaker) ▪ Severe hypotension.
Use Cautiously in: ▪ Severe hepatic disease (dosage reduction may be required) ▪ Congestive heart failure ▪ Pregnancy, lactation, or children (safety not established).

ADVERSE REACTIONS AND SIDE EFFECTS*

CNS: headache, fatigue, dizziness.
Resp: shortness of breath.
CV: peripheral edema, palpitations, angina, tachycardia.
GI: nausea, diarrhea, abdominal discomfort, vomiting.
Derm: rashes, flushing.

INTERACTIONS

Drug-Drug: ▪ **Beta-adrenergic blockers** may increase the risk of myocardial depression ▪ **Fentanyl** increases the risk of hypotension.

ROUTE AND DOSAGE

- **PO (Adults):** 2.5 mg twice daily, may be increased at 2–4 wk intervals by 5 mg/day (not to exceed 20 mg/day).

PHARMACODYNAMICS (antihypertensive effect)

	ONSET	PEAK	DURATION
PO	<2 hr	2–3 hr	12 hr

*Maximum antihypertensive effects may require 2–4 wk of therapy.

NURSING IMPLICATIONS

ASSESSMENT

- Monitor blood pressure and pulse prior to and periodically throughout therapy. Monitor ECG periodically in patients receiving prolonged therapy.
- Monitor intake and output ratios and daily weight. Assess patient for signs of congestive heart failure (peripheral edema, rales/crackles, dyspnea, weight gain, jugular venous distention).

*Underlines indicate most frequent; **CAPITALS** indicate life-threatening.

- **Lab Test Considerations:** Monitor hepatic function periodically in patients receiving long-term therapy. May cause elevated liver function tests.

Potential Nursing Diagnoses
- Cardiac output, decreased (indications).
- Knowledge deficit related to medication regimen (patient/family teaching).

Implementation
- **PO:** Administration with food significantly increases the time to peak effects by about 1 hr, but has no effect on the total bioavailability of isradipine.

Patient/Family Teaching
- Advise patient to take medication exactly as directed, not to skip or double up on missed doses. Isradipine may need to be discontinued gradually.
- Caution patients to make position changes slowly to minimize orthostatic hypotension.
- Isradipine may cause dizziness. Advise patient to avoid driving or other activities requiring alertness until response to the medication is known.
- Instruct patient to avoid concurrent use of alcohol or over-the-counter medications without consulting physician or pharmacist.
- Advise patient to notify the physician if irregular heart beats, dyspnea, swelling of hands and feet, pronounced dizziness, nausea, constipation, or hypotension occur.

Evaluation
Effectiveness of therapy can be demonstrated by: ▪ Decrease in blood pressure. Antihypertensive response may be seen in 2–3 hr, but maximal response may require 2–4 wk.

KANAMYCIN
Kan-a-**mye**-sin)
Kantrex

CLASSIFICATION(S):
Anti-infective—aminoglycoside
Pregnancy Category D

INDICATIONS
▪ Treatment of gram-negative bacillary infections and infections due to staphylococci when penicillins or other less toxic drugs are contraindicated ▪ Treatment of the following infections due to susceptible organisms: ▫ Bone infections ▫ Respiratory tract infections ▫ Skin and soft tissue infections ▫ Abdominal infections ▫ Complicated urinary tract infections ▫ Endocarditis ▫ Septicemia ▪ Treatment of enterococcal infections requires synergy with a penicillin ▪ Adjunct therapy in the management of hepatic encephalopathy.

ACTION
▪ Inhibits protein synthesis in bacteria at the level of the 30S ribosome. **Therapeutic Effect:** ▪ Bactericidal action against susceptible bacteria. **Spectrum:** ▪ *Pseudomonas aeruginosa* ▪ *Klebsiella pneumoniae* ▪ *Escherichia coli* ▪ *Proteus* ▪ *Serratia* ▪ *Acenitobacter.*

PHARMACOKINETICS
Absorption: Poorly absorbed following oral administration. Well absorbed after IM administration. Some absorption follows intraperitoneal instillation.
Distribution: Widely distributed into extracellular fluids following IM or IV administration. Crosses the placenta. Poor penetration into CSF.
Metabolism and Excretion: Excretion is mainly (>90%) renal. Minimal amounts metabolized by the liver.
Half-life: 2–4 hr (increased in renal impairment).

CONTRAINDICATIONS AND PRECAUTIONS
Contraindicated in: ▪ Hypersensitivity ▪ Cross-sensitivity with other aminoglycosides may exist ▪ Hypersensitivity to bisulfites (parenteral only).
Use Cautiously in: ▪ Renal impairment of any kind (dosage adjustments necessary) ▪ Pregnancy and lactation (safety not established) ▪ Neuromuscular disases, such as myasthenia gravis.

ADVERSE REACTIONS AND SIDE EFFECTS*

EENT: ototoxicity (vestibular and cochlear).
GU: nephrotoxicity.
Neuro: enhanced neuromuscular blockade.
Misc: hypersensitivity reactions.

INTERACTIONS

Drug–Drug: ▪ Inactivated by penicillins when coadministered to patients with renal insufficiency ▪ Possible respiratory paralysis after **inhalation anesthetics (ether, cyclopropane, halothane,** or **nitrous oxide)** or **neuromuscular blockers (tubocurarine, succinylcholine, decamethonium)** ▪ Increased incidence of ototoxicity with **loop diuretics (ethacrynic acid, furosemide)** ▪ Increased incidence of nephrotoxicity with other **nephrotoxic drugs.**

ROUTE AND DOSAGE

Note: Not to exceed 1.5 g/day by any route.

Parenteral Therapy for Infections

- **IM, IV (Adults):** 15 mg/kg/day in divided doses q 8–12 hr.
- **IM, IV (Children and Infants):** 15 mg/kg/day in divided doses q 8–12 hr.

Preoperative Intestinal Antisepsis

- **PO (Adults):** 1 g q 4–6 hr for 36–72 hr.

Intraperitoneal Instillation

- **Intraperitoneal (Adults):** 500 mg in 20 ml sterile water.

Irrigation of Pleural, Ventricular, or Abscess Cavities

- **Irrigation (Adults):** 0.25% soln.

Inhalation

- **Inhaln (Adults):** 250 mg by nebulization 2–4 times daily.

Adjunct in the Treatment of Hepatic Encephalopathy

- **PO (Adults):** 8–12 g/day, in divided doses.

PHARMACODYNAMICS (blood levels)

	ONSET	PEAK
IM	rapid	0.5–2 hr
IV	rapid	end of infusion

NURSING IMPLICATIONS

Assessment

- Assess patient for infection (vital signs; appearance of wound, sputum, urine, and stool; WBC) at beginning and throughout course of therapy.
- Obtain specimens for culture and sensitivity prior to initiating therapy. First dose may be given before receiving results.
- Evaluate eighth cranial nerve function by audiometry prior to and throughout course of therapy. Hearing loss is usually of the high-frequency type. Prompt recognition and intervention is essential in preventing permanent damage. Also monitor for vestibular dysfunction (vertigo, ataxia, nausea, vomiting). Eighth cranial nerve dysfunction is associated with persistently elevated peak kanamycin levels.
- Monitor intake and output and daily weight to assess hydration status and renal function.
- Assess patient for signs of superinfection (fever, upper respiratory infection, vaginal itching or discharge, increasing malaise, diarrhea). Report to physician.
- **Lab Test Considerations:** Monitor renal function by urinalysis, specific gravity, BUN, creatinine, and creatinine clearance prior to and throughout therapy.
- May cause increased SGOT (AST), SGPT (ALT), LDH, bilirubin, and serum alkaline phosphatase levels.
- May cause decreased serum calcium, magnesium, sodium, and potassium levels.
- **Toxicity and Overdose:** Blood levels should be monitored periodically during therapy. Timing of blood lev-

*Underlines indicate most frequent; **CAPITALS** indicate life-threatening.

els is important in interpreting results. Draw blood for peak levels 30–60 min after IM injection and immediately after IV infusion is completed. Trough levels should be drawn just prior to next dose. Acceptable peak level is 15–30 mcg/ml; trough level should not exceed 5–10 mcg/ml.

POTENTIAL NURSING DIAGNOSES

- Infection, high risk for (indications).
- Sensory-perceptual alteration: auditory (side effects).
- Knowledge deficit related to medication regimen (patient/family teaching).

IMPLEMENTATION

- **General Info:** Keep patient well-hydrated (1500–2000 ml/day) during therapy.
- **PO:** May be taken without regard to meals.
- **IM:** Administration should be deep into a well-developed muscle.
- **Intermittent Infusion:** Dilute each 500 mg of kanamycin in 100–200 ml or each 1 g in 200–400 ml of D5W, D10W, D5/0.9% NaCl, 0.9% NaCl, or lactated Ringer's soln. Darkening of soln does not alter potency.
  - Administer separately, manufacturer does not recommend admixing. Give aminoglycosides and penicillins at least 1 hr apart to prevent inactivation.
  - *Rate:* Infuse slowly over 30–60 min. Flush IV line with D5W or 0.9% NaCl following administration.
- **Syringe Incompatibility:** heparin.
- **Y-Site Compatibility:** cyclophosphamide, furosemide, heparin with hydrocortisone sodium succinate, hydromorphone, magnesium sulfate, meperidine, morphine, perphenazine, or potassium chloride.
- **Additive Compatibility:** ascorbic acid, cefoxitin, chloramphenicol, clindamycin, dopamine, furosemide, polymyxin B, sodium bicarbonate, or tetracycline.
- **Additive Incompatibility:** amphotericin B, cephalothin, cephapirin, chlorpheniramine, colistimethate, heparin, or methohexital.
- **Intraperitoneal:** Dilute each 500-mg vial with 20 ml of sterile water for injection. May be instilled postoperatively via polyethylene catheter sutured into wound at closure. Hold instillation until patient has fully recovered from anesthesia to prevent neuromuscular blockade.
- **Irrigation:** May be administered as an irrigation in a concentration of 0.25%.
- **Inhaln:** Reconstitute 250 mg in 3 ml of 0.9% NaCl for nebulization.

PATIENT/FAMILY TEACHING

- **General Info:** Instruct patient to report signs of hypersensitivity, tinnitus, vertigo, or hearing loss.
- **PO:** Instruct patient to take kanamycin as directed. Missed doses should be taken as soon as remembered if not almost time for next dose; do not double doses.

EVALUATION

Clinical response can be evaluated by:
- Resolution of the signs and symptoms of infection. If no response is seen within 3–5 days, new cultures should be taken. Length of time for resolution depends on the organism and site of infection.

KAOLIN/PECTIN

(**kay**-oh-lin **pek**-tin)
{Donnagel-MB}, K-C, K-P, K-Pek, {Kao-Con}, Kaopectate, Kaopectate Concentrate, Kaotin, Kapectolin

CLASSIFICATION(S):
Antidiarrheal
Pregnancy Category UK

INDICATIONS

- Adjunctive therapy in the treatment of mild to moderate diarrhea.

ACTION

- Acts as an adsorbent and protectant
- Decreases stool fluid content, al-

K

though total water loss does not change. **Therapeutic Effect:** ▪ Relief of diarrhea.

PHARMACOKINETICS

Absorption: Action is local, not systemically absorbed.
Distribution: Distribution not known.
Metabolism and Excretion: Pectin decomposes in the GI tract.
Half-life: UK.

CONTRAINDICATIONS AND PRECAUTIONS

Contraindicated in: ▪ Severe abdominal pain of unknown cause, especially when associated with fever ▪ Children <3 yr.
Use Cautiously in: ▪ Elderly patients (>60 yr) ▪ Diarrhea continuing >48 hr (physician should be consulted).

ADVERSE REACTIONS AND SIDE EFFECTS*

GI: constipation.

INTERACTIONS

Drug-Drug: ▪ Decreases the absorption of **digoxin** and **chloroquine**.

ROUTE AND DOSAGE

Note: Kaolin/pectin suspension contains 0.65–0.98 g kaolin/5 ml and 21.7–43.5 mg pectin/5 ml. Concentrated suspension contains 1.46 g kaolin/5 ml and 32.4 mg pectin/5 ml.

- **PO (Adults):** 60–120 ml (45–90 ml concentrate) after each loose stool.
- **PO (Children 6–11 yr):** 30–60 ml (30 ml concentrate) after each loose stool.
- **PO (Children 3–5 yr):** 15–30 ml (15 ml concentrate) after each loose stool.

PHARMACODYNAMICS (relief of diarrhea)

	ONSET	PEAK	DURATION
PO	30 min	UK	4–6 hr

NURSING IMPLCATIONS

Assessment

- □ Assess the frequency and consistency of stools and bowel sounds prior to and throughout course of therapy.
- □ Assess fluid and electrolyte balance and skin turgor for dehydration.

Potential Nursing Diagnoses

- ▪ Bowel elimination, altered: diarrhea (indications).
- ▪ Bowel elimination, altered: constipation (side effects).
- ▪ Knowledge deficit related to medication regimen (patient/family teaching).

Implementation

- ▪ **General Info:** Administer after each loose bowel movement until diarrhea is controlled.
- □ Available in combination with other drugs (see Appendix A).
- ▪ **PO:** Shake suspension well prior to administration.

Patient/Family Teaching

- □ Instruct patient to notify physician if diarrhea persists longer than 48 hr or if fever or abdominal pain develops.

Evaluation

Effectiveness of therapy can be demonstrated by: ▪ Decrease in frequency of loose stools □ Return to soft, formed stools.

KETAMINE

(**ket**-a-meen)
Ketalar

CLASSIFICATION(S):
Anesthetic—general
Pregnancy Category UK

INDICATIONS

▪ Provides anesthesia for short-term procedures ▪ As induction prior to the use of other anesthetics ▪ As a supplement to other anesthetics.

*Underlines indicate most frequent; **CAPITALS** indicate life-threatening.

ACTION

▪ Blocks afferent impulses of pain perception ▪ Suppresses spinal cord activity ▪ Effects CNS transmitter systems.
Therapeutic Effects: ▪ Anesthesia with profound analgesia, minimal respiratory depression, and minimal skeletal muscle relaxation.

PHARMACOKINETICS

Absorption: Rapidly absorbed following IM administration.
Distribution: Rapidly distributed, enters the CNS. Crosses the placenta.
Metabolism and Excretion: Mostly metabolized by the liver. Some conversion to another active compound.
Half-life: 2.5 hr.

CONTRAINDICATIONS AND PRECAUTIONS

Contraindicated in: ▪ Hypersensitivity ▪ Psychiatric disturbances ▪ Hypertension ▪ Pregnancy or lactation.
Use Cautiously in: ▪ Cardiovascular disease ▪ Procedures involving larynx, pharynx, or bronchial tree (muscle relaxants required) ▪ History of alcohol abuse ▪ Cerebral trauma ▪ Intracerebral mass or hemorrhage ▪ Hyperthyroidism ▪ History of psychiatric problems ▪ Increased CSF pressure ▪ Increased intraocular pressure ▪ Severe eye trauma.

ADVERSE REACTIONS AND SIDE EFFECTS*

CNS: emergence reactions.
EENT: diplopia, nystagmis, increased introcular pressure.
Resp: respiratory depression and apnea (rapid IV administration of large doses), laryngospasm.
CV: hypertension, tachycardia, hypotension, bradycardia, arrhythmias.
GI: nausea, vomiting, excessive salivation.
Derm: erythema, rash.
Local: pain at injection site.
MS: increased skeletal muscle tone.

INTERACTIONS

Drug-Drug: ▪ Use with **barbiturates** or **narcotic analgesics** may result in prolonged recovery time ▪ Use with **halothane** may result in decreased blood pressure, cardiac output, and heart rate ▪ Use with **tubocurarine** or **nondepolarizing neuromuscular blocking agents** may result in prolonged respiratory depression ▪ Concurrent use with **thyroid hormone** increases the risk of tachycardia and hypertension ▪ Concurrent administration with **diazepam** may decrease the incidence of emergence reaction ▪ Concurrent administration with **atropine** may increase the incidence of unpleasant dreams.

ROUTE AND DOSAGE

- **IV (Adults and Children):** *Induction*—1–4.5 mg/kg (average dose—2 mg/kg produces 5–10 min of surgical anesthesia) or 1–2 mg/kg (at rate of 0.5 mg/kg/min) with diazepam. *Maintenance*—one half to the full induction dose may be repeated as needed to maintain anesthesia or 0.01–0.05 mg/kg as an infusion at 1–2 mg/min. If given with concurrent diazepam, an infusion of 0.1–0.5 mg/min may be used, augmented by 2–5-mg doses of diazepam.
- **IM (Adults and Children):** 5–10 mg/kg (10 mg/kg produces 12–25 min of surgical anesthesia).

PHARMACODYNAMICS (anesthesia)

	ONSET	PEAK	DURATION
IV	30 sec	UK	5–10 min
IM	3–4 min	UK	12–25 min

NURSING IMPLICATIONS

ASSESSMENT

□ Assess level of consciousness frequently throughout therapy. Ketamine produces a dissociative state. The patient does not appear to be asleep and experiences a feeling of dissociation from the environment.

*Underlines indicate most frequent; **CAPITALS** indicate life-threatening.

K

- ▫ Monitor blood pressure, ECG, and respiratory status frequently throughout therapy. May cause hypertension and tachycardia. May cause increased cerebrospinal fluid pressure and increased intraocular pressure.
- ▪ **Toxicity and Overdose:** Respiratory depression or apnea may be treated with mechanical ventilation or analeptics.

Potential Nursing Diagnoses

- ▪ Injury, high risk for (side effects).
- ▪ Sensory-perceptual alteration (adverse reactions).
- ▪ Knowledge deficit related to medication regimen (patient/family teaching).

Implementation

- ▪ **General Info:** Administer on an empty stomach to prevent vomiting and aspiration.
- ▫ May be administered concurrently with a drying agent (atropine, scopolamine), as ketamine increases salivary and tracheobronchial mucous gland secretions. Atropine may also increase the incidence of unpleasant dreams.
- ▫ Patients may experience a state of confusion (emergence delirium) during recovery from ketamine. Administration of a benzodiazepine and minimizing verbal, tactile, and visual stimulation may prevent emergence delirium. Severe emergence delirium may be treated with short- or ultrashort-acting barbiturates.
- ▪ **Direct IV:** Dilute 100 mg/ml concentration with equal parts of sterile water for injection, 0.9% NaCl, or D5W.
- ▫ *Rate:* Administer over 60 sec unless a rapid-sequence induction technique is indicated. More rapid administration may cause respiratory depression, apnea, and hypertension.
- ▪ **Continuous Infusion:** Dilute 10 ml of 50 mg/ml concentration or 5 ml of 100 mg/ml concentration with 500 ml of 0.9% NaCl or D5W and mix well, for a concentration of 1 mg/ml. Dilution with 250 ml may be used if fluid restriction is needed.
- ▫ *Rate:* Administer at a rate of 1–2 mg/min. Dosage must be titrated according to individual patient requirements. Tonic-clonic movements during anesthesia do not indicate the need for more ketamine.
- ▪ **Syringe Compatibility:** benzquinamide.
- ▪ **Syringe Incompatibility:** barbiturates, diazepam, or doxipram.

Patient/Family Teaching

- ▫ Psychomotor impairment may last for 24 hr following anesthesia. Caution patient to avoid driving or other activities requiring alertness until response to medication is known.
- ▫ Advise patient to avoid alcohol or other CNS depressants for 24 hr following anesthesia.

Evaluation

Effectiveness of therapy can be demonstrated by: ▪ Sense of dissociation and general anesthesia without muscle relaxation.

KETOCONAZOLE

(kee-toe-**koe**-na-zole)

Nizoral

CLASSIFICATION(S):

Antifungal

Pregnancy Category C

INDICATIONS

▪ **PO:** Treatment of the following fungal infections: ▫ Candidiasis (disseminated and mucocutaneous) ▫ Chromomycosis ▫ Coccidiomycosis ▫ Histoplasmosis ▫ Paracoccidiomycosis ▪ **Top:** Treatment of fungal dermatologic infections caused by: ▫ *Tinea corporis* ▫ *Tinea cruris* ▫ *Tinea versicolor* ▪ **Shampoo:** Treatment of seborrheic dermatitis and dandruff due to *Pityrosporum ovale*. **Unlabeled Uses:** ▪ *PO:* Treatment of advanced prostate cancer ▪ Treatment of Cushing's syndrome.

ACTION

▪ Disrupts fungal cell wall ▪ Interferes with fungal metabolism ▪ Also inhibits the production of adrenal steroids. **Therapeutic Effect:** ▪ Fungistatic or fungicidal action against susceptible organisms, depending on organism and site of infection. **Spectrum:** ▪ Active against many pathogenic fungi, including: ▫ Blastomycoses ▫ *Candida* ▫ *Coccidioides* ▫ *Cryptococcus* ▫ *Histoplasma* ▫ Many dermatophytes.

PHARMACOKINETICS

Absorption: Absorption from the GI tract is pH dependent; increasing pH decreases absorption. Negligable absorption following topical administration.
Distribution: Widely distributed. CNS penetration is unpredictable and minimal. Crosses the placenta and enters breast milk.
Metabolism and Excretion: Partially metabolized by the liver. Excreted in feces via biliary excretion.
Half-life: 8 hr.

CONTRAINDICATIONS AND PRECAUTIONS

Contraindicated in: ▪ Hypersensitivity ▪ Pregnancy or lactation.
Use Cautiously in: ▪ History of liver disease ▪ Achlorhydria ▪ Alcoholism.

ADVERSE REACTIONS AND SIDE EFFECTS*

Note: For oral ketoconazole, unless indicated.

EENT: photophobia.
GI: HEPATITIS, <u>nausea</u>, <u>vomiting</u>, abdominal pain, flatulence, constipation, diarrhea.
Derm: PO—rashes; Top—stinging, burning, irritation; Shampoo—increased hair loss, altered hair or scalp texture.
Endo: gynecomastia.

INTERACTIONS

Note: For oral ketoconazole, unless indicated.

Drug-Drug: ▪ Drugs that increase gastric pH, including **antacids, nizatadine, famotidine, ranitidine, cimetidine,** or **omeprazole** may decrease absorption ▪ Additive hepatoxicity with other **hepatotoxic agents,** including **alcohol** ▪ **Rifampin** or **isoniazid** may decrease serum levels and effectiveness ▪ May enhance the activity of **oral anticoagulants** ▪ May increase blood levels and toxicity of **cyclosporine** or **glucocorticoids** ▪ May alter the metabolism of **phenytoin** ▪ May decrease serum levels and effectiveness of **theophylline** ▪ Increased risk of arrhythmias with **terfenadine.**

ROUTE AND DOSAGE

- **PO (Adults):** 200–400 mg/day, single dose.
- **PO (Children >2 yr):** 3.3–6.6 mg/kg/day, single dose.
- **Top (Adults and Children):** 2% cream applied 1–2 times daily.
- **Shampoo (Adults):** Massage 2% shampoo into scalp for 1 min, rinse, then reapply for 3 min, then rinse and dry. Shampoo twice weekly for 4 wk waiting at least 3 days between treatments.

PHARMACODYNAMICS (blood levels)

	ONSET	PEAK
PO	rapid	1–4 hr

NURSING IMPLICATIONS

Assessment

- ▫ Assess infected area prior to and periodically throughout therapy.
- ▫ Specimens for culture should be taken prior to instituting therapy. Therapy may be started before results are obtained.
- ▪ **Lab Test Considerations:** Hepatic function tests should be monitored prior to and periodically throughout course of therapy. May cause increased SGOT (ALT), SGPT (AST), serum alkaline phosphatase, and bilirubin concentrations.

*<u>Underlines</u> indicate most frequent; **CAPITALS** indicate life-threatening.

K

□ May cause decreased serum testosterone concentrations.

Potential Nursing Diagnoses

▪ Infection, high risk for (indications).

▪ Knowledge deficit related to medication regimen (patient/family teaching).

Implementation

▪ **PO:** Administer with meals or snacks to minimize nausea and vomiting.

□ Shake suspension well prior to administration.

□ Do not administer histamine H_2 antagonists within 2 hr of ketoconazole.

□ For patients with achlorhydria, dissolve each tablet in 4 ml of aqueous soln of 0.2 N hydrochloric acid. Use a glass or plastic straw to avoid contact with teeth and follow with a glass of water, swished in mouth and swallowed. Patients with AIDS may be at increased risk for achlorhydria.

▪ **Top:** Apply enough medication to cover affected and surrounding areas and rub in gently.

Patient/Family Teaching

▪ **General Info:** Instruct patient to take medication exactly as directed, even if feeling better. Doses should be taken at the same time each day. If a dose is missed, take as soon as remembered; if almost time for next dose, space missed dose and next dose 10–12 hr apart.

□ Advise patient to avoid taking over-the-counter antacids within 2 hr of ketoconazole.

□ Caution patient to wear sunglasses and to avoid prolonged exposure to bright light to prevent photophobic reactions.

□ Advise patient to avoid concurrent use of alcohol while taking ketoconazole.

□ Instruct patient to notify physician if abdominal pain, fever, or diarrhea become pronounced or if signs and symptoms of liver dysfunction (unusual fatigue, anorexia, nausea, vomiting, jaundice, dark urine, or pale stools) occur.

▪ **Top:** Caution patient to avoid contact of medication with eyes.

□ Advise patient to use a bland, absorbent or antifungal powder on the skin between administration times for cream.

□ Instruct patient with tinea cruris to wear loose-fitting cotton underwear and to avoid tight-fitting or synthetic clothing.

□ Instruct patient with tinea pedis to dry feet, especially between toes, after bathing. Sandals or well-ventilated shoes with cotton socks should be worn and socks changed daily or more often if feet perspire excessively. Avoid wool or synthetic socks.

□ Advise patient to notify physician if skin irritation develops or if no improvement is seen in 2–4 wk.

▪ **Shampoo:** Moisten hair and scalp with water and apply enough shampoo to lather scalp and hair. Gently massage over entire scalp for 1 min. Rinse thoroughly with warm water. Repeat, leaving shampoo on scalp for an additional 3 min and rinse.

□ Shampoo twice weekly for 4 wk with at least 3 days between shampooing, then intermittently prn.

Evaluation

Effectiveness of therapy can be demonstrated by: ▪ Resolution of clinical and laboratory indications of fungal infections □ Minimal treatment for candidiasis is 1–2 wk and for other systemic mycoses is 6 mon □ Chronic mucocutaneous candidiasis usually requires maintenance therapy □ Tinea infections should be treated for at least 2–4 wk ▪ Reduction of scaling due to dandruff.

KETOPROFEN

(kee-toe-**proe**-fen)

Orudis, {Orudis-E}

CLASSIFICATION(S):

Nonsteroidal anti-inflammatory agent

Pregnancy Category B

{} = Available in Canada only.

INDICATIONS

■ Management of inflammatory disorders, including: □ Rheumatoid arthritis □ Osteoarthritis ■ Management of mild to moderate pain, including dysmenorrhea.

ACTION

■ Inhibits prostaglandin synthesis. **Therapeutic Effects:** ■ Suppression of pain and inflammation.

PHARMACOKINETICS

Absorption: Well absorbed from the GI tract.
Distribution: Distribution not known.
Metabolism and Excretion: Mostly (60%) metabolized by the liver. Some renal excretion.
Half-life: 2–4 hr.

CONTRAINDICATIONS AND PRECAUTIONS

Contraindicated in: ■ Hypersensitivity ■ Cross-sensitivity may exist with other nonsteroidal anti-inflammatory agents, including aspirin ■ Active GI bleeding ■ Ulcer disease.
Use Cautiously in: ■ Severe cardiovascular, renal, or hepatic disease. ■ History of ulcer disease ■ Pregnancy, lactation, or children (safety not established) ■ Renal impairment (dosage reduction suggested).

ADVERSE REACTIONS AND SIDE EFFECTS*

CNS: headache, drowsiness, dizziness.
EENT: blurred vision, tinnitus.
CV: edema.
GI: nausea, dyspepsia, vomiting, diarrhea, constipation, GI BLEEDING, discomfort, HEPATITIS, flatulence, anorexia.
GU: renal failure, hematuria, cystitis.
Derm: rashes.
Endo: gynecomastia.
Hemat: blood dyscrasias, prolonged bleeding time.
MS: myalgia.
Misc: allergic reactions, including ANAPHYLAXIS, fever.

INTERACTIONS

Drug-Drug: ■ Aspirin alters distribution, metabolism, and excretion of ketoprofen (concurrent use not recommended) ■ Additive adverse GI effects with other **nonsteroidal anti-inflammatory agents, potassium supplements, glucocorticoids,** or **alcohol** ■ Chronic use with **acetaminophen may increase the risk of adverse renal reactions** ■ May decrease the effectiveness of **diuretics** or **antihypertensive** therapy ■ May increase the hypoglycemic effects of **insulin** or **oral hypoglycemic agents** ■ May increase serum **lithium** levels and increase the risk of toxicity ■ Increases the risk of toxicity from **methotrexate** ■ **Probenecid** increases risk of toxicity from ketoprofen (concurrent use not recommended) ■ Increased risk of bleeding with **cefamandole, cefotetan, cefoperazone, moxalactam** or **plicamycin, heparin, thrombolytic agents,** or **oral anticoagulants** ■ Increased risk of adverse hematologic reactions with **antineoplastic agents** or **radiation therapy**.

ROUTE AND DOSAGE

■ **PO (Adults):** 150–300 mg/day in 3–4 divided doses.

PHARMACODYNAMICS

	ONSET	PEAK	DURATION
PO (analgesic)	1–2 days	UK	UK
PO (anti-inflammatory)	few days–1 wk	UK	UK

NURSING IMPLICATIONS

Assessment

■ **General Info:** Patients who have asthma, aspirin-induced allergy, and nasal polyps are at increased risk for developing hypersensitivity reactions. Assess for rhinitis, wheezing, and urticaria.
■ **Arthritis:** Assess pain and range of motion prior to and 1 hr following administration.

*Underlines indicate most frequent; **CAPITALS** indicate life-threatening.

- **Pain:** Assess pain (note type, location, and intensity) prior to and 1 hr following administration.
- **Lab Test Considerations:** BUN, serum creatinine, CBC, and liver function tests should be evaluated periodically in patients receiving prolonged courses of therapy.
  - May prolong bleeding time by 3–4 min.
  - May cause decreased hemoglobin and hematocrit.
  - May cause increased SGOT (AST), SGPT (ALT), LDH, and serum alkaline phosphatase.

Potential Nursing Diagnoses
- Comfort, altered: pain (indications).
- Mobility, impaired physical (indications).
- Knowledge deficit related to medication regimen (patient/family teaching).

Implementation
- **General Info:** Coadministration with narcotic analgesics may have additive analgesic effects and may permit lower narcotic doses.
  - Analgesic is more effective if given before pain becomes severe.
- **PO:** For rapid initial effect, administer 30 min before or 2 hr after meals. Capsules may be administered with food, milk, or antacids containing aluminum hydroxide and magnesium hydroxide to decrease GI irritation. Food slows but does not reduce the extent of absorption.
- **Dysmenorrhea:** Administer as soon as possible after the onset of menses. Prophylactic treatment has not been proved effective.

Patient/Family Teaching
- Advise patient to take this medication with a full glass of water and to remain in an upright position for 15–30 min after administration.
- Instruct patient to take medication exactly as directed. If a dose is missed, it should be taken as soon as remembered but not if almost time for the next dose. Do not double doses.
- Medication may occasionally cause drowsiness or dizziness. Advise patient to avoid driving or other activities requiring alertness until response to medication is known.
- Caution patient to avoid the concurrent use of alcohol, aspirin, acetaminophen, or other over-the-counter medications without consulting a physician.
- Advise patient to wear sunscreen and protective clothing to prevent photosensitivity reactions.
- Instruct patient to notify physician if rash, itching, chills, fever, muscle aches, visual disturbances, weight gain, edema, black stools, or persistent headache occurs.
- Advise patient to notify physician or dentist of medication regimen prior to treatment or surgery.

Evaluation
Effectiveness of therapy can be demonstrated by: ▪ Improved joint mobility ▪ Decrease in severity of moderate pain ▫ Improvement in arthritis may be seen in a few days to 1 wk; 2–3 wk may be required for maximum effectiveness. Patients who do not respond to one nonsteroidal anti-inflammatory agent may respond to another.

KETOROLAC
(kee-**toe**-role-ak)
Toradol

CLASSIFICATION(S):
Non-narcotic analgesic, Nonsteroidal anti-inflammatory agent
Pregnancy Category B

INDICATIONS
- Short-term management of pain.

ACTION
- Inhibits prostaglandin synthesis producing peripherally mediated analgesia ▪ Also has antipyretic and anti-inflammatory properties. **Therapeutic Effect:** ▪ Relief of pain.

PHARMACOKINETICS

Absorption: Rapidly and completely absorbed following IM administration.
Distribution: Enters breast milk in low concentrations. >99% bound to plasma proteins.
Metabolism and Excretion: <50% metabolized by the liver. Ketorolac and its metabolites are excreted primarily by the kidneys (92%). 6% excreted in feces.
Half-life: 4.5 hr (range 3.8–6.3; increased in elderly patients and patients with impaired renal function).

CONTRAINDICATIONS AND PRECAUTIONS

Contraindicated in: ▪ Hypersensitivity ▪ Cross-sensitivity with other nonsteroidal anti-inflammatory agents may exist.
Use Cautiously in: ▪ Pregnancy and children (use not recommended) ▪ Lactation (use with caution) ▪ History of GI bleeding ▪ Renal impairment (dosage reduction may be required) ▪ Cardiovascular disease.

ADVERSE REACTIONS AND SIDE EFFECTS*

CNS: drowsiness, dizziness, headache, abnormal thinking, euphoria.
EENT: abnormal vision.
Resp: dyspnea, asthma.
CV: edema, vasodilation, pallor.
GI: abnormal taste, dry mouth, nausea, dyspepsia, GI pain, diarrhea, BLEEDING.
GU: urinary frequency, oliguria, renal toxicity.
Hemat: prolonged bleeding time.
Derm: sweating, pruritus, urticaria, purpura.
Local: injection site pain.
Neuro: paresthesia.

INTERACTIONS

Drug–Drug: ▪ May increase blood levels and risk of toxicity from **lithium** ▪ May decrease clearance and increase risk of toxicity with **methotrexate** ▪ Risk of additive toxicity with other **NSAIDs** or **aspirin**.

ROUTE AND DOSAGE

- **IM (Adults):** 30–60 mg initially, followed by 15–30 mg q 6 hr (not to exceed 150 mg/day on first day or 120 mg/day thereafter).

PHARMACODYNAMICS (analgesic effects)

	ONSET	PEAK	DURATION
IM	about 10 min	75–150 min	3–6 hr

NURSING IMPLICATIONS

Assessment

- □ Patients who have asthma, aspirin-induced allergy, and nasal polyps are at increased risk for developing hypersensitivity reactions. Assess for rhinitis, asthma, and urticaria.
- □ Assess pain (note type, location, and intensity) prior to and 1–2 hr following administration.
- ▪ **Lab Test Considerations:** Liver function tests, especially SGOT (AST) and SGPT (ALT) should be evaluated periodically in patients receiving prolonged courses of therapy. May cause increased levels.
- □ May cause prolonged bleeding time that may persist for 24–48 hr following discontinuation of therapy.

Potential Nursing Diagnoses

- ▪ Comfort, altered: pain (indications).
- ▪ Knowledge deficit related to medication regimen (patient/family teaching).

Implementation

- □ Coadministration with narcotic analgesics may have additive analgesic effects and may permit lower narcotic doses.
- □ Ketorolac may be administered as a routine or prn schedule depending on the type and severity of the pain.

Patient/Family Teaching

- □ Instruct patients taking medication at home on correct technique for IM injection. Instruct patient to take medication exactly as prescribed. If dose is missed it should be taken as soon as

*Underlines indicate most frequent; **CAPITALS** indicate life-threatening.

remembered but not if almost time for next dose. Do not double dose.

- This medication may cause drowsiness or dizziness. Advise patient to avoid driving or other activities requiring alertness until response to the medication is known.
- Caution patient to avoid the concurrent use of alcohol, aspirin, acetaminophen, or other over-the-counter medications without consultation with physician or pharmacist.
- Advise patient to inform physician or dentist of medication regimen prior to treatment or surgery.
- Instruct patient to notify physician if rash, itching, visual disturbances, weight gain, edema, black stools, or persistent headache occur.

Evaluation

Effectiveness of therapy can be demonstrated by: ▪ Decrease in severity of pain. Patients who do not respond to one nonsteroidal anti-inflammatory agent may respond to another.

LABETALOL
(la-**bet**-a-lole)
Normodyne, Trandate

CLASSIFICATION(S):
Beta-adrenergic blocker—nonselective, Antihypertensive-beta-adrenergic blocker
Pregnancy Category C

INDICATIONS

▪ **PO:** Used alone or in combination with other agents in the treatment of hypertension ▪ **IV:** Treatment of severe hypertension. **Unlabeled Uses:** ▪ ***PO:*** Angina pectoris ▪ ***IV:*** Production of controlled hypotension during surgery.

ACTION

▪ Blocks stimulation of $beta_1$ (myocardial) and $beta_2$ (pulmonary, vascular, or uterine) receptor sites ▪ Has alpha-adrenergic blocking activity, which results in peripheral vasodilation and orthostatic hypotension. **Therapeutic Effects:** ▪ Decreased heart rate and blood pressure.

PHARMACOKINETICS

Absorption: Although absorbed following oral administration, rapid metabolism results in low systemic bioavailability (25%).

Distribution: Moderate penetration of the CNS. Crosses the placenta and enters breast milk.

Metabolism and Excretion: Undergoes extensive hepatic metabolism.

Half-life: 3–8 hr.

CONTRAINDICATIONS AND PRECAUTIONS

Contraindicated in: ▪ Hypersensitivity to labetolol ▪ Hypersensitivity to parabens (IV only) ▪ Uncompensated congestive heart failure ▪ Pulmonary edema ▪ Cardiogenic shock ▪ Bradycardia ▪ Heart block ▪ Pregnancy or lactation (may cause apnea, low Apgar scores, bradycardia, and hypoglycemia in the newborn).

Use Cautiously in: ▪ Thyrotoxicosis or hypoglycemia (may mask symptoms) ▪ Do not withdraw abruptly ▪ Renal impairment (dosage reduction recommended) ▪ Children (safety not established).

ADVERSE REACTIONS AND SIDE EFFECTS*

CNS: <u>fatigue</u>, <u>weakness</u>, dizziness, depression, memory loss, mental changes, nightmares.

CV: BRADYCARDIA, CONGESTIVE HEART FAILURE, PULMONARY EDEMA, <u>orthostatic hypotension</u>, peripheral vasoconstriction.

EENT: dry eyes, blurred vision.

GI: constipation, diarrhea, nausea, change in taste.

GU: impotence, diminished libido, urinary retention.

Derm: rash, itching.

Endo: hyperglycemia, hypoglycemia.

*<u>Underlines</u> indicate most frequent; **CAPITALS** indicate life-threatening.

MS: joint pain, arthralgia.
Resp: bronchospasm, wheezing.

INTERACTIONS

Drug–Drug: ▪ **Halothane** anesthesia may produce severe myocardial depression ▪ Additive bradycardia may occur with concurrent use of **cardiac glycosides** ▪ Additive hypotension may occur with other **antihypertensive agents, nitrates,** and acute ingestion of **alcohol** ▪ Concurrent **thyroid** administration may decrease effectiveness ▪ May antagonize **beta-adrenergic bronchodilators** ▪ **Cimetidine** decreases metabolism and may increase toxicity ▪ **Glutethimide** may decrease the effects of labetolol ▪ May blunt tachycardia produced by **nitroglycerin** ▪ Avoid concurrent **MAO inhibitor** therapy (may produce hypertension for up to 14 days following discontinuation of MAO inhibitor).

Drug–Food: ▪ Food increases oral absorption.

ROUTE AND DOSAGE

- **PO (Adults):** 100 mg bid, increase by 100 mg bid q 2–3 days until desired response is obtained. Usual maintenance dose is 200–400 mg bid.
- **IV (Adults):** 20 mg, may give an additional 40–80 mg at 10-min intervals until desired response is obtained or 2-mg/min infusion (total dose should not exceed 300 mg).

PHARMACODYNAMICS (antihypertensive effect)

	ONSET	PEAK	DURATION
PO	20 min–2 hr	1–4 hr	8–12 hr
IV	2–5 min	5–15 min	2–4 hr (up to 24 hr)

NURSING IMPLICATIONS

Assessment

- □ Monitor blood pressure and pulse frequently during period of adjustment and periodically throughout therapy. Confer with physician prior to giving drug if pulse is <50 bpm.
- □ Patients receiving labetolol IV must be supine during and for 3 hr after administration. Vital signs should be monitored every 5–15 min during and for several hrs after administration. Assess for orthostatic hypotension when assisting patient up from supine position.
- □ Monitor intake and output ratios and daily weight. Assess patient routinely for evidence of congestive heart failure (peripheral edema, dyspnea, rales/crackles, fatigue, weight gain, jugular venous distension).
- ▪ **Lab Test Considerations:** Hepatic and renal function and CBC should be monitored routinely in patients receiving prolonged therapy.
- □ May cause elevations in serum potassium, uric acid, LDH, SGOT (AST), SGPT (ALT), alkaline phosphatase, ANA titers, BUN, serum lipoprotein, and triglyceride concentrations.

Potential Nursing Diagnoses

- ▪ Cardiac output, decreased (indications, adverse reactions).
- ▪ Knowledge deficit related to medication regimen (patient/family teaching).
- ▪ Noncompliance (patient/family teaching).

Implementation

- ▪ **PO:** Administer with meals or directly after eating to enhance absorption.
- ▪ **IV:** Soln ranges from clear, colorless to slight yellow in color.
- ▪ **Direct IV:** Administer by injecting 20 mg over 2 min; increase dose to 40–80 mg every 10 min until desired response is achieved.
- ▪ **Continuous Infusion:** Add 200 mg to 160 ml of diluent (1 mg/1 ml soln) or 200 mg to 250 ml of diluent (2 mg/3 ml soln). Compatible diluents include D5W, 0.9% NaCl, D5/0.25% NaCl, D5/0.9% NaCl, D5/Ringer's soln, D5/LR, Ringer's and lactated Ringer's soln.
- □ *Rate:* Administer at a rate of 2 mg/min and titrate for desired response. Infuse via infusion pump to ensure accurate dosage of medication.

L

- **Y-Site Compatibility:** amikacin, aminophylline, ampicillin, butorphanol, calcium gluconate, cefazolin, ceftazidine, ceftizoxime, chloramphenicol, cimetidine, clindamycin, co-trimoxazole, dopamine, enalaprilat, erythromycin lactobionate, famotidine, fentanyl, gentamycin, heparin, lidocaine, magnesium sulfate, metronidazole, morphine, oxycillin, penicillin G potassium, piperacillin, potassium chloride, potassium phosphate, ranitidine, sodium acetate, tobramycin, or vancomycin.
- **Y-Site Incompatibility:** cefoperazone or nafcillin.
- **Additive Incompatibility:** sodium bicarbonate.

Patient/Family Teaching

- Instruct patient to take medication exactly as directed, even if feeling better. If a dose is missed, it may be taken as soon as remembered up to 8 hr before next dose. Abrupt withdrawal may precipitate a severe reaction and result in arrhythmias, hypertension, or myocardial ischemia. Labetolol controls but does not cure hypertension.
- Teach patient and family how to check pulse and blood pressure. Instruct them to take pulse daily and blood pressure biweekly. Advise patient to hold dose and contact physician if pulse is <50 bpm or blood pressure changes significantly.
- Caution patient to make position changes slowly and to avoid standing in a stationary position for long periods to minimize orthostatic hypotension. Patient should also be instructed to call for assistance when ambulating during period of dose adjustment.
- Reinforce need to continue additional therapies for hypertension (weight loss, restricted sodium intake, stress reduction, regular exercise, moderation of alcohol consumption, and cessation of smoking).
- Caution patient that this medication may cause increased sensitivity to cold.
- Advise patient to consult physician or pharmacist before taking any over-the-counter drugs concurrently with this medication.
- Diabetics should monitor serum glucose closely, especially if weakness, fatigue, or irritability occurs.
- Instruct patient to notify physician or dentist of medication regimen prior to treatment or surgery.
- Advise patient to carry identification describing disease process and medication regimen at all times.

Evaluation

Effectiveness of therapy can be demonstrated by: ▪ Decrease in blood pressure.

LACTULOSE
(**lak**-tyoo-lose)
Cephulac, Cholac, Chronulac, Constilac, {Lactulax}

CLASSIFICATION(S):
Laxative—hyperosmotic
Pregnancy Category UK

INDICATIONS

▪ Treatment of chronic constipation in adults and in the elderly ▪ Adjunct in the management of hepatic encephalopathy.

ACTION

▪ Increases water content and softens the stool ▪ Inhibits the diffusion of ammonia from the colon into the blood, thereby reducing blood ammonia levels. **Therapeutic Effects:** ▪ Relief of constipation and decreased blood ammonia levels.

PHARMACOKINETICS

Absorption: Less than 3% absorbed following oral administration.
Distribution: Distribution not known.
Metabolism and Excretion: Absorbed

lactulose is excreted unchanged in the urine. Unabsorbed lactulose is metabolized by colonic bacteria to lactic, acetic, and formic acids.
Half-life: UK.

CONTRAINDICATIONS AND PRECAUTIONS

Contraindicated in: ▪ Patients on low-galactose diets.
Use Cautiously in: ▪ Diabetes mellitus ▪ Pregnancy, lactation, or children (safety not established) ▪ Excessive or prolonged use (may lead to dependence).

ADVERSE REACTIONS AND SIDE EFFECTS*

GI: cramps, distention, flatulence, belching, diarrhea.
Endo: hyperglycemia (diabetic patients).

INTERACTIONS

Drug-Drug: ▪ Do not use with **other laxatives** in the treatment of hepatic encephalopathy ▪ Use with **neomycin** in hepatic encephalopathy may diminish effectiveness.

ROUTE AND DOSAGE

Note: Contains 10 g lactulose/15 ml.

Constipation

- **PO (Adults):** 10–20 g (15–30 ml)/day.

Hepatic Encephalopathy

- **PO (Adults):** 20–30 g (30–45 ml) 3–4 times/day.
- **Rect (Adults):** 200 g (300 ml) diluted and administered as a retention enema.

PHARMACODYNAMICS (relief of constipation)

	ONSET	PEAK	DURATION
PO	24–48 hr	UK	UK

NURSING IMPLICATIONS

Assessment

- **General Info:** Assess patient for abdominal distention, presence of bowel sounds, and normal pattern of bowel function.
  - Assess color, consistency, and amount of stool produced.
- **Hepatic Encephalopathy:** Assess mental status (orientation, level of consciousness) prior to and periodically throughout course of therapy.
- **Lab Test Considerations:** Decreases blood ammonia concentrations by 25–50%.
  - May cause increased blood glucose levels in diabetic patients.
  - Monitor serum electrolytes periodically when used chronically. May cause diarrhea with resulting hypokalemia and hypernatremia.

Potential Nursing Diagnoses

- Bowel elimination, altered: constipation (indications).
- Knowledge deficit related to medication regimen (patient/family teaching).

Implementation

- **General Info:** Darkening of soln does not alter potency.
- **PO:** Mix with fruit juice, water, milk, or carbonated citrus beverage to improve flavor. Administer with a full glass of water or juice. May be administered on an empty stomach for more rapid results.
- **Rect:** To administer enema, use rectal balloon catheter. Mix 300 ml of lactulose with 700 ml of water or 0.9% NaCl. Enema should be retained for 30–60 min. If inadvertently evacuated, may repeat administration.

Patient/Family Teaching

- Encourage patients to utilize other forms of bowel regulation, such as increasing bulk in the diet, increasing fluid intake, increasing mobility. Normal bowel habits are individualized and may vary from 3 times/day to 3 times/wk.
- Caution patients that this medication may cause belching, flatulence, or abdominal cramping. Physician should be notified if this becomes bothersome or if diarrhea occurs.

*Underlines indicate most frequent; **CAPITALS** indicate life-threatening.

L

EVALUATION

Effectiveness of therapy can be demonstrated by: ▪ Passage of a soft, formed bowel movement, usually within 24–48 hr ▪ Clearing of confusion, apathy, and irritation and improved mental status in hepatic encephalopathy ▫ When used in hepatic encephalopathy, dosage will be adjusted until patient averages 2–3 soft bowel movements per day. Improvement may occur within 2 hr following enema and 24–48 hr following oral administration.

LEUCOVORIN CALCIUM

(loo-koe-**vor**-in)

Citrovorum factor, 5-formyl tetrahydrofolate, Folinic acid, Wellcovorin

CLASSIFICATION(S):
Antidote for methotrexate and folic acid antagonists, Vitamin—folic acid analog
Pregnancy Category C

INDICATIONS

▪ Used to minimize the hematologic effects of high-dose methotrexate therapy ("leucovorin rescue") ▪ Management of overdoses of folic acid antagonists (pyrimethamine or trimethoprim) ▪ Treatment of folic acid deficiency unresponsive to oral replacement.

ACTION

▪ The reduced form of folic acid that serves as a cofactor in the synthesis of DNA and RNA. **Therapeutic Effects:** ▪ Reversal of toxic effects of folic acid antagonists, such as methotrexate and trimethoprim ▪ Reversal of folic acid deficiency.

PHARMACOKINETICS

Absorption: Rapidly absorbed following oral administration. Bioavailability decreases with increasing dose.

Distribution: Widely distributed. Concentrates in the CNS and liver.

Metabolism and Excretion: Extensively converted to tetrahydrofolic derivatives, including 5-methyltetrahydrofolate, a major storage form.

Half-life: 3.5 hr.

CONTRAINDICATIONS AND PRECAUTIONS

Contraindicated in: ▪ Hypersensitivity ▪ Hypersensitivity to alcohol (liquid preparation only).

Use Cautiously in: ▪ Undiagnosed anemia (may mask the progression of pernicious anemia) ▪ Pregnancy and lactation (safety not established but has been used safely to treat megaloblastic anemia in pregnancy) ▪ Coadministration with high-dose methotrexate requires crucial timing of dosing and knowledge of methotrexate levels ▪ Ascites ▪ Renal failure ▪ Dehydration ▪ Pleural effusions ▪ Urine pH <7.

ADVERSE REACTIONS AND SIDE EFFECTS*

Hemat: thrombocytosis (intra-arterial methotrexate only).

Misc: allergic reactions (rash, urticaria, wheezing).

INTERACTIONS

Drug-Drug: ▪ May decrease the anticonvulsant effect of **barbiturates, phenytoin,** or **primidone** ▪ High doses of the oral liquid contain significant amounts of **alcohol** and may result in additive CNS depression when used with **other CNS depressants**.

ROUTE AND DOSAGE

High-Dose Methotrexate-Leucovorin Rescue

Note: Must begin leucovorin within 24 hr of methotrexate.

▪ **PO, IM, IV (Adults and Children):** 10 mg/m^2, followed by 10 mg/m^2 PO q 6 hr for 72 hr. If serum creatinine at 24 hr is 50% greater than premethotrexate level, dosage should be increased to 100 mg/m^2 q 3 hr until serum methotrexate level is $<5 \times 10^{-8}$ M. (Daily doses of the liquid preparation

*Underlines indicate most frequent; **CAPITALS** indicate life-threatening.

should not exceed 25 mg due to high alcohol content of preparation). Many other rescue protocols are used.

Megaloblastic Anemia

- **PO, IM, IV (Adults and Children):** up to 1 mg/day.

Treatment of Hematologic Toxicity of other Folic Acid Antagonists

- **PO, IM, IV (Adults and Children):** 5–15 mg.

Prevention of Hematologic Toxicity of other Folic Acid Antagonists

- **IM, IV (Adults and Children):** 0.4–0.5 mg with each dose of folic acid antagonist.

PHARMACODYNAMICS (serum folate levels)

	ONSET	PEAK	DURATION
PO	<5 min	UK	3–6 hr
IM	<5 min	UK	3–6 hr
IV	<5 min	UK	3–6 hr

NURSING IMPLICATIONS

Assessment

- **General Info:** Assess patient for nausea and vomiting secondary to methotrexate therapy or folic acid antagonists (pyrimethamine and trimethoprim) overdose; if present, notify physician. Parenteral route may be necessary to ensure that patient receives dose.
  - Monitor for development of allergic reactions (rash, urticaria, wheezing). Notify physician if these occur.
- **Megaloblastic Anemia:** Assess degree of weakness and fatigue.
- **Leucovorin Rescue:** Monitor serum methotrexate levels to determine dosage and effectiveness of therapy. Leucovorin calcium levels should be equal to or greater than methotrexate level. Rescue continues until serum methotrexate level is $<5 \times 10^{-8}$M.
  - Monitor creatinine clearance and serum creatinine prior to and every 24 hr during therapy to detect methotrexate toxicity. An increase >50% over the pretreatment concentration at 24 hr is associated with severe renal toxicity.
  - Monitor urine pH every 6 hr throughout therapy. pH should be maintained >7 to decrease nephrotoxic effects of high-dose methotrexate. Sodium bicarbonate or acetazolamide may be ordered to alkalinize urine.
- **Megaloblastic Anemia:** Monitor plasma folic acid levels, hemoglobin, hematocrit, and reticulocyte count prior to and periodically during course of therapy.

Potential Nursing Diagnoses

- Injury, high risk for (indications).
- Nutrition, altered: less than body requirements (indications).
- Knowledge deficit related to medication regimen (patient/family teaching).

Implementation

- **General Info:** Make sure leucovorin calcium is available before administering high-dose methotrexate. Administration must be initiated within 24 hr of methotrexate therapy.
  - Administer as soon as possible after toxic dose of folic acid antagonists (pyrimethamine and trimethoprim). Effectiveness of therapy begins to decrease 1 hr after overdose.
- **PO:** Available as a tablet or oral soln.
  - For oral concentrate, mix contents of 60-mg vial with 60 ml aromatic elixir to yield final concentration 1 mg/ml. Stable for 14 days if refrigerated, 7 days at room temperature. Contains 21–33% ethanol. Maximum dose of concentrate is usually 25 mg to limit ethanol intake.
- **IM:** IM route is preferred for treatment of megaloblastic anemia. Ampules of leucovorin calcium injection for IM use do not require reconstitution.
- **IV:** To reconstitute 50-mg vial of leucovorin calcium for injection, add 5 ml of bacteriostatic water or sterile water for injection, to yield a concentration of 10 mg/ml. Use 10 ml diluent for 100-mg vial. Use immediately if reconstituted with sterile water for in-

jection. Stable for 7 days when reconstituted with bacteriostatic water.
- **Direct IV:** Rate of direct IV infusion should not exceed 16 ml/min.
- **Intermittent Infusion:** May be diluted in 100–500 ml of D5W, D10W, 0.9% NaCl, Ringer's or lactated Ringer's soln. Stable for 24 hr.
- **Syringe/Y-Site Compatibility:** bleomycin, cisplatin, cyclophosphamide, doxorubicin, fluorouracil, furosemide, heparin, methotrexate, metoclopramide, mitomycin, vinblastine, or vincristine.
- **Syringe/Y-Site Incompatibility:** droperidol.
- **Additive Compatibility:** floxuridine.

PATIENT/FAMILY TEACHING

- **General Info:** Explain purpose of medication to patient. Emphasize need to take exactly as ordered. Advise patient to contact physician if a dose is missed.
- □ Instruct patient to drink at least 3 liters of fluid each day during leucovorin rescue.
- **Folic Acid Deficiency:** Encourage patient to eat a diet high in folic acid (meat proteins, bran, dried beans, and green leafy vegetables).

EVALUATION

Effectiveness of therapy can be demonstrated by: ▪ Reversal of bone marrow and GI toxicity in patients receiving methotrexate or in overdose of folic acid antagonists. ▪ Increased sense of well-being and increased production of normoblasts in patients with megaloblastic anemia.

LEUPROLIDE

(loo-**proe**-lide)
Leuprorelin, Lupron

CLASSIFICATION(S):
Antineoplastic—hormone
Pregnancy Category X (depot only)

INDICATIONS

▪ **SC:** Palliative treatment of advanced prostate cancer in patients who are unable to tolerate orchiectomy or estrogen therapy ▪ **IM:** Treatment of endometriosis.

ACTION

▪ A synthetic analog of luteinizing hormone releasing hormone (LHRH) ▪ Initially causes a transient increase in testosterone; however, with continuous administration testosterone levels are decreased. **Therapeutic Effects:** ▪ Decreased testosterone levels and resultant decrease in spread of prostate cancer ▪ Decreased pain and lesions in endometriosis.

PHARMACOKINETICS

Absorption: Rapidly and almost completely absorbed following SC administration. More slowly absorbed following IM administration of depot form.
Distribution: Distribution not known.
Metabolism and Excretion: Metabolism and elimination not known.
Half-life: 3 hr.

CONTRAINDICATIONS AND PRECAUTIONS

Contraindicated in: ▪ Intolerance to synthetic analogs of LHRH.
Use Cautiously in: ▪ Hypersensitivity to benzyl alcohol (results in induration and erythema at SC site).

ADVERSE REACTIONS AND SIDE EFFECTS*

CNS: dizziness, headache.
EENT: blurred vision.
CV: edema of the lower extremities.
GI: constipation, anorexia, nausea, vomiting.
GU: decreased libido, impotence, gonadal suppression.
Endo: gynecomastia.
Local: burning, itching, redness at SC site.
MS: transient increase in bone pain, myalgia.

*Underlines indicate most frequent; **CAPITALS** indicate life-threatening.

Neuro: numbness or tingling in hands or feet.
Misc: hot flashes, transient increase in tumor pain.

INTERACTIONS

Drug–Drug: ▪ Additive antineoplastic effects with **antiandrogens (megestrol, flutamide).**

ROUTE AND DOSAGE

- **SC (Adults):** 1 mg/day.
- **IM (Adults):** 7.5 mg/mon.

PHARMACODYNAMICS (decline in serum testosterone concentrations)

	ONSET	PEAK	DURATION
SC	1–2 wk*	2–4 wk	UK

*Follows a transient increase in the first wk of therapy.

NURSING IMPLICATIONS

Assessment

- **Prostate Cancer:** Monitor patients with vertebral metastases for increased back pain and decreased sensory/motor function.
- Monitor intake and output ratios, assess for bladder distention in patients with urinary tract obstruction during initiation of therapy.
- **Endometriosis:** Assess patient for endometrial pain prior to and periodically throughout therapy.
- **Lab Test Considerations:** Initially increases, then decreases, luteinizing hormone (LH) and follicle stimulating hormone (FSH). This leads to castration levels of testosterone in males 2–4 wk after initial increase in concentrations.
- Monitor acid phosphate to evaluate response to therapy. Transient increase in levels may occur during the first mon of therapy for prostate cancer.

Potential Nursing Diagnoses

- Sexual dysfunction (indications, side effects).
- Knowledge deficit related to medication regimen (patient/family teaching).

Implementation

- **SC/IM:** Use syringe supplied by manufacturer. Rotate sites.
- Leuprolide depot is *only* for IM injections.

Patient/Family Teaching

- **General Info:** Advise patient that medication may cause hot flashes. Notify physician if these become bothersome.
- **Prostate Cancer:** Instruct patient/family on SC injection technique. Review patient insert provided with leuprolide patient administration kit.
- Instruct patient to take medication exactly as directed. If a dose is missed, take as soon as remembered unless not remembered until next day.
- Advise patient that bone pain may increase at initiation of therapy. This will resolve with time. Patient should discuss with physician use of analgesics to control pain.
- Instruct patient to notify physician promptly if difficulty urinating, weakness, or numbness occurs.
- **Endometriosis:** Advise patient to use a form of contraception other than oral contraceptives during therapy. Inform patient that amenorrhea is expected but does not guarantee contraception.

Evaluation

Effectiveness of therapy can be demonstrated by: ▪ Decrease in the spread of prostate cancer ▪ Decrease in lesions and pain in endometriosis.

LEVAMISOLE

(lee-**vam**-i-sole)
Ergamisole

CLASSIFICATION(S):
Antineoplastic—immunomodulator
Pregnancy Category C

INDICATIONS

▪ Adjunctive treatment following surgery of Dukes C colorectal carcinoma in combination with fluorouracil. **Unlabeled Use:** ▪ Advanced malignant melanoma.

ACTION

▪ Restores depressed immune function including formation of antibodies, T-cell response, phagocytosis, and chemotaxis ▪ Also has cholinergic activity. **Therapeutic Effect:** ▪ Enhanced immunologic response to presence of tumor when used in conjunction with fluorouracil.

PHARMACOKINETICS

Absorption: Rapidly absorbed following oral administratin.
Distribution: Distribution not known.
Metabolism and Excretion: Extensively metabolized by the liver.
Half-life: 3–4 hr.

CONTRAINDICATIONS AND PRECAUTIONS

Contraindicated in: ▪ Hypersensitivity ▪ Pregnancy
Use Cautiously in: ▪ Bone marrow depression ▪ Other chronic debilitating illnesses ▪ Patients with childbearing potential ▪ Lactation or children (safety not established).

ADVERSE REACTIONS AND SIDE EFFECTS*

Note: As occurring in combination with fluorouracil.

CNS: fatigue, dizziness, headache, somnolence, depression, nervousness, insomnia, anxiety, forgetfulness.
EENT: altered sense of smell, abnormal tearing, conjunctivitis, blurred vision.
GI: nausea, vomiting, stomatitis, diarrhea, anorexia, abdominal pain, flatulence, dyspepsia, abnormal taste.
Derm: dermatitis, alopecia, pruritis, skin discoloration.
Hemat: anemia, leukopenia, thrombocytopenia, AGRANULOCYTOSIS.
MS: arthralgia, myalgia.
Neuro: paresthesia, ataxia.
Misc: fever, chills.

INTERACTIONS

Drug-Drug: ▪ Increased bone marrow depression with other **antineoplastic agents** or **radiation therapy** ▪ Ingestion of **alcohol** may produce disulfiram-like reaction ▪ May increase blood levels and risk of toxicity with **phenytoin**.

ROUTE AND DOSAGE

▪ **PO (Adults):** 50 mg q 8 hr for 3 days every 2 wk with fluorouracil 450 mg/m^2/day for 5 days initially then followed 28 days later by fluorouracil 450 mg/m^2 once weekly.

PHARMACODYNAMICS (blood levels)

	ONSET	PEAK	DURATION
PO	UK	1.5–2 hr	UK

NURSING IMPLICATIONS

Assessment

□ Assess mucous membranes, number and consistency of stools, and frequency of vomiting. Assess for fever, chills, sore throat, and signs of infection. Assess for bleeding (bleeding gums, bruising, petechiae; guaiac stools, urine, and emesis). Avoid IM injections and rectal temperatures. Apply pressure to venipuncture sites for 10 min. Notify physician if symptoms of toxicity (stomatitis, uncontrollable vomiting, diarrhea, gastrointestinal bleeding, leukocyte count of less than 3500/mm^3, platelet count $<$100,000/mm^3, or hemorrhage from any site) occur as drug will need to be discontinued.

▪ **Lab Test Considerations:** Hematologic functions should be monitored prior to and throughout therapy. CBC with differential and platelets, electrolytes, and liver function tests should be performed on the first day of therapy with levamisole and fluorouracil. Then, a CBC with differential should be performed weekly prior to each treatment with fluorouracil.

*Underlines indicate most frequent; **CAPITALS** indicate life-threatening.

Electrolytes and liver function should be monitored every 3 mon for 1 yr. If WBC is 2500–3500/mm^3, withhold fluorouracil until WBC >3500/mm^3; if WBC <2500/mm^3 withhold fluorouracil until WBC >3500/mm^3 and decrease dose by 20%; if WBC remains <2500/mm^3 for >10 days despite withholding fluorouracil, discontinue levamisole. Withhold both levamisole and fluorouracil if platelet count <100,000/mm^3. Neutropenia is usually reversible upon discontinuation of therapy.

Potential Nursing Diagnoses

- Infection, high risk for (side effects).
- Nutrition, altered: less than body requirements (side effects).
- Knowledge deficit related to medication regimen (patient/family teaching).

Implementation

- **General Info:** Levamisole therapy should be initiated no earlier than 7 days and no later than 30 days following surgery. Fluorouracil therapy should be initiated no earlier than 21 days and no later than 35 days following surgery in patients who are out of the hospital, ambulatory, maintaining oral nutrition, have well-healed wounds, and are fully recovered from postoperative complications. If levamisole has been initiated 7–20 days postop, begin fluorouracil therapy with the second course of levamisole therapy; if levamisole is initiated 21–30 days postop, initiate fluorouracil with first course of levamisole therapy.
- □ Refer to fluorouracil monograph for specific information on administration of fluorouracil.
- **PO:** Administer levamisole every 8 hr for 3 days. Repeat course every 14 days for 1 yr.

Patient/Family Teaching

- □ Instruct patient to notify physician immediately if flu-like symptoms or malaise occurs. Physician should also be notified if fever, chills, sore throat, signs of infection, bleeding gums, bruising, petechiae, or blood in urine, stool, or emesis occurs. Caution patient to avoid crowds and persons with known infections. Instruct patient to use soft toothbrush and electric razor. Patients should be cautioned not to take aspirin-containing products.
- □ Caution patient that concurrent use of alcohol may cause a disulfiram-like reaction (abdominal cramps, nausea, headache, flushing, hypoglycemia).
- □ Advise patient to rinse mouth with clear water after eating and drinking and to avoid flossing to minimize stomatitis. Consult physician if mouth pain interferes with eating.
- □ Discuss with patient the possibility of hair loss. Explore methods of coping.
- □ Instruct patient not to receive any vaccinations without advice of physician.
- □ Review with patient the need for contraception during therapy.
- □ Emphasize the importance of routine follow-up lab tests to monitor progress and check for side effects.

Evaluation

Effectiveness of therapy can be demonstrated by: ▪ Enhanced immunologic response to presence of tumor when used in conjunction with fluorouracil.

LEVOBUNOLOL

(lee-voe-**byoo**-noe-lole)
Betagan

CLASSIFICATION(S):
Ophthalmic—beta-adrenergic blocker, Antiglaucoma
Pregnancy Category C

INDICATIONS

- Used to decrease intraocular pressure in patients with chronic open-angle glaucoma.

ACTION

▪ Blockade of beta-adrenergic receptors in the eye decreases the production of aqueous humor ▪ Although systemic effects are minimal, blockade of $beta_1$ (myocardial) and $beta_2$ (pulmonary) receptors may occur. **Therapeutic Effect:** ▪ Decreased intraocular pressure.

PHARMACOKINETICS

Absorption: Systemic absorption following ophthalmic administration is minimal but may occur.
Distribution: Well distributed throughout ocular tissues following ophthalmic administration.
Metabolism and Excretion: Mostly metabolized by the liver.
Half-life: 60–90 min (in eye), 5–6 hr (in plasma).

CONTRAINDICATIONS AND PRECAUTIONS

Contraindicated in: ▪ Hypersensitivity to levobunolol or bisulfites ▪ Uncompensated congestive heart failure ▪ Pulmonary edema ▪ Cardiogenic shock ▪ Bradycardia ▪ Heart block.
Use Cautiously in: ▪ Cardiac failure ▪ Diabetes mellitus ▪ Underlying pulmonary disease, including asthma ▪ Myasthenia gravis or thyrotoxicosis ▪ Pregnancy, lactation, or children (safety not established).

ADVERSE REACTIONS AND SIDE EFFECTS*

CV: bradycardia, pulmonary edema.
EENT: ocular stinging, conjunctivitis, erythema, blepharitis, decreased visual acuity.
Resp: bronchospasm.
Derm: rashes.

INTERACTIONS

Drug-Drug: ▪ Additive beta-adrenergic blockade may occur with concurrent **systemic beta-adrenergic blocking agents (acebutolol, atenolol, labetolol, metoprolol, nadolol, pindolol, propranolol,** or **timolol)** ▪ If systemic absorption occurs, concurrent use with **antihypertensives** or **nitrates** will result in additive hypotensive effects ▪ Additive effects with other **intraocular hypotensive agents**.

ROUTE AND DOSAGE

- **Ophth (Adults):** 1 drop of 0.5% soln 1–2 times daily.

PHARMACODYNAMICS

	ONSET	PEAK	DURATION
Ophth	1 hr	2–6 hr	24 hr

NURSING IMPLICATIONS

Assessment

- □ Intraocular pressure should be monitored periodically during therapy.
- □ Monitor heart rate and blood pressure periodically throughout therapy. May reduce cardiac output if systemically absorbed.
- **Lab Test Considerations:** May cause increased or decreased blood glucose levels.

Potential Nursing Diagnoses

- Sensory-perceptual alteration: visual (indications, side effects).
- Knowledge deficit related to medication regimen (patient/family teaching).

Implementation

- **Ophth:** Administer ophthalmic soln by having patient tilt head back and look up, gently depress lower lid with index finger until conjunctival sac is exposed, and instill medication. After instillation, maintain gentle pressure on the inner canthus for 1 min to avoid systemic absorption of the drug. Wait at least 5 min before administering other types of eyedrops.
- □ When using levobunolol to replace other antiglaucoma agents, discontinue administration of single-agent antiglaucoma therapy. If beta blockers are used with multiple agents, discontinue beta blocker before starting levobunolol therapy. To control intraocular pressure, levobunolol may be used concurrently with muscarinic agents (pilocarpine, echothiopate, carbachol), beta agonists (ophthalmic epinephrine, dipivefrin),

*Underlines indicate most frequent; **CAPITALS** indicate life-threatening.

and/or systemic carbonic anhydrase inhibitors (acetazolamide).

Patient/Family Teaching

- Advise patient to take medication exactly as directed. Do not take more than the prescribed amount. Missed doses should be taken as soon as remembered unless almost time for the next dose; administer next dose at scheduled time. If dosing schedule is once daily, do not administer if not remembered until next day.
- Instruct patient in proper technique for instillation of ophthalmic medications. Emphasize the importance of not touching the applicator tip to any surface.
- Inform diabetic patient that levobunolol may mask some signs of hypoglycemia and may cause decreased or increased blood glucose levels if systemically absorbed.
- Advise patient to inform physician or dentist of medication regimen prior to treatment or surgery. Gradual withdrawal of levobunolol may be necessary.
- Instruct patient to inform patient if eye irritation or inflammation, decreased vision, rash, or itching occurs.
- Emphasize the importance of regular follow-up examinations to monitor progress.

Evaluation

Effectiveness of therapy may be demonstrated by: ▪ Decreased intraocular pressure.

LEVOCARNITINE

(lee-voe-**car**-ni-teen)
Carnitor, L-carnitine, VitaCarn

CLASSIFICATION(S):
Amino acid derivative
Pregnancy Category C

INDICATIONS

▪ Treatment of primary systemic carnitine deficiency.

ACTION

▪ An amino acid compound made from methionine and lysine that facilitates the use of fatty acids in cellular metabolism and energy production. **Therapeutic Effect:** ▪ Lowering of free fatty acid levels and triglycerides with resultant prevention of end organ damage in carnitine deficiency.

PHARMACOKINETICS

Absorption: Well absorbed following oral administration.
Distribution: Present in breast milk.
Metabolism and Excretion: Used up during cellular metabolism.
Half-life: UK.

CONTRAINDICATIONS AND PRECAUTIONS

Contraindicated in: ▪ No known contraindications.
Use Cautiously in: ▪ Avoid use of D, L-carnitine, which exaggerates L-carnitine deficiency.

ADVERSE REACTIONS AND SIDE EFFECTS*

GI: nausea, vomiting, abdominal cramps, diarrhea.
Misc: drug-related body odor.

INTERACTIONS

Drug–Drug: ▪ **Valproic acid** may increase carnitine requirements ▪ Avoid use of **D, L-carnitine,** which exaggerates levocarnitine deficiency.

ROUTE AND DOSAGE

- **PO (Adults):** Start with 1 g/day (990 mg if tablets), increase gradually as tolerated to 3 g/day in divided doses q 3–4 hr.
- **PO (Children):** 50 mg/kg/day initially, increase as tolerated to 100 mg/kg/day in divided doses q 3–4 hr (not to exceed 3 g/day).

PHARMACODYNAMICS

	ONSET	PEAK	DURATION
PO	UK	UK	UK

*Underlines indicate most frequent; CAPITALS indicate life-threatening.

L

NURSING IMPLICATIONS

Assessment

- ▫ Monitor vital signs periodicaly throughout therapy.
- ▫ Assess patient for signs of carnitine deficiency (elevated triglycerides and free fatty acids, hypoglycemia, hypotonia, lethargy, encephalopathy, cardiomegaly, congestive heart failure).
- ▪ **Lab Test Considerations:** Monitor blood chemistries and plasma carnitine concentrations throughout therapy.

Potential Nursing Diagnoses

- ▪ Nutrition, altered: less than body requirements (indications).
- ▪ Knowledge deficit related to medication regimen (patient/family teaching).

Implementation

- ▪ **PO:** Administer soln alone or dissolve in drinks or liquid food. Doses should be spaced evenly, every 3–4 hr, and given with or after meals.

Patient/Family Teaching

- ▫ Instruct patient to take levocarnitine exactly as directed. Soln should be consumed slowly to maximize tolerance.
- ▫ Advise patient that D, L-carnitine, which is sold in health food stores as vitamin B_T, may exaggerate deficiency.

Evaluation

Effectiveness of therapy can be demonstrated by: ▪ Decrease in triglyceride and free fatty acid levels ▫ Prevention of end organ deficiency in chronic levocarnitine deficiency.

LEVODOPA

(**lee**-voe-doe-pa)

Dopar, Larodopa, L-Dopa

CLASSIFICATION(S):

Antiparkinsonian—dopamine agonist

Pregnancy Category UK

INDICATIONS

▪ Treatment of Parkinson's syndrome. Not useful for drug-induced extrapyramidal reactions.

ACTION

▪ Levodopa is converted to dopamine in the CNS, where it serves as a neurotransmitter. **Therapeutic Effect:** ▪ Relief of tremor and rigidity in Parkinson's syndrome.

PHARMACOKINETICS

Absorption: Well absorbed following oral administration.

Distribution: Widely distributed. When administered alone, enters the CNS in small concentrations. Enters breast milk.

Metabolism and Excretion: Mostly metabolized by the GI tract and liver.

Half-life: 1 hr.

CONTRAINDICATIONS AND PRECAUTIONS

Contraindicated in: ▪ Hypersensitivity ▪ Narrow-angle glaucoma ▪ Patients receiving MAO inhibitors ▪ Malignant melanoma ▪ Undiagnosed skin lesions ▪ Lactation.

Use Cautiously in: ▪ History of cardiac, psychiatric, or ulcer disease ▪ Pregnancy or children <18 yr (safety not established).

ADVERSE REACTIONS AND SIDE EFFECTS*

CNS: <u>involuntary movements</u>, memory loss, anxiety, psychiatric problems, hallucinations, dizziness.

EENT: mydriasis, blurred vision.

CV: hypertension, hypotension.

GI: <u>nausea</u>, <u>vomiting</u>, anorexia, dry mouth, hepatotoxicity.

Derm: melanoma.

Hemat: hemolytic anemia, leukopenia.

Misc: darkening of sweat or urine.

INTERACTIONS

Drug-Drug: ▪ Use with **MAO inhibitors** may result in hypertensive reactions ▪ **Phenothiazines, haloperidol,**

*<u>Underlines</u> indicate most frequent; **CAPITALS** indicate life-threatening.

papaverine, phenytoin, and **reserpine** may antagonize the beneficial effect of levodopa ▪ Large doses of **pyridoxine** may reverse the effect of levodopa ▪ Concurrent use with **methyldopa** may alter the effectiveness of levodopa and increase the risk of CNS side effects ▪ Additive hypotension may result with concurrent **antihypertensives** ▪ **Anticholinergics** may decrease absorption of levodopa ▪ Increased risk of adverse reactions (dyskinesias, nausea, hypotension, confusion, hallucinations) with **selegiline** (decrease dose of levodopa) ▪ Increased risk of arrhythmias with **cocaine.**

Drug–Food: ▪ Ingestion of foods containing large amounts of **pyridoxine** may reverse the effect of levodopa.

ROUTE AND DOSAGE

- **PO (Adults):** 500–1000 mg given in divided doses q 6–12 hr initially. Increase by 100–750 mg/day q 3–7 days until response occurs or 8000 mg/day is reached. Usual maintenance dose is 2000–8000 mg/day.

PHARMACODYNAMICS (antiparkinson effects)

	ONSET	PEAK	DURATION
PO	10–15 min	UK	5–24 hr or more

NURSING IMPLICATIONS

Assessment

- Assess parkinsonian symptoms (akinesia, rigidity, tremors, gait, facial expression, and drooling) prior to and throughout course of therapy. "On-off phenomena" may cause symptoms to appear or to improve suddenly.
- Assess blood pressure and pulse frequently during period of dose adjustment.
- **Toxicity and Overdose:** Assess for signs of toxicity (involuntary muscle twitching, facial grimacing, spasmodic eye winking, exaggerated protrusion of tongue, or behavioral changes). Consult physician promptly if these symptoms occur.
- **Lab Test Considerations:** May cause false-positive Coombs' test, serum and urine uric acid, serum gonadotropin, urine norepinephrine, and urine protein concentrations.
- May interfere with results of urine glucose and urine ketone tests. Copper reduction method (Clinitest) of testing urine glucose and dipstick (Ketostix) for urine ketones may reveal false-positive results. Glucose oxidase method (Tes-Tape) of testing urine glucose may yield false-negative results.
- Patients on long-term therapy should have hepatic and renal functions and CBC monitored periodically. May cause elevated BUN, SGPT (ALT), SGOT (AST), bilirubin, alkaline phosphatase, LDH, and serum protein-bound iodine.

Potential Nursing Diagnoses

- Mobility, impaired physical (indications).
- Injury, high risk for (indications).
- Knowledge deficit related to medication regimen (patient/family teaching).

Implementation

- **General Info:** In preoperative patients or patients who are NPO, confer with physician regarding continuing medication administration.
- Wait 8 hr after last levodopa dose before switching patient to carbidopa/levodopa. Carbidopa reduces the need for levodopa by 75%. Administering carbidopa shortly after a full dose of levodopa may result in toxicity.
- **PO:** Administer food shortly after medication to minimize GI irritation; taking food before or concurrently may retard levodopa's effects but may be necessary to minimize GI irritation. If patient has difficulty swallowing, confer with pharmacist.

Patient/Family Teaching

- Instruct patient to take this drug exactly as prescribed. If a dose is missed, take as soon as remembered unless next scheduled dose is within 2 hr; do not double doses.

- ▫ Explain that gastric irritation may be decreased by taking food shortly after medication but that high-protein meals may impair levodopa's effects. Dividing the daily protein intake between all meals may help ensure adequate protein intake and drug effectiveness. Do not drastically alter diet during levodopa therapy without consulting physician.
- ▫ May cause drowsiness or dizziness. Advise patient to avoid driving or other activities that require alertness until response to drug is known.
- ▫ Caution patient to make position changes slowly to minimize orthostatic hypotension. Physician should be notified if orthostatic hypotension occurs.
- ▫ Instruct patient that frequent rinsing of mouth, good oral hygiene, and sugarless gum or candy may decrease dry mouth.
- ▫ Advise patient to confer with physician or pharmacist prior to taking over-the-counter medications, especially cold remedies. Patients receiving only levodopa should avoid multivitamins. Large amounts of vitamin B_6 (pyridoxine) may interfere with levodopa's action.
- ▫ Inform patient that harmless darkening of urine or sweat may occur.
- ▫ Advise patient to notify physician if palpitations, urinary retention, involuntary movements, behavioral changes, severe nausea and vomiting, or new skin lesions occur.

Evaluation

Effectiveness of therapy can be demonstrated by: ▪ Resolution of parkinsonian signs and symptoms ▫ Therapeutic effects usually become evident after 2–3 wk of therapy but may require up to 6 mon ▫ Patients who take this medication for several yr may experience a decrease in the effectiveness of this drug ▫ Effectiveness of therapy may sometimes be restored after a "drug holiday."

LEVORPHANOL

(lee-**vor**-fan-ole)
Levo-Dromoran, Levorphan

CLASSIFICATION(S):
Narcotic analgesic—agonist
Schedule II
Pregnancy Category UK

INDICATIONS

▪ Management of moderate to severe pain.

ACTION

▪ Binds to opiate receptors in the CNS, altering perception of and response to pain ▪ Produces generalized CNS depression. **Therapeutic Effect:** ▪ Decreased pain.

PHARMACOKINETICS

Aborption: Well absorbed following oral and SC administration.
Distribution: Distribution not known.
Metabolism and Excretion: Mostly metabolized by the liver.
Half-life: 12–16 hr.

CONTRAINDICATIONS AND PRECAUTIONS

Contraindicated in: ▪ Hypersensitivity ▪ Avoid chronic use during pregnancy or lactation.
Use Cautiously in: ▪ Head trauma ▪ Increased intracranial pressure ▪ Severe renal, hepatic, or pulmonary disease ▪ Hypothyroidism ▪ Adrenal insufficiency ▪ Alcoholism ▪ Undiagnosed abdominal pain ▪ Prostatic hypertrophy ▪ Elderly or debilitated patients (dosage reduction suggested) ▪ Patients who may have been addicted to narcotics previously.

ADVERSE REACTIONS AND SIDE EFFECTS*

CNS: sedation, confusion, headache, euphoria, floating feeling, unusual dreams, hallucinations, dysphoria.
EENT: miosis, diplopia, blurred vision.
Resp: respiratory depression.
CV: hypotension, bradycardia.
GI: nausea, vomiting, constipation, dry mouth.
GU: urinary retention.
Derm: sweating, flushing.
Misc: tolerance, physical dependence, psychological dependence.

INTERACTIONS

Drug–Drug: ▪ Use with extreme caution in patients receiving **MAO inhibitors** (may result in unpredictable, severe reactions—decrease initial dose of levorphanol to 25% of usual dose) ▪ Additive CNS depression with **alcohol, antihistamines, antidepressants,** and **sedative/hypnotics** ▪ Administration of **partial-antagonist narcotic analgesics** may precipitate narcotic withdrawal in physically dependent patients ▪ **Nalbuphine** or **pentazocine** may decrease analgesia.

ROUTE AND DOSAGE

- **PO (Adults):** 2 mg initially q 4–5 hr, may be increased to 3–4 mg if necessary.
- **SC, IV (Adults):** 2 mg q 4–5 hr, may be increased to 3 mg if pain is severe.

PHARMACODYNAMICS (analgesic effect)

	ONSET	PEAK	DURATION
PO	10–60 min	90–120 min	4–5 hr
SC	UK	60–90 min	4–5 hr
IV	UK	within 20 min	4–8 hr

NURSING IMPLICATIONS

Assessment

- Assess type, location, and intensity of pain prior to and 60 min following administration.
- Assess blood pressure, pulse, and respiratory rate before and periodically during administration.
- Prolonged use may lead to physical and psychological dependence and tolerance. This should not prevent patient from receiving adequate analgesia. Most patients who receive levorphanol for medical reasons do not develop psychological dependency. Progressively higher doses may be required to relieve pain with long-term therapy.
- Assess bowel function routinely. Increased intake of fluids and bulk, stool softeners, and laxatives may minimize constipating effects.
- Monitor intake and output ratios. If significant discrepancies occur, assess for urinary retention and inform physician.
- **Lab Test Considerations:** May increase plasma amylase and lipase levels.
- **Toxicity and Overdose:** If overdosage occurs, naloxone (Narcan) is the antidote.

Potential Nursing Diagnoses

- Comfort, altered: pain (indications).
- Sensory-perceptual alteration: visual, auditory (side effects).
- Injury, high risk for (side effects).

Implementation

- **General Info:** Explain therapeutic value of medication prior to administration to enhance the analgesic effect.
- Regularly administered doses may be more effective than prn administration. Analgesic is more effective if given before pain becomes severe.
- Coadministration with non-narcotic analgesics may have additive analgesic effects and permit lower narcotic doses.
- Encourage patient to turn, cough, and breathe deeply every 2 hr to prevent atelectasis.
- Medication should be discontinued gradually after long-term use to prevent withdrawal symptoms.

*Underlines indicate most frequent; **CAPITALS** indicate life-threatening.

L

- Available in tablet and injectable forms.
- **PO:** May be administered with food or milk to minimize GI irritation.
- **SC/IV:** Patients receiving parenteral therapy should be lying down and remain recumbent to minimize side effects for at least 30–60 min.
- **Direct IV:** Administer slowly, over 3–5 min. Rapid administration may lead to increased respiratory depression, hypotension, and circulatory collapse. Do not use IV administration without antidote available.
- **Syringe Compatibility:** glycopyrrolate.
- **Additive Incompatibility:** aminophylline, ammonium chloride, amobarbital, chlorothiazide, heparin, methicillin, pentobarbital, phenobarbital, phenytoin, secobarbital, sodium bicarbonate, sodium iodide, or thiopental.

Patient/Family Teaching

- Instruct patient on how and when to ask for prn pain medication.
- Instruct patient to take levorphanol exactly as directed. If dose is less effective after a few wks, do not increase dose without consulting physician.
- Medication may cause drowsiness or dizziness. Advise patient to call for assistance when ambulating or smoking. Caution patient to avoid driving or other activities that require alertness until response to the medication is known.
- Advise patient to make position changes slowly to minimize orthostatic hypotension.
- Caution patient to avoid concurrent use of alcohol or other CNS depressants.
- Advise ambulatory patients that nausea and vomiting may be decreased by lying down.

Evaluation

Effectiveness of therapy can be demonstrated by: ▪ Decrease in severity of pain without a significant alteration in level of consciousness, respiratory status, or blood pressure.

LEVOTHYROXINE

(lee-voe-thye-**rox**-een)
{Eltroxin}, Levoid, Levothroid, Levoxine, Synthroid, T_4

CLASSIFICATION(S):
Hormone—thyroid
Pregnancy Category A

INDICATIONS

▪ Replacement or substitution therapy in diminished or absent thyroid function of many causes. Provides a standardized and predictable effect.

ACTION

▪ Principal effect is increasing metabolic rate of body tissues ▪ Promotes gluconeogenesis, increases utilization and mobilization of glycogen stores, and stimulates protein synthesis ▪ Promotes cell growth and differentiation and aids in the development of the brain and CNS. **Therapeutic Effects:** ▪ Replacement in deficiency states ▪ Restoration of normal hormonal balance.

PHARMACOKINETICS

Absorption: Variably (50–80%) absorbed from the GI tract.
Distribution: Distributed into most body tissues. Thyroid hormones do not readily cross the placenta; minimal amounts enter breast milk.
Metabolism and Excretion: Metabolized by the liver. Undergoes enterohepatic recirculation. Excreted in the feces via the bile.
Half-life: 6–7 days.

CONTRAINDICATIONS AND PRECAUTIONS

Contraindicated in: ▪ Hypersensitivity ▪ Recent myocardial infarction ▪ Thyrotoxicosis.
Use Cautiously in: ▪ Cardiovascular

disease ▪ Severe renal insufficiency ▪ Uncorrected adrenocortical disorders ▪ Elderly and myxedematous patients (extremely sensitive to thyroid hormones; initial dosage should be markedly reduced) ▪ Has been used safely in pregnancy.

ADVERSE REACTIONS AND SIDE EFFECTS*

CNS: irritability, insomnia, nervousness, headache.
CV: tachycardia, arrhythmias, increased cardiac output, angina pectoris, increased blood pressure, CARDIOVASCULAR COLLAPSE, hypotension.
GI: diarrhea, cramps, vomiting.
Derm: increased sweating, hair loss (children only).
Endo: menstrual irregularities.
Metab: weight loss, heat intolerance.
MS: accelerated bone maturation in children.

INTERACTIONS

Drug-Drug: ▪ **Cholestyramine** and **colestipol** decrease oral absorption ▪ **IV phenytoin** causes the release of thyroid hormone ▪ Thyroid hormones increase the effect of **oral anticoagulants** ▪ May cause an increase in the requirement for **insulin** or **oral hypoglycemic agents** in diabetics ▪ Additive CNS and cardiac stimulation with **sympathomimetic agents (amphetamines, vasopressors, decongestants)** ▪ May decrease some effects of **beta-adrenergic blockers**.

ROUTE AND DOSAGE

Hypothyroidism

- **PO (Adults):** 12.5–50 mcg as a single daily dose initially, may be increased q 2–4 wk. Usual maintenance dose 75–125 mcg/day.
- **PO (Children >10 yr):** 2–3 mcg/kg/day as a single daily dose.
- **PO (Children 6–12 yr):** 4–5 mcg/kg/day as a single daily dose.
- **PO (Children 1–5 yr):** 5–6 mcg/kg/day as a single dose.
- **PO (Children 6–12 mon):** 6–8 mcg/kg/day as a single daily dose.
- **PO (Children 0–6 mon):** 8–10 mcg/kg/day as a single dose.
- **IM, IV (Adults):** 50–100 mcg/day as a single dose.
- **IM, IV (Children):** 75% of the calculated oral dose.

Myxedema Coma

- **IV (Adults):** 200–500 mcg, if no response in 24 hr, may give additional 100–300 mcg.

PHARMACODYNAMICS (effects on thyroid function testing)

	ONSET	PEAK	DURATION
PO	UK	1–3 wk	1–3 wk
IV	6–8 hr	24 hr	UK

NURSING IMPLICATIONS

Assessment

- **General Info:** Assess apical pulse and blood pressure prior to and periodically during therapy. Assess for tachyarrhythmias and chest pain.
- **Children:** Monitor height, weight, and psychomotor development.
- **Lab Test Considerations:** Thyroid function studies should be monitored prior to and throughout course of therapy.
- □ Monitor blood and urine glucose in diabetic patients. Insulin or oral hypoglycemic dose may need to be increased.
- **Toxicity and Overdose:** Overdose is manifested as hyperthyroidism (tachycardia, chest pain, nervousness, insomnia, diaphoresis, tremors, weight loss). Usual treatment is to withhold dose for 2–6 days. Acute overdose is treated by induction of emesis or gastric lavage, followed by activated charcoal. Sympathetic overstimulation may be controlled by antiadrenergic drugs, such as propranolol. Oxygen and supportive measures to control symptoms such as fever are also used.

*Underlines indicate most frequent; **CAPITALS** indicate life-threatening.

L

Potential Nursing Diagnoses
- Knowledge deficit related to medication regimen (patient/family teaching).

Implementation
- **General Info:** Administer as a single dose, preferably before breakfast to prevent insomnia.
- **IV:** For IV levothyroxine, dilute each 500 mcg in 5 ml of 0.9% NaCl without preservatives (diluent usually provided), for a concentration of 100 mcg/ml. Shake well to dissolve completely. Administer soln immediately after preparation; discard unused portion.
  - *Rate:* Administer at a rate of 100 mcg over 1 min. Do not add to IV infusions; may be administered through Y-tubing or a 3-way stopcock.

Patient/Family Teaching
- **General Info:** Instruct patient to take medication exactly as directed at the same time each day. If a dose is missed, take as soon as remembered unless almost time for next dose. If more than 2–3 doses are missed, notify physician. Do not discontinue without consulting physician.
  - Instruct patient and family on correct technique for checking pulse. Dose should be withheld and physician notified if resting pulse >100 bpm.
  - Explain to patient that levothyroxine does not cure hypothyroidism, it provides a thyroid hormone; therapy is lifelong.
  - Caution patient not to change brands of this medication, as this may effect drug bioavailability.
  - Advise patient to notify physician if headache, nervousness, diarrhea, excessive sweating, heat intolerance, chest pain, increased pulse rate, palpitations, weight loss >2 lb/wk, or any unusual symptoms occur.
  - Caution patient to avoid taking other medications concurrently with levothyroxine unless instructed by physician.
  - Instruct patient to inform physician or dentist of thyroid therapy.
  - Emphasize importance of follow-up examinations to monitor effectiveness of therapy. Thyroid function tests are performed at least yearly.
- **Children:** Discuss with parents need for routine follow-up studies to ensure correct development. Inform patient that partial hair loss may be experienced by children on thyroid therapy. This is usually temporary.

Evaluation
Clinical response can be evaluated by:
- Resolution of symptoms of hypothyroidism. Response includes: □ Diuresis □ Weight loss □ Increased sense of well-being □ Increased energy, pulse rate, appetite, psychomotor activity □ Normalization of skin texture and hair □ Correction of constipation □ Increased T_3 and T_4 levels ▪ In children, effectiveness of therapy is determined by: □ Appropriate physical and psychomotor development.

LIDOCAINE
(**lye**-doe-kane)
Anestacon, Baylocaine, L-Caine, LidoPen, Xylocaine, {Xylogard}

CLASSIFICATION(S):
Antiarrhythmic—class IB, Anesthetic—local
Pregnancy Category B

INDICATIONS
- **IV:** Acute treatment of ventricular arrhythmias ▪ **IM:** Given as a self-injection or when IV unavailable (during transport to hospital facilities) ▪ **Local:** Used as a local or infiltration anesthetic.

ACTION
- Suppresses automaticity of conduction tissue and spontaneous depolarization of the ventricles during diastole by altering the flux of sodium ions across cell membranes. Has little or no

effect on heart rate. **Therapeutic Effects:** ▪ Control of ventricular arrhythmias ▪ Local anesthetic activity.

PHARMACOKINETICS

Absorption: Well absorbed following IM administration into the deltoid muscle. Some absorption may follow topical application.
Distribution: Widely distributed. Concentrates in adipose tissue. Crosses the blood-brain barrier and placenta.
Metabolism and Excretion: Mostly metabolized by the liver.
Half-life: Biphasic—initial phase 7–30 min; terminal phase—90–120 min.

CONTRAINDICATIONS AND PRECAUTIONS

Contraindicated in: ▪ Hypersensitivity ▪ Advanced AV block.
Use Cautiously in: ▪ Liver disease, congestive heart failure, patients weighing <50 kg, and elderly patients (dosage reduction required) ▪ Respiratory depression, shock, or heart block ▪ Pregnancy or lactation (safety not established).

ADVERSE REACTIONS AND SIDE EFFECTS*

CNS: drowsiness, dizziness, lethargy, confusion, nervousness, SEIZURES, tremor.
CV: hypotension, arrhythmias, bradycardia, CARDIAC ARREST.
GI: nausea, vomiting.
Local: burning, stinging, erythema (Top or infiltration use).

INTERACTIONS

Drug-Drug: ▪ Additive cardiac depression and toxicity with **phenytoin, quinidine, procainamide,** or **propranolol** ▪ **Cimetidine** and **beta-adrenergic blockers** may decrease metabolism and increase risk of toxicity.

ROUTE AND DOSAGE

Note: See infusion rate table in Appendix D.

- **IV (Adults):** 50–100 mg bolus (or 1 mg/kg, repeat ½ of dose in 5 min), then 1–4 mg/min (20–50 mcg/kg/min) infusion (up to 200–300 mg in 1 hr).
- **IV (Children):** 0.5–1 mg/kg bolus, repeat as needed (not to exceed 3–5 mg/kg total dose), 10–50 mcg/kg/min infusion.
- **IM (Adults):** 300 mg (4.3 mg/kg), may be repeated in 60–90 min.
- **Top (Adults and Children):** Apply to affected area as needed (increased amount and frequency of use increases likelihood of systemic absorption and adverse reactions).

PHARMACODYNAMICS (IV, IM = antiarrhythmic effects, Top = local anesthetic effects)

	ONSET	PEAK	DURATION
IV	immediate	immediate	10–20 min
IM	5–15 min	20–30 min	60–90 min
Top	UK	2–5 min	30–60 min

NURSING IMPLICATIONS

Assessment

- **General Info:** Serum electrolyte levels should be monitored periodically throughout prolonged therapy.
- **Antiarrhythmic:** Monitor ECG continuously and blood pressure and respiratory status frequently throughout administration.
- **Anesthetic:** Assess degree of numbness of affected part. If spray or viscous lidocaine was used on the throat, assess gag reflex before giving food or fluids.
- **Lab Test Considerations:** IM administration may cause increased CPK levels.
- **Toxicity and Overdose:** Serum lidocaine levels should be monitored periodically throughout prolonged or high-dose therapy. Therapeutic serum lidocaine levels range from 1.5 to 5 mcg/ml.
  - ☐ Signs and symptoms of toxicity include confusion, excitation, blurred or double vision, nausea, vomiting, ringing in ears, tremors, twitching,

*Underlines indicate most frequent; **CAPITALS** indicate life-threatening.

convulsions, difficulty breathing, severe dizziness or fainting, and unusually slow heart rate.

- If symptoms of overdose occur, stop infusion and monitor patient closely.

POTENTIAL NURSING DIAGNOSES

- Cardiac output, decreased (indications).
- Comfort, altered: pain (indications).
- Knowledge deficit related to medication regimen (patient/family teaching).

IMPLEMENTATION

- **General Info:** Available in spray, topical soln, jelly, and injectable forms.
- **IM:** IM injections are recommended only when ECG monitoring is not available and physician feels benefits outweigh risks. Administer IM injections only into deltoid muscle while frequently aspirating to prevent IV injection.
- **IV:** Available in 1%, 2%, 4%, 10%, and 20% soln. Only 1% and 2% soln are used for direct IV injection.
- **Direct IV:** Administer undiluted IV loading dose of 1 mg/kg at a rate of 25–50 mg over 1 min. May follow with second loading dose of ½ to ⅓ of original dose after 5 min. Follow by IV infusion. Do not use lidocaine with preservatives or other medications, such as epinephrine, for IV injection.
- **Continuous Infusion:** To prepare for IV infusion add 1 g lidocaine to 250, 500, or 1000 ml of D5W. Soln is stable for 24 hr. Other compatible solns include D5/LR, D5/0.45% NaCl, D5/0.9% NaCl, 0.45% NaCl, 0.9% NaCl, and lactated Ringer's soln.
  - *Rate:* Administer via infusion pump for accurate dose at a rate of 1–4 mg/min (see Appendix D for infusion rate table).
- **Syringe Compatibility:** glycopyrrolate, heparin, hydroxyzine, methicillin, metoclopramide, moxalactam, or nalbuphine.
- **Syringe Incompatibility:** amphotericin, cefazolin, or dacarbazine.
- **Y-Site Compatibility:** altaplase, amrinone, cefazolin, dobutamine, enalaprilat, famotidine, heparin with hydrocortisone sodium succinate, labetalol, nitroglycerine, nitroprusside, potassium chloride, or streptokinase.
- **Additive Compatibility:** aminophylline, bretylium, calcium chloride, calcium gluceptate, calcium gluconate, chloramphenicol, chlorothiazide, cimetidine, dexamethasone, digoxin, diphenhydramine, dobutamine, dopamine, ephedrine, erythromycin lactobionate, heparin, hydrocortisone sodium succinate, hydroxyzine, insulin, metaraminol, nitroglycerin, oxytetracycline, penicillin G potassium, pentobarbital, phenylephrine, potassium chloride, procainamide, prochlorperazine, promazine, ranitidine, sodium bicarbonate, tetracycline, or verapamil.
- **Additive Incompatibility:** methohexital or phenytoin. Do not admix with blood transfusions.
- **Infiltration:** Physician may order lidocaine with epinephrine to minimize systemic absorption and prolong local anesthesia.

PATIENT/FAMILY TEACHING

- **General Info:** May cause drowsiness and dizziness. Advise patient to call for assistance during ambulation and transfer.
- **IM:** Available in LidoPen Auto-Injector for use outside the hospital setting. Advise patient to telephone physician immediately if symptoms of a heart attack occur. Do not administer unless instructed by physician. To administer, remove safety cap and place back end on thickest part of thigh. Press hard until needle prick is felt. Hold in place for 10 sec, then massage area for 10 sec. Do not drive after administration unless absolutely necessary.

EVALUATION

Effectiveness of therapy can be demonstrated by: ▪ Decrease in ventricular arrhythmias ▪ Local anesthesia.

LINDANE

(lin-dane)
Gamma-benzene-hexachloride, {gBh}, G-well, Kwell, Kwildane, Scabene

CLASSIFICATION(S):
Antiparasitic
Pregnancy Category B

INDICATIONS

▪ Treatment of: ▫ Scabies ▫ Head lice ▫ Body lice ▫ Crab lice.

ACTION

▪ Causes seizures and death in parasitic arthropods. **Therapeutic Effect:** ▪ Cure of infestion by parasitic arthropods (scabies and lice).

PHARMACOKINETICS

Absorption: Significant systemic absorption (9–13%) occurs slowly following topical application.
Distribution: Stored in fat.
Metabolism and Excretion: Metabolized by the liver.
Half-life: 18 hr (infants and children).

CONTRAINDICATIONS AND PRECAUTIONS

Contraindicated in: ▪ Hypersensitivity.
Use Cautiously in: ▪ Children $<$10 yr (increased risk of systemic absorption and CNS side effects) ▪ Pregnancy or lactation (do not exceed recommended dose; do not use $>$2 courses of therapy).

ADVERSE REACTIONS AND SIDE EFFECTS*

CNS: SEIZURES.
Derm: local irritation, contact dermatitis.

INTERACTIONS

Drug–Drug: ▪ Simultaneous topical use of **skin, scalp,** or **hair preparations** may increase systemic absorption.

ROUTE AND DOSAGE

Scabies

▪ **Top (Adults and Children):** 1% cream or lotion applied to all skin surfaces from neck to toes; treatment may be repeated in 1 wk.

Lice

▪ **Top (Adults and Children):** 1% cream or lotion applied to hairy affected and adjacent areas.

Head Lice

▪ **Top (Adults and Children):** 15–30 ml of 1% shampoo, apply and lather for 4–5 min (may need 60 ml for long hair), rinse thoroughly.

PHARMACODYNAMICS (antiparasitic action)

	ONSET	PEAK	DURATION
Top	rapid	rapid	UK

NURSING IMPLICATIONS

Assessment

▫ Assess skin and hair for signs of infestation before and after treatment.
▫ Examine family members and close contacts for infestation. When used in treatment of pediculosis pubis or scabies, sexual partners should receive concurrent therapy.

Potential Nursing Diagnoses

▪ Skin integrity, impaired: actual (indications).
▪ Knowledge deficit related to medication regimen (patient/family teaching).

Implementation

▪ **Top:** When applying medication to another person, wear gloves to prevent systemic absorption.
▫ Do not apply to open wounds (scratches, cuts, sores on skin or scalp) to minimize systemic absorption. Avoid contact with the eyes. If eye contact occurs, flush thoroughly with water and notify physician.
▫ Institute appropriate isolation techniques.

{} = Available in Canada only.
*Underlines indicate most frequent; **CAPITALS** indicate life-threatening.

- **Cream/Lotion:** Instruct patient to bathe with soap and water. Dry skin well and allow to cool prior to application. Apply cream or lotion in amount sufficient to cover entire body surface with a thin film from neck down (60 ml for an adult). Leave medication on for 8–12 hr, then remove by washing. If rash, burning, or itching develops, wash off medication and notify physician.
- **Shampoo:** Use a sufficient amount of shampoo to wet hair and scalp (30 ml for short hair, 45 ml for medium hair, 60 ml for long hair). Rub thoroughly into hair and scalp and leave in place for 4 min. Then use enough water to work up a good lather; follow with thorough rinsing and drying. When hair is dry, use fine-toothed comb to remove remaining nits or nit shells. Shampoo may also be used on combs and brushes to prevent spread of infestation.

Patient/Family Teaching

- **General Info:** Instruct patient on application technique. Patient should repeat therapy only at the recommendation of the physician. Discuss hygienic measures to prevent and to control infestation. Discuss potential for infectious contacts with patient. Explain why household members should be examined and sexual partners treated simultaneously.
- □ Instruct patient to wash all recently worn clothing and used bed linens and towels in very hot water or to dry clean to prevent reinfestation or spreading.
- □ Instruct patient not to apply other oils or creams during therapy, as these increase the absorption of lindane and may lead to toxicity.
- □ Explain to patient that itching may persist after treatment; repeat treatment is necessary only if live mites are found.
- **Shampoo:** Advise patient that shampoo should not be used as a regular shampoo in the absence of infestation. Emphasize need to avoid eye contact.
- **Children:** Advise parents to monitor young children closely for evidence of CNS toxicity during and immediately after treatment. Infestation in children <10 yr should be managed with alternate therapy.

Evaluation

Effectiveness of therapy can be demonstrated by: ▪ Resolution of signs of infestation with scabies or lice.

LIOTHYRONINE

(lye-oh-**thye**-roe-neen)

Cytomel, L-triiodothyronine, T_3

CLASSIFICATION(S):
Hormone—thyroid
Pregnancy Category A

INDICATIONS

▪ Replacement or substitution therapy in diminished or absent thyroid function of many causes.

ACTION

▪ Principal effect is increasing metabolic rate of body tissues ▪ Promotes gluconeogenesis, increases utilization and mobilization of glycogen stores, and stimulates protein synthesis ▪ Promotes cell growth and aids in the development of the brain and CNS. **Therapeutic Effects:** ▪ Replacement in deficiency states ▪ Restoration of normal hormonal balance.

PHARMACOKINETICS

Absorption: 95% absorbed following oral administration.

Distribution: Distributed into many body tissues. Thyroid hormones do not readily cross the placenta; minimal amounts enter breast milk.

Metabolism and Excretion: Metabolized by the liver and other tissues.

Half-life: 1–2 days (increased in hypothyroidism).

CONTRAINDICATIONS AND PRECAUTIONS

Contraindicated in: ▪ Hypersensitivity ▪ Recent myocardial infarction ▪ Thyrotoxicosis.

Use Cautiously in: ▪ Cardiovascular disease ▪ Severe renal insufficiency ▪ Uncorrected adrenocortical disorders ▪ Elderly and myxedematous patients (extremely sensitive to thyroid hormones, initial dosage should be markedly reduced).

ADVERSE REACTIONS AND SIDE EFFECTS*

CNS: irritability, nervousness, insomnia, headache.

CV: tachycardia, arrhythmias, increased cardiac output, angina pectoris, increased blood pressure, CARDIOVASCULAR COLLAPSE, hypotension.

GI: diarrhea, cramps, vomiting.

Derm: increased sweating, hair loss (in children).

Endo: menstrual irregularities.

Metab: weight loss, heat intolerance.

MS: accelerated bone maturation in children.

INTERACTIONS

Drug-Drug: ▪ **Colestipol** and **cholestyramine** decrease absorption ▪ **IV phenytoin** causes release of thyroid hormone ▪ May increase the effectiveness of **oral anticoagulants** ▪ May alter the requirements for **insulin** or **oral hypoglycemic agents** in diabetics ▪ Additive CNS and cardiac stimulation with **sympathomimetic agents (amphetamines, vasopressors, decongestants)** ▪ May decrease some cardiac effects of **beta-adrenergic blockers**.

ROUTE AND DOSAGE

Mild Hypothyroidism

- **PO (Adults):** 25 mcg once daily, may increase by 12.5–25 mcg/day at 1–2 wk intervals; usual maintenance dose is 25–75 mcg/day.

Severe Hypothyroidism

- **PO (Adults):** 5 mcg once daily initially, increase by 5 mcg/day at 1–2-wk intervals.

Congenital Hypothyroidism

- **PO (Infants and Children):** 5 mcg once daily, increase by 5 mcg/day at 3–4-day intervals until desired effect is achieved.

Simple Goiter

- **PO (Adults):** 5 mcg once daily initially, increase by 5–10 mcg/day at 1–2-wk intervals until daily dose is 25 mcg, then increase by 12.5–25 mcg/day at 1–2-wk intervals until effect is obtained.

T_3 Suppression Test

- **PO (Adults):** 75–100 mcg daily for 7 days. Radioactive I^{131} is administered before and after 7-day course.

PHARMACODYNAMICS (effects on thyroid function tests)

	ONSET	PEAK	DURATION
PO	UK	24–72 hr	72 hr

NURSING IMPLICATIONS

Assessment

- **General Info:** Assess apical pulse and blood pressure prior to and periodically during therapy. Assess for tachyarrhythmias and chest pain.
  - ▫ Thyroid function studies should be monitored prior to and throughout course of therapy.
  - ▫ Monitor blood and urine glucose in diabetic patients: Insulin or oral hypoglycemic dose may need to be increased.
- **Children:** Monitor height, weight, and psychomotor development.
- **Toxicity and Overdose:** Overdose is manifested as hyperthyroidism (tachycardia, chest pain, nervousness, insomnia, diaphoresis, tremors, weight loss). Usual treatment is to withhold dose for 2–6 days.

Potential Nursing Diagnoses

- Knowledge deficit related to medication regimen (patient/family teaching).

*Underlines indicate most frequent; **CAPITALS** indicate life-threatening.

L

Implementation

- **General Info:** Administer as a single dose, preferably before breakfast to prevent insomnia.
- □ Initial dose is low, especially in elderly and cardiac patients. Dosage is increased gradually based on thyroid function tests. Side effects occur more rapidly with liothyronine because of its rapid onset of effect.

Patient/Family Teaching

- **General Info:** Instruct patient to take medication exactly as prescribed at the same time each day. If a dose is missed, take as soon as remembered, unless almost time for next dose. If more than 2–3 doses are missed, notify physician. Do not discontinue without consulting physician.
- □ Instruct patient and family on correct technique for checking pulse. Dose should be withheld and physician notified if resting pulse >100 bpm.
- □ Explain to patient that liothyronine does not cure hypothyroidism, it provides a thyroid hormone; therapy is lifelong.
- □ Advise patient to notify physician if headache, nervousness, diarrhea, excessive sweating, heat intolerance, chest pain, increased pulse rate, palpitations, weight loss >2 lb/wk, or any unusual symptoms occur.
- □ Caution patient to avoid taking other medications concurrently with levothyroxine unless instructed by physician.
- □ Instruct patient to inform physician or dentist of thyroid therapy.
- □ Emphasize importance of follow-up examinations to monitor effectiveness of therapy. Thyroid function tests are performed at least yearly.
- **Children:** Discuss with parents need for routine follow-up studies to ensure correct development. Inform parents that partial hair loss may be experienced by children on thyroid therapy. This is usually temporary.

Evaluation

Clinical response can be determined by: ▪ Resolution of symptoms of hypothyroidism. Response includes: □ Diuresis □ Weight loss □ Increased sense of well-being □ Increased energy, pulse rate, appetite, psychomotor activity □ Normalization of skin texture and hair □ Correction of constipation □ Increased T_3 and T_4 levels ▪ In children, effectiveness of therapy is determined by: □ Appropriate physical and psychomotor development.

LIOTRIX

(**lye**-oh-trix)
Euthroid, T_3/T_4, Thyrolar

CLASSIFICATION(S):
Hormone—thyroid
Pregnancy Category A

INDICATIONS

▪ Replacement or substitution therapy in diminished or absent thyroid function of many causes.

ACTION

▪ A synthetic mixture of T_3 (liothyronine) and T_4 (levothyroxine) in a fixed ratio ▪ Principal effect is increasing metabolic rate of body tissues ▪ Promotes gluconeogenesis, increases utilization and mobilization of glycogen stores, and stimulates protein synthesis ▪ Promotes cell growth and aids in the development of the brain and CNS. **Therapeutic Effects:** ▪ Replacement in deficiency states ▪ Restoration of normal hormonal balance.

PHARMACOKINETICS

Absorption: Liothyronine (T_3) is 95% absorbed following oral administration; levothyroxine (T_4) is variably (50–80%) absorbed following oral administration.

Distribution: Distributed into many body tissues. Thyroid hormones do not readily cross the placenta; minimal amounts enter breast milk.

Metabolism and Excretion: Metabolized by the liver and other tissues.

Half-life: Liothyronine 1–2 days; levothyroxine 6–7 days (increased in hypothyroidism).

CONTRAINDICATIONS AND PRECAUTIONS

Contraindicated in: ▪ Hypersensitivity ▪ Recent myocardial infarction ▪ Thyrotoxicosis.

Use Cautiously in: ▪ Cardiovascular disease ▪ Severe renal insufficiency ▪ Uncorrected adrenocortical disorders ▪ Elderly and myxedematous patients (extremely sensitive to thyroid hormones; initial dosage should be markedly reduced) ▪ Has been used safely in pregnancy.

ADVERSE REACTIONS AND SIDE EFFECTS*

CNS: irritability, nervousness, insomnia, headache.

CV: tachycardia, arrhythmias, increased cardiac output, angina pectoris, increased blood pressure, CARDIOVASCULAR COLLAPSE, hypotension.

Derm: increased sweating, hair loss in children.

Endo: menstrual irregularities.

GI: diarrhea, cramps, vomiting.

Metab: weight loss, heat intolerance.

INTERACTIONS

Drug-Drug: ▪ **Colestipol** and **cholestyramine** decrease absorption ▪ **IV phenytoin** causes release of thyroid hormone ▪ May increase the effectiveness of **oral anticoagulants** ▪ May alter the requirements for **insulin** or **oral hypoglycemic agents** in diabetic patients ▪ Additive CNS and cardiac stimulation with **sympathomimetic agents (amphetamines, vasopressors, decongestants)** ▪ May decrease some cardiac effects of **beta-adrenergic blockers**.

ROUTE AND DOSAGE

Note: Thyrolar contains T_3 and T_4 in fixed ratios, representing thyroid hormone equivalents (ex: Thyrolar ½ contains the equivalent of ½ grain or 30 mg of thyroid hormone)

Product	Thyroid equivalent (mg)	T_3 (mcg)	T_4 (mcg)
Euthroid ½	30	7.5	30
Euthroid 1	60	15	60
Euthroid 2	120	30	120
Euthroid 3	180	45	180
Thyrolar ¼	15	3.1	12.5
Thyrolar ½	30	6.25	25
Thyrolar 1	60	12.5	50
Thyrolar 2	120	25	100
Thyrolar 3	180	37.5	150

Hypothyroidism

- **PO (Adults):** Thyrolar—¼, Thyrolar—½, or Euthroid—½ initially; dosage may be increased at 2–3-wk intervals.

PHARMACODYNAMICS (effects on thyroid function testing)

	ONSET	PEAK	DURATION
PO (liothyronine)	UK	24–72 hr	72 hr
PO (levothyroxine)	UK	1–3 wk	1–3 wk

NURSING IMPLICATIONS

Assessment

- **General Info:** Assess apical pulse and blood pressure prior to and periodically during therapy. Assess for tachyarrhythmias and chest pain.
  - Thyroid function studies should be monitored prior to and throughout course of therapy.
  - Monitor blood and urine glucose in diabetic patients; insulin or oral hypoglycemic dose may need to be increased.
- **Children:** Monitor height, weight, and psychomotor development.
- **Toxicity and Overdose:** Overdose is manifested as hyperthyroidism (tachycardia, chest pain, nervousness, insomnia, diaphoresis, tremors,

*Underlines indicate most frequent; **CAPITALS** indicate life-threatening.

weight loss). Usual treatment is to withhold dose for 2–6 days.

Potential Nursing Diagnoses

- Knowledge deficit related to medication regimen (patient/family teaching).

Implementation

- **General Info:** Administer as a single dose, preferably before breakfast to prevent insomnia.
- □ Initial dose is low, especially in elderly patients and patients with cardiovascular disease. Dosage is increased in small increments based on thyroid function test results.

Patient/Family Teaching

- **General Info:** Instruct patient to take medication exactly as directed at the same time each day. If a dose is missed, take as soon as remembered, unless almost time for next dose. If more than 2–3 doses are missed, notify physician. Do not discontinue without consulting physician.
- □ Instruct patient and family on correct technique for checking pulse. Dose should be withheld and physician notified if resting pulse >100 bpm.
- □ Explain to patient that liotrix does not cure hypothyroidism but provides a thyroid hormone; therapy is lifelong.
- □ Caution patient not to change brands of this medication, as this may affect drug bioavailability.
- □ Advise patient to notify physician if headache, nervousness, diarrhea, excessive sweating, heat intolerance, chest pain, increased pulse rate, palpitations, weight loss >2 lb/wk, or any unusual symptoms occur.
- □ Caution patient to avoid taking other medications concurrently with liotrix unless instructed by physician.
- □ Instruct patient to inform physician or dentist of thyroid therapy.
- □ Emphasize importance of follow-up examinations to monitor effectiveness of therapy. Thyroid function tests are performed at least yearly.
- **Children:** Discuss with parents need for routine follow-up studies to ensure correct development. Inform parents that partial hair loss may be experienced by children on thyroid therapy. This is usually temporary.

Evaluation

Clinical response is indicated by:

- Resolution of symptoms of hypothyroidism. Response includes: □ Diuresis Weight loss □ Increased sense of well-being □ Increased energy, pulse rate, appetite, psychomotor activity □ Normalization of skin texture and hair □ Correction of constipation □ Increased T_3 and T_4 levels □ Normal thyroid stimulating hormone (TSH) levels ▪ In children effectiveness of therapy is determined by: □ Appropriate physical and psychomotor development.

LISINOPRIL

(lyse-**in**-oh-pril)
Privinil, Zestril

CLASSIFICATION(S):
Antihypertensive—angiotensin converting enzyme (ACE) inhibitor
Pregnancy Category C

INDICATIONS

- Used alone or in combination with other antihypertensives in the management of hypertension.

ACTION

- Prevents the production of angiotensin II, a potent vasoconstrictor that stimulates the production of aldosterone by blocking its conversion to the active form. Result is systemic vasodilation. **Therapeutic Effect:** ▪ Lowering of blood pressure in hypertensive patients.

PHARMACOKINETICS

Absorption: 25% absorbed following oral administration; much variability.
Distribution: Distribution not known.
Metabolism and Excretion: Excreted entirely unchanged by the kidneys.
Half-life: 12 hr.

CONTRAINDICATIONS AND PRECAUTIONS

Contraindicated in: ▪ Hypersensitivity.

Use Cautiously in: ▪ Renal impairment (dosage reduction required) ▪ Pregnancy, lactation, or children (safety not established) ▪ Surgery/anesthesia (hypotension may be exaggerated) ▪ Aortic stenosis, cerebrovascular or cardiac insufficiency.

ADVERSE REACTIONS AND SIDE EFFECTS*

CNS: <u>headache</u>, <u>dizziness</u>, <u>fatigue</u>, insomnia.
Resp: cough, dyspnea.
CV: hypotension, tachycardia, angina pectoris.
GI: anorexia, diarrhea, nausea, altered taste, stomatitis.
GU: impotence, increased BUN.
Derm: rashes.
F and E: hyperkalemia.
Hemat: neutropenia.
Neuro: paresthesias.
Misc: fever, ANGIODEMA with laryngospasm.

INTERACTIONS

Drug–Drug: ▪ Additive hypotension with other **antihypertensives, nitrates,** or acute ingestion of **alcohol** ▪ Hyperkalemia may result with concurrent **potassium supplements** or **potassium-sparing diuretics** ▪ Antihypertensive response may be blunted by **nonsteroidal anti-inflammatory agents** ▪ Incidence of hypersensitivity reactions may be increased with **allopurinol** ▪ May increase serum **lithium** or **digoxin** levels and risk of toxicity.

Drug–Food: ▪ Hyperkalemia may result from a **high-potassium** diet.

ROUTE AND DOSAGE

- **PO (Adults):** 10 mg once daily (5 mg if on diuretics), can be increased up to 20–40 mg day.

PHARMACODYNAMICS (antihypertensive effect)

	ONSET	PEAK	DURATION
PO	1 hr	7 hr	24 hr

NURSING IMPLICATIONS

Assessment

- ▫ Monitor blood pressure and pulse frequently during initial dosage adjustment and periodically throughout course of therapy. Notify physician of significant changes.
- ▫ Monitor weight and signs of congestive heart failure (peripheral edema, rales/crackles, dyspnea, weight gain).
- ▪ **Lab Test Considerations:** Monitor BUN, creatinine, and electrolyte levels periodically. Serum potassium may be increased and BUN and creatinine transiently increased, while sodium levels may be decreased.

Potential Nursing Diagnoses

- ▪ Cardiac output, decreased (indications, side effects).
- ▪ Knowledge deficit related to medication regimen (patient/family teaching).
- ▪ Noncompliance (patient/family teaching).

Implementation

- ▪ **General Info:** Patients treated with diuretics should discontinue diuretic therapy for 2–3 days, if possible, prior to initial dose of lisinopril to prevent hypotension. If this is not possible, decreased dose of lisinopril may be necessary.
- ▫ If blood pressure is not controlled with lisinopril, diuretic therapy may be added.

Patient/Family Teaching

- ▫ Instruct patient to take lisinopril exactly as directed, even if feeling well. Medication controls but does not cure hypertension. Advise patients not to discontinue lisinopril therapy unless directed by physician.

*<u>Underlines</u> indicate most frequent; **CAPITALS** indicate life-threatening.

L

- Encourage patient to comply with additional interventions for hypertension (low-sodium diet, weight reduction, discontinuation of smoking, moderation of alcohol consumption, regular exercise, and stress management).
- Instruct patient and family on proper technique for blood pressure monitoring. Advise them to check blood pressure at least weekly and to report significant changes to physician.
- Caution patient to avoid salt substitutes or foods containing high levels of potassium or sodium, unless directed by physician (see Appendix K).
- Advise patient that lisinopril may cause an impairment of taste, which generally reverses itself within 8–12 wk.
- Caution patient to change position slowly to minimize orthostatic hypotension, particularly after initial dose. Patient should also be advised that exercising or hot weather may increase hypotensive effects.
- Advise patient to consult physician or pharmacist before taking any over-the-counter medications, especially cold remedies. Patient should also avoid excessive amounts of tea, coffee, or cola.
- Advise patient to inform physician or dentist of medication regimen prior to treatment or surgery.
- Instruct patient to notify physician if cough, rash, mouth sores, sore throat, fever, swelling of hands or feet, irregular heart beat, chest pain, swelling of face, eyes, lips, or tongue, persistent fatigue, headache, or difficulty breathing occurs.
- Emphasize the importance of follow-up examinations to monitor progress.

Evaluation

Effectiveness of therapy can be demonstrated by: ▪ Decrease in blood pressure without appearance of side effects. Several wks may be necessary before full effects of the drug are recognized.

LITHIUM
(**lith**-ee-um)
{Carbolith}, Cibalith-S, {Duralth}, Eskalith, Lithane, {Lithizine}, Lithobid, Lithonate, Lithotabs

CLASSIFICATION(S):
Antimanic
Pregnancy Category D

INDICATIONS

▪ Treatment of a variety of psychiatric disorders, particularly bipolar affective disorders, both to treat acute manic episodes and as prophylaxis against their recurrence.

ACTION

▪ Alters cation transport in nerve and muscle ▪ May also influence re-uptake of neurotransmitters. **Therapeutic Effects:** ▪ Antimanic and antidepressant properties.

PHARMACOKINETICS

Absorption: Completely absorbed following oral administration.
Distribution: Widely distributed into many tissues and fluids; CSF levels are 50% of plasma levels. Crosses the placenta and enters breast milk.
Metabolism and Excretion: Excreted almost entirely unchanged by the kidneys.
Half-life: 20–27 hr.

CONTRAINDICATIONS AND PRECAUTIONS

Contraindicated in: ▪ Hypersensitivity ▪ Severe cardiovascular or renal disease ▪ Dehydrated or debilitated patients ▪ Pregnancy or lactation ▪ Should be used only where therapy, including blood levels, may be closely monitored.
Use Cautiously in: ▪ Elderly patients ▪ Any degree of cardiac, renal, or thyroid disease ▪ Diabetes mellitus ▪ Children (safety not established).

ADVERSE REACTIONS AND SIDE EFFECTS*

CNS: tremors, headache, impaired memory, lethargy, fatigue, drowsiness, confusion, seizures, ataxia, dizziness, psychomotor retardation, restlessness, stupor.
EENT: tinnitus, blurred vision, dysarthria, aphasia.
CV: ECG changes, hypotension, arrhythmias, edema.
GI: nausea, anorexia, epigastric bloating, diarrhea, abdominal pain, dry mouth, metallic taste.
GU: polyuria, nephrogenic diabetes insipidus, glycosuria, renal toxicity.
Derm: acneiform erruption, folliculitis, pruritis, diminished sensation, alopecia.
Endo: hypothyroidism, goiter, hyperglycemia, hyperthyroidism.
F and E: hyponatremia.
Hemat: leukocytosis.
Metab: weight gain.
MS: muscle weakness, rigidity, hyperirritability.

INTERACTIONS

Drug–Drug: ▪ May prolong the action of **neuromuscular blocking agents** ▪ Encephalopathic syndrome may occur with **haloperidol** ▪ **Diuretics, methyldopa, probenecid, indomethacin,** and other **nonsteroidal anti-inflammatory agents** may increase the risk of toxicity ▪ **Aminophylline, phenothiazines, sodium bicarbonate,** and **sodium chloride** may hasten excretion and lead to decreased effect ▪ Lithium may decrease the effects of **chlorpromazine** ▪ **Chlorpromazine** may mask early signs of lithium toxicity ▪ Hypothyroid effects may be additive with **potassium iodide** or **antithyroid drugs** ▪ Drugs containing large amounts of **sodium (ticarcillin)** may increase the renal elimination and decrease the effectiveness of lithium.

Drug–Food: ▪ Large changes in **sodium** intake may alter the renal elimination of lithium. Increasing sodium intake will increase renal excretion.

ROUTE AND DOSAGE

- **PO (Adults):** 900–1200 mg/day in 3–4 divided doses (usual dose 300 mg 3–4 times daily). Blood level monitoring necessary to determine proper dose. Extended-release dosage forms (Eskalith-CR, Lithobid) may be given bid.

PHARMACODYNAMICS (antimanic effects)

	ONSET	PEAK	DURATION
PO	5–7 days	10–21 days	days
PO liq	5–7 days	10–21 days	days
PO ER caps	5–7 days	10–21 days	days

NURSING IMPLICATIONS

Assessment

- □ Assess mood, ideation, and behaviors frequently. Initiate suicide precautions if indicated.
- □ Monitor intake and output ratios. Notify physician of significant changes in totals. Unless contraindicated, fluid intake of at least 2000–3000 ml/day should be maintained. Weight should also be monitored at least every 3 mon.
- ▪ **Lab Test Considerations:** Renal and thyroid function, WBC with differential, serum electrolytes, and glucose should be evaluated periodically throughout therapy.
- ▪ **Toxicity and Overdose:** Serum lithium levels should be monitored twice weekly during initiation of therapy and every 2–3 mon during chronic therapy. Blood samples should be drawn in the morning immediately prior to next dose. Therapeutic levels range from 0.5 to 1.5 mEq/liter.
- □ Assess patient for signs and symptoms of lithium toxicity (vomiting, diarrhea, slurred speech, decreased coordination, drowsiness, muscle weakness, or twitching). If these occur, inform physician prior to administering next dose.

*Underlines indicate most frequent; **CAPITALS** indicate life-threatening.

Potential Nursing Diagnoses

- Thought processes, altered: (indications).
- Violence, high risk for: directed at self/others (indications).
- Knowledge deficit related to medication regimen (patient/family teaching).
- Noncompliance (patient/family teaching).

Implementation

- **General Info:** Available in tablet, capsule, extended-release preparations, and syrup.
- **PO:** Administer with food or milk to minimize GI irritation. Extended-release preparations should be swallowed whole; do not break, crush, or chew.

Patient/Family Teaching

- Instruct patient to take medication exactly as ordered, even if feeling well. If a dose is missed, take as soon as remembered unless within 2 hr of next dose (6 hr if extended-release).
- Medication may cause dizziness or drowsiness. Caution patient to avoid driving or other activities requiring alertness until response to medication is known.
- Low sodium levels may predispose patient to toxicity. Advise patient to drink 2000–3000 ml fluid each day and eat a diet with liberal sodium intake. Excessive amounts of coffee, tea, and cola should be avoided because of diuretic effect. Avoid activities that cause excess sodium loss (heavy exertion, exercise in hot weather, saunas). Notify physician of vomiting and diarrhea, which also cause sodium loss.
- Advise patient that weight gain may occur. Review principles of a low-calorie diet.
- Instruct patient to consult physician or pharmacist prior to taking over-the-counter medications concurrently with this therapy.
- Advise patient to use contraception and to consult physician if pregnancy is suspected.
- Review side effects and symptoms of toxicity with patient. Inform patient of the importance of reporting adverse effects to physician promptly.
- Explain to patients with cardiovascular disease or >40 yr the need for ECG evaluation prior to and periodically during therapy. Patient should inform physician if fainting, irregular pulse, or difficulty breathing occurs.
- Emphasize the importance of periodic lab tests to monitor for lithium toxicity.

Evaluation

Effectiveness of therapy can be demonstrated by: ▪ Resolution of the symptoms of mania (hyperactivity, pressured speech, poor judgment, need for little sleep) ▪ Decreased incidence of mood swings in bipolar disorders ▪ Improved affect in unipolar disorders. Improvement in condition may require 1–3 wk.

LOMUSTINE
(loe-**mus**-teen)
CCNU, CeeNu

CLASSIFICATION(S):
Antineoplastic agent—nitrosourea
Pregnancy Category UK

INDICATIONS

▪ Used alone or with other treatment modalities in the management of primary and metastatic brain tumors and Hodgkin's disease. **Unlabeled Uses:** ▪ Bronchogenic carcinoma ▪ Non-Hodgkin's lymphoma ▪ Malignant melanoma ▪ Breast carcinoma ▪ Renal cell carcinoma ▪ GI tract carcinoma.

ACTION

▪ Inhibits DNA and RNA synthesis by alkylation (cell cycle phase-nonspecific. **Therapeutic Effect:** ▪ Death of rapidly replicating cells, particularly malignant ones.

PHARMACOKINETICS

Absorption: Rapidly absorbed following oral administration.
Distribution: Widely distributed. Active metabolites enter the CSF well. Enters breast milk.
Metabolism and Excretion: Mostly metabolized by the liver. Some metabolites are active antineoplastic agents.
Half-life: 1–2 days.

CONTRAINDICATIONS AND PRECAUTIONS

Contraindicated in: ▪ Hypersensitivity ▪ Pregnancy or lactation.
Use Cautiously in: ▪ Patients with childbearing potential ▪ Active infections ▪ Decreased bone marrow reserve ▪ Other chronic debilitating illnesses ▪ Impaired liver function.

ADVERSE REACTIONS AND SIDE EFFECTS*

CNS: disorientation, lethargy, ataxia, dysarthria.
GI: nausea, vomiting, stomatitis, hepatotoxicity, anorexia.
GU: azotemia, renal failure.
Endo: gonadal suppression.
Hemat: anemia, leukopenia, thrombocytopenia.
Metab: hyperuricemia.
Resp: pulmonary infiltrates, fibrosis.

INTERACTIONS

Drug-Drug: ▪ Additive bone marrow depression with other **antineoplastic agents** or **radiation therapy** ▪ May decrease antibody response to **live virus vaccines** and increase risk of adverse reactions.

ROUTE AND DOSAGE

- **PO (Adults and Children):** 130 mg/m^2 as a single dose. Dosage adjustments are required for concurrent therapy or decreased blood counts.

PHARMACODYNAMICS (effects on blood counts)

	ONSET	PEAK	DURATION
PO	UK	4–7 wk	1–2 wk

NURSING IMPLICATIONS

ASSESSMENT

- Assess for fever, sore throat, and signs of infection. Notify physician if these symptoms occur.
- Assess for bleeding (bleeding gums, bruising, petechiae; guaiac stools, urine, and emesis). Avoid IM injections and rectal temperatures. Apply pressure to venipuncture sites for 10 min.
- Assess for nausea and vomiting, which usually begins within 3 hr of administration and persists for 24 hr. Confer with physician regarding prophylactic use of an antiemetic. Monitor intake and output, daily weight, and appetite. Adjust diet as tolerated for anorexia.
- **Lab Test Considerations:** Monitor CBC and differential prior to and periodically throughout therapy. The nadir of leukopenia occurs in 6 wk. Notify physician if leukocyte count is <4000/mm^3. The nadir of thrombocytopenia occurs in 4 wk. Notify physician if platelet count is <100,000/mm^3. Recovery of leukopenia and thrombocytopenia occurs in 1–2 wk. Myelosuppression is cumulative; subsequent courses of therapy should be delayed until recovery occurs.
- Monitor liver function studies (SGOT [AST], SGPT [ALT], LDH, bilirubin) and renal function studies (BUN, creatinine) prior to and periodically throughout therapy to detect hepatotoxicity and nephrotoxicity.
- May cause increased uric acid. Monitor periodically during therapy.

POTENTIAL NURSING DIAGNOSES

- Infection, high risk for (side effects).
- Nutrition, altered: less than body requirements (side effects).
- Knowledge deficit related to medication regimen (patient/family teaching).

IMPLEMENTATION

- **PO:** Administer on empty stomach at bedtime. Preadministration of an an-

*Underlines indicate most frequent; **CAPITALS** indicate life-threatening.

tiemetic and a hypnotic may help control nausea.

Patient/Family Teaching

- Instruct patient to take lomustine exactly as directed, even if nausea and vomiting occurs. If vomiting occurs shortly after dose is taken, consult physician.
- Inform patient that several different types of capsules may be found in medication container. Patient should take all the capsules at one time in order to receive the correct dose.
- Advise patient to notify physician promptly if fever, chills, sore throat, signs of infection, bleeding gums, bruising, petechiae, or blood in urine, stool, or emesis occurs. Caution patient to avoid crowds and persons with known infections. Instruct patient to use soft toothbrush and electric razor. Patient should be cautioned not to drink alcoholic beverages or take aspirin-containing products.
- Instruct patient to notify physician if abdominal pain, yellow skin, weakness, cough, slurred speech, or decreased urine output occurs.
- Instruct patient to inspect oral mucosa for redness and ulceration. If ulceration occurs, advise patient to use sponge brush and rinse mouth with water after eating and drinking. Physician may order viscous lidocaine swishes if pain interferes with eating.
- Discuss with patient the possibility of hair loss. Explore coping strategies.
- Advise patient that although lomustine may cause infertility, contraception is necessary because of potential teratogenic effects in the fetus.
- Instruct patient not to receive any vaccinations without advice of physician.
- Emphasize need for periodic lab tests to monitor for side effects.

Evaluation

Effectiveness of therapy can be demonstrated by: ▪ Decrease in size and spread of malignant tissue.

LOPERAMIDE
(loe-**per**-a-mide)
Imodium, Imodium A-D

CLASSIFICATION(S):
Antidiarrheal
Pregnancy Category B

INDICATIONS

▪ Adjunctive therapy in the treatment of acute diarrhea ▪ Treatment of chronic diarrhea associated with inflammatory bowel disease ▪ Used to decrease the volume of ileostomy drainage.

ACTION

▪ Inhibits peristalsis and prolongs transit time by a direct effect on nerves in the intestinal muscle wall ▪ Reduces fecal volume, increases fecal viscosity and bulk while diminishing loss of fluid and electrolytes. **Therapeutic Effect:** ▪ Relief of diarrhea.

PHARMACOKINETICS

Absorption: Not well absorbed following oral administration.
Distribution: Distribution not known. Does not cross the blood-brain barrier.
Metabolism and Excretion: Metabolized partially by the liver, undergoes enterohepatic recirculation. 30% eliminated in the feces. Minimal excretion in the urine.
Half-life: 10.8 hr.

CONTRAINDICATIONS AND PRECAUTIONS

Contraindicated in: ▪ Hypersensitivity ▪ Patients in whom constipation must be avoided ▪ Abdominal pain of unknown cause, especially if associated with fever. Alcohol intolerance (liquid only).
Use Cautiously in: ▪ Hepatic dysfunction ▪ Pregnancy, lactation, or children <2 yr (safety not established).

ADVERSE REACTIONS AND SIDE EFFECTS*

CNS: drowsiness, dizziness.
GI: constipation, nausea, dry mouth.

*Underlines indicate most frequent; **CAPITALS** indicate life-threatening.

INTERACTIONS

Drug–Drug: ▪ Additive CNS depression with other **CNS depressants,** including **alcohol, antihistamines, narcotics,** and **sedative/hypnotics** ▪ Additive anticholinergic properties with other **drugs having anticholinergic properties,** including **antidepressants** and **antihistamines**.

ROUTE AND DOSAGE

- **PO (Adults):** 4 mg initially, then 2 mg after each loose stool. Maintenance dose usually 4–8 mg/day (not to exceed 16 mg/day).
- **PO (Children 8–12 yr or >30 kg):** 2 mg, may be repeated 3 times in first 24 hr, then 0.1 mg/kg after each loose stool or 2 mg initially, then 1 mg with each loose stool (not to exceed 6 mg/24 hr).
- **PO (Children 5–8 yr or 20–30 kg):** 2 mg, may be repeated twice in first 24 hr, then 0.1 mg/kg after each loose stool or 2 mg initially then 1 mg with each loose stool (not to exceed 4 mg/24 hr).
- **PO (Children 2–5 yr or 13–20 kg):** 1 mg, may be repeated 3 times in first 24 hr, then 0.1 mg/kg after each loose stool.

PHARMACODYNAMICS (relief of diarrhea)

	ONSET	PEAK	DURATION
PO	1 hr	2.5–5 hr	10 hr

NURSING IMPICATIONS

Assessment

- ▫ Assess frequency and consistency of stools and bowel sounds prior to and throughout course of therapy.
- ▫ Assess fluid and electrolyte balance and skin turgor for dehydration.

Potential Nursing Diagnoses

- Bowel elminiation, altered: diarrhea (indications).
- Injury, high risk for (side effects).
- Knowledge deficit related to medication regimen (patient/family teaching).

Implementation

- **PO:** Available in capsule and liquid forms.

Patient/Family Teaching

- ▫ Instruct patient to take medication exactly as directed. Do not take missed doses, and do not double doses. In acute diarrhea, medication may be ordered after each unformed stool. Advise patient of the maximum number of doses.
- ▫ Medication may cause drowsiness. Advise patient to avoid driving or other activities requiring alertness until response to drug is known.
- ▫ Advise patient that frequent mouth rinses, good oral hygiene, and sugarless gum or candy may relieve dry mouth.
- ▫ Caution patient to avoid using alcohol and other CNS depressants concurrently with this medication.
- ▫ Instruct patient to notify physician if diarrhea persists or if fever occurs.

Evaluation

Effectiveness of therapy can be determined by: ▪ Decrease in diarrhea ▫ In acute diarrhea, treatment should be discontinued if no improvement is seen in 48 hr ▫ In chronic diarrhea, if no improvement has occurred after at least 10 days of treatment with maximum dose, loperamide is unlikely to be effective.

LORAZEPAM

(lor-**az**-e-pam)
{Apo-Lorazepam}, Alzapam, Ativan, Loraz, {Novolorazrem}

CLASSIFICATION(S):
Sedative/hypnotic—benzodiazepine, Antianxiety agent
Schedule IV
Pregnancy Category D—parenteral only, UK for oral

L

INDICATIONS

■ Adjunct in the management of anxiety or insomnia ■ Provides preoperative sedation ■ Relieves preoperative anxiety and provides amnesia.

ACTION

■ Depresses the CNS, probably by potentiating gamma-aminobutyric acid (GABA), an inhibitory neurotransmitter. **Therapeutic Effects:** ■ Sedation ■ Relief of anxiety.

PHARMACOKINETICS

Absorption: Well absorbed following oral administration. Rapidly and completely absorbed following IM administration.
Distribution: Widely distributed. Crosses the blood-brain barrier. Crosses the placenta and enters breast milk.
Metabolism and Excretion: Highly metabolized by the liver.
Half-life: 10–20 hr.

CONTRAINDICATIONS AND PRECAUTIONS

Contraindicated in: ■ Hypersensitivity ■ Cross-sensitivity with other benzodiazepines may exist ■ Comatose patients or those with pre-existing CNS depression ■ Uncontrolled severe pain ■ Narrow-angle glaucoma ■ Pregnancy and lactation.
Use Cautiously in: ■ Severe hepatic or renal impairment ■ Patients who may be suicidal or who may have been addicted to drugs previously ■ Elderly or debilitated patients (dosage reduction suggested) ■ Hypnotic use—should be short-term.

ADVERSE REACTIONS AND SIDE EFFECTS*

CNS: dizziness, drowsiness, lethargy, hangover, paradoxical excitation, headache, mental depression.
EENT: blurred vision.
Resp: respiratory depression.
GI: nausea, vomiting, diarrhea, constipation.
Derm: rashes.
Misc: tolerance, psychological dependence, physical dependence.

INTERACTIONS

Drug-Drug: ■ Additive CNS depression with other **CNS depressants,** including **alcohol, antihistamines, antidepressants, narcotic analgesics,** and other **sedative/hypnotics** ■ May decrease the efficacy of **levodopa** ■ **Smoking** may increase metabolism and decrease effectiveness ■ **Probenecid** may decrease metabolism of lorazepam, enhancing its actions ■ May decrease the efficacy of **lepodopa**.

ROUTE AND DOSAGE

Anxiety

■ **PO (Adults):** 2–3 mg/day in 2–3 divided doses (usual dosage range 2–6 mg/day, up to 10 mg/day).

Insomnia

■ **PO (Adults):** 2–4 mg at bedtime.

Preoperative Sedation

■ **IV (Adults):** 0.044 mg/kg (not to exceed 2 mg) 15–20 min before surgery.
■ **IM (Adults):** 0.05 mg/kg 2 hr before surgery (not to exceed 4 mg).

Operative Amnesia

■ **IV (Adults):** up to 0.05 mg/kg (not to exceed 4 mg).

PHARMACODYNAMICS (sedation)

	ONSET	PEAK*	DURATION
PO	15–45 min	1–6 hr	up to 48 hr
IM	15–30 min	1–1.5 hr	up to 48 hr
IV	5–15 min	UK	up to 48 hr

*Peak plasma levels.

NURSING IMPLICATIONS

Assessment

□ Assess degree and manifestations of anxiety prior to and periodically throughout therapy.
□ Prolonged high-dose therapy may lead to psychological or physical de-

*Underlines indicate most frequent; **CAPITALS** indicate life-threatening.

pendence. Restrict amount of drug available to patient.

- **Lab Test Considerations:** Patients on high-dose therapy should receive routine evaluation of renal, hepatic, and hematologic function.

POTENTIAL NURSING DIAGNOSES

- Anxiety (indications).
- Injury, high risk for (indications, side effects).
- Knowledge deficit related to medication regimen (patient/family teaching).

IMPLEMENTATION

- **General Info:** Following parenteral administration, keep patient supine for at least 8 hr and observe closely.
- **IM:** Administer IM doses deep into muscle mass.
- **Direct IV:** Dilute immediately before use with an equal amount of sterile water, D5W, or 0.9% NaCl for injection. Do not use if soln is colored or contains a precipitate.
- □ *Rate:* Administer direct IV, through Y-site injection or via 3-way stopcock at a rate of 2 mg over 1 min. Rapid IV administration may result in apnea, hypotension, bradycardia, or cardiac arrest.
- **Syringe Compatibility:** cimetidine.
- **Y-Site Compatibility:** acyclovir, atracurium, pancuronium, vecuronium, or zidovudine.
- **Y-Site Incompatibility:** foscarnet or ondansetron.

PATIENT/FAMILY TEACHING

- □ Instruct patient to take medication exactly as directed, not to skip or double up on missed doses. Abrupt withdrawal may cause tremors, nausea, vomiting, and abdominal and muscle cramps.
- □ Medication may cause drowsiness or dizziness. Advise patient to avoid driving or other activities requiring alertness until response to medication is known.
- □ Caution patient to avoid taking alcohol or other CNS depressants concurrently with this medication.
- □ Instruct patient to contact physician immediately if pregnancy is suspected or planned.
- □ Emphasize the importance of follow-up examinations to determine effectiveness of the medication.

EVALUATION

Effectiveness of therapy can be demonstrated by: ■ Increase in sense of well-being □ Decrease in subjective feelings of anxiety without excessive sedation ■ Reduction of preoperative anxiety ■ Postoperative amnesia.

LOVASTATIN

(**loe**-va-sta-tin)
Mevacor, Mevinolin

CLASSIFICATION(S):
Lipid-lowering agent
Pregnancy Category X

INDICATIONS

- Adjunct to dietary therapy in the management of primary hypercholesterolemia.

ACTION

- Inhibits the enzyme (HMG-CoA reductase) responsible for catalyzing an early step in the synthesis of cholesterol. **Therapeutic Effect:** ■ Lowering of total and LDL cholesterol. Increases HDL and decreases VLDL cholesterol and triglycerides.

PHARMACOKINETICS

Absorption: Poorly and variably absorbed followed oral administration.
Distribution: Crosses the blood-brain barrier and placenta.
Metabolism and Excretion: Highly metabolized by the liver. Excreted in bile and feces. Small amounts (10%) excreted unchanged by the kidneys.
Half-life: UK.

CONTRAINDICATIONS AND PRECAUTIONS

Contraindicated in: ▪ Hypersensitivity ▪ Pregnancy or lactation ▪ Active liver disease.

Use Cautiously in: ▪ History of liver disease ▪ Alcoholism ▪ Severe acute infection ▪ Hypotension ▪ Major surgery ▪ Trauma ▪ Severe metabolic, endocrine, or electrolyte problems ▪ Uncontrolled seizures ▪ Visual disturbances ▪ Children (safety not established).

ADVERSE REACTIONS AND SIDE EFFECTS*

CNS: dizziness, headache.

EENT: blurred vision.

GI: constipation, diarrhea, dyspepsia, flatus, abdominal cramps, heartburn, nausea, hepatitis, altered taste.

Derm: rashes, pruritus.

MS: muscle cramps, myalgia, myopathy.

INTERACTIONS

Drug–Drug: ▪ Cholesterol-lowering effect may be additive with **bile acid sequestrants (cholestyramine, colestipol)** ▪ Increased risk of myopathy with concurrent **niacin, gemfibrozil,** or **cyclosporine.**

ROUTE AND DOSAGE

- **PO (Adults):** 20 mg once daily with evening meal. Dosage may be increased at 4-wk intervals to a maximum of 80 mg/day in single or divided doses.

PHARMACODYNAMICS (cholesterol-lowering effect)

	ONSET	PEAK	DURATION
PO	2 wk	4–6 wk	UK

NURSING IMPLICATIONS

Assessment

- Obtain a diet history, especially in regard to fat consumption.
- Ophthalmic examinations are recommended prior to and yearly throughout therapy.
- **Lab Test Considerations:** Serum cholesterol levels should be evaluated before initiating and periodically throughout course of therapy.
- Liver function tests, including SGOT (AST), should be monitored prior to and monthly during the first 15 mon of therapy, and then periodically. If SGOT (AST) levels increase to 3 times normal, lovastatin therapy should be discontinued.
- If patient develops muscle tenderness during therapy, CPK levels should be monitored. If CPK levels are markedly increased or myopathy occurs, lovastatin therapy should be discontinued.

Potential Nursing Diagnoses

- Knowledge deficit related to diet and medication regimen (patient/family teaching).
- Noncompliance (patient/family teaching).

Implementation

- **PO:** Administer lovastatin with food. Administration on an empty stomach decreases absorption by approximately 30%. Initial once-daily dose is administered with the evening meal.

Patient/Family Teaching

- Instruct patient to take medication exactly as directed, not to skip doses or double up on missed doses. Lovastatin helps control but does not cure elevated serum cholesterol levels. Consult physician prior to discontinuing lovastatin therapy; serum lipid levels may increase significantly. Therapy may be long-term.
- Advise patient that this medication should be used in conjunction with diet restrictions (fat, cholesterol, carbohydrates, alcohol), exercise, and cessation of smoking.
- Instruct female patients to notify physician promptly if pregnancy is planned or suspected.
- Advise patient to notify physician or

*Underlines indicate most frequent; **CAPITALS** indicate life-threatening.

dentist of medication regimen prior to treatment or surgery.

- Emphasize the importance of follow-up examinations to determine effectiveness and to monitor for side effects.

Evaluation

Effectiveness of therapy can be demonstrated by: ▪ Decrease in serum LDL, VLDL, and total cholesterol levels ▪ Increase in HDL cholesterol levels.

LOXAPINE

(**lox**-a-peen)
{Loxapac}, Loxitane, Loxitane-C, Loxitane IM

CLASSIFICATION(S):
Antipsychotic
Pregnancy Category C

INDICATIONS

▪ Management of psychoses. **Unlabeled Use:** ▪ Management of depression and anxiety associated with depression.

ACTION

▪ Appears to block dopamine at postsynaptic receptors sites in the CNS. **Therapeutic Effect:** ▪ Diminution of psychotic behavior.

PHARMACOKINETICS

Absorption: Well absorbed following oral or IM administration.
Distribution: Distribution in humans not known.
Metabolism and Excretion: Extensively metabolized by the liver. Some conversion to active antipsychotic compounds.
Half-life: 19 hr.

CONTRAINDICATIONS AND PRECAUTIONS

Contraindicated in: ▪ Hypersensitivity or intolerance to loxapine or amoxapine ▪ Coma ▪ CNS depression ▪ Pregnancy or lactation.

Use Cautiously in: ▪ Glaucoma ▪ Elderly men or patients with prostatic hypertrophy (more prone to urinary retention) ▪ Elderly patients (more susceptible to adverse reactions) ▪ Intestinal obstruction ▪ History of seizures ▪ Alcoholism ▪ Cardiovascular disease ▪ Impaired liver function ▪ Children <16 yr (safety not established).

ADVERSE REACTIONS AND SIDE EFFECTS*

CNS: drowsiness, extrapyramidal syndromes, including NEUROLEPTIC MALIGNANT SYNDROME, tardive dyskinesia, insomnia, dizziness, lethargy, lightheadedness, syncope, headache, ataxia, weakness, confusion.
EENT: nasal congestion, blurred vision, lens opacities.
CV: tachycardia, hypotension.
GI: constipation, dry mouth, hepatitis, nausea, vomiting, ileus.
GU: urinary retention.
Derm: rashes, dermatitis, facial photosensitivity, edema, seborrhea, pigment changes.
Endo: galactorrhea.
Hemat: AGRANULOCYTOSIS.
Misc: allergic reactions, NEUROLEPTIC MALIGNANT SYNDROME.

INTERACTIONS

Drug-Drug: ▪ Decreases the antihypertensive effects of **guanethidine** or **guanadrel** ▪ Blocks the alpha-adrenergic effects of **epinephrine** (may result in hypotension and tachycardia) ▪ Additive CNS depression with other **CNS depressants,** including **alcohol, antihistamines, narcotic analgesics,** and **sedative/hypnotics** ▪ **Antacids** or **adsorbent antidiarrheals** may decrease absorption ▪ Use with **antidepressants** or **MAO inhibitors** may result in prolonged CNS depression and increased anticholinergic effects.

ROUTE AND DOSAGE

- **PO (Adults):** 10 mg bid, may be increased gradually over the first 7–10

{} = Available in Canada only.
*Underlines indicate most frequent; **CAPITALS** indicate life-threatening.

days as needed and tolerated. Usual maintenance dose is 15–25 mg 2–4 times daily. Severely ill patients may require up to 50 mg initially and maintenance doses up to 250 mg/day.
- **IM (Adults):** 12.5–50 mg q 4–6 hr as needed and tolerated.

PHARMACODYNAMICS (antipsychotic effect)

	ONSET	PEAK	DURATION
PO	30 min	1.5–3 hr	12 hr
IM	UK	UK	UK

NURSING IMPLICATIONS

Assessment

- Monitor patient's mental status (delusions, hallucinations, and behavior) prior to and periodically throughout therapy.
- Monitor blood pressure (sitting, standing, lying) and pulse rate prior to and frequently during the period of dosage adjustment.
- Observe patient carefully when administering medication to ensure medication is actually taken and not hoarded.
- Monitor patient for onset of extrapyramidal side effects (akathisia—restlessness; dystonia—muscle spasms and twisting motions; or pseudoparkinsonism—mask facies, rigidity, tremors, drooling, shuffling gait, dysphagia). Notify physician if these symptoms occur, as reduction in dosage or discontinuation of medication may be necessary. Physician may also order antiparkinson agents (trihexyphenidyl, benztropine) to control these symptoms.
- Monitor for tardive dyskinesia (rhythmic movement of mouth, face, and extremities). Notify physician immediately if these symptoms occur, as these side effects may be irreversible.
- Monitor frequency and consistency of bowel movement. Increasing bulk and fluids in the diet may help minimize constipation.
- Loxapine lowers the seizure threshold. Institute seizure precautions for patients with history of seizure disorder.
- Monitor for development of neuroleptic malignant syndrome (fever, respiratory distress, tachycardia, convulsions, diaphoresis, hypertension or hypotension, pallor, tiredness). Notify physician immediately if these symptoms occur.
- **Lab Test Considerations:** Monitor CBC and differential prior to and periodically throughout therapy.
- Monitor liver function studies prior to and periodically during therapy.
- **Toxicity and Overdose:** Antiemetic effects of loxapine may block the action of ipecac. Overdose is treated by gastric lavage, barbiturates to control seizures, and supportive care for fluctuations in body temperature. Hypotension may be corrected by use of IV fluids, norepinephrine, or phenylephrine. Avoid use of epinephrine, as it may worsen hypotension.

Potential Nursing Diagnoses

- Thought processes, altered (indications).
- Injury, high risk for (side effects).
- Knowledge deficit related to medication regimen (patient/family teaching).

Implementation

- **General Info:** Available as capsule, oral soln, and parenteral injection.
- **PO:** Administer capsules with food or milk to decrease gastric irritation.
- Dilute oral solution with orange or grapefruit juice immediately prior to administration. Measure dose with provided dropper.
- **IM:** Do not inject SC. Inject slowly into deep, well-developed muscle. Light amber color does not alter potency of soln. Do not administer soln that is markedly discolored or that contains a precipitate.
- Keep patient recumbent for at least 30 min following parenteral administra-

tion to minimize hypotensive effects.

Patient/Family Teaching

- Instruct patient on need to take medication exactly as ordered. If a dose is missed, it should be taken as soon as remembered, up to 1 hr before next scheduled dose. Patients on long-term high-dose therapy may need to discontinue gradually to avoid withdrawal symptoms (dyskinesia, tremors, dizziness, nausea, and vomiting).
- Instruct patient receiving oral soln on correct method of measuring dose with provided dropper.
- Inform patient of possibility of extrapyramidal symptoms and tardive dyskinesia. Instruct patient to report these symptoms immediately to physician.
- Advise patient to make position changes slowly to minimize orthostatic hypotension.
- May cause drowsiness. Caution patient to avoid driving or other activities requiring alertness until response to the medication is known.
- Caution patient to use sunscreen and protective clothing to prevent photosensitivity reactions.
- Caution patient to avoid concurrent use of alcohol, other CNS depressants, and over-the-counter medications without prior approval of physician.
- Instruct patient to use frequent mouth rinses, good oral hygiene, and sugarless gum or candy to minimize dry mouth. Consult physician or dentist if dry mouth continues >2 wk.
- Advise patient to notify physician or dentist of medication regimen prior to treatment or surgery.
- Instruct patient to notify physician promptly if sore throat, fever, unusual bleeding or bruising, rash, weakness, tremors, visual disturbances, dark-colored urine, or clay-colored stools occur.
- Advise patient of need for continued medical follow-up for psychotherapy, eye examinations, and laboratory tests.

Evaluation

Effectiveness of therapy can be demonstrated by: ▪ Decreased psychotic ideation.

LUBRICANTS, OCULAR

Akwa Tears, Artificial Tears, Duolube, Duratears, Hypotears, Lacri-Lube N.P., Lacri-Lube SOP, Refresh PM

CLASSIFICATION(S):
Ophthalmic—lubricant
Pregnancy Category UK

INDICATIONS

▪ Provide ocular lubrication and protection in the following conditions: ▫ Exposure keratitis ▫ Decreased corneal sensitivity ▫ Corneal erosions ▫ Keratitis sicca (nighttime use) ▫ During and following surgery ▫ Following removal of a foreign body.

ACTION

▪ All contain sterile petrolatum and mineral oil, which act as lubricants and emollients. **Therapeutic Effect:** ▪ Protection and lubrication of the eye.

PHARMACOKINETICS

Absorption: No systemic absorption; action is primarily local.
Distribution: Distribution does not occur.
Metabolism and Excretion: Metabolism and excretion not known.
Half-life: UK.

CONTRAINDICATIONS AND PRECAUTIONS

Contraindicated in: ▪ Hypersensitivity to petrolatum or mineral oil ▪ Hypersensitivity to chlorobutanol (Lacri-Lube SOP only).
Use Cautiously in: ▪ Undiagnosed or suspected ocular infections.

ADVERSE REACTIONS AND SIDE EFFECTS*

EENT: blurred vision, eye discomfort.

*Underlines indicate most frequent; **CAPITALS** indicate life-threatening.

M

INTERACTIONS

Drug–Drug: ▪ May alter the action of concurrently administered **ophthalmic medications**.

ROUTE AND DOSAGE

▪ **Ophth (Adults):** Small amount instilled into the conjunctival sac several times daily.

PHARMACODYNAMICS (emollient effect)

	ONSET	PEAK	DURATION
Ophth	rapid	UK	UK

NURSING IMPLICATIONS

Assessment

□ Monitor patient for changes in vision and eye irritation and inflammation.

Potential Nursing Diagnoses

▪ Sensory-perceptual alteration: visual (indications, side effects).
▪ Knowledge deficit related to medication regimen (patient/family teaching).

Implementation

▪ **Eyedrops:** Wash hands. Have patient lie down or tilt head back and look at ceiling. Pull down on lower lid, creating a small pocket. Place prescribed number of drops in pocket. Gently close lids and roll eyes around in all directions to ensure even distribution. Wait 5 min before applying other prescribed eyedrops. Do not touch cap or tip of container to eye, fingers, or any surface.
□ Discard soln if it becomes cloudy.
▪ **Ointment:** Hold tube in hand for several mins to warm. Apply ribbon of ointment to lower conjunctival sac at bedtime immediately before retiring. Recap tightly after use. Wait 10 min before instilling any other ophthalmic ointment.
□ Ointment may be refrigerated or kept for 8 wk at room temperature.

Patient/Family Teaching

□ Instruct patient in correct method of application of drops or ointment. If a dose is missed, it should be taken as soon as remembered. Patient should confer with physician before wearing contact lenses.
□ Caution patient that vision may be blurred. Advise patient not to drive until response to medication is known. Increased sensitivity to light may occur; sunglasses should provide relief.
□ Discuss the possibility of matting of eyelashes. Instruct patient in correct technique for washing lids from inner to outer canthus.
□ Instruct patient to notify physician if eye irritation or discomfort increases or if blurred vision persists.
□ Advise patients using over-the-counter preparations to seek medical help if condition does not resolve within 3 days.

Evaluation

Effectiveness of therapy can be demonstrated by: ▪ Increased tear film in dry eye conditions.

MAGALDRATE

(**mag**-al-drate)
{Antiflux}, Lowsium, Riopan

CLASSIFICATION(S):
Antacid
Pregnancy Category UK

INDICATIONS

▪ Adjunctive therapy in the treatment of peptic ulcer pain and to promote healing of duodenal and gastric ulcers ▪ Also useful in a variety of GI complaints, including: □ Hyperacidity □ Indigestion □ Reflux esophagitis.

ACTION

▪ A chemically combined form of magnesium and aluminum ▪ Neutralizes gastric acid following dissolution in gastric contents. Inactivates pepsin if pH >4. **Therapeutic Effect:** ▪ Neutral-

{} = Available in Canada only.

ization of gastric acid with subsequent healing of ulcers and diminution of associated pain.

PHARMACOKINETICS

Absorption: In general, during routine use, antacids are nonabsorbable. With chronic use, 15–30% of magnesium and smaller amounts of aluminum may be absorbed.
Distribution: Small amounts of magnesium and aluminum are widely distributed, cross the placenta and enter breast milk. Aluminum concentrates in the CNS.
Metabolism and Excretion: Excreted by the kidneys.
Half-life: UK.

CONTRAINDICATIONS AND PRECAUTIONS

Contraindicated in: ▪ Severe abdominal pain of unknown cause, especially if accompanied by fever.
Use Cautiously in: ▪ Magnesium-containing antacids should be used cautiously in patients with renal insufficiency.

ADVERSE REACTIONS AND SIDE EFFECTS*

GI: constipation (aluminum salts), diarrhea (magnesium salts).
F and E: hypermagnesemia (magnesium), hypophosphatemia (aluminum).

INTERACTIONS

Drug-Drug: ▪ Magnesium and aluminum salts change the absorptive characteristics of **many orally administered drugs** ▪ Absorption of **tetracyclines, phenothiazines, iron salts, ketoconazole, fluoroquinolones,** and **isoniazid** may be decreased by concurrent magaldrate ▪ If urine pH is increased by large doses, **salicylate** blood levels may be decreased, **quinidine,** flecainide, and **amphetamine** blood levels may be increased.

ROUTE AND DOSAGE

Note: Dosages vary depending on concentration of ingredients in product chosen. Generally 5–30 ml or 1–2 tab is given 1 and 3 hr after meals and at bedtime. In the early healing phase of peptic ulcer more frequent administration may be necessary.

Duodenal Ulcer

- **PO (Adults):** 80–160 mEq neutralizing capacity/dose.

Gastric Ulcer

- **PO (Adults):** 40–80 mEq neutralizing capacity/dose.

PHARMACODYNAMICS (acid neutralization)

ONSET	PEAK	DURATION	
		Empty Stomach	After Meals
Aluminum PO (slightly delayed)	30 min	30 min–1 hr	3 hr
Magnesium PO (immediate)	30 min	30 min–1 hr	3 hr

NURSING IMPLICATIONS

Assessment

- □ Assess for heartburn; indigestion; and location, duration, character, and precipitating factors of gastric pain.

Potential Nursing Diagnoses

- Comfort, altered: pain (indications).
- Knowledge deficit related to medication regimen (patient/family teaching).

Implementation

- **General Info:** Available in tablet and liquid forms. Some tablets must be chewed thoroughly before swallowing (Lowsium, Riopan); others are designed to be swallowed whole (Riopan). Follow with ½ glass of water. Shake suspension well.
- **PO:** Administer between meals and at bedtime.

Patient/Family Teaching

- □ Caution patient to consult physician

*Underlines indicate most frequent; **CAPITALS** indicate life-threatening.

before taking antacids for more than 2 wk or if problem is recurring. Advise patient to consult physician if relief is not obtained or if symptoms of gastric bleeding (black tarry stools, coffee-ground emesis) occur.

EVALUATION

Effectiveness of therapy can be demonstrated by: ▪ Relief of gastric pain and irritation.

MAGNESIUM CITRATE

(mag-**nee**-zhum **si**-trate)
Citrate of Magnesia, Citroma, {Citromag}, Citro-Nesia, Evac-Q-Mag

CLASSIFICATION(S):
Laxative—saline
Pregnancy Category UK

INDICATIONS

▪ Used as a laxative and to evacuate the bowel in preparation for surgical or radiographic procedures.

ACTION

▪ Is osmotically active in GI tract, drawing water into the lumen and causing peristalsis. **Therapeutic Effect:** ▪ Evacuation of the colon.

PHARMACOKINETICS

Absorption: 15–30% of magnesium may be absorbed orally.
Distribution: Magnesium is widely distributed. Crosses the placenta and is present in breast milk.
Metabolism and Excretion: Magnesium is excreted primarily by the kidneys.
Half-life: UK.

CONTRAINDICATIONS AND PRECAUTIONS

Contraindicated in: ▪ Hypermagnesemia ▪ Hypocalcemia ▪ Anuria ▪ Heart block ▪ Active labor.
Use Cautiously in: ▪ Any degree of renal insufficiency.

ADVERSE REACTIONS AND SIDE EFFECTS*

Note: Non-GI adverse reactions are seen only in patients who receive large doses over prolonged periods and have underlying renal disease.

CNS: drowsiness.
Resp: decreased respiratory rate.
CV: bradycardia, arrhythmias, hypotension.
GI: diarrhea.
Derm: flushing, sweating.
Metab: hypothermia.
Neuro: decreased deep-tendon reflexes, PARALYSIS.

INTERACTIONS

Drug-Drug: ▪ If systemic absorption occurs, may potentiate **neuromuscular blocking agents.**

ROUTE AND DOSAGE

Note: Contains 77 mEq magnesium/100 ml.

▪ **PO (Adults):** 100–240 ml.
▪ **PO (Children 6–12 yr):** 50–100 ml.
▪ **PO (Children 2–5 yr):** 4–12 ml.

PHARMACODYNAMICS (laxative effect)

	ONSET	PEAK	DURATION
PO	3–6 hr	UK	UK

NURSING IMPLICATIONS

ASSESSMENT

□ Assess patient for abdominal distention, presence of bowel sounds, and usual pattern of bowel function.
□ Assess color, consistency, and amount of stool produced.

POTENTIAL NURSING DIAGNOSES

▪ Bowel elimination, altered: constipation (indications).
▪ Knowledge deficit related to medication regimen (patient/family teaching).

IMPLEMENTATION

▪ **General Info:** Refrigerate magnesium citrate soln to increase palatability.

{} = Available in Canada only.
*Underlines indicate most frequent; **CAPITALS** indicate life-threatening.

May be served over ice. An open container of magnesium citrate may become flat upon standing; this will not affect potency but may decrease palatability.

- For laxative effect, administer on empty stomach for more rapid results. Follow all oral laxative doses with a full glass of liquid to prevent dehydration and for faster effect. Do not administer at bedtime or late in the day.

Patient/Family Teaching

- Advise patients that laxatives should be used only for short-term therapy. Long-term therapy may cause electrolyte imbalance and dependence.
- If administered as part of a bowel preparation kit, explain the schedule in regard to other laxatives, suppository, and diet modification.
- Encourage patient to utilize other forms of bowel regulation, such as increasing bulk in the diet, increasing fluid intake, increasing mobility. Normal bowel habits are individualized and may vary from 3 times/day to 3 times/wk.
- Advise patient to notify physician if unrelieved constipation, rectal bleeding, or symptoms of electrolyte imbalance (muscle cramps or pain, weakness, dizziness, etc.) occur.

Evaluation

Effectiveness of therapy can be demonstrated by: ▪ Evacuation of colon ▪ Passage of a soft, formed bowel movement.

MAGNESIUM HYDROXIDE

(mag-**nee**-zhum hye-**drox**-ide)
Magnesia tablets, Milk of Magnesia, MOM

CLASSIFICATION(S):
Laxative—saline, Antacid
Pregnancy Category UK

INDICATIONS

▪ Used as a laxative and to evacuate the bowel in preparation for surgical or radiographic procedures ▪ Has also been used as an antacid.

ACTION

▪ Is osmotically active in GI tract, drawing water into the lumen and causing peristalsis ▪ Also has acid-neutralizing activity. **Therapeutic Effects:** ▪ Evacuation of the colon ▪ Neutralization of gastric acid.

PHARMACOKINETICS

Absorption: 15–30% of magnesium may be absorbed orally.
Distribution: Magnesium is widely distributed. Crosses the placenta and is present in breast milk.
Metabolism and Excretion: Magnesium is excreted primarily by the kidneys.
Half-life: UK.

CONTRAINDICATIONS AND PRECAUTIONS

Contraindicated in: ▪ Hypermagnesemia ▪ Hypocalcemia ▪ Anuria ▪ Heart block ▪ Active labor.
Use Cautiously in: ▪ Any degree of renal insufficiency.

ADVERSE REACTIONS AND SIDE EFFECTS*

Note: Non-GI adverse reactions are seen only in patients who receive large doses over prolonged periods and have underlying renal disease.

CNS: drowsiness.
Resp: decreased respiratory rate.
CV: bradycardia, arrhythmias, hypotension.
GI: diarrhea.
Derm: flushing, sweating.
Metab: hypothermia.
Neuro: decreased deep-tendon reflexes, PARALYSIS.

INTERACTIONS

Drug–Drug: ▪ If systemically absorbed, may potentiate **neuromuscular blocking agents** ▪ May decrease absorption of **fluoroquinolones**.

*Underlines indicate most frequent; **CAPITALS** indicate life-threatening.

ROUTE AND DOSAGE

Laxative

(82 mEq magnesium/30 ml milk of magnesia)

- **PO (Adults):** 15–40 ml milk of magnesia (10–20 ml of concentrate).
- **PO (Children 2–5 yr):** ¼–½ adult dose.

Antacid

- **PO (Adults and Children >12 yr):** 5 ml liquid or 650–1300 mg as tablets 4 times daily.

PHARMACODYNAMICS (laxative effect)

	ONSET	PEAK	DURATION
PO	3–6 hr	UK	UK

NURSING IMPLICATIONS

Assessment

- **Laxative:** Assess patient for abdominal distention, presence of bowel sounds, and usual pattern of bowel function.
- □ Assess color, consistency, and amount of stool produced.
- **Antacid:** Assess for heartburn; indigestion; and location, duration, character, and precipitating factors of gastric pain.

Potential Nursing Diagnoses

- Bowel elimination, altered: constipation (indications).
- Comfort, altered: pain (indications).
- Knowledge deficit related to medication regimen (patient/family teaching).

Implementation

- **General Info:** Available in tablet and liquid forms.
- **PO:** Tablet must be chewed thoroughly before swallowing to prevent entering small intestine in undissolved form. Follow with ½ glass of water.
- □ Shake suspension well before administration.
- **Laxative:** For more rapid results, administer on empty stomach and follow dose with a full glass of liquid to prevent dehydration. Do not administer at bedtime or late in the day when used for laxative effect.

Patient/Family Teaching

- **General Info:** Advise patient not to take this medication within 2 hr of other medications.
- **Laxative:** Advise patient that laxatives should be used only for short-term therapy. Long-term therapy may cause electrolyte imbalance and dependence.
- □ Encourage patient to utilize other forms of bowel regulation, such as increasing bulk in the diet, increasing fluid intake, increasing mobility. Normal bowel habits are individualized and may vary from 3 times/day to 3 times/wk.
- □ Advise patient to notify physician if unrelieved constipation, rectal bleeding, or symptoms of electrolyte imbalance (muscle cramps or pain, weakness, dizziness) occur.
- **Antacid:** Caution patient to consult physician before taking antacids for more than 2 wk or if problem is recurring. Advise patient to consult physician if relief is not obtained or if symptoms of gastric bleeding (black tarry stools, coffee-ground emesis) occur.

Evaluation

Effectiveness of therapy can be demonstrated by: ▪ Relief of gastric pain and irritation ▪ Passage of a soft, formed bowel movement, usually within 3–6 hr.

MAGNESIUM HYDROXIDE/ ALUMINUM HYDROXIDE

(mag-**nee**-zhum hye-**drox**-ide/ a-**loo**-mi-num hye-**drox**-ide)

Alamag, {Algenic Alka Improved}, Aludrox, Alumid, {Amphogel 500}, Creamalin, Delcid, {Diovol Ex}, Gelamal, Gelusil-M, Gelusil-II, Kudrox Double Strength, Maalox, Maalox No. 1, Maalox No. 2, Maalox TC, Magmalín, Mintox, Mylanta, Mylanta-II, {Neutralca-S}, Rolox, Rulox, Rulox No. 1, Rulox No. 2, {Univol}, WinGel

CLASSIFICATION(S):
Antacid, Antiulcer
Pregnancy Category UK

INDICATIONS

▪ Adjunctive therapy in the treatment of peptic ulcer pain and to promote healing of duodenal and gastric ulcers ▪ Useful in a variety of GI complaints, including: ▫ Hyperacidity ▫ Indigestion ▫ Reflux esophagitis.

ACTION

▪ Neutralize gastric acid following dissolution in gastric contents. Pepsin is inactivated if pH ≥4. **Therapeutic Effect:** ▪ Neutralization of gastric acid with subsequent healing of ulcers and diminution of associated pain.

PHARMACOKINETICS

Absorption: In general, during routine use, antacids are nonabsorbable. With chronic use, 15–30% of magnesium and smaller amounts of aluminum may be absorbed.
Distribution: Small amounts of magnesium and aluminum absorbed are widely distributed, cross the placenta and enter breast milk. Aluminum concentrates in the CNS.
Metabolism and Excretion: Excreted by the kidneys.
Half-life: UK.

CONTRAINDICATIONS AND PRECAUTIONS

Contraindicated in: ▪ Severe abdominal pain of unknown cause, especially if accompanied by fever ▪ Magnesium is contraindicated in anuria.
Use Cautiously in: ▪ Magnesium-containing antacids should be used cautiously in patients with any degree of renal insufficiency.

ADVERSE REACTIONS AND SIDE EFFECTS*

GI: <u>constipation</u>; (aluminum salts), <u>diarrhea</u> (magnesium salts).
F and E: hypermagnesemia (magnesium); hypophosphatemia (aluminum).

INTERACTIONS

Drug-Drug: ▪ Magnesium and aluminum salts change the absorptive characteristics of **many orally administered drugs** ▪ The absorption of **tetracyclines, phenothiazines, iron salts, isoniazid,** and **fluoroquinolones** may be decreased ▪ If urine pH is increased by large doses, **salicylate** blood levels may be decreased and **quinidine** and **amphetamine** levels may be increased.

ROUTE AND DOSAGE

Note: Dosages vary depending on concentration of ingredients in product chosen. Generally 5–30 ml or 1–2 tab is given 1 and 3 hr after meals and at bedtime. In the early healing phase of peptic ulcer more frequent administration may be necessary.

Duodenal Ulcer

▪ **PO (Adults):** 80–160 mEq neutralizing capacity/dose.

Gastric Ulcer

▪ **PO (Adults):** 40–80 mEq neutralizing capacity/dose.

PHARMACODYNAMICS (acid neutralization)

ONSET	PEAK	DURATION	
		Empty Stomach	After Meals
Aluminum PO (slightly delayed)	30 min	30 min–1 hr	3 hr
Magnesium PO (immediate)	30 min	30 min–1 hr	3 hr

{} = Available in Canada only.
*<u>Underlines</u> indicate most frequent; **CAPITALS** indicate life-threatening.

NURSING IMPLICATIONS

Assessment

- ▫ Assess for heartburn; indigestion; and location, duration, character, and precipitating factors of gastric pain.

Potential Nursing Diagnoses

- ▪ Comfort, altered: pain (indications).
- ▪ Knowledge deficit related to medication regimen (patient/family teaching).

Implementation

- ▪ **General Info:** Magnesium and aluminum are combined as antacids to balance the constipating effects of aluminum with the diarrheal effects of magnesium.
- ▫ Available in tablet and liquid forms. Liquid forms are considered more effective.
- ▪ **PO:** Tablet must be chewed thoroughly before swallowing to prevent entering small intestine in undissolved form. Follow with ½ glass of water.
- ▫ Shake suspensions well before administration.
- ▫ For an antacid effect, administer 1–3 hr after meals and at bedtime.

Patient/Family Teaching

- ▫ Caution patient to consult physician before taking antacids for more than 2 wk or if problem is recurring. Advise patient to consult physician if relief is not obtained or if symptoms of gastric bleeding (black tarry stools, coffee-ground emesis) occur.
- ▫ Advise patient not to take this medication within 2 hr of other medication.
- ▫ Some antacids contain large amounts of sodium. Caution patients on a sodium-restricted diet to check sodium content when on long-term, high-dose therapy.

Evaluation

Effectiveness of therapy can be demonstrated by: ▪ Relief of gastric pain and irritation.

MAGNESIUM SULFATE

(mag-**nee**-zhum **sul**-fate)
Bilagog, Epsom salt

CLASSIFICATION(S):
Electrolyte modifier—magnesium supplement, Laxative—saline, Anticonvulsant
Pregnancy Category UK

INDICATIONS

▪ Treatment and prevention of hypomagnesemia ▪ As an anticonvulsant in severe eclampsia or pre-eclampsia ▪ Used as a laxative and to evacuate the bowel in preparation for surgical or radiographic procedures.

ACTION

▪ Essential for the activity of many enzymes ▪ Plays an important role in neurotransmission and muscular excitability ▪ Is osmotically active in GI tract, drawing water into the lumen and causing peristalsis. **Therapeutic Effects:** ▪ Replacement in deficiency states, resolution of eclampsia, and evacuation of the colon.

PHARMACOKINETICS

Absorption: 15–30% may be absorbed orally. Well absorbed from IM sites.
Distribution: Widely distributed. Crosses the placenta and is present in breast milk.
Metabolism and Excretion: Excreted primarily by the kidneys.
Half-life: UK.

CONTRAINDICATIONS AND PRECAUTIONS

Contraindicated in: ▪ Hypermagnesemia ▪ Hypocalcemia ▪ Anuria ▪ Heart block ▪ Active labor.
Use Cautiously in: ▪ Any degree of renal insufficiency.

ADVERSE REACTIONS AND SIDE EFFECTS*

Note: Serious reactions are associated with parenteral use only.

CNS: drowsiness.
Resp: decreased respiratory rate.
CV: bradycardia, arrhythmias, hypotension.
GI: diarrhea.
Derm: flushing, sweating.
Metab: hypothermia.
Neuro: decreased deep-tendon reflexes, PARALYSIS.

INTERACTIONS

Drug–Drug: ▪ Potentiates **neuromuscular blocking agents** ▪ Orally administered magnesium decreases absorption of **fluoroquinolones.**

ROUTE AND DOSAGE

Note: Each g magnesium sulfate contains 8 mEq magnesium.

Hypomagnesemia

- **PO (Adults):** 3 g q 6 hr for 4 doses.
- **IM (Adults):** 1 g q 6 hr for 4 doses, up to 250 mg/kg over a 4-hr period.
- **IV (Adults):** up to 5 g diluted and infused slowly over 3 hr.

Eclampsia, Pre-Eclampsia

- **IV (Adults):** 4 g IV initially, then IM or 1–2 g/hr infusion.
- **IM (Adults):** 4–5 g q 4 hr.

Anticonvulsant

- **IM, IV (Adults):** 1–4 g.

Laxative

- **PO (Adults):** 10–30 g.
- **PO (Children 6–12 yr):** 5–10 g.
- **PO (Children 2–5 yr):** 2.5–5 g.

PHARMACODYNAMICS (PO = laxative effect; IM, IV = anticonvulsant effect)

	ONSET	PEAK	DURATION
PO	3–6 hr	UK	UK
IM	60 min	UK	3–4 hr
IV	immediate	UK	30 min

NURSING IMPLICATIONS

Assessment

- **General Info:** Serum magnesium levels and renal function should be monitored periodically throughout administration of parenteral magnesium sulfate.
- **Hypomagnesemia / Anticonvulsant:** Monitor pulse, blood pressure, respirations, and ECG frequently throughout administration of parenteral magnesium sulfate. Respirations should be at least 16/min prior to each dose.
  - Monitor neurologic status prior to and throughout course of therapy. Institute seizure precautions. Patellar reflex (knee jerk) should be tested before each parenteral dose of magnesium sulfate. If response is absent, no additional doses should be administered until positive response is obtained.
  - Monitor newborn for hypotension, hyporeflexia, and respiratory depression if mother has received magnesium sulfate.
  - Monitor intake and output ratios. Urine output should be maintained at a level of at least 100 ml every 4 hr.
- **Laxative:** Assess patient for abdominal distention, presence of bowel sounds, and usual pattern of bowel function.
  - Assess color, consistency, and amount of stool produced.
- **Toxicity and Overdose:** Toxicity is manifested by a prolonged P-Q and widened QRS interval, loss of deep tendon reflexes, heart block, respiratory paralysis, and cardiac arrest. Treatment includes IV calcium gluconate to antagonize the effects of magnesium.

Potential Nursing Diagnoses

- Injury, high risk for (indications, side effects).
- Bowel elimination, altered: constipation (indications).
- Knowledge deficit related to medica-

*Underlines indicate most frequent; **CAPITALS** indicate life-threatening.

tion regimen (patient/family teaching).

IMPLEMENTATION

- **PO:** For laxative effect, administer on empty stomach for more rapid results. Dissolve magnesium sulfate in a full glass of water; may use lemon-flavored carbonated beverage to mask bitter taste. Follow with a full glass of liquid to prevent dehydration and for faster effect. Do not administer at bedtime or late in the day.
- ▫ Available in many concentrations.
- **IM:** Administer deep IM using gluteal sites. Administer subsequent injections in alternate sides.
- ▫ Use 25–50% concentrations for adults, 20% concentrations for children <14 yr.
- **Direct IV:** Administer undiluted at a rate of 1.5 ml of a 10% soln (or its equivalent) over 1 min.
- **Continuous Infusion:** When given as an anticonvulsant, dilute 4 g in 250 ml of D5W or 0.9% NaCl.
- ▫ *Rate:* Administer at a rate not to exceed 4 ml/min.
- ▫ When given for hypomagnesemia, may dilute 5 g in 1 liter of D5W, 0.9% NaCl, Ringer's or lactated Ringer's soln and administer slowly over 3 hr.
- ▫ Use infusion pump to regulate rate accurately.
- **Syringe Compatibility:** metoclopramide.
- **Y-Site Compatibility:** acyclovir, amikacin, ampicillin, cefamandole, cefazolin, cefoperazone, ceforanide, cefotaxime, cefoxitin, cephalothin, cephapirin, chloramphenicol, clindamycin, co-trimoxazole, dobutamine, doxycycline, enalaprilat, erythromycin lactobionate, esmolol, famotidine, gentamicin, heparin, hydrocortisone, kanamycin, labetalol, metronidazole, minocycline, moxalactam, nafcillin, ondanstron, oxacillin, penicillin G potassium, piperacillin, potassium chloride, tetracycline, ticarcillin, tobramycin, or vancomycin.
- **Additive Compatibility:** calcium gluconate, cephalothin, chloramphenicol, cisplatin, hydrocortisone sodium succinate, isoproterenol, methyldopate, norepinephrine, penicillin G potassium, potassium phosphate, or verapamil.
- **Additive Incompatibility:** calcium gluceptate, dobutamine, polymyxin, procaine hydrochloride, sodium bicarbonate, streptomycin, or tobramycin.

PATIENT/FAMILY TEACHING

- **Laxative:** Advise patient that laxatives should be used only for short-term therapy. Long-term therapy may cause electrolyte imbalance and dependence.
- ▫ Encourage patient to utilize other forms of bowel regulation, such as increasing bulk in the diet, increasing fluid intake, increasing mobility. Normal bowel habits are individualized and may vary from 3 times/day to 3 times/wk.
- ▫ Advise patient to notify physician if unrelieved constipation, rectal bleeding, or symptoms of electrolyte imbalance (muscle cramps or pain, weakness, dizziness) occur.

EVALUATION

Effectiveness of therapy can be demonstrated by: ▪ Normal serum magnesium concentrations ▪ Control of seizures associated with toxemias of pregnancy ▪ Passage of a soft, formed bowel movement, usually within 3–6 hr.

MANNITOL

(**man**-i-tol)
Osmitrol

CLASSIFICATION(S):
Diuretic—osmotic
Pregnancy Category C

INDICATIONS

▪ Adjunct in the treatment of acute oliguric renal failure ▪ Adjunct in the treatment of edema ▪ Reduction of intracranial or intraocular pressure ▪ To promote the excretion of certain toxic substances.

ACTION

▪ Increases the osmotic pressure of the glomerular filtrate, thereby inhibiting reabsorption of water and electrolytes ▪ Causes excretion of: ▫ Water ▫ Sodium ▫ Potassium ▫ Chloride ▫ Calcium ▫ Phosphorus ▫ Magnesium ▫ Urea ▫ Uric acid.

PHARMACOKINETICS

Absorption: Administered IV only, resulting in complete bioavailability.
Distribution: Confined to the extracellular space. Does not usually cross the blood-brain barrier or eye.
Metabolism and Excretion: Excreted by the kidneys. Minimal metabolism by the liver.
Half-life: 100 min.

CONTRAINDICATIONS AND PRECAUTIONS

Contraindicated in: ▪ Hypersensitivity ▪ Anuria ▪ Dehydration ▪ Active intracranial bleeding.
Use Cautiously in: ▪ Pregnancy and lactation (safety not established).

ADVERSE REACTIONS AND SIDE EFFECTS*

CNS: headache, confusion.
EENT: blurred vision, rhinitis.
CV: transient volume expansion, tachycardia, chest pain, congestive heart failure, pulmonary edema.
GI: thirst, nausea, vomiting.
GU: renal failure, urinary retention.
F and E: hyponatremia, hypernatremia, hypokalemia, hyperkalemia, dehydration.
Local: phlebitis at IV site.

INTERACTIONS

Drug-Drug: ▪ Enhances **lithium** excretion; may decrease effectiveness.

ROUTE AND DOSAGE

Edema, Oliguric Renal Failure

- **IV (Adults):** 50–100 g as a 5–25% soln.
- **IV (Children):** 2 g/kg as a 15–20% soln over 2–6 hr.

Reduction of Intracranial or Intraocular Pressure

- **IV (Adults):** 1.5–2 g/kg as 15–25% soln over 30–60 min.
- **IV (Children):** 2 g/kg as a 15–20% soln over 30–60 min (500 mg/kg may be sufficient in small or debilitated patients).

Diuresis in Drug Intoxications

- **IV (Adults):** 50–200 g as a 5–25% soln titrated to maintain urine flow of 100–500 ml/hr.
- **IV (Children):** 2 g/kg as a 5–10% soln.

PHARMACODYNAMICS (diuretic effect)

	ONSET	PEAK	DURATION
IV	30–60 min	1 hr	6–8 hr

NURSING IMPLICATIONS

Assessment

- **General Info:** Monitor vital signs, urine output, CVP, and pulmonary artery pressures (PAP) prior to and hourly throughout administration. Assess patient for signs and symptoms of dehydration (decreased skin turgor, fever, dry skin and mucous membranes, thirst) or signs of fluid overload (increased CVP, dyspnea, rales/crackles, edema).
  - ▫ Assess patient for anorexia, muscle weakness, numbness, tingling, paresthesia, confusion, and excessive thirst. Notify physician promptly if these signs of electrolyte imbalance occur.
- **Increased Intracranial Pressure:** Monitor neurologic status and intracranial pressure readings in patients receiving this medication to decrease cerebral edema.

*Underlines indicate most frequent; **CAPITALS** indicate life-threatening.

M

- **Increased Intraocular Pressure:** Monitor for persistent or increased eye pain or decreased visual acuity.
- **Lab Test Considerations:** Renal function and serum electrolytes should be monitored routinely throughout course of therapy.

Potential Nursing Diagnoses
- Fluid volume excess (indications).
- Fluid volume deficit, potential (side effects).

Implementation
- **General Info:** Observe infusion site frequently for infiltration. Extravasation may cause tissue irritation and necrosis.
- □ Do not administer electrolyte-free mannitol soln with blood. If blood must be administered simultaneously with mannitol, add at least 20 mEq NaCl to each liter of mannitol.
- □ Confer with physician regarding placement of an indwelling foley catheter (except when used to decrease intraocular pressure).
- **IV:** Administer by IV infusion undiluted. If soln contains crystals, warm bottle in hot water and shake vigorously. Do not administer soln in which crystals remain undissolved. Cool to body temperature. Use an in-line filter for 15%, 20%, and 25% infusions.
- **Test Dose:** Administer over 3–5 min to produce a urine output of 30–50 ml/hr. If urine flow does not increase, administer second test dose. If urine output is not at least 30–50 ml/hr for 2–3 hr after second test dose, patient should be re-evaluated.
- **Oliguria:** Administration rate should be titrated to produce a urine output of 30–50 ml/hr.
- **Increased Intracranial Pressure:** Infuse dose over 30–60 min.
- **Intraocular Pressure:** Administer dose over 30 min. When used preoperatively, administer 60–90 min prior to surgery.
- **Y-Site Compatability:** ondansetron.
- **Additive Compatibility:** amikacin, bretylium, cefamandole, cefoxitin, cimetidine, cisplatin, dopamine, gentamicin, metoclopramide, netilmicin, tobramycin, or verapamil.
- **Additive Incompatibility:** blood products or imipenem/cilastatin.

Patient/Family Teaching
- □ Explain purpose of therapy to patient.

Evaluation

Effectiveness of therapy can be demonstrated by: ▪ Urine output of at least 30–50 ml/hr or an increase in urine output in accordance with parameters set by physician ▪ Reduction in intracranial pressure ▪ Reduction of intraocular pressure ▪ Excretion of certain toxic substances.

MAPROTILINE
(ma-**proe**-ti-leen)
Ludiomil

CLASSIFICATION(S):
Antidepressant—tetracyclic
Pregnancy Category B

INDICATIONS
- Treatment of various forms of depression and anxiety associated with depression, often in conjunction with psychotherapy.

ACTION
▪ Potentiates the effects of serotonin and norepinephrine ▪ Has significant anticholinergic properties. **Therapeutic Effect:** ▪ Antidepressant action, which may develop only over several wks.

PHARMACOKINETICS
Absorption: Slowly but completely absorbed from the GI tract.

Distribution: Widely distributed. Probably crosses the placenta. Enters breast milk in concentrations similar to those in plasma.

Metabolism and Excretion: Slowly and extensively metabolized by the

liver. Some conversion to active compounds. 30% excreted in the feces.
Half-life: 51 hr.

CONTRAINDICATIONS AND PRECAUTIONS

Contraindicated in: ▪ Narrow-angle glaucoma ▪ Pregnancy and lactation ▪ Acute myocardial infarction ▪ Seizure disorders (may lower seizure threshold).
Use Cautiously in: ▪ Elderly patients (increased risk of adverse reactions, dosage reduction suggested) ▪ Patients with pre-existing cardiovascular disease ▪ Elderly men with prostatic hypertrophy (more susceptible to urinary retention).

ADVERSE REACTIONS AND SIDE EFFECTS*

CNS: drowsiness, sedation, lethargy, fatigue, confusion, agitation, hallucinations, SEIZURES.
EENT: dry mouth, dry eyes, blurred vision.
CV: hypotension, ECG changes, ARRHYTHMIAS.
GI: constipation, paralytic ileus.
GU: urinary retention.
Derm: photosensitivity.
Endo: gynecomastia.
Hemat: blood dyscrasias.

INTERACTIONS

Drug-Drug: ▪ May cause hyperpyrexia, seizures, hypertension and death when used with **MAO inhibitors** (avoid concurrent use—discontinue 2 wk prior to maprotiline) ▪ May prevent the therapeutic response to **antihypertensives** ▪ Additive CNS depression with other **CNS depressants,** including **alcohol, antihistamines, narcotic analgesics, clonidine,** and **sedative/hypnotics** ▪ Adrenergic effects may be additive with other **adrenergic agents,** including **vasoconstrictors** and **decongestants** ▪ Additive anticholinergic effects with other **drugs possessing anticholinergic properties,** including **antihistamines, atropine, haloperidol, phenothiazines, quinidine,** and **disopyramide** ▪ **Cimetidine** or **oral contraceptives** increase levels and may cause toxicity ▪ **Sympathomimetics** increase risk of adverse cardiovascular reactions ▪ Increased risk of seizures with **phenothiazines.**

ROUTE AND DOSAGE

- **PO (Adults):** 75 mg/day initially, may increase by 25 mg q 2 wk to a maximum of 150 mg/day. Some patients may require up to 225 mg/day. May be given in 3 divided doses or single daily dose.

PHARMACODYNAMICS (antidepressant effect)

	ONSET	PEAK	DURATION
PO	3–7 days	2–3 wk	UK

NURSING IMPLICATIONS

Assessment

- □ Assess mental status frequently. Confusion, agitation, and hallucinations may occur during initiation of therapy and may require dosage reduction. Monitor mood changes. Assess for suicidal tendencies, especially during early therapy. Restrict amount of drug available to patient.
- □ Monitor blood pressure and pulse rate periodically during initial therapy. Notify physician of significant changes.
- □ Monitor for seizure activity in patients with a history of convulsions or alcohol abuse. Institute seizure precautions.
- ▪ **Lab Test Considerations:** Assess CBC and hepatic function prior to and periodically during therapy.

Potential Nursing Diagnoses

- ▪ Coping, ineffective individual (indications).
- ▪ Anxiety (indications).
- ▪ Knowledge deficit related to medication regimen (patient/family teaching).

Implementation

- ▪ **General Info:** May be given as a single

*Underlines indicate most frequent; **CAPITALS** indicate life-threatening.

dose at bedtime to minimize excessive drowsiness or dizziness.

Patient/Family Teaching

- □ Instruct patient to take medication exactly as directed. If a dose is missed, take as soon as remembered; if almost time for next dose, skip missed dose and return to regular schedule. If single bedtime dose regimen is used, do not take missed dose in morning, but consult physician.
- □ May cause drowsiness and blurred vision. Caution patient to avoid driving and other activities requiring alertness until response to drug is known.
- □ Caution patient to make position changes slowly to minimize orthostatic hypotension.
- □ Advise patient to avoid alcohol or other CNS depressant drugs during and for at least 3–7 days after therapy has been discontinued.
- □ Advise patient to notify physician if dry mouth, urinary retention, or constipation occurs. Frequent rinses, good oral hygiene, and sugarless candy or gum may diminish dry mouth. An increase in fluid intake, fiber, and exercise may prevent constipation.
- □ Caution patient to use sunscreen and protective clothing to prevent photosensitivity reactions.
- □ Advise patient to consult physician or pharmacist before taking any over-the-counter cold remedies with this medication.
- □ Advise patient to notify physician or dentist of medication regimen prior to treatment or surgery.
- □ Therapy for depression may be prolonged. Emphasize the importance of follow-up examination to monitor effectiveness and side effects.

Evaluation

Effectiveness of therapy can be demonstrated by: ▪ Resolution of the symptoms of depression: □ Increased sense of well-being □ Renewed interest in surroundings □ Increased appetite □ Improved energy level □ Improved sleep ▪ Decrease in anxiety associated with depression. Therapeutic effects are sometimes seen in 3–7 days, although 2–3 wk is usually necessary before improvement is observed.

MEBENDAZOLE

(me-**ben**-da-zole)
{Nemasole}, Vermox

CLASSIFICATION(S):
Antihelmintic
Pregnancy Category C

INDICATIONS

▪ Treatment of: □ Whipworm (trichuriasis) □ Pinworm (enterobiasis) □ Roundworm (ascariasis) □ Hookworm (uncinariasis) infections. **Unlabeled Uses:** ▪ Tapeworm ▪ Threadworm ▪ Strongyloidiasis ▪ Larvae migrans ▪ Capillariasis ▪ Toxocariasis.

ACTION

▪ Inhibits the uptake of glucose and other nutrients by susceptible helminths. **Therapeutic Effect:** ▪ Death of parasites, eggs, and hydatid cysts (vermicidal and ovacidal).

PHARMACOKINETICS

Absorption: Minimally (2–10%) absorbed following oral administration.
Distribution: Distribution not known.
Metabolism and Excretion: >95% eliminated in feces. Absorbed drug is mostly metabolized by the liver; small amounts excreted unchanged by the kidneys.
Half-life: 2.5–9 hr (increased in liver impairment).

CONTRAINDICATIONS AND PRECAUTIONS

Contraindicated in: ▪ Hypersensitivity.
Use Cautiously in: ▪ Pregnancy, lactation, or children <2 yr (safety not es-

tablished) ▪ Impaired liver function ▪ Crohn's ileitis ▪ Ulcerative colitis.

ADVERSE REACTIONS AND SIDE EFFECTS*

Note: Most side effects and adverse reactions are seen with high-dose therapy only.

CNS: headache, dizziness.
EENT: tinnitus.
GI: diarrhea, abdominal pain, nausea, vomiting.
Hemat: reversible myelosuppression (leukopenia, thrombocytopenia).
Neuro: numbness.
Misc: fever.

INTERACTIONS

Drug-Drug: ▪ **Carbamazepine** and **phenytoin** may increase the metabolism and decrease effectiveness of therapy in patients receiving high-dose therapy.
Drug-Food: ▪ Absorption may be increased by **fatty foods**.

ROUTE AND DOSAGE

Enterobiasis

- **PO (Adults and Children >2 yr):** 100 mg as a single dose.

Trichuriasis, Ascariasis, Hookworm, or Mixed Infections

- **PO (Adults and Children >2 yr):** 200 mg/day in 2 divided doses for 3 days. If not cured in 3–4 wk, a second course is given.

Capillariasis

- **PO (Adults and Children >2 yr):** 200 mg bid for 20–30 days.

Toxocariasis

- **PO (Adults):** 200–400 mg daily for 4–5 days.

Hydatid Disease

- **PO (Adults and Children >2 yr):** 40 mg/kg daily for 6 mon or 50 mg/kg/day for 2 wk, then 200 mg/kg/day for 2 wk, then 50 mg/kg/day for 2 wk.

Trichinosis

- **PO (Adults):** 200–400 mg tid for 3 days, then 400–500 mg tid for 10 days.

PHARMACODYNAMICS

	ONSET	PEAK	DURATION
PO	UK	UK	UK

NURSING IMPLICATIONS

Assessment

- **Pinworm:** Perianal examinations should be performed to detect the presence of adult worms in the perianal area, and cellophane tape swabs of the perianal area should be taken prior to and starting 1 wk following treatment to detect the presence of ova. Swabs should be taken each morning prior to defecation or bathing for at least 3 days. Patients are not considered cured unless perianal swabs have been negative for 7 days.
- **Roundworm:** Stool examinations should be monitored prior to and 1–3 wk following treatment.
- **Lab Test Considerations:** May cause transient increase in serum BUN, SGPT (ALT), SGOT (AST), and alkaline phosphatase levels.
  - CBC should be monitored prior to therapy and 2–3 times a wk from day 10 to 25 and weekly thereafter in patients receiving high-dose therapy. Mebendazole may cause reversible leukopenia and thrombocytopenia.
  - May cause decreased serum hemoglobin concentrations.

Potential Nursing Diagnoses

- Infection, high risk for (indications).
- Home maintenance management, impaired (indications).
- Knowledge deficit related to disease process and medication regimen (patient/family teaching).

Implementation

- **General Info:** No special diets, fasting, or enemas are required prior to administration of mebendazole.
- **PO:** Mebendazole tablet may be chewed, swallowed whole, or crushed and mixed with food. Patients on high-dose therapy should take tablets

*Underlines indicate most frequent; **CAPITALS** indicate life-threatening.

M

with high-fat meals to increase absorption.
- **Pinworm:** All members of the household should be treated concurrently, with treatment repeated in 2–3 wk.
- **Hookworm and Whipworm:** Patient may be required to take an iron supplement daily during treatment and for 6 mon following treatment if anemia occurs.

PATIENT/FAMILY TEACHING
- **General Info:** Instruct patient to take medication exactly as directed and to continue medication for full course of therapy, even if feeling better. If a dose is missed, take as soon as remembered; if on 2 doses/day schedule, space missed dose and next dose 4–5 hr apart or double next dose; if on 8 dose/day schedule, space missed dose and next dose 1½ hr apart or double next dose. A second course of therapy may be required.
  - Advise patient of hygienic precautions to minimize reinfection (wash hands with soap prior to eating and after using the toilet, disinfect toilet daily, keep hands away from mouth, wash all fruits and vegetables, wear shoes).
  - Medication may cause dizziness. Caution patient to avoid driving or activities requiring alertness until response to medication is known.
  - Advise patient to consult physician if no improvement is seen within a few days.
  - Emphasize the importance of follow-up examinations to determine effectiveness, especially with high-dose therapy.
- **Pinworm:** Instruct patient to wash (do not shake) all bedding, undergarments, towels, and nightclothes after treatment to prevent reinfection.

EVALUATION
Effectiveness of therapy can be demonstrated by: ▪ Resolution of the signs and symptoms of infection or when stool specimens and perianal swabs are negative. Length of time for complete resolution depends on the parasite.

MECHLORETHAMINE
(me-klor-**eth**-a-meen)
Mustargen, Nitrogen mustard

CLASSIFICATION(S):
Antineoplastic—alkylating agent
Pregnancy Category UK

INDICATIONS
▪ As part of combination therapy of Hodgkin's disease and malignant lymphomas ▪ Used palliatively in: ▫ Bronchogenic carcinoma ▫ Breast carcinoma ▫ Ovarian carcinoma ▫ Leukemias ▪ Administered into cavities (pleural, peritoneal) to prevent reaccumulation of malignant effusions.

ACTION
▪ Interferes with DNA and RNA synthesis by cross-linking strands (cell cycle-phase nonspecific). **Therapeutic Effect:** ▪ Death of rapidly replicating cells, particularly malignant ones.

PHARMACOKINETICS
Absorption: Administered IV and intracavitary only. Some absorption occurs following intracavitary instillation.
Distribution: Distribution not known.
Metabolism and Excretion: Rapidly degraded in body tissues and fluids.
Half-life: UK.

CONTRAINDICATIONS AND PRECAUTIONS
Contraindicated in: ▪ Hypersensitivity ▪ Pregnancy or lactation.
Use Cautiously in: ▪ Patients with childbearing potential ▪ Infections ▪ Decreased bone marrow reserve ▪ Other chronic debilitating illnesses ▪ Prior radiotherapy (dosage reduction required).

ADVERSE REACTIONS AND SIDE EFFECTS*
CNS: weakness, headache, drowsiness, vertigo, seizures.

*Underlines indicate most frequent; **CAPITALS** indicate life-threatening.

GI: nausea, vomiting, diarrhea, anorexia.
GU: gonadal suppression.
Hemat: anemia, leukopenia, thrombocytopenia.
Derm: rashes, alopecia.
Local: phlebitis at IV site, tissue necrosis.
Metab: hyperuricemia.
Misc: reactivation of herpes zoster.

INTERACTIONS

Drug–Drug: ▪ Additive myelosuppression with other **antineoplastic agents** or **radiation therapy** ▪ May decrease antibody response to **live virus vaccines** and increase the risk of adverse reactions.

ROUTE AND DOSAGE

- **IV (Adults):** 0.4 mg/kg or 6–10 mg/m^2 as single dose or divided doses repeated q 3–6 wk.
- **Intracavitary (Adults):** 10–20 mg.

PHARMACODYNAMICS (effects on blood counts)

	ONSET	PEAK	DURATION
WBCs	24 hr	7–14 days	10–21 days
Platelets	UK	9–16 days	20 days

NURSING IMPLICATIONS

Assessment

- Monitor blood pressure, pulse, and respiratory rate frequently during administration. Notify physician if significant changes occur.
- Assess injection site frequently for redness, irritation, or inflammation. If extravasation occurs, infusion must be stopped and restarted elsewhere to avoid damage to SC tissue. Infiltrate affected area promptly with isotonic sodium thiosulfate 1% or lidocaine and apply ice compresses for 6–12 hr as directed by physician.
- Monitor intake and output, appetite, and nutritional intake. Nausea and vomiting may occur 1–3 hr after therapy. Vomiting may persist for 8 hr; nausea may last 24 hr. Parenteral antiemetic agents should be administered 30–45 min prior to therapy and routinely around the clock for the next 24 hr as indicated. Adjust diet as tolerated to help maintain fluid and electrolyte balance and nutritional status.
- Assess for fever, chills, sore throat, and signs of infection. Notify physician if these symptoms occur.
- Assess for bleeding (bleeding gums, bruising, petechiae; guaiac stools, urine, and emesis). Avoid IM injections and rectal temperatures. Apply pressure to venipuncture sites for 10 min.
- Anemia may occur. Monitor for increased fatigue and dyspnea.
- Monitor for symptoms of gout (increased uric acid, joint pain, edema). Encourage patient to drink at least 2 liters of fluid each day. Allopurinol may be given to decrease uric acid levels. Alkalinization of urine may be ordered to increase excretion of uric acid.
- **Lab Test Considerations:** Monitor CBC and differential prior to and periodically throughout therapy. The nadir of leukopenia occurs in 7–14 days. Notify physician if leukocyte count is <1000/mm^3. The nadir of thrombocytopenia occurs in 9–16 days. Notify physician if platelet count is <75,000/mm^3. Recovery of leukopenia and thrombocytopenia occurs in 20 days.
- Monitor liver function studies (SGOT [AST], SGPT [ALT], LDH, bilirubin) and renal function studies (BUN, creatinine) prior to and periodically throughout therapy to detect hepatotoxicity and nephrotoxicity.
- May cause increased uric acid levels.

Potential Nursing Diagnoses

- Infection, high risk for (adverse reactions).
- Nutrition, altered: less than body requirements (adverse reactions).
- Knowledge deficit related to medication regimen (patient/family teaching).

M

Implementation

- **General Info:** Soln should be prepared in a biologic cabinet. Wear gloves, gown, and mask while handling medication. All equipment in contact with this medication must be decontaminated prior to disposal. Soak gloves, IV tubing, syringes, etc. in soln of 5% sodium thiosulfate and 5% sodium bicarbonate for 45 min. Unused portions of the drug must be mixed with equal amounts of this soln.
- □ Discard all contaminated equipment in specially designated containers. If medication comes in contact with skin, flush with large volume of water for 15 min, followed by a 2% sodium thiosulfate soln. If eye contact occurs, flush eye with 0.9% NaCl and notify physician immediately (see Appendix I.)
- **Direct IV:** Discard vial if droplets of water appear to be present prior to reconstitution. Dilute each 10 mg with 10 ml of 0.9% NaCl or sterile water for injection. Do not remove the needle from the vial stopper prior to agitating soln. Allow soln to dissolve completely. Reconstituted soln decomposes in 15 min. Administer immediately. Do not use a discolored soln or one that contains precipitates.
- □ *Rate:* Withdraw desired amount of drug and administer over 3–5 min via Y-tubing or 3-way stopcock into a free-flowing soln of 0.9% NaCl.
- **Intracavitary:** May be further diluted in 100 ml of 0.9% NaCl. Assist physician in paracentesis prior to installation of mechlorethamine. Confer with physician regarding analgesia and schedule for repositioning patient to ensure mechlorethamine comes in contact with entire cavity surface. Remaining fluid may be removed after 24–36 hr.

Patient/Family Teaching

- □ Advise patient to notify physician if fever, chills, sore throat, signs of infection, bleeding gums, bruising, petechiae, or blood in urine, stool, or emesis occurs. Caution patient to avoid crowds and persons with known infections. Instruct patient to use soft toothbrush and electric razor. Caution patient not to drink alcoholic beverages or take aspirin-containing products.
- □ This drug may cause irreversible gonadal suppression; however, patient should still practice birth control during and for at least 4 mon after therapy, as it may have teratogenic effects.
- □ Discuss with patient the possibility of hair loss. Explore methods of coping.
- □ Instruct patient not to receive any vaccinations without advice of physician.
- □ Instruct patient to notify physician if skin rash occurs. Rash may indicate idiosyncratic reaction or reactivation of herpes zoster.
- □ Emphasize the need for periodic lab tests to monitor for side effects.

Evaluation

Effectiveness of therapy can be demonstrated by: ▪ Decrease in size or spread of malignancies in solid tumors or ▪ Improvement of hematologic status in leukemias.

MECLIZINE
(**mek**-li-zeen)
Antivert, {Bonamine}, Bonine, Ru-vert M

CLASSIFICATION(S):
Antiemetic, Antihistamine
Pregnancy Category B

INDICATIONS

▪ Management and prevention of motion sickness ▪ Used to treat labyrinthitis or Meniere's disease.

ACTION

▪ Has central anticholinergic, CNS depressant, and antihistaminic properties

■ Decreases excitability of the middle ear labyrinth and depresses conduction in middle ear vestibular-cerebellar pathways. **Therapeutic Effects:** ■ Decreased motion sickness ■ Decreased vertigo due to vestibular pathology.

PHARMACOKINETICS

Absorption: Appears to be absorbed following oral administration.
Distribution: Distribution not known.
Metabolism and Excretion: Metabolism and excretion not known.
Half-life: 6 hr.

CONTRAINDICATIONS AND PRECAUTIONS

Contraindicated in: ■ Hypersensitivity ■ Pregnancy.
Use Cautiously in: ■ Prostatic hypertrophy ■ Narrow-angle glaucoma. ■ Children or lactation (safety not established).

ADVERSE REACTIONS AND SIDE EFFECTS*

CNS: drowsiness, fatigue.
EENT: blurred vision.
GI: dry mouth.

INTERACTIONS

Drug-Drug: ■ Additive CNS depression with other **CNS depressants,** including **alcohol,** other **antihistamines, narcotic analgesics,** and **sedative/hypnotics** ■ Additive anticholinergic effects with other **drugs possessing anticholinergic properties,** including **antihistamines, antidepressants, atropine, haloperidol, phenothiazines, quinidine,** and **disopyramide.**

ROUTE AND DOSAGE

Motion Sickness

- **PO (Adults):** 25–50 mg 1 hr before exposure, may repeat in 24 hr.

Labrynthitis or Meniere's Disease

- **PO (Adults):** 25–100 mg/day in divided doses.

PHARMACODYNAMICS (antihistaminic effects)

	ONSET	PEAK	DURATION
PO	1 hr	UK	8–24 hr

NURSING IMPLICATIONS

Assessment

- **General Info:** Assess patient for level of sedation following administration.
- **Motion Sickness:** Assess patient for nausea and vomiting prior to and 60 min following administration.
- **Vertigo:** Assess degree of vertigo periodically in patients receiving meclizine for labyrinthitis.
- **Lab Test Considerations:** May cause false-negative results in skin tests using allergen extracts. Discontinue meclizine 72 hr prior to testing.

Potential Nursing Diagnoses

- Injury, high risk for (side effects).
- Knowledge deficit related to medication regimen (patient/family teaching).

Implementation

- **PO:** Administer oral doses with food, water, or milk to minimize GI irritation. Chewable tablet may be chewed or swallowed whole.

Patient/Family Teaching

- **General Info:** Meclizine may cause drowsiness. Caution patient to avoid driving or other activities requiring alertness until response to the medication is known.
- □ Advise patient that frequent mouth rinses, good oral hygiene, and sugarless gum or candy may decrease dryness of mouth.
- □ Caution patient to avoid concurrent use of alcohol and other CNS depressants with this medication.
- **Motion Sickness:** When used as prophylaxis for motion sickness, advise patient to take medication at least 1 hr prior to exposure to conditions that may cause motion sickness.

*Underlines indicate most frequent; **CAPITALS** indicate life-threatening.

Evaluation

Effectiveness of therapy can be demonstrated by: ▪ Prevention and relief of symptoms in motion sickness ▪ Prevention and treatment of vertigo due to vestibular pathology.

MECLOFENAMATE

(me-kloe-**fen**-am-ate)
Meclomen

CLASSIFICATION(S):
Nonsteroidal anti-inflammatory agent, Non-narcotic analgesic
Pregnancy Category UK

INDICATIONS

▪ Management of inflammatory disorders, including: ▫ Rheumatoid arthritis ▫ Osteoarthritis ▪ Management of mild to moderate pain.

ACTION

▪ Inhibits prostaglandin synthesis. **Therapeutic Effects:** ▪ Suppression of pain and inflammation.

PHARMACOKINETICS

Absorption: Well absorbed from the GI tract.
Distribution: Distribution not known.
Metabolism and Excretion: Mostly metabolized by the liver.
Half-life: 40 min–2 hr.

CONTRAINDICATIONS AND PRECAUTIONS

Contraindicated in: ▪ Hypersensitivity ▪ Cross-sensitivity may exist with other nonsteroidal anti-inflammatory agents, including aspirin ▪ Active GI bleeding or ulcer disease.
Use Cautiously in: ▪ Severe cardiovascular, renal, or hepatic disease ▪ History of ulcer disease ▪ Pregnancy, lactation, or children (safety not established).

ADVERSE REACTIONS AND SIDE EFFECTS*

CNS: headache, drowsiness, dizziness.
EENT: visual disturbances, tinnitus.
CV: edema.
GI: nausea, dyspepsia, vomiting, diarrhea, constipation, GI BLEEDING, discomfort, HEPATITIS, flatulence, anorexia, stomatitis.
GU: renal failure.
Derm: hives, itching.
Hemat: blood dyscrasias, prolonged bleeding time.
Misc: allergic reactions, including ANAPHYLAXIS and STEVENS-JOHNSON SYNDROME, drug-induced systemic lupus erythematosus-like syndrome.

INTERACTIONS

Drug–Drug: ▪ Concurrent use with **aspirin** may decrease meclofenamate blood levels and may decrease effectiveness ▪ May increase risk of bleeding with **anticoagulants, thrombolytics, cefamandole, cefoperazone, cefotetan, moxalactam,** or **plicamycin** ▪ Additive adverse GI side effects with **aspirin, alcohol, colchicine, glucocorticoids, potassium supplements,** and other **nonsteroidal anti-inflammatory agents** ▪ **Probenecid** increases blood levels and may increase toxicity ▪ Chronic use with **acetaminophen** or **gold compounds** may increase the risk of adverse renal reactions ▪ May decrease the effectiveness of **antihypertensive agents** or **diuretics** ▪ May increase hypoglycemia from **oral hypoglycemic agents** or **insulin** ▪ Increased risk of hematologic adverse reactions with **antineoplastic agents** or **radiation therapy** ▪ May increase blood levels and toxicity of **lithium** or **methotrexate**.

ROUTE AND DOSAGE

Anti-Inflammatory

- **PO (Adults):** 200–300 mg/day in 3–4 divided doses (not to exceed 400 mg/day).

*Underlines indicate most frequent; **CAPITALS** indicate life-threatening.

Analgesic
- **PO (Adults):** 50–100 mg q 4–6 hr.

PHARMACODYNAMICS (anti-inflammatory activity)

	ONSET	PEAK	DURATION
PO	days	2–3 wk	days

NURSING IMPLICATIONS

Assessment

- **General Info:** Patients who have asthma, aspirin-induced allergy, and nasal polyps are at increased risk for developing hypersensitivity reactions. Monitor for rhinitis, asthma, and urticaria.
- **Arthritis:** Assess pain and range of movement prior to and 1–2 hr following administration.
- **Pain:** Assess location, duration, and intensity of pain prior to and 1 hr following administration.
- **Lab Test Considerations:** Serum BUN, creatinine, potassium, SGOT (AST), SGPT (AST), LDH, and alkaline phosphatase concentrations may be increased.
- □ May cause decreased hemoglobin and hematocrit levels.

Potential Nursing Diagnoses

- Comfort, altered: pain (indications).
- Mobility, impaired physical (indications).
- Knowledge deficit related to medication regimen (patient/family teaching).

Implementation

- **PO:** For rapid initial effect, administer 30 min before or 2 hr after meals. May be administered with food, milk, or antacids to decrease GI irritation. Food slows but does not reduce the extent of absorption.

Patient/Family Teaching

- □ Advise patients to take this medication with a full glass of water and to remain in an upright position for 15–30 min after administration.
- □ Instruct patient to take medication exactly as prescribed. If a dose is missed, take as soon as remembered but not if almost time for next dose. Do not double doses.
- □ This medication may occasionally cause drowsiness or dizziness. Advise patient to avoid driving or other activities requiring alertness until response to the medication is known.
- □ Caution patient to avoid the concurrent use of alcohol, aspirin, acetaminophen, or other over-the-counter medications without consulting physician or pharmacist.
- □ Instruct patient to notify physician if rash, itching, chills, fever, visual disturbances, tinnitus, weight gain, edema, black stools, persistent or severe diarrhea, or persistent headache occurs.
- □ Advise patient to inform physician or dentist of medication regimen prior to treatment or surgery.

Evaluation

Effectiveness of therapy can be demonstrated by: ▪ Decrease in severity of pain ▪ Improved joint mobility □ Partial arthritic relief is usually seen within a few days, but maximum effectiveness may require 2–3 wk of continuous therapy. Patients who do not respond to one nonsteroidal anti-inflammatory agent may respond to another.

MEDROXYPROGESTERONE

(me-**drox**-ee-proe-jess-te-rone)
Amen, Curretab, Cycrin, Depo-Provera, Provera

CLASSIFICATION(S):
Hormone—progestin, Antineoplastic agent—hormone
Pregnancy Category UK

INDICATIONS

▪ Treatment of secondary amenorrhea and abnormal uterine bleeding caused by hormonal imbalance ▪ Treatment of advanced unresponsive endometrial or renal carcinoma. **Unlabeled Uses:** ▪ Long-acting contraceptive ▪ Management of sexual deviance ▪ Management of the postmenopausal syndrome ▪ Obesity-hypoventilation (Pickwickian) syndrome ▪ Sleep apnea ▪ Hypersomnolence ▪ Precocious puberty ▪ Hirsutism ▪ Homozygous sickle cell disease.

ACTION

▪ A synthetic form of progesterone—actions include secretory changes in the endometrium, increases in basal body temperature, histologic changes in vaginal epithelium, relaxation of uterine smooth muscle, mammary alveolar tissue growth, pituitary inhibition, and withdrawal bleeding in the presence of estrogen. **Therapeutic Effect:** ▪ Restoration of hormonal balance with control of uterine bleeding.

PHARMACOKINETICS

Absorption: UK.
Distribution: Enters breast milk.
Metabolism and Excretion: UK.
Half-life: UK.

CONTRAINDICATIONS AND PRECAUTIONS

Contraindicated in: ▪ Hypersensitivity ▪ Hypersensitivity to parabens (IM suspension only) ▪ Pregnancy ▪ Missed abortion ▪ Thromboembolic disease ▪ Cerebrovascular disease ▪ Severe liver disease ▪ Breast or genital cancer ▪ Porphyria.
Use Cautiously in: ▪ History of liver disease ▪ Renal disease ▪ Cardiovascular disease ▪ Seizure disorders ▪ Mental depression.

ADVERSE REACTIONS AND SIDE EFFECTS*

CNS: depression.
EENT: retinal thrombosis.
CV: THROMBOEMBOLISM, PULMONARY EMBOLISM, thrombophlebitis.
GI: gingival bleeding, hepatitis.
GU: cervical erosions.
Endo: breakthrough bleeding, spotting, amenorrhea, breast tenderness, galactorrhea, changes in menstrual flow.
Derm: rashes, melasma, chloasma.
F and E: edema.
Misc: weight gain, weight loss, allergic reactions, including ANAPHYLAXIS and ANGIOEDEMA.

INTERACTIONS

Drug-Drug: ▪ May decrease the effectiveness of **bromocriptine** when used concurrently for galactorrhea/amenorrhea.

ROUTE AND DOSAGE

Secondary Amenorrhea

- **PO (Adults):** 5–10 mg/day for 5–10 days, start at any time in cycle.

Functional Uterine Bleeding

- **PO (Adults):** 5–10 mg/day for 5–10 days, start on calculated day 16 or day 21 of menstrual cycle.

Induction of Secretory Endometrium Following Estrogen Priming

- **PO (Adults):** 10 mg/day for 10 days.

Renal or Endometrial Carcinoma

- **IM (Adults):** 400–1000 mg, may be repeated weekly; if improvement occurs, attempt to decrease dosage to 400 mg weekly.

Contraceptive

- **IM (Adults):** 150 mg every 3 mon.

PHARMACODYNAMICS (IM = antineoplastic effects)

	ONSET	PEAK	DURATION
PO	UK	UK	UK
IM	wks–mons	mon	UK

NURSING IMPLICATIONS

Assessment

- **General Info:** Monitor blood pressure periodically throughout therapy.
- Assess patient's usual menstrual history. Administration of drug may begin on any day of cycle in patients with amenorrhea and on day 16 or 21 of cycle in patients with dysfunctional bleeding.
- Monitor intake and output ratios and

*Underlines indicate most frequent; **CAPITALS** indicate life-threatening.

weekly weight. Report significant discrepancies or steady weight gain to physician.

- **Lab Test Considerations:** Monitor hepatic function prior to and periodically throughout therapy.
  - May cause increased alkaline phosphatase, prothrombin, and factors VII, IX, and X levels. May decrease pregnanediol excretion concentrations.
  - May cause increased serum concentrations of low-density lipoproteins and decreased concentrations of high-density lipoproteins.
  - May alter thyroid hormone assays.

Potential Nursing Diagnoses
- Sexual dysfunction (indications).
- Tissue perfusion, altered (side effects).
- Knowledge deficit related to medication regimen (patient/family teaching).

Implementation
- **General Info:** Available as a tablet for oral route and as a suspension for IM injection.
- **IM:** Shake vial before preparing IM dose. Administer deep IM.
  - In patients with cancer, IM dose may initially be required weekly. Once stabilized, IM dose may be required only monthly.
  - As a contraceptive, IM dose may need to be administered only every 3 mon.

Patient/Family Teaching
- **General Info:** Explain the dosage schedule. Instruct patient to take medication at the same time each day. If a dose is missed, patient should make up dose as soon as remembered, but do not double doses.
  - Advise patients receiving medroxyprogesterone for menstrual dysfunction to anticipate withdrawal bleeding 3–7 days after discontinuing medication.
  - Review patient package insert (PPI) with patient. Emphasize the importance of notifying physician if the following side effects occur: visual changes, sudden weakness, incoordination, difficulty with speech, headache, leg or calf pain, shortness of breath, chest pain, changes in vaginal bleeding pattern, yellow skin, swelling of extremities, depression, or rash. Patients receiving medroxyprogesterone for cancer may not receive PPI.
  - Advise patient to keep a 1-mon supply of medroxyprogesterone available at all times.
  - Instruct patient in correct method of monthly breast self-examination. Increased breast tenderness may occur.
  - Advise patient that gingival bleeding may occur. Instruct patient to use good oral hygiene and to receive regular dental care and examinations.
  - Instruct patient to notify physician if menstrual period is missed or if pregnancy is suspected. Patient should not attempt conception for 3 mon after discontinuing medication, in order to decrease risk to fetus.
  - Medroxyprogesterone may cause melasma (brown patches of discoloration) on face when patient is exposed to sunlight. Advise patient to avoid sun exposure and to wear sunscreen or protective clothing when outdoors.
  - Emphasize the importance of routine follow-up physical examinations, including blood pressure; breast, abdomen, and pelvic examinations; and PAP smears every 6–12 mon.

Evaluation
Effectiveness of therapy can be demonstrated by: ■ Regular menstrual periods ■ Prevention of pregnancy ■ Control of the spread of endometrial or renal cancer.

MEGESTROL
(me-**jess**-trole)
Megace

CLASSIFICATION(S):
Antineoplastic agent—hormone
Pregnancy Category UK

M

INDICATIONS

▪ Palliative treatment of endometrial and breast carcinoma, either alone or with surgery or radiation. **Unlabeled Use:** ▪ Treatment of anorexia, weight loss, and cachexia associated with AIDS.

ACTION

▪ Antineoplastic effect may result from inhibition of pituitary function. **Therapeutic Effect:** ▪ Regression of tumor.

PHARMACOKINETICS

Absorption: Well absorbed from the GI tract.
Distribution: Distribution not known.
Metabolism and Excretion: Completely metabolized by the liver.
Half-life: UK.

CONTRAINDICATIONS AND PRECAUTIONS

Contraindicated in: ▪ Hypersensitivity ▪ Pregnancy, missed abortion, or lactation ▪ Undiagnosed vaginal bleeding ▪ Severe liver disease.
Use Cautiously in: ▪ Diabetes ▪ Mental depression ▪ Renal disease ▪ History of thrombophlebitis ▪ Cardiovascular disease ▪ Seizure disorders.

ADVERSE REACTIONS AND SIDE EFFECTS*

GI: GI irritation.
Derm: alopecia.
Hemat: thrombophlebitis.
MS: carpal tunnel syndrome.

INTERACTIONS

Drug–Drug: ▪ None significant.

ROUTE AND DOSAGE

Breast Carcinoma

▪ **PO (Adults):** 160 mg/day in 4 divided doses.

Endometrial and Ovarian Carcinoma

▪ **PO (Adults):** 40–320 mg/day in divided doses.

PHARMACODYNAMICS (antineoplastic activity)

	ONSET	PEAK	DURATION
PO	wk–mons	2 mon	UK

NURSING IMPLICATIONS

Assessment

□ Assess patient for swelling, pain, or tenderness in legs. Notify physician if these signs of deep vein thrombophlebitis occur.

Potential Nursing Diagnoses

▪ Knowledge deficit related to medication regimen (patient/family teaching).

Implementation

▪ **PO:** May be administered with meals if GI irritation becomes a problem.

Patient/Family Teaching

□ Instruct patient to take medication exactly as prescribed by physician; do not skip or double up on missed doses. Missed doses may be taken as long as it is not right before next dose.
□ Advise patient to report to physician any unusual vaginal bleeding.
□ Advise patient that this medication may have teratogenic effects. Contraception should be practiced during therapy and for at least 4 mon after therapy is completed.
□ Discuss with patient the possibility of hair loss. Explore methods of coping.

Evaluation

Effectiveness of therapy can be demonstrated by: ▪ Slowing or arresting the spread of endometrial or breast malignancy. Therapeutic effects usually occur within 2 mon of initiating therapy.

MELPHALAN

(**mel**-fa-lan)
Alkeran, L-PAM, L-Sarcolysin, Phenylalanine mustard

*Underlines indicate most frequent; **CAPITALS** indicate life-threatening.

CLASSIFICATION(S):
Antineoplastic agent—alkylating agent
Pregnancy Category UK

INDICATIONS

▪ Used alone or with other treatment modalities in the management of: ▫ Multiple myeloma ▫ Ovarian cancer. **Unlabeled Uses:** ▪ Breast cancer ▪ Prostate cancer ▪ Testicular carcinoma ▪ Chronic myelogenous leukemia ▪ Osteogenic sarcoma.

ACTION

▪ Inhibits DNA and RNA synthesis by alkylation (cell cycle-phase nonspecific). **Therapeutic Effects:** ▪ Death of rapidly replicating cells, particularly malignant ones ▪ Also has immunosuppressive properties.

PHARMACOKINETICS

Absorption: Incompletely and variably absorbed following oral administration.
Distribution: Rapidly distributed throughout total body water.
Metabolism and Excretion: Rapidly metabolized in the bloodstream. Small amounts (10%) excreted unchanged by the kidneys.
Half-life: 1.5 hr.

CONTRAINDICATIONS AND PRECAUTIONS

Contraindicated in: ▪ Hypersensitivity to melphelan or chlorambucil ▪ Pregnancy or lactation.
Use Cautiously in: ▪ Patients with childbearing potential ▪ Active infections ▪ Decreased bone marrow reserve ▪ Other chronic debilitating illnesses ▪ Impaired renal function ▪ Children (safety not established).

ADVERSE REACTIONS AND SIDE EFFECTS*

Resp: pulmonary fibrosis, bronchopulmonary dysplasia.
GI: nausea, vomiting, stomatitis, diarrhea.
GU: gonadal suppression.
Derm: rashes, pruritus, alopecia.
Endo: menstrual irregularities.
Hemat: leukopenia, thrombocytopenia, anemia.
Metab: hyperuricemia.
Misc: allergic reactions, including ANAPHYLAXIS.

INTERACTIONS

Drug-Drug: ▪ Additive bone marrow depression with other **antineoplastic agents** or **radiation therapy** ▪ May decrease antibody response to **live virus vaccines** and increase the risk of adverse reactions.

ROUTE AND DOSAGE

Multiple Myeloma

▪ **PO (Adults):** 6 mg/day initially for 2–3 wk, then stop for up to 4 wk to allow recovery of bone marrow, then 2 mg/day or 0.15 mg/kg/day for 7 days or 0.25 mg/kg/day for 4 days given every 4–6 wk.

Ovarian Carcinoma

▪ **PO (Adults):** 0.2 mg/kg/day for 5 days given every 4–5 wk.

PHARMACODYNAMICS (effects on blood counts)

	ONSET	PEAK	DURATION
PO	5 days	2–3 wk	5–6 wk

NURSING IMPLICATIONS

Assessment

▫ Assess for fever, sore throat, and signs of infection. Notify physician if these symptoms occur.
▫ Assess for bleeding (bleeding gums, bruising, petechiae; guaiac stools, urine, and emesis). Avoid IM injections and rectal temperatures. Apply pressure to venipuncture sites for 10 min.
▫ May cause nausea and vomiting. Monitor intake and output, appetite, and nutritional intake. Confer with physician regarding prophylactic use

*Underlines indicate most frequent; **CAPITALS** indicate life-threatening.

of an antiemetic. Adjust diet as tolerated.

- Monitor for symptoms of gout (increased uric acid, joint pain, edema). Encourage patient to drink at least 2 liters of fluid per day. Allopurinol may be given to decrease uric acid levels.
- Anemia may occur. Monitor for increased fatigue and dyspnea.
- Assess patient for allergy to chlorambucil. Patients may have cross-sensitivity.
- **Lab Test Considerations:** Monitor CBC and differential weekly throughout therapy. The nadir of leukopenia occurs in 2–3 wk. Notify physician if leukocyte count is $<3000/mm^3$. The nadir of thrombocytopenia occurs in 2–3 wk. Notify physician if platelet count is $<100,000/mm^3$. Recovery of leukopenia and thrombocytopenia occurs in 5–6 wk.
- Monitor liver function studies (SGOT [AST], SGPT [ALT], LDH, bilirubin) and renal function studies (BUN, creatinine) prior to and periodically throughout therapy to detect hepatotoxicity and nephrotoxicity.
- May cause increased uric acid. Monitor periodically during therapy.
- May cause elevated 5-hydroxyindoleacetic acid (5-HIAA) concentrations as a result of tumor breakdown.

Potential Nursing Diagnoses

- Injury, high risk for (side effects).
- Infection, high risk for (side effects).
- Knowledge deficit related to medication regimen (patient/family teaching).

Implementation

- **PO:** Available in tablet only. May be ordered in divided doses or as a single daily dose.

Patient/Family Teaching

- Instruct patient to take melphalan exactly as directed, even if nausea and vomiting occurs. If vomiting occurs shortly after dose is taken, consult physician. If a dose is missed, do not take at all.
- Advise patient to notify physician if fever, chills, sore throat, signs of infection, bleeding gums, bruising, petechiae, or blood in urine, stool, or emesis occurs. Caution patient to avoid crowds and persons with known infections. Instruct patient to use soft toothbrush and electric razor. Caution patient not to drink alcoholic beverages or take aspirin-containing products.
- Instruct patient to notify physician if rash, itching, joint pain, or swelling occurs.
- Instruct patient to inspect oral mucosa for redness and ulceration. If ulceration occurs, advise patient to use sponge brush and to rinse mouth with water after eating and drinking. Consult physician regarding the use of viscous xylocaine swishes if pain interferes with eating.
- Advise patient that although fertility may be decreased, contraception should be used during melphalan therapy because of potential teratogenic effects on the fetus.
- Instruct patient not to receive any vaccinations without advice of physician.
- Emphasize need for periodic lab tests to monitor for side effects.

Evaluation

Effectiveness of therapy can be demonstrated by: ▪ Decrease in size and spread of malignant tissue.

MENADIOL

(men-a-**dye**-ole)
Synkayvite, vitamin K_3

CLASSIFICATION(S):
Vitamin—fat-soluble
Pregnancy Category UK

INDICATIONS

- Prevention and treatment of hypoprothrombinemia.

ACTION

- Required for hepatic synthesis of blood coagulation factors II (prothrombin), VII, IX, and X. **Therapeutic Effect:** ▪ Prevention of bleeding due to hypoprothrombinemia.

PHARMACOKINETICS

Absorption: Well absorbed following oral and IM administration.
Distribution: Distribution not known.
Metabolism and Excretion: Metabolism and excretion not known.
Half-life: Half-life not known.

CONTRAINDICATIONS AND PRECAUTIONS

Contraindicated in: ▪ Hypersensitivity to bisulfites (parenteral form only).
Use Cautiously in: ▪ Glucose-6-phosphate dehydrogenase (G6-PD) deficiency ▪ Severe liver disease ▪ Premature infants (increased risk of hyperbilirubinemia, kernicterus, and hemolytic anemia).

ADVERSE REACTIONS AND SIDE EFFECTS*

GI: gastric upset (oral only).
Derm: rash, urticaria, flushing.
Hemat: hemolysis (in G6-PD-deficient patients).
Local: erythema, swelling, pain at injection site.
Misc: hemolytic anemia, kernicterus, hyperbilirubinemia (large doses in very premature infants), allergic reactions.

INTERACTIONS

Drug–Drug: ▪ Large doses will counteract the effect of **oral anticoagulants** ▪ Increased risk of hemolysis with **primaquine** ▪ **Anticonvulsants** or large doses of **salicylates** or broad-spectrum **anti-infectives** may increase vitamin K requirements ▪ **Cholestyramine, colestipol, mineral oil,** and **sucralfate** may decrease vitamin K absorption.

ROUTE AND DOSAGE

- **PO (Adults):** 5–10 mg/day.
- **PO (Children):** 50–100 mcg/day.
- **IV, SC, IM (Adults):** 5–15 mg 1–2 times daily.
- **IV, SC, IM (Children):** 5–10 mg 1–2 times daily.

PHARMACODYNAMICS (effects on prothrombin time)

	ONSET	PEAK	DURATION
PO	UK	UK	UK
SC, IM	1–2 hr	8–24 hr	UK
IV	UK	UK	UK

NURSING IMPLICATIONS

Assessment

- □ Monitor for frank and occult bleeding (guaiac stools, urine, and emesis). Monitor pulse and blood pressure frequently; notify physician immediately if symptoms of internal bleeding or hypovolemic shock develop. Inform all personnel of patient's bleeding tendency to prevent further trauma. Apply pressure to all venipuncture sites for at least 5 min; avoid unnecessary IM injections.
- □ Monitor prothrombin time (PT) before and after therapy to assess effectiveness of therapy.
- ▪ **Lab Test Considerations:** May cause falsely elevated urinary 17-hydroxycorticosteroid values.

Potential Nursing Diagnoses

- Nutrition, altered: less than body requirements (indications).
- Tissue perfusion, altered: potential (indications).
- Knowledge deficit related to medication regimen (patient/family teaching).

Implementation

- **General Info:** Menadiol is *not* indicated for treatment of anticoagulant (warfarin sodium) overdose.
- **SC/IM:** SC and IM route provide longer duration of action than IV route.
- **Direct IV:** Administer through IV line

*Underlines indicate most frequent; **CAPITALS** indicate life-threatening.

of D5W, 0.9% NaCl, Ringer's soln, lactated Ringer's soln, or D5/LR over 1 min.
- **Y-Site Compatibility:** heparin, hydrocortisone sodium succinate, or potassium chloride.

PATIENT/FAMILY TEACHING
- Instruct patient to take menadiol as ordered. If a dose is missed, take as soon as remembered unless almost time for next dose. Notify physician of missed doses.
- Review foods high in vitamin K (green leafy vegetables, meat, and dairy products); see Appendix K. Inform patient that cooking does not destroy substantial amounts of vitamin K.
- Caution patient to avoid IM injections and activities leading to injury. Use a soft toothbrush, do not floss, and shave with an electric razor until coagulation defect is corrected.
- Advise patient to report any symptoms of unusual bleeding or bruising (bleeding gums, nose bleed, black tarry stools, hematuria, excessive menstrual flow) to physician.
- Instruct patient not to take over-the-counter medications, especially those containing aspirin, or alcohol without advice of physician or pharmacist.
- Advise patient to inform physician or dentist of the use of this medication prior to treatment or surgery.
- Advise patient to carry identification describing disease process at all times.
- Emphasize the importance of frequent lab tests to monitor coagulation factors.

EVALUATION
Effectiveness of therapy can be demonstrated by: ▪ Prevention of spontaneous bleeding or cessation of bleeding in patients with hypoprothrombinemia secondary to impaired intestinal absorption or salicylate or antibiotic therapy.

MENOTROPINS
(men-oh-**troe**-pins)
HMG, Pergonal

CLASSIFICATION(S):
Hormone—gonadotropin
Pregnancy Category UK

INDICATIONS
▪ Used in conjunction with chorionic gonadotropin to stimulate ovulation in patients with ovarian dysfunction and resultant infertility ▪ Used in conjunction with chorionic gonadotropin to stimulate spermatogenesis in male patients with hypogonadotropic hypogonadism and resultant infertility.

ACTION
▪ A purified form of human pituitary gonadotropins consisting of follicle-stimulating hormone (FSH) and luteinizing hormone (LH). In females, FSH causes growth and maturation of the ovarian follicle. LH causes ovulation and development of the corpeus luteum. In male patients, LH causes spermatogenesis. **Therapeutic Effect:** ▪ Ovulation or spermatogenesis, with resultant fertility.

PHARMACOKINETICS
Absorption: Appears to be well absorbed following IM administration.
Distribution: Distribution not known.
Metabolism and Excretion: 8% excreted unchanged in the urine.
Half-life: FSH—70 hr; LH—4 hr.

CONTRAINDICATIONS AND PRECAUTIONS
Contraindicated in: ▪ Vaginal bleeding of unknown cause ▪ Uterine fibroid tumors ▪ Ovarian cysts.
Use Cautiously in: ▪ Asthma ▪ Cardiovascular disease ▪ Seizure disorders ▪ Migraine headaches ▪ Polycystic ovaries ▪ Pituitary hypertrophy or tumor ▪ Severe renal impairment.

ADVERSE REACTIONS AND SIDE EFFECTS*

CV: thrombophlebitis, THROMBOEMBOLISM, PULMONARY EMBOLISM.
GI: bloating, abdominal pain, nausea, vomiting, diarrhea.
GU: pelvic pain, ovarian enlargement, multiple pregnancies.
Endo: gynecomastia (males).
F and E: edema.
Misc: fever.

INTERACTIONS

Drug–Drug: ▪ None significant.

ROUTE AND DOSAGE

Induction of Ovulation and Pregnancy

- **IM (Adults):** 75 IU FSH and 75 IU LH daily for 9–12 days, followed by chorionic gonadotropin. Course may be repeated 2 more times. If pregnancy does not occur, dosage can be increased to 150 IU FSH and 150 IU LH daily for 9–12 days, followed by chorionic gonadotropin. If pregnancy does not occur, 2 more courses may be attempted (not to exceed doses of 150 IU FSH and 150 IU LH).

Stimulation of Spermatogenesis

- **IM (Adults):** Following pretreatment with chorionic gonadotropins, 75 IU FSH and 75 IU LH 3 times weekly with chorionic gonadotropins; therapy is continued for at least 4 mon. If there is no evidence of increased spermatogenesis after 4 mon, dosage may be increased to 150 IU FSH and 150 IU LH with chorionic gonadotropins.

PHARMACODYNAMICS (females—peak = ovulation after chorionic gonadotropins; males—peak = increased spermatogenesis)

	ONSET	PEAK	DURATION
IM (females)	UK	18 hr	UK
IM (males)	UK	4 mon	UK

NURSING IMPLICATIONS

Assessment

- **Female Infertility:** A gynecologic and endocrine examination to determine the cause of infertility should be completed prior to course of therapy. The patient's partner should also be evaluated for possible decreased fertility. An endometrial biopsy should be done in older patients to rule out the presence of endometrial carcinoma.
- **Male Infertility:** A urologic and endocrine examination to determine the cause of infertility should be completed prior to the course of therapy.
- **Lab Test Considerations:** In female infertility, cervical mucus volume and character, urinary excretion of estrogen or serum estrogen levels, and ultrasound may be used to determine whether follicular maturation has occurred.
  - In male infertility, serum testosterone and sperm count and motility should be evaluated prior to and after course of therapy.

Potential Nursing Diagnoses

- Sexual dysfunction (indications).
- Body image disturbance (indications).
- Knowledge deficit related to medication regimen (patient/family teaching).

Implementation

- **General Info:** Female infertility—chorionic gonadotropin is usually administered 1 day following course of human menotropins. Male infertility—chorionic gonadotropin is administered alone until secondary sex characteristics develop, then administered concurrently with menotropins.
- **IM:** Reconstitute powder with 2-ml vial of 0.9% NaCl for injection provided by manufacturer. Use immediately; discard any unused portion of dose.

*Underlines indicate most frequent; **CAPITALS** indicate life-threatening.

PATIENT/FAMILY TEACHING

- **General Info:** Instruct patient in correct technique for medication reconstitution and administration of IM injection. Ensure that patient understands medication administration schedule.
- **Female Infertility:** Instruct patient in the correct method for measuring basal body temperature. A record of the daily basal body temperature should be maintained prior to and throughout course of therapy.
  - Reinforce physician's instructions regarding timing of sexual intercourse (usually daily beginning 1 day after administration of chorionic gonadotropin).
  - Emphasize the importance of close monitoring by the physician throughout course of therapy (daily pelvic examinations are indicated after estrogen levels rise and for 2 wk after chorionic gonadotropin therapy).
  - Inform patient prior to therapy of the potential for multiple births.
  - Instruct patient to notify physician immediately if pregnancy is suspected (menses do not occur when expected and basal body temperature is biphasic).
  - Advise patient to report to physician signs and symptoms of fluid retention (swelling of ankles and feet, weight gain), thromboembolic disorders (pain, swelling, tenderness in extremities, headache, chest pain, blurred vision), or abdominal or pelvic pain or bloating.
- **Male Infertility:** Inform patient that breast enlargement may occur. Physician should be consulted if this is problematic.

EVALUATION

Effectiveness of therapy can be demonstrated by: ▪ Follicular maturation in females. Menotropin therapy is followed by human chorionic gonadotropin, which should lead to ovulation with subsequent pregnancy ▪ Increased spermatogenesis after 4 mon of therapy in males.

M

MEPERIDINE

(me-**per**-i-deen)
Demerol, Pethidine

CLASSIFICATION(S):
Narcotic analgesic—agonist
Schedule II
Pregnancy Category UK

INDICATIONS

▪ Used alone and in combination with non-narcotic analgesics in the management of moderate to severe pain ▪ Has been used as: ▫ An adjunct to anesthesia ▫ An analgesic during labor ▫ Preoperative sedation.

ACTION

▪ Binds to opiate receptors in the CNS. Alters the perception of and response to painful stimuli, while producing generalized CNS depression. **Therapeutic Effect:** ▪ Decrease in severity of pain.

PHARMACOKINETICS

Absorption: Moderately absorbed (50%) from the GI tract. Well absorbed from IM sites. Oral and parenteral doses are not equal.

Distribution: Widely distributed. Crosses the placenta and enters breast milk.

Metabolism and Excretion: Mostly metabolized by the liver. Some converted to normperidine, which has a long half-life (15–20 hr), and CNS stimulatory effects. 5% excreted unchanged by the kidneys.

Half-life: 3–8 hr (prolonged in impaired renal or hepatic function).

CONTRAINDICATIONS AND PRECAUTIONS

Contraindicated in: ▪ Hypersensitivity ▪ Pregnancy or lactation (chronic use) ▪ Recent (14–21 days) MAO inhibitor therapy.

Use Cautiously in: ▪ Head trauma ▪ Increased intracranial pressure ▪ Severe renal, hepatic, or pulmonary disease ▪ Hypothyroidism ▪ Adrenal insufficiency ▪ Alcoholism ▪ Elderly or debilitated patients (dosage reduction suggested) ▪ Undiagnosed abdominal pain or prostatic hypertrophy ▪ Labor (respiratory depression may occur in the newborn).

ADVERSE REACTIONS AND SIDE EFFECTS*

CNS: sedation, confusion, headache, euphoria, floating feeling, unusual dreams, hallucinations, dysphoria.
EENT: miosis, diplopia, blurred vision.
CV: hypotension, bradycardia.
GI: nausea, vomiting, constipation.
GU: urinary retention.
Derm: sweating, flushing.
Resp: respiratory depression.
Misc: tolerance, physical dependence, psychological dependence.

INTERACTIONS

Drug-Drug: ▪ Use with extreme caution in patients receiving **MAO inhibitors** or **procarbazine** (may result in unpredictable fatal reaction—contraindicated within 14–21 days of MAO inhibitor therapy) ▪ Additive CNS depression with **alcohol, antihistamines,** and **sedative/hypnotics** ▪ Administration of **partial-antagonist narcotic analgesics** may precipitate narcotic withdrawal in physically dependent patients ▪ **Nalbuphine** or **pentazocine** may decrease analgesia.

ROUTE AND DOSAGE

Analgesia

- **PO, IM, SC (Adults):** 50–150 mg q 3–4 hr.
- **PO, IM, SC (Children):** 1.1–1.8 mg/kg q 3–4 hr (not to exceed 100 mg dose).
- **IV (Adults):** 15–35 mg/hr as a continuous infusion.

Analgesia During Labor

- **IM, SC (Adults):** 50–100 mg when contractions become regular, may repeat q 1–3 hr.

Preoperative Sedation

- **IM, SC (Adults):** 50–100 mg 30–90 min before anesthesia.
- **IM, SC (Children):** 1–2.2 mg/kg 30–90 min before anesthesia (not to exceed adult dose).

PHARMACODYNAMICS (analgesia)

	ONSET	PEAK	DURATION
PO	15 min	60 min	2–4 hr
IM	10–15 min	30–50 min	2–4 hr
SC	10–15 min	40–60 min	2–4 hr
IV	immediate	5–7 min	2–4 hr

NURSING IMPLICATIONS

Assessment

- □ Assess blood pressure, pulse, and respiratory rate before and periodically during administration.
- □ Assess type, location, and intensity of pain prior to and 30–60 min following administration.
- □ Prolonged use may lead to physical and psychological dependence and tolerance. This should not prevent patient from receiving adequate analgesia. Most patients who receive meperidine for medical reasons do not develop psychological dependence. Progressively higher doses may be required to relieve pain with long-term therapy.
- □ Assess bowel function routinely. Increased intake of fluids and bulk, stool softeners, and laxatives may minimize constipating effects.
- ▪ **Lab Test Considerations:** May increase plasma amylase and lipase concentrations.
- ▪ **Toxicity and Overdose:** If overdosage occurs, naloxone (Narcan) is the antidote. Monitor patient closely; dose may need to be repeated or naloxone infusion administered.

Potential Nursing Diagnoses

- Comfort, altered: pain (indications).
- Sensory-perceptual alteration: visual, auditory (side effects).
- Injury, high risk for (side effects).

Implementation

- **General Info:** Explain therapeutic value of medication prior to adminis-

*Underlines indicate most frequent; **CAPITALS** indicate life-threatening.

tration to enhance the analgesic effect.

- Regularly administered doses may be more effective than prn administration. Analgesic is more effective if given before pain becomes severe.
- Coadministration with non-narcotic analgesics may have additive analgesic effects and permit lower doses.
- Oral dose is <50% as effective as parenteral. When changing to oral administration, dose may need to be increased.
- Medication should be discontinued gradually after long-term use to prevent withdrawal symptoms.
- Available in tablet, syrup, and injectable forms. Also available in combination with promethazine, acetaminophen, or atropine (see Appendix A).
- May be administered via patient-controlled analgesia (PCA) pump.
- **PO:** Doses may be administered with food or milk to minimize GI irritation. Syrup should be diluted in ½ glass of water.
- **IM:** IM is the preferred parenteral route for repeated doses. SC administration may cause local irritation.
- **Direct IV:** Dilute for IV administration to a concentration of 10 mg/ml with sterile water or 0.9% NaCl for injection.
- *Rate:* Administer slowly, at a rate not to exceed 25 mg over 1 min. Rapid administration may lead to increased respiratory depression, hypotension, and circulatory collapse. Do not use IV without antidote available.
- **Continuous Infusion:** Dilute to a concentration of 1 mg/ml with D5W, D10W, dextrose/saline combinations, dextrose/Ringer's or lactated Ringer's injection combinations, 0.45% NaCl, 0.9% NaCl, Ringer's or lactated Ringer's soln. Administer via infusion pump. Titrate according to patient needs.
- **Syringe Compatibility:** atropine, benzquinamide, butorphanol, chlorpromazine, cimetidine, dimenhydrinate, diphenhydramine, droperidol, fentanyl, glycopyrrolate, hydroxyzine, metoclopramide, midazolam, pentazocine, perphenazine, prochlorperazine, promazine, promethazine, ranitidine, or scopolamine.
- **Syringe Incompatibility:** heparin, morphine, or pentobarbital.
- **Y-Site Compatibility:** acyclovir, amikacin, ampicillin, ampicillin/sulbactam, cefamandole, cefazolin, cefonicid, cefotaxime, cefotetan, cefoxitin, ceftizoxime, cefuroxime, cephalothin, cephapirin, chloramphenicol, clindamycin, co-trimoxazole, doxycycline, erythromycin lactobionate, gentamicin, heparin, insulin, kanamycin, metronidazole, moxalactam, ondansetron, oxacillin, oxytocin, penicillin G potassium, piperacillin, ranitidine, ticarcillin, ticarcillin/clavulanate, tobramycin, or vancomycin.
- **Y-Site Incompatibility:** cefoperazone, mezlocillin, minocycline, or tetracycline.
- **Additive Compatibility:** dobutamine, scopolamine, succinylcholine, triflupromazine, or verapamil.
- **Additive Incompatibility:** aminophylline, amobarbital, heparin, methicillin, morphine, phenobarbital, sodium iodide, or thiopental.

Patient/Family Teaching

- Instruct patient on how and when to ask for prn pain medication.
- Medication may cause drowsiness or dizziness. Advise patient to call for assistance when ambulating or smoking. Caution patient to avoid driving or other activities requiring alertness until response to medication is known.
- Advise patient to make position changes slowly to minimize orthostatic hypotension.
- Instruct patient to avoid concurrent use of alcohol or other CNS depressants.
- Encourage patient to turn, cough, and breathe deeply every 2 hr to prevent atelectasis.

EVALUATION

Effectiveness of therapy can be demonstrated by: ▪ Decrease in severity of pain without a significant alteration in level of consciousness or respiratory status.

MEPROBAMATE

(me-proe-**ba**-mate)
{Apo-Meprobamate}, Equanil, {Meditran}, Meprospan, Miltown, Neuramate, {Novomepro}, Sedabamate, Tranmep

CLASSIFICATION(S):
Sedative/hypnotic—miscellaneous
Schedule IV
Pregnancy Category UK

INDICATIONS

▪ Used as a sedative in the management of anxiety disorders.

ACTION

▪ Produces CNS depression by acting at multiple sites in the CNS. **Therapeutic Effect:** ▪ Sedation.

PHARMACOKINETICS

Absorption: Well absorbed following oral administration.
Distribution: Widely distributed. Crosses the placenta and enters breast milk in high concentrations.
Metabolism and Excretion: Metabolized by the liver.
Half-life: 6–16 hr.

CONTRAINDICATIONS AND PRECAUTIONS

Contraindicated in: ▪ Hypersensitivity ▪ Comatose patients or those with pre-existing CNS depression ▪ Uncontrolled severe pain ▪ Pregnancy and lactation.
Use Cautiously in: ▪ Hepatic dysfunction or severe renal impairment ▪ Patients who may be suicidal or who may have been addicted to drugs previously ▪ Elderly patients (dosage reduction suggested).

ADVERSE REACTIONS AND SIDE EFFECTS*

CNS: drowsiness, ataxia.
EENT: blurred vision.
CV: hypotension.
GI: anorexia, nausea, vomiting, diarrhea.
Derm: pruritus, urticaria, rashes.
Misc: hypersensitivity reactions, tolerance, psychological dependence, physical dependence.

INTERACTIONS

Drug-Drug: ▪ Additive CNS depression with other **CNS depressants,** including **alcohol, antihistamines, narcotic analgesics,** and other **sedative/hypnotics.**

ROUTE AND DOSAGE

- **PO (Adults):** 1200–1600 mg/day in 2–4 divided doses or in 2 divided doses as extended-release capsules (maximum 2400 mg/day).
- **PO (Children 6–12 yr):** 100–200 mg 2–3 times daily or 200 mg as extended-release capsules bid.

PHARMACODYNAMICS (sedation)

	ONSET	PEAK	DURATION
PO	<1 hr	1–3 hr	6–12 hr
PO	UK	UK	12 hr

NURSING IMPLICATIONS

ASSESSMENT

- ▫ Assess degree and manifestations of anxiety prior to and periodically throughout therapy.
- ▫ Monitor blood pressure and pulse rate prior to and during initial therapy.
- ▫ Prolonged high-dose therapy may lead to psychological or physical dependence. Restrict amount of drug available to patient.
- ▪ **Lab Test Considerations:** Assess CBC periodically during course of therapy.

{} = Available in Canada only.
*Underlines indicate most frequent; **CAPITALS** indicate life-threatening.

M

□ May cause false elevations in urinary steroid concentrations.

Potential Nursing Diagnoses
- Anxiety (indications).
- Injury, high risk for (side effects).
- Knowledge deficit related to medication regimen (patient/family teaching).

Implementation
- **PO:** May be administered with food to minimize GI irritation.

□ Do not crush, break, or chew sustained-release capsules.

Patient/Family Teaching

□ Instruct patient to take medication exactly as directed. If a dose is missed, take if remembered within 1 hr; if remembered later, do not take. Do not double doses. Abrupt discontinuation of medication may precipitate pre-existing symptoms or withdrawal reactions within 12–48 hr (vomiting, ataxia, muscle twitching, confusion, hallucinations, convulsions). Symptoms usually subside within 12–48 hr.

□ Meprobamate may cause drowsiness and blurred vision. Caution patient to avoid driving and other activities requiring alertness until effects of drug are known.

□ Caution patient to make position changes slowly to minimize orthostatic hypotension.

□ Advise patient to avoid concurrent use of alcohol or other CNS depressants.

□ Instruct patient to notify physician if pregnancy is planned or suspected.

□ Advise patient to notify physician if skin rash, sore throat, or fever occurs.

□ Emphasize the importance of participation in psychotherapy if ordered by physician and follow-up examinations to evaluate progress.

Evaluation

Effectiveness of therapy can be demonstrated by: ▪ Decrease in the signs and symptoms of anxiety ▪ Sedation. Medication's efficacy should be reassessed periodically. Therapy is generally of less than 4 mon duration.

MERCAPTOPURINE
(mer-kap-toe-**pyoor**-een)
6-MP, Purinethol

CLASSIFICATION(S):
Antineoplastic—antimetabolite
Pregnancy Category UK

INDICATIONS
▪ Used in combination regimens in the treatment of leukemias. **Unlabeled Uses:** ▪ Treatment of: □ Some lymphomas □ Polycythemia vera □ Inflammatory bowel disease □ Psoriatic arthritis.

ACTION
▪ Disrupts DNA and RNA synthesis (cell cycle-S phase specific). **Therapeutic Effects:** ▪ Death of rapidly proliferating cells, especially malignant ones ▪ Also has immunosuppressant properties.

PHARMACOKINETICS
Absorption: Variably and incompletely (5–50%) absorbed after oral administration.
Distribution: Widely distributed throughout total body water.
Metabolism and Excretion: Mostly metabolized by liver. Some metabolism by the GI mucosa. Small amounts excreted unchanged by the kidneys.
Half-life: UK.

CONTRAINDICATIONS AND PRECAUTIONS
Contraindicated in: ▪ Hypersensitivity ▪ Pregnancy or lactation ▪ Severe liver disease.
Use Cautiously in: ▪ Patients with childbearing potential ▪ Infections ▪ Decreased bone marrow reserve ▪ Other chronic debilitating illnesses.

ADVERSE REACTIONS AND SIDE EFFECTS*

CNS: weakness.
Derm: hyperpigmentation, rashes.
Endo: gonadal suppression.
GI: nausea, vomiting, anorexia, diarrhea, HEPATOTOXICITY.
GU: gonadal suppression.
Hemat: anemia, leukopenia, thrombocytopenia.
Metab: hyperuricemia.
Misc: fever.

INTERACTIONS

Drug–Drug: ▪ **Allopurinol** decreases the metabolism and increases the potential of toxicity from mercaptopurine (reduce dosage of mercaptopurine to 25–33% of the usual dose) ▪ Additive hepatotoxicity with other **hepatotoxic agents** ▪ Additive bone marrow depression with other **antineoplastic agents** or **radiation therapy** ▪ May alter the effect of **warfarin** (increase or decrease effectiveness) ▪ Decreases the antibody response to **live virus vaccines** and increases the risk of adverse reactions.

ROUTE AND DOSAGE

- **PO (Adults):** 1.5–2.5 mg/kg/day, single dose (80–100 mg/m^2).
- **PO (Children):** 70 mg/m^2/day, single dose.

PHARMACODYNAMICS (effects on blood counts)

	ONSET	PEAK	DURATION
PO	7–10 days	14 days	21 days

NURSING IMPLICATIONS

Assessment

- Monitor blood pressure, pulse, respiratory rate, and temperature frequently during course of therapy. Notify physician of significant changes.
- Assess for fever, chills, sore throat, and signs of infection. Notify physician if these symptoms occur.
- Assess for bleeding (bleeding gums, bruising, petechiae; guaiac stools, urine, and emesis). Avoid IM injections and rectal temperatures. Apply pressure to venipuncture sites for 10 min.
- Monitor intake and output ratios and inform physician if significant discrepancies occur. Encourage fluid intake of 2000–3000 ml/day. Physician may also order allopurinol and alkalinization of the urine to decrease serum uric acid levels and to help prevent urate stone formation.
- Assess patient's nutritional status. Anorexia and weight loss can be decreased by feeding light, frequent meals. Nausea and vomiting can be minimized by administering an antiemetic at least 1 hr prior to receiving medication.
- Anemia may occur. Monitor for increased fatigue and dyspnea.
- **Lab Test Considerations:** CBC and differential should be monitored prior to and weekly throughout course of therapy. May cause leukopenia, thrombocytopenia, and anemia. Notify physician if a sudden drop in values occurs.
- Monitor hepatic function (serum transaminase, alkaline phosphatase, and bilirubin) weekly throughout therapy.
- May cause increased uric acid. Monitor levels periodically during therapy.
- Serum glucose and uric acid levels may show false increases when sequential multiple analyzer is used to determine values.

Potential Nursing Diagnoses

- Infection, high risk for (adverse reactions).
- Nutrition, altered: less than body requirements (adverse reactions).
- Knowledge deficit related to medication regimen (patient/family teaching).

Implementation

- **General Info:** The dose of mercaptopurine should be reduced to ⅓ to ¼ the usual dose in patients receiving concurrent allopurinol to decrease

*Underlines indicate most frequent; **CAPITALS** indicate life-threatening.

the risk of toxic effects of mercaptopurine.

- **PO:** Administer medication with meals. Tablets may be crushed if patient has difficulty swallowing.

Patient/Family Teaching

- ▫ Instruct patient to take medication exactly as ordered. If a dose is missed, it should be omitted.
- ▫ Advise patient to notify physician if fever, chills, sore throat, signs of infection, bleeding gums, bruising, petechiae, or blood in urine, stool, or emesis occurs. Caution patient to avoid crowds and persons with known infections. Instruct patient to use soft toothbrush and electric razor. Patient should be cautioned not to drink alcoholic beverages or take aspirin-containing products, as these may precipitate gastric bleeding.
- ▫ Instruct patient to report yellowing of skin or eyes, dark-colored urine, or clay-colored stools to physician promptly.
- ▫ Advise patient that this medication may have teratogenic effects. Contraception should be practiced during therapy and for at least 4 mon after therapy is concluded.
- ▫ Instruct patient not to receive any vaccinations without advice of physician.
- ▫ Emphasize the need for periodic lab tests to monitor for side effects.

Evaluation

Effectiveness of therapy can be demonstrated by: ▪ Remission of acute leukemia. Patients may receive subsequent doses if hematologic profiles are within normal ranges and patients do not demonstrate serious side effects.

MESALAMINE
(me-**sal**-a-meen)
Rowasa, {Salofalk}

CLASSIFICATION(S):
Anti-inflammatory—local, GI
Pregnancy Category B

INDICATIONS

▪ Management of: ▫ Active distal ulcerative colitis ▫ Proctitis ▫ Proctosigmoiditis.

ACTION

▪ Locally acting anti-inflammatory in the colon, where activity is probably due to inhibition of prostaglandin synthesis. **Therapeutic Effect:** ▪ Reduction of symptoms of ulcerative colitis, proctitis, or proctosigmoiditis.

PHARMACOKINETICS

Absorption: 10–30% absorbed from the colon, depending on retention time of the enema formulation.
Distribution: Distribution not known.
Metabolism and Excretion: Some metabolism occurs, site unknown. Mostly eliminated unchanged in the feces.
Half-life: 0.5–1.5 hr.

CONTRAINDICATIONS AND PRECAUTIONS

Contraindicated in: ▪ Hypersensitivity to mesalamine or sulfites ▪ Cross-sensitivity with sulfonamides or salicylates may exist.
Use Cautiously in: ▪ Renal impairment ▪ Previous hypersensitivity to sulfasalazine ▪ Pregnancy, lactation, or children (safety not established).

ADVERSE REACTIONS AND SIDE EFFECTS*

CNS: malaise, headache.
Derm: hair loss, rash.
GI: flatulence, nausea.
Local: anal irritation.
Misc: acute intolerance syndrome, ANAPHYLAXIS.

INTERACTIONS

Drug-Drug: ▪ None significant.

{} = Available in Canada only.
*Underlines indicate most frequent; **CAPITALS** indicate life-threatening.

ROUTE AND DOSAGE

- **Rect (Adults):** 4-g enema (60 ml) at bedtime, retained for 8 hr for 3–6 wk.

PHARMACODYNAMICS (signs of improvement)

	ONSET	PEAK	DURATION
Rect	3–21 days	UK	UK

NURSING IMPLICATIONS

Assessment

- Assess abdominal pain and frequency, quantity, and consistency of stools at the beginning of and throughout therapy.
- Assess patient for allergy to sulfonamides and salicylates. Patients allergic to sulfasalazine may take mesalamine without difficulty, but therapy should be discontinued if rash or fever occurs.
- **Lab Test Considerations:** Monitor urinalysis, BUN, and serum creatinine closely for signs of renal toxicity.

Potential Nursing Diagnoses

- Comfort, altered: pain (indications).
- Bowel elimination, altered: diarrhea (indications).
- Knowledge deficit related to medication regimen (patient/family teaching).

Implementation

- **Rect:** Administer 60-ml retention enema once daily at bedtime. Soln should be retained for approximately 8 hr.
- Prior to administration, shake bottle well and remove the protective cap. Have patient lie on left side with the lower leg extended and the upper leg flexed for support or place the patient in knee-chest position. Gently insert the applicator tip into the rectum, pointing toward the umbilicus. Squeeze the bottle steadily to discharge most of the preparation.

Patient/Family Teaching

- Instruct patient on the correct method of administration for mesalamine. Advise patient to take medication as directed, even if feeling better.
- Advise patient to notify physician if hives, itching, wheezing, rash, or fever occur.
- Instruct patient to notify physician if symptoms worsen or do not improve. If symptoms of acute intolerance (cramping, acute abdominal pain, bloody diarrhea, fever, headache, rash) occur, discontinue therapy and notify physician immediately.
- Inform patient that proctoscopy and sigmoidoscopy may be required periodically during treatment to determine response.

Evaluation

Clinical response can be evaluated by:
- Decrease in diarrhea and abdominal pain
- Return to normal bowel pattern. Effects may be seen within 3–21 days. The usual course of therapy is 3–6 wk.

MESNA
(**mes**-na)
Mesnex

CLASSIFICATION(S):
Antidote—detoxifying agent
Pregnancy Category B

INDICATIONS

- Prevention of ifosfamide-induced hemorrhagic cystitis. **Unlabeled Use:**
- May also prevent hemorrhagic cystitis from cyclophosamide.

ACTION

- Binds to the toxic metabolites of ifosfamide in the kidneys, thereby preventing hemorrhagic cystitis.

PHARMACOKINETICS

Absorption: Administered IV only, resulting in complete bioavailability.
Distribution: Distribution not known.
Metabolism and Excretion: Rapidly converted to mesna disulfide, then converted back to mesna in the kidneys,

where it is able to bind to the toxic metabolites of ifosfamide.
Half-life: Mesna—0.36 hr; mesdan disulfide—1.17 hr.

CONTRAINDICATIONS AND PRECAUTIONS

Contraindicated in: ▪ Hypersensitivity to mesna or other thiol (rubber) compounds.
Use Cautiously in: ▪ Pregnancy or lactation (safety not established).

ADVERSE REACTIONS AND SIDE EFFECTS*

GI: nausea, vomiting, diarrhea, unpleasant taste.

INTERACTIONS

Drug–Drug: ▪ None significant.

ROUTE AND DOSAGE

- **IV (Adults):** Give a dose of mesna equal to 20% of the ifosfamide dose at the same time as ifosfamide and 4 and 8 hr later.

PHARMACODYNAMICS

	ONSET	PEAK	DURATION
IV	rapid	UK	4 hr

NURSING IMPLICATIONS

Assessment

- ▫ Monitor for development of hemorrhagic cystitis in patients receiving ifosfamide.
- **Lab Test Considerations:** Causes a false-positive result when testing urinary ketones.

Potential Nursing Diagnoses

- Knowledge deficit related to medication regimen (patient/family teaching).

Implementation

- **General Info:** Initial bolus is to be given at time of ifosfamide administration, second dose is given 4 hr later, third dose is given 8 hr after initial dose. This schedule must be repeated with each subsequent dose of ifosfamide.
- **Direct IV:** Available in 2-, 4-, and 10-ml ampules, each containing a concentration of 100 mg/ml. Dilute in 8 ml, 16 ml, or 50 ml, respectively, of D5W, 0.9% NaCl, D5/0.9% NaCl, or lactated Ringer's soln, to yield a final concentration of 20 mg/ml. Refrigerate to store. Use within 6 hr.
- **Syringe Compatibility:** ifosfamide.
- **Y-Site Compatibility:** ondansetron.
- **Additive Compatibility:** hydroxyzine or ifosfamide.
- **Additive Incompatibility:** cisplatin.

Patient/Family Teaching

- ▫ Inform patient that unpleasant taste may occur during administration.
- ▫ Advise patient to notify physician if nausea, vomiting, or diarrhea persists or is severe.

Evaluation

Effectiveness of therapy can be demonstrated by: ▪ Prevention of hemorrhagic cystitis associated with ifosfamide therapy.

MESORIDAZINE

(mez-oh-**rid**-a-zeen)
Serentil

CLASSIFICATION(S):
Antipsychotic—phenothiazine
Pregnancy Category UK

INDICATIONS

▪ Treatment of acute and chronic psychoses.

ACTION

▪ Alters the effects of dopamine in the CNS ▪ Possesses anticholinergic and alpha-adrenergic blocking activity.
Therapeutic Effect: ▪ Diminished signs and symptoms of psychoses.

PHARMACOKINETICS

Absorption: Appears to be well absorbed following oral administration.
Distribution: Widely distributed. Crosses the placenta. Crosses the

*Underlines indicate most frequent; **CAPITALS** indicate life-threatening.

blood-brain barrier and probably enters breast milk.
Metabolism and Excretion: Mostly metabolized by the liver.
Half-life: UK.

CONTRAINDICATIONS AND PRECAUTIONS

Contraindicated in: ▪ Hypersensitivity ▪ Cross-sensitivity with other phenothiazines may exist ▪ Narrow-angle glaucoma ▪ Bone marrow depression ▪ Severe liver or cardiovascular disease.
Use Cautiously in: ▪ Elderly or debilitated patients (dosage reduction may be necessary) ▪ Pregnancy or lactation (safety not established) ▪ Diabetes mellitus ▪ Respiratory disease ▪ Prostatic hypertrophy ▪ CNS tumors ▪ Epilepsy ▪ Intestinal obstruction.

ADVERSE REACTIONS AND SIDE EFFECTS*

CNS: sedation, extrapyramidal reactions, tardive dyskinesia, NEUROLEPTIC MALIGNANT SYNDROME.
EENT: dry eyes, blurred vision, lens opacities.
CV: hypotension, tachycardia.
GI: constipation, dry mouth, ileus, anorexia, hepatitis.
GU: urinary retention.
Derm: rashes, photosensitivity, pigment changes.
Endo: galactorrhea.
Hemat: AGRANULOCYTOSIS, leukopenia.
Misc: allergic reactions, hyperthermia.

INTERACTIONS

Drug-Drug: ▪ Additive hypotension with acute ingestion of **alcohol, antihypertensive agents,** or **nitrates** ▪ Additive CNS depression with other **CNS depressants,** including **alcohol, antidepressants, antihistamines, MAO inhibitors, narcotic analgesics, sedative/hypnotics,** or **general anesthetics** ▪ Concurrent use with **lithium** may produce any of the following—acute encephalopathy, decreased mesoridazine absorption, increased excretion of lithium, increased risk of extrapyramidal reactions, or masking of the early signs of lithium toxicity ▪ **Antacids** or **adsorbent antidiarrheals (kaolin)** may decrease absorption ▪ Increased risk of agranulocytoses with **antithyroid drugs** ▪ May decrease antiparkinson activity of **levodopa** and **bromocriptine** ▪ Decreases vasopressor response to **epinephrine** and **norepinephrine** ▪ Decreases antihypertensive effect of **guanethidine** ▪ Concurrent use with **beta blockers** may result in inhibition of metabolism of one or both drugs producing an increased response ▪ Increased risk of anticholinergic effects with other **agents having anticholinergic properties,** including **antihistamines, tricyclic antidepressants, quinidine,** or **disopyramide.**

ROUTE AND DOSAGE

- **PO (Adults and Children >12 yr):** 30–150 mg/day in 2–3 divided doses.
- **IM (Adults):** 25 mg, may be repeated in 30 min–1 hr if needed and tolerated.

PHARMACODYNAMICS (sedation)

	ONSET	PEAK	DURATION
PO	UK	UK	UK

NURSING IMPLICATIONS

Assessment

- ▫ Monitor patient's mental status (orientation to reality, anxiety, and behavior) prior to and periodically throughout therapy.
- ▫ Monitor blood pressure (sitting, standing, lying), pulse, and respiratory rate prior to and frequently during the period of dosage adjustment.
- ▫ Observe patient carefully when administering oral medication to ensure medication is actually taken and not hoarded.
- ▫ Assess patient for level of sedation following administration.
- ▫ Monitor patient for onset of extrapyramidal side effects (akathisia—rest-

*Underlines indicate most frequent; **CAPITALS** indicate life-threatening.

lessness, dystonia—muscle spasms and twisting motions, or pseudoparkinsonism—mask facies, rigidity, tremors, drooling, shuffling gait, dysphagia). Risk of extrapyramidal effects is lower with mesoridazine than with most phenothiazines. Notify physician if these symptoms occur as reduction in dosage or discontinuation of medication may be necessary. Physician may also order antiparkinsonian agents (trihexyphenidyl or benztropine) to control these symptoms.

- Monitor for tardive dyskinesia (rhythmic movement of mouth, face, and extremities). Notify physician immediately if these symptoms occur, as these side effects may be irreversible.
- Monitor for development of neuroleptic malignant syndrome (fever, respiratory distress, tachycardia, convulsions, diaphoresis, hypertension or hypotension, pallor, tiredness). Notify physician immediately if these symptoms occur.
- **Lab Test Considerations:** Monitor CBC and differential prior to and periodically throughout therapy. May cause blood dyscrasias.
- Monitor liver function studies prior to and periodically during therapy.
- May cause increased serum prolactin levels.

Potential Nursing Diagnoses

- Thought processes, altered (indications).
- Injury, high risk for (side effects).
- Knowledge deficit related to medication regimen (patient/family teaching).

Implementation

- **General Info:** Available as tablet, oral soln, and parenteral injection.
- To prevent contact dermatitis, avoid getting liquid preparations on hands and wash hands thoroughly if spillage occurs.
- **PO:** Administer capsules with food or milk to decrease gastric irritation.
- Dilute oral soln with 120 ml of acidified water, distilled water, or orange or grapefruit juice. Measure dose with provided dropper. Use just after diluting.
- **IM:** Should be administered deep into well-developed muscle. Do not use if precipitate is present; soln may be slightly yellow.

Patient/Family Teaching

- Instruct patient receiving parenteral mesoridazine to remain supine for 30 min after administration. Position changes should be made slowly to prevent orthostatic hypotension.
- Instruct patient on need to take medication exactly as directed. If a dose is missed, medication should be taken as soon as remembered unless almost time for next dose. Patients on long-term high-dose therapy may need to discontinue medication gradually to avoid withdrawal symptoms (dyskinesia, tremors, dizziness, nausea, and vomiting).
- Instruct patient receiving oral soln on correct method of measuring dose with provided dropper.
- Drowsiness may occur. Caution patient to avoid driving or other activities requiring alertness until response to medication is known.
- Advise patient that good oral hygiene, frequent rinsing of mouth with water, and sugarless gum or candy may help relieve dryness of mouth. Physician or dentist should be notified if dryness persists beyond 2 wk.
- Caution patient to use sunscreen and protective clothing to prevent photosensitivity reactions.
- Caution patient to avoid concurrent use of alcohol, other CNS depressants, and over-the-counter medications without consulting physician or pharmacist.
- Instruct patient to notify physician promptly if sore throat, fever, unusual bleeding or bruising, skin rashes, weakness, tremors, visual disturbances, dark-colored urine, or clay-colored stools are noted.

- ▫ Advise patient to notify physician or dentist of medication regimen prior to treatment or surgery.
- ▫ Inform patient of possibility of extrapyramidal symptoms and tardive dyskinesia. Caution patient to report these symptoms to physician immediately.
- ▫ Caution patient to avoid exercising in hot weather and taking very hot baths or showers.
- ▫ Inform patient that increasing bulk and fluids in the diet and exercising regularly may minimize the constipating effects of this medication.
- ▫ Advise patient of need for continued medical follow-up for psychotherapy, eye examinations, and laboratory tests.

EVALUATION

Effectiveness of therapy can be demonstrated by: ▪ Decreased psychotic ideation.

METAPROTERENOL

(met-a-pro-**ter**-e-nole)

Alupent, Arm-a-Med Metaproterenol, Metaprel

CLASSIFICATION(S):
Bronchodilator—beta-adrenergic agonist
Pregnancy Category C

INDICATIONS

▪ Used as a bronchodilator in reversible airway obstruction due to asthma or COPD.

ACTION

▪ A beta-adrenergic agonist that results in the accumulation of cyclic adenosine monophosphate (cAMP) ▪ Results of increased levels of cAMP at beta-adrenergic receptors include bronchodilation, CNS and cardiac stimulation, diuresis, and gastric acid secretion. Relatively selective for $beta_2$ (pulmonary) receptors. **Therapeutic Effect:** ▪ Bronchodilation.

PHARMACOKINETICS

Absorption: Well absorbed following oral administration, but rapidly undergoes extensive metabolism.

Distribution: Distribution not known.

Metabolism and Excretion: Extensively metabolized by the liver and other tissues.

Half-life: UK.

CONTRAINDICATIONS AND PRECAUTIONS

Contraindicated in: ▪ Hypersensitivity to adrenergic amines or any ingredients in preparations (fluorocarbons in inhaler, parabens in syrup, edetate sodium and benzalkonium chloride in soln for nebulization).

Use Cautiously in: ▪ Elderly patients (more susceptible to adverse reactions; dosage reduction suggested) ▪ Pregnancy or lactation (safety not established) ▪ Cardiac disease ▪ Hypertension ▪ Hyperthyroidism ▪ Diabetes mellitus ▪ Glaucoma ▪ Excessive use of inhalers (may lead to tolerance and paradoxical bronchospasm).

ADVERSE REACTIONS AND SIDE EFFECTS*

CNS: nervousness, restlessness, insomnia, tremor, headache.

CV: hypertension, arrhythmias, angina.

Endo: hyperglycemia.

GI: nausea, vomiting.

INTERACTIONS

Drug-Drug: ▪ Additive adrenergic effects with other **adrenergic amines (sympathomimetics)** ▪ Use with **MAO inhibitors** may lead to hypertensive crisis ▪ **Beta-adrenergic blockers** may block therapeutic effect.

ROUTE AND DOSAGE

- ▪ **PO (Adults and Children >9 yr and >27 kg):** 20 mg 3–4 times daily.
- ▪ **PO (Children 6–9 yr and <27 kg):** 10 mg 3–4 times daily.
- ▪ **Inhaln (Adults and Children >12 yr):** *Metered-dose inhaler* (650 mcg/

*Underlines indicate most frequent; **CAPITALS** indicate life-threatening.

spray)—2–3 inhaln q 3–4 hr (not to exceed 12 inhaln/day. *Hand-bulb nebulizer*—5–15 inhaln of undiluted 5% soln 3–4 times daily (not to exceed q 4 hr use). *IPPB*—0.2–0.3 ml of 5% soln or 2.5 ml of 0.4% or 0.6% soln for nebulization 3–4 times daily (not to exceed q 4 hr use).

PHARMACODYNAMICS (bronchodilation)

	ONSET	PEAK	DURATION
PO	15 min	1 hr	4 hr
Inhaln	1–5 min	1 hr	3–4 hr

NURSING IMPLICATIONS

Assessment
- □ Assess blood pressure, pulse, respiratory pattern, lung sounds, and character of secretions prior to and after treatment.
- □ Observe patient for appearance of drug tolerance and rebound bronchospasm.
- ■ **Lab Test Considerations:** May cause decreased serum potassium concentrations.

Potential Nursing Diagnoses
- ■ Airway clearance, ineffective (indications).
- ■ Knowledge deficit related to medication regimen (patient/family teaching).
- ■ Noncompliance (patient/family teaching).

Implementation
- ■ **General Info:** Available in tablet, syrup, as an aerosol, and in soln for nebulization or IPPB.
- ■ **PO:** Administer oral preparations with food if GI irritation becomes a problem.
- ■ **Inhaln:** For IPPB administration, dilute each dose in 2.5 ml of 0.9% NaCl.

Patient/Family Teaching
- ■ **General Info:** Instruct patient to take medication exactly as prescribed. Taking more often than prescribed may lead to paradoxical bronchospasm. If a dose is missed, take right away if remembered within 1 hr; do not take if remembered later. Do not double doses.
- □ Advise patient to maintain adequate fluid intake to help liquify tenacious secretions.
- □ Advise patient to consult physician if respiratory symptoms are not relieved or worsen after treatment. Patient should also inform physician if chest pain, headache, severe dizziness, palpitations, nervousness, or weakness occurs.
- ■ **Inhaln:** Instruct patient to shake inhaler well, clear airways before taking medication, exhale deeply before placing inhaler in mouth, close lips tightly around mouthpiece, inhale deeply while administering medication, and hold breath for several secs after receiving dose. Wait 1–2 min before administering next dose. Mouthpiece should be washed after each use.
- □ Patient taking inhalant glucocorticoids concurrently with metaproterenol should be advised to use metaproterenol first and to allow 5 min to elapse between using the 2 aerosols, unless directed by physician.

Evaluation
Effectiveness of therapy can be demonstrated by: ■ Decrease in bronchospasm □ Increased ease of breathing.

METARAMINOL
(me-ta-**ram**-i-nole)
Aramine

CLASSIFICATION(S):
Vasopressor
Pregnancy Category UK

INDICATIONS
- ■ Management of hypotension and circulatory shock unresponsive to fluid volume replacement, which may occur as a consequence of hemorrhage, drug reactions, or anesthesia.

ACTION

▪ Stimulates alpha- and $beta_1$-adrenergic receptors, producing vasoconstriction and cardiac stimulation (inotropic effect) ▪ Releases norepinephrine from storage sites; prolonged use may lead to depletion and tachyphylaxis (tolerance developing over a short period of time). ▪ Minimal effect on $beta_2$ (pulmonary receptors). **Therapeutic Effect:** ▪ Maintenance of blood pressure with perfusion of vital organs.

PHARMACOKINETICS

Absorption: Well absorbed following IM or SC administration.
Distribution: Does not cross the blood-brain barrier; remainder of distribution not known.
Metabolism and Excretion: Metabolized by tissue uptake.
Half-life: UK.

CONTRAINDICATIONS AND PRECAUTIONS

Contraindicated in: ▪ Hypersensitivity to metaraminol, parabens, or bisulfites ▪ Peripheral or mesenteric vascular thrombosis ▪ Hypoxia ▪ Hypercapnea ▪ Cyclopropane or halogenated hydrocarbon anesthesia.
Use Cautiously in: ▪ Hyperthyroidism ▪ Hypertension ▪ Heart disease ▪ Diabetes mellitus ▪ Severe liver disease ▪ Pregnancy or lactation (safety not established) ▪ Concurrent acidosis (may decrease effectiveness) ▪ Peripheral vascular disease ▪ History of malaria.

ADVERSE REACTIONS AND SIDE EFFECTS*

CNS: apprehension, anxiety, restlessness, dizziness, faintness, headache, nervousness.
Resp: respiratory distress.
CV: arrhythmias, bradycardia, peripheral and visceral vasoconstriction, precordial pain.
Derm: flushing, pallor, sweating.
GI: nausea.
GU: decreased urine output.
Local: irritation, sloughing, tissue necrosis at IV site.
Misc: tachyphylaxis.

INTERACTIONS

Drug–Drug: ▪ Pressor effect may be partially antagonized by **alpha-adrenergic blocking agents (labetalol, phenoxybenzamine, phentolamine, prazosin,** or **tolazoline)** or **agents with alpha-adrenergic blocking properties (haloperidol, loxapine, phenothiazines,** or **thioxanthenes)** ▪ Cardiac effects may be decreased by **beta-adrenergic blockers** ▪ Use with **cyclopropane** or other **halogenated hydrocarbon anesthetics, tricyclic antidepressants, maprotiline,** or **cardiac glycosides** increases the risk of arrhythmias ▪ Increased risk of hypertension and cardiac arrhythmias with **guanethidine, guanadrel, and MAO inhibitors** ▪ Pressor response may be enhanced by **atropine** ▪ **Diuretics** may decrease arterial responsiveness to metaraminol ▪ Use with **beta-adrenergic blocking agents** may result in excessive hypertension and bradycardia ▪ Additive vasoconstriction may occur with **ergotamine, ergonovine, methylergonovine, methysergide,** or **oxytocin.**

ROUTE AND DOSAGE

Acute Treatment of Hypotension

- **IV (Adults):** 15–100 mg in 500 ml of soln infused at rate necessary to maintain desired blood pressure.
- **IV (Children):** 0.4 mg/kg or 12 mg/m^2 diluted and infused at rate necessary to maintain desired blood pressure.

Acute Prophylaxis of Hypotension

- **SC, IM (Adults):** 2–10 mg; do not repeat for at least 10 min.
- **SC, IM (Children):** 0.1 mg/kg or 3 mg/m^2; do not repeat for at least 10 min.

Treatment of Severe Shock

- **IV (Adults):** 0.5–5 mg followed by IV infusion at rate necessary to maintain blood pressure.

*<u>Underlines</u> indicate most frequent; **CAPITALS** indicate life-threatening.

M

- **IV (Children):** 0.01 mg/kg or 0.3 mg/m^2.

PHARMACODYNAMICS (pressor response)

	ONSET	PEAK	DURATION
SC	5–20 min	UK	1 hr (variable)
IM	10 min	UK	1 hr (variable)
IV	1–2 min	UK	20 min

NURSING IMPLICATIONS

Assessment

- Monitor blood pressure, pulse, respiration, ECG, and hemodynamic parameters every 5–15 min during and after administration until stable for at least 1 hr. Notify physician if significant changes in vital signs or arrhythmias occur. Consult physician regarding parameters (pulse, blood pressure, or ECG changes) for adjusting dosage or discontinuing medication.
- Monitor urinary output hourly. May decrease initially and then increase as blood pressure normalizes. Notify physician if urinary output remains decreased.
- Assess IV administration site frequently. Extravasation may cause necrosis and sloughing of tissue. If extravasation occurs, discontinue metaraminol and infiltrate affected area with 10–15 ml of 0.9% NaCl containing 5–10 mg of phentolamine.
- **Toxicity and Overdose:** Symptoms of overdose include convulsions, severe hypertension, and arrhythmias.
- For excessive hypertension, rate of infusion should be decreased or temporarily discontinued until blood pressure is decreased. While additional measures are usually not necessary due to short duration of metaraminol, phentolamine may be administered IV if hypertension continues.

Potential Nursing Diagnoses

- Cardiac output, decreased (indications).
- Tissue perfusion, altered: (indications, adverse effects).

Implementation

- **General Info:** Hypovolemia should be corrected prior to administration of metaraminol.
- Discontinue metaraminol gradually to prevent recurrent hypotension. Monitor patient closely following discontinuation, in the event that further metaraminol therapy is necessary. Therapy should be reinstated if systolic blood pressure falls below 70–80 mmHg.
- **IM/SC:** The IV route is preferred over the IM and SC routes. If IM or SC route must be used, choose a site with good circulation to increase patient response and to decrease the chance of tissue necrosis, sloughing, or abscess formation. Do not massage site following injection.
- Following IM or SC injection observe patient response for at least 10 min before repeating the dose, as the maximum effect may not be immediately evident.
- **IV:** IV metaraminol should be administered via a large vein; avoid veins in the ankle or dorsum of hand.
- **Direct IV:** Direct IV injections should be followed by a continuous infusion.
- *Rate:* In severe shock may be administered slowly, each 0.5 mg over at least 1 min.
- **Continuous Infusion:** For adults, dilute 15–100 mg in 500 ml of 0.9% NaCl, D5W, D10W, D20W, D5/LR, D5/0.9% NaCl, or Ringer's soln. Dilution for pediatric patients may contain 1 mg in 25 ml. Soln is stable for 24 hr.
- *Rate:* Titrate rate of administration to maintain the desired blood pressure. Infusion must be administered via infusion pump to ensure precise amount delivered.
- **Y-Site Compatibility:** amrinone.
- **Additive Compatibility:** amino acids, amikacin, cephalothin, cephapirin, chloramphenicol, cimetidine, cyanocobalamin, dobutamine, ephedrine, epinephrine, hydrocortisone sodium phosphate, lidocaine, oxytocin, po-

tassium chloride, promazine, sodium bicarbonate, tetracycline, or verapamil.

- **Additive Incompatibility:** amphotericin B, barbiturates, dexamethasone, erythromycin lactobionate, fibrinogen, methicillin, methylprednisolone, penicillin G potassium, phenytoin, prednisolone sodium phosphate, or warfarin.

Patient/Family Teaching

- ☐ Instruct patient to inform nurse immediately of pain or discomfort at site of administration or if coldness of extremities or paresthesia occurs.

Evaluation

Effectiveness of therapy can be demonstrated by: ▪ Increase in systolic blood pressure to 80–100 mmHg for normotensive patients or 30–40 mmHg below the usual systolic blood pressure in hypertensive patients.

METHADONE
(**meth**-a-done)
Dolophine, Methadose

CLASSIFICATION(S):
Narcotic analgesic—agonist
Schedule II
Pregnancy Category UK

INDICATIONS

▪ Used alone and in combination with non-narcotic analgesics (acetaminophen or aspirin) in the management of severe pain ▪ Replaces heroin or other narcotic analgesics in detoxification/maintenance programs.

ACTION

▪ Binds to opiate receptors in the CNS ▪ Alters the perception of and response to painful stimuli, while producing generalized CNS depression. **Therapeutic Effects:** ▪ Decrease in severity of pain ▪ Heroin detoxification/maintenance.

PHARMACOKINETICS

Absorption: Well absorbed from the GI tract and IM and SC sites.
Distribution: Widely distributed. Crosses the placenta and enters breast milk.
Metabolism and Excretion: Mostly metabolized by the liver.
Half-life: 25 hr.

CONTRAINDICATIONS AND PRECAUTIONS

Contraindicated in: ▪ Hypersensitivity ▪ Pregnancy or lactation (chronic use).
Use Cautiously in: ▪ Head trauma ▪ Increased intracranial pressure ▪ Severe renal, hepatic, or pulmonary disease ▪ Hypothyroidism ▪ Adrenal insufficiency ▪ Alcoholism ▪ Elderly or debilitated patients (dosage reduction suggested) ▪ Undiagnosed abdominal pain ▪ Prostatic hypertrophy.

ADVERSE REACTIONS AND SIDE EFFECTS*

CNS: <u>sedation</u>, <u>confusion</u>, headache, euphoria, floating feeling, unusual dreams, hallucinations, dysphoria, dizziness.
EENT: miosis, diplopia, blurred vision.
Resp: respiratory depression.
CV: <u>hypotension</u>, bradycardia.
GI: nausea, vomiting, <u>constipation</u>.
GU: urinary retention.
Derm: sweating, flushing.
Misc: tolerance, physical dependence, psychological dependence.

INTERACTIONS

Drug-Drug: ▪ Use with extreme caution in patients receiving **MAO inhibitors** (may result in severe, unpredictable reactions—reduce initial dose of methadone to 25% of usual dose) ▪ Additive CNS depression with **alcohol, antihistamines,** and **sedative/hypnotics** ▪ Administration of **partial-antagonist narcotic analgesics** may precipitate narcotic withdrawal in physically dependent patients ▪ **Nalbuphine** or **pentazocine** may decrease analgesia.

*<u>Underlines</u> indicate most frequent; **CAPITALS** indicate life-threatening.

M

ROUTE AND DOSAGE

Analgesia

- **PO, IM, SC (Adults):** 2.5–10 mg q 3–4 hr, up to 5–20 mg q 6–12 hr.

Detoxification

- **PO (Adults):** 15–40 mg/day.

Maintenance

- **PO (Adults):** 20–120 mg/day.

PHARMACODYNAMICS (analgesic effect)

	ONSET	PEAK	DURATION
PO	30–60 min	90–120 min	4–12 hr
IM	10–20 min	60–120 min	4–6 hr
SC	10–20 min	60–120 min	4–6 hr

NURSING IMPLICATIONS

Assessment

- Assess type, location, and intensity of pain prior to and 60 min after administration. Cumulative effects of this medication may require periodic dosage adjustments.
- Assess blood pressure, pulse, and respiratory rate before and periodically during administration.
- Prolonged use may lead to physical and psychological dependence and tolerance. This should not prevent patient from receiving adequate analgesia. Most patients who receive methadone for medical reasons do not develop psychological dependency.
- Assess bowel function routinely. Increased intake of fluids and bulk, stool softeners, and laxatives may minimize constipating effects.
- **Lab Test Considerations:** May increase plasma amylase and lipase levels.
- **Toxicity and Overdose:** If overdosage occurs, naloxone (Narcan) is the antidote.

Potential Nursing Diagnoses

- Comfort, altered: pain (indications).
- Sensory-perceptual alteration: visual, auditory (side effects).
- Injury, high risk for (side effects).

Implementation

- **General Info:** Explain therapeutic value of medication prior to administration to enhance the analgesic effect.
- Regularly administered doses may be more effective than prn administration. Analgesic is more effective if administered before pain becomes severe.
- Coadministration with non-narcotic analgesics may have additive analgesic effects and may permit lower doses.
- Medication should be discontinued gradually after long-term use to prevent withdrawal symptoms.
- Available in tablet, soln, concentrate, diskette (dispersible tablets to be dissolved and used in detoxification and maintenance treatment only), and injectable forms.
- **PO:** Doses may be administered with food or milk to minimize GI irritation.
- For patients in chronic severe pain the oral soln containing 5 or 10 mg/5 ml is recommended on a fixed dosage schedule.
- The 10-mg/ml oral concentrate is used only as a suppressant in methadone detoxification and maintenance programs. Dilute each dose with at least 30 ml of water or other liquid prior to administration.
- **IM/SC:** IM is the preferred parenteral route for repeated doses. SC administration may cause tissue irritation.

Patient/Family Teaching

- Instruct patient on how and when to ask for prn pain medication.
- Methadone may cause drowsiness or dizziness. Advise patient to call for assistance when ambulating or smoking and to avoid driving or other activities requiring alertness until response to medication is known.
- Advise patient to make position changes slowly to minimize orthostatic hypotension.
- Caution patient to avoid concurrent use of alcohol or other CNS depressants with this medication.

□ Encourage patient to turn, cough, and breathe deeply every 2 hr to prevent atelectasis.

Evaluation

Effectiveness of therapy can be demonstrated by: ▪ Decrease in severity of pain without a significant alteration in level of consciousness or respiratory status ▪ Prevention of withdrawal symptoms in detoxification from heroin and other narcotic analgesics.

METHAZOLAMIDE
(meth-a-**zole**-a-mide)
Neptazane

CLASSIFICATION(S):
Antiglaucoma agent—carbonic anhydrase inhibitor
Pregnancy Category UK

INDICATIONS

▪ Used to lower intraocular pressure in the treatment of glaucoma.

ACTION

▪ Inhibition of the enzyme carbonic anhydrase in the eye decreases the secretion of aqueous humor. Also inhibits renal carbonic anhydrase, resulting in self-limiting urinary excretion of sodium, potassium, bicarbonate, and water. **Therapeutic Effect:** ▪ Reduction of intraocular pressure.

PHARMACOKINETICS

Absorption: Slowly but completely absorbed following oral administration.
Distribution: Widely distributed into various tissues and fluids, including aqueous humor. Crosses the placenta.
Metabolism and Excretion: Partially metabolized by the liver. 20–30% excreted by the kidneys.
Half-life: 14 hr.

CONTRAINDICATIONS AND PRECAUTIONS

Contraindicated in: ▪ Hypersensitivity to methazolamide or other sulfonamides ▪ Chronic use in noncongestive angle-closure glaucoma ▪ Severe hepatic or renal disease ▪ Adrenal insufficiency.
Use Cautiously in: ▪ Chronic respiratory disease ▪ Electrolyte abnormalities ▪ Diabetes mellitus ▪ Pregnancy and lactation (safety not established).

ADVERSE REACTIONS AND SIDE EFFECTS*

CNS: dizziness, drowsiness, headache, SEIZURES, malaise, depression.
EENT: transient myopia.
GI: diarrhea, nausea, vomiting, metallic taste, anorexia.
GU: crytalluria, renal calculi.
Derm: rash.
Endo: hyperglycemia.
F and E: hyperchloremic acidosis, hypokalemia.
Hemat: anemia, leukopenia, thrombocytopenia, APLASTIC ANEMIA.
Metab: hyperuricemia.
Neuro: paresthesias.
Misc: allergic reactions, weight loss.

INTERACTIONS

Drug-Drug: ▪ Excretion of **barbiturates, aspirin,** and **lithium** is increased and may lead to decreased effectiveness ▪ Excretion of **amphetamines, flecainide, quinidine, procainamide,** and possibly **tricyclic antidepressants** is decreased and may lead to toxicity ▪ Decreases the effectiveness of **methanamine**.

ROUTE AND DOSAGE

▪ **PO (Adults):** 25–100 mg 2–3 times daily.

PHARMACODYNAMICS (effects on intraocular pressure)

	ONSET	PEAK	DURATION
PO	2–4 hr	6–8 hr	10–18 hr

NURSING IMPLICATIONS

Assessment

□ Assess for eye discomfort or decrease in visual acuity.

*Underlines indicate most frequent; CAPITALS indicate life-threatening.

M

- ▫ Monitor intake and output and daily weight.
- ▫ Observe patient for signs of hypokalemia (muscle weakness, malaise, fatigue, ECG changes, vomiting).
- ▫ Assess patient for allergy to sulfonamides
- ▪ **Lab Test Considerations:** CBC should be evaluated initially and periodically during the course of prolonged therapy. May cause leukopenia and thrombocytopenia.
- ▫ May cause transient mild decrease in potassium, sodium, and bicarbonate. May cause mild transient increase in serum chloride.
- ▫ May cause decrease in serum citrate and uric acid excretion.
- ▫ May cause false-positive results for urine protein.

POTENTIAL NURSING DIAGNOSES

- ▪ Knowledge deficit related to medication regimen (patient/family teaching).

IMPLEMENTATION

- ▪ **General Info:** Encourage fluids to 2000–3000 ml per day, unless contraindicated, to prevent crystalluria and stone formation.
- ▪ **PO:** Give with food to minimize GI irritation.

PATIENT/FAMILY TEACHING

- ▫ Instruct patient to take medication as directed. If a dose is missed, it should be taken as soon as remembered unless almost time for next dose.
- ▫ Inform patient that metallic taste may occur. Taking medication with meals may decrease GI upset. Physician should be notified if anorexia, nausea, vomiting, or diarrhea persists.
- ▫ Advise patient to report numbness or tingling of extremities, weakness, rash, sore throat, unusual bleeding, or fever.
- ▫ Methazolamide may cause drowsiness. Caution patient to avoid driving and other activities that require alertness until response to the drug is known.
- ▫ Advise patient of need for periodic ophthalmologic examinations, as chronic open-angle glaucoma is painless and loss of vision is gradual. Intraocular pressure will be assessed by the physician.

EVALUATION

Effectiveness of therapy can be demonstrated by: ▪ Decrease in intraocular pressure.

METHICILLIN
(meth-i-**sill**-in)
Staphcillin

CLASSIFICATION(S):
Anti-infective—penicillinase-resistant penicillin
Pregnancy Category B

INDICATIONS

▪ Treatment of the following infections due to susceptible strains of penicillinase-producing staphylococci: ▫ Respiratory tract infections ▫ Skin and skin structure infections ▫ Bone and joint infections ▫ Urinary tract infections ▫ Endocarditis ▫ Septicemia ▫ Meningitis.

ACTION

▪ Binds to bacterial cell wall, leading to cell death ▪ Resists the action of penicillinase, an enzyme capable of inactivating penicillin. **Therapeutic Effect:** ▪ Bactericidal action against susceptible bacteria. **Spectrum:** ▪ Active against most gram-positive aerobic cocci, but less so than penicillin ▪ Spectrum is notable for activity against penicillinase-producing strains of: ▫ *Staphylococcus aureus* ▫ *Staphyloccoccus epidermidis* ▪ Not active against methicillin-resistant staphylococci.

PHARMACOKINETICS

Absorption: Poorly absorbed from the GI tract. Well absorbed from IM sites.
Distribution: Widely distributed. Penetration into CSF is minimal but sufficient in the presence of inflamed meninges. Crosses the placenta and enters breast milk.

Metabolism and Excretion: Excreted unchanged by the kidneys.
Half-life: 20–30 min (increased in renal impairment).

CONTRAINDICATIONS AND PRECAUTIONS

Contraindicated in: ▪ Hypersensitivity to penicillins.
Use Cautiously in: ▪ Severe renal impairment (dosage reduction recommended) ▪ Pregnancy or lactation (safety not established) ▪ Previous hypersensitivity reactions.

ADVERSE REACTIONS AND SIDE EFFECTS*

CNS: SEIZURES (high doses).
Derm: rashes, urticaria.
GI: nausea, vomiting, diarrhea, hepatitis.
GU: interstitial nephritis.
Hemat: blood dyscrasias.
Local: phlebitis at IV site, pain at IM site.
Misc: superinfection, allergic reactions, including ANAPHYLAXIS and serum sickness.

INTERACTIONS

Drug-Drug: ▪ **Probenecid** decreases renal excretion and increases blood levels ▪ May alter the effect of **oral anticoagulants.**

ROUTE AND DOSAGE

Note: 1 g contains 2.6–3.1 mEq of sodium.

- **IM (Adults):** 1 g q 4–6 hr (up to 24 g/day).
- **IM (Children):** 25 mg/kg q 6 hr (up to 300 mg/kg/day).
- **IV (Adults):** 1–2 g q 4 hr (up to 24 g/day).
- **IV (Children):** 100–300 mg/kg/day in divided doses q 4–6 hr.

PHARMACODYNAMICS (blood levels)

	ONSET	PEAK	DURATION
IM	rapid	30–60 min	4–6 hr
IV	rapid	end of infusion	4–6 hr

NURSING IMPLICATIONS

ASSESSMENT

- Assess patient for infection (vital signs; appearance of wound, sputum, urine, and stool; WBC) at beginning and throughout course of therapy.
- Obtain a history before initiating therapy to determine previous use of and reactions to penicillins or cephalosporins. Persons with a negative history of penicillin sensitivity may still have an allergic response.
- Obtain specimens for culture and sensitivity prior to initiating therapy. First dose may be given before receiving results.
- Observe patient for signs and symptoms of anaphylaxis (rash, pruritus, laryngeal edema, wheezing). Discontinue the drug and notify physician immediately if these occur. Keep epinephrine, an antihistamine, and resuscitation equipment close by in the event of an anaphylactic reaction.
- Assess vein for signs of irritation and phlebitis. Change IV site every 48 hr to prevent phlebitis.
- **Lab Test Considerations:** Renal function tests should be monitored periodically during prolonged therapy.
- May cause positive direct Coombs' test result.

POTENTIAL NURSING DIAGNOSES

- Infection, high risk for (indications, side effects).
- Knowledge deficit related to medication regimen (patient/family teaching).

IMPLEMENTATION

- **General Info:** To reconstitute for IM or IV use add 1.5 ml of sterile water or 0.9% NaCl for injection to each 1-g vial, 5.7 ml to each 5-g vial, and 8.6 ml to each 6-g vial for a concentration of 500 mg/ml. Soln is straw-colored.
- **IM:** Administer slowly by deep intragluteal injection.
- **Direct IV:** Each ml (500 mg) of reconstituted soln should be further diluted in 20–25 ml of sterile water or 0.9% NaCl for injection.

*Underlines indicate most frequent; **CAPITALS** indicate life-threatening.

- *Rate:* Administer at a rate of 10 ml over 1 min.
- **Intermittent Infusion:** Dilute in 0.9% NaCl, D5W, D10W, D5/0.9% NaCl, D5/LR, Ringer's or lactated Ringer's soln. Diluted concentrations of 2–60 mg/ml are stable for 8 hr at room temperature. Manufacturer recommends that methicillin not be admixed with other drugs.
- *Rate:* Infuse over 30 min–8 hr.
- **Syringe Compatibility:** chloramphenicol, colistimethate, erythromycin lactobionate, gentamicin, lidocaine, polymyxin B, or procaine.
- **Syringe Incompatibility:** heparin, kanamycin, oxytetracycline, or tetracycline.
- **Y-Site Compatibility:** heparin, hydrocortisone sodium succinate, potassium chloride, or verapamil.
- **Additive Compatibility:** aminophylline, ascorbic acid, calcium chloride, calcium gluconate, cephalothin, chloramphenicol, colistimethate, corticotropin, dimenhydrinate, diphenhydramine, erythromycin, gentamicin, penicillin G, polymyxin B, potassium chloride, prednisolone, procaine, or verapamil.
- **Additive Incompatibility:** amikacin, chlorpromazine, codeine, levorphanol, meperidine, metaraminol, methadone, methohexital, morphine, oxytetracycline, promethazine, tetracycline, or vancomycin.

PATIENT/FAMILY TEACHING

- Advise patient to report to physician signs of superinfection (black, furry overgrowth on the tongue, vaginal itching or discharge, loose or foul-smelling stools) and allergy promptly.
- Instruct patient to notify physician if fever and diarrhea develop, especially if stool contains blood, pus, or mucus. Advise patient not to treat diarrhea without consulting physician or pharmacist.

EVALUATION

Clinical response can be evaluated by:
- Resolution of the signs and symptoms of infection. Length of time for complete resolution depends on the organism and site of infection.

METHIMAZOLE
(meth-**im**-a-zole)
Tapazole

CLASSIFICATION(S):
Antithyroid agent
Pregnancy Category D

INDICATIONS

- Palliative treatment of hyperthyroidism - Used as an adjunct to control hyperthyroidism in preparation for thyroidectomy or radioactive iodine therapy.

ACTION

- Inhibits the synthesis of thyroid hormones. **Therapeutic Effect:** - Decreased signs and symptoms of hyperthyroidism.

PHARMACOKINETICS

Absorption: Rapidly absorbed following oral administration.
Distribution: Crosses the placenta and enters breast milk in high concentrations.
Metabolism and Excretion: Mostly metabolized by the liver, <10% eliminated unchanged by the kidneys.
Half-life: 3–5 hr.

CONTRAINDICATIONS AND PRECAUTIONS

Contraindicated in: - Hypersensitivity - Lactation.
Use Cautiously in: - Patients with decreased bone marrow reserve - Pregnancy (may be used cautiously; however, thyroid problems may result in the fetus) - Patients >40 yr (increased risk of agranulocytosis).

ADVERSE REACTIONS AND SIDE EFFECTS*

CNS: headache, drowsiness, vertigo.
GI: diarrhea, nausea, vomiting, hepatitis, parotitis, loss of taste.
Hemat: AGRANULOCYTOSIS, anemia, leukopenia, thrombocytopenia.
Derm: rash, urticaria, skin discoloration.
MS: arthralgia.
Misc: fever, lymphadenopathy.

INTERACTIONS

Drug–Drug: ▪ Additive bone marrow depression with **antineoplastic agents** or **radiation therapy** ▪ Antithyroid effect may be intensified by **potassium iodide** or **lithium** ▪ Increased risk of agranulocytosis with **phenothiazines**.

ROUTE AND DOSAGE

- **PO (Adults):** 5–20 mg q 8 hr.
- **PO (Children):** 0.2–0.4 mg/kg/day in divided doses q 8 hr.

PHARMACODYNAMICS (effect on thyroid status)

	ONSET	PEAK	DURATION
PO	1 wk	4–10 wk	wks

NURSING IMPLICATIONS

Assessment

- Monitor response for symptoms of hyperthyroidism or thyrotoxicosis (tachycardia, palpitations, nervousness, insomnia, fever, diaphoresis, heat intolerance, tremors, weight loss, diarrhea).
- Assess patient for development of hypothyroidism (intolerance to cold, constipation, dry skin, headache, listlessness, tiredness, or weakness). Dosage adjustment may be required.
- Assess patient for skin rash or swelling of cervical lymph nodes. Treatment may be discontinued if this occurs.
- **Lab Test Considerations:** Thyroid function studies should be monitored prior to therapy, monthly during initial therapy, and every 2–3 mon throughout therapy.
- WBC and differential counts should be monitored periodically throughout course of therapy. Agranulocytosis may develop rapidly; it usually occurs during the first 2 mon and is more common in patients >40 yr and those receiving >40 mg/day. This necessitates discontinuation of therapy.
- May cause increased SGOT (AST), SGPT (ALT), LDH, alkaline phosphatase, serum bilirubin, and prothrombin time.

Potential Nursing Diagnoses

- Knowledge deficit related to medication regimen (patient/family teaching).
- Noncompliance (patient/family teaching).

Implementation

- **PO:** Administer at same time in relation to meals every day. Food may either increase or decrease absorption.

Patient/Family Teaching

- Instruct patient to take medication exactly as directed, around the clock. If a dose is missed, take as soon as remembered; take both doses together if almost time for next dose; check with physician if more than 1 dose is missed. Consult physician prior to discontinuing medication.
- Instruct patient to monitor weight 2–3 times weekly. Notify physician of significant changes.
- May cause drowsiness. Caution patient to avoid driving or other activities requiring alertness until response to medication is known.
- Advise patient to consult physician regarding dietary sources of iodine (iodized salt, shellfish).
- Advise patient to report sore throat, fever, chills, headache, malaise, weakness, yellowing of eyes or skin, unusual bleeding or bruising, rash, or symptoms of hyperthyroidism or hypothyroidism to physician promptly.
- Instruct patient to consult physician

*Underlines indicate most frequent; **CAPITALS** indicate life-threatening.

M

or pharmacist before taking any over-the-counter medications.

- ▫ Advise patient to carry identification describing medication regimen at all times.
- ▫ Advise patient to notify physician or dentist of medication regimen prior to treatment or surgery.
- ▫ Emphasize the importance of routine examinations to monitor progress and to check for side effects.

EVALUATION

Effectiveness of therapy can be demonstrated by: ▪ Decrease in severity of symptoms of hyperthyroidism ▫ Lowered pulse rate ▫ Weight gain) ▪ Return of thyroid function studies to normal ▪ May be used as short-term adjunctive therapy to prepare patient for thyroidectomy or radiation therapy or may be used in treatment of hyperthyroidism. Treatment of 6 mon to several yrs may be necessary, usually averaging 1 yr.

METHOCARBAMOL

(meth-oh-**kar**-ba-mole)
Delaxin, Marbaxin, Robaxin, Robomol

CLASSIFICATION(S):
Skeletal muscle relaxant—centrally acting
Pregnancy Category UK

INDICATIONS

▪ Adjunct to rest and physical therapy in the treatment of muscle spasm associated with acute painful musculoskeletal conditions ▪ Adjunct in the management of tetanus.

ACTION

▪ Skeletal muscle relaxation, probably due to CNS depression. **Therapeutic Effect:** ▪ Skeletal muscle relaxation.

PHARMACOKINETICS

Absorption: Rapidly absorbed from the GI tract.

Distribution: Widely distributed. Crosses the placenta.

Metabolism and Excretion: Metabolized by the liver.

Half-life: 1–2 hr.

CONTRAINDICATIONS AND PRECAUTIONS

Contraindicated in: ▪ Hypersensitivity ▪ Hypersensitivity to polyethylene glycol (parenteral only) ▪ Renal impairment (parenteral form).

Use Cautiously in: ▪ Pregnancy, lactation, and children (safety not established) ▪ Seizure disorders (parenteral form).

ADVERSE REACTIONS AND SIDE EFFECTS*

CNS: SEIZURES (IV, IM only), <u>drowsiness</u>, <u>dizziness</u>, <u>lightheadedness</u>.

EENT: blurred vision, nasal congestion.

CV: IV—hypotension, bradycardia.

GI: <u>nausea</u>, <u>anorexia</u>, <u>GI upset</u>.

GU: brown, black, or green urine.

Derm: urticaria, pruritis, rashes, flushing (IV only).

Local: pain at IM site, phlebitis at IV site.

Misc: fever, allergic reactions including ANAPHYLAXIS (IM, IV use only).

INTERACTIONS

Drug-Drug: ▪ Additive CNS depression with other **CNS depressants,** including **alcohol, antihistamines, narcotic analgesics,** and **sedative/hypnotics**.

ROUTE AND DOSAGE

Muscle Spasm

- **PO (Adults):** 1.5 g qid initially (up to 8 g/day), for 2–3 days then 4–4.5 g/day in 3–6 divided doses.
- **IM, IV (Adults):** 1 g, if PO not feasible can give up to 1 g q 8 hr for up to 3 days.

Tetanus

- **PO (Adults):** up to 24 g/day in divided doses.

*<u>Underlines</u> indicate most frequent; **CAPITALS** indicate life-threatening.

- **IV (Adults):** 1–2 g, additional 1–2 g may be given (total initial dose not to exceed 3 g), repeat 1–2 g q 6 hr until nasogastric tube is inserted, then change to PO.
- **IV (Children):** 15 mg/kg, may be repeated q 6 hr.

PHARMACODYNAMICS (skeletal muscle relaxation)

	ONSET	PEAK	DURATION
PO	30 min	2 hr	UK
IM	rapid	UK	UK
IV	immediate	end of infusion	UK

NURSING IMPLICATIONS

Assessment

- □ Assess patient for pain, muscle stiffness, and range of motion prior to and periodically throughout therapy.
- □ Monitor pulse and blood pressure every 15 min during parenteral administration.
- □ Assess patient for allergic reactions (skin rash, asthma, hives, wheezing, hypotension) following parenteral administration. Keep epinephrine and oxygen on hand in the event of a reaction.
- □ Monitor IV site. Injection is hypertonic and may cause thrombophlebitis. Avoid extravasation.
- **Lab Test Considerations:** Monitor renal function periodically during prolonged parenteral therapy (>3 days), as polyethylene glycol 300 vehicle is nephrotoxic.

Potential Nursing Diagnoses

- Comfort, altered (indications).
- Mobility, impaired physical (indications).
- Injury, high risk for (side effects).

Implementation

- **General Info:** Provide safety measures as indicated. Supervise ambulation and transfer of patients.
- **PO:** May be administered with food to minimize GI irritation. Tablets may be crushed and mixed with food or liquids to facilitate swallowing. For administration via nasogastric tube crush tablet and suspend in water or saline.
- **IM:** Do not administer SC. IM injections should contain no more than 5 ml (500 mg) in the gluteal region at a time.
- **Direct IV:** May be given undiluted at a rate of 3 ml (300 mg) over 1 min.
- **Intermittent Infusion:** Dilute each dose in no more than 250 ml of 0.9% NaCl or D5W for injection. Do not refrigerate after dilution.
- □ Have patient remain recumbent during and for at least 10–15 min following infusion to avoid orthostatic hypotension.

Patient/Family Teaching

- □ Advise patient to take medication exactly as directed. Missed doses should be taken within 1 hr, if not, return to regular dosing schedule. Do not double doses.
- □ Encourage patient to comply with additional therapies prescribed for muscle spasm (rest, physical therapy, heat).
- □ Medication may cause dizziness, drowsiness, and blurred vision. Advise patient to avoid driving and other activities requiring alertness until response to drug is known.
- □ Instruct patient to make position changes slowly to minimize orthostatic hypotension.
- □ Advise patient to avoid concurrent use of alcohol and other CNS depressants while taking this medication.
- □ Inform patient that urine may turn black, brown, or green, especially if left standing.
- □ Instruct patient to notify physician if skin rash, itching, fever, or nasal congestion occurs.
- □ Emphasize the importance of routine follow-up examinations to monitor progress.

Evaluation

Effectiveness of therapy can be demonstrated by: ▪ Decreased musculoskeletal pain and muscle spasticity □ Increased range of motion.

M

METHOHEXITAL
(meth-o-**hex**-i-tal)
Brevital, {Brietal}

CLASSIFICATION(S):
Anesthetic—general, Barbiturate—ultra-short-acting
Schedule IV
Pregnancy Category C

INDICATIONS

▪ Induction of general anesthesia ▪ Sole anesthesia in short (<15 min), minimally painful procedures ▪ Supplement with other anesthetic agents ▪ To produce unconsciousness during balanced anesthesia.

ACTION

▪ Produces anesthesia by depressing the CNS, probably by potentiating gamma-aminobutyric acid (GABA), an inhibitory neurotransmitter. **Therapeutic Effects:** ▪ Unconsciousness and general anesthesia.

PHARMACOKINETICS

Absorption: Well absorbed following IM administration.
Distribution: Accumulates and may be slowly re-released from lipoid tissues. Excreted in breast milk following large doses.
Metabolism and Excretion: Mostly metabolized by the liver. Some metabolism in kidneys and brain.
Half-life: 4 hr (increased in elderly patients).

CONTRAINDICATIONS AND PRECAUTIONS

Contraindicated in: ▪ Hypersensitivity ▪ Porphyria ▪ Lactation.
Use Cautiously in: ▪ Addison's disease ▪ Severe anemia ▪ Severe cardiovascular or hepatic disease ▪ Myxedema ▪ Shock or hypotension ▪ Pulmonary disease ▪ Elderly or debilitated patients ▪ Obesity ▪ Pregnancy (safety not established).

ADVERSE REACTIONS AND SIDE EFFECTS*

CNS: **SEIZURES**, restlessness, anxiety, headache, emergence delerium.
EENT: rhinitis.
Resp: coughing, **LARYNGOSPASM**, **APNEA**, respiratory depression, dyspnea, bronchospasm.
CV: **CARDIORESPIRATORY ARREST**, hypotension.
GI: hiccoughs, salivation, nausea, vomiting, abdominal pain.
Derm: erythema, pruritus, urticaria.
MS: muscle twitching.
Local: phlebitis at IV site, pain at IM site.
Misc: shivering, allergic reactions.

INTERACTIONS

Drug-Drug: ▪ Additive CNS depression with **alcohol**, **antihistamines**, **narcotic analgesics**, and **sedative/hypnotics**.

ROUTE AND DOSAGE

Note: All doses must be individualized.

Induction

- **IV (Adults and Children):** 1–2 mg/kg.
- **IM (Children):** 5–10 mg/kg as needed.

Maintenance

- **IV (Adults):** 0.25–1 mg/kg as needed or continuous infusion of 0.2% soln, usually at rate of 3 ml/min (6 mg/min), with additional doses of 20–40 mg q 4–7 min as needed.

Basal Anesthesia in Children

- **Rect (Children):** 15–30 mg/kg as a 10% soln (decrease dosage in inactive or debilitated patients). Rectal product not commercially available, must be compounded.

PHARMACODYNAMICS (anesthesia)

	ONSET	PEAK	DURATION
IM	UK	UK	UK
IV	within 60 sec	UK	5–7 min

{} = Available in Canada only.
*Underlines indicate most frequent; **CAPITALS** indicate life-threatening.

NURSING IMPLICATIONS

Assessment

- □ Assess blood pressure, ECG, heart rate, and respiratory status continuously throughout methohexital therapy. Methohexital should be used only by individuals qualified to administer anesthesia and experienced in endotracheal intubation. Equipment for this procedure should be immediately available. Apnea may occur immediately after IV injection, especially in the presence of narcotic premedication.
- □ Monitor IV site carefully. Extravasation may cause pain, swelling, ulceration, and necrosis. Intra-arterial injection may cause arteritis, vasospasm, edema, thrombosis, and gangrene of the extremity.
- ■ **Toxicity and Overdose:** Overdose may occur from rapid injection (drop in blood pressure, possibly to shock levels) or excessive or repeated injections (respiratory distress, laryngospasm, apnea).

Potential Nursing Diagnoses

- ■ Breathing pattern, ineffective (side effects).
- ■ Injury, high risk for (side effects).

Implementation

- ■ **General Info:** Dose is individualized according to depth of anesthesia desired; concurrent use of other medications and/or nitrous oxide; patient's condition, age, weight, and sex.
- □ Middle-aged or elderly patients may require smaller doses than young patients. Tolerance may develop with repeated use, such as for burns. Individuals tolerant to alcohol or barbiturates may require higher doses.
- ■ **Rect:** May be administered via rectal suspension. To prepare a 10% rectal soln, dissolve the appropriate amount of methohexital in warm tap water. Discard soln that is cloudy or that contains a precipitate.
- ■ **IV:** Repeated doses or continuous infusion of methohexital may cause prolonged somnolence and respiratory and circulatory depression. If the patient requires a second anesthetic in the same day, reduction in the dose of methohexital may be required.
- □ Methohexital may be given in doses sufficient to produce deep surgical anesthesia, but such doses may cause dangerous respiratory and circulatory depression.
- □ Premedication with anticholinergics (atropine, glycopyrrolate) may be used to decrease mucus secretions. Narcotics may be administered preoperatively to enhance the poor analgesic effects of methohexital. Preoperative medications should be given so that peak effect is attained shortly before induction of anesthesia. Muscle relaxants, if required, should be administered separately.
- □ Dilute methohexital with sterile water for injection, D5W, or 0.9% NaCl. Soln should be freshly prepared and used within 24 hr of reconstitution. Refrigerate and keep sealed. Do not administer soln containing a precipitate.
- ■ **Direct IV:** Induction dose is administered at a rate not to exceed 1 ml (10 mg) over 5 sec. Anesthesia is maintained by intermittent injections every 4–7 min or by continuous infusion.
- ■ **Continuous Infusion:** To prepare a 1% (10 mg/ml) soln, reconstitute each 2.5-g vial with 15 ml or each 5-g vial with 30 ml of sterile water, D5W, or 0.9% NaCl. Initial soln will be yellow. Further dilute the 2.5-g vial in 250 ml or the 5-g vial in 500 ml. Soln should be used only if clear and colorless.
- □ To prepare a 0.2% soln, dilute 500 mg in 250 ml of D5W or 0.9% NaCl. Do not dilute with sterile water to avoid hypotonicity.
- □ Soln is stable for 24 hr.
- ■ **Syringe Incompatibility:** glycopyrrolate.
- ■ **Additive Incompatibility:** atropine, chlorpromazine, cimetidine, clindamycin, droperidol, fentanyl, hydralazine, kanamycin, lidocaine, mechlorethamine, metaraminol, methicillin, methyldopate, metocurine, oxytetracycline, pancuronium, penicillin G

M

potassium, pentazocine, prochlorperazine, promazine, promethazine, propiomazine, scopolamine, succinylcholine, streptomycin, tetracycline, or tubocurarine.

Patient/Family Teaching

- ▫ Methohexital may cause psychomotor impairment for 24 hr following administration. Caution patient to avoid driving or other activities requiring alertness for 24 hr.
- ▫ Advise patient to avoid use of alcohol or other CNS depressants for 24 hr following anesthesia, unless directed by physician or dentist.

Evaluation

Effectiveness of therapy can be demonstrated by: ▪ Loss of consciousness ▪ Maintenance of desired level of anesthesia without complications.

METHOTREXATE

(meth-o-**trex**-ate)
Amethopterin, Folex, Folex PFS, Mexate, Mexate-AQ,

CLASSIFICATION(S):
Antineoplastic—antimetabolite, Immunosuppressant
Pregnancy Category X

INDICATIONS

▪ Alone or in combination with other treatment modalities (other antineoplastic agents, surgery, or radiation therapy) in the treatment of: ▫ Trophoblastic neoplasms (choriocarcinoma, chorioadenoma destruens, hydatidiform mole) ▫ Leukemias ▫ Breast carcinoma ▫ Head carcinoma ▫ Neck carcinoma ▫ Lung carcinoma ▪ Treatment of severe psoriasis and rheumatoid arthritis unresponsive to conventional therapy ▪ Treatment of mycosis fungoides.

ACTION

▪ Interferes with folic acid metabolism. Result is inhibition of DNA synthesis and cell reproduction (cell cycle-S phase specific) ▪ Also has immunosuppressive activity. **Therapeutic Effects:** ▪ Death of rapidly replicating cells, particularly malignant ones, and immunosuppression.

PHARMACOKINETICS

Absorption: Small doses are well absorbed from the GI tract. Larger doses incompletely absorbed.

Distribution: Actively transported across cell membranes, widely distributed. Does not reach therapeutic concentrations in the CSF. Crosses the placenta. Enters breast milk in low concentrations.

Metabolism and Excretion: Excreted mostly unchanged by the kidneys.

Half-life: 2–4 hr (increased in renal impairment).

CONTRAINDICATIONS AND PRECAUTIONS

Contraindicated in: ▪ Hypersensitivity ▪ Pregnancy or lactation.

Use Cautiously in: ▪ Renal impairment (dosage reduction required) ▪ Childbearing potential ▪ Active infections ▪ Decreased bone marrow reserve ▪ Other chronic debilitating illnesses.

ADVERSE REACTIONS AND SIDE EFFECTS*

CNS: arachnoiditis (IT use only), headaches, blurred vision, drowsiness, malaise, dizziness.

GI: stomatitis, anorexia, nausea, vomiting, hepatotoxicity.

GU: gonadal suppression.

Derm: rashes, urticaria, photosensitivity, pruritus, alopecia.

Hemat: anemia, leukopenia, thrombocytopenia.

Metab: hyperuricemia.

Misc: nephropathy, chills, fever.

INTERACTIONS

Drug-Drug: ▪ The following drugs may increase the toxicity of methotrexate: high-dose **salicylates, nonsteroidal anti-inflammatory agents, sulfonyl-**

*Underlines indicate most frequent; **CAPITALS** indicate life-threatening.

ureas (oral hypoglycemic agents), phenytoin, phenylbutazone, tetracyclines, probenecid, and chloramphenicol ▪ Additive hepatotoxicity with other hepatotoxic drugs ▪ Additive nephrotoxicity with other nephrotoxic drugs ▪ Additive bone marrow depression with other antineoplastic agents or radiation therapy ▪ May decrease antibody response to live virus vaccines and increase the risk of adverse reactions ▪ Increased risk of neurologic reactions with acyclovir (IT methotrexate only) ▪ Asparaginase may decrease effects of methotrexate.

ROUTE AND DOSAGE

Trophoblastic Neoplasms

- **PO, IM (Adults):** 15–30 mg/day for 5 days, repeat after 1 or more wks for 3–5 courses.

Leukemia—Induction

- **PO (Adults and Children):** 3.3 mg/m^2/day, usually with prednisone.
- **IT (Adults and Children):** 12 mg/m^2 or 15 mg.

Leukemia—Maintenance

- **PO, IM (Adults and Children):** 20–30 mg/m^2 weekly.
- **IV (Adults and Children):** 2.5 mg/kg q 2 wk.

Osteosarcoma

- **IV (Adults and Children):** 12 g/m^2 as a 4-hr infusion followed by leucovorin rescue, usually as part of a combination chemotherapeutic regimen.

Psoriasis

(Precede therapy with 5–10 mg test dose.)

- **PO (Adults):** 2.5–5 mg q 12 hr for 3 doses once weekly, or q 8 hr for 4 doses; may increase by 2.5 mg/wk up to 30 mg/wk.
- **PO, IM, IV (Adults):** 10 mg once weekly; may be increased up to 25 mg/weekly.

Arthritis

(Precede therapy with 5–10 mg test dose.)

- **PO (Adults):** 7.5 mg weekly (2.5 mg q 12 hr for 3 doses; not to exceed 20 mg/wk).

Mycosis Fungoides

- **PO (Adults):** 2.5–10 mg/day for several wks–mons.
- **IM (Adults):** 50 mg once weekly or 25 mg twice weekly.

PHARMACODYNAMICS (effects on blood counts)

	ONSET	PEAK	DURATION
PO, IM, IV	4–7 days	7–14 days	21 days

NURSING IMPLICATIONS

Assessment

- **General Info:** Monitor blood pressure, pulse, and respiratory rate periodically during administration. Notify physician if significant changes occur.
  - Monitor for abdominal pain, diarrhea, or stomatitis. Inform physician if these occur, as therapy may need to be discontinued.
  - Assess for fever, sore throat, and signs of infection. If these symptoms occur, notify physician immediately.
  - Assess for bleeding (bleeding gums; bruising; petechiae; guaiac stools, urine, emesis). Avoid IM injections and rectal temperatures. Hold pressure on all venipuncture sites for at least 10 min.
  - Monitor intake and output ratios and daily weights. Notify physician if significant changes in totals occur.
  - Monitor for symptoms of gout (increased uric acid, joint pain, edema). Encourage patient to drink at least 2 liters of fluid each day. Allopurinol and alkalinization of urine may be used to decrease uric acid levels.
  - Assess patient's nutritional status. Administering an antiemetic prior to and periodically throughout therapy and adjusting diet as tolerated may help maintain fluid and electrolyte balance and nutritional status.
  - Anemia may occur. Monitor for increased fatigue, dyspnea, and orthostatic hypotension.
- **IT:** Assess for development of nuchal rigidity, headache, fever, confusion,

M

drowsiness, dizziness, weakness, or seizures.

- **Lab Test Considerations:** Monitor CBC and differential prior to and frequently throughout therapy. The nadir of leukopenia and thrombocytopenia occurs in 7–14 days. Leukocyte and thrombocyte counts usually recover 7 days after the nadirs. Notify physician of any sudden drop in values.
- □ Renal (BUN and creatinine) and hepatic function (SGPT [ALT], SGOT [AST], bilirubin, and LDH) should be monitored prior to and routinely throughout course of therapy. Urine pH should be monitored prior to high-dose methotrexate therapy and every 6 hr during leucovorin rescue. Urine pH should be kept above 7.0 to prevent renal damage.
- □ Serum methotrexate levels should be monitored every 12–24 hr during high-dose therapy until levels are $<5 \times 10^{-8}$ M. This monitoring is essential to plan correct leucovorin dose and determine duration of rescue therapy.
- □ May cause elevated serum uric acid concentrations, especially during initial treatment of leukemia and lymphoma.
- **Toxicity and Overdose:** With high-dose therapy, patient must receive folinic acid or citrovorum factor (leucovorin rescue) exactly when ordered to prevent fatal toxicity.

Potential Nursing Diagnoses

- Infection, high risk for (adverse reactions).
- Nutrition, altered: less than body requirements (adverse reactions).
- Knowledge deficit related to medication regimen (patient/family teaching).

Implementation

- **General Info:** May be given PO, IM, IV, intra-arterially, or IT. Injectable forms available as powder or preservative-free soln. Reconstitute immediately before use. Discard unused portion.
- □ Soln for injection should be prepared in a biologic cabinet. Wear gloves, gown, and mask while handling medication. Discard equipment in specially designated containers (see Appendix I).
- **PO:** Administer doses 1 hr before or 2 hr after meals.
- **Direct IV:** Reconstitute each vial with 2–10 ml of sterile preservative-free 0.9% NaCl for injection. Do not use preparations that are discolored or that contain a precipitate.
- □ *Rate:* Administer at a rate of 10 mg/min into Y-site or 3-way stopcock of a free-flowing IV.
- **Intermittent/Continuous Infusion:** May be diluted in D5W, D5/0.9% NaCl, or 0.9% NaCl and infused as intermittent or continuous infusion.
- **Syringe Compatibility:** bleomycin, cisplatin, cyclophosphamide, doxapram, doxorubicin, fluorouracil, furosemide, leucovorin, mitomycin, vinblastine, or vincristine.
- **Syringe Incompatibility:** droperidol or ranitidine.
- **Y-Site Compatibility:** bleomycin, cisplatin, cyclophosphamide, doxorubicin, fluorouracil, furosemide, heparin, leucovorin, metoclopramide, mitomycin, ondansetron, vinblastine, or vincristine.
- **Y-Site Incompatibility:** droperidol.
- **Additive Compatibility:** cephalothin, cytarabine, hydroxyzine, sodium bicarbonate, or vincristine.
- **Additive Incompatibility:** bleomycin, fluorouracil, or prednisolone.
- **IT:** Reconstitute preservative-free methotrexate with preservative-free 0.9% NaCl, Elliot's B soln, or patient's CSF to a concentration of 1 mg/ml. May be administered via lumbar puncture or Ommaya reservoir. To prevent bacterial contamination use immediately.

Patient/Family Teaching

- □ Instruct patient to take medication exactly as directed. If a dose is missed, it should be omitted. Physician should be consulted if vomiting occurs shortly after a dose is taken.

- ▫ Caution patient to avoid crowds and persons with known infections. Physician should be informed immediately if symptoms of infection occur.
- ▫ Instruct patient to report unusual bleeding. Advise patient of thrombocytopenia precautions (use soft toothbrush and electric razor; avoid falls; do not drink alcoholic beverages or take medication containing aspirin, as these may precipitate gastric bleeding).
- ▫ Instruct patient to inspect oral mucosa for erythema and ulceration. If ulceration occurs, advise patient to use sponge brush and to rinse mouth with water after eating and drinking. Physician may order viscous lidocaine swishes if mouth pain interferes with eating.
- ▫ Instruct patient to avoid the use of over-the-counter drugs without first consulting physician or pharmacist.
- ▫ Advise patient that this medication may have teratogenic effects. Contraception should be practiced during therapy and for at least 8 wk after completion of therapy.
- ▫ Discuss the possibility of hair loss with patient. Explore methods of coping.
- ▫ Instruct patient not to receive any vaccinations without advice of physician.
- ▫ Caution patient to use sunscreen and protective clothing to prevent photosensitivity reactions.
- ▫ Emphasize the need for periodic lab tests to monitor for side effects.

EVALUATION

Effectiveness of therapy can be demonstrated by: ▪ Improvement of hematopoietic values in leukemia ▫ Decrease in symptoms of meningeal involvement in leukemia ▪ Decrease in size and spread of non-Hodgkin's lymphomas and other solid cancers ▪ Resolution of skin lesions in severe psoriasis ▪ Decreased joint pain and swelling ▫ Improved mobility in patients with rheumatoid arthritis ▪ Regression of lesions in mycosis fungoides.

METHOTRIMEPRAZINE

(meth-oh-try-**mep**-ra-zeen)
{Nozinan}, Levoprome

CLASSIFICATION(S):
Non-narcotic analgesic—phenothiazine
Pregnancy Category UK

INDICATIONS

▪ Management of moderate to severe pain in patients who are not ambulatory ▪ Used as an obstetric analgesic in situations where respiratory depression should not occur ▪ Used as a preoperative sedative. **Unlabeled Uses:** ▪ Treatment of psychotic disorders.

ACTION

▪ Alters the effects of dopamine in the CNS ▪ Suppresses sensory impulses resulting in increased pain threshold ▪ Produces amnesia ▪ Has alpha-adrenergic blocking activity that results in orthostatic hypotension. **Therapeutic Effects:** ▪ Reduction in severity of pain ▪ Sedation.

PHARMACOKINETICS

Absorption: Well absorbed following IM administration.
Distribution: Enters CSF and crosses the placenta. Minimal amounts enter breast milk.
Metabolism and Excretion: Mostly metabolized by the liver. Some metabolites are active. 1% excreted unchanged by the kidneys.
Half-life: 15–30 hr.

CONTRAINDICATIONS AND PRECAUTIONS

Contraindicated in: ▪ Hypersensitivity to methotrimeprazine, benzyl alcohol, or sulfites ▪ Comatose patients ▪ Severe renal, cardiac, or hepatic disease ▪ Patients who have overdosed on CNS depressants ▪ Premature labor.

Use Cautiously in: ▪ History of seizures ▪ Children or lactation (safety not established) ▪ Prolonged use (>30 days) ▪ Elderly or debilitated patients (initial dosage reduction recommended).

ADVERSE REACTIONS AND SIDE EFFECTS*

CNS: drowsiness, excess sedation, amnesia, disorientation, euphoria, headache, weakness, slurred speech, extrapyramidal reactions, SEIZURES.
EENT: nasal congestion.
CV: orthostatic hypotension, tachycardia, bradycardia, palpitations.
GI: abdominal discomfort, dry mouth, nausea, vomiting.
GU: difficulty in urination.
Local: pain at injection site.
Misc: chills.

INTERACTIONS

Drug-Drug: ▪ Additive CNS depression with other **CNS depressants** including **alcohol, antihistamines, antidepressants, narcotic analgesics,** or **sedative/hypnotics** ▪ Additive anticholinergic effects with **antihistamines, antidepressants, phenothiazines, quinidine, disopyramide, atropine,** or **scopolamine** (reduce doses of concurrent atropine or scopolamine) ▪ Reverses vasopressor effects of **epinephrine** (avoid concurrent use—if vasopressor required use phenylephrine, methoxamine, or norepinephrine) ▪ Additive hypotension with acute ingestion of **alcohol, nitrates, MAO inhibitors,** or **antihypertensives.**

ROUTE AND DOSAGE

Analgesia

- **IM (Adults):** 10–20 mg q 4–6 hr (range 5–40 mg given q 1–24 hr).

Preoperative Sedation

- **IM (Adults):** 2–20 mg 45 min–3 hr before surgery, if also used postoperatively, initial dose should be 2.5–7.5 mg.

Obstetric Analgesia

- **IM (Adults):** 15–20 mg

PHARMACODYNAMICS (analgesia)

	ONSET	PEAK	DURATION
IM	UK	20–40 min	4 hr

NURSING IMPLICATIONS

Assessment

- □ Assess type, location, and intensity of pain prior to and 30 min following administration.
- □ Monitor blood pressure frequently following injection. Orthostatic hypotension, fainting, syncope, and weakness frequently occur from 10 min to 12 hr after administration. Patient should remain supine for 6–12 hr following injection.
- □ Observe patient carefully for extrapyramidal symptoms (pill-rolling motions, drooling, tremors, rigidity, shuffling gait).
- ▪ **Lab Test Considerations:** CBC and liver function tests should be evaluated periodically throughout long-term (>30 days) therapy.

Potential Nursing Diagnoses

- ▪ Comfort, altered: pain (indications).
- ▪ Injury, high risk for (side effects).
- ▪ Knowledge deficit related to medication regimen (patient/family teaching).

Implementation

- ▪ **General Info:** To prevent contact dermatitis avoid getting soln on hands.
- □ Phenothiazines should be discontinued 48 hr before and not resumed for 24 hr following metrizamide myelography as they lower the seizure threshold.
- ▪ **IM:** Do not inject SC or IV. Inject slowly into deep, well-developed muscle. Rotate injection sites.
- ▪ **Syringe Compatibility:** atropine or scopolamine.

Patient/Family Teaching

- □ Instruct patient on how and when to ask for prn pain medication.
- □ Advise patients to make position

*Underlines indicate most frequent; **CAPITALS** indicate life-threatening.

changes slowly and to remain recumbent for 6–12 hr after administration to minimize orthostatic hypotension.

- Medication may cause drowsiness. Caution patient to request assistance with ambulation and transfer and to avoid driving or other activities requiring alertness until response to the medication is known.
- Caution patient to avoid taking alcohol or other CNS depressants concurrently with this medication.
- Instruct patient to use frequent mouth rinses, good oral hygiene, and sugarless gum or candy to minimize dry mouth.
- Instruct patient to notify physician promptly if sore throat, fever, unusual bleeding or bruising, rash, weakness, tremors, dark-colored urine, or clay-colored stools occur.

Evaluation

Effectiveness of therapy can be demonstrated by: ▪ Decrease in severity of pain ▪ Sedation.

METHYLDOPA (oral)

(meth-ill-**doe**-pa)
Aldomet, {Apo-Methyldopa}, {Dopamet}, {Novamedopa}

METHYLDOPATE (intravenous)

(meth-ill-**doe**-pate)
Aldomet

CLASSIFICATION(S):
Antihypertensive—centrally acting alpha-adrenergic agonist
Pregnancy Category UK

INDICATIONS

▪ Used in combination with other antihypertensives in the management of moderate to severe hypertension ▪ Due to delayed onset, parenteral form should not be used in emergencies.

ACTION

▪ Stimulates central alpha-adrenergic receptors, resulting in decreased sympathetic outflow. Result is inhibition of cardioacceleration and vasoconstrictor center ▪ Overall effect is decrease in total peripheral resistance, with little change in heart rate or cardiac output.
Therapeutic Effect: ▪ Lowering of blood pressure.

PHARMACOKINETICS

Absorption: 50% absorbed from the GI tract. Parenteral form, methyldopate hydrochloride, is slowly converted to methyldopa.
Distribution: Crosses the blood-brain barrier. Crosses the placenta and small amounts enter breast milk.
Metabolism and Excretion: Partially metabolized by the liver, partially excreted unchanged by the kidneys.
Half-life: 1.7 hr.

CONTRAINDICATIONS AND PRECAUTIONS

Contraindicated in: ▪ Hypersensitivity ▪ Active liver disease.
Use Cautiously in: ▪ Previous history of liver disease ▪ Pregnancy (has been used safely) ▪ Lactation.

ADVERSE REACTIONS AND SIDE EFFECTS*

CNS: <u>sedation</u>, depression, decreased mental acuity.
EENT: nasal stuffiness.
CV: orthostatic hypotension, bradycardia, **MYOCARDITIS**, edema.
GI: diarrhea, dry mouth, **HEPATITIS**.
GU: <u>impotence</u>.
Hemat: hemolytic anemia.
Misc: fever.

INTERACTIONS

Drug-Drug: ▪ Additive hypotension with other **antihypertensive agents,** acute **ingestion of alcohol,** and **nitrates** ▪ **Amphetamines, tricyclic antidepressants, nonsteroidal anti-inflammatory agents,** and **phenothiazines** may de-

{} = Available in Canada only.
*Underlines indicate most frequent; **CAPITALS** indicate life-threatening.

crease antihypertensive effect of methyldopa ▪ May increase **lithium** toxicity ▪ Additive hypotension and CNS toxicity with **levodopa**.

ROUTE AND DOSAGE

- **PO (Adults):** 500–2000 mg/day in 2–3 divided doses (not to exceed 3000 mg/24 hr).
- **PO (Children):** 10–65 mg/kg/day in 2–4 divided doses (not to exceed 3000 mg/24 hr).
- **IV (Adults):** 250–1000 mg q 6 hr.
- **IV (Children):** 20–40 mg/kg/24 hr given in divided doses q 6 hr (not to exceed 3000 mg/24 hr).

PHARMACODYNAMICS (antihypertensive effect)

	ONSET	PEAK	DURATION
PO	12–24 hr	4–6 hr	24–48 hr
IV	4–6 hr	UK	10–16 hr

NURSING IMPLICATIONS

Assessment

- □ Monitor blood pressure and pulse frequently during initial dosage adjustment and periodically throughout course of therapy. Notify physician of significant changes.
- □ Monitor intake and output ratios and weight and assess for edema daily, especially at beginning of therapy. Notify physician if weight gain or edema occurs, as sodium and water retention may be treated with diuretics.
- □ Assess patient for depression or other alterations in mental status. Notify physician promptly if these symptoms develop.
- ▪ **Lab Test Considerations:** Renal and hepatic function and CBC should be monitored prior to and periodically throughout therapy.
- □ May cause a positive direct Coombs' test, rarely associated with hemolytic anemia.
- □ May cause increased BUN, serum potassium, sodium, prolactin, uric acid, SGOT (AST), SGPT (ALT), alkaline phosphatase, and bilirubin concentrations.
- □ May interfere with serum creatinine and SGOT (AST) measurements.
- ▪ **Toxicity and Overdose:** If overdose occurs, monitor blood pressure frequently. Treatment includes elevation of legs, replacement of volume with IV fluids, and administration of vasopressors if hypotension is severe.

Potential Nursing Diagnoses

- ▪ Injury, high risk for (side effects).
- ▪ Knowledge deficit related to medication regimen (patient/family teaching).
- ▪ Noncompliance (patient/family teaching).

Implementation

- ▪ **General Info:** Fluid retention and expanded volume may cause tolerance to develop within 2–3 mon after initiation of therapy. Diuretics may be added to regimen at this time to maintain control.
- □ Dosage increases should be made with the evening dose to minimize drowsiness.
- □ When changing from IV to oral forms, dosage should remain consistent.
- □ Available in tablet, oral suspension, and injectable forms. Also available in combination with thiazide diuretics (see Appendix A).
- ▪ **PO:** Shake suspension prior to administration.
- ▪ **Intermittent Infusion:** Dilute in 100 ml of D5W, 0.9% NaCl, D5/0.9% NaCl, 5% sodium bicarbonate, or Ringer's soln.
- □ *Rate:* Infuse slowly over 30–60 min.
- ▪ **Y-Site Compatibility:** esmolol.
- ▪ **Additive Compatibility:** aminophylline, ascorbic acid, chloramphenicol, diphenhydramine, heparin, magnesium sulfate, multivitamins, netilmicin, oxytetracycline, potassium chloride, promazine, sodium bicarbonate, succinylcholine, or verapamil.
- ▪ **Additive Incompatibility:** barbiturates or sulfonamides.

Patient/Family Teaching

- Emphasize the importance of continuing to take this medication, even if feeling better. Instruct patient to take medication at the same time each day; last dose of the day should be taken at bedtime. If a dose is missed, take as soon as remembered, but not if almost time for next dose. Do not double doses. Methyldopa controls but does not cure hypertension.
- Encourage patient to comply with additional interventions for hypertension (weight reduction, low-sodium diet, discontinuation of smoking, moderation of alcohol consumption, regular exercise, and stress management).
- Instruct patient and family on proper technique for monitoring blood pressure. Advise them to check blood pressure at least weekly and to report significant changes to physician.
- Inform patient that urine may darken or turn red-black when left standing.
- Methyldopa may cause drowsiness. Advise patient to avoid driving or other activities requiring alertness until response to medication is known. Drowsiness usually subsides after 7–10 days of continuous use.
- Caution patient to avoid sudden changes in position to decrease orthostatic hypotension.
- Advise patient that frequent mouth rinses, good oral hygiene, and sugarless gum or candy may minimize dry mouth. Notify physician or dentist if dry mouth continues for >2 wk.
- Caution patient to avoid concurrent use of alcohol or other CNS depressants.
- Advise patient to consult physician or pharmacist before taking any cough, cold, or allergy remedies. Patient should also avoid excessive amounts of coffee, tea, and cola.
- Advise patient to notify physician or dentist of medication regimen prior to treatment or surgery.
- Instruct patient to notify physician if fever, muscle aches, or flu-like syndrome occurs.

Evaluation

Effectiveness of therapy can be demonstrated by: ▪ Decrease in blood pressure without appearance of side effects.

METHYLERGONOVINE
(meth-ill-er-goe-**noe**-veen)
Methergine, Methylergometrine

CLASSIFICATION(S):
Oxytocic
Pregnancy Category C

INDICATIONS

▪ Prevention and treatment of postpartum or postabortion hemorrhage caused by uterine atony or subinvolution.

ACTION

▪ Directly stimulates uterine and vascular smooth muscle. **Therapeutic Effect:** ▪ Uterine contraction.

PHARMACOKINETICS

Absorption: Well absorbed following oral or IM administration.
Distribution: Distribution not known. Enters breast milk in small quantities.
Metabolism and Excretion: Metabolic fate unknown. Probably metabolized by the liver.
Half-life: 30–120 min.

CONTRAINDICATIONS AND PRECAUTIONS

Contraindicated in: ▪ Hypersensitivity ▪ Hypersensitivity to phenol (injection only) ▪ Should not to be used to induce labor.
Use Cautiously in: ▪ Hypertensive or eclamptic patients (more susceptible to hypertensive and arrhythmogenic side effects) ▪ Severe hepatic or renal disease ▪ Sepsis.
Extreme Caution in: ▪ Third stage of labor.

ADVERSE REACTIONS AND SIDE EFFECTS*

CNS: dizziness, headache.
EENT: tinnitus.
Resp: dyspnea.
CV: palpitations, HYPOTENSION, chest pain, hypertension, arrhythmias.
GI: nausea, vomiting.
GU: cramps.
Derm: diaphoresis.
Misc: allergic reactions.

INTERACTIONS

Drug–Drug: ▪ Excessive vasoconstriction may result when used with heavy cigarette smoking **(nicotine)** or other **vasopressors,** such as **dopamine.**

ROUTE AND DOSAGE

- **PO (Adults):** 0.2–0.4 mg q 6–12 hr for 2–7 days.
- **IM, IV (Adults):** 0.2 mg q 2–4 hr for up to 5 doses, then change to PO.

PHARMACODYNAMICS (effects on uterine contractions)

	ONSET	PEAK	DURATION
PO	5–15 min	UK	3 hr
IM	2–5 min	UK	3 hr
IV	immediate	UK	45 min–3 hr

NURSING IMPLICATIONS

Assessment

- □ Monitor blood pressure, heart rate, and uterine response frequently during medication administration. Notify physician promptly if uterine relaxation becomes prolonged or character of vaginal bleeding changes.
- □ Assess for signs of ergotism (cold, numb fingers and toes; chest pain; nausea; vomiting; headache; muscle pain; weakness).
- ▪ **Lab Test Considerations:** If no response to methylergonovine, calcium levels may need to be assessed. Effectiveness of medication is decreased with hypocalcemia.
- □ May cause decreased serum prolactin levels.

Potential Nursing Diagnoses

- ▪ Comfort, altered: pain (side effects).
- ▪ Knowledge deficit related to medication regimen (patient/family teaching).

Implementation

- ▪ **IV:** IV administration is used for emergencies only. Oral and IM routes are preferred.
- ▪ **Direct IV:** May be given undiluted or diluted in 5 ml of 0.9% NaCl and administered through Y-site or 3-way stopcock. Do not add to IV soln. Do not mix in syringe with any other drug. Refrigerate; stable for storage at room temperature for 60 days; deteriorates with age. Only use soln that is clear and colorless and that contains no precipitate.
- □ *Rate:* Administer at a rate of 0.2 mg over 1 min.
- ▪ **Y-Site Compatibility:** heparin, hydrocortisone sodium succinate, or potassium chloride.

Patient/Family Teaching

- □ Instruct patient to take medication as directed; do not skip or double up on missed doses. If a dose is missed, omit it and return to regular dosage schedule.
- □ Advise patient that medication may cause menstrual-like cramps.
- □ Caution patient to avoid smoking, as nicotine constricts blood vessels.
- □ Instruct patient to notify physician if infection develops, as this may cause increased sensitivity to the medication.

Evaluation

Effectiveness of therapy can be demonstrated by: ▪ Contractions that maintain uterine tone and prevent postpartum hemorrhage.

*Underlines indicate most frequent; **CAPITALS** indicate life-threatening.

METHYLPHENIDATE
(meth-ill-**fen**-i-date)
Ritalin, Ritalin-SR

CLASSIFICATION(S):
CNS stimulant
Schedule II
Pregnancy Category UK

INDICATIONS
▪ Adjunct in the treatment of: ▫ Attention deficit disorder (ADD) ▫ Hyperkinetic syndrome of childhood ▫ Minimal brain dysfunction ▪ Symptomatic treatment of narcolepsy.

ACTION
▪ Produces CNS and respiratory stimulation with weak sympathomimetic activity. **Therapeutic Effects:** ▪ Increased attention span in ADD ▪ Increased motor activity, mental alertness, and diminished fatigue in narcoleptic patients.

PHARMACOKINETICS
Absorption: Well absorbed following oral administration, although absorption of extended-release tablet (SR) is delayed.
Distribution: Distribution not known.
Metabolism and Excretion: Mostly metabolized (80%) by the liver.
Half-life: 1–3 hr.

CONTRAINDICATIONS AND PRECAUTIONS
Contraindicated in: ▪ Hypersensitivity ▪ Pregnancy or lactation ▪ Hyperexcitable states ▪ Hyperthyroidism ▪ Patients with psychotic personalities, suicidal or homicidal tendencies ▪ Glaucoma ▪ Motor tics.
Use Cautiously in: ▪ History of cardiovascular disease ▪ Hypertension ▪ Diabetes mellitus ▪ Elderly or debilitated patients ▪ Continual use (may result in psychological or physical dependence) ▪ Seizure disorders (may lower seizure threshold).

ADVERSE REACTIONS AND SIDE EFFECTS*
CNS: restlessness, tremor, hyperactivity, insomnia, irritability, dizziness, headache.
EENT: blurred vision.
CV: tachycardia, palpitations, hypertension, hypotension.
GI: nausea, vomiting, anorexia, dry mouth, cramps, diarrhea, constipation, metallic taste.
Derm: rashes.
Neuro: akathisia, dyskinesia.
Misc: hypersensitivity reactions, fever.

INTERACTIONS
Drug-Drug: ▪ Additive sympathomimetic effects with other **sympathomimetics,** including **vasoconstrictors** and **decongestants** ▪ Use with **MAO inhibitors** or **vasopressors** may result in hypertensive crisis ▪ May antagonize the hypotensive effect of **guanethidine** ▪ Metabolism of **oral anticoagulants, anticonvulsants,** and **tricyclic antidepressants** may be inhibited and effects increased.
Drug-Food: ▪ Excessive use of **caffeine**-containing foods or beverages (coffee, cola, tea) may cause additive CNS stimulation.

ROUTE AND DOSAGE
Attention Deficit Disorder
▪ **PO (Children >6 yr):** 5 mg before breakfast and lunch, increase by 5–10 mg at weekly intervals (not to exceed 60 mg/day).

Narcolepsy
▪ **PO (Adults):** 10 mg 2–3 times daily (50 mg/day maximum).

PHARMACODYNAMICS (CNS stimulation)

	ONSET	PEAK	DURATION
PO	UK	1–3 hr	4–6 hr
PO-ER	UK	UK	up to 8 hr

*Underlines indicate most frequent; **CAPITALS** indicate life-threatening.

NURSING IMPLICATIONS

Assessment

- **General Info:** Monitor blood pressure, pulse, and respiration before administering and periodically throughout course of therapy.
- □ Monitor growth, both height and weight, in children on long-term therapy.
- □ May produce a false sense of euphoria and well-being. Provide frequent rest periods and observe patient for rebound depression after the effects of the medication have worn off.
- □ Methylphenidate has high dependence and abuse potential. Tolerance to medication occurs rapidly; do not increase dose.
- **Attention Deficit Disorders:** Assess attention span, impulse control, and interactions with others in children. Therapy may be interrupted at intervals to determine if symptoms are sufficient to continue therapy.
- **Narcolepsy:** Observe and document frequency of episodes.
- **Lab Test Considerations:** Monitor CBC, differential, and platelet count periodically in patients receiving prolonged therapy.

Potential Nursing Diagnoses

- Thought processes, altered (side effects).
- Knowledge deficit related to medication regimen (patient/family teaching).

Implementation

- **PO:** Administer 30–45 min before meals. Extended-release tablets should be swallowed whole; do not crush, break, or chew.

Patient/Family Teaching

- **General Info:** Instruct patient to take medication exactly as directed. If a dose is missed, take the remaining doses for that day at regularly spaced intervals; do not double doses. Take the last dose before 6 PM to minimize the risk of insomnia. Instruct patient not to alter dosage without consulting physician. Abrupt cessation with high doses may cause extreme fatigue and mental depression.
- □ Advise patient to check weight 2–3 times weekly and report weight loss to physician.
- □ May cause dizziness or blurred vision. Caution patient to avoid driving or activities requiring alertness until response to medication is known.
- □ Advise patient to avoid using caffeine-containing beverages concurrently with this therapy.
- □ Advise patient to notify physician if nervousness, insomnia, palpitations, vomiting, skin rash, or fever occur.
- □ Inform patient that physician may order periodic holidays from the drug to assess progress and to decrease dependence.
- □ Emphasize the importance of routine follow-up examinations to monitor progress.
- **Attention Deficit Disorder:** Advise parents to notify school nurse of medication regimen.

Evaluation

Effectiveness of therapy can be demonstrated by: ▪ Decreased frequency of narcoleptic symptoms ▪ Improved attention span and social interactions.

METHYLPREDNISOLONE
(meth-ill-pred-**niss**-oh-lone)
Medrol

METHYLPREDNISOLONE ACETATE
dep Medalone, Depoject, Depo-Medrol, Depopred, D-Med, Duralone, Dura-meth, Medralone, Medrol Enpak, Medrone, M-Prednisol, Rep-Pred

METHYLPREDNISOLONE SODIUM SUCCINATE
A-Methapred, Solu-Medrol

CLASSIFICATION(S):
Glucocorticoid—intermediate-acting
Pregnancy Category UK

INDICATIONS

▪ Used systemically and locally in a wide variety of: ▫ Chronic inflammatory diseases ▫ Allergic diseases ▫ Hematologic diseases ▫ Neoplastic diseases ▫ Autoimmune diseases ▪ Suitable for alternate-day dosing.

ACTION

▪ Suppresses inflammation and the normal immune response ▪ Has numerous intense metabolic effects ▪ Suppresses adrenal function at chronic doses of 4 mg/day ▪ Practically devoid of mineralocorticoid (sodium-retaining) activity. **Therapeutic Effects:** ▪ Suppression of inflammation and modification of the normal immune response.

PHARMACOKINETICS

Absorption: Well absorbed following oral and IM administration. Chronic high-dose topical application may also lead to systemic absorption. IM acetate salt is long-acting.

Distribution: Widely distributed. Crosses the placenta and small amounts enter breast milk.

Metabolism and Excretion: Mostly metabolized by the liver; small amounts excreted unchanged by the kidneys.

Half-life: 80–190 min. Adrenal suppression lasts 1.25–1.5 days.

CONTRAINDICATIONS AND PRECAUTIONS

Contraindicated in: ▪ Active untreated infections, except for some forms of meningitis ▪ Lactation (avoid chronic use) ▪ Hypersensitivity to additives (parabens, benzyl alcohol).

Use Cautiously in: ▪ Chronic treatment (will lead to adrenal suppression) ▪ Should never be abruptly discontinued ▪ Stress (surgery, infection)—supplemental doses needed during chronic therapy ▪ Pregnancy or lactation (safety not established) ▪ Children (chronic use will result in decreased growth) ▪ Infections (may mask fever, inflammation).

ADVERSE REACTIONS AND SIDE EFFECTS*

CNS: headache, restlessness, psychoses, <u>depression</u>, <u>euphoria</u>, personality changes, increased intracranial pressure (children only).

EENT: cataracts, increased intraocular pressure.

CV: <u>hypertension</u>.

GI: <u>nausea</u>, vomiting, <u>anorexia</u>, peptic ulceration.

Hemat: thromboembolism, thrombophlebitis.

Derm: <u>decreased wound healing</u>, <u>petechiae</u>, <u>ecchymoses</u>, <u>fragility</u>, <u>hirsutism</u>, <u>acne</u>.

Endo: <u>adrenal suppression</u>, hyperglycemia.

F and E: hypokalemia, hypokalemic alkalosis, fluid retention (long-term high doses).

Metab: weight loss, weight gain.

MS: <u>muscle wasting</u>, muscle pain, aseptic necrosis of joints, <u>osteoporosis</u>.

Misc: <u>increased susceptibility to infection</u>, <u>cushingoid appearance (moon face, buffalo hump)</u>.

INTERACTIONS

Drug-Drug: ▪ Additive hypokalemia with **diuretics, amphotericin B, mezlocillin, piperacillin,** or **ticarcillin** ▪ Hypokalemia may increase the risk of **cardiac glycoside** toxicity ▪ May increase requirement for **insulin** or **hypoglycemic agents** ▪ May decrease antibody response to **live virus vaccines** and increase the risk of adverse reactions.

ROUTE AND DOSAGE

- **PO (Adults):** 2–60 mg/day in 1–4 divided doses.
- **PO (Children):** 0.117–1.66 mg/kg/day in 3–4 divided doses.
- **IM (Adults):** 40–120 mg/day (acetate).
- **IM (Children):** 0.139–1.66 mg/kg/day in 1–2 divided doses.
- **IM, IV (Adults):** 10–250 mg q 4 hr (succinate).
- **IA, IL (Adults):** 4–30 mg (acetate).

*<u>Underlines</u> indicate most frequent; **CAPITALS** indicate life-threatening.

- **Top (Adults):** 0.25–1% oint 1–4 times daily.

PHARMACODYNAMICS (anti-inflammatory activity)

	ONSET	PEAK	DURATION
PO	hr	1–2 hr	1.25–1.5 days
IM acetate	6–48 hr	4–8 days	1–4 wk
IM succinate	rapid	UK	UK
IV succinate	rapid	UK	UK
IA, IL acetate	very slow	7 days	1–5 wk

NURSING IMPLICATIONS

Assessment

- **General Info:** This drug is indicated for many conditions. Assess involved systems prior to and periodically throughout course of therapy.
- Assess patient for signs of adrenal insufficiency (hypotension, weight loss, weakness, nausea, vomiting, anorexia, lethargy, confusion, restlessness) prior to and periodically throughout course of therapy.
- Monitor intake and output ratios and daily weights. Observe patient for the appearance of peripheral edema, steady weight gain, rales/crackles, or dyspnea. Notify physician should these occur.
- Children should also have periodic evaluations of growth.
- **Intra-articular:** Monitor pain, edema, and range of motion of affected joints.
- **Top Intralesional:** Assess affected skin prior to and daily during therapy. Note degree of inflammation, pruritus, lesion characteristics, and size.
- **Lab Test Considerations:** Patients on prolonged courses of therapy should routinely have hematologic values, serum electrolytes, serum and urine glucose evaluated. May cause decreased WBC counts. May cause hyperglycemia, especially in persons with diabetes. May decrease serum potassium and calcium and increase serum sodium concentrations.
- Promptly report presence of guaiac-positive stools.
- Periodic adrenal function tests may be ordered to assess degree of hypothalamic-pituitary-adrenal (HPA) axis suppression in systemic and chronic topical therapy.
- May increase serum cholesterol and lipid values.
- May decrease serum protein-bound iodine and thyroxine concentrations.
- Suppresses reactions to allergy skin tests.

Potential Nursing Diagnoses

- Infection, high risk for (side effects).
- Knowledge deficit related to medication regimen (patient/family teaching).

Implementation

- **General Info:** If dose is ordered daily or every other day, administer in the morning to coincide with the body's normal secretion of cortisol.
- Available in oral, topical, and injectable forms. Injectable forms are for IM, IV, intra-articular, and intralesional administration.
- **PO:** Administer with meals to minimize gastric irritation.
- **IM:** Shake suspension well before drawing up. IM doses should not be administered when rapid effect is desirable.
- **Direct IV:** Reconstitute with provided soln (Act-O-Vials) or 2 ml of bacteriostatic water (with benzyl alcohol) for injection.
- *Rate:* May be administered direct IV push over 1 to several mins.
- **Intermittent/Continuous Infusion:** May be diluted further in D5W, 0.9% NaCl, or D5/0.9% NaCl and administered as intermittent or continuous infusion at the prescribed rate. Soln may form a haze upon dilution.

Methylprednisolone Sodium Succinate

- **Syringe Compatibility:** metoclopramide.
- **Y-Site Compatibility:** acyclovir, amrinone, or famotidine.
- **Additive Compatibility:** chloramphenicol, cimetidine, clindamycin, dopamine, heparin, norepinephrine,

penicillin G potassium, theophylline, or verapamil.

- **Additive Incompatibility:** calcium gluconate, glycopyrrolate, insulin, metaraminol, nafcillin, penicillin G sodium, or tetracycline.
- **Top:** Apply to clean, slightly moist skin. Wear gloves. Apply occlusive dressing only with physician's order.

PATIENT/FAMILY TEACHING

- Instruct patient on correct technique of administration for prescribed form. Patient should take medication exactly as directed and not skip doses or double up on missed doses. Stopping the medication suddenly may result in adrenal insufficiency (anorexia, nausea, fatigue, weakness, hypotension, dyspnea, and hypoglycemia). If these signs appear, notify physician immediately. This can be life-threatening.
- Encourage patient on long-term therapy to eat a diet high in protein, calcium, and potassium, and low in sodium and carbohydrates (see Appendix K for foods included).
- This drug causes immunosuppression and may mask symptoms of infection. Instruct patient to avoid people with known contagious illnesses and to report possible infections.
- Review side effects with patient. Instruct patient to inform physician promptly if severe abdominal pain or tarry stools occur. Patient should also report unusual swelling, weight gain, tiredness, bone pain, bruising, nonhealing sores, visual disturbances, or behavior changes.
- Instruct patient to inform physician if symptoms of underlying disease return or worsen.
- Advise patient to carry identification in the event of an emergency in which patient cannot relate medical history.
- Caution patient to avoid vaccinations without consulting physician.
- Emphasize the importance of follow-up examinations to monitor progress and side effects.

EVALUATION

Effectiveness of therapy can be demonstrated by: ▪ Suppression of the inflammatory and immune responses in autoimmune disorders and allergic reactions ▪ Resolution of the symptoms of adrenal insufficiency.

METHYSERGIDE
(meth-i-**ser**-jide)
Sansert

CLASSIFICATION(S):
Vascular headache suppressant
Pregnancy Category UK

INDICATIONS

▪ Prevention of vascular headaches, including migraine headaches and cluster headaches.

ACTION

▪ Antiserotonin activity on smooth muscle produces direct vasoconstriction. **Therapeutic Effect:** ▪ Prevention of vascular headaches.

PHARMACOKINETICS

Absorption: Rapidly absorbed following oral administration.
Distribution: Widely distributed. Probably enters breast milk.
Metabolism and Excretion: Metabolized by the liver. Some conversion to methylergonovine (an active compound).
Half-life: 10 hr.

CONTRAINDICATIONS AND PRECAUTIONS

Contraindicated in: ▪ Hypersensitivity ▪ Hypersensitivity to tartrazine (FDC yellow dye #5) ▪ Pulmonary disease ▪ Severe cardiovascular disease ▪ Valvular heart disease ▪ Sepsis ▪ Peripheral vascular disease ▪ Pregnancy, lactation, or children.
Use Cautiously in: ▪ Impaired renal or hepatic function ▪ Peptic ulcer disease

M

■ Pruritus ■ Rheumatoid arthritis and related conditions.

ADVERSE REACTIONS AND SIDE EFFECTS*

CNS: insomnia, drowsiness, mild euphoria, lethargy, depression, vertigo, dizziness, ataxia, lightheadedness, restlessness, nervousness, rapid speech, confusion, hallucinations, psychoses.
EENT: visual disturbances.
Resp: pulmonary fibrosis.
CV: myocardial fibrosis, peripheral vasoconstriction, hypotension, tachycardia, edema.
GI: GI irritation.
Derm: flushing, rashes, dermatitis, thickened skin, itching.
Neuro: peripheral neuropathy.
Misc: retroperitoneal fibrosis.

INTERACTIONS

Drug–Drug: ■ Additive vasoconstriction with **cocaine,** other **vasopressors,** and heavy **cigarette smoking**.

ROUTE AND DOSAGE

- **PO (Adults):** 4–8 mg/day in divided doses (not to be given for more than 6 mon without a 3–4 wk rest period).

PHARMACODYNAMICS (headache prophylaxis)

	ONSET	PEAK	DURATION
PO	1–2 days	UK	1–2 days

NURSING IMPLICATIONS

Assessment

- □ Assess frequency, location, duration, and characteristics (pain, nausea, vomiting, visual disturbances) of chronic headaches.
- □ Monitor blood pressure and peripheral pulses periodically during therapy. Inform physician if signs of vascular insufficiency or peripheral neuropathy occur.
- □ Assess for signs of ergotism (cold, numb fingers and toes; nausea; vomiting; headache; muscle pain; weakness).

Potential Nursing Diagnoses

- Comfort, altered: pain, acute (indications).
- Injury, high risk for (side effects).
- Knowledge deficit related to medication regimen (patient/family teaching).

Implementation

- **PO:** Administer with milk or meals to minimize GI irritation.

Patient/Family Teaching

- □ Instruct patient to take methysergide exactly as directed. If a dose is missed, omit; do not double doses.
- □ Do not discontinue without consulting with physician, as gradual withdrawal over 2–3 wk may be required to prevent rebound headaches. Methysergide should not be used continuously for more than 6 mon.
- □ Methysergide may cause dizziness, lightheadedness, or drowsiness. Caution patient to avoid driving or other activities requiring alertness until response to medication is known.
- □ Instruct patient to report signs of infection to physician promptly.
- □ Advise patient to make position changes slowly to minimize dizziness or lightheadedness.
- □ Caution patient not to smoke and to avoid exposure to cold, as these vasoconstrictors may further impair peripheral circulation.
- □ Advise patient to avoid alcohol, as it may precipitate vascular headaches.

Evaluation

Effectiveness of therapy can be demonstrated by: ■ Prevention of vascular headaches.

METIPRANOLOL

(me-tee-**pran**-o-lole)
OptiPranolol

CLASSIFICATION(S):
Ophthalmic—beta adrenergic blocker, Antiglaucoma
Pregnancy Category C

*Underlines indicate most frequent; **CAPITALS** indicate life-threatening.

INDICATIONS

■ Used to lower intraocular pressure in patients with chronic open angle glaucoma or ocular hypertension.

ACTION

■ Blockade of beta-adrenergic receptors in the eye decreases the production of aqueous humor ■ Although systemic effects are minimal, blockade of $beta_1$ (myocardial) and $beta_2$ (pulmonary) receptors may occur. **Therapeutic Effect:** ■ Decreased intraocular pressure.

PHARMACOKINETICS

Absorption: Systemic absorption following ophthalmic administration is minimal, but may occur.
Distribution: Well distributed throughout ocular tissues following ophthalmic administration.
Metabolism and Excretion: UK.
Half-life: UK.

CONTRAINDICATIONS AND PRECAUTIONS

Contraindicated in: ■ Hypersensitivity to metipranolol or benzalkonium chloride ■ Uncompensated congestive heart failure ■ Pulmonary edema ■ Cardiogenic shock ■ Bradycardia ■ Heart block.
Use Cautiously in: ■ Cardiac failure ■ Diabetes mellitus (if systemic absorption occurs may mask some symptoms of hypoglycemia) ■ Underlying pulmonary disease, including asthma ■ Myasthenia gravis or thyrotoxicosis ■ Pregnancy, lactation, or children (safety not established).

ADVERSE REACTIONS AND SIDE EFFECTS*

CV: bradycardia, pulmonary edema, hypotension.
CNS: fatigue.
EENT: ocular stinging, conjunctivitis, erythema, blepharitis, decreased visual acuity, conjunctival leukoplakia, tearing, browache, eyelid dermatitis, photophobia.
Resp: bronchospasm.
Derm: rashes.

INTERACTIONS

Drug-Drug: ■ Additive beta-adrenergic blockade may occur with concurrent **systemic beta-adrenergic blocking agents (acebutolol, atenolol, betaxolol, carteolol, labetalol, metoprolol, nadolol, pindolol, propranolol,** or **timolol)** ■ If systemic absorption occurs, concurrent use with **antihypertensives** or **nitrates** will result in additive hypotensive effects ■ Additive effects with other **intraocular hypotensive agents.**

ROUTE AND DOSAGE

■ **Ophth (Adults):** 1 drop of 0.3% soln twice daily.

PHARMACODYNAMICS (effects on intraocular pressure)

	ONSET	PEAK	DURATION
Ophth	30 min	2 hr	12–24 hr

NURSING IMPLICATIONS

Assessment

□ Intraocular pressure should be monitored periodically during therapy.
□ Monitor heart rate and blood pressure periodically throughout therapy. May reduce cardiac output if systemically absorbed.

Potential Nursing Diagnoses

■ Sensory-perceptual alteration: visual (indications, side effects).
■ Knowledge deficit related to medication regimen (patient/family teaching).

Implementation

■ **Ophth:** Administer ophthalmic soln by having patient tilt head back and look up, gently depress lower lid with index finger until conjunctival sac is exposed and instill medication. After instillation, maintain gentle pressure on the inner canthus for 1 min to avoid systemic aborption of the drug. Wait at least 5 min before administering other types of eyedrops.

*Underlines indicate most frequent; **CAPITALS** indicate life-threatening.

M

Patient/Family Teaching

- □ Advise patient to take medication exactly as directed. Do not take more than the prescribed amount. Missed doses should be taken as soon as remembered unless almost time for the next dose; administer next dose at scheduled time.
- □ Instruct patient in proper technique for instillation of ophthalmic medications. Emphasize the importance of not touching the applicator tip to any surface.
- □ Advise patient to inform physician or dentist of medication regimen prior to treatment or surgery. Gradual withdrawal of metipranolol may be necessary.
- □ Instruct patient to inform physician if eye irritation or inflammation, decreased vision, rash, or itching occur.
- □ Emphasize the importance of regular follow-up examinations to monitor progress.

Evaluation

Effectiveness of therapy can be demonstrated by: ▪ Decreased intraocular pressure.

METOCLOPRAMIDE

(met-oh-kloe-**pra**-mide)
{Emex}, Clopra, {Maxeran}, Maxolon, Octamide, Recomide, Reglan

CLASSIFICATION(S):
Antiemetic, GI stimulant
Pregnancy Category B

INDICATIONS

▪ Prevention of chemotherapy-induced emesis ▪ Treatment of postsurgical and diabetic gastric stasis ▪ Facilitation of small bowel intubation in radiographic procedures ▪ Management of esophageal reflux ▪ Treatment and prevention of postoperative nausea and vomiting when nasogastric suctioning is undesirable.

ACTION

▪ Blocks dopamine receptors in chemoreceptor trigger zone of the CNS ▪ Stimulates motility of the upper GI tract and accelerates gastric emptying. **Therapeutic Effects:** ▪ Decreased nausea and vomiting ▪ Decreased symptoms of gastric stasis.

PHARMACOKINETICS

Absorption: Well absorbed from the GI tract and from IM sites.
Distribution: Widely distributed into body tissues and fluids. Crosses blood-brain barrier and placenta. Enters breast milk in concentrations greater than plasma.
Metabolism and Excretion: Partially metabolized by the liver. 25% eliminated unchanged in the urine.
Half-life: 2.5–5 hr.

CONTRAINDICATIONS AND PRECAUTIONS

Contraindicated in: ▪ Hypersensitivity ▪ Possible GI obstruction or hemorrhage ▪ History of seizure disorders ▪ Pheochromocytoma.
Use Cautiously in: ▪ Children and the elderly (increased incidence of extrapyramidal reactions) ▪ Pregnancy and lactation (safety not established).

ADVERSE REACTIONS AND SIDE EFFECTS*

CNS: <u>restlessness</u>, <u>drowsiness</u>, <u>fatigue</u>, <u>extrapyramidal reactions</u>, depression, irritability, anxiety.
CV: arrhythmias.
GI: constipation, diarrhea, nausea, dry mouth.
Endo: gynecomastia.

INTERACTIONS

Drug-Drug: ▪ Additive CNS depression with other **CNS depressants**, including **alcohol, antidepressants, antihistamines, narcotic analgesics,** and **sedative/hypnotics** ▪ Diabetics may require adjustments in **insulin** dosing ▪ May affect the GI absorption of other

{} = Available in Canada only.
*<u>Underlines</u> indicate most frequent; **CAPITALS** indicate life-threatening.

orally administered drugs as a result of effect on GI motility ▪ May exaggerate hypotension during **general anesthesia** ▪ Increased risk of extrapyramidal reactions with agents such as **haloperidol** or **phenothiazines**.

ROUTE AND DOSAGE

Prevention of Postoperative Nausea and Vomiting

- **IM (Adults):** 10–20 mg at end of procedure and q 4–6 hr as needed.

Facilitation of Small Bowel Intubation (Stimulation of Peristalsis, Improvement of Gastric Emptying)

- **IV (Adults):** 10 mg.
- **IV (Children 6–14 yr):** 2.5–5 mg (dose should not exceed 0.5 mg/kg).
- **IV (Children <6 yr):** 0.1 mg/kg.

Diabetic Gastroparesis

- **PO, IM, IV (Adults):** 10 mg 30 min before meals and at bedtime.

Gastroesophageal Reflux

- **PO (Adults):** 10–15 mg 30 min before meals and at bedtime (up to 4 times daily, not to exceed 0.5 mg/kg/day).

Postoperative Nausea and Vomiting

- **IM (Adults):** 10–20 mg at end of procedure and q 4–6 hr as needed.

PHARMACODYNAMICS (effects on peristalsis)

	ONSET	PEAK	DURATION
PO	30–60 min	UK	1–2 hr
IM	10–15 min	UK	1–2 hr
IV	1–3 min	immediate	1–2 hr

NURSING IMPLICATIONS

Assessment

- Assess patient for nausea, vomiting, abdominal distention, and bowel sounds prior to and following administration.
- Assess patient for extrapyramidal effects (involuntary movements, facial grimacing, rigidity, shuffling walk, trembling of hands) periodically throughout course of therapy. Extrapyramidal effects are more common in children and the elderly. May be treated with IM diphenhydramine.

Potential Nursing Diagnoses

- Nutrition, altered: less than body requirements (indications).
- Injury, high risk for (side effects).
- Knowledge deficit related to medication regimen (patient/family teaching).

Implementation

- **PO:** Administer doses 30 min before meals and at bedtime.
- Also available as a syrup.
- **Direct IV:** Administer IV dose 30 min prior to administration of chemotherapeutic agent.
- *Rate:* Doses may be given slowly over 1–2 min. Rapid administration causes a transient but intense feeling of anxiety and restlessness followed by drowsiness.
- **Intermittent Infusion:** May be diluted for IV infusion in 50 ml of D5W, 0.9% NaCl, D5/0.45% NaCl, Ringer's soln, or lactated Ringer's soln. Diluted soln is stable for 48 hr if protected from light, or 24 hr under normal light.
- *Rate:* Infuse slowly over at least 15 min.
- **Syringe Compatibility:** aminophylline, ascorbic acid, atropine, benztropine, bleomycin, chlorpromazine, cisplatin, cyclophosphamide, cytarabine, dexamethasone, dimenhydrinate, diphenhydramine, doxorubicin, droperidol, fentanyl, fluorouracil, heparin, hydrocortisone, hydroxyzine, regular insulin, leucovorin, lidocaine, magnesium sulfate, meperidine, methylprednisolone sodium succinate, midazolam, mitomycin, morphine, pentazocine, perphenazine, prochlorperazine, promazine, promethazine, ranitidine, scopolamine, vinblastine, or vincristine.
- **Syringe Incompatibility:** ampicillin, calcium gluconate, cephalothin, chloramphenicol, furosemide, penicillin G potassium, or sodium bicarbonate.
- **Y-Site Compatibility:** acyclovir, bleomycin, cisplatin, cyclophosphamide,

doxorubicin, droperidol, famotidine, foscarnet, fluorouracil, heparin, leucovorin, methotrexate, mitomycin, ondansetron, vinblastine, vincristine, or zidovudine.

- **Y-Site Incompatibility:** furosemide.
- **Additive Compatibility:** clindamycin, multivitamins, potassium acetate, potassium chloride, potassium phosphate, or verapamil.
- **Additive Incompatibility:** cisplatin, erythromycin lactobionate, or tetracycline.

Patient/Family Teaching

- Instruct patient to take metoclopramide exactly as directed. If a dose is missed, take as soon as remembered if not almost time for next dose.
- Metoclopramide may cause drowsiness. Caution patient to avoid driving or other activities requiring alertness until response to medication is known.
- Advise patient to avoid concurrent use of alcohol and other CNS depressants while taking this medication.
- Advise patient to notify physician immediately if involuntary movement of eyes, face, or limbs occurs.

Evaluation

Effectiveness of therapy can be demonstrated by: ▪ Relief of nausea and vomiting ▪ Decreased symptoms of gastric stasis.

METOCURINE

(me-toe-**cure**-een)
Metubine

CLASSIFICATION(S):
Neuromuscular blocking agent—nondepolarizing
Pregnancy Category C

INDICATIONS

▪ Production of skeletal muscle paralysis after induction of anesthesia in surgical procedures ▪ Adjunct to electroconvulsive therapy.

ACTION

▪ Prevents neuromuscular transmission by blocking the effect of acetylcholine at the myoneural junction. **Therapeutic Effect:** ▪ Skeletal muscle paralysis. Has no anxiolytic or analgesic effects.

PHARMACOKINETICS

Absorption: Administered IV only, resulting on complete bioavailability.
Distribution: Extensively distributed. Crosses the placenta.
Metabolism and Excretion: 50% excreted unchanged in urine.
Half-life: 3.6 hr.

CONTRAINDICATIONS AND PRECAUTIONS

Contraindicated in: ▪ Hypersensitivity to metocurine, iodides, or phenol.
Use Cautiously in: ▪ History of pulmonary disease, renal or hepatic impairment ▪ Elderly patients (recovery time may be increased, dosage requirements may vary) ▪ Myasthenia gravis or myasthenic syndromes (prolonged respiratory paralysis).

ADVERSE REACTIONS AND SIDE EFFECTS*

EENT: excess salivation.
Resp: bronchospasm, APNEA.
CV: hypotension, arrhythmias.
GI: decreased GI tone, decreased GI motility.
MS: muscle weakness.
Misc: allergic reactions.

INTERACTIONS

Drug-Drug: ▪ Intensity and duration of paralysis may be prolonged by pretreatment with **succinylcholine, general anesthesia, aminoglycoside antibiotics, polymixin B, colistin, clindamycin, lidocaine, quinidine, procainamide, beta-adrenergic blocking agents, potassium-losing diuretics,** and **magnesium** ▪ **Ether, methoxyflurane, halothane, enflurane,** or **isoflurane** increase intensity and duration of action (dosage reduction recommended) ▪ **Doxapram** masks residual effects ▪ **Succinylcho-**

*Underlines indicate most frequent; **CAPITALS** indicate life-threatening.

line pretreatment increases muscle paralysis.

ROUTE AND DOSAGE

Surgery

- **IV (Adults):** 0.15–0.4 mg initially, may give additional doses of 0.5–1 mg.

Adjunct to Electroconvulsive Therapy

- **IV (Adults):** 2–3 mg (range 1.75–5.5 mg)

PHARMACODYNAMICS (skeletal muscle paralysis)

	ONSET	PEAK	DURATION
IV	within min	6 min	25–90 min*

*Total recovery of function may take several hrs.

NURSING IMPLICATIONS

Assessment

- Assess respiratory status continuously throughout metocurine therapy. Metocurine should be used only by individuals experienced in endotracheal intubation, and equipment for this procedure should be immediately available.
- Neuromuscular response to metocurine should be monitored with a peripheral nerve stimulator. Paralysis is initially selective and usually occurs consecutively in the following muscles: levator muscles of eyelids, muscles of mastication, limb muscles, abdominal muscles, muscles of the glottis, intercostal muscles, and the diaphragm. Recovery of muscle function usually occurs in reverse order.
- Observe the patient for residual muscle weakness and respiratory distress during the recovery period.
- **Toxicity and Overdose:** If overdose occurs use peripheral nerve stimulator to determine the degree of neuromuscular blockade. Maintain airway patency and ventilation until recovery of normal respirations occur.
- Administration of anticholinesterase agents (edrophonium, neostigmine, pyridostigmine) may be used to antagonize the action of metocurine. Atropine is usually administered prior to or concurrently with anticholinesterase agents to counteract the muscarinic effects.
- Administration of fluids and vasopressors may be necessary to treat severe hypotension or shock.

Potential Nursing Diagnoses

- Breathing pattern, ineffective (indications).
- Communication, impaired: verbal (side effects).
- Fear (side effects).

Implementation

- **General Info:** Dose is titrated to patient response.
- Metocurine has no effect on consciousness or the pain threshold. Adequate anesthesia should *always* be used when metocurine is used as an adjunct to surgical procedures.
- **Direct IV:** Administer over 30–60 sec. Relaxation from initial dose lasts 25–90 min (average 60 min), administer supplemental doses of 0.5–1 mg as needed.
- **Syringe Incompatibility:** barbiturates, meperidine, morphine, or sodium bicarbonate.

Patient/Family Teaching

- Explain all procedures to patient receiving metocurine therapy without anesthesia, as consciousness is not affected by metocurine alone.
- Reassure patient that communication abilities will return as the medication wears off.

Evaluation

Effectiveness of therapy can be demonstrated by: ▪ Adequate suppression of the twitch response when tested with peripheral nerve stimulation and subsequent muscle paralysis.

M

METOLAZONE
(me-**tole**-a-zone)
Diulo, Mykrox, Zaroxolyn

CLASSIFICATION(S):
Diuretic—thiazidelike, Antihypertensive—diuretic
Pregnancy Category B

INDICATIONS

▪ Used alone or in combination with other agents in the management of mild to moderate hypertension ▪ Used alone or in combination in the treatment of edema associated with congestive heart failure or the nephrotic syndrome ▪ May continue to be effective in renal impairment.

ACTION

▪ Increases excretion of sodium and water by inhibiting sodium reabsorption in the distal tubule ▪ Promotes excretion of chloride, potassium, magnesium, and bicarbonate ▪ May produce arteriolar dilation. **Therapeutic Effects:** ▪ Lowering of blood pressure in hypertensive patients ▪ Diuresis with subsequent mobilization of edema.

PHARMACOKINETICS

Absorption: Absorption is more rapid and more complete with prompt tablet (Mykrox). Absorption is more variable with extended tablet (Zaroxolyn, Diulo).
Distribution: Distribution not known.
Metabolism and Excretion: Excreted mainly unchanged by the kidneys.
Half-life: Extended tablet—8 hr, prompt tablet—14 hr.

CONTRAINDICATIONS AND PRECAUTIONS

Contraindicated in: ▪ Hypersensitivity ▪ Cross-sensitivity with other sulfonamides may exist ▪ Anuria ▪ Lactation.
Use Cautiously in: ▪ Severe hepatic impairment ▪ Pregnancy or children (safety not established).

ADVERSE REACTIONS AND SIDE EFFECTS*

CNS: drowsiness, lethargy.
CV: hypotension, palpitations, chest pain.
Derm: rashes, photosensitivity.
Endo: hyperglycemia.
F and E: <u>hypokalemia</u>, hypochloremic alkalosis, hyponatremia, hypercalcemia, hypophosphatemia, hypomagnesemia, dehydration, hypovolemia.
GI: anorexia, nausea, vomiting, cramping, hepatitis, bloating.
Hemat: blood dyscrasias.
Metab: <u>hyperuricemia</u>.
MS: muscle cramps.
Misc: pancreatitis, chills.

INTERACTIONS

Drug-Drug: ▪ Additive hypotension with **nitrates, acute ingestion of alcohol** or other **antihypertensives** ▪ Additive hypokalemia with **glucocorticoids, amphotericin B, azlocillin, carbenicillin, mezlocillin, piperacillin,** or **ticarcillin** ▪ By causing hypokalemia, may increase the risk of **cardiac glycoside** toxicity ▪ Decreases the excretion of **lithium,** may cause toxicity ▪ May decrease the effectiveness of **methenamine.**
Drug-Food: ▪ **Food** may increase extent of absorption.

ROUTE AND DOSAGE

Note: Zaroxolyn and Diulo are extended tablets; Mykrox is a prompt tablet.

Diuretic

- **PO (Adults):** 5–20 mg/day single dose as extended tablets.

Antihypertensive

- **PO (Adults):** 2.5–5 mg/day single dose as extended tablet or 0.5–1 mg/day single dose as prompt tablet.

PHARMACODYNAMICS (noted for diuretic effect, full antihypertensive effect may take days–wk)

	ONSET	PEAK	DURATION
PO (extended tab)	1 hr	2 hr	12–24 hr
PO (prompt tab)	UK	2 hr	12–24 hr

*<u>Underlines</u> indicate most frequent; **CAPITALS** indicate life-threatening.

NURSING IMPLICATIONS

Assessment

- □ Monitor blood pressure, intake and output, and daily weight and assess feet, legs, and sacral area for edema daily.
- □ Assess patient, especially if taking cardiac glycosides, for anorexia, nausea, vomiting, muscle cramps, paresthesia, and confusion. Patients receiving cardiac glycosides are at increased risk of digitalis toxicity due to the potassium-depleting effect of the diuretic.
- □ Assess patient for allergy to sulfonamides.
- ■ **Lab Test Considerations:** Monitor electrolytes (especially potassium), blood glucose, BUN, and serum uric acid levels prior to and periodically throughout course of therapy.
- □ May cause increase in serum and urine glucose in diabetic patients. May cause an increase in serum bilirubin, calcium, and uric acid and a decrease in serum magnesium, potassium, and sodium levels.

Potential Nursing Diagnoses

- ■ Fluid volume excess (indications).
- ■ Fluid volume deficit (side effects).
- ■ Knowledge deficit related to medication regimen (patient/family teaching).

Implementation

- ■ **General Info:** Administer in the morning to prevent disruption of sleep cycle.
- □ Intermittent dose schedule may be used for continued control of edema.
- □ Extended and prompt metolazone tablets are not equal. Do not substitute.
- ■ **PO:** May give with food or milk to minimize GI irritation.

Patient/Family Teaching

- □ Instruct patient to take this medication at the same time each day. If a dose is missed, take as soon as remembered, but not just before next dose is due. Do not double doses. Advise patients using metolazone for hypertension to continue taking the medication even if feeling better. Medication controls but does not cure hypertension.
- □ Encourage patient to comply with additional interventions for hypertension (weight reduction, low sodium diet, regular exercise, discontinuation of smoking, moderation of alcohol consumption, and stress management).
- □ Instruct patient to monitor weight biweekly and to notify physician of significant changes. Instruct patients with hypertension in correct technique for monitoring weekly blood pressure.
- □ Caution patient to make position changes slowly to minimize orthostatic hypotension. This may be potentiated by alcohol.
- □ Advise patient to use sunscreen (avoid those containing PABA) and protective clothing when in the sun to prevent photosensitivity reactions.
- □ Instruct patient to follow a diet high in potassium (see Appendix K).
- □ Advise patient to consult physician or pharmacist before taking over-the-counter medication concurrently with this therapy.
- □ Advise patient to report muscle weakness, cramps, nausea, or dizziness to the physician.
- □ Instruct patient to notify physician or dentist of medication regimen prior to treatment or surgery.
- □ Emphasize the importance of routine follow-up examinations.

Evaluation

Effectiveness of therapy can be demonstrated by: ■ Decrease in blood pressure ■ Increase in urine output □ Decrease in edema.

METOPROLOL

(me-**toe**-proe-lole)
{Apo-Metoprolol}, {Betaloc}, Lopressor, {Novometoprol}

M

CLASSIFICATION(S):
Antihypertensive–beta-adrenergic blocker, Antianginal, Beta-adrenergic blocker—selective
Pregnancy Category B

INDICATIONS

▪ **PO:** Used alone or in combination with other agents in the treatment of hypertension and angina pectoris ▪ **PO, IV:** Prevention of myocardial infarction. **Unlabeled Uses:** ▪ Prophylaxis and treatment of arrhythmias ▪ Treatment of hypertrophic cardiomyopathy ▪ Mitral valve prolapse ▪ Tremors ▪ Symptomatic treatment of pheochromocytoma ▪ Prevention of vascular headaches ▪ Management of aggressive behavior.

ACTION

▪ Blocks stimulation of $beta_1$ (myocardial) adrenergic receptors with less effect on $beta_2$ (pulmonary, vascular, or uterine) receptor sites. **Therapeutic Effects:** ▪ Decreased heart rate ▪ Decreased blood pressure.

PHARMACOKINETICS

Absorption: Well absorbed following oral administration.
Distribution: Crosses the blood-brain barrier. Crosses the placenta, and small amounts enter breast milk.
Metabolism and Excretion: Mostly metabolized by the liver, mostly on first pass through.
Half-life: 3–7 hr.

CONTRAINDICATIONS AND PRECAUTIONS

Contraindicated in: ▪ Uncompensated congestive heart failure ▪ Pulmonary edema ▪ Cardiogenic shock ▪ Bradycardia or heart block.
Use Cautiously in: ▪ Pregnancy (may cause apnea, low Apgar scores, bradycardia, and hypoglycemia in the newborn) ▪ Hyperthyroidism (may mask symptoms) ▪ Diabetes mellitus (may mask signs of hypoglycemia) ▪ Lactation or children (safety not established).

ADVERSE REACTIONS AND SIDE EFFECTS*

CNS: fatigue, weakness, dizziness, depression, memory loss, mental changes, nightmares.
EENT: blurred vision.
Resp: bronchospasm, wheezing.
CV: BRADYCARDIA, CONGESTIVE HEART FAILURE, PULMONARY EDEMA, peripheral vasoconstriction.
GI: constipation, diarrhea, nausea.
GU: impotence, diminished libido.
Endo: hyperglycemia, hypoglycemia.

INTERACTIONS

Drug–Drug: ▪ **General anesthesia, IV phenytoin,** and **verapamil** may cause additive myocardial depression ▪ Additive bradycardia may occur with concurrent use of **cardiac glycosides** ▪ Additive hypotension may occur with other **antihypertensive agents,** acute ingestion of **alcohol,** or **nitrates** ▪ Concurrent use with **amphetamines, cocaine, ephedrine, epinephrine, norepinephrine, phenylephrine,** or **pseudoephedrine** may result in excess alpha-adrenergic stimulation, hypertension, and bradycardia ▪ May produce hypertension within 14 days of **MAO inhibitor** therapy ▪ May negate the beneficial $beta_1$ cardiac effects of **dopamine** or **dobutamine** ▪ Concurrent **thyroid** administration may decrease effectiveness ▪ Use with **insulin** may result in prolonged hypoglycemia.

ROUTE AND DOSAGE

Chronic Treatment of Hypertension, Angina; Myocardial Infarction Prophylaxis

▪ **PO (Adults):** 100–450 mg/day—single dose or bid.

Myocardial Infarction Prophylaxis—Acute Treatment

▪ **IV (Adults):** 5 mg q 2 min for 3 doses.

*Underlines indicate most frequent; **CAPITALS** indicate life-threatening.

PHARMACODYNAMICS (PO = hypotensive effects, IV = beta-adrenergic blockade)

	ONSET	PEAK	DURATION
PO*	15 min	UK hr	6–12 hr
IV	immediate	20 min	5–8 hr

*Maximal effects on blood pressure during chronic therapy may not occur for 1 wk. Hypotensive effects may persist for up to 4 wk after discontinuation.

NURSING IMPLICATIONS

Assessment

- **General Info:** Monitor intake and output ratios and daily weight. Assess patient routinely for evidence of fluid overload (peripheral edema, dyspnea, rales/crackles, fatigue, weight gain, jugular venous distention).
- **Hypertension:** Monitor blood pressure and pulse frequently during period of adjustment and periodically throughout therapy. Confer with physician prior to giving drug if pulse is <50 bpm. Vital signs and ECG should be monitored every 5–15 min during and for several hrs after parenteral administration.
- **Angina:** Assess frequency and duration of episodes of chest pain throughout therapy.
- **Lab Test Considerations:** May occasionally cause elevations in serum potassium, uric acid, lipoprotein levels, and BUN.
- □ Hepatic and renal function and CBC should be monitored periodically in patients receiving prolonged therapy.

Potential Nursing Diagnoses

- Cardiac output, decreased (indications, adverse reactions).
- Knowledge deficit related to medication regimen (patient/family teaching).
- Noncompliance (patient/family teaching).

Implementation

- **PO:** Administer medication with meals or directly after eating.
- **Direct IV:** May be administered by injecting 5 mg slowly over 2 min.

Patient/Family Teaching

- □ Instruct patient to take medication exactly as directed, even if feeling well. If a dose is missed, it may be taken as soon as remembered up to 4 hr before next dose. Abrupt withdrawal may result in life-threatening arrhythmias, hypertension, or myocardial ischemia.
- □ Teach patient and family how to check pulse and blood pressure. Instruct them to take pulse daily and blood pressure biweekly. Advise patient to withhold dose and contact physician if pulse is <50 bpm or blood pressure changes significantly.
- □ Reinforce need to continue additional therapies for hypertension (weight loss, restricted sodium intake, stress reduction, regular exercise, moderation of alcohol consumption, and cessation of smoking). Metoprolol controls but does not cure hypertension.
- □ Caution patient that this medication may cause increased sensitivity to cold.
- □ Advise patient to consult physician before taking any over-the-counter drugs, especially cold remedies, concurrently with this medication. Patients on antihypertensive therapy should also avoid excessive amounts of coffee, tea, and cola.
- □ Diabetics should monitor serum glucose closely, especially if weakness, fatigue, or irritability occurs. Medication does not block sweating as a sign of hypoglycemia.
- □ Instruct patient to inform physician or dentist of this therapy prior to treatment or surgery.
- □ Advise patient to carry identification describing medication regimen at all times.
- □ Instruct patient to notify physician if slow pulse rate, dizziness, lightheadedness, or depression occurs.

Evaluation

Effectiveness of therapy can be demonstrated by: ▪ Decrease in blood pressure ▪ Reduction in frequency of anginal attacks and improved exercise tolerance ▪ Prevention of myocardial infarction.

M

METRONIDAZOLE

(me-troe-**ni**-da-zole)

{Apo-Metronidazole}, Flagyl, Flagyl IV, Flagyl IV RTU, Metizol, Metric 21, MetroGel, Metro IV, Metryl, Metryl IV, {Neo-Metric}, {Novonidazol}, {PMS Metronidazole}, Protostat, Satric

CLASSIFICATION(S):

Anti-infective—miscellaneous

Pregnancy Category B

INDICATIONS

▪ Treatment of the following anaerobic infections: ▫ Intra-abdominal infections ▫ Gynecologic infections ▫ Skin and skin structure infections ▫ Lower respiratory tract infections ▫ Bone and joint infections ▫ CNS infections ▫ Septicemia ▫ Endocarditis ▪ Perioperative prophylactic agent in colorectal surgery ▪ Used topically in the treatment of acne rosacea. **Unlabeled Uses:** ▪ Treatment of acute intestinal amebiasis and amebic liver abscesses due to *Entamoeba histolytica* and giardiasis.

ACTION

▪ Disrupts DNA and protein synthesis in susceptible organisms. **Therapeutic Effect:** ▪ Bactericidal, trichomonacidal, or amebicidal action. **Spectrum:** ▪ Most notable for activity against anaerobic bacteria, including: ▫ *Bacteroides* ▫ *Clostridium* ▪ In addition, is active against: ▫ *Trichomonas vaginalis* ▫ *Entamoeba histolytica* ▫ *Giardia lambaia.*

PHARMACOKINETICS

Absorption: 80% absorbed following oral administration. Minimal absorption following topical application.

Distribution: Widely distributed into most tissues and fluids, including CSF. Crosses the placenta and enters breast milk in concentrations equal to plasma levels.

Metabolism and Excretion: Partially metabolized by the liver (30–60%), partially excreted unchanged in the urine, 6–15% eliminated in the feces.

Half-life: 6–8 hr.

CONTRAINDICATIONS AND PRECAUTIONS

Contraindicated in: ▪ Hypersensitivity ▪ Hypersensitivity to parabens (topical only) ▪ First trimester of pregnancy.

Use Cautiously in: ▪ History of blood dyscrasias. ▪ Children (safe use of IV form not established; safety of oral form for infections other than amebiasis in children not established) ▪ Pregnancy (although safety not established, has been used to treat trichomoniasis in second- and third-trimester pregnancy—but not as single-dose regimen) ▪ Lactation (if needed, use single dose and interrupt nursing for 24 hr thereafter) ▪ History of seizures or neurologic problems ▪ Severe hepatic impairment (dosage reduction suggested).

ADVERSE REACTIONS AND SIDE EFFECTS*

CNS: headache, vertigo, SEIZURES, dizziness.

EENT: tearing (top only).

GI: nausea, vomiting, abdominal pain, anorexia, dry mouth, diarrhea, unpleasant taste, furry tongue, glossitis.

Derm: transient redness, mild dryness, burning, skin irritation (top only), urticaria, rashes.

Hemat: leukopenia.

Local: phlebitis at IV site.

Neuro: peripheral neuropathy.

Misc: superinfection.

INTERACTIONS

Drug-Drug: ▪ **Cimetidine** may decrease the metabolism of metronidazole ▪ **Phenobarbital** increases metabolism and may decrease effectiveness ▪ Metronidazole increases the effects of **oral anticoagulants** ▪ Disulfiram-like reaction may occur with **alcohol** ingestion ▪ May cause acute psychosis and confusion

{} = Available in Canada only.

*Underlines indicate most frequent; **CAPITALS** indicate life-threatening.

with **disulfiram** ▪ Increased risk of leukopenia with **fluorouracil** or **azathioprine**.

ROUTE AND DOSAGE

Note: Flagyl IV RTU contains 14 mEq of sodium/500 mg metronidazole.

Anaerobic Infections

- **PO (Adults):** 7.5 mg/kg q 6 hr (not to exceed 4 g/day).
- **IV (Adults):** Initial dose 15 mg/kg, then 7.5 mg/kg q 6 hr (not to exceed 4 g/day).

Trichomoniasis

- **PO (Adults):** 250 mg q 8 hr for 7 days (single 2 g dose may be used).
- **PO (Children):** 15 mg/kg/day in 3 divided doses q 8 hr for 7–10 days.

Perioperative Prophylaxis

- **IV (Adults):** Initial dose 15 mg/kg 1 hr prior to surgery, then 7.5 mg/kg 6 and 12 hr later.

Amebiasis

- **PO (Adults):** 500–750 mg q 8 hr for 5–10 days.
- **PO (Children):** 35–50 mg/kg/day in 3 divided doses q 8 hr for 5–10 days.
- **IV (Adults):** 500–750 mg q 8 hr for 5–7 days.

Acne Rosacea

- **Top (Adults):** Apply thin film to affected area bid.

PHARMACODYNAMICS (PO, IV = blood levels, Top = improvement in rosacea)

	ONSET	PEAK
PO	rapid	1–3 hr
IV	rapid	end of infusion
Top	3 wk	9 wk

NURSING IMPLICATIONS

Assessment

- **General Info:** Assess patient for infection (vital signs; appearance of wound, sputum, urine, and stool; WBC) at beginning and throughout course of therapy.
- □ Obtain specimens for culture and sensitivity prior to initiating therapy. First dose may be given before receiving results.
- □ Monitor neurologic status during and after IV infusions. Inform physician if numbness, paresthesia, weakness, ataxia, or convulsions occur.
- □ Monitor intake and output and daily weight, especially for patients on sodium restriction. Each 500 mg of Flagyl IV for dilution contains 5 mEq of sodium; each 500 mg of Flagyl RTU contains 14 mEq of sodium.
- **Giardiasis:** Monitor 3 stool samples taken several days apart beginning 1–2 wk following treatment.
- **Lab Test Considerations:** May cause low serum SGOT (AST) levels.

Potential Nursing Diagnoses

- Infection, high risk for (indications).
- Bowel elimination, altered: diarrhea (indications).
- Knowledge deficit related to medication regimen (patient/family teaching).

Implementation

- **PO:** Administer with food or milk to minimize GI irritation. Tablets may be crushed for patients with difficulty swallowing.
- **Intermittent Infusion:** Flagyl IV RTU is prediluted and ready to use (5 mg/ml). Prefilled plastic minibags should not be used in series connections, as air embolism may result. Crystals may form during refrigeration but will dissolve when warmed to room temperature.
- □ Preparation of Flagyl IV requires a specific process. Do not use aluminum needles or hubs; color will turn orange/rust. Add 4.4 ml of sterile or bacteriostatic sterile water, or 0.9% or bacteriostatic 0.9% NaCl for injection (100 mg/ml). Soln should be clear, pale yellow-green. Do not use cloudy or precipitated soln. Dilute further to at least 8 mg/ml with 0.9% NaCl, D5W, or lactated Ringer's soln. Neutralize soln with 5 mEq sodium bicarbonate for each 500 mg. Mix thoroughly. Carbon dioxide gas will be generated and may require venting.

Do not refrigerate. Stable for 24 hr at room temperature.

- *Rate:* Administer IV doses as a slow infusion, each single dose over 1 hr. Do not admix with other medications. Discontinue primary IV during metronidazole infusion.
- **Y-Site Compatibility:** acyclovir, cyclophosphamide, enalaprilat, esmolol, foscarnet, hydromorphone, labetalol, magnesium sulfate, meperidine, morphine, or perphenazine.
- **Additive Compatibility:** amikacin, aminophylline, cefazolin, cefotaxime, ceftazidime, cefuroxime, chloramphenicol, ciprofloxacin, clindamycin, gentamicin, heparin, moxalactam, multivitamins, netilmicin, or tobramycin.
- **Additive Incompatibility:** amino acids, aztronam, or dopamine.
- **Top:** Cleanse affected area prior to application. Apply and rub in a thin film twice daily, morning and evening. Avoid contact with eyes.

Patient/Family Teaching

- Instruct patient to take medication exactly as prescribed with evenly spaced times between doses, even if feeling better. Do not skip doses or double up on missed doses. If a dose is missed, take as soon as remembered if not almost time for next dose.
- Advise patients treated for trichomoniasis that sexual partners may be asymptomatic sources of reinfection and should be treated concurrently. Patient should also refrain from intercourse or use a condom to prevent reinfection.
- Caution patients to avoid intake of alcoholic beverages or alcohol-containing preparations during and for at least 1 day following treatment with metronidazole. May cause a disulfiram-like reaction (flushing, nausea, vomiting, headache, abdominal cramps).
- May cause dizziness or lightheadedness. Caution patient to avoid driving or other activities requiring alertness until response to medication is known.
- Advise patient not to take over-the-counter medications concurrently without advice of the physician or pharmacist.
- Advise patient that frequent mouth rinses, good oral hygiene, and sugarless gum or candy may minimize dry mouth. Notify physician or dentist if dry mouth persists for more than 2 wk.
- Advise patient to inform physician if pregnancy is suspected prior to taking this medication.
- Inform patient that medication may cause urine to turn dark.
- Advise patient to consult physician if no improvement in a few days or if signs and symptoms of superinfection (black, furry overgrowth on tongue; vaginal itching or discharge; loose or foul-smelling stools) and allergy develop.
- **Top:** Instruct patient on correct technique for application of topical gel. Cosmetics may be used following application of gel.

Evaluation

Effectiveness of therapy can be demonstrated by: ▪ Resolution of the signs and symptoms of infection. Length of time for complete resolution depends on organism and site of infection ▫ Significant results should be seen in 3 wk of application of topical gel. Application may be continued for 9 wk.

MEXILETINE

(mex-il-e-teen)

Mexitil

CLASSIFICATION(S):

Antiarrhythmic—type IB

Pregnancy Category C

INDICATIONS

- Prophylaxis and treatment of serious ventricular arrhythmias, including VT and PVCs.

ACTION

▪ Decreases the duration of the action potential and effective refractory period in cardiac conduction tissue by altering transport of sodium across myocardial cell membranes ▪ Has little or no effect on heart rate. **Therapeutic Effect:** ▪ Control of ventricular arrhythmias.

PHARMACOKINETICS

Absorption: Well absorbed from the GI tract.

Distribution: Enters breast milk in concentrations similar to plasma.

Metabolism and Excretion: Mostly metabolized by the liver. 10% excreted unchanged by the kidneys.

Half-life: 10–12 hr.

CONTRAINDICATIONS AND PRECAUTIONS

Contraindicated in: ▪ Hypersensitivity ▪ Cardiogenic shock ▪ 2nd- or 3rd-degree heart block (if a pacemaker has not been inserted) ▪ Lactation.

Use Cautiously in: ▪ Sinus node or intraventricular conduction abnormalities ▪ Hypotension ▪ Congestive heart failure ▪ Severe hepatic impairment (dosage reduction suggested) ▪ Pregnancy or children (safety not established).

ADVERSE REACTIONS AND SIDE EFFECTS*

CNS: dizziness, lightheadedness, nervousness.

EENT: blurred vision, tinnitus.

CV: arrhythmias, palpitations, chest pain, headache, change in sleep habits, fatigue, confusion, edema.

GI: **HEPATIC NECROSIS**, nausea, vomiting, heartburn.

Derm: rashes.

Hemat: blood dyscrasias.

Neuro: tremor, coordination difficulties, paresthesia.

Resp: dyspnea.

INTERACTIONS

Drug-Drug: ▪ **Narcotics, atropine,** and **antacids** may slow absorption ▪ **Metoclopramide** may speed absorption ▪ **Phenytoin, rifampin, cigarette smoking,** or **phenobarbital** may increase metabolism and decrease effectiveness ▪ **Cimetidine** may slow metabolism and increase toxicity ▪ Additive cardiac effects may occur with other **antiarrythmics** ▪ **Drugs that drastically alter urine pH** may alter blood levels (alkalinization increases reabsorption and blood levels; acidification increases excretion and decreases blood levels).

Drug-Food: ▪ **Foods that drastically alter urine pH** (see Appendix K) may alter blood levels. Alkalinization increases reabsorption and increases blood levels. Acidification increases excretion and may decrease effectiveness (see Appendix K).

ROUTE AND DOSAGE

▪ **PO (Adults):** 400 mg loading dose initially, then 200 mg 8 hr later, then 200–400 mg q 8 hr. If controlled on less than 300 mg q 8 hr, can give same daily dose at 12 hr intervals (not to exceed 1200 mg/day).

PHARMACODYNAMICS (antiarrhythmic effects, provided a loading dose has been given)

	ONSET	PEAK	DURATION
PO	30 min–2 hr	2–3 hr	8–12 hr

NURSING IMPLICATIONS

Assessment

- Monitor pulse, blood pressure, and ECG periodically throughout course of therapy. Continuous Holter monitoring and chest x-ray examinations may be necessary to determine efficacy and aid in dosage adjustment.
- **Lab Test Considerations:** May occasionally cause a positive ANA test result.
- May cause a transient increase in SGOT (AST) concentrations.
- May cause thrombocytopenia within a few days after initiation of therapy. Blood counts usually return to normal

*Underlines indicate most frequent; CAPITALS indicate life-threatening.

within 1 mon after discontinuation of therapy.

- **Toxicity and Overdose:** Serum mexiletine concentrations may be determined during dosage adjustment. Incidence of side effects is greater with concentrations >2 mcg/ml.

POTENTIAL NURSING DIAGNOSES

- Cardiac output, decreased (indications).
- Knowledge deficit related to medication regimen (patient/family teaching).

IMPLEMENTATION

- **General Info:** When changing from other antiarrhythmic therapy, give the first dose of mexiletine 6–12 hr after the last dose of quinidine, 3–6 hr after last dose of procainamide, or 8–12 hr after last dose of tocainide. When changing from parenteral lidocaine, decrease lidocaine dose or discontinue lidocaine 1–2 hr after administration of mexiletine or administer lower initial doses of mexiletine.
  - Transfer of patients with life-threatening arrhythmias from other antiarrhythmic agents to mexiletine should be managed in the hospital.
- **PO:** Administer with food or antacids to minimize GI irritation.

PATIENT/FAMILY TEACHING

- Advise patient to take medication exactly as directed, at evenly spaced intervals, even if feeling well. Missed doses should be taken within 4 hr or omitted. Do not skip or double up on missed doses.
- Teach patients to monitor pulse. Advise patient to contact physician if pulse rate is <50 bpm or becomes irregular.
- Mexiletine may cause dizziness and lightheadedness. Caution patient to avoid driving and other activities requiring alertness until response to medication is known.
- Instruct patient to avoid changes in diet that may drastically acidify or alkalinize the urine (see Appendix K for foods included).
- Advise patient to notify physician or dentist of disease process and medication regimen prior to treatment or surgery.
- Advise patient to notify physician if general tiredness, yellowing of the skin or eyes, fever, sore throat, or persistent side effects occur.
- Patient should carry identification describing disease process and medication regimen at all times.

EVALUATION

Effectiveness of therapy can be demonstrated by: ▪ Decrease in frequency or resolution of serious ventricular arrhythmias.

MEZLOCILLIN
(mez-loe-**sill**-in)
Mezlin

CLASSIFICATION(S):
Anti-infective—extended-spectrum pencillin
Pregnancy Category B

INDICATIONS

▪ Treatment of serious infections due to susceptible organisms, including: ▫ Skin and skin structure infections ▫ Bone and joint infections ▫ Septicemia ▫ Respiratory tract infections ▫ Intra-abdominal, gynecologic, and urinary tract infections ▪ Combination with an aminoglycoside may be synergistic against *Pseudomonas* ▪ Has been combined with other antibiotics in the treatment of infections in immunosuppressed patients.

ACTION

▪ Binds to bacterial cell wall membrane, causing cell death. **Therapeutic Effect:** ▪ Bactericidal against susceptible bacteria. **Spectrum:** ▪ Spectrum similar to penicillin but greatly extended to include several important gram-negative aerobic pathogens, notably: ▫ *Pseudomonas aeruginosa* ▫ *Escherichia coli* ▫ *Proteus mirabilis* ▫ *Providencia rettgeri* ▪ Also active against some anaerobic bacteria, including *Bacteroides* ▪ Not active against penicillinase-producing staphylococci or beta-lactamase–producing Enterobacteriaceae.

PHARMACOKINETICS

Absorption: Well absorbed from IM sites.
Distribution: Widely distributed. Enters CSF well only when meninges are inflamed. Crosses the placenta and enters breast milk in low concentrations.
Metabolism and Excretion: 40–70% excreted unchanged by the kidneys. Small amounts metabolized by the liver. 15–30% excreted in the bile.
Half-life: 0.7–1.3 hr (increased in renal impairment).

CONTRAINDICATIONS AND PRECAUTIONS

Contraindicated in: ▪ Hypersensitivity to penicillins or cephalosporins.
Use Cautiously in: ▪ Renal impairment (dosage reduction suggested) ▪ Pregnancy and lactation (safety not established) ▪ Severe liver disease.

ADVERSE REACTIONS AND SIDE EFFECTS*

CNS: confusion, lethargy, SEIZURES (high doses).
CV: congestive heart failure, arrhythmias.
GI: nausea, diarrhea.
GU: hematuria (children only).
Derm: rashes, urticaria.
F and E: hypokalemia, hypernatremia.
Hemat: bleeding, blood dyscrasias, increased bleeding time.
Local: phlebitis at IV site, pain at IM site.
Metab: metabolic alkalosis.
Misc: superinfection, hypersensitivity reactions, including ANAPHYLAXIS and serum sickness.

INTERACTIONS

Drug-Drug: ▪ **Probenecid** decreases renal excretion and increases blood levels ▪ May alter excretion of **lithium** ▪ **Diuretics** may increase the risk of hypokalemia ▪ Hypokalemia increases the risk of **cardiac glycoside** toxicity.

ROUTE AND DOSAGE

Note: Contains 1.85 mEq sodium/g.

- **IV (Adults):** 6–24 g/day in divided doses q 4–6 hr.
- **IM (Adults):** 1.5–2 g q 6 hr.
- **IV (Children 1 mon–12 yr):** 50 mg/kg q 4 hr.
- **IM, IV (Children 1 mon–12 yr):** 50 mg/kg q 4 hr.
- **IM, IV (Neonates ≥8 days and >2 kg):** 75 mg/kg q 6 hr.
- **IM, IV (Neonates ≥8 days and <2 kg):** 75 mg/kg q 8 hr.
- **IM, IV (Neonates 0–7 days):** 75 mg/kg q 12 hr.

PHARMACODYNAMICS (blood levels)

	ONSET	PEAK
IM	rapid	45–90 min
IV	rapid	end of infusion

NURSING IMPLICATIONS

Assessment

- □ Assess patient for infection (vital signs; appearance of wound, sputum, urine, and stool; WBC) at beginning and throughout course of therapy.
- □ Obtain a history before initiating therapy to determine previous use of and reactions to penicillins or cephalosporins. Persons with a negative history of penicillin sensitivity may still have an allergic response.
- □ Obtain specimens for culture and sensitivity prior to initiating therapy. First dose may be given before receiving results.
- □ Observe patient for signs and symptoms of anaphylaxis (rash, pruritus, laryngeal edema, wheezing). Discontinue the drug and notify the physician immediately if these occur. Keep epinephrine, an antihistamine, and resuscitation equipment close by in the event of an anaphylactic reaction.
- ▪ **Lab Test Considerations:** Renal and

*Underlines indicate most frequent; CAPITALS indicate life-threatening.

hepatic function, CBC, and serum potassium should be evaluated prior to and routinely throughout course of therapy.
- May cause false-positive urine protein test results.
- May cause elevated serum creatinine, SGOT (AST), SGPT (ALT), bilirubin, and alkaline phosphatase. May also cause elevated serum sodium and decreased serum potassium levels.
- May cause positive direct Coombs' test result.

POTENTIAL NURSING DIAGNOSES
- Infection, high risk for (indications, side effects).
- Knowledge deficit related to medication regimen (patient/family teaching).

IMPLEMENTATION
- **General Info:** Reconstituted soln is stable for 48 hr at room temperature and 72 hr if refrigerated. Soln is colorless to pale yellow; darkened soln does not affect potency.
- **IM:** To constitute for IM use, add 3–4 ml of sterile water for injection or 0.5 or 1% lidocaine hydrochloride injection (without epinephrine) to each 1-g vial and shake vigorously. Inject deep into a well-developed muscle mass over 12–15 sec to minimize discomfort and massage well. IM injections should not exceed 2 g at each site.
- **IV:** The initial reconstitution is made with at least 10 ml of sterile water for injection, 0.9% NaCl or D5W.
  - Change IV sites every 48 hr to prevent phlebitis.
- **Direct IV:** Inject slowly, 1 g over 3–5 min to minimize vein irritation.
- **Intermittent Infusion:** Dilute in 50–100 ml of 0.9% NaCl, D5W, D10W, D5/0.25% NaCl, D5/0.45% NaCl, Ringer's or lactated Ringer's soln.
  - *Rate:* Administer over 30 min via Y-site or direct IV. If Y-site is used, temporarily discontinue primary infusion during mezlocillin administration.
- **Syringe Compatibility:** heparin.
- **Y-Site Compatibility:** cyclophosphamide, famotadine, hydromorphone, morphine, or perphenazine.
- **Y-Site Incompatibility:** ciprofloxacin, meperidine, ondansetron, or verapamil.
- **Additive Incompatibility:** ciprofloxacin. Incompatible with aminoglycosides; do not admix, administer at least 1 hr apart.

PATIENT/FAMILY TEACHING
- Advise patient to report the signs of superinfection (black, furry overgrowth on the tongue; vaginal itching or discharge; loose or foul-smelling stools) and allergy.
- Advise patient to notify physician if fever and diarrhea develop, especially if stool contains blood, pus, or mucus. Instruct patient not to treat diarrhea without consulting physician or pharmacist.

EVALUATION

Clinical response can be evaluated by:
- Resolution of the signs and symptoms of infection. Length of time for complete resolution depends on the organism and site of infection.

MICONAZOLE
(mi-**kon**-a-zole)
Micatin, {Monistat}, Monistat IV, Monistat-Derm

CLASSIFICATION(S):
Antifungal
Pregnancy Category UK

INDICATIONS

- **IV:** Treatment of severe fungal infections, such as: Pulmonary infections Disseminated infections - **IV, Intrathecal:** Meningitis - **IV, Bladder Irrigation:** Candida bladder infections caused by susceptible organisms - **Top, Vag:** Treatment of a variety of skin and mucous membrane fungal infections.

ACTION

■ Alters permeability of fungal cell membrane and function of fungal enzymes. **Therapeutic Effect:** ■ Fungistatic or fungicidal action. **Spectrum:** ■ Active against all pathogenic fungi and gram-positive bacteria ■ Spectrum notable for activity against: □ *Aspergillus* □ *Coccidioides* □ *Cryptococcus* □ *Candida albicans* □ *Histoplasma* □ *Dermatophytes.*

PHARMACOKINETICS

Absorption: Poorly (50%) absorbed following oral administration. Small amounts systemically absorbed after topical application.

Distribution: Following IV administration is widely distributed. CSF penetration is poor, necessitating intrathecal administration in the treatment of meningitis.

Metabolism and Excretion: Mostly metabolized by the liver.

Half-life: 24 hr.

CONTRAINDICATIONS AND PRECAUTIONS

Contraindicated in: ■ Hypersensitivity ■ Hypersensitivity to castor oil or parabens (IV only).

Use Cautiously in: ■ Pregnancy, lactation, or children <1 yr (safety of IV form not established; vaginal miconazole has been used during pregnancy).

ADVERSE REACTIONS AND SIDE EFFECTS*

Note: All adverse reactions listed except local irritation are for IV dosage form.

CNS: drowsiness, dizziness, anxiety, headache.

EENT: blurred vision, dry eyes.

CV: arrhythmias.

GI: nausea, vomiting, diarrhea, bitter taste.

F and E: hyponatremia.

Hemat: anemia.

Local: IV—phlebitis, pruritus ; Top—irritation.

Misc: hyperlipidemia, fever, increased libido, allergic reaction, including ANAPHYLAXIS.

INTERACTIONS

Drug-Drug: ■ Parenteral miconazole enhances the anticoagulant effect of **warfarin** ■ Concurrent use with **rifampin** or **isoniazid** decreases blood levels and effectiveness of miconazole.

ROUTE AND DOSAGE

- **IV (Adults):** 200–3600 mg/day in divided doses q 8 hr.
- **IV (Children):** 20–40 mg/kg/day in divided doses q 8 hr (not to exceed 15 mg/kg dose).
- **Intrathecal (Adults):** 20 mg q 3–7 days if not (q 1–2 days if ventricular reservoir placed).
- **Bladder Irrigation (Adults):** 200 mg q 6–12 hr by continuous irrigation.
- **Vag (Adults):** 100 mg suppository once daily into vagina for 7 days or 200–400 mg once daily for 3 days or 1 applicatorful of vaginal cream once daily for 7 days.
- **Top (Adults and Children):** 2% cream, lotion, powder, soln, aerosol, apply 1–2 times daily.

PHARMACODYNAMICS (blood levels)

	ONSET	PEAK
IV	rapid	end of infusion
Vag	UK	UK

NURSING IMPLICATIONS

ASSESSMENT

- □ Assess patient for infection prior to and throughout course of therapy.
- □ Obtain specimens for culture prior to treatment. First dose may be given before receiving results.
- □ Monitor IV site closely for phlebitis.
- ■ **Lab Test Considerations:** Hemoglobin, hematocrit, serum electrolytes, and lipids should be monitored periodically throughout IV therapy.

*Underlines indicate most frequent; **CAPITALS** indicate life-threatening.

- ▫ May cause abnormalities in tests of serum lipid concentrations.

POTENTIAL NURSING DIAGNOSES

- ▪ Infection, high risk for (indications).
- ▪ Skin integrity, impaired: actual (indications).
- ▪ Knowledge deficit related to medication regimen (patient/family teaching).

IMPLEMENTATION

- ▪ **General Info:** Available in topical aerosol powder, cream, topical powder, topical aerosol soln, vaginal cream or suppositories, and injectable forms.
- ▪ **Intermittent Infusion:** Dilute each dose in at least 200 ml of 0.9% NaCl or D5W. Soln is stable at room temperature for 48 hr. Darkened color of soln shows deterioration; discard. Manufacturer does not recommend admixing miconazole with other medications.
- ▫ Initial dose of 200 mg should be administered under physician's supervision to determine hypersensitivity.
- ▫ *Rate:* Administer over 30–60 min. Rapid administration may cause transient tachycardia or arrhythmias.
- ▫ Nausea and vomiting may be minimized by reducing dose, slowing infusion rate, avoiding administration at mealtime, or administering antiemetics or antihistamines prior to IV miconazole infusion.
- ▪ **Y-Site Compatibility:** foscarnet or ondansetron.
- ▪ **Bladder Irrigation:** Bladder irrigation may be used concurrently with IV administration for bladder mycoses.

PATIENT/FAMILY TEACHING

- ▪ **General Info:** Instruct patient to apply topical miconazole exactly as directed. Missed doses should be applied as soon as remembered, unless almost time for next dose.
- ▪ **Vag:** Instruct patient to use vaginal preparations at bedtime unless otherwise directed. Applicator for cream is included in package. Instruct patient to insert high into vagina and to use a sanitary napkin to prevent staining of clothing or bedding. Patient should remain recumbent for at least 30 min after administration. Advise patient not to douche without consulting physician.
- ▫ Advise patients treated for vaginal infection to avoid intercourse during therapy to prevent reinfection.
- ▪ **Top:** Instruct patient using topical cream or lotion to apply sufficient amount to cover affected area and rub in gently. Avoid contact with eyes. Do not use occlusive dressings unless directed by physician.
- ▫ Advise patient to consult physician if no improvement is seen in 4 wk.

EVALUATION

Effectiveness of therapy can be demonstrated by: ▪ Resolution of the signs and symptoms of infection ▫ Vaginal application should be continued for 3–7 days ▫ Topical application may require 2 wk to 1 mon to prevent recurrence.

MIDAZOLAM
(mid-ay-zoe-lam)
Versed

CLASSIFICATION(S):
Sedative/hypnotic—benzodiazepine
Schedule IV
Pregnancy Category D

INDICATIONS

▪ Used to produce sedation preoperatively and amnesia postoperatively ▪ To aid in the induction of anesthesia ▪ Provides conscious sedation before diagnostic or radiographic procedures.

ACTION

▪ Acts at many levels of the CNS to produce generalized CNS depression ▪ Effects may be mediated by gamma-aminobutyric acid (GABA), an inhibitory neurotransmitter. **Therapeutic Effects:** ▪ Short-term sedation ▪ Postoperative amnesia.

PHARMACOKINETICS

Absorption: Well absorbed following IM administration.

Distribution: Crosses the blood-brain barrier and placenta.

Metabolism and Excretion: Almost exclusively metabolized by the liver.

Half-life: 1–12 hr (increased in renal impairment or congestive heart failure).

CONTRAINDICATIONS AND PRECAUTIONS

Contraindicated in: ▪ Hypersensitivity ▪ Cross-sensitivity with other benzodiazepines may exist ▪ Shock ▪ Comatose patients or those with pre-existing CNS depression ▪ Controlled severe pain ▪ Pregnancy or lactation.

Use Cautiously in: ▪ Pulmonary disease ▪ Congestive heart failure ▪ Renal impairment ▪ Severe hepatic impairment ▪ Elderly or debilitated patients (more susceptible to depressant effects; dosage reduction required) ▪ Children (safety not established).

ADVERSE REACTIONS AND SIDE EFFECTS*

CNS: headache, excess sedation, drowsiness, agitation.

EENT: blurred vision.

Resp: coughing, LARYNGOSPASM, bronchospasm, RESPIRATORY DEPRESSION, APNEA.

CV: arrhythmias, CARDIAC ARREST.

GI: hiccoughs, nausea, vomiting.

Derm: rashes.

Local: pain at IM site, <u>phlebitis</u> at IV site.

INTERACTIONS

Drug–Drug: ▪ Additive CNS depression with **alcohol, antihistamines, narcotic analgesics,** and **sedative/hypnotics** (decrease midazolam dose by 30–50% if used concurrently) ▪ Increased risk of hypotension with **antihypertensives,** acute ingestion of **alcohol,** or **nitrates.**

ROUTE AND DOSAGE

Note: Dosage must be individualized, taking caution to reduce dosage in elderly patients and those who are already sedated.

Preoperative Sedation

- **IM (Adults):** 70–80 mcg/kg 1 hr before surgery (usual dose 5 mg).

Pre-Endoscopy or Cardiovascular Procedures

- **IV (Adults):** 1–2.5 mg initially, dosage may be increased further as needed, doses >5 mg are rarely needed. In elderly (>60 yr) or debilitated patients initial dose should not exceed 1.5 mg with doses >3.5 mg rarely needed.

Induction of Anesthesia

- **IV (Adults):** 150–350 mcg/kg, may give additional doses in increments of 25% of initial dose (up to 600 mcg/kg). If >55 yr, debilitated, or sedated start with 150 mcg/kg.

PHARMACODYNAMICS (sedation)

	ONSET	PEAK	DURATION
IM	15 min	30–60 min	2–6 hr
IV	1.5–5 min	rapid	2–6 hr

NURSING IMPLICATIONS

Assessment

- ▫ Assess level of sedation and level of consciousness throughout and for 2–6 hr following administration.
- ▫ Monitor blood pressure, pulse, and respiration continuously throughout IV administration. Oxygen and resuscitative equipment should be immediately available.
- ▪ **Toxicity and Overdose:** If overdose occurs, monitor pulse, respiration, and blood pressure continuously. Maintain patent airway and assist ventilation as needed. If hypotension occurs, treatment includes IV fluids, repositioning, and vasopressors.

Potential Nursing Diagnoses

- ▪ Breathing pattern, ineffective (adverse reactions).

*<u>Underlines</u> indicate most frequent; **CAPITALS** indicate life-threatening.

M

- Injury, high risk for (side effects).
- Knowledge deficit related to medication regimen (patient/family teaching).

Implementation

- **IM:** Administer IM doses deep into muscle mass.
- **Direct IV:** Administer undiluted or diluted with D5W, 0.9% NaCl, or lactated Ringer's injection through Y-site or 3-way stopcock.
  - When administered concurrently with narcotic analgesics, dose should be reduced by 30–50%.
  - *Rate:* Administer each dose slowly over at least 2 min. Monitor IV site closely to avoid extravasation. Titrate dose to patient response.
- **Syringe Compatibility:** atropine, benzquinamide, buprenorphine, butorphanol, chlorpromazine, cimetadine, diphenhydramine, droperidol, fentanyl, glycopyrrolate, hydromorphine, hydroxyzine, meperidine, metoclopramide, morphine, nalbuphine, promazine, promethazine, scopolamine, thiethylperazine, or trimethobenzamide.
- **Syringe Incompatibility:** dimenhydrinate, pentobarbital, perphenazine, prochlorperazine, or ranitidine.
- **Y-Site Compatibility:** atracurium, pancuronium, or vecuronium.
- **Y-Site Incompatibility:** foscarnet.

Patient/Family Teaching

- Inform patient that this medication will decrease mental recall of the procedure.
- Medication may cause drowsiness or dizziness. Advise patient to request assistance prior to ambulation and transfer, and to avoid driving or other activities requiring alertness for 24 hr following administration.
- Instruct patient to inform physician prior to administration if pregnancy is suspected.
- Advise patient to avoid alcohol or other CNS depressants for 24 hr following administration of midazolam.

Evaluation

Effectiveness of therapy can be demonstrated by: ▪ Sedation during and amnesia following surgical, diagnostic, and radiologic procedures.

MINERAL OIL

Agarol Plain, Fleet Mineral Oil, {Kondremul}, Kondremul Plain, Milkinol, {Lansoyl}, Neo-Cultol, Nujol, Petrogalar

CLASSIFICATION(S):
Laxative—lubricant
Pregnancy Category UK

INDICATIONS

▪ Used to soften impacted feces in the management of constipation.

ACTION

▪ Coats surface of stool and intestine with lubricant film to allow passage of stool through intestine ▪ Improves water retention of stool. **Therapeutic Effect:** ▪ Softening of fecal mass and subsequent passage.

PHARMACOKINETICS

Absorption: Minimally absorbed following oral administration.
Distribution: Distributes into mesenteric lymph nodes, intestinal mucosa, liver, and spleen.
Metabolism and Excretion: Metabolism and excretion not known. Action is primarily local; unabsorbed mineral oil is passed with fecal mass.
Half-life: UK.

CONTRAINDICATIONS AND PRECAUTIONS

Contraindicated in: ▪ Hypersensitivity ▪ Children <6 yr (oral) ▪ Children <2 yr (rect).
Use Cautiously in: ▪ Children, elderly or debilitated patients (increased risk of lipid pneumonia) ▪ Pregnancy (chronic use decreases absorption of

fat-soluble vitamins, may cause hypoprothrombinemia in newborn).

ADVERSE REACTIONS AND SIDE EFFECTS*

Resp: lipid pneumonia.

GI: rectal seepage of mineral oil, anal irritation.

INTERACTIONS

Drug–Drug: ▪ Decreases absorption of **fat-soluble vitamins (A, D, E, K).**

Drug–Food: ▪ Decreases absorption of **fat-soluble vitamins (A, D, E, K).**

ROUTE AND DOSAGE

- **PO (Adults and Children >12 yr):** 15–45 ml as a single dose or divided doses.
- **PO (Children 6–12 yr):** 5–15 ml as a single dose or divided doses.
- **Rect (Adults and Children >12 yr):** 60–150 ml as a single dose.
- **Rect (Children 2–11 yr):** 30–60 ml as a single dose.

PHARMACODYNAMICS (laxation)

	ONSET	PEAK	DURATION
PO	6–8 hr	UK	UK
Rect	2–15 min	UK	UK

NURSING IMPLICATIONS

Assessment

- □ Assess patient for abdominal distention, presence of bowel sounds, and usual pattern of bowel function.
- □ Assess color, consistency, and amount of stool produced.

Potential Nursing Diagnoses

- ▪ Bowel elmination, altered: constipation (indications).
- ▪ Knowledge deficit related to medication regimen (patient/family teaching).

Implementation

- ▪ **General Info:** Available in combination with other products (see Appendix A).
- □ This medication does not stimulate intestinal peristalsis.
- □ Administer carefully to bedridden patients or children to prevent lipid pneumonia from aspiration of mineral oil. Do not administer to patients in a reclining position.
- ▪ **PO:** Usually administered at bedtime. Do not administer within 2 hr of meals; may interfere with absorption of nutrients and vitamins.
- □ Do not administer within 2 hr of stool softeners; may cause increased absorption of mineral oil.
- ▪ **Rect:** Do not lubricate suppositories containing mineral oil, as this may interfere with the action of the suppository. Moisten with water by placing under tap for 30 sec or in a cup of water for at least 10 sec prior to insertion.

Patient/Family Teaching

- □ Advise patients that laxatives should be used only for short-term therapy. Long-term therapy may interfere with absorption of nutrients and vitamins A, D, E, and K.
- □ Advise patient not to take this medication within 2 hr of food or other medications.
- □ Encourage patients to use other forms of bowel regulation, such as increasing bulk in the diet, increasing fluid intake, increasing mobility. Normal bowel habits are variable and may vary from 3 times/day to 3 times/wk.
- □ Instruct patients with cardiac disease to avoid straining during bowel movements (Valsalva maneuver).
- □ Advise patients that large doses of mineral oil may cause leakage of mineral oil from the rectum; protection of clothing may be necessary. This may be prevented by reducing or dividing the dose or by administration of emulsified form.
- □ Advise patient not to use laxatives when abdominal pain, nausea, vomiting, or fever is present.

Evaluation

Effectiveness of therapy can be demonstrated by: ▪ Soft, formed bowel move-

*Underlines indicate most frequent; **CAPITALS** indicate life-threatening.

ment, usually within 6–8 hr ▫ Results are usually obtained from rectal doses in 2–15 min.

MINOCYCLINE
(min-oh-**sye**-kleen)
Minocin

CLASSIFICATION(S):
Anti-infective—tetracycline
Pregnancy Category UK

INDICATIONS

▪ Used most commonly in the treatment of infections due to unusual (atypical) organisms, including: ▫ *Mycoplasma* ▫ *Chlamydia* ▫ *Rickettsia* ▪ Treatment of gonorrhea in patients who cannot tolerate conventional therapy ▪ Management of inflammatory acne ▪ Eradication of the asymptomatic carrier of *Neisseria meningitidis* in patients who cannot tolerate rifampin.

ACTION

▪ Inhibits bacterial protein synthesis at the level of the 30S ribosome. **Therapeutic Effect:** ▪ Bacteriostatic action against susceptible bacteria. **Spectrum:** ▪ Active against a wide variety of gram-positive, gram-negative, and atypical organisms, including: ▫ *Neisseria meningitidis* ▫ *Neisseria gonorrhea* ▫ *Treponema pallidum* ▫ *Chlamydia trachomatis* ▫ *Ureaplasma urealyticum* ▫ *Mycoplasma pneumoniae* ▫ Norcardia.

PHARMACOKINETICS

Absorption: Well absorbed from the GI tract.
Distribution: Widely distributed, some penetration into CSF. Crosses the placenta and enters breast milk.
Metabolism and Excretion: 5–20% excreted unchanged by the urine. Some metabolism by the liver with enterohepatic circulation and excretion in bile and feces.
Half-life: 11–26 hr.

CONTRAINDICATIONS AND PRECAUTIONS

Contraindicated in: ▪ Hypersensitivity ▪ Children <8 (permanent staining of teeth) ▪ Pregnancy or lactation.
Use Cautiously in: ▪ Cachectic or debilitated patients ▪ Hepatic or renal disease.

ADVERSE REACTIONS AND SIDE EFFECTS*

CNS: lightheadedness, dizziness, vertigo.
EENT: vestibular reactions.
GI: nausea, vomiting, diarrhea, pancreatitis, hepatotoxicity.
Derm: rashes, photosensitivity.
Hemat: blood dyscrasias.
Local: phlebitis at IV site.
Misc: superinfection, hypersensitivity reactions.

INTERACTIONS

Drug–Drug: ▪ May enhance the effect of **oral anticoagulants** ▪ May decrease the effectiveness of **oral contraceptives** ▪ **Calcium, iron,** and **magnesium** form chelates and may decrease absorption ▪ **Kaolin/pectin antidiarrheals** may decrease absorption.

ROUTE AND DOSAGE

Treatment of Infections, Eradication of Meningococcal Carriers
- **PO, IV (Adults):** 200 mg initially, then 100 mg q 12 hr.

Inflammatory Acne
- **PO (Adults):** 50 mg 1–3 times daily.

PHARMACODYNAMICS (blood levels)

	ONSET	PEAK
PO	rapid	2–3 hr
IV	rapid	end of infusion

NURSING IMPLICATIONS

ASSESSMENT

▫ Assess patient for infection (vital signs; appearance of wound, sputum, urine, and stool; WBC) at beginning and throughout course of therapy.

*Underlines indicate most frequent; **CAPITALS** indicate life-threatening.

- Obtain specimens for culture and sensitivity prior to initiating therapy. First dose may be given before receiving results.
- **Lab Test Considerations:** May cause increased SGOT (AST), SGPT (ALT), serum alkaline phosphatase, bilirubin, and amylase concentrations.

Potential Nursing Diagnoses

- Infection, high risk for (indications, side effects).
- Knowledge deficit related to medication regimen (patient/family teaching).
- Noncompliance related to medication regimen (patient/family teaching).

Implementation

- **General Info:** May cause yellow-brown discoloration and softening of teeth and bones if administered prenatally or prior to 8 yrs of age.
- Available in tablet, capsule, oral suspension, and injectable forms.
- **PO:** Administer around the clock. May be taken with food or milk. Take with a full glass of liquid and take at least 1 hr before going to bed. Use calibrated measuring for liquid preparations. Shake liquid preparations well.
- Do not administer within 1–3 hr of other medications.
- Avoid administration of calcium salts, antacids, magnesium-containing medications, or iron supplements within 1–3 hr of oral minocycline.
- **SC/IM:** Do not administer SC or IM.
- **Intermittent Infusion:** Dilute each 100 mg with 5–10 ml of sterile water for injection. Dilute further in 500–1000 ml of 0.9% NaCl, D5W, D5/0.9% NaCl, Ringer's or lactated Ringer's soln. Soln is stable for 24 hr at room temperature.
- *Rate:* Administer at prescribed rate immediately following dilution. Avoid rapid infusions. May cause thrombophlebitis; avoid extravasation.
- **Y-Site Compatibility:** cyclophosphamide, heparin, hydrocortisone sodium succinate, magnesium sulfate, perphenazine, or potassium chloride.
- **Y-Site Incompatibility:** hydromorphone, meperidine, or morphine.

Patient/Family Teaching

- Instruct patients to take medication around the clock and to finish the drug completely as directed, even if feeling better. Missed doses should be taken as soon as remembered unless almost time for next dose. Advise patients that sharing of this medication may be dangerous.
- Commonly causes dizziness, lightheadedness, or unsteadiness. Caution patient to avoid driving or other activities requiring alertness until response to medication is known. Notify physician if these symptoms occur.
- Caution patient to use sunscreen and protective clothing to prevent photosensitivity reactions.
- Advise patient to use a nonhormonal method of contraception while taking minocycline.
- Instruct patient to notify physician or dentist of medication regimen prior to treatment or surgery.
- Advise patient to report the signs of superinfection (black, furry overgrowth on the tongue; vaginal itching or discharge; loose or foul-smelling stools). Skin rash, pruritus, and urticaria should also be reported.
- Instruct the patient to notify the physician if symptoms do not improve.
- Caution patient to discard outdated or decomposed products as they may be toxic.

Evaluation

Clinical response can be evaluated by:
- Resolution of the signs and symptoms of infection. Length of time for complete resolution depends on the organism and site of infection ▪ Improvement in acne.

M

MINOXIDIL
(mi-**nox**-i-dill)
Loniten, Minodyl, Rogaine

CLASSIFICATION(S):
Antihypertensive—vasodilator, Dermatologic—hair growth stimulant
Pregnancy Category C (PO)

INDICATIONS
▪ **PO:** Management of severe symptomatic hypertension or hypertension associated with end-organ damage that has failed to respond to combinations of more conventional therapy ▪ **Top:** Management of androgenic alopecia.

ACTION
▪ Directly relaxes vascular smooth muscle, probably by inhibiting the enzyme phosphodiesterase. Results in vasodilation, which is more pronounced on arterioles than veins ▪ Hair regrowth may be due to increased cutaneous blood flow or stimulation of hair follicles from resting phase to growing phase. **Therapeutic Effects:** ▪ Lowering of blood pressure ▪ Hair regrowth.

PHARMACOKINETICS
Absorption: Well absorbed from the GI tract following oral administration. Minimal absorption follows topical use (<2%), but is enhanced by increasing dose or applying to larger surface area.
Distribution: Widely distributed. Enters breast milk.
Metabolism and Excretion: 90% metabolized by the liver.
Half-life: 4.2 hr.

CONTRAINDICATIONS AND PRECAUTIONS
Contraindicated in: ▪ Hypersensitivity ▪ Pheochromocytoma ▪ Patients currently receiving guanethidine.
Use Cautiously in: ▪ **PO:** Recent myocardial infarction ▪ Pregnancy or lactation (safety not established) ▪ Severe renal impairment (can be used in moderate renal impairment) ▪ **Top:** Cardiovascular disease ▪ Abraded or irritated skin (increased risk of systemic absorption).

ADVERSE REACTIONS AND SIDE EFFECTS*
CNS: PO—headache.
Resp: PO—pulmonary edema.
CV: PO—edema, **CONGESTIVE HEART FAILURE,** <u>tachycardia</u>, <u>ECG changes</u> (alteration in T waves), pericardial effusion, angina.
GI: PO—nausea.
Derm: PO—<u>hypertrichosis</u>, pigment changes, rashes; Top—burning or itching of scalp, skin rash, swelling of face.
Endo: PO—breast tenderness, gynecomastia, menstrual irregularities.
F and E: PO—<u>sodium and water retention</u>.
Misc: PO—intermittent claudication.

INTERACTIONS
Note: For oral minoxidil, unless indicated.

Drug-Drug: ▪ Additive hypotensive effects with other **antihypertensive agents,** acute ingestion of **alcohol,** or **nitrates** ▪ Severe hypotension may occur with **guanethidine** ▪ **Nonsteroidal anti-inflammatory agents** may decrease the antihypertensive effectiveness of minoxidil ▪ **Top:** Topical **glucocorticoids, petrolatum,** or **retinoids** may enhance absorption and lead to systemic side effects.

ROUTE AND DOSAGE
Hypertension
- **PO (Adults and Children >12 yr):** 5 mg once daily initially, increase at 3-day intervals (for rapid control with careful monitoring, doses may be adjusted q 6 hr) to 10 mg/day, then 20 mg/day, then 40 mg/day given in 2 divided doses. Usual dose required is 10–40 mg/day. Doses up to 100 mg have been used.
- **PO (Children <12 yr):** 0.2 mg/kg/day

*<u>Underlines</u> indicate most frequent; **CAPITALS** indicate life-threatening.

(5 mg maximum) initially, may be gradually increased at 3-day intervals in increments of 50–100% until response is obtained. Usual dose required is 0.25–1 mg/kg/day in 1–2 divided doses. For rapid control, doses may be adjusted q 6 hr (daily dose not to exceed 50 mg).

Alopecia

- **Top (Adults):** Apply 1 ml of 2% soln to affected area bid (up to 2 ml/day).

PHARMACODYNAMICS (PO = antihypertensive effect, Top = hair regrowth)

	ONSET	PEAK	DURATION
PO	30 min	2–8 hr	2–5 days
Top	4 mon	UK	3–4 mon

NURSING IMPLICATIONS

Assessment

- **Hypertension:** Monitor blood pressure and pulse frequently during initial dosage adjustment and periodically throughout course of therapy. Notify physician of significant changes.
- Monitor intake and output ratios and daily weight and assess for edema daily, especially at beginning of therapy. Notify physician of weight gain or edema, as sodium and water retention may be treated with diuretics.
- **Lab Test Considerations:** Renal and hepatic function, CBC, and electrolytes should be monitored prior to and periodically throughout therapy.
- May cause increased BUN, serum creatinine, alkaline phosphatase, and sodium levels. May also cause decreased RBC, hemoglobin, and hematocrit counts.

Potential Nursing Diagnoses

- Tissue perfusion, altered (indications).
- Body image disturbance (indications, side effects).
- Knowledge deficit related to medication regimen (patient/family teaching).

Implementation

- **Hypertension:** Medication may need to be discontinued gradually to prevent rebound hypertension.
- Minoxidil is given concurrently with a diuretic unless patient is on hemodialysis.
- Dosage adjustments should not be made more frequently than every 3 days to allow for maximum effectiveness, unless rapid control is necessary.
- **PO:** May be administered without regard to meals or food.
- **Top:** The same 1-ml dose is used regardless of the size of the balding area. More than 2 ml/day does not speed up process of hair growth and may increase side effects.
- Available with pump spray, extended tip, or rub-on applicators.

Patient/Family Teaching

- **Hypertension:** Emphasize the importance of continuing to take this medication, even if feeling well. Instruct patient to take medication at the same time each day. If a dose is missed, take as soon as remembered if within a few hours; otherwise omit dose and return to regular dosage schedule. Do not double doses. Advise patient not to discontinue minoxidil without consulting physician. Minoxidil helps control but does not cure hypertension.
- Encourage patient to comply with additional interventions for hypertension (weight reduction, low-sodium diet, discontinuation of smoking, moderation of alcohol consumption, regular exercise, and stress management).
- Instruct patient and family on proper technique for pulse and blood pressure monitoring. Advise them to check blood pressure at least weekly and to report significant changes to physician. Physician should also be notified if resting pulse increases more than 20 bpm above baseline.
- Advise patient to check weight daily and to notify physician of rapid

weight gain of >5 lb or if signs of fluid retention occur.

- Caution patient to make position changes slowly to minimize orthostatic hypotension.
- Advise patient to consult physician or pharmacist before taking any cough, cold, or allergy remedies. Patient should also avoid excessive amounts of coffee, tea, or cola.
- Inform patient that depilatory creams may minimize increased hair growth. This is temporary and is reversible within 1–6 mon following discontinuation of minoxidil.
- **Top:** Instruct patient to use minoxidil exactly as directed. Do not use more medication or more frequently to avoid systemic side effects. Missed doses should be applied as soon as remembered if not almost time for next dose.
- Instruct patient to apply only to scalp, not to other parts of the body, to minimize side effects. Do not use with other topical scalp medications or if scalp is sunburned. Hair should be dry prior to application.
- Inform patient that first hair growth may be soft, colorless, and barely visable. With further treatment hair should be same color and thickness as other hair on scalp.
- Caution patient that if treatment is stopped, new hair may be shed within mons.
- Shampoo hair each morning before first daily application. Apply to affected area beginning at center of balding area. Wash hands immediately after application. Do not use hairdryer to speed drying. Do not lie down within 30 min of application to prevent transfer of medication to pillow.
- Advise patient to avoid contact of minoxidil with eyes, nose, or mouth. Flush area with water if accidental contact occurs.
- Advise patient to notify physician if itching, burning, rash, or swelling of face; chest pain; weight gain; or tachycardia occurs.

EVALUATION

Effectiveness of therapy can be demonstrated by: ▪ Decrease in blood pressure without appearance of serious side effects ▪ Hair regrowth in androgenic alopecia. Evidence of hair growth usually requires 4 mon or longer.

MISOPROSTOL

(mye-soe-**prost**-ole)
Cytotec

CLASSIFICATION(S):
Gastrointestinal—antiulcer
Pregnancy Category X

INDICATIONS

▪ Prevention of gastric mucosal injury from nonsteroidal anti-inflammatory agents, including aspirin, in high-risk patients (elderly or debilitated patients, or those with a history of ulcers). **Unlabeled Use:** ▪ Treatment of duodenal ulcers.

ACTION

▪ Acts as a prostaglandin analog, decreasing gastric acid secretion (antisecretory effect) and increasing the production of protective mucus (cytoprotective effect). **Therapeutic Effect:** ▪ Prevention of gastic ulceration from nonsteroidal anti-inflammatory agents.

PHARMACOKINETICS

Absorption: Well absorbed following oral administration and rapidly converted to its active form (misoprostol acid).
Distribution: Distribution not known.
Metabolism and Excretion: Undergoes some metabolism and is then excreted by the kidneys.
Half-life: 20–40 min.

CONTRAINDICATIONS AND PRECAUTIONS

Contraindicated in: ▪ Hypersensitivity to prostaglandins ▪ Pregnancy or lactation.
Use Cautiously in: ▪ Women with child-

bearing potential ▪ Children <18 yr (safety not established).

ADVERSE REACTIONS AND SIDE EFFECTS*

CNS: headache.

GI: diarrhea, abdominal pain, nausea, flatulence, dyspepsia, vomiting, constipation.

GU: menstrual disorders, miscarriage.

INTERACTIONS

Drug–Drug: ▪ Increased risk of diarrhea with **magnesium-containing antacids**.

ROUTE AND DOSAGE

- **PO (Adults):** 200 mcg 4 times daily with or after meals and at bedtime, or 400 mcg twice daily, last dose at bedtime. If intolerance occurs, dosage may be decreased to 100 mcg.

PHARMACODYNAMICS (gastric acid secretion)

	ONSET	PEAK	DURATION
PO	30 min	UK	3 hr

NURSING IMPLICATIONS

Assessment

- □ Assess patient routinely for epigastric or abdominal pain and frank or occult blood in the stool, emesis, or gastric aspirate.
- □ Assess women of childbearing age for pregnancy. Medication is usually begun on second or third day of menstrual period following a negative pregnancy test.

Potential Nursing Diagnoses

- Comfort, altered: pain (indications).
- Knowledge deficit related to medication regimen (patient/family teaching).

Implementation

- **PO:** Administer medication with meals and at bedtime to reduce severity of diarrhea.

Patient/Family Teaching

- □ Instruct patient to take medication as prescribed for the full course of therapy, even if feeling better. Emphasize that sharing of this medication may be dangerous.
- □ Inform patient that misoprostol will cause abortion of a fetus. Women of childbearing age must be informed of this effect through verbal and written information and must practice contraception throughout course of therapy. If pregnancy is suspected, the woman should stop taking misoprostol and immediately notify her physician.
- □ Inform patient that diarrhea may occur. The physician should be notified if diarrhea persists for more than 1 wk. Also advise patient to report onset of black, tarry stools or severe abdominal pain.
- □ Advise patient to avoid alcohol and foods that may cause an increase in GI irritation.

Evaluation

Effectiveness of therapy can be demonstrated by: ▪ The prevention of gastric ulcers in patients receiving chronic nonsteroidal anti-inflammatory drug therapy.

MITOMYCIN

(mye-toe-**mye**-sin)
Mutamycin

CLASSIFICATION(S):
Antineoplastic agent—antitumor antibiotic
Pregnancy Category UK

INDICATIONS

▪ Used with other agents in the management of disseminated adenocarcinoma of the stomach or pancreas. **Unlabeled Uses:** ▪ Palliative treatment of: □ Carcinoma of the colon or breast □ Head and neck tumors □ Advanced biliary, lung, and cervical squamous cell carcinomas.

*Underlines indicate most frequent; **CAPITALS** indicate life-threatening.

M

ACTION

▪ Primarily inhibits DNA synthesis by causing cross-linking, also inhibits RNA and protein synthesis (cell cycle-phase nonspecific, but is most active in S and G phases). **Therapeutic Effect:** ▪ Death of rapidly replicating cells, particularly malignant ones.

PHARMACOKINETICS

Absorption: Administered IV only, resulting in complete bioavailability.
Distribution: Widely distributed, concentrates in tumor tissue. Does not enter CSF.
Metabolism and Excretion: Mostly metabolized by the liver. Small amounts (<10%) excreted unchanged by the kidneys and in bile.
Half-life: 50 min.

CONTRAINDICATIONS AND PRECAUTIONS

Contraindicated in: ▪ Hypersensitivity ▪ Pregnancy or lactation.
Use Cautiously in: ▪ Patients with childbearing potential ▪ Active infections ▪ Decreased bone marrow reserve ▪ Other chronic debilitating illnesses ▪ Impaired liver function ▪ History of pulmonary problems.

ADVERSE REACTIONS AND SIDE EFFECTS*

Resp: pulmonary toxicity (hemoptysis, dyspnea, coughing, pneumonia).
CV: edema.
GI: nausea, vomiting, anorexia, stomatitis.
GU: renal failure, gonadal suppression.
Derm: alopecia, desquamation.
Hemat: anemia, leukopenia, thrombocytopenia.
Local: phlebitis at IV site.
Misc: prolonged malaise, fever, HEMOLYTIC UREMIC SYNDROME.

INTERACTIONS

Drug-Drug: ▪ Additive bone marrow depression with other **antineoplastic agents** or **radiation therapy** ▪ May decrease antibody response to **live virus vaccines** and increase the risk of adverse reactions.

ROUTE AND DOSAGE

▪ **IV (Adults):** 10–20 mg/m^2 every 6–8 wk.

PHARMACODYNAMICS (effects on blood counts)

	ONSET	PEAK	DURATION
IV	3–8 wk	4–8 wk	up to 3 mon

NURSING IMPLICATIONS

Assessment

- Monitor vital signs periodically during administration.
- Assess for fever, sore throat, and signs of infection due to leukopenia. Notify physician if these symptoms occur.
- Assess for bleeding (bleeding gums, bruising, petechiae; guaiac stools, urine, and emesis) due to thrombocytopenia. Avoid IM injections and rectal temperatures. Apply pressure to venipuncture sites for 10 min.
- Monitor intake and output, appetite, and nutritional intake. Nausea and vomiting usually occur within 1–2 hr. Vomiting may stop within 3–4 hr; nausea may persist for 2–3 days. Physician may order prophylactic use of an antiemetic. Adjust diet as tolerated to help maintain fluid and electrolyte balance and nutritonal status.
- Assess respiratory status and chest x-ray examination prior to and periodically throughout course of therapy. Notify physician if cough, bronchospasm, or dyspnea develops.
- Monitor for potentially fatal hemolytic uremia syndrome in patients receiving long-term therapy. Symptoms include microangiopathic hemolytic anemia, thrombocytopenia, renal failure, and hypertension.

▪ **Lab Test Considerations:** Monitor CBC and differential prior to and pe-

*Underlines indicate most frequent; **CAPITALS** indicate life-threatening.

riodically throughout course of therapy and for several mons following therapy.

- ▫ Monitor liver function studies (SGOT [AST], SGPT [ALT], LDH, bilirubin) and renal function studies (BUN, creatinine) prior to and periodically throughout therapy to detect hepatotoxicity and nephrotoxicity. Notify physician if creatinine is greater than 1.7 mg/dl.
- ▫ The nadir of leukopenia occurs in 4 wk. Notify physician if leukocyte count is <4000/mm^3. The nadir of thrombocytopenia occurs in 4 wk. Notify physician if the platelet count is <150,000/mm^3 or is progressively declining. Recovery of leukopenia and thrombocytopenia occurs within 10 wk after cessation of therapy. Myelosuppression is cumulative and may be irreversible. Repeat courses of therapy are held until leukocyte count is >3000/mm^3 and platelet count is >75,000/mm^3.

Potential Nursing Diagnoses

- ▪ Injury, high risk for (side effects).
- ▪ Infection, high risk for (side effects).
- ▪ Body image disturbance (side effects).

Implementation

- ▪ **General Info:** Soln should be prepared in a biologic cabinet. Wear gloves, gown, and mask while handling medication. Discard equipment in designated containers (see Appendix I).
- ▫ Ensure patency of IV. Extravasation may cause severe tissue necrosis. If patient complains of discomfort at IV site, discontinue immediately and restart infusion at another site. Promptly notify physician of extravasation.
- ▪ **Direct IV:** Reconstitute 5-mg vial with 10 ml and 10-mg vial with 40 ml of sterile water for injection. Shake the vial; may need to stand at room temperature for additional time to dissolve. Final soln is blue-gray. Reconstituted soln is stable for 7 days at room temperature, 14 days if refrigerated.
- ▫ *Rate:* May be administered IV push over 5–10 min through free-flowing IV of 0.9% NaCl or D5W.
- ▪ **Syringe Compatibility:** bleomycin, cisplatin, cyclophosphamide, doxorubicin, droperidol, fluorouracil, furosemide, heparin, leucovorin, methotrexate, metoclopramide, vinblastine, or vincristine.
- ▪ **Y-Site Compatibility:** bleomycin, cisplatin, cyclophosphamide, doxorubicin, droperidol, fluorouracil, furosemide, heparin, leucovorin, methotrexate, metoclopramide, ondansetron, vinblastine, or vincristine.
- ▪ **Additive Compatibility:** sodium lactate.
- ▪ **Additive Incompatibility:** bleomycin.

Patient/Family Teaching

- ▫ Advise patient to notify physician promptly if fever, chills, sore throat, signs of infection, bleeding gums, bruising, petechiae, or blood in urine, stool, or emesis occurs. Caution patient to avoid crowds and persons with known infections. Instruct patient to use soft toothbrush and electric razor. Patients should be cautioned not to drink alcoholic beverages or take aspirin-containing products.
- ▫ Instruct patient to notify physician if decreased urine output, edema in lower extremities, shortness of breath, skin ulceration, or persistent nausea occurs.
- ▫ Instruct patient to inspect oral mucosa for redness and ulceration. If ulceration occurs, advise patient to use sponge brush and rinse mouth with water after eating and drinking. Physician may order viscous lidocaine swishes if pain interferes with eating.
- ▫ Discuss with patient the possibility of hair loss. Explore coping strategies.
- ▫ Advise patient that although mitomycin may cause infertility, contraception during therapy is necessary because of teratogenic effects.
- ▫ Instruct patient not to receive any vac-

cinations without advice of physician.

- Emphasize need for periodic lab tests to monitor for side effects.

Evaluation

Effectiveness of therapy can be demonstrated by: ▪ Decrease in size and spread of malignant tissue.

MITOTANE
(**mye**-toe-tane)
o, p′-DDD, Lysodren

CLASSIFICATION(S):
Antineoplastic agent—miscellaneous
Pregnancy Category C

INDICATIONS

▪ Treatment of carcinoma of the adrenal cortex. **Unlabeled Use:** ▪ Cushing's syndrome due to pituitary disorders.

ACTION

▪ Suppresses the adrenal function ▪ Has a direct cytotoxic effect on adrenal tumors ▪ Structurally related to DDT (an insecticide). **Therapeutic Effect:** ▪ Regression of adrenal cortical tumors.

PHARMACOKINETICS

Absorption: 30–40% absorbed following oral administration.
Distribution: Widely distributed to all body tissues. Accumulates in fatty tissue.
Metabolism and Excretion: Slowly released from fatty tissue. Mostly metabolized by the liver. 10% excreted by the kidneys. 15% excreted in bile.
Half-life: 18–159 days.

CONTRAINDICATIONS AND PRECAUTIONS

Contraindicated in: ▪ Hypersensitivity.
Use Cautiously in: ▪ Pregnancy or lactation (especially first trimester; safety not established) ▪ Obesity (increased risk of adverse reactions).

ADVERSE REACTIONS AND SIDE EFFECTS*

CNS: brain damage, functional impairment (high-dose, long-term therapy), lethargy, somnolence, dizziness, vertigo, mental depression, headache, irritability, tremors, weakness, fatigue.
EENT: blurred vision, diplopia, lens opacities, optic neuritis, toxic retinopathy, decreased hearing.
Resp: wheezing, shortness of breath.
CV: hypotension, hypertension.
GI: anorexia, nausea, vomiting, diarrhea, increased salivation.
GU: hemorrhagic cystitis, hematuria, albuminuria.
Derm: maculopapular rash, flushing.
Endo: adrenal suppression, gynecomastia.
Metab: hypouricemia, hypercholesterolemia.
MS: arthralgia, myalgia, aching.
Misc: fever.

INTERACTIONS

Drug-Drug: ▪ Stimulates hepatic drug–metabolizing enzymes, which may decrease the effectiveness of **drugs that are highly metabolized (warfarin, phenytoin)** ▪ Additive CNS depression with other **CNS depressants,** including **alcohol, antihistamines, antidepressants, narcotic analgesics,** or **sedative/hypnotics** ▪ **Spironolactone** may block the effects of mitotane in Cushing's disease.

ROUTE AND DOSAGE

Adrenocortical Carcinoma

- **PO (Adults):** 8–10 g/day in 3–4 divided doses, may be increased as tolerated (range 2–16 g/day).
- **PO (Children):** 0.1–0.5 mg/kg/day or 1–2 g/day in divided doses. May be increased gradually to 5–7 g/day in divided doses.

Cushing's Disease

- **PO (Adults):** 3–6 g/day in 3–4 divided doses initially, decreased to maintenance dose of 500 mg twice weekly—2 g/day.

*Underlines indicate most frequent; **CAPITALS** indicate life-threatening.

PHARMACODYNAMICS (onset = inhibition of adrenocortical function, peak = tumor response)

	ONSET	PEAK	DURATION
PO	2–4 wk	6 wk	UK

NURSING IMPLICATIONS

Assessment

- □ Monitor for symptoms of adrenal insufficiency (anorexia, nausea and vomiting, diarrhea, fatigue, weakness, hypotension, darkening of skin). Obese patients are at increased risk for this side effect.
- □ Monitor for development of dose-limiting side effects (severe nausea, vomiting, anorexia, or diarrhea). Physician may order an antiemetic. Adjust diet as tolerated to maintain nutritional intake and fluid and electrolyte balance.
- □ Monitor neurologic status; report depression, lethargy, and complaints of dizziness.
- ▪ **Lab Test Considerations:** 8-hr plasma cortisol concentations and 24-hr urine tests for 17-hydroxycorticosteroid (OHCS) concentrations should be obtained prior to and periodically throughout therapy to determine degree of adrenal suppression.
- □ May decrease serum uric acid and protein bound iodine (PBI) concentrations.

Potential Nursing Diagnoses

- ▪ Knowledge deficit related to medication regimen (patient/family teaching).

Implementation

- ▪ **PO:** Premedication with an antiemetic may be necessary.

Patient/Family Teaching

- □ Instruct patient to take medication exactly as directed. If a dose is missed, it should be taken as soon as remembered unless almost time for next dose. Notify physician of missed doses.
- □ Explain to patient that this drug suppresses the adrenal glands and therefore impairs the body's ability to cope with stress. Concurrent glucocorticoid and mineralocorticoid therapy may be ordered to ensure that adequate amounts of adrenal hormones are present. The physician should be notified if an infection, illness, or injury occurs because supplemental steroids may be necessary or mitotane may need to be discontinued in the event of severe trauma or shock.
- □ Advise patient to carry identification describing medication regimen in the event of an emergency in which patient cannot relate medical history.
- □ Mitotane may cause drowiness. Caution patient to avoid driving or other activities requiring alertness until response to medication is known.
- □ Instruct patient to notify physician if depression; lethargy; dizziness; or persistent nausea, vomiting, or diarrhea occurs; or if skin rashes develop.
- □ Caution patient to avoid taking alcohol or other CNS depressants with this medication.
- □ Explain need for continued medical follow-up, including neurologic examination to assess effectiveness and possible side effects of medication.

Evaluation

Effectiveness of therapy can be demonstrated by: ▪ Decrease in the size and spread of adrenal malignancy as evidenced by a decrease in pain and symptoms of excess adrenal function.

MITOXANTRONE

(mye-toe-**zan**-trone)
Novantrone

CLASSIFICATION(S):
Antineoplastic—antitumor antibiotic
Pregnancy Category D

INDICATIONS

▪ Used in combination with other antineoplastic agents in the treatment of acute nonlymphocytic leukemia (ANLL)

M

in adults. **Unlabeled Uses:** ▪ Breast cancer, liver cancer, and non-Hodgkin's lymphoma.

ACTION

▪ Inhibits DNA synthesis (cell cycle-phase nonspecific. **Therapeutic Effect:** ▪ Death of rapidly replicating cells, particularly malignant ones.

PHARMACOKINETICS

Absorption: Administered IV only, resulting in complete bioavailability.
Distribution: Widely distributed. Limited penetration of CSF.
Metabolism and Excretion: Small amounts (<10%) excreted unchanged by the kidneys. Mostly eliminated by hepatobiliary clearance.
Half-life: 5.8 days.

CONTRAINDICATIONS AND PRECAUTIONS

Contraindicated in: ▪ Hypersensitivity ▪ Pregnancy or lactation.
Use Cautiously in: ▪ Previous cardiac disease ▪ Patients with childbearing potential ▪ Active infections ▪ Depressed bone marrow reserve ▪ Previous mediastinal radiation ▪ Other chronic debilitating illness ▪ Children (safety not established) ▪ Impaired hepatobiliary function or decreased blood counts (dosage reduction required).

ADVERSE REACTIONS AND SIDE EFFECTS*

CNS: headache, SEIZURES.
EENT: conjunctivitis, blue-green sclera.
Resp: cough, dyspnea.
CV: cardiotoxicity, ECG changes, arrhythmias.
GI: nausea, vomiting, diarrhea, abdominal pain, stomatitis, hepatic toxicity.
GU: renal failure, gonadal suppression, blue-green urine.
Derm: alopecia, rashes.
Hemat: anemia, leukopenia, thrombocytopenia.
Metab: hyperuricemia.
Misc: fever, hypersensitivity reactions.

INTERACTIONS

Drug–Drug: ▪ Additive bone marrow depression with other **antineoplastics** or **radiation therapy** ▪ Risk of cardiomyopathy increased by previous **anthracycline antineoplastic** therapy or **mediastinal radiation** ▪ May decrease antibody response to **live virus vaccines** and increase the risk of adverse reactions.

ROUTE AND DOSAGE

▪ **IV (Adults):** *Induction*—12 mg/m²/day for 3 days as IV infusion (usually given with cytosine arabinoside 100 mg/m²/day for 7 days as continuous IV infusion); if incomplete remission occurs, a second induction may be given. *Consolidation*—12 mg/m²/day for 2 days as IV infusion (usually given with cytosine arabinoside 100 mg/m²/day for 5 days as continous IV infusion), given 6 wk after induction, with another course 4 wk later.

PHARMACODYNAMICS (effects on blood counts)

	ONSET	PEAK	DURATION
IV	UK	10–14 days	28 days

NURSING IMPLICATIONS

Assessment

- ▫ Monitor for hypersensitivity reaction (rash, urticaria, bronchospasm, tachycardia, hypotension). If these occur, stop infusion and notify physician. Keep epinephrine, an antihistamine, and resuscitation equipment close by in the event of an anaphylactic reaction.
- ▫ Assess for fever, sore throat, and signs of infection caused by leukopenia. Notify physician if these symptoms occur.
- ▫ Assess for bleeding (bleeding gums, bruising, petechiae; guaiac stools, urine, and emesis) caused by thrombocytopenia. Avoid IM injections and rectal temperatures. Apply pressure to venipuncture sites for 10 min.

*Underlines indicate most frequent; **CAPITALS** indicate life-threatening.

- Monitor intake and output, appetite, and nutritional intake. Assess patient for nausea and vomiting. Confer with physician regarding prophylactic use of an antiemetic. Adjust diet as tolerated to help maintain fluid and electrolyte balance and nutritional status.
- May cause cardiotoxicity, especially in patients who have received daunorubicin or doxorubicin. Assess for rales/crackles, dyspnea, edema, jugular vein distention, ECG changes, arrhythmias, and chest pain.
- Monitor for symptoms of gout (increased uric acid levels and joint pain and swelling). Encourage patient to drink at least 2 liters of fluid per day. Allopurinol may be given to decrease serum uric acid levels.
- **Lab Test Considerations:** Monitor CBC and differential prior to and periodically throughout therapy.
- Monitor liver function studies (SGOT [AST], SGPT [ALT], LDH, bilirubin) and renal function studies (BUN, creatinine) prior to and periodically throughout therapy to detect hepatotoxicity and nephrotoxicity.
- May cause increased uric acid. Monitor periodically during therapy.

Potential Nursing Diagnoses

- Injury, high risk for (side effects).
- Infection, high risk for (side effects).
- Body image disturbance (side effects).

Implementation

- **General Info:** Soln should be prepared in a biologic cabinet. Wear gloves, gown, and mask while handling medication. Discard equipment in designated containers (see Appendix I).
- Avoid contact with skin. Use Luer Loc tubing to prevent accidental leakage. If contact with skin occurs, immediately wash skin with soap and water.
- Clean all spills with an aqueous soln of calcium hypochlorite. Mix soln by adding 5.5 parts (per weight) of calcium hypochlorite to 13 parts water.
- **IV:** Monitor IV site. If extravasation occurs, discontinue IV and restart at another site. Mitoxantrane is not a vesicant.
- **Direct IV:** Dilute soln in at least 50 ml of 0.9% NaCl or D5W. Discard unused soln appropriately.
- *Rate:* Administer slowly over at least 3 min into the tubing of a free-flowing IV of 0.9% NaCl or D5W.
- **Intermittent IV:** May be further diluted in D5W, 0.9% NaCl, or D5/0.9% NaCl and used immediately.
- **Y-Site Compatibility:** ondansetron.
- **Additive Compatibility:** hydrocortisone sodium succinate.
- **Additive Incompatibility:** heparin.

Patient/Family Teaching

- Advise patient to notify physician promptly if fever, chills, sore throat, signs of infection, bleeding gums, bruising, petechiae, or blood in urine, stool, or emesis occurs.
- Caution patient to avoid crowds and persons with known infections. Instruct patient to use soft toothbrush and electric razor. Patients should be cautioned not to drink alcoholic beverages or take aspirin-containing products.
- Instruct patient to notify physician if abdominal pain, yellow skin, cough, diarrhea, or decreased urine output occurs.
- Inform patient that medication may cause the urine and sclera to turn blue-green.
- Instruct patient to inspect oral mucosa for redness and ulceration. If mouth sores occur, advise patient to use sponge brush and rinse mouth with water after eating and drinking. Physician may order viscous lidocaine swishes if pain interferes with eating.
- Discuss with patient the possibility of hair loss. Explore coping strategies.
- Advise patient that although mitoxantrone may cause infertility, contraception during therapy is necessary because of possible teratogenic effects.
- Instruct patient not to receive any vaccinations without advice of physician.

M

- Emphasize need for periodic lab test to monitor for side effects.

Evaluation

Effectiveness of therapy can be demonstrated by: ▪ Decrease in the production and spread of leukemic cells.

MOLINDONE
(**moe**-lin-done)
Moban

CLASSIFICATION(S):
Antipsychotic
Pregnancy Category UK

INDICATIONS
▪ Treatment of schizophrenia.

ACTION
▪ Blocks the effects of dopamine in the reticular activating and limbic systems in the brain. **Therapeutic Effect:** ▪ Diminished psychoses associated with schizophrenic behavior.

PHARMACOKINETICS
Absorption: Rapidly absorbed following oral administration.
Distribution: Appears to be widely distributed; probably enters the CNS and enters breast milk.
Metabolism and Excretion: Mainly (>90%) metabolized by the liver. Small (<3%) amounts excreted unchanged by the kidneys.
Half-life: 1.5 hr.

CONTRAINDICATIONS AND PRECAUTIONS
Contraindicated in: ▪ Hypersensitivity to molindone ▪ Cross-sensitivity with other antipsychotics may exist ▪ Hypersensitivity to bisulfites, parabens, or alcohol (in liquid) or povidone (in tablets).
Use Cautiously in: ▪ Elderly or debilitated patients ▪ Diabetes mellitus ▪ Respiratory disease ▪ Prostatic hypertrophy ▪ CNS tumors ▪ Epilepsy ▪ Intestinal obstruction ▪ Pregnancy, lactation, or children (safety not established).

ADVERSE REACTIONS AND SIDE EFFECTS*
CNS: sedation, extrapyramidal reactions, tardive dyskinesia, headache, dizziness, insomnia, depression, euphoria, **NEUROLEPTIC MALIGNANT SYNDROME.**
EENT: dry eyes, blurred vision, nasal congestion.
CV: hypotension, tachycardia.
GI: constipation, dry mouth, nausea, anorexia, hepatitis.
Derm: rashes, photosensitivity.
Endo: galactorrhea, irregular menses, increased libido.
Misc: allergic reactions.

INTERACTIONS
Drug-Drug: ▪ Calcium in the formulation may decrease absorption of **phenytoin** or **tetracycline** ▪ Additive CNS depression with other **CNS depressants**, including **alcohol, antihistamines, antidepressants, MAO inhibitors, narcotic analgesics,** and **sedative/hypnotics** ▪ Additive anticholinergic properties with **agents having anticholinergic effects,** including **phenothiazines, haloperidol, antihistamines, MAO inhibitors,** or **disopyramide** ▪ Encephalopathy may occur with **lithium** ▪ Molindone may mask early signs of **lithium** toxicity ▪ May negate the beneficial effects of **levodopa**.

ROUTE AND DOSAGE
- **PO (Adults):** 50–75 mg/day in 3–4 divided doses initially in acute schizophrenia. Dosage may be increased to 100 mg/day after 3–4 days (not to exceed 225 mg/day). Usual maintenance dose is 5–15 mg 3–4 times daily. (Doses up to 225 mg/day in divided doses have been used in severe psychoses).

*Underlines indicate most frequent; **CAPITALS** indicate life-threatening.

PHARMACODYNAMICS (peak = blood levels, duration = antipsychotic effects)

	ONSET	PEAK	DURATION
PO	UK	1.5 hr	24–36 hr

NURSING IMPLICATIONS

Assessment

- Assess patient's mental status (orientation, mood, behavior, degree of sedation) prior to and periodically throughout therapy.
- Observe patient carefully when administering medication to ensure medication is actually taken and not hoarded.
- Assess fluid intake and bowel function. Increased bulk and fluids in the diet help minimize the constipating effects of this medication.
- Observe patient carefully for extrapyramidal symptoms (pill-rolling motions, drooling, tremors, rigidity, shuffling gait) and tardive dyskinesia (uncontrolled movements of face, mouth, tongue, or jaw and involuntary movements of extremities). Notify physician immediately at the onset of these symptoms.
- Monitor patient for akathisia (restlessness or need to keep moving). This may appear during first few days of treatment and may increase with increase in dosage. Elderly patients are more susceptible to akathisia. Treatment may include antiparkinsonian agents, propranolol, diazepam, or decrease in molindone dosage.
- Molindone may lower seizure threshold. Institute seizure precautions for patients with a history of a seizure disorder.
- Monitor patient for development of neuroleptic malignant syndrome (fever, respiratory distress, tachycardia, convulsions, diaphoresis, hypertension or hypotension, pallor, tiredness). Notify physician immediately if these symptoms occur.
- Ocular examinations may be required periodically during high-dose or prolonged therapy to monitor for deposition of particulate matter on the lens or cornea.

- **Lab Test Considerations:** Monitor WBC periodically throughout therapy. WBC may be increased or decreased, but molindone therapy may be continued unless clinical symptoms of leukocytosis or leukopenia occur. However, if the WBC is <4000 without clinical symptoms, it is recommended that therapy be discontinued until WBC increases. Therapy should then be re-evaluated.
  - Liver function tests should be monitored periodically during therapy.
  - May cause alterations in BUN, RBC counts, and serum glucose. These alterations are not clinically significant.
  - May cause elevated serum prolactin concentrations during chronic use.

Potential Nursing Diagnoses

- Thought processes, altered (indications).
- Bowel elimination, altered: constipation (side effects).
- Knowledge deficit related to medication regimen (patient/family teaching).

Implementation

- **General Info:** Available in tablet and oral solution.
- **PO:** Administer molindone with food or a full glass of milk or water to minimize gastric irritation. Liquid form may be administered undiluted or mixed with water, milk, fruit juice, or carbonated beverage.

Patient/Family Teaching

- Instruct patient to take medication exactly as directed and not to take more or less than prescribed. If a dose is missed, take as soon as remembered but not within 2 hr of next dose; do not double up on missed doses. Consult physician prior to discontinuing molindone; gradual withdrawal may be necessary.
- Inform patient of possibility of extra-

pyramidal symptoms and tardive dyskinesia. Caution patient to report these symptoms immediately to physician.
- Instruct patient not to take molindone within 2 hr of antacids or medications for treating diarrhea.
- Advise patient to make position changes slowly to minimize orthostatic hypotension. Exercise, hot weather, or hot baths may increase hypotensive effects.
- Medication may cause drowsiness. Caution patient to avoid driving or other activities requiring alertness until response to medication is known.
- Caution patient to avoid taking alcohol or other CNS depressants concurrently with this medication.
- Advise patient to use frequent mouth rinses, good oral hygiene, and sugarless gum or candy to minimize dry mouth.
- Advise patient to use sunscreen and protective clothing to prevent photosensitivity reactions.
- Instruct patient to notify physician promptly if tremors, involuntary muscle twitching, or visual disturbances occur.
- Emphasize the importance of routine follow-up examinations.

Evaluation

Effectiveness of therapy can be demonstrated by: ▪ Decrease in hallucinations, insomnia, agitation, hostility, and delusions. May require several wks of therapy to obtain optimal effects.

MONOAMINE OXIDASE INHIBITORS (MAO INHIBITORS)

isocarboxazid
(eye-soe-kar-**box**-a-zid)
Marplan

phenelzine
(**fen**-el-zeen)
Nardil

tranylcypromine
(tran-ill-**sip**-roe-meen)
Parnate

CLASSIFICATIONS:
Antidepressants—monoamine oxidase inhibitors
Pregnancy Category UK

INDICATIONS

▪ Treatment of neurotic or atypical depression, usually in conjunction with psychotherapy, in patients who may not tolerate other more conventional modes of therapy (tricyclic antidepressants or electroconvulsive therpy).

ACTION

▪ Inhibits the enzyme monoamine oxidase resulting in an accumulation of various neurotransmitters (dopamine, epinephrine, norepinephrine, and serotonin) in the body. **Therapeutic Effect:** ▪ Improved mood in depressed patients.

PHARMACOKINETICS

Absorption: All are well absorbed from the GI tract.
Distribution: All cross the placenta and probably enter breast milk.
Metabolism and Excretion: All are mostly metabolized by the liver.
Half-life: UK

CONTRAINDICATIONS AND PRECAUTIONS

Contraindicated in: ▪ Hypersensitivity ▪ Liver disease ▪ Severe renal disease ▪ Cerebrovascular disease ▪ Pheochromocytoma ▪ Congestive heart failure ▪ History of headache ▪ Patients >60 yr ▪ Concurrent meperidine administration.
Use Cautiously in: ▪ Patients who may be suicidal or have a history of drug dependency ▪ Symptomatic cardiovascular disease ▪ Hyperthyroidism ▪ Seizure disorders ▪ Pregnancy, lactation, or children (safety not established) ▪ Surgery (should be discontinued several wks prior to surgery if possible due to increased risk of unpredictable reactions).

ADVERSE REACTIONS AND SIDE EFFECTS*

CNS: restlessness, insomnia, dizziness, headache, confusion, **SEIZURES**, weakness, drowsiness.
EENT: glaucoma, nystagmus, blurred vision.
CV: **HYPERTENSIVE CRISIS**, orthostatic hypotension, arrhythmias, edema.
GI: constipation, anorexia, nausea, vomiting, diarrhea, abdominal pain, dry mouth.
GU: dysuria, urinary incontinence, urinary retention.
Derm: rashes.
Endo: hypoglycemia.
MS: arthralgia.

INTERACTIONS

Drug–Drug: ▪ Hypertensive crisis may occur with **amphetamines, methyldopa, levodopa, dopamine, epinephrine, norepinephrine, desipramine, imipramine, guanethidine, reserpine,** or **vasoconstrictors** ▪ Hyper- or hypotension, coma, convulsions, and death may occur with **narcotic analgesics** (avoid use of meperidine within 14–21 days of MAO inhibitor therapy—decrease initial dose of other agents to 25% of usual dose) ▪ Additive hypotension with **antihypertensives** or **spinal anesthesia** ▪ Additive hypoglycemia with **insulin** or **oral hypoglycemic agents**.
Drug–Food: ▪ Hypertensive crisis may occur with ingestion of foods containing high concentrations of **tyramine** (see Appendix K).

ROUTE AND DOSAGE

Isocarboxazid

- **PO (Adults):** 10–20 mg/day in single or divided doses (not to exceed 30 mg/day)

Phenylzine

- **PO (Adults):** 15 mg 3 times daily, increase to 60 mg/day in divided doses, then gradually reduce to smallest effective dose.

Tranylcypromine

- **PO (Adults):** 20 mg/day in 2 divided doses (morning and afternoon); can increase after 2–3 wk to 30 mg/day (20 mg in the morning and 10 mg in the afternoon).

PHARMACODYNAMICS (antidepressant effect)

	ONSET	PEAK	DURATION
isocarboxazid	1–4 wk	3–4 wk	2 wk
phenelzine	1–4 wk	2–6 wk	2 wk
tranylcypromine	several days	2–3 wk	3–5 days

NURSING IMPLICATIONS

Assessment

- □ Assess mental status and mood changes and anxiety level frequently. Assess for suicidal tendencies, especially during early therapy. Restrict amount of drug available to patient.
- □ Monitor blood pressure and pulse rate prior to and frequently throughout therapy. Notify physician promptly of significant changes.
- □ Monitor intake and output ratios and daily weight. Assess patient for peripheral edema and urinary retention.
- ▪ **Lab Test Considerations:** Assess hepatic function periodically during prolonged or high-dose therapy.
- □ Monitor serum or urine glucose closely in diabetic patients; hypoglycemia may occur.
- ▪ **Toxicity and Overdose:** Concurrent ingestion of tyramine-rich foods and many medications may result in a life-threatening hypertensive crisis. Signs and symptoms of hypertensive crisis include chest pain, severe headache, nausea and vomiting, photosensitivity, and enlarged pupils. Treatment includes IV phentolamine.
- □ Symptoms of overdose include anxiety, irritability, tachycardia, hypertension or hypotension, respiratory distress, dizziness, drowsines, hallucinations, confusion, seizures, fever, and diaphoresis. Treatment includes

*Underlines indicate most frequent; **CAPITALS** indicate life-threatening.

induction of vomiting or gastric lavage and supportive therapy as symptoms arise.

Potential Nursing Diagnoses

- Coping, ineffective individual (indications)
- Knowledge deficit related to medication regimen (patient/family teaching)
- Noncompliance (patient/family teaching)

Implementation

- **General Info:** Do not administer these medications in the evening because the psychomotor stimulating effects may cause insomnia or other sleep disturbances.
- **PO:** Tablets may be crushed and mixed with food or fluids for patients with difficulty swallowing.

Patient/Family Teaching

- Instruct patient to take medication exactly as directed. If a dose is missed, take if remembered within 2 hours; otherwise omit and return to regular dosage schedule. Medication should not be abruptly discontinued as withdrawal symptoms (confusion, hallucinations, nightmares, headache, nausea, diaphoresis, shivering, tachycardia, slurred speech, unsteady gait) may occur.
- Caution patient to avoid alcohol, CNS depressants, over-the-counter drugs, and foods or beverages containing tyramine (see Appendix K) during and for at least 2 wk after therapy has been discontinued; they may precipitate a hypertensive crisis. Physician should be contacted immediately if symptoms of hypertensive crisis develop.
- Medication may occasionally cause dizziness or drowsiness. Caution patient to avoid driving and other activities requiring alertness until response to medication is known.
- Caution patient to make position changes slowly to minimize orthostatic hypotension. Elderly patients are at increased risk for this side effect.
- Advise patient to notify physisican if dry mouth, urinary retention, or constipation occurs. Frequent rinses, good oral hygiene, and sugarless candy or gum may diminish dry mouth. An increase in fluid intake, fiber, and exercise may prevent constipation.
- Instruct patient to notify physician if severe headache, skin rash, diarrhea, swelling of feet, palpitations, or increased nervousness occur.
- Advise patient to notify physician or dentist of medication regimen prior to treatment or surgery. If possible, therapy should be discontinued at least 2 wk prior to surgery.
- Instruct patient to carry identification describing medication regimen at all times.
- Emphasize the importance of participation in psychotherapy if ordered by physician and follow-up examinations to evaluate progress. Ophthalmic testing should also be done periodically during long-term therapy.

Evaluation

Effectiveness of therapy can be demonstrated by: ▪ Improved mood in depressed patients ▫ Decreased anxiety ▫ Increased appetite ▫ Improved energy level ▫ Improved sleep. Patients may require 1–4 wk of therapy before therapeutic effects of medication are seen.

MORICIZINE

(more-i-siz-een)
Ethmozine

CLASSIFICATION(S):
Antiarrhythmic—class I
Pregnancy Category B

INDICATIONS

- Treatment of life-threatening ventricular arrhythmias, including sustained ventricular tachycardia.

ACTION

- Suppresses abnormal automaticity and prolongs PR and QRS interval by blocking fast sodium channel in myocardial tissue ▪ Also has membrane stabilizing and local anesthetic properties. **Therapeutic Effect:** ▪ Suppression of life-threatening arrhythmias.

PHARMACOKINETICS

Absorption: Well absorbed, but rapidly metabolized following oral administration.
Distribution: 95% bound to plasma proteins. Enters breast milk.
Metabolism and Excretion: Extensively metabolized, <1% excreted unchanged in the urine. Metabolites may be active.
Half-life: 1.5–3.5 hr.

CONTRAINDICATIONS AND PRECAUTIONS

Contraindicated in: ▪ Hypersensitivity ▪ Cardiogenic shock ▪ 2nd- or 3rd-degree AV block or bundle branch block (unless a pacemaker has been placed).
Use Cautiously in: ▪ Electrolyte disturbances ▪ Severe renal or hepatic impairment (dosage reduction may be necessary) ▪ Pregnancy, lactation, or children (safety not established) ▪ Congestive heart failure.
Extreme Caution in: ▪ Sick-sinus syndrome.

ADVERSE REACTIONS AND SIDE EFFECTS*

CNS: dizziness, headache, fatigue, weakness, nervousness, sleep disorders.
EENT: blurred vision.
Resp: dyspnea.
CV: ARRHYTHMIAS, chest pain, congestive heart failure, palpitations.
GI: nausea, vomiting, dyspepsia, diarrhea, dry mouth.
Derm: sweating.
MS: musculoskeletal pain.
Neuro: paresthesia.
Misc: drug fever.

INTERACTIONS

Drug-Drug: ▪ Decreases blood levels of **theophylline** ▪ **Cimetidine** increases blood levels of moricizine.

ROUTE AND DOSAGE

- **PO (Adults):** 600–900 mg/day given q 8–12 hr. May increase by 150 mg/day every 3 days as required and tolerated.

PHARMACODYNAMICS

	ONSET	PEAK*	DURATION
PO	UK	0.5–2 hr	8–12 hr

*Blood levels.

NURSING IMPLICATIONS

Assessment

- Monitor ECG or Holtor monitor prior to and periodically throughout therapy. May cause PR prolongation and QT prolongation.
- Monitor blood pressure and pulse periodically throughout course of therapy.
- Monitor intake and output ratios and daily weight. Assess patient for signs of congestive heart failure (peripheral edema, rales/crackles, dyspnea, weight gain, jugular venous distension).
- **Lab Test Considerations:** Renal, pulmonary, and hepatic function, and CBC should be evaluated periodically on patients receiving long-term therapy.

Potential Nursing Diagnoses

- Cardiac output, decreased (indications).
- Knowledge deficit related to medication regimen (patient/family teaching).

Implementation

- **General Info:** Moricizine therapy should be initiated in a hospital with facilities for cardiac rhythm monitoring.
- Previous antiarrhythmic therapy should be withdrawn 1–2 half-lives before starting moricizine.
- Dosage adjustments should be at

*Underlines indicate most frequent; **CAPITALS** indicate life-threatening.

least 3 days apart due to the long half-life of moricizine.

- Pre-existing hypokalemia, hyperkalemia, or hypomagnesemia should be corrected prior to instituting therapy.
- **PO:** Tablets are usually administered every 8 hr. Total daily dose may be divided and administered every 12 hr for greater compliance, but risk of adverse reactions is greater with higher single dose.

Patient/Family Teaching

- Instruct patient to take medication around the clock exactly as directed, even if feeling better. Missed doses should be taken as soon as remembered if within 6 hr; omit if remembered later. Gradual dosage reduction may be necessary.
- Medication may cause dizziness or visual disturbances. Caution patient to avoid driving and other activities requiring alertness until response to medication is known.
- Advise patient to notify physician or dentist of medication regimen prior to treatment or surgery.
- Instruct patient to notify physician if chest pain, shortness of breath, fever, or diaphoresis occurs.
- Advise patient to carry identification describing disease process and medication regimen at all times.
- Emphasize the importance of follow-up examinations to monitor progress.

Evaluation

Effectiveness of therapy can be demonstrated by: ▪ Decrease in frequency of ventricular arrhythmias.

MORPHINE

(**mor**-feen)

Astramorph, Duramorph, {Epimorph}, {Morphine H.P.}, {Morphitec}, {M.O.S.}, {M.O.S.-S.R.}, MS, MSO_4, MS Contin, MSIR, Oramorph SR RMS, Roxanol, Roxanol SR, {Statex}

CLASSIFICATION(S):
Narcotic analgesic—agonist
Schedule II
Pregnancy Category C

INDICATIONS

▪ Management of severe pain ▪ Management of pulmonary edema ▪ Management of pain associated with myocardial infarction.

ACTION

▪ Binds to opiate receptors in the CNS. Alters the perception of and response to painful stimuli, while producing generalized CNS depression. **Therapeutic Effect:** ▪ Decrease in severity of pain.

PHARMACOKINETICS

Absorption: Variably absorbed following oral administration. More reliably absorbed from Rect, SC, and IM sites.
Distribution: Widely distributed. Crosses the placenta and enters breast milk in small amounts.
Metabolism and Excretion: Mostly metabolized by the liver.
Half-life: 2–3 hr.

CONTRAINDICATIONS AND PRECAUTIONS

Contraindicated in: ▪ Hypersensitivity ▪ Pregnancy or lactation (avoid chronic use).

Use Cautiously in: ▪ Head trauma ▪ Increased intracranial pressure ▪ Severe renal, hepatic, or pulmonary disease ▪ Hypothyroidism ▪ Adrenal insufficiency ▪ Alcoholism ▪ Elderly or debilitated patients (dosage reduction suggested) ▪ Undiagnosed abdominal pain ▪ Prostatic hypertrophy ▪ During labor (has been used to relieve pain; may cause respiratory depression in the newborn).

ADVERSE REACTIONS AND SIDE EFFECTS*

CNS: <u>sedation</u>, <u>confusion</u>, headache, euphoria, floating feeling, unusual

{} = Available in Canada only.
*Underlines indicate most frequent; **CAPITALS** indicate life-threatening.

dreams, hallucinations, dysphoria, dizziness.
EENT: miosis, diplopia, blurred vision.
Resp: respiratory depression.
CV: hypotension, bradycardia.
GI: nausea, vomiting, constipation.
GU: urinary retention.
Derm: sweating, flushing.
Misc: tolerance, physical dependence, psychological dependence.

INTERACTIONS

Drug-Drug: ▪ Use with **extreme caution** in patients receiving **MAO inhibitors** (may result in unpredictable, severe reactions—decrease initial dose of morphine to 25% of usual dose) ▪ Additive CNS depression with **alcohol, sedative/hypnotics,** and **antihistamines** ▪ Administration of **partial-antagonist narcotic analgesics** may precipitate narcotic withdrawal in physically dependent patients ▪ May increase risk of **zidovudine** toxicity ▪ **Nalbuphine** or **pentazocine** may decrease analgesia.

ROUTE AND DOSAGE

- **PO (Adults):** 10–30 mg q 4 hr or 30 mg q 8–12 hr as extended-release preparations (q 8 hr for Roxanol or q 12 hr for MS Contin or Oramorph SR).
- **IM, SC (Adults):** 5–20 mg q 4 hr as needed.
- **SC (Children):** 0.1–0.2 mg/kg q 4 hr (not to exceed 15 mg/dose).
- **IV (Adults):** 2.5–15 mg q 4 hr or IV infusion initiated with a loading dose of 15 mg followed by infusion at 0.8–10 mg/hr, rate increased as needed. Doses of 20–150 mg/hr have been used.
- **IM, IV (Children):** 50–100 mcg/kg (not to exceed 10 mg/dose).
- **Rect (Adults):** 10–30 mg q 4 hr.
- **Epidural (Adults):** 2–10 mg/day (increased as needed) or up to 0.6–0.8 mg/kg/day as a continuous infusion.
- **Intrathecal (Adults):** 0.2–1 mg as a single dose.

PHARMACODYNAMICS (analgesia)

	ONSET	PEAK	DURATION
PO	UK	60 min	4–5 hr
PO-ER	UK	UK	8–12 hr
IM	10–30 min	30–60 min	4–5 hr
SC	20 min	50–90 min	4–5 hr
Rect	UK	20–60 min	4–5 hr
IV	rapid	20 min	4–5 hr
Epidural	6–30 min	UK	up to 24 hr
IT	rapid (min)	UK	up to 24 hr

NURSING IMPLICATIONS

Assessment

- □ Assess type, location, and intensity of pain prior to and 30–60 min following administration.
- □ Assess blood pressure, pulse, and respiratory rate before and periodically during administration.
- □ Prolonged use may lead to physical and psychological dependence and tolerance. This should not prevent patient from receiving adequate analgesia. Most patients who receive morphine for medical reasons do not develop psychological dependency. Progressively higher doses may be required to relieve pain with long-term therapy.
- □ Assess bowel function routinely. Increased intake of fluids and bulk, stool softeners, and laxatives may minimize constipating effects.
- □ Monitor intake and output ratios. If significant discrepancies occur, assess for urinary retention and inform physician.
- ▪ **Lab Test Considerations:** May increase plasma amylase and lipase levels.
- ▪ **Toxicity and Overdose:** If overdosage occurs, naloxone (Narcan) is the antidote. Monitor patient closely; dose may need to be repeated or may need to be administered as an infusion.

Potential Nursing Diagnoses

- ▪ Comfort, altered: pain (indications).
- ▪ Sensory-perceptual alteration: visual, auditory (side effects).

- Injury, high risk for (side effects).
- Knowledge deficit related to medication regimen (patient/family teaching).

Implementation

- **General Info:** Explain therapeutic value of medication prior to administration to enhance the analgesic effect.
  - Regularly administered doses may be more effective than prn administration. Analgesic is more effective if given before pain becomes severe.
  - Coadministration with non-narcotic analgesics may have additive analgesic effects and may permit lower doses.
  - When transferring from other narcotics or other forms of morphine to extended-release tablets, administer a total daily dose of oral morphine equivalent to previous daily dose (see Appendix B) and divided every 8 hr (Roxanol SR) or every 12 hr (MS Contin, Oramorph SR).
  - Medication should be discontinued gradually after long-term use, to prevent withdrawal symptoms.
  - Available in tablet, long-acting tablet, soln, concentrated soln, suppository, and injectable forms.
- **PO:** Doses may be administered with food or milk to minimize GI irritation.
  - Extended-release tablet should be swallowed whole; do not crush, break, or chew.
  - Soln may be diluted in a glass of fruit juice just prior to administration to improve taste.
- **SC/IM:** Use IM route for repeated doses, as morphine is irritating to SC tissues.
- **IV:** Soln is colorless; do not administer discolored soln.
- **Direct IV:** Dilute with at least 5 ml of sterile water or 0.9% NaCl for injection.
  - *Rate:* Administer 2.5–15 mg over 4–5 min. Rapid administration may lead to increased respiratory depression, hypotension, and circulatory collapse.
  - Do not use IV administration without antidote available.
- **Continuous Infusion:** May be added to D5W, D10W, 0.9% NaCl, 0.45% NaCl, Ringer's or lactated Ringer's soln, dextrose/saline soln, or dextrose/Ringer's or lactated Ringer's soln in a concentration of 0.1–1 mg/ml or greater for continuous infusion.
  - *Rate:* Administer via infusion pump to control the rate. Dose should be titrated to ensure adequate pain relief without excessive sedation, respiratory depression, or hypotension.
  - May be administered via patient-controlled analgesia (PCA) pump.
- **Syringe Compatibility:** atropine, benzquinamide, butorphanol, chlorpromazine, cimetidine, dimenhydrinate, diphenhydramine, droperidol, fentanyl, glycopyrrolate, hydroxyzine, metoclopramide, midazolam, pentazocine, perphenazine, promazine, ranitidine, or scopolamine.
- **Syringe Incompatibility:** meperidine or thiopental.
- **Y-Site Compatibility:** acyclovir, amikacin, aminophylline, ampicillin, ampicillin/sulbactam, atracurium, calcium chloride, cefamandole, cefazolin, cefoperazone, ceforanide, cefotaxime, cefotetan, cefoxitin, ceftizoxime, cefuroxime, cephalothin, cephapirin, chloramphenicol, clindamycin, co-trimoxazole, doxycycline, enalaprilat, erythromycin lactobionate, esmolol, famotidine, foscarnet, gentamicin, heparin, hydrocortisone sodium succinate, insulin, kanamycin, labetalol, metronidazole, mezlocillin, moxalactam, nafcillin, ondansetron, oxacillin, oxytocin, pancuronium, penicillin G potassium, piperacillin, potassium chloride, ranitidine, sodium bicarbonate, ticarcillin, ticarcillin/clavulanate, tobramycin, vancomycin, vecuronium.
- **Y-Site Incompatibility:** minocycline or tetracycline.
- **Additive Compatibility:** dobutamine, succinylcholine, or verapamil.
- **Additive Incompatibility:** aminophyl-

line, amobarbital, chlorothiazide, heparin, meperidine, methicillin, phenobarbital, phenytoin, sodium bicarbonate, sodium iodide, or thiopental.

Patient/Family Teaching

- □ Instruct patient on how and when to ask for prn pain medication.
- □ Medication may cause drowsiness or dizziness. Caution patient to call for assistance when ambulating or smoking, and to avoid driving or other activities requiring alertness until response to medication is known.
- □ Advise patient to make position changes slowly to minimize orthostatic hypotension.
- □ Caution patient to avoid concurrent use of alcohol or other CNS depressants with this medication.
- □ Encourage patient to turn, cough, and breathe deeply every 2 hr to prevent atelectasis.

Evaluation

Effectiveness of therapy can be demonstrated by: ▪ Decrease in severity of pain without a significant alteration in level of consciousness, respiratory status, or blood pressure.

MOXALACTAM

(**mox**-a-lak-tam)

Lamoxactam, Latamoxef, Moxam

CLASSIFICATION(S):
Anti-infectives—third generation cephalosporin
Pregnancy Category C

INDICATIONS

▪ Treatment of the following conditions: □ Skin and skin structure infections □ Bone and joint infections □ Urinary and gynecologic infections □ Respiratory tract infections □ Intra-abdominal infections □ Septicemia □ Meningitis.

ACTION

▪ Binds to the bacterial cell wall membrane, causing cell death. **Therapeutic Effect:** ▪ Bactericidal action against susceptible bacteria. **Spectrum:** ▪ Spectrum is similar to that of second generation cephalosporins; however, activity against staphylococci is diminished in comparison while activity against gram-negative pathogens is enhanced, even for organisms resistant to first and second generation agents ▪ Notable is increased action against: □ *Citrobacter* □ *Enterobacter* □ *Escherichia coli* □ *Klebsiella pneumoniae* □ *Niesseria* □ *Proteus* □ *Providencia* □ *Serratia* □ *Pseudomonas aeruginosa* ▪ Has some activity against anaerobes, including *Bacteroides fragilis*.

PHARMACOKINETICS

Absorption: Well absorbed following IM administration.
Distribution: Widely distributed. Crosses the placenta and enters breast milk in low concentrations. CSF penetration is better than with first and second generation agents.
Metabolism and Excretion: Primarily renally excreted (>90%).
Half-life: 2.0–3.5 hr.

CONTRAINDICATIONS AND PRECAUTIONS

Contraindicated in: ▪ Hypersensitivity to cephalosporins ▪ Serious hypersensitivity to penicillins.
Use Cautiously in: ▪ Renal impairment (dosage reduction required) ▪ Pregnancy or lactation (safety not established).

ADVERSE REACTIONS AND SIDE EFFECTS*

CNS: SEIZURES (high doses).
GI: <u>nausea</u>, <u>vomiting</u>, <u>diarrhea</u>, cramps, PSEUDOMEMBRANOUS COLITIS.
Derm: <u>rashes</u>, urticaria.
Hemat: blood dyscrasias, hemolytic anemia, bleeding.

*<u>Underlines</u> indicate most frequent; **CAPITALS** indicate life-threatening.

Local: phlebitis at IV site, pain at IM site.
Misc: superinfection, allergic reactions, including ANAPHYLAXIS and serum sickness.

INTERACTIONS

Drug–Drug: ▪ **Probenecid** decreases excretion and increases serum levels ▪ Ingestion of **alcohol** within 48–72 hr may result in a disulfiram-like reaction ▪ Increased risk of bleeding with **anticoagulants, thrombolytic agents, plicamycin,** or **nonsteroidal anti-inflammatory agents.**

ROUTE AND DOSAGE

- **IM, IV (Adults):** 2–4 g daily in divided doses q 8 hr (12 g/day maximum); as little as 250 mg q 12 hr may be used for urinary tract infections.
- **IM, IV (Children 1–14 yr):** 50 mg/kg q 6–8 hr.
- **IM, IV (1 mon–1 yr):** 50 mg/kg q 6 hr.
- **IM, IV (Neonates 1–4 wk):** 50 mg/kg q 8 hr.
- **IM, IV (Neonates <1 wk):** 50 mg/kg q 12 hr.

PHARMACODYNAMICS (blood levels)

	ONSET	PEAK
IM	rapid	0.5–1 hr
IV	rapid	end of infusion

NURSING IMPLICATIONS

Assessment

- Assess patient for infection (vital signs; appearance of wound, sputum, urine, and stool; WBC) at beginning and throughout course of therapy.
- Obtain a history before initiating therapy to determine previous use of and reactions to penicillins or cephalosporins. Persons with a negative history of penicillin sensitivity may still have an allergic response.
- Obtain specimens for culture and sensitivity prior to initiating therapy. First dose may be given before receiving results.
- Observe patient for signs and symptoms of anaphylaxis (rash, pruritus, laryngeal edema, wheezing). Discontinue the drug and notify physician immediately if these occur. Keep epinephrine, an antihistamine, and resuscitation equipment close by in the event of an anaphylactic reaction.
- Monitor prothrombin time and assess patient for bleeding (guaiac stools; check for hematuria, bleeding gums, ecchymosis) daily in patients receiving moxalactam, as it may cause hypoprothrombinemia. Elderly or debilitated patients are at greater risk of developing hypoprothrombinemia. If bleeding occurs, it can be reversed with vitamin K, or prophylactic vitamin K 10 mg/wk may be given.
- **Lab Test Considerations:** Peak and trough blood levels should be drawn periodically on patients with renal dysfunction.
- May cause false-positive results for Coombs' test and may interfere with cross-matching of blood.

Potential Nursing Diagnoses

- Infection, high risk for (indications, side effects).
- Bowel elimination, altered: diarrhea (adverse reactions).
- Knowledge deficit related to medication regimen (patient/family teaching).

Implementation

- **General Info:** Soln may range from colorless to a light straw color.
- **IM:** Reconstitute doses with 3 ml of sterile or bacteriostatic water for injection or 0.9% NaCl to each 1-g vial. Shake well to dissolve. Physician may order dilution with 0.5% lidocaine HCl to minimize injection discomfort.
- Inject deep into a well-developed muscle mass; massage well.
- **IV:** Change sites every 48–72 hr to prevent phlebitis. Discontinue other IV soln during IV administration of cephalosporins.
- **Direct IV:** Add 10 ml of sterile water, D5W, or 0.9% NaCl to each 1 g of moxalactam.

- ▫ *Rate:* Administer slowly over 3–5 min (15–20 min for children).
- ▪ **Intermittent Infusion:** Each 1 g in soln should be further diluted in at least 20 ml of 0.9% NaCl, D5W, D10W, D5/0.25% NaCl, D5/0.45% NaCl, D5/0.9% NaCl, D5/LR, Ringer's or lactated Ringer's soln. Soln is stable for 24 hr at room temperature and 96 hr if refrigerated.
- ▫ *Rate:* Administer over 30 min. Monitor for phlebitis.
- ▪ **Continuous Infusion:** May be diluted in 500–1000 ml for continuous infusion.
- ▪ **Syringe Compatibility:** heparin.
- ▪ **Y-Site Compatibility:** cyclophosphamide, hydromorphone, magnesium sulfate, meperidine, morphine, or perphenazine.
- ▪ **Additive Compatibility:** metronidazole, ranitidine, or verapamil.
- ▪ **Additive Incompatibility:** Do not admix with aminoglycosides.

Patient/Family Teaching

- ▫ Advise patient to report the signs of superinfection (furry overgrowth on the tongue, vaginal itching or discharge, loose or foul-smelling stools) and allergy.
- ▫ Caution patient that concurrent use of alcohol with moxalactam may cause a disulfiram-like reaction (abdominal cramps, nausea, vomiting, hypotension, palpitations, dyspnea, tachycardia, sweating, flushing). Alcohol and medications containing alcohol should be avoided during and for several days after therapy.
- ▫ Instruct patient to notify physician if diarrhea and fever develop, especially if loose stools contain blood, pus, or mucus. Advise patient not to treat diarrhea without consulting physician or pharmacist.

Evaluation

Clinical response can be evaluated by: ▪ Resolution of the signs and symptoms of infection. Length of time for complete resolution depends on the organism and site of infection.

MULTIPLE VITAMINS—ORAL

Abdec, Day-Vite, Multi-Thera, One-A-Day, Optilets 500, Poly-Vi-Sol, Quintabs, Theragran, Theravee, Unicap, Vi-Daylin

MULTIVITAMIN INFUSION

Berocca Parenteral Nutrition, M.V.C. 9 + 3, M.V.C. Plus, M.V.I.-12, M.V.I. Pediatric

CLASSIFICATION(S):
Vitamins—multiple, parenteral, Vitamins—multiple, oral
Pregnancy Category UK

INDICATIONS

▪ **PO:** Treatment and prevention of vitamin deficiencies. Special formulations are available for patients with particular needs, including: ▫ Prenatal multiple vitamins (with larger doses of folic acid) ▫ Multiple vitamins with iron ▫ Multiple vitamins with fluoride ▫ Multiple vitamins with minerals or trace elements ▪ **Parenteral:** Treatment and prevention of vitamin deficiencies in patients who are unable to ingest oral feedings or vitamins.

ACTION

▪ Contain fat-soluble vitamins (A, D, and E) and water-soluble vitamins (B-complex vitamins B_1, B_2, B_3, B_5, B_6, B_{12}, vitamin C, biotin, and folic acid). These vitamins are a diverse group of compounds necessary for normal growth and development that act as coenzymes or catalysts in numerous metabolic processes. **Therapeutic Effect:** ▪ ***PO:*** Prevention of deficiency or replacement in patients whose nutritional status is questionable ▪ ***Parenteral:*** Replacement in patients who are unable to ingest oral feedings or vitamins.

PHARMACOKINETICS

Absorption: Well absorbed from the GI tract following oral administration; some processes are active, some are passive. Absorption of water-soluble vi-

tamins generally increases in deficiency states. Absorption of some lipid-soluble vitamins may require bile acids.
Distribution: Widely distributed, cross the placenta and enter breast milk. Fat-soluble vitamins (A, D, and E) are stored in fatty tissues and the liver.
Metabolism and Excretion: Utilized in various biologic processes. Excess amounts of water-soluble vitamins (B vitamins, vitamin C, and folic acid) are excreted unchanged by the kidneys.
Half-life: UK.

CONTRAINDICATIONS AND PRECAUTIONS

Contraindicated in: ▪ Hypersensitivity to preservatives, colorants, or additives, including tartrazine, saccharin, and aspartame (oral forms) ▪ Hypersensitivity to preservatives, including polysorbates, propylene glycol, EDTA, or benzyl alcohol (parenteral forms).

ADVERSE REACTIONS AND SIDE EFFECTS*

Note: In recommended doses, adverse reactions are extremely rare.

Misc: allergic reactions to preservatives, additives, or colorants.

INTERACTIONS

Drug–Drug: ▪ Large amounts of vitamin B_6 may interfere with the beneficial effect of **levodopa**.

ROUTE AND DOSAGE

- **PO (Adults and Children):** 1 dosage unit (tablet/capsule/dropperful)/day or amount recommended by individual manufacturer.
- **IV (Adults and Children):** Amount sufficient to meet RDA (Recommended Daily Allowances—see Appendix L). for age group. Usually added to large volume of parenteral or total parenteral nutrition (hyperalimentation) soln.

PHARMACODYNAMICS

	ONSET	PEAK	DURATION
PO	UK	UK	UK
IV	UK	UK	UK

NURSING IMPLICATIONS

Assessment

- □ Assess patient for signs of nutritional deficiency prior to and throughout therapy. Patients at risk include those who are elderly, debilitated, burned, unable to take oral nutrition, and those with malabsorption syndromes or chronic alcoholism.
- ▪ **Toxicity and Overdose:** Toxicity rarely occurs with multivitamin preparations due to the small amounts per unit of fat-soluble vitamins. For symptoms, see individual vitamin entries.
- □ If overdose occurs, treatment includes induction of emesis or gastric lavage, calcium gluconate IV if hypocalcemic, and maintenance of high urine output.

Potential Nursing Diagnoses

- ▪ Nutrition, altered: less than body requirements (indications).
- ▪ Knowledge deficit related to dietary needs and medication regimen (patient/family teaching).

Implementation

- ▪ **General Info:** Vitamins are usually given orally but may be given parenterally to patients in whom oral administration is not feasible.
- □ Available in many combinations with folic acid, fluoride, minerals, and trace elements. Combinations with >1 mg folic acid require a prescription.
- ▪ **PO:** Forms are not standardized.
- □ Chewable tablets should be crushed or chewed prior to swallowing.
- □ Liquid preparations may be dropped directly into mouth or mixed with juice or cereal.
- ▪ **IV:** Administer multivitamin infusion

*Underlines indicate most frequent; **CAPITALS** indicate life-threatening.

by infusion only; do not use direct IV injection.
- □ Soln is bright yellow and will color IV soln.
- ▪ **Continuous Infusion:** Dilute each 5- or 10-ml ampule in 500–1000 ml of D5/LR, D5/0.9% NaCl, D5W, D10W, D20W, lactated Ringer's injection, 0.9% NaCl, 3% NaCl, or ⅙ M sodium lactate. Do not administer soln that has crystallized.
- ▪ **Y-Site Compatibility:** acyclvoir, ampicillin, cefazolin, cephalothin, cephapirin, erythromycin lactobionate, gentamicin, or tetracycline.
- ▪ **Additive Compatibility:** cefoxitin, isoproterenol, methyldopate, metoclopramide, metronidazole with sodium bicarbonate, netilmicin, norepinephrine, sodium bicarbonate, or verapamil.
- ▪ **Additive Incompatibility:** Incompatible in soln with many antibiotics or bleomycin.

PATIENT/FAMILY TEACHING

- □ Encourage patient to comply with physician's recommendations. Explain that the best source of vitamins is a well-balanced diet with foods from the 4 basic food groups.
- □ Advise parents not to refer to chewable multivitamins for children as candy.

EVALUATION

Effectiveness of therapy can be demonstrated by: ▪ Prevention or decrease in the symptoms of vitamin deficiency.

MUPIROCIN

(myoo-**peer**-oh-sin)
Bactroban, Pseudomonic acid A

CLASSIFICATION(S):
Anti-infective—topical
Pregnancy Category B

INDICATIONS

▪ Treatment of impetigo.

ACTION

▪ Inhibits bacterial protein synthesis. **Therapeutic Effect:** ▪ Inhibition of bacterial growth and reproduction. **Spectrum:** ▪ Greatest activity against gram-positive organisms, including: □ *Staphylococcus aureus* □ Beta hemolytic streptococci.

PHARMACOKINETICS

Absorption: Minimal systemic absorption.
Distribution: Remains in the stratum corneum for prolonged periods of time (72 hr).
Metabolism and Excretion: Metabolized in the skin, removed by desquamation.
Half-life: UK.

CONTRAINDICATIONS AND PRECAUTIONS

Contraindicated in: ▪ Hypersensitivity to mupirocin or polyethylene glycol.
Use Cautiously in: ▪ Pregnancy or lactation (safety not established).

ADVERSE REACTIONS AND SIDE EFFECTS*

Derm: burning, stinging, pain, erythema, dry skin, tenderness, contact dermatitis, increased exudate.
GI: nausea.

INTERACTIONS

Drug–Drug: ▪ None known.

ROUTE AND DOSAGE

- ▪ **Top (Adults and Children):** 2% ointment applied tid.

PHARMACODYNAMICS

	ONSET	PEAK	DURATION
Top	UK	3–5 days	72 hr

NURSING IMPLICATIONS

ASSESSMENT

- □ Assess lesions prior to and daily during therapy.

*Underlines indicate most frequent; **CAPITALS** indicate life-threatening.

POTENTIAL NURSING DIAGNOSES

- Skin integrity, impaired: actual (indications).
- Infection, high risk for (indications, patient/family teaching).
- Knowledge deficit related to medication regimen (patient/family teaching).

IMPLEMENTATION

- **Top:** Apply a small amount of mupirocin ointment to the affected area tid. Treated area may be covered with gauze if desired.

PATIENT/FAMILY TEACHING

- Instruct patient on the correct application of mupirocin. Advise patient to apply medication exactly as directed for the full course of therapy.
- Teach patient and family appropriate hygienic measures to prevent spread of impetigo.
- Instruct parents to notify school nurse for screening and prevention of transmission.
- Patient should consult physician if symptoms have not improved in 3–5 days.

EVALUATION

Effectiveness of therapy can be demonstrated by: ▪ Healing of skin lesions. If no clinical response is seen in 3–5 days, condition should be re-evaluated.

MUROMONAB-CD3

(myoor-oh-**mon**-ab CD3)
Orthoclone OKT3

CLASSIFICATION(S):
Immunosuppressant—monoclonal antibody
Pregnancy Category C

INDICATIONS

▪ Treatment of acute renal allograft rejection reactions in transplant patients that have occurred despite conventional antirejection therapy. **Unlabeled Use:** ▪ Treatment of acute hepatic or cardiac allograft rejection reactions in transplant patients that have occurred despite conventional antirejection therapy.

ACTION

▪ A purified immunoglobulin antibody that acts as an immunosuppressant by interfering with normal T cell function. **Therapeutic Effect:** ▪ Reversal of graft rejection in transplant patients.

PHARMACOKINETICS

Absorption: Administered IV only, resulting in complete bioavailability.
Distribution: UK.
Metabolism and Excretion: UK.
Half-life: UK.

CONTRAINDICATIONS AND PRECAUTIONS

Contraindicated in: ▪ Hypersensitivity to muromonab-CD3, murine (mouse) proteins, or polysorbate ▪ Previous muromonab therapy ▪ Fluid overload ▪ Fever >37.8°C or 110°F ▪ Chickenpox or recent exposure to chickenpox ▪ Herpes zoster.
Use Cautiously in: ▪ Active infections ▪ Depressed bone marrow reserve ▪ Chronic debilitating illnesses ▪ Congestive heart failure ▪ Pregnancy, lactation, or children <2 yr (safety not established).

ADVERSE REACTIONS AND SIDE EFFECTS*

CNS: <u>tremor</u>, aseptic meningitis, dizziness.
Resp: <u>dyspnea</u>, <u>shortness of breath</u>, <u>wheezing</u>, PULMONARY EDEMA.
CV: <u>chest pain</u>.
GI: <u>vomiting</u>, <u>nausea</u>, <u>diarrhea</u>.
Misc: <u>fever</u>, <u>chills</u>, INFECTIONS, increased risk of lymphoma, <u>hypersensitivity reactions</u>.

INTERACTIONS

Drug-Drug: ▪ Additive immunosuppression with other **immunosuppressive agents** ▪ Concurrent **prednisone** and **azathioprine** dosages should be

*<u>Underlines</u> indicate most frequent; **CAPITALS** indicate life-threatening.

reduced during muromonab therapy (increased risk of infection and lymphoproliferative disorders) ▪ **Cyclosporine** should be reduced or discontinued during muromonab-CD3 therapy (increased risk of infection and lymphoproliferative disorders).

ROUTE AND DOSAGE

- **IV (Adults):** 5 mg/day for 10–14 days (pretreatment with glucocorticoids, acetaminophen, and antihistamines may be necessary to decrease febrile reactions).

PHARMACODYNAMICS (noted as levels of circulating CD3-positive T cells)

	ONSET	PEAK	DURATION
IV	min	2–7 days	1 wk

NURSING IMPLICATIONS

Assessment

- Assess for fluid overload (monitor weight and intake and output, assess for edema and rales/crackles). Notify physician if patient has experienced 3% or more weight gain in the previous wk. Chest x-ray examination should be obtained prior to beginning therapy. Fluid-overloaded patients are at high risk of developing pulmonary edema. Monitor vital signs and breath sounds closely.
- Assess for fever and chills, nausea and vomiting, chest pain, shortness of breath, dizziness, diarrhea, and trembling of hands. The severity of this reaction is greatest with initial dose. Reaction occurs within 45–60 min and may persist for up to 6 hr. Prophylactic glucocorticoids, antihistamines, and acetaminophen may be ordered prior to administration of muromonab-CD3, especially with the initial doses. Hydrocortisone IV may also be ordered 30 min after the first and possibly second dose to control respiratory side effects.
- Monitor for infection (fever, chills, rash, sore throat, purulent discharge, dysuria). Notify physician immediately if these symptoms occur, as they may necessitate discontinuation of therapy.
- Monitor for development of aseptic meningitis. Onset is usually within 3 days of beginning therapy. Assess for fever, headache, nuchal rigidity, and photophobia.
- **Lab Test Considerations:** Monitor CBC and differential prior to and periodically throughout therapy.
- Monitor assays of T cell with CD3 antigen daily.

Potential Nursing Diagnoses

- Infection, high risk for (side effects).
- Fluid volume excess (side effects).
- Knowledge deficit related to medication regimen (patient/family teaching).

Implementation

- **General Info:** Physician will reduce dosage of glucocorticoids and azathioprine and discontinue cyclosporine during 10–14 day course of muromonab-CD3. Cyclosporine may be resumed 3 days before end of therapy.
- Initial dose is administered during hospitalization; patient should be monitored closely for 48 hr. Subsequent doses may be administered on outpatient basis.
- Keep medication refrigerated at 2–8°C. Do not shake vial.
- **Direct IV:** Draw soln into syringe via low-protein-binding 0.2- or 22-micrometer filter to ensure removal of translucent protein particles that may be present. Discard filter and attach 20-gauge needle for IV administration.
- Do not administer as an infusion; do not admix; do not administer in IV line containing other medications.
- *Rate:* Administer IV push over <1 min.

Patient/Family Teaching

- Explain purpose of medication to patient. Inform patient of possible initial-dose side effects, which are markedly reduced in subsequent doses. Explain that patient will need

to resume lifelong therapy with other immunosuppressive drugs after completion of muromonab course.
- Instruct patient not to receive any vaccinations and to avoid contact with persons receiving oral polio vaccine without advice of physician.
- Instruct patient to continue to avoid crowds and persons with known infections, as this drug also suppresses the immune system.

Evaluation

Effectiveness of therapy can be demonstrated by: ▪ Reversal of the symptoms of acute organ rejection.

NADOLOL
(nay-doe-lole)
Corgard

CLASSIFICATION(S):
Beta-adrenergic blocker—nonselective, Antihypertensive, Antianginal
Pregnancy Category C

INDICATIONS

▪ Used alone or in combination with other agents in the treatment of hypertension ▪ Used alone or with other agents in the management of angina pectoris. **Unlabeled Uses:** ▪ Treatment of: ▫ Tachyarrhythmias ▫ Anxiety ▫ Aggressive behavior ▫ Tremors ▫ Rebleeding of esophageal vances ▫ Migraine prophylaxis.

ACTION

▪ Blocks stimulation of $beta_1$ (myocardial) and $beta_2$ (pulmonary, vascular, or uterine) receptor sites. **Therapeutic Effects:** ▪ Decreased heart rate and blood pressure.

PHARMACOKINETICS

Absorption: Variably (30%) absorbed following oral administration.
Distribution: Minimal penetration of the CNS. Crosses the placenta and enters breast milk.
Metabolism and Excretion: 70% excreted unchanged by the kidneys.
Half-life: 10–24 hr (increased in renal failure).

CONTRAINDICATIONS AND PRECAUTIONS

Contraindicated in: ▪ Uncompensated congestive heart failure ▪ Pulmonary edema ▪ Cardiogenic shock ▪ Bradycardia ▪ Heart block ▪ COPD or asthma.
Use Cautiously in: ▪ Thyrotoxicosis or hypoglycemia (may mask symptoms) ▪ Renal impairment (dosage reduction suggested) ▪ Pregnancy or lactation (may cause apnea, low Apgar scores, bradycardia, and hypoglycemia in the newborn) ▪ Children (safety not established).

ADVERSE REACTIONS AND SIDE EFFECTS*

CNS: fatigue, weakness, depression, memory loss, mental change, drowsiness.
EENT: dry eyes, blurred vision, nasal stuffiness.
Resp: bronchospasm, wheezing.
CV: BRADYCARDIA, CONGESTIVE HEART FAILURE, PULMONARY EDEMA, hypotension, peripheral vasoconstriction.
GI: constipation, diarrhea, nausea, vomiting.
GU: impotence, diminished libido.
Derm: rash, itching.
Endo: hyperglycemia, hypoglycemia.
Misc: Raynaud's phenomenon.

INTERACTIONS

Drug-Drug: ▪ **General anesthesia, IV phenytoin,** or **verapamil** may cause additive myocardial depression ▪ Additive bradycardia may occur with concurrent use of **cardiac glycosides** ▪ Additive hypotension may occur with other **antihypertensive agents,** acute ingestion of **alcohol,** or **nitrates** ▪ May negate the benefical effects of **beta-adrenergic bronchodilators, dopamine,** or **dobutamine** ▪ **Nonsteroidal anti-inflam-**

*Underlines indicate most frequent; CAPITALS indicate life-threatening.

matory agents or **thyroid** may decrease effectiveness ▪ Concurrent use of **amphetamines, cocaine, ephedrine, epinephrine, norepinephrine, phenylephrine,** or **pseudoephedrine** may cause excess alpha-adrenergic stimulation, hypertension, and bradycardia ▪ Use with **insulin** may produce prolonged hypoglycemia ▪ May produce hypertension when used within 14 days of **MAO inhibitor** therapy.

ROUTE AND DOSAGE

- **PO (Adults):** 40–80 mg once daily (doses up to 240 mg/day have been used).

PHARMACODYNAMICS (antihypertensive effect)

	ONSET	PEAK	DURATION
PO	up to 5 days	6–9 days	24 hr

NURSING IMPLICATIONS

Assessment

- **General Info:** Monitor blood pressure and pulse frequently during period of adjustment and periodically throughout therapy. Confer with physician prior to giving drug if pulse is <50 bpm. Assess for orthostatic hypotension when assisting patient up from supine position.
- □ Monitor intake and output ratios and daily weight. Assess patient routinely for evidence of congestive heart failure (peripheral edema, dyspnea, rales/crackles, fatigue, weight gain, jugular venous distention).
- **Angina:** Assess frequency and duration of episodes of chest pain periodically throughout therapy.
- **Lab Test Considerations:** Hepatic and renal function and CBC should be monitored routinely in patients receiving prolonged therapy.
- □ May cause elevations in serum potassium, uric acid, triglyceride, LDH, alkaline phosphatase levels, and BUN.

Potential Nursing Diagnoses

- Cardiac output, decreased (indications, adverse reactions).
- Knowledge deficit related to medication regimen (patient/family teaching).
- Noncompliance (patient/family teaching).

Implementation

- **PO:** May be administered with food or on an empty stomach. May be crushed and mixed with food or fluid if patient has difficulty swallowing.

Patient/Family Teaching

- □ Instruct patient to take medication exactly as directed, even if feeling well. If a dose is missed, it may be taken as soon as remembered up to 8 hr before next dose. Abrupt withdrawal may result in life-threatening arrhythmias, hypertension, or myocardial ischemia.
- □ Teach patient and family how to check pulse and blood pressure. Instruct them to take pulse daily and blood pressure biweekly. Advise patient to withhold dose and contact physician if pulse is <50 bpm or blood pressure changes significantly.
- □ Reinforce need to continue additional therapies for hypertension (weight loss, restricted sodium intake, stress reduction, regular exercise, moderation of alcohol consumption, and cessation of smoking). Nadolol helps control but does not cure hypertension.
- □ May occasionally cause drowsiness. Caution patient to avoid driving or other activities that require alertness until response to drug is known.
- □ Caution patient that nadolol may cause increased sensitivity to cold.
- □ Advise patient to consult physician or pharmacist before taking any over-the-counter drugs, especially cold remedies, concurrently with this medication. Patient should also avoid excessive amounts of coffee, tea, and cola.
- □ Diabetic patients should monitor se-

rum glucose closely, especially if weakness, fatigue, or irritability occurs.

- Instruct patient to inform physician or dentist of this therapy prior to treatment or surgery.
- Advise patient to carry identification describing medication regimen at all times.
- Instruct patient to notify physician if slow pulse rate, depression, or skin rash occurs.

Evaluation

Effectiveness of therapy can be demonstrated by: ▪ Decrease in blood pressure ▪ Reduction in frequency of anginal attacks ▫ Improved exercise tolerance. May require up to 5 days before therapeutic effects are seen.

NAFARELIN

(na-**fare**-e-lin)

Synarel

CLASSIFICATION(S):
Hormone—gonadotropin-releasing hormone
Pregnancy Category X

INDICATIONS

▪ Management of endometriosis.

ACTION

▪ Acts as a synthetic analogue of gonadotropin-releasing hormone (GnRH). Initially increases pituitary production of luteinizing hormone (LH) and follicle-stimulating hormone (FSH), which cause ovarian steroid production. Chronic administration leads to decreased production. Endometriotic lesions are sensitive to ovarian hormones. **Therapeutic Effects:** ▪ Reduction in lesions and associated pain in endometriosis.

PHARMACOKINETICS

Absorption: Well absorbed following intransal administration.
Distribution: Distribution not known.
Metabolism and Excretion: 20–40% excreted in feces. 3% excreted unchanged by the kidneys.
Half-life: 3 hr.

CONTRAINDICATIONS AND PRECAUTIONS

Contraindicated in: ▪ Hypersensitivity to gonadotropin-releasing hormone, its analogues, benzalkonium chloride, galcial acetic acid, or sorbitol ▪ Pregnancy or lactaion.
Use Cautiously in: ▪ Children (safety not established) ▪ Rhinitis

ADVERSE REACTIONS AND SIDE EFFECTS*

CNS: headaches, emotional instability, insomnia, depression.
EENT: nasal irritation.
CV: edema.
GU: vaginal dryness.
Derm: acne, seborrhea, hirsutism.
Endo: reduced breast size, impaired fertility, cessation of menses.
MS: myalgia, decreased bone density.
Misc: hot flashes, decreased libido, weight gain, hypersensitivity reactions.

INTERACTIONS

Drug–Drug: ▪ Concurrent **topical nasal decongestants** may reduce absorption of nafarelin (administer decongestant at least 30 min after nafarelin).

ROUTE AND DOSAGE

Note: Each spray contains 200 mcg of nafarelin.

- **Intranasal (Adults):** 1 spray in one nostril in the morning and 1 spray in the other nostril in the evening.

PHARMACODYNAMICS (decreased ovarian steroid production)

	ONSET	PEAK	DURATION
Intranasal	UK	4 wk	UK

NURSING IMPLICATIONS

Assessment

- Assess patient for endometriotic pain periodically throughout therapy.

*Underlines indicate most frequent; **CAPITALS** indicate life-threatening.

Potential Nursing Diagnoses
- Comfort, altered: pain (indications).
- Sexual dysfunction (side effects).
- Knowledge deficit related to medication regimen (patient/family teaching).

Implementation
- **General Info:** Treatment should be started between day 2 and 4 of the menstrual cycle.

Patient/Family Teaching
- Instruct patient on the correct technique for nasal spray. One spray should be administered into one nostril in the morning and one spray into the other nostril in the evening. One bottle should provide a 30-day supply.
- Advise patient to use a form of contraception other than oral contraceptives during therapy. Inform patient that amenorrhea is expected. Instruct patient to notify physician if regular menstruation persists or if successive doses are missed.
- Advise patient to consult physician if rhinitis occurs during therapy. If a topical decongestant is needed, do not use decongestant until 30 min after nafarelin dosing.
- Advise patient that medication may cause hot flashes. Notify physician if these become bothersome.

Evaluation
Effectiveness of therapy can be demonstrated by: ▪ Reduction in lesions and associated pain in endometriosis.

NAFCILLIN
(naf-**sill**-in)
Nafcil, Nallpen, Unipen

CLASSIFICATION(S):
Anti-infective—penicillinase-resistant penicillin
Pregnancy Category B

INDICATIONS
▪ Treatment of the following infections due to susceptible strains of penicillinase-producing staphylococci: ▫ Respiratory tract infections ▫ Skin and skin structure infections ▫ Bone and joint infections ▫ Urinary tract infections ▫ Endocarditis ▫ Septicemia ▫ Meningitis.

ACTION
▪ Binds to bacterial cell wall, leading to cell death ▪ Resists the action of penicillinase, an enzyme capable of inactivating penicillin. **Therapeutic Effect:** ▪ Bactericidal action against susceptible bacteria. **Spectrum:** ▪ Active against most gram-positive aerobic cocci, but less so than penicillin ▪ Notable for activity against penicillinase-producing strains of: ▫ *Staphylococcus aureus* ▫ *Staphylococcus epidermidis* ▪ Not active against methicillin-resistant staphylococci.

PHARMACOKINETICS
Absorption: Poorly and erratically absorbed from the GI tract. Well absorbed from IM sites.
Distribution: Widely distributed. Penetration into CSF is minimal but sufficient in the presence of inflamed meninges. Crosses the placenta and enters breast milk.
Metabolism and Excretion: Excreted unchanged by the kidneys.
Half-life: 30–90 min (increased in renal impairment).

CONTRAINDICATIONS AND PRECAUTIONS
Contraindicated in: ▪ Hypersensitivity to penicillins.
Use Cautiously in: ▪ Severe renal impairment (dosage reduction required) ▪ Pregnancy or lactation (safety not established) ▪ History of previous hypersensitivity reactions.

ADVERSE REACTIONS AND SIDE EFFECTS*

CNS: SEIZURES (high doses).

GI: nausea, vomiting, diarrhea, hepatitis.

GU: interstitial nephritis.

Derm: rashes, urticaria.

Hemat: blood dyscrasias.

Local: phlebitis at IV site, pain at IM site.

Misc: superinfection, allergic reactions, including **ANAPHYLAXIS** and serum sickness.

INTERACTIONS

Drug–Drug: ▪ **Probenecid** decreases renal excretion and increases blood levels ▪ May alter the effect of **oral anticoagulants**.

Drug–Food: ▪ **Food, acidic juices,** or **carbonated beverages** decrease absorption of nafcillin.

ROUTE AND DOSAGE

Note: Parenteral nafcillin contains 2.9 mEq sodium/g.

- **PO (Adults):** 250–1000 mg q 4–6 hr.
- **PO (Children and Infants):** 50–100 mg/kg/day in divided doses q 6 hr.
- **PO (Neonates):** 30–40 mg/kg/day in divided doses q 6–8 hr.
- **IM (Adults):** 500 mg q 4–6 hr.
- **IM (Children and Infants):** 25 mg/kg q 12 hr.
- **IM (Neonates):** 10 mg/kg q 12 hr.
- **IV (Adults):** 500–1000 mg q 4 hr.
- **IV (Children):** 50–200 mg/kg/day in divided doses q 4–6 hr.

PHARMACODYNAMICS (blood levels)

	ONSET	PEAK
PO	30 min	1–2 hr
IM	30 min	1–2 hr
IV	rapid	end of infusion

NURSING IMPLICATIONS

Assessment

- Assess patient for infection (vital signs; appearance of wound, sputum, urine, and stool; WBC) at beginning and throughout course of therapy.
- Obtain a history before initiating therapy to determine previous use of and reactions to penicillins or cephalosporins. Persons with a negative history of penicillin sensitivity may still have an allergic response.
- Obtain specimens for culture and sensitivity prior to initiating therapy. First dose may be given before receiving results.
- Observe patient for signs and symptoms of anaphylaxis (rash, pruritus, laryngeal edema, wheezing). Discontinue the drug and notify physician immediately if these occur. Keep epinephrine, an antihistamine, and resuscitation equipment close by in the event of an anaphylactic reaction.
- **Lab Test Considerations:** May cause positive direct Coombs' test results.

Potential Nursing Diagnoses

- Infection, high risk for (indications, side effects).
- Knowledge deficit related to medication regimen (patient/family teaching).
- Noncompliance related to medication regimen (patient/family teaching).

Implementation

- **PO:** Administer around the clock on an empty stomach, at least 1 hr before or 2 hr after meals. Take with a full glass of water; acidic juices or carbonated beverages may decrease absorption of penicillins. Use calibrated measuring device for liquid preparations. Shake well. Soln is stable for 14 days if refrigerated.
- **IM/IV:** To reconstitute, add 1.7–1.8 ml of sterile water or bacteriostatic water for injection to each 500-mg vial, 3.4 ml to each 1-g vial, or 6.6–6.8 ml to each 2-g vial, for a concentration of 250 mg/ml. Stable for 2–7 days if refrigerated.
- **Direct IV:** Dilute reconstituted soln of with 15–30 ml of sterile water or 0.9% NaCl for injection.
  - *Rate:* Administer over 5–10 min.

*Underlines indicate most frequent; **CAPITALS** indicate life-threatening.

- **Intermittent Infusion:** Dilute to a concentration of 2–40 mg/ml with sterile water for injection, 0.9% NaCl, D5W, D10W, D5/0.25% NaCl, D5/0.45% NaCl, D5/0.9% NaCl, D5/LR, Ringer's or lactated Ringer's soln. Stable for 24 hr at room temperature, 96 hr if refrigerated.
  - *Rate:* Infuse over at least 30–60 min to avoid vein irritation.
- **Syringe Compatibility:** cimetidine or heparin
- **Y-Site Compatibility:** acyclovir, atropine, cyclophosphamide, diazepam, esmolol, famotidine, fentanyl, hydromorphone, magnesium sulfate, morphine, perphenazine, or zidovudine.
- **Y-Site Incompatibility:** droperidol, droperidol/fentanyl, labetalol, nalbuphine, pentazocine, or verapamil.
- **Additive Compatibility:** chloramphenicol, chlorothiazide, dexamethasone, diphenhydramine, ephedrine, heparin, hydroxyzine, potassium chloride, prochlorperazine, sodium bicarbonate, or sodium lactate.
- **Additive Incompatibility:** ascorbic acid, aztreonam, bleomycin, cytarabine, hydrocortisone sodium succinate, methylprednisolone sodium succinate, or promazine.

Patient/Family Teaching

- Instruct patient to take medication around the clock and to finish the drug completely as directed, even if feeling better. If a dose is missed, it should be taken as soon as remembered. Advise patient that sharing of this medication may be dangerous.
- Advise patient to report the signs of superinfection (black, furry overgrowth on the tongue; vaginal itching or discharge; loose or foul-smelling stools) and allergy to physician promptly.
- Instruct patient to notify physician if symptoms do not improve.

Evaluation

Clinical response can be evaluated by:

- Resolution of the signs and symptoms of infection. Length of time for complete resolution depends on the organism and site of infection.

NAFTIFINE

(**naf**-ti-feen)
Naftin

CLASSIFICATION(S):
Antifungal—topical
Pregnancy Category B

INDICATIONS

- Treatment of tinea cruris and tinea corporis.

ACTION

- Inhibits fungal sterol synthesis. **Therapeutic Effects:** ▪ Fungicidal and fungistatic activity. **Spectrum:** ▪ Broad antifungal spectrum includes fungicidal activity against: ▫ *Trichophyton rubrum* ▫ *T. mentagrophytes* ▫ *T. tonsurans* ▫ *Epidermophyton floccosum* ▫ *Microsporum canis* ▫ *M. audouini* ▫ *M. gypseum* ▪ Also has fungistatic action against *Candida* species, including *C. albicans.*

PHARMACOKINETICS

Absorption: 6% of topically applied naftifine reaches systemic circulation.
Distribution: Penetrates stratum corneum.
Metabolism and Excretion: Metabolism not known.
Half-life: 2–3 days.

CONTRAINDICATIONS AND PRECAUTIONS

Contraindicated in: ▪ Hypersensitivity to naftifine or any components.
Use Cautiously in: ▪ Pregnancy, lactation, or children (safety not established).

ADVERSE REACTIONS AND SIDE EFFECTS*

Derm: burning, stinging, dryness, erythema, itching, irritation.

*Underlines indicate most frequent; **CAPITALS** indicate life-threatening.

N

INTERACTIONS

Drug–Drug: ▪ None known.

ROUTE AND DOSAGE

- **Top (Adults):** Apply 1% cream once daily, or 1% gel twice daily (morning and evening).

PHARMACODYNAMICS (response of skin lesions)

	ONSET	PEAK	DURATION
Top	1–4 wk	UK	UK

NURSING IMPLICATIONS

ASSESSMENT

□ Assess lesions prior to and daily during therapy.

POTENTIAL NURSING DIAGNOSES

- Skin integrity, impaired: actual (indications).
- Infection, high risk for (indications, patient/family teaching).
- Knowledge deficit related to medication regimen (patient/family teaching).

IMPLEMENTATION

- **Top:** Wash and dry affected area prior to application. Gently massage a sufficient quantity into the affected area and surrounding skin once a day with the cream, and twice a day with the gel (morning and evening). Wash hands after application. Do not apply occlusive dressings or wrappings unless directed.

□ Clinical improvement should be seen within the first wk of therapy. Continue treatment for 1–2 wk after symptoms have subsided to ensure healing and prevent recurrence.

PATIENT/FAMILY TEACHING

□ Instruct patient on the correct application of naftifine. Advise patient to apply medication exactly as directed for the full course of therapy.

□ Patient should consult physician if symptoms have not improved within the first wk of treatment.

EVALUATION

Effectiveness of therapy can be demonstrated by: ▪ Healing of skin lesions. If no clinical improvement is seen after 4 wk of treatment, condition should be re-evaluated.

NALBUPHINE
(**nal**-byoo-feen)
Nubain

CLASSIFICATION(S):
Narcotic analgesic—agonist/antagonist
Pregnancy Category C

INDICATIONS

▪ Management of moderate to severe pain ▪ Also used as an analgesic during labor, as a sedative prior to surgery, and as a supplement in balanced anesthesia.

ACTION

▪ Binds to opiate receptors in the CNS ▪ Alters the perception of and response to painful stimuli, while producing generalized CNS depression ▪ In addition, has partial antagonist properties, which may result in narcotic withdrawal in physically dependent patients. **Therapeutic Effect:** ▪ Decrease in moderate to severe pain.

PHARMACOKINETICS

Absorption: Well absorbed following IM and SC administration.
Distribution: Probably crosses the placenta and enters breast milk.
Metabolism and Excretion: Mostly metabolized by the liver and eliminated in the feces via biliary excretion. Minimal amounts excreted unchanged by the kidneys.
Half-life: 5 hr.

CONTRAINDICATIONS AND PRECAUTIONS

Contraindicated in: ▪ Hypersensitivity to nalbuphine or bisulfites ▪ Narcotic-dependent patients who have not been detoxified (may precipitate withdrawal).

Use Cautiously in: ▪ Head trauma ▪ Increased intracranial pressure ▪ Severe renal, hepatic, or pulmonary disease ▪ Hypothyroidism ▪ Adrenal insufficiency ▪ Alcoholism ▪ Elderly or debilitated patients (dosage reduction suggested) ▪ Undiagnosed abdominal pain ▪ Prostatic hypertrophy ▪ Pregnancy (has been used during labor, but may cause respiratory depression in the newborn) ▪ Lactation or children (safety not established).

ADVERSE REACTIONS AND SIDE EFFECTS*

CNS: sedation, confusion, headache, euphoria, floating feeling, unusual dreams, hallucinations, dysphoria, dizziness, vertigo.
EENT: miosis (high doses), blurred vision, diplopia.
Resp: respiratory depression.
CV: orthostatic hypotension, hypertension, palpitations.
GI: nausea, vomiting, constipation, ileus, dry mouth.
GU: urinary urgency.
Derm: sweating, clammy feeling.
Misc: tolerance, physical dependence, psychological dependence.

INTERACTIONS

Drug-Drug: ▪ Use with extreme caution in patients receiving **MAO inhibitors** (may result in unpredictable, severe reactions—reduce initial dose of nalbuphine to 25% of usual dose) ▪ Additive CNS depression with **alcohol, antihistamines,** and **sedative/hypnotics** ▪ May precipitate narcotic withdrawal in patients who are physically dependent on **narcotic analgesic-agonists** and have not been detoxified ▪ Avoid concurrent use with other **narcotic analgesic-agonists** (may diminish analgesic effect).

ROUTE AND DOSAGE

Analgesia

- **IM, SC, IV (Adults):** Usual dose is 10 mg q 3–6 hr (0.14 mg/kg) in patients not dependent on narcotic agonists (single dose not to exceed 20 mg, total daily dose not to exceed 160 mg).

Supplement To Balanced Anesthesia

- **IV (Adults):** 0.3–3 mg/kg over 10–15 min initially. Maintenance dose 0.25–0.5 mg/kg as needed.

PHARMACODYNAMICS (analgesia)

	ONSET	PEAK	DURATION
IM	<15 min	60 min	3–6 hr
SC	<15 min	UK	3–6 hr
IV	2–3 min	30 min	3–6 hr

NURSING IMPLICATIONS

Assessment

- □ Assess type, location, and intensity of pain prior to and 60 min following IM and 30 min following IV administration.
- □ Assess blood pressure, pulse, and respirations before and periodically during administration. Nalbuphine produces respiratory depression, but this does not markedly increase with increased doses.
- □ Although this drug has a low potential for dependence, prolonged use may lead to physical and psychological dependence and tolerance. This should not prevent patient from receiving adequate analgesia. Most patients who receive nalbuphine for medical reasons do not develop psychological dependence. Progressively higher doses may be required to relieve pain with long-term therapy.
- □ Assess prior analgesic history. Antagonistic properties may induce withdrawal symptoms (vomiting, restlessness, abdominal cramps, increased blood pressure, and temperature) in narcotic-dependent patients.

▪ **Lab Test Considerations:** May cause

*Underlines indicate most frequent; **CAPITALS** indicate life-threatening.

elevated serum amylase and lipase levels.

- **Toxicity and Overdose:** If overdose occurs, respiratory depression may be partially reversed by naloxone (Narcan), the antidote.

POTENTIAL NURSING DIAGNOSES

- Comfort, altered: pain (indications).
- Injury, high risk for (side effects).
- Sensory-perceptual alteration: visual, auditory (side effects).

IMPLEMENTATION

- **General Info:** Explain therapeutic value of medication prior to administration to enhance the analgesic effect.
- □ Regularly administered doses may be more effective than prn administration. Analgesic is more effective if administered before pain becomes severe.
- □ Coadministration with non-narcotic analgesics may have additive effects and permit lower narcotic doses.
- **IM:** Administer deep into well-developed muscle. Rotate sites of injections.
- **Direct IV:** May give IV undiluted.
- □ *Rate:* Administer slowly, each 10 mg over 3–5 min.
- **Syringe Compatibility:** atropine, cimetidine, droperidol, hydroxyzine, lidocaine, midazolam, prochlorperazine, promethazine, ranitidine, scopolamine, or trimethobenzamide.
- **Syringe Incompatibility:** diazepam or pentobarbital.
- **Y-Site Incompatibility:** nafcillin.

PATIENT/FAMILY TEACHING

- □ Instruct patient on how and when to ask for prn pain medication.
- □ Nalbuphine may cause drowsiness or dizziness. Advise patient to call for assistance when ambulating and to avoid driving or other activities requiring alertness until response to the medication is known.
- □ Caution patient to make position changes slowly to minimize orthostatic hypotension.
- □ Advise patient that frequent mouth rinses, good oral hygiene, and sugarless gum or candy may decrease dry mouth.
- □ Encourage patient to turn, cough, and breathe deeply every 2 hr to prevent atelectasis.
- □ Advise patient to avoid concurrent use of alcohol or other CNS depressants with this medication.

EVALUATION

Effectiveness of therapy can be demonstrated by: ■ Decrease in severity of pain without a significant alteration in level of consciousness or respiratory status.

NALOXONE

(nal-**ox**-one)

Narcan

CLASSIFICATION(S):

Narcotic antagonist, Antidote—narcotic analgesics

Pregnancy Category B

INDICATIONS

- Reversal of CNS depression and respiratory depression due to suspected narcotic overdosage.

ACTION

- Competitively blocks the effects of narcotics, including CNS and respiratory depression, without producing any agonist (narcotic-like) effects. **Therapeutic Effect:** ■ Reversal of signs of narcotic excess.

PHARMACOKINETICS

Absorption: Well absorbed following IM or SC administration.

Distribution: Rapidly distributed to tissues. Crosses the placenta.

Metabolism and Excretion: Metabolized by the liver.

Half-life: 60–90 min (up to 3 hr in neonates).

CONTRAINDICATIONS AND PRECAUTIONS

Contraindicated in: ■ Hypersensitivity.

Use Cautiously in: ▪ Cardiovascular disease ▪ Patients physically dependent on narcotic analgesics (may precipitate severe withdrawal) ▪ Pregnancy (may cause withdrawal in mother and fetus if mother is narcotic-dependent) ▪ Lactation (safety not established) ▪ Neonates of narcotic-dependent mothers.

ADVERSE REACTIONS AND SIDE EFFECTS*

CV: ventricular tachycardia, ventricular fibrillation, hypotension, hypertension.
GI: nausea, vomiting.

INTERACTIONS

Drug-Drug: ▪ Can precipitate withdrawal in patients who are physically dependent on **narcotic analgesics** ▪ May antagonize postoperative **analgesia**.

ROUTE AND DOSAGE

Narcotic-Induced Respiratory or CNS Depression

- **IV, IM, SC (Adults):** 0.4 mg or 10 mcg/kg, may repeat q 2–3 min (IV route is preferred); some patients may require up to 2 mg. If patient is suspected of being narcotic-dependent, initial dose should be decreased to 0.1–0.2 mg. May also be given by IV infusion at rate adjusted to patient's response.
- **IV, IM, SC (Children):** 0.01 mg/kg in inadequate response increase to 0.1 mg/kg, may repeat IV dose q 2–3 min as needed.

Postoperative Respiratory Depression

- **IV (Adults):** 0.1–0.2 mg q 2–3 min until response obtained, may repeat q 1–2 hr later if needed or continuous infusion of 3.7 mcg/kg/hr.
- **IV (Children):** 5–10 mcg, may repeat q 2–3 min until response obtained with additional doses q 2–3 hr later if needed.

PHARMACODYNAMICS (reversal of narcotic effects)

	ONSET	PEAK	DURATION
IV	1–2 min	UK	45 min
IM/SC	2–5 min	UK	>45 min

*Underlines indicate most frequent; **CAPITALS** indicate life-threatening.

NURSING IMPLICATIONS

Assessment

- ▫ Monitor respiratory rate, rhythm, and depth, pulse, ECG, blood pressure, and level of consciousness frequently until effects of narcotic wear off. The effects of some narcotics may last longer than the effects of naloxone, and repeat doses may be necessary.
- ▫ Assess patient for level of pain following administration when used to treat postoperative respiratory depression. Naloxone decreases respiratory depression but also reverses analgesia.
- ▫ Assess patient for signs and symptoms of narcotic withdrawal (vomiting, restlessness, abdominal cramps, increased blood pressure, and temperature). Symptoms may occur within a few mins to 2 hr. Severity depends on dose of naloxone, narcotic involved, and degree of physical dependence.
- ▫ Lack of significant improvement indicates that symptoms are due to a disease process or to other non-narcotic CNS depressants not affected by naloxone.

Potential Nursing Diagnoses

- Breathing pattern, ineffective (indications).
- Coping, ineffective individual (indications).
- Comfort, altered: pain (interactions).

Implementation

- **General Info:** Larger doses of naloxone may be necessary when used to antagonize the effects of buprenorphine, butorphanol, nalbuphine, pentazocine, and propoxyphene.
- ▫ Resuscitation equipment, oxygen, vasopressors, and mechanical ventilation should be available to supplement naloxone therapy as needed.
- **Direct IV:** Administer undiluted at a rate of 0.4 mg over 15 sec. Titrate to patient response.
- **Continuous Infusion:** Dilute in D5W or 0.9% NaCl for injection. Naloxone 2

mg in 500 ml equals a concentration of 4 mcg/ml. Mixture is stable for 24 hr; discard unused soln.

- *Rate:* Titrate dose according to patient response. Supplemental doses, administered IM, or a continuous infusion may provide longer-lasting effects.
- Doses should be titrated carefully in postoperative patients to avoid interference with control of postoperative pain.
- **Syringe Compatibility:** benzquinamide or heparin.
- **Additive Compatibility:** verapamil.
- **Additive Incompatibility:** Incompatible with preparations containing bisulfite, sulfite, and solns with an alkaline pH.

PATIENT/FAMILY TEACHING

- As medication becomes effective, explain purpose and effects of naloxone to patient.

EVALUATION

Clinical response can be demonstrated by: ▪ Adequate ventilation ▫ Alertness without significant pain.

NANDROLONE
(**nan**-droe-lone)

NANDROLONE DECANOATE
Anabolin LA, Androlone-D, Deca-Durabolin, Hybolin Decanoate, Kabolin, Nandrobolic L.A., Neo-Durabolic

NANDROLONE PHENPROPIONATE
Anabolin IM, Durabolin, Hybolin Improved, Nandrobolic

CLASSIFICATION(S):
Hormone—anabolic steroid
Schedule III
Pregnancy Category X

INDICATIONS

▪ With iron therapy in the treatment of anemia associated with chronic renal failure (decanoate) ▪ Palliative treatment of advanced metastatic breast carcinoma known to be hormone-sensitive.

ACTION

▪ Promotes protein anabolism, resulting in reversal of catabolism and negative nitrogen balance ▪ Stimulates production of erythropoietin ▪ Has antineoplastic effect in hormone-sensitive breast cancer. **Therapeutic Effects:** ▪ Increased appetite and weight gain (if calories are provided) ▪ Increased RBC indices ▪ Tumor regression.

PHARMACOKINETICS

Absorption: Slowly absorbed from IM sites.
Distribution: Distribution not known.
Metabolism and Excretion: Metabolism and excretion not known.
Half-life: UK.

CONTRAINDICATIONS AND PRECAUTIONS

Contraindicated in: ▪ Hypersensitivity to nandrolone, benzyl alcohol, or sesame oil ▪ Pregnancy, lactation, or infancy ▪ Prostatic hypertrophy ▪ Pituitary insufficiency ▪ History of myocardial infarction ▪ Hepatic dysfunction ▪ Nephrosis ▪ Nephrotic phase of nephritis ▪ Hypercalcemia ▪ Some forms of breast carcinoma.
Use Cautiously in: ▪ Children (safety not established).

ADVERSE REACTIONS AND SIDE EFFECTS*

CNS: excitation, insomnia, toxic confusion.
EENT: deepening of the voice in females.
CV: edema, congestive heart failure.
GI: <u>hepatotoxicity</u>, HEPATIC NECROSIS, HEPATIC TUMORS, nausea, vomiting, diarrhea, abdominal fullness, decreased appetite, burning tongue.
Derm: acne, hirsutism, increased pigmentation.
Endo: gynecomastia; females and pre-

*<u>Underlines</u> indicate most frequent; **CAPITALS** indicate life-threatening.

pubertal males—virilization; postpubertal males—oligospermia, testicular atrophy, decreased libido.
F and E: hypercalcemia.
Metab: increased blood lipids, weight gain, growth disturbances in children.
MS: muscle cramps, premature epiphyseal closure in children.
Misc: chills.

INTERACTIONS

Drug-Drug: ▪ Increased risk of edema with **glucocorticoids** ▪ May increase the effectiveness of **oral anticoagulants** ▪ May decrease requirements for **insulin** or **oral hypoglycemic agents**.

ROUTE AND DOSAGE

Anemia of Chronic Renal Failure

- **IM (Adults):** Men—100–200 mg/wk of decanoate; Women—50–100 mg/wk of decanoate.
- **IM (Children 2–13 yr):** 50–50 mg/wk of decanoate.

Antineoplastic—Metastatic Breast Carcinoma

- **IM (Adults):** 25–100 mg/wk of phenpropionate.

PHARMACODYNAMICS (blood levels)

	ONSET	PEAK	DURATION
IM—decanoate	UK	3–6 days	UK
IM—phenpropionate	UK	1–2 days	UK

NURSING IMPLICATIONS

Assessment

- **Females:** Monitor for masculinizing side effects (acne, deepening of the voice, irregular menses, unusual hair growth or loss, increased clitoral size). In women with metastatic breast cancer, monitor for symptoms of hypercalcemia (nausea, vomiting, unusual weakness or tiredness).
- **Males:** Monitor for precocious puberty in boys (acne, darkening of skin, development of male secondary sex characteristics—increase in penis size, frequent erections, growth of body hair).
  - Monitor for breast enlargement, persistent erections, and increased urge to urinate in men. Monitor for difficulty urinating in elderly men, as prostate enlargement may occur.
- **Lab Test Considerations:** May cause hepatotoxicity. Monitor liver function tests. May increase SGOT (AST), SGPT (ALT), alkaline phosphatase, and bilirubin. May increase prothrombin time and decrease levels of clotting factors II, V, VII, and X.
  - Monitor serum cholesterol and lipids. May cause increased low-density lipoprotein (LDL) levels and decreased high-density lipoprotein levels (HDL). May decrease serum triglycerides.
  - May increase serum calcium, inorganic phosphates, potassium, and sodium.
  - Monitor serum iron and iron-binding capacity.
  - May cause decreased levels in 24-hr urine tests for 17-ketosteroid concentrations.
  - May alter results of fasting blood sugar, glucose tolerance tests, thyroid function tests, and metyrapone tests.

Potential Nursing Diagnoses

- Sexual dysfunction (side effect).
- Knowledge deficit related to medication regimen (patient/family teaching).

Implementation

- **IM:** Administer deep IM into gluteal site.

Patient/Family Teaching

- Review diet alterations with patient. Diet should be high in protein and calories. Improvement in appetite may occur.
- Instruct patient to notify physician if unexpected weight gain, swelling of feet, unusual bleeding or bruising, abdominal pain, nausea, light-colored stools, or darkening of urine occur. Review side effects specific to client's age and sex. Instruct patient to notify physician if these occur.
- Explain need for continued medical follow-up to assess effectiveness and

possible side effects of medication. Children need semiannual x-ray examinations to detect premature closure of epiphyseal plates.

Evaluation

Effectiveness of therapy can be demonstrated by: ▪ Improvement in hematologic parameters in anemia ▪ Decrease in size and spread of breast malignancy in postmenopausal women.

NAPHAZOLINE

(naf-**az**-oh-leen)

Ak-Con, Albalon, Allerest, Allergy Drops, Clear Eyes, Degest-2, I-Naphline, Muro's Opcon, Naphcon, Naphcon Forte, VasoClear, {Vasocon}, Vasocon Regular

CLASSIFICATION(S):
Decongestant—local
Pregnancy Category C

INDICATIONS

▪ Symptomatic relief of ocular redness or nasal congestion due to minor irritation associated with: ▫ Rhinitis ▫ Sinusitus ▫ Environmental pollutants ▫ Allergies ▫ Wind ▫ Swimming ▫ Contact lenses.

ACTION

▪ An alpha-adrenergic agonist that produces local vaconstriction following ocular instillation. **Therapeutic Effects:** ▪ Ocular or nasal decongestion and relief of redness.

PHARMACOKINETICS

Absorption: Minimal systemic absorption follows ocular instillation.
Distribution: Distribution not known.
Metabolism and Excretion: Metabolism and excretion not known.
Half-life: UK.

CONTRAINDICATIONS AND PRECAUTIONS

Contraindicated in: ▪ Hypersensitivity to naphazoline, benzalkonium chloride, or edetate disodium.
Use Cautiously in: ▪ Cardiovascular disease, including hypertension ▪ Hyperthyroidism ▪ Diabetes mellitus ▪ Children (Ophth—safety not established).

ADVERSE REACTIONS AND SIDE EFFECTS*

CNS: headache, nervousness, dizziness, weakness.
EENT: rebound congestion (with prolonged use), conjunctival or nasal irritation, liberation of iris pigment granules (ocular use in elderly patients), blurred vision, sneezing.
CV: hypertension.
Derm: sweating.

INTERACTIONS

Drug-Drug: ▪ Pressor effect may be increased by concurrent **tricyclic antidepressants, maprotiline,** or **MAO inhibitor** therapy.

ROUTE AND DOSAGE

- **Ophth (Adults):** 1 drop of 0.012% soln to conjunctiva qid as needed or 1 drop of 0.1% soln q 3–4 hr as needed.
- **Nasal (Adults and Children >12 yr):** 2 sprays or drops of 0.05% soln in each nostril q 3–6 hr as needed.
- **Nasal (Adults and Children 6–12 yr):** 2 sprays or drops of 0.025% soln in each nostril q 3–6 hr as needed.

PHARMACODYNAMICS (local decongestion)

	ONSET	PEAK	DURATION
Ophth	within 10 min	UK	2–6 hr
Nasal	within 10 min	UK	2–6 hr

NURSING IMPLICATIONS

Assessment

▪ **General Info:** Monitor patient for signs of systemic side effects (in-

{} = Available in Canada only.
*Underlines indicate most frequent; **CAPITALS** indicate life-threatening.

creased pulse, blood pressure, and blood sugar in diabetic patients). Notify physician if these symptoms occur.

- **Ocular Irritation:** Assess degree of ocular irritation prior to and periodically throughout course of therapy.
- **Rhinitis:** Assess severity of nasal congestion prior to and periodically throughout course of therapy.

Potential Nursing Diagnoses

- Sensory-perceptual alteration: visual (indications, side effects).
- Airway clearance, ineffective (indications).
- Knowledge deficit related to medication regimen (patient/family teaching).

Implementation

- **General Info:** Available in combination with antihistamines (see Appendix A).

Patient/Family Teaching

- **General Info:** Instruct patient to avoid known allergens.
- **Eyedrops:** Instruct patient on correct method of application of drops. Wash hands. Lie down or tilt head back and look at ceiling. Pull down on lower lid, creating a small pocket. Place prescribed number of drops in pocket. Apply pressure to the inner canthus for 1–2 min to confine effects to the eye. Wait 5 min before applying other prescribed eyedrops. Do not touch cap or tip of container to eye, fingers, or any surface.
  - Instruct patient not to use soln if it becomes cloudy or discolored.
- **Nasal:** Emphasize need to take only as directed. Rebound congestion may occur if used too frequently or for prolonged duration.
- **Nasal Soln:** Squeeze bulb until dropper contains correct amount of medication. Tilt head back and place 2 drops of soln into 1 nostril. Tilt head forward and turn head to the opposite side and inhale through the nostril. Repeat the process with the other side.
- **Nasal Spray:** Keep head upright and squeeze bottle prescribed number of times briskly while sniffing through nostril.
  - Instruct patient to contact physician if no improvement is seen or if condition worsens.

Evaluation

Effectiveness of therapy can be demonstrated by: ▪ Decrease in ocular redness ▪ Decrease in nasal congestion.

NAPROXEN

(na-**prox**-en)
{Apo-Naproxen}, Naprosyn, {Naxen}, {Novonaprox}

NAPROXEN SODIUM

(na-**prox**-en **soe**-dee-um)
Anaprox

CLASSIFICATION(S):
Non-narcotic analgesic, Nonsteroidal anti-inflammatory agent
Pregnancy Category C

INDICATIONS

▪ Management of inflammatory disorders, including: ▫ Rheumatoid arthritis ▫ Osteoarthritis ▪ Management of mild to moderate pain ▪ Treatment of dysmenorrhea.

ACTION

▪ Inhibits prostaglandin synthesis. **Therapeutic Effects:** ▪ Suppression of inflammation ▪ Decreased pain.

PHARMACOKINETICS

Absorption: Completely absorbed from the GI tract. Sodium salt (Anaprox) is more rapidly absorbed.
Distribution: Crosses the placenta and enters breast milk in low concentrations.
Metabolism and Excretion: Mostly metabolized by the liver.
Half-life: 10–20 hr.

{} = Available in Canada only.

CONTRAINDICATIONS AND PRECAUTIONS

Contraindicated in: ▪ Hypersensitivity ▪ Cross-sensitivity may exist with other nonsteroidal anti-inflammatory agents, including aspirin ▪ Active GI bleeding ▪ Ulcer disease.

Use Cautiously in: ▪ Severe cardiovascular, renal, or hepatic disease ▪ History of ulcer disease ▪ Pregnancy or lactation (safety not established).

ADVERSE REACTIONS AND SIDE EFFECTS*

CNS: headache, drowsiness, dizziness.
CV: edema, palpitations, tachycardia.
EENT: tinnitus.
Resp: dyspnea.
GI: nausea, dyspepsia, vomiting, diarrhea, constipation, **GI BLEEDING**, discomfort, **HEPATITIS**, flatulence, anorexia.
GU: renal failure, hematuria, cystitis.
Derm: rashes, sweating, photosensitivity.
Hemat: blood dyscrasias, prolonged bleeding time.
Misc: allergic reactions, including **ANAPHYLAXIS**.

INTERACTIONS

Drug-Drug: ▪ Concurrent use with **aspirin** decreases naproxen blood levels and may decrease effectiveness ▪ Increased risk of bleeding with **anticoagulants, thrombolytic agents, cefamandole, cefotetan, cefoperazone, moxalactam,** or **plicamycin** ▪ Additive adverse GI side effects with **aspirin, glucocorticoids,** and other **nonsteroidal anti-inflammatory agents** ▪ **Probenecid** increases blood levels and may increase toxicity ▪ Increased risk of photosensitivity with other **photosensitizing agents** ▪ May increase the risk of toxicity from **methotrexate, antineoplastic agents,** or **radiation therapy** ▪ May increase serum levels and risk of toxicity from **lithium** ▪ Increased risk of adverse renal effects with **gold compounds** or chronic use of **acetaminophen** ▪ May decrease response to **antihypertensives** or **diuretics** ▪ May increase risk of hypoglycemia with **insulin** or **oral hypoglycemic agents**.

ROUTE AND DOSAGE

Note: 275 mg naproxen sodium is equivalent to 250 mg naproxen.

Inflammatory Diseases

- **PO (Adults):** 250–500 mg naproxen bid or 275 mg naproxen sodium in the morning and 550 mg in the evening.
- **PO (Children):** 10 mg/kg/day of naproxen in 2 divided doses.

Pain, Dysmenorrhea

- **PO (Adults):** 500 mg naproxen initially followed by 250 mg q 6–8 hr, or 550 mg naproxen sodium initially followed by 275 mg q 6–8 hr (not to exceed 1.25 g naproxen or 1.375 g naproxen sodium/day).

PHARMACODYNAMICS

	ONSET	PEAK	DURATION
PO (analgesic)	1 hr	UK	up to 7 hr
PO (anti-inflammatory)	14 days	4 wk	UK

NURSING IMPLICATIONS

Assessment

- **General Info:** Patients who have asthma, aspirin-induced allergy, and nasal polyps are at increased risk for developing hypersensitivity reactions. Assess for rhinitis, asthma, and urticaria.
- **Arthritis:** Assess pain and range of motion prior to and 1–2 hr following administration.
- **Pain:** Assess pain (note type, location, and intensity) prior to and 1–2 hr following administration.
- **Lab Test Considerations:** BUN, serum creatinine, CBC, and liver function tests should be evaluated periodically in patients receiving prolonged courses of therapy.
- ▫ Serum potassium, BUN, serum creati-

*Underlines indicate most frequent; **CAPITALS** indicate life-threatening.

nine, SGOT (AST), and SGPT (ALT) may show increased levels.

- Bleeding time may be prolonged up to 4 days following discontinuation of therapy.

Potential Nursing Diagnoses

- Comfort, altered: pain (indications).
- Mobility, impaired physical (indications).
- Knowledge deficit related to medication regimen (patient/family teaching).

Implementation

- **General Info:** Coadministration with narcotic analgesics may have additive analgesic effects and may permit lower narcotic doses. Analgesic is more effective if administered before pain becomes severe.
- **PO:** For rapid initial effect, administer 30 min before or 2 hr after meals. May be administered with food, milk, or antacids to decrease GI irritation. Food slows but does not reduce the extent of absorption. Do not mix suspension with antacid or other liquid prior to administration.
- **Dysmenorrhea:** Administer as soon as possible after the onset of menses. Prophylactic treatment has not been shown to be effective.

Patient/Family Teaching

- Advise patient to take this medication with a full glass of water and to remain in an upright position for 15–30 min after administration.
- Instruct patient to take medication exactly as directed. If a dose is missed, it should be taken as soon as remembered but not if almost time for the next dose. Do not double doses.
- Naproxen may cause drowsiness or dizziness. Advise patient to avoid driving or other activities requiring alertness until response to the medication is known.
- Caution patient to avoid the concurrent use of alcohol, aspirin, acetaminophen, or other over-the-counter medications without consulting physician or pharmacist.
- Advise patient to use sunscreen and protective clothing to prevent photosensitivity reactions.
- Advise patient to inform physician or dentist of medication regimen prior to treatment or surgery.
- Instruct patient to notify physician if rash, itching, muscle aches, tinnitus, weight gain, edema, black stools, or persistent headache occurs.

Evaluation

Effectiveness of therapy may be determined by: ▪ Relief of pain ▪ Improved joint mobility. Partial arthritic relief is usually seen within 2 wk, but maximum effectiveness may require 2–4 wk of continuous therapy. Patients who do not respond to one nonsteroidal anti-inflammatory agent may respond to another.

NATAMYCIN

(na-ta-**mye**-sin)
Natacyn, Pimaricin

CLASSIFICATION(S):
Ophthalmic—antifungal
Pregnancy Category UK

INDICATIONS

▪ Treatment of fungal eye infections due to susceptible fungi, including: ▫ Blepharitis ▫ Conjunctivitis ▫ Keratitis.

ACTION

▪ Binds to fungal cell membrane, allowing leakage of cellular contents. **Therapeutic Effect:** ▪ Fungicidal action against susceptible organisms. **Spectrum:** ▪ Active against: ▫ *Aspergillus* ▫ *Cephalosporium* ▫ *Curvularia* ▫ *Fusarium solani* ▫ *Penicillium* ▫ *Microsporum* ▫ *Epidermophyton* ▫ *Blastomyces dermatidis* ▫ *Coccidioides immitis* ▫ *Cryptococcus neoformans* ▫ *Histoplasma capsulatum* ▫ *Sporothrix schenckii.*

PHARMACOKINETICS

Absorption: Negligible systemic absorption.

Distribution: Adheres to areas of corneal ulceration and is retained in the conjunctival fornices. Does not penetrate deep ocular fluids or structures.
Metabolism and Excretion: Metabolism and excretion not known.
Half-life: UK.

CONTRAINDICATIONS AND PRECAUTIONS

Contraindicated in: ▪ Hypersensitivity to natamycin or benzalkonium chloride ▪ Concurrent ocular glucocorticoids.
Use Cautiously in: ▪ No known cautions.

ADVERSE REACTIONS AND SIDE EFFECTS*

EENT: ocular irritation not previously present.

INTERACTIONS

Drug-Drug: ▪ Avoid use with concurrent **ocular glucocorticoids** (increased risk of spreading infection).

ROUTE AND DOSAGE

Fungal Conjunctivitis or Keratitis

- **Ophth (Adults):** 1 drop of 5% suspension instilled into the conjunctival sac 4–6 times daily.

Fungal Keratitis

- **Ophth (Adults):** 1 drop of 5% suspension instilled into the conjunctival sac q 1–2 hr for 3–4 days, then may be decreased to 1 drop 6–8 times daily and then gradually decreased every 4–7 days, continued for total of 14–21 days.

PHARMACODYNAMICS (resolution of fungal infection)

	ONSET	PEAK
Ophth	2 days	2–4 wk*

*Complete healing.

NURSING IMPLICATIONS

Assessment

- □ Assess degree of ocular inflammation and irritation, and character and amount of discharge throughout course of therapy.
- ▪ **Lab Test Considerations:** Physician will obtain culture prior to therapy.

Potential Nursing Diagnoses

- ▪ Sensory-perceptual alteration: visual (indications, side effects).
- ▪ Infection, high risk for (indications).
- ▪ Knowledge deficit related to medication regimen (patient/family teaching).

Implementation

- ▪ **General Info:** Shake container well prior to instillation of drops.
- □ Wash hands before and after instillation of drops. Wear gloves to help prevent the spread of infection.

Patient/Family Teaching

- □ Instruct patient to take as ordered for the full course of therapy and not to discontinue without physician's approval, even if feeling better. If a dose is missed, it should be taken as soon as remembered. Sharing this medication may lead to the spread of infection.
- □ Instruct patient on correct method of application of drops. Wash hands. Lie down or tilt head back and look at ceiling. Pull down on lower lid, creating a small pocket. Place prescribed number of drops in pocket. Wait 5 min before applying other prescribed eyedrops. Wash hands again after instilling eyedrops.
- □ Instruct patient to contact physician if no improvement is seen in 7–10 days, if condition worsens, or if irritation of the eye persists.
- □ Advise patient with ophthalmic infection to avoid wearing contact lenses until the infection is resolved and physician approves.
- □ Emphasize need for follow-up to ensure resolution of infection.

Evaluation

Effectiveness of therapy can be demonstrated by: ▪ Resolution of fungal ocular infections.

NEOMYCIN
(nee-oh-**mye**-sin)
Myciguent

CLASSIFICATION(S):
Anti-infective—aminoglycoside
Pregnancy Category D

INDICATIONS
▪ **IM:** Used only for the treatment of serious gram-negative bacillary urinary tract infections due to susceptible organisms where resistance patterns or patient characteristics contraindicate the use of safer anti-infectives ▪ **PO:** Used to prepare the GI tract for surgery or to decrease the population of ammonia-producing bacteria in the management of hepatic encephalopathy ▪ **PO:** Treatment of diarrhea caused by enteropathogenic *Escherichia coli* ▪ **Top:** Treatment of minor skin infections.

ACTION
▪ Inhibits protein synthesis in bacteria at the level of the 30S ribosome. **Therapeutic Effect:** ▪ Bactericidal action against susceptible bacteria.

PHARMACOKINETICS
Absorption: Minimally absorbed (<3%) following oral or topical administration. Well absorbed after IM administration.
Distribution: Distribution not known.
Metabolism and Excretion: If systemically absorbed, eliminated unchanged by the kidneys. Orally administered neomycin is eliminated unchanged in the feces.
Half-life: 2–3 hr.

CONTRAINDICATIONS AND PRECAUTIONS
Contraindicated in: ▪ Hypersensitivity ▪ Cross-sensitivity with other aminoglycosides may exist ▪ Renal impairment (chronic use of high-dose oral therapy).
Use Cautiously in: ▪ Renal impairment of any degree (dosage reduction required) ▪ Pregnancy and lactation (safety not established) ▪ Neuromuscular diseases, such as myasthenia gravis.

ADVERSE REACTIONS AND SIDE EFFECTS*
EENT: ototoxicity (vestibular and cochlear).
GU: nephrotoxicity.
Derm: Top—rashes.
Neuro: enhanced neuromuscular blockade (parenteral).
Misc: hypersensitivity reactions.

INTERACTIONS
Drug-Drug: ▪ Possible respiratory paralysis after **inhalation anesthetics (ether, cyclopropane, halothane,** or **nitrous oxide)** or **neuromuscular blockers (tubocurarine, succinylcholine, decamethonium)** ▪ Increased risk of ototoxicity with **loop diuretics (ethacrynic acid, furosemide)** ▪ Increased risk of nephrotoxicity with other **nephrotoxic drugs (cisplatin).**

ROUTE AND DOSAGE
Serious Urinary Tract Infections
- **IM (Adults):** 15 mg/kg/day in divided doses q 6 hr (not to exceed 1 g/day).

Preparation for GI Surgery
- **PO (Adults):** 1 g q hr for 4 hr, then 1 g q 4 hr for 24 hr prior to surgery.
- **PO (Children):** 88 mg/kg/day in divided doses q 4 hr for 24 hr prior to surgery.

Hepatic Encephalopathy
- **PO (Adults):** 4–12 g/day in divided doses q 6 hr.
- **PO (Children):** 40–100 mg/kg/day in divided doses q 4–6 hr.
- **Rect (Adults):** 100–200 ml of 1–2% soln retained for 20–60 min.

Diarrhea Caused by Enterpathogenic *E. Coli*
- **PO (Adults):** 50 mg/kg/day in divided doses q 6 hr.

Minor Skin Infections
- **Top (Adults and Children):** 0.5% cream or ointment 1–3 times daily.

*Underlines indicate most frequent; **CAPITALS** indicate life-threatening.

N

PHARMACODYNAMICS (blood levels)

	ONSET	PEAK	DURATION
IM	rapid	1–4 hr	6–8 hr

NURSING IMPLICATIONS

Assessment

- **General Info:** Assess patient for infection (vital signs; appearance of infected skin) at beginning and throughout course of therapy.
- Obtain specimens for culture and sensitivity prior to initiating therapy. First dose may be given before receiving results.
- **Hepatic Encephalopathy:** Monitor neurologic status. Prior to administering oral medication assess patient's ability to swallow.
- **Lab Test Considerations:** Monitor urinalysis, specific gravity, BUN, creatinine, and creatinine clearance prior to and throughout prolonged therapy.

Potential Nursing Diagnoses

- Infection, high risk for (indications).
- Knowledge deficit related to medication regimen (patient/family teaching).

Implementation

- **General Info:** Available in combination with other topical antibiotics or anti-inflammatory agents for skin, ear, and eye infections (see Appendix A).
- **Preoperative Bowel Prep:** Usually used in conjunction with erythromycin, a low-residue diet, and a cathartic or enema.
- **Rect:** When used as an enema in hepatic encephalopathy, dilution should be 100–200 ml of 1–2% soln. Enema should be retained 20–60 min.
- **IM:** Parenteral route is no longer recommended. If necessary, dilute 500-mg vial with 2 ml of 0.9% NaCl. Administer deep into a well-developed muscle.

Patient/Family Teaching

- **General Info:** Advise patient to take medication for full course of therapy, even if feeling better.
- Instruct patient to inform physician if rash, diarrhea, tinnitus, vertigo, or hearing loss occurs.
- **Top Therapy:** Instruct patient to wash affected skin gently and pat dry. Apply a thin film of ointment. Apply occlusive dressing only if ordered by physician. Patient should assess skin and inform physician if skin irritation develops or infection worsens.

Evaluation

Effectiveness of therapy can be demonstrated by: ▪ Resolution of the signs and symptoms of infection ▪ Prevention of infection in intestinal surgery ▪ Improved neurologic status in hepatic encephalopathy.

NEOSTIGMINE

(nee-oh-**stig**-meen)
Prostigmin

CLASSIFICATION(S):
Cholinergic—anticholinesterase agent
Pregnancy Category C

INDICATIONS

▪ Used to increase muscle strength in symptomatic treatment of myasthenia gravis ▪ Prevention and treatment of postoperative bladder distention and urinary retention or ileus ▪ Reversal of nondepolarizing neuromuscular blockers.

ACTION

▪ Inhibits the breakdown of acetylcholine so that it accumulates and has a prolonged effect ▪ Effects include miosis, increased intestinal and skeletal muscle tone, bronchial and ureteral constriction, bradycardia, increased salivation, lacrimation, and sweating. **Therapeutic Effects:** ▪ Improved muscular function in patients with myasthenia gravis, bladder emptying in patients with urinary retention, or reversal of nondepolarizing neuromuscular blockers.

PHARMACOKINETICS

Absorption: Poorly absorbed following oral administration, necessitating large oral doses as compared to parenteral doses.
Distribution: Does not appear to cross the placenta or enter breast milk.
Metabolism and Excretion: Metabolized by plasma cholinesterases and the liver.
Half-life: PO, IV—40–60 min; IM—50–90 min.

CONTRAINDICATIONS AND PRECAUTIONS

Contraindicated in: ▪ Hypersensitivity ▪ Mechanical obstruction of the GI or GU tract.
Use Cautiously in: ▪ History of asthma ▪ Ulcer disease ▪ Cardiovascular disease ▪ Epilepsy ▪ Hyperthyroidism ▪ Pregnancy (may cause uterine irritability after IV administration near term; newborns may display muscle weakness) ▪ Lactation.

ADVERSE REACTIONS AND SIDE EFFECTS*

CNS: dizziness, weakness, SEIZURES.
EENT: miosis, lacrimation.
Resp: excess secretions, bronchospasm.
CV: bradycardia, hypotension.
GI: abdominal cramps, nausea, vomiting, diarrhea, excess salivation.
Derm: rashes, sweating.

INTERACTIONS

Drug-Drug: ▪ Action may be antagonized by **drugs possessing anticholinergic properties,** including **antihistamines, antidepressants, atropine, haloperidol, phenothiazines, quinidine,** and **disopyramide** ▪ Prolongs action of **depolarizing muscle-relaxing agents (succinylcholine, decamethonium).**

ROUTE AND DOSAGE

Myasthenia Gravis

- **PO (Adults):** 15–30 mg tid initially, increase at daily intervals until optimal response is achieved. Usual maintenance dose is 150 mg/day (up to 375 mg/day may be needed).
- **PO (Children):** 7.5–15 mg 3–4 times daily.
- **IV, IM (Adults):** 0.5–2 mg q 1–3 hr.

Bladder Atony, Abdominal Distention: Prevention

- **IM, SC (Adults):** 0.25 mg q 4–6 hr for 2–3 days.

Bladder Atony, Abdominal Distention: Treatment

- **IM, SC (Adults):** 0.5–1 mg q 4–6 hr (may repeat if no response after 1 hr). Repeat q 3 hr for 5 doses after bladder has been emptied.

Antidote for Nondepolarizing Neuromuscular Blockers

- **IV (Adults):** 0.5–2 mg slowly; pretreat with 0.6–1.2 mg atropine IV.

PHARMACODYNAMICS (cholinergic effects, increased muscle tone)

	ONSET	PEAK	DURATION
PO	45–75 min	UK	2–4 hr
IM	10–30 min	20–30 min	2–4 hr
IV	10–30 min	20–30 min	2–4 hr

NURSING IMPLICATIONS

Assessment

- **General Info:** Assess pulse, respiratory rate, and blood pressure prior to administration. Notify physician of significant changes in heart rate.
- **Myasthenia Gravis:** Assess neuromuscular status, including vital capacity, ptosis, diplopia, chewing, swallowing, hand grasp, and gait, prior to administering and at peak effect. Patients with myasthenia gravis may be advised to keep a daily record of their condition and the effects of this medication.

*Underlines indicate most frequent; **CAPITALS** indicate life-threatening.

- Assess patient for overdosage and underdosage or resistance. Both have similar symptoms (muscle weakness, dyspnea, dysphagia), but symptoms of overdosage usually occur within 1 hr of administration, whereas underdosage symptoms occur 3 or more hr after administration. Overdosage (cholinergic crisis) symptoms may also include increased respiratory secretions and saliva, bradycardia, nausea, vomiting, cramping, diarrhea, and diaphoresis. A Tensilon test (edrophonium chloride) may be used to distinguish between overdosage and underdosage.
- **Postoperative Ileus:** Monitor abdominal status (assess for distention, auscultate bowel sounds). A rectal tube may be inserted to facilitate expulsion of flatus.
- **Postoperative Urinary Retention:** Assess for bladder distention. Monitor intake and output. If patient is unable to void within 1 hr of neostigmine administration, confer with physician about catheterization.
- **Antidote to Nondepolarizing Neuromuscular Blocking Agents:** Monitor reversal of effects of neuromuscular blocking agents with a peripheral nerve stimulator. Recovery usually occurs consecutively in the following muscles: diaphragm, intercostal muscles, muscles of the glottis, abdominal muscles, limb muscles, muscles of mastication, and levator muscles of the eyelids. Closely observe the patient for residual muscle weakness and respiratory distress throughout the recovery period. Maintain airway patency and ventilation until recovery of normal respirations occurs.
- **Toxicity and Overdose:** If overdose occurs, atropine is the antidote.

Potential Nursing Diagnoses
- Mobility, impaired physical (indications).
- Breathing pattern, ineffective (indications).
- Knowledge deficit related to medication regimen (patient/family teaching).

Implementation
- **General Info:** Oral and parenteral doses are not interchangeable.
- When used as an antidote to nondepolarizing neuromuscular blocking agents, atropine may be ordered prior to or currently with neostigmine to prevent or treat bradycardia.
- **PO:** Administer with food or milk to minimize side effects. For patients who have difficulty chewing, neostigmine may be ordered 30 min before meals.
- **Direct IV:** Administer doses undiluted. Do not add to IV soln. May be given through Y-site or 3-way stopcock of an IV of D5W, 0.9% NaCl, Ringer's soln, or lactated Ringer's soln.
- *Rate:* Administer each 0.5 mg over 1 min.
- **Syringe Compatibility:** glycopyrrolate, heparin, pentobarbital, or thiopental.
- **Y-Site Compatibility:** heparin, hydrocortisone sodium succinate, or potassium chloride.
- **Additive Compatibility:** netilmicin.

Patient/Family Teaching
- Instruct patient to take medication exactly as directed. Do not skip or double up on missed doses. Patients with a history of dysphagia should have a nonelectric or battery-operated backup alarm clock to remind them of exact dose time. Patients with dysphagia may not be able to swallow the medication if the dose is not taken exactly on time. Taking the dose late may result in myasthenic crisis. Taking the dose early may result in a cholinergic crisis. Patients with myasthenia gravis must continue this regimen as a lifelong therapy.
- Instruct patient with myasthenia gravis to space activities to avoid fatigue.
- Advise patient to carry identification describing disease and medication regimen at all times.

EVALUATION

Effectiveness of therapy can be demonstrated by: ▪ Relief of ptosis and diplopia ▫ Improved chewing, swallowing, extremity strength, and breathing without the appearance of cholinergic symptoms in myasthenia gravis ▪ Relief or prevention of postoperative gastrointestinal ileus ▪ Relief of nonobstructive postoperative urinary retention ▪ Reversal of nondepolarizing neuromuscular blocking agents in general anesthesia.

NETILMICIN
(ne-till-**mye**-sin)
Netromycin

CLASSIFICATION(S):
Anti-infective—aminoglycoside
Pregnancy Category D

INDICATIONS

▪ Useful in the treatment of gram-negative bacillary infections and infections due to staphylococci when penicillins or other less toxic drugs are contraindicated or resistance to other aminoglycosides has occurred ▪ Used in the treatment of the following infections due to susceptible organisms: ▫ Bone infection ▫ CNS infections (IT administration required) ▫ Respiratory tract infections ▫ Skin and soft tissue infections ▫ Abdominal infections ▫ Complicated urinary tract infections ▫ Endocarditis ▫ Septicemia.

ACTION

▪ Inhibits protein synthesis in bacteria at the level of the 30S ribosome. **Therapeutic Effect:** ▪ Bactericidal action against susceptible bacteria. **Spectrum:** ▪ Especially useful in serious gram-negative bacillary infections due to *Pseudomonas aeruginosa* and many Enterobacteriaceae, including: ▫ *Citrobacter diversus* ▫ *C. freundii* ▫ *Enterobacter aerogenes* ▫ *E. cloacae* ▫ *Escherichia coli* ▫ *Klebsiella* ▫ *Morganella morganii* ▫ *Proteus* ▫ *Providencia* ▫ *Salmonella* ▫ *Shigella*.

PHARMACOKINETICS

Absorption: Well absorbed after IM administration.
Distribution: Widely distributed in extracellular fluids following IM or IV administration. Crosses the placenta. Enters breast milk. Poor penetration into CSF.
Metabolism and Excretion: Excretion is mainly (>90%) renal. Dosage adjustments are required for any decrease in renal function. Minimal amounts metabolized by the liver.
Half-life: 2–3.4 hr (increased in renal impairment).

CONTRAINDICATIONS AND PRECAUTIONS

Contraindicated in: ▪ Hypersensitivity to netilmicin, bisulfites, or benzyl alcohol ▪ Cross-sensitivity with other aminoglycosides may exist.
Use Cautiously in: ▪ Renal impairment of any degree (dosage reduction required) ▪ Pregnancy and lactation (safety not established) ▪ Neuromuscular diseases, such as myasthenia gravis.

ADVERSE REACTIONS AND SIDE EFFECTS*

EENT: <u>ototoxicity</u> (vestibular and cochlear).
GU: <u>nephrotoxicity</u>.
Neuro: enhanced neuromuscular blockade.
Misc: hypersensitivity reactions, superinfection.

INTERACTIONS

Drug-Drug: ▪ Inactivated by **penicillins** when coadministered to patients with renal insufficiency ▪ Possible respiratory paralysis after **general anesthetics** or **neuromuscular blockers (tubocurarine, succinylcholine, decamethonium)** ▪ Increased risk of ototoxicity with **loop diuretics** ▪ Risk of neph-

*<u>Underlines</u> indicate most frequent; **CAPITALS** indicate life-threatening.

rotoxicity may be increased with other potentially **nephrotoxic drugs (cisplatin).**

ROUTE AND DOSAGE

Note: All doses after initial loading dose should be determined by renal function/blood level monitoring.

- **IM, IV (Adults):** 4–6.5 mg/kg/day individual doses q 8–12 hr (3–4 mg/kg/day in divided doses q 12 hr) for urinary tract infection.
- **IM, IV (Children 6 wk–12 yr):** 1.83–2.67 mg/kg q 12 hr or 2.75–4 mg/kg q 12 hr.
- **IM, IV (Premature or Full-Term Neonates <6 wk):** 2–3.25 mg/kg q 12 hr.

PHARMACODYNAMICS (blood levels)

	ONSET	PEAK
IM	rapid	30–90 min
IV	rapid	end of infusion

NURSING IMPLICATIONS

Assessment

- Assess patient for infection (vital signs; wound appearance, sputum, urine, and stool; WBC) at beginning and throughout course of therapy.
- Obtain specimens for culture and sensitivity prior to initiating therapy. First dose may be given before receiving results.
- Evaluate eighth cranial nerve function by audiometry prior to and throughout course of therapy. Hearing loss is usually in the high-frequency range. Prompt recognition and intervention is essential in preventing permanent damage. Also monitor for vestibular dysfunction (vertigo, ataxia, nausea, vomiting). Eighth cranial nerve dysfunction is associated with persistently elevated peak netilmicin levels.
- Monitor intake and output and daily weight to assess hydration status and renal function.
- Assess patient for signs of superinfection (fever, upper respiratory infection, vaginal itching or discharge, increasing malaise, diarrhea). Report to physician.
- **Lab Test Considerations:** Monitor renal function by urinalysis, specific gravity, BUN, creatinine, and creatinine clearance prior to and throughout therapy.
- May cause increased serum BUN, SGPT (ALT), SGOT (AST), LDH, alkaline phosphatase, bilirubin, and creatinine concentrations.
- May cause decreased serum calcium, magnesium, potassium, and sodium concentrations.
- **Toxicity and Overdose:** Blood levels should be monitored periodically during therapy. Timing of blood levels is important in interpreting results. Draw blood for peak levels 1 hr after IM injection and 15–30 min after IV infusion is completed. Trough levels should be drawn just prior to next dose. Acceptable peak level is 6–10 mcg/ml; trough level should not exceed 4 mcg/ml.

Potential Nursing Diagnoses

- Infection, high risk for (indications).
- Sensory-perceptual alteration: auditory (side effects).

Implementation

- **General Info:** Keep patient well hydrated (1500–2000 ml/day) during therapy.
- Soln is clear and colorless to pale yellow.
- **Intermittent Infusion:** Dilute each dose in 50–200 ml of D5/LR, D5/0.9% NaCl, D5W, D10W, Ringer's or lactated Ringer's soln, 0.9% NaCl, 3% NaCl, or 5% NaCl. Dilute in a proportionately smaller volume for pediatric patients. Stable for 72 hr at room temperature.
- *Rate:* Infuse slowly over 30 min–2 hr.
- **Y-Site Compatibility:** aminophylline or calcium gluconate.
- **Y-Site Incompatibility:** furosemide or heparin.
- **Additive Incompatibility:** Manufacturer recommends administering separately; do not admix. Give aminogly-

cosides and penicillins at least 1 hr apart to prevent inactivation.

Patient/Family Teaching

□ Instruct patient to report signs of hypersensitivity, tinnitus, vertigo, or hearing loss.

Evaluation

Clinical response can be evaluated by: ▪ Resolution of the signs and symptoms of infection. Length of time for complete resolution depends on the organism and site of infection. If no response is seen within 3–5 days, new cultures should be obtained.

NIACIN

(**nye**-a-sin)
Niac, Niacels, Nico-400, Nicobid, Nicolar, Nicotinex, Nicotinic acid, Span Niacin, Tega-Span, {Tri-B3}, vitamin B_3

NIACINAMIDE

(nye-a-**sin**-a-mide)
Nicotinamide

CLASSIFICATION(S):
Lipid-lowering agent, Vitamin—water-soluble
Pregnancy Category C

INDICATIONS

▪ Treatment and prevention of niacin deficiency (pellagra) ▪ Adjunctive therapy in certain hyperlipidemias (niacin only).

ACTION

▪ Required as coenzymes (for lipid metabolism, glycogenolysis, and tissue respiration) ▪ Large doses decrease lipoprotein and triglyceride synthesis by inhibiting the release of free fatty acids from adipose tissue and decreasing hepatic lipoprotein synthesis (niacin only) ▪ Causes peripheral vasodilation in large doses (niacin only). **Therapeutic Effects:** ▪ Decreased blood lipids (niacin only) ▪ Supplementation in deficiency states.

PHARMACOKINETICS

Absorption: Well absorbed following oral administration.
Distribution: Widely distributed following conversion to niacinamide. Enters breast milk.
Metabolism and Excretion: Amounts required for metabolic processes are converted to niacinamide. Large doses of niacin are excreted unchanged in the urine.
Half-life: 45 min.

CONTRAINDICATIONS AND PRECAUTIONS

Contraindicated in: ▪ Hypersensitivity to niacin ▪ Some products may contain tartazine (FDC yellow dye #5) and should be avoided in patients with aspirin allergy ▪ Hypersensitivity to chlorobutanol (parenteral niacinamide) ▪ Alcohol intolerance (Nicotinex only).
Use Cautiously in: ▪ Liver disease ▪ Arterial bleeding ▪ History of peptic ulcer disease ▪ Gout ▪ Glaucoma ▪ Diabetes mellitus.

ADVERSE REACTIONS AND SIDE EFFECTS*

Note: Adverse reactions and side effects refer to IV administration or doses used to treat hyperlipidemias.

CNS: nervousness, panic.
CV: orthostatic hypotension.
EENT: toxic amblyopia, blurred vision, proptosis, loss of central vision.
GI: metallic taste (IV only), GI upset, nausea, bloating, flatulence, hunger pains, heartburn, diarrhea, dry mouth, peptic ulceration, hepatotoxicity (SR oral form only).
Derm: flushing of the face and neck, pruritus, burning, stinging or tingling of skin, increased sebaceous gland activity, rashes, hyperpigmentation, dry skin.
Hemat: activation of fibrinolysis (IV only).

{} = Available in Canada only.
*Underlines indicate most frequent; **CAPITALS** indicate life-threatening.

N

Metab: hyperuricemia, hyperglycemia, glycosuria.
Misc: ANAPHYLACTIC SHOCK (IV only).

INTERACTIONS

Drug–Drug: ▪ Increased risk of myopathy with concurrent use of **lovastatin** ▪ Additive hypotension with **ganglionic blocking agents (guanethidine, guanedrel)** ▪ Large doses may decrease the uricosuric effects of **probenecid** or **sulfinpyrazone**.

ROUTE AND DOSAGE

Niacin—Dietary Supplementation

- **PO (Adults and Children):** 10–20 mg/day.

Niacin—Hyperlipidemias

- **PO (Adults):** 1–2 g tid.

Niacin—Pellagra

- **PO (Adults):** 300–500 mg/day in divided doses.
- **PO (Children):** 100–300 mg/day in divided doses.
- **IM, SC (Adults):** 50–100 mg 5 or more times daily.
- **IV (Adults):** 25–100 mg slowly.

Niacinamide

- **PO (Adults):** 50 mg 3–10 times daily.
- **IM (Adults):** 50–100 mg 5 or more times daily (up to 3 g/day).
- **IV (Adults):** 25–100 mg 2 or more times daily.
- **IV (Children):** <100–300 mg/day in divided doses.

PHARMACODYNAMICS (effects on blood lipids)

	ONSET	PEAK	DURATION
PO (cholesterol)	several days	UK	UK
PO (triglycerides)	several hrs	UK	UK
IV	UK	UK	UK

NURSING IMPLICATIONS

Assessment

- **Vitamin Deficiency:** Assess patient for signs of niacin deficiency (pellagra—dermatitis, stomatitis, glossitis, anemia, nausea, and vomiting, confusion, memory loss, and delirium) prior to and periodically throughout therapy.
- **Hyperlipidemia:** Obtain a diet history, especially in regard to fat consumption.
- **Lab Test Considerations:** Serum glucose and uric acid levels and hepatic function tests should be monitored periodically during prolonged high-dose therapy. Notify physician if SGOT (AST), SGPT (ALT), or LDH becomes elevated. May increase prothrombin times and decrease serum albumin.
  - □ High-dose therapy may cause elevated serum glucose and uric acid levels. May also cause falsely elevated urine glucose when measured with copper sulfate method (Clinitest) and catecholamine levels during high-dose therapy. Use glucose oxidase method (Tes-Tape) to measure urine glucose.
  - □ When niacin is used as a lipid-lowering agent, serum cholesterol and triglyceride levels should be monitored prior to and periodically throughout course of therapy.

Potential Nursing Diagnoses

- Nutrition, altered: less than body requirements (indications).
- Knowledge deficit related to medication regimen (patient/family teaching).
- Noncompliance (patient/family teaching).

Implementation

- **General Info:** Because of infrequency of single B-vitamin deficiencies, combinations are commonly administered.
- **PO:** Administer with meals or milk to minimize GI irritation.
  - □ Extended-release tablet and capsules should be swallowed whole, without crushing, breaking, or chewing. Use calibrated measuring device to ensure accurate dosage of soln.

- **Direct IV:** Dilute to a strength of 2 mg/ml
  - *Rate:* Administer at a rate not exceeding 2 mg/min.
- **Intermittent/Continuous Infusion:** Add to 500 ml of 0.9% NaCl.
  - *Rate:* Administer at a rate not exceeding 2 mg/min.
- **Additive Compatibility:** TPN soln.
- **Additive Incompatibility:** erythromycin, kanamycin, streptomycin, alkalis, or strong acids.

Patient/Family Teaching

- **General Info:** Inform patient that cutaneous flushing and a sensation of warmth, especially in the face, neck, and ears, and itching or tingling and headache may occur within the first 2 hr after taking the drug (immediately after IV doses). These effects are usually transient and subside with continued therapy.
  - Emphasize the importance of follow-up examinations to evaluate progress.
- **Vitamin Deficiency:** Encourage patient to comply with diet recommendations of physician. Explain that the best source of vitamins is a well-balanced diet with foods from the 4 basic food groups.
  - Foods high in niacin include meats, eggs, milk, and dairy products; little is lost during ordinary cooking.
  - Patients self-medicating with vitamin supplements should be cautioned not to exceed RDA (see Appendix L). The effectiveness of megadoses for treatment of various medical conditions is unproven and may cause side effects.
- **Hyperlipidemia:** Advise patient that this medication should be used in conjunction with diet restrictions (fat, cholesterol, carbohydrates, alcohol), exercise, and cessation of smoking.

Evaluation

Effectiveness of therapy can be demonstrated by: ▪ Prevention and treatment of niacin deficiency ▪ Decrease in serum cholesterol and triglyceride levels.

NICARDIPINE

(nye-**kar**-de-peen)
Cardene

CLASSIFICATION(S):
Calcium channel blocker, Antianginal, Coronary vasodilator, Antihypertensive
Pregnancy Category C

INDICATIONS

▪ Management of angina pectoris ▪ Alone or with other agents in the management of hypertension.

ACTION

▪ Inhibits the transport of calcium into myocardial and vascular smooth muscle cells, resulting in inhibition of excitation-contraction coupling and subsequent contraction. **Therapeutic Effects:** ▪ Coronary vasodilation and subsequent decrease in frequency and severity of attacks of angina pectoris ▪ Lowering of blood pressure.

PHARMACOKINETICS

Absorption: Well absorbed following oral administration. Large amounts are rapidly metabolized, resulting in decreased bioavailability (35%).
Distribution: Distribution not known.
Metabolism and Excretion: Mostly metabolized by the liver. Negligible amounts excreted by the kidneys.
Half-life: 2–4 hr.

CONTRAINDICATIONS AND PRECAUTIONS

Contraindicated in: ▪ Hypersensitivity ▪ Aortic stenosis ▪ Lactation.
Use Cautiously in: ▪ Hepatic impairment ▪ Congestive heart failure ▪ Pregnancy or children (safety not established).

ADVERSE REACTIONS AND SIDE EFFECTS*

CNS: dizziness, lightheadedness, headache, nervousness, somnolence, weakness.

*Underlines indicate most frequent; **CAPITALS** indicate life-threatening.

N

Resp: dyspnea.
CV: peripheral edema, palpitations, angina, tachycardia, orthostatic hypotension.
GI: nausea, abdominal pain, dry mouth, constipation.
Derm: flushing, rash.
Neuro: paresthesia.

INTERACTIONS

Drug–Drug: ▪ Increased risk of bradycardia, conduction defects, or congestive heart failure when used with **beta-adrenergic blockers, disopyramide,** or **digoxin** ▪ **Phenytoin** and **phenobarbital** may hasten metabolism and decrease effectiveness ▪ **Cimetidine** and **propranolol** may slow metabolism and lead to toxicity ▪ May increase blood levels and toxicity of **cyclosporine** ▪ Antihypertensive effect may be decreased by **nonsteroidal anti-inflammatory agents** ▪ Additive hypertension with acute ingestion of **alcohol, nitrates,** and other **antihypertensives.**
Drug–Food: ▪ Absorption may be decreased by concurrent administration with a **high-fat** meal.

ROUTE AND DOSAGE

- **PO (Adults):** 20 mg tid, may be increased at 3-day intervals (range 20–40 mg tid).

PHARMACODYNAMICS (hypotensive effects)

	ONSET	PEAK	DURATION
PO	20 min	1–2 hr	8 hr

NURSING IMPLICATIONS

Assessment

- **Angina:** Assess location, duration, intensity, and precipitating factors of patient's anginal pain.
- **Hypertension:** Monitor blood pressure and pulse before administering medication. Measurements taken 1–2 hr following administration demonstrate peak effectiveness; measurements 8 hr after administration demonstrate adequacy of dose.
- ▫ Monitor intake and output ratios and daily weight. Assess patient for peripheral edema periodically throughout therapy

Potential Nursing Diagnoses

- Cardiac output, decreased (indications).
- Comfort, altered: pain (indications).
- Knowledge deficit related to medication regimen (patient/family teaching).

Implementation

- **General Info:** Dosage adjustments should be made no more frequently than every 3 days.
- **PO:** Administer on an empty stomach, 1 hr before or 3 hr after meals. Food with especially high-fat content decreases absorption.

Patient/Family Teaching

- **General Info:** Advise patient to take medication exactly as prescribed, not to skip or double up on missed doses.
- ▫ May cause dizziness and drowsiness. Advise patient to avoid driving or other activities requiring alertness until response to the medication is known.
- ▫ Instruct patient to avoid concurrent use of alcohol or over-the-counter medications without consulting physician or pharmacist.
- ▫ Advise patient to notify physician if irregular heartbeats, dyspnea, swelling of hands and feet, pronounced dizziness, nausea, constipation, or hypotension occurs.
- **Angina:** Inform patient that anginal attacks may occur 30 min after administration due to reflex tachycardia. This is usually temporary and is not an indication for discontinuation.
- ▫ Instruct patient on concurrent nitrate or beta-blocker therapy to continue taking both medications as ordered and using SL nitroglycerin as needed for anginal attacks.
- ▫ Advise patient to contact physician if chest pain does not improve or worsens after therapy or is accompanied by diaphoresis or shortness of breath

or if severe, persistent headache occurs.

- **Hypertension:** Encourage patient to comply with additional interventions for hypertension (weight reduction, low-sodium diet, discontinuation of smoking, moderation of alcohol consumption, regular exercise, and stress management).

EVALUATION

Effectiveness of therapy can be demonstrated by: ▪ Decrease in frequency and severity of anginal attacks ▫ Decrease in need for nitrate therapy ▫ Increase in activity tolerance and sense of well-being ▪ Decrease in blood pressure.

NICOTINE POLACRILEX CHEWING GUM

(**nik**-o-teen)
Nicorette

CLASSIFICATION(S):
Smoking deterrent
Pregnancy Category X

INDICATIONS

▪ Adjunct therapy (with behavior modification) in the management of nicotine withdrawal in patients desiring to give up cigarette smoking.

ACTION

▪ Provides a source of nicotine during controlled withdrawal from cigarette smoking. **Therapeutic Effect:** ▪ Lessened sequelae of nicotine withdrawal (irritability, insomnia, somnolence, headache, and increased appetite).

PHARMACOKINETICS

Absorption: Slowly absorbed from buccal mucosa during chewing.
Distribution: Distribution not known.
Metabolism and Excretion: Mostly metabolized by the liver. Small amounts metabolized by kidneys and lungs.
Half-life: 30–60 min.

CONTRAINDICATIONS AND PRECAUTIONS

Contraindicated in: ▪ Severe cardiovascular disease ▪ Temporomandibular joint disease ▪ Pregnancy ▪ Children.
Use Cautiously in: ▪ Cardiovascular disease, including hypertension ▪ Diabetes mellitus ▪ Pheochromocytoma ▪ Peripheral vascular diseases ▪ Dental problems ▪ Hyperthyroidism ▪ Esophagitis, stomatitis, or pharyngitis ▪ Lactation (potential for adverse effects in the newborn).

ADVERSE REACTIONS AND SIDE EFFECTS*

CNS: headache, dizziness, lightheadedness, irritability, insomnia.
EENT: <u>pharyngitis</u>, hoarseness.
Resp: coughing.
CV: atrial fibrillation, <u>tachycardia</u>, hypotension.
GI: <u>oral injury</u>, <u>belching</u>, <u>sore mouth</u>, <u>increased salivation</u>, <u>increased appetite</u>, constipation, dry mouth, hiccoughs, loss of appetite, diarrhea, nausea, vomiting, abdominal pain.
MS: <u>jaw muscle ache</u>.

INTERACTIONS

Drug-Drug: ▪ **Insulin** requirements may decrease during nicotine withdrawal ▪ Effects of **propranolol, theophylline,** or **propoxyphene** may be increased during nicotine withdrawal (decreased metabolism).

ROUTE AND DOSAGE

- **Chew (Adults):** 2 mg (1 piece of gum) as needed, amount determined by smoking urge and rate of chewing. Usual initial requirement 20 mg (10 pieces of gum)/day. Not to exceed 100 mg/day.

PHARMACODYNAMICS (nicotine blood levels)

	ONSET	PEAK	DURATION
Chew	UK	15–30 min	UK

*<u>Underlines</u> indicate most frequent; **CAPITALS** indicate life-threatening.

N

NURSING IMPLICATIONS

Assessment

- ▫ Prior to therapy, assess smoking history (number of cigarettes smoked daily, smoking patterns, nicotine content of preferred brand, degree to which patient inhales smoke).
- ▫ Assess patient for history of temporomandibular joint pain or dysfunction.
- ▪ **Toxicity and Overdose:** Monitor for nausea, vomiting, diarrhea, increased salivation, abdominal pain, headache, dizziness, auditory and visual disturbances, weakness, dyspnea, hypotension, and irregular pulse.

Potential Nursing Diagnoses

- ▪ Coping, ineffective (indications).
- ▪ Knowledge deficit related to medication regimen (patient/family teaching).

Implementation

- ▪ **General Info:** Protect gum from light; exposure to light causes gum to turn brown.

Patient/Family Teaching

- ▫ Explain purpose of nicotine gum to patient. The patient should chew 1 piece of gum whenever a craving for nicotine occurs. The gum should be chewed slowly until a tingling sensation is felt (after about 15 chews). Then patient should stop chewing and store the gum between the cheek and gums until the tingling sensation disappears (after about 1 min). The process of stopping then resuming chewing should be repeated for approximately 30 min. Rapid, vigorous chewing may result in side effects similar to those of smoking too many cigarettes (headache, dizziness, nausea, increased salivation, heartburn, and hiccoughs).
- ▫ Explain to patient that the gum has a slight tobacco/pepperlike taste. Many patients initially find it unpleasant and slightly irritating to the mouth. This usually resolves after several days of therapy.
- ▫ The gum usually can be chewed by denture wearers. Contact dentist if the gum adheres to bridgework.
- ▫ Use of the gum may be discontinued when 1–2 pieces/day is sufficient to control the craving for nicotine. The duration of treatment is limited to 6 mon because physical and psychological dependence can occur. Discontinuing the gum too soon may result in withdrawal symptoms (anxiety, irritability, GI distress, headache, drowsiness, or tobacco craving).
- ▫ Instruct patient not to swallow gum.
- ▫ Emphasize need to keep nicotine gum out of the reach of children. Call the poison control center, emergency department, or physician immediately if a child ingests the gum.
- ▫ Emphasize the need to discontinue the gum and inform the physician if pregnancy occurs.
- ▫ Review the patient instruction sheet enclosed in the package of gum.

Evaluation

Effectiveness of therapy can be demonstrated by: ▪ Decrease in nicotine withdrawal symptoms in patients participating in a supervised smoking cessation program. Therapy is limited to 6 mon; most patients begin a gradual withdrawal after 3 mon of therapy.

NIFEDIPINE

(nye-**fed**-i-peen)
Adalat, {Adalat P. A.}, {Apo-Nifed}, {Novo-Nifedin}, Procardia, Procardia XL

CLASSIFICATION(S):
Calcium channel blocker, Antianginal, Coronary vasodilator
Pregnancy Category C

INDICATIONS

▪ **PO:** Management of angina pectoris due to coronary insufficiency or vasospasm (Prinzmetal's angina) ▪ Treatment of hypertension. **Unlabeled Uses:** ▪ *SL:* Acute treatment of hypertension ▪ *PO:* Management of migraine headache, Raynaud's syndrome, and congestive heart failure.

ACTION

▪ Acts on slow calcium channels in vascular smooth muscle and myocardium, producing coronary vasodilation. **Therapeutic Effects:** ▪ Coronary vasodilation and subsequent decrease in frequency and severity of attacks of angina pectoris ▪ Lowering of blood pressure.

PHARMACOKINETICS

Absorption: Well absorbed after oral administration, but large amounts are rapidly metabolized resulting in decreased bioavailability (45–70%). Bioavailability increased with sustained-release (XL) form (80%).
Distribution: Distribution not known.
Metabolism and Excretion: Mostly metabolized by the liver.
Half-life: 2–5 hr.

CONTRAINDICATIONS AND PRECAUTIONS

Contraindicated in: ▪ Hypersensitivity ▪ Severe hypotension.
Use Cautiously in: ▪ Severe hepatic disease (dosage reduction required) ▪ Congestive heart failure ▪ Edema ▪ Aortic stenosis ▪ Pregnancy, lactation, or children (safety not established).

ADVERSE REACTIONS AND SIDE EFFECTS*

CNS: dizziness, lightheadedness, giddiness, headache, nervousness.
EENT: nasal congestion, sore throat.
Resp: dyspnea, cough, wheezing.
CV: hypotension, syncope, CONGESTIVE HEART FAILURE, MYOCARDIAL INFARCTION, ventricular arrhythmias, tachycardia.
GI: nausea, heartburn, abdominal discomfort, hepatitis, diarrhea, constipation, flatulence.
MS: muscle cramps.
Derm: flushing, warmth, rashes, sweating.
Misc: fever.

INTERACTIONS

Drug-Drug: ▪ Increased risk of bradycardia, conduction defects, or congestive heart failure when used with **beta-adrenergic blockers, disopyramide,** or **digoxin** ▪ **Cimetidine** may slow metabolism and lead to toxicity ▪ Severe hypotension may occur when used with **fentanyl** ▪ Additive hypotension with **antihypertensives,** acute ingestion of **alcohol,** or **nitrates** ▪ May increase blood levels and risk of toxicity with **digoxin** ▪ **NSAIDs** may decrease antihypertensive effects.

ROUTE AND DOSAGE

- **PO (Adults):** 10–40 mg 3–4 times daily (not to exceed 180 mg/day) or 30–60 mg once daily as sustained release (XL) form (not to exceed 90–120 mg/day).
- **SL (Adults):** 10 mg, repeated in 20–30 min (unlabeled).

PHARMACODYNAMICS (effects on blood pressure)

	ONSET	PEAK	DURATION
PO	20 min	UK	6–8 hr
PO-SR	UK	UK	24 hr

NURSING IMPLICATIONS

Assessment

- **General Info:** Monitor blood pressure and pulse before administering medication. Monitor ECG periodically in patients receiving prolonged therapy. Blood pressure should be monitored closely when nifedipine is administered for hypertension.
- Monitor intake and output ratios and daily weight. Assess patient for signs of congestive heart failure (peripheral edema, rales/crackles, dyspnea, weight gain, jugular venous distention).
- Patients receiving cardiac glycosides

*Underlines indicate most frequent; **CAPITALS** indicate life-threatening.

concurrently with nifedipine should have routine serum digitalis levels and be monitored for signs and symptoms of cardiac glycoside toxicity.

- ▫ Monitor renal and hepatic function periodically in patients receiving long-term therapy.
- ▪ **Angina:** Assess location, duration, intensity, and precipitating factors of patient's anginal pain.
- ▪ **Lab Test Considerations:** May cause elevated alkaline phosphatase, CPK, LDH, SGOT (AST), and SGPT (ALT) levels.
- ▫ May cause positive direct Coombs' test results.

Potential Nursing Diagnoses

- ▪ Cardiac output, decreased (indications).
- ▪ Comfort, altered: pain (indications).
- ▪ Knowledge deficit related to medication regimen (patient/family teaching).

Implementation

- ▪ **PO:** May be administered with meals if gastric irritation becomes a problem. Capsules and XL tablets should be swallowed whole; do not crush, break, or chew.
- ▪ **SL:** May be administered by puncturing the capsule with a sterile needle and squeezing to administer the liquid into the buccal pouch. The dose used is the same as the oral dose. Chewing capsule has shown similar effectiveness as SL route for hypertensive emergencies.

Patient/Family Teaching

- ▪ **General Info:** Advise patient to take medication exactly as prescribed, not to skip or double up on missed doses. May need to be discontinued gradually.
- ▫ Caution patient to make position changes slowly to minimize orthostatic hypotension.
- ▫ May cause dizziness. Advise patient to avoid driving or other activities requiring alertness until response to the medication is known.
- ▫ Instruct patient to avoid concurrent use of alcohol or over-the-counter medications without consulting physician or pharmacist.
- ▫ Advise patient to notify physician if irregular heart beats, dyspnea, swelling of hands and feet, pronounced dizziness, nausea, constipation, or hypotension occur.
- ▪ **Angina:** Inform patient that anginal attacks may occur 30 min after administration due to reflex tachycardia. This is usually temporary and is not an indication for discontinuation.
- ▫ Instruct patient on concurrent nitrate or beta-blocker therapy to continue taking both medications as ordered and using SL nitroglycerin as needed for anginal attacks.
- ▫ Advise patient to contact physician if chest pain does not improve or worsens after therapy or is accompanied by diaphoresis or shortness of breath or if severe, persistent headache occurs.
- ▪ **Hypertension:** Encourage patient to comply with additional interventions for hypertension (weight reduction, low-sodium diet, discontinuation of smoking, moderation of alcohol consumption, regular exercise, and stress management).

Evaluation

Effectiveness of therapy can be demonstrated by: ▪ Decrease in frequency and severity of anginal attacks ▫ Decrease in need for nitrate therapy ▫ Increase in activity tolerance and sense of well-being ▪ Decrease in blood pressure.

NIMODIPINE

(ni-**moe**-dip-een)
Nimotop

CLASSIFICATION(S):
Calcium channel blocker
Pregnancy Category C

INDICATIONS

- ▪ Prevention of cerebral vasospasm in the management of subarachnoid hemorrhage following ruptured congenital intracranial aneurysm.

ACTION

▪ Acts on slow calcium channels in vascular smooth muscle, producing vasodilation ▪ High CNS concentrations may have specific spasmolytic effect on cerebral arteries. **Therapeutic Effect:** ▪ Prevention of vascular spasm after subarachnoid hemorrhage, resulting in decreased neurologic impairment.

PHARMACOKINETICS

Absorption: Although well absorbed following oral administration, rapid hepatic metabolism leads to decreased bioavailability.
Distribution: Crosses the blood-brain barrier. Remainder of distribution not known.
Metabolism and Excretion: Mostly metabolized by the liver.
Half-life: 1–2 hr.

CONTRAINDICATIONS AND PRECAUTIONS

Contraindicated in: ▪ Hypersensitivity.
Use Cautiously in: ▪ Severe hypertension.

ADVERSE REACTIONS AND SIDE EFFECTS*

CNS: psychiatric disturbances, headache, dizziness.
Resp: shortness of breath, dyspnea, wheezing.
CV: hypotension, tachycardia, bradycardia, peripheral edema.
GI: nausea, constipation, hepatitis, abdominal discomfort.
Derm: dermatitis, rash, flushing.
MS: muscle cramps.

INTERACTIONS

Drug-Drug: ▪ Additive hypotension with **antihypertensive agents,** acute ingestion of **alcohol,** or **nitrates** ▪ May produce additive myocardial depression with **beta-adrenergic blockers** ▪ May result in severe hypotension with **fentanyl.**

ROUTE AND DOSAGE

- **PO (Adults):** 60 mg q 4 hr for 21 days; therapy should be started within 96 hr of subarachnoid hemorrhage.

PHARMACODYNAMICS

	ONSET	PEAK	DURATION
PO	UK	UK	UK

NURSING IMPLICATIONS

Assessment

- ▫ Assess patient's neurologic status (level of consciousness, movement) prior to and periodically following administration.
- ▫ Monitor blood pressure before and during administration of medication.
- ▫ Monitor intake and output ratios and daily weight. Assess patient for peripheral edema periodically throughout therapy.
- ▪ **Lab Test Considerations:** May occasionally cause decreased platelet count.
- ▫ May cause elevated alkaline phosphatase, LDH, SGPT (ALT), and serum glucose levels.

Potential Nursing Diagnoses

- Injury, high risk for (indications).
- Knowledge deficit related to medication regimen (patient/family teaching).

Implementation

- **General Info:** Begin administration within 96 hr of subarachnoid hemorrhage and continue every 4 hr for 21 consecutive days.
- **PO:** If patient is unable to swallow capsule, make a hole in both ends of the capsule with a sterile 18-gauge needle and extract the contents into a syringe. Empty contents into water or nasogastric tube and flush with 30 ml normal saline.

*Underlines indicate most frequent; **CAPITALS** indicate life-threatening.

N

PATIENT/FAMILY TEACHING

- Advise patient to take medication exactly as prescribed, not to skip or double up on missed doses.
- Caution patients to make position changes slowly to minimize orthostatic hypotension.
- Advise patient to notify physician if irregular heart beat, dyspnea, swelling of hands and feet, pronounced dizziness, nausea, constipation, hypotension, or persistent headache occurs.

EVALUATION

Effectiveness of therapy can be demonstrated by: ▪ Improvement in neurologic deficits due to vasospasm following subarachnoid hemorrhage.

NITROFURANTOIN

(nye-troe-fyoor-**an**-toyn)

{Apo-Nitrofurantoin}, Furadantin, Furalan, Furan, Macpac, Macrodantin, {Nephronex}, {Novofuran}

CLASSIFICATION(S):

Anti-infective—miscellaneous

Pregnancy Category UK

INDICATIONS

▪ Treatment of urinary tract infections due to susceptible organisms. Not effective in systemic bacterial infections ▪ Chronic suppressive therapy of urinary tract infections.

ACTION

▪ Interferes with bacterial enzymes. **Therapeutic Effect:** ▪ Bactericidal or bacteriostatic action against susceptible organisms. **Spectrum:** ▪ Many gram-negative and some gram-positive organisms, specifically: □ *Citrobacter* □ *Corynebacterium* □ *Enterobacter* □ *Escherichia coli* □ *Klebsiella* □ *Neisseria* □ *Salmonella* □ *Shigella* □ *Staphylococcus aureus* □ *Staphylococcus epidermidis* □ *Enterococcus.*

PHARMACOKINETICS

Absorption: Readily absorbed following oral administration. Absorption is slower, but more complete with macrocrystals (Macrodantin).

Distribution: Crosses the placenta and enters breast milk.

Metabolism and Excretion: Partially metabolized by the liver. 30–50% excreted unchanged by the kidneys.

Half-life: 20 min (increased in renal impairment).

CONTRAINDICATIONS AND PRECAUTIONS

Contraindicated in: ▪ Hypersensitivity ▪ Hypersensitivity to parabens (suspension) ▪ Oliguria or anuria ▪ Infants <1 mon and pregnancy near term (increased risk of hemolytic anemia in newborn) ▪ Glucose-6-phosphate dehydrogenase (G6-PD) deficiency.

Use Cautiously in: ▪ Diabetics or debilitated patients (neuropathy may be more common) ▪ Pregnancy and lactation (although safety not established, has been used in pregnant women).

ADVERSE REACTIONS AND SIDE EFFECTS*

CNS: dizziness, headache, drowsiness.
EENT: nystagmus.
Resp: pneumonitis.
CV: chest pain.
GI: nausea, vomiting, anorexia, diarrhea, abdominal pain, hepatitis.
GU: rust/brown discoloration of urine.
Derm: photosensitivity.
Hemat: blood dyscrasias, hemolytic anemia.
Neuro: peripheral neuropathy.

INTERACTIONS

Drug-Drug: ▪ **Probenecid** and **sulfinpyrazone** prevent high urinary concentrations, may decrease effectiveness ▪ **Antacids** may decrease absorption ▪ Increased risk of neurotoxicity with

{} = Available in Canada only.
*Underlines indicate most frequent; **CAPITALS** indicate life-threatening.

neurotoxic drugs ■ Increased risk of hepatoxicity with **hepatotoxic drugs** ■ Increased risk of pneumonitis with **drugs having pulmonary toxicity** ■ Nitrofurantoin decreases the anti-infective action of **fluoroquinolones**.

ROUTE AND DOSAGE

Active Infection

- **PO (Adults):** 50–100 mg in divided doses q 6 hr.
- **PO (Children >1 mon):** 5–7 mg/kg/day in divided doses q 6 hr.

Chronic Suppression

- **PO (Adults):** 50–100 mg, single evening dose.
- **PO (Children):** 1 mg/kg/day as single dose or 2 divided doses.

PHARMACODYNAMICS (urine levels)

	ONSET	PEAK
PO	UK	30 min

NURSING IMPLICATIONS

Assessment

- Assess patient for signs and symptoms of urinary tract infection (frequency, urgency, pain, and burning on urination, fever, cloudy or foul-smelling urine) prior to and periodically throughout course of therapy.
- Obtain specimens for culture and sensitivity prior to and during drug administration.
- Monitor intake and output ratios. Notify physician of significant discrepancies in totals.
- **Lab Test Considerations:** CBC should be routinely monitored with patients on prolonged therapy.
- May cause elevated serum glucose, bilirubin, alkaline phosphatase, BUN, and creatinine.
- May cause a false-positive result with copper sulfate urine glucose tests (Clinitest). Use glucose oxidase method (Ketodiastix or Tes-Tape) to test for urine glucose.

Potential Nursing Diagnoses

- Infection, high risk for (indications).
- Comfort, altered: pain (indications).
- Knowledge deficit related to medication regimen (patient/family teaching).

Implementation

- **PO:** Administer with food or milk to minimize GI irritation, to delay and increase absorption, to increase peak concentration, and to prolong duration of therapeutic concentration in the urine.
- Do not crush tablets or open capsules.
- Administer liquid preparations with calibrated measuring device. Shake well prior to administration. Oral suspension may be mixed with water, milk, fruit juices, or infant's formula. Rinse mouth with water following administration of oral suspension to avoid staining teeth.

Patient/Family Teaching

- Instruct patient to take medication around the clock, exactly as directed. If a dose is missed, take as soon as remembered and space next dose 2–4 hr apart. Do not skip or double up on missed doses.
- May cause dizziness or drowsiness. Caution patient to avoid driving or other activities requiring alertness until response to medication is known.
- Inform patient that medication may cause a rust-yellow to brown discoloration of urine, which is not significant.
- Advise patient to notify physician if fever, chills, cough, chest pain, dyspnea, skin rash, numbness or tingling of the fingers or toes, or intolerable GI upset occurs. Signs of superinfection (milky, foul-smelling urine; perineal irritation; dysuria) should also be reported.
- Instruct patient to consult physician if no improvement is seen within a few days after initiation of therapy.

Evaluation

Effectiveness of therapy can be demonstrated by: ■ Resolution of the signs and symptoms of infection. Therapy should be continued for a minimum of 7 days and for at least 3 days after the urine has become sterile ▪ Decrease in the frequency of infections in chronic suppressive therapy.

NITROGLYCERIN
(nye-tro-**gli**-ser-in)
NITROGLYCERIN EXTENDED-RELEASE CAPSULES
Nitrobid, Nitrocap T.D., Nitrocine, Nitroglyn, Nitrolin
NITROGLYCERIN EXTENDED-RELEASE TABLETS
Klavikordal, Niong, Nitronet, Nitrong
NITROGLYCERIN EXTENDED-RELEASE BUCCAL TABLETS
Nitrogard, {Nitrogard SR}
NITROGLYCERIN INTRAVENOUS
Nitro-bid, Nitrol, Nitrostat, Tridil
NITROGLYCERIN LINGUAL SPRAY
Nitrolingual
NITROGLYCERIN OINTMENT
Nitro-bid, Nitrol, Nitrong
NITROGLYCERIN SUBLINGUAL
Nitrostat
NITROGLYCERIN TRANSDERMAL SYSTEM
Deponit, Nitrocine, Nitro-Dur, Nitro-Dur II, NTS, Transderm-Nitro

CLASSIFICATION(S):
Vasodilator—nitrate, Antianginal/coronary vasodilator
Pregnancy Category C

INDICATIONS

▪ **Lingual, SL:** Acute treatment of angina pectoris ▪ **Lingual, SL, extended-release tablet, buccal tablet, capsules, ointment, transdermal:** Long-term prophylactic management of angina pectoris ▪ **PO, transdermal, ointment:** Adjunct treatment of congestive heart failure ▪ **IV:** Adjunct treatment of acute myocardial infarction ▪ **IV:** Production of controlled hypotension during surgical procedures.

ACTION

▪ Increases coronary blood flow by dilating coronary arteries and improving collateral flow to ischemic regions ▪ Produces vasodilation (venous greater than arterial) ▪ Decreases left ventricular end-diastolic pressure and left ventricular end-diastolic volume (preload) ▪ Reduces myocardial oxygen consumption. **Therapeutic Effects:** ▪ Relief or prevention of anginal attacks ▪ Increased cardiac output.

PHARMACOKINETICS

Absorption: Well absorbed following oral, buccal, and sublingual administration. Also absorbed through skin. Orally administered nitroglycerin is rapidly metabolized, leading to decreased bioavailability.
Distribution: Distribution not known.
Metabolism and Excretion: Undergoes rapid and almost complete metabolism by the liver. Also metabolized by enzymes in bloodstream.
Half-life: 1–4 min.

CONTRAINDICATIONS AND PRECAUTIONS

Contraindicated in: ▪ Hypersensitivity ▪ Severe anemia ▪ Pericardial tamponade ▪ Constrictive pericarditis ▪ Alcohol intolerance (large IV doses only).
Use Cautiously in: ▪ Head trauma or cerebral hemorrhage ▪ Pregnancy (may compromise maternal/fetal circulation) ▪ Children or lactation (safety not established) ▪ Glaucoma ▪ Hypertrophic cardiomyopathy ▪ Severe liver impairment ▪ Malabsorption or hypermotility (PO) ▪ Hypovolemia (IV) ▪ Normal or decreased pulmonary capillary wedge

{} = Available in Canada only.

pressure (IV) ▪ Cardioversion (remove transdermal patch prior to).

ADVERSE REACTIONS AND SIDE EFFECTS*

CNS: headache, apprehension, weakness, dizziness, lightheadedness, restlessness.
EENT: blurred vision.
CV: hypotension, tachycardia, syncope.
GI: nausea, vomiting, abdominal pain.
Derm: contact dermatitis (transdermal or oint).
Misc: flushing, tolerance, cross-tolerance, alcohol intoxication (large IV doses only).

INTERACTIONS

Drug-Drug: ▪ Additive hypotension with **antihypertensives,** acute ingestion of **alcohol, beta-adrenergic blocking agents, calcium channel blockers, haloperidol,** or **phenothiazines** ▪ **Agents having anticholinergic properties (tricyclic antidepressants, antihistamines, phenothiazines)** may decrease absorption of sublingual or buccal nitroglycerin.

ROUTE AND DOSAGE

Note: See Appendix D for infusion rate chart.

- **SL (Adults):** 0.15–0.6 mg, may repeat q 5 min for 15 min for acute attack.
- **Lingual Spray (Adults):** (0.4 mg/spray) 1–2 sprays, may be repeated q 3–5 min for a total of 3 sprays.
- **Buccal (Adults):** 1 mg buccal transmucosal tablet placed on oral mucosa (under upper lip or between cheek and gums) q 5 hr; dosage and frequency may be increased as needed.
- **PO (Adults):** 2.5–9 mg 3–4 times daily as extended-release capsules or 1.3–6.5 mg q 12 hr as extended-release tab (may be increased to q 8 hr as needed).
- **IV (Adults):** 5 mcg/min, increase by 5 mcg/min q 3–5 min to 20 mcg/min, then increase by 10 mcg/min q 3–5 min (dosing determined by hemodynamic parameters.)
- **Oint (Adults):** (1 in = 15 mg) ½–4 in q 8 hr (up to 5 in q 4 hr).
- **Transdermal Patch:** 2.5–15 mg/24 hr.

PHARMACODYNAMICS (cardiovascular effects)

	ONSET	PEAK	DURATION
SL	1–3 min	UK	30–60 min
Buccal-ER	UK	UK	5 hr
PO	40–60 min	UK	8–12 hr
Oint	20–60 min	UK	4–8 hr
Patch	40–60 min	UK	8–24 hr
IV	immediate	UK	several min

NURSING IMPLICATIONS

Assessment

- □ Assess location, duration, intensity, and precipitating factors of patient's anginal pain.
- □ Monitor blood pressure and pulse prior to and following administration. Patients receiving IV nitroglycerin require continuous ECG and blood pressure monitoring. Additional hemodynamic parameters may be ordered.
- ▪ **Lab Test Considerations:** May cause increased urine catecholamine and urine vanillylmandelic concentrations.
- □ Excessive doses may cause increased methemoglobin concentrations.
- □ May cause falsely elevated serum cholesterol levels.

Potential Nursing Diagnoses

- Comfort, altered: pain (indications).
- Tissue perfusion, altered (indications).
- Knowledge deficit related to medication regimen (patient/family teaching).

Implementation

- **General Info:** Available in extended-release buccal tablet, lingual aerosol, extended-release tablet and capsule,

*Underlines indicate most frequent; **CAPITALS** indicate life-threatening.

SL tablet, ointment, transdermal systems, and intravenous forms.

- **PO:** Administer dose 1 hr before or 2 hr after meals with a full glass of water for faster absorption. Extended-release preparations should be swallowed whole; do not crush, break, or chew.
- **SL:** Tablet should be held under tongue until dissolved. Avoid eating, drinking, or smoking until tablet is dissolved.
- **Buccal:** Place tablet under upper lip or between cheek and gum. Onset of action may be increased by touching the tablet with the tongue or by drinking hot liquids.
- **IV:** Doses must be diluted and administered as an infusion. Standard infusion sets made of polyvinyl chloride (PVC) plastic may absorb up to 80% of the nitroglycerin in soln. Use glass bottles only and special tubing provided by manufacturer.
- **Continuous Infusion:** Dilute in D5W or 0.9% NaCl in a concentration of 25–40 mcg/ml, dependent upon patient fluid tolerance (see Appendix D for infusion rate chart). Soln is stable for 48 hr at room temperature. Soln is not explosive either before or after dilution.
  - *Rate:* Administer via infusion pump to ensure accurate rate. Titrate rate according to patient response.
- **Syringe Compatibility:** heparin.
- **Y-Site Compatibility:** amrinone, atracurium, dobutamine, dopamine, famotidine, lidocaine, nitroprusside, pancuronium, ranitidine, streptokinase, or vecuronium.
- **Additive Incompatibility:** Manufacturer recommends that nitroglycerin not be admixed with other medications.
- **Top:** Sites of topical application should be rotated to prevent skin irritation. Remove patch or ointment from previous site before application.
  - Doses may be increased to the highest dose that does not cause symptomatic hypotension.
  - Apply ointment by using dose-measuring application papers supplied with ointment. Squeeze ointment onto measuring scale printed on paper. Use paper to spread ointment onto nonhairy area of skin (chest, abdomen, thighs; avoid distal extremities) in a thin, even layer, covering a 2–3-in area. Do not allow ointment to come in contact with hands. Do not massage or rub in ointment, as this will increase absorption and interfere with sustained action. Apply occlusive dressing if ordered.
  - Transdermal patches may be applied to any hairless site (avoid distal extremities or areas with cuts or calluses). Apply firm pressure over patch to ensure contact with skin, especially around edges. Apply a new dosage unit if the first one becomes loose or falls off. Units are waterproof and not affected by showering or bathing. Do not cut or trim system to adjust dosage. Do not alternate between brands of transdermal products; dosage may not be equivalent. Remove patches before cardioversion or defibrillation to prevent patient burns. Physician may recommend removing patch at night to prevent development of tolerance.

Patient/Family Teaching

- **General Info:** Instruct patient to take medication exactly as directed, even if feeling better. If a dose is missed, take as soon as remembered unless next dose is scheduled within 2 hr (6 hr with extended-release preparations). Do not double doses. Do not discontinue abruptly; gradual dosage reduction may be necessary to prevent rebound angina.
  - Caution patient to make position changes slowly to minimize orthostatic hypotension.
  - Advise patient to avoid concurrent use of alcohol with this medication. Patient should also consult physician or pharmacist before taking over-the-counter medications while taking nitroglycerin.
  - Inform patient that headache is a

common side effect that should decrease with continuing therapy. Aspirin or acetaminophen may be ordered to treat headache. Notify physician if headache is persistent or severe.

- Advise patient to notify physician if dry mouth or blurred vision occurs.
- **Acute Anginal Attacks:** Advise patient to sit down and use medication at first sign of attack. Relief usually occurs within 5 min. Dose may be repeated if pain is not relieved in 5–10 min. Call physician or go to nearest emergency room if anginal pain is not relieved by 3 tablets in 15 min.
- **SL:** Inform patient that tablets should be kept in original glass container or in specially made metal containers, with cotton removed to prevent absorption. Tablets lose potency in containers made of plastic or cardboard or when mixed with other capsules or tablets. Exposure to air, heat, and moisture also causes loss of potency. Instruct patient not to open bottle frequently, handle tablets, or keep bottle of tablets next to body (i.e., shirt pocket) or in automobile glove compartment. Advise patient that tablets should be replaced 6 mon after opening to maintain potency.
- **Lingual Spray:** Instruct patient to lift tongue and spray dose under tongue.

Evaluation

Effectiveness of therapy can be demonstrated by: ▪ Decrease in frequency and severity of anginal attacks ▫ Increase in activity tolerance. During chronic therapy, tolerance may be minimized by intermittent administration of 12 hr on/12 hr off intervals ▪ Controlled hypotension during surgical procedures.

NITROPRUSSIDE

(nye-troe-**pruss**-ide)
Nipride, Nitropress

CLASSIFICATION(S):
Antihypertensive—vasodilator
Pregnancy Category C

INDICATIONS

▪ Management of hypertensive crises ▪ Production of controlled hypotension during anesthesia ▪ Treatment of cardiac pump failure or cardiogenic shock (alone or with dopamine).

ACTION

▪ Produces peripheral vasodilation by direct action on venous and arteriolar smooth muscle. **Therapeutic Effects:** ▪ Rapid lowering of blood pressure ▪ Decreased cardiac preload and afterload.

PHARMACOKINETICS

Absorption: Administered IV only, resulting in complete bioavailability.
Distribution: Distribution not known.
Metabolism and Excretion: Rapidly metabolized in RBCs and tissues to cyanide and subsequently by the liver to thiocyananate.
Half-life: UK.

CONTRAINDICATIONS AND PRECAUTIONS

Contraindicated in: ▪ Hypersensitivity ▪ Decreased cerebral perfusion.
Use Cautiously in: ▪ Renal disease (increased risk of thiocyanate accumulation) ▪ Hepatic disease (increased risk of cyanide accumulation) ▪ Hypothyroidism ▪ Hyponatremia ▪ Pregnancy or lactation (safety not established) ▪ Vitamin B_{12} deficiency.

ADVERSE REACTIONS AND SIDE EFFECTS*

CNS: <u>headache</u>, <u>dizziness</u>, restlessness.
EENT: tinnitus, blurred vision.
CV: palpitations, dyspnea, excessive hypotension.
GI: <u>nausea</u>, vomiting, <u>abdominal pain</u>.
F and E: acidosis.
Local: phlebitis at IV site.
Misc: thiocyanate toxicity, cyanide toxicity.

INTERACTIONS

Drug-Drug: ▪ Increased hypotensive effect with **ganglionic blocking agents,**

*<u>Underlines</u> indicate most frequent; **CAPITALS** indicate life-threatening.

general anesthetics, and other **antihypertensives.**

ROUTE AND DOSAGE

Note: See infusion rate chart in Appendix D.

- **IV (Adults and Children):** 0.5–10 mcg/kg/min. Not to exceed 10 min of therapy at 10 mcg/kg/min infusion rate.

PHARMACODYNAMICS (hypotensive effect)

	ONSET	PEAK	DURATION
IV	immediate	rapid	1–10 min

NURSING IMPLICATIONS

Assessment

- Monitor blood pressure, heart rate, and ECG frequently throughout course of therapy; continuous monitoring is preferred. Consult physician for parameters. Monitor for rebound hypertension following discontinuation of nitroprusside.
- Pulmonary capillary wedge pressures (PCWP) may be monitored in patients with myocardial infarction or congestive heart failure.
- **Lab Test Considerations:** May cause decrease in bicarbonate concentrations, pCO_2, and pH.
- May cause increased lactate concentrations.
- May cause increased serum cyanate and thiocyanate concentrations.
- **Toxicity and Overdose:** If severe hypotension occurs, drug effects are quickly reversed by decreasing rate or temporarily discontinuing infusion.
- Plasma cyanide and thiocyanate levels should be monitored every 48–72 hr. Levels should not exceed 100 mcg of thiocyanate per ml or 3 micromoles of cyanide per ml.
- Signs and symptoms of thiocyanate toxicity include tinnitus, blurred vision, dyspnea, dizziness, headache, syncope, and metabolic acidosis.
- Treatment may include amyl nitrate inhalation and infusions of sodium nitrite and sodium thiosulfate.

Potential Nursing Diagnoses

- Tissue perfusion, altered (indications).

Implementation

- **General Info:** If infusion of 10 mcg/kg/min for 10 min does not produce adequate reduction in blood pressure, manufacturer recommends nitroprusside be discontinued.
- May be administered in left ventricular congestive heart failure concurrently with an inotropic agent (dopamine, dobutamine) when effective doses of nitroprusside restore pump function and cause excessive hypotension.
- **Continuous Infusion:** Reconstitute each 50 mg with 2–3 ml of D5W for injection. Dilute further in 250–1000 ml of D5W. Do not use other diluents for reconstitution or infusion. Wrap infusion bottle in aluminum foil to protect from light; administration set tubing need not be covered. Freshly prepared soln has a slight brownish tint; discard if soln is dark brown, orange, blue, green, or dark red. Soln must be used within 24 hr of preparation.
- *Rate:* Administer via infusion pump to ensure accurate dosage rate (see Appendix D for dosage rate chart).
- Avoid extravasation.
- **Additive Incompatibility:** Do not admix with other medications.

Patient/Family Teaching

- Advise patient to report the onset of tinnitus, dyspnea, dizziness, headache, or blurred vision immediately.

Evaluation

Effectiveness of therapy is indicated by: ▪ Decrease in blood pressure without the appearance of side effects ▪ Treatment of cardiac pump failure or cardiogenic shock.

NIZATIDINE
(ni-**za**-ti-deen)
Axid

CLASSIFICATION(S):
Histamine H_2 antagonist—antiulcer
Pregnancy Category C

INDICATIONS

▪ Short-term treatment and maintenance preventive treatment of active duodenal ulcers. **Unlabeled Uses:** ▪ Short-term treatment of benign gastric ulcers ▪ Management of gastroesophageal reflux disease (GERD).

ACTION

▪ Inhibits the action of histamine at the H_2 receptor site located primarily in gastric parietal cells ▪ Inhibits gastric acid secretion. **Therapeutic Effects:** ▪ Healing and prevention of ulcers.

PHARMACOKINETICS

Absorption: Well absorbed following oral administration.
Distribution: Distribution not known. Probably enters breast milk.
Metabolism and Excretion: 60% excreted unchanged by the kidneys. Some hepatic metabolism; one metabolite is active.
Half-life: 1.6 hr (increased in renal failure).

CONTRAINDICATIONS AND PRECAUTIONS

Contraindicated in: ▪ Hypersensitivity.
Use Cautiously in: ▪ Pregnancy, lactation, or children (safety not established) ▪ Impaired liver function ▪ Elderly patients (increased risk of adverse reactions) ▪ Renal impairment (dosage reduction recommended).

ADVERSE REACTIONS AND SIDE EFFECTS*

CNS: somnolence, dizziness.
CV: arrhythmias.
Derm: sweating, urticaria.
GI: hepatitis.
Metab: hyperuricemia.

INTERACTIONS

Drug–Drug: ▪ May increase salicylate serum levels in patients on high-dose (>3900 mg/day) **aspirin** therapy ▪ Concurrently administered **antacids** may decrease absorption of nizatidine.

ROUTE AND DOSAGE

Active Duodenal Ulcers

▪ **PO (Adults):** 150 mg bid or 300 mg at bedtime.

Maintenance Therapy of Duodenal Ulcers

▪ **PO (Adults):** 150 mg at bedtime.

PHARMACODYNAMICS (inhibition of gastric acid secretion)

	ONSET	PEAK	DURATION
PO	UK	UK	8–12 hr

NURSING IMPLICATIONS

Assessment

□ Assess patient routinely for epigastric or abdominal pain and frank or occult blood in the stool, emesis, or gastric aspirate.
▪ **Lab Test Considerations:** Monitor liver function test periodically throughout therapy.
□ May cause elevated SGOT (AST), SGPT (ALT), and alkaline phosphatase concentrations.
□ May cause false-positive tests for urobilinogen.

Potential Nursing Diagnoses

▪ Comfort, altered: pain (indications).
▪ Knowledge deficit related to medication regimen (patient/family teaching).

Implementation

▪ **General Info:** Diagnosis of malignant GI neoplasm should be ruled out prior to initiation of nizatidine therapy.
□ If antacids are used concurrently with

*Underlines indicate most frequent; **CAPITALS** indicate life-threatening.

nizatidine for relief of pain, avoid administration within 2 hr of nizatidine, as they decrease the absorption of nizatidine.

- **PO:** Usually administered once daily at bedtime to prolong effect. May also be divided into 2 daily doses.

Patient/Family Teaching

- Instruct patient to take medication as directed for the full course of therapy, even if feeling better. If a dose is missed, it should be taken as soon as remembered, but not if almost time for next dose. Do not double doses. Nizatidine therapy is not recommended for >8 wk.
- Inform patient that smoking interferes with the action of nizatidine. Encourage patient to quit smoking or at least not to smoke after last dose of the day.
- Nizatidine may cause drowsiness. Caution patient to avoid driving or other activities requiring alertness until response to drug is known.
- Advise patient to avoid alcohol, products containing aspirin, and foods that may cause an increase in GI irritation.
- Advise patient to report onset of black, tarry stools or dizziness to physician promptly.

Evaluation

Effectiveness of therapy can be demonstrated by: ▪ Decrease in abdominal pain ▪ Prevention of gastric irritation and bleeding ▫ Healing of duodenal ulcers is demonstrated by x-rays or endoscopy.

NOREPINEPHRINE

(**nor**-ep-i-nef-rin)
Levarterenol, Levophed

CLASSIFICATION(S):
Vasopressor
Pregnancy Category C

INDICATIONS

▪ Produces vasoconstriction and myocardial stimulation, which may be required after adequate fluid replacement in the treatment of shock.

ACTION

▪ Stimulates alpha-adrenergic receptors located mainly in blood vessels causing constriction of both capacitance and resistance vessels ▪ Also has minor $beta_1$-adrenergic activity (myocardial stimulation). **Therapeutic Effects:** ▪ Increased blood pressure ▪ Increased cardiac output.

PHARMACOKINETICS

Absorption: Administered IV only, resulting in complete bioavailability.
Distribution: Concentrates in sympathetic nervous tissue. Does not cross the blood-brain barrier, but readily crosses the placenta.
Metabolism and Excretion: Taken up and metabolized rapidly by sympathetic nerve endings.
Half-life: UK.

CONTRAINDICATIONS AND PRECAUTIONS

Contraindicated in: ▪ Vascular, mesenteric, or peripheral thrombosis ▪ Pregnancy (reduces uterine blood flow) ▪ Hypoxia ▪ Hypercarbia ▪ Hypotension secondary to hypovolemia ▪ Hypersensitivity to bisulfites.
Use Cautiously in: ▪ Hypertension ▪ Hyperthyroidism ▪ Cardiovascular disease ▪ Lactation (safety not established).

ADVERSE REACTIONS AND SIDE EFFECTS*

CNS: headache, anxiety, dizziness, weakness, tremor, restlessness, insomnia.
Resp: dyspnea.
CV: bradycardia, hypertension, arrhythmias, chest pain.
GU: decreased urine output, renal failure.

*Underlines indicate most frequent; **CAPITALS** indicate life-threatening.

Endo: hyperglycemia.
F and E: metabolic acidosis.
Local: phlebitis at IV site.
Misc: fever.

INTERACTIONS

Drug–Drug: ▪ Use with **cyclopropane or halothane anesthesia, cardiac glycosides, doxapram,** or **local use of cocaine** may result in increased myocardial irritability ▪ Use with **MAO inhibitors, guanethidine, methyldopa, doxapram,** or **tricyclic antidepressants** may result in severe hypertension ▪ **Alpha-adrenergic blockers** can prevent pressor responses ▪ **Beta-adrenergic blockers** may exaggerate hypertension or block cardiac stimulation ▪ Concurrent use with **ergot alkaloids (ergotamine, ergonovine, methylergonovine, methysergide)** or **oxytocin** may result in enhanced vasoconstriction.

ROUTE AND DOSAGE

Note: See infusion rate chart in Appendix D.

- **IV (Adults):** 8–12 mcg/min initially, then 2–4 mcg/min maintenance infusion rate, titrated by blood pressure response.
- **IV (Children):** 2 mcg/min initially or 2 mcg/m^2/min maintenance infusion rate, titrated by blood pressure response. In severe hypotension during cardiac arrest use initial dose of 0.1 mcg/kg/min; maintenance infusion rate titrated by blood pressure response.

PHARMACODYNAMICS (effects on blood pressure)

	ONSET	PEAK	DURATION
IV	immediate	rapid	1–2 min

NURSING IMPLICATIONS

Assessment

- □ Monitor blood pressure every 2–3 min until stabilized and every 5 min thereafter. Systolic blood pressure is usually maintained at 80–100 mmHg or 30–40 mmHg below the previously existing systolic pressure in previously hypertensive patients. Consult physician for parameters. Continue to monitor blood pressure frequently for hypotension following discontinuation of norepinephrine.
- □ ECG should be monitored continuously. CVP, intra-arterial pressure, pulmonary artery diastolic pressure, pulmonary capillary wedge pressure (PCWP), and cardiac output may also be monitored.
- □ Monitor urine output and notify physician if it decreases to <30 ml/hr.
- □ Assess IV site frequently throughout infusion. The antecubital or other large vein should be used to minimize risk of extravasation, which may cause tissue necrosis. Phentolamine 5–10 mg may be added to each liter of soln to prevent sloughing of tissue in extravasation. If extravasation occurs, the site should be infiltrated promptly with 10–15 ml of 0.9% NaCl soln containing 5–10 mg of phentolamine to prevent necrosis and sloughing. If prolonged therapy is required or blanching along the course of the vein occurs, change injection sites to provide relief from vasoconstriction.

Potential Nursing Diagnoses

- Cardiac output, decreased (indications).
- Tissue perfusion, altered (indications).

Implementation

- **General Info:** Volume depletion should be corrected, if possible, prior to initiation of norepinephrine.
- □ Heparin may be added to each 500 ml of soln to prevent thrombosis in the infused vein, perivenous reactions, and necrosis in patients with severe hypotension following myocardial infarction.
- □ Norepinephrine may deplete plasma volume and cause ischemia of vital organs, resulting in hypotension when discontinued, if used for prolonged periods. Prolonged or large

doses may also decrease cardiac output.

- ▫ Infusion should be discontinued gradually, upon adequate tissue perfusion and maintenance of blood pressure, to prevent hypotension. Do not resume therapy unless blood pressure falls to 70–80 mmHg.
- ▪ **Continuous Infusion:** Dilute 4 mg in 1000 ml of D5W or D5/0.9% NaCl, for a concentration of 4 mcg/ml. Do not dilute in 0.9% NaCl without dextrose. Do not use discolored soln (pink, yellow, brown) or those containing a precipitate.
- ▫ *Rate:* Titrate infusion rate according to patient response, using slowest possible ratc to correct hypotension (see Appendix D for infusion rate chart). Administer via infusion pump to ensure accurate dosage.
- ▪ **Y-Site Compatibility:** amrinone, famotidine, heparin, hydrocortisone sodium succinate, potassium chloride, or ranitidine.
- ▪ **Additive Compatibility:** amikacin, calcium chloride, calcium gluceptate, calcium gluconate, cimetidine, dimenhydrinate, dobutamine, heparin, hydrocortisone sodium succinate, magnesium sulfate, methylprednisolone sodium succinate, multivitamins, netilmicin, ranitidine, potassium chloride, succinylcholine, tetracycline, or verapamil.
- ▪ **Additive Incompatibility:** blood or plasma, aminophylline, amobarbital, cephapirin, chlorothiazide, chlorpheniramine, lidocaine, pentobarbital, phenobarbital, phenytoin, secobarbital, sodium bicarbonate, sodium iodide, streptomycin, or thiopental.

Patient/Family Teaching

- ▫ Instruct patient to report headache, dizziness, dyspnea, chest pain, or pain at infusion site promptly.

Evaluation

Effectiveness of therapy can be demonstrated by: ▪ Increase in blood pressure to normal range ▫ Increased tissue perfusion

NORFLOXACIN

(nor-**flox**-a-sin)
Chibroxin, Noroxin

CLASSIFICATION(S):
Anti-infective—fluoroquinolone
Pregnancy Category C

INDICATIONS

▪ **PO:** Treatment of urinary tract infections due to susceptible organisms ▪ **Ophth:** Treatment of superficial occular infections due to susceptible organisms.

ACTION

▪ Inhibits bacterial DNA synthesis by inhibiting DNA gyrase. **Therapeutic Effect:** ▪ Bactericidal action against susceptible organisms. **Spectrum:** ▪ Broad spectrum of activity includes many gram-positive pathogens: ▫ Staphylococci (including *Staphylococcus epidermidis* and methicillin-resistant strains of *Staphylococcus aureus*) ▫ Group D streptococci ▪ Gram-negative spectrum notable for activity against: ▫ *E. coli* ▫ *Klebsiella pneumoniae* ▫ *Enterobacter cloacae* ▫ *Proteus mirabilis* ▫ Indole positive *Proteus* (including *P. vulgaris, Providencia retgerii,* and *Morganella morganii*) ▫ *Pseudomonas aeruginosa* ▫ *Citrobacter freundii.*

PHARMACOKINETICS

Absorption: 30–40% absorbed following oral administration.
Distribution: High urinary concentrations are achieved.
Metabolism and Excretion: Small amount (10%) metabolized by the liver. 30% excreted unchanged by the kidneys, 30% excreted in feces.
Half-life: 6.5 hr (increased in renal disease).

CONTRAINDICATIONS AND PRECAUTIONS

Contraindicated in: ▪ Hypersensitivity ▪ Cross-sensitivity with other fluoroquinolones may exist ▪ Pregnancy, lactation, or children <18 yr.

Use Cautiously in: ▪ Underlying CNS pathology ▪ History of seizure disorders ▪ Severe renal impairment (dosage reduction recommended).

ADVERSE REACTIONS AND SIDE EFFECTS*

Note: For oral norfloxacin, unless indicated.

CNS: dizziness, headache, somnolence, fatigue, depression, SEIZURES.

EENT: tinnitus, photophobia; Ophth—conjunctival hyperemia, conjunctival edema, photophobia.

GI: nausea, abdominal pain, dyspepsia, constipation, flatulence, heartburn, dry mouth, diarrhea, vomiting; Ophth—bitter taste in mouth.

GU: crystalluria.

Derm: rash, erythema.

MS: joint swelling, tendonitis.

Misc: fever.

INTERACTIONS

Note: Listed for oral norfloxacin.

Drug-Drug: ▪ Concurrent use with **probenecid** decreases urinary levels of norfloxacin ▪ **Nitrofurantoin** may negate the anti-infective activity of norfloxacin ▪ **Agents that akalinize the urine** may increase the risk of crystalluria ▪ **Antacids, sucralfate, iron salts,** or **zinc salts** decrease absorption; do not use concurrently ▪ May increase serum **theophylline** levels ▪ May increase the effects of **oral anticoagulants**.

ROUTE AND DOSAGE

- **PO (Adults):** 400 mg q 12 hr for 7–10 days in uncomplicated infections; continue for 10–21 days in complicated infections.
- **Ophth (Adults):** 1–2 drops of 3 mg/ml soln q 15–30 min initially, then decrease frequency as infection responds, to 1–2 drops q 4–6 hr.

PHARMACODYNAMICS (urine levels)

	ONSET	PEAK
PO	UK	2–3 hr

NURSING IMPLICATIONS

Assessment

- **Urinary Tract Infections:** Assess patient for infection (vital signs, urinalysis, frequency and urgency of urination, WBC, fever, cloudy or foul-smelling urine) at beginning and throughout course of therapy.
  - Obtain specimens for culture and sensitivity prior to initiating therapy. First dose may be given before receiving results
- **Ophth:** Assess patient for conjunctival swelling, redness, and pain prior to and throughout therapy.
- **Lab Test Considerations:** May cause increased serum BUN, SGOT (AST), SGPT (ALT), LDH, alkaline phosphatase, and creatinine concentrations.
  - May cause decreased WBC, neutrophils, and hematocrit concentrations.

Potential Nursing Diagnoses

- Infection, high risk for (indications, side effects).
- Knowledge deficit related to medication regimen (patient/family teaching).
- Noncompliance related to medication regimen (patient/family teaching).

Implementation

- **PO:** Administer around the clock on an empty stomach, at least 1 hr before or 2 hr after meals, with a full glass of water.
- **Ophth:** See appendix H for instillation of ophthalmic soln.

Patient/Family Teaching

- **PO:** Instruct patient to take medication around the clock and to finish the drug completely as directed, even if feeling better. If a dose is missed, take as soon as remembered unless almost time for next dose; do not double doses. Advise patient that sharing of this medication may be dangerous.
  - Encourage patient to maintain a fluid intake of at least 1200–1500 ml/day to prevent crystalluria.
  - Advise patient that antacids will decrease absorption and should not be

*Underlines indicate most frequent; **CAPITALS** indicate life-threatening.

taken within 2 hr of this medication.

- □ May cause dizziness and drowsiness. Caution patient to avoid driving or other activities requiring alertness until response to medication is known.
- □ Caution patient to use sunglasses and avoid prolonged exposure to bright light to prevent photophobia.
- □ Advise patient that frequent mouth rinses, good oral hygiene, and sugarless gum or candy may minimize dry mouth.
- □ Instruct patient to notify physician if symptoms do not improve within a few days of therapy.
- ▪ **Ophth:** Instruct patient on correct technique for instillation of eye drops (see Appendix H).

EVALUATION

Clinical response can be evaluated by: ▪ Resolution of the signs and symptoms of urinary tract infection □ Negative urine culture ▪ Resolution of the signs and symptoms of ophthalmic infections.

NORTRIPTYLINE

(nor-**trip**-ti-leen)
Aventyl, Pamelor

CLASSIFICATION(S):
Antidepressant—tricyclic
Pregnancy Category UK

INDICATIONS

▪ Treatment of various forms of depression, often in conjunction with psychotherapy. **Unlabeled Use:** ▪ Adjunct in the management of chronic neurogenic pain.

ACTION

▪ Potentiates the effect of serotonin and norepinephrine ▪ Has significant anticholinergic properties. **Therapeutic Effect:** ▪ Antidepressant action that develops slowly over several wks.

PHARMACOKINETICS

Absorption: Well absorbed following oral administration.

Distribution: Widely distributed. Enters breast milk in small amounts. Probably crosses the placenta.

Metabolism and Excretion: Extensively metabolized by the liver, much of it on its first pass through the liver. Some is converted to active compounds. Undergoes enterohepatic recirculation and secretion into gastric juices.

Half-life: 18–28 hr.

CONTRAINDICATIONS AND PRECAUTIONS

Contraindicated in: ▪ Hypersensitivity ▪ Narrow-angle glaucoma ▪ Pregnancy and lactation.

Use Cautiously in: ▪ Elderly patients (more susceptible to adverse reactions; dosage reduction recommended) ▪ Children (more susceptible to adverse reactions) ▪ Pre-existing cardiovascular disease ▪ Elderly men with prostatic hypertrophy (more susceptible to urinary retention) ▪ Seizures or history of seizure disorder ▪ Asthma.

ADVERSE REACTIONS AND SIDE EFFECTS*

CNS: <u>drowsiness</u>, <u>sedation</u>, <u>lethargy</u>, <u>fatigue</u>, confusion, agitation, hallucinations, insomnia, headache, extrapyramidal reactions.

CV: <u>hypotension</u>, ECG changes, ARRHYTHMIAS.

Derm: photosensitivity.

EENT: <u>dry mouth</u>, <u>dry eyes</u>, <u>blurred vision</u>.

Endo: gynecomastia.

GI: <u>constipation</u>, paralytic ileus, nausea, unpleasant taste.

GU: urinary retention.

Hemat: blood dyscrasias, weight gain.

INTERACTIONS

Drug-Drug: ▪ May cause hypertension, hyperpyrexia, seizures, and death when used with **MAO inhibitors** (avoid concurrent use—discontinue 2 wk prior

*<u>Underlines</u> indicate most frequent; **CAPITALS** indicate life-threatening.

to nortriptyline) ▪ May prevent the therapeutic response to most **antihypertensives** ▪ Hypertensive crisis may occur with **clonidine** ▪ Additive CNS depression with other **CNS depressants,** including **alcohol, antihistamines, narcotics,** and **sedative/hypnotics** ▪ Sympathomimetic effects may be additive with other **adrenergic agents,** including **vasoconstrictors** and **decongestants** ▪ Additive anticholinergic effects with other **drugs possessing anticholinergic properties,** including **antihistamines, antidepressants, atropine, haloperidol, phenothiazines, quinidine,** and **disopyramide** ▪ **Cimetidine** or **oral contraceptives** increase blood levels and risk of toxicity ▪ Increased risk of agranulocytosis with **antithyroid agents** ▪ **Fluoxetine** increases risk of toxicity.

ROUTE AND DOSAGE

- **PO (Adults):** 25 mg 3–4 times daily (not to exceed 150 mg/day).
- **PO (Children—Adolescents):** 25–50 mg/day or 1–3 mg/kg/day in divided doses.
- **PO (Children 6–12 yr):** 10–20 mg/day or 1–3 mg/kg/day in divided doses.

PHARMACODYNAMICS (antidepressant effect)

	ONSET	PEAK	DURATION
PO	2–3 wk	6 wk	UK

NURSING IMPLICATIONS

Assessment

- **General Info:** Monitor mental status and affect. Assess for suicidal tendencies, especially during early therapy. Restrict amount of drug available to patient.
  - Monitor blood pressure and pulse rate prior to and during initial therapy. Notify physician of significant decreases in blood pressure or a sudden increase in pulse rate.
  - Monitor baseline and periodic ECGs in elderly patients or patients with heart disease. May cause prolonged PR and QT intervals and may flatten T waves.
- **Pain:** Assess type, location, and severity of pain prior to and periodically throughout therapy
- **Lab Test Considerations:** Assess leukocyte and differential blood counts and renal and hepatic functions prior to and periodically during prolonged or high-dose therapy.
  - Serum levels may be monitored in patients who fail to respond to usual therapeutic dose. Therapeutic plasma concentration range is 50–150 ng/ml.
  - May cause alterations in blood glucose levels.

Potential Nursing Diagnoses

- Coping, ineffective individual (indications).
- Injury, high risk for (side effects).
- Knowledge deficit related to medication regimen (patient/family teaching).

Implementation

- **PO:** Administer medication with meals to minimize gastric irritation.
  - May be given as a single dose at bedtime to minimize sedation during the day. Dose increases should be made at bedtime because of sedation.

Patient/Family Teaching

- Instruct patient to take medication exactly as prescribed. Do not skip or double up on missed doses. If a dose is missed, it should be taken as soon as remembered unless almost time for next dose. Inform patient that at least 2 wk are needed before drug effects may be noticed. Abrupt discontinuation after long-term therapy may cause nausea, headache, vivid dreams, and malaise.
- May cause drowsiness and blurred vision. Caution patient to avoid driving and other activities requiring alertness until response to drug is known.
- Instruct patient to notify physician if visual changes occur. Inform patient that physician may order periodic glaucoma testing during long-term therapy.

N

□ Caution patient to make position changes slowly to minimize orthostatic hypotension. (This side effect is less pronounced with this medication than with other tricyclic antidepressants.)
□ Advise patient to avoid alcohol or other CNS depressant drugs during therapy and for at least 3–7 days after therapy has been discontinued.
□ Instruct patient to notify physician if urinary retention, uncontrolled movements, or fever occur or if dry mouth or constipation persists. Sugarless candy or gum may diminish dry mouth, and an increase in fluid intake or bulk may prevent constipation.
□ Caution patient to use sunscreen and protective clothing to prevent photosensitivity reactions.
□ Advise patient to notify physician or dentist of medication regimen prior to treatment or surgery.
□ Therapy for depression is usually prolonged. Emphasize the importance of follow-up examinations and participation in prescribed psychotherapy.

EVALUATION

Effectiveness of therapy can be demonstrated by: ▪ Increased sense of well-being □ Renewed interest in surroundings □ Increased appetite □ Improved energy level □ Improved sleep ▪ Decrease in severity of chronic neurogenic pain. Patients may require 2–6 wk of therapy before full therapeutic effects of medication are seen.

NYSTATIN

(nye-**stat**-in)
Mycostatin, Mykinac, {Nadostine}, Nilstat, {Nyaderm}, Nystex

CLASSIFICATION(S):
Antifungal
Pregnancy Category A (Vaginal), UK (Others)

INDICATIONS

▪ **PO, Top, Vag:** Local treatment of *Candida* infections ▪ **PO:** Treatment of intestinal candidiasis ▪ **PO:** Preparation of bowel for GI surgery.

ACTION

▪ Binds to fungal cell membrane, allowing leakage of cellular contents. **Therapeutic Effect:** ▪ Fungistatic or fungicidal action. **Spectrum:** ▪ Active against most pathogenic *Candida* species, including *Candida albicans*.

PHARMACOKINETICS

Absorption: Poorly absorbed. Action is local. Not absorbed through intact skin or mucous membranes.
Distribution: Distribution not known.
Metabolism and Excretion: Excreted unchanged in the feces following oral administration.
Half-life: UK.

CONTRAINDICATIONS AND PRECAUTIONS

Contraindicated in: ▪ Hypersensitivity ▪ Some products may contain povidone, propylene glycol, alcohol, parabens, or benzyl alcohol—avoid use in patients who may be hypersensitive to these additives.
Use Cautiously in: ▪ Children <5 yr (lozenges) ▪ Denture wearers (dentures require soaking in nystatin suspension).

ADVERSE REACTIONS AND SIDE EFFECTS*

GI: PO—nausea, vomiting, diarrhea, stomach pain (large doses).

INTERACTIONS

Drug-Drug: ▪ None significant.

ROUTE AND DOSAGE

Mucocutaneous Fungal Infection

▪ **Top (Adults and Children):** Cream, ointment, powder—apply several times daily.

{} = Available in Canada only.
*Underlines indicate most frequent; CAPITALS indicate life-threatening.

Oral Monilia
- **PO (Adults and Children):** 400,000–600,000 units q 6–8 hr.
- **PO (Infants):** 200,000 units q 6–8 hr.
- **PO (Premature and Low-Birth-Weight Infants):** 100,000 units q 6–8 hr.

Vaginal *Candida* Infections
- **Vag (Adults):** Vag Tab—insert 1–2 times daily.

Intestinal Infections
- **PO (Adults):** 500,000–1,000,000 units q 8 hr.

PHARMACODYNAMICS (antifungal effects)

	ONSET	PEAK	DURATION
PO	rapid	UK	6–12 hr
Top, Vag	24–72 hr	UK	UK

NURSING IMPLICATIONS

Assessment
- Inspect involved areas of skin or mucous membranes prior to and frequently throughout course of therapy. Increased skin irritation may indicate need to discontinue medication.

Potential Nursing Diagnoses
- Skin integrity, impaired: actual (indications).
- Infection, high risk for (indications).
- Knowledge deficit related to medication regimen (patient/family teaching).

Implementation
- **PO:** Suspension should be administered by placing ½ of dose in each side of mouth. Patient should hold suspension in mouth or swish throughout mouth for several mins prior to swallowing. Use calibrated measuring device for liquid doses. Shake well prior to administration.
- Nystatin Vaginal tablets can be administered orally for treatment of oral candidiasis. Also available as a lozenge (Pastilles).
- **Top:** Consult physician for proper cleansing technique prior to applying medication. Use a glove to apply sufficient medication to cover affected area. Do not apply occlusive dressing. Avoid using tight-fitting diapers or plastic pants on diaper area of children.
- Cream is usually preferred in candidiasis involving intertriginous areas; very moist lesions are best treated with powder. When powder is used for infections of the feet, dust freely on feet as well as in socks and shoes.
- **Vag:** Applicators are supplied for vaginal administration.
- Vaginal tablets may be administered to patients with candidal vaginitis for 3–6 wk prior to delivery to prevent thrush in the newborn.

Patient/Family Teaching
- **General Info:** Instruct patient to take medication as directed. If a dose is missed, take as soon as remembered, but not if almost time for next dose. Do not double doses.
- Advise patient to report increased skin irritation or lack of therapeutic response to physician.
- **Vag:** Instruct patient on proper use of vaginal applicator for vaginal tablets. Patient should remain recumbent for at least 30 min following administration. Advise use of sanitary napkins to prevent staining of clothing or bedding. Vaginal treatment should be continued during menstruation. Avoid use of tampons during therapy.
- Advise patient to consult physician regarding douching and intercourse during therapy. Advise patient to refrain from sexual contact during therapy or to have male partner wear a condom to prevent reinfection.

Evaluation
Effectiveness of therapy can be demonstrated by: ▪ Decrease in skin irritation and discomfort ▫ To prevent relapse following oral therapy, therapy should be continued for 48 hr after symptoms have disappeared and cultures are negative ▫ With topical or vaginal therapy, symptomatic relief usually occurs within 24–72 hr after initiation of therapy. Therapy for a period of 2 wk is

usually sufficient, but more prolonged therapy may be necessary. Persistent candidiasis may be a sign of undetected diabetes mellitus and requires evaluation of serum and urine glucose.

OCTREOTIDE
(ok-**tree**-oh-tide)
Sandostatin

CLASSIFICATION(S):
Hormone—gastrointestinal, Antidiarrheal
Pregnancy Category B

INDICATIONS

▪ Treatment of severe diarrhea and flushing episodes in patients with GI endocrine tumors including metastatic carcinoid tumors and Vasoactive Intestinal Peptide Tumors (VIPomas). **Unlabeled Use:** ▪ Relief of symptoms and suppressed tumor growth in patients with pituitary tumors associated with acromegaly.

ACTION

▪ Suppresses secretion of serotonin and gastroenterohepatic peptides ▪ Increases absorption of fluid and electrolytes from the GI tract and increases transit time ▪ Decreased levels of serotonin metabolites ▪ Also suppresses growth hormone, insulin, and glucagon. **Therapeutic Effect:** ▪ Control of severe flushing and diarrhea associated with GI endocrine tumors.

PHARMACOKINETICS

Absorption: Well absorbed following SC administration.
Distribution: Distribution not known.
Metabolism and Excretion: 32% excreted unchanged in urine.
Half-life: 1.5 hr.

CONTRAINDICATIONS AND PRECAUTIONS

Contraindicated in: ▪ Hypersensitivity.

Use Cautiously in: ▪ Gallbladder disease (increased risk of stone formation) ▪ Renal impairment (dosage reduction may be necessary) ▪ Pregnancy or lactation (safety not established) ▪ Hyper- or hypoglycemia (changes in blood sugar may occur) ▪ Fat malabsorption (may be aggravated).

ADVERSE REACTIONS AND SIDE EFFECTS*

CNS: headache, dizziness, fatigue, weakness, drowsiness.
EENT: visual disturbances.
CV: edema, palpitations, orthostatic hypotension.
GI: nausea, diarrhea, abdominal pain, vomiting, fat malabsorption, cholelithiasis.
Derm: flushing.
Endo: hyperglycemia, hypoglycemia.
Local: injection site pain.

INTERACTIONS

Drug-Drug: ▪ May alter requirements for **insulin** or **oral hypoglycemic agents** ▪ **Glucagon** or **growth hormone** may produce hypo- or hyperglycemia ▪ May reduce blood levels of **cyclosporine**.

ROUTE AND DOSAGE

Carcinoid Tumors

▪ **SC (Adults):** 100–600 mcg/day in 2–4 divided doses during first 2 wk of therapy (range 50–1500 mcg/day).

VIPomas

▪ **SC (Adults):** 100–200 mcg/day in 2–4 divided doses during first 2 wk of therapy (range 150–750 mcg/day).

PHARMACODYNAMICS

	ONSET	PEAK	DURATION
SC	UK	UK	up to 12 hr

NURSING IMPLICATIONS

Assessment

□ Assess frequency and consistency of stools and bowel sounds throughout therapy.
□ Monitor pulse and blood pressure

*Underlines indicate most frequent; **CAPITALS** indicate life-threatening.

prior to and periodically throughout therapy.

- ▫ Assess patient's fluid and electrolyte balance and skin turgor for dehydration.
- ▫ Monitor diabetic patients for signs of hypoglycemia. May require reduction in requirements for insulin, sulfonureas, and diazoxide.
- ▫ Assess patient for gallbladder disease; assess for pain and monitor ultrasound examinations of gallbladder and bile ducts prior to and periodically throughout prolonged therapy.
- ▪ **Lab Test Considerations:** Monitor 5-HIAA (urinary 5-hydroxyindole acetic acid), plasma serotonin, plasma substance P in patients with carcinoid; VIP (plasma vasoactive intestinal peptide) in patients with VIPoma; and free T_4, and serum glucose concentrations prior to and periodically throughout therapy in all patients taking octreotide.
- ▫ Monitor quantitative 72-hr fecal fat and serum carotene determinations periodically for possible drug-induced aggravations of fat malabsorption.
- ▫ May cause a slight increase in liver enzymes.

Potential Nursing Diagnoses

- ▪ Bowel elimination, altered: diarrhea (indications).
- ▪ Knowledge deficit related to medication regimen (patient/family teaching).

Implementation

- ▪ **General Info:** Do not use soln that is discolored or contains particulate matter. Ampules should be refrigerated, but may be stored at room temperature for days they will be used.
- ▪ **SC:** Rotate injection sites; avoid multiple injections in same site within short periods of time.

Patient/Family Teaching

- ▫ Instruct patients administering octreotide at home on correct technique for injection, storage, and disposal of equipment.
- ▫ May cause dizziness, drowsiness, or visual disturbances. Caution patient to avoid driving or other activities requiring alertness until response to medication is known.
- ▫ Advise patient to make position changes slowly to minimize orthostatic hypotension.

Evaluation

Effectiveness of therapy can be demonstrated by: ▪ Decrease in severity of diarrhea and improvement of electrolyte imbalances in patients with carcinoid or VIP-secreting tumors.

OFLOXACIN

(oh-**flox**-a-sin)

Floxin

CLASSIFICATION(S):

Anti-infective—fluoroquinolone

Pregnancy Category C

INDICATIONS

▪ Treatment of the following infections due to susceptible organisms: ▫ Lower respiratory infections ▫ Skin and skin structure infections ▫ Urinary tract infections including prostatitis, gonorrhea, cervicitis, and urethritis.

ACTION

▪ Inhibits bacterial DNA synthesis by inhibiting DNA gyrase. **Therapeutic Effect:** ▪ Death of susceptible bacteria. **Spectrum:** ▪ Broad activity includes many gram-positive pathogens: ▫ Staphylococci (including *Staphylococcus epidermidis* and methicillin-resistant strains of *Staphylococcus aureus*) ▫ *Streptococcus pyogenes* ▫ *Streptococcus pneumoniae* ▪ Gram-negative spectrum notable for activity against: ▫ *E. coli* ▫ Klebsiella species ▫ Enterobacter ▫ Salmonella ▫ Shigella ▫ *Proteus vulgaris* ▫ *Providencia stuartii* ▫ *Providencia retgerii* ▫ *Morganella morganii* ▫ *Pseudomonas aeruginosa* ▫ Serratia ▫ Haemophilus species ▫ Acenitobacter ▫ *Neisseria gonorrhea* and *meningitidis* ▫ *Branhamella ca-*

tarrhalis ▫ Yersinia, Vibrio, Brucella, Campylobacter, and Aeromonas species ▪ Active against the following anaerobic pathogens: ▫ *Bacteroides fragilis* and *intermedius* ▫ Clostridium perfrigens and *welchii* ▫ *Gardnerella vaginalis* ▫ *Peptococcus niger* ▫ *Peptostreptococcus* sp ▪ Additional spectrum includes: ▫ *Chlamydia pneumoniae* and *trachomatis* ▫ *Legionella pneumoniae* ▫ *Mycobacterium tuberculosis* ▫ *Mycoplasma pneumoniae* ▫ *Urea urealyticum* ▪ Not active against *T. pallidum*.

PHARMACOKINETICS

Absorption: Well absorbed following oral administration (89% bioavailability.)

Distribution: Widely distributed to body tissue and fluids.

Metabolism and Excretion: 70–80% excreted unchanged by the kidneys.

Half-life: 5–7 hr (increased in renal disease).

CONTRAINDICATIONS AND PRECAUTIONS

Contraindicated in: ▪ Hypersensitivity to ofloxacin or other fluoroquinolones ▪ Children ▪ Pregnancy.

Use Cautiously in: ▪ Underlying CNS pathology ▪ Lactation (high milk concentrations achieved, safety not established) ▪ Severe renal impairment (dosage reduction required).

ADVERSE REACTIONS AND SIDE EFFECTS*

CNS: tremors, restlessness, confusion, sleep disorders, nervousness, drowsiness, hallucinations, SIEZURES, dizziness.

EENT: photophobia.

CV: chest pain.

GI: nausea, diarrhea, vomiting, abdominal pain, unpleasant taste, decreased appetite, dry mouth.

GU: crystalluria, cylinduria, hematuria, vaginal discharge, genital pruritus.

Derm: rash.

INTERACTIONS

Drug-Drug: ▪ Increases serum **theophylline** levels and may lead to toxicity ▪ Administration with **antacids, iron salts, sucralfate,** or **zinc salts** decreases absorption of ofloxacin ▪ **Drugs that alkalinize the urine** increase the risk of crystalluria ▪ May increase the effects of **oral anticoagulants**.

ROUTE AND DOSAGE

▪ **PO (Adults):** 200–400 mg q 12 hr.

PHARMACODYNAMICS (blood levels)

	ONSET	PEAK
PO	rapid	1–2 hr

NURSING IMPLICATIONS

Assessment

▫ Assess patient for infection (vital signs, urinalysis, frequency, urgency, cloudy or foul-smelling urine; sputum, fever, WBC) at beginning and throughout course of therapy.

▫ Obtain specimens for culture and sensitivity prior to initiating therapy. First dose may be given before receiving results.

▪ **Lab Test Considerations:** May cause increased serum SGOT (AST), SGPT (ALT). May cause decreased WBC; increased or decreased serum glucose; and glucosuria, hematuria, proteinuria, and albuminuria.

Potential Nursing Diagnoses

▪ Infection, high risk for (indications, side effects).

▪ Knowledge deficit related to medication regimen (patient/family teaching).

▪ Noncompliance related to medication regimen (patient/family teaching).

Implementation

▪ **PO:** Administer around the clock on an empty stomach at least 1 hr before or 2 hr after meals with a full glass of water. Do not administer with food.

*Underlines indicate most frequent; **CAPITALS** indicate life-threatening.

PATIENT/FAMILY TEACHING

- □ Instruct patient to take medication around the clock and to finish the drug completely as directed, even if feeling better. If a dose is missed, take as soon as remembered unless almost time for next dose; do not double doses. Advise patients that sharing of this medication may be dangerous.
- □ Encourage patient to maintain a fluid intake of at least 1200–1500 ml/day to prevent crystalluria.
- □ Advise patient that antacids or iron preparations will decrese absorption of ofloxacin and should not be taken within 2 hr of ofloxacin.
- □ May cause dizziness and drowsiness. Caution patient to avoid driving or other activities requiring alertness until response to medication is known.
- □ Caution patient to use sunglasses and avoid prolonged exposure to bright light to prevent photophobia.
- □ Advise patient that frequent mouth rinses, good oral hygiene, and sugarless gum or candy may minimize dry mouth.
- □ Instruct the patient to notify the physician if symptoms do not improve within a few days of therapy.

EVALUATION

Clinical response to therapy can be evaluated by: ▪ Resolution of the signs and symptoms of infection.

OLSALAZINE

(ole-**sal**-a-zeen)
Dipentum

CLASSIFICATION(S):
Gastrointestinal—anti-inflammatory
Pregnancy Category C

INDICATIONS

▪ Management of ulcerative colitis in patients who cannot tolerate sulfasalazine.

ACTION

▪ Locally acting anti-inflammatory in the colon, where activity is probably due to inhibition of prostaglandin synthesis. **Therapeutic Effect:** ▪ Reduction of symptoms of ulcerative colitis, proctitis, or proctosigmoiditis.

PHARMACOKINETICS

Absorption: Acts locally in colon where 98–99% is converted to mesalamine (5-aminosalicylic acid).
Distribution: Action is primarily local and remains in the colon.
Metabolism and Excretion: 2% absorbed into systemic circulation is rapidly metabolized. Mostly eliminated as mesalamine in the feces.
Half-life: 0.9 hr.

CONTRAINDICATIONS AND PRECAUTIONS

Contraindicated in: ▪ Hypersensitivity to mesalamine, olsalazine, or salicylates.
Use Cautiously in: ▪ Renal impairment (increased risk of renal tubular damage) ▪ Pregnancy, lactation, or children (safety not established).

ADVERSE REACTIONS AND SIDE EFFECTS*

CNS: vertigo, depression.
GI: diarrhea, exacerbation of colitis, hepatitis, abdominal pain, loss of appetite, nausea, vomiting.
Hemat: blood dyscrasias.
Derm: rash, itching.

INTERACTIONS

Drug–Drug: ▪ None significant.

ROUTE AND DOSAGE

▪ **PO (Adults):** 500 mg twice daily.

PHARMACODYNAMICS

	ONSET	PEAK	DURATION
PO	UK	1hr* (4–8 hr†)	UK

*For olsalazine.
†For mesalamine.

*Underlines indicate most frequent; **CAPITALS** indicate life-threatening.

O

NURSING IMPLICATIONS

Assessment

- ▫ Assess abdominal pain and frequency, quantity, and consistency of stools at the beginning and throughout therapy.
- ▫ Assess patient for allergy to salicylates. Patients allergic to sulfasalazine may take olsalazine without difficulty, but therapy should be discontinued if rash or fever occur.
- ▪ **Lab Test Considerations:** Monitor urinalysis, BUN, and serum creatinine closely for signs of renal toxicity.
- ▫ May cause elevated SGOT (AST) and SGPT (ALT) levels.

Potential Nursing Diagnoses

- ▪ Comfort, altered: pain (indications).
- ▪ Bowel elimination, altered: diarrhea (indications).
- ▪ Knowledge deficit related to medication regimen (patient/family teaching).

Implementation

- ▪ **PO:** Administer with food in evenly divided doses every 12 hr.

Patient/Family Teaching

- ▫ Instruct patient to take medication as directed, even if feeling better.
- ▫ Advise patient to notify physician if hives, itching, wheezing, rash, or fever occur.
- ▫ Instruct patient to notify physician if symptoms worsen or do not improve or if diarrhea occurs.
- ▫ Inform patient that proctoscopy and sigmoidoscopy may be required periodically during treatment to determine response.

Evaluation

Clinical response can be evaluated by:
▪ Decrease in diarrhea and abdominal pain ▫ Return to normal bowel pattern.

OMEPRAZOLE

(o-**mep**-ra-zole)
{Losec}, PriLosec

CLASSIFICATION(S):
Gastrointestinal—antiulcer, Gastric acid pump inhibitor
Pregnancy Category C

INDICATIONS

▪ Treatment of gastroesophageal reflux disease (GERD) which has not responded to conventional therapy with histamine H_2-receptor blocking agents ▪ Treatment of gastric hypersecretory conditions associated with Zollinger-Ellison Syndrome, systemic mastocytosis, or multiple endocrine adenomas ▪ Short-term management of active duodenal ulcers.

ACTION

▪ Binds to an enzyme on gastric parietal cells in the presence of acidic gastric pH, preventing the final transport of hydrogen ions into the gastric lumen. **Therapeutic Effect:** ▪ Diminished accumulation of acid in the gastric lumen with lessened gastroesophageal reflux.

PHARMACOKINETICS

Absorption: Rapidly absorbed following oral administration.
Distribution: Good distribution into gastric parietal cells.
Metabolism and Excretion: Extensively metabolized by the liver.
Half-life: 0.5–1 hr (increased in liver disease).

CONTRAINDICATIONS AND PRECAUTIONS

Contraindicated in: ▪ Hypersensitivity.
Use Cautiously in: ▪ Pregnancy, lactation, or children (safety not established).

ADVERSE REACTIONS AND SIDE EFFECTS*

CNS: weakness, dizziness, headache, somnolence, fatigue.
CV: chest pain.
GI: abdominal pain, acid regurgitation,

{} = Available in Canada only.
*Underlines indicate most frequent; **CAPITALS** indicate life-threatening.

constipation, diarrhea, flatulence, nausea, vomiting.
Derm: rash, itching.

INTERACTIONS

Drug-Drug: ▪ Decreases metabolism and may increase effects of **phenytoin, diazepam,** and **warfarin** ▪ May interfere with absorption of drugs requiring acidic gastric pH including **ketoconazole,** esters of **ampicillin,** and **iron salts** ▪ Has been used safely with **antacids**.

ROUTE AND DOSAGE

Gastroesophageal Reflux Disease

- **PO (Adults):** 20 mg once daily for 4–8 wk.

Gastric Hypersecretory Conditions

- **PO (Adults):** 60 mg once daily initially, may be increased up to 120 mg 3 times daily. Doses >80 mg/day should be given in divided doses.

PHARMACODYNAMICS

	ONSET	PEAK	DURATION
PO	within 1 hr	within 2 hr	72–96 hr

NURSING IMPLICATIONS

Assessment

- Assess patient routinely for epigastric or abdominal pain and frank or occult blood in the stool, emesis, or gastric aspirate.
- **Lab Test Considerations:** CBC with differential should be monitored periodically throughout therapy.
- May cause elevated SGOT (AST), SGPT (ALT), alkaline phosphatase, and bilirubin.

Potential Nursing Diagnoses

- Comfort, altered: pain (indications).
- Knowledge deficit related to medication regimen (patient/family teaching).

Implementation

- **PO:** Administer doses before meals, preferably in the morning. Capsules should be swallowed whole; do not crush, open, or chew.
- May be administered concurrently with antacids.

Patient/Family Teaching

- Instruct patient to take medication as prescribed for the full course of therapy, even if feeling better. If a dose is missed it should be taken as soon as remembered, but not if almost time for next dose. Do not double doses.
- May cause drowsiness or dizziness. Caution patient to avoid driving or other activities requiring alertness until response to medication is known.
- Advise patient to avoid alcohol, products containing aspirin or ibuprofen, and foods that may cause an increase in GI irritation.
- Advise patient to report onset of black, tarry stools, diarrhea, abdominal pain, or persistent headache to the physician promptly.

Evaluation

Effectiveness of therapy can be demonstrated by: ▪ Decrease in abdominal pain or prevention of gastric irritation and bleeding. Healing of duodenal ulcers can be seen on x-ray examination or endoscopy. Therapy is continued for 4–8 wk after initial episode.

ONDANSETRON

(on-**dan**-se-tron)
Zofran

CLASSIFICATION(S):
Antiemetic—miscellaneous
Pregnancy Category B

INDICATIONS

▪ Prevention of nausea and vomiting associated with chemotherapy.

ACTION

▪ Blocks the effects of serotonin at 5-HT_3 receptor sites (selective antagonist) located in vagal nerve terminals and the chemoreceptor trigger zone in the CNS. **Therapeutic Effect:** ▪ Decreased incidence and severity of nausea and vomiting following chemotherapy.

PHARMACOKINETICS

Absorption: IV administration results in complete bioavailability.
Distribution: Distribution not known.
Metabolism and Excretion: Extensively metabolized by the liver. 5% excreted unchanged by the kidneys.
Half-life: 3.5–5.5 hr.

CONTRAINDICATIONS AND PRECAUTIONS

Contraindicated in: ▪ Hypersensitivity.
Use Cautiously in: ▪ Pregnancy, lactation, or children ≤3 yr (safety not established).

ADVERSE REACTIONS AND SIDE EFFECTS*

CNS: headache.
GI: diarrhea.
Neuro: extrapyramidal reactions.

INTERACTIONS

Drug–Drug: ▪ None significant.

ROUTE AND DOSAGE

- **IV (Adults and Children:** 3 doses of 0.15 mg/kg/dose. Administer first dose 15–30 min before chemotherapy. Administer second and third doses 4 and 8 hr after first dose.

PHARMACODYNAMICS

	ONSET	PEAK	DURATION
IV	rapid	15–30 min	4 hr

NURSING IMPLICATIONS

Assessment

- □ Assess patient for nausea, vomiting, abdominal distention, and bowel sounds prior to and following administration.
- □ Assess patient for extrapyramidal effects (involuntary movements, facial grimacing, rigidity, shuffling walk, trembling of hands) periodically throughout course of therapy.
- ▪ **Lab Test Considerations:** May cause transient elevations in SGOT (AST) and SGPT (ALT) levels.

Potential Nursing Diagnoses

- ▪ Nutrition, altered: less than body requirements (indications).
- ▪ Bowel elimination, altered: diarrhea or constipation (side effects).
- ▪ Knowledge deficit related to medication regimen (patient/family teaching).

Implementation

- ▪ **Intermittent Infusion:** Dilute in 50 ml of D5W or 0.9% NaCl. Stable for 48 hr following dilution.
- □ *Rate:* Administer each of 3 doses as IV infusion over 15 min. Infuse first dose 30 min prior to start of emetogenic chemotherapy. Administer subsequent doses 4 and 8 hr after first dose.
- ▪ **Solution Compatibility:** May also be diluted with D5/0.9% NaCl, D5/0.45% NaCl, and 3% NaCl.

Patient/Family Teaching

- □ Advise patient to notify physician immediately if involuntary movement of eyes, face, or limbs occurs.

Evaluation

Effectiveness of therapy can be demonstrated by: ▪ Prevention of nausea and vomiting associated with initial and repeat courses of emetogenic cancer chemotherapy.

OXACILLIN
(ox-a-**sill**-in)
Bactocill, Prostaphilin

CLASSIFICATION(S):
Anti-infective—penicillinase-resistant penicillin
Pregnancy Category B

INDICATIONS

▪ Treatment of the following infections due to susceptible strains of penicillinase-producing staphylococci: □ Respiratory tract infections □ Skin and skin structure infections □ Bone and joint infections □ Urinary tract infections □ Endocarditis □ Septicemia □ Meningitis.

*Underlines indicate most frequent; **CAPITALS** indicate life-threatening.

ACTION

▪ Binds to bacterial cell wall, leading to cell death ▪ Resists the action of penicillinase, an enzyme capable of inactivating penicillin. **Therapeutic Effect:** ▪ Bactericidal action against susceptible bacteria. **Spectrum:** ▪ Active against most gram-positive aerobic cocci, but less so than penicillin ▪ Notable for activity against penicillinase-producing strains of: ▫ *Staphylococcus aureus* ▫ *Staphylococcus epidermidis* ▪ Not active against methicillin-resistant stapylococci.

PHARMACOKINETICS

Absorption: Rapidly but incompletely absorbed from the GI tract. Well absorbed from IM sites.
Distribution: Widely distributed. Penetration into CSF is minimal but sufficient in the presence of inflamed meninges. Crosses the placenta and enters breast milk.
Metabolism and Excretion: Partially metabolized by the liver (49%), partially excreted unchanged by the kidneys.
Half-life: 20–50 min (increased in severe hepatic impairment).

CONTRAINDICATIONS AND PRECAUTIONS

Contraindicated in: ▪ Hypersensitivity to penicillins.
Use Cautiously in: ▪ Severe hepatic impairment (dosage reduction recommended) ▪ Seriously ill patients or patients who are experiencing nausea or vomiting (use parenteral dosage form) ▪ Pregnancy or lactation (safety not established) ▪ History of previous hypersensitivity reactions.

ADVERSE REACTIONS AND SIDE EFFECTS*

CNS: SEIZURES (high doses).
GI: nausea, vomiting, diarrhea, hepatitis.
GU: interstitial nephritis.
Derm: rashes, urticaria.
Hemat: blood dyscrasias.
Local: phlebitis at IV site, pain at IM site.
Misc: superinfection, allergic reactions, including ANAPHYLAXIS and serum sickness.

INTERACTIONS

Drug-Drug: ▪ **Probenecid** decreases renal excretion and increases blood levels ▪ May alter the effects of **oral anticoagulants**.
Drug-Food: ▪ **Food, acidic juices,** or **carbonated beverages** decrease absorption.

ROUTE AND DOSAGE

Note: Contains 2.5–3.1 mEq sodium/g.

- **PO (Adults):** 500 mg q 4–6 hr.
- **PO (Children >1 mon and <40 kg):** 50–100 mg/kg/day in divided doses q 4–6 hr.
- **IM, IV (Adults):** 250–2000 mg q 4–6 hr.
- **IM, IV (Children >1 mon and <40 kg):** 50–200 mg/kg/day in divided doses q 4–6 hr.

PHARMACODYNAMICS (blood levels)

	ONSET	PEAK
PO	rapid	30–60 min
IM	rapid	30 min
IV	rapid	end of infusion

NURSING IMPLICATIONS

Assessment

▫ Assess patient for infection (vital signs; appearance of wound, sputum, urine, and stool; WBC) at beginning and throughout course of therapy.
▫ Obtain a history before initiating therapy to determine previous use of and reactions to penicillins or cephalosporins. Persons with a negative history of penicillin sensitivity may still have an allergic response.
▫ Obtain specimens for culture and sensitivity prior to initiating therapy. First dose may be given before receiving results.
▫ Observe patient for signs and symp-

*Underlines indicate most frequent; **CAPITALS** indicate life-threatening.

toms of anaphylaxis (rash, pruritus, laryngeal edema, wheezing). Discontinue the drug and notify physician immediately if these occur. Keep epinephrine, an antihistamine, and resuscitation equipment close by in the event of an anaphylactic reaction.

- **Lab Test Considerations:** CBC, BUN, creatinine, urinalysis, and liver function tests should be monitored periodically during therapy.
  - May cause elevations in SGOT (AST) and SGPT (ALT).
  - May cause positive direct Coombs' test results.

Potential Nursing Diagnoses

- Infection, high risk for (indications, side effects).
- Knowledge deficit related to medication regimen (patient/family teaching).
- Noncompliance related to medication regimen (patient/family teaching).

Implementation

- **PO:** Administer around the clock on an empty stomach, at least 1 hr before or 2 hr after meals. Take with a full glass of water; acidic juices or carbonated beverages may decrease absorption of penicillins.
  - Use calibrated measuring device for liquid preparations. Shake well. Soln is stable for 14 days if refrigerated.
- **IM/IV:** To reconstitute for IM or IV use, add 1.4 ml of sterile water for injection to each 250-mg vial, 2.7–2.8 ml to each 500-mg vial, 5.7 ml to each 1-g vial, 11.4–11.5 ml to each 2-g vial, and 21.8–23 ml to each 4-g vial, for a concentration of 250 mg/1.5 ml. Stable for 3 days at room temperature or 7 days if refrigerated.
- **Direct IV:** Further dilute each reconstituted 250-mg or 500-mg vial with 5 ml of sterile water or 0.9% NaCl for injection, 10 ml for each 1-g vial, 20 ml for each 2-g vial, and 40 ml for each 4-g vial.
  - *Rate:* Administer slowly over 10 min.
- **Intermittent Infusion:** Dilute to a concentration of 0.5–40 mg/ml with 0.9% NaCl, D5W, D5/0.9% NaCl, or lactated Ringer's soln.
  - *Rate:* May be infused for up to 6 hr.
- **Y-Site Compatibility:** acyclovir, cyclophosphamide, famotidine, foscarnet, heparin, hydrocortisone sodium succinate, hydromorphone, labetalol, magnesium sulfate, meperidine, morphine, perphenazine, potassium chloride, or zidovudine.
- **Y-Site Incompatibility:** verapamil.
- **Additive Compatibility:** cephapirin, chloramphenicol, dopamine, potassium chloride, or sodium bicarbonate.
- **Additive Incompatibility:** cytarabine, oxytetracycline, or tetracycline.

Patient/Family Teaching

- Instruct patient to take medication around the clock and to finish the drug completely as directed, even if feeling better. If a dose is missed, it should be taken as soon as remembered. Advise patient that sharing of this medication may be dangerous.
- Advise patient to report signs of superinfection (black, furry overgrowth on the tongue; vaginal itching or discharge; loose or foul-smelling stools) and allergy promptly to physician.
- Instruct patient to notify physician if symptoms do not improve.

Evaluation

Clinical response can be evaluated by:

- Resolution of the signs and symptoms of infection. Length of time for complete resolution depends on the organism and site of infection.

OXAZEPAM

(ox-**az**-e-pam)
{Apo-Oxazepam}, {Novoxapam}, {Ox-Pam}, Serax, {Zapex}

CLASSIFICATION(S):
Sedative/hypnotic—benzodiazepine
Schedule IV
Pregnancy Category UK

{} = Available in Canada only.

INDICATIONS

■ Management of anxiety ■ Symptomatic treatment of alcohol withdrawal.

ACTION

■ Depresses the CNS, probably by potentiating gamma-aminobutyric acid (GABA), an inhibitory neurotransmitter. **Therapeutic Effects:** ■ Relief of anxiety ■ Diminished symptoms of alcohol withdrawal.

PHARMACOKINETICS

Absorption: Well absorbed following oral administration. Absorption is slower than with other benzodiazepines.
Distribution: Widely distributed. Crosses the blood-brain barrier. May cross the placenta and enter breast milk.
Metabolism and Excretion: Metabolized by the liver to inactive compounds.
Half-life: 5–15 hr.

CONTRAINDICATIONS AND PRECAUTIONS

Contraindicated in: ■ Hypersensitivity ■ Cross-sensitivity with other benzodiazepines may exist ■ Comatose patients or those with pre-existing CNS depression ■ Uncontrolled severe pain ■ Narrow-angle glaucoma ■ Pregnancy and lactation.
Use Cautiously in: ■ Hepatic dysfunction ■ Patients who may be suicidal or who may have been addicted to drugs previously ■ Elderly or debilitated patients (dosage reduction recommended) ■ Severe chronic obstructive pulmonary disease ■ Myasthenia gravis.

ADVERSE REACTIONS AND SIDE EFFECTS*

CNS: <u>dizziness</u>, <u>drowsiness</u>, <u>lethargy</u>, confusion, impaired memory, hangover, paradoxical excitation, mental depression, headache, slurred speech.
EENT: blurred vision.
Resp: respiratory depression.
CV: tachycardia.
GI: nausea, vomiting, diarrhea, constipation, hepatitis.
GU: urinary problems.
Hemat: leukopenia.
Derm: rashes.
Misc: tolerance, psychological dependence, physical dependence.

INTERACTIONS

Drug-Drug: ■ Additive CNS depression with other **CNS depressants**, including **alcohol, antihistamines, antidepressants, narcotic analgesics,** and other **sedative/hypnotics** ■ May decrease the therapeutic effectiveness of **levodopa** ■ **Oral contraceptives** or **phenytoin** may decrease effectiveness ■ **Theophylline** may decrease sedative effects of oxazepam.

ROUTE AND DOSAGE

Mild to Moderate Anxiety

■ **PO (Adults):** 15–30 mg 3–4 times daily.

Severe Anxiety, Alcohol Withdrawal

■ **PO (Adults):** 15–30 mg 3–4 times daily.

PHARMACODYNAMICS (sedation)

	ONSET	PEAK	DURATION
PO	45–90 min	UK	6–12 hr

NURSING IMPLICATIONS

Assessment

□ Assess patient for anxiety and level of sedation (ataxia, dizziness, slurred speech) periodically throughout course of therapy.
□ Prolonged high-dose therapy may lead to psychological or physical dependence. Restrict the amount of drug available to patient.
■ **Lab Test Considerations:** Monitor CBC and liver function tests periodically during prolonged therapy.
□ May cause an increase in serum bilirubin, SGOT (AST), and SGPT (ALT).

*<u>Underlines</u> indicate most frequent; **CAPITALS** indicate life-threatening.

Potential Nursing Diagnoses

- Anxiety (indications).
- Injury, high risk for (side effects).
- Knowledge deficit related to medication regimen (patient/family teaching).

Implementation

- **General Info:** Medication should be tapered at the completion of therapy. Sudden cessation of medication may lead to withdrawal (insomnia, irritability, nervousness, tremors).
- **PO:** Administer with food if GI irritation becomes a problem.

Patient/Family Teaching

- Instruct patient to take oxazepam exactly as directed. Missed doses should be taken within 1 hr; if remembered later, omit and return to regular dosing schedule. Do not double or increase doses. If dose is less effective after a few wks, notify physician.
- Oxazepam may cause drowsiness or dizziness. Caution patient to avoid driving or other activities requiring alertness until response to medication is known.
- Advise patient to avoid the use of alcohol and to consult physician or pharmacist prior to the use of over-the-counter preparations that contain antihistamines or alcohol.
- Advise patient to inform physician if pregnancy is planned or suspected.

Evaluation

Effectiveness of therapy can be demonstrated by: ▪ Decreased sense of anxiety ▫ Increased ability to cope ▪ Prevention or relief of acute agitation, tremor, and hallucinations during alcohol withdrawal.

OXICONAZOLE

(oxy-**kon**-a-zole)
Oxistat

CLASSIFICATION(S):
Antifungal—topical
Pregnancy Category B

INDICATIONS

▪ Treatment of superficial fungal infections, including: ▫ Tinea pedis ▫ Tinea cruris ▫ Tinea corporis.

ACTION

▪ Inhibits the synthesis of sterols in fungal cells, resulting in decreased membrane integrity. **Therapeutic Effect:** ▪ Fungicidal activity against susceptible isolates. **Spectrum:** ▪ Broad antifungal spectrum, including: ▫ *Trichophyton rubrum* ▫ *Trichophyton mentagrophytes.*

PHARMACOKINETICS

Absorption: Minimal systemic absorption following topical application.
Distribution: Appears to concentrate in epidermis, with lesser concentrations in upper and lower corneum.
Metabolism and Excretion: Metabolism and excretion not known.
Half-life: UK.

CONTRAINDICATIONS AND PRECAUTIONS

Contraindicated in: ▪ Hypersensitivity.
Use Cautiously in: ▪ Pregnancy, lactation, or children (safety not established).

ADVERSE REACTIONS AND SIDE EFFECTS

Derm: itching, burning, irritation, erythema, maceration, fissuring.

INTERACTIONS

Drug-Drug: ▪ None significant.

ROUTE AND DOSAGE

- **Top (Adults):** Apply to affected areas once daily, in the evening.

PHARMACODYNAMICS (antifungal activity)

	ONSET	PEAK	DURATION
Top	UK	2–4 wk	UK

NURSING IMPLICATIONS

Assessment

- Assess patient for infection prior to and throughout course of therapy.
- Obtain specimens for culture prior to treatment. First dose may be given before receiving results.

Potential Nursing Diagnoses

- Infection, high risk for (indications).
- Skin integrity, impaired: actual (indications).
- Knowledge deficit related to medication regimen (patient/family teaching).

Implementation

- **Top:** Apply to affected area once daily, in the evening. Completely cover affected area with oxiconazole cream.

Patient/Family Teaching

- **General Info:** Instruct patient to apply topical oxiconazole exactly as directed. Missed doses should be applied as soon as remembered, unless almost time for next dose.
- **Top:** Instruct patient to wash and dry affected area thoroughly prior to application. Avoid contact with eyes
- Advise patient to consult physician if no improvement is seen in 2–4 wk.

Evaluation

Effectiveness of therapy can be demonstrated by: ▪ Resolution of the signs and symptoms of infection ▫ Treatment of tinea corporis and tinea cruris requires 2 wk ▫ Treatment of tinea pedis requires 1 mon to prevent recurrence.

OXTRIPHYLLINE

(ox-**trye**-fi-lin)
{Apo-Oxtriphylline}, Choledyl, Choledyl SA, {Novotriphyl}

CLASSIFICATION(S):
Bronchodilator—phosphodiesterase inhibitor
Pregnancy Category C

INDICATIONS

- Bronchodilator in reversible airway obstruction due to asthma or COPD.

ACTION

- Inhibits phosphodiesterase, producing increased tissue concentrations of cyclic adenosine monophosphate (cAMP). Increased levels of cAMP result in bronchodilation, CNS stimulation, positive inotropic and chronotropic effects, diuresis, and gastric acid secretion ▪ Oxtriphylline is the choline salt of theophylline and releases theophylline following administration. **Therapeutic Effect:** ▪ Bronchodilation.

PHARMACOKINETICS

Absorption: Well absorbed following oral administration. Absorption of enteric-coated and sustained-release forms may be delayed, unpredictable, or unreliable.

Distribution: Widely distributed as theophylline. Crosses the placenta. Breast milk concentrations are 70% of plasma levels.

Metabolism and Excretion: Mostly metabolized by the liver (90%), some conversion to caffeine. Metabolites are renally excreted. 10% excreted unchanged by the kidneys (up to 50% in neonates).

Half-life: 3–13 hr (theophylline). Increased in the elderly (>60 yr), neonates, and patients with congestive heart failure or liver disease. Shortened in cigarette smokers and children.

CONTRAINDICATIONS AND PRECAUTIONS

Contraindicated in: ▪ Uncontrolled arrhythmias ▪ Hyperthyroidism.

Use Cautiously in: ▪ Elderly patients (>60 yr) ▪ CHF or liver disease—decrease dosage ▪ Pregnancy (although safety not established, has been used safely during pregnancy) ▪ Lactation (may cause irritability in the newborn) ▪ Alcohol intolerance (Choledyl elixir only).

O

ADVERSE REACTIONS AND SIDE EFFECTS*

CNS: nervousness, anxiety, headache, insomnia, SEIZURES.
CV: tachycardia, palpitations, arrhythmias, angina pectoris.
GI: nausea, vomiting, anorexia, cramps.
Neuro: tremor.

INTERACTIONS

Drug–Drug: ▪ Additive CV and CNS side effects with **adrenergic agents** ▪ May decrease the therapeutic effect of **lithium** ▪ **Smoking, adrenergic agents, phenobarbital, rifampin, ketoconazole, phenytoin,** and **carbamazepine** increase metabolism and may decrease effectiveness ▪ **Erythromycin, beta blockers, cimetidine, influenza vaccination, oral contraceptives, glucocorticoids, disulfiram, interferon, mexiletine, thiabendazole, fluoroquinolones,** and large doses of **allopurinol** decrease metabolism and may lead to toxicity ▪ Increased risk of arrhythmias with **halothane**.
Drug–Food: ▪ Large amounts of **caffeine (cola, chocolate, coffee, tea)** may increase serum theophylline levels and risk of toxicity ▪ Chronic ingestion of **charcoal-broiled beef** may increase metabolism and decrease effectiveness.

ROUTE AND DOSAGE

Note: Dosage should be determined by theophylline serum level monitoring. Dosage expressed in mg of oxtriphylline. Oxtriphylline contains 64% theophylline.

- **PO (Adults):** 4.6 mg/kg q 8 hr. If daily dose is 800 or 1200 mg may be given as sustained-action tablets q 12 hr.
- **PO (Adult Smokers and Children 9–16 yr):** 4.7 mg/kg q 6 hr. If daily dose is 800 or 1200 mg may be given as sustained-action tablets q 12 hr.
- **PO (Children 1–9 yr):** 6.2 mg/kg q 6 hr.

PHARMACODYNAMICS
(onset = onset of bronchodilation, peak = peak plasma levels, duration = duration of bronchodilation)

	ONSET	PEAK	DURATION
PO (liquid)	UK	1 hr	UK
PO (tab)	15–60 min	5 hr	6–8 hr
PO-SA tab	UK	4–7 hr	12 hr

NURSING IMPLICATIONS

Assessment

- ▫ Assess blood pressure, pulse, respiration, and lung sounds before administering medication and throughout therapy.
- ▫ Monitor intake and output ratios for an increase in diuresis.
- ▫ Patients with cardiovascular problems should be monitored for ECG changes.
- ▪ **Lab Test Considerations:** Caffeine ingestion may falsely elevate drug concentration levels.
- ▪ **Toxicity and Overdose:** Observe patient closely for drug toxicity (anorexia, nausea, vomiting, restlessness, insomnia, tachycardia, arrhythmias, seizures). Notify physician immediately if these occur.
- ▫ Monitor drug levels routinely. Peak levels should be evaluated 1–2 hr after rapid-acting forms and 4–12 hr after extended-release forms.
- ▫ Therapeutic plasma levels range from 10 to 20 mcg/ml. Drug levels >20 mcg/ml are associated with toxicity.

Potential Nursing Diagnoses

- ▪ Airway clearance, ineffective (indications).
- ▪ Activity intolerance (indications).
- ▪ Knowledge deficit related to medication regimen (patient/family teaching).

Implementation

- ▪ **General Info:** Administer around the clock to maintain therapeutic plasma levels.
- ▫ Determine if patient has had another

*Underlines indicate most frequent; **CAPITALS** indicate life-threatening.

form of theophylline prior to administering loading dose.
- □ Available in enteric-coated tablets, extended-release tablets, and elixir forms.
- ■ **PO:** Administer with food or a full glass of water to minimize GI irritation. Food slows but does not reduce the extent of absorption. Do not crush, break, or chew enteric-coated or extended-release tablets.

Patient/Family Teaching
- □ Emphasize the importance of taking only the prescribed dose at the prescribed time intervals. Missed doses should be taken as soon as remembered unless almost time for the next dose.
- □ Encourage patient to drink adequate liquids (2000 ml/day minimum) to decrease the viscosity of the airway secretions.
- □ Advise patient to avoid over-the-counter cough, cold, or breathing preparations without consulting physician or pharmacist. These medications may increase side effects and cause arrhythmias.
- □ Encourage patients not to smoke. A change in smoking habits may necessitate a change in dosage.
- □ Advise patient to minimize intake of xanthine-containing foods or beverages (cola, coffee, chocolate) and not to eat charcoal-broiled foods daily.
- □ Instruct patient not to change brands or dosage forms without consulting physician.
- □ Advise patient to contact physician promptly if the usual dose of medication fails to produce the desired results, symptoms worsen after treatment, or toxic effects occur.
- □ Emphasize the importance of having serum levels routinely tested every 6–12 mon.

Evaluation
Effectiveness of therapy can be demonstrated by: ■ Increased ease in breathing □ Clearing of lung fields on auscultation.

OXYBUTYNIN
(ox-i-**byoo**-ti-nin)
Ditropan

CLASSIFICATION(S):
Antispasmodic—urinary
Pregnancy Category UK

INDICATIONS
■ Treatment of the following urinary symptoms that may be associated with neurogenic bladder: □ Frequent urination □ Urgency □ Nocturia □ Incontinence.

ACTION
■ Inhibits the action of acetylcholine at postganglionic receptors ■ Has direct spasmolytic action on smooth muscle, including smooth muscle lining the GU tract, without affecting vascular smooth muscle. **Therapeutic Effects:** ■ Increased bladder capacity ■ Delayed desire to void.

PHARMACOKINETICS
Absorption: Rapidly absorbed following oral administration.
Distribution: Distribution not known.
Metabolism and Excretion: Metabolism and excretion not known.
Half-life: UK.

CONTRAINDICATIONS AND PRECAUTIONS
Contraindicated in: ■ Hypersensitivity ■ Glaucoma ■ Intestinal obstruction or atony ■ Toxic megacolon ■ Paralytic ileus ■ Severe colitis ■ Myasthenia gravis ■ Acute hemorrhage with shock ■ Obstructive uropathy.
Use Cautiously in: ■ Pregnancy or children <5 yr (safety not established) ■ Lactation (may inhibit lactation) ■ Cardiovascular disease ■ Reflux esophagitis.

ADVERSE REACTIONS AND SIDE EFFECTS*
CNS: drowsiness, dizziness, insomnia, weakness, hallucinations.

*Underlines indicate most frequent; **CAPITALS** indicate life-threatening.

O

EENT: blurred vision, mydriasis, increased intraocular pressure, cycloplegia, photophobia.
CV: tachycardia, palpitations.
GI: dry mouth, nausea, vomiting, bloated feeling, constipation.
GU: urinary hesitancy, urinary retention, impotence.
Derm: decreased sweating, urticaria.
Endo: suppressed lactation.
Metab: hyperthermia.
Misc: allergic reactins, hot flashes, fever.

INTERACTIONS

Drug–Drug: ▪ Additive anticholinergic effects with other **agents having anticholinergic properties,** including **antidepressants, phenothiazine, disopyramide,** and **haloperidol** ▪ Additive CNS depression with other **CNS depressants,** including **alcohol, antihistamines, antidepressants, narcotic analgesics,** and **sedative/hypnotics**.

ROUTE AND DOSAGE

- **PO (Adults):** 5 mg qid.
- **PO (Children <5 yr):** 5 mg 2–3 times daily (not to exceed 15 mg/day).

PHARMACODYNAMICS (urinary spasmolytic effect)

	ONSET	PEAK	DURATION
PO	30–60 min	3–6 hr	6–10 hr

NURSING IMPLICATIONS

Assessment

- Monitor voiding pattern and intake and output ratios and assess abdomen for bladder distention prior to and periodically throughout therapy. Physician may order catheterization to assess postvoid residual. Cystometry, to diagnose type of bladder dysfunction, is usually performed prior to prescription of oxybutynin.

Potential Nursing Diagnoses

- Urinary elimination, altered patterns (indications).
- Comfort, altered (indications).
- Knowledge deficit related to medication regimen (patient/family teaching).

Implementation

- **PO:** May be administered on an empty stomach or with meals or milk to prevent gastric irritation.

Patient/Family Teaching

- Instruct patient to take medication exactly as directed. If a dose is missed, it should be taken as soon as remembered unless almost time for next dose.
- Medication may cause drowsiness or blurred vision. Advise patient to avoid driving and other activities requiring alertness until response to medication is known.
- Advise patient to avoid concurrent use of alcohol and other CNS depressants while taking this medication.
- Instruct patient that frequent rinsing of mouth, good oral hygiene, and sugarless gum or candy may decrease dry mouth. Physician or dentist should be notified if mouth dryness persists >2 wk.
- Inform patient that oxybutynin decreases the body's ability to perspire. The patient should avoid strenuous activity in a warm environment because overheating may occur.
- Advise patient to wear sunglasses when out in bright sunlight, as increased sensitivity to light may occur.
- Advise patient to notify physician if urinary retention occurs or if constipation persists. Discuss with patient methods of preventing constipation, such as increasing bulk in the diet, increasing fluid intake, and increasing mobility.
- Discuss need for continued medical follow-up. Physician may order periodic cystometry to evaluate effectiveness of medication and periodic ophthalmic examinations to detect glaucoma, especially in patients over 40 yrs of age.

Evaluation

Effectiveness of therapy can be demonstrated by: ▪ Relief of bladder spasm and associated symptoms (frequency, urgency, nocturia, and incontinence) in patients with a neurogenic bladder.

OXYCODONE
(ox-i-**koe**-done)
Roxicodone, {Supeudol}

OXYCODONE/ACETAMINOPHEN
{Endocet}, Oxycet, {Oxycocet}, Percocet, Roxicet, Tylox

OXYCODONE/ASPIRIN
Codoxy, {Endodan}, {Oxycodan}, Percodan, Percodan-Demi, Roxiprin

CLASSIFICATION(S):
Narcotic analgesic—agonist
Schedule II
Pregnancy Category UK

INDICATIONS

- Used alone and in combination with non-narcotic analgesics in the management of moderate to severe pain.

ACTION

- Binds to opiate receptors in the CNS
- Alters the perception of and response to painful stimuli, while producing generalized CNS depression. **Therapeutic Effect:**
- Decrease in severity of moderate to severe pain.

PHARMACOKINETICS

Absorption: Well absorbed from the GI tract.
Distribution: Widely distributed. Crosses the placenta and enters breast milk.
Metabolism and Excretion: Mostly metabolized by the liver.
Half-life: 2–3 hr.

CONTRAINDICATIONS AND PRECAUTIONS

Contraindicated in: ▪ Hypersensitivity ▪ Pregnancy or lactation (avoid chronic use).

Use Cautiously in: ▪ Head trauma ▪ Increased intracranial pressure ▪ Severe renal, hepatic, or pulmonary disease ▪ Hypothyroidism ▪ Adrenal insufficiency ▪ Alcoholism ▪ Elderly or debilitated patients (dosage reduction recommended) ▪ Undiagnosed abdominal pain ▪ Prostatic hypertrophy.

ADVERSE REACTIONS AND SIDE EFFECTS*

CNS: sedation, confusion, headache, euphoria, floating feeling, unusual dreams, hallucinations, dysphoria, dizziness.
EENT: miosis, diplopia, blurred vision.
Resp: respiratory depression.
CV: orthostatic hypotension.
GI: nausea, vomiting, constipation, dry mouth.
GU: urinary retention.
Derm: sweating, flushing.
Misc: tolerance, physical dependence, psychological dependence.

INTERACTIONS

Drug–Drug: ▪ Use with caution in patients receiving **MAO inhibitors** (may result in unpredictable reactions—decrease initial dose of oxycodone to 25% of usual dose) ▪ Additive CNS depression with **alcohol, antihistamines,** and **sedative/hypnotics** ▪ Administration of **partial-antagonist narcotic analgesics** may precipitate narcotic withdrawal in physically dependent patients ▪ **Nalbuphine** or **pentazocine** may decrease analgesia.

ROUTE AND DOSAGE

- **PO (Adults):** 5 mg q 3–6 hr as needed or 10 mg 3–4 times daily as needed.
- **PO (Children >12 yr):** 2.5 mg q 6 hr as needed.
- **PO (Children 6–12 yr):** 1.25 mg q 6 hr as needed.

{} = Available in Canada only.
*Underlines indicate most frequent; **CAPITALS** indicate life-threatening.

O

PHARMACODYNAMICS (analgesic effects)

	ONSET	PEAK	DURATION
PO	10–15 min	60–90 min	3–6 hr

NURSING IMPLICATIONS

Assessment

- Assess type, location, and intensity of pain prior to and 60 min following administration.
- Assess blood pressure, pulse, and respiratory rate before and periodically during administration.
- Prolonged use may lead to physical and psychological dependence and tolerance. This should not prevent patient from receiving adequate analgesia. Most patients who receive oxycodone for medical reasons do not develop psychological dependence. Progressively higher doses may be required to relieve pain with long-term therapy.
- Assess bowel function routinely. Increased intake of fluids and bulk, stool softeners, and laxatives may minimize constipating effects.
- **Lab Test Considerations:** May increase plasma amylase and lipase levels.
- **Toxicity and Overdose:** If overdose occurs, naloxone (Narcan) is the antidote.

Potential Nursing Diagnoses

- Comfort, altered: pain (indications).
- Sensory-perceptual alteration: visual, auditory (side effects).
- Injury, high risk for (side effects).

Implementation

- **General Info:** Explain therapeutic value of medication prior to administration to enhance the analgesic effect.
- Regularly administered doses may be more effective than prn administration. Analgesic is more effective if given before pain becomes severe.
- Coadministration with non-narcotic analgesics may have additive analgesic effects and may permit lower doses.
- Medication should be discontinued gradually after long-term use to prevent withdrawal symptoms.
- **PO:** May be administered with food or milk to minimize GI irritation.

Patient/Family Teaching

- Instruct patient on how and when to ask for prn pain medication.
- Medication may cause drowsiness or dizziness. Advise patient to call for assistance when ambulating or smoking. Caution patient to avoid driving and other activities requiring alertness until response to medication is known.
- Advise patient to make position changes slowly to minimize orthostatic hypotension.
- Advise patient to avoid concurrent use of alcohol or other CNS depressants with this medication.
- Encourage patient to turn, cough, and breathe deeply every 2 hr to prevent atelectasis.

Evaluation

Effectiveness of therapy can be demonstrated by: ▪ Decrease in severity of pain without a significant alteration in level of consciousness or respiratory status.

OXYMORPHONE

(ox-i-**mor**-fone)
Numorphan

CLASSIFICATION(S):
Narcotic analgesic—agonist
Schedule II
Pregnancy Category UK

INDICATIONS

▪ Used in the management of moderate to severe pain ▪ As a supplement in balanced anesthesia.

ACTION

▪ Binds to opiate receptors in the CNS ▪ Alters the perception of and response to painful stimuli, while producing generalized CNS depression. **Therapeutic Effect:** ▪ Decrease in moderate to severe pain.

PHARMACOKINETICS

Absorption: Well absorbed following IM, SC, or rectal administration.
Distribution: Widely distributed. Crosses the placenta and enters breast milk.
Metabolism and Excretion: Mostly metabolized by the liver.
Half-life: 2.6–4 hr.

CONTRAINDICATIONS AND PRECAUTIONS

Contraindicated in: ▪ Hypersensitivity ▪ Hypersensitivity to bisulfites (injection only) ▪ Pregnancy or lactation (avoid chronic use) ▪ Children <12 yr.
Use Cautiously in: ▪ Head trauma ▪ Increased intracranial pressure ▪ Severe renal, hepatic, or pulmonary disease ▪ Hypothyroidism ▪ Adrenal insufficiency ▪ Alcoholism ▪ Elderly or debilitated patients (dosage reduction recommended) ▪ Undiagnosed abdominal pain ▪ Prostatic hypertrophy.

ADVERSE REACTIONS AND SIDE EFFECTS*

CNS: sedation, confusion, headache, euphoria, floating feeling, unusual dreams, hallucinations, dysphoria, dizziness.
EENT: miosis, diplopia, blurred vision.
Resp: respiratory depression.
CV: orthostatic hypotension.
GI: nausea, vomiting, constipation, dry mouth.
GU: urinary retention.
Derm: sweating, flushing.
Misc: tolerance, physical dependence, psychological dependence.

INTERACTIONS

Drug-Drug: ▪ Use with caution in patients receiving **MAO inhibitors** (may result in unpredictable reactions—decrease initial dose of oxymorphone to 25% of usual dose) ▪ Additive CNS depression with **alcohol, antihistamines,** and **sedative/hypnotics** ▪ Administration of **partial-antagonist narcotic analgesics** may precipitate narcotic withdrawal in physically dependent patients ▪ **Nalbuphine** or **pentazocine** may decrease analgesia.

ROUTE AND DOSAGE

Analgesia—Moderate to Severe Pain

- **SC, IM (Adults):** 1–1.5 mg q 3–6 hr as needed.
- **IV (Adults):** 0.5 mg q 3–6 hr as needed, increase as needed.
- **Rect (Adults):** 5 mg q 4–6 hr as needed.

Analgesia During Labor

- **IM (Adults):** 0.5–1 mg.

PHARMACODYNAMICS (analgesic effects)

	ONSET	PEAK	DURATION
IM	10–15 min	30–90 min	3–6 hr
IV	5–10 min	15–30 min	3–4 hr
SC	10–20 min	UK	3–6 hr
Rect	15–30 min	120 min	3–6 hr

NURSING IMPLICATIONS

Assessment

- Assess type, location, and intensity of pain prior to and 60 min following administration.
- Assess blood pressure, pulse, and respiratory rate before and periodically during administration.
- Prolonged use may lead to physical and psychological dependence and tolerance. This should not prevent patient from receiving adequate analgesia. Most patients who receive oxymorphone for medical reasons do not develop psychological dependence. Progressively higher doses may be required to relieve pain with long-term therapy.
- Assess bowel function routinely. Increased intake of fluids and bulk, stool softeners, and laxatives may minimize constipating effects.

*Underlines indicate most frequent; **CAPITALS** indicate life-threatening.

- **Lab Test Considerations:** May increase plasma amylase and lipase levels.
- **Toxicity and Overdose:** If overdose occurs, naloxone (Narcan) is the antidote.

Potential Nursing Diagnoses
- Comfort, altered: pain (indications).
- Sensory-perceptual alteration: visual, auditory (side effects).
- Injury, high risk for (side effects).

Implementation
- **General Info:** Explain therapeutic value of medication prior to administration to enhance the analgesic effect.
  - Regularly administered doses may be more effective than prn administration. Analgesic is more effective if given before pain becomes severe.
  - Coadministration with non-narcotic analgesics may have additive analgesic effects and may permit lower doses.
  - Medication should be discontinued gradually after long-term use to prevent withdrawal symptoms.
- **Rect:** Suppositories should be stored in the refrigerator.
- **Direct IV:** Administer undiluted over 2–3 min.
- **Y-Site Compatibility:** glycopyrrolate, hydroxyzine, or ranitidine.

Patient/Family Teaching
- Instruct patient on how and when to ask for prn pain medication.
- Medication may cause drowsiness or dizziness. Advise patient to call for assistance when ambulating or smoking. Caution patient to avoid driving and other activities requiring alertness until response to medication is known.
- Advise patient to make position changes slowly to minimize orthostatic hypotension.
- Advise patient to avoid concurrent use of alcohol or other CNS depressants with this medication.
- Encourage patient to turn, cough, and breathe deeply every 2 hr to prevent atelectasis.

Evaluation

Effectiveness of therapy can be demonstrated by: ▪ Decrease in severity of pain without a significant alteration in level of consciousness or respiratory status.

OXYTOCIN
(ox-i-**toe**-sin)
Pitocin, Syntocinon

CLASSIFICATION(S):
Hormone—oxytocic
Pregnancy Category UK

INDICATIONS
▪ Induction of labor at term ▪ Facilitation of uterine contractions at term ▪ Facilitation of threatened abortion ▪ Postpartum control of bleeding after expulsion of the placenta ▪ Nasal preparation used to promote milk letdown in lactating women. **Unlabeled Use:** ▪ Evaluation of fetal competence (fetal stress test).

ACTION
▪ Stimulates uterine smooth muscle, producing uterine contractions similar to those in spontaneous labor ▪ Stimulates mammary gland smooth muscle, facilitating lactation ▪ Has vasopressor and antidiuretic effects. **Therapeutic Effects:** ▪ Induction of labor (IV) ▪ Milk letdown (intranasal).

PHARMACOKINETICS
Absorption: Well absorbed from the nasal mucosa.
Distribution: Widely distributed in extracellular fluid. Small amounts reach fetal circulation.
Metabolism and Excretion: Rapidly metabolized by liver and kidneys.
Half-life: 3–9 min.

CONTRAINDICATIONS AND PRECAUTIONS
Contraindicated in: ▪ Hypersensitivity ▪ Hypersensitivity to chlorobutanol (IV

only) ▪ Anticipated nonvaginal delivery ▪ Pregnancy (intranasal).

Use Cautiously in: ▪ First and second stages of labor.

ADVERSE REACTIONS AND SIDE EFFECTS*

Maternal

Seen following IV use only.

CNS: SEIZURES, COMA.

CV: hypotension.

F and E: water intoxication, hyponatremia, hypochloremia.

Hemat: afibrinogenemia, thrombocytopenia.

Misc: abruptio placenta, hypersensitivity, painful contractions, decreased uterine blood flow, increased uterine motility.

Fetal

CNS: INTRACRANIAL HEMORRHAGE.

Resp: hypoxia, asphyxia.

CV: arrhythmias.

INTERACTIONS

Drug-Drug: ▪ Severe hypertension may occur if oxytocin follows administration of **vasopressors** ▪ Concurrent use with **cyclopropane anesthesia** may result in excessive hypotension.

ROUTE AND DOSAGE

Induction of Labor

- **IV (Adults):** 1–2 milliunits/min, increase by 1–2 milliunits q 15–30 min until pattern established (maximum 20 milliunits/min), then decrease dose.

Postpartum

- **IV (Adults):** 10 units infused at 10–20 milliunits/min.

Promotion of Milk Letdown

- **Intranasal (Adults):** 1 spray or 1 drop in one or both nostrils 2–3 min before breast feeding or pumping breasts.

Fetal Stress Test

- **IV (Adults):** 0.5 milliunits/min, may be increased q 15 min until 3 moderate contractions occur in one 10-min period, to a maximum of 20 milliunits with maternal/fetal monitoring.

PHARMACODYNAMICS (IV = uterine contractions, Intranasal = milk letdown)

	ONSET	PEAK	DURATION
IV	immediate	UK	1 hr
Intranasal	few mins	UK	20 min

NURSING IMPLICATIONS

Assessment

- Fetal maturity, presentation, and pelvic adequacy should be assessed prior to administration of oxytocin for induction of labor.
- Assess character, frequency, and duration of uterine contractions; resting uterine tone; and fetal heart rate frequently throughout administration. If contractions occur <2 min apart and are >50–65 mmHg on monitor, if they last 60–90 sec or longer, or if a significant change in fetal heart rate develops, stop infusion and turn patient on her left side to prevent fetal anoxia. Notify physician immediately.
- Monitor maternal blood pressure and pulse frequently and fetal heart rate continuously throughout administration.
- This drug occasionally causes water intoxication. Monitor patient for signs and symptoms (drowsiness, listlessness, confusion, headache, anuria) and notify physician if they occur.
- Monitor maternal electrolytes. Water retention may result in hypochloremia or hyponatremia.

Potential Nursing Diagnoses

- Knowledge deficit related to medication regimen (patient/family teaching).

Implementation

- **Continuous Infusion:** Rotate infusion container to ensure thorough mixing. Store soln in refrigerator, but do not freeze.

*Underlines indicate most frequent; **CAPITALS** indicate life-threatening.

- □ Infuse via infusion pump for accurate dosage. Oxytocin should be connected via Y-site injection or 3-way stopcock to an IV of 0.9% NaCl for use during adverse reactions.
- □ Magnesium sulfate should be available if needed for relaxation of the myometrium.
- ■ **Induction of Labor:** Dilute 1 ml (10 units) in 1 liter of compatible infusion fluid for a concentration of 10 milliunits/ml.
- □ *Rate:* Begin infusion at 1–2 milliunits//min (0.1–0.2 ml), increase in increments of 1–2 milliunits/min at 15–30 min intervals until contractions simulate normal labor.
- ■ **Postpartum Bleeding:** For control of postpartum bleeding, dilute 1–4 ml (10–40 units) in 1 liter of compatible infusion fluid (10–40 milliunits/ml).
- □ *Rate:* Begin infusion at a rate of 10–20 milliunits/min to control uterine atony. Adjust rate as indicated.
- ■ **Incomplete or Inevitable Abortion:** For incomplete or inevitable abortion, dilute 1 ml (10 units) in 500 ml of compatible infusion fluid, for a concentration of 20 milliunits/ml.
- □ *Rate:* Infuse at a rate of 10–20 milliunits/min.
- ■ **Y-Site Compatibility:** heparin, hydrocortisone sodium succinate, meperidine, morphine, or potassium chloride.
- ■ **Additive/Solution Compatibility:** chloramphenicol, metaraminol, netilimicin, sodium bicarbonate, tetracycline, thiopental, or verapamil. Compatible infusion fluids include dextrose/Ringer's or lactated Ringer's combinations, dextrose/saline combinations, Ringer's or lactated Ringer's injection, D5W, D10W, 0.45% NaCl, or 0.9% NaCl.
- ■ **Additive Incompatibility:** fibrinolysin or warfarin sodium.
- ■ **Intranasal:** Hold squeeze bottle upright while patient is in sitting position. Patient should clear nasal passages prior to administration.

Patient/Family Teaching

- ■ **General Info:** Advise patient to expect contractions similar to menstrual cramps after administration has started.
- ■ **Nasal Spray:** Advise patient to administer nasal spray 2–3 min prior to planned breast feeding. Patient should notify physician if milk drips from non-nursed breast or if uterine cramps occur.

Evaluation

Effectiveness of therapy can be demonstrated by: ■ Onset of effective contractions ■ Increase in uterine tone ■ Effective letdown reflex.

PANCRELIPASE

(pan-kree-li-pase)
Cotazym, {Cotazym E.C.S.}, Cotazym-S, {Cotazym-65 B}, Creon, Entolase, Entolase HP, Ilozyme, Ku-Zyme HP, Pancrease, Pancrease MT, Viokase, Zymase

CLASSIFICATION(S):
Enzyme
Pregnancy Category C

INDICATIONS

■ Treatment of pancreatic insufficiency associated with: □ Chronic pancreatitis □ Pancreatectomy □ Cystic fibrosis □ GI bypass surgery □ Ductal obstruction secondary to tumor.

ACTION

■ Contains lipolytic, amylolytic, and proteolytic activity. **Therapeutic Effect:** ■ Increased digestion of fats, carbohydrates, and proteins in the GI tract.

PHARMACOKINETICS

Absorption: Absorption not known.
Distribution: Distribution not known.
Metabolism and Excretion: Metabolism and excretion not known.
Half-life: UK.

CONTRAINDICATIONS AND PRECAUTIONS

Contraindicated in: ▪ Hypersensitivity to hog proteins ▪ Hypersensitivity to additives (povidone iodine, benzyl alcohol, parabens).

Use Cautiously in: ▪ Pregnancy or lactation (safety not established).

ADVERSE REACTIONS AND SIDE EFFECTS*

EENT: nasal stuffiness.

Resp: shortness of breath, wheezing, dyspnea.

GI: diarrhea, nausea, stomach cramps, abdominal pain (high doses only), oral irritation.

GU: hematuria.

Derm: rash, hives.

Metab: hyperuricemia.

Misc: allergic reactions.

INTERACTIONS

Drug–Drug: ▪ **Antacids (calcium carbonate** or **magnesium hydroxide)** may decrease effectiveness of pancrelipase ▪ May decrease the absorption of concurrently administered **iron preparations**.

Drug–Food: ▪ **Alkaline foods** destroy coating on enteric-coated products.

ROUTE AND DOSAGE

- **PO (Adults):** 1–3 capsule(s) before or with meals, dosage may be increased as needed (up to 8 capsules may be needed), or 1–2 delayed-release capsule(s) (Pancrease MT, Cotazym S, Cotazym E.C.S., Entolase, Entolase HP, Zymase) or 0.7 g powder.
- **PO (Children):** 1–3 capsule(s) before or with meals, dosage may be increased as needed, or 1–2 delayed-release capsule(s) (Pancrease, Cotazym S, Cotazym E.C.S. or 0.7 g powder.

PHARMACODYNAMICS (digestant effects)

	ONSET	PEAK	DURATION
PO	rapid	UK	UK

NURSING IMPLICATIONS

Assessment

- Assess patient's nutritional status (height, weight, skin-fold thickness, arm muscle circumference, and lab values) prior to and periodically throughout therapy.
- Monitor stools for high fat content (steatorrhea). Stools will be foul-smelling and frothy.
- Assess patient for allergy to pork; sensitivity to pancrelipase may exist.
- **Lab Test Considerations:** May cause elevated serum and urine uric acid concentrations.

Potential Nursing Diagnoses

- Nutrition, altered: less than body requirements (indications).
- Knowledge deficit related to medication regimen (patient/family teaching).

Implementation

- **PO:** Administer immediately before or with meals and snacks.
- Capsules may be opened and sprinkled on foods. Capsules filled with enteric-coated beads should not be chewed (sprinkle on soft foods that can be swallowed without chewing, such as apple sauce or jello).
- Pancrelipase is destroyed by acid. Physician may order concurrent sodium bicarbonate or aluminum-containing antacids with non-enteric-coated preparations to neutralize gastric pH. Enteric-coated beads are designed to withstand the acid pH of the stomach. These medications should not be chewed or mixed with alkaline foods prior to ingestion or coating will be destroyed.

Patient/Family Teaching

- Encourage patients to comply with diet recommendations of physician (generally high-calorie, high-protein, low-fat). Dosage should be adjusted for fat content of diet. Usually 300 mg of pancrelipase is necessary to digest every 17 g of dietary fat. If a dose is missed, it should be omitted.
- Instruct patient not to chew tablets

*Underlines indicate most frequent; **CAPITALS** indicate life-threatening.

and to swallow them quickly with plenty of liquid to prevent mouth and throat irritation. Patient should be sitting upright to enhance swallowing. Eating immediately after taking medication helps further assure that the medication is swallowed and does not remain in contact with mouth and esophagus for a prolonged period. Patient should avoid sniffing powdered contents of capsules, as sensitization of nose and throat may occur (nasal stuffiness or respiratory distress).

□ Instruct patient to notify physician if joint pain, swelling of legs, gastric distress, or rash occurs.

EVALUATION

Effectiveness of therapy can be demonstrated by: ▪ Improved nutritional status in patients with pancreatic insufficiency □ Normalization of stools in patients with steatorrhea.

PANCURONIUM
(pan-cure-**oh**-nee-yum)
Pavulon

CLASSIFICATION(S):
Neuromuscular blocking agent—nondepolarizing
Pregnancy Category C

INDICATIONS

▪ Production of skeletal muscle paralysis and facilitation of intubation after induction of anesthesia in surgical procedures ▪ Used during mechanical ventilation to increase pulmonary compliance.

ACTION

▪ Prevents neuromuscular transmission by blocking the effect of acetylcholine at the myoneural junction ▪ Has no analgesic or anxiolytic effects. **Therapeutic Effect:** ▪ Skeletal muscle paralysis.

PHARMACOKINETICS

Absorption: Administered IV only, resulting in complete bioavailability.
Distribution: Rapidly distributes into extracellular fluid. Small amounts cross the placenta.
Metabolism and Excretion: Excreted mostly unchanged by the kidneys; small amounts are eliminated in bile.
Half-life: 2 hr.

CONTRAINDICATIONS AND PRECAUTIONS

Contraindicated in: ▪ Hypersensitivity to pancuronium or benzyl alcohol ▪ Avoid use of benzyl alcohol-containing preparations in neonates.
Use Cautiously in: ▪ Patients with any history of pulmonary disease or renal or liver impairment ▪ Elderly or debilitated patients ▪ Electrolyte disturbances ▪ Patients receiving cardiac glycosides ▪ Pregnancy (has been used during caesarian section).
Extreme Caution in: Myasthenia gravis or myasthenic syndromes.

ADVERSE REACTIONS AND SIDE EFFECTS*

Note: Almost all adverse reactions to pancuronium are extensions of pharmacologic effects.
CV: mild tachycardia.
EENT: excessive salivation (children).
Resp: apnea, wheezing.
Local: burning sensation along vein.
MS: muscle weakness.
Derm: excessive sweating (children), rashes.
Misc: allergic reactions.

INTERACTIONS

Drug-Drug: ▪ Intensity and duration of paralysis may be prolonged by pretreatment with **succinylcholine, general anesthesia, aminoglycoside antibiotics, polymyxin B, colistin, clindamycin, lidocaine, quinidine, procainamide, beta-adrenergic blocking agents, potassium-losing diuretics,** and **magnesium.**

ROUTE AND DOSAGE

▪ **IV (Adults and Children >1 mon):** 0.04–0.1 mg/kg initially, supplemental doses of 0.01 mg/kg may be given q

*Underlines indicate most frequent; **CAPITALS** indicate life-threatening.

25–60 min to maintain paralysis or 0.015 mg/kg to allow mechanical ventilation.

PHARMACODYNAMICS (skeletal muscle relaxation)

	ONSET	PEAK	DURATION
IV	30–45 sec	3–4.5 min	35–45 min

NURSING IMPLICATIONS

Assessment

- Assess respiratory status continuously throughout pancuronium therapy. Pancuronium should be used only for intubated patients. Assess patient for increased respiratory secretions; suction as necessary.
- Neuromuscular response to pancuronium should be monitored with a peripheral nerve stimulator intraoperatively. Monitor deep tendon reflexes during prolonged administration. Paralysis is initially selective and usually occurs consecutively in the following muscles: levator muscles of eyelids, muscles of mastication, limb muscles, abdominal muscles, muscles of the glottis, intercostal muscles, and diaphragm. Recovery of muscle function usually occurs in reverse order.
- Monitor heart rate, ECG, and blood pressure periodically throughout pancuronium therapy. May cause a slight increase in heart rate and blood pressure.
- Observe patient for residual muscle weakness and respiratory distress during the recovery period.
- **Toxicity and Overdose:** If overdose occurs, use peripheral nerve stimulator to determine the degree of neuromuscular blockade. Maintain airway patency and ventilation until recovery of normal respirations occurs.
- Administration of anticholinesterase agents (edrophonium, neostigmine, pyridostigmine) may be used to antagonize the action of pancuronium. Atropine is usually administered prior to or concurrently with anticholinesterase agents.

Potential Nursing Diagnoses

- Breathing pattern, ineffective (indications).
- Communication, impaired: verbal (side effects).
- Fear (patient/family teaching).

Implementation

- **General Info:** Pancuronium is approximately 5 times as potent as tubocurarine.
- Pancuronium has no effect on consciousness or the pain threshold. Adequate anesthesia should *always* be used when pancuronium is used as an adjunct to surgical procedures or when painful procedures are performed. Benzodiazepines and/or analgesics should be administered concurrently when prolonged pancuronium therapy is used for ventilator patients, as patient is awake and able to feel all sensations.
- If eyes remain open throughout prolonged administration, protect corneas with artificial tears.
- To prevent absorption by plastic, pancuronium should not be stored in plastic syringes. May be administered in plastic syringes.
- **Direct IV:** Incremental doses may be administered every 20–60 min as needed. Dose is titrated to patient response.
- **Intermittent Infusion:** May be diluted in 0.9% NaCl, D5W, D5/0.9% NaCl, and lactated Ringer's injection. Soln is stable for 48 hr.
- *Rate:* Titrate rate according to patient response.
- **Syringe Compatibility:** heparin.
- **Y-Site Compatibility:** aminophylline, cefazolin, cefuroxime, cimetidine, co-trimoxazole, dobutamine, dopamine, epinephrine, esmolol, fentanyl, gentamicin, heparin, hydrocortisone sodium succinate, isoproterenol, lorazepam, midazolam, morphine, nitroglycerin, nitroprusside, ranitidine, or vancomycin.
- **Y-Site Incompatibility:** diazepam.

P

PATIENT/FAMILY TEACHING

- Explain all procedures to patient receiving pancuronium therapy without anesthesia, as consciousness is not affected by pancuronium alone. Provide emotional support.
- Reassure patient that communication abilities will return as the medication wears off.

EVALUATION

Effectiveness of therapy can be demonstrated by: ▪ Adequate suppression of the twitch response when tested with peripheral nerve stimulation and subsequent muscle paralysis.

PANTOTHENIC ACID
(pan-toe-**then**-ik **as**-id)

PANTOTHENIC ACID
Dexor T.D., Vitamin B_5

CALCIUM PANTOTHENATE
Durasil, Pantholin

DEXPANTHENOL
Dexol, D-Pantothenyl, Ilopan, Panthoderm

CLASSIFICATION(S):
Vitamin—water-soluble
Pregnancy Category UK

INDICATIONS

▪ **PO:** Treatment and prevention of deficiencies of the B-complex vitamins associated with poor nutritional status or chronic debilitating illnesses ▪ **IM, IV:** Used to promote GI peristalsis ▪ **Top:** Management of various dermatoses (dexpanthenol only).

ACTION

▪ Converted to co-enzyme A, which is required for intermediary metabolism of proteins, carbohydrates, and lipids. **Therapeutic Effects:** ▪ Treatment and prevention of deficiencies ▪ Stimulation of GI peristalsis.

PHARMACOKINETICS

Absorption: Appears to be well absorbed following oral administration.
Distribution: Widely distributed as coenzyme A. Concentrates in liver, adrenals, heart, and kidneys.
Metabolism and Excretion: 70% excreted unchanged by the kidneys. 30% eliminated in feces.
Half-life: UK.

CONTRAINDICATIONS AND PRECAUTIONS

Contraindicated in: ▪ Mechanical obstruction of the GI tract (dexpanthenol) ▪ Hemophilia (dexpanthenol).
Use Cautiously in: ▪ Pregnancy, lactation, or children (dexpanthenol only, safety not established).

ADVERSE REACTIONS AND SIDE EFFECTS*

GI: GI cramps.
Misc: allergic reactions (dexpanthenol only).

INTERACTIONS

Drug-Drug: ▪ None significant.

ROUTE AND DOSAGE

Dietary Supplement (Pantothenic Acid, Calcium Pantothenate)

- **PO (Adults):** 5–10 mg.

Stimulation of Intestinal Peristalsis (Dexpanthenol)

- **IM (Adults):** 250–500 mg, may repeat in 2 hr and again q 4–12 hr.
- **IM (Children):** 11–12.5 mg/kg, may repeat in 2 hr and again q 4–12 hr.
- **IV (Adults):** 500 mg, infused slowly.

Dermatoses (Dexpanthenol)

- **Top (Adults and Children):** 2% cream applied 1–2 times daily.

PHARMACODYNAMICS

	ONSET	PEAK	DURATION
PO	UK	UK	UK
IV	UK	UK	UK

*Underlines indicate most frequent; **CAPITALS** indicate life-threatening.

NURSING IMPLICATIONS

Assessment

- Assess patient for signs of vitamin deficiency prior to and periodically throughout therapy. Solitary pantothenic acid (B_5) deficiency is very rare and is characterized by burning paresthesia in the feet.

Potential Nursing Diagnoses

- Nutrition, altered: less than body requirements (indications).
- Knowledge deficit related to medication regimen (patient/family teaching).

Implementation

- **General Info:** Because of infrequency of single B-vitamin deficiencies, combinations are commonly administered.
- **Intermittent Infusion:** Dilute in 500 ml or more of D5W or lactated Ringer's soln. Do not administer soln that is discolored or that contains a precipitate.
- *Rate:* Infuse slowly over 3–6 hr.
- **Top:** Wash affected area and dry thoroughly prior to application.

Patient/Family Teaching

- Encourage patient to comply with diet recommendations of physician. Explain that the best source of vitamins is a well-balanced diet with foods from the 4 basic food groups.
- Foods high in pantothenic acid include organ meats (liver, kidney) and whole-grain cereal. There is slight loss of pantothenic acid from foods with cooking.
- Patients self-medicating with vitamin supplements should be cautioned not to exceed RDA (see Appendix L). The effectiveness of megadoses for treatment of various medical conditions is unproven and may cause side effects.
- Emphasize the importance of follow-up examinations to evaluate progress.

Evaluation

Effectiveness of therapy can be demonstrated by: ▪ Prevention of or decrease in the symptoms of vitamin B_5 deficiency ▪ Stimulation of GI peristalsis.

PAPAVERINE

(pa-**pav**-er-een)

Cerespan, Genabid, Pavabid, Pavabid HP, Pavacap, Pavacen, Pavagen, Pava Par, Pavarine, Pavased, Pavatine, Pavatym, Paverolan

CLASSIFICATION(S):

Vasodilator

Pregnancy Category C

INDICATIONS

▪ Although FDA-designated as ineffective for these indications, has been used in the following: ▫ Management of cerebral and peripheral ischemia, usually associated with arterial spasm ▫ Treatment of myocardial ischemia complicated by arrhythmias ▫ Improvement of collateral circulation in acute vascular occlusion ▫ Management of ureteral, biliary, or GI colic. **Unlabeled Use:** ▪ Adjunct treatment (with alpha-adrenergic blockers) in the management of male impotence due to organic causes (intracavernosal injection).

ACTION

▪ Claimed to dilate coronary, cerebral, pulmonary, and peripheral arteries by a direct spasmolytic action on vascular smooth muscle. **Therapeutic Effect:** ▪ Claimed arterial vasodilation.

PHARMACOKINETICS

Absorption: Variably (50%) absorbed following oral administration, absorption from extended-release formulations may be less. Slowly absorbed following intracavernosal administration.

Distribution: Distribution not known.

Metabolism and Excretion: Mainly metabolized by the liver.

Half-life: 0.5–2 hr (highly variable—may be as long as 24 hr).

CONTRAINDICATIONS AND PRECAUTIONS

Contraindicated in: ▪ Hypersensitivity or complete AV block.

Use Cautiously in: ▪ Glaucoma ▪ Depressed cardiac conduction ▪ Priapism ▪ Sickle cell disease ▪ Impaired liver function ▪ Severe coagulation defects ▪ Pregnancy, lactation, or children (safety not established).

ADVERSE REACTIONS AND SIDE EFFECTS*

CNS: depression, dizziness, vertigo, headache, drowsiness, sedation.
CV: arrhythmias (IV only), hypotension, slight hypertension.
Derm: flushing, sweating.
EENT: dry throat, visual changes.
GI: dry mouth, constipation, nausea, diarrhea, abdominal distress, anorexia, hepatitis.
GU: priapism (intracavernosal only).
Local: thrombosis at IV site.
Resp: APNEA (IV only).

INTERACTIONS

Drug-Drug: ▪ May prevent response to **levodopa** in patients with Parkinson's disease ▪ **Alpha-adrenergic agonists (metaraminol, epinephrine,** or **phenylephrine)** or **cigarette smoking** may reverse the vasodilating effects of papaverine.

ROUTE AND DOSAGE

- **PO (Adults):** 100–300 mg 3–5 times daily or 150 mg of extended-release formulation (Cerespan, Genabid, Pavabid, Pavacap, Pavacen, Pavagen, Pava Par, Pavarine, Pavased, Pavatine, Pavatym, Paverolan) q 8–12 hr or 300 mg of extended-release formulation q 12 hr.
- **IM, IV (Adults):** 30 mg initially, 30–120 mg may be repeated q 3 hr if necessary.
- **Intracavernosal (Adults):** 30 mg with 0.5–1 mg of phentolamine or 60 mg alone (not to exceed 60 mg/dose, not to be repeated more than 3 times/wk.

PHARMACODYNAMICS (PO, IM, IV = vasodilating effects, Intracavernosal = penile erection)

	ONSET	PEAK	DURATION
PO	UK	UK	4–8 hr
PO-ER	UK	UK	8–12 hr
IM	UK	UK	3 hr
IV	UK	UK	3 hr
Intracavernosal	10 min	UK	4 hr

NURSING IMPLICATIONS

Assessment

- ▫ Monitor blood pressure and pulse prior to and periodically throughout course of therapy.
- ▫ Monitor ECG in patients receiving IV papaverine. Withhold dose and notify physician if AV block is present.
- ▫ Monitor IV site for thrombosis (erythema, pain, edema).
- ▪ **Lab Test Considerations:** Monitor liver function studies. May cause elevated SGOT (AST), SGPT (ALT), alkaline phosphatase, and bilirubin levels. Notify physician of these symptoms of hepatic sensitivity. Eosinophils may also be elevated.

Potential Nursing Diagnoses

- ▪ Tissue perfusion, altered: (indications).
- ▪ Knowledge deficit related to medication regimen (patient/family teaching).

Implementation

- ▪ **PO:** Tablets may be administered with milk, meals, or antacids if nausea occurs.
- ▫ The oral form is available in regular and extended-release tablets. The extended-release form should not be crushed or chewed.
- ▪ **Direct IV:** Soln should be clear to light yellow. Do not refrigerate.
- ▫ *Rate:* Administer dose undiluted over at least 2 min. Rapid administration may cause hypotension, tachycardia, dizziness, and facial flushing.

*Underlines indicate most frequent; **CAPITALS** indicate life-threatening.

- **Syringe Compatibility:** phentolamine.
- **Solution/Additive Compatibility** 0.9% NaCl, 0.45% NaCl, D5W, D10W, D5/0.9% NaCl, D5/0.45% Nacl, D5/0.25% NaCl, Ringer's injection, or phentolamine.
- **Solution/Additive Incompatibility:** lactated Ringer's injection, aminophylline, alkaline solns, bromides, or iodides.
- **Impotence:** Has been used with phentolamine to treat men with impotence associated with spinal cord injury. This method requires special training. Produces an erection following injection into corpus cavernosum. Risk of priapism exists.

Patient/Family Teaching

- Instruct patient to take medication as ordered. If a dose is missed, patient should take dose as soon as remembered, but not if almost time for next dose. Do not double doses. Instruct patient not to discontinue medication without conferring with physician.
- Encourage patient not to smoke, as nicotine will cause vasoconstriction.
- May cause dizziness or drowsiness. Advise patient to avoid driving or other activities requiring alertness until response to medication is known.
- Caution patient to make position changes slowly to minimize orthostatic hypotension.
- Instruct patient to notify physician if dizziness, drowsiness, jaundice, or vision changes occur.
- Advise patients with a history of glaucoma to have regular eye examinations.

Evaluation

Effectiveness of therapy can be demonstrated by: ▪ Absence of symptoms of cerebral, peripheral, or myocardial ischemia ▪ Relief of ureteral, biliary, or GI colic ▪ Erection in men with impotence, beginning 10 min after injection into corpus cavernosum and sustained for up to 4 hr.

PAREGORIC

(par-e-**gor**-ik)
Camphorated opium tincture

CLASSIFICATION(S):
Antidiarrheal
Schedule III
Pregnancy Category UK

INDICATIONS

▪ Symptomatic treatment of diarrhea.

ACTION

▪ Morphine contained in paregoric inhibits normal GI peristalsis. **Therapeutic Effect:** ▪ Decreased frequency of bowel movements in patients with diarrhea.

PHARMACOKINETICS

Absorption: Variably absorbed from the GI tract.
Distribution: Distribution not known. Small amounts of morphine probably cross the placenta and enter breast milk.
Metabolism and Excretion: Morphine is metabolized by the liver.
Half-life: Morphine—2–3 hr.

CONTRAINDICATIONS AND PRECAUTIONS

Contraindicated in: ▪ Hypersensitivity ▪ Severe undiagnosed abdominal pain, especially when accompanied by fever.
Use Cautiously in: ▪ Asthma ▪ Severe prostatic hypertrophy ▪ Severe liver disease ▪ History of drug dependence (prolonged use may result in physical dependence).

ADVERSE REACTIONS AND SIDE EFFECTS*

CNS: drowsiness, dizziness, lightheadedness (high dose).
CV: hypotension (high dose).
GI: constipation.
GU: urinary retention.

INTERACTIONS

Drug-Drug: ▪ Additive CNS depression with other **CNS depressants,**

*Underlines indicate most frequent; **CAPITALS** indicate life-threatening.

including **alcohol, antihistamines, narcotic analgesics,** and **sedative/hypnotics**.

ROUTE AND DOSAGE

Note: Contains 2 mg anhydrous morphine/5 ml.

- **PO (Adults):** 5–10 ml 1–4 times daily.
- **PO (Children):** 0.25–0.5 ml/kg 1–4 times daily.

PHARMACODYNAMICS (antidiarrheal effects)

	ONSET	PEAK	DURATION
PO	1–2 hr	2–4 hr	4–6 hr

NURSING IMPLICATIONS

Assessment

- Assess frequency and consistency of stools and bowel sounds prior to and throughout course of therapy.
- Assess fluid and electrolyte balance and skin turgor for dehydration.
- Monitor respiratory rate, especially in infants and elderly and severely ill patients, as respiratory depression may occur.
- **Lab Test Considerations:** May cause elevations in serum amylase and lipase levels.

Potential Nursing Diagnoses

- Bowel elimination, altered: diarrhea (indications).
- Injury, high risk for (side effects).
- Knowledge deficit related to medication regimen (patient/family teaching).

Implementation

- **General Info:** The effect of 4 ml of paregoric is similar to that of 2.5 mg of diphenoxylate.
- Do not confuse with deodorized opium tincture, which is 25 times more potent.
- **PO:** Administer with food or meals if GI irritation occurs. Shake well. Mix with enough water to facilitate passage to stomach. Mixture will be milky in appearance. Do not refrigerate.

Patient/Family Teaching

- Instruct patient to take medication exactly as directed. If a dose is missed, it should be taken as soon as remembered unless almost time for next dose. Dosage may need to be gradually reduced after prolonged therapy to prevent withdrawal symptoms (tachycardia, irritability, tremors, difficulty sleeping, diaphoresis, shivering, stomach cramps, nausea, or vomiting). Physical or psychological dependence may occur.
- Caution patient to make position changes slowly to minimize orthostatic hypotension.
- Paregoric may cause drowsiness in large doses. Advise patient to avoid driving or other activities requiring alertness until response to drug is known.
- Caution patient to avoid using alcohol and other CNS depressants concurrently with this medication.
- Instruct patient to notify physician if diarrhea persists or if fever occurs.

Evaluation

Effectiveness of therapy can be demonstrated by: ▪ Decrease in diarrhea ▫ Return to normal bowel habits.

PEMOLINE

(**pem**-oh-leen)
Cylert

CLASSIFICATION(S):
CNS stimulant
Schedule IV
Pregnancy Category B

INDICATIONS

▪ Adjunct in the managment of attention deficit disorder (ADD) in children >6 yr. **Unlabeled Uses:** ▪ Treatment of fatigue or mental depression ▪ Schizophrenia ▪ As a stimulant in geriatric patients.

ACTION

▪ Produces CNS stimulation, which may be mediated by dopamine ▪ Causes increased motor activity and mental alertness, decreased fatigue, mild euphoria, and decreased appetite. **Therapeutic Effect:** ▪ Increased attention span in children with attention deficit disorder.

PHARMACOKINETICS

Absorption: Absorbed from the GI tract.
Distribution: Distribution not known.
Metabolism and Excretion: Partially (50%) metabolized by the liver. 40% excreted unchanged by the kidneys.
Half-life: 9–14 hr.

CONTRAINDICATIONS AND PRECAUTIONS

Contraindicated in: ▪ Hypersensitivity ▪ Liver disease.
Use Cautiously in: ▪ Renal impairment ▪ Pregnancy or lactation (safety not established) ▪ Unstable emotional status or psychoses ▪ History of seizure disorders ▪ Tics.

ADVERSE REACTIONS AND SIDE EFFECTS*

CNS: insomnia, SEIZURES, dyskinetic movements, dizziness, headache, depression, irritability, nervousness (large doses).
CV: tachycardia (large doses).
GI: anorexia, hepatitis.
Derm: rash, sweating.
Metab: weight loss.
Misc: fever.

INTERACTIONS

Drug-Drug: ▪ May have additive CNS stimulation with other **CNS stimulants** or **adrenergics**, including **decongestants**.

ROUTE AND DOSAGE

- **PO (Children >6 yr):** 37.5 mg initially as single morning dose, may be increased 18.75 mg at weekly intervals until optimum response is achieved. Usual maintenance dose is 56.25–75 mg/day.

PHARMACODYNAMICS (ADD = effects in attention deficit disorder)

	ONSET	PEAK	DURATION
PO (ADD)	days–wks	2–3 wk	days
PO (CNS stimulation)	UK	4 hr	8 hr

NURSING IMPLICATIONS

Assessment

- Assess attention span, impulse control, and interactions with others in children with attention deficit disorders. Therapy may be interrupted at intervals to determine if symptoms are sufficient to continue therapy.
- Monitor growth, both height and weight, in children on long-term therapy. Inform physician if growth inhibition occurs.
- **Lab Test Considerations:** Hepatic function should be monitored prior to and periodically throughout course of therapy. May cause elevated LDH, alkaline phosphatase, SGOT (AST), and SGPT (ALT) levels.

Potential Nursing Diagnoses

- Sleep pattern disturbance (side effects).
- Knowledge deficit related to medication regimen (patient/family teaching).

Implementation

- **General Info:** Administer daily dose in the morning. Chewable tablets must be chewed well before swallowing.

Patient/Family Teaching

- **General Info:** Instruct patient to take medication in morning to avoid sleep disturbances. If a dose is missed, take as soon as remembered; if remembered the next day, omit and continue on dosage schedule. Do not double doses. Pemoline has a high dependence and abuse potential. Tolerance occurs rapidly; do not increase dose. Consult physician before discontinu-

*Underlines indicate most frequent; **CAPITALS** indicate life-threatening.

ing. In long-term therapy, dosage should be reduced gradually to prevent withdrawal symptoms. Abrupt cessation of high doses may cause extreme fatigue and mental depression.

- Pemoline may cause dizziness. Caution patient to avoid driving or other activities requiring alertness until response to medication is known.
- Advise patient to avoid intake of large amounts of caffeine.
- Advise patient to notify physician if yellow skin or sclera, pale stools or dark urine, palpitations, sweating, fever, or uncontrolled tremors develop or if nervousness, restlessness, insomnia, dizziness, or anorexia becomes severe.
- Inform patient that physician may order periodic holidays from the drug to assess progress and to decrease dependence.
- Emphasize the importance of routine follow-up examinations to monitor progress.
- **Attention Deficit Disorder:** Advise parents to notify school nurse of medication regimen.

EVALUATION

Effectiveness of therapy can be demonstrated by: ▪ Calming effect with decreased hyperactivity and prolonged attention span in children with an attention deficit disorder. Significant beneficial effects may not be evident until the third or fourth wk of therapy, because clinical improvement is gradual.

PENBUTOLOL

(pen-**byoo**-toe-lole)
Levatol

CLASSIFICATION(S):
Antihypertensive, Beta-adrenergic blocker—nonselective
Pregnancy Category C

INDICATIONS

▪ Alone or with other agents in the treatment of hypertension.

ACTION

▪ Blocks stimulation of $beta_1$ (myocardial) and $beta_2$ (pulmonary, vascular, or uterine) receptor sites. Has minor intrinsic sympathomimetic activity (ISA), which may result in less bradycardia. **Therapeutic Effects:** ▪ Decreased heart rate ▪ Decreased blood pressure.

PHARMACOKINETICS

Absorption: Well absorbed following oral administration.
Distribution: Distribution not known.
Metabolism and Excretion: Mostly metabolized by the liver.
Half-life: 5 hr.

CONTRAINDICATIONS AND PRECAUTIONS

Contraindicated in: ▪ Uncompensated congestive heart failure ▪ Pulmonary edema ▪ Cardiogenic shock ▪ Bradycardia ▪ Heart block ▪ COPD or asthma.
Use Cautiously in: ▪ Thyroxicosis or hypoglycemia (may mask symptoms) ▪ Liver disease ▪ Pregnancy or lactation (may cause apnea, low Apgar scores, bradycardia, and hypoglycemia in the newborn) ▪ Children (safety not established).

ADVERSE REACTIONS AND SIDE EFFECTS*

CNS: fatigue, weakness, depression, memory loss, mental change.
EENT: dry eyes, blurred vision, nasal stuffiness.
Resp: bronchospasm, wheezing.
CV: BRADYCARDIA, CONGESTIVE HEART FAILURE, PULMONARY EDEMA, hypotension, peripheral vasoconstriction.
GI: constipation, diarrhea, nausea, vomiting.
GU: impotence, diminished libido.
Derm: rash, itching.
Endo: hyperglycemia, hypoglycemia.
Misc: Raynaud's phenomenon.

*Underlines indicate most frequent; **CAPITALS** indicate life-threatening.

INTERACTIONS

Drug–Drug: ▪ **General anesthesia,** IV **phenytoin,** or **verpamil** may cause additive myocardial depression ▪ Concurrent use with **amphetamines, cocaine, ephedrine, norepinephrine, phenylephrine,** or **pseudoephedrine** may result in excess alpha-adrenergic stimulation, hypertension, and bradycardia ▪ Additive bradycardia may occur with concurrent use of **cardiac glycosides** ▪ Additive hypotension may occur with other **antihypertensive agents,** acute ingestion of **alcohol,** and **nitrates** ▪ Concurrent **thyroid** administration may decrease effectiveness ▪ May antagonize **beta-adrenergic bronchodilators** ▪ **Nonsteroidal anti-inflammatory agents** may decrease antihypertensive effectiveness ▪ May prolong **insulin**-induced hypoglycemia ▪ May negate the beneficial $beta_1$ cardiac effects of **dopamine** or **dobutamine** ▪ May produce hypertension within 14 days of **MAO inhibitor** therapy.

ROUTE AND DOSAGE

- **PO (Adults):** Usual dose—20 mg/day (not to exceed 80 mg/day).

PHARMACODYNAMICS (full antihypertensive effect)

	ONSET	PEAK	DURATION
PO	UK	2–6 wk	UK

NURSING IMPLICATIONS

Assessment

- Monitor blood pressure and pulse frequently during period of adjustment and periodically throughout therapy. Confer with physician prior to giving drug if pulse is <50 bpm.
- Monitor intake and output ratios and daily weight. Assess patient routinely for evidence of fluid overload (peripheral edema, dyspnea, rales/crackles, fatigue, weight gain, jugular venous distension).

Potential Nursing Diagnoses

- Cardiac output, decreased (indications, adverse reactions).
- Knowledge deficit related to medication regimen (patient/family teaching).
- Noncompliance (patient/family teaching).

Implementation

- **PO:** Administered as a single daily dose. Doses >20 mg do not usually increase effectiveness.

Patient/Family Teaching

- Instruct patient to take medication exactly as directed, even if feeling well. If a dose is missed, it may be taken as soon as remembered up to 4 hr before next dose. Abrupt withdrawal may result in life-threatening arrhythmias, hypertension, or myocardial ischemia.
- Teach patient and family how to check pulse and blood pressure. Instruct them to take pulse daily and blood pressure biweekly. Advise patient to withhold dose and contact physician if pulse is <50 bpm or blood pressure changes significantly.
- Reinforce need to continue additional therapies for hypertension (weight loss, restricted sodium intake, stress reduction, regular exercise, moderation of alcohol consumption, and cessation of smoking). Penbutolol controls but does not cure hypertension.
- Caution patient that this medication may cause increased sensitivity to cold.
- Advise patient to consult physician before taking any over-the-counter drugs, especially cold remedies, concurrently with this medication. Patients on antihypertensive therapy should also avoid excessive amounts of coffee, tea, and cola.
- Instruct patient to inform physician or dentist of this therapy prior to treatment or surgery.
- Advise patient to carry identification describing medication regimen at all times.
- Instruct patient to notify physician if slow pulse rate, depression, or skin rash occurs.

P

Evaluation

Effectiveness of therapy can be demonstrated by: ▪ Decrease in blood pressure. Maximum antihypertensive effects of the 20-mg or 40-mg/day dose are usually seen by the end of second wk. Full effects of lower doses may not be seen for 4–6 wk.

PENICILLAMINE
(pen-i-**sill**-a-meen)
Cuprimine, Depen

CLASSIFICATION(S):
Anti-inflammatory agent, Chelating agent, Antiurolithic
Pregnancy Category UK

INDICATIONS

▪ Treatment of progressive rheumatoid arthritis resistant to conventional therapy ▪ Prophylaxis and treatment of copper deposition in Wilson's disease ▪ Management of recurrent cystine calculi. **Unlabeled Use:** ▪ Adjunct in the treatment of heavy metal poisoning.

ACTION

▪ Antirheumatic effect, probably due to enhanced lymphocyte function ▪ Chelates heavy metals, including copper, mercury, lead, and iron, into complexes that are excreted by the kidneys ▪ Forms a soluble complex with cystine that is readily excreted by the kidneys. **Therapeutic Effects:** ▪ Decreased disease progression in rheumatoid arthritis ▪ Decreased copper deposition in Wilson's disease ▪ Decreased cystine renal calculi formation.

PHARMACOKINETICS

Absorption: Well absorbed following oral administration.
Distribution: Crosses the placenta.
Metabolism and Excretion: Some excreted in urine as heavy metal-penicillamine complex, some excreted in urine as cystine-penicillamine complex, some metabolized by the liver.
Half-life: UK.

CONTRAINDICATIONS AND PRECAUTIONS

Contraindicated in: ▪ Hypersensitivity ▪ Cross-sensitivity with penicillin may exist.

Use Cautiously in: ▪ Elderly patients (increased risk of hematologic toxicity; dosage reduction recommended) ▪ Renal impairment (increased risk of adverse renal reactions in patients with rheumatoid arthritis) ▪ Pregnancy (limit daily dose to <1 g. If cesarean section is planned, decrease daily dose to 250 mg for last 6 wk of pregnancy and until incision is healed) ▪ History of aplastic anemia due to penicillamine ▪ Lactation (safety not established) ▪ Patients requiring surgery (may impair wound healing).

ADVERSE REACTIONS AND SIDE EFFECTS*

EENT: eye pain, blurred vision.
Resp: coughing, wheezing, shortness of breath.
GI: oral ulceration, anorexia, nausea, vomiting, epigastric pain, dyspepsia, diarrhea, decreased taste sensation, hepatic dysfunction, cholestatic jaundice, pancreatitis.
GU: proteinuria.
Derm: pemphigus, rashes, hives, itching, ecchymoses, wrinkling.
Hemat: APLASTIC ANEMIA, leukopenia, thrombocytopenia, eosinophilia, thrombocytosis, anemia.
MS: arthralgia, migratory polyarthritis.
Neuro: myasthenia gravis syndrome.
Misc: allergic reactions, fever, lymphadenopathy, systemic lupus erythematosus-like syndrome, GOODPASTURE'S SYNDROME (glomerulonephritis and intra-alveolar hemorrhage).

INTERACTIONS

Drug-Drug: ▪ Increased risk of adverse hematologic effects with **antineoplastic agents, immunosuppresive**

*Underlines indicate most frequent; **CAPITALS** indicate life-threatening.

agents, or **gold salts** ▪ Concurrent administration of **iron supplements** may decrease absorption of penicillamine.

Drug–Food: ▪ May increase requirements for **pyridoxine** (vitamin B_6).

ROUTE AND DOSAGE

Antirheumatic

- **PO (Adults):** 125–250 mg/day as a single dose. May be slowly increased up to 1.5 g/day.

Chelating Agent (Wilson's Disease)

- **PO (Adults and Older Children):** 250 mg qid.
- **PO (Children >6 mon):** 250 mg/day as a single dose.

Antiurolithic

- **PO (Adults):** 500 mg qid.
- **PO (Children):** 7.5 mg/kg qid.

PHARMACODYNAMICS

	ONSET	PEAK	DURATION
PO (antirheumatic)	1–3 mon	UK	1–3 mon
PO (Wilson's disease)	1–3 mon	UK	UK

NURSING IMPLICATIONS

Assessment

- **General Info:** Monitor intake and output and daily weight and assess patient for edema throughout therapy. Notify physician if edema or weight gain occurs.
- **Arthritis:** Assess pain and range of motion periodically throughout course of therapy.
- **Cystinuria:** X-ray examinations for renal calculi should be monitored annually for stone formation.
- **Lab Test Considerations:** Monitor CBC with differential, platelet counts, and urinalysis (especially for protein and cells) at least every 2 wk during the first 6 mon of therapy or following dose increases, and monthly thereafter. May cause leukopenia, anemia, and thrombocytopenia.
  - ▫ Monitor liver function tests every 6 mon during the first 18 mon of therapy.
  - ▫ *Arthritis:* Monitor 24-hr urinary protein levels every 1–2 wk in patients with moderate proteinuria.
  - ▫ *Wilson's Disease:* Monitor urinary copper levels prior to and soon after initiation of therapy and every 3 mon during continued therapy.
  - ▫ *Cystinuria:* Monitor urinary cystine levels. Urinary cystine excretion should be maintained at <100 mg in patients with a history of pain or calculi, or 100–200 mg in patients without a history of calculi.

Potential Nursing Diagnoses

- Comfort, altered: pain (indications).
- Knowledge deficit related to medication regimen (patient/family teaching).

Implementation

- **PO:** Administer on an empty stomach, at least 1 hr before or 2 hr after meals. Other medications should be administered at least 1 hr apart from penicillamine to maximize absorption.
  - ▫ Do not administer concurrently with iron-containing products.
  - ▫ Penicillamine increases the daily requirements for pyridoxine. Supplemental doses of pyridoxine 25 mg/day (vitamin B_6) may be ordered in patients with impaired nutrition.
- **Arthritis:** Dosage adjustments may be required every 2–3 mon during therapy.
  - ▫ If no improvement is seen after 3–4 mon of therapy with doses of 1–1.5 g daily, medication should be discontinued.
- **Wilson's Disease:** Sulfurated potash (10–40 mg) may be administered with meals to minimize copper absorption.

Patient/Family Teaching

- **General Info:** Instruct patient to take penicillamine exactly as directed. If on once-daily schedule, missed doses should be taken as soon as remembered unless remembered the next day; if on twice-daily schedule, take missed doses as soon as remembered unless almost time for next dose; if on more than twice-daily dosing schedule, take missed doses within 1 hr or omit. Do not double doses.

- □ Consult physician prior to discontinuation of therapy, as interruption of therapy may cause sensitivity reactions when therapy is resumed. Therapy should be resumed starting with smaller dose and increasing gradually.
- □ Inform patient that penicillamine may alter taste acuity, which may be restored by administration of copper 5–10 mg daily. Cupric sulfate 4% soln 5–10 drops may be mixed in fruit juice and taken bid. This is contraindicated in patients with Wilson's disease.
- □ Advise patient to notify physician or dentist of medication regimen prior to surgery or treatment. Dose of penicillamine should be reduced until wound healing is complete.
- □ Instruct patient to notify physician if skin rash, unusual bleeding or bruising, sore throat, exertional dyspnea, unexplained coughing or wheezing, fever, chills, or any unusual effects occur.
- □ Emphasize the importance of follow-up examinations to check progress.
- ▪ **Wilson's Disease:** Advise patient to discuss dietary restrictions with physician. A low-copper diet may be required. Chocolate, nuts, shellfish, mushrooms, liver, molasses, broccoli, and cereals enriched with copper should be avoided. If drinking water contains >100 mcg/liter of copper, distilled or demineralized water should be used.
- ▪ **Crystinuria:** Advise patient to maintain a fluid intake of at least 2000–3000 ml/day, with increased fluids at night.
- □ Advise patient to discuss dietary restrictions with physician. Low-methionine diet may be required to minimize cystine production but is contraindicated in growing children or pregnancy due to low protein content.

Evaluation

Effectiveness of therapy can be demonstrated by: ▪ Decreased pain and increased range of motion in patients with rheumatoid arthritis ▪ Prevention and treatment of symptoms of Wilson's disease ▪ Prevention and treatment of renal calculi in patients with excessive urinary cystine levels.

PENICILLIN G BENZATHINE

(pen-i-**sill**-in jee **ben**-za-theen)
Bicillin, Bicillin L-A, Permapen

CLASSIFICATION(S):
Anti-infective—penicillin
Pregnancy Category B

INDICATIONS

▪ Treatment of a wide variety of infections, including: □ Pneumococcal pneumonia □ Streptococcal pharyngitis □ Syphilis ▪ Prevention of rheumatic fever.

ACTION

▪ Binds to bacterial cell wall, resulting in cell death. **Therapeutic Effect:** ▪ Bactericidal action against susceptible bacteria. **Spectrum:** ▪ Active against most gram-positive organisms, including: □ Streptococci (*Streptococcus pneumoniae,* group A beta-hemolytic streptococci) □ Staphylococci (non-penicillinase-producing strains) □ Some gram-negative organisms, such as *Neisseria meningitis* and *Neisseria gonorrheae* □ Some anaerobic bacteria and spirochetes.

PHARMACOKINETICS

Absorption: IM absorption is delayed and prolonged, resulting in sustained therapeutic blood levels.
Distribution: Widely distributed, although CNS penetration is poor in the presence of uninflamed meninges. Crosses the placenta and enters breast milk.

Metabolism and Excretion: Minimally metabolized by the liver, excreted mainly unchanged by the kidneys.
Half-life: 30–60 min.

CONTRAINDICATIONS AND PRECAUTIONS

Contraindicated in: ▪ Previous hypersensitivity to penicillins ▪ Cross-sensitivity may exist with cephalosporins ▪ Hypersensitivity to benzathine.
Use Cautiously in: ▪ Severe renal insufficiency (dosage reduction recommended) ▪ Pregnancy (although safety not established, has been used safely) ▪ Lactation.

ADVERSE REACTIONS AND SIDE EFFECTS*

CNS: SEIZURES.
GI: nausea, vomiting, diarrhea, epigastric distress.
GU: interstitial nephritis.
Derm: rashes, urticaria.
Hemat: eosinophilia, hemolytic anemia, leukopenia.
Local: pain at IM site.
Misc: superinfection, allergic reactions, including ANAPHYLAXIS and serum sickness.

INTERACTIONS

Drug-Drug: ▪ **Probenecid** decreases renal excretion and increases blood levels of penicillin. Therapy may be combined for this purpose ▪ Effectiveness of penicillin may be decreased by concurrent use of **chloramphenicol** ▪ Half-life of **chloramphenicol** may be increased by concurrent use of penicillin.

ROUTE AND DOSAGE

Note: 1 mg = 1600 units.

Streptococcal Infections

- **IM (Adults):** 1.2 million units single dose.
- **IM (Children >27 kg):** 900,000 units single dose.
- **IM (Children <27 kg):** 300,000–600,000 units single dose.

Syphilis

- **IM (Adults):** 2.4 million units single dose (primary, secondary, or latent syphilis); repeated q wk for 3 wk (tertiary or neurosyphilis).
- **IM (Children <2 yr):** 50,000 units/kg single dose (congenital syphilis).

Prevention of Rheumatic Fever

- **IM (Adults and Children):** 1.2 million units/mon or 600,000 units twice a mon.

PHARMACODYNAMICS (blood levels)

	ONSET	PEAK	DURATION
IM	delayed	12–24 hr	1–4 wk

NURSING IMPLICATIONS

Assessment

- ▫ Assess patient for infection (vital signs; appearance of wound, sputum, urine, and stool; WBC) at beginning and throughout course of therapy.
- ▫ Obtain a history before initiating therapy to determine previous use of and reactions to penicillins or cephalosporins. Persons with a negative history of penicillin sensitivity may still have an allergic response.
- ▫ Obtain specimens for culture and sensitivity prior to initiating therapy. First dose may be given before receiving results.
- ▫ Observe patient for signs and symptoms of anaphylaxis (rash, pruritus, laryngeal edema, wheezing). Discontinue drug and notify physician immediately if these occur. Keep epinephrine, an antihistamine, and resuscitation equipment close by in the event of an anaphylactic reaction.
- ▪ **Lab Test Considerations:** Patients receiving penicillin G may have false-positive results for urine glucose using the copper sulfate method (Clinitest). Use glucose oxidase method (Keto-Diastix, Tes-Tape) to test urine glucose.
- ▫ May cause positive direct Coombs' test results.

Potential Nursing Diagnoses

- ▪ Infection, high risk for (indications, side effects).

*Underlines indicate most frequent; **CAPITALS** indicate life-threatening.

P

- Knowledge deficit related to medication regimen (patient/family teaching).
- Noncompliance related to medication regimen (patient/family teaching).

Implementation

- **IM:** Reconstitute according to manufacturer's directions with sterile water for injection, D5W, or 0.9% NaCl.
  - Shake medication well prior to injection. Inject deep into a well-developed muscle mass at a slow, consistent rate to prevent blockage of the needle. Massage well. Accidental injection near or into a nerve can result in severe pain and dysfunction. Do not inject SC, as this may cause pain and induration.
  - Never give penicillin G benzathine suspension IV. May cause embolism or toxic reactions.

Patient/Family Teaching

- Advise patient to report the signs of superinfection (black, furry overgrowth on the tongue; vaginal itching or discharge; loose or foul-smelling stools) and allergy.
- Instruct patient to notify the physician if symptoms do not improve.
- Patients with an allergy to penicillin should be instructed to carry an identification card with this information at all times.

Evaluation

Clinical response to therapy can be evaluated by: ▪ Resolution of the signs and symptoms of infection. Length of time for complete resolution depends on the organism and site of infection.

PENICILLIN G POTASSIUM

(pen-i-**sill**-in jee poe-**tass**-ee um)
{Crystapen}, {Megacillin}, {Novapen-G}, {P-50}, Pentids, Pfizerpen, Pfizerpen G

CLASSIFICATION(S):
Anti-infective—penicillin
Pregnancy Category B

INDICATIONS

▪ Treatment of a wide variety of infections, including: □ Pneumococcal pneumonia □ Streptococcal pharyngitis □ Syphilis □ Gonorrhea □ Lyme disease ▪ Treatment of enterococcal infections (requires the addition of an aminoglycoside) ▪ Prevention of rheumatic fever.

ACTION

▪ Binds to bacterial cell wall, resulting in cell death. **Therapeutic Effect:** ▪ Bactericidal action against susceptible bacteria. **Spectrum:** ▪ Active against most gram-positive organisms, including: □ Streptococci (*Streptococcus pneumoniae,* group A beta-hemolytic streptococci) □ Staphylococci (non-penicillinase-producing strains) □ Some gram-negative organisms, such as *Neisseria meningitis* and *Neisseria gonorrheae* □ Some anaerobic bacteria and spirochetes (including *Treponema pallidum* and *Borrelia burgdorferi*).

PHARMACOKINETICS

Absorption: Variably absorbed from the GI tract due to acid lability. Well absorbed following IM administration.

Distribution: Widely distributed, although CNS penetration is poor in the presence of uninflamed meninges. Crosses the placenta and enters breast milk.

Metabolism and Excretion: Minimally metabolized by the liver, excreted mainly unchanged by the kidneys.

Half-life: 30–60 min.

CONTRAINDICATIONS AND PRECAUTIONS

Contraindicated in: ▪ Previous hypersensitivity to penicillins ▪ Cross-sensitivity with cephalosporins may exist ▪ Some products may contain tartrazine (Pentids)—avoid use in patients with tartrazine (FDC yellow dye #5) hypersensitivity.

Use Cautiously in: ▪ Severe renal insufficiency (dosage reduction recommended) ▪ Pregnancy (although safety

not established, has been used safely)
- Lactation.

ADVERSE REACTIONS AND SIDE EFFECTS*

CNS: SEIZURES.
GI: nausea, vomiting, diarrhea, epigastric distress.
GU: interstitial nephritis.
Derm: rashes, urticaria.
Hemat: eosinophilia, hemolytic anemia, leukopenia.
Local: phlebitis at IV site, pain at IM site.
Misc: superinfection, allergic reactions, including ANAPHYLAXIS and serum sickness.

INTERACTIONS

Drug-Drug: ▪ **Probenecid** decreases renal excretion and increases blood levels of penicillin. Therapy may be combined for this purpose ▪ **Cholestyramine** and **colestipol** may decrease the absorption of penicillin G ▪ Effectiveness of penicillin may be decreased by concurrent use of **chloramphenicol** ▪ Half-life of **chloramphenicol** may be increased by concurrent use of penicillin.
Drug-Food: ▪ **Food, acidic juices,** or **carbonated beverages** decrease absorption.

ROUTE AND DOSAGE

Note: 1 mg = 1600 units. Contains 1.7 mEq potassium and 0.3 mEq sodium/million units.

- **PO (Adults):** 200,000–500,000 units q 6–8 hr.
- **PO (Infants and Children <12 yr):** 25,000–90,000 units/kg/day in 3–6 divided doses (4167–15,000 units/kg q 4 hr; 6250–22,500 units/kg q 6 hr; or 8333–30,000 units/kg q 8 hr). Doses up to 400,000 units/kg/day have been used.
- **IM, IV (Adults):** 1 million–5 million units q 4–6 hr.
- **IM, IV (Children):** 4167–16,667 units/kg q 4 hr or 6250–25,000 units/kg q 6 hr.
- **IM, IV (Neonates):** 30,000 units/kg q 12 hr (up to 1 million units/day for Listeria infections).

PHARMACODYNAMICS (blood levels)

	ONSET	PEAK
PO	rapid	0.5–1 hr
IM	rapid	0.25–0.5 hr
IV	rapid	rapid

NURSING IMPLICATIONS

Assessment

- ▫ Assess patient for infection (vital signs; appearance of wound, sputum, urine, and stool; WBC) at beginning and throughout course of therapy.
- ▫ Obtain a history before initiating therapy to determine previous use of and reactions to penicillins or cephalosporins. Persons with a negative history of penicillin sensitivity may still have an allergic response.
- ▫ Obtain specimens for culture and sensitivity prior to initiating therapy. First dose may be given before receiving results.
- ▫ Observe patient for signs and symptoms of anaphylaxis (rash, pruritus, laryngeal edema, wheezing). Discontinue drug and notify physician immediately if these occur. Keep epinephrine, an antihistamine, and resuscitation equipment close by in the event of an anaphylactic reaction.
- ▪ **Lab Test Considerations:** Patients receiving penicillin G may have false-positive results for urine glucose using the copper sulfate method (Clinitest). Use glucose oxidase method (Keto-Diastix, Tes-Tape) to test urine glucose.
- ▫ May cause positive direct Coombs' test results.
- ▫ Hyperkalemia may develop following large doses of penicillin G potassium.

*Underlines indicate most frequent; **CAPITALS** indicate life-threatening.

P

Potential Nursing Diagnoses

- Infection, high risk for (indications, side effects).
- Knowledge deficit related to medication regimen (patient/family teaching).
- Noncompliance related to medication regimen (patient/family teaching).

Implementation

- **PO:** Administer around the clock. Penicillin G should be administered on an empty stomach, at least 1 hr before or 2 hr after meals. Acidic juices or carbonated beverages may decrease absorption of penicillin G potassium.
  - Use calibrated measuring device for liquid preparations. Soln is stable for 14 days if refrigerated.
- **IM/IV:** Reconstitute according to manufacturer's directions with sterile water for injection, D5W, or 0.9% NaCl.
- **IM:** Shake medication well prior to injection. Inject deep into a well-developed muscle mass at a slow, consistent rate to prevent blockage of the needle. Massage well. Accidental injection near or into a nerve can result in severe pain and dysfunction. Do not inject SC, as this may cause pain and induration.
  - Penicillin G potassium may be diluted with lidocaine 1% or 2% (without epinephrine) to minimize pain from IM injection.
- **IV:** Change sites every 48 hr to prevent phlebitis.
  - Administer IV form of penicillin slowly and observe patient closely for signs of hypersensitivity.
- **Intermittent Infusion:** Doses of 3 million units or less should be diluted in at least 50 ml; doses of more than 3 million units should be diluted with 100 ml of D5W, D10W, 0.45% NaCl, 0.9% NaCl, Ringer's or lactated Ringer's soln, dextrose/saline combinations, or dextrose/Ringer's or lactated Ringer's combinations.
  - *Rate:* Infuse over 1–2 hr in adults, 15–30 min in children.
- **Continuous Infusion:** May be diluted and infused over 24 hr.
- **Syringe Compatibility:** heparin.
- **Syringe Incompatibility:** metoclopramide.
- **Y-Site Compatibility:** acyclovir, cyclophosphamide, enalaprilat, esmolol, foscarnet, heparin with hydrocortisone sodium succinate, hydromorphone, labetalol, magnesium sulfate, meperidine, morphine, perphenazine, potassium chloride, or verapamil.
- **Additive Compatibility:** ascorbic acid, calcium chloride, calcium gluconate, cephapirin, chloramphenicol, cimetidine, clindamycin, colistimethate, corticotropin, dimenhydrinate, diphenhydramine, ephedrine, erythromycin, hydrocortisone sodium succinate, kanamycin, lidocaine, magnesium sulfate, methicillin, methylprednisolone sodium succinate, polymyxin B, prednisolone sodium phosphate, potassium chloride, procaine, prochlorperazine edisylate, sodium iodide, or verapamil.
- **Additive Incompatibility:** aminophylline, amphotericin B, chlorpromazine, dopamine, hydroxyzine, metaraminol, oxytetracycline, pentobarbital, prochlorperazine mesylate, promazine, tetracycline, or thiopental. Incompatible with aminoglycosides; do not admix.

Patient/Family Teaching

- Instruct patient to take medication around the clock and to finish the drug completely as directed, even if feeling better. Advise patient that sharing of this medication may be dangerous.
- Advise patient to report the signs of superinfection (black, furry overgrowth on the tongue; vaginal itching or discharge; loose or foul-smelling stools) and allergy.
- Instruct the patient to notify physician if symptoms do not improve.
- Patients with an allergy to penicillin should be instructed to carry an iden-

tification card with this information at all times.

Evaluation

Clinical response to therapy can be evaluated by: ▪ Resolution of the signs and symptoms of infection. Length of time for complete resolution depends on the organism and site of infection.

PENICILLIN G PROCAINE

(pen-i-**sill**-in jee **proe**-cane)
{Ayercillin}, Crysticillin, Duracillin A.S., Pfizerpen-AS, Wycillin

CLASSIFICATION(S):
Anti-infective—penicillin
Pregnancy Category B

INDICATIONS

▪ Treatment of a wide variety of infections, including: ▫ Pneumococcal pneumonia ▫ Streptococcal pharyngitis ▫ Syphilis ▫ Gonorrhea ▪ Treatment of enterococcal infections (requires the addition of an aminoglycoside).

ACTION

▪ Binds to bacterial cell wall, resulting in cell death. **Therapeutic Effect:** ▪ Bactericidal action against susceptible bacteria. **Spectrum:** ▪ Active against most gram-positive organisms, including: ▫ Streptococci (*Streptococcus pneumoniae,* group A beta-hemolytic streptococci) ▫ Staphylococci (non-penicillinase-producing strains) ▫ Some gram-negative organisms, such as *Neisseria meningitis* and *Neisseria gonorrheae* ▫ Some anaerobic bacteria and spirochetes.

PHARMACOKINETICS

Absorption: IM absorption is delayed and prolonged, resulting in sustained therapeutic blood levels.

Distribution: Widely distributed, although CNS penetration is poor in the presence of uninflamed meninges. Crosses the placenta and enters breast milk.

Metabolism and Excretion: Minimally metabolized by the liver, excreted mainly unchanged by the kidneys.

Half-life: 30–60 min.

CONTRAINDICATIONS AND PRECAUTIONS

Contraindicated in: ▪ Previous hypersensitivity to penicillins ▪ Cross-sensitivity with cephalosporins may exist ▪ Hypersensitivity to procaine.

Use Cautiously in: ▪ Severe renal insufficiency (dosage reduction recommended) ▪ Pregnancy (although safety not established, has been used safely) ▪ Lactation.

ADVERSE REACTIONS AND SIDE EFFECTS*

CNS: SEIZURES.

GI: <u>nausea</u>, <u>vomiting</u>, <u>diarrhea</u>, <u>epigastric distress</u>.

GU: interstitial nephritis.

Derm: <u>rashes</u>, urticaria.

Hemat: eosinophilia, hemolytic anemia, leukopenia.

Local: <u>pain</u> at IM site.

Misc: superinfection, allergic reactions, including ANAPHYLAXIS and serum sickness.

INTERACTIONS

Drug-Drug: ▪ **Probenecid** decreases renal excretion and increases blood levels of penicillin. Therapy may be combined for this purpose ▪ Effectiveness of penicillin may be decreased by concurrent use of **chloramphenicol** ▪ Half-life of **chloramphenicol** may be increased by concurrent use of penicillin.

ROUTE AND DOSAGE

Note: 1 mg = 1600 units.

Moderate to Severe Infections

- **IM (Adults):** 600,000–1.2 million units/day, single dose.
- **IM (Children):** 300,000 units/day, single dose.

{} = Available in Canada only.
*<u>Underlines</u> indicate most frequent; **CAPITALS** indicate life-threatening.

P

Uncomplicated Gonorrhea

- **IM (Adults):** 4.8 million units divided into 2 injection sites, preceded by 1 g probenecid PO.

PHARMACODYNAMICS (blood levels)

	ONSET	PEAK	DURATION
IM	delayed	1–4 hr	1–2 days

NURSING IMPLICATIONS

Assessment

- Assess patient for infection (vital signs; appearance of wound, sputum, urine, and stool; WBC) at beginning and throughout course of therapy.
- Obtain a history before initiating therapy to determine previous use of and reactions to penicillins or cephalosporins. Persons with a negative history of penicillin sensitivity may still have an allergic response.
- Obtain specimens for culture and sensitivity prior to initiating therapy. First dose may be given before receiving results.
- Observe patient for signs and symptoms of anaphylaxis (rash, pruritus, laryngeal edema, wheezing). Discontinue drug and notify physician immediately if these occur. Keep epinephrine, an antihistamine, and resuscitation equipment close by in the event of an anaphylactic reaction.
- **Lab Test Considerations:** Patients receiving penicillin G may have false-positive results for urine glucose using the copper sulfate method (Clinitest). Use glucose oxidase method (Keto-Diastix, Tes-Tape) to test urine glucose.
- May cause positive direct Coombs' test results.

Potential Nursing Diagnoses

- Infection, high risk for (indications, side effects).
- Knowledge deficit related to medication regimen (patient/family teaching).

Implementation

- **IM:** Reconstitute according to manufacturer's directions with sterile water for injection, D5W, or 0.9% NaCl.
- Shake medication well prior to injection. Inject deep into a well-developed muscle mass at a slow, consistent rate to prevent blockage of the needle. Massage well. Accidental injection near or into a nerve can result in severe pain and dysfunction.
- Patient may experience a transient toxic reaction to procaine (anxiety, confusion, agitation, combativeness, depression, seizures, hallucinations, expressed fear of impending death).
- Never give penicillin G procaine suspension IV. May cause embolism or toxic reactions.

Patient/Family Teaching

- Advise patient to report the signs of superinfection (black, furry overgrowth on the tongue; vaginal itching or discharge; loose or foul-smelling stools) and allergy.
- Instruct patient to notify physician if symptoms do not improve.
- Patients with an allergy to penicillin should be instructed to carry an identification card with this information at all times.

Evaluation

Clinical response to therapy can be evaluated by: ▪ Resolution of the signs and symptoms of infection. Length of time for complete resolution depends on the organism and site of infection.

PENICILLIN G SODIUM

(pen-i-**sill**-in jee **soe**-dee-um)
{Crystapen}

CLASSIFICATION(S):
Anti-infective—penicillin
Pregnancy Category B

INDICATIONS

- Treatment of a wide variety of infections, including: ▫ Pneumococcal pneumonia ▫ Streptococcal pharyngitis

{} = Available in Canada only.

□ Syphilis □ Gonorrhea ▪ Treatment of enterococcal infections (requires the addition of an aminoglycoside) ▪ Prevention of rheumatic fever.

ACTION

▪ Binds to bacterial cell wall, resulting in cell death. **Therapeutic Effect:** ▪ Bactericidal action against susceptible bacteria. **Spectrum:** ▪ Active against most gram-positive organisms, including: □ Streptococci (*Streptococcus pneumoniae,* group A beta-hemolytic streptococci) □ Staphylococci (non-penicillinase-producing strains) □ Some gram-negative organisms, such as *Neisseria meningitis* and *Neisseria gonorrheae* □ Some anaerobic bacteria and spirochetes.

PHARMACOKINETICS

Absorption: Well absorbed following IM administration.
Distribution: Widely distributed, although CNS penetration is poor in the presence of uninflamed meninges. Crosses the placenta and enters breast milk.
Metabolism and Excretion: Minimally metabolized by the liver, excreted mainly unchanged by the kidneys.
Half-life: 30–60 min.

CONTRAINDICATIONS AND PRECAUTIONS

Contraindicated in: ▪ Previous hypersensitivity to penicillins ▪ Cross-sensitivity with cephalosporins may exist.
Use Cautiously in: ▪ Severe renal insufficiency (dosage reduction recommended) ▪ Pregnancy (although safety not established, has been used safely) ▪ Lactation.

ADVERSE REACTIONS AND SIDE EFFECTS*

CNS: SEIZURES.
GI: nausea, vomiting, diarrhea, epigastric distress.
GU: interstitial nephritis.
Derm: rashes, urticaria.
Hemat: eosinophilia, hemolytic anemia, leukopenia.
Local: phlebitis at IV site, pain at IM site.
Misc: superinfection, allergic reactions, including ANAPHYLAXIS and serum sickness.

INTERACTIONS

Drug-Drug: ▪ May decrease the effectiveness of **oral contraceptive agents** ▪ **Probenecid** decreases renal excretion and increases blood levels of penicillin. Therapy may be combined for this purpose ▪ **Cholestyramine** and **colestipol** may decrease the absorption of penicillin G ▪ Effectiveness of penicillin may be decreased by concurrent **chloramphenicol** ▪ Half-life of **chloramphenicol** may be increased by concurrent penicillin.

ROUTE AND DOSAGE

Note: 1 mg = 1600 units. Contains 2 mEq sodium/million units.

- **IM, IV (Adults):** 1 million–5 million units q 4–6 hr (up to 40 million units/day).
- **IM, IV (Children):** 4167–16,667 units/kg q 4 hr or 6250–25,000 units/kg q 6 hr (up to 400,000 units/kg/day).
- **IM, IV (Neonates):** 30,000 units/kg q 12 hr (50,000–150,000 units/kg/day; up to 1 million units/day for Listeria infections).

PHARMACODYNAMICS (blood levels)

	ONSET	PEAK
IM	rapid	0.25–0.5 hr
IV	rapid	rapid

NURSING IMPLICATIONS

ASSESSMENT

□ Assess patient for infection (vital signs; appearance of wound, sputum, urine, and stool; WBC) at beginning and throughout course of therapy.
□ Obtain a history before initiating therapy to determine previous use of and

*Underlines indicate most frequent; **CAPITALS** indicate life-threatening.

reactions to penicillins or cephalosporins. Persons with a negative history of penicillin sensitivity may still have an allergic response.

- ▫ Obtain specimens for culture and sensitivity prior to initiating therapy. First dose may be given before receiving results.
- ▫ Observe patient for signs and symptoms of anaphylaxis (rash, pruritus, laryngeal edema, wheezing). Discontinue drug and notify physician immediately if these occur. Keep epinephrine, an antihistamine, and resuscitation equipment close by in the event of an anaphylactic reaction.
- ▪ **Lab Test Considerations:** Patients receiving penicillin G may have false-positive results for urine glucose using the copper sulfate method (Clinitest). Use glucose oxidase method (Keto-Diastix, Tes-Tape) to test urine glucose.
- ▫ May cause positive direct Coombs' test results.
- ▫ Monitor sodium concentrations in patients with hypertension or congestive heart failure. Hypernatremia may develop following large doses of penicillin G sodium.

Potential Nursing Diagnoses

- ▪ Infection, high risk for (indications, side effects).
- ▪ Knowledge deficit related to medication regimen (patient/family teaching).

Implementation

- ▪ **IM/IV:** Reconstitute according to manufacturer's directions with sterile water for injection, D5W, or 0.9% NaCl.
- ▪ **IM:** Shake medication well prior to injection. Inject penicillin deep into a well-developed muscle mass at a slow, consistent rate to prevent blockage of the needle. Massage well. Accidental injection near or into a nerve can result in severe pain and dysfunction. Do not inject SC, as this may cause pain and induration.
- ▫ Penicillin G sodium may be diluted with lidocaine 1% or 2% (without epinephrine) to minimize pain from IM injection.
- ▪ **IV:** Change sites every 48 hr to prevent phlebitis.
- ▫ Administer slowly and observe patient closely for signs of hypersensitivity.
- ▪ **Intermittent Infusion:** Doses of 3 million units or less should be diluted with at least 50 ml; doses of >3 million units should be diluted with 100 ml of D5W or 0.9% NaCl.
- ▫ *Rate:* Infuse over 1–2 hr in adults, 15–30 min in children.
- ▪ **Continuous Infusion:** May be diluted and infused over 24 hr.
- ▪ **Syringe Compatibility:** chloramphenicol, cimetidine, colistimethate, heparin, lincomycin, or polymyxin B.
- ▪ **Syringe Incompatibility:** oxytetracycline or tetracycline.
- ▪ **Additive Compatibility:** calcium chloride, calcium gluconate, chloramphenicol, clindamycin, colistimethate, diphenhydramine, erythromycin lactobionate, hydrocortisone sodium succinate, methicillin, polymyxin B, prednisolone sodium phosphate, procaine, ranitidine, or verapamil.
- ▪ **Additive Incompatibility:** amphotericin B, bleomycin, cephalothin, chlorpromazine, cytarabine, hydroxyzine, methylprednisolone sodium succinate, oxytetracycline, prochlorperazine mesylate, or promethazine. Incompatible with aminoglycosides; do not admix.

Patient/Family Teaching

- ▫ Advise patient to report the signs of superinfection (black, furry overgrowth on the tongue; vaginal itching or discharge; loose or foul-smelling stools) and allergy.
- ▫ Instruct patient to notify physician if symptoms do not improve.
- ▫ Patients with an allergy to penicillin should be instructed to carry an identification card with this information at all times.

EVALUATION

Clinical response to therapy can be evaluated by: ▪ Resolution of the signs and symptoms of infection. Length of time for complete resolution depends on the organism and site of infection.

PENICILLIN V

(pen-i-**sill**-in vee)

{Apo-Pen-VK}, Beepen-VK, Betapen-VK, Ledercillin VK, {Nadopen-V}, {Novopen-VK}, Pen-Vee-K, {PVF K}, Robicillin-VK, {VC-K}, V-Cillin VK, Veetids

CLASSIFICATION(S):
Anti-infective—penicillin
Pregnancy Category B

INDICATIONS

▪ Treatment of a wide variety of infections, including: ▫ Pneumococcal pneumonia ▫ Erisipelas ▫ Skin and soft tissue infections ▫ Streptococcal pharyngitis ▪ Prevention of rheumatic fever.

ACTION

▪ Binds to bacterial cell wall, resulting in cell death. **Therapeutic Effect:** ▪ Bactericidal action against susceptible bacteria. **Spectrum:** ▪ Active against most gram-positive organisms, including: ▫ Streptococci (*Streptococcus pneumoniae,* group A beta-hemolytic streptococci) ▫ Staphylococci (non-penicillinase-producing strains) ▫ Some gram-negative organisms, such as *Neisseria meningitis* and *Neisseria gonorrheae* ▫ Some anaerobic bacteria and spirochetes

PHARMACOKINETICS

Absorption: Penicillin V resists acid degradation in the GI tract and is absorbed better than penicillin G.

Distribution: Widely distributed, although CNS penetration is poor in the presence of uninflamed meninges. Crosses the placenta and enters breast milk.

Metabolism and Excretion: Minimally metabolized by the liver, excreted mainly unchanged by the kidneys.

Half-life: 30–60 min.

CONTRAINDICATIONS AND PRECAUTIONS

Contraindicated in: ▪ Previous hypersensitivity to penicillins ▪ Cross-sensitivity with cephalosporins may exist ▪ Hypersensitivity to procaine or benzathine (procaine and benzathine preparations only) ▪ Some products may contain tartrazine (Veetids 125 liquid)—avoid use in patients with tartrazine (FDC yellow dye #5) hypersensitivity.

Use Cautiously in: ▪ Severe renal insufficiency (dosage reduction recommended) ▪ Pregnancy (although safety not established, has been used safely) ▪ Lactation.

ADVERSE REACTIONS AND SIDE EFFECTS*

CNS: SEIZURES.

GI: nausea, vomiting, diarrhea, epigastric distress.

GU: interstitial nephritis.

Derm: rashes, urticaria.

Hemat: eosinophilia, hemolytic anemia, leukopenia.

Misc: superinfection, allergic reactions, including ANAPHYLAXIS and serum sickness.

INTERACTIONS

Drug-Drug: ▪ May decrease the effectiveness of **oral contraceptive agents** ▪ **Probenecid** decreases renal excretion and increases blood levels of penicillin. Therapy may be combined for this purpose ▪ **Neomycin** may decrease the absorption of penicillin V ▪ Effectiveness of penicillin may be decreased by concurrent use of **chloramphenicol** ▪ Half-life of **chloramphenicol** may be increased by concurrent use of penicillin.

{} = Available in Canada only.

*Underlines indicate most frequent; **CAPITALS** indicate life-threatening.

P

ROUTE AND DOSAGE

Note: 1 mg = 1600 units.

Infections Due to Susceptible Organisms

- **PO (Adults):** 250–500 mg q 6 hr.
- **PO (Children):** 15–50 mg/kg/day in divided doses q 6–8 hr.

Rheumatic Fever Prophylaxis

- **PO (Adults):** 125–250 mg q 12 hr.

PHARMACODYNAMICS (blood levels)

	ONSET	PEAK
PO	rapid	0.5–1 hr

NURSING IMPLICATIONS

Assessment

- Assess patient for infection (vital signs; appearance of wound, sputum, urine, and stool; WBC) at beginning and throughout course of therapy.
- Obtain a history before initiating therapy to determine previous use of and reactions to penicillins or cephalosporins. Persons with a negative history of penicillin sensitivity may still have an allergic response.
- Obtain specimens for culture and sensitivity prior to initiating therapy. First dose may be given before receiving results.
- Observe patient for signs and symptoms of anaphylaxis (rash, pruritus, laryngeal edema, wheezing). Discontinue drug and notify physician immediately if these occur. Keep epinephrine, an antihistamine, and resuscitation equipment close by in the event of an anaphylactic reaction.
- **Lab Test Considerations:** May cause positive direct Coombs' test results.

Potential Nursing Diagnoses

- Infection, high risk for (indications, side effects).
- Knowledge deficit related to medication regimen (patient/family teaching).
- Noncompliance related to medication regimen (patient/family teaching).

Implementation

- **PO:** Administer around the clock. Penicillin V may be administered without regard for meals.
- Use calibrated measuring device for liquid preparations. Soln is stable for 14 days if refrigerated.

Patient/Family Teaching

- Instruct patient to take medication around the clock and to finish the drug completely as directed, even if feeling better. Advise patient that sharing of this medication may be dangerous.
- Advise patient to report the signs of superinfection (black, furry overgrowth on the tongue; vaginal itching or discharge; loose or foul-smelling stools) and allergy.
- Instruct patient to notify physician if symptoms do not improve.
- Advise patients taking oral contraceptives to use additional nonhormonal methods of contraception during therapy with penicillin V and until next menstrual period.
- Patients with an allergy to penicillin should be instructed to carry an identification card with this information at all times.

Evaluation

Clinical response to therapy can be evaluated by: ▪ Resolution of the signs and symptoms of infection. Length of time for complete resolution depends on the organism and site of infection.

PENTAMIDINE

(pen-**tam**-i-deen)
Nebupent, Pentam

CLASSIFICATION(S):
Anti-infective—antiprotozoal
Pregnancy Category C

INDICATIONS

▪ **IM, IV:** Treatment of *Pneumocystis carinii* pneumonia (PCP) ▪ **Inhaln:** Prevention of *Pneumocystis carinii* pneu-

monia (PCP) in AIDS or HIV-positive patients who have had PCP or who have a peripheral CD4 lymphocyte (T_4 helper/inducer) count of $\leq 200/mm^3$.
Unlabeled Uses: ▪ Management of: ▫ African trypanosomiasis ▫ Leishmaniasis ▫ Babesiosis.

ACTION

▪ Appears to disrupt DNA or RNA synthesis in protozoa ▪ Also has a direct toxic effect on pancreatic islet cells.
Therapeutic Effect: ▪ Death of susceptible protozoa.

PHARMACOKINETICS

Absorption: Well absorbed following deep IM administration. Minimal systemic absorption occurs following inhalation.
Distribution: Widely and extensively distributed. Does not appear to enter the CSF. Concentrates in liver, kidneys, lungs, and spleen, with prolonged storage in some tissues.
Metabolism and Excretion: 1–30% excreted unchanged by the kidneys. Remainder of metabolic fate unknown.
Half-life: 6.4–9.4 hr (increased in renal impairment).

CONTRAINDICATIONS AND PRECAUTIONS

Contraindicated in: ▪ History of previous anaphylactic reaction to pentamidine.
Use Cautiously in: ▪ Hypotension ▪ Hypertension ▪ Hypoglycemia ▪ Hyperglycemia ▪ Hypocalcemia ▪ Leukopenia ▪ Thrombocytopenia ▪ Anemia ▪ Renal impairment (dosage reduction required) ▪ Diabetes mellitus ▪ Liver impairment ▪ Pregnancy or lactation (safety not established) ▪ Cardiovascular disease ▪ Bone marrow depression, previous antineoplastic therapy, or radiation therapy.

ADVERSE REACTIONS AND SIDE EFFECTS*

Note: For parenteral form, unless indicated.

CNS: dizziness, confusion, hallucinations, anxiety, headache.
EENT: burning in throat (inhaln only).
CV: HYPOTENSION, ARRHYTHMIAS.
GI: nausea, vomiting, abdominal pain, unpleasant metallic taste, anorexia, PANCREATITIS, hepatitis.
GU: nephrotoxicity.
Derm: rash, pallor.
Endo: HYPOGLYCEMIA, hyperglycemia.
F and E: hypocalcemia, hyperkalemia.
Hemat: leukopenia, thrombocytopenia, anemia.
Local: pain, induration, sterile abscesses at IM site, necrosis at IM site, phlebitis, pruritus, urticaria at IV site.
Resp: bronchospasm, cough (inhaln only).
Misc: fever, chills, STEVENS-JOHNSON SYNDROME, allergic reactions, including ANAPHYLAXIS.

INTERACTIONS

Note: Listed for parenteral administration.

Drug-Drug: ▪ Additive nephrotoxicity with other **nephrotoxic agents,** including **aminoglycosides, amphotericin B,** and **vancomycin** ▪ Additive bone marrow depression with **antineoplastic agents** or previous **radiation therapy**.

ROUTE AND DOSAGE

Pneumocystis Carinii Pneumonia—Treatment

- **IM, IV (Adults):** 4 mg/kg once daily for 14 days (treatment up to 21 days or longer may be required in AIDS patients).
- **IM, IV (Children):** 4 mg/kg once daily for 14 days or 150 mg/m^2 for 5 days, then 100 mg/m^2 for 9 days (treatment up to 21 days or longer may be required in AIDS patients).

Pneumocystis Carinii Pneumonia—Prevention

- **Inhaln (Adults):** 300 mg q 4 wk, administered using a Respirgard II Nebulizer.

*Underlines indicate most frequent; **CAPITALS** indicate life-threatening.

PHARMACODYNAMICS (blood levels)

	ONSET	PEAK
IM	UK	0.5–1 hr
IV	UK	end of infusion
Inhaln	UK	UK

NURSING IMPLICATIONS

Assessment

- Assess patient for infection (vital signs, sputum, WBC) and monitor respiratory status (rate, character, lung sounds, dyspnea, sputum) at beginning and throughout course of therapy.
- Obtain specimens for culture and sensitivity prior to initiating therapy. First dose may be given before receiving results.
- Monitor blood pressure frequently during and following IM or IV administration of pentamidine. Patient should be lying down during administration. Sudden, severe hypotension may occur following a single dose. Resuscitation equipment should be immediately available.
- Assess patient for signs of hypoglycemia (anxiety, chills, diaphoresis, cold pale skin, headache, increased hunger, nausea, nervousness, shakiness) and hyperglycemia (drowsiness, flushed dry skin, fruit-like breath odor, increased thirst, increased urination, loss of appetite), which may occur up to several mons after therapy is discontinued.
- Pulse and ECG should be monitored prior to and periodically during course of therapy. Fatalities due to cardiac arrhythmias, tachycardia, and cardiotoxicity have been reported.
- **Lab Test Considerations:** Blood glucose concentrations should be monitored prior to, daily during, and for several mons following course of therapy.
- Monitor BUN and serum creatinine prior to and daily during therapy to monitor for nephrotoxicity.
- Monitor CBC and platelet count prior to and periodically during course of therapy. Pentamidine may cause leukopenia, anemia, and thrombocytopenia.
- May cause elevated serum bilirubin, alkaline phosphatase, SGOT (AST), and SGPT (ALT) concentrations. These liver function tests should be monitored prior to and every 3 days during course of therapy.
- Serum calcium concentrations should be monitored prior to and every 3 days during therapy, as pentamidine may cause hypocalcemia.
- May cause elevated serum potassium concentrations.

Potential Nursing Diagnoses

- Infection, high risk for (indications, side effects).
- Knowledge deficit related to medication regimen (patient/family teaching).

Implementation

- **General Info:** Pentamidine must be given on a regular schedule for the full course of therapy. If a dose is missed, administer as soon as remembered. If almost time for the next dose, skip the missed dose and return to the regular schedule. Do not double doses.
- **IM:** To reconstitute, add 3 ml of sterile water for injection to each 300-mg vial. Administer deep into well-developed muscle. May cause hardness or pain at injection site.
- **Intermittent Infusion:** To reconstitute, add 3, 4, or 5 ml of sterile water for injection or D5W to each 300-mg vial for a concentration of 100, 75, or 60 mg/ml, respectively. Withdraw dose and dilute further in 50–250 ml of D5W. Soln is stable for 48 hr at room temperature. Discard unused portions.
- *Rate:* Administer slowly over at least 60 min.

- **Y-Site Compatibility:** zidovudine.
- **Y-Site Incompatibility:** foscarnet.
- **Inhaln:** Dilute 300 mg in 600 ml of sterile water for injection. Place reconstituted soln into Respirgard II nebulizer. Do not dilute with 0.9% NaCl or admix with other medications, as soln will form a precipitate. Soln is stable for 48 hr at room temperature if protected from light. Do not use Respirgard II nebulizer for other medications.
- □ Administer inhalation dose through nebulizer until chamber is empty, approximately 30–45 min.

Patient/Family Teaching

- □ Inform patient of the importance of completing the full course of pentamidine therapy, even if feeling better.
- □ Instruct patient to notify physician promptly if fever, sore throat, signs of infection, bleeding of gums, unusual bruising, petechiae, or blood in stool, urine, or emesis occurs. Caution patient to avoid crowds and persons with known infections. Instruct patient to use soft toothbrush and electric razor and to avoid falls. Patient should not be given IM injections or rectal thermometers. Patient should also be cautioned not to drink alcoholic beverages or take medication containing aspirin, as these may precipitate gastric bleeding.
- □ Caution patient to make position changes slowly to minimize orthostatic hypotension.
- □ Advise patient that an unpleasant metallic taste may occur with pentamidine administration but is not significant.

Evaluation

Clinical response to therapy can be evaluated by: ▪ Prevention or resolution of the signs and symptoms of protozoan infections, especially *Pneumocystis carinii* pneumonia in patients with HIV infections.

PENTAZOCINE

pen-**taz**-oh-seen
Talwin, Talwin NX

CLASSIFICATION(S):
Narcotic analgesic—agonist/antagonist
Schedule IV
Pregnancy Category C

INDICATIONS

▪ Management of moderate to severe pain ▪ Has also been used as: □ An analgesic during labor □ A sedative prior to surgery □ A supplement in balanced anesthesia.

ACTION

▪ Binds to opiate receptors in the CNS ▪ Alters perception of and response to painful stimuli, while producing generalized CNS depression ▪ Has partial antagonist properties, which may result in narcotic withdrawal in physically dependent patients. **Therapeutic Effect:** ▪ Decrease in moderate to severe pain.

PHARMACOKINETICS

Absorption: Well absorbed following oral, IM, and SC administration. Small amount (0.5 mg) of naloxone in tablets included to prevent parenteral abuse.
Distribution: Widely distributed. Crosses the placenta.
Metabolism and Excretion: Mostly metabolized by the liver. Small amounts excreted unchanged by the kidneys.
Half-life: 2–3 hr.

CONTRAINDICATIONS AND PRECAUTIONS

Contraindicated in: ▪ Hypersensitivity ▪ Narcotic-dependent patients who have not been detoxified (may precipitate withdrawal).
Use Cautiously in: ▪ Head trauma ▪ Increased intracranial pressure ▪ Severe

P

renal, hepatic, or pulmonary disease ▪ Hypothyroidism ▪ Adrenal insufficiency ▪ Alcoholism ▪ Elderly, debilitated patients or patients with severe liver impairment (dosage reduction recommended) ▪ Undiagnosed abdominal pain ▪ Prostatic hypertrophy ▪ Pregnancy (has been used during labor, but may cause respiratory depression in the newborn) ▪ Lactation or children (safety not established).

ADVERSE REACTIONS AND SIDE EFFECTS*

CNS: sedation, confusion, headache, euphoria, floating feeling, unusual dreams, hallucinations, dysphoria, dizziness, vertigo.

EENT: miosis (high doses), blurred vision, diplopia.

Resp: respiratory depression.

CV: hypotension, hypertension, palpitations.

GI: nausea, vomiting, constipation, ileus, dry mouth.

GU: urinary retention.

Derm: sweating, clammy feeling.

Misc: tolerance, physical dependence, psychological dependence.

INTERACTIONS

Drug-Drug: ▪ Use with caution in patients receiving **MAO inhibitors** (may result in unpredictable reactions—decrease initial dose of pentazocine to 25% of usual dose) ▪ Additive CNS depression with **alcohol, antihistamines,** and **sedative/hypnotics** ▪ May precipitate narcotic withdrawal in patients who are physically dependent on **narcotic analgesic agonists** and have not been detoxified ▪ May diminish analgesic effects of other **narcotic analgesics**.

ROUTE AND DOSAGE

Moderate to Severe Pain

- **PO (Adults):** 50–100 mg q 3–4 hr (not to exceed 600 mg/day).
- **IV (Adults):** 30 mg q 3–4 hr as needed (not to exceed 360 mg/day).
- **IM, SC (Adults):** 30–60 mg q 3–4 hr as needed (not to exceed 360 mg/day).

Obstetric Use

- **IM (Adults):** 30 mg when contractions become regular, may be repeated 2–3 times at 2–3-hr intervals.
- **IV (Adults):** 20 mg when contractions become regular, may be repeated 2–3 times at 2–3-hr intervals.

PHARMACODYNAMICS (analgesia)

	ONSET	PEAK	DURATION
PO	15–30 min	1–3 hr	3 hr
IM, SC	15–20 min	1 hr	2 hr
IV	2–3 min	15 min	1 hr

NURSING IMPLICATIONS

Assessment

- Assess type, location, and intensity of pain prior to and 60 min following IM and oral doses, and 15 min following IV administration.
- Assess blood pressure, pulse, and respirations before and periodically during administration.
- While this drug has a low potential for dependence, prolonged use may lead to physical and psychological dependence and tolerance. This should not prevent patient from receiving adequate analgesia. Most patients receiving pentazocine for medical reasons do not develop psychological dependence. Progressively higher doses may be required to relieve pain with long-term therapy.
- Assess prior analgesic history. Antagonistic properties may induce withdrawal symptoms (vomiting, restlessness, abdominal cramps, increased blood pressure and temperature) in narcotic-dependent patients.
- **Lab Test Considerations:** May cause elevated serum amylase and lipase levels.
- **Toxicity and Overdose:** If overdose occurs, respiratory depression may be partially reversed with naloxone (Narcan).

*Underlines indicate most frequent; **CAPITALS** indicate life-threatening.

Potential Nursing Diagnoses
- Comfort, altered: pain (indications).
- Injury, high risk for (side effects).
- Sensory-perceptual alteration: visual, auditory (side effects).

Implementation
- **General Info:** Explain therapeutic value of medication prior to administration to enhance the analgesic effect.
- □ Regularly administered doses may be more effective than prn administration. Analgesic is more effective if administered before pain becomes severe.
- □ Coadministration with non-narcotic analgesics may have additive effects and may permit lower narcotic doses.
- □ Also available in combination with aspirin and acetaminophen (see Appendix A).
- **PO:** Talwin NX contains 0.5 mg of naloxone, which has no pharmacologic activity when administered orally. If the product is abused by injection, naloxone antagonizes pentazocine. Parenteral use of oral pentazocine may lead to severe, potentially fatal reactions (pulmonary emboli, vascular occlusion, ulceration and abscess, and withdrawal symptoms in narcotic-dependent individuals).
- **IM/SC:** Administer IM injections deep into well-developed muscle. Rotate sites of injections. SC route may cause tissue damage with repeated injections.
- **Direct IV:** Manufacturer recommends diluting each 5 mg with at least 1 ml of sterile water for injection.
- □ *Rate:* Administer slowly, each 5 mg over at least 1 minute.
- **Syringe Compatibility:** atropine, benzquinamide, butorphanol, chlorpromazine, cimetidine, dimenhydrinate, diphenhydramine, droperidol, hydroxyzine, metoclopramide, perphenazine, prochlorperazine edisylate, promazine, promethazine, propiomazine, ranitidine, or scopolamine.
- **Syringe Incompatibility:** glycopyrrolate, heparin, or pentobarbital.
- **Y-Site Compatibility:** heparin, hydrocortisone sodium succinate, or potassium chloride.
- **Y-Site Incompatibility:** nafcillin.
- **Additive Incompatibility:** aminophylline, amobarbital, pentobarbital, phenobarbital, secobarbital, or sodium bicarbonate.

Patient/Family Teaching
- □ Instruct patient on how and when to ask for prn pain medication.
- □ Medication may cause drowsiness, dizziness, or hallucinations. Advise patient to call for assistance when ambulating and to avoid driving or other activities requiring alertness until response to medication is known.
- □ Encourage patient to turn, cough, and breathe deeply every 2 hr to prevent atelectasis.
- □ Caution patient to make position changes slowly to minimize orthostatic hypotension.
- □ Advise patient to avoid concurrent use of alcohol and other CNS depressants.
- □ Advise patient that frequent mouth rinses, good oral hygiene, and sugarless gum or candy may decrease dry mouth.

Evaluation
Effectiveness of therapy can be demonstrated by: ■ Decrease in severity of pain without a significant alteration in level of consciousness or respiratory status.

PENTOBARBITAL
(pen-toe-**bar**-bi-tal)
Nembutal, {Novopentobarb}

CLASSIFICATION(S):
Sedative/hypnotic—barbiturate
Schedule II
Pregnancy Category D

P

INDICATIONS

▪ Hypnotic agent (short-term use) ▪ As a preoperative sedation and in other situations where sedation is required. **Unlabeled Uses:** ▪ ***IV:*** Induction of coma in selected patients with cerebral ischemia and management of increased intracranial pressure.

ACTION

▪ Depresses the CNS, probably by potentiating gamma-aminobutyric acid (GABA), an inhibitory neurotransmitter ▪ Produces all levels of CNS depression, including the sensory cortex, motor activity, and altered cerebellar function ▪ May decrease cerebral blood flow, cerebral edema, and intracranial pressure (IV only). **Therapeutic Effect:** ▪ Sedation and/or induction of sleep.

PHARMACOKINETICS

Absorption: Well absorbed following oral, rectal, or IM administration.
Distribution: Widely distributed, highest concentrations in brain and liver. Crosses the placenta, small amounts enter breast milk.
Metabolism and Excretion: Metabolized by the liver. Minimal amounts excreted unchanged by the kidneys.
Half-life: 35–50 hr.

CONTRAINDICATIONS AND PRECAUTIONS

Contraindicated in: ▪ Hypersensitivity ▪ Hypersensitivity to propylene glycol ▪ Comatose patients or those with pre-existing CNS depression (unless used to induce coma) ▪ Uncontrolled severe pain ▪ Pregnancy or lactation.
Use Cautiously in: ▪ Hepatic dysfunction ▪ Severe renal impairment ▪ Patients who may be suicidal or who may have been addicted to drugs previously ▪ Elderly patients (dosage reduction recommended) ▪ Hypnotic use should be short-term (chronic use may lead to dependence).

ADVERSE REACTIONS AND SIDE EFFECTS*

CNS: drowsiness, lethargy, vertigo, depression, hangover, excitation, delirium.
Resp: respiratory depression, LARYNGOSPASM (IV only), bronchospasm (IV only).
CV: hypotension (IV only).
GI: nausea, vomiting, diarrhea, constipation.
Derm: rashes, urticaria.
Local: phlebitis at IV site.
MS: myalgia, arthralgia, neuralgia.
Misc: hypersensitivity reactions, including ANGIODEDEMA and serum sickness; psychological dependence, physical dependence.

INTERACTIONS

Drug–Drug: ▪ Additive CNS depression with other **CNS depressants**, including **alcohol, antihistamines, narcotic analgesics**, and other **sedative/hypnotics** ▪ May induce hepatic enzymes, which metabolize other drugs, decreasing their effectiveness, including **oral contraceptives, oral anticoagulants, chloramphenicol, cyclosporine, dacarbazine, glucocorticoids, tricyclic antidepressants**, and **quinidine** ▪ May increase the risk of hepatic toxicity of **acetaminophen** ▪ **MAO inhibitors, valproic acid**, or **divalproex** may decrease the metabolism of pentobarbital, increasing sedation.

ROUTE AND DOSAGE

Sedation

- **PO (Adults):** 20–40 mg 2–4 times daily.
- **PO (Children):** 6 mg/kg/day in divided doses.

Insomnia

- **PO (Adults):** 100–200 mg at bedtime.
- **IM (Adults):** 150–200 mg at bedtime.
- **IM (Children):** 3–5 mg/kg (up to 100 mg).
- **IV (Adults):** 100 mg initially (up to 500 mg).

*Underlines indicate most frequent; **CAPITALS** indicate life-threatening.

- **Rect (Adults):** 120–200 mg at bedtime.
- **Rect (Children 12–14 yr):** 60–120 mg at bedtime.
- **Rect (Children 5–12 yr):** 60 mg at bedtime.
- **Rect (Children 1–4 yr):** 30–60 mg at bedtime.

Preoperative Sedation

- **PO, IM (Adults):** 2–6 mg/kg (100–200 mg).

PHARMACODYNAMICS (sedation)*

	ONSET	PEAK	DURATION
PO	15–60 min	3–4 hr	1–4 hr
Rect	15–60 min	UK	1–4 hr
IM	10–25 min	UK	1–4 hr
IV	immediate	1 min	15 min

*Noted as hypnotic effect; sedative effects are longer-lasting.

NURSING IMPLICATIONS

Assessment

- **General Info:** Assess sleep patterns prior to and periodically throughout course of therapy. Hypnotic doses of pentobarbital suppress REM sleep. Patient may experience an increase in dreaming upon discontinuation of medication.
  - Monitor respiratory status, pulse, and blood pressure frequently in patients receiving pentobarbital IV. Equipment for resuscitation and artificial ventilation should be readily available. Respiratory depression is dose-dependent.
  - Prolonged therapy may lead to psychological or physical dependence. Restrict amount of drug available to patient, especially if depressed, suicidal, or previously addicted.
  - Assess postoperative patients for pain. Pentobarbital may increase responsiveness to painful stimuli.
- **Cerebral Edema:** Monitor intracranial pressure and level of consciousness in patients in barbiturate coma.

Potential Nursing Diagnoses

- Sleep pattern disturbance (indications).
- Injury, high risk for (side effects).
- Knowledge deficit related to medication regimen (patient/family teaching).

Implementation

- **General Info:** Supervise ambulation and transfer of patients following administration. Remove cigarettes. Side rails should be raised and call bell within reach at all times. Keep bed in low position.
- **PO:** Elixir may be administered undiluted or diluted in water, milk, or fruit juice. Use calibrated measuring device for accurate dosage. Do not use cloudy soln.
- **IM:** Do not administer SC. IM injections should be given deep into the gluteal muscle to minimize tissue irritation. Do not inject more than 5 ml into any one site, because of tissue irritation.
- **Direct IV:** Doses may be given undiluted or diluted with sterile water, 0.45% NaCl, 0.9% NaCl, D5W, D10W, Ringer's or lactated Ringer's soln, dextrose/saline combinations or dextrose/Ringer's or lactated Ringer's combinations. Do not use soln that is discolored or that contains particulate matter.
  - Soln is highly alkaline; avoid extravasation, which may cause tissue damage and necrosis. If extravasation occurs, infiltration of 5% procaine soln into affected area and application of moist heat may be ordered.
  - *Rate:* Administer each 50 mg over at least 1 min. Titrate slowly for desired response. Rapid administration may result in respiratory depression, apnea, laryngospasm, bronchospasm, or hypertension.
- **Syringe Compatibility:** aminophylline, ephedrine, hydromorphone, neostigmine, scopolamine, sodium bicarbonate, sodium iodide, or thiopental.
- **Syringe Incompatibility:** benzquinamide, butorphanol, chlorpromazine, cimetidine, dimenhydrinate, diphenhydramine, droperidol, fentanyl, glycopyrrolate, hydroxyzine, meperidine,

midazolam, nalbuphine, pentazocine, perphenazine, prochlorperazine edisylate, promazine, promethazine, or ranitidine.

- **Y-Site Compatibility:** acyclovir or regular insulin.
- **Additive Compatibility:** amikacin, aminophylline, calcium chloride, cephapirin, chloramphenicol, dimenhydrinate, erythromycin lactobionate, lidocaine, thiopental, or verapamil.
- **Additive Incompatibility:** chlorpheniramine, codeine, ephedrine, erythromycin gluceptate, hydrocortisone, hydroxyzine, insulin, levorphanol, methadone, norepinephrine, oxytetracycline, penicillin G potassium, pentazocine, phenytoin, promazine, promethazine, streptomycin, triflupromazine, or vancomycin.
- **Rect:** To ensure accurate dose, do not divide rectal suppository. Suppositories should be refrigerated.

PATIENT/FAMILY TEACHING

- □ Advise patient to take medication exactly as prescribed. Do not increase dose of the drug without consulting physician.
- □ Discuss the importance of preparing environment for sleep (dark room, quiet, avoidance of nicotine and caffeine).
- □ Advise patients on prolonged therapy not to discontinue medication without consulting physician. Abrupt withdrawal may precipitate withdrawal symptoms.
- □ May cause daytime drowsiness. Caution patient to avoid driving and other activities requiring alertness until response to medication is known.
- □ Caution patient to avoid taking alcohol or other CNS depressants concurrently with this medication.
- □ Instruct patient to contact physician immediately if pregnancy is suspected.

EVALUATION

Effectiveness of therapy can be demonstrated by: ▪ Improvement in sleep pattern without excessive daytime sedation. Therapy is usually limited to a 2 wk period ▪ Prevention of cerebral anoxia.

PENTOXIFYLLINE

(pen-tox-**if**-i-lin)
Trental

CLASSIFICATION(S):
Hemorrheologic agent
Pregnancy Category C

INDICATIONS

▪ Management of symptomatic peripheral vascular disease (intermittent claudication).

ACTION

▪ Increases the flexibility of red blood cells by increasing levels of cyclic adenosine monophosphate (cAMP) ▪ Decreases blood viscosity by inhibiting platelet aggregation and decreasing fibrinogen. **Therapeutic Effect:** ▪ Increased blood flow.

PHARMACOKINETICS

Absorption: Well absorbed following oral administration.
Distribution: Distribution not known.
Metabolism and Excretion: Metabolized by red blood cells and the liver.
Half-life: 25–50 min.

CONTRAINDICATIONS AND PRECAUTIONS

Contraindicated in: ▪ Hypersensitivity ▪ Intolerance to other xanthine derivatives (caffeine and theophylline).
Use Cautiously in: ▪ Coronary artery or cerebrovascular disease ▪ Pregnancy, lactation, or children (safety not established).

ADVERSE REACTIONS AND SIDE EFFECTS*

CNS: headache, tremor, dizziness, agitation, nervousness, drowsiness, insomnia.
EENT: blurred vision.

*Underlines indicate most frequent; **CAPITALS** indicate life-threatening.

Resp: dyspnea.
CV: angina, hypotension, arrhythmias, flushing, edema.
GI: dyspepsia, nausea, vomiting, belching, flatus, bloating, abdominal discomfort, diarrhea.

INTERACTIONS

Drug–Drug: ▪ Additive hypotension may occur with **antihypertensives** and **nitrates**.

ROUTE AND DOSAGE

- **PO (Adults):** 400 mg tid.

PHARMACODYNAMICS (improvement in blood flow)

	ONSET	PEAK	DURATION
PO	2–4 wk	8 wk	UK

NURSING IMPLICATIONS

Assessment

- Assess patient for intermittent claudication prior to and periodically throughout course of therapy.
- Monitor blood pressure periodically in patients on concurrent antihypertensive therapy.

Potential Nursing Diagnoses

- Comfort, altered: pain (indications).
- Activity intolerance (indications).
- Knowledge deficit related to medication regimen (patient/family teaching).

Implementation

- **PO:** Administer with meals to minimize GI irritation. Tablets should be swallowed whole; do not crush, break, or chew.

Patient/Family Teaching

- Instruct patient to take medication exactly as prescribed. If a dose is missed, it should be taken as soon as remembered unless almost time for next dose. Consult physician before discontinuing medication, as it may need to be taken for several wks before effects are seen.
- Medication may cause dizziness and blurred vision. Caution patient to avoid driving and other activities requiring alertness until response to medication is known.
- Advise patient to avoid smoking, as nicotine constricts blood vessels.
- Instruct patient to notify physician if nausea, vomiting, GI upset, drowsiness, dizziness, or headache persists, as the dose may need to be reduced.

Evaluation

Effectiveness of therapy can be demonstrated by: ▪ Relief from cramping in calf muscles, buttocks, thighs, and feet during exercise ▫ Improvement in walking endurance.

PERGOLIDE

(**per**-goe-lide)
Permax

CLASSIFICATION(S):
Antiparkinson agent—dopamine agonist
Pregnancy Category B

INDICATIONS

▪ Management of Parkinson's disease in conjunction with levodopa/carbidopa.

ACTION

▪ Acts as a dopamine agonist, directly stimulating postsynaptic dopaminergic receptors in the CNS. **Therapeutic Effect:** ▪ Continued relief of symptoms of Parkinson's disease at a lower dosage of levodopa/carbidopa.

PHARMACOKINETICS

Absorption: Well absorbed following oral administration.
Distribution: Distribution not known.
Metabolism and Excretion: Highly metabolized by the liver. Metabolites are excreted by the kidneys.
Half-life: UK.

CONTRAINDICATIONS AND PRECAUTIONS

Contraindicated in: ▪ Hypersensitivity to pergolide or ergot derivatives.

P

Use Cautiously in: ▪ Arrhythmias ▪ Pregnancy or children (safety not established) ▪ Lactation (may inhibit lactation, safety not established).

ADVERSE REACTIONS AND SIDE EFFECTS*

CNS: hallucinations, dyskinesia, somnolence, insomnia, confusion.
EENT: rhinitis.
Resp: dyspnea.
CV: orthostatic hypotension, palpitations, arrhythmias (atrial premature contractions, sinus tachycardia).
GI: nausea, constipation, diarrhea, abdominal pain, dyspepsia.

INTERACTIONS

Drug-Drug: ▪ **Phenothiazines, metoclopramide,** or **haloperidol** may decrease effectiveness by antagonizing the effects of dopamine.

ROUTE AND DOSAGE

- **PO (Adults):** 50 mcg/day in divided doses for 2 days, increase by 100–150 mcg/day every third day for 12 days, then may increase by 250 mcg/day every third day until optimal response is obtained. Usual dose is 3 mg/day in divided doses tid, not to exceed 5 mg/day.

PHARMACODYNAMICS (antiparkinson effects)

	ONSET	PEAK	DURATION
PO	UK	UK	UK

NURSING IMPLICATIONS

Assessment

- Assess patient for signs and symptoms of Parkinson's disease (tremor, muscle weakness and rigidity, ataxic gait) prior to and throughout therapy.
- Assess patient for confusion or hallucinations. Notify physician if these occur.
- Monitor ECG frequently during dosage adjustment and periodically throughout therapy.

Potential Nursing Diagnoses

- Mobility, impaired physical (indications).
- Injury, high risk for (indications, side effects).
- Knowledge deficit related to medication regimen (patient/family teaching).

Implementation

- **PO:** An attempt to reduce the dose of levodopa/carbidopa may be made cautiously during pergolide therapy.

Patient/Family Teaching

- Instruct patient to take medication exactly as directed.
- May cause drowsiness. Caution patient to avoid driving or other activities requiring alertness until response to medication is known.
- Advise patient to make position changes slowly to minimize orthostatic hypotension.

Evaluation

Effectiveness of therapy can be demonstrated by: ▪ Improved response to levodopa/carbidopa in patients with Parkinson's disease.

PERMETHRIN

(per-**meth**-rin)
Elimite, Nix

CLASSIFICATION(S):
Anti-infective—pediculocide
Pregnancy Category B

INDICATIONS

▪ Nix®: Eradication of *Pediculus humanus capitis* (head lice and their eggs) ▪ Elimite®: Eradication of *Sarcoptes scabiei* (scabies).

ACTION

▪ Causes repolarization and paralysis in lice by disrupting normal nerve cell-sodium transport. **Therapeutic Effect:** ▪ Death of parasites.

*Underlines indicate most frequent; **CAPITALS** indicate life-threatening.

PHARMACOKINETICS

Absorption: Small amounts (<2%) systemically absorbed. Remains on hair for 10 days.
Distribution: Distribution not known.
Metabolism and Excretion: Rapidly inactivated by enzymes.
Half-life: UK.

CONTRAINDICATIONS AND PRECAUTIONS

Contraindicated in: ▪ Hypersensitivity to permethrins, pyrethrins (insecticides or veterinary pesticides), chrysanthemums, or isopropyl alcohol.
Use Cautiously in: ▪ Pregnancy or lactation ▪ Children <2 yr (Nix®) ▪ Children <2 mon (Elimite®).

ADVERSE REACTIONS AND SIDE EFFECTS*

Derm: itching, redness, swelling, rash, stinging, burning.
Neuro: numbness, tingling.

INTERACTIONS

Drug–Drug: ▪ No significant interactions.

ROUTE AND DOSAGE

Pediculus Humanus Capitis Infestation

- **Top (Adults and Children >2 yr):** 1% lotion applied to the hair, left on for 10 min, then rinsed, for 1 application. If live lice are observed 7 days after initial treatment, a second application may be necessary.

Sarcoptes Scabiei Infestation

- **Top (Adults and Children):** Massage 5% cream into all skin surfaces. Leave on for 8–14 hr, then wash off.
- **Top (Infants >2 mon):** Massage 5% cream into hairline, scalp, neck, temple, and forehead. Leave on for 8–14 hr, then wash off.

PHARMACODYNAMICS (pediculocidal action)

	ONSET	PEAK	DURATION
Top	10 min	UK	14 days

NURSING IMPLICATIONS

Assessment

- **Head Lice:** Assess scalp for presence of lice and their ova (nits) prior to and 1 wk after application of permethrin.
- **Scabies:** Assess skin for scabies prior to and following therapy.

Potential Nursing Diagnoses

- Home maintenance management, impaired (indications).
- Self-care deficit (indications).
- Knowledge deficit related to medication regimen (patient/family teaching).

Implementation

- **Top:** For topical application only.

Patient/Family Teaching

- **General Info:** Instruct patient to notify physician if scalp itching, numbness, redness, or rash occurs.
- Instruct patient to avoid getting lotion in eyes. If this occurs, eyes should be flushed thoroughly with water. Physician should be contacted if eye irritation persists.
- Advise patient that others residing in the home should also be checked for lice.
- Instruct patient on methods of preventing reinfestation. All clothes, including outdoor apparel, and household linens should be machine-washed using very hot water and dried for at least 20 min in a hot dryer. Nonwashable clothes should be dry-cleaned. Brushes and combs should be soaked in hot (130°F), soapy water for 5–10 min. Remind patient that brushes and combs should not be shared. Wigs and hairpieces should be shampooed. Rugs and upholstered furniture should be vacuumed. Toys should be washed in hot, soapy water. Items that cannot be washed should be sealed in a plastic bag for 2 wk.
- If patient is a child, instruct parents to notify school nurse or day care center so that classmates and playmates can be checked.

*Underlines indicate most frequent; **CAPITALS** indicate life-threatening.

P

- **Head Lice:** Instruct patient to wash hair with regular shampoo, rinse, and towel dry. Each container holds enough medication for 1 treatment. The patient should use as much of the soln as necessary to coat entire head of hair, then discard the remainder of the soln. Shake the container well. Thoroughly wet scalp and hair with the lotion. Allow lotion to remain on hair for 10 min, then thoroughly rinse hair and towel dry with a clean towel. Comb hair with a fine-toothed comb to remove dead lice and eggs.
- Explain to patient that permethrin will protect from reinfestation for 2 wk. These effects continue even when the patient resumes regular shampooing.
- **Scabies:** Instruct patient to massage thoroughly into the skin from head to soles of feet. Treat infants on the hairline, neck, scalp, temple, and forehead. Remove the cream by washing after 8–14 hr.

Evaluation

Effectiveness of therapy can be demonstrated by: ▪ Absence of lice and nits 1 wk after therapy. A second application is indicated if lice are detected at this time ▪ Eradication of scabies following one application.

PERPHENAZINE

(per-**fen**-a-zeen)
{Apo-Perphenazine}, {Phenazine}, Trilafon

CLASSIFICATION(S):
Antipsychotic—phenothiazine, Antiemetic—phenothiazine
Pregnancy Category UK

INDICATIONS

▪ Treatment of acute and chronic psychoses ▪ Management of nausea and vomiting.

ACTION

▪ Alters the effects of dopamine in the CNS ▪ Possesses significant anticholinergic and alpha-adrenergic blocking activity ▪ Blocks dopamine in the chemoreceptor trigger zone (CTZ). **Therapeutic Effects:** ▪ Diminished signs and symptoms of psychoses ▪ Decreased nausea and vomiting.

PHARMACOKINETICS

Absorption: Absorption from tablet is variable; may be better with oral liquid formulations. Well absorbed following IM administration.
Distribution: Widely distributed, high concentrations in the CNS. Crosses the placenta and enters breast milk.
Metabolism and Excretion: Highly metabolized by the liver and GI mucosa. Some conversion to active compounds.
Half-life: UK.

CONTRAINDICATIONS AND PRECAUTIONS

Contraindicated in: ▪ Hypersensitivity ▪ Cross-sensitivity with other phenothiazines may exist ▪ Narrow-angle glaucoma ▪ Bone marrow depression ▪ Severe liver or cardiovascular disease ▪ Intestinal obstruction.
Use Cautiously in: ▪ Elderly or debilitated patients ▪ Pregnancy or lactation (safety not established) ▪ Diabetes mellitus ▪ Respiratory disease ▪ Prostatic hypertrophy ▪ CNS tumors ▪ History of seizure disorder.

ADVERSE REACTIONS AND SIDE EFFECTS*

CNS: sedation, extrapyramidal reactions, tardive dyskinesia, NEUROLEPTIC MALIGNANT SYNDROME.
CV: hypotension, tachycardia.
EENT: dry eyes, blurred vision, lens opacities.
GI: constipation, dry mouth, ileus, anorexia, hepatitis.
GU: urinary retention.

{} = Available in Canada only.
*Underlines indicate most frequent; **CAPITALS** indicate life-threatening.

Derm: rashes, photosensitivity, pigment changes.
Endo: galactorrhea.
Hemat: AGRANULOCYTOSIS, leukopenia.
Metab: hyperthermia.
Misc: allergic reactions.

INTERACTIONS

Drug-Drug: ▪ Additive hypotension with **antihypertensive agents,** acute ingestion of **alcohol,** or **nitrates** ▪ Additive CNS depression with **MAO inhibitors** or other **CNS depressants,** including **alcohol, antihistamines, narcotic analgesics, sedative/hypnotics,** and **general anesthetics** ▪ Additive anticholinergic effects with other **drugs possessing anticholinergic properties,** including **antihistamines, antidepressants, atropine, disopyramide, haloperidol,** and **other phenothiazines** ▪ Hypotension and tachycardia may occur with **epinephrine** ▪ Increased risk of agranulocytosis with **antithyroid agents** ▪ Increased risk of extrapyramidal reactions with **lithium** ▪ May mask **lithium** toxicity ▪ **Antacids** or **lithium** may decrease absorption of perphenazine ▪ May decrease antiparkinson effect of **levodopa.**

ROUTE AND DOSAGE

Psychoses

- **PO (Adults):** 8–16 mg 2–4 times daily.
- **PO (Children >12 yr):** 6–12 mg/day in divided doses.
- **IM (Adults and Children >12 yr):** 5 mg initially (can use up to 10 mg), may repeat 5 mg in 6 hr.

Nausea and Vomiting

- **PO (Adults):** 8–16 mg/day in divided doses (up to 24 mg/day) or 8 mg ER tablet bid.
- **IM (Adults):** 5–10 mg.

Severe Nausea, Vomiting

- **IV (Adults):** 1 mg at 1–2-min intervals to a total of 5 mg or as an infusion at a rate not to exceed 1 mg/min.

PHARMACODYNAMICS (PO, IM = antipsychotic effect,* IV = antiemetic effect)

	ONSET	PEAK	DURATION
PO	2–6 hr	UK	6–12 hr
IM	2–6 hr	UK	6–12 hr
IV	rapid	UK	UK

*Optimal antipsychotic response may not occur for several wks.

NURSING IMPLICATIONS

Assessment

- **General Info:** Assess patient's mental status (orientation, mood, behavior) prior to and periodically throughout therapy.
- Monitor blood pressure (sitting, standing, lying), pulse, and respiratory rate prior to and frequently during the period of dosage adjustment.
- Observe patient carefully when administering medication to ensure that medication is actually taken and not hoarded.
- Observe patient carefully for extrapyramidal symptoms (akathesia—restlessness; dystonia—muscle spasm and twisting motions; or pseudoparkinsonism—mask facies, pill-rolling motions, drooling, tremors, rigidity, shuffling gait, dysphagia). Notify physician immediately at the onset of these symptoms, as a reduction of dosage or discontinuation of medication may be necessary. Physician may also order antiparkinsonian agents (trihexylphenidyl or benztropine) to control these symptoms.
- Monitor for tardive dyskinesia (uncontrolled movements of face, mouth, tongue, or jaw and involuntary movements of extremities). Notify physician immediately if these symptoms occur, as these side effects may be irreversible.
- Monitor for development of neuroleptic malignant syndrome (fever, respiratory distress, tachycardia, convulsions, diaphoresis, hypertension or

hypotension, pallor, tiredness). Notify physician immediately if these symptoms occur.

- **Antiemetic:** Assess nausea and vomiting prior to and following perphenazine administration.
- Monitor intake and output. Patients with severe nausea and vomiting may require IV fluids with electrolytes in addition to antiemetics.
- **Lab Test Considerations:** May cause false-positive and false-negative pregnancy tests.
- May cause blood dyscrasias; monitor CBC periodically throughout course of therapy.
- Monitor liver function tests, urine bilirubin, and bile for evidence of hepatic toxicity periodically throughout course of therapy. Urine bilirubin may be falsely elevated.

Potential Nursing Diagnoses

- Thought processes, altered (indications).
- Knowledge deficit related to medication regimen (patient/family teaching).
- Noncompliance (patient/family teaching).

Implementation

- **General Info:** Available in tablet, repetabs, oral concentrate, and injectable forms.
- Available in combination with amitriptyline (see Appendix A).
- To prevent contact dermatitis, avoid getting liquid preparations on hands, and wash hands thoroughly if spillage occurs.
- **PO:** Do not crush or chew extended-release tablets.
- Dilute concentrate just prior to administration in 120 ml of water, milk, carbonated beverage, soup, or tomato or fruit juice. Do not mix with beverages containing caffeine (cola, coffee), tannics (tea), or pectinates (apple juice).
- **IM:** Inject deep into well-developed muscle. Keep patient in recumbent position and monitor for at least 30 min following injection. Slight yellow color will not alter potency; do not use if soln is dark or contains a precipitate.
- **Direct IV:** Dilute to a concentration of 0.5 mg/ml with 0.9% NaCl.
- *Rate:* Administer each 1 mg over at least 1 min.
- **Syringe Compatibility:** atropine, butorphanol, chlorpromazine, cimetidine, dimenhydrinate, diphenhydramine, droperidol, fentanyl, meperidine, metoclopramide, morphine, pentazocine, prochlorperazine, promethazine, ranitidine, or scopolamine.
- **Syringe Incompatibility:** midazolam, pentobarbital, or thiethylperazine.
- **Y-Site Compatibility:** acyclovir, amikacin, ampicillin, azlocillin, cefamandole, cefazoline, ceforanide, cefotaxime, cefoxitin, cefuroxime, cephalothin, cephapirin, chloramphenicol, clindamycin, co-trimoxazole, doxycycline, erythromycin lactobionate, famotidine, gentamicin, kanamycin, metronidazole, mezlocillin, minocycline, moxalactam, nafcillin, oxacillin, penicillin G potassium, piperacillin, tetracycline, ticarcillin, ticarcillin/clavulanate, tobramycin, or vancomycin.
- **Y-Site Incompatibility:** cefoperazone.

Patient/Family Teaching

- Advise patient to take medication exactly as directed and not to skip doses or double up on missed doses. If a dose is missed, it should be taken as soon as remembered unless almost time for the next dose. If more than 2 doses a day are ordered, the missed dose should be taken within 1 hr of the scheduled time or omitted. Abrupt withdrawal may lead to gastritis, nausea, vomiting, dizziness, headache, tachycardia, and insomnia.
- Inform patient of possibility of extrapyramidal symptoms and tardive dys-

kinesia. Caution patient to report these symptoms immediately to physician.

- □ Advise patient to make position changes slowly to minimize orthostatic hypotension.
- □ Medication may cause drowsiness. Caution patient to avoid driving or other activities requiring alertness until response to medication is known.
- □ Caution patient to avoid taking alcohol or other CNS depressants concurrently with this medication.
- □ Advise patient to use sunscreen and protective clothing when exposed to the sun. Exposed surfaces may develop a blue-gray pigmentation, which may fade following discontinuation of the medication. Extremes in temperature should also be avoided, as this drug impairs body temperature regulation.
- □ Instruct patient to notify physician if urinary retention, uncontrolled movements, rash, fever, or yellow coloration of skin occurs or if dry mouth or constipation persists. Sugarless candy or gum may diminish dry mouth, and an increase in fluid intake, bulk, or exercise may prevent constipation.
- □ Advise patient to notify physician or dentist of medication regimen prior to treatment or surgery.
- □ Inform patient that this medication may turn urine pink to reddish-brown.
- □ Emphasize the importance of routine follow-up examinations, including ocular examinations, with long-term therapy and continued participation in psychotherapy.

EVALUATION

Effectiveness of therapy can be demonstrated by: ▪ Decrease in excitable, paranoic, or withdrawn behavior ▪ Relief of nausea and vomiting.

PHENAZOPYRIDINE

(fen-az-oh-**peer**-i-deen)
Azo-Standard, Baridium, Eridium, Geridium, {Phenazo}, Phenazodine, Pyrazodine, Pyridiate, Pyridin, Pyridium, {Pyronium}, Urodine, Urogesic, Viridium

CLASSIFICATION(S):
Non-narcotic analgesic—urinary tract analgesic
Pregnancy Category B

INDICATIONS

▪ Provides relief from the following urinary tract symptoms, which may occur in association with infection or following urologic procedures: □ Pain □ Itching □ Burning □ Urgency □ Frequency.

ACTION

▪ Acts locally on the urinary tract mucosa to produce analgesic or local anesthetic effects ▪ Has no antimicrobial activity. **Therapeutic Effect:** Diminished urinary tract discomfort.

PHARMACOKINETICS

Absorption: Appears to be well absorbed following oral administration.
Distribution: Distribution not known. Small amounts cross the placenta.
Metabolism and Excretion: Rapidly excreted unchanged in the urine.
Half-life: UK.

CONTRAINDICATIONS AND PRECAUTIONS

Contraindicated in: ▪ Hypersensitivity ▪ Glomerulonephritis ▪ Pregnancy or lactation ▪ Severe hepatitis, uremia, or renal failure.
Use Cautiously in: ▪ Renal insufficiency ▪ Hepatitis.

ADVERSE REACTIONS AND SIDE EFFECTS*

CNS: headache, vertigo.
GI: nausea, hepatotoxicity.

{} = Available in Canada only.

*Underlines indicate most frequent; **CAPITALS** indicate life-threatening.

GU: renal failure, bright-orange urine.
Derm: rash.
Hemat: methemoglobinemia, hemolytic anemia.

INTERACTIONS

Drug–Drug: ▪ None significant.

ROUTE AND DOSAGE

- **PO (Adults):** 200 mg tid.
- **PO (Children):** 12 mg/kg/day in 3 divided doses.

PHARMACODYNAMICS (urinary analgesia)

	ONSET	PEAK	DURATION
PO	UK	5–6 hr	6–8 hr

NURSING IMPLICATIONS

Assessment

- □ Assess patient for urgency, frequency, and pain on urination prior to and throughout therapy.
- ▪ **Lab Test Considerations:** Renal function should be monitored periodically during course of therapy.
- □ Interferes with urine tests based on color reactions (glucose, ketones, bilirubin, steroids, protein). Use Clinitest to test urine glucose concentration.

Potential Nursing Diagnoses

- ▪ Comfort, altered: pain (indications).
- ▪ Urinary elimination, altered patterns (indications).
- ▪ Knowledge deficit related to medication regimen (patient/family teaching).

Implementation

- ▪ **General Info:** Medication should be discontinued after pain or discomfort is relieved (usually 2 days for treatment of urinary tract infection). Concurrent antibiotic therapy should continue for full prescribed duration.
- ▪ **PO:** Administer medication with or following meals to decrease GI irritation.

Patient/Family Teaching

- □ Instruct patient to take medication exactly as directed. If a dose is missed, take as soon as remembered unless almost time for next dose.
- □ Advise patient that while phenazopyridine administration is stopped once pain or discomfort is relieved, concurrent antibiotic therapy must be continued for full duration of therapy.
- □ Inform patient that drug causes reddish-orange discoloration of urine that may stain clothing or bedding. Sanitary napkin may be worn to avoid clothing stains.
- □ Instruct patient to notify physician if rash, skin discoloration, or unusual tiredness occurs.

Evaluation

Effectiveness of therapy can be demonstrated by: ▪ Decrease in pain and burning on urination.

PHENOBARBITAL

(fee-noe-**bar**-bi-tal)
Barbita, Luminal, Solfoton

CLASSIFICATION(S):
Anticonvulsant—barbiturate, Sedative/hypnotic—barbiturate
Schedule IV
Pregnancy Category D

INDICATIONS

▪ Anticonvulsant in tonic-clonic (grand mal), partial, and febrile seizures in children ▪ Preoperative sedative and in other situations in which sedation may be required ▪ Hypnotic. **Unlabeled Uses:** ▪ Prevention and treatment of neonatal hyperbilirubinemia ▪ Lowering of bilirubin and lipid levels in chronic cholestasis.

ACTION

▪ Produces all levels of CNS depression ▪ Depresses the sensory cortex, decreases motor activity, and alters cerebellar function ▪ Inhibits transmission in the nervous system and raises the seizure threshold ▪ Capable of inducing (speeding up) enzymes in the liver that metabolize drugs, bilirubin, and other compounds. **Therapeutic Effects:** ▪ Anticonvulsant activity ▪ Sedation.

PHARMACOKINETICS

Absorption: Absorption is slow but relatively complete (70–90%).
Distribution: Distribution not known.
Metabolism and Excretion: 75% metabolized by the liver, 25% excreted unchanged by the kidneys.
Half-life: 2–6 days.

CONTRAINDICATIONS AND PRECAUTIONS

Contraindicated in: ▪ Hypersensitivity ▪ Comatose patients or those with pre-existing CNS depression ▪ Uncontrolled severe pain ▪ Lactation.
Use Cautiously in: ▪ Pregnancy (chronic use results in drug dependency in the infant; may result in coagulation defects and fetal malformation; acute use at term may result in respiratory depression in the newborn) ▪ Hepatic dysfunction ▪ Severe renal impairment ▪ Patients who may be suicidal or who may have been addicted to drugs previously ▪ Elderly patients (dosage reduction recommended) ▪ Hypnotic use should be short-term. Chronic use may lead to dependence.

ADVERSE REACTIONS AND SIDE EFFECTS*

CNS: drowsiness, lethargy, vertigo, depression, <u>hangover</u>, excitation, delirium.
Resp: respiratory depression, LARYNGOSPASM (IV only), bronchospasm (IV only).
CV: hypotension (IV only).
GI: nausea, vomiting, diarrhea, constipation.
Derm: rashes, urticaria, photosensitivity.
Local: phlebitis at IV site.
MS: mylagia, arthralgia, neuralgia.
Misc: hypersensitivity reactions, including ANGIOEDEMA and serum sickness; physical dependence, psychological dependence.

INTERACTIONS

Drug-Drug: ▪ Additive CNS depression with other **CNS depressants,** including **alcohol, antihistamines, narcotic analgesics,** and other **sedative/hypnotics** ▪ May induce hepatic enzymes that metabolize other drugs, decreasing their effectiveness, including **oral contraceptives, oral anticoagulants, chloramphenicol, cyclosporine, dacarbazine, glucocorticoids, tricyclic antidepressants,** and **quinidine** ▪ May increase the risk of hepatic toxicity of **acetaminophen** ▪ **MAO inhibitors, valproic acid,** or **divalproex** may decrease the metabolism of phenobarbital, increasing sedation ▪ May increase the risk of hemotologic toxicity with **cyclophosphamide**.

ROUTE AND DOSAGE

Anticonvulsant

- **PO (Adults):** 100–300 mg/day, single dose or 2–3 divided doses.
- **PO (Children):** 3–5 mg/kg/day, single dose or divided doses.
- **IV (Adults):** 200–600 mg (total of 600 mg/24 hr period).
- **IV (Children):** 100–400 mg.

Status Epilepticus

- **IV (Adults):** 10–20 mg/kg, may be repeated.
- **IV (Children):** 15–20 mg/kg.

Sedation

- **PO (Adults):** 30–120 mg/day in 2–3 divided doses.
- **PO (Children):** 2 mg/kg 3 times daily.
- **IM (Adults):** 30–120 mg/day in 2–3 divided doses.

Preoperative Sedation

- **IM (Adults):** 130–200 mg 60–90 min preop.
- **PO, IM, IV (Children):** 1–3 mg/kg.

Hypnotic

- **PO (Adults):** 100–320 mg at bedtime.
- **IV, IM, SC (Adults):** 100–325 mg at bedtime.
- **IV, IM, SC (Children):** 3–5 mg/kg at bedtime.

*<u>Underlines</u> indicate most frequent; **CAPITALS** indicate life-threatening.

P

Hyperbilirubinemia

- **PO (Adults):** 30–60 mg 3 times daily.
- **PO (Children up to 12 yr):** 1–4 mg/kg 3 times daily.
- **PO, IM (Neonates):** 5–10 mg/kg/day.

PHARMACODYNAMICS (noted as sedation; full anticonvulsant effects occur after 2–3 wk of chronic dosing)

	ONSET	PEAK	DURATION
PO	30–60 min	UK	>6 hr
IM, SC	10–30 min	UK	4–6 hr
IV	5 min	30 min	4–6 hr

NURSING IMPLICATIONS

Assessment

- **General Info:** Monitor respiratory status, pulse, and blood pressure frequently in patients receiving phenobarbital IV. Equipment for resuscitation and artificial ventilation should be readily available. Respiratory depression is dose-dependent.
- □ Prolonged therapy may lead to psychological or physical dependence. Restrict amount of drug available to patient, especially if depressed, suicidal, or previously addicted.
- **Seizures:** Assess location, duration, and characteristics of seizure activity.
- **Sedation:** Assess level of consciousness and anxiety when used as a preoperative sedative.
- □ Assess postoperative patients for pain. Phenobarbital may increase responsiveness to painful stimuli.
- **Lab Test Considerations:** Patients on prolonged therapy should have hepatic and renal function and CBC evaluated periodically.
- **Toxicity and Overdose:** Serum phenobarbital levels should be routinely monitored when used as an anticonvulsant. Therapeutic blood levels are 10–40 mcg/ml. Symptoms of toxicity include confusion, drowsiness, dyspnea, slurred speech, and staggering.

Potential Nursing Diagnoses

- Injury, high risk for (indications, side effects).
- Knowledge deficit related to medication regimen (patient/family teaching).

Implementation

- **General Info:** Supervise ambulation and transfer of patients following administration. Remove cigarettes. Side rails should be raised and call bell within reach at all times. Keep bed in low position. Institute seizure precautions.
- □ When changing from phenobarbital to another anticonvulsant, gradually decrease phenobarbital dose while concurrently increasing dose of replacement medication to maintain anticonvulsant effects.
- □ Available in capsule, tablet, oral soln, elixir, and injectable forms. Also available in combination with many other drugs (see Appendix A).
- **PO:** Tablets may be crushed and mixed with food or fluids (do not administer dry) for patients with difficulty swallowing. Oral soln may be taken undiluted or mixed with water, milk, or fruit juice. Use calibrated measuring device for accurate measurement of liquid doses.
- **SC:** Sterile phenobarbital sodium may be administered SC after reconstitution, but phenobarbital sodium injection is not recommended for SC use.
- **IM:** Injections should be given deep into the gluteal muscle to minimize tissue irritation. Do not inject >5 ml into any one site, because of tissue irritation.
- **IV:** Doses may require 15–30 min to reach peak concentrations in the brain. Administer minimal dose and wait for effectiveness before administering second dose to prevent cumulative barbiturate-induced depression.
- **Direct IV:** Reconstitute sterile powder for IV dose with a minimum of 10 ml of sterile water for injection. Dilute further with 10 ml of sterile water. Do not use soln that is not absolutely clear within 5 min after reconstitution or that contains a precipitate. Discard

powder or soln that has been exposed to air for >30 min.

- Soln is highly alkaline; avoid extravasation, which may cause tissue damage and necrosis. If extravasation occurs, injection of 5% procaine soln into affected area and application of moist heat may be ordered.
- *Rate:* Administer each 1 grain (60 mg) over at least 1 min. Titrate slowly for desired response. Rapid administration may result in respiratory depression.
- **Syringe Compatibility:** heparin.
- **Syringe Incompatibility:** benzquinamide, dimenhydrinate, diphenhydramine, erythromycin gluceptate, hydroxyzine, kanamycin, oxytetracycline, phenytoin, prochlorperazine, promazine, promethazine, ranitidine, or tetracycline.
- **Solution/Additive Compatibility:** D5W, D10W, 0.45% NaCl, 0.9% NaCl, Ringer's and lactated Ringer's soln, dextrose/saline combinations, dextrose/Ringer's or dextrose/lactated Ringer's combinations, amikacin, aminophylline, calcium chloride, calcium gluceptate, cephapirin, colistimethate, dimenhydrinate, polymyxin B, sodium bicarbonate, thiopental, or verapamil.
- **Additive Incompatibility:** cephalothin, chlorpromazine, codeine, ephedrine, hydralazine, hydrocortisone sodium succinate, hydroxyzine, insulin, levorphanol, meperidine, methadone, morphine, norepinephrine, pentazocine, procaine, prochlorperazine mesylate, promazine, promethazine, streptomycin, or vancomycin.

Patient/Family Teaching

- Advise patient to take medication exactly as prescribed. If a dose is missed, take as soon as remembered if not almost time for next dose; do not double doses.
- Advise patients on prolonged therapy not to discontinue medication without consulting physician. Abrupt withdrawal may precipitate seizures or status epilepticus.
- Medication may cause daytime drowsiness. Caution patient to avoid driving and other activities requiring alertness until response to medication is known. Do not resume driving until physician gives clearance based on control of seizure disorder.
- Caution patient to avoid taking alcohol or other CNS depressants concurrently with this medication.
- Instruct patient to contact physician immediately if pregnancy is suspected.
- Advise patient to notify physician if fever, sore throat, mouth sores, unusual bleeding or bruising, nosebleeds, or petechiae occur.

Evaluation

Effectiveness of therapy can be demonstrated by: ▪ Decrease or cessation of seizure activity without excessive sedation. Several wks may be required to achieve maximum anticonvulsant effects ▪ Preoperative sedation ▪ Improvement in sleep patterns.

PHENOLPHTHALEIN

(fee-nole-**thay**-leen)

Alophen Pills, Correctol, Espotabs, Evac-U-Gen, Evac-U-Lax, Ex-Lax, Ex-Lax Pills, Feen-a-Mint, Feen-a-Mint Gum, Lax-Pills, Modane, Modane Mild, No. 973, Phenolax

CLASSIFICATION(S):
Laxative—stimulant
Pregnancy Category UK

INDICATIONS

- Treatment of constipation (short-term).

ACTION

▪ Initiates peristalsis by acting directly on mucosa, stimulating myenteric plexus ▪ Alters fluid and electrolyte

P

transport, producing fluid accumulation in the small intestine ▪ Action requires the presence of bile. **Therapeutic Effect:** ▪ Evacuation of the colon.

PHARMACOKINETICS

Absorption: 15% absorbed following oral administration. Action is primarily local in intestine.
Distribution: Small amounts excreted in breast milk.
Metabolism and Excretion: Eliminated by kidneys and in feces.
Half-life: UK.

CONTRAINDICATIONS AND PRECAUTIONS

Contraindicated in: ▪ Hypersensitivity ▪ Abdominal pain of unknown cause, especially if associated with fever ▪ Rectal fissures ▪ Ulcerated hemorrhoids.
Use Cautiously in: ▪ Chronic use (may lead to laxative dependence) ▪ Pregnancy or lactation (safety not established) ▪ Possibility of intestinal obstruction.

ADVERSE REACTIONS AND SIDE EFFECTS*

GI: nausea, abdominal cramps, diarrhea, rectal burning.
MS: muscle weakness (chronic use).
F and E: hypokalemia (chronic use).
Misc: protein-losing enteropathy, tetany (chronic use).

INTERACTIONS

Drug–Drug: ▪ May decrease the absorption of other **orally administered drugs** because of increased motility and decreased transit time.

ROUTE AND DOSAGE

- **PO (Adults and Children >12 yr):** 30–270 mg/day as a single dose or in divided doses.
- **PO (Children 6–11 yr):** 30–60 mg/day as a single dose or in divided doses.
- **PO (Children 2–5 yr):** 15–30 mg/day as a single dose or in divided doses.

PHARMACODYNAMICS (laxative effect)

	ONSET	PEAK	DURATION
PO	6–10 hr	UK	several days

NURSING IMPLICATIONS

Assessment

- Assess patient for abdominal distention, presence of bowel sounds, and usual pattern of bowel function.
- Assess color, consistency, and amount of stool produced.

Potential Nursing Diagnoses

- Bowel elimination, altered: constipation (indications).
- Bowel elimination, altered: diarrhea (side effects).
- Knowledge deficit related to medication regimen (patient/family teaching).

Implementation

- **General Info:** Available in tablet, liquid, chewing gum, and wafers. Available in combination with docusate, cascara, and mineral oil (see Appendix A).
- **PO:** Take with a full glass of water. Administer at bedtime for bowel movement 6–12 hr later. Administer on an empty stomach for more rapid results.
- Chewable tablets should not be swallowed whole. Chew well before swallowing.

Patient/Family Teaching

- Advise patient that laxatives should be used only for short-term therapy. Long-term therapy may cause electrolyte imbalance and dependence.
- Encourage patient to utilize other forms of bowel regulation, such as increasing bulk in the diet, fluid intake, and mobility. Normal bowel habits are individualized and may vary from 3 times/day to 3 times/wk.
- Inform patient that this medication may cause a color change in feces and

*Underlines indicate most frequent; **CAPITALS** indicate life-threatening.

urine to pink, red, yellow, or brown.
- Instruct patient with cardiac disease to avoid straining during bowel movements (Valsalva maneuver).
- Advise patient not to use laxatives when abdominal pain, nausea, vomiting, or fever is present.

EVALUATION

Effectiveness of therapy can be demonstrated by: ▪ Soft, formed bowel movement. Laxative effects may last for up to 3 days.

PHENOXYBENZAMINE

(fen-ox-ee-**ben**-za-meen)
Dibenzyline

CLASSIFICATION(S):
Antihypertensive—alpha-adrenergic blocking agent
Pregnancy Category UK

INDICATIONS

▪ Management of symptoms of pheochromocytoma (particularly hypertension and sweating) due to adrenergic (sympathomimetic) excess ▪ Treatment of hypertension associated with adrenergic excess, including that produced by tyramine-containing foods in patients receiving MAO inhibitor therapy. **Unlabeled Uses:** ▪ Treatment of peripheral vascular disease.

ACTION

▪ Produces long-lasting blockade of alpha-adrenergic receptors in smooth muscle and exocrine glands ▪ Blocks epinephrine- and norepinephrine-induced vasoconstriction, resulting in hypotension and tachycardia. **Therapeutic Effect:** ▪ Reduction of symptoms of pheochromocytoma.

PHARMACOKINETICS

Absorption: Variably absorbed from the GI tract.
Distribution: Distribution not known.
Metabolism and Excretion: Mostly metabolized by the liver.
Half-life: 24 hr.

CONTRAINDICATIONS AND PRECAUTIONS

Contraindicated in: ▪ Shock (if fluid deficits have not been corrected).
Use Cautiously in: ▪ Coronary or cerebral arteriosclerosis ▪ Renal impairment ▪ Pregnancy (although safety not established, has been used safely in the third trimester of pregnancy) ▪ Lactation or children ▪ Elderly patients (more susceptible to hypotensive effects; dosage reduction recommended) ▪ Peptic ulcer disease ▪ Respiratory infection.

ADVERSE REACTIONS AND SIDE EFFECTS*

CNS: drowsiness, sedation, tiredness, weakness, malaise, confusion, headache, dizziness.
EENT: miosis, nasal congestion.
CV: hypotension, tachycardia, congestive heart failure, angina.
GI: nausea, vomiting, diarrhea, dry mouth.
GU: inhibition of ejaculation.

INTERACTIONS

Drug-Drug: ▪ Antagonizes the effects of **alpha-adrenergic stimulants** ▪ May decrease the pressor response to **ephedrine, phenylephrine,** or **methoxamine** ▪ Hypotension, vasodilation, and tachycardia may be exaggerated by **drugs that stimulate both alpha and beta receptors,** such as **epinephrine** ▪ Use with **guanethidine** or **guanadrel** may result in exaggerated hypotension and bradycardia ▪ Decreases peripheral vasoconstriction from high doses of **dopamine** ▪ Additive CNS depression may occur with concurrent use of **antihistamines, antidepressants, alcohol, narcotic analgesics,** or **sedative/hypnotics**.

ROUTE AND DOSAGE

Note: Requires individual titration.

▪ **PO (Adults):** 10 mg once daily, increase by 10 mg/day at 4-day inter-

*Underlines indicate most frequent; **CAPITALS** indicate life-threatening.

P

vals. Usual maintenance dose is 20–40 mg/day, 2–3 times daily.

- **PO (Children):** 0.2 mg/kg or 6 mg/m^2 daily, initial dose not to exceed 10 mg. Usual pediatric maintenance dose is 0.4–1.2 mg/kg/day or 12–36 mg/m^2/day in 3–4 divided doses (not labeled for use in children).

PHARMACODYNAMICS (alpha-adrenergic blockade)

	ONSET	PEAK	DURATION
PO	1–4 hr	1 wk	3–4 days

NURSING IMPLICATIONS

Assessment

- Monitor blood pressure (sitting and lying), pulse, respiratory status, and diaphoretic episodes frequently, especially during initiation of therapy.
- **Lab Test Considerations:** Urinary catecholamine measurements should be made periodically to determine maximal dose.

Potential Nursing Diagnoses

- Tissue perfusion, altered (indications).
- Injury, high risk for (side effects).
- Knowledge deficit related to medication regimen (patient/family teaching).

Implementation

- **General Info:** Concurrent use of a beta-adrenergic blocker may be necessary to control reflex tachycardia.
- **PO:** May be administered with meals or milk if GI irritation becomes a problem. Dosage reduction may be required.

Patient/Family Teaching

- Instruct patient to take medication exactly as directed at the same time each day. Do not skip or double up on missed doses. Consult physician prior to discontinuation.
- Medication may cause drowsiness or dizziness. Caution patient to avoid driving or other activities requiring alertness until response to medication is known.
- Caution patient to make position changes slowly to minimize orthostatic hypotension. Standing for long periods or exercising during hot weather may also induce orthostatic hypotension.
- Inform patient that good oral hygiene, frequent mouth rinses, and sugarless gum or candy may reduce dryness of mouth. The physician or dentist should be notified if dryness persists >2 wk. Regular dental care is recommended, as a dry mouth may increase risk of caries and periodontal disease.
- Advise patient to avoid use of alcohol or over-the-counter cold preparations without consulting physician or pharmacist.
- Inform patient that medication may cause nasal congestion, inhibition of ejaculation, and constriction of pupils, which may interfere with night vision. These effects usually decrease with continued therapy. Notify physician if these side effects persist.
- Advise patient to inform physician or dentist of medication regimen prior to treatment or surgery.

Evaluation

Effectiveness of therapy can be demonstrated by: ▪ Decrease in blood pressure, pulse, and sweating in patients with pheochromocytoma ▪ Decrease in blood pressure due to adrenergic excess. May require 1 wk of therapy for full therapeutic effects to be apparent.

PHENTOLAMINE

(fen-**tole**-a-meen)
Regitine, {Rogitine}

CLASSIFICATION(S):
Alpha-adrenergic blocking agent
Pregnancy Category UK

INDICATIONS

- Treatment of hypertension associated with pheochromocytoma or adrenergic (sympathetic) excess, such as administration of phenylephrine, tyramine-containing foods in patients on MAO inhibitor therapy, or clonidine withdrawal ▪ Control of blood pressure during surgical removal of a pheochromocytoma ▪ Prevention and treatment of dermal necrosis and sloughing following extravasation of norepinephrine, phenylephrine, or dopamine. **Unlabeled Use:** ▪ Adjunct therapy of impotence (intracavernosal).

ACTION

▪ Produces incomplete and short-lived blockade of alpha-adrenergic receptors located primarily in smooth muscle and exocrine glands ▪ Induces hypotension by direct relaxation of vascular smooth muscle and by alpha blockade. **Therapeutic Effects:** ▪ Reduction of blood pressure in situations in which hypertension is due to adrenergic (sympathetic) excess. ▪ When infiltrated locally, reverses vasoconstriction caused by norepinephrine or dopamine.

PHARMACOKINETICS

Absorption: Well absorbed following IM administration.
Distribution: Distribution not known.
Metabolism and Excretion: 10% excreted unchanged by kidneys.
Half-life: UK.

CONTRAINDICATIONS AND PRECAUTIONS

Contraindicated in: ▪ Hypersensitivity ▪ Coronary or cerebral arteriosclerosis ▪ Renal impairment.
Use Cautiously in: ▪ Pregnancy or lactation (safety not established) ▪ Peptic ulcer disease ▪ Elderly patients (more susceptible to hypotensive effects; dosage reduction recommended).

ADVERSE REACTIONS AND SIDE EFFECTS*

CNS: CEREBROVASCULAR SPASM, weakness, dizziness.
CV: HYPOTENSION, tachycardia, arrhythmias, angina, MYOCARDIAL INFARCTION.
Derm: flushing.
EENT: nasal stuffiness.
GI: abdominal pain, nausea, vomiting, diarrhea, aggravation of peptic ulcer.

INTERACTIONS

Drug-Drug: ▪ Antagonizes the effects of **alpha-adrenergic stimulants** ▪ May decrease the pressor response to **ephedrine, phenylephrine,** or **methoxamine** ▪ Hypotension, vasodilation, and tachycardia may be exaggerated by **drugs that stimulate both alpha and beta receptors,** such as **epinephrine** ▪ Use with **guanethidine** or **guanedrel** may result in exaggerated hypotension and bradycardia ▪ Decreases peripheral vasoconstriction from high doses of **dopamine**.

ROUTE AND DOSAGE

Diagnosis of Pheochromocytoma

- **IM, IV (Adults):** 5 mg (may be given IM, but IV is preferred).
- **IV (Children):** 1 mg or 3 mg/m^2 or 0.1 mg/kg.
- **IM (Children):** 3 mg.

Hypertension Associated with Pheochromocytoma—During Surgery

- **IV, IM (Adults):** 5 mg given 1–2 hr preop, repeated as necessary.
- **IV, IM (Children):** 1 mg or 0.1 mg/kg or 3 mg/m^2 given 1–2 hr preop, repeated as necessary.

Prevention of Dermal Necrosis Following Extravasation of Norepinephrine, Phenylephrine, or Dopamine

- **Infiltrate:** 5–10 mg phentolamine in 10 ml of 0.9% NaCl within 12 hr of extravasation.

Prevention of Dermal Necrosis During Infusion of Norepinephrine

- Add 10 mg phentolamine to every 1000 ml of fluid containing norepinephrine.

Adjunct Therapy of Impotence

- **Intracavernosal (Adults):** 0.5–1 mg with 30–60 mg papaverine (not to exceed 3 treatments/wk).

*Underlines indicate most frequent; **CAPITALS** indicate life-threatening.

PHARMACODYNAMICS (IM, IV = alpha-adrenergic blockade, Intracavernosal = erection)

	ONSET	PEAK	DURATION
IM	UK	20 min	30–45 min
IV	immediate	2 min	15–30 min
Intra-cavernosal	10 min	UK	4 hr

NURSING IMPLICATIONS

Assessment

- Monitor blood pressure, pulse, and ECG every 2 min until stable during IV administration. If hypotensive crisis occurs, epinephrine is contraindicated and may cause paradoxical further decrease in blood pressure; norepinephrine may be used.

Potential Nursing Diagnoses

- Tissue perfusion, altered (indications).
- Injury, high risk for (indications).
- Knowledge deficit related to medication regimen (patient/family teaching).

Implementation

- **General Info:** Patient should remain supine throughout parenteral administration.
- **IV:** Reconstitute each 5 mg with 1 ml of sterile water for injection or 0.9% NaCl. Discard unused soln.
- **Direct IV:** Inject each 5 mg over 1 min.
- **Continuous Infusion:** Dilute 5–10 mg in 500 ml of D5W.
- *Rate:* Titrate infusion rate according to patient response.
- May also add 10 mg to every 1000 ml of fluid containing norepinephrine for prevention of dermal necrosis and sloughing. Does not affect pressor effect of norepinephrine.
- **Syringe Compatibility:** papaverine.
- **Additive Compatibility:** dobutamine or verapamil.
- **Infiltration:** Dilute with 5–10 ml of 0.9% NaCl. Infiltrate site of extravasation promptly. Must be given within 12 hr of extravasation to be effective.
- **Impotence:** Has been used with papaverine to treat men with impotence, usually associated with spinal cord injury. This method requires special training. Administration is by injection into the corpus cavernosum, producing an erection. Risk of priapism exists.

Patient/Family Teaching

- Advise patient to make position changes slowly to minimize orthostatic hypotension.
- Instruct patient to notify physician if chest pain occurs during IV infusion.

Evaluation

Clinical response to therapy is indicated by: ▪ Decrease in blood pressure ▪ Prevention of dermal necrosis and sloughing in extravasation of norepinephrine, dopamine, and phenylephrine ▪ Erection in men with impotence, beginning 10 min after injection into corpus cavernosum and sustained for up to 4 hr.

PHENYLEPHRINE
(fen-il-**eff**-rin)

PHENYLEPHRINE NASAL
Alcon-Efrin, Coricidin Nasal Mist, Doktors, Duration Mild, Neo-Synephrine, Nostril, Rhinall, Sinex

PHENYLEPHRINE OPHTHALMIC
Ak-Dilate, Ak-Nefrin, I-Liqui-Tears-Plus, I-Phrine, Isopto Frin, {Minims Phenylephrine}, Mydfrin, Neo-Synephrine, Prefrin Liquifilm, Relief

PHENYLEPHRINE PARENTERAL
Neo-Synephrine

CLASSIFICATION(S):
Vasopressor, Decongestant, Ophthalmic—mydriatic
Pregnancy Category C (Ophth, Parenteral)

{} = Available in Canada only.

INDICATIONS

■ **SC, IM, IV:** Adjunct in the treatment of shock—to correct hypotension that may persist after adequate fluid replacement ■ **Ophth:** Mydriatic ■ **Nasal, Ophth:** Decongestant ■ As an adjunct in spinal anesthesia (to prolong duration of anesthesia) ■ As an adjunct in regional anesthesia (to localize effect).

ACTION

■ Constricts blood vessels by stimulating alpha-adrenergic receptors. **Therapeutic Effects:** ■ ***SC, IM, IV:*** Increased blood pressure ■ ***Ophth:*** Mydriasis ■ ***Nasal, Ophth:*** Decreased congestion.

PHARMACOKINETICS

Absorption: Erratically absorbed and rapidly metabolized in the GI tract following oral administration. Well absorbed from IM sites. Minimal absorption following nasal and ophthalmic application.
Distribution: Distribution not known.
Metabolism and Excretion: Metabolized by the liver and other tissues.
Half-life: UK.

CONTRAINDICATIONS AND PRECAUTIONS

Contraindicated in: ■ Uncorrected fluid volume deficits ■ Tachyarrhythmias ■ Pheochromocytoma ■ Angle-closure glaucoma ■ Hypersensitivity to bisulfites (parenteral) ■ Hypersensitivity to benzalkonium chloride, bisulfites, cetylpyridium, EDTA, phenylmercurin acetate, sorbitol, benzalkonium, menthol, camphor, eucalyptol, thimerisol, chlorobutanol (nasal and ophthalmic preparations).
Use Cautiously in: ■ Occlusive vascular disease ■ Cardiovascular disease ■ Elderly patients ■ Hyperthyroidism ■ Pregnancy and lactation (safety not established) ■ Diabetes mellitus.

ADVERSE REACTIONS AND SIDE EFFECTS*

Note: Seen mainly with parenteral administration.

CNS: dizziness, trembling, restlessness, anxiety, nervousness, weakness, dizziness, tremor, insomnia, headache.
EENT: Ophth—<u>burning</u>, <u>stinging</u>, <u>browache</u>, <u>photophobia</u>, <u>lacrimation</u>, irritation; Nasal—burning, stinging, dry nasal mucosa, rebound congestion.
Resp: respiratory distress, dyspnea.
CV: tachycardia, **ARRHYTHMIAS**, hypertension, chest pain, bradycardia, vasoconstriction.
Derm: blanching, piloerection, pallor, sweating.
Local: phlebitis, sloughing at IV sites.

INTERACTIONS

Drug-Drug: ■ Use with **MAO inhibitors, ergot alkaloids (ergonovine, methylergonovine),** or **oxytocics** results in severe hypertension ■ Use with **general anesthetics** may result in myocardial irritability ■ **Alpha-adrenergic blockers (phenoxybenzamine, phentolamine)** may antagonize vasopressor effects ■ **Atropine** blocks bradycardia from phenylephrine and enhances pressor effects.

ROUTE AND DOSAGE

Note: See infusion rate chart in Appendix D.

Hypotension

- **SC, IM (Adults):** 2–5 mg, may repeat in 1–2 hr.
- **SC (Children):** 0.1 mg/kg, may repeat in 1–2 hr.
- **IV (Adults):** 0.1–0.18 mg/min initially, 0.04–0.06 mg/min maintenance.

Mydriasis

- **Ophth (Adult):** 1 drop of 2.5% or 10% soln.

Decongestant

- **Ophth (Adults and Children >2 yr):** 2 drops of 0.08%–0.25% soln, may repeat q 3–4 hr.
- **Nasal (Adults):** 2–3 drops or sprays of 0.25%–1% soln, may be repeated in 4 hr, or small amount of 0.5% jelly placed in each nostril and sniffed

*<u>Underlines</u> indicate most frequent; **CAPITALS** indicate life-threatening.

well back into nasal passage q 3–4 hr as needed.
- **Nasal (Children 6–12 yr):** 2–3 drops or sprays of 0.25% soln, may be repeated in 4 hr.
- **Nasal (Children <6 yr):** 2–3 drops or sprays of 0.125% soln, may be repeated in 4 hr.

PHARMACODYNAMICS (IV, IM, SC = vasopressor effects, Ophth = mydriasis, Nasal = decongestant action)

	ONSET	PEAK	DURATION
IV	immediate	UK	15–20 min
IM	10–15 min	UK	30 min–2 hr
SC	10–15 min	UK	50–60 min
Nasal	UK	UK	30 min–4 hr
Ophth	several mins	10–90 min	3–7 hr

NURSING IMPLICATIONS

Assessment
- **Hypotension:** Monitor blood pressure every 2–3 min until stabilized and every 5 min thereafter during IV administration.
  - Monitor ECG continuously for arrhythmias during IV administration.
  - Assess IV site frequently throughout infusion. Antecubital or other large vein should be used to minimize risk of extravasation, which may cause tissue necrosis. If extravasation occurs, the site should be infiltrated promptly with 10–15 ml of 0.9% NaCl soln containing 5–10 mg of phentolamine to prevent necrosis and sloughing.
- **Decongestant:** Assess patient for allergic symptoms prior to and periodically throughout therapy. Chronic, excessive use can lead to rebound congestion.

Potential Nursing Diagnoses
- Cardiac output, decreased (indications).
- Tissue perfusion, altered (indications).
- Knowledge deficit related to medication regimen (patient/family teaching).

Implementation
- **General Info:** Available in ophthalmic soln, nasal soln, nasal jelly, and parenteral forms. Available in combination with many other drugs for symptomatic treatment of colds and allergies (see Appendix A).
  - Available in several concentrations. Carefully check label for percentage of soln prior to administration.
- **IV:** Blood volume depletion should be corrected, if possible, prior to initiation of IV phenylephrine.
- **Direct IV:** Dilute each 1 mg with 9 ml of sterile water for injection.
  - *Rate:* Administer each single dose over 1 min.
- **Continuous Infusion:** Dilute 10 mg in 500 ml of dextrose/Ringer's or lactated Ringer's combination, dextrose/saline combinations, D5W, D10W, Ringer's or lactated Ringer's soln, 0.45% NaCl, or 0.9% NaCl to provide a 1:50,000 soln.
  - *Rate:* Titrate rate according to patient response. Infuse via infusion pump to ensure accurate dosage rate.
- **Y-Site Compatibility:** amrinone, famotidine, or zidovudine.
- **Additive Compatibility:** chloramphenicol, dobutamine, lidocaine, potassium chloride, or sodium bicarbonate.
- **Anesthesia:** Phenylephrine 2–5 mg may be added to spinal anesthetic soln to prolong anesthesia.
  - Phenylephrine 1 mg may be added to each 20 ml of local anesthetic to produce vasoconstriction.

Patient/Family Teaching
- **IV:** Instruct patient to report headache, dizziness, dyspnea, or pain at IV infusion site promptly.
- **Ophth:** Instruct patient on correct procedure to instill ophthalmic preparations. Tilt head back, look at ceiling, pull down on lower lid, and instill eyedrops. Apply pressure to the inner canthus for 1 min to prevent systemic absorption. Soln may cause stinging or burning.

- Inform patient that ophthalmic preparations will dilate pupils and may make eyes more sensitive to light. Dark glasses will minimize this sensitivity.
- **Nasal:** Instruct patient to blow nose gently prior to instilling nasal preparations. For instillation of nasal drops, instruct patient to tilt head back or lie on bed and hang head over the side. After instillation, remain in this position to allow medication to be distributed throughout nose. After using, wash dropper in hot water and dry with clean tissues.
- For nasal spray, hold head upright and squeeze bottle quickly and firmly. Wait 3–5 min, blow nose, and repeat.
- For nasal jelly, place a small amount of 0.5% jelly into each nostril and sniff well back into nasal passages.
- Soln that is brown or has formed a precipitate has lost potency and should be discarded.
- Advise patient that prolonged or excessive use may cause rebound congestion. Use the weakest strength that is effective. Use only as directed.

Evaluation

Effectiveness of therapy can be demonstrated by: ▪ Increase in blood pressure to normal range ▪ Mydriasis ▪ Decongestant effects in nose and eyes ▪ Prolonged duration of spinal anesthesia ▪ Localization of regional anesthesia.

PHENYLPROPANOLAMINE

(fen-il-proe-pa-**nole**-a-meen)
Acutrim, Control, Dex-A-Diet, Dexatrim, Diadax, Efed-II Yellow, Help, PPA, Prolamine, Propagest, Rhinedecon, Unitrol, Westrim, Westrim-LA

CLASSIFICATION(S):
Appetite suppressant, Decongestant
Pregnancy Category UK

INDICATIONS

▪ Short-term adjunct therapy in the management of exogenous obesity in conjunction with behavior modification, diet, and exercise ▪ Short-term management of nasal congestion.

ACTION

▪ Acts as an agonist of dopamine and norepinephrine ▪ Suppresses appetite by depressing CNS appetite control center ▪ Stimulates alpha-adrenergic receptors in nasal mucosa, producing vasoconstriction. **Therapeutic Effects:** ▪ Decreased appetite ▪ Nasal decongestion.

PHARMACOKINETICS

Absorption: Well absorbed following oral administration.
Distribution: Distribution not known.
Metabolism and Excretion: 80–90% excreted unchanged by the kidneys. Small amounts metabolized by the liver.
Half-life: 3–4 hr.

CONTRAINDICATIONS AND PRECAUTIONS

Contraindicated in: ▪ Hypersensitivity ▪ Children <12 yr (appetite suppressant use only) ▪ Pregnancy or lactation.
Use Cautiously in: ▪ Glaucoma ▪ Prostatic hypertrophy ▪ Hyperthyroidism ▪ Cardiovascular disease, including hypertension ▪ Diabetes mellitus.

ADVERSE REACTIONS AND SIDE EFFECTS*

CNS: nervousness, restlessness, insomnia, dizziness, headache, drowsiness.
EENT: rebound congestion (decongestant use).
CV: chest pain, arrhythmias, hypertension.
GI: nausea.
Misc: tachyphylaxis (decongestant use).

*Underlines indicate most frequent; **CAPITALS** indicate life-threatening.

P

INTERACTIONS

Drug–Drug: ▪ Additive sympathomimetic effects with other **adrenergic (sympathomimetic) agents** ▪ Vasopressor effects are increased by concurrent administration of **MAO inhibitors** ▪ Increased risk of arrhythmias with **some general anesthetics** ▪ Increased risk of hypertension with **rauwolfia alkaloids (reserpine), tricyclic antidepressants,** or **ganglionic blocking agents.**

ROUTE AND DOSAGE

Appetite Suppressant

- **PO (Adults):** 25 mg tid or 37.5 mg bid or 50–75 mg of extended-release preparation once daily.

Decongestant

- **PO (Adults):** 25–50 mg q 4 hr (not to exceed 150 mg/day) or 75 mg of extended-release preparation q 12 hr.
- **PO (Children 6–12 yr):** 10–12.5 mg q 4 hr (not to exceed 75 mg/day).
- **PO (Children 2–6 yr):** 6.25 mg q 4 hr (not to exceed 37.5 mg/day).

PHARMACODYNAMICS (nasal decongestion)

	ONSET	PEAK	DURATION
PO	15–30 min	UK	3 hr
PO-ER	UK	UK	12–16 hr

NURSING IMPLICATIONS

Assessment

- **Obesity:** Monitor patient's weight and nutritional intake periodically throughout therapy.
- **Nasal Congestion:** Assess patient for nasal congestion periodically throughout therapy.

Potential Nursing Diagnoses

- Nutrition, altered: more than body requirements (indications).
- Knowledge deficit related to medication regimen (patient/family teaching).

Implementation

- **General Info:** Administer last dose a few hrs prior to sleep (12 hr with extended-release forms) to minimize insomnia.
  - Available in combination with many cold and allergy products (see Appendix A).
- **PO:** Administer extended-release tablets once daily, in the morning after breakfast. Extended-release tablets should be swallowed whole; do not crush or chew.
- **Obesity:** Do not administer to children <12 yr. Administer to children 12–18 yr according to physician's recommendations.

Patient/Family Teaching

- **General Info:** Instruct patient to take only as directed. Do not take more medication or for a longer time than directed; tolerance may develop.
  - Advise patient not to drink large amounts of coffee, tea, or colas containing caffeine.
- **Obesity:** Instruct patient on modification of caloric intake and exercise program.
- **Nasal Decongestant:** Missed doses should be taken as soon as remembered if within 2 hr (12 hr with extended-release tablets) of next scheduled dose. Do not double doses.
  - Advise patient to consult physician if symptoms do not improve within 7 days or if a fever is present.

Evaluation

Effectiveness of therapy can be demonstrated by: ▪ Decrease in appetite and subsequent decrease in weight when used for obesity. Should be used no longer than a few wks for obesity ▪ Decrease in nasal congestion.

PHENYTOIN

(**fen**-i-toyn)
diphenylhydantoin, DPH, Dilantin, Diphenylan

CLASSIFICATION(S):
Anticonvulsant—hydantoin, Antiarrhythmic—class IB
Pregnancy Category UK

INDICATIONS

■ Treatment and prevention of tonic–clonic (grand mal) seizures and complex partial seizures. **Unlabeled Uses:** ■ As an antiarrhythmic, particularly for arrhythmias associated with cardiac glycoside toxicity ■ Management of painful syndromes, including trigeminal neuralgia.

ACTION

■ Limits seizure propagation by altering ion transport ■ Antiarrhythmic properties as a result of improvement in AV conduction ■ May also decrease synaptic transmission. **Therapeutic Effects:** ■ Diminished seizure activity ■ Control of arrhythmias ■ Decreased pain.

PHARMACOKINETICS

Absorption: Absorbed slowly from the GI tract. Erratically and unreliably absorbed from IM sites. Bioavailability differs among products. Only Dilantin preparation is considered to be extended release. Other products are considered to be prompt release.
Distribution: Distribution not known. Crosses the placenta and enters breast milk.
Metabolism and Excretion: Mostly metabolized by the liver; minimal amounts excreted in the urine.
Half-life: 22 hr.

CONTRAINDICATIONS AND PRECAUTIONS

Contraindicated in: ■ Hypersensitivity ■ Hypersensitivity to propylene glycol (injection only) ■ Alcohol intolerance (injection only) ■ Sinus bradycardia and heart block (antiarrhythmic use).
Use Cautiously in: ■ Severe liver disease (dosage reduction recommended) ■ Pregnancy (safety not established; may result in "fetal hydantoin syndrome" if used chronically or hemorrhage in the newborn if used at term) ■ Lactation (safety not established) ■ Elderly patients or those with severe cardiac or respiratory disease (parenteral use—increased risk of serious adverse reactions).

ADVERSE REACTIONS AND SIDE EFFECTS*

CNS: nystagmus, ataxia, diplopia, drowsiness, lethargy, coma, dizziness, headache, nervousness, dyskinesia.
EENT: gingival hyperplasia.
CV: hypotension (IV only).
GI: nausea, vomiting, anorexia, weight loss, constipation, hepatitis.
GU: pink, red, reddish-brown discoloration of urine.
Derm: hypertrichosis, rashes, exfoliative dermatitis.
F and E: hypocalcemia.
Hemat: **APLASTIC ANEMIA, AGRANULOCYTOSIS,** leukopenia, thrombocytopenia, megaloblastic anemia.
MS: osteomalacia.
Misc: lymphadenopathy, fever, allergic reactions, including **STEVENS–JOHNSON SYNDROME.**

INTERACTIONS

Drug–Drug: ■ **Phenylbutazone, disulfiram, isoniazid, chloramphenicol,** and **cimetidine** may decrease phenytoin metabolism and increase blood levels ■ **Barbiturates, alcohol,** and **warfarin** may stimulate phenytoin metabolism and decrease blood levels ■ Phenytoin may stimulate the metabolism and decrease the effectiveness of **digitoxin** and **oral contraceptives** ■ IV phenytoin and **dopamine** may cause additive hypotension ■ Additive CNS depression with other **CNS depressants,** including **alcohol, antihistamines, antidepressants, narcotic analgesics,** and **sedative/hypnotics** ■ Phenytoin may alter the effect of **oral anticoagulants** ■ **Antacids** may decrease absorption of orally administered phenytoin.
Drug–Food: ■ Phenytoin may decrease absorption of **folic acid.**

ROUTE AND DOSAGE

Note: IM administration should be a last resort. Dosage should be increased

*Underlines indicate most frequent; **CAPITALS** indicate life-threatening.

P

by 50% over previously established daily oral dosage.

Anticonvulsant

- **PO (Adults):** Loading dose 10–15 mg/kg, maintenance dose 300–400 mg/day (once daily as extended-release capsule or in 3–4 divided doses). Usual maximum dose 600 mg/day.
- **PO (Children):** Initially 5 mg/kg, maintenance dose 4–8 mg/kg/day in divided doses q 8–12 hr.

Status Epilepticus

- **IV (Adults):** 150–250 mg, or up to 15–18 mg/kg (rate not to exceed 25-50 mg/min).
- **IV (Children):** 250 mg/m^2 or up to 10–15 mg/kg (at a rate of 0.5–1.5 mg/kg/min).

Antiarrhythmic

- **IV (Adults):** 100 mg q 5 min or 50–100 mg q 10–15 min until arrhythmia is abolished, 1000 mg has been given, or toxicity occurs.
- **PO (Adults):** 100 mg 2–4 times daily.

PHARMACODYNAMICS (anticonvulsant effect)

	ONSET*	PEAK	DURATION
PO	2–24 hr (1 wk)	1.5–3 hr	6–12 hr
PO-ER	2–24 hr (1 wk)	4–12 hr	12–36 hr
IV	1–2 hr (1 wk)	rapid	12–24 hr
IM	UK (erratic)	erratic	12–24 hr

*( ) = time required for onset of action without a loading dose.

NURSING IMPLICATIONS

Assessment

- **General Info:** Assess oral hygiene. Vigorous cleaning beginning within 10 days of initiation of phenytoin therapy may help control gingival hyperplasia.
- **Seizures:** Assess location, duration, and characteristics of seizure activity.
- **Arrhythmias:** Monitor ECG continuously during treatment of arrhythmias.
- **Trigeminal Neuralgia:** Assess pain (location, duration, intensity, precipitating factors) prior to and periodically throughout therapy.
- **Lab Test Considerations:** CBC and platelet count, serum calcium, urinalysis, and hepatic and thyroid function tests should be monitored prior to and monthly for the first several mons, then periodically throughout course of therapy.
  - May cause increased serum alkaline phosphatase and glucose levels.
- **Toxicity and Overdose:** Serum phenytoin levels should be routinely monitored. Therapeutic blood levels are 10–20 mcg/ml.
  - Progressive signs and symptoms of phenytoin toxicity include nystagmus, ataxia, confusion, nausea, slurred speech, dizziness.

Potential Nursing Diagnoses

- Injury, high risk for (indications).
- Oral mucous membranes, altered: (side effects).
- Knowledge deficit related to medication regimen (patient/family teaching).

Implementation

- **General Info:** Implement seizure precautions.
  - When transferring from phenytoin to another anticonvulsant, dosage adjustments are made gradually over several wks.
  - Available in combination with phenobarbital (see Appendix A).
- **PO:** Administer with or immediately after meals to minimize GI irritation. Shake liquid preparations well before pouring. Use a calibrated measuring device for accurate dosage. Chewable tablets must be crushed or chewed well before swallowing. Capsules may be opened and mixed with food or fluids for patients with difficulty swallowing. To prevent direct contact of alkaline drug with mucosa, have patient swallow a liquid first, follow with mixture of medication, then follow with a full glass of water, milk, or with food.
  - Do not interchange 100-mg tablets

with capsules, as capsules contain 92 mg of phenytoin and are not equal to two 50-mg tablets or capsules.

- Capsules labeled "extended" may be used for once-a-day dosage (Dilantin Kapseals only); those labeled "prompt" may result in toxic serum levels if used for once-a-day dosage.
- **IV:** Slight yellow color will not alter soln potency. If refrigerated, may form precipitate, which dissolves after warming to room temperature. Discard soln that is not clear.
- **Direct IV:** Administer at a rate not to exceed 50 mg over 1 min (25 mg/min in elderly patients; 1–3 mg/kg/min in neonates). Rapid administration may result in severe hypotension or CNS depression.
- **Intermittent Infusion:** Administer by mixing with 0.9% NaCl in a concentration of 1–10 mg/ml. Administer immediately following admixture. Use tubing with a 0.22-micron in-line filter.
- To prevent precipitation and minimize local venous irritation, follow infusion with 0.9% NaCl. Avoid extravasation; phenytoin is caustic to tissues.
- *Rate:* Complete infusion within 4 hr at a rate not to exceed 50 mg/min. Monitor cardiac function and blood pressure throughout infusion.
- **Y-Site Compatibility:** esmolol, famotidine, or foscarnet.
- **Y-Site Incompatibility:** potassium chloride.
- **Additive Incompatibility:** Do not admix with other solns or medications, especially dextrose, as precipitation will occur.

Patient/Family Teaching

- Instruct patient to take medication every day exactly as directed. Consult physician if doses are missed for 2 consecutive days. Abrupt withdrawal may lead to status epilepticus.
- Phenytoin may cause drowsiness or dizziness. Caution patient to avoid driving or other activities requiring alertness until response to medication is known. Do not resume driving until physician gives clearance based on control of seizure disorder.
- Caution patient to avoid taking alcohol or over-the-counter medications concurrently with phenytoin without consulting physician or pharmacist.
- Instruct patient on importance of maintaining good dental hygiene and seeing dentist frequently for teeth cleaning to prevent tenderness, bleeding, and gingival hyperplasia. Institution of oral hygiene program within 10 days of initiation of phenytoin therapy may minimize growth rate and severity of gingival enlargement. Patients under 23 yrs of age and those taking doses >500 mg/day are at increased risk for gingival hyperplasia.
- Advise patient that brands of phenytoin may not be equivalent. Check with physician or pharmacist if brand or dosage form is changed.
- Inform patient that phenytoin may color urine pink, red, or reddish brown, but color change is not significant.
- Advise diabetic patients to monitor urine glucose carefully and to notify physician of significant changes.
- Instruct patient to notify physician or dentist of medication regimen prior to treatment or surgery.
- Advise patient not to take phenytoin within 2–3 hr of antacids.
- Advise patient to carry identification describing disease process and medication regimen at all times.
- Advise patient to notify physician if skin rash, severe nausea or vomiting, drowsiness, slurred speech, unsteady gait, swollen glands, bleeding or tender gums, yellow skin or eyes, joint pain, fever, sore throat, unusual bleeding or bruising, persistent headache, or pregnancy occurs.
- Emphasize the importance of routine examinations to monitor progress. Patient should have routine physical examinations, especially monitoring skin and lymph nodes, and EEG testing.

Evaluation

Effectiveness of therapy can be demonstrated by: ▪ Decrease or cessation of seizures without excessive sedation ▪ Suppression of arrhythmias ▪ Relief of pain due to trigeminal neuralgia.

PHOSPHATE/BIPHOSPHATE

(**foss**-fate/bye-**foss**-fate)
Fleet Enema, Phospho-Soda

CLASSIFICATION(S):
Laxative—saline
Pregnancy Category UK

INDICATIONS

▪ Preparation of the bowel prior to surgery or radiologic studies. May be used intermittently in the treatment of chronic constipation.

ACTION

▪ Osmotically active in the lumen of the GI tract ▪ Produces laxative effect by causing water retention and stimulation of peristalsis ▪ Stimulates motility and inhibits fluid and electrolyte absorption from the small intestine. **Therapeutic Effects:** ▪ Relief of constipation ▪ Emptying of the bowel.

PHARMACOKINETICS

Absorption: 1–20% of rectal administered sodium and phosphate may be absorbed.
Distribution: Distribution not known.
Metabolism and Excretion: Excreted by the kidneys.
Half-life: UK.

CONTRAINDICATIONS AND PRECAUTIONS

Contraindicated in: ▪ Abdominal pain, nausea, or vomiting, especially when associated with fever or other signs of an acute abdomen ▪ Pregnancy (at term) ▪ Renal disease ▪ Severe cardiac disease ▪ Intestinal obstruction.
Use Cautiously in: ▪ Excessive or chronic use (may lead to dependence) ▪ Pregnancy (may cause sodium retention and edema).

ADVERSE REACTIONS AND SIDE EFFECTS*

GI: <u>cramping</u>, <u>nausea</u>.
F and E: sodium retention, hyperphosphatemia, hypocalcemia.

INTERACTIONS

Drug-Drug: ▪ None significant.

ROUTE AND DOSAGE

Note: Each Fleet Enema contains 4.4 g sodium/118 ml. Each 5 ml of Fleet Phospho-Soda oral soln contains 24.1 mEq sodium/5 ml.

- **PO (Adults):** 9–16 g biphosphate/3–6 g phosphate (15–30 ml).
- **PO (Children >10 yr):** 50% of the adult dose (7.5–15 ml Phospho-Soda).
- **PO (Children 5–10 yr):** 25% of the adult dose (3.25–7.5 ml Phospho-Soda).
- **Rect (Adults):** 19 g biphosphate/7 g phosphate (60–120 ml Fleet).
- **Rect (Children >2 yr):** 50% of the adult rectal dose (30–60 ml Fleet).

PHARMACODYNAMICS (laxative effect)

	ONSET	PEAK	DURATION
PO	0.5–3 hr	UK	UK
Rect	2–5 min	UK	UK

NURSING IMPLICATIONS

Assessment

- ▫ Assess patient for fever, abdominal distention, presence of bowel sounds, and usual pattern of bowel function.
- ▫ Assess color, consistency, and amount of stool produced.
- ▪ **Lab Test Considerations:** May cause increased serum sodium and phosphorus levels, decreased serum calcium levels, and acidosis.

Potential Nursing Diagnoses

- ▪ Bowel elimination, altered: constipation (indications).
- ▪ Knowledge deficit related to medica-

*<u>Underlines</u> indicate most frequent; **CAPITALS** indicate life-threatening.

tion regimen (patient/family teaching).

IMPLEMENTATION

- **General Info:** Do not administer at bedtime or late in the day.
- **PO:** Administer on an empty stomach for more rapid results. Mix dose in at least ½ glass cold water. May be followed by carbonated beverage or fruit juice to improve flavor.
- **Rect:** Position patient on left side with knee slightly flexed. Insert prelubricated tip about 2 inches into rectum, aiming toward the umbilicus. Gently squeeze bottle until empty. Discontinue if resistance is met, as perforation may occur if contents are forced into rectum.

PATIENT/FAMILY TEACHING

- □ Advise patient that laxatives should be used only for short-term therapy. Long-term therapy may cause electrolyte imbalance and dependence.
- □ Caution patient on sodium restriction that this product has a high sodium content.
- □ Advise patient not to take oral form of this medication within 2 hr of other medications.
- □ Encourage patient to use other forms of bowel regulation, such as increasing bulk in the diet, fluid intake, mobility. Normal bowel habits are variable and may vary from 3 times/day to 3 times/wk.
- □ Advise patient to notify physician if unrelieved constipation, rectal bleeding, or symptoms of electrolyte imbalance (muscle cramps or pain, weakness, dizziness, and so forth) occur.

EVALUATION

Effectiveness of therapy can be demonstrated by: ▪ Soft, formed bowel movement.

PHYSOSTIGMINE

(fi-zoe-**stig**-meen)

Antilerium, Isopto-Eserine

CLASSIFICATION(S):
Cholinergic—anticholinesterase agent, Ophthalmic—antiglaucoma
Pregnancy Category C (Ophth)

INDICATIONS

▪ **IM, IV, SC:** Reversal of CNS effects due to overdose of drugs capable of causing the anticholinergic syndrome, including: □ Belladonna or other plant alkaloids □ Phenothiazines □ Tricyclic antidepressants □ Antihistamines (reverses delerium, hallucinations, coma, and some arrhythmias, but not completely effective in reversing cardiac conduction defects or tachycardia) ▪ **Ophth:** As miotic to decrease intraocular pressure in treatment of glaucoma.

ACTION

▪ Inhibits the breakdown of acetylcholine so that it accumulates and has a prolonged effect. Result is generalized cholinergic response, including: □ Miosis □ Increased tone of intestinal and skeletal musculature □ Bronchial and ureteral constriction □ Bradycardia □ Increased salivation □ Lacrimation □ Sweating □ CNS stimulation. **Therapeutic Effects:** ▪ ***IM, IV, SC:*** Reversal of anticholinergic excess ▪ ***Ophth:*** Miosis with decreased intraocular pressure.

PHARMACOKINETICS

Absorption: Readily absorbed from SC and IM sites. Some absorption may occur following ophthalmic use.

Distribution: Widely distributed, crosses the blood-brain barrier.

Metabolism and Excretion: Metabolized by cholinesterases present in many tissues. Small amounts excreted unchanged in the urine.

Half-life: UK.

CONTRAINDICATIONS AND PRECAUTIONS

Contraindicated in: ▪ Hypersensitivity ▪ Mechanical obstruction of the GI or GU tract ▪ Pregnancy or lactation (10–

P

20% of newborns will suffer from muscle weakness).

Use Cautiously in: ▪ History of asthma ▪ Ulcer disease ▪ Cardiovascular disease ▪ Epilepsy ▪ Hyperthyroidism ▪ Uveitis or corneal injury (ophth only).

ADVERSE REACTIONS AND SIDE EFFECTS*

CNS: dizziness, weakness, restlessness, hallucinations, SEIZURES.

EENT: miosis, lacrimation; Ophth—blurred vision, eye pain, eye irritation, brow ache, twitching of eyelids.

Resp: excess respiratory secretions, bronchospasm.

CV: bradycardia, hypotension.

GI: abdominal cramps, nausea, vomiting, diarrhea, excess salivation.

Derm: rash.

INTERACTIONS

Drug-Drug: ▪ Cholinergic effects may be antagonized by other **drugs possessing anticholinergic properties,** including **antihistamines, antidepressants, atropine, haloperidol, phenothiazines, quinidine,** and **disopyramide** ▪ Prolongs action of **depolarizing muscle-relaxing agents (succinylcholine, decamethonium)** ▪ Beneficial ophthalmic effects may be decreased by concurrent **ophthalmic belladonna alkaloids (atropine, scopolamine)** ▪ May decrease the duration of action of **echothiophate** or **isoflurophate** if administered before physostigmine.

ROUTE AND DOSAGE

- **IM, IV, SC, (Adults):** 0.5–2 mg initially, can repeat q 20 min until response, then may give 1–4 mg q 30–60 min as symptoms recur.
- **IV (Children):** 0.02 mg/kg may repeat every 5–10 minutes as needed.
- **Ophth (Adults and Children):** 1–2 drops of 0.25–0.5% soln qid, ointment at bedtime.

PHARMACODYNAMICS (SC, IM, IV = systemic cholinergic effects; Ophth = miosis)

	ONSET	PEAK	DURATION
SC	UK	UK	45–60 min*
IM	3–8 min	UK	45–60 min*
IV	3–8 min	UK	45–60 min*
Ophth	1–30 min	UK	12–48 hr

*May be up to 5 hr.

NURSING IMPLICATIONS

Assessment

- **General Info:** Monitor pulse, respiratory rate, and blood pressure frequently throughout parenteral administration. Monitor ECG during IV administration.
- **Anticholinergic Excess:** Monitor neurologic status frequently. Institute seizure precautions. Protect patient from self-injury due to CNS effects of overdose.
- **Glaucoma:** Monitor patient for changes in vision, eye irritation, and persistent headache.
- **Toxicity and Overdose:** Overdose is manifested by bradycardia, respiratory distress, seizures, weakness, nausea, vomiting, stomach cramps, diarrhea, diaphoresis, and increased salivation and tearing.
  - ▫ Atropine is the antidote.
  - ▫ Treatment of overdose includes establishing an airway and supporting ventilation, atropine sulfate 2–4 mg (may be repeated every 3–10 min to control muscarinic effects), pralidoxime chloride 50–100 mg/min (to control neurologic and skeletal muscle effects), and supportive therapy.

Potential Nursing Diagnoses

- Sensory-perceptual alteration: visual (indications, side effects).
- Injury, high risk for (indications).
- Knowledge deficit related to medication regimen (patient/family teaching).

*Underlines indicate most frequent; **CAPITALS** indicate life-threatening.

IMPLEMENTATION

- **Direct IV:** Repeated doses may be needed due to short duration of action.
  - *Rate:* May be given through Y-site or 3-way stopcock at a rate of 1 mg over 1 min (0.5 mg over 1 min for children). Rapid administration may cause bradycardia; increased salivation, which can lead to respiratory distress; or seizures.
- **Additive Incompatibility:** Do not add to IV solns.

PATIENT/FAMILY TEACHING

- **Anticholinergic Excess:** Explain purpose of medication and need for close monitoring.
- **Ophth:** Instruct patient to take as ordered and not to discontinue without physician's approval. Lifelong therapy may be required. A missed dose of eyedrops should be taken as soon as remembered unless almost time for next dose. If dose of ointment is missed, patient should take it as soon as remembered. If not remembered until next day, patient should wait until usual time for dose.
  - Instruct patient on correct method of application of drops or ointment. Wash hands. Lie down or tilt head back and look at ceiling. Pull down on lower lid creating a small pocket. Place prescribed number of drops in pocket waiting 5 min between instillation of each drop. Apply pressure to the inner canthus for 1–2 min to confine effects to the eye. Wait 5 min before applying other prescribed eyedrops.
  - For instillation of ointment, instruct patient to hold tube in hand for several mins to warm. Apply ribbon of ointment to lower conjunctival sac at bedtime immediately before retiring. Close eye gently and roll eyeball around in all directions with eye closed. Recap tightly after use. Wait 10 min before installing any other ophthalmic ointment. Ointment may be refrigerated or kept for 8 wk at room temperature.
  - Do not touch cap or tip of container to eye, fingers, or any surface.
  - Explain to patient that pupil constriction and temporary stinging and blurring of vision are expected. Physician should be notified if blurred vision and brow ache persist.
  - Caution patient that night vision may be impaired. Advise patient not to drive at night until response to medication is known. To prevent injury at night, patient should use a night light and keep environment uncluttered.
  - Instruct patient to report signs of systemic side effects (sweating, increased salivation, nausea, vomiting, diarrhea, bradycardia, weakness, and respiratory distress).
  - Advise patient of the need for regular eye examinations to monitor intraocular pressure and visual fields.

EVALUATION

Effectiveness of therapy can be demonstrated by: ▪ Reversal of CNS symptoms secondary to anticholinergic excess resulting from drug overdose or ingestion of poisonous plants ▪ Control of elevated intraocular pressure.

PHYTONADIONE

(fye-toe-na-**dye**-one)
AquaMEPHYTON, Konakion, Mephyton, vitamin K_1

CLASSIFICATION(S):
Vitamin—fat-soluble
Pregnancy Category UK

INDICATIONS

▪ Prevention and treatment of hypoprothrombinemia, which may be associated with: ▫ Excessive doses of oral anticoagulants ▫ Salicylates ▫ Certain anti-infective agents ▫ Nutritional deficiencies ▫ Prolonged total parenteral nutrition ▪ Prevention of hemorrhagic disease of the newborn.

ACTION

▪ Required for hepatic synthesis of blood coagulation factors II (prothrombin), VII, IX, and X. **Therapeutic Effect:** ▪ Prevention of bleeding due to hypoprothrombinemia.

PHARMACOKINETICS

Absorption: Well absorbed following oral, IM, or SC administration. Oral absorption requires presence of bile salts. Some vitamin K is produced by bacteria in the GI tract.
Distribution: Crosses the placenta. Does not enter breast milk.
Metabolism and Excretion: Rapidly metabolized by the liver.
Half-life: UK.

CONTRAINDICATIONS AND PRECAUTIONS

Contraindicated in: ▪ Hypersensitivity ▪ Hypersensitivity to benzyl alcohol (AquaMEPHYTON only), phenol, propylene glycol, or polysorbate 80 (Konakion only).
Use Cautiously in: ▪ Impaired liver function.

ADVERSE REACTIONS AND SIDE EFFECTS*

GI: gastric upset, unusual taste.
Derm: rash, urticaria, flushing.
Local: erythema, swelling, pain at injection site.
Misc: hemolytic anemia, kernicterus, hyperbilirubinemia (large doses in very premature infants), allergic reactions.

INTERACTIONS

Drug–Drug: ▪ Large doses will counteract the effect of **oral anticoagulants** ▪ Large doses of **salicylates** or broad-spectrum **anti-infectives** may increase vitamin K requirements ▪ **Cholestyramine, colestipol, mineral oil,** and **sucralfate** may decrease vitamin K absorption.

ROUTE AND DOSAGE

Treatment of Hypoprothrombinemia

- **PO, SC, IM (Adults):** 2.5–10 mg, repeat in 12–48 hr if necessary after oral dose or 6–8 hr after parenteral dose (up to 25 mg).
- **SC, IM (Children):** 5–10 mg.
- **IM, SC (Infants):** 1–2 mg.

Prevention of Hypoprothrombinemia During Total Parenteral Nutrition

- **IM (Adults):** 5–10 mg once weekly.
- **IM (Children):** 2–5 mg once weekly.

Prevention of Hemorrhagic Disease of Newborn

- **SC, IM (Neonates):** 0.5–1 mg, may be repeated in 6–8 hr if needed.

PHARMACODYNAMICS

	ONSET	PEAK*	DURATION†
PO	6–12 hr	UK	UK
IM, SC	1–2 hr	3–6 hr	12–14 hr

* = Control of hemorrhage.
† = Normal prothrombin time achieved.

NURSING IMPLICATIONS

Assessment

- □ Monitor for frank and occult bleeding (guaiac stools, hematest urine and emesis). Monitor pulse and blood pressure frequently; notify physician immediately if symptoms of internal bleeding or hypovolemic shock develop. Inform all personnel of patient's bleeding tendency to prevent further trauma. Apply pressure to all venipuncture sites for at least 5 min; avoid unnecessary IM injections.
- **Lab Test Considerations:** Prothrombin time should be monitored prior to and throughout vitamin K therapy to determine response to and need for further therapy.

Potential Nursing Diagnoses

- Nutrition, altered: less than body requirements (indications).
- Tissue perfusion, altered: (indications).
- Knowledge deficit related to medication regimen (patient/family teaching).

Implementation

- **General Info:** The parenteral route is preferred for phytonadione therapy, but because of severe hypersensitvity

reactions, IV vitamin K is not recommended.
- □ Administration of whole blood or plasma may also be required in severe bleeding because of the delayed onset of this medication.
- □ Phytonadione is an antidote for warfarin overdose but does not counteract the anticoagulant activity of heparin.

PATIENT/FAMILY TEACHING

- □ Instruct patient to take this medication as ordered. If a dose is missed, take as soon as remembered unless almost time for next dose. Notify physician of missed doses.
- □ Foods high in vitamin K include leafy green vegetables, meat, and dairy products. Cooking does not destroy substantial amounts of vitamin K. Patient should not drastically alter diet while taking vitamin K.
- □ Caution patient to avoid IM injections and activities leading to injury. Use a soft toothbrush, do not floss, and shave with an electric razor until coagulation defect is corrected.
- □ Advise patient to report any symptoms of unusual bleeding or bruising (bleeding gums, nosebleed, black tarry stools, hematuria, excessive menstrual flow) to physician.
- □ Patients receiving vitamin K therapy should be cautioned not to take over-the-counter medications without advice of physician or pharmacist.
- □ Advise patient to inform physicians and dentists of the use of this medication prior to treatment or surgery.
- □ Advise patient to carry identification describing disease process at all times.
- □ Emphasize the importance of frequent lab tests to monitor coagulation factors.

EVALUATION

Effectiveness of therapy can be demonstrated by: ▪ Prevention of spontaneous bleeding or cessation of bleeding in patients with hypoprothrombinemia secondary to impaired intestinal absorption or oral anticoagulant, salicylate, or antibiotic therapy ▪ Prevention of hemorrhagic disease in the newborn.

PILOCARPINE

(pye-loe-**kar**-peen)
Adsorbocarpine, Akarpine, Almocarpine, I-Pilopine, {Minims Pilocarpine}, {Miocarpine}, Ocusert Pilo, Pilocar, Pilokair, Pilopine HS, P.V. Carpine Liquifilm

CLASSIFICATION(S):
Ophthalmic—antiglaucoma agent, Ophthalmic—miotic
Pregnancy Category C

INDICATIONS

▪ Alone or with other agents in the treatment of glaucoma ▪ As a miotic in the postoperative period or following cycloplegics and mydriatics.

ACTION

▪ Directly stimulates cholinergic receptors, resulting in: □ Miosis □ Increased accommodation □ Constricted pupils □ Reduced intraocular pressure secondary to increased aqueous outflow. **Therapeutic Effects:** ▪ Decreased intraocular pressure ▪ Miosis.

PHARMACOKINETICS

Absorption: Some systemic absorption may follow ophthalmic administration.
Distribution: Binds to ocular tissues.
Metabolism and Excretion: Metabolism and excretion not known.
Half-life: UK.

CONTRAINDICATIONS AND PRECAUTIONS

Contraindicated in: ▪ Hypersensitivity ▪ Risk or history of retinal detachment ▪ Acute ocular inflammation ▪ Posterior synechiae (adhesion between the iris and the lens).

Use Cautiously in: ▪ Corneal abrasion ▪ Asthma ▪ Hypertension ▪ Hyperthyroidism ▪ Cardiovascular disease ▪ Epilepsy ▪ Parkinsonism ▪ Bradycardia ▪ Ulcer disease ▪ Urinary tract obstruction ▪ Hypotension ▪ GI obstruction.

ADVERSE REACTIONS AND SIDE EFFECTS*

CNS: headache.
EENT: blurred vision, eye pain, eye irritation, brow ache.
Resp: dyspnea, wheezing.
GI: nausea, vomiting, diarrhea, salivation.
Derm: increased sweating.
MS: muscle tremor.

INTERACTIONS

Drug-Drug: ▪ Additive intraocular pressure-lowering effects with ophthalmic administration of **epinephrine, beta-adrenergic blockers,** and systemic **carbonic anhydrase inhibitors** ▪ Counteracts mydriasis from **cyclopentolate** or **ophthalmic belladonna alkaloids (atropine, scopolamine).**

ROUTE AND DOSAGE

Chronic Treatment of Glaucoma

- **Ophth (Adults):** 1 drop of 0.5–4% soln to conjunctiva qid or 1.5 cm of 4% gel to conjunctiva once daily at bedtime or one 20- or 40-mg ocular system to conjunctiva once weekly.

Acute Treatment of Angle-Closure Glaucoma

- **Ophth (Adults):** 1 drop of 1% or 2% soln q 5–10 min for 3–6 doses then 1 drop q 3–6 hr until intraocular pressure is decreased (nonaffected eye may be treated with 1 drop of 1% or 2% soln q 6–8 hr).

Miosis

- **Ophth (Adults):** 1 drop of 1% or 2% soln.

PHARMACODYNAMICS

	ONSET	PEAK	DURATION
Ophth (miosis)	10–30 min	UK	4–8 hr
Ophth (reduced intraocular pressure)	UK	75 min	4–14 hr
Ophth (Ocusert) (reduced intraocular pressure)	UK	1.5–2 hr	7 days

NURSING IMPLICATIONS

Assessment

- Monitor patient for changes in vision, eye irritation, and persistent headache.
- Monitor patient for signs of systemic side effects (sweating, increased salivation, nausea, vomiting, diarrhea, and respiratory distress). Notify physician if these signs occur.
- **Toxicity and Overdose:** Toxicity is manifested as systemic side effects. Atropine is the antidote.

Potential Nursing Diagnoses

- Sensory-perceptual alteration: visual (indications, side effects).
- Knowledge deficit related to medication regimen (patient/family teaching).

Implementation

- **Ophth:** Available in several concentrations. Carefully check percentage on label prior to administration.

Patient/Family Teaching

- Instruct patient to take as ordered and not to discontinue without physician's approval. Lifelong therapy may be required. A missed dose of eyedrops should be taken as soon as remembered unless almost time for next dose. If dose of ointment is missed, patient should take it as soon as remembered. If not remembered until next day, patient should wait until usual time for dose.

*Underlines indicate most frequent; **CAPITALS** indicate life-threatening.

- Instruct patient on correct method of application of drops or ointment. Wash hands. Lie down or tilt head back and look at ceiling. Pull down on lower lid, creating a small pocket. Place prescribed number of drops in pocket waiting 5 min between instillatin of each drop. Apply pressure to the inner canthus for 1–2 min to confine effects to the eye. Wait 5 min before applying other prescribed eyedrops.
- For instillation of ointment, instruct patient to hold tube in hand for several mins to warm. Apply ribbon of ointment to lower conjunctival sac at bedtime immediately before retiring. Close eye gently and roll eyeball around in all directions with eye closed. Recap tightly after use. Wait 10 min before installing any other ophthalmic ointment. Ointment may be refrigerated or kept for 8 wk at room temperature. Do not touch cap or tip of container to eye, fingers, or any surface.
- Instruct patient on correct method of using pilocarpine ocular system (Ocusert). Store Ocusert in refrigerator prior to use. New system is inserted once a wk at bedtime. Bedtime application minimizes initial visual effects (myopia). Ocusert may be placed in upper or lower conjunctival sac. The system is less likely to fall out at night if placed in upper conjunctival sac. The system may be removed from eye by gently pressing Ocusert through closed lids or by directly pushing it with clean hands. If Ocusert falls out, it may be washed with cool tap water and reinserted. Do not insert if contaminated or damaged. If an Ocusert is lost, patient wearing bilateral Ocuserts may replace both systems to maintain similar changing schedule. Review systemic side effects and instruct patient to remove system and notify physician if these occur.
- Explain to patient that pupil constriction and temporary stinging and blurring of vision are expected. Physician should be notified if blurred vision and brow ache persist.
- Caution patient that night vision may be impaired. Advise patient not to drive at night until response to medication is known. To prevent injury at night, patient should use a night light and keep environment uncluttered.
- Advise patient of the need for regular eye examinations to monitor intraocular pressure and visual fields.

Evaluation

Effectiveness of therapy can be demonstrated by: ▪ Control of elevated intraocular pressure ▪ Reversal of mydriatic agents.

PINDOLOL
(**pin**-doe-lole)
Visken

CLASSIFICATION(S):
Antihypertensive—beta-adrenergic blocker, Beta-adrenergic blocker—nonselective
Pregnancy Category B

INDICATIONS

▪ Used alone or in combination with other agents in the treatment of hypertension. **Unlabeled Uses:** ▪ Chronic treatment of angina pectoris ▪ Hypertrophic cardiomyopathy ▪ Tremors ▪ Mitral valve prolapse syndrome.

ACTION

▪ Blocks stimulation of $beta_1$ (myocardial) adrenergic receptors and $beta_2$ (pulmonary, vascular, or uterine) receptor sites ▪ Possesses mild intrinsic sympathomimetic activity (ISA) which may result in less bradycardia. **Therapeutic Effects:** ▪ Decreased heart rate ▪ Decreased blood pressure.

PHARMACOKINETICS

Absorption: Well absorbed following oral administration.
Distribution: Moderate penetration of the CNS. Crosses the placenta and enters breast milk.

P

Metabolism and Excretion: Partially metabolized by the liver, up to 50% excreted unchanged by the kidneys.
Half-life: 3–4 hr.

CONTRAINDICATIONS AND PRECAUTIONS

Contraindicated in: ▪ Uncompensated congestive heart failure ▪ Pulmonary edema ▪ Cardiogenic shock ▪ Bradycardia ▪ Heart block ▪ Pregnancy or lactation (may cause apnea, low Apgar scores, bradycardia, and hypoglycemia in the newborn) ▪ Asthma or COPD.
Use Cautiously in: ▪ Thyrotoxicosis or hypoglycemia (may mask symptoms) ▪ Renal impairment (dosage reduction recommended) ▪ Children (safety not established).

ADVERSE REACTIONS AND SIDE EFFECTS*

CNS: fatigue, weakness, depression, insomnia, memory loss, mental changes, nightmares, anxiety, nervousness, dizziness.
CV: BRADYCARDIA, CONGESTIVE HEART FAILURE, PULMONARY EDEMA, peripheral vasoconstriction, hypotension, edema.
EENT: dry eyes, blurred vision.
Resp: bronchospasm, wheezing.
GI: diarrhea, nausea.
GU: impotence, diminished libido.
Derm: rash.
Endo: hyperglycemia, hypoglycemia.
MS: joint pain, arthralgia.

INTERACTIONS

Drug-Drug: ▪ **General anesthesia, IV phenytoin,** and **verapamil** may cause additive myocardial depression ▪ Additive bradycardia may occur with concurrent use of **cardiac glycosides** ▪ Additive hypotension may occur with other **antihypertensive agents,** acute ingestion of **alcohol,** and **nitrates** ▪ Use with **epinephrine, cocaine, amphetamines, ephedrine, norepinephrine, phenylephrine,** or **pseudophedrine** may result in unopposed alpha-adrenergic stimulation, hypertension, or bradycardia ▪ Concurrent **thyroid** administration may decrease effectiveness ▪ Use with **insulin** may result in prolonged hypoglycemia ▪ May antagonize **beta-adrenergic bronchodilators** ▪ May negate the beneficial $beta_1$ cardiac effects of **dopamine** or **dobutamine.**

ROUTE AND DOSAGE

- **PO (Adults):** 5 mg bid initially, increase by 10 mg/day at 2–3 wk intervals. Usual dose maintenance is 10–15 mg/day in 2–3 divided doses. Single daily dosing may be used when response is determined. Up to 60 mg/day has been used.

PHARMACODYNAMICS (antihypertensive effect)

	ONSET	PEAK	DURATION
PO	7 days	2 wk	8–24 hr

NURSING IMPLICATIONS

Assessment

- Monitor blood pressure and pulse frequently during period of adjustment and periodically throughout therapy. Confer with physician prior to giving drug if pulse is <50 bpm. Assess for orthostatic hypotension when assisting patient up from supine position.
- Monitor intake and output ratios and daily weight. Assess patient routinely for evidence of congestive heart failure (peripheral edema, dyspnea, rales/crackles, fatigue, weight gain, jugular venous distention).
- **Lab Test Considerations:** Hepatic and renal function and CBC should be monitored routinely in patients receiving prolonged therapy.
- May cause elevations in serum potassium, uric acid, triglyceride and lipoprotein levels, and BUN. May also cause elevated antinuclear antibody (ANA) titers.

Potential Nursing Diagnoses

- Cardiac output, decreased (indications, adverse reactions).
- Knowledge deficit related to medica-

*Underlines indicate most frequent; CAPITALS indicate life-threatening.

tion regimen (patient/family teaching).

- Noncompliance (patient/family teaching).

IMPLEMENTATION

- **PO:** May be administered with food or on an empty stomach. May be crushed and mixed with food or fluid if patient has difficulty swallowing.

PATIENT/FAMILY TEACHING

- Instruct patient to take medication exactly as directed, even if feeling well. If a dose is missed, it may be taken as soon as remembered up to 4 hr before next dose. Abrupt withdrawal may precipitate life-threatening arrhythmias, hypertension, and myocardial ischemia.
- Teach patient and family how to check pulse and blood pressure. Instruct them to take pulse daily and blood pressure biweekly. Advise patient to withhold dose and contact physician if pulse is <50 bpm or blood pressure changes significantly.
- Caution patients to make position changes slowly and to avoid standing in a stationary position for long periods to minimize orthostatic hypotension.
- Reinforce need to continue additional therapies for hypertension (weight loss, restricted sodium intake, stress reduction, regular exercise, moderation of alcohol consumption, and cessation of smoking). Pindolol helps control but does not cure hypertension.
- Caution patient that this medication may cause increased sensitivity to cold.
- Advise patient to consult physician or pharmacist before taking any over-the-counter drugs, especially cold remedies, concurrently with this medication. Patients should also avoid excessive amounts of coffee, tea, and cola.
- Diabetic patient should monitor serum glucose closely, especially if weakness, fatigue, or irritability occurs.
- Instruct patient to inform physician or dentist of this therapy prior to treatment or surgery.
- Advise patient to carry identification describing medication regimen at all times.
- Instruct patient to notify physician if slow pulse rate, dizziness, depression, or skin rash occurs.

EVALUATION

Effectiveness of therapy can be demonstrated by: ▪ Decrease in blood pressure. Hypotensive effects may begin within 7 days, but maximum effect is reached in approximately 2 wk.

PIPECURONIUM

(pip-e-**kyoor**-oh-nee-um)
Arduan

CLASSIFICATION(S):
Neuromuscular blocking agent—nondepolarizing
Pregnancy Category C

INDICATIONS

- Production of skeletal muscle paralysis and facilitation of intubation after induction of anesthesia in surgical procedures lasting ≥90 min.

ACTION

▪ Prevents neuromuscular transmission by blocking the effect of acetylcholine at the myoneural junction ▪ Has no analgesic or anxiolytic effects. **Therapeutic Effect:** ▪ Skeletal muscle paralysis.

PHARMACOKINETICS

Absorption: Administered IV only, resulting in complete absorption.
Distribution: Distribution not known.
Metabolism and Excretion: >75% excreted by the kidneys, mostly as unmetabolized drug.
Half-life: 1.7 hr (prolonged in renal impairment).

P

CONTRAINDICATIONS AND PRECAUTIONS

Contraindicated in: ▪ Hypersensitivity to pipecuronium or bromides ▪ ICU patients requiring prolonged mechanical ventilation ▪ Avoid concurrent use with other nondepolarizing neuromuscular blocking agents ▪ Not recommended for use before succinylcholine (may be used following recovery).

Use Cautiously in: ▪ Cardiovascular disease, edematous states, elderly patients (delays onset time) ▪ Obesity (prolongs duration of paralysis; base dose on ideal body weight) ▪ Electrolyte disturbances ▪ Myasthenia gravis or myasthenic syndromes (extreme caution; duration may be dangerously prolonged) ▪ Patients with renal impairment ▪ Pregnancy or lactation (safety not established).

ADVERSE REACTIONS AND SIDE EFFECTS*

Note: Almost all adverse reactions to pipecuronium are extensions of pharmacologic effects.

Resp: apnea, respiratory insufficiency.
CV: hypotension, bradycardia.
MS: muscle weakness.
Misc: allergic reactions.

INTERACTIONS

Drug-Drug: ▪ Intensity and duration of paralysis may be prolonged by pretreatment with **aminoglycoside antibiotics, polymyxin B, tetracycline, colistin, clindamycin, lidocaine, quinidine,** or **procainamide** ▪ Additive neuromuscular blockade (prolonged duration and recovery) with **inhalation anesthetics (enflurane, isoflurane, halothane)**.

ROUTE AND DOSAGE

Note: Doses are listed for nonobese patients with normal renal function.

- **IV (Adults):** 70–85 mcg/kg (dosage adjustments required for obesity or renal impairment). If given following recovery from succinlycholine during intubation decrease dose to 50 mcg/kg. Additional doses of 10–15 mcg/kg may be required as maintenance (dosage reduction recommended if using concurrent inhalation anesthetics).
- **IV (Children 1–14 yr):** 57 mcg/kg
- **IV (Infants 3 mon–1 yr):** 40 mcg/kg.

PHARMACODYNAMICS

	ONSET	PEAK	DURATION
IV	2.5–3 min	5 min	1–2 hr

NURSING IMPLICATIONS

Assessment

- ▫ Assess respiratory status continuously throughout pipecuronium therapy. Pipecuronium should be used only by individuals experienced in endotracheal intubation, and equipment for this procedure should be readily available.
- ▫ Neuromuscular response to pipecuronium should be monitored with a peripheral nerve stimulator. Paralysis is initially selective and usually occurs sequentially in the following muscles: levator muscles of eyelids, muscles of mastication, limb muscles, abdominal muscles, muscles of the glottis, intercostal muscles, and the diaphragm. Recovery of muscle function usually occurs in reverse order.
- ▫ Observe the patient for residual muscle weakness and respiratory distress during the recovery period.
- ▪ **Toxicity and Overdose:** If overdose occurs use peripheral nerve stimulator to determine the degree of neuromuscular blockade. Maintain airway patency and ventilation until recovery of normal respirations occur.
- ▫ Administration of anticholinesterase agents (neostigmine, pyridostigmine) may be used to antagonize the action of pipecuronium once patient has demonstrated some spontaneous recovery from neuromuscular block.
- ▫ Administration of fluids and vasopressors may be necessary to treat severe hypotension or shock.

*Underlines indicate most frequent; **CAPITALS** indicate life-threatening.

Potential Nursing Diagnoses

- Breathing pattern, ineffective (indications).
- Communication, impaired: verbal (side effects).
- Fear (side effects).

Implementation

- **General Info:** Dose is titrated to patient response.
  - Pipecuronium has no effect on consciousness or the pain threshold. Adequate anesthesia should *always* be used when pipecuronium is used as an adjunct to surgical procedures.
  - Store at room temperature.
- **Direct IV:** Reconstitute with 0.9% NaCl, D5W, D5/0.9% NaCl, LR, sterile water for injection, or bacteriostatic water for injection. Soln reconstituted with bacteriostatic water contains benzyl alcohol and should not be used for newborns; use within 5 days. Soln reconstituted with sterile water or other IV solns should be refrigerated and used within 24 hr. Do not dilute into or administer from large volume IV solns.

Patient/Family Teaching

- Explain all procedures to patient receiving pipecuronium therapy without anesthesia, as consciousness is not affected by pipecuronium alone.
- Reassure patient that communication abilities will return as the medication wears off.

Evaluation

Effectiveness of therapy can be demonstrated by: ■ Adequate suppression of the twitch response when tested with peripheral nerve stimulation and subsequent muscle paralysis.

PIPERACILLIN

(pi-**per**-a-sill-in)
Pipracil

CLASSIFICATION(S):
Anti-infective—extended-spectrum penicillin
Pregnancy Category B

INDICATIONS

■ Treatment of serious infections due to susceptible organisms, including: □ Skin and skin structure infections □ Bone and joint infections □ Septicemia □ Respiratory tract infections □ Intra-abdominal infections □ Gynecologic and urinary tract infections ■ Combination with an aminoglycoside may be synergistic against *Pseudomonas* ■ Has been combined with other antibiotics in the treatment of infections in immunosuppressed patients ■ Perioperative prophylactic anti-infective in abdominal, genitourinary, and head and neck surgery.

ACTION

■ Binds to bacterial cell wall membrane, causing cell death. Spectrum is extended when compared with other penicillins. **Therapeutic Effect:** ■ Death of susceptible bacteria. **Spectrum:** ■ Spectrum similar to penicillin but greatly extended, including several important gram-negative aerobic pathogens, notably: □ *Pseudomonas aeruginosa* □ *Escherichia coli* □ *Proteus mirabilis* □ *Providencia rettgeri* ■ Also active against some anaerobic bacteria, including *Bacteroides* ■ Not active against penicillinase-producing staphylococci or beta-lactamase–producing *Enterobacteriaceae*.

PHARMACOKINETICS

Absorption: Well absorbed (80%) from IM sites.
Distribution: Widely distributed. Enters CSF well only when meninges are inflamed. Crosses the placenta and enters breast milk in low concentrations.
Metabolism and Excretion: Mostly (90%) excreted unchanged by the kidneys. 10% excreted in bile.
Half-life: 0.7–1.3 hr.

CONTRAINDICATIONS AND PRECAUTIONS

Contraindicated in: ■ Hypersensitivity to penicillins or cephalosporins.
Use Cautiously in: ■ Renal impair-

P

ment (dosage reduction recommended) ▪ Pregnancy and lactation (safety not established) ▪ Sodium restriction.

ADVERSE REACTIONS AND SIDE EFFECTS*

CNS: confusion, lethargy, SEIZURES (high doses).
CV: congestive heart failure, arrhythmias.
Derm: rashes, urticaria.
F and E: hypokalemia, hypernatremia.
GI: nausea, diarrhea, hepatitis.
GU: hematuria (children only), interstitial nephritis.
Hemat: bleeding, bloody dyscrasias, increased bleeding time.
Local: phlebitis at IV site, pain at IM site.
Metab: metabolic alkalosis.
Misc: superinfection, hypersensitivity reactions, including ANAPHYLAXIS and serum sickness.

INTERACTIONS

Drug-Drug: ▪ **Probenecid** decreases renal excretion and increases blood levels ▪ May alter excretion of **lithium** ▪ **Diuretics, glucocorticoids,** or **amphotericin B** may increase the risk of hypokalemia ▪ Additive risk of hepatotoxicity with other **hepatotoxic agents** ▪ May decrease the half-life of **aminoglycosides** (given by different routes) when used concurrently in patients with renal impairment.

ROUTE AND DOSAGE

Note: Contains 1.85 mEq sodium/g of piperacillin.

- **IM (Adults):** 1.5–4 g q 6–12 hr.
- **IV (Adults):** 1.5–4 g q 6–12 hr (up to 4 g q 4 hr, maximum of 24 g/day)

PHARMACODYNAMICS (blood levels)

	ONSET	PEAK
IM	rapid	30–50 min
IV	rapid	end of infusion

NURSING IMPLICATIONS

Assessment

- □ Assess patient for infection (vital signs; appearance of wound, sputum, urine, and stool; WBC) at beginning and throughout course of therapy.
- □ Obtain a history before initiating therapy to determine previous use of and reactions to penicillins or cephalosporins. Persons with a negative history of penicillin sensitivity may still have an allergic response.
- □ Obtain specimens for culture and sensitivity prior to initiating therapy. First dose may be given before receiving results.
- □ Observe patient for signs and symptoms of anaphylaxis (rash, pruritus, laryngeal edema, wheezing). Discontinue the drug and notify the physician immediately if these occur. Keep epinephrine, an antihistamine, and resuscitation equipment close by in the event of an anaphylactic reaction.
- ▪ **Lab Test Considerations:** Renal and hepatic function, CBC, serum potassium, and bleeding times should be evaluated prior to and routinely throughout course of therapy.
- □ May cause positive direct Coombs' test results.
- □ May cause elevated BUN, creatinine, SGOT (AST), SGPT (ALT), serum bilirubin, and LDH.
- □ May cause elevated serum sodium and decreased serum potassium concentrations.

Potential Nursing Diagnoses

- Infection, high risk for (indications, side effects).
- Knowledge deficit related to medication regimen (patient/family teaching).

Implementation

- **IM:** To constitute for IM use, add 4 ml of sterile water, bacteriostatic water, 0.9% NaCl for injection, or 0.5 or 1% lidocaine hydrochloride injection (without epinephrine) to each 2-g vial, 6 ml to each 3-g vial, and 7.8 ml

*Underlines indicate most frequent; **CAPITALS** indicate life-threatening.

to each 4-g vial for a concentration of 1 g/2.5 ml.

- ▫ Inject deep into a well-developed muscle mass and massage well. IM injections should not exceed 2 g at each site.
- ▪ **IV:** The initial reconstitution for IV use is made with at least 5 ml of sterile water for injection, 0.9% NaCl, or bacteriostatic water. Shake well until dissolved. Reconstituted soln is stable for 24 hr at room temperature and 7 days if refrigerated.
- ▫ Change IV sites every 48 hr to prevent phlebitis.
- ▪ **Direct IV:** Inject slowly, over 3–5 min, to minimize vein irritation.
- ▪ **Intermittent Infusion:** Dilute in at least 50 ml of 0.9% NaCl, D5W, D5/0.9% NaCl, or lactated Ringer's soln.
- ▫ *Rate:* Administer over 20–30 min via Y-site injection. Manufacturer recommends temporarily discontinuing primary infusion during piperacillin administration.
- ▪ **Syringe Compatibility:** heparin.
- ▪ **Y-Site Compatibility:** acyclovir, ciprofloxacin, cyclophosphamide, enalaprilat, esmolol, famotidine, foscarnet, hydromorphone, labetalol, magnesium sulfate, meperidine, morphine, perphenazine, verapamil, or zidovudine.
- ▪ **Y-Site Incompatibility:** ondansetron.
- ▪ **Additive Compatibility:** ciprofloxacin, clindamycin, hydrocortisone sodium succinate, potassium chloride, or verapamil.
- ▪ **Additive Incompatibility:** Incompatible with aminoglycosides; do not admix; administer at least 1 hr apart.

PATIENT/FAMILY TEACHING

- ▫ Advise patient to report the signs of superinfection (black, furry overgrowth on the tongue; vaginal itching or discharge; loose or foul-smelling stools) and allergy.

EVALUATION

Clinical response can be evaluated by:
▪ Resolution of the signs and symptoms of infection. Length of time for complete resolution depends on the organism and site of infection.

PIRBUTEROL
(peer-**byoo**-ter-ole)
Maxair

CLASSIFICATION(S):
Bronchodilator—beta-adrenergic agonist
Pregnancy Category C

INDICATIONS

▪ Used as a bronchodilator in reversible airway obstruction due to asthma or COPD.

ACTION

▪ Results in the accumulation of cyclic adenosine monophosphate (cAMP) at beta-adrenergic receptors, producing: ▫ Bronchodilation ▫ CNS and cardiac stimulation ▫ Diuresis ▫ Gastric acid secretion ▪ Relatively selective for $beta_2$ (pulmonary) receptors. **Therapeutic Effect:** ▪ Bronchodilation.

PHARMACOKINETICS

Absorption: Minimal systemic absorption following inhalation.
Distribution: Not known.
Metabolism and Excretion: Metabolized by the liver.
Half-life: 2 hr.

CONTRAINDICATIONS AND PRECAUTIONS

Contraindicated in: ▪ Hypersensitivity to adrenergic amines.
Use Cautiously in: ▪ Cardiac disease ▪ Hypertension ▪ Hyperthyroidism ▪ Diabetes mellitus ▪ Glaucoma ▪ Pregnancy (near term) ▪ Elderly patients (more susceptible to adverse reactions; dosage reduction recommended) ▪ Lactation and children (safety not established) ▪ Excessive use (may lead to tolerance and paradoxical bronchospasm).

P

ADVERSE REACTIONS AND SIDE EFFECTS*

CNS: nervousness, insomnia, tremor, headache.
EENT: dry mouth.
Resp: cough, paradoxical bronchospasm.
CV: palpitations, tachycardia.
GI: nausea.

INTERACTIONS

Drug–Drug: ▪ Increased risk of adverse cardiovascular effects (hypertension, arrhythmias) with concurrent use of **inhalation anesthetics, cocaine, antidepressants, cardiac glycosides, decongestants, CNS stimulants,** and **vasopressors** ▪ Use with **MAO inhibitors** may lead to hypertensive crisis ▪ **Beta-adrenergic blockers** may decrease effectiveness ▪ Although frequently used in combination with **theophylline-type bronchodilators,** CNS and cardiovascular toxicity may be additive.

ROUTE AND DOSAGE

- **Inhaln (Adults and Children >12 yr):** 1–2 inhaln (200 mcg/spray) q 4–6 hr, not to exceed 12 inhaln/24 hr.

PHARMACODYNAMICS

	ONSET	PEAK	DURATION
Inhaln	5–15 min	60–90 min	4–6 hr

NURSING IMPLICATIONS

Assessment

- Assess blood pressure, pulse, respiratory pattern, lung sounds, and character of secretions before administration and during peak of medication.
- Monitor pulmonary function tests before initiating therapy and periodically throughout course to determine effectiveness of medication.
- Observe patient for paradoxical bronchospasm (wheezing). If this condition occurs, withhold medication and notify physician immediately.

Potential Nursing Diagnoses

- Airway clearance, ineffective (indications).
- Knowledge deficit related to medication regimen (patient/family teaching).

Implementation

- **Inhaln:** Allow at least 1 min between inhalation of aerosol medications. Have patient rinse mouth with water following each inhalation to decrease dry mouth and throat.

Patient/Family Teaching

- Instruct patient in the proper use of the inhaler. Shake well, exhale, close lips firmly around mouthpiece, administer during second half of inhalation, and hold breath as long as possible after treatment to ensure deep instillation of medication. Do not take more than 2 inhalations at one time; allow 1–2 min between inhalations. Wash inhalation assembly at least daily in warm running water.
- Caution patient not to exceed recommended dose; may cause adverse effects or loss of effectiveness of medication.
- Patients using inhalation glucocorticoids and pirbuterol should be advised to use pirbuterol first and allow 5 min to elapse between using other aerosols, unless otherwise directed by physician.
- Advise patient to contact physician immediately if shortness of breath is not relieved by medication or is accompanied by diaphoresis, dizziness, palpitations, or chest pain.
- Instruct patient to maintain an adequate fluid intake (2000–3000 ml/day) to help liquefy tenacious secretions.
- Advise patient to consult physician or pharmacist before taking any over-the-counter medications or alcoholic beverages concurrently with this therapy.

Evaluation

Effectiveness of therapy can be demonstrated by: ▪ Decrease in bronchocon-

*Underlines indicate most frequent; **CAPITALS** indicate life-threatening.

striction and bronchospasm ▫ Increased ease of breathing.

PIROXICAM
(peer-**ox**-i-kam)
{Apo-Piroxicam}, Feldene, {Novopirocam}

CLASSIFICATION(S):
Nonsteroidal anti-inflammatory agent
Pregnancy Category UK

INDICATIONS
▪ Management of inflammatory disorders, including: ▫ Rheumatoid arthritis ▫ Osteoarthritis.

ACTION
▪ Inhibits prostaglandin synthesis. **Therapeutic Effects:** ▪ Suppression of pain and inflammation.

PHARMACOKINETICS
Absorption: Well absorbed from the GI tract.
Distribution: Distribution not known. Enters breast milk in small amounts.
Metabolism and Excretion: Mostly metabolized by the liver. Minimal amounts excreted unchanged by the kidneys.
Half-life: 50 hr.

CONTRAINDICATIONS AND PRECAUTIONS
Contraindicated in: ▪ Hypersensitivity ▪ Cross-sensitivity may exist with other nonsteroidal anti-inflammatory agents, including aspirin ▪ Active GI bleeding or ulcer disease ▪ Pregnancy.
Use Cautiously in: ▪ Severe cardiovascular or hepatic disease ▪ History of ulcer disease ▪ Lactation or children (safety not established) ▪ Renal impairment (dosage reduction recommended).

ADVERSE REACTIONS AND SIDE EFFECTS*
CNS: <u>headache</u>, <u>drowsiness</u>, dizziness.
EENT: blurred vision, tinnitus.
CV: edema.
GI: <u>nausea</u>, <u>dyspepsia</u>, <u>vomiting</u>, diarrhea, constipation, **GI BLEEDING**, <u>discomfort</u>, **HEPATITIS**, flatulence, anorexia.
GU: renal failure.
Derm: rashes.
Hemat: blood dyscrasias, prolonged bleeding time.
Misc: allergic reactions, including **ANAPHYLAXIS**.

INTERACTIONS
Drug-Drug: Concurrent use with **aspirin** decreases piroxicam blood levels and may decrease effectiveness ▪ Increased risk of bleeding with **oral anticoagulants, cefamandole, cefoperazone, cefotetan, moxalactam, heparin, thrombolytic agents,** or **plicamycin** ▪ Additive adverse GI side effects with **aspirin, glucocorticoids,** and other **nonsteroidal anti-inflammatory agents** ▪ **Probenecid** increases blood levels and may increase toxicity ▪ May decrease response to **antihypertensives** or **diuretics** ▪ May increase serum levels and risk of toxicity from **lithium** ▪ Increased risk of photosensitivity with other **photosensitizing agents** ▪ May increase risk of hypoglycemia from **insulin** or **oral hypoglycemic agents** ▪ Increased risk of adverse renal effects with **gold compounds** or chronic use of **acetaminophen** ▪ May increase the risk of hematologic toxicity from **antineoplastic agents** or **radiation therapy**.

ROUTE AND DOSAGE
▪ **PO (Adults):** 20 mg/day, may be given as single dose or divided bid.

PHARMACODYNAMICS

	ONSET	PEAK	DURATION
PO (analgesic effect)	1 hr	UK	48–72 hr
PO (anti-inflammatory effect)	7–12 days	2–3 wk*	UK

*May take up to 12 wk.

{} = Available in Canada only.
*<u>Underlines</u> indicate most frequent; **CAPITALS** indicate life-threatening.

P

NURSING IMPLICATIONS

Assessment

- **General Info:** Patients who have asthma, aspirin-induced allergy, and nasal polyps are at increased risk for developing hypersensitivity reactions. Monitor for rhinitis, asthma, and urticaria.
- **Arthritis:** Assess pain and range of motion prior to and 1–2 hr following administration.
- **Lab Test Considerations:** BUN, serum creatinine, CBC, serum potassium, and liver function tests should be evaluated periodically in patients receiving prolonged courses of therapy.
  - Serum potassium, alkaline phosphatase, LDH, SGOT (AST), and SGPT (ALT) levels may be increased.
  - Hematocrit, hemoglobin, and uric acid concentrations may be decreased. Blood glucose concentrations may be increased or decreased.
  - Bleeding time may be prolonged for up to 2 wk following discontinuation of therapy.

Potential Nursing Diagnoses

- Comfort, altered: pain (indications).
- Mobility, impaired physical (indications).
- Knowledge deficit related to medication regimen (patient/family teaching).

Implementation

- **PO:** Administered with meals or antacids (preferably magnesium-containing or aluminum-containing) to decrease GI irritation.

Patient/Family Teaching

- Advise patients to take this medication with a full glass of water and to remain in an upright position for 15–30 min after administration.
- Instruct patient to take medication exactly as prescribed. If a dose is missed, it should be taken as soon as remembered but not if almost time for the next dose. Do not double doses.
- This medication may cause drowsiness or dizziness. Advise patient to avoid driving or other activities requiring alertness until response to the medication is known.
- Caution patient to avoid the concurrent use of alcohol, aspirin, acetaminophen, or other over-the-counter medications without consultation with physician or pharmacist.
- Advise patient to notify physician or dentist of medication regimen prior to treatment of surgery.
- Instruct patient to notify physician if rash, itching, chills, fever, muscle aches, visual disturbances, weight gain, edema, black stools, or persistent headache occurs.

Evaluation

Effectiveness of therapy can be demonstrated by: ▪ Decreased pain and improved joint mobility. Partial arthritic relief is usually seen within 2 wk, but maximum effectiveness may require up to 12 wk of continuous therapy. Patients who do not respond to one nonsteroidal anti-inflammatory agent may respond to another.

PLASMA PROTEIN FRACTION

(**plaz**-ma **proe**-teen **frak**-shun)
Plasmanate, Plasma-Plex, Plasmatein, Protenate

CLASSIFICATION(S):
Volume expander
Pregnancy Category C

INDICATIONS

▪ Expansion of plasma volume and maintenance of cardiac output in situations associated with deficiencies in circulatory volume, including: ▫ Shock ▫ Hemorrhage ▫ Burns ▪ Temporary replacement therapy in edema associated with low plasma proteins, such as the nephrotic syndrome and end-stage liver disease.

ACTION

▪ Provides colloidal osmotic pressure (in the form of albumin and globulins)

within the intravascular space, causing the shift of water from extravascular tissues back into the intravascular space.
Therapeutic Effect: ▪ Mobilization of fluid from extravascular tissue into intravascular space.

PHARMACOKINETICS

Absorption: Administered IV only, resulting in complete bioavailability.
Distribution: Stays mainly in the intravascular space.
Metabolism and Excretion: UK.
Half-life: UK.

CONTRAINDICATIONS AND PRECAUTIONS

Contraindicated in: ▪ Allergic reactions to albumin ▪ Severe anemia ▪ Congestive heart failure ▪ Normal or increased intravascular volume ▪ Cardiopulmonary bypass procedures.
Use Cautiously in: ▪ Severe hepatic or renal disease ▪ Rapid infusion (may cause hypotension or hypertension) ▪ Dehydration (additional fluids may be required) ▪ Large doses (may cause anemia, requiring transfusion).

ADVERSE REACTIONS AND SIDE EFFECTS*

CNS: headache.
CV: tachycardia, hypotension, vascular overload.
GI: nausea, vomiting, excess salivation.
Derm: erythema, urticaria.
MS: back pain.
Misc: fever, chills, flushing.

INTERACTIONS

Drug–Drug: ▪ None significant.

ROUTE AND DOSAGE

Note: Dose is highly individualized and depends on condition being treated. Contains 130–160 mEq sodium/L.

Hypovolemia

- **IV (Adults):** 250–500 ml (12.5–25 g protein).
- **IV (Infants and Young Children):** 6.3–33 ml/kg (0.33–1.65 g/kg protein).

Hypoproteinemia

- **IV (Adults):** 1000–1500 ml (50–75 g protein).

PHARMACODYNAMICS (intravascular volume expansion)

	ONSET	PEAK	DURATION
IV	15–30 min	UK	UK

NURSING IMPLICATIONS

Assessment

- Monitor vital signs, CVP, pulmonary capillary wedge pressure (PCWP), and intake and output prior to and frequently throughout therapy. Hypotension may result from too rapid infusion.
- Assess patient for signs of vascular overload (elevated CVP, elevated PCWP, rales/crackles, dyspnea, hypertension, jugular venous distention) during and following administration.
- Assess surgical patients for increased bleeding following administration caused by increased blood pressure and circulating blood volume. Plasma protein fraction does not contain clotting factors.
- **Lab Test Considerations:** Monitor hemoglobin, hematocrit, serum protein, and electrolytes throughout course of therapy.

Potential Nursing Diagnoses

- Cardiac output, decreased (indications).
- Fluid volume deficit (indications).
- Fluid volume excess (side effects).

Implementation

- **General Info:** Administer through a large-gauge (at least 20-G) needle. Use administration set provided by manufacturer.
- Soln may vary from nearly colorless to straw to brownish. Do not use cloudy soln. Each liter of plasma protein fraction contains 130–160 mEq of so-

*Underlines indicate most frequent; **CAPITALS** indicate life-threatening.

P

dium. Store at room temperature. Do not administer more than 250 g (5000 ml 5%) in 48 hr.

- □ There is no danger of serum hepatitis from plasma protein fraction. Cross-matching is not required.
- □ Dehydration should be corrected by additional IV fluids.
- ▪ **Intermittent Infusion:** Administer plasma protein fraction undiluted by IV infusion. Infusion must be completed within 4 hr.
- □ *Rate:* Rate of administration is determined by blood volume, indication, and patient response but should not exceed 10 ml/min, to minimize the possibility of hypotension. As the plasma volume approaches normal, the rate of administration should not exceed 5–8 ml/min. The rate for infants and children should not exceed 5–10 ml/min. Monitor the patient for signs of hypervolemia.
- ▪ **Additive Compatibility:** carbohydrate and electrolyte solns, whole blood, packed red blood cells, chloramphenicol, or tetracycline.
- ▪ **Additive Incompatibility:** solns containing protein hydrolysates, amino acids, alcohol, or norepinephrine.

Patient/Family Teaching

- □ Explain the rationale for use of this soln to the patient.

Evaluation

Effectiveness of therapy can be demonstrated by: ▪ Increase in blood pressure and blood volume when used to treat shock ▪ Elevated serum plasma protein in patients with hypoproteinemia.

PLICAMYCIN

(plye-ka-**mye**-sin)
mithramycin, Mithracin

CLASSIFICATION(S):
Antineoplastic—antitumor antibiotic, Electrolyte/Electrolyte modifier—hypocalcemic agent
Pregnancy Category X

INDICATIONS

▪ Treatment of advanced unresponsive testicular carcinoma ▪ Management of hypercalcemia and hypercalciuria associated with malignancy.

ACTION

▪ Forms a complex with DNA that subsequently inhibits RNA synthesis ▪ Antagonizes the action of vitamin D and inhibits the action of parathyroid hormone on osteoclasts. **Therapeutic Effects:** ▪ Death of rapidly replicating cells, particularly malignant ones ▪ Lowering of serum calcium.

PHARMACOKINETICS

Absorption: Administered IV only, resulting in complete bioavailability.
Distribution: Appears to concentrate in the liver, renal tubule, and bone surface. Crosses the blood-brain barrier.
Metabolism and Excretion: Excreted primarily by the kidneys.
Half-life: UK.

CONTRAINDICATIONS AND PRECAUTIONS

Contraindicated in: ▪ Hypersensitivity ▪ Bleeding disorders ▪ Depressed bone-marrow reserve ▪ Hypocalcemia ▪ Severe renal or liver disease ▪ Pregnancy or lactation.
Use Cautiously in: ▪ Patients with childbearing potential ▪ Active infections ▪ Other chronic debilitating illnesses ▪ Renal or hepatic impairment (dosage reduction required) ▪ Children (safety not established).

ADVERSE REACTIONS AND SIDE EFFECTS*

CNS: drowsiness, weakness, lethargy, malaise, headache, depression, nervousness, irritability, dizziness, fatigue.
EENT: epistaxis.
GI: anorexia, nausea, vomiting, stomatitis, diarrhea, hepatitis.
GU: renal failure, gonadal suppression.
Derm: facial flushing, rashes.
F and E: hypocalcemia, hypophospha-

*Underlines indicate most frequent; **CAPITALS** indicate life-threatening.

temia, hypokalemia, rebound hypercalcemia.
Hemat: BLEEDING, thrombocytopenia, leukopenia, anemia.
Local: phlebitis at IV site.
Misc: fever.

INTERACTIONS

Drug-Drug: ▪ Additive myelosuppression with other **antineoplastic agents** or **radiation therapy** ▪ Increased risk of bleeding with **aspirin, oral anticoagulants, thrombolytic agents, heparin, some cephalosporins, nonsteroidal anti-inflammatory agents, sulfinpyrazone, valproic acid,** or **dextran** ▪ Increased risk of hepatotoxicity with other **hepatotoxic agents** ▪ Increased risk of renal toxicity with other **nephrotoxic agents**.

ROUTE AND DOSAGE

Testicular Tumors

- **IV (Adults):** 25–30 mcg/kg once daily for 8–10 days or until toxicity occurs (not to exceed 30 mcg/kg/day or more than 10 days or 2.5–50 mcg/kg every other day for 8 doses). May be repeated monthly.

Hypercalcemia, Hypercalciuria

- **IV (Adults):** 15–25 mcg/kg once daily for 3–4 days, may be repeated q 3–7 days.

PHARMACODYNAMICS

	ONSET	PEAK	DURATION
IV (hematologic effects)	UK	7–10 days	3–4 wk
IV (hypocalcemic effects)	24–48 hr	UK	3–15 days

NURSING IMPLICATIONS

Assessment

- **General Info:** Monitor closely for bleeding (bleeding gums, bruising, petechiae; guaiac stools, urine, and emesis). May begin as epistaxis and progress to severe generalized or GI bleeding. May require blood transfusions, fresh frozen plasma, vitamin K, or aminocaproic acid to control bleeding. Avoid IM injections and rectal temperatures. Apply pressure to venipuncture sites for 10 min.
- □ Monitor intake and output, appetite, and nutritional intake. May cause nausea and vomiting. Confer with physician regarding prophylactic use of an antiemetic. Adjust diet as tolerated to help maintain fluid and electrolyte balance and nutritional status.
- □ Assess for fever, sore throat, and signs of infection. Notify physician if these symptoms occur.
- **Hypercalcemia:** Monitor symptoms of hypercalcemia (nausea, vomiting, anorexia, thirst, weakness, constipation, paralytic ileus, and bradycardia). Observe patient for evidence of hypocalcemia (paresthesia, muscle twitching, laryngospasm, colic, cardiac arrhythmias, and Chvostek's or Trousseau's sign).
- **Lab Test Considerations:** Monitor platelet count, prothrombin time, and bleeding time prior to and periodically throughout therapy. Notify physician if platelet count is $<150,000/mm^3$ or prothrombin time is elevated 4 or more secs above control.
- □ Monitor CBC and differential prior to and periodically throughout therapy. Notify physician if leukocyte count is $<4000/mm^3$.
- □ Monitor serum electrolytes prior to and daily during course of therapy. May cause hypocalcemia, hypokalemia, and hypophosphatemia. Correct electrolyte imbalances before beginning therapy. Calcium and phosphate levels may rebound after therapy.
- □ Monitor liver function studies (SGOT [AST], SGPT [ALT], LDH, bilirubin) and renal function studies (BUN, creatinine, urinalysis) prior to and periodically throughout therapy to detect hepatotoxicity and nephrotoxicity.

Potential Nursing Diagnoses

- Injury, high risk for (side effects).
- Infection, high risk for (side effects).

- Body image disturbance (side effects).

Implementation

- **General Info:** Soln should be prepared in a biologic cabinet. Wear gloves, gown, and mask while handling medication. Discard equipment in designated containers (see Appendix I).
- Ensure patency of the IV. If patient complains of discomfort at the IV site or if extravasation occurs, discontinue IV and restart at another site. Extravasation may cause irritation and cellulitis. Apply ice to site to prevent pain and swelling. If swelling occurs, confer with physician regarding application of moderate heat to site.
- **Intermittent Infusion:** To reconstitute, add 4.9 ml of sterile water for injection to the 2.5-mg vial of plicamycin to yield a final concentration of 500 mcg/ml. Use immediately after reconstitution.
- *Rate:* Add to 1000 ml of D5W or 0.9% NaCl and infuse over 4–6 hr. Rapid infusion rate will increase GI side effects.

Patient/Family Teaching

- Advise patient to notify physician promptly if fever, chills, sore throat, signs of infection, bleeding gums, bruising, petechiae, or blood in urine, stool, or emesis occurs. Caution patient to avoid crowds and persons with known infections. Instruct patient to use soft toothbrush and electric razor. Patients should be cautioned not to drink alcoholic beverages or take aspirin-containing products.
- Instruct patient to notify physician if weakness, rash, persistent nausea or vomiting, or depression occurs.
- Instruct patient to inspect oral mucosa for redness and ulceration. If mouth sores occur, advise patient to use sponge brush and rinse mouth with water after eating and drinking. Physician may order viscous lidocaine swishes if pain interferes with eating.
- Advise patient that although fertility may be decreased with plicamycin, contraception should be used during therapy because of potential teratogenic effects on the fetus.
- Instruct patient not to receive any vaccinations without advice of physician.
- Emphasize need for periodic lab tests to monitor for side effects.

Evaluation

Effectiveness of therapy can be demonstrated by: ▪ Decrease in size and spread of malignant tissue ▪ Normalization of elevated calcium levels in hypercalcemia and hypercalciuria within 24–48 hr.

POLYCARBOPHIL

(pol-i-**kar**-boe-fil)

Equalactin, FiberCon, Mitrolan

CLASSIFICATION(S):

Laxative—bulk-forming agent, Antidiarrheal

Pregnancy Category UK

INDICATIONS

- Treatment of constipation or diarrhea.

ACTION

▪ Acts as a bulk laxative by keeping water within the bowel lumen ▪ Acts as an antidiarrheal by taking on water within the bowel lumen to create a formed stool. **Therapeutic Effect:** ▪ Normalization of bowel water content while adding bulk, treating both diarrhea and constipation.

PHARMACOKINETICS

Absorption: Minimal systemic absorption.

Distribution: Distribution not known.

Metabolism and Excretion: Complex plus absorbed water is excreted in the feces.

Half-life: UK.

CONTRAINDICATIONS AND PRECAUTIONS

Contraindicated in: ▪ Hypersensitivity ▪ Abdominal pain ▪ Nausea or vomiting (especially when associated with fever or other signs of acute abdomen) ▪ Serious intra-abdominal adhesions ▪ Dysphagia.

Use Cautiously in: ▪ Pregnancy or lactation (has been used safely).

ADVERSE REACTIONS AND SIDE EFFECTS*

GI: abdominal fullness.

INTERACTIONS

Drug–Drug: ▪ May decrease the absorption of concurrently administered **tetracycline**.

ROUTE AND DOSAGE

- **PO (Adults):** 1 g qid, or as needed, not to exceed 6 g/24 hr.
- **PO (Children 6–12 yr):** 500 mg 1–3 times daily or as needed, not to exceed 3 g/24 hr.
- **PO (Children 2–6 yr):** 500 mg 1–2 times daily, or as needed, not to exceed 1.5 g/24 hr.

PHARMACODYNAMICS (effect on bowel function)

	ONSET	PEAK	DURATION
PO	12–24 hr*	UK	UK

*May take as long as 72 hr.

NURSING IMPLICATIONS

Assessment

- **General Info:** Assess for fever, nausea, vomiting, abdominal distention, and pain. Notify physician if present. Auscultate bowel sounds. Inquire about patient's usual diet, fluid intake, activity level, and bowel function.
- □ Monitor for color, consistency, and amount of stool produced.
- **Diarrhea:** Monitor for signs of dehydration (decreased skin turgor, dry mucous membranes, weight loss, decreased urine output, tachycardia, and hypotension).

Potential Nursing Diagnoses

- Bowel elimination, altered: constipation (indications).
- Bowel elimination, altered: diarrhea (indications).
- Knowledge deficit related to medication regimen (patient/family teaching).

Implementation

- **General Info:** Administer 1 hr before or 2 hr after tetracycline.
- **Diarrhea:** For treatment of severe diarrhea, dose may be repeated every 30 min. Do not exceed total daily prescribed dose.
- **Constipation:** For treatment of constipation, administer with 8 oz of water or juice.

Patient/Family Teaching

- □ Encourage patients with constipation to use other forms of bowel regulation, such as increasing bulk in diet, fluid intake, and mobility. Normal bowel habits are individualized and may vary from 3 times/day to 3 times/wk.
- □ Instruct patients with sudden onset of constipation to notify physician, as medical evaluation may be necessary.
- □ Instruct patients with diarrhea to notify physician if fever or bloody stools occur or if diarrhea persists or worsens. Discuss need for fluids and diet modifications during episode of diarrhea.

Evaluation

Effectiveness of therapy can be demonstrated by: ▪ Soft, formed bowel movement. May require 3 days for therapeutic effect to occur.

POLYETHYLENE GLYCOL/ELECTROLYTE

(po-lee-**eth**-e-leen **glye**-kole/e-**lek**-troe-lite)

Colovage, CoLyte, GoLYTELY, NuLytely, OCL, PEG-ES

*Underlines indicate most frequent; **CAPITALS** indicate life-threatening.

P

CLASSIFICATION(S):
Laxative—osmotic
Pregnancy Category C

INDICATIONS

▪ Bowel cleansing in preparation for GI examination. **Unlabeled Use:** ▪ Treatment of acute iron overdose in children.

ACTION

▪ Polyethylene glycol (PEG) in soln acts as an osmotic agent, drawing water into the lumen of the GI tract. **Therapeutic Effect:** ▪ Evacuation of the GI tract without water or electrolyte imbalance.

PHARMACOKINETICS

Absorption: Ions in the soln are nonabsorbable.
Distribution: Distribution not known.
Metabolism and Excretion: Soln is excreted in fecal contents.
Half-life: UK.

CONTRAINDICATIONS AND PRECAUTIONS

Contraindicated in: ▪ GI obstruction ▪ Gastric retention ▪ Toxic colitis ▪ Megacolon.
Use Cautiously in: ▪ Patients with absent or diminished gag reflex ▪ Unconscious or semicomatose states, in which administration is via nasogastric tube ▪ Barium enema using double-contrast technique (may not allow proper barium coating of mucosa) ▪ Abdominal pain of uncertain cause, particularly if accompanied by fever ▪ Children (safety not established).

ADVERSE REACTIONS AND SIDE EFFECTS*

GI: abdominal fullness, nausea, bloating, cramps, vomiting.

INTERACTIONS

Drug–Drug: ▪ Interferes with the absorption of **orally administered medications** by decreasing transit time. (Do not administer within 1 hr of start of therapy.)

ROUTE AND DOSAGE

▪ **PO (Adults):** 4 liters of soln, given as 240 ml q 10 min.

PHARMACODYNAMICS

	ONSET	PEAK	DURATION
PO	1 hr	UK	4 hr

NURSING IMPLICATIONS

Assessment

- Assess patient for abdominal distention, presence of bowel sounds, and usual pattern of bowel function.
- Assess color, consistency, and amount of stool produced.
- Monitor semiconscious or unconscious patients closely for regurgitation when administering via nasogastric tube.

Potential Nursing Diagnoses

▪ Bowel elimination, altered: diarrhea (side effects).
▪ Knowledge deficit related to medication regimen (patient/family teaching).

Implementation

▪ **General Info:** Do not add flavorings or additional ingredients to soln prior to administration.
- Patient should fast for 3–4 hr prior to administration and should not have solid food within 2 hr of administration.
- Patient should be allowed only clear liquids after administration.

▪ **PO:** Soln may be reconstituted with tap water. Shake vigorously until powder is dissolved.

Patient/Family Teaching

- Instruct patient to drink 240 ml every 10 min until 4 liters have been consumed. Rapidly drinking each 240 ml is preferred over drinking small amounts continuously.

*Underlines indicate most frequent; **CAPITALS** indicate life-threatening.

Evaluation

Effectiveness of therapy can be demonstrated by: ▪ Diarrhea, which cleanses the bowel within 4 hr. The first bowel movement usually occurs within 1 hr of administration.

POLYMYXIN B

(pol-ee-**mix**-in bee)
Aerosporin

CLASSIFICATION(S):
Anti-infective—miscellaneous
Pregnancy Category UK

INDICATIONS

▪ **IM, IV:** Treatment of the following serious infections due to susceptible organisms in patients who are unable to tolerate less toxic anti-infectives: ▫ Urinary tract infections ▫ Meningitis (requires additional intrathecal administration) ▫ Septicemia ▪ **Ophth:** Ophthalmic infections ▪ **Top:** Used locally in combination with other anti-infectives in a wide variety of dosage forms for the treatment and prevention of superficial infections.

ACTION

▪ Binds to bacterial cell wall, resulting in death of the organism. **Therapeutic Effect:** ▪ Bactericidal action. **Spectrum:** ▪ Limited to some gram-negative pathogens that may be resistant to other anti-infectives, including: ▫ *Haemophilus influenzae* ▫ *Pseudomonas aeruginosa* ▫ *Enterobacter aerogenes* ▫ *Klebsiella pneumoniae* ▪ Not active against *Proteus* or *Neisseria* species.

PHARMACOKINETICS

Absorption: Poorly absorbed following oral administration (up to 10% in neonates). Well absorbed following IM administration. Minimal systemic absorption following topical use.
Distribution: Widely distributed. Does not enter the CNS or cross the placenta.
Metabolism and Excretion: 60% excreted unchanged by the kidneys.
Half-life: 4.3–6 hr (increased in renal impairment).

CONTRAINDICATIONS AND PRECAUTIONS

Contraindicated in: ▪ Hypersensitivity.
Use Cautiously in: ▪ Neuromuscular diseases, including myasthenia gravis ▪ Renal impairment (dosage reduction recommended) ▪ Pregnancy or lactation (safety not established).

ADVERSE REACTIONS AND SIDE EFFECTS*

CNS: neurotoxicity; IT—headache.
EENT: Ophth—blurred vision, stinging, burning, itching.
Resp: RESPIRATORY PARALYSIS.
GU: nephrotoxicity.
Derm: flushing of the face, rashes; Top—allergic contact dermatitis.
Local: pain at IM site, phlebitis at IV site.
MS: IT—stiff neck.
Neuro: neuromuscular blockade.
Misc: fever, hypersensitivity reactions, including ANAPHYLAXIS, fungal superinfection.

INTERACTIONS

Drug-Drug: ▪ Increased risk of neuromuscular blockade with **general anesthetics** or **neuromuscular blocking agents, aminoglycoside anti-infectives, procainamide,** or **quinidine**.

ROUTE AND DOSAGE

Note: 1 mg = 10,000 units.

- **IV (Adults and Children >2 yr):** 15,000–25,000 units/kg/day in divided doses q 12 hr (not to exceed 25,000 units/kg/day in adults).
- **IM (Adults and Children >2 yr):** 25,000–30,000 units/kg/day in divided doses q 4–6 hr (not to exceed 25,000 units/kg/day in adults).
- **IV, IM (Infants):** up to 40,000 units/kg/day in divided doses.
- **IT (Adults and Children >2 yr):**

*Underlines indicate most frequent; **CAPITALS** indicate life-threatening.

50,000 units/day for 3–4 days, then every other day for 2 wk after negative CSF cultures and normal CSF glucose.

- **Intratrathecal (Children <2 yr):** 20,000 units/day for 3–4 days then 25,000 units every other day for 2 wk after negative CSF cultures and normal CSF glucose; or 25,000 units every other day continued for 2 wk after negative CSF cultures and normal CSF glucose.
- **Ophth:** 1–3 drops of soln (soln contains 10,000–25,000 units/ml) q 1 hr; dosage interval may be increased as response occurs.

PHARMACODYNAMICS (blood levels)

	ONSET	PEAK
IV	rapid	end of infusion
IM	rapid	within 2 hr

NURSING IMPLICATIONS

Assessment

- Assess patient for infection (vital signs; appearance of wound, sputum, urine, and stool; WBC) at beginning and throughout course of therapy.
- Obtain specimens for culture and sensitivity prior to initiating therapy. First dose may be given before receiving results.
- Monitor intake and output and daily weight to assess hydration status and renal function. Notify physician if a decrease in urine output occurs.
- Assess patient for neurotoxic reaction (irritability, weakness, ataxia, drowsiness, perioral paresthesia, numbness of extremities, blurred vision) throughout course of therapy. Neurotoxicity is usually associated with high serum levels.
- Assess patient for signs of superinfection (fever, upper respiratory infection, vaginal itching or discharge, increasing malaise, diarrhea). Report occurrence to physician.
- Monitor IV site for thrombophlebitis throughout therapy.
- **Lab Test Considerations:** Monitor renal function by urinalysis, specific gravity, BUN, creatinine, and creatinine clearance prior to and throughout therapy.

Potential Nursing Diagnoses

- Infection, high risk for (indications).
- Injury, high risk for (side effects).

Implementation

- **General Info:** Keep patient well hydrated (1500–2000 ml/day) during therapy.
- Available in ophthalmic soln and injectable forms. Also available in combination with other antibiotics in other dosage forms (see Appendix A).
- **IM:** Reconstitute each 500,000-unit vial with 2 ml of sterile water for injection, 0.9% NaCl, or procaine 1%.
- IM administration is not routinely recommended because of severe pain at injection site. Administer deep into a well-developed muscle.
- **Intermittent Infusion:** Dilute each 500,000 units in 300–500 ml of D5W. Soln should be refrigerated; discard unused portions after 72 hr.
- *Rate:* Infuse slowly over 60–90 min.
- **Syringe Compatibility:** methicillin or penicillin G sodium.
- **Y-Site Compatibility:** esmolol.
- **Additive Compatibility:** amikacin, ascorbic acid, colistimethate, diphenhydramine, erythromycin lactobionate, hydrocortisone sodium succinate, kanamycin, methicillin, penicillin G potassium and sodium, or phenobarbital.
- **Additive Incompatibility:** amphotericin B, cefazolin, cephalothin, chloramphenicol, chlorothiazide, heparin, magnesium sulfate, prednisolone sodium phosphate, or tetracycline.
- **IT:** Dissolve 500,000 units of polymyxin B in 10 ml of 0.9% NaCl for a concentration of 50,000 units/ml.
- **Ophth:** See Appendix H for administration of ophthalmic preparations.

Patient/Family Teaching

- **IM/IV:** Advise patient to notify physician or nurse if symptoms of superinfection occur.
- **Ophth:** Instruct patient on correct

method for instillation of ophthalmic preparation. Soln may cause temporary blurring of vision or burning.
- Advise patient to notify physician if stinging, burning, or itching becomes pronounced or if redness, irritation, swelling, or pain becomes pronounced or persists.

EVALUATION

Clinical response to therapy can be evaluated by: ▪ Resolution of the signs and symptoms of infection. Length of time for complete resolution depends on the organism and site of infection.

POTASSIUM AND SODIUM PHOSPHATES
(**foss**-fates)

Monobasic Potassium and Sodium Phosphates
K-Phos M.F., K-Phos Neutral, K-Phos No. 2

Potassium and Sodium Phosphates
Uro-KP Neutral, Neutra-Phos

CLASSIFICATION(S):
Electrolyte—phosphate supplement, Electrolyte modifier—urinary acidifier, Antiurolithic
Pregnancy Category C

INDICATIONS
▪ Treatment and prevention of phosphate depletion in patients who are unable to ingest adequate dietary potassium ▪ Adjunct therapy of urinary tract infections with methenamine hippurate or mandelate (potassium and sodium phosphates or monobasic potassium phosphate) ▪ Prevention of calcium urinary stones (potassium and sodium phosphates or monobasic potassium phosphate) ▪ Phosphate salts of potassium may be used in hypokalemic patients with metabolic acidosis or coexisting phosphorus deficiency.

ACTION
▪ Phosphate is present in bone and is involved in energy transfer and carbohydrate metabolism ▪ Serves as a buffer for the excretion of hydrogen ions by the kidneys ▪ Dibasic potassium phosphate is converted in renal tubule to monobasic salt by hydrogen ions, resulting in urinary acidification ▪ Acidification of urine is required for methenamine hippurate or mendelate to be active as a urinary anti-infective ▪ Acidification of urine increases solubility of calcium, decreasing calcium stone formation. **Therapeutic Effects:** ▪ Replacement of phosphorus in deficiency states ▪ Urinary acidification ▪ Increased efficacy of methenamine ▪ Decreased formation of calcium urinary tract stones.

PHARMACOKINETICS
Absorption: Well absorbed following oral administration. Vitamin D promotes GI absorption of phosphates.
Distribution: Phosphates enter extracellular fluids and are then actively transported to sites of action.
Metabolism and Excretion: Excreted mainly (>90%) by the kidneys.
Half-life: UK.

CONTRAINDICATIONS AND PRECAUTIONS
Contraindicated in: ▪ Hyperkalemia (potassium salts) ▪ Hyperphosphatemia ▪ Hypocalcemia ▪ Severe renal impairment ▪ Untreated Addison's disease (potassium salts) ▪ Severe tissue trauma (potassium salts) ▪ Hyperkalemic familial periodic paralysis (potassium salts).
Use Cautiously in: ▪ Hyperparathyroidism ▪ Cardiac disease ▪ Hypernatremia (sodium phosphate only) ▪ Hypertension (sodium phosphate only) ▪ Renal impairment.

ADVERSE REACTIONS AND SIDE EFFECTS*
Note: Related to hyperphosphatemia, unless indicated.

*Underlines indicate most frequent; **CAPITALS** indicate life-threatening.

CNS: listlessness, confusion, weakness.
CV: ARRHYTHMIAS, ECG changes (absent P waves, widening of the QRS complex with biphasic curve), CARDIAC ARREST, hypotension; hyperkalemia—ARRHYTHMIAS, ECG changes (prolonged PR interval, ST segment depression, tall-tented T waves); hypernatremia—edema.
F and E: hypomagnesemia, hyperphosphatemia, hyperkalemia, hypocalcemia, hypernatremia.
GI: diarrhea, nausea, vomiting, abdominal pain.
Local: phlebitis, irritation at IV site.
MS: hypocalcemia—tremors; hyperkalemia—muscle cramps.
Neuro: paresthesias of extremities, flaccid paralysis, heaviness of legs.

INTERACTIONS

Drug-Drug: ▪ Concurrent use of **potassium-sparing diuretics** or **angiotensin converting enzyme (ACE) inhibitors** with potassium phosphates may result in hyperkalemia ▪ Concurrent use of **glucocorticoids** with sodium phosphate may result in hypernatremia ▪ Concurrent administration of **calcium-, magnesium-,** or **aluminum**-containing compounds decreases absorption of phosphates by formation of insoluble complexes ▪ **Vitamin D** enhances the absorption of phosphates.
Drug-Food: ▪ **Oxalates** (in spinach and rhubarb) and **phytates** (in bran and whole grains) may decrease the absorption of phosphates by binding them in the GI tract.

ROUTE AND DOSAGE

Monobasic Potassium and Sodium Phosphates

Note: Each 155 mg of monobasic potassium phosphate and 350 mg of anhydrous monobasic sodium phosphate contains 125.6 mg (4 millimoles) phosphorus, 1.14 mEq potassium, and 2.9 mEq sodium. Each 155 mg of monobasic potassium phosphate and 130 mg of hydrous monobasic sodium phosphate and 852 mg of anhydrous dibasic sodium phosphate contains 250 mg (8 millimoles) phosphorus, 1.15 mEq potassium, and 12.9 mEq sodium.

- **PO (Adults):** 250 mg (8 millimoles) qid; may be increased to 250 mg (8 millimoles) q 2 hr (not to exceed 2 g phosphorus/24 hr).

Potassium and Sodium Phosphates

Note: Each 173-mg tablet contains 173 mg (5.5 millimoles) phosphorus, 1.28 mEq potassium, and 9.8 mEq sodium. Each 1.25-g capsule contains 250 mg (8 millimoles) phosphorus, 7.125 mEq potassium, and 7.125 mEq sodium.

- **PO (Adults and Children >4 yr):** 250 mg (8 millimoles) phosphorus qid or 346 mg (11 millimoles) tid.
- **PO (Children <4 yr):** 200 mg (6.4 millimoles) qid.

PHARMACODYNAMICS (effects on serum phosphate levels)

	ONSET	PEAK	DURATION
PO	UK	UK	UK

NURSING IMPLICATIONS

Assessment

- ☐ Assess patient for signs and symptoms of hypokalemia (weakness, fatigue, arrhythmias, presence of U waves on ECG, polyuria, polydipsia), hypophosphatemia (anorexia, weakness, decreased reflexes, bone pain, confusion, blood dyscrasias) throughout course of therapy.
- ☐ Monitor intake and output ratios and daily weight. Report significant discrepancies to physician.
- ▪ **Lab Test Considerations:** Monitor serum phosphate, potassium, sodium, and calcium levels prior to and periodically throughout therapy. Increased phosphate may cause hypocalcemia.
- ☐ Monitor renal function studies prior to and periodically throughout course of therapy.
- ☐ Monitor urinary pH in patients receiv-

ing potassium and sodium phosphate as a urinary acidifier.

Potential Nursing Diagnoses

- Nutrition, altered: less than body requirements (indications).
- Knowledge deficit related to medication regimen (patient/family teaching).

Implementation

- **PO:** Tablets should be dissolved in a full glass of water. Capsules should be opened and mixed thoroughly in ⅓ cup of water each. Allow mixture to stand for 2–5 min to ensure it is fully dissolved. Solns prepared by pharmacy should not be further diluted.
  - Medication should be administered after meals to minimize gastric irritation and laxative effect.
  - Do not administer simultaneously with antacids containing aluminum, magnesium, or calcium.

Patient/Family Teaching

- Explain to the patient the purpose of the medication and the need to take as directed. If a dose is missed, it should be taken as soon as remembered unless within 1 or 2 hr of the next dose. Explain that the tablets and capsules should not be swallowed whole. Tablets should be dissolved in water; capsules should be opened and the contents mixed in water.
- Instruct patients in low-sodium diet (see Appendix K).
- Instruct the patient to promptly report diarrhea, weakness, fatigue, muscle cramps, unexplained weight gain, swelling of lower extremities, shortness of breath, unusual thirst, or tremors.

Evaluation

Effectiveness of therapy can be demonstrated by: ▪ Prevention and correction of serum phosphate and potassium deficiencies ▪ Maintenance of acid urine ▪ Decreased urine calcium, which prevents formation of renal calculi.

POTASSIUM BICARBONATE

(poe-**tass**-ee-um bye-kar-boe-nate)

Klor-Con/EF

CLASSIFICATION(S):

Electrolyte/Electrolyte modifier—potassium supplement

Pregnancy Category C

INDICATIONS

▪ Treatment or prevention of potassium depletion in patients who are unable to ingest adequate dietary potassium.

ACTION

▪ Maintains the following cell characteristics: ▫ Acid-base balance ▫ Isotonicity ▫ Electrophysiology ▪ Serves as an activator in many enzymatic reactions and is essential to many processes, including: ▫ Transmission of nerve impulses ▫ Contraction of cardiac skeletal, and smooth muscle ▫ Gastric secretion ▫ Renal function ▫ Tissue synthesis ▫ Carbohydrate metabolism. **Therapeutic Effects:** ▪ Replacement in deficiency states ▪ Prevention of deficiency.

PHARMACOKINETICS

Absorption: Well absorbed following oral administration of liquid form.

Distribution: Enters extracellular fluid and is then actively transported into cells.

Metabolism and Excretion: Excreted by the kidneys.

Half-life: UK.

CONTRAINDICATIONS AND PRECAUTIONS

Contraindicated in: ▪ Hyperkalemia ▪ Severe renal impairment ▪ Untreated Addison's disease ▪ Severe tissue trauma ▪ Hyperkalemic familial periodic paralysis.

Use Cautiously in: ▪ Cardiac disease ▪ Renal impairment.

ADVERSE REACTIONS AND SIDE EFFECTS*

CNS: paresthesias, restlessness, confusion, weakness, paralysis.
CV: arrhythmias, ECG changes (prolonged PR interval, ST segment depression, tall-tented T waves).
GI: nausea, vomiting, diarrhea, abdominal pain, gastric ulceration (tab only).

INTERACTIONS

Drug–Drug: ▪ Use with **potassium-sparing diuretics** or **angiotensin converting enzyme (ACE) inhibitors** may lead to hyperkalemia.

ROUTE AND DOSAGE

Note: Contains 10 mEq potassium/g.

Prevention of Hypokalemia

- **PO (Adults):** 20 mEq/day in 2–4 divided doses.

Treatment of Hypokalemia

- **PO (Adults):** 40–100 mEq/day in 2–4 divided doses.
- **PO (Infants and Children):** 2–3 mEq/kg/day or 40 mEq/m^2/day.

PHARMACODYNAMICS (increase in serum potassium levels)

	ONSET	PEAK	DURATION
PO	UK	1–2 hr	UK

NURSING IMPLICATIONS

Assessment

- □ Assess patient for signs and symptoms of hypokalemia (weakness, fatigue, U wave on ECG, arrhythmias, polyuria, polydipsia) and hyperkalemia (fatigue, muscle weakness, paresthesia, confusion, dyspnea, peaked T waves, depressed ST segments, prolonged QT segments, widened QRS complexes, loss of P waves and cardiac arrhythmias).
- ▪ **Lab Test Considerations:** Monitor serum potassium levels prior to and periodically throughout therapy.
- □ Monitor renal function, serum bicarbonate, and pH. Serum magnesium level should be determined in refractory hypokalemia, as hypomagnesemia should be corrected to facilitate effectiveness of potassium replacement. Monitor serum chloride levels, as hypochloremia may occur when chloride is not replaced concurrently with potassium.

Potential Nursing Diagnoses

- ▪ Nutrition, altered: less than body requirements (indications).
- ▪ Knowledge deficit related to medication regimen (patient/family teaching).

Implementation

- ▪ **General Info:** Available in combination with other potassium salts.
- ▪ **PO:** Administer with or after meals to decrease GI irritation.
- □ Dissolve effervescent tablets and powders in 8 oz cold water or juice. Ensure that effervescent tablet is fully dissolved. Instruct patient to drink slowly.

Patient/Family Teaching

- □ Explain to patient purpose of the medication and the need to take as directed, especially when concurrent cardiac glycosides or diuretics are ordered. A missed dose should be taken as soon as remembered within 2 hr; if not, return to regular dosage schedule. Do not double dose.
- □ Emphasize correct method of administration. GI irritation or ulceration may result from insufficient dilution of effervescent.
- □ Instruct patient to avoid salt substitutes unless approved by physician.
- □ Advise patient regarding sources of dietary potassium (see Appendix K). Encourage compliance with recommended diet.
- □ Instruct patient to report promptly dark, tarry, or bloody stools; weakness; unusual fatigue; or tingling of extremities. Physician should be notified if nausea, vomiting, diarrhea, or stomach discomfort persists. Dose may require adjustment.
- □ Emphasize the importance of regular

*Underlines indicate most frequent; **CAPITALS** indicate life-threatening.

follow-up examinations to monitor serum levels and monitor progress.

EVALUATION

Effectiveness of therapy can be demonstrated by: ▪ Prevention or treatment of serum potassium depletion.

POTASSIUM CHLORIDE

(poe-**tass**-ee-um **klor**-ide)

Apo-K, Cena-K, K-10, {Kalium Durules}, Kaochlor, Kaochlor S-F, Kaon CL, Kato, Kay Ciel, KCl, K-Dur, {K-Long}, K-Lor, Klor-10%, Klor-Con, Klor-Con/25, Klorvess, Klotrix, K-Lyte/Cl Powder, K-Norm, K-Tab, Micro-K, {Novolente-K}, Potachlor, Potasalane, {Roychlor}, Rum-K, {Slo-Pot}, Slow-K, Ten-K

CLASSIFICATION(S):
Electrolyte/Electrolyte modifier—potassium supplement
Pregnancy Category C

INDICATIONS

▪ **PO, IV:** Treatment or prevention of potassium depletion in patients who are unable to ingest adequate dietary potassium ▪ **IV:** Treatment of some arrhythmias due to cardiac glycoside toxicity.

ACTION

▪ Maintains the following cell characteristics: □ Acid-base balance □ Isotonicity □ Electrophysiology ▪ Serves as an activator in many enzymatic reactions and is essential to many processes, including: □ Transmission of nerve impulses □ Contraction of cardiac, skeletal, and smooth muscle □ Gastric secretion □ Renal function □ Tissue synthesis □ Carbohydrate metabolism. **Therapeutic Effects:** ▪ Replacement in deficiency states ▪ Prevention of deficiency.

PHARMACOKINETICS

Absorption: Well absorbed following oral administration of liquid form. Absorption is slow but complete from wax matrix extended-release formulations.
Distribution: Enters extracellular fluid and is then actively transported into cells.
Metabolism and Excretion: Excreted by the kidneys.
Half-life: UK.

CONTRAINDICATIONS AND PRECAUTIONS

Contraindicated in: ▪ Hyperkalemia ▪ Severe renal impairment ▪ Untreated Addison's disease ▪ Severe tissue trauma ▪ Hyperkalemic familial periodic paralysis ▪ Elixirs may contain alcohol—avoid use in alcohol-intolerant patients ▪ Some products may contain tartrazine (FDC yellow dye #5)—avoid use in patients with aspirin allergy.
Use Cautiously in: ▪ Cardiac disease ▪ Renal impairment ▪ GI hypomotility, including dysphagia or esophageal compression due to left atrial enlargement (tab, enteric-coated tab, extended-release tab or cap) ▪ Diabetes mellitus (liquid products may contain sugar).

ADVERSE REACTIONS AND SIDE EFFECTS*

CNS: paresthesias, restlessness, confusion, weakness, paralysis.
CV: arrhythmias, ECG changes (prolonged PR interval, ST segment depression, tall-tented T waves).
GI: nausea, vomiting, diarrhea, abdominal pain, gastric ulceration (tab only).
Local: irritation at IV site.

INTERACTIONS

Drug-Drug: ▪ Use with **potassium-sparing diuretics** or **angiotensin converting enzyme (ACE) inhibitors** may lead to hyperkalemia ▪ **Anticholinergics** may increase GI mucosal lesions in patients taking wax-matrix potassium chloride preparations.

ROUTE AND DOSAGE

Note: Contains 13.4 mEq potassium/g.

{} = Available in Canada only.

*Underlines indicate most frequent; **CAPITALS** indicate life-threatening.

Prevention of Hypokalemia
- **PO (Adults):** 20 mEq/day in 2–4 divided doses.

Treatment of Hypokalemia
- **PO (Adults):** 40–100 mEq/day in 2–4 divided doses.
- **IV (Adults):** 10–20 mEq/hr (not to exceed 150 mEq/day).
- **PO, IV, (Infants and Children):** 2–3 mEq/kg/day or 40 mEq/m^2/day

PHARMACODYNAMICS (increase in serum potassium levels)

	ONSET	PEAK	DURATION
PO (liquid)	UK	1–2 hr	UK
PO (wax matrix)	UK	30 min	UK
IV	rapid	UK	UK

NURSING IMPLICATIONS

Assessment

- Assess patient for signs and symptoms of hypokalemia (weakness, fatigue, U wave on ECG, arrhythmias, polyuria, polydipsia) and hyperkalemia (see Toxicity and Overdose section).
- Monitor pulse, blood pressure, and ECG periodically throughout IV therapy.
- **Lab Test Considerations:** Monitor serum potassium levels prior to and periodically throughout therapy.
- Monitor renal function, serum bicarbonate, and pH. Serum magnesium level should be determined in refractory hypokalemia; hypomagnesemia should be corrected to facilitate effectiveness of potassium replacement.
- **Toxicity and Overdose:** Symptoms of toxicity are those of hyperkalemia (fatigue, muscle weakness, paresthesia, confusion, dyspnea, peaked T waves, depressed ST segments, prolonged QT segments, widened QRS complexes, loss of P waves, and cardiac arrhythmias).
- Treatment includes discontinuation of potassium, administration of sodium bicarbonate to correct acidosis, dextrose and insulin to facilitate passage of potassium into cells, calcium salts to reverse ECG effects (in patients who are not receiving cardiac glycosides), sodium polystyrene used as an exchange resin, and/or dialysis in patients with impaired renal function.

Potential Nursing Diagnoses

- Nutrition, altered: less than body requirements (indications).
- Knowledge deficit related to medication regimen (patient/family teaching).

Implementation

- **General Info:** Available in tablet, capsule, controlled-release tablets and capsules, effervescent tablet for oral soln, powder, and IV forms. Sugarless oral preparations are also available.
- Available in combination with other potassium salts.
- **PO:** Administer with or after meals to decrease GI irritation.
- Tablets should be administered with full glass of water. Do not chew or crush extended-release tablets or capsules.
- Dissolve effervescent tablets, powders, and soln in 8 oz cold water or juice. Ensure that effervescent tablet is fully dissolved. Instruct patient to drink slowly.
- **IV:** Do not administer IM or SC. Avoid extravasation, as severe pain and tissue necrosis may occur.
- **Intermittent Infusion:** Do not administer undiluted. Each single dose must be diluted and thoroughly mixed in 100–1000 ml of IV soln. Usually limited to 40 mEq/liter of IV soln. In severe hypokalemia may be as concentrated as 80 mEq/liter.
- *Rate:* Infuse at a rate of 10–20 mEq/hr.
- **Solution Compatibility:** May be diluted in dextrose, saline, Ringer's soln, lactated Ringer's soln, dextrose/saline, dextrose/Ringer's soln, and dextrose/lactated Ringer's soln combinations. Commercially available premixed with many of the above IV solns.

- **Y-Site Compatibility:** acyclovir, aminophylline, ampicillin, amrinone, atropine, betamethasone, calcium gluconate, cephalothin, cephapirin, chlordiazepoxide, chlorpromazine, cyanocobalamin, deslanoside, dexamethasone, digoxin, diphenhydramine, dobutamine, dopamine, droperidol, droperidol/fentanyl, edrophonium, enalaprilat, epinephrine, esmolol, conjugated estrogens, ethacrynate sodium, famotidine, fentanyl, fluorouracil, furosemide, hydralazine, insulin, isoproterenol, kanamycin, labetalol, lidocaine, magnesium sulfate, menadiol, methicillin, methoxamine, methylergonovine, minocycline, morphine, neostigmine, norepinephrine, ondansetron, oxacillin, oxytocin, penicillin G potassium, pentazocine, phytonadione, prednisolone, procaine, prochlorperazine, propranolol, pyridostigmine, scopolamine, sodium bicarbonate, succinylcholine, trimethaphan, trimethobenzamide, or zidovudine.
- **Y-Site Incompatibility:** diazepam, ergotamine tartrate, or phenytoin.
- **Additive Compatibility:** aminophylline, bretylium, calcium gluconate, cephalothin, cephapirin, chloramphenicol, cimetidine, clindamycin, corticotropin, dimenhydrinate, dopamine, erythromycin gluceptate, erythromycin lactobionate, heparin, hydrocortisone sodium succinate, isoproterenol, lidocaine, metaraminol, methicillin, methyldopate, methylprednisolone sodium succinate, metoclopramide, nafcillin, netilmicin, norepinephrine, oxacillin, oxytetracycline, penicillin G potassium, phenylephrine, piperacillin, ranitidine, sodium bicarbonate, tetracycline, thiopental, vancomycin, or verapamil.
- **Additive Incompatibility:** amphotericin B.

Patient/Family Teaching

- ☐ Explain to patient purpose of the medication and the need to take as directed, especially when concurrent cardiac glycosides or diuretics are taken. A missed dose should be taken as soon as remembered within 2 hr; if not, return to regular dosage schedule. Do not double dose.
- ☐ Emphasize correct method of administration. GI irritation or ulceration may result from chewing enteric-coated tablets or insufficient dilution of liquid or effervescent forms.
- ☐ Extended-release tablets contain potassium chloride in a wax matrix, which may be expelled in the stool. This is not significant.
- ☐ Instruct patient to avoid salt substitutes unless approved by physician.
- ☐ Advise patient regarding sources of dietary potassium (see Appendix K). Encourage compliance with recommended diet.
- ☐ Instruct patient to report dark, tarry, or bloody stools; weakness; unusual fatigue; or tingling of extremities promptly.
- ☐ Physician should be notified if nausea, vomiting, diarrhea, or stomach discomfort persists. Dosage may require adjustment.
- ☐ Emphasize the importance of regular follow-up examinations to monitor serum levels and to monitor progress.

Evaluation

Effectiveness of therapy can be demonstrated by: ▪ Prevention or treatment of serum potassium depletion.

POTASSIUM GLUCONATE

(poe-**tass**-ee-um **glu**-koe-nate)
Bayon, Kaon, K-G Elixir, {Potassium-Rougier}, {Royonate}

CLASSIFICATION(S):
Electrolyte/Electrolyte modifier—potassium supplement
Pregnancy Category C

INDICATIONS

▪ Treatment or prevention of potassium depletion in patients who are unable to ingest adequate dietary potassium.

ACTION

▪ Maintains the following cell characteristics: ▫ Acid-base balance ▫ Isotonicity ▫ Electrophysiology ▪ Serves as an activator in many enzymatic reactions and is essential to many processes, including: ▫ Transmission of nerve impulses ▫ Contraction of cardiac, skeletal, and smooth muscle ▫ Gastric secretion ▫ Renal function ▫ Tissue synthesis ▫ Carbohydrate metabolism. **Therapeutic Effects:** ▪ Replacement in deficiency states ▪ Prevention of deficiency.

PHARMACOKINETICS

Absorption: Well absorbed following oral administration.
Distribution: Enters extracellular fluid and is then actively transported into cells.
Metabolism and Excretion: Excreted by the kidneys.
Half-life: UK.

CONTRAINDICATIONS AND PRECAUTIONS

Contraindicated in: ▪ Hyperkalemia ▪ Severe renal impairment ▪ Untreated Addison's disease ▪ Severe tissue trauma ▪ Hyperkalemic familial periodic paralysis ▪ Elixirs may contain alcohol—avoid use in alcohol-intolerant patients ▪ Some products may contain tartrazine (FDC yellow dye #5)—avoid use in patients with aspirin allergy.
Use Cautiously in: ▪ Cardiac disease ▪ Renal impairment ▪ Diabetes mellitus (liquid products may contain sugar) ▪ GI hypomotility, including dysphagia or esophageal compression due to left atrial enlargement (tablets only).

ADVERSE REACTIONS AND SIDE EFFECTS*

CNS: paresthesias, restlessness, confusion, weakness, paralysis.
CV: arrhythmias, ECG changes (prolonged PR interval, ST segment depression, tall-tented T waves).
GI: nausea, vomiting, diarrhea, abdominal pain, gastric ulceration (tablets only).

INTERACTIONS

Drug-Drug: ▪ Use with **potassium-sparing diuretics** or **angiotensin converting enzyme (ACE) inhibitors** may lead to hyperkalemia.

ROUTE AND DOSAGE

Note: Contains 4.3 mEq potassium/g.

Prevention of Hypokalemia

- **PO (Adults):** 20 mEq/day in 2–4 divided doses.

Treatment of Hypokalemia

- **PO (Adults):** 40–100 mEq/day in 2–4 divided doses.
- **PO (Infants and Children):** 2–3 mEq/kg/day or 40 mEq/m^2/day.

PHARMACODYNAMICS (increase in serum potassium levels)

	ONSET	PEAK	DURATION
PO	UK	1–2 hr	UK

NURSING IMPLICATIONS

Assessment

▫ Assess patient for signs and symptoms of hypokalemia (weakness, fatigue, U wave on ECG, arrhythmias, polyuria, polydipsia) and hyperkalemia (fatigue, muscle weakness, paresthesia, confusion, dyspnea, peaked T waves, depressed ST segments, prolonged QT segments, widened QRS complexes, loss of P waves, and cardiac arrhythmias).

▪ **Lab Test Considerations:** Monitor serum potassium levels prior to and periodically throughout therapy.

▫ Monitor renal function, serum bicarbonate, and pH. Serum magnesium level should be determined in refractory hypokalemia; hypomagnesemia should be corrected to facilitate effectiveness of potassium replacement. Monitor serum chloride levels; hypochloremia may occur when chloride is not replaced concurrently with potassium.

*Underlines indicate most frequent; **CAPITALS** indicate life-threatening.

Potential Nursing Diagnoses

- Nutrition, altered: less than body requirements (indications).
- Knowledge deficit related to medication regimen (patient/family teaching).

Implementation

- **General Info:** Available in combination with other potassium salts.
- **PO:** Administer with or after meals to decrease GI irritation.
  - Tablets should be administered with full glass of water. Do not chew or crush.
  - Use calibrated measuring device to ensure accurate dosage of elixir. Mix in 120 ml of cold water or juice.

Patient/Family Teaching

- Explain to patient purpose of the medication and the need to take as directed, especially when concurrent cardiac glycosides or diuretics are taken. A missed dose should be taken as soon as remembered within 2 hr; if not, return to regular dosage schedule. Do not double dose.
- Emphasize correct method of administration: GI irritation or ulceration may result from chewing tablets or insufficient dilution of liquid forms .
- Instruct patient to avoid salt substitutes unless approved by physician.
- Advise patient regarding sources of dietary potassium (see Appendix K). Encourage compliance with recommended diet.
- Instruct patient to report dark, tarry, or bloody stools; weakness; unusual fatigue; or tingling of extremities promptly. Physician should be notified if nausea, vomiting, diarrhea, or stomach discomfort persists. Dosage may require adjustment.
- Emphasize the importance of regular follow-up examinations to monitor serum levels and progress.

Evaluation

Effectiveness of therapy can be demonstrated by: ▪ Prevention or treatment of serum potassium depletion.

POTASSIUM IODIDE, SATURATED SOLUTION (SSKI)

(poe-**tass**-ee-um **eye**-oh-dide)
Iostat, Pima, Thyro-Block

CLASSIFICATION(S):
Antithyroid
Pregnancy Category UK

INDICATIONS

▪ Adjunct with other antithyroid drugs in preparation for thyroidectomy ▪ Treatment of thyrotoxic crisis or neonatal thyrotoxicosis ▪ Radiation protectant following radiation emergencies.

ACTION

▪ Rapidly inhibits the release and synthesis of thyroid hormones ▪ Decreases the vascularity of the thyroid gland ▪ Prevents thyroidal uptake of radioactive iodine following radiation emergencies. **Therapeutic Effects:** ▪ Control of hyperthyroidism ▪ Decreased bleeding during thyroid surgery ▪ Prevention of thyroid cancers following radiation emergencies.

PHARMACOKINETICS

Absorption: Converted in the GI tract and enters circulation as iodine.
Distribution: Concentrates in the thyroid gland. Crosses the placenta and enters breast milk.
Metabolism and Excretion: Taken up by the thyroid gland.
Half-life: UK.

CONTRAINDICATIONS AND PRECAUTIONS

Contraindicated in: ▪ Hypersensitivity.
Use Cautiously in: ▪ Tuberculosis ▪ Bronchitis ▪ Hyperkalemia ▪ Impaired renal function ▪ Pregnancy and lactation (although iodine has been used safely in pregnancy, thyroid abnormalities in the newborn may be seen).

ADVERSE REACTIONS AND SIDE EFFECTS*

EENT: parotitis.
Derm: acneform eruptions.
Endo: thyroid hyperplasia, hypothyroidism, hyperthyroidism.
GI: gastric irritation, diarrhea.
Misc: hypersensitivity, iodism.

INTERACTIONS

Drug–Drug: ▪ Use with **lithium** may cause additive hypothyroidism ▪ Increases the antithyroid effect of **antithyroid agents (methimazole, propylthiouracil)** ▪ Additive hyperkalemia may result from combined use of potassium iodide with **potassium-sparing diuretics** or **angiotensin converting enzyme (ACE) inhibitors.**

ROUTE AND DOSAGE

Note: Potassium iodide contains 6 mEq potassium/g; SSKI = 1 g iodine/ml; doses expressed in mg of potassium iodide.

Preparation for Thyroidectomy

- **PO (Adults and Children):** 250 mg (5 drops of SSKI diluted in liquid) tid for 10 days prior to thyroidectomy, usually given with antithyroid drugs.

Radiation Protectant

- **PO (Adults):** 100–150 mg (2–3 drops of SSKI) 24 hr prior to and daily for 3–10 days following exposure to radioactive isotopes of iodine.
- **PO (Infants and Children >1 yr):** 130 mg daily for 10 days following exposure to radioactive isotopes of iodine.
- **PO (Infants and Children ≤1 yr):** 65 mg daily for 10 days following exposure to radioactive isotopes of iodine.

PHARMACODYNAMICS (effects on thyroid function testing)

	ONSET	PEAK	DURATION
PO	24 hr	10–15 days	variable

NURSING IMPLICATIONS

Assessment

- **General Info:** Assess for signs and symptoms of iodism (metallic taste, stomatitis, skin lesions, cold symptoms, severe GI upset). Report these symptoms promptly to physician.
- **Hyperthyroidism:** Monitor response symptoms of hyperthyroidism (tachycardia, palpitations, nervousness, insomnia, diaphoresis, heat intolerance, tremors, weight loss).
- **Lab Test Considerations:** Monitor thyroid function tests prior to and periodically during course of therapy.
  - ▫ Monitor serum potassium periodically during course of therapy.

Potential Nursing Diagnoses

- Airway clearance, ineffective (indications).
- Knowledge deficit related to medication regimen (patient/family teaching).

Implementation

- **General Info:** Available in soln, tablet, and enteric-coated tablet forms.
  - ▫ Available in combination with various cough and cold products.
- **PO:** Mix soln in 8 oz fruit juice, water, or milk. Dissolve tablets in 4 oz water or milk. Administer after meals to minimize GI irritation.
  - ▫ Oral soln is normally clear and colorless. Darkening upon standing does not affect potency of drug.
- **Radiation Protectant:** Administer exactly when ordered. In a nuclear emergency 90–99% protection is provided if administered immediately after exposure, 50% protection if administered within 3–4 hr. Protection is limited to the thyroid gland and does not include other effects of radiation exposure.

Patient/Family Teaching

- **Hyperthyroidism:** Instruct patient to take medication exactly as ordered. Missing a dose may precipitate hyperthyroidism. If a dose is missed, take as soon as remembered unless almost time for next dose.
  - ▫ Instruct patient to report suspected pregnancy to physician before therapy is initiated.
  - ▫ Advise patient to confer with physi-

*Underlines indicate most frequent; **CAPITALS** indicate life-threatening.

cian regarding avoidance of foods high in iodine (seafood, iodized salt, cabbage, kale, turnips).

- Advise patient to consult physician or pharmacist prior to using over-the-counter cold remedies. Some cold remedies contain iodide as an expectorant.

Evaluation

Effectiveness of therapy can be demonstrated by: ▪ Resolution of the symptoms of thyroid crisis ▪ Decrease in size and vascularity of the gland prior to thyroid surgery ▪ Protection of the thyroid gland from the effects of radiation emergencies.

POTASSIUM PHOSPHATES

(poe-**tass**-ee-um **foss**-fates)

Monobasic potassium phosphate
K-Phos Original

Potassium phosphates
Neutra-Phos-K

Potassium phosphate

CLASSIFICATION(S):
Electrolyte—phosphate supplement, Electrolyte modifier—urinary acidifier, Antiurolithic
Pregnancy Category C

INDICATIONS

▪ Treatment and prevention of phosphate depletion in patients who are unable to ingest adequate dietary potassium ▪ Adjunct therapy of urinary tract infections with methenamine hippurate or mandelate (potassium and sodium phosphates or monobasic potassium phosphate) ▪ Prevention of calcium urinary stones (potassium and sodium phosphates or monobasic potassium phosphate) ▪ Phosphate salts of potassium may be used in hypokalemic patients with metabolic acidosis or coexisting phosphorous deficiency.

ACTION

▪ Phosphate is present in bone and is involved in energy transfer and carbohydrate metabolism ▪ Serves as a buffer for the excretion of hydrogen ions by the kidney ▪ Dibasic potassium phosphate is converted in renal tubule to monobasic salt by hydrogen ions, resulting in urinary acidification ▪ Acidification of urine is required for methenamine hippurate or mendelate to be active as a urinary anti-infective ▪ Acidification of urine increases solubility of calcium, decreasing calcium stone formation. **Therapeutic Effects:** ▪ Replacement of phosphorus in deficiency states ▪ Urinary acidification ▪ Increased efficacy of methenamine ▪ Decreased formation of calcium urinary tract stones.

PHARMACOKINETICS

Absorption: Well absorbed following oral administration. Vitamin D promotes GI absorption of phosphates.

Distribution: Phosphates enter extracellular fluids and are then actively transported to sites of action.

Metabolism and Excretion: Excreted mainly (>90%) by the kidneys.

Half-life: UK.

CONTRAINDICATIONS AND PRECAUTIONS

Contraindicated in: ▪ Hyperkalemia ▪ Hyperphosphatemia ▪ Hypocalcemia ▪ Severe renal impairment ▪ Untreated Addison's disease ▪ Severe tissue trauma ▪ Hyperkalemic familial periodic paralysis.

Use Cautiously in: ▪ Hyperparathyroidism ▪ Cardiac disease ▪ Renal impairment.

ADVERSE REACTIONS AND SIDE EFFECTS*

Note: Related to hyperphosphatemia, unless indicated.

CNS: listlessness, confusion, weakness.

CV: ARRHYTHMIAS, ECG changes (absent P waves, widening of the QRS com-

*Underlines indicate most frequent; **CAPITALS** indicate life-threatening.

plex with biphasic curve), CARDIAC ARREST, hypotension; hyperkalemia—ARRHYTHMIAS, ECG changes (prolonged PR interval, ST segment depression, tall-tented T waves).

F and E: hypomagnesemia, hyperphosphatemia, hyperkalemia, hypocalcemia.

GI: diarrhea, nausea, vomiting, abdominal pain.

Local: phlebitis, irritation at IV site.

MS: hyperkalemia—muscle cramps; hypercalcemia—tremors.

Neuro: paresthesias of extremities, flaccid paralysis, heaviness of legs.

INTERACTIONS

Drug-Drug: ▪ Concurrent use of **potassium-sparing diuretics** or **angiotensin converting enzyme (ACE) inhibitors** may result in hyperkalemia ▪ Concurrent administration of **calcium-** or **aluminum-**containing compounds decreases absorption of phosphates by formation of insoluble complexes ▪ **Vitamin D** enhances the absorption of phosphates.

Drug-Food: ▪ **Oxalates** (in spinach and rhubarb) and **phytates** (in bran and whole grains) may decrease the absorption of phosphates by binding them in the GI tract.

ROUTE AND DOSAGE

Monobasic Potassium Phosphate

Note: 500 mg of monobasic potassium phosphate contains 114 mg (3.7 millimoles) phosphorus and 3.7 mEq (144 mg) potassium.

- **PO (Adults):** 1 g in water qid.

Potassium Phosphates

Note: Each 1.45-g capsule contains 250 mg (8 millimoles) phosphorus and 14.25 mEq potassium. Each 75 ml of soln contains 250 mg (8 millimoles) phosphorus and 14.25 mEq potassium. Each ml of injection contains 283.5 mg phosphate (3 millimoles or 93 mg phosphorus) and 4.4 mEq potassium.

- **PO (Adults and Children >4 yr):** 250 mg phosphorus qid.
- **PO (Children <4 yr):** 200 mg phosphorus qid.
- **IV (Adults):** 10 millimoles phosphorus/day as an infusion.
- **IV (Children):** 1.5–2 millimoles phosphorus/day as an infusion.

PHARMACODYNAMICS (effects on serum phosphate levels)

	ONSET	PEAK	DURATION
PO	UK	UK	UK
IV	rapid (min–hr)	end of infusion	UK

NURSING IMPLICATIONS

Assessment

- ▫ Assess patient for signs and symptoms of hypokalemia (weakness, fatigue, arrhythmias, presence of U waves on ECG, polyuria, polydipsia) and hypophosphatemia (anorexia, weakness, decreased reflexes, bone pain, confusion, blood dyscrasias) throughout course of therapy.
- ▫ Monitor pulse, blood pressure, and ECG prior to and periodically throughout IV therapy.
- ▫ Monitor intake and output ratios and daily weight. Report significant discrepancies to physician.
- ▪ **Lab Test Considerations:** Monitor serum phosphate, potassium, and calcium levels prior to and periodically throughout therapy. Increased phosphate may cause hypocalcemia.
- ▫ Monitor renal function studies prior to and periodically throughout course of therapy.
- ▫ Monitor urinary pH in patients receiving potassium phosphate as a urinary acidifier.
- ▪ **Toxicity and Overdose:** Symptoms of toxicity are those of hyperkalemia (fatigue, muscle weakness, paresthesia, confusion, dyspnea, peaked T waves, depressed ST segments, prolonged QT segments, widened QRS complexes, loss of P waves, and cardiac arrhythmias) and hyperphosphatemia or hypocalcemia (paresthesia,

muscle twitching, laryngospasm, colic, cardiac arrhythmias, or Chvostek's or Trousseau's sign).

- Treatment includes discontinuation of infusion, calcium replacement, and lowering serum potassium (dextrose and insulin to facilitate passage of potassium into cells, sodium polystyrene as an exchange resin, and/or dialysis in patients with impaired renal function).

Potential Nursing Diagnoses

- Nutrition, altered: less than body requirements (indications).
- Knowledge deficit related to medication regimen (patient/family teaching).

Implementation

- **General Info:** Available in combination with sodium phosphates for acidification of urine and to decrease urine calcium.
- **PO:** Tablets should be administered with full glass of water. Capsules should be opened and mixed thoroughly in ⅓ cup water each. Allow mixture to stand for 2–5 min to ensure that it is fully dissolved.
  - Medication should be administered after meals to minimize gastric irritation and laxative effect.
  - Do not administer simultaneously with antacids containing aluminum, magnesium, or calcium.
- **IV:** Administer only in dilute concentration. Common component of total parenteral nutrition. Do not administer IM.
- **Continuous Infusion:** Dilute to a concentration no greater than 160 mEq/liter with 0.45% NaCl, 0.9% NaCl, D5W, D10W, D5/0.45% NaCl, D5/0.9% NaCl, or TPN solns.
  - *Rate:* Infuse as a continuous infusion at a slow rate.
- **Y-Site Compatibility:** enalaprilat, esmolol, famotidine, or labetalol.
- **Additive Compatibility:** magnesium sulfate, metoclopramide, or verapamil.
- **Solution/Additive Incompatibility:** Ringer's or lactated Ringer's soln, D10/0.9% NaCl, D5/LR, or dobutamine.

Patient/Family Teaching

- Explain to patient purpose of the medication and the need to take as directed. If a dose is missed, it should be taken as soon as remembered unless within 1–2 hr of the next dose. Explain that the tablets and capsules should not be swallowed whole. Tablets should be dissolved in water; capsules should be opened and the contents mixed in water.
- Instruct the patient to report diarrhea, weakness, fatigue, muscle cramps, or tremors promptly.

Evaluation

Effectiveness of therapy can be demonstrated by: ▪ Prevention and correction of serum phosphate and potassium deficiencies ▪ Maintenance of acid urine ▪ Decreased urine calcium, which prevents formation of renal calculi.

PRALIDOXIME

(pra-li-**dox**-eem)
Protopam

CLASSIFICATION(S):
Antidote—anticholinesterase poisoning
Pregnancy Category UK

INDICATIONS

▪ Early (first 24–36 hr) treatment of organophosphate anticholinesterase insecticide poisoning, usually with atropine and supportive measures, including mechanical ventilation, if necessary ▪ Management of anticholinesterase (neostigmine, pyridostigmine, ambemonium, or nerve gas) overdosage.

ACTION

▪ Reactivates cholinesterase following poisoning with anticholinesterase agents ▪ May also directly inactivate organophosphates. **Therapeutic Effect:**

▪ Reversal of muscle paralysis following organophosphate poisoning.

PHARMACOKINETICS

Absorption: Variably and incompletely absorbed following oral administration. Well absorbed following IM administration.
Distribution: Widely distributed throughout extracellular water. Does not appear to enter the CNS.
Metabolism and Excretion: 80–90% excreted unchanged by the kidneys.
Half-life: 0.8–2.7 hr.

CONTRAINDICATIONS AND PRECAUTIONS

Contraindicated in: ▪ Hypersensitivity.
Use Cautiously in: ▪ Myasthenia gravis (may precipitate myasthenic crisis) ▪ Renal impairment (dosage reduction required) ▪ Pregnancy, lactation, or children (safety not established) ▪ Efficacy in carbamate insecticide poisoning is not known (may increase toxicity).

ADVERSE REACTIONS AND SIDE EFFECTS*

CNS: dizziness, headache, drowsiness.
EENT: diplopia, blurred vision, impaired accommodation.
Resp: hyperventilation, LARYNGOSPASM.
CV: tachycardia.
GI: nausea.
Derm: rash.
Local: pain at IM site.
MS: muscle weakness, muscle rigidity, neuromuscular blockade.

INTERACTIONS

Drug-Drug: ▪ Avoid concurrent use with **succinylcholine, morphine, aminophylline, theophylline, reserpine,** and **respiratory depressants,** including **barbiturates, narcotic analgesics,** and **sedative/hypnotics** in patients with anticholinesterase poisoning.

ROUTE AND DOSAGE

Note: IV route is preferred.

Organophosphate Poisoning

Atropine 2–6 mg IV is given concurrently. If patient is cyanotic, give atropine IM while improving ventilatory status. Atropine is repeated q 5–60 min until toxicity is encountered and is then continued for at least 48 hr.

- **PO (Adults):** 1–2 g, may be repeated in 1 hr if muscle paralysis is still present. In the absence of severe GI symptoms 1–3 g may be given q 5 hr if continued GI absorption is suspected.
- **SC, IM, IV (Adults):** 1–2 g, may be repeated in 1 hr if muscle paralysis is still present, or as a continuous IV infusion at 500 mg/hr. If exposure continues, additional doses may be given q 3–8 hr.
- **PO, SC, IM, IV (Children):** 20–40 mg/kg, may be repeated in 1 hr if muscle paralysis is still present. If exposure continues, additional doses may be given q 3–8 hr.
- **Subconjunctival:** 0.1–0.2 ml 5% soln.

Anticholinesterase Overdose

- **IV (Adults):** 1 g, followed by 250-mg increments q 5 min as needed.

PHARMACODYNAMICS (plasma levels)

	ONSET	PEAK	DURATION
PO	UK	2–3 hr	UK
IM	UK	10–20 min	UK
IV	UK	5–15 min	UK

NURSING IMPLICATIONS

Assessment

- ▫ Determine insecticide to which patient was exposed and time of exposure. Therapy should begin as soon as possible within 24 hr. Contact poison control center for complete information on the specific insecticide.
- ▫ Monitor neuromuscular status prior to and periodically throughout therapy. Document skeletal muscle strength, tidal volume, and vital capacity. Note presence of nicotinic effects of anticholinesterases (twitch-

*Underlines indicate most frequent; **CAPITALS** indicate life-threatening.

ing, muscle cramps, fasiculations, weakness, pallor, tachycardia, increased blood pressure).

- □ Closely monitor respirations, pulse, and blood pressure. Rapid IV infusion rate may cause tachycardia, laryngospasm, muscle rigidity, and hypertension. Notify physician immediately if hypertension occurs. Physician may order decrease in infusion rate or discontinuation of infusion. Phentolamine may be required to control blood pressure.
- ▪ **Lab Test Considerations:** May cause elevated SGOT (AST), SGPT (ALT), and CPK levels. These usually return to normal in 2 wk.

Potential Nursing Diagnoses

- ▪ Injury, high risk for (indications).
- ▪ Airway clearance, ineffective (indications).

Implementation

- ▪ **General Info:** Concurrent atropine and supportive measures (suctioning, intubation, and ventilation) may be ordered. Atropine is used to reverse muscarinic effects (bronchoconstriction, dyspnea, cough, increased bronchial secretions, nausea, vomiting, abdominal cramps, diarrhea, increased sweating, salivation, lacrimation, bradycardia, decreased blood pressure, miosis, blurred vision, urinary frequency, incontinence) of anticholinesterases. Pralidoxime is effective only against nicotinic effects.
- □ Dosage may need to be repeated every 3–8 hr if insecticide was ingested; absorption from bowel may continue.
- □ Emergency kit containing pralidoxime, sterile water for injection, 20-ml syringe, needle, and alcohol swab is commercially available for SC, IM, or IV injection.
- □ Physician may administer pralidoxime subconjunctivally when insecticide splashed into eye.
- □ If dermal exposure has occurred, remove clothing and thoroughly wash hair and skin in sodium bicarbonate or alcohol as soon as possible. Health care workers should wear gloves to prevent self-exposure. Carefully dispose of clothing to prevent contamination of others.
- □ Also available as an auto-injector for nerve gas emergencies.
- ▪ **PO:** Available in tablet form.
- ▪ **SC/IM:** May be administered IM or SC in patients unable to tolerate IV infusion.
- ▪ **IV:** Reconstitute vial containing 1 g of powdered pralidoxime with 20 ml of sterile water for injection.
- ▪ **Direct IV:** May be administered undiluted (50 mg/ml) over at least 5 min in patients who cannot tolerate IV infusion (for example, pulmonary edema).
- ▪ **Intermittent Infusion:** Further dilute in 100 ml of 0.9% NaCl.
- □ *Rate:* Infuse over 15–30 min.

Patient/Family Teaching

- □ Explain purpose of medication to patient.

Evaluation

Effectiveness of therapy can be demonstrated by: ▪ Reversal of respiratory and skeletal muscle weakness caused by exposure to organophosphate anticholinesterase insecticides or anticholesterase overdose.

PRAVASTATIN

(**pra**-va-sta-tin)
Pravachol

CLASSIFICATION(S):
Lipid-lowering agent
Pregnancy Category X

INDICATIONS

▪ Adjunct to dietary therapy in the management of primary hypercholesterolemia.

ACTION

▪ Inhibits the enzyme (HMG-CoA reductase) responsible for catalyzing an early step in the synthesis of cholesterol. **Therapeutic Effects:** ▪ Lowering of total and low-density lipoprotein (LDL) cholesterol, VLDL cholesterol, and triglycerides ▪ Increased high-density lipoproteins (HDL).

PHARMACOKINETICS

Absorption: Poor absorption following oral administration and rapid hepatic metabolism result in decreased bioavailability (18%).

Distribution: Does not cross the blood-brain barrier. Small amounts appear in breast milk. Enters hepatocytes where action takes place. Remainder of distribution not known.

Metabolism and Excretion: Highly metabolized by the liver. 71% eliminated in the feces. Small amounts (8%) excreted unchanged by the kidneys.

Half-life: 1.8 hr.

CONTRAINDICATIONS AND PRECAUTIONS

Contraindicated in: ▪ Hypersensitivity ▪ Pregnancy or lactation ▪ Active liver disease.

Use Cautiously in: ▪ Women of child-bearing age ▪ History of liver disease ▪ Alcoholism ▪ Children <18 yr (safety not established).

ADVERSE REACTIONS AND SIDE EFFECTS*

CNS: headache.

Derm: rashes.

MS: myalgia.

INTERACTIONS

Drug-Drug: ▪ Cholesterol-lowering effect may be additive with **bile acid sequestrants (cholestyramine, colestipol)**, but absorption of pravastatin is decreased if administered concurrently (give 1 hr before or 4 hr after bile acid sequestrant) ▪ Risk of myopathy may be increased by concurrent **niacin, gemfibrozil, erythromycin**, or **cyclosporine**.

ROUTE AND DOSAGE

- **PO (Adults):** 10–20 mg once daily at bedtime.

PHARMACODYNAMICS (lipid-lowering effect)

	ONSET	PEAK	DURATION
PO	1 wk	4 wks	UK

NURSING IMPLICATIONS

Assessment

- ▫ Obtain a diet history, especially in regard to fat consumption.
- ▫ Ophthalmic examinations are recommended prior to and yearly throughout therapy.
- ▪ **Lab Test Considerations:** Serum cholesterol and triglyceride levels should be evaluated before initiating and periodically throughout course of therapy.
- ▫ Liver function tests, including SGOT (AST), should be monitored prior to and every 6 wk during the first 3 mon of therapy, every 8 wk for the remainder of the first yr, and then every 6 mon. If SGOT (AST) levels increase to 3 times normal, pravastatin therapy should be discontinued.
- ▫ If patient develops muscle tenderness during therapy, CPK levels should be monitored. If CPK levels are markedly increased or myopathy occurs, pravastatin therapy should be discontinued.

Potential Nursing Diagnoses

- ▪ Knowledge deficit related to diet and medication regimen (patient/family teaching).
- ▪ Noncompliance (patient/family teaching).

Implementation

- ▪ **PO:** Administer once daily at bedtime. May be administered without regard to food.
- ▫ If administered in conjunction with bile acid sequestrants (cholestyramine, colestipol), administer pravastatin 1 hour before or at least 4 hours after bile acid sequestrant.

Patient/Family Teaching

- ▫ Instruct patient to take medication exactly as directed, not to skip doses or double up on missed doses. Pravastatin helps control but does not cure elevated serum cholesterol levels.
- ▫ Advise patient that pravastatin should be used in conjunction with diet restrictions (fat, cholesterol, car-

*Underlines indicate most frequent; **CAPITALS** indicate life-threatening.

bohydrates, alcohol), exercise, and cessation of smoking.

- Instruct patient to notify physician if unexplained muscle pain, tenderness, or weakness occur, especially if accompanied by fever or malaise. Instruct female patients to notify physician promptly if pregnancy is planned or suspected.
- Advise patient to notify physician or dentist of medication regimen prior to treatment or surgery.
- Emphasize the importance of follow-up examinations to determine effectiveness and monitor for side effects.

EVALUATION

Effectiveness of therapy can be demonstrated by: ▪ Decrease in low-density lipoprotein (LDL), very low-density lipoprotein (VLDL), and total cholesterol levels ▪ Increase in high-density lipoprotein levels ▪ Decrease in serum triglyceride levels.

PRAZEPAM

(**praz**-e-pam)
Centrax

CLASSIFICATION(S):
Sedative/hypnotic—benzodiazepine
Schedule IV
Pregnancy Category UK

INDICATIONS

▪ Used as an adjunct in the management of anxiety.

ACTION

▪ Depresses the CNS, probably by potentiating gamma-aminobutyric acid (GABA), an inhibitory neurotransmitter. **Therapeutic Effects:** ▪ Sedation ▪ Relief of anxiety.

PHARMACOKINETICS

Absorption: Slowly absorbed but is rapidly metabolized following oral administration.

Distribution: Widely distributed. Crosses the blood-brain barrier. Crosses the placenta and enters breast milk.

Metabolism and Excretion: Highly metabolized by the liver and converted to active benzodiazepines (desmethyldiazepam and oxazepam).

Half-life: Oxazepam—5–15 hr; desmethyldiazepam—30–100 hr.

CONTRAINDICATIONS AND PRECAUTIONS

Contraindicated in: ▪ Hypersensitivity ▪ Cross-sensitivity with other benzodiazepines may exist ▪ Comatose patients or those with pre-existing CNS depression ▪ Uncontrolled severe pain ▪ Narrow-angle glaucoma ▪ Pregnancy and lactation.

Use Cautiously in: ▪ Hepatic dysfunction ▪ Severe renal impairment ▪ Patients who may be suicidal or who may have been addicted to drugs previously ▪ Elderly or debilitated patients (dosage reduction recommended) ▪ Children (safety not established).

ADVERSE REACTIONS AND SIDE EFFECTS*

CNS: dizziness, drowiness, lethargy, hangover, paradoxical excitation, headache.

EENT: blurred vision.

Resp: respiratory depression.

GI: nausea, vomiting, diarrhea, constipation.

Derm: rashes.

Misc: tolerance, psychological dependence, physical dependence.

INTERACTIONS

Drug-Drug: ▪ Additive CNS depression with other **CNS depressants,** including **alcohol, antihistamines, antidepressants, narcotic analgesics,** and other **sedative/hypnotics** ▪ **Cimetidine, oral contraceptives, disulfiram, fluoxetine, isoniazid, ketoconazole, metoprolol, propoxyphene, propranolol,** and **valproic acid** may decrease metabolism and increase CNS depression

*Underlines indicate most frequent; **CAPITALS** indicate life-threatening.

■ May decrease the efficacy of **levodopa** ■ **Rifampin** or **barbiturates** may increase metabolism and decrease effectiveness of prazepam ■ Sedative effects may be decreased by **theophylline**.

ROUTE AND DOSAGE

- **PO (Adults):** 30 mg/day in divided doses (usual range 20–60 mg/day) or give as single bedtime dose of 20 mg (up to 50 mg).

PHARMACODYNAMICS (antianxiety effects)

	ONSET	PEAK	DURATION
PO	UK	days–wks	days

NURSING IMPLICATIONS

Assessment

- □ Assess patient for anxiety and level of sedation (ataxia, dizziness, slurred speech) periodically throughout course of therapy.
- □ Prolonged high-dose therapy may lead to psychological or physical dependence. Restrict the amount of drug available to patient.
- ■ **Lab Test Considerations:** Monitor CBC and liver function tests periodically during prolonged therapy.
- □ May cause an increase in serum bilirubin, SGOT (AST), and SGPT (ALT).

Potential Nursing Diagnoses

- ■ Anxiety (indications).
- ■ Injury, high risk for (side effects).
- ■ Knowledge deficit related to medication regimen (patient/family teaching).

Implementation

- ■ **General Info:** Available in tablets and capsules.
- ■ **PO:** Administer with food if GI irritation becomes a problem.
- □ Medication should be tapered at the completion of long-term therapy. Sudden cessation of medication may lead to withdrawal (insomnia, irritability, nervousness, tremors).

Patient/Family Teaching

- □ Instruct patient to take prazepam exactly as directed. Do not take more than amount prescribed or increase dose if less effective after a few wks of therapy. Consult physician prior to adjusting dose or discontinuing.
- □ Prazepam may cause drowsiness or dizziness. Caution patient to avoid driving or other activities requiring alertness until response to medication is known.
- □ Advise patient to avoid the use of alcohol and to consult physician or pharmacist prior to the use of over-the-counter preparations that contain antihistamines or alcohol.
- □ Advise patient to inform physician if pregnancy is planned or suspected.
- □ Emphasize the importance of follow-up appointments to monitor progress.

Evaluation

Effectiveness of therapy can be demonstrated by: ■ Decreased sense of anxiety □ Increased ability to cope. Maximum therapeutic effects are usually seen within 1–2 wk. Effectiveness should be re-evaluated after 4 mon.

PRAZOSIN

(pra-zoe-sin)
Minipress

CLASSIFICATION(S):
Antihypertensive—peripherally acting antiadrenergic
Pregnancy Category UK

INDICATIONS

■ Treatment of mild to moderate hypertension. **Unlabeled Use:** ■ Management of congestive heart failure unresponsive to cardiac glycosides and diuretics ■ Management of peripheral vascular disorders including peripheral vasospasm and Raynaud's phenomenon.

ACTION

■ Dilates both arteries and veins by blocking postsynaptic $alpha_1$-adrenergic receptors. **Therapeutic Effects:** ▪ Lowering of blood pressure ▪ Decreased cardiac preload and afterload.

PHARMACOKINETICS

Absorption: 60% absorbed following oral administration.
Distribution: Widely distributed.
Metabolism and Excretion: Extensively metabolized by the liver. Minimal (5–10%) renal excretion of unchanged drug.
Half-life: 2–3 hr.

CONTRAINDICATIONS AND PRECAUTIONS

Contraindicated in: ▪ Hypersensitivity.
Use Cautiously in: ▪ Renal insufficiency (increased sensitivity to effects; dosage reduction may be required) ▪ Pregnancy, lactation, or children (safety not established) ▪ Angina pectoris.

ADVERSE REACTIONS AND SIDE EFFECTS*

CNS: dizziness, drowsiness, syncope, depression, headache, weakness.
EENT: blurred vision.
CV: first-dose orthostatic hypotension, palpitations, angina, edema.
GI: dry mouth, nausea, vomiting, diarrhea, abdominal cramps.
GU: impotence, priapism.

INTERACTIONS

Drug–Drug: ▪ Additive hypotension with acute ingestion of **alcohol,** other **antihypertensive agents,** or **nitrates** ▪ Antihypertensive effects may be decreased by **nonsteroidal anti-inflammatory agents.**

ROUTE AND DOSAGE

▪ **PO (Adults):** Initial dose 1 mg at bedtime; usual maintenance dose 2–20 mg/day in 2–3 divided doses.

PHARMACODYNAMICS (antihypertensive effects)

	ONSET	PEAK	DURATION
PO	2 hr	2–4 hr*	10 hr

*Following single dose; maximal antihypertensive effects occur after 3–4 wk of chronic dosing.

NURSING IMPLICATIONS

Assessment

□ Monitor blood pressure and pulse frequently during initial dosage adjustment and periodically throughout course of therapy. Notify physician of significant changes.
□ Monitor intake and output ratios and daily weight and assess for edema daily, especially at beginning of therapy. Notify physician of weight gain or edema.
▪ **Lab Test Considerations:** May cause elevated serum sodium levels.

Potential Nursing Diagnoses

▪ Injury, high risk for (side effects).
▪ Knowledge deficit related to medication regimen (patient/family teaching).
▪ Noncompliance (patient/family teaching).

Implementation

▪ **General Info:** Following initial dose, patient may develop "first-dose orthostatic hypotensive reaction," which most frequently occurs 30 min–2 hr after initial dose and may be manifested by dizziness, weakness, lightheadedness, and syncope. Observe patient closely during this period and take precautions to prevent injury. The first dose may be given at bedtime to minimize this reaction.
□ Commonly administered concurrently with a thiazide diuretic or a beta-adrenergic blocker.
□ Available in combination with polythiazide (Minizide); see Appendix A.

Patient/Family Teaching

□ Emphasize the importance of continuing to take this medication, even if

*Underlines indicate most frequent; **CAPITALS** indicate life-threatening.

feeling well. Instruct patient to take medication at the same time each day. If a dose is missed, take as soon as remembered unless almost time for next dose. Do not double doses.

- Encourage patient to comply with additional interventions for hypertension (weight reduction, low-sodium diet, discontinuation of smoking, moderation of alcohol consumption, regular exercise, and stress management).
- Instruct patient and family on proper technique for blood pressure monitoring. Advise them to check blood pressure at least weekly and to report significant changes to physician.
- Prazosin may cause drowsiness or dizziness. Advise patient to avoid driving or other activities requiring alertness until response to medication is known.
- Caution patient to avoid sudden changes in position to decrease orthostatic hypotension.
- Advise patient to consult physician or pharmacist before taking any cough, cold, or allergy remedies. Patient should also avoid excessive amounts of coffee, tea, or cola.
- Emphasize the importance of follow-up visits to determine effectiveness of therapy.

EVALUATION

Effectiveness of therapy can be demonstrated by: ▪ Decrease in blood pressure without appearance of side effects.

PREDNISOLONE

(pred-**niss**-oh-lone)

Articulose, Cortalone, Delta-Cortef, Hydeltra-T.B.A., Hydeltrasol, Key-Pred, Metalone T.B.A., Nor-Pred T.B.A., Pediapred, Predaject, Predalone, Predalone T.B.A., Predate, Predate-S, Predate T.B.A., Predcor, Predicort, Predicort-RP, Predicort T.B.A., Prelone

CLASSIFICATION(S):
Glucocorticoid—intermediate-acting
Pregnancy Category UK

INDICATIONS

▪ Used systemically and locally in a wide variety of chronic diseases including: ▫ Inflammatory ▫ Allergic ▫ Hematologic ▫ Neoplastic ▫ Autoimmune ▪ Replacement therapy in adrenal insufficiency.

ACTION

▪ Suppresses inflammation and the normal immune response. Has numerous intense metabolic effects ▪ Suppresses adrenal function at chronic doses of 5 mg/day ▪ Has minimal mineralocorticoid (sodium-retaining) activity. **Therapeutic Effects:** ▪ Suppression of inflammation and modification of the normal immune response ▪ Replacement therapy in adrenal insufficiency.

PHARMACOKINETICS

Absorption: Well absorbed following oral and IM administration. Chronic high-dose topical application may also lead to systemic absorption. IM acetate salt is long-acting.

Distribution: Widely distributed. Crosses the placenta and probably enters breast milk.

Metabolism and Excretion: Mostly metabolized by the liver and other tissues. Small amounts excreted unchanged by the kidneys.

Half-life: 115–212 min; adrenal suppression lasts 1.25–1.5 days.

CONTRAINDICATIONS AND PRECAUTIONS

Contraindicated in: ▪ Active untreated infections, except for tuberculous meningitis ▪ Lactation (chronic use).

Use Cautiously in: ▪ Chronic treatment (will lead to adrenal suppression) ▪ Should never be abruptly discontinued ▪ Supplemental doses may be needed during stress (surgery, infection) ▪ Pregnancy (safety not established) ▪ Children (chronic use will result in decreased growth) ▪ May mask signs of infections (fever, inflammation) ▪ Use lowest possible dose for shortest period of time.

ADVERSE REACTIONS AND SIDE EFFECTS*

CNS: headache, restlessness, psychoses, depression, euphoria, personality changes, increased intracranial pressure (children only).
EENT: cataracts, increased intraocular pressure.
CV: hypertension.
GI: nausea, vomiting, anorexia, peptic ulceration.
Derm: decreased wound healing, petechiae, ecchymoses, fragility, hirsutism, acne.
Endo: adrenal suppression, hyperglycemia.
F and E: hypokalemia, hypokalemic alkalosis, fluid retention (long-term high doses).
Hemat: thromboembolism, thrombophlebitis.
Metab: weight loss, weight gain.
MS: muscle wasting, muscle pain, aseptic necrosis of joints, osteoporosis.
Misc: increased susceptibility to infection, cushingoid appearance (moon face, buffalo hump).

INTERACTIONS

Drug-Drug: ▪ Additive hypokalemia with **diuretics, amphotericin B, mezlocillin, piperacillin,** or **ticarcillin** ▪ Hypokalemia may increase the risk of **cardiac glycoside** toxicity ▪ May increase requirement for **insulin** or **oral hypoglycemic agents** ▪ Increased risk of adverse GI effects with **alcohol, aspirin,** or **nonsteroidal anti-inflammatory agents**.

ROUTE AND DOSAGE

- **PO (Adults):** 2.5–15 mg 2–4 times daily (maintenance doses may be given as a single dose or every other day).
- **IM (Adults):** 2–30 mg q 12 hr (acetate, phosphate), doses up to 400 mg/day (phosphate) have been given.
- **IV (Adults):** 2–30 mg q hr (phosphate), doses up to 400 mg/day have been given.
- **Ophth (Adults and Children):** 1–2 drops q 1–2 hr (acetate, phosphate) or oint 1–4 times daily (phosphate).
- **Otic (Adults and Children):** 3–4 drops 2–3 times daily (phosphate).
- **IA, IL (Adults):** 2–30 mg (phosphate), 4–40 mg (tebutate), 4–100 mg (acetate).
- **IA (Adults):** 0.25–1 ml (acetate/phosphate suspension).

PHARMACODYNAMICS (anti-inflammatory effects)

	ONSET	PEAK	DURATION
PO	hr	1–2	1.25–1.5 days
IM (phosphate)	rapid	1 hr	UK
IM (acetate)	slow	UK	up to 4 wk
IV	rapid	1 hr	UK
IA, IL	slow	UK	3 days–4 wk

NURSING IMPLICATIONS

Assessment

- **General Info:** This drug is indicated for many conditions. Assess involved systems prior to and periodically throughout course of therapy.
  - Assess patient for signs of adrenal insufficiency (hypotension, weight loss, weakness, nausea, vomiting, anorexia, lethargy, confusion, restlessness) prior to and periodically throughout course of therapy.
  - Monitor intake and output ratios and daily weight. Observe patient for the appearance of peripheral edema, steady weight gain, rales/crackles, or dyspnea. Notify physician should these occur.
  - Children should have periodic evaluations of growth.
- **Intra-articular:** Monitor pain, edema, and range of motion of affected joints.
- **Intralesional:** Assess affected area prior to and daily during therapy. Note lesion size and degree of inflammation.

*Underlines indicate most frequent; **CAPITALS** indicate life-threatening.

- **Lab Test Considerations:** Patients on prolonged courses of therapy should routinely have hematologic values, serum electrolytes, serum and urine glucose evaluated. May cause decreased WBC counts. May cause hyperglycemia, especially in persons with diabetes. May cause decreased serum potassium and calcium and increased serum sodium concentrations.
- ◻ Promptly report presence of guaiac-positive stools.
- ◻ May increase serum cholesterol and lipid values. May decrease serum protein-bound iodine and thyroxine concentrations.
- ◻ Suppresses reactions to skin tests.
- ◻ Periodic adrenal function tests may be ordered to assess degree of hypothalamic-pituitary-adrenal (HPA) axis suppression.

Potential Nursing Diagnoses

- Infection, high risk for (side effects).
- Body image disturbance (side effects).
- Knowledge deficit related to medication regimen (patient/family teaching).

Implementation

- **General Info:** Available in many forms: tablet; oral syrup, soln, and suspension; ophthalmic suspension, soln, and ointment; otic soln; and as parenteral soln for IM and IV injection, infusion, and direct injection into joints and soft tissue lesions.
- ◻ If dose is ordered daily or every other day, administer in the morning to coincide with the body's normal secretion of cortisol.
- **PO:** Administer with meals to minimize gastric irritation.
- ◻ Use calibrated measuring device to ensure accurate dosage of liquid forms.
- **IM:** Shake suspension well before drawing up. Do not administer suspension IV. IM doses should not be administered when rapid effect is desirable.
- **Direct IV:** Do not use the acetate form of this drug for IV administration.
- ◻ *Rate:* Prednisolone sodium phosphate IV may be administered direct IV push at a rate of no more than 10 mg/min.
- **Intermittent Infusion:** May be added to 50–1000 ml of D5W or 0.9% NaCl. Stable for 24 hr.
- ◻ *Rate:* Administer infusions at prescribed rate.
- **Y-Site Compatibility:** heparin with hydrocortisone sodium succinate or potassium chloride.
- **Additive Compatibility:** ascorbic acid, cephalothin, cytarabine, erythromycin lactobionate, fluorouracil, heparin, methicillin, penicillin G potassium, penicillin G sodium, or tetracycline.
- **Additive Incompatibility:** calcium gluceptate, metaraminol, methotrexate, or polymyxin B sulfate.
- **Ophth:** Have patient tilt head back and look up, gently depress lower lid with index finger until conjunctival sac is exposed, and instill medication. Wait at least 5 min before instilling other types of eyedrops.

Patient/Family Teaching

- ◻ Instruct patient to take medication exactly as directed. Do not skip doses or double up on missed doses. Stopping the medication suddenly may result in adrenal insufficiency (anorexia, nausea, fatigue, weakness, hypotension, dyspnea, and hypoglycemia). If these signs appear, notify physician immediately. This can be life-threatening.
- ◻ Encourage patients on long-term therapy to eat a diet high in protein, calcium, and potassium and low in sodium and carbohydrates (see Appendix K for foods included).
- ◻ This drug causes immunosuppression and may mask symptoms of infection. Instruct patient to avoid people with known contagious illnesses and to report possible infections.
- ◻ Review side effects with patient. In-

struct patient to inform physician promptly if severe abdominal pain or tarry stools occur. Patient should also report unusual swelling, weight gain, tiredness, bone pain, bruising, nonhealing sores, visual disturbances, or behavior changes.

- Discuss possible effects on body image. Explore coping mechanisms.
- Instruct patient to inform physician if symptoms of underlying disease return or worsen.
- Advise patient to carry identification describing disease process and medication regimen in the event of an emergency in which patient cannot relate medical history.
- Caution patient to avoid vaccinations without consulting physician.
- Explain need for continued medical follow-up to assess effectiveness and possible side effects of medication. Physician may order periodic lab tests and eye examinations.

Evaluation

Effectiveness of therapy can be demonstrated by: ▪ Suppression of inflammatory and immune responses in autoimmune disorders, allergic reactions, and organ transplants ▪ Management of symptoms in adrenal insufficiency.

PREDNISONE

(**pred**-ni-sone)
{Apo-Prednisone}, Deltasone, Liquid Pred, Meticorten, Orasone, Panasol, Prednicen-M, Sterapred, {Winpred}

CLASSIFICATIONS(S):
Glucocorticoid—intermediate-acting
Pregnancy Category UK

INDICATIONS

▪ Used systemically and locally in a wide variety of chronic diseases including: ▫ Inflammatory ▫ Allergic ▫ Hematologic ▫ Neoplastic ▫ Autoimmune ▪ Suitable for alternate-day dosing in the management of chronic illness ▪ Replacement therapy in adrenal insufficiency.

ACTION

▪ Suppresses inflammation and the normal immune response ▪ Has numerous intense metabolic effects ▪ Suppresses adrenal function at chronic doses of 5 mg/day ▪ Has minimal mineralocorticoid (sodium-retaining) activity. **Therapeutic Effects:** ▪ Suppression of inflammation and modification of the normal immune response ▪ Replacement therapy in adrenal insufficiency.

PHARMACOKINETICS

Absorption: Well absorbed following oral administration.
Distribution: Widely distributed. Crosses the placenta and probably enters breast milk.
Metabolism and Excretion: Converted by the liver to prednisolone, which is then metabolized by the liver.
Half-life: 3.4–3.8 hr; adrenal suppression lasts 1.25–1.5 days.

CONTRAINDICATIONS AND PRECAUTIONS

Contraindicated in: ▪ Active untreated infections ▪ Lactation (avoid chronic use).
Use Cautiously in: ▪ Chronic treatment (will lead to adrenal suppression) ▪ Should never be abruptly discontinued ▪ Supplemental doses may be needed during stress (surgery, infection) ▪ Pregnancy (safety not established) ▪ Children (chronic use will result in decreased growth) ▪ May mask signs of infections (fever, inflammation) ▪ Use lowest possible dose for shortest period of time.

ADVERSE REACTIONS AND SIDE EFFECTS*

CNS: headache, restlessness, psychoses, depression, euphoria, personality

{} = Available in Canada only.
*Underlines indicate most frequent; **CAPITALS** indicate life-threatening.

P

changes, increased intracranial pressure (children only).
EENT: cataracts, increased intraocular pressure.
CV: hypertension.
GI: nausea, vomiting, anorexia, peptic ulceration.
Derm: decreased wound healing, petechiae, ecchymoses, fragility, hirsutism, acne.
Endo: adrenal suppression, hyperglycemia.
F and E: hypokalemia, hypokalemic alkalosis, fluid retention (long-term high doses).
Hemat: thromboembolism, thrombophlebitis.
Metab: weight loss, weight gain.
MS: muscle wasting, muscle pain, aseptic necrosis of joints, osteoporosis.
Misc: increased susceptibility to infection, cushingoid appearance (moon face, buffalo hump).

INTERACTIONS

Drug–Drug: ▪ Additive hypokalemia with **diuretics, amphotericin B, mezlocillin, piperacillin,** or **ticarcillin** ▪ Hypokalemia may increase the risk of **cardiac glycoside** toxicity ▪ May increase requirement for **insulin** or **oral hypoglycemic agents** ▪ Increased risk of adverse GI effects with **alcohol, aspirin,** or **nonsteroidal anti-inflammatory agents**.

ROUTE AND DOSAGE

Note: Maintenance doses may be given once daily or every other day.

- **PO (Adults):** 2.5–15 mg 2–4 times daily.
- **PO (Children):** 0.14–2 mg/kg/day in 4 divided doses.

PHARMACODYNAMICS (anti-inflammatory effects)

	ONSET	PEAK	DURATION
PO	hr	UK	1.25–1.5 days

NURSING IMPLICATIONS

Assessment

- This drug is indicated for many conditions. Assess involved systems prior to and periodically throughout course of therapy.
- Assess patient for signs of adrenal insufficiency (hypotension, weight loss, weakness, nausea, vomiting, anorexia, lethargy, confusion, restlessness) prior to and periodically throughout course of therapy.
- Monitor intake and output ratios and daily weight. Observe patient for the appearance of peripheral edema, steady weight gain, rales/crackles, or dyspnea. Notify physician should these occur.
- Children should have periodic evaluations of growth.
- **Lab Test Considerations:** Patients on prolonged courses of therapy should routinely have hematologic values, serum electrolytes, serum and urine glucose evaluated. May cause decreased WBC counts. May cause hyperglycemia, especially in persons with diabetes. May cause decreased serum potassium and calcium and increased serum sodium concentrations.
- Promptly report presence of guaiac-positive stools.
- May increase serum cholesterol and lipid values. May decrease serum protein-bound iodine and thyroxine concentrations.
- Suppresses reactions to skin tests.
- Periodic adrenal function tests may be ordered to assess degree of hypothalamic-pituitary-adrenal (HPA) axis suppression.

Potential Nursing Diagnoses

- Infection, high risk for (side effects).
- Body image disturbance (side effects).
- Knowledge deficit related to medication regimen (patient/family teaching).

Implementation

- **General Info:** Available in soln, syrup, and tablet forms.
- If dose is ordered daily or every other day, administer in the morning to co-

incide with the body's normal secretion of cortisol.

- **PO:** Administer with meals to minimize gastric irritation.
- □ Use calibrated measuring device to ensure accurate dosage of liquid forms.

PATIENT/FAMILY TEACHING

- □ Instruct patient to take medication exactly as directed. Do not skip doses or double up on missed doses. Stopping the medication suddenly may result in adrenal insufficiency (anorexia, nausea, fatigue, weakness, hypotension, dyspnea, and hypoglycemia). If these signs appear, notify physician immediately. This can be life-threatening.
- □ Encourage patients on long-term therapy to eat a diet high in protein, calcium, and potassium and low in sodium and carbohydrates (see Appendix K for foods included).
- □ This drug causes immunosuppression and may mask symptoms of infection. Instruct patient to avoid people with known contagious illnesses and to report possible infections.
- □ Review side effects with patient. Instruct patient to inform physician promptly if severe abdominal pain or tarry stools occur. Patient should also report unusual swelling, weight gain, tiredness, bone pain, bruising, nonhealing sores, visual disturbances, or behavior changes.
- □ Discuss possible effects on body image. Explore coping mechanisms.
- □ Instruct patient to inform physician if symptoms of underlying disease return or worsen.
- □ Advise patient to carry identification describing disease process and medication regimen in the event of an emergency in which patient cannot relate medical history.
- □ Caution patient to avoid vaccinations without consulting physician.
- □ Explain need for continued medical follow-up to assess effectiveness and possible side effects of medication. Physician may order periodic lab tests and eye examinations.

EVALUATION

Effectiveness of therapy can be demonstrated by: ▪ Suppression of inflammatory and immune responses in autoimmune disorders, allergic reactions, and organ transplants ▪ Management of symptoms in adrenal insufficiency.

PRIMIDONE

(**pri**-mi-done)

{Apo-Primidone}, Myidone, Mysoline, {Sertan}

CLASSIFICATION(S):
Anticonvulsant—miscellaneous

Pregnancy Category UK

INDICATIONS

▪ Management of tonic-clonic, complex partial, and focal seizures.

ACTION

▪ Decreases neuron excitability ▪ Increases the threshold of electric stimulation of the motor cortex. **Therapeutic Effect:** ▪ Prevention of seizures.

PHARMACOKINETICS

Absorption: 60–80% absorbed from the GI tract.

Distribution: Widely distributed. Crosses the placenta and enters breast milk.

Metabolism and Excretion: Converted to phenobarbital and another active anticonvulsant compound (PEMA) by the liver.

Half-life: 3–24 hr.

CONTRAINDICATIONS AND PRECAUTIONS

Contraindicated in: ▪ Previous hypersensitivity ▪ Porphyria.

Use Cautiously in: ▪ Severe liver disease (dosage adjustment required)

{} = Available in Canada only.

P

▪ Pregnancy and lactation (safety not established; may cause hemorrhage in the newborn).

ADVERSE REACTIONS AND SIDE EFFECTS*

CNS: drowsiness, ataxia, vertigo, lethargy, excitement (children).
EENT: visual changes.
Resp: dyspnea.
CV: edema, orthostatic hypotension.
GI: nausea, anorexia, vomiting, hepatitis.
Derm: rashes, alopecia.
Hemat: blood dyscrasias, megaloblastic anemia.
Misc: folic acid deficiency.

INTERACTIONS

Drug–Drug: ▪ Induces liver enzymes and may hasten metabolism and decrease the effectiveness of other drugs metabolized by the liver, including **oral contraceptives, chloramphenicol, acebutolol, propranolol, metoprolol, timolol, doxycycline, glucocorticoids, tricyclic antidepressants, phenothiazines, phenylbutazone,** and **quinidine** ▪ Additive CNS depression with other **CNS depressants,** including **alcohol, antihistamines, narcotic analgesics,** and **sedative/hypnotics** ▪ Concurrent use with **phenobarbital** may lead to phenobarbital toxicity.
Drug–Food: ▪ Decreases the absorption of **folic acid.**

ROUTE AND DOSAGE

- **PO (Adults and Children >8 yr):** Initial dose of 100–125 mg hs for 3 days, then 100–125 mg bid for 3 days, then 100–125 mg tid for 3 days, then maintenance dose of 250 mg 3–4 times daily (not to exceed 2 g/day).
- **PO (Children <8 yr):** Initial dose of 50 mg hs for 3 days, then 50 mg bid for next 3 days, 100 mg bid for 3 days, then maintenance dose of 125–250 mg tid (10–25 mg/kg/day).

PHARMACODYNAMICS (anticonvulsant effect)

	ONSET	PEAK	DURATION
PO	4–7 days	7–10 days	8–12 hr

NURSING IMPLICATIONS

Assessment

- □ Assess location, duration, and characteristics of seizure activity. Institute seizure precautions.
- □ Assess patient for allergy to phenobarbital, as it is a primidone metabolite.
- □ Assess patient for signs of folic acid deficiency (mental dysfunction, unusual tiredness or weakness, psychiatric disorders, neuropathy, megaloblastic anemia). May be treated with folic acid.
- ▪ **Lab Test Considerations:** Serum primidone and phenobarbital (a major metabolite of primidone) levels should be routinely monitored. Therapeutic blood levels for primidone: 5–10 mcg/ml; for phenobarbital: 15–40 mcg/ml.
- □ CBC and Sequential Multiple Analyzer-12 (SMA-12) tests should be monitored every 6 mon throughout course of therapy. May cause leukopenia and thrombocytopenia. May cause decreased serum bilirubin concentrations.
- ▪ **Toxicity and Overdose:** Signs of primidone toxicity include ataxia, lethargy, changes in vision, confusion, and dyspnea.

Potential Nursing Diagnoses

- ▪ Injury, high risk for (indications).
- ▪ Knowledge deficit related to medication regimen (patient/family teaching).

Implementation

- ▪ **General Info:** When switching from alternative anticonvulsant medication to primidone or adding primidone to regimen, increase primidone dose gradually while decreasing or continuing other anticonvulsant dos-

*Underlines indicate most frequent; **CAPITALS** indicate life-threatening.

ages to maintain seizure control. The switch to primidone alone should take at least 2 wk. Dosage adjustment is usually done at bedtime.

- **PO:** May be administered with food to minimize GI irritation. Tablets may be crushed and mixed with food or fluids for patients with difficulty swallowing. Shake liquid preparations well before pouring. Use calibrated measuring device to ensure accurate dosage.

Patient/Family Teaching

- Instruct patient to take medication every day exactly as directed. If a dose is missed, take as soon as remembered unless within 1 hr of next dose. Abrupt withdrawal may lead to status epilepticus.
- Primidone may cause drowsiness or dizziness. Caution patient to avoid driving or other activities requiring alertness until response to medication is known. These symptoms usually diminish in frequency and intensity with continued use of the medication. Do not resume driving until physician gives medical clearance based on control of seizure disorder.
- Caution patient to avoid taking alcohol or other CNS depressants concurrently with this medication.
- Caution patient to avoid sudden changes in position to decrease orthostatic hypotension.
- Instruct patient to notify physician or dentist of medication regimen prior to treatment or surgery.
- Advise patient to carry identification describing medication regimen at all times.
- Advise patient to notify physician if skin rash, unsteady gait, joint pain, fever, changes in vision, dyspnea, pregnancy, or paradoxical excitement (especially in children or the elderly) occurs.
- Emphasize the importance of routine examinations to monitor progress.

Evaluation

Effectiveness of therapy can be demonstrated by: ▪ Decrease or cessation of seizures without excessive sedation. May require 1 wk or more of therapy before therapeutic response is seen.

PROBENECID

(proe-**ben**-e-sid)
Benemid, {Benuryl}, Parbenem, Probalan

CLASSIFICATION(S):
Antigout agent—uricosuric
Pregnancy Category UK

INDICATIONS

▪ Prevention recurrences of gouty arthritis ▪ Treatment of hyperuricemia secondary to thiazide therapy ▪ Used to increase and prolong serum levels of penicillin and related anti-infectives.

ACTION

▪ Inhibits renal tubular reabsorption of uric acid, thus promoting its renal excretion. **Therapeutic Effect:** ▪ Reduction of serum uric acid levels.

PHARMACOKINETICS

Absorption: Well absorbed following oral administration.
Distribution: Crosses the placenta.
Metabolism and Excretion: Metabolized by the liver. Small amounts (10%) excreted unchanged in the urine.
Half-life: 4–17 hr.

CONTRAINDICATIONS AND PRECAUTIONS

Contraindicated in: ▪ Hypersensitivity ▪ Chronic high-dose salicylate therapy.
Use Cautiously in: ▪ Peptic ulcer ▪ Blood dyscrasias ▪ Uric acid kidney stones ▪ Pregnancy (has been used safely) ▪ Renal impairment (dosage reduction recommended).

P

ADVERSE REACTIONS AND SIDE EFFECTS*

CNS: headache, dizziness.
GI: nausea, vomiting, diarrhea, sore gums, hepatitis, abdominal pain.
GU: urinary frequency, uric acid stones.
Derm: flushing, rashes.
Hemat: anemia, APLASTIC ANEMIA.

INTERACTIONS

Drug-Drug: ▪ Increases blood levels of **penicillins, cephalosporins** and **fluoroquinolones** ▪ Blocks excretion and may increase toxicity or effectiveness of **nonsteroidal anti-inflammatory agents, methotrexate,** and **nitrofurantoin** ▪ Large doses of **aspirin** may decrease uricosuric activity.

ROUTE AND DOSAGE

Hyperuricemia

- **PO (Adults):** 250 mg bid for 1 wk, increase to 500 mg bid, then may increase by 500 mg/day every 4 wk (not to exceed 2–3 g/day).

To Augment Penicillin or Cephalosporin Therapy

- **PO (Adults):** 500 mg qid.
- **PO (Children):** 25 mg/kg initially; then 40 mg/kg/day in 4 divided doses.

Single-Dose Therapy of Gonorrhea

- **PO (Adults):** 1 g with amoxicillin or penicillin G procaine.

PHARMACODYNAMICS (effects on serum uric acid levels)

	ONSET	PEAK	DURATION
PO	30 min	2–4 hr	8 hr

NURSING IMPLICATIONS

Assessment

- **Gout:** Assess involved joints for pain, mobility, and edema throughout course of therapy.
- □ Monitor intake and output ratios. Fluids should be encouraged to prevent urate stone formation (2000–3000 ml/day). Alkalinization of the urine with sodium bicarbonate, potassium citrate, or acetazolamide may also be ordered for this purpose.
- **Lab Test Considerations:** May cause false-positive results in copper sulfate urine glucose tests (Clinitest). Use glucose oxidase method (Keto-Diastix, Test-Tape) to monitor urine glucose. CBC, serum uric acid levels, and renal function should be monitored routinely during long-term therapy.
- □ Serum and urine uric acid determinations may be measured periodically when probenecid is used to treat hyperuricemia.

Potential Nursing Diagnoses

- Comfort, altered: pain (indications).
- Mobility, impaired physical (indications).
- Knowledge deficit related to medication regimen (patient/family teaching).

Implementation

- **General Info:** Available in combination with colchicine (see Appendix A).
- □ Probenecid therapy is not used to treat gouty arthritis but rather, for prevention. If acute attacks occur during therapy, probenecid is usually continued at full dose along with colchicine or nonsteroidal anti-inflammatory agents.
- **PO:** Administer with food or antacid to minimize gastric irritation.

Patient/Family Teaching

- □ Instruct patient to take medication exactly as directed, not to discontinue without consulting physician. Irregular dosage schedules may cause elevation of uric acid levels and precipitate an acute gout attack.
- □ Explain purpose of the medication to patients taking probenecid with penicillin.
- □ Advise patient to follow physician's recommendations regarding weight loss, diet, and alcohol consumption.
- □ Caution patient not to take aspirin or

*Underlines indicate most frequent; **CAPITALS** indicate life-threatening.

other salicylates, as they decrease the effects of probenecid.

- Instruct patient to report nausea, vomiting, abdominal pain, unusual bleeding or bruising, sore throat, fatigue, malaise, or yellowing of the skin or eyes to physician promptly.

Evaluation

Therapeutic effects can be demonstrated by: ▪ Decrease in pain and swelling in affected joints and subsequent decrease in frequency of gout attacks. May require several mons of continuous therapy for maximum effects ▪ Prolonged serum levels of penicillins and other related antibiotics.

PROBUCOL
(proe-byoo-kole)
Lorelco

CLASSIFICATION(S):
Lipid-lowering agent
Pregnancy Category B

INDICATIONS

▪ Adjunct therapy of primary hypercholesterolemia.

ACTION

▪ May decrease transport of cholesterol from intestine or interfere with cholesterol synthesis ▪ May also increase fecal excretion of cholesterol and bile acids ▪ Lowers high-density lipoprotein (HDL) cholesterol. **Therapeutic Effects:** ▪ Lowers serum cholesterol levels ▪ Lowers low-density lipoprotein (LDL) cholesterol.

PHARMACOKINETICS

Absorption: Limited and variable absorption following oral administration (2–8%). Absorption is increased by concurrent administration of food.
Distribution: Accumulates in fatty tissue during chronic administration.
Metabolism and Excretion: Appears to be excreted in feces following biliary elimination.
Half-life: 20 days.

CONTRAINDICATIONS AND PRECAUTIONS

Contraindicated in: ▪ Hypersensitivity ▪ Pregnancy (continue contraception for 6 mon following therapy with probucol) ▪ Lactation ▪ Primary biliary cirrhosis.
Use Cautiously in: ▪ Cardiac arrhythmias ▪ Untreated congestive heart failure ▪ Children (safety not established).

ADVERSE REACTIONS AND SIDE EFFECTS*

CNS: dizziness, headache, insomnia.
EENT: blurred vision, tinnitus, decreased sense of smell, conjunctivitis, lacrimation.
CV: arrhythmias, ECG changes (prolonged QT interval), **SUDDEN DEATH**.
GI: <u>diarrhea</u>, <u>bloating</u>, flatulence, <u>abdominal pain</u>, <u>nausea</u>, <u>vomiting</u>, indigestion, GI bleeding, decreased taste.
Derm: rashes, pruritus, sweating.
Endo: enlargement of goiter.
Hemat: eosinophilia, anemia, thrombocytopenia.
Neuro: paresthesia, peripheral neuritis.

INTERACTIONS

Drug–Drug: ▪ Increased risk of adverse cardiovascular effects with concurrent use of **tricyclic antidepressants, anticholinergics, class I and II antiarrhythmics, phenothiazines, beta-adrenergic blocking agents,** or **cardiac glycosides** ▪ Concurrent use with **clofibrate** may further decrease high-density lipoprotein (HDL) cholesterol.
Drug–Food: ▪ Concurrent administration of **food** increases absorption.

ROUTE AND DOSAGE

▪ **PO (Adults):** 500 mg bid (not to exceed 1 g/day).

*<u>Underlines</u> indicate most frequent; **CAPITALS** indicate life-threatening.

P

PHARMACODYNAMICS (lipid-lowering effects)

	ONSET	PEAK	DURATION
PO	UK	20–50 days	1–3 mon

NURSING IMPLICATIONS

Assessment

- Obtain a diet history, especially regarding fat and alcohol consumption.
- **Lab Test Considerations:** May cause slight increase in serum bilirubin, blood glucose, BUN, creatine phosphokinase, SGOT (AST), SGPT (ALT), alkaline phosphatase, and uric acid concentrations.
- Serum triglyceride and cholesterol levels should be monitored prior to therapy, after 1 mon of therapy, and then every 3–6 mon. Medication should be discontinued if serum triglycerides increase despite low-fat diet.
- May decrease hemoglobin, hematocrit, and eosinophil concentrations.

Potential Nursing Diagnoses

- Knowledge deficit related to medication regimen (patient/family teaching).
- Noncompliance (patient/family teaching).
- Bowel elimination, altered: diarrhea (side effects).

Implementation

- **PO:** Administer with meals to enhance absorption.

Patient/Family Teaching

- Instruct patient to take medication as directed. If a dose is missed, take as soon as remembered unless almost time for next dose.
- Advise patient that this medication should be used in conjunction with dietary restrictions (fat, cholesterol, carbohydrates, alcohol), exercise, and cessation of smoking.
- Probucol may occasionally cause dizziness. Avoid driving or other activities requiring coordination until response to medication is known.
- Instruct patient to notify physician if abdominal discomfort, nausea, diarrhea, or bloating persists. GI side effects are usually transient.
- Explain need for medical follow-up to monitor response to therapy and to detect side effects. Patients with a history of cardiac arrhythmias should have periodic ECGs, and therapy should be withdrawn if QT intervals become prolonged or arrhythmias increase.

Evaluation

Effectiveness of therapy can be demonstrated by: ▪ Decrease in serum cholesterol levels. If a response is not seen within 4 mon, medication is usually discontinued.

PROCAINAMIDE

(proe-**kane**-ah-mide)
Procan SR, Promine, Pronestyl, Pronestyl-SR, Rhythmin

CLASSIFICATION(S):
Antiarrhythmic—class IA
Pregnancy Category C

INDICATIONS

▪ Treatment of a wide variety of ventricular and atrial arrhythmias, including: ▫ Atrial premature contractions ▫ Premature ventricular contractions ▫ Ventricular tachycardia ▫ Paroxysmal atrial tachycardia ▪ Maintenance of normal sinus rhythm after conversion from atrial fibrillation or flutter.

ACTION

▪ Decreases myocardial excitability ▪ Slows conduction velocity ▪ May depress myocardial contractility. **Therapeutic Effect:** ▪ Suppression of arrhythmias.

PHARMACOKINETICS

Absorption: Well absorbed (75–90%) following oral and IM administration. Sustained-release oral preparation is more slowly absorbed.

Distribution: Rapidly and widely distributed.
Metabolism and Excretion: Converted by the liver to n-acetylprocainamide (NAPA), an active antiarrhythmic compound. Remainder (40–70%) excreted unchanged by the kidneys.
Half-life: 2.5–4.7 hr (NAPA—7 hr), prolonged in renal impairment.

CONTRAINDICATIONS AND PRECAUTIONS

Contraindicated in: ▪ Hypersensitivity ▪ AV block ▪ Myasthenia gravis.
Use Cautiously in: ▪ Myocardial infarction or cardiac glycoside toxicity ▪ Congestive heart failure, renal and hepatic insufficiency (dosage reduction may be necessary) ▪ Pregnancy, lactation, or children (safety not established).

ADVERSE REACTIONS AND SIDE EFFECTS*

CNS: confusion, seizures, dizziness.
CV: hypotension, ventricular arrhythmias, asystole, heart block.
GI: nausea, vomiting, bitter taste.
Derm: rashes.
Hemat: leukopenia, thrombocytopenia, AGRANULOCYTOSIS, eosinophilia.
Misc: drug-induced systemic lupus syndrome, fever, chills.

INTERACTIONS

Drug–Drug: ▪ May have additive or antagonistic effects with other **antiarrhythmics** ▪ Additive neurologic toxicity (confusion, seizures) with **lidocaine** ▪ **Antihypertensives** and **nitrates** may potentiate hypotensive effect ▪ Potentiates **neuromuscular blocking agents** ▪ May partially antagonize the therapeutic effects of **anticholinesterase agents** in myasthenia gravis ▪ Additive anticholinergic effects with other **drugs possessing anticholinergic properties,** including **antihistamines, antidepressants, atropine, haloperidol,** and **phenothiazines**.

ROUTE AND DOSAGE

Note: See infusion rate chart in Appendix D.

- **PO (Adults):** 500–1000 mg q 3–6 hr (sustained-release preparations given q 6 hr).
- **IM (Adults):** 500–1000 mg q 4–8 hr.
- **IV Bolus (Adults):** 100 mg over 2 min, repeat q 5 min until toxicity, response, or total of 1000 mg.
- **IV Infusion (Adults):** 2–6 mg/min.

PHARMACODYNAMICS (antiarrhythmic effects)

	ONSET	PEAK	DURATION
PO	30 min	60–90 min	3–4 hr
PO-ER	UK	UK	6 hr
IV	immediate	25–60 min	3–4 hr
IM	10–30 min	15–60 min	3–4 hr

NURSING IMPLICATIONS

ASSESSMENT

- ◻ Monitor ECG, pulse, and blood pressure continuously throughout IV administration. Parameters should be monitored periodically during oral administration. IV administration is usually discontinued if any of the following occur: arrhythmia is resolved, QRS complex widens by 50%, PR interval is prolonged, blood pressure drops >15 mmHg, or toxic side effects develop. Patient should remain supine throughout IV administration to minimize hypotension.
- ▪ **Lab Test Consideration:** CBC should be monitored every 2 wk during the first 3 mon of therapy. Rarely causes decreased leukocyte, neutrophil, and platelet counts. Therapy may be discontinued if leukopenia occurs.
- ◻ Antinuclear antibody (ANA) should be periodically monitored during prolonged therapy or if symptoms of lupus-like reaction occur. Therapy is discontinued if a steady increase in ANA titer occurs.
- ◻ May cause an increase in SGOT (AST), SGPT (ALT), alkaline phos-

*Underlines indicate most frequent; **CAPITALS** indicate life-threatening.

phatase, LDH, and bilirubin, and a positive Coombs' test result.

- **Toxicity and Overdose:** Serum procainamide and NAPA levels may be monitored periodically during dosage adjustment. Therapeutic blood level of procainamide is 4–8 mcg/ml.
  - Toxicity may occur with procainamide blood levels of 8–16 mcg/ml or greater.
  - Signs of toxicity include confusion, dizziness, drowsiness, decreased urination, nausea, vomiting, and tachyarrhythmias.

Potential Nursing Diagnoses

- Cardiac output, decreased (indications).
- Knowledge deficit related to medication regimen (patient/family teaching).

Implementation

- **General Info:** When converting from IV to oral dose regimen, allow 3–4 hr to elapse between last IV dose and administration of first oral dose.
- **PO:** Administer with a full glass of water on an empty stomach either 1 hr before or 2 hr after meals for faster absorption. If GI irritation becomes a problem, may be administered with or immediately after meals. Tablets may be crushed and capsules opened and mixed with food or fluids for patients with difficulty swallowing. Do not break, crush, or chew extended-release tablets (Procan SR, Pronestyl-SR). Wax matrix of extended-release tablets may be found in stool but is not significant.
- **IM:** Used only when oral and IV routes are not feasible.
- **Direct IV:** Dilute each 100 mg with 10 ml of D5W or sterile water for injection.
  - *Rate:* Administer at a rate not to exceed 50 mg/min. Rapid administration may cause ventricular fibrillation or asystole.
- **Intermittent Infusion:** Prepare IV infusion by adding 200 mg–1 g to 50–500 ml of D5W, for a concentration of 2–4 mg/ml. Slight yellow color of soln will not alter potency; do not use when darker than light amber or if soln contains a precipitate.
  - *Rate:* Administer initial infusion over 30 min. Maintenance infusion should infuse at 2–6 mg/min to maintain control of arrhythmia. Use infusion pump to ensure accurate dosage (see Appendix D for infusion rate chart).
- **Y-Site Compatibility:** amrinone, famotidine, heparin, hydrocortisone sodium succinate, potassium chloride, or ranitidine.
- **Additive Compatibility:** dobutamine, lidocaine, netilmicin, or verapamil.
- **Additive Incompatibility:** esmolol or ethacrynate.

Patient/Family Teaching

- Instruct patient to take medication around the clock, exactly as directed, even if feeling better. If a dose is missed, take as soon as remembered within 2 hr (4 hr for extended-release tablets); omit if remembered later. Do not double doses. Consult physician prior to discontinuing medication, as gradual reduction in dosage may be needed to prevent worsening of condition.
- Instruct patient or family member on how to take pulse. Advise patient to report changes in pulse rate or rhythm to physician.
- Procainamide may cause dizziness. Caution patient to avoid driving or other activities requiring alertness until response to medication is known.
- Advise patient to notify physician immediately if signs of drug-induced lupus syndrome (fever, chills, joint pain or swelling, pain with breathing, skin rash), leukopenia (sore throat, mouth, or gums), or thrombocytopenia (unusual bleeding or bruising) occur. Medication may be discontinued if these occur.
- Caution patient not to take over-the-counter medications with procainamide without consulting physician or pharmacist.
- Advise patient to inform physician or

dentist of medication regimen prior to treatment or surgery.

- Advise patient to carry identification describing disease process and medication regimen at all times.
- Emphasize the importance of routine follow-up examinations to monitor progress.

Evaluation

Effectiveness of therapy can be demonstrated by: ▪ Resolution of cardiac arrhythmias without detrimental side effects.

PROCARBAZINE

(proe-**kar**-ba-zeen)
Matulane, {Natulan}

CLASSIFICATION(S):
Antineoplastic—alkylating agent
Pregnancy Category D

INDICATIONS

▪ In combination with other antineoplastic agents and modalities in the treatment of Hodgkin's disease. **Unlabeled Uses:** ▪ Other lymphomas ▪ Brain and lung tumors ▪ Multiple myeloma ▪ Malignant melanoma ▪ Polycythemia vera.

ACTION

▪ Appears to inhibit DNA, RNA, and protein synthesis (cell cycle-S phase specific). **Therapeutic Effect:** ▪ Death of rapidly replicating cells, particularly malignant ones.

PHARMACOKINETICS

Absorption: Well absorbed following oral administration.
Distribution: Widely distributed. Crosses the blood-brain barrier.
Metabolism and Excretion: Metabolized by the liver.
Half-life: 1 hr.

CONTRAINDICATIONS AND PRECAUTIONS

Contraindicated in: ▪ Hypersensitivity ▪ Pregnancy or lactation ▪ Alcoholism ▪ Severe renal or liver impairment ▪ Pheochromocytoma ▪ Congestive heart failure.
Use Cautiously in: ▪ Patients with childbearing potential ▪ Infections ▪ Decreased bone marrow reserve ▪ Other chronic debilitating illnesses ▪ Headaches ▪ Psychiatric illness ▪ Liver impairment ▪ Cardiovascular disease.

ADVERSE REACTIONS AND SIDE EFFECTS*

CNS: neuropathy, confusion, depression, psychosis, mania, headache, hallucinations, nightmares, tremor, seizures, syncope, drowsiness, dizziness.
EENT: retinal hemorrhage, nystagmus, photophobia.
Resp: cough, pleural effusions.
CV: edema, tachycardia, hypotension.
GI: nausea, vomiting, anorexia, stomatitis, dry mouth, dysphagia, diarrhea, hepatic dysfunction.
GU: gonadal suppression.
Derm: rashes, pruritus, alopecia, photosensitivity.
Endo: gynecomastia.
Hemat: anemia, leukopenia, thrombocytopenia.
Neuro: neuropathies, paresthesias.
Misc: ascites.

INTERACTIONS

Drug-Drug: ▪ Additive CNS depression with other **CNS depressants,** including **alcohol, antidepressants, antihistamines, narcotic analgesics,** and **sedative/hypnotics** ▪ Disulfiram-like reaction may occur with **alcohol** ▪ **Sympathomimetic amines, local anesthetics, levodopa, reserpine, guanethidine, guanedrel, vasoconstrictors,** and **antidepressants** should be avoided, since procarbazine has some MAO inhibitory properties (increased risk of hypertensive reactions) ▪ Severe paradoxical reactions may occur with **meperidine** and

{} = Available in Canada only.
*Underlines indicate most frequent; **CAPITALS** indicate life-threatening.

P

other **narcotic analgesics** (avoid concurrent meperidine—decrease initial dose of other narcotic analgesics to 25% of usual dose) ▪ Seizure and hyperpyrexia may occur with concurrent use of **MAO inhibitors** or **carbamazepine** ▪ Additive bone marrow depression with other **antineoplastic agents** or **radiation therapy**.

Drug–Food: ▪ Ingestion of foods high in **tyramine** content (see Appendix K) may result in hypertension.

ROUTE AND DOSAGE

- **PO (Adults):** 100–150 mg/m²/day for 10 days, maintenance dose of 50–100 mg/day; or 2–4 mg/kg/day for 1 wk, then 4–6 mg/kg/day until response is obtained, maintenance dose of 1–2 mg/kg/day.
- **PO (Children):** 50 mg/day for 7 days, then 100 mg/m²/day, maintenance dose of 50 mg/day.

PHARMACODYNAMICS (effects on blood counts)

	ONSET	PEAK	DURATION
PO	14 days	2–8 wk	28 days or more (up to 6 wk)

NURSING IMPLICATIONS

Assessment

- ▫ Monitor blood pressure, pulse, and respiratory rate periodically during course of therapy. Notify physician if significant changes occur.
- ▫ Assess patient's nutritional status (appetite, intake and output ratios, weight, frequency and amount of emesis). Anorexia and weight loss can be decreased by feeding light, frequent meals. Nausea and vomiting can be minimized by administering an antiemetic at least 1 hr prior to receiving medication.
- ▪ **Lab Test Considerations:** Renal and hepatic function, CBC, and urinalysis should be monitored prior to and routinely throughout course of therapy. Inform physician if WBC $<4000/mm^3$ or platelet count $<100,000/mm^3$. The nadir of leukopenia and thrombocytopenia occurs in approximately 4 wk and recovery usually occurs in about 6 wk. Anemia may also occur.
- ▫ Closely monitor serum glucose in diabetic patients. Oral hypoglycemics or insulin dosage may need to be reduced, as hypoglycemic effects are enhanced.
- ▪ **Toxicity and Overdose:** Concurrent ingestion of tyramine-rich foods and many medications may result in life-threatening hypertensive crisis. Signs and symptoms of hypertensive crisis include chest pain, severe headache, nausea and vomiting, photosensitivity, and enlarged pupils. Treatment includes IV phentolamine.

Potential Nursing Diagnoses

- ▪ Infection, high risk for (adverse reactions).
- ▪ Nutrition, altered: less than body requirements (adverse reactions).
- ▪ Knowledge deficit related to medication regimen (patient/family teaching).

Implementation

- ▪ **PO:** Administer with food or fluids if GI irritation occurs. Confer with pharmacist regarding opening of capsules if patient has difficulty swallowing.

Patient/Family Teaching

- ▫ Emphasize the need to take medication exactly as directed. If a dose is missed, it should be taken as soon as remembered unless almost time for next dose. Physician should be consulted if vomiting occurs shortly after a dose is taken.
- ▫ Instruct patient to notify physician promptly if fever, sore throat, signs of infection, bleeding gums, bruising, petechiae, or blood in stool, urine, or emesis occurs. Caution patient to avoid crowds and persons with known infections. Instruct patient to use soft toothbrush and electric razor and to avoid falls. Patient should not receive IM injections or rectal temperatures. Patient should also be cautioned not to drink alcoholic beverages or take medication containing

aspirin, as these may precipitate gastric bleeding.

- Caution patient to avoid alcohol, caffeinated beverages, CNS depressants, over-the-counter drugs, and foods or beverages containing tyramine (see Appendix K for foods included) during therapy and for at least 2 wk after therapy has been discontinued, as they may precipitate a hypertensive crisis.
- Advise patient that an additional interaction of alcohol with procarbazine is a disulfiram-like reaction (flushing, nausea, vomiting, headache, abdominal cramps).
- Instruct patient to inspect oral mucosa for erythema and ulceration. If ulceration occurs, advise patient to use sponge brush and rinse mouth with water after eating and drinking. Physician may order viscous lidocaine swishes if mouth pain interferes with eating.
- Medication may cause drowsiness or dizziness. Caution patient to avoid driving or other activities that require alertness until response to medication is known.
- Advise patient that this medication may have teratogenic effects. Contraception should be practiced during therapy and for at least 4 mon after therapy is concluded.
- Discuss the possibility of hair loss with patient. Explore methods of coping.
- Caution patient to use sunscreen and protective clothing to prevent photosensitivity reactions.
- Instruct patient not to receive any vaccinations without advice of physician.
- Advise patient to notify physician or dentist of medication regimen prior to treatment or surgery. This therapy usually should be withdrawn at least 2 wk prior to surgery.
- Emphasize the need for periodic lab tests to monitor for side effects.
- Instruct patient to inform physician if confusion, hallucinations, cough, paresthesia, unsteady gait, severe headache, skin rash, jaundice, or diarrhea occurs.

Evaluation

Effectiveness of therapy can be demonstrated by: ▪ Decrease in size and spread of malignant tissue in Hodgkin's disease.

PROCHLORPERAZINE

(proe-klor-**pair**-a-zeen)
Chlorpazine, Compazine, {Stemetil}

CLASSIFICATION(S):
Antiemetic—phenothiazine, Antipsychotic—phenothiazine
Pregnancy Category UK

INDICATIONS

▪ Management of nausea and vomiting ▪ Treatment of acute and chronic psychoses.

ACTION

▪ Alters the effects of dopamine in the CNS ▪ Possesses significant anticholinergic and alpha-adrenergic blocking activity ▪ Depresses the chemoreceptor trigger zone (CTZ) in the CNS. **Therapeutic Effects:** ▪ Diminished nausea and vomiting ▪ Diminished signs and symptoms of psychoses.

PHARMACOKINETICS

Absorption: Absorption from tablet is variable; may be better with oral liquid formulations. Well absorbed following IM administration.

Distribution: Widely distributed, high concentrations in the CNS. Crosses the placenta and probably enters breast milk.

Metabolism and Excretion: Highly metabolized by the liver and GI mu-

{} = Available in Canada only.

cosa. Converted to some compounds with antipsychotic activity.
Half-life: UK.

CONTRAINDICATIONS AND PRECAUTIONS

Contraindicated in: ▪ Hypersensitivity ▪ Cross-sensitivity with other phenothiazines may exist ▪ Narrow-angle glaucoma ▪ Bone marrow depression ▪ Severe liver or cardiovascular disease ▪ Hypersensitivity to bisulfites or benzyl alcohol (some parenteral products).
Use Cautiously in: ▪ Elderly or debilitated patients (dosage reduction recommended) ▪ Pregnancy or lactation (safety not established; may cause adverse reactions in newborns) ▪ Diabetes mellitus ▪ Respiratory disease ▪ Prostatic hypertrophy ▪ CNS tumors ▪ Epilepsy ▪ Intestinal obstruction.

ADVERSE REACTIONS AND SIDE EFFECTS*

CNS: sedation, extrapyramidal reactions, tardive dyskinesia, NEUROLEPTIC MALIGNANT SYNDROME.
EENT: dry eyes, blurred vision, lens opacities.
CV: hypotension, tachycardia, ECG changes.
GI: constipation, dry mouth, ileus, anorexia, hepatitis.
GU: urinary retention, pink or reddish-brown discoloration of urine.
Derm: rashes, photosensitivity, pigment changes.
Endo: galactorrhea.
Hemat: AGRANULOCYTOSIS, leukopenia.
Metab: hyperthermia.
Misc: allergic reactions.

INTERACTIONS

Drug-Drug: ▪ Additive hypotension with **antihypertensive agents, nitrates,** or acute ingestion of **alcohol** ▪ Additive CNS depression with other **CNS depressants,** including **alcohol, antidepressants, antihistamines, narcotic analgesics, sedative/hypnotics,** or **general anesthetics** ▪ Additive anticholinergic effects with other **drugs possessing anticholinergic properties,** including **antihistamines, antidepressants, atropine, haloperidol,** and other **phenothiazines** ▪ **Lithium** decreases absorption and increases the risk of extrapyramidal reactions ▪ May mask early signs of **lithium** toxicity ▪ Increased risk of agranulocytosis with **antithyroid agents** ▪ Decreases the beneficial effects of **levodopa** ▪ **Antacids** may decrease absorption.

ROUTE AND DOSAGE

Antiemetic, Mild to Moderate Emotional Disturbances

- **PO (Adults):** 5–10 mg 3–4 times daily or 15 mg/day of extended-release preparation or 10 mg bid of extended-release preparation (not to exceed 40 mg/day).
- **IM (Adults):** 5–10 mg q 3–4 hr (not to exceed 40 mg/day).
- **Rect (Adults):** 25 mg bid.
- **PO, Rect (Children 18–39 kg):** 2.5 mg tid or 5 mg bid (not to exceed 15 mg/day).
- **PO, Rect (Children 14–17 kg):** 2.5 mg 2–3 times daily (not to exceed 10 mg/day).
- **PO, Rect (Children 9–13 kg):** 2.5 mg 1–2 times daily (not to exceed 7.5 mg/day).
- **IM (Children >2 yr):** 0.13 mg/kg, single dose.
- **IV (Adults):** 2.5–10 mg, rate not to exceed 5 mg/min, may be repeated in 30 min; single dose not to exceed 10 mg (not to exceed 40 mg/day).

Psychomotor Agitation, Psychoses

- **PO (Adults):** 5–10 mg qid adjusted and increased as needed (not to exceed 150 mg/day).
- **IM (Adults):** 10–20 mg q 4–6 hr as needed (not to exceed 150–200 mg/day).

*Underlines indicate most frequent; **CAPITALS** indicate life-threatening.

PHARMACODYNAMICS (antiemetic effect)

	ONSET	PEAK	DURATION
PO	30–40 min	UK	3–4 hr
PO-ER	30–40 min	UK	10–12 hr
Rect	60 min	UK	3–4 hr
IM	10–20 min	UK	3–4 hr
IV	rapid (min)	UK	3–4 hr

NURSING IMPLICATIONS

Assessment

- **General Info:** Monitor blood pressure (sitting, standing, lying), pulse, and respiratory rate prior to and frequently during the period of dosage adjustment.
- Assess patient for level of sedation following administration.
- Monitor patient for onset of extrapyramidal side effects (akathisia—restlessness; dystonia—muscle spasms and twisting motions; pseudoparkinsonism—mask facies, rigidity, tremors, drooling, shuffling gait, dysphagia). Notify physician if these symptoms occur, as reduction in dosage or discontinuation of medication may be necessary. Physician may also order antiparkinsonian agents (trihexyphenidyl or benztropine) to control these symptoms.
- Monitor for tardive dyskinesia (rhythmic movement of mouth, face, and extremities). Notify physician immediately if these symptoms occur, as these side effects may be irreversible.
- Monitor for development of neuroleptic malignant syndrome (fever, respiratory distress, tachycardia, convulsions, diaphoresis, hypertension or hypotension, pallor, tiredness). Notify physician immediately if these symptoms occur.
- **Antiemetic:** Assess patient for nausea and vomiting prior to and 30–60 min following administration.
- **Antipsychotic:** Monitor patient's mental status (orientation to reality and behavior) prior to and periodically throughout therapy.
- Observe patient carefully when administering oral medication to ensure that medication is actually taken and not hoarded.
- **Lab Test Considerations:** CBC and liver function tests should be evaluated periodically throughout course of therapy. May cause blood dyscrasias, especially between wks 4–10 of therapy. Hepatotoxicity is more likely to occur between 14 and 30 days of therapy.
- May cause false-positive or false-negative pregnancy tests and false-positive urine bilirubin test results.
- May cause increased serum prolactin levels and interfere with gonadorelin test results.
- May cause Q-wave and T-wave changes in ECG.

Potential Nursing Diagnoses

- Fluid volume deficit (indications).
- Thought processes, altered (indications).
- Knowledge deficit related to medication regimen (patient/family teaching).

Implementation

- **General Info:** Available in tablet, extended-release capsule, syrup, oral soln, suppository, and injectable forms.
- To prevent contact dermatitis avoid getting soln on hands.
- Phenothiazines should be discontinued 48 hr before and not resumed for 24 hr following metrizamide myelography, as they lower seizure threshold.
- **PO:** Do not crush or chew sustained-release capsules. Administer with food, milk, or a full glass of water to minimize gastric irritation.
- Dilute syrup in citrus or chocolate-flavored drinks.
- **IM:** Do not inject SC. Inject slowly, deep into well-developed muscle. Keep patient recumbent for at least 30 min following injection to minimize hypotensive effects. Slight yellow color will not alter potency. Do not administer soln that is markedly discolored or that contains a precipitate.

P

- **Direct IV:** Dilute to a concentration of 1 mg/ml.
  - □ *Rate:* Administer no faster than 1 mg/min.
- **Intermittent Infusion:** Dilute 20 mg in up to 1 liter dextrose, saline, Ringer's or lactated Ringer's soln, dextrose/saline, dextrose/Ringer's, or lactated Ringer's combinations.
- **Syringe Compatibility:** Manufacturer does not recommend mixing prochlorperazine with other medications in syringe. Prochlorperazine has been found to be compatible in syringe for a limited period (15 min) with atropine, butorphanol, chlorpromazine, cimetidine, diphenhydramine, droperidol, fentanyl, glycopyrrolate, hydroxyzine, meperidine, metoclopramide, morphine, nalbuphine, pentazocine, perphenazine, promazine, promethazine, ranitidine, or scopolamine.
- **Syringe Incompatibility:** dimenhydrinate, midazolam, pentobarbital, or thiopental.
- **Y-Site Compatibility:** heparin, hydrocortisone sodium succinate, ondansetron, or potassium chloride.
- **Y-Site Incompatibility:** foscarnet.
- **Additive Compatibility:** amikacin, ascorbic acid, dexamethasone sodium phosphate, erythromycin lactobionate, ethacrynate sodium, lidocaine, nafcillin, or sodium bicarbonate.
- **Additive Incompatibility:** aminophylline, amphotericin B, ampicillin, calcium gluceptate, cephalothin, chloramphenicol, chlorothiazide, hydrocortisone sodium succinate, methohexital, penicillin G sodium, phenobarbital, or thiopental.

Patient/Family Teaching

- □ Instruct patient to take medication exactly as directed, not to skip doses or double up on missed doses. If a dose is missed, it should be taken as soon as remembered unless almost time for next dose. If more than 2 doses are scheduled each day, missed dose should be taken within about 1 hr of the ordered time. Abrupt withdrawal may lead to gastritis, nausea, vomiting, dizziness, headache, tachycardia, and insomnia.
- □ Inform patient of possibility of extrapyramidal symptoms and tardive dyskinesia. Caution patient to report these symptoms immediately to physician.
- □ Advise patient to make position changes slowly to minimize orthostatic hypotension.
- □ Medication may cause drowsiness. Caution patient to avoid driving or other activities requiring alertness until response to medication is known.
- □ Caution patient to avoid taking alcohol or other CNS depressants concurrently with this medication.
- □ Advise patient to use sunscreen and protective clothing when exposed to the sun to prevent photosensitivity reactions. Extremes in temperature should also be avoided, as this drug impairs body temperature regulation.
- □ Instruct patient to use freqent mouth rinses, good oral hygiene, and sugarless gum or candy to minimize dry mouth. Consult physician or dentist if dry mouth continues >2 wk.
- □ Advise patient that increasing bulk and fluids in the diet and exercise may help minimize the constipating effects of this medication.
- □ Inform patient that this medication may turn urine pink to reddish-brown.
- □ Advise patient to notify physician or dentist of medication regimen prior to treatment or surgery.
- □ Instruct patient to notify physician promptly if sore throat, fever, unusual bleeding or bruising, skin rashes, weakness, tremors, visual disturbances, dark-colored urine, or clay-colored stools are noted.
- □ Emphasize the importance of routine follow-up examinations to monitor response to medication and detect side effects. Periodic ocular examinations are indicated. Encourage continued

participation in psychotherapy as ordered by physician.

EVALUATION

Effectiveness of therapy can be demonstrated by: ▪ Relief of nausea and vomiting ▪ Decrease in excitable, paranoic, or withdrawn behavior when used as an antipsychotic.

PROGESTERONE

(proe-**jess**-te-rone)
Femotrone, Gestrol, {Progestilin}

CLASSIFICATION(S):
Hormone—progestin
Pregnancy Category UK

INDICATIONS

▪ Treatment of secondary amenorrhea and abnormal uterine bleeding caused by hormonal imbalance. **Unlabeled Use:** ▪ Corpus luteum dysfunction.

ACTION

▪ Produces secretory changes in the endometrium: ▫ Increases in basal body temperature ▫ Histologic changes in vaginal epithelium ▫ Relaxation of uterine smooth muscle ▫ Mammary alveolar tissue growth ▫ Pituitary inhibition ▫ Withdrawal bleeding in the presence of estrogen. **Therapeutic Effect:** ▪ Restoration of hormonal balance with control of uterine bleeding.

PHARMACOKINETICS

Absorption: UK.
Distribution: Enters breast milk.
Metabolism and Excretion: UK.
Half-life: UK.

CONTRAINDICATIONS AND PRECAUTIONS

Contraindicated in: ▪ Hypersensitivity ▪ Hypersensitivity to parabens (IM suspension only) ▪ Pregnancy (except corpus luteum dysfunction) ▪ Missed abortion ▪ Thromboembolic disease ▪ Cerebrovascular disease ▪ Severe liver disease ▪ Breast or genital cancer ▪ Porphyria.
Use Cautiously in: ▪ History of liver disease ▪ Renal disease ▪ Cardiovascular disease ▪ Seizure disorders ▪ Mental depression.

ADVERSE REACTIONS AND SIDE EFFECTS*

CNS: depression.
EENT: retinal thrombosis.
CV: THROMBOEMBOLISM, PULMONARY EMBOLISM, thrombophlebitis.
GI: gingival bleeding, hepatitis.
GU: cervical erosions.
Endo: breakthrough bleeding, spotting, amenorrhea, breast tenderness, galactorrhea, changes in menstrual flow.
Derm: rashes, melasma, chloasma.
F and E: edema.
Local: pain, irritation at IM injection site.
Misc: weight gain, weight loss, allergic reactions, including ANAPHYLAXIS and ANGIOEDEMA.

INTERACTIONS

Drug-Drug: ▪ May decrease the effectiveness of **bromocriptine** when used concurrently for galactorrhea/amenorrhea.

ROUTE AND DOSAGE

Secondary Amenorrhea

▪ **IM (Adults):** 50–100 mg (single dose) or 5–10 mg daily for 6–8 days given 8–10 days prior to expected menstrual period.

Abnormal Uterine Bleeding

▪ **IM (Adults):** 50–100 mg (single dose) or 5–10 mg daily for 6 days.

Corpus Luteum Insufficiency

▪ **IM (Adults):** 12.5 mg at onset of ovulation for 2 wk (may continue until 11th wk of gestation).

PHARMACODYNAMICS

	ONSET	PEAK	DURATION
IM	UK	UK	UK

{} = Available in Canada only.
*Underlines indicate most frequent; **CAPITALS** indicate life-threatening.

P

NURSING IMPLICATIONS

ASSESSMENT

- **General Info:** Blood pressure should be monitored periodically throughout therapy.
- □ Monitor intake and output ratios and weekly weight. Report significant discrepancies or steady weight gain to physician.
- **Amenorrhea:** Assess patient's usual menstrual history. Administration of drug usually begins 8–10 days before anticipated menstruation. Withdrawal bleeding usually occurs 48–72 hr after course of therapy. Therapy should be discontinued if menses occur during injection series.
- **Dysfunctional Bleeding:** Monitor pattern and amount of vaginal bleeding (pad count). Bleeding should end by 6th day of therapy. Therapy should be discontinued if menses occur during injection series.
- **Lab Test Considerations:** Monitor hepatic function prior to and periodically throughout therapy.
- □ May cause increased plasma amino acid and alkaline phosphatase levels.
- □ May decrease pregnanediol excretion concentrations.
- □ High doses may increase sodium and chloride excretion.
- □ May alter thyroid function test results.

POTENTIAL NURSING DIAGNOSES

- Sexual dysfunction (indications).
- Knowledge deficit related to medication regimen (patient/family teaching).

IMPLEMENTATION

- **IM:** Shake vial before preparing IM dose. Administer deep IM. Rotate sites.

PATIENT/FAMILY TEACHING

- □ Advise patient to report signs and symptoms of fluid retention (swelling of ankles and feet, weight gain), thromboembolic disorders (pain, swelling, tenderness in extremities, headache, chest pain, blurred vision), mental depression, or hepatic dysfunction (yellowed skin or eyes, pruritus, dark urine, light-colored stools) to physician.
- □ Instruct patient to notify physician if change in vaginal bleeding pattern or spotting occurs.
- □ Instruct patient to stop taking medication and notify physician if pregnancy is suspected.
- □ Caution patient to use sunscreen and protective clothing to prevent photosensitivity reactions.
- □ Advise patient to notify physician or dentist of medication regimen prior to treatment or surgery.
- □ Emphasize the importance of routine follow-up physical examinations, including blood pressure; breast, abdomen, and pelvic examinations; and PAP smears.

EVALUATION

Effectiveness of therapy can be demonstrated by: ▪ Development of normal cyclic menses.

PROMAZINE

(**proe**-ma-zeen)
Sparine

CLASSIFICATION(S):
Antipsychotic—phenothiazine
Pregnancy Category UK

INDICATIONS

- Treatment of acute and chronic psychoses.

ACTION

▪ Alters the effects of dopamine in the CNS ▪ Possesses significant anticholinergic and alpha-adrenergic blocking activity. **Therapeutic Effect:** ▪ Diminished signs and symptoms of psychoses.

PHARMACOKINETICS

Absorption: Absorption from tablets is variable; may be better with oral liquid formulations. Well absorbed following IM administration.
Distribution: Widely distributed, high concentrations in the CNS. Crosses the

placenta and probably enters breast milk.
Metabolism and Excretion: Highly metabolized by the liver and GI mucosa.
Half-life: UK.

CONTRAINDICATIONS AND PRECAUTIONS

Contraindicated in: ▪ Hypersensitivity ▪ Cross-sensitivity with other phenothiazines may exist ▪ Narrow-angle glaucoma ▪ Bone marrow depression ▪ Severe liver or cardiovascular disease ▪ Hypersensitivity to bisulfites or formaldehyde (injection only).
Use Cautiously in: ▪ Elderly or debilitated patients (dosage reduction may be required) ▪ Pregnancy or lactation (safety not established) ▪ Diabetes mellitus ▪ Respiratory disease ▪ Prostatic hypertrophy ▪ CNS tumors ▪ Epilepsy ▪ Intestinal obstruction.

ADVERSE REACTIONS AND SIDE EFFECTS*

CNS: sedation, extrapyramidal reactions, tardive dyskinesia, NEUROLEPTIC MALIGNANT SYNDROME.
EENT: dry eyes, blurred vision, lens opacities.
CV: hypotension, tachycardia.
GI: constipation, dry mouth, ileus, anorexia, hepatitis.
GU: urinary retention.
Derm: rashes, photosensitivity, pigment changes.
Endo: galactorrhea.
Hemat: AGRANULOCYTOSIS, leukopenia.
Metab: hyperthermia.
Misc: allergic reactions.

INTERACTIONS

Drug-Drug: ▪ Additive hypotension with **antihypertensive agents, nitrates,** or acute ingestion of **alcohol** ▪ Additive CNS depression with other **CNS depressants,** including **alcohol, antihistamines, narcotic analgesics, sedative/hypnotics,** or **general anesthetics** ▪ Additive anticholinergic effects with other **drugs possessing anticholinergic properties,** including **antihistamines, antidepressants, atropine, haloperidol,** and other **phenothiazines** ▪ **Lithium** decreases absorption and increases the risk of extrapyramidal reactions ▪ May mask early signs of **lithium** toxicity ▪ Decreases beneficial effects of **levodopa** ▪ Increased risk of agranulocytosis with **antithyroid agents.**

ROUTE AND DOSAGE

Psychoses

- **PO, IM (Adults):** 10–200 mg q 4–6 hr up to 1000 mg/day.
- **PO, (Children >12 yr):** 10–25 mg q 4–6 hr.

Severe Agitation

- **IM (Adults):** 50–150 mg initially; if required, additional doses may be given after 30 min up to a total dose of 300 mg, then maintenance dose of 10–200 mg q 4–6 hr as needed (not to exceed 1 g/24 hr).
- **IV (Adults):** 50–150 mg initially; if required, additional doses may be given after 30 min, up to a total dose of 300 mg.

PHARMACODYNAMICS (antipsychotic effects)

	ONSET	PEAK	DURATION
PO	30 min	UK	4–6 hr
IM	within 30 min	UK	UK
IV	within 30 min	UK	UK

NURSING IMPLICATIONS

Assessment

- ▫ Monitor patient's mental status (orientation to reality and behavior) prior to and periodically throughout therapy.
- ▫ Monitor blood pressure (sitting, standing, lying), pulse, and respiratory rate prior to and frequently during the period of dosage adjustment.
- ▫ Observe patient carefully when administering oral medication to ensure medication is actually taken and not hoarded.

*Underlines indicate most frequent; **CAPITALS** indicate life-threatening.

- Assess patient for level of sedation following administration.
- Monitor patient for onset of extrapyramidal side effects (akathisia—restlessness; dystonia—muscle spasms and twisting motions; pseudoparkinsonism—mask facies, rigidity, tremors, drooling, shuffling gait, dysphagia). Notify physician if these symptoms occur, as reduction in dosage or discontinuation of medication may be necessary. Physician may also order antiparkinsonian agents (trihexyphenidyl or benztropine) to control these symptoms.
- Monitor for tardive dyskinesia (rhythmic movement of mouth, face, and extremities). Notify physician immediately if these symptoms occur, as these side effects may be irreversible.
- Monitor for development of neuroleptic malignant syndrome (fever, respiratory distress, tachycardia, convulsions, diaphoresis, hypertension or hypotension, pallor, tiredness). Notify physician immediately if these symptoms occur.
- Assess fluid intake and bowel function. Increased bulk and fluids in the diet help minimize the constipating effects of this medication.
- **Lab Test Considerations:** CBC and liver function tests should be evaluated periodically throughout course of therapy. May cause blood dyscrasias especially between wks 4–10 of therapy.
- May cause false-positive or false-negative pregnancy test results and false-positive urine bilirubin test results.
- May cause increased serum prolactin levels, thereby interfering with gonadorelin test results.
- May cause Q-wave and T-wave changes in ECG.

Potential Nursing Diagnoses

- Thought processes, altered (indications).
- Knowledge deficit related to medication regimen (patient/family teaching).
- Noncompliance (patient/family teaching).

Implementation

- **General Info:** Available in tablet, syrup, and injectable forms.
- To prevent contact dermatitis, avoid getting soln on hands.
- Phenothiazines should be discontinued 48 hr before and not resumed for 24 hr following metrizamide myelography, as they lower the seizure threshold.
- **PO:** Administer with food, milk, or a full glass of water to minimize gastric irritation.
- Dilute syrup in citrus or chocolate-flavored drinks.
- **IM:** Do not inject SC. Inject slowly into deep, well-developed muscle. Keep patient recumbent for at least 30 min following injection to minimize hypotensive effects. Slight yellow color will not alter potency. Do not administer soln that is markedly discolored or that contains a precipitate.
- **Direct IV:** Use concentration of 25 mg/ml or less.
- *Rate:* Administer each 25 mg over at least 1 min through IV tubing with infusion of dextrose, saline, Ringer's or lactated Ringer's soln, dextrose/saline, dextrose/Ringer's, or lactated Ringer's combinations.
- **Syringe Compatibility:** atropine, chlorpromazine, cimetidine, diphenhydramine, droperidol, fentanyl, glycopyrrolate, hydroxyzine, meperidine, metoclopramide, midazolam, morphine, pentazocine, prochlorperazine, promethazine, or scopolamine.
- **Syringe Incompatibility:** dimenhydrinate or pentobarbital.
- **Additive Compatibility:** chloramphenicol, erythromycin lactobionate, ethacrynate, heparin, lidocaine, metaraminol, methyldopate, or tetracycline.
- **Additive Incompatibility:** aminophylline, chlorothiazide, fibrinogen, fibrinolysin, methohexital, nafcillin, penicillin G potassium, pentobar-

bital, phenobarbital, thiopental, or warfarin.

Patient/Family Teaching

- Advise patient to take medication exactly as directed, not to skip doses or double up on missed doses. If a dose is missed, it should be taken as soon as remembered unless almost time for the next dose. If more than 2 doses are scheduled each day, the missed dose should be taken within about 1 hr of the ordered time. Abrupt withdrawal may lead to gastritis, nausea, vomiting, dizziness, headache, tachycardia, and insomnia.
- Inform patient of possibility of extrapyramidal symptoms, tardive dyskinesia, and neuroleptic malignant syndrome. Caution patient to report these symptoms immediately to physician.
- Advise patient to make position changes slowly to minimize orthostatic hypotension.
- Medication may cause drowsiness. Caution patient to avoid driving or other activities requiring alertness until response to medication is known.
- Caution patient to avoid taking alcohol or other CNS depressants concurrently with this medication.
- Advise patient to use sunscreen and protective clothing when exposed to the sun to prevent photosensitivity reactions. Extremes in temperature should also be avoided, as this drug impairs body temperature regulation.
- Instruct patient to use frequent mouth rinses, good oral hygiene, and sugarless gum or candy to minimize dry mouth. Consult physician or dentist if dry mouth continues >2 wk.
- Advise patient to notify physician or dentist of medication regimen prior to treatment or surgery.
- Instruct patient to notify physician promptly if sore throat, fever, unusual bleeding or bruising, skin rashes, weakness, tremors, visual disturbances, dark-colored urine, or clay-colored stools are noted.
- Emphasize the importance of routine follow-up examinations to monitor response to medication and detect side effects. Periodic ocular examinations are indicated. Encourage continued participation in psychotherapy as ordered by physician.

Evaluation

Effectiveness of therapy can be demonstrated by: ▪ Decrease in excitable, paranoic, or withdrawn behavior.

PROMETHAZINE

(proe-**meth**-a-zeen)
Anergan 25, Anergan 50, {Histanil}, K-Phen, Mallergan, Pentazine, Phenameth, Phenazine 25, Phenazine 50, Phencen-50, Phenergan, Phenergan Fortis, Phenergan Plain, Phenoject-50, PMS Promethazine, Pro-50, Prometh-25, Prometh-50, Promethegan, Prorex-25, Prorex-50, Protazine, Prothazine Plain, Remsed, V-Gan-25, V-Gan-50

CLASSIFICATION(S):
Antihistamine—phenothiazine, Antiemetic—phenothiazine, Sedative/hypnotic—phenothiazine
Pregnancy Category UK

INDICATIONS

▪ Treatment of various allergic conditions and motion sickness ▪ Preoperative sedation ▪ Treatment and prevention of nausea and vomiting ▪ Adjunct to anesthesia and analgesia.

ACTION

▪ Blocks the effects of histamine ▪ Has inhibitory effect on the chemoreceptor trigger zone in the medulla, resulting in antiemetic properties ▪ Alters the effects of dopamine in the CNS ▪ Possesses significant anticholinergic activity ▪ Produces CNS depression by indirectly decreased stimulation of the CNS reticular system. **Therapeutic Effects:** ▪ Relief of symptoms of histamine

{} = Available in Canada only.

excess usually seen in allergic conditions ▪ Diminished nausea or vomiting ▪ Sedation.

PHARMACOKINETICS

Absorption: Well absorbed following oral and IM administration. Rectal administration may be less reliable.
Distribution: Widely distributed. Crosses the blood-brain barrier and the placenta.
Metabolism and Excretion: Metabolized by the liver.
Half-life: UK.

CONTRAINDICATIONS AND PRECAUTIONS

Contraindicated in: ▪ Hypersensitivity ▪ Comatose patients ▪ Prostatic hypertrophy ▪ Bladder neck obstruction ▪ Narrow-angle glaucoma.
Use Cautiously in: ▪ Hypertension ▪ Sleep apnea ▪ Epilepsy ▪ Pregnancy (has been used safely during labor; avoid chronic use during pregnancy) ▪ Lactation (safety not established; may cause drowsiness in infant).

ADVERSE REACTIONS AND SIDE EFFECTS*

CNS: excess sedation, confusion, disorientation, dizziness, fatigue, extrapyramidal reactions, nervousness, insomnia.
CV: tachycardia, bradycardia, hypotension, hypertension.
Derm: rashes, photosensitivity.
EENT: blurred vision, tinnitus, diplopia.
GI: dry mouth, hepatitis, constipation.
Hemat: blood dyscrasias.

INTERACTIONS

Drug–Drug: ▪ Additive CNS depression with other **CNS depressants,** including **alcohol, antianxiety agents,** other **antihistamines, narcotic analgesics,** and other **sedative/hypnotics** ▪ Additive anticholinergic effects with other **drugs possessing anticholinergic properties,** including other **antihistamines, antidepressants, atropine, haloperidol,** other **phenothiazines, quinidine,** and **disopyramide.**

ROUTE AND DOSAGE

Allergic Conditions

- **PO (Adults):** 25 mg at bedtime or 12.5 mg tid and at bedtime.
- **PO (Children):** 25 mg at bedtime or 12.5 mg tid or 0.5 mg/kg at bedtime or 0.125 mg/kg as needed.
- **IM, IV, Rect (Adults):** 25 mg, may repeat in 2 hr.

Motion Sickness

- **PO (Adults):** 25 mg 30–60 min prior to departure, may be repeated in 8–12 hr. Additional doses may be given in the morning and at bedtime for duration of travel.
- **PO (Children):** 12.5–25 mg or 0.5 mg/kg 30–60 min prior to departure, may be repeated in 8–12 hr. Additional doses may be given in the morning and at bedtime for duration of travel.

Sedation

- **PO, Rect, IM, IV (Adults):** 25–50 mg.
- **PO, Rect, IM, IV (Children):** 12.5–25 mg or 0.5–1.1 mg/kg.

Sedation During Labor

- **IM, IV (Adults):** 50 mg in early labor; 25–75 mg may be given when labor is established and additional doses of 25–50 mg may be given 1–2 times at 4-hr intervals (24-hr dose should not exceed 100 mg).

Antiemetic

- **PO, Rect, IM, IV (Adults):** 12.5–25 mg q 4 hr as needed.
- **PO, Rect, IM, IV (Children):** 0.25–0.5 mg/kg 4–6 times daily.

PHARMACODYNAMICS (noted as antihistaminic effects; sedative effects last 2–8 hr)

	ONSET	PEAK	DURATION
PO	20 min	UK	up to 12 hr
IM	20 min	UK	up to 12 hr
Rect	20 min	UK	up to 12 hr
IV	3–5 min	UK	up to 12 hr

*Underlines indicate most frequent; **CAPITALS** indicate life-threatening.

NURSING IMPLICATIONS

Assessment

- **General Info:** Monitor blood pressure, pulse, and respiratory rate frequently in patients receiving IV doses.
  - Assess patient for level of sedation following administration.
  - Monitor patient for onset of extrapyramidal side effects (akathisia—restlessness; dystonia—muscle spasms and twisting motions; pseudoparkinsonism—mask facies, rigidity, tremors, drooling, shuffling gait, dysphagia). Notify physician if these symptoms occur.
- **Antiemetic:** Assess patient for nausea and vomiting prior to and following administration.
- **Allergy:** Assess allergy symptoms (rhinitis, conjunctivitis, hives) prior to and periodically throughout course of therapy.
- **Lab Test Considerations:** May cause false-positive or false-negative pregnancy tests.
  - CBC should be evaluated periodically during chronic therapy, as blood dyscrasias may occur.
  - May cause increased serum glucose.
  - May cause false-negative results in skin tests using allergen extracts. Promethazine should be discontinued 72 hr prior to the test.

Potential Nursing Diagnoses

- Fluid volume deficit (indications).
- Injury, high risk for (side effects).
- Knowledge deficit related to medication regimen (patient/family teaching).

Implementation

- **General Info:** Available in tablet, syrup, suppository, and injectable forms. Also available in combination preparations (see Appendix A).
  - When administering promethazine concurrently with narcotic analgesics, supervise ambulation closely to prevent injury secondary to increased sedation.
- **PO:** Administer with food, water, or milk to minimize GI irritation. Tablets may be crushed and mixed with food or fluids for patients with difficulty swallowing.
- **IM:** Administer deep into well-developed muscle. SC administration may cause tissue necrosis.
- **Direct IV:** Doses should not exceed a concentration of 25 mg/ml. Slight yellow color does not alter potency. Do not use if precipitate present.
  - *Rate:* Administer each 25 mg slowly, over at least 1 min. Rapid administration may produce a transient fall in blood pressure.
- **Solution Compatibility:** dextrose, saline, Ringer's or lactated Ringer's soln, dextrose/saline, dextrose/Ringer's, or lactated Ringer's combinations.
- **Syringe Compatibility:** atropine, butorphanol, chlorpromazine, cimetadine, diphenhydramine, droperidol, fentanyl, glycopyrrolate, hydromorphone, hydroxyzine, meperidine, metoclopramide, midazolam, morphine, pentazocine, perphenazine, prochlorperazine, promazine, ranitidine, or scopolamine.
- **Syringe Incompatibility:** dimenhydrinate, heparin, pentobarbital, or thiopental.
- **Y-Site Compatibility:** ondansetron.
- **Y-Site Incompatibility:** cefoperazone, foscarnet, heparin, hydrocortisone sodium succinate, or potassium chloride.
- **Additive Compatibility:** amikacin, ascorbic acid, or netilmicin.
- **Additive Incompatibility:** aminophylline, chloramphenicol, chlorothiazide, heparin, hydrocortisone sodium succinate, methicillin, methohexital, penicillin G, pentobarbital, phenobarbital, or thiopental.

Patient/Family Teachng

- **General Info:** Review dosage schedule with patient. If medication is ordered regularly and a dose is missed, take as soon as remembered unless time for next dose.
  - Promethazine may cause drowsiness. Caution patient to avoid driving or other activities requiring alertness

until response to medication is known.

- Advise patient that frequent mouth rinses, good oral hygiene, and sugarless gum or candy may decrease dry mouth. Dentist or physician should be notified if dry mouth persists >2 wk.
- Caution patient to use sunscreen and protective clothing to prevent photosensitivity reactions.
- Advise patient to make position changes slowly to minimize orthostatic hypotension. Elderly patients are at increased risk for this side effect.
- Caution patient to avoid concurrent use of alcohol and other CNS depressants with this medication.
- Instruct patient to notify physician if sore throat, fever, jaundice, or uncontrolled movements are noted.
- **Motion Sickness:** When used as prophylaxis for motion sickness, advise patient to take medication at least 30 min and preferably 1–2 hr prior to exposure to conditions that may cause motion sickness.

Evaluation

Effectiveness of therapy can be demonstrated by: ▪ Relief from nausea and vomiting ▪ Prevention of motion sickness ▪ Sedation ▪ Relief from allergic symptoms.

PROPAFENONE

(proe-**paff**-e-nown)
Rhythmol

CLASSIFICATION(S):
Antiarrhythmic—class IC
Pregnancy Category C

INDICATIONS

▪ Treatment of life-threatening ventricular arrhythmias including ventricular tachycardia.

ACTION

▪ Slows conduction in cardiac tissue by altering transport of ions across cell membranes. **Therapeutic Effect:** ▪ Suppression of ventricular arrhythmias.

PHARMACOKINETICS

Absorption: Although well absorbed following oral administration undergoes rapid hepatic metabolism (bioavailability 3–11%).
Distribution: Distribution not known.
Metabolism and Excretion: Extensively metabolized by the liver, some metabolites have antiarrhythmic activity. >90% of patients are considered extensive metabolizers. Others metabolize propafenone more slowly.
Half-life: 2–10 hr in extensive metabolizers, 10–32 hr in slow metabolizers.

CONTRAINDICATIONS AND PRECAUTIONS

Contraindicated in: ▪ Hypersensitivity ▪ Cardiogenic shock ▪ Conduction disorders including sick-sinus syndrome and AV block (without a pacemaker) ▪ Bradycardia ▪ Severe hypotension ▪ Nonallergic bronchospasm ▪ Electrolyte disturbances ▪ Uncontrolled congestive heart failure.
Use Cautiously in: ▪ Pregnancy, lactation, or children (safety not established) ▪ Severe hepatic or renal impairment (dosage reduction may be necessary) ▪ Elderly patients (lower doses may be necessary).

ADVERSE REACTIONS AND SIDE EFFECTS*

CNS: dizziness, shaking, WEAKNESS.
EENT: blurred vision.
CV: VENTRICULAR ARRHYTHMIAS, SUPRAVENTRICULAR ARRHYTHMIA, conduction disturbances, angina, hypotension, bradycardia.
GI: altered taste, nausea, vomiting, constipation, diarrhea, dry mouth.
Derm: rash.
MS: joint pain.

*Underlines indicate most frequent; **CAPITALS** indicate life-threatening.

INTERACTIONS

Drug–Drug: ▪ Increases serum **digoxin** levels (dosage reduction may be required) ▪ Increases blood levels of **metoprolol** and **propranolol** (dosage reduction may be required) ▪ Concurrent use of **local anesthetics** may increase the risk of CNS adverse reactions ▪ May increase the effects of **warfarin**.

ROUTE AND DOSAGE

- **PO (Adults):** 150 mg q 8 hr, may be increased at 3–4 day intervals as required up to 300 mg q 8 hr.

PHARMACODYNAMICS (antiarrhythmic effects)

	ONSET	PEAK	DURATION
PO	hrs–days	4–5 days*	hrs

*Following chronic dosing.

NURSING IMPLICATIONS

Assessment

- Monitor ECG or Holter monitor prior to and periodically throughout therapy. May cause PR prolongation and QT prolongation.
- Monitor blood pressure and pulse periodically throughout course of therapy.
- Monitor intake and output ratios and daily weight. Assess patients for signs of congestive heart failure (peripheral edema, rales/crackles, dyspnea, weight gain, jugular venous distension).
- **Lab Test Considerations:** May cause elevated antinuclear antibody (ANA) titer, which is usually asymptomatic and reversible.

Potential Nursing Diagnoses

- Cardiac output, decreased (indications).
- Knowledge deficit related to medication regimen (patient/family teaching).

Implementation

- **General Info:** Propafenone therapy should be initiated in a hospital with facilities for cardiac rhythm monitoring. Most serious proarrhythmic effects are seen in the first 2 wk of therapy.
- Previous antiarrhythmic therapy should be withdrawn 2–5 half-lives before starting propafenone.
- Dosage adjustments should be at least 3–4 days apart due to the long half-life of propafenone.
- Pre-existing hypokalemia or hyperkalemia should be corrected prior to instituting therapy.

Patient/Family Teaching

- Instruct patient to take medication around the clock exactly as directed, even if feeling better. Missed doses should be taken as soon as remembered if within 4 hr; omit if remembered later. Gradual dosage reduction may be necessary.
- Medication may cause dizziness. Caution patient to avoid driving and other activities requiring alertness until response to medication is known.
- Advise patient to notify physician or dentist of medication regimen prior to treatment or surgery.
- Instruct patient to notify physician if chest pain, shortness of breath, or diaphoresis occurs.
- Advise patient to carry identification describing disease process and medication regimen at all times.
- Emphasize the importance of follow-up examinations to monitor progress.

Evaluation

Effectiveness of therapy can be demonstrated by: ▪ Decrease in frequency of ventricular arrhythmias.

PROPANTHELINE

(proe-**pan**-the-leen)
Norpanth, {Probanthel}, Pro-Banthine

CLASSIFICATION(S):
Anticholinergic—antimuscarinic
Pregnancy Category C

P

INDICATIONS

- Adjunctive therapy in the treatment of peptic ulcer disease.

ACTION

- Competitively inhibits the muscarinic action of acetylcholine, resulting in decreased GI secretions. **Therapeutic Effect:** - Reduction of signs and symptoms of peptic ulcer disease.

PHARMACOKINETICS

Absorption: Incompletely absorbed from the GI tract.
Distribution: Distribution not known. Does not cross the blood-brain barrier.
Metabolism and Excretion: Inactivated in the upper small intestine.
Half-life: UK.

CONTRAINDICATIONS AND PRECAUTIONS

Contraindicated in: - Hypersensitivity - Narrow-angle glaucoma - Tachycardia secondary to cardiac insufficiency or thyrotoxicosis - Myasthenia gravis.
Use Cautiously in: - Elderly patients (dosage reduction required) - Prostatic hypertrophy - Chronic renal, cardiac, or pulmonary disease - Patients who may have intra-abdominal infections - Pregnancy, lactation, or children (safety not established).

ADVERSE REACTIONS AND SIDE EFFECTS*

CNS: drowsiness, confusion, excitement, dizziness.
EENT: blurred vision, mydriasis, photophobia.
CV: palpitations, tachycardia, orthostatic hypotension.
GI: dry mouth, constipation.
GU: urinary hesitancy, urinary retention.
Derm: rash.
Misc: decreased sweating.

INTERACTIONS

Drug-Drug: - Additive anticholinergic effects with other **drugs possessing anticholinergic properties,** including **antihistamines, antidepressants, atropine, haloperidol, phenothiazines, quinidine,** and **disopyramide** - May alter the absorption of other **orally administered drugs** by slowing motility of the GI tract - **Antacids** and **adsorbent antidiarrheals** decrease the absorption of anticholinergics - May increase GI mucosal lesions in patients taking **wax-matrix potassium chloride preparations.**

ROUTE AND DOSAGE

- **PO (Adults):** 15 mg tid, 30 mg hs.

PHARMACODYNAMICS (anticholinergic effects)

	ONSET	PEAK	DURATION
PO	30–60 min	2–6 hr	6 hr

NURSING IMPLICATIONS

Assessment

- Assess for abdominal pain prior to and periodically throughout therapy.
- **Lab Test Considerations:** Antagonizes effects of pentagastrin and histamine during gastric acid secretion test. Avoid administration for 24 hr preceding the test.

Potential Nursing Diagnoses

- Comfort, altered: pain (indications).
- Bowel elimination, altered: constipation (side effects).
- Knowledge deficit related to medication regimen (patient/family teaching).

Implementation

- **PO:** Administer 30 min before meals. Bedtime dose should be administered at least 2 hr after last meal of the day.
- Do not administer within 1 hr of antacids or antidiarrheal medications.

Patient/Family Teaching

- Instruct patient to take medication as directed. If a dose is missed take as soon as remembered unless almost time for next dose. Do not double doses.
- May cause drowsiness or blurred vi-

*Underlines indicate most frequent; **CAPITALS** indicate life-threatening.

sion. Caution patient to avoid driving or other activities requiring alertness until response to medication is known.

- Instruct patient that frequent oral rinses, sugarless gum or candy, and good oral hygiene may help relieve dry mouth. Consult physician or dentist regarding use of saliva substitute if dry mouth persists >2 wk.
- Advise patient that increasing fluid intake, adding bulk to the diet, and exercise may help alleviate the constipating effects of the drug.
- Advise elderly patients to make position changes slowly to minimize the effects of drug-induced orthostatic hypotension.
- Caution patient to avoid extremes of temperature. This medication decreases the ability to sweat and may increase the risk of heat stroke.
- Instruct patient to notify physician if confusion, excitement, dizziness, rash, difficulty with urination, or eye pain occurs. Physician may order periodic ophthalmic examinations to monitor intraocular pressure, especially in the elderly.

Evaluation

Effectiveness of therapy can be demonstrated by: ▪ Decrease in GI pain in patients with peptic ulcer disease.

PROPOFOL

(**proe**-poe-fol)
disoprofol, Diprivan

CLASSIFICATION(S):
Anesthetic—general
Pregnancy Category B

INDICATIONS

▪ Induction of general anesthesia ▪ Maintenance of balanced anesthesia when used with other agents. **Unlabeled Use:** ▪ Production of sedation and amnesia as a supplement to regional anesthesia.

ACTION

▪ Short-acting hypnotic. Mechanism of action is unknown ▪ Produces amnesia ▪ Has no analgesic properties. **Therapeutic Effect:** ▪ Induction and maintenance of anesthesia.

PHARMACOKINETICS

Absorption: Administered IV only, resulting in complete absorption.
Distribution: Rapidly and widely distributed. Crosses the blood-brain barrier well. Rapidly redistributed to other tissues. Crosses the placenta and enters breast milk.
Metabolism and Excretion: Rapidly metabolized by the liver.
Half-life: 3–12 hr (blood-brain equilibration half-life 2.9 min).

CONTRAINDICATIONS AND PRECAUTIONS

Contraindicated in: ▪ Hypersensitivity to propofol, soybean oil, egg lecithin, or glycerol ▪ Labor and delivery.
Use Cautiously in: ▪ Cardiovascular disease ▪ Lipid disorders (emulsion may have detrimental effect) ▪ Increased intracranial pressure ▪ Cerebrovascular disorders ▪ Elderly, debilitated, or hypovolemic patients (dosage reduction recommended) ▪ Children or lactation (safety not established).

ADVERSE REACTIONS AND SIDE EFFECTS*

CNS: dizziness, headache.
Resp: APNEA, cough.
CV: bradycardia, hypotension, hypertension.
GI: nausea, vomiting, abdominal cramping, hiccups.
Derm: flushing.
Local: pain, burning, stinging, tingling, numbness, coldness at IV site.
MS: perioperative myoclonia, involuntary muscle movements.
Misc: fever.

INTERACTIONS

Drug-Drug: ▪ Additive CNS and respiratory depression with **alcohol, antihis-**

*Underlines indicate most frequent; **CAPITALS** indicate life-threatening.

tamines, narcotic analgesics, and **sedative/hypnotics** (dosage reduction may be required).

ROUTE AND DOSAGE

Induction

- **IV (Adults <55 yr):** 2–2.5 mg/kg given as 40 mg q 10 sec until induction achieved.
- **IV (Adults >55 yr, Debilitated, or Hypovolemic Patients):** 1–1.5 mg/kg given as 20 mg q 10 sec until induction achieved.

Maintenance

- **IV (Adults <55 yr):** 100–200 mcg (0.1–0.2 mg)/kg/min maintenance. Rates of 150–200 mcg (0.15–0.2 mg)/kg/min are usually required during first 10–15 min after induction, then decreased by 30–50% during first 30 min of maintenance. Rates of 50–100 mcg (0.05–0.1 mg)/kg/min are associated with optimal recovery time. May also be given intermittently in increments of 20–50 mg.
- **IV (Adults >55 yr, Debilitated, or Hypovolemic Patients):** 50–100 mcg (0.5–1 mg)/kg/min).

PHARMACODYNAMICS

	ONSET	PEAK	DURATION*
IV	40 sec	UK	3–5 min

*Time to recovery is 8 min (up to 19 min if narcotic analgesics have been used).

NURSING IMPLICATIONS

Assessment

- Assess respiratory status, pulse, and blood pressure continuously throughout propofol therapy. Propofol should be used only by individuals experienced in endotracheal intubation, and equipment for this procedure should be readily available.
- Assess level of sedation and level of consciousness throughout and following administration.
- **Toxicity and Overdose:** If overdose occurs monitor pulse, respiration, and blood pressure continuously. Maintain patent airway and assist ventilation as needed. If hypotension occurs, treatment includes IV fluids, repositioning, and vasopressors.

Potential Nursing Diagnoses

- Breathing pattern, ineffective (adverse reaction).
- Injury, high risk for (side effects).
- Knowledge deficit related to medication regimen (patient/family teaching).

Implementation

- **General Info:** Dose is titrated to patient response.
- Propofol has no effect on the pain threshold. Adequate anesthesia should *always* be used when propofol is used as an adjunct to surgical procedures.
- **Direct IV:** Shake well before use. If diluted prior to administration use only D5W and dilute to a concentration not less than 2 mg/ml. Soln is opaque, making detection of contaminates difficult. Do not use if separation of the emulsion is evident. Contains no preservatives; maintain sterile technique and administer immediately after preparation. Discard unused portions and IV lines at the end of procedure or within 6 hr.
- Frequently causes pain, burning, and stinging at injection site; use larger veins of the forearm of antecubital fossa or a dedicated IV catheter. Physician may order lidocaine 10–20 mg IV prior to injection to minimize pain.
- **Solution Compatibility:** D5W, LR, D5/0.45% NaCl, or D5/0.2% NaCl.
- **Y-Site Incompatibility:** blood or plasma.
- **Additive Incompatibility:** Manufacturer does not recommend admixing propofol with other medications.

Patient/Family Teaching

- Inform patient that this medication will decrease mental recall of the procedure.
- Medication may cause drowsiness or dizziness. Advise patient to request assistance prior to ambulation and transfer and to avoid driving or other activities requiring alertness for 24 hr following administration.

□ Advise patient to avoid alcohol or other CNS depressants for 24 hr following administration of propofol.

Evaluation

Effectiveness of therapy can be demonstrated by: ▪ Induction and maintenance of anesthesia □ Amnesia.

PROPOXYPHENE

(pro-**pox**-i-feen)

Darvon, Darvon-N, Dextropropoxyphene, Dolene, Doraphen, Doxaphene, {Novopropoxyn}, Profene, Pro-Pox, Propoxycon

PHROPOXYPHENE/ACETAMINOPHEN

Darvocet-N, Dolene AP, Doxapap-N, D-Rex, Genagesic, Pancet, Propacet, Pro-Pox with APAP, Propoxyphene with APAP, Pro-x/Apap, Wygesic, {642}

PROPOXYPHENE/ASPIRIN/CAFFEINE

Bexophene, Cotanal, Darvon Compound-65, {Darvon-N Compound}, Dolene Compound, Doraphen Compound, Doxaphene Compound, Margesic A-C, {Novopropoxyn Compound}, Pro-Pox Plus, {692}

CLASSIFICATION(S):
Narcotic analgesic—agonist
Schedule IV
Pregnancy Category C

INDICATIONS

▪ Management of mild to moderate pain.

ACTION

▪ Binds to opiate receptors in the CNS ▪ Alters the perception of and response to painful stimuli, while producing generalized CNS depression. **Therapeutic Effect:** ▪ Decrease in mild to moderate pain.

PHARMACOKINETICS

Absorption: Well absorbed following oral administration. Napsylate salt is more slowly absorbed.
Distribution: Widely distributed. Probably crosses the placenta. Enters breast milk in small amounts.
Metabolism and Excretion: Mostly metabolized by the liver.
Half-life: 6–12 hr.

CONTRAINDICATIONS AND PRECAUTIONS

Contraindicated in: ▪ Hypersensitivity ▪ Pregnancy or lactation (avoid chronic use).
Use Cautiously in: ▪ Head trauma ▪ Increased intracranial pressure ▪ Severe renal, hepatic, or pulmonary disease ▪ Hypothyroidism ▪ Adrenal insufficiency ▪ Alcoholism ▪ Elderly or debilitated patients (dosage reduction recommended) ▪ Undiagnosed abdominal pain ▪ Prostatic hypertrophy ▪ Lactation (has been used safely).

ADVERSE REACTIONS AND SIDE EFFECTS*

CNS: dizziness, lightheadedness, headache, weakness, sedation, drowsiness, insomnia, euphoria, dysphoria, paradoxical excitement.
EENT: blurred vision.
CV: hypotension.
GI: nausea, vomiting, abdominal pain, constipation.
Derm: rashes.
Misc: tolerance, physical dependence, psychological dependence.

INTERACTIONS*

Drug-Drug: ▪ Use with extreme caution in patients receiving **MAO inhibitors** (may result in unpredicatable, severe, and potentially fatal reactions—decrease initial dose to 25% of usual dose ▪ Additive CNS depression with **al-**

{} = Available in Canada only.
*Underlines indicate most frequent; **CAPITALS** indicate life-threatening.

cohol, antidepressants, and **sedative/hypnotics** ▪ **Smoking (nicotine)** increases metabolism and may decrease analgesic effectiveness ▪ Administration of **partial-antagonist narcotic analgesics** may precipitate narcotic withdrawal in physically dependent patients ▪ **Nalbuphine** or **pentazocine** may decrease analgesic effects.

ROUTE AND DOSAGE

Note: 100 mg propoxyphene napsylate = 65 mg propoxyphene hydrochloride.

- **PO (Adults):** 65 mg q 4 hr (hydrochloride—Darvon, Dolene) or 100 mg q 4 hr (napsylate—Darvocet-N with acetaminophen, Darvon-N) as needed.

PHARMACODYNAMICS (analgesic effect)

	ONSET	PEAK	DURATION
PO	15–60 min	2–3 hr	4–6 hr

NURSING IMPLICATIONS

Assessment

- Assess type, location, and intensity of pain prior to and 60 min following administration.
- Prolonged, high-dose therapy may lead to physical and psychological dependence and tolerance, but propoxyphene has less risk of dependence than other narcotic agonists. This should not prevent patient from receiving adequate analgesia. Most patients who receive propoxyphene for medical reasons do not develop psychological dependence. Progressively higher doses may be required to relieve pain with long-term therapy.
- **Lab Test Considerations:** May cause elevated serum amylase and lipase levels.
- May cause increased SGOT (AST), SGPT (ALT), serum alkaline phosphatase, LDH, and bilirubin concentrations.
- **Toxicity and Overdose:** If overdose occurs, naloxone (Narcan) is the antidote.

Potential Nursing Diagnoses

- Comfort, altered: pain (indications).
- Sensory-perceptual alteration: visual, auditory (side effects).
- Injury, high risk for (side effects).

Implementation

- **General Info:** Explain therapeutic value of medication prior to administration to enhance the analgesic effect.
- Regularly administered doses may be more effective than prn administration.
- Analgesic is more effective if given before pain becomes severe.
- Coadministration with non-narcotic analgesics may have additive analgesic effects and may permit lower narcotic doses.
- Medication should be discontinued gradually after long-term use to prevent withdrawal symptoms.
- **PO:** Doses may be administered with food or milk to minimize GI irritation.

Patient/Family Teaching

- Instruct patient on how and when to ask for prn pain medication.
- Medication may cause drowsiness or dizziness. Caution patient to avoid driving and other activities requiring alertness until response to the drug is known.
- Advise patient to make position changes slowly to minimize orthostatic hypotension.
- Caution patient to avoid concurrent use of alcohol or other CNS depressants with this medication.
- Encourage patient to turn, cough, and breathe deeply every 2 hr to prevent atelectasis.
- Advise patient that increased intake of fluids and bulk, increased activity, stool softeners, and laxatives may minimize constipating effects.

Evaluation

Effectiveness of therapy can be demonstrated by: ▪ Decrease in severity of pain without a significant alteration in level of consciousness.

PROPRANOLOL

(proe-**pran**-oh-lole)
{Apo-Propranolol}, {Detensol}, Inderal, Inderal-LA, {Novopranol}, {PMS Propranolol}

CLASSIFICATION(S):
Antihypertensive—beta-adrenergic blocker, Antianginal, Beta-adrenergic blocker—nonselective, Antiarrhythmic—class II
Pregnancy Category C

INDICATIONS

▪ Treatment of the following: ▫ Hypertension (alone or with other agents) ▫ Angina pectoris (alone or with other agents) ▫ Supraventricular tachyarrhythmias, ventricular tachycardia, and other tachyarrhythmias ▪ Symptoms associated with hypertrophic subaortic stenosis (angina, palpitations, syncope) ▫ Tremors ▪ Prevention of myocardial infarction ▪ Migraine prophylaxis ▪ Management of pheochromocytoma. **Unlabeled Uses:** ▪ Management of arrhythmias associated with thyrotoxicosis ▪ Treatment of symptoms associated with mitral value prolapse syndrome ▪ Adjunct in the management of anxiety.

ACTION

▪ Blocks stimulation of $beta_1$ (myocardial) and $beta_2$ (pulmonary, vascular, or uterine) receptor sites. **Therapeutic Effects:** ▪ Decreased heart rate ▪ Decreased blood pressure ▪ Decreased AV conduction.

PHARMACOKINETICS

Absorption: Well absorbed following oral administration. Absorption of sustained-release capsules is slow.
Distribution: Widely distributed. Crosses the blood-brain barrier and the placenta. Enters breast milk.
Metabolism and Excretion: Almost completely metabolized by the liver.
Half-life: 3.4–6 hr.

CONTRAINDICATIONS AND PRECAUTIONS

Contraindicated in: ▪ Uncompensated congestive heart failure ▪ Pulmonary edema ▪ Cardiogenic shock ▪ Bradycardia ▪ Heart block.
Use Cautiously in: ▪ Thyrotoxicosis or hypoglycemia (may mask symptoms) ▪ Pregnancy or lactation (may cause apnea, low Apgar scores, bradycardia, and hypoglycemia in the newborn) ▪ Do not withdraw abruptly ▪ Hepatic impairment (dosage reduction recommended) ▪ Children (safety not established).

ADVERSE REACTIONS AND SIDE EFFECTS*

CNS: fatigue, weakness, depression, memory loss, mental changes, insomnia, drowsiness, confusion, dizziness.
EENT: dry eyes, blurred vision, nasal stuffiness.
Resp: bronchospasm, wheezing.
CV: BRADYCARDIA, CONGESTIVE HEART FAILURE, PULMONARY EDEMA, hypotension, edema.
GI: constipation, diarrhea, nausea, vomiting.
GU: impotence, diminished libido.
Derm: rash.
Endo: hyperglycemia, hypoglycemia.
Misc: Raynaud's phenomenon.

INTERACTIONS

Drug–Drug: ▪ **General anesthesia,** IV **phenytoin,** and **verapamil** may cause additive myocardial depression ▪ Additive bradycardia may occur with concurrent use of **cardiac glycosides** ▪ Additive hypotension may occur with other **antihypertensive agents,** acute ingestion of **alcohol,** or **nitrates** ▪ Concurrent use with **amphetamines, cocaine, ephedrine, epinephrine, norepinephrine, phenylephrine,** or **pseudoephedrine** may result in excess alpha-adrenergic stimulation, hypertension, and bradycardia ▪ May negate the beneficial $beta_1$ cardiac effects of **dopamine** or **dobu-**

{} = Available in Canada only.
*Underlines indicate most frequent; CAPITALS indicate life-threatening.

tamine ▪ Use with **insulin** may result in prolonged hypoglycemia ▪ May produce hypertension within 14 days of **MAO inhibitor** therapy ▪ Concurrent **thyroid** administration may decrease effectiveness ▪ **Nonsteroidal anti-inflammatory agents** may decrease antihypertensive effectiveness ▪ May antagonize **beta-adrenergic bronchodilators** ▪ **Cimetidine** may decrease metabolism and increase the effects of propranolol.

ROUTE AND DOSAGE

Hypertension

- **PO (Adults):** 40 mg bid initially or 80 mg extended-release preparation, increase at 3–7-day intervals until response is obtained. Usual maintenance dose is 160–480 mg/day in 2 divided doses or 120–160 mg/day of extended-release preparation. Up to 640 mg/day may be needed. Some patients may need 3 daily doses.

Angina

- **PO (Adults):** 10–20 mg 3–4 times daily initially or 80 mg once daily of extended-release preparation. Increase at 3–7-day intervals until response is obtained. Usual maintenance dose is 160–240 mg/day. Up to 320 mg may be required.

Tachyarrhythmias

- **PO (Adults):** 10–30 mg 3–4 times daily.
- **IV (Adults):** 0.5–3 mg, may repeat in 2 min if needed; subsequent doses may be repeated q 4 hr.

Myocardial Infarction Prophylaxis

- **PO (Adults):** 180–240 mg/day in 2–4 divided doses starting 5–21 days after myocardial infarction.

Migraine Prophylaxis

- **PO (Adults):** 80 mg/day in divided doses or once daily of extended-release preparation, increase gradually until response is obtained. Usual dose is 160–240 mg/day.

Pheochromocytoma

- **PO (Adults):** 30–60 mg/day in 2–4 divided doses.

Hypertrophic Subaortic Stenosis

- **PO (Adults):** 20–40 mg 3–4 times daily or 80–160 mg single dose of extended-release preparation.

Tremors

- **PO (Adults):** 40 mg 3–4 times daily, subsequent dosage adjustments as required (range 120–320 mg/day).

PHARMACODYNAMICS (PO, PO-ER = antihypertensive effects; IV = antiarrhythmic effects)

	ONSET	PEAK	DURATION
PO	30 min	60–90 min	6–12 hr
PO-ER	UK	6 hr	24 hr
IV	immediate	1 min	4–6 hr

NURSING IMPLICATIONS

Assessment

- **General Info:** Monitor blood pressure and pulse frequently when adjusting dose and periodically throughout therapy. Confer with physician prior to giving drug if pulse <50 bpm. Patients receiving propranolol IV must have continuous ECG monitoring and may have pulmonary capillary wedge pressure (PCWP) or central venous pressure (CVP) monitoring during and for several hrs after administration. Assess for orthostatic hypotension when assisting patient up from supine position.
- □ Monitor intake and output ratios and daily weight. Assess patient routinely for evidence of congestive heart failure (peripheral edema, dyspnea, rales/crackles, fatigue, weight gain, jugular venous distension).
- **Angina:** Assess frequency and duration of episodes of chest pain periodically throughout therapy.
- **Migraine Prophylaxis:** Assess frequency and severity of migraine headaches periodically throughout therapy.
- **Lab Test Considerations:** Hepatic and renal function, and CBC should be monitored routinely in patients receiving prolonged therapy.

- May cause elevations in serum potassium, uric acid, LDH, glucose, lipoprotein, triglyceride levels, and BUN.

Potential Nursing Diagnoses

- Cardiac output, decreased (indications, adverse reactions).
- Knowledge deficit related to medication regimen (patient/family teaching).
- Noncompliance (patient/family teaching).

Implementation

- **General Info:** Available in tablets, extended-release capsule, oral soln, and injectable forms.
- Oral and parenteral doses are not interchangeable. Check dose carefully.
- **PO:** Administer medication with meals or immediately after eating. Tablets may be crushed and mixed with food or fluids for patients with difficulty swallowing. Long-acting capsules should be swallowed whole; do not crush, break, or chew.
- **Direct IV:** Administer undiluted or dilute each 1 mg in 10 ml of D5W for injection.
- *Rate:* Administer over at least 1 min.
- **Intermittent Infusion:** May also be diluted for infusion in 50 ml of 0.9% NaCl, D5W, D5/0.45% NaCl, D5/0.9% NaCl, or lactated Ringer's injection.
- *Rate:* Infuse over 10–15 min.
- **Syringe Compatibility:** benzquinamide.
- **Y-Site Compatibility:** heparin, hydrocortisone sodium succinate, or potassium chloride.
- **Additive Compatibility:** dobutamine or verapamil.

Patient/Family Teaching

- **General Info:** Instruct patient to take medication exactly as directed, even if feeling well. If dose is missed, it may be taken as soon as remembered up to 8 hr before next dose. Abrupt withdrawal may precipitate life-threatening arrhythmias, hypertension, or myocardial ischemia.
- Teach patient and family how to check pulse and blood pressure. Instruct them to take pulse daily and blood pressure at least weekly. Advise patient to withhold dose and contact physician if pulse <50 bpm or blood pressure changes significantly.
- Reinforce need to continue additional therapies for hypertension (weight loss, restricted sodium intake, stress reduction, regular exercise, moderation of alcohol consumption, and cessation of smoking). Propranolol helps control but does not cure hypertension.
- Propranolol may cause drowsiness. Caution patient to avoid driving or other activities that require alertness until response to the drug is known.
- Caution patient that this medication may cause increased sensitivity to cold.
- Advise patient to consult physician or pharmacist before taking any over-the-counter drugs concurrently with this medication. Patient should also avoid excessive amounts of coffee, tea, or cola.
- Diabetic patients should monitor serum glucose closely, especially if weakness, fatigue, or irritability occurs.
- Advise patient to notify physician if slow pulse, dizziness, lightheadedness, confusion, depression, or skin rash occur.
- Instruct patient to inform physician or dentist of medication regimen prior to treatment or surgery.
- Advise patient to carry identification describing medication regimen at all times.
- **Migraine Prophylaxis:** Caution patient that sharing of this medication may be dangerous.

Evaluation

Effectiveness of therapy can be demonstrated by: ▪ Decrease in blood pressure ▪ Decrease in frequency of anginal attacks ▪ Decrease in arrhythmias ▪ Decrease in frequency and severity of migraine headaches ▪ Decrease in tremors.

P

PROPYLTHIOURACIL
(proe-pill-thye-oh-**yoor**-a-sill)
{Propyl-Thyracil}, PTU

CLASSIFICATION(S):
Antithyroid agent
Pregnancy Category D

INDICATIONS

▪ Palliative treatment of hyperthyroidism ▪ Adjunct in the control of hyperthyroidism in preparation for thyroidectomy or radioactive iodine therapy.

ACTION

▪ Inhibits the synthesis of thyroid hormones. **Therapeutic Effect:** ▪ Decreased signs and symptoms of hyperthyroidism.

PHARMACOKINETICS

Absorption: Rapidly absorbed from the GI tract.
Distribution: Concentrates in the thyroid gland. Crosses the placenta and enters breast milk in low concentrations.
Metabolism and Excretion: Metabolized by the liver.
Half-life: 1–2 hr.

CONTRAINDICATIONS AND PRECAUTIONS

Contraindicated in: ▪ Hypersensitivity.
Use Cautiously in: ▪ Decreased bone marrow reserve ▪ Pregnancy (may be used safely; however, fetus may develop thyroid problems) ▪ Lactation (safety not established).

ADVERSE REACTIONS AND SIDE EFFECTS*

CNS: headache, drowsiness, vertigo.
GI: diarrhea, <u>nausea</u>, <u>vomiting</u>, hepatitis, loss of taste.
Derm: <u>rash</u>, urticaria, skin discoloration.
Hemat: AGRANULOCYTOSIS, leukopenia, thrombocytopenia.
MS: arthralgia.
Misc: fever, parotitis, lymphadenopathy.

INTERACTIONS

Drug-Drug: ▪ Additive bone marrow depression with **antineoplastic agents** or **radiation therapy** ▪ Additive antithyroid effects with **lithium, potassium iodide,** or **sodium iodide** ▪ Increased risk of agranulocytosis with **phenothiazines**.

ROUTE AND DOSAGE

- **PO (Adults):** 100–300 mg tid (up to 1200 mg/day; 200 mg q 4–6 hr has been used in thyrotoxic crisis).
- **PO (Children >10 yr):** 150 mg/day in divided doses q 8 hr.
- **PO (Children 6–10 yr):** 50–150 mg/day in divided doses q 8 hr.

PHARMACODYNAMICS (effects on clinical thyroid status)

	ONSET	PEAK	DURATION
PO	10–21 days*	6–10 wk	wks

*Effects on serum thyroid hormone concentration may occur within 60 min of a single dose.

NURSING IMPLICATIONS

Assessment

- ▫ Monitor response of symptoms of hyperthyroidism or thyrotoxicosis (tachycardia, palpitations, nervousness, insomnia, fever, diaphoresis, heat intolerance, tremors, weight loss, diarrhea).
- ▫ Assess patient for development of hypothyroidism (intolerance to cold, constipation, dry skin, headache, listlessness, tiredness, or weakness). Dosage adjustment may be required.
- ▫ Assess patient for skin rash or swelling of cervical lymph nodes. Treatment may be discontinued if this occurs.
- ▪ **Lab Test Considerations:** Thyroid function studies should be monitored prior to therapy, monthly during

{} = Available in Canada only.
*<u>Underlines</u> indicate most frequent; **CAPITALS** indicate life-threatening.

initial therapy, and every 2–3 mon throughout therapy.
- □ WBC and differential counts should be monitored periodically throughout course of therapy. Agranulocytosis may develop rapidly and usually occurs during first 2 mon. This necessitates discontinuation of therapy.
- □ May cause increased SGOT (AST), SGPT (ALT), LDH, alkaline phosphatase, serum bilirubin, and prothrombin time.

Potential Nursing Diagnoses
- ■ Knowledge deficit related to medication regimen (patient/family teaching).
- ■ Noncompliance (patient/family teaching).

Implementation
- ■ **PO:** Administer at same time in relation to meals every day. Food may either increase or decrease absorption.

Patient/Family Teaching
- □ Instruct patient to take medication exactly as directed, around the clock. If a dose is missed, take as soon as remembered; take both doses together if almost time for next dose; check with physician if more than 1 dose is missed. Consult physician prior to discontinuing medication.
- □ Instruct patient to monitor weight 2–3 times weekly. Notify physician of significant changes.
- □ Medication may cause drowsiness. Caution patient to avoid driving or other activities requiring alertness until response to medication is known.
- □ Advise patient to consult physician regarding dietary sources of iodine (iodized salt, shellfish).
- □ Advise patient to report sore throat, fever, chills, headache, malaise, weakness, yellowing of eyes or skin, unusual bleeding or bruising, symptoms of hyperthyroidism or hypothyroidism, or rash to physician promptly.
- □ Instruct patient to consult physician or pharmacist before taking any over-the-counter medications containing iodine concurrently with this medication.
- □ Advise patient to carry identification describing medication regimen at all times and to notify physician or dentist of medication regimen prior to treatment or surgery.
- □ Emphasize the importance of routine examinations to monitor progress and to check for side effects.

Evaluation
Effectiveness of therapy can be demonstrated by: ■ Decrease in severity of symptoms of hyperthyroidism (lowered pulse rate and weight gain) □ Return of serum thyroid levels to normal. Treatment of 6 mon to several yrs may be necessary, usually averages 1 yr.

PROTAMINE SULFATE
(**proe**-ta-meen)

CLASSIFICATION(S):
Antidote—antiheparin agent
Pregnancy Category UK

INDICATIONS
■ Acute management of severe heparin overdosage ■ Used to neutralize heparin received during dialysis, cardiopulmonary bypass, and other procedures.

ACTION
■ A strong base that forms a complex with heparin (an acid). **Therapeutic Effect:** ■ Inactivation of heparin.

PHARMACOKINETICS
Absorption: Administered IV only, resulting in complete bioavailability.
Distribution: Distribution not known.
Metabolism and Excretion: Metabolic fate not known. Protamine-heparin complex eventually degrades.
Half-life: UK.

CONTRAINDICATIONS AND PRECAUTIONS

Contraindicated in: ▪ Hypersensitivity to protamine or fish ▪ Avoid reconstitution with diluents containing benzyl alcohol if used in neonates.

Use Cautiously in: ▪ Patients who have received previous protamine-containing insulin or vasectomized males (increased risk of hypersensitivity reactions) ▪ Pregnancy, lactation, and children (safety not established).

ADVERSE REACTIONS AND SIDE EFFECTS*

CV: hypertension, hypotension, bradycardia, pulmonary hypertension.
Resp: dyspnea.
GI: nausea, vomiting.
Derm: warmth, flushing.
Hemat: bleeding.
MS: back pain.
Misc: hypersensitivity reactions, including angioedema, pulmonary edema, and ANAPHYLAXIS.

INTERACTIONS

Drug-Drug: ▪ None significant.

ROUTE AND DOSAGE

Within Minutes of IV Heparin

- **IV (Adults):** 1–1.5 mg protamine/100 units heparin administered.

30–60 Minutes Following IV Heparin

- **IV (Adults):** 0.5–0.75 mg protamine/100 units heparin administered.

2 Hr or More Following IV Heparin

- **IV (Adults):** 0.25–0.375 mg protamine/100 units heparin administered.

Following IV Infusion of Heparin

- **IV (Adults):** 25–50 mg protamine.

Following Deep SC Heparin

- **IV (Adults):** 1–1.5 mg protamine/100 units heparin administered or loading dose of 25–50 mg protamine, remainder infused over 8–16 hr.

PHARMACODYNAMICS (reversal of heparin effect)

	ONSET	PEAK	DURATION
IV	30 sec–1 min	UK	2 hr*

*Depends on body temperature.

NURSING IMPLICATIONS

Assessment

- □ Assess for bleeding and hemorrhage throughout course of therapy. Hemorrhage may recur 8–9 hr after therapy due to rebound effects of heparin. Rebound may occur as late as 18 hr after therapy in patients heparinized for cardiopulmonary bypass.
- □ Assess for allergy to fish (salmon), previous reaction to or use of protamine insulin or protamine sulfate. Vasectomized and infertile men also have higher risk of hypersensitivity reaction.
- □ Observe patient for signs and symptoms of hypersensitivity reaction (hives, edema, coughing, wheezing). Keep epinephrine, an antihistamine, and resuscitative equipment close by in the event of anaphylaxis.
- □ Assess for hypovolemia prior to initiation of therapy. Failure to correct hypovolemia may result in cardiovascular collapse from peripheral vasodilating effects of protamine sulfate.
- ▪ **Lab Test Considerations:** Monitor clotting factors activated clotting time (ACT), activated partial thromboplastin time (aPTT), and thrombin time (TT) 5–15 min after therapy and again as necessary.

Potential Nursing Diagnoses

- ▪ Injury, high risk for (indications).
- ▪ Tissue perfusion, altered (indications).

Implementation

- ▪ **General Info:** Discontinue heparin infusion. In milder cases overdosage may be treated by heparin withdrawal alone.

*Underlines indicate most frequent; **CAPITALS** indicate life-threatening.

- In severe cases, fresh frozen plasma or whole blood may also be required to control bleeding.
- Dosage varies with type of heparin, route of heparin therapy, and amount of time elapsed since discontinuation of heparin.
- Do not administer >100 mg in 2 hr without rechecking clotting studies, as protamine sulfate has its own anticoagulant properties.
- **IV:** Reconstitute 50-mg vial with 5 ml sterile water for injection or bacteriostatic water for injection. Reconstitute 250-mg vial with 25 ml. Shake vigorously. Soln reconstituted with sterile water for injection should be discarded after dose is withdrawn. Soln reconstituted with bacteriostatic water is stable for 24 hr when refrigerated.
- **Direct IV:** May be administered slow IV push over 1–3 min.
- **Intermittent Infusion:** May be diluted in D5W or 0.9% NaCl.
- *Rate:* Infuse no faster than 50 mg over 10 min. Rapid infusion rate may result in hypotension, bradycardia, flushing, or feeling of warmth. If these symptoms occur, stop infusion and notify physician. For accurate administration do not admix.
- **Additive Compatibility:** cimetidine or verapamil.
- **Additive Incompatibility:** cephalosporins or penicillins.

Patient/Family Teaching

- Explain purpose of the medication to patient. Instruct patient to report recurrent bleeding immediately.
- Advise patient to avoid activities that may result in bleeding (shaving, brushing teeth, receiving injections or rectal temperatures, or ambulation) until risk of hemorrhage has passed.

Evaluation

Effectiveness of therapy can be demonstrated by: ▪ Control of bleeding ▪ Normalization of clotting factors in heparinized patients.

PSEUDOEPHEDRINE

(soo-doe-e-**fed**-rin)

Afrinol, Cenafed, Decofed, Dorcol Children's Decongestant, {Eltor}, Gebafed, Halofed, Neofed, Novafed, {Ornex Cold}, PediaCare Infant's Oral Decongestant Drops, {Pseudofrin}, Pseudogest, {Robidrine}, Sinufed, Sudafed, Sudrin, Sufedrin

CLASSIFICATION(S):

Decongestant

Pregnancy Category B

INDICATIONS

▪ Symptomatic management of nasal congestion associated with acute viral upper respiratory tract infections ▪ Used in combination with antihistamines in the management of allergic conditions ▪ Used to open obstructed eustachian tubes in chronic otic inflammation or infection.

ACTION

▪ Stimulates alpha- and beta-adrenergic receptors ▪ Produces vasoconstriction in the respiratory tract mucosa (alpha-adrenergic stimulation) and possibly bronchodilation ($beta_2$-adrenergic stimulation). **Therapeutic Effects:** ▪ Reduction of nasal congestion, hyperemia, and swelling in nasal passages.

PHARMACOKINETICS

Absorption: Well absorbed following oral administration.

Distribution: Appears to enter the CSF. Probably crosses the placenta and enters breast milk.

Metabolism and Excretion: Partially metabolized by the liver. 55–75% excreted unchanged by the kidneys (depends on urine pH).

Half-life: 7 hr (depends on urine pH).

CONTRAINDICATIONS AND PRECAUTIONS

Contraindicated in: ▪ Hypersensitivity to sympathomimetic amines ▪ Hyper-

{} = Available in Canada only.

P

tension, severe coronary artery disease ▪ Concurrent MAO inhibitor therapy.

Use Cautiously in: ▪ Hyperthyroidism ▪ Diabetes mellitus ▪ Prostatic hypertrophy ▪ Ischemic heart disease ▪ Pregnancy or lactation (safety not established) ▪ Glaucoma.

ADVERSE REACTIONS AND SIDE EFFECTS*

CNS: nervousness, excitability, restlessness, weakness, dizziness, insomnia, headache, drowsiness, fear, anxiety, hallucinations, SEIZURES.

CV: CARDIOVASCULAR COLLAPSE, tachycardia, palpitations, hypertension.

GI: anorexia, dry mouth.

GU: dysuria.

Resp: respiratory difficulty.

INTERACTIONS

Drug-Drug: ▪ Additive sympathomimetic effects with other **sympathomimetic agents** ▪ Concurrent use with **MAO inhibitors** may cause hypertensive crisis ▪ Concurrent use with **beta-adrenergic blockers** may result in hypertension or bradycardia ▪ **Drugs that acidify the urine (ammonium chloride)** may decrease effectiveness ▪ **Drugs that alkalinize the urine (sodium bicarbonate, high-dose antacid therapy)** may intensify effectiveness.

Drug-Food: ▪ **Foods that acidify the urine** may decrease effectiveness ▪ **Foods that alkalinize the urine** may intensify effectiveness (see lists in Appendix K).

ROUTE AND DOSAGE

- **PO (Adults and Children >12 yr):** 60 mg q 4–6 hr as needed (not to exceed 240 mg/day) or 120 mg of extended-release preparation q 12 hr.
- **PO (Children 6–11 yr):** 30 mg q 4–6 hr as needed (not to exceed 120 mg/day) or 4 mg/kg/day or 125 mg/m²/day in 4 divided doses.
- **PO (Children 2–5 yr):** 15 mg q 4–6 hr (not to exceed 60 mg/day) or 4 mg/kg/day or 125 mg/m²/day in 4 divided doses.

PHARMACODYNAMICS (decongestant effects)

	ONSET	PEAK	DURATION
PO	30 min	UK	4–8 hr
PO-ER	60 min	UK	12 hr

NURSING IMPLICATIONS

Assessment

- ▫ Assess congestion (nasal, sinus, eustachian tube) prior to and periodically throughout course of therapy.
- ▫ Monitor pulse and blood pressure before beginning therapy and periodically throughout therapy.
- ▫ Assess lung sounds and character of bronchial secretions. Maintain fluid intake of 1500–2000 ml/day to decrease viscosity of secretions.

Potential Nursing Diagnoses

- ▪ Airway clearance, ineffective (indications).
- ▪ Knowledge deficit related to medication regimen (patient/family teaching).

Implementation

- ▪ **General Info:** Administer pseudoephedrine at least 2 hr before bedtime to minimize insomnia.
- ▫ Available in tablets, oral soln, and extended-release tablets and capsules. Also available in combination with many other medications (see Appendix A).
- ▪ **PO:** Extended-release tablets and capsules should be swallowed whole; do not crush, break, or chew. Contents of the capsule can be mixed with jam or jelly and swallowed without chewing for patients with difficulty swallowing.

Patient/Family Teaching

- ▫ Instruct patient to take medication exactly as directed and not to take more than recommended. If a dose is missed, take within 1 hr; if remembered later, omit. Do not double doses.
- ▫ Instruct patient to notify physician if

*Underlines indicate most frequent; **CAPITALS** indicate life-threatening.

nervousness, slow or fast heart rate, breathing difficulties, hallucinations, or seizures occur, as these symptoms may indicate overdosage.
- Instruct patient to contact physician if symptoms do not improve within 5 days or if fever is present.

Evaluation

Effectiveness of therapy can be demonstrated by: ▪ Decreased nasal, sinus, or eustachian tube congestion.

PSYLLIUM

(**sill**-i-yum)

Cillium, Correctol Powder, Effer-Syllium, Fiberall, Hydrocil, {Karacil}, Konsyl-D, Metamucil, Modane Bulk, Naturacil, Natural Vegetable, Perdiem Plain, {Prodiem Plain}, Pro-Lax, Reguloid, Serutan, Sibilin, Syllact, V-Lax

CLASSIFICATION(S):
Laxative—bulk-forming agent
Pregnancy Category UK

INDICATIONS

▪ Management of simple or chronic constipation, particularly if associated with a low-fiber diet ▪ Useful in situations where straining should be avoided (after myocardial infarction or rectal surgery, prolonged bedrest) ▪ Used in the management of chronic watery diarrhea.

ACTION

▪ Combines with water in the intestinal contents to form an emollient gel or viscous soln, which promotes peristalsis and reduces transit time. **Therapeutic Effect:** ▪ Relief and prevention of constipation.

PHARMACOKINETICS

Absorption: Not absorbed from the GI tract.

Distribution: No distribution occurs.

Metabolism and Excretion: Excreted in feces.

Half-life: UK.

CONTRAINDICATIONS AND PRECAUTIONS

Contraindicated in: ▪ Hypersensitivity ▪ Abdominal pain, nausea, or vomiting (especially when associated with fever) ▪ Serious adhesions ▪ Dysphagia.

Use Cautiously in: ▪ Some dosage forms contain sugar, aspartame, or excessive sodium and should be avoided in patients on restricted diets ▪ Pregnancy and lactation (has been used safely).

ADVERSE REACTIONS AND SIDE EFFECTS*

GI: nausea, vomiting, cramps, intestinal or esophageal obstruction.

Resp: bronchospasm.

INTERACTIONS

Drug-Drug: ▪ May decrease the absorption of **oral anticoagulants, salicylates,** or **cardiac glycosides.**

ROUTE AND DOSAGE

- **PO (Adults):** 1–2 tsp or packets (3–4 g psyllium) in a full glass of liquid 2–3 times daily (wafers or chewable forms should be taken with ½ glass of liquid).
- **PO (Children >6 yr):** 1 tsp or packet (1.5–2 g psyllium) in ½ glass of liquid 2–3 times daily (wafers or chewable forms should be taken with ½ glass of liquid).

PHARMACODYNAMICS (laxative effect)

	ONSET	PEAK	DURATION
PO	12–24 hr	2–3 days	UK

{} = Available in Canada only.

*Underlines indicate most frequent; **CAPITALS** indicate life-threatening.

P

NURSING IMPLICATIONS

Assessment

- Assess patient for abdominal distention, presence of bowel sounds, and usual pattern of bowel function.
- Assess color, consistency, and amount of stool produced.
- **Lab Test Considerations:** May cause elevated blood glucose levels with prolonged use of preparations containing sugar.

Potential Nursing Diagnoses

- Bowel elimination, altered: constipation (indications).
- Knowledge deficit related to medication regimen (patient/family teaching).

Implementation

- **General Info:** Available in sugar-free, flavored, effervescent, and wafer forms. Packets are not standardized for volume, but each contains 3–4 g of psyllium.
- **PO:** Administer with a full glass of water or juice, followed by an additional glass of liquid. Soln should be taken immediately after mixing, as it will congeal. Do not administer without sufficient fluid and do not chew granules.

Patient/Family Teaching

- Encourage patient to use other forms of bowel regulation, such as increasing bulk in the diet, increasing fluid intake, and increasing mobility. Normal bowel habits are individualized and may vary from 3 times/day to 3 times/wk.
- May be used for long-term management of chronic constipation.
- Instruct patients with cardiac disease to avoid straining during bowel movements (Valsalva maneuver).
- Advise patient not to use laxatives when abdominal pain, nausea, vomiting, or fever is present.

Evaluation

Effectiveness of therapy can be demonstrated by: ▪ A soft, formed bowel movement, usually within 12–24 hr. May require 3 days of therapy for results.

PYRAZINAMIDE

(peer-a-**zin**-a-mide)
{PMS Pyrazinamide}, {Tebrazid}

CLASSIFICATION(S):
Antitubercular
Pregnancy Category UK

INDICATIONS

▪ Used in combination with other agents in the treatment of active tuberculosis.

ACTION

▪ Mechanism not known. **Therapeutic Effect:** ▪ Bacteriostatic action against susceptible mycobacterium. **Spectrum:** ▪ Active only against mycobacterium.

PHARMACOKINETICS

Absorption: Well absorbed following oral administration.

Distribution: Widely distributed. Reaches high concentrations in the CNS (same as plasma). Excreted in breast milk.

Metabolism and Excretion: Mostly metabolized by the liver. Metabolite (pyrazinoic acid) has antimycobacterial activity. 3–4% excreted unchanged by the kidneys.

Half-life: Pyrazinamide—9.5 hr. Pyrazinoic acid—12 hr. Both are prolonged in renal impairment.

CONTRAINDICATIONS AND PRECAUTIONS

Contraindicated in: ▪ Hypersensitivity ▪ Cross-sensitivity with ethionamide, isoniazid, niacin, or nicotinic acid may exist ▪ Severe liver impairment.

Use Cautiously in: ▪ Gout ▪ Diabetes mellitus ▪ Acute intermittent porphyria ▪ Pregnancy (safety not established).

{} = Available in Canada only.

ADVERSE REACTIONS AND SIDE EFFECTS*

GI: HEPATOTOXICITY, nausea, vomiting, diarrhea, anorexia.
GU: dysuria.
Derm: itching, skin rash, photosensitivity, acne.
Hemat: anemia, thrombocytopenia.
Metab: hyperuricemia.
MS: gouty arthritis, arthralgia.

INTERACTIONS

Drug–Drug: ▪ None significant.

ROUTE AND DOSAGE

- **PO (Adults):** 15–35 mg/kg/day in 3–4 divided doses. 20–30 mg/kg/day is required in HIV-positive (AIDS) patients for the first 2 mon of treatment. Up to 60 mg/kg/day has been used in isoniazid-resistant tuberculosis. (Not to exceed 3 g/day).
- **PO (Children):** 15–30 mg/kg/day in divided doses (up to 2 g/day).

PHARMACODYNAMICS (blood levels)

	ONSET	PEAK
PO	UK	1–2 hr (4–5 hr*)

*For pyrazinoic acid.

NURSING IMPLICATIONS

Assessment

- □ Mycobacterial studies and susceptibility tests should be performed prior to and periodically throughout therapy to detect possible resistance.
- ▪ **Lab Test Considerations:** Hepatic function should be evaluated prior to and every 2–4 wk during therapy. Increased SGOT (AST) and SGPT (ALT) may not be predictive of clinical hepatitis and may return to normal levels during treatment. Patients with impaired liver function should only receive pyrazinamide therapy if crucial to treatment.
- □ Monitor serum uric acid concentrations during therapy. May cause elevations resulting in precipitation of acute gout.
- □ May interfere with urine ketone determinations.

Potential Nursing Diagnoses

- ▪ Infection, high risk for (indications).
- ▪ Knowledge deficit related to medication regimen (patient/family teaching).
- ▪ Noncompliance (patient/family teaching).

Implementation

- ▪ **General Info:** May be given concurrently with isoniazid and/or rifampin.

Patient/Family Teaching

- □ Advise patient to take medication exactly as directed, not to skip doses or double up on missed doses. Missed doses should be taken as soon as remembered unless almost time for next dose. Emphasize the importance of continuing therapy even after symptoms have subsided. May require 6 mon–2 yr of continuous therapy.
- □ Inform diabetic patients that pyrazinamide may interfere with urine ketone measurements.
- □ Advise patients to notify physician if no improvement is noticed after 2–3 wk of therapy.
- □ Emphasize the importance of regular follow-up examinations to monitor progress and check for side effects.

Evaluation

Effectiveness of therapy can be demonstrated by: ▪ Resolution of signs and symptoms of tuberculosis □ Negative sputum cultures.

PYRIDOSTIGMINE

(peer-id-oh-**stig**-meen)
Mestinon, {Mestinon Supraspan}, Mestinon Timespan, Regonol

CLASSIFICATION(S):
Cholinergic—anticholinesterase, Antimyasthenic
Pregnancy Category UK

{} = Available in Canada only.

*Underlines indicate most frequent; **CAPITALS** indicate life-threatening.

P

INDICATIONS

■ Used to increase muscle strength in the symptomatic treatment of myasthenia gravis ■ Reversal of nondepolarizing neuromuscular blockers.

ACTION

■ Inhibits the breakdown of acetylcholine and prolongs its effects ■ Effects include: □ Miosis □ Increased intestinal and skeletal muscle tone □ Bronchial and ureteral constriction □ Bradycardia □ Increased salivation □ Lacrimation □ Sweating. **Therapeutic Effects:** ■ Improved muscular function in patients with myasthenia gravis ■ Reversal of nondepolarizing neuromuscular blocking agents.

PHARMACOKINETICS

Absorption: Poorly absorbed following oral administration, necessitating large oral doses as compared to parenteral doses. Extended-release oral preparations release 50% of drug for immediate absorption; remainder is poorly absorbed.
Distribution: Appears to cross the placenta.
Metabolism and Excretion: Metabolized by plasma cholinesterases and the liver.
Half-life: PO—3.7 hr; IV—1.9 hr.

CONTRAINDICATIONS AND PRECAUTIONS

Contraindicated in: ■ Hypersensitivity ■ Mechanical obstruction of the GI or GU tract.
Use Cautiously in: ■ Pregnancy or lactation (may cause uterine irritability following IV administration near term; 20% of newborns may display transient muscle weakness) ■ History of asthma ■ Ulcer disease ■ Cardiovascular disease ■ Epilepsy ■ Hyperthyroidism.

ADVERSE REACTIONS AND SIDE EFFECTS*

CNS: SEIZURES, dizziness, weakness.
EENT: miosis, lacrimation.
Resp: excessive secretions, bronchospasm.
CV: bradycardia, hypotension.
GI: abdominal cramps, nausea, vomiting, diarrhea, excessive salivation.
Derm: sweating, rashes.

INTERACTIONS

Drug-Drug: ■ Cholinergic effects may be antagonized by other **drugs possessing anticholinergic properties,** including **antihistamines, antidepressants, atropine, haloperidol, phenothiazines, procainamide, quinidine,** or **disopyramide** ■ Prolongs the action of **depolarizing muscle-relaxing agents (succinylcholine, decamethonium)** ■ Additive toxicity with other **cholinesterase inhibitors,** including **demecarium, echothiophate,** and **isoflurophate** ■ Antimyasthenic effects may be decreased by concurrent **guanadrel, guanethidine,** or **trimethophan.**

ROUTE AND DOSAGE

Myasthenia Gravis

- **PO (Adults):** 60–180 mg 2–4 times daily (up to 1500 mg/day).
- **PO (Children):** 7 mg/kg/day in 5–6 divided doses.
- **IM, IV (Adults):** 2 mg or 1/30 of oral dose; may be repeated q 2–3 hr.

Antidote for Nondepolarizing Neuromuscular Blockers

- **IV (Adults):** 10–20 mg; pretreat with 0.6–1.2 mg atropine IV.

PHARMACODYNAMICS (cholinergic effects)

	ONSET	PEAK	DURATION
PO	30–35 min	UK	3–6 hr
PO-ER	30–60 min	UK	6–12 hr
IM	15 min	UK	2–4 hr
IV	2–5 min	UK	2–3 hr

NURSING IMPLICATIONS

Assessment

- **General Info:** Assess pulse, respiratory rate, and blood pressure prior to

*Underlines indicate most frequent; CAPITALS indicate life-threatening.

administration. Notify physician of significant changes in heart rate.

- **Myasthenia Gravis:** Assess neuromuscular status, including vital capacity, ptosis, diplopia, chewing, swallowing, hand grasp, and gait prior to administering and at peak effect. Patients with myasthenia gravis may be advised to keep a daily record of their condition and the effects of this medication.
- □ Assess patient for overdosage and underdosage or resistance. Both have similar symptoms (muscle weakness, dyspnea, dysphagia), but symptoms of overdosage usually occur within 1 hr of administration, while symptoms of underdosage occur ≥3 hr after administration. Overdosage (cholinergic crisis) symptoms may also include increased respiratory secretions and saliva, bradycardia, nausea, vomiting, cramping, diarrhea, and diaphoresis. A Tensilon test (edrophonium chloride) may be used to differentiate between overdosage and underdosage.
- **Antidote to Nondepolarizing Neuromuscular Blocking Agents:** Monitor reversal of effect of neuromuscular blocking agents with a peripheral nerve stimulator. Recovery usually occurs consecutively in the following muscles: diaphragm, intercostal muscles, muscles of the glottis, abdominal muscles, limb muscles, muscles of mastication, and levator muscles of eyelids. Closely observe patient for residual muscle weakness and respiratory distress throughout the recovery period. Maintain airway patency and ventilation until recovery of normal respirations occurs.
- **Toxicity and Overdose:** Atropine is the antidote.

Potential Nursing Diagnoses

- Mobility, impaired physical (indications).
- Breathing pattern, ineffective (indications).
- Knowledge deficit related to medication regimen (patient/family teaching).

Implementation

- **General Info:** For patients who have difficulty chewing, pyridostigmine may be administered 30 min before meals.
- □ Oral dose is not interchangeable with IV dose. Parenteral form is 30 times more potent.
- □ When used as an antidote to nondepolarizing neuromuscular blocking agents, atropine may be ordered prior to or currently with large doses of pyridostigmine to prevent or to treat bradycardia and other side effects.
- **PO:** Administer with food or milk to minimize side effects. Extended-release tablets should be swallowed whole; do not crush, break, or chew. Regular tablets or syrup may be administered with extended-release tablets for optimum control of symptoms. Mottled appearance of extended-release tablet does not affect potency.
- **Direct IV:** Administer undiluted. Do not add to IV solns. May be given through Y-site or 3-way stopcock of soln of D5W, 0.9% NaCl, lactated Ringer's soln, D5/Ringer's soln, or D5/LR.
- □ *Rate:* For reversal of nondepolarizing neuromuscular blocking agents, administer each 0.5 mg over 1 min.
- □ For muscle relaxant antagonist, administer each 5 mg over 1 min.
- **Syringe Compatibility:** glycopyrrolate.
- **Y-Site Compatibility:** heparin, hydrocortisone sodium succinate, or potassium chloride.

Patient/Family Teaching

- □ Instruct patient to take medication exactly as directed. Do not skip or double up on missed doses. Patients with a history of dysphagia should have a nonelectric or battery-back-up alarm clock to remind them of exact dose time. Patients with dysphagia may not be able to swallow medication if the dose is not taken exactly on time. Taking dose late may result in myasthenic crisis. Taking dose early may result in cholinergic crisis. Patients with myasthenia gravis must continue this regimen as a lifelong therapy.

- Advise patient to carry identification describing disease and medication regimen at all times.
- Instruct patient to space activities to avoid fatigue.

Evaluation

Effectiveness of therapy can be demonstrated by: ▪ Relief of ptosis and diplopia; improved chewing, swallowing, extremity strength, and breathing without the appearance of cholinergic symptoms ▪ Reversal of nondepolarizing neuromuscular blocking agents in general anesthesia.

PYRIDOXINE

(peer-i-**dox**-een)

Beesix, Rodex, TexSix T.R., vitamin B_6

CLASSIFICATION(S):

Vitamin—water-soluble

Pregnancy Category UK

INDICATIONS

▪ Treatment and prevention of pyridoxine deficiency (may be associated with poor nutritional status or chronic debilitating illnesses) ▪ Treatement and prevention of neuropathy, which may develop from isoniazid, penicillamine, or hydralazine therapy.

ACTION

▪ Required for amino acid, carbohydrate, and lipid metabolism ▪ Used in the transport of amino acids, formation of neurotransmitters, and synthesis of heme. **Therapeutic Effects:** ▪ Prevention of pyridoxine deficiency ▪ Prevention or reversal of neuropathy associated with hydralazine, penicillamine, or isoniazid therapy.

PHARMACOKINETICS

Absorption: Well absorbed from the GI tract.

Distribution: Stored in liver, muscle, and brain. Crosses the placenta and enters breast milk.

Metabolism and Excretion: Amounts in excess of requirements are excreted unchanged by the kidneys.

Half-life: 15–20 days.

CONTRAINDICATIONS AND PRECAUTIONS

Contraindicated in: ▪ No known contraindications.

Use Cautiously in: ▪ Parkinson's disease (treatment with levodopa only) ▪ Pregnancy (chronic ingestion of large doses may produce pyridoxine-dependency syndrome in newborn).

ADVERSE REACTIONS AND SIDE EFFECTS*

Note: Adverse reactions listed are seen with excessive doses only.

Neuro: sensory neuropathy.

Misc: pyridoxine-dependency syndrome.

INTERACTIONS

Drug–Drug: ▪ Interferes with the therapeutic response to **levodopa** ▪ Requirements are increased by **isoniazid, hydralazine, chloramphenicol, penicillamine, estrogens,** and **immunosuppressants.**

ROUTE AND DOSAGE

Pyridoxine Deficiency

- **PO, IM, IV, SC (Adults):** 2.5–10 mg/day.

Dietary Supplementation

- **PO (Adults and Children):** 2 mg (2.5–10 mg/day during pregnancy).

Drug-Induced Deficiency (isoniazid, hydralazine, penicillamine)—Prevention

- **PO (Adults):** 10–50 mg/day (penicillamine), 100–300 mg/day (hydralazine or isoniazid).

Drug-Induced Deficiency (isoniazid, hydralazine, penicillamine)—Treatment

- **PO, IM, IV (Adults):** 50–200 mg/day for 3 wk, then 25–100 mg/day.

*Underlines indicate most frequent; **CAPITALS** indicate life-threatening.

Drug-Induced Deficiency (Chronic Alcoholism)
- **PO (Adults):** 50 mg/day for 2–4 wk, may be continued indefinitely.

Pyridoxine-Dependency Syndrome
- **PO (Adults):** 30–600 mg/day initially, then 50 mg/day for life.
- **PO, IM, IV (Infants):** 10–100 mg initially, followed by PO therapy of 2–100 mg/day, followed by 2–10 mg/day PO for life.
- **IM, IV (Adults):** 30–600 mg/day (initial treatment).

PHARMACODYNAMICS

	ONSET	PEAK	DURATION
PO	UK	UK	UK
IM	UK	UK	UK
IV	UK	UK	UK

NURSING IMPLICATIONS

Assessment
- Assess patient for signs of vitamin B_6 deficiency (anemia, dermatitis, cheilosis, irritability, seizures, nausea, and vomiting) prior to and periodically throughout therapy. Institute seizure precautions in pyridoxine-dependent infants.
- **Lab Test Considerations:** May cause false elevations in urobilinogen concentrations.

Potential Nursing Diagnoses
- Nutrition, altered: less than body requirements (indications).
- Knowledge deficit related to medication regimen (patient/family teaching).

Implementation
- **General Info:** Pyridoxine is available in tablet, capsule, extended-release tablet and capsule, and injectable forms.
- Because of infrequency of single B-vitamin deficiencies, combinations are commonly administered.
- Administration of parenteral vitamin B_6 is limited to patients who are NPO, have nausea and vomiting, or have malabsorption syndromes.
- Protect parenteral soln from light, as decomposition will occur.
- **PO:** Extended-release capsules and tablets should be swallowed whole, without crushing, breaking, or chewing. For patients unable to swallow capsule, contents of capsules may be mixed with jam or jelly.
- **SC/IM:** Rotate sites; burning or stinging at site may occur.
- **IV:** May be administered direct IV or as infusion in standard IV solns.
- B_6-dependent seizures should cease within 2–3 min of IV administration of pyridoxine.
- **Additive Incompatibility:** alkaline solns, erythromycin, iron salts, kanamycin, riboflavin, or streptomycin.

Patient/Family Teaching
- Instruct patient to take medication as ordered. If a dose is missed, it may be omitted, as an extended period of time is required to become deficient in vitamin B_6.
- Encourage patient to comply with physician's diet recommendations. Explain that the best source of vitamins is a well-balanced diet with foods from the 4 basic food groups. Foods high in vitamin B_6 include bananas, whole-grain cereals, potatoes, lima bean, and meats.
- Patients self-medicating with vitamin supplements should be cautioned not to exceed RDA (see Appendix L). The effectiveness of megadoses for treatment of various medical conditions is unproven and may cause side effects, such as unsteady gait, numbness in feet, and difficulty with hand coordination.
- Emphasize the importance of follow-up examinations to evaluate progress.

Evaluation
Effectiveness of therapy may be demonstrated by: ▪ Decrease in the symptoms of vitamin B_6 deficiency.

P

PYRIMETHAMINE
(peer-i-**meth**-a-meen)
Daraprim

CLASSIFICATION(S):
Antimalarial, Antiprotozoal
Pregnancy Category C

INDICATIONS

■ Used alone or with other agents as chemoprophylaxis against malaria ■ Used in combination with other antimalarials in the treatment of chloroquine-resistant malaria ■ Used in combination with a sulfonamide in the treatment of toxoplasmosis. **Unlabeled Use:** ■ Used in combination with other agents (sulfonamides, dapsone) in the treatment of *Pneumocystis carinii* pneumonia.

ACTION

■ Binds to an enzyme in the protozoa, which results in depletion of folic acid. **Therapeutic Effect:** ■ Death and arrested growth of susceptible organisms (protozoa).

PHARMACOKINETICS

Absorption: Well absorbed following oral administration.
Distribution: Widely distributed with high concentrations achieved in blood cells, kidneys, lungs, liver, and spleen. Some enters CSF (13–26% of serum levels). Crosses the placenta and enters breast milk.
Metabolism and Excretion: Mostly metabolized by the liver. 20–30% excreted unchanged by the kidneys.
Half-life: 4 days (shortened in patients with AIDS).

CONTRAINDICATIONS AND PRECAUTIONS

Contraindicated in: ■ Hypersensitivity ■ First 14–16 wk of pregnancy ■ Megaloblastic anemia due to folate deficiency ■ Concurrent folate antagonist therapy (due to risk of megaloblastic anemia).
Use Cautiously in: ■ History of seizures (high doses) ■ Underlying anemia or bone marrow depression ■ Impaired liver function ■ Pregnancy >16 wk (may require concurrent leucovorin) ■ Lactation (large doses to mother may cause folic and acid deficiency in infant) ■ G6-PD deficiency.

ADVERSE REACTIONS AND SIDE EFFECTS*

CNS: SEIZURES (high doses), insomnia, headache, lightheadedness, malaise, depression.
Resp: dry throat, pulmonary eosinophilia.
CV: arrhythmias (large doses).
GI: anorexia, nausea, atrophic glossitis (high doses), diarrhea.
GU: hematuria.
Derm: dermatitis, abnormal pigmentation.
Hemat: megaloblastic anemia (high doses), thrombocytopenia, pancytopenia.
Misc: fever.

INTERACTIONS

Drug-Drug: ■ Increased risk of bone marrow depression with other **bone marrow depressants** including **antineoplastic agents** or **radiation therapy** ■ Increased risk of megaloblastic anemia with **folate antagonists (methotrexate)**; concurrent use should be avoided.

ROUTE AND DOSAGE

Antimalarial Chemoprophylaxis

- **PO (Adults and Children ≥10 yr):** 25 mg once weekly or 12.5 mg once weekly with dapsone for prophylaxis against chloroquine-resistant malaria.
- **PO (Children 4–10 yr):** 12.5 mg once weekly or 0.25 mg/kg once weekly with dapsone for prophylaxis against chloroquine-resistant malaria.
- **PO (Children <4 yr):** 6.25 mg once weekly or 0.25 mg/kg once weekly with dapsone for prophylaxis against chloroquine-resistant malaria.

Treatment of Malaria

- **PO (Adults):** 25 mg once daily for 2

*Underlines indicate most frequent; **CAPITALS** indicate life-threatening.

days or 25 mg twice daily for 3 days with quinine and sulfadiazine for chloroquine-resistant malaria.

- **PO (Children 20–40 kg):** 25 mg once daily for 3 days with quinine and sulfadiazine for chloroquine-resistant malaria.
- **PO (Children 10–20 kg):** 12.5 mg once daily for 3 days with quinine and sulfadiazine for chloroquine-resistant malaria.
- **PO (Children <10 kg):** 6.25 mg once daily for 3 days with quinine and sulfadiazine for chloroquine-resistant malaria.

Toxoplasmosis (with a sulfonamide or clindamycin)

- **PO (Adults):** 50–75 mg/day for 1–3 wk, then decrease dose by 50% and continue for additional 4–5 wk or 25 mg/day for 3–4 wk. Higher doses may be required for HIV-positive (AIDS) patients.
- **PO (Children):** 1 mg/kg/day in 2 divided doses for 2–4 days, then 0.5 mg/kg for 1 mon or 2 mg/kg for 3 days followed by 1 mg/kg for 4 wk.

PHARMACODYNAMICS (blood levels)

	ONSET	PEAK	DURATION
PO	UK	3 hr	2 wk*

*Suppressive levels.

NURSING IMPLICATIONS

Assessment

- Assess patient for improvement in signs and symptoms of infection daily throughout course of therapy.
- **Lab Test Considerations:** Monitor CBC and platelet count periodically throughout therapy. May cause decreased WBC and platelet counts.

Potential Nursing Diagnoses

- Infection, high risk for (indications).
- Knowledge deficit related to medication regimen (patient/family teaching).

Implementation

- **PO:** Administer with milk or meals to minimize GI distress.

Patient/Family Teaching

- Instruct patient to take medication exactly as directed and continue full course of therapy, even if feeling better.
- Review methods of minimizing exposure to mosquitos with patients receiving pyrimethamine prophylactically (use repellant, wear long-sleeved shirt and long trousers, use screen or netting).
- Advise patient to notify physician promptly if sore throat, pallor, purpura, or glossitis occur. Instruct patients to stop taking pyrimethamine and notify physician immediately at the first sign of a skin rash.
- Emphasize the importance of lab tests at scheduled intervals, especially in patients taking high doses. Tests should not be delayed or missed.

Evaluation

Effectiveness of therapy can be demonstrated by: ▪ Prevention of or improvement in signs and symptoms of malaria ▪ Improvement in signs and symptoms of toxoplasmosis ▪ Improvement in the signs and symptoms of *Pneumocystis carinii* pneumonia.

QUAZEPAM

(kway-ze-pam)
Doral

CLASSIFICATION(S):
Sedative/hypotic—benzodiazepine
Schedule IV
Pregnancy Category X

INDICATIONS

- Short-term (up to 4 wk) management of insomnia

ACTION

- Depresses the CNS, probably by potentiating gamma-aminobutyric acid (GABA), an inhibitory neurotransmitter. **Therapeutic Effect:** ▪ Relief of insomnia.

Q

PHARMACOKINETICS

Absorption: Well absorbed following oral administration.
Distribution: >95% bound to plasma proteins.
Metabolism and Excretion: Mostly metabolized by the liver. Two metabolites have CNS depressant activity (2-oxoquazepam and N-desalkylflurazepam).
Half-life: Quazepam—39 hr (increased in elderly); 2-oxoquazepam—39 hr; N-desalkylflurazepam—70–75 hr.

CONTRAINDICATIONS AND PRECAUTIONS

Contraindicated in: ▪ Hypersensitivity ▪ Cross-sensitivity with other benzodiazepines may exist ▪ Pre-existing CNS depression ▪ Severe uncontrolled pain ▪ Narrow-angle glaucoma ▪ Pregnancy or lactation.
Use Cautiously in: ▪ Hepatic dysfunction, elderly, very small or debilitated patients (dosage reduction may be necessary) ▪ Patients who are suicidal or who may have been previously addicted to drugs ▪ Children <18 yr (safety not established).

ADVERSE REACTIONS AND SIDE EFFECTS*

CNS: daytime drowsiness, dizziness, weakness, confusion, hallucinations, trouble sleeping, nervousness, false sense of well-being, headache, slurred speech.
EENT: blurred vision.
CV: palpitations.
GI: dry mouth, abdominal pain, constipation, diarrhea, nausea, vomiting.
GU: urinary frequency, urinary hesitancy.
Derm: skin rash, itching.
MS: muscle spasm.
Neuro: ataxia, trembling.
Misc: allergic reactions, changes in libido, physical dependence, psychological dependence.

INTERACTIONS

Drug-Drug: ▪ Additive CNS depression with **alcohol, antihistamines, antidepressants, MAO inhibitors,** other **sedative/hypnotics,** or **narcotic analgesics** ▪ **Cimetidine** or **oral contraceptives** may decrease metabolism and increase effects of quazepam ▪ May decrease efficacy of **levodopa** ▪ **Rifampin** or **cigarette smoking** increase metabolism and may decrease effectiveness.

ROUTE AND DOSAGE

- **PO (Adults):** 7.5–15 mg (start with 7.5 mg in elderly patients) at bedtime.

PHARMACODYNAMICS

	ONSET	PEAK	DURATION
PO	30 min	2 hr	8 hr

NURSING IMPLICATIONS

Assessment

- ▫ Assess sleep patterns prior to and periodically throughout course of therapy.
- ▫ Prolonged therapy may lead to psychological or physical dependence. Restrict amount of drug available to patient, especially if patient is depressed, suicidal, or has a history of addiction.

Potential Nursing Diagnoses

- Sleep pattern disturbance (indications).
- Injury, high risk for (side effects).
- Knowledge deficit related to medication regimen (patient/family teaching).

Implementation

- **General Info:** Supervise ambulation and transfer of patients following administration. Remove cigarettes. Side rails should be raised and call bell within reach at all times.

Patient/Family Teaching

- ▫ Advise patient to take medication exactly as directed. Discuss the importance of preparing environment for sleep (dark room, quiet, avoidance of

*Underlines indicate most frequent; **CAPITALS** indicate life-threatening.

nicotine and caffeine). Gradual discontinuation may be required following prolonged therapy. May cause disturbed sleep for the first 2 nights following discontinuation of quazepam.

- □ Medication may cause daytime drowsiness. Caution patient to avoid driving and other activities requiring alertness until response to medication is known.
- □ Caution patients to avoid taking alcohol or other CNS depressants concurrently with this medication.
- □ Instruct patient to contact physician immediately if pregnancy is planned or suspected.

EVALUATION

Effectiveness of therapy can be demonstrated by: ▪ Improvement in sleep pattern.

QUINAPRIL

(**kwin**-a-pril)
Accupril

CLASSIFICATION(S):
Antihypertensive—angiotensin converting enzyme (ACE) inhibitor
Pregnancy Category UK

INDICATIONS

▪ Alone or in combination with thiazide diuretics in the management of hypertension.

ACTION

▪ Prevents the production of angiotensin II, a potent vasoconstrictor that stimulates the production of aldosterone, by blocking its conversion to the active form. Result is systemic vasodilation. **Therapeutic Effect:** ▪ Lowering of blood pressure in hypertensive patients.

PHARMACOKINETICS

Absorption: Well absorbed following oral administration.

Distribution: Distribution not known. Appears to cross the placenta. Small amounts may enter breast milk.

Metabolism and Excretion: UK.

Half-life: UK.

CONTRAINDICATIONS AND PRECAUTIONS

Contraindicated in: ▪ Hypersensitivity ▪ Cross-sensitivity with other ACE inhibitors may exist ▪ Lactaion.

Use Cautiously in: ▪ Renal impairment, hypovolemia, hyponatremia, elderly patients (dosage reduction required) ▪ Aortic stenosis ▪ Cerebrovascular or cardiac insufficiency ▪ Pregnancy (may cause fetal hypotension, oliguria, renal failure, skull hypoplasia, other fetal abnormalities, and death) ▪ Children (safety not established) ▪ Surgery/anesthesia (hypotension may be exaggerated).

ADVERSE REACTIONS AND SIDE EFFECTS*

CNS: headache, dizziness, fatigue, insomnia, weakness.

EENT: ANGIOEDEMA.

Resp: cough.

CV: hypotension, palpitations, chest pain.

GI: nausea, diarrhea.

GU: renal failure, proteinuria, impotence.

Derm: rash.

Hemat: leukopenia, eosinophilia.

INTERACTIONS

Drug-Drug: ▪ Additive or possibly excessive hypotension with other **antihypertensives, diuretics, nitrates,** and acute ingestion of **alcohol** ▪ Hyperkalemia may result with concurrent **potassium supplements** or **potassium-sparing diuretics** ▪ Antihypertensive response may be blunted by **nonsteroidal anti-inflammatory agents** ▪ Increases blood levels and risk of toxicity from **lithium** ▪ Increased risk of hypersensitivity reaction with **allopurinol**.

*Underlines indicate most frequent; **CAPITALS** indicate life-threatening.

Q

ROUTE AND DOSAGE

- **PO (Adults):** 10 mg given once daily. If given with diuretics, initiate therapy with 5 mg once daily. Doses up to 80 mg/day have been used. Larger doses may be divided and given twice daily. Dosage increments should be made at 2-wk intervals.

PHARMACODYNAMICS (antihypertensive effect)

	ONSET	PEAK	DURATION
PO	UK	2–6 hr	12–24 hr

NURSING IMPLICATIONS

Assessment

- Monitor blood pressure and pulse frequently during initial dosage adjustment and periodically throughout course of therapy. Notify physician of significant changes.
- **Lab Test Considerations:** Monitor BUN, creatinine, and electrolyte levels periodically. Serum potassium may be increased, and BUN and creatinine transiently increased while sodium levels may be decreased.

Potential Nursing Diagnoses

- Cardiac output, decreased (indications, side effects).
- Knowledge deficit related to medication regimen (patient/family teaching).
- Noncompliance (patient/family teaching).

Implementation

- **PO:** Precipitous drop in blood pressure following first dose may occur. Discontinuing diuretic therapy 2–3 days prior to initiation of quinapril may decrease risk of hypotension. Resume diuretics if blood pressure is not controlled with quinapril.
- Dose is adjusted at 2-wk intervals based on blood pressure response at peak (2–6 hr) and trough (predose) blood levels.

Patient/Family Teaching

- Instruct patient to take quinapril exactly as directed, even if feeling well. Missed doses should be taken as soon as possible but not if almost time for next dose. Do not double doses. Medication controls but does not cure hypertension. Warn patients not to discontinue quinapril therapy unless directed by the physician.
- Encourage patient to comply with additional interventions for hypertension (weight reduction, discontinuation of smoking, moderation of alcohol consumption, regular exercise, and stress management).
- Instruct patient and family on proper technique for blood pressure monitoring. Advise them to check blood pressure at least weekly and report significant changes to physician.
- Caution patient to avoid salt substitutes or foods containing high levels of potassium or sodium unless directed by physician (see Appendix K).
- Caution patient to change positions slowly to minimize orthostatic hypotension, particularly after initial dose. Patients should also be advised that exercising or hot weather may increase hypotensive effects.
- Advise patient to consult physician or pharmacist before taking any over-the-counter medicaitons, especially cold remedies. Patients should also avoid excessive amounts of tea, coffee, or cola.
- May cause dizziness. Caution patient to avoid driving and other activities requiring alertness until response to medication is known.
- Advise patient to inform physician or dentist of medication regimen prior to treatment or surgery.
- Instruct patient to notify physician if rash, mouth sores, sore throat, fever, swelling of hands or feet, irregular heart beat, chest pain, dry cough, swelling of face, eyes, lips, or tongue, or difficulty breathing occurs or if taste impairment persists.
- Emphasize the importance of follow-up examinations to monitor progress.

EVALUATION

Effectiveness of therapy can be demonstrated by: ▪ Decrease in blood pressure without appearance of side effects.

QUINIDINE
(**kwin**-i-deen)

quinidine gluconate
Duraquin, Quinaglute, Quinalan, {Quinate}, Quinatime, Quin-Release

quinidine polygalacturonate
Cardioquin

quinidine sulfate
{Apo-Quinidine}, Cin-Quin, {Novoquinidin}, Quinidex, Quinidex Extentabs, Quinora

CLASSIFICATION(S):
Antiarrhythmic—class IA
Pregnancy Category C

INDICATIONS

▪ Used in the management of a wide variety of atrial and ventricular arrhythmias, including: ▫ Atrial premature contractions ▫ Premature ventricular contractions ▫ Ventricular tachycardia ▫ Paroxysmal atrial tachycardia ▫ Maintenance of normal sinus rhythm after conversion from atrial fibrillation or flutter. **Unlabeled Use:** ▪ Treatment of malaria (IV gluconate only).

ACTION

▪ Decreases myocardial excitability ▪ Slows conduction velocity. **Therapeutic Effect:** ▪ Suppression of arrhythmias.

PHARMACOKINETICS

Absorption: Well absorbed from the GI tract and IM sites. Extended-release quinidine sulfate (Quinidex Extentabs) or gluconate (Duraquin, Quinaglute, Quinalan, Quinatime, Quin-Release) oral preparations and polygalacturonate salt are absorbed more slowly following oral administration.

Distribution: Widely distributed. Crosses the placenta and enters breast milk.

Metabolism and Excretion: Metabolized by the liver; 10–30% excreted unchanged by the kidneys.

Half-life: 6–8 hr (increased in congestive heart failure or severe liver impairment).

CONTRAINDICATIONS AND PRECAUTIONS

Contraindicated in: ▪ Hypersensitivity ▪ Conduction defects ▪ Cardiac glycoside toxicity.

Use Cautiously in: ▪ Congestive heart failure or severe liver disease (dosage reduction recommended) ▪ Pregnancy, lactation, or children (safety not established; extended-release preparations should not be used in children).

ADVERSE REACTIONS AND SIDE EFFECTS*

CNS: vertigo, headache, dizziness.

EENT: tinnitus, blurred vision, photophobia, mydriasis, diplopia.

CV: HYPOTENSION, tachycardia, arrhythmias.

GI: <u>diarrhea</u>, <u>nausea</u>, <u>cramping</u>, <u>anorexia</u>, bitter taste, hepatitis.

Derm: rashes.

Hemat: thrombocytopenia, hemolytic anemia.

Misc: fever.

INTERACTIONS

Drug-Drug: ▪ Increases serum **digoxin** levels and may cause toxicity (dosage reduction recommended) ▪ **Phenytoin, phenobarbital,** or **rifampin** may increase metabolism and decrease effectiveness ▪ **Cimetidine** decreases metabolism and may increase blood levels ▪ Potentiates **neuromuscular blocking agents** and **oral anticoagulants** ▪ Additive hypotension with **antihypertensives, nitrates,** and acute ingestion of

{} = Available in Canada only.

*<u>Underlines</u> indicate most frequent; **CAPITALS** indicate life-threatening.

Q

alcohol ▪ May antagonize **anticholinesterase therapy** in patients with myasthenia gravis ▪ **Drugs that alkalinize the urine,** including high-dose **antacid** therapy or **sodium bicarbonate** increase blood levels and the risk of toxicity.

Drug–Food: ▪ **Foods that alkalinize the urine** (see Appendix K) may increase serum quinidine levels and the risk of toxicity.

ROUTE AND DOSAGE

Quinidine Gluconate (62% Quinidine)

- **PO (Adults):** 324–660 mg q 6–12 hr of extended-release tablets.
- **IM (Adults):** 600 mg initially, followed by up to 400 mg q 2 hr.
- **IV (Adults):** Infuse at 16 mg/min.

Quinidine Polygalacturonate (60% Quinidine)

- **PO (Adults):** 275–825 mg initially, may repeat in 3–4 hr; may increase by 137.5–275 mg and repeat 3–4 times until arrhythmia is controlled. Usual maintenance dose is 275 mg q 8–12 hr.
- **PO (Children):** 8.25 mg/kg or 247.5 mg/m^2 5 times daily.

Quinidine Sulfate (83% Quinidine)

Premature Atrial or Ventricular Contractions

- **PO (Adults):** 200–300 mg q 6–8 hr or 300–600 mg of extended-release preparation every 8–12 hr maintenance (not to exceed 4 g/day).
- **PO (Children):** 6 mg/kg or 180 mg/m^2 5 times daily.

Paroxysmal Atrial Tachycardia

- **PO (Adults):** 400–600 mg q 2–3 hr until arrhythmia is terminated, then 200–300 mg q 6–8 hr or 300–600 mg of extended-release preparation every 8–12 hr maintenance (not to exceed 4 g/day).

Conversion of Atrial Fibrillation

- **PO (Adults):** 200 mg q 2–3 hr for 5–8 doses, may increase dose daily as needed, then 200–300 mg q 6–8 hr or 300–600 mg of extended-release preparation every 8–12 hr maintenance (not to exceed 4 g/day).

PHARMACODYNAMICS (antiarrhythmic effects)

	ONSET	PEAK	DURATION
PO (sulfate)	30 min	1–1.5 hr	6–8 hr
PO (sulfate-ER)	UK	4 hr	8–12 hr
PO (gluconate)	UK	3–4 hr	6–8 hr
PO (polygalacturonate)	UK	6 hr	8–12 hr
IM	30 min	30–90 min	6–8 hr
IV	1–5 min	rapid	6–8 hr

NURSING IMPLICATIONS

Assessment

- ☐ Monitor ECG, pulse, and blood pressure continuously throughout IV administration. Parameters should be monitored periodically during oral administration. IV administration is usually discontinued if any of the following occurs: arrhythmia is resolved, QRS complex widens by 50%, PR or QT intervals are prolonged, frequent ventricular ectopic beats or tachycardia develops. Patient should remain supine throughout IV administration to minimize hypotension.
- ▪ **Lab Test Considerations:** Hepatic and renal function, CBC, and serum potassium levels should be periodically monitored during prolonged therapy.
- ▪ **Toxicity and Overdose:** Serum quinidine levels may be monitored periodically during dosage adjustment. Therapeutic serum concentrations are 3–6 mcg/ml. Toxic effects usually occur at concentrations >8 mcg/ml.
- ☐ Signs and symptoms of toxicity or cinchonism include tinnitus, visual disturbances, headache, and dizziness.
- ☐ Cardiac signs of toxicity include QRS widening, cardiac asystole, ventricular ectopic beats, idioventricular rhythms (ventricular tachycardia,

ventricular fibrillation), paradoxical tachycardia, and arterial embolism.

Potential Nursing Diagnoses

- Cardiac output, decreased (indications).
- Knowledge deficit related to medication regimen (patient/family teaching).

Implementation

- **General Info:** A test dose of one regular oral tablet may be administered prior to quinidine therapy to check for intolerance.
  - Higher doses may be required to correct atrial arrhythmias than those required for ventricular arrhythmias.
  - Available in tablets, capsules, extended-release tablets, and injectable forms.
- **PO:** Administer with a full glass of water on an empty stomach either 1 hr before or 2 hr after meals for faster absorption. If GI irritation becomes a problem, may be administered with or immediately after meals. Extended-release preparations (Duraquin, Quinaglute, Quinatime, Quinidex Extentabs, Quin-Release) should be swallowed whole; do not break, crush, or chew.
- **IV:** Use only clear, colorless soln.
- **Intermittent Infusion:** Dilute 800 mg of quinidine gluconate (10 ml) in at least 40 ml of D5W for injection for a maximum concentration of 16 mg/ml. Soln is stable for 24 hr at room temperature.
  - Dilute 600 mg of quinidine sulfate in 40 ml of D5W.
  - *Rate:* Administer either quinidine gluconate or quinidine sulfate at a rate not to exceed 1 ml/min. Administer via infusion pump to ensure accurate dose. Rapid administration may cause hypotension.
- **Y-Site Compatibility:** ▫ QUINIDINE GLUCONATE with diazepam.
- **Y-Site Incompatibility:** ▫ QUINIDINE GLUCONATE with furosemide.
- **Additive Compatibility:** ▫ QUINIDINE GLUCONATE with bretylium, cimetidine, or verapamil.

Patient/Family Teaching

- Instruct patient to take medication around the clock, exactly as directed, even if feeling better. If a dose is missed, take as soon as remembered if within 2 hr; if remembered later, omit. Do not double doses.
- Instruct patient or family member on how to take pulse. Advise patient to report changes in pulse rate or rhythm to physician.
- Quinidine may cause dizziness or blurred vision. Caution patient to avoid driving or other activities requiring alertness until response to medication is known.
- Inform patient that quinidine may cause increased sensitivity to light. Dark glasses may minimize this effect.
- Advise patient to inform physician or dentist of medication regimen prior to treatment or surgery.
- Instruct patient not to take over-the-counter medications with quinidine without consulting physician or pharmacist.
- Advise patient to consult physician if diarrhea is severe or persistent.
- Advise patient to carry identification describing disease process and medication regimen at all times.
- Emphasize the importance of routine follow-up examinations to monitor progress.

Evaluation

Effectiveness of therapy can be demonstrated by: ▪ Resolution of cardiac arrhythmias without detrimental side effects.

RAMIPRIL

(**ram**-i-pril)
Altace

CLASSIFICATION(S):
Antihypertensive—angiotensin converting enzyme (ACE) inhibitor
Pregnancy Category D

INDICATIONS

▪ Alone or in combination with thiazide diuretics in the management of hypertension.

ACTION

▪ Prevents the production of angiotensin II, a potent vasoconstrictor that stimulates the production of aldosterone, by blocking its conversion to the active form. Result is systemic vasodilation. **Therapeutic Effect:** ▪ Lowering of blood pressure in hypertensive patients.

PHARMACOKINETICS

Absorption: Well absorbed following oral administration.
Distribution: Distribution not known. Appears to cross the placenta. Small amounts may enter breast milk.
Metabolism and Excretion: Mostly metabolized by the liver. Some converted to ramiprilat, an active hypotensive compound.
Half-life: Ramipril—5 hr, ramiprilat—23.5 hr.

CONTRAINDICATIONS AND PRECAUTIONS

Contraindicated in: ▪ Hypersensitivity ▪ Cross-sensitivity with other ACE inhibitors may exist ▪ Lactation.
Use Cautiously in: ▪ Renal impairment, hypovolemia, hyponatremia, elderly patients (dosage reduction required) ▪ Aortic stenosis ▪ Cerebrovascular or cardiac insufficiency ▪ Pregnancy (may cause fetal hypotension, oliguria, renal failure, skull hypoplasia, other fetal abnormalities, and death) ▪ Children (safety not established) ▪ Surgery/anesthesia (hypotension may be exaggerated).

ADVERSE REACTIONS AND SIDE EFFECTS*

CNS: <u>headache</u>, dizziness, fatigue, insomnia, weakness.
EENT: ANGIOEDEMA.
Resp: <u>cough</u>.
CV: hypotension, palpitations, chest pain.
GI: nausea, diarrhea.
GU: renal failure, proteinuria, impotence.
Derm: rash.
Hemat: leukopenia, eosinophilia.

INTERACTIONS

Drug-Drug: ▪ Additive or possibly excessive hypotension with other **antihypertensives, diuretics, nitrates,** and acute ingestion of **alcohol** ▪ Hyperkalemia may result with concurrent **potassium supplements** or **potassium-sparing diuretics** ▪ Antihypertensive response may be blunted by **nonsteroidal anti-inflammatory agents** ▪ Increases blood levels and risk of toxicity from **lithium** ▪ Increased risk of hypersensitivity reactions with **allopurinol**.

ROUTE AND DOSAGE

▪ **PO (Adults):** 2.5–20 mg given once daily or in 2 divided doses.

PHARMACODYNAMICS (antihypertensive effect)

	ONSET	PEAK	DURATION
PO	1.5–2 hr	6–8 hr	24–72 hr

NURSING IMPLICATIONS

Assessment

□ Monitor blood pressure and pulse frequently during initial dosage adjustment and periodically throughout course of therapy. Notify physician of significant changes.
▪ **Lab Test Considerations:** Monitor BUN, creatinine, and electrolyte levels periodically. Serum potassium may be increased and BUN and creatinine transiently increased while sodium levels may be decreased.

Potential Nursing Diagnoses

▪ Cardiac output, decreased (indications, side effects).
▪ Knowledge deficit related to medica-

*<u>Underlines</u> indicate most frequent; **CAPITALS** indicate life-threatening.

tion regimen (patient/family teaching).

- Noncompliance (patient/family teaching).

IMPLEMENTATION

- **PO:** Precipitous drop in blood pressure following first dose may occur. Discontinuing diuretic therapy 2–3 days prior to initiation of ramipril may decrease risk of hypotension. Resume diuretics if blood pressure is not controlled with ramipril.

PATIENT/FAMILY TEACHING

- Instruct patient to take ramipril exactly as directed, even if feeling better. Missed doses should be taken as soon as remembered but not if almost time for next dose. Do not double doses. Medication controls but does not cure hypertension. Warn patients not to discontinue ramipril therapy unless directed by the physician.
- Encourage patient to comply with additional interventions for hypertension (weight reduction, discontinuation of smoking, moderation of alcohol consumption, regular exercise, and stress management).
- Instruct patient and family on proper technique for blood pressure monitoring. Advise them to check blood pressure at least weekly and report significant changes to physician.
- Caution patient to avoid salt substitutes or foods containing high levels of potassium or sodium unless directed by physician.
- Caution patient to change positions slowly to minimize orthostatic hypotension, particularly after initial dose. Patients should also be advised that exercising or hot weather may increase hypotensive effects.
- Advise patient to consult physician or pharmacist before taking any over-the-counter medications, especially cold remedies. Patients should also avoid excessive amounts of tea, coffee, or cola.
- Ramipril may cause dizziness. Caution patient to avoid driving and other activities requiring alertness until response to medication is known.
- Advise patient to inform physician or dentist of medication regimen prior to treatment or surgery.
- Instruct patient to notify physician if rash, mouth sores, sore throat, fever, swelling of hands or feet, irregular heart beat, chest pain, dry cough, swelling of face, eyes, lips, or tongue, or difficulty breathing occurs.
- Emphasize the importance of follow-up examinations to monitor progress.

EVALUATION

Effectiveness of therapy can be demonstrated by: ▪ Decrease in blood pressure without appearance of side effects.

RANITIDINE
(ra-**nit**-ti-deen)
Zantac

CLASSIFICATION(S):
Histamine H_2 Antagonist, Gastrointestinal—antiulcer
Pregnancy Category B

INDICATIONS

▪ Treatment (short-term) and prevention (long-term) of active duodenal ulcers ▪ Short-term treatment of benign gastric ulcers ▪ Management of gastroesophageal reflux disease (GERD) ▪ Treatment of gastric hypersecretory states (Zollinger-Ellison syndrome).

ACTION

▪ Inhibits the action of histamine at the H_2-receptor site located primarily in gastric parietal cells ▪ Inhibits gastric acid secretion. **Therapeutic Effect:** ▪ Healing and prevention of ulcers.

PHARMACOKINETICS

Absorption: Well absorbed following oral and IM administration.

Distribution: Widely distributed. Enters breast milk and probably crosses

R

the placenta. Crosses the blood-brain barrier only in small amounts.

Metabolism and Excretion: Metabolized by the liver, mostly on first pass. 30% eliminated unchanged by the kidneys following oral administration. Up to 70–80% may be eliminated unchanged by the kidneys following parenteral dosing.

Half-life: 1.7–3 hr (increased in renal impairment).

CONTRAINDICATIONS AND PRECAUTIONS

Contraindicated in: ▪ Hypersensitivity.

Use Cautiously in: ▪ Elderly patients ▪ Renal impairment ▪ Hepatic impairment (increased risk of confusion; dosage reduction recommended) ▪ Pregnancy, lactation, or children (safety not established).

ADVERSE REACTIONS AND SIDE EFFECTS*

CNS: confusion, dizziness, headache, malaise, drowsiness.

CV: bradycardia, tachycardia, premature ventricular contractions.

Derm: rashes.

EENT: ocular pain, blurred vision.

Endo: gynecomastia.

GI: nausea, constipation, hepatitis, abdominal pain, diarrhea.

GU: impotence.

INTERACTIONS

Drug–Drug: ▪ **Antacids** may decrease the absorption of ranitidine ▪ **Smoking** may decrease the effectiveness of ranitidine ▪ Reduces absorption of **ketoconazole**.

ROUTE AND DOSAGE

Short-Term Treatment of Active Ulcers

- **PO (Adults):** 150 mg bid or 300 mg at bedtime.
- **IM (Adults):** 50 mg q 6–8 hr (up to 400 mg/day).
- **IV (Adults):** 50 mg q 6–8 hr or 6.25 mg/hr infusion.

Prevention of Duodenal Ulcers

- **PO (Adults):** 150 mg once daily, at bedtime.

Management of Gastroesophageal Reflux

- **PO (Adults):** 150 mg bid.

Gastric Hypersecretory Conditions (Zollinger-Ellison Syndrome)

- **PO (Adults):** 150 mg bid (up to 6 g/day).
- **IV (Adults):** 1 mg/kg/hr initially by continuous infusion. Based on gastric acid output after 4 hr, may increase by 0.5 mg/kg/hr up to 2.5 mg/kg/hr.

PHARMACODYNAMICS (inhibition of gastric acid secretion)

	ONSET	PEAK	DURATION
PO	UK	1–3 hr	8–12 hr
IM	UK	15 min	8–12 hr
IV	UK	15 min	8–12 hr

NURSING IMPLICATIONS

Assessment

- ▫ Assess patient routinely for epigastric or abdominal pain and frank or occult blood in the stool, emesis, or gastric aspirate.
- ▫ Assess elderly and severely ill patients routinely for confusion. Notify physician promptly should this occur.
- ▪ **Lab Test Considerations:** CBC with differential should be monitored periodically throughout therapy.
- ▫ May cause transient increase in serum transaminase and serum creatinine.
- ▫ Antagonizes the effects of pentagastrin and histamine during gastric acid secretion test. Avoid administration during the 24 hr preceding the test.
- ▫ May cause false-negative results for urine protein.
- ▫ May cause false-negative results in

*Underlines indicate most frequent; **CAPITALS** indicate life-threatening.

skin tests using allergen extracts. Ranitidine should be discontinued 24 hr prior to the test.

Potential Nursing Diagnoses

- Comfort, altered: pain (indications).
- Knowledge deficit related to medication regimen (patient/family teaching).

Implementation

- **PO:** Food does not affect absorption; may be given without regard to meals.
- If administering oral doses concurrently with antacids, give at least 1 hr apart.
- **Direct IV:** Dilute each 50 mg in 20 ml of 0.9% NaCl or D5W for injection.
- *Rate:* Administer over at least 5 min. Rapid administration may cause hypotension and arrhythmias.
- **Intermittent Infusion:** Dilute each 50 mg in 100 ml of 0.9% NaCl or D5W. Diluted soln is stable for 48 hr at room temperature. Do not use soln that is discolored or that contains precipitate.
- *Rate:* Administer over 15–20 min.
- **Continuous Infusion:** Add ranitidine to D5W for a concentration of 150 mg/250 ml (no greater than 2.5 mg/ml for Zollinger-Ellison patients).
- *Rate:* Administer at a rate of 6.25 mg/hr. In patients with Zollinger-Ellison syndrome start infusion at 1 mg/kg/hr. If gastric acid output is >10 mEq/hr or patient becomes symptomatic after 4 hr, adjust dose by 0.5 mg/kg/hr increments and remeasure gastric output.
- **Syringe Compatibility:** atropine, cyclizine, dexamethasone, dimenhydrinate, diphenhyramine, dobutamine, dopamine, fentanyl, glycopyrrolate, hydromorphone, isoproterenol, meperidine, metoclopramide, morphine, nalbuphine, oxymorphone, pentazocine, perphenazine, prochlorperazine edisylate, promethazine, scopolamine, or thiethylperazine.
- **Syringe Incompatibility:** hydroxyzine, methotrimeprazine, midazolam, pentobarbital, or phenobarbital.
- **Y-Site Compatibility:** acyclovir, aminophylline, atracurium, bretylium, dobutamine, dopamine, enalaprilat, esmolol, heparin, labetalol, meperidine, nitroglycerin, ondansetron, pancuronium, procainamide, vecuronium, or zidovudine.
- **Additive Compatibility:** amikacin, aminophylline, chloramphenicol, dobutamine, dopamine, doxycycline, gentamicin, heparin, lidocaine, moxalactam, nitroprusside, norepinephrine, penicillin G sodium, potassium chloride, ticarcillin, tobramycin, or vancomycin.
- **Additive Incompatibility:** amphotericin B or clindamycin.

Patient/Family Teaching

- Instruct patient to take medication as prescribed for the full course of therapy, even if feeling better. If a dose is missed, it should be taken as soon as remembered, but not if almost time for next dose. Do not double doses.
- Inform patient that smoking interferes with the action of ranitidine. Encourage patient to quit smoking or at least not to smoke after last dose of the day.
- Ranitidine may cause drowsiness or dizziness. Caution patient to avoid driving or other activities requiring alertness until response to the drug is known.
- Advise patient to avoid alcohol, products containing aspirin, and foods that may cause an increase in GI irritation.
- Advise patient to report onset of black, tarry stools; diarrhea; dizziness; rash; or confusion to physician promptly.

Evaluation

Effectiveness of therapy can be demonstrated by: ▪ Decrease in abdominal pain ▪ Prevention of gastric irritation and bleeding. Healing of duodenal ulcers can be seen on x-ray examinations or endoscopy. Therapy is continued for at least 6 wk after initial episode.

R

RESERPINE
(re-**ser**-peen)
{Novoreseroine}, {Reserfia}, Serpalan, Serpasil

CLASSIFICATION(S):
Antihypertensive—peripherally acting antiadrenergic
Pregnancy Category C

INDICATIONS

- Used in combination with other antihypertensives (thiazide diuretics) in the management of mild to moderate hypertension.

ACTION

- Depletes stores of norepinephrine and inhibits uptake in postganglionic adrenergic nerve endings. **Therapeutic Effect:** ▪ Lowering of blood pressure.

PHARMACOKINETICS

Absorption: 40–50% absorbed following oral administration.
Distribution: Widely distributed. Crosses the placenta and enters breast milk.
Metabolism and Excretion: Metabolized by the liver. At least 50% lost in feces as unabsorbed drug following oral administration. Small amounts excreted unchanged by the kidneys.
Half-life: 11 days.

CONTRAINDICATIONS AND PRECAUTIONS

Contraindicated in: ▪ Hypersensitivity ▪ Active peptic ulcer, ulcerative colitis ▪ Gallstones ▪ Mental depression ▪ Electroconvulsive therapy.
Use Cautiously in: ▪ Cardiac, cerebrovascular, or renal insufficiency ▪ Pregnancy or lactation (safety not established).

ADVERSE REACTIONS AND SIDE EFFECTS*

CNS: drowsiness, fatigue, lethargy, depression, headache, nervousness, anxiety, nightmares.
EENT: nasal stuffiness, miosis, blurred vision, conjunctival congestion.
CV: bradycardia, arrhythmias, angina, edema.
GI: diarrhea, dry mouth, cramps, nausea, vomiting, GI bleeding.
GU: impotence.
Derm: flushing.
Endo: galactorrhea, gynecomastia.
F and E: sodium and water retention.

INTERACTIONS

Drug-Drug: ▪ Additive hypotension with other **antihypertensive agents, nitrates,** or acute ingestion of **alcohol** ▪ Increased risk of arrhythmias with **cardiac glycosides, quinidine, procainamide,** or other **antiarrhythmics** ▪ Excitement and hypertension may result from concurrent **MAO inhibitor** therapy ▪ May decrease the therapeutic response to **ephedrine** or **levodopa** ▪ May increase responsiveness to **direct-acting sympathomimetic amines (dopamine, dobutamine, metaraminol, phenylephrine)** ▪ Additive CNS depression with other **CNS depressants,** including **alcohol, antihistamines, antidepressants, narcotic analgesics,** or **sedative/hypnotics.**

ROUTE AND DOSAGE

- **PO (Adults):** 0.1–0.25 mg/day in 1–2 divided doses.
- **PO (Children):** 5–20 mcg/kg/day in 1–2 divided doses.

PHARMACODYNAMICS (antihypertensive effect)

	ONSET	PEAK	DURATION
PO	several days–3 wk	3–6 wk	1–6 wk

{} = Available in Canada only.
*Underlines indicate most frequent; **CAPITALS** indicate life-threatening

NURSING IMPLICATIONS

Assessment

- ▫ Monitor blood pressure and pulse frequently during initial dosage adjustment and periodically throughout course of therapy. Notify physician of significant changes.
- ▫ Monitor intake and output ratios and daily weight and assess for edema daily, especially at beginning of therapy. Notify physician of weight gain or edema. Reserpine is commonly administered concurrently with diuretics.
- ▫ Assess patient for depression, early morning insomnia, anorexia, impotence, and self-depreciation. Notify physician promptly if these symptoms develop, as this may necessitate discontinuation of the medication. Mental depression may have an insidious onset and may be severe enough to cause suicide. Risk of depression may persist for several mons following discontinuation of therapy.
- ▪ **Lab Test Considerations:** May cause an increase in serum prolactin concentrations.
- ▫ May cause a decrease in urinary catecholamine excretion and urinary vanillylmandelic acid excretion.

Potential Nursing Diagnoses

- ▪ Coping, ineffective individual (side effects).
- ▪ Knowledge deficit related to medication regimen (patient/family teaching).
- ▪ Noncompliance (patient/family teaching).

Implementation

- ▪ **General Info:** Available in combination with thiazide diuretics (see Appendix A).
- ▪ **PO:** Administer with meals or milk to minimize GI irritation.

Patient/Family Teaching

- ▫ Emphasize the importance of continuing to take this medication, even if feeling better. Instruct patient to take medication at the same time each day. If a dose is missed, omit and return to regular dosage schedule. Do not double doses. Consult physician prior to discontinuing medication.
- ▫ Encourage patient to comply with additional interventions for hypertension (weight reduction, low-sodium diet, discontinuation of smoking, moderation of alcohol consumption, regular exercise, and stress management). Reserpine helps control but does not cure hypertension.
- ▫ Instruct patient and family on proper technique for blood pressure monitoring. Advise them to check blood pressure at least weekly and to report significant changes to physician.
- ▫ Reserpine may cause drowsiness. Advise patient to avoid driving or other activities requiring alertness until response to medication is known.
- ▫ If dry mouth occurs, frequent mouth rinses, good oral hygiene, or sugarless gum or candy may decrease effect. Notify dentist if dry mouth persists >2 wk.
- ▫ Caution patient to avoid concurrent use of alcohol or other CNS depressants with this medication.
- ▫ May cause nasal stuffiness. Advise patient to consult physician or pharmacist before taking any cough, cold, decongestant, or allergy remedies. Patient should also avoid excessive amounts of coffee, tea, or cola.
- ▫ Advise patient to inform physician or dentist of medication regimen prior to treatment or surgery.
- ▫ Instruct patient to notify physician promptly if abdominal pain, depression, or change in sleep patterns occurs.
- ▫ Emphasize the importance of follow-up examinations to monitor progress.

Evaluation

Effectiveness of therapy can be demonstrated by: ▪ Decrease in blood pressure without appearance of side effects.

R

Rh_o (D) IMMUNE GLOBULIN
(arr aych oh dee im-**yoon** **glob**-yoo-lin)
Rh_o (D) IMMUNE GLOBULIN STANDARD DOSE
Gamulin Rh, HypRho-D, Rhesonativ, RhoGAM
Rh_o (D) GLOBULIN MICRODOSE
HypRho-D Mini-Dose, MICRho-GAM, Mini-Gamulin Rh

CLASSIFICATION(S):
Serum immune globulin
Pregnancy Category C

INDICATIONS

▪ Administered to Rh_o(D)-negative patients who have beeen exposed to Rh_o(D)-positive blood by: ▫ Delivering an Rh_o(D)-positive infant ▫ Miscarrying or aborting a Rh_o(D)-positive fetus ▫ Having amniocentesis or intra-abdominal trauma while carrying an Rh_o(D)-positive fetus ▪ Following accidental transfusion of Rh_o(D)-positive blood to an Rh_o(D)-negative patient.

ACTION

▪ Prevents the production of anti-Rh_o(D) antibodies in Rh_o(D)-negative patients who have been exposed to Rh_o(D)-positive blood. **Therapeutic Effects:** ▪ Prevention of antibody response and subsequent prevention of hemolytic disease of the newborn (erythroblastosis fetalis) in future pregnancies of women who have conceived an Rh_o(D)-positive fetus ▪ Prevention of Rh_o(D) sensitization following transfusion accident.

PHARMACOKINETICS

Absorption: Well absorbed from IM sites.
Distribution: Distribution not known.
Metabolism and Excretion: Metabolism and excretion are not known.
Half-life: UK.

CONTRAINDICATIONS AND PRECAUTIONS

Contraindicated in: ▪ Rh_o(D)- or D^u-positive patients ▪ Patients previously sensitized to Rh_o(D) or D^u ▪ Hypersensitivity to thimerisol (some products).
Use Cautiously in: ▪ Patients with previous hypersensitivity reactions to immune globulins.

ADVERSE REACTIONS AND SIDE EFFECTS*

Local: pain at IM site.
Misc: fever.

INTERACTIONS

Drug–Drug: ▪ May decrease antibody response to some **live virus vaccines (measles, mumps, rubella)**.

ROUTE AND DOSAGE

Following Delivery

▪ **IM (Adults):** 1 vial standard dose within 72 hr of delivery.

Prior to Delivery

▪ **IM (Adults):** 1 vial standard dose at 28 wk, 1 vial standard dose 72 hr after delivery.

Termination of Pregnancy (<13 wk Gestation)

▪ **IM (Adults):** 1 vial standard dose of *microdose* within 72 hr.

Termination of Pregnancy (>13 wk Gestation)

▪ **IM (Adults):** 1 vial standard dose within 72 hr.

Large Fetal-Maternal Hemorrhage

▪ **IM (Adults):** Packed red blood cell volume of hemorrhage/15 = number of vials of standard dose preparation (round to next whole number of vials).

Transfusion Accident

▪ **IM (Adults):** (Volume of Rh-positive blood administered × Hct of donor blood)/15 = number of vials of standard dose preparation (round to next whole number of vials).

*Underlines indicate most frequent; **CAPITALS** indicate life-threatening.

PHARMACODYNAMICS

	ONSET	PEAK	DURATION
IM	rapid	UK	UK

NURSING IMPLICATIONS

Assessment

- **Lab Test Considerations:** Type and cross-match of mother's and newborn's cord blood must be performed to determine need for medication. Mother must be $Rh_o(D)$-negative and D^{u}-negative. Infant must be $Rh_o(D)$-positive. If there is doubt regarding infant's blood type or if father is $Rh_o(D)$-positive, medication should be given.
- □ An infant born to a woman treated with $Rh_o(D)$ immune globulin antepartum may have a weakly positive direct Coombs' test result on cord or infant blood.

Potential Nursing Diagnoses

- Knowledge deficit related to medication regimen (patient/family teaching).

Implementation

- **General Info:** Do not give to infant, to $Rh_o(D)$-positive individual, or to $Rh_o(D)$-negative individual previously sensitized to the $Rh_o(D)$ antigen.
- **IM:** Administer into the deltoid muscle. Dose should be given within 3 hr but may be given up to 72 hr after delivery, miscarriage, abortion, or transfusion. Do not administer IV.

Patient/Family Teaching

- □ Explain to patient that the purpose of this medication is to protect future $Rh_o(D)$-positive infants.

Evaluation

Effectiveness of therapy can be demonstrated by: ▪ Prevention of erythroblastosis fetalis in future $Rh_o(D)$-positive infants ▪ Prevention of $Rh_o(D)$ sensitization following transfusion accident.

RIBAVIRIN

(rye-ba-**vye**-rin)
Virazole

CLASSIFICATION(S):
Antiviral
Pregnancy Category X

INDICATIONS

▪ Treatment of severe lower respiratory tract infections caused by the respiratory syncytial virus (RSV) in infants and young children. **Unlabeled Use:** ▪ Early (within 24 hr of symptoms) secondary treatment of influenza A or B in young adults.

ACTION

▪ Inhibits viral DNA and RNA synthesis and subsequent replication ▪ Must be phosphorylated intracellularly to be active. **Therapeutic Effect:** ▪ Virustatic action.

PHARMACOKINETICS

Absorption: Systemic absorption occurs following nasal and oral inhalation.
Distribution: 70% of inhaled drug is deposited in the respiratory tract. Appears to concentrate in the respiratory tract and red blood cells. Enters breast milk.
Metabolism and Excretion: Eliminated from the respiratory tract by distribution across membranes, macrophages, and ciliary motion. Metabolized primarily by the liver.
Half-life: 9.5 hr (40 days in red blood cells).

CONTRAINDICATIONS AND PRECAUTIONS

Contraindicated in: ▪ Hypersensitivity ▪ Women with childbearing potential.
Use Cautiously in: ▪ Patients receiving mechanically assisted ventilation ▪ Underlying anemia ▪ Adults (safety not established).

ADVERSE REACTIONS AND SIDE EFFECTS*

CNS: dizziness, faintness.
CV: CARDIAC ARREST, hypotension.
Derm: rash.
EENT: ocular irritation, erythema of the eyelids, conjunctivitis, photosensitivity, blurred vision.
Hemat: reticulocytosis.

INTERACTIONS

Drug–Drug: ▪ May antagonize the antiviral action of **zidovudine** ▪ May potentiate the hematologic toxicity of **zidovudine** ▪ May increase the risk of **cardiac glycoside** toxicity.

ROUTE AND DOSAGE

- **Inhaln (Infants and Young Children):** Mist of 190 mcg/liter via SPAG-2 aerosol generator and oxygen hood, face mask, or oxygen tent at a rate of 12.5 liter mist/min for 12–18 hr/day for 3–7 days or 15 liter/min when using an oxygen hood or tent or 12 liter/min when using a face mask.

PHARMACODYNAMICS (blood levels)

	ONSET	PEAK	DURATION
Inhaln	UK	end of inhaln	UK

NURSING IMPLICATIONS

Assessment

- □ Assess patient for infection (vital signs, sputum, WBC) at beginning and throughout course of therapy.
- □ Obtain specimens for culture and sensitivity prior to initiating therapy. First dose may be given before receiving results.
- □ Assess respiratory status (lung sounds, quality and rate of respirations) prior to and throughout therapy.

Potential Nursing Diagnoses

- ▪ Infection, high risk for (indications, side effects).
- ▪ Gas exchange, impaired (indications).
- ▪ Knowledge deficit related to medication regimen (patient/family teaching).

Implementation

- ▪ **General Info:** Do not administer ribavirin to infants requiring assisted ventilation, because precipitation of the drug in the respiratory equipment may interfere with safe and effective patient ventilation.
- □ Ribavirin treatment should begin within the first 3 days of respiratory syncytial virus (RSV) infection to be effective.
- ▪ **Inhaln:** Ribavirin aerosol should be administered using the Viratek SPAG model SPAG-2 only. Do not administer via other aerosol-generating devices. Usually administered using an infant oxygen hood attached to the SPAG-2 aerosol generator. Administration by face mask may be used if the oxygen hood cannot be used.
- □ Reconstitute ribavirin 6-g vial with preservative-free sterile water for injection or inhalation. Transfer to clean, sterilized Erlenmeyer flask of the SPAG-2 reservoir and dilute to a final volume of 300 ml. This recommended concentration (20 mg/ml) in the reservoir provides a concentration of aerosol ribavirin of 190 mcg/liter of air over a 12-hr period. Soln should be discarded and replaced every 24 hr.
- □ Frequency of aerosol treatments may vary from continuous aerosolization for 3–7 days to aerosolization for a 4-hr period 3 times/day for 3 days.

Patient/Family Teaching

- □ Explain the purpose and route of treatment to the patient and parents.
- □ Inform patient and parents that ribavirin may cause blurred vision and photosensitivity.
- □ Emphasize the importance of receiving ribavirin for the full course of therapy and on a regular or continuous schedule.

*Underlines indicate most frequent; **CAPITALS** indicate life-threatening.

EVALUATION

Clinical response can be evaluated by: ▪ Resolution of the signs and symptoms of respiratory syncytial virus.

RIBOFLAVIN

(rye-boe-flay-vin)
vitamin B_2

CLASSIFICATION(S):
Vitamin–water-soluble
Pregnancy Category UK

INDICATIONS

▪ Treatment and prevention of riboflavin deficiency, which may be associated with poor nutritional status or chronic debilitating illnesses.

ACTION

▪ Serves as a coenzyme for metabolic reactions involving transfer of hydrogen ions ▪ Necessary for normal red blood cell function. **Therapeutic Effect:** ▪ Replacement in or prevention of deficiency.

PHARMACOKINETICS

Absorption: Well absorbed from the upper GI tract by an active transport process.
Distribution: Widely distributed. Crosses the placenta and enters breast milk.
Metabolism and Excretion: Amounts in excess of requirements are excreted unchanged by the kidneys.
Half-life: 66–84 min.

CONTRAINDICATIONS AND PRECAUTIONS

Contraindicated in: ▪ No known contraindications.
Use Cautiously in: ▪ No known precautions.

ADVERSE REACTIONS AND SIDE EFFECTS*

GU: yellow discoloration of urine (large doses only).

INTERACTIONS

Drug–Drug: ▪ **Phenothiazines, tricyclic antidepressants, probenecid,** and chronic ingestion of **alcohol** increase ribloflavin requirements.

ROUTE AND DOSAGE

Treatment of Deficiency

- **PO (Adults):** 5–30 mg/day in divided doses.
- **PO (Children):** 3–10 mg/day.

Dietary Supplement

- **PO (Adults and Children):** 1–4 mg/day.

PHARMACODYNAMICS

	ONSET	PEAK	DURATION
PO	UK	UK	UK

NURSING IMPLICATIONS

ASSESSMENT

- □ Assess patient for signs of vitamin B_2 deficiency (dermatoses, stomatitis, ocular inflammation and irritation, photophobia, and cheilosis) prior to and periodically throughout therapy.
- ▪ **Lab Test Considerations:** May cause false elevations in urobilinogen and urinary catecholamine measurements.

POTENTIAL NURSING DIAGNOSES

- ▪ Nutrition, altered: less than body requirements (indications).
- ▪ Knowledge deficit related to medication regimen (patient/family teaching).

IMPLEMENTATION

- ▪ **General Info:** Because of infrequency of single B-vitamin deficiencies, combinations are commonly administered.

PATIENT/FAMILY TEACHING

- □ Instruct patient to take as ordered. If a dose is missed, it may be omitted, as an extended period of time is required to become deficient in riboflavin.
- □ Encourage patient to comply with physician's diet recommendations. Explain that the best source of vita-

*Underlines indicate most frequent; **CAPITALS** indicate life-threatening.

R

mins is a well-balanced diet with foods from the 4 basic food groups. Foods high in riboflavin include dairy products, enriched flour, nuts, meats, and green leafy vegetables; little is lost from cooking.
- Patients self-medicating with vitamin supplements should be cautioned not to exceed RDA (see Appendix L). The effectiveness of megadoses for treatment of various medical conditions is unproven and may cause side effects.
- Advise patient to avoid alcoholic beverages, as alcohol impairs the absorption of riboflavin.
- Explain to patient that medically insignificant increase in yellow coloration of urine may occur.
- Emphasize the importance of follow-up examinations to evaluate progress.

Evaluation

Effectiveness of therapy can be demonstrated by: ▪ Prevention of decrease in the symptoms of riboflavin deficiency.

RIFAMPIN

(rif-**am**-pin)

Rifadin, Rifampicin, Rimactane, {Rofact}

CLASSIFICATION(S):
Antitubercular
Pregnancy Category UK

INDICATIONS

▪ Used in combination with other agents in the management of active tuberculosis ▪ Used to eliminate carriers of meningococcal disease ▪ Prophylaxis *Hemophilus influenzae* type B infection.

ACTION

▪ Inhibits RNA synthesis by blocking RNA transcription in susceptible organisms. **Therapeutic Effect:** ▪ Bactericidal action against susceptible organisms. **Spectrum:** ▪ Broad spectrum notable for activity against: ▫ *Mycobacteria* ▫ *Staphylococcus aureus* ▫ *Hemophilus influenzae* ▫ *Legionella pneumophila* ▫ *Neisseria meningitidis.*

PHARMACOKINETICS

Absorption: Well absorbed following oral administration.

Distribution: Widely distributed into many body tissues and fluids, including CSF. Crosses the placenta and enters breast milk.

Metabolism and Excretion: Mostly metabolized by the liver. 60% eliminated in the feces via biliary elimination.

Half-life: 3 hr.

CONTRAINDICATIONS AND PRECAUTIONS

Contraindicated in: ▪ Hypersensitivity ▪ Pregnancy or lactation.

Use Cautiously in: ▪ History of liver disease ▪ Concurrent use of other hepatotoxic agents.

ADVERSE REACTIONS AND SIDE EFFECTS*

CNS: headache, drowsiness, confusion, fatigue, ataxia, weakness.

GI: nausea, vomiting, heartburn, abdominal pain, flatulence, diarrhea, hepatitis.

Hemat: hemolytic anemia, thrombocytopenia.

MS: myalgia, arthralgia.

Misc: flu-like syndrome, red discoloration of all body fluids.

INTERACTIONS

Drug-Drug: ▪ Rifampin stimulates liver enzymes, which may increase metabolism and decrease the effectiveness of other drugs, including **glucocorticoids, disopyramide, quinidine, narcotic analgesics, oral hypoglycemic agents, oral anticoagulants, estrogens,** and **oral contraceptive agents** ▪ Increased risk of hepatotoxicity with other

{} = Available in Canada only.

*Underlines indicate most frequent; **CAPITALS** indicate life-threatening.

hepatotoxic agents, including **alcohol, isoniazid, ketoconazole,** and **miconazole.**

ROUTE AND DOSAGE

Tuberculosis

- **PO (Adults):** 10 mg/kg/day (usual dose 600 mg/day); may also be given twice weekly.
- **PO (Children):** 10–20 mg/kg/day (not to exceed 600 mg/day).

Asymptomatic Carriers of Meningococcus

- **PO (Adults):** 600 mg bid for 2 days.
- **PO (Children 1–12 yr):** 10 mg/kg bid for 2 days.
- **PO (Infants 3 mon–1 yr):** 5 mg/kg bid for 2 days.

Prophylaxis of Hemophilus Influenzae Type B Infection

- **PO (Adults and Children):** 20 mg/kg/day (up to 600 mg) as a single dose for 4 days.

PHARMACODYNAMICS (blood levels)

	ONSET	PEAK	DURATION
PO	rapid	2–4 hr	24 hr

NURSING IMPLICATIONS

Assessment

- Mycobacterial studies and susceptibility tests should be performed prior to and periodically throughout therapy to detect possible resistance.
- Assess lung sounds and character and amount of sputum periodically throughout therapy.
- **Lab Test Considerations:** Hepatic and renal function, CBC, and urinalysis should be evaluated periodically throughout course of therapy.
- May cause increased BUN, SGOT (AST), SGPT (ALT), and serum alkaline phosphatase, bilirubin, and uric acid concentrations.
- May cause false-positive direct Coombs' test results. May interfere with folic acid and vitamin B_{12} assays.

Potential Nursing Diagnoses

- Infection, high risk for (indications).
- Knowledge deficit related to medication regimen (patient/family teaching).
- Noncompliance (patient/family teaching).

Implementation

- **General Info:** Available in combination with isoniazid. (See Appendix A.)
- **PO:** Administer medication on an empty stomach, at least 1 hr before or 2 hr after meals. If GI irritation becomes a problem, may be administered with food. Antacids may also be taken 1 hr prior to administration. Capsules may be opened and contents mixed with applesauce or jelly for patients with difficulty swallowing.
- Pharmacist can compound a syrup for patients unable to swallow solids.

Patient/Family Teaching

- Advise patient to take medication once daily (unless biweekly regimens are used), exactly as directed; not to skip doses or double up on missed doses. Emphasize the importance of continuing therapy even after symptoms have subsided. Course of therapy commonly lasts for 1–2 yr. Patients on short-term prophylactic therapy should also be advised of the importance of compliance with therapy.
- Advise patient to notify physician promptly if signs and symptoms of hepatitis (yellow eyes and skin, nausea, vomiting, anorexia, unusual tiredness, weakness) or thrombocytopenia (unusual bleeding or bruising) occur.
- Caution patient to avoid the use of alcohol during this therapy, as this may increase the risk of hepatotoxicity.
- Instruct patient to report the occurrence of flu-like symptoms (fever, chills, myalgia, headache) promptly.
- Rifampin may occasionally cause drowsiness. Caution patient to avoid driving or other activities requiring

alertness until response to medication is known.

- □ Inform patient that saliva, sputum, sweat, tears, urine, and feces may become red-orange to red-brown, and that soft contact lenses may become permanently discolored.
- □ Advise patient that this medication has teratogenic properties. Counsel patient to use a nonhormonal form of contraception throughout therapy.
- □ Emphasize the importance of regular follow-up examinations to monitor progress and to check for side effects.

Evaluation

Effectiveness of therapy can be demonstrated by: ▪ Decreased fever and night sweats □ Diminished cough and sputum production □ Negative sputum cultures □ Increased appetite □ Weight gain □ Reduced fatigue □ Sense of well-being in patients with tuberculosis ▪ Prevention of meningococcal meningitis ▪ Prevention of *Hemophilus influenzae* type B infection. Prophlactic course is usually short-term.

SALIVA SUBSTITUTES

(sa-**lye**-va **sub**-sti-toot)

Moi-Stir, Orex, Salivart, Xero-Lube

CLASSIFICATION(S):
Saliva substitutes
Pregnancy Category UK

INDICATIONS

▪ Management of dry mouth or throat, which may occur as a consequence of: □ Medications (tricyclic antidepressants, antihistamines, anticholinergics) □ Radiation therapy □ Chemotherapy □ Other illnesses.

ACTION

▪ Composition is similar to saliva ▪ Contains electrolytes in a thickening agent (carboxymethylcellulose). **Therapeutic Effect:** ▪ Relief of dry mouth.

PHARMACOKINETICS

Absorption: Electrolytes may be absorbed through oral mucosa.
Distribution: Distribution not known.
Metabolism and Excretion: Metabolism and excretion not known.
Half-life: UK.

CONTRAINDICATIONS AND PRECAUTIONS

Contraindicated in: ▪ Hypersensitivity to carboxymethylcellulose, parabens, or other components.
Use Cautiously in: ▪ Situations in which absorption of electrolytes may compromise the patient's condition, such as potassium and magnesium in patients with renal failure or sodium in patients with congestive heart failure or hypertension.

ADVERSE REACTIONS AND SIDE EFFECTS*

F and E: excessive absorption of electrolytes.

INTERACTIONS

Drug–Drug: ▪ None significant.

ROUTE AND DOSAGE

- ▪ **PO (Adults):** Spray or apply to oral mucosa as needed.

PHARMACODYNAMICS (relief of dry mouth)

	ONSET	PEAK	DURATION
PO	upon application	UK	UK

NURSING IMPLICATIONS

Assessment

- □ Assess patient for xerostomia (dry mouth) or dry throat prior to and periodically throughout therapy.
- □ Assess gingiva and oral mucosa for stomatitis.

Potential Nursing Diagnoses

- ▪ Oral mucous membranes, altered (indications).
- ▪ Knowledge deficit related to medica-

*Underlines indicate most frequent; **CAPITALS** indicate life-threatening.

tion regimen (patient/family teaching).

Implementation

- **General Info:** Administer as necessary for xerostomia or dry throat.

Patient/Family Teaching

- Instruct patient to swish saliva substitute around in mouth following spray or application.
- Advise patient of the importance of good oral hygiene in addition to the use of saliva substitutes.
- Emphasize the importance of routine dental examinations throughout course of therapy.

Evaluation

Effectiveness of therapy can be demonstrated by: ▪ Decrease in dry mouth and throat.

SALSALATE

(**sal**-sa-late)

salicylsalycylic acid, Arthra-G, Dilsalcid, Mono-Gesic, Salflex, Salsitab

CLASSIFICATION(S):

Non-narcotic analgesic, Nonsteroidal anti-inflammatory agent, Antipyretic

Pregnancy Category C

INDICATIONS

▪ Treatment of mild to moderate pain ▪ Management of inflammatory disorders including: ▫ Rheumatoid arthritis ▫ Osteoarthritis ▪ Treatment of fever.

ACTION

▪ Produces analgesia and reduces inflammation by inhibiting the production of prostaglandins ▪ Unlike aspirin, has no effect on platelet function. **Therapeutic Effects:** ▪ Analgesia resulting in reduction of mild to moderate pain ▪ Reduction of inflammation ▪ Reduction of fever.

PHARMACOKINETICS

Absorption: Splits into 2 molecules of salicylic acid following oral administration. Absorbed in the small intestine.

Distribution: Rapidly and widely distributed. Crosses the placenta and enters breast milk.

Metabolism and Excretion: Amount excreted unchanged by the kidneys depends on urine pH. As pH increases, amount excreted unchanged increases from 2–3% up to 80%.

Half-life: 2–3 hr for low doses. For larger doses, half-life may increase up to 15–30 hr due to saturation of liver metabolism.

CONTRAINDICATIONS AND PRECAUTIONS

Contraindicated in: ▪ Hypersensitivity to aspirin or other nonsteroidal anti-inflammatory agents (less cross-sensitivity than aspirin).

Use Cautiously in: ▪ Renal insufficiency (magnesium toxicity may occur) ▪ Severe liver impairment ▪ Pregnancy (may have adverse effects on fetus and mother) ▪ Lactation (safety not established) ▪ Children or adolescents with viral infections (may increase the risk of Reye's Syndrome).

ADVERSE REACTIONS AND SIDE EFFECTS*

EENT: tinnitus, hearing loss.

GI: dyspepsia, heartburn, epigastric distress, nausea, vomiting, anorexia, abdominal pain, GI BLEEDING, hepatotoxicity.

Misc: noncardiogenic pulmonary edema; allergic reactions, including ANAPHYLAXIS or LARYNGEAL EDEMA.

INTERACTIONS

Drug-Drug: ▪ May enhance the activity of **penicillins, phenytoin, methotrexate, oral hypoglycemic agents, valproic acid,** and **sulfonamides** ▪ May antagonize the beneficial effects of **probenecid** or **sulfinpyrazone** ▪ **Glucocorticoids** may decrease serum salicylate levels. ▪ **Urinary acidification** enhances re-

*Underlines indicate most frequent; **CAPITALS** indicate life-threatening.

S

absorption and may increase serum salicylate levels ▪ **Alkalinization of the urine** or the ingestion of large amounts of **antacids** promotes excretion and decreases serum salicylate levels ▪ May blunt the therapeutic response to **diuretics** or **antihypertensives** ▪ May increase the risk of bleeding with **anticoagulants, thrombolytic agents, cefamandole, cefoperazone, cefotetan, moxalactam, valproic acid,** or **plicamycin** (effect less than aspirin) ▪ Increased risk of GI irritation with **nonsteroidal anti-inflammatory agents** (effect less than aspirin) ▪ Increased risk of ototoxicity with **vancomycin**.

Drug–Food: ▪ **Foods capable of acidifying the urine** (see Appendix K) may enhance reabsorption and increase serum salicylate levels.

ROUTE AND DOSAGE

- **PO (Adults):** 3000 mg/day in divided doses.

PHARMACODYNAMICS (analgesia and fever reduction)*

	ONSET	PEAK	DURATION
PO	5–30 min	1–3 hr	3–6 hr

*Antirheumatic effect may take 2–3 wk of chronic dosing.

NURSING IMPLICATIONS

Assessment

- **General Info:** Patients who have asthma, allergies, and nasal polyps or who are allergic to tartrazine dyes are at an increased risk for developing hypersensitivity reactions.
- **Pain:** Assess pain and limitation of movement; note type, location, and intensity prior to and 1–3 hr following administration.
- **Fever:** Assess fever and note associated signs (diaphoresis, tachycardia, malaise, chills).
- **Toxicity and Overdose:** Observe patient for the onset of tinnitus, hyperventilation, agitation, mental confusion, lethargy, diarrhea, and sweating. If these symptoms appear, withhold medication and notify physician immediately.

Potential Nursing Diagnoses

- Comfort, altered: pain (indications).
- Mobility, impaired physical (indications).
- Knowledge deficit related to medication regimen (patient/family teaching).

Implementation

- **PO:** Administer after meals or with food or an antacid to minimize gastric irritation. Food slows but will not alter the total amount absorbed.

Patient/Family Teaching

- Instruct patient to take with a full glass of water and to remain in an upright position for 15–30 min after administration.
- Advise patient to report tinnitus, unusual bleeding of gums, bruising, or black, tarry stools, or fever lasting longer than 3 days.
- Caution patient to avoid concurrent use of alcohol with this medication to minimize possible gastric irritation.
- Advise patients on long-term therapy to inform physician or dentist of medication regimen prior to surgery.
- Centers for Disease Control warn against giving salicylates to children or adolescents with varicella (chickenpox) or influenza-like or viral illnesses because of a possible association with Reye's syndrome.

Evaluation

Effectiveness of therapy can be demonstrated by: ▪ Decrease in severity of mild to moderate discomfort ▪ Increased ease of joint movement ▪ Reduction of fever.

SARGRAMOSTIM

(sar-**gram**-oh-stim)

Leukine, Prokine, rhu GM-CSF, recombinant human—granulocyte/macrophage colony stimulating factor

CLASSIFICATION(S):

Colony stimulating factor

Pregnancy Category C

INDICATIONS

▪ Acceleration of bone marrow recovery following autologous bone marrow transplantation in patients with non-Hodgkin's lymphoma, acute lymphoblastic leukemia, or Hodgkin's disease.

ACTION

▪ Consists of a glycoprotein produced by recombinant DNA technique that is capable of binding to and stimulating the production, division, differentiation, and activation of granulocytes and macrophages. **Therapeutic Effect:** ▪ Accelerated recovery of bone marrow following autologous bone marrow transplantation resulting in decreased risk of infection and other complications.

PHARMACOKINETICS

Absorption: Following IV administration absorption is essentially complete.
Distribution: Distribution not known.
Metabolism and Excretion: Metabolism and excretion not known.
Half-life: UK.

CONTRAINDICATIONS AND PRECAUTIONS

Contraindicated in: ▪ Presence of ≥10% leukemic myeloid blast cells in bone marrow or peripheral blood ▪ Hypersensitivity to GM-CSF, yeast products, or additives (mannitol, tromethamine, or sucrose).
Use Cautiously in: ▪ Pre-existing fluid retention, congestive heart failure, or pulmonary infiltrates ▪ Pre-existing cardiac disease ▪ Myeloid malignancies ▪ Previous extensive radiation or chemotherapy (response may be limited) ▪ Pregnancy (use only if clearly needed) ▪ Lactation or children (safety not established).

ADVERSE REACTIONS AND SIDE EFFECTS*

CNS: weakness, malaise.
Resp: dyspnea.
CV: transient supraventricular tachycardia, peripheral edema, pericardial effusion.
GI: diarrhea.
Derm: rash.
MS: bone pain.
Misc: fever, chills.

INTERACTIONS

Drug-Drug: ▪ **Lithium** or **glucocorticoids** may potentiate myeloproliferative effects of sargramostim.

ROUTE AND DOSAGE

- **IV (Adults):** 250 mcg/m²/day for 21 days as a 2-hr infusion. Begin 2–4 hr after bone marrow infusion, and not less than 24 hr after last chemotherapy or 12 hr after last radiation. Dosage modification or discontinuation required if WBC >50,000 cells/mm³ or ANC >20,000 cells/mm³.

PHARMACODYNAMICS (noted as effects on blood counts)

	ONSET	PEAK	DURATION
IV	rapid	UK	3–7 days

NURSING IMPLICATIONS

Assessment

□ Monitor heart rate, blood pressure, and respiratory status during and immediately following infusion. If dyspnea develops, slow infusion rate by half; may require discontinuation of medication. Assess for peripheral edema daily throughout therapy.

▪ **Lab Test Considerations:** Obtain a CBC and platelet count prior to chemotherapy and twice weekly during therapy to avoid leukocytosis. Monitor absolute neutrophil count (ANC), may increase rapidly. If ANC >20,000/mm³, WBC >50,000/mm³, or platelet count >500,000/mm³, interrupt administration and reduce dose by half. Excessive blood levels usually return to baseline 3–7 days following discontinuation of therapy.

□ Monitor renal and hepatic function

*Underlines indicate most frequent; **CAPITALS** indicate life-threatening.

prior to and biweekly throughout therapy in patients with renal or hepatic dysfunction.

Potential Nursing Diagnoses

- Infection, high risk for (indications).
- Knowledge deficit related to medication regimen (patient/family teaching).

Implementation

- **General Info:** Administer 2–4 hr after bone marrow transplant and no earlier than 24 hr following cytotoxic chemotherapy or 12 hr after last dose of radiotherapy.
- □ Refrigerate, but do not freeze powder, reconstituted soln, or diluted soln. Do not shake. Discard if left at room temperature for >6 hr. Vial is for one time use only.
- **Intermittent Infusion:** Reconstitute with 1 ml of sterile water without preservatives injected toward side of vial. Swirl gently to avoid foaming. Soln should be clear and colorless.
- □ Dilute in 0.9% NaCl. If final concentration is <10 mcg/ml, add a final concentration of 0.1% human albumin to 0.9% NaCl prior to addition of sargramostim to prevent absorption of the components of the drug delivery system. Do not admix with other medications.
- □ *Rate:* Infuse over 2 hr.

Patient/Family Teaching

- □ Instruct patient to notify nurse or physician if dyspnea or palpitations occur.

Evaluation

Effectiveness of therapy can be demonstrated by: ▪ Decreased incidence of infection in patients following autologous bone marrow transplantation.

SCOPOLAMINE

(scoe-**pol**-a-meen)
{Bucospan}, Isopto Hyoscine, TransdermScōp, {Transderm-V}, Triptone

CLASSIFICATION(S):
Anticholinergic–antimuscarinic, Antiemetic–anticholinergic, Ophthalmic–mydriatic
Pregnancy Category C

INDICATIONS

▪ **Transdermal:** Prevention of motion sickness ▪ **IM, IV, SC:** Preoperatively to produce amnesia and to decrease salivation and excessive respiratory secretions ▪ **Ophth:** Mydriatic.

ACTION

▪ Inhibits the muscarinic activity of acetylcholine ▪ Corrects the imbalance of acetylcholine and norepinephrine in the CNS, which may be responsible for motion sickness. **Therapeutic Effects:** ▪ Reduction of nausea and vomiting associated with motion sickness ▪ Preoperative amnesia and decreased secretions ▪ Mydriasis.

PHARMACOKINETICS

Absorption: Well absorbed following IM, SC, and transdermal administration.
Distribution: Crosses the placenta and blood-brain barrier.
Metabolism and Excretion: Mostly metabolized by the liver.
Half-life: 8 hr.

CONTRAINDICATIONS AND PRECAUTIONS

Contraindicated in: ▪ Hypersensitivity ▪ Narrow-angle glaucoma ▪ Acute hemorrhage ▪ Tachycardia secondary to cardiac insufficiency or thyrotoxicosis.
Use Cautiously in: ▪ Elderly patients, infants, and children (increased risk of adverse reactions) ▪ Possible intestinal obstruction ▪ Prostatic hypertrophy ▪ Chronic renal, hepatic, pulmonary, or cardiac disease ▪ Pregnancy or lactation (safety not established).

ADVERSE REACTIONS AND SIDE EFFECTS*

CNS: drowsiness, confusion.
EENT: blurred vision, mydriasis, photophobia.
CV: palpitations, tachycardia.
GI: dry mouth, constipation.
GU: urinary hesitancy, urinary retention.
Derm: decreased sweating.

INTERACTIONS

Drug-Drug: ▪ Additive anticholinergic effects with **antihistamines, antidepressants, quinidine,** or **disopyramide** ▪ Additive CNS depression with **alcohol, antidepressants, antihistamines, narcotic analgesics,** or **sedative/hypnotics** ▪ May alter the absorption of other **orally administered drugs** by slowing motility of the GI tract ▪ May increase GI mucosal lesions in patients taking oral **wax-matrix potassium chloride preparations.**

ROUTE AND DOSAGE

Prevention of Motion Sickness

- **Transdermal (Adults):** 1.5-mg system (delivers 0.5 mg over 72 hr) applied at least 4 hr prior to travel. Canadian product (Transderm-V) delivers 1 mg over 72 hr and should be applied 12 hr prior to travel.

Parenteral Doses

- **IM, IV, SC (Adults):** 0.3–0.65 mg, may be repeated 3–4 times daily (0.2–1 mg for antiemetic effect; 0.2–0.6 mg for inhibition of salivation; 0.32–0.65 mg for amnesic effects; 0.6 mg for sedation).
- **IM, IV, SC (Children):** 0.006 mg/kg or 0.2 mg/m^2.

Ophthalmic Use

- **Ophth (Adults):** 1–2 drops of 0.25% soln.
- **Ophth (Children):** 1 drop of 0.25% soln.

PHARMACODYNAMICS (PO, IM, IV, SC, Transdermal = antiemetic, sedative properties, Ophth = mydriasis)

	ONSET	PEAK	DURATION
PO, IM, SC	30 min	1 hr	4–6 hr
IV	10 min	1 hr	2–4 hr
Transdermal	4 hr	UK	72 hr
Ophth	10–30 min	30–45 min	several days

NURSING IMPLICATIONS

Assessment

- □ Assess patient for signs of urinary retention periodically throughout course of therapy.
- □ Monitor heart rate periodically throughout parenteral therapy.
- □ Assess patient for pain prior to administration. Scopolamine may act as a stimulant in the presence of pain, producing delirium if used without morphine or meperidine.

Potential Nursing Diagnoses

- Oral mucous membranes, altered (indications, side effects).
- Injury, high risk for (side effects).
- Knowledge deficit related to medication regimen (patient/family teaching).

Implementation

- **Direct IV:** Scopolamine should be diluted with sterile water for injection prior to IV administration. Inject slowly.
- **Syringe Compatibility:** atropine, benzquinamide, butorphanol, chlorpromazine, cimetidine, dimenhydrinate, diphenhydramine, droperidol, fentanyl, glycopyrrolate, hydromorphone, hydroxyzine, meperidine, metoclopramide, midazolam, morphine, nalbuphine, pentazocine, pentobarbital, perphenazine, prochlorperazine edisylate, promazine, promethazine, ranitidine, or thiopental.
- **Y-Site Compatibility:** heparin, hydrocortisone sodium succinate, or potassium chloride.

*Underlines indicate most frequent; **CAPITALS** indicate life-threatening.

S

- **Additive Compatibility:** meperidine or succinylcholine.
- **Ophth:** Instruct patient to lie down or tilt head back and look at ceiling. Pull down on lower lid, creating a small pocket, and instill soln into pocket. Apply pressure to the inner canthus for 1–2 min to prevent systemic absorption. Wait 5 min before instilling other ophthalmic solns.

Patient/Family Teaching

- **General Info:** Instruct patient to take medication exactly as prescribed. If a dose is missed, take as soon as remembered. Do not double doses.
  - Medication may cause drowsiness or blurred vision. Caution patient to avoid driving or other activities requiring alertness until response to medication is known.
  - Patient should use caution when exercising and in hot weather; overheating may result in heatstroke.
  - Advise patient to avoid concurrent use of alcohol and other CNS depressants with this medication.
  - Inform patient that frequent mouth rinses, good oral hygiene, and sugarless gum or candy may minimize dry mouth.
- **Transdermal:** Instruct patient on application of transdermal patches. Apply at least 4 hr before exposure to travel to prevent motion sickness. Wash hands and dry thoroughly before and after application. Apply to hairless, clean, dry area behind ear; avoid areas with cuts or irritation. Apply pressure over system to ensure contact with skin. System is effective for 3 days. If system becomes dislodged, replace with a new system on another site behind the ear. System is waterproof and not affected by bathing or showering.
- **Ophth:** Caution patient that this medication may increase sensitivity of eyes to light. Dark glasses may minimize this effect. Notify physician if this lasts longer than 7 days after discontinuation.

Evaluation

Effectiveness of therapy can be demonstrated by: ▪ Decrease in salivation and respiratory secretion preoperatively ▪ Postoperative amnesia ▪ Prevention of motion sickness ▪ Mydriasis.

SECOBARBITAL

(see-koe-**bar**-bi-tal)
{Novosecobarb}, Seconal

CLASSIFICATION(S):
Sedative/hypnotic–barbiturate
Schedule II (oral, parenteral); III (rectal)
Pregnancy Category C

INDICATIONS

▪ Hypnotic agent (short-term use) ▪ Preoperative or other sedative ▪ Adjunct to regional or spinal anesthesia (IV only).

ACTION

▪ Produces all levels of CNS depression. **Therapeutic Effects:** ▪ Induction of sleep ▪ Sedation.

PHARMACOKINETICS

Absorption: Well absorbed following oral, IM, or rectal administration.
Distribution: Widely distributed, highest concentration in brain and liver. Crosses the placenta; small amounts enter breast milk.
Metabolism and Excretion: Metabolized by the liver.
Half-life: 30 hr.

CONTRAINDICATIONS AND PRECAUTIONS

Contraindicated in: ▪ Hypersensitivity ▪ Pre-existing CNS depression ▪ Uncontrolled severe pain ▪ Pregnancy or lactation.
Use Cautiously in: ▪ Hepatic or renal impairment ▪ Patients who may be suicidal or have been previously addicted to drugs ▪ Elderly patients (dosage reduction recommended) ▪ Chronic ob-

{} = Available in Canada only.

structive pulmonary disease ▪ Prolonged use (may lead to physical dependence).

ADVERSE REACTIONS AND SIDE EFFECTS*

CNS: drowsiness, lethargy, vertigo, depression, hangover, excitation, delirium.
Resp: respiratory depression; IV—LARYNGOSPASM, bronchospasm.
CV: hypotension (IV only).
GI: nausea, vomiting, diarrhea, constipation.
Derm: rashes, urticaria, photosensitivity.
Local: phlebitis at IV site.
MS: arthralgia, myalgia.
Neuro: neuralgia.
Misc: hypersensitivity reactions, including ANGIOEDEMA and serum sickness; psychological dependence, physical dependence.

INTERACTIONS

Drug–Drug: ▪ Additive CNS depression with other **CNS depressants,** including **alcohol, antihistamines, antidepressants, narcotic analgesics,** and other **sedative/hypnotics** ▪ **Valproates** may decrease metabolism and increase CNS depression ▪ Stimulates hepatic enzymes, which metabolize other drugs, resulting in decreased effectiveness of **oral contraceptives, chloramphenicol, cyclosporine, glucocorticoids, dacarbazine, levothyroxine,** and **quinidine**.

ROUTE AND DOSAGE

Hypnotic

- **PO, IM (Adults):** 100–200 mg.
- **IM (Children):** 3–5 mg/kg (not to exceed 100 mg).

Preoperative (Sedation)

- **PO (Adults):** 100–300 mg 1–2 hr preop.
- **PO (Children):** 50–100 mg 1–2 hr preop.
- **Rect (Children >3 yr):** 60–120 mg.
- **Rect (Children 6 mon–3 yr):** 60 mg.
- **Rect (Children <6 mon):** 30–60 mg.

Sedation

- **PO, Rect (Adults):** 100–300 mg/day in 3 divided doses.
- **PO, Rect (Children):** 6 mg/kg/day in 3 divided doses.

Adjunct to Regional or Spinal Anesthesia

- **IV (Adults):** 50–100 mg.

PHARMACODYNAMICS (hypnotic effect)

	ONSET	PEAK	DURATION
PO	15 min	15–30 min	1–4 hr
IM	UK	7–10 min	1–4 hr
IV	rapid	1–3 min	15 min
Rect	UK	15–30 min	1–4 hr

NURSING IMPLICATIONS

Assessment

- Assess sleep patterns prior to and periodically throughout course of therapy. Hypnotic doses of secobarbital suppress REM sleep. Patient may experience an increase in dreaming upon discontinuation of medication.
- Monitor respiratory status, pulse, and blood pressure frequently in patients receiving secobarbital IV. Equipment for resuscitation and artificial ventilation should be readily available.
- Prolonged therapy may lead to psychological or physical dependence. Restrict amount of drug available to patient, especially if depressed, suicidal, or with a history of addiction.
- Assess postoperative patients for pain. Secobarbital may increase responsiveness to painful stimuli.

Potential Nursing Diagnoses

- Sleep pattern disturbance (indications).
- Injury, high risk for (side effects).
- Knowledge deficit related to medication regimen (patient/family teaching).

Implementation

- **General Info:** Supervise ambulation and transfer of patients following administration. Remove cigarettes. Side

*Underlines indicate most frequent; **CAPITALS** indicate life-threatening.

S

rails should be raised and call bell within reach at all times.

- **IM:** Do not administer SC. Injections should be given deep into the gluteal muscle to minimize tissue irritation. Do not inject more than 5 ml into any one site because of tissue irritation.
- **Direct IV:** May be administered undiluted or diluted with sterile water for injection, 0.9% NaCl, or Ringer's soln. Do not dilute with lactated Ringer's soln. Do not use soln that is discolored or that contains particulate matter.
- □ Soln is highly alkaline; avoid extravasation, which may cause tissue damage and necrosis. If extravasation occurs, infiltration with 5% procaine soln into affected area and application of moist heat may be ordered.
- □ *Rate:* Administer each 50 mg over at least 1 min. Titrate slowly for desired response. Rapid administration may result in respiratory depression, apnea, laryngospasm, bronchospasm, or hypertension.
- **Syringe Incompatibility:** benzquinamide, cimetidine, glycopyrrolate, or pentazocine.
- **Additive Compatibility:** amikacin or aminophylline.
- **Additive Incompatibility:** atracurium, chlorpromazine, clindamycin, codeine, droperidol, ephedrine, erythromycin gluceptate, hydrocortisone sodium succinate, insulin, levorphanol, methadone, norepinephrine, pancuronium, pentazocine, phenytoin, procaine, sodium bicarbonate, streptomycin, succinylcholine, tetracycline, or vancomycin.
- **Rect:** To ensure accurate dose, do not divide rectal suppository. Suppositories should be refrigerated.

PATIENT/FAMILY TEACHING

- □ Advise patient to take medication exactly as prescribed. Do not increase dose without consulting physician.
- □ Discuss the importance of preparing environment for sleep (dark room, quiet, avoidance of nicotine and caffeine).
- □ Advise patients on prolonged therapy not to discontinue medication without consulting physician. Abrupt withdrawal may precipitate withdrawal symptoms.
- □ Medication may cause daytime drowsiness. Caution patient to avoid driving and other activities requiring alertness until response to medication is known.
- □ Caution patient to avoid taking alcohol or other CNS depressants concurrently with this medication.
- □ Instruct patient to contact physician immediately if pregnancy is planned or suspected.

EVALUATION

Effectiveness of therapy can be demonstrated by: ▪ Improvement in sleep pattern without excessive daytime sedation. Therapy is usually limited to a 2-wk period ▪ Sedation

SELEGILINE

(se-**le**-ji-leen)

Eldepryl, L-deprenyl

CLASSIFICATION(S):

Antiparkinson agent

Pregnancy Category C

INDICATIONS

▪ Management of Parkinson's disease in conjunction with levodopa/carbidopa therapy in patients who fail to respond to levodopa/carbidopa alone.

ACTION

▪ Following conversion by monoamine oxidase to its active form, selegiline inactivates monoamine oxidase by irreversibly binding to it at type B (brain) sites ▪ Inactivation of monoamine oxidase leads to increased amounts of dopamine available in the CNS. **Therapeutic Effect:** ▪ Increased response to levodopa/dopamine therapy in Parkinson's disease.

PHARMACOKINETICS

Absorption: Appears to be well absorbed following oral administration.
Distribution: Widely distributed.
Metabolism and Excretion: Metabolism involves some conversion to amphetamine and methamphetamine. 45% excreted in urine as metabolites.
Half-life: UK.

CONTRAINDICATIONS AND PRECAUTIONS

Contraindicated in: ▪ Hypersensitivity ▪ Concurrent meperidine or narcotic analgesic therapy (possible fatal reactions).
Use Cautiously in: ▪ Doses >10 mg/day (increased risk of hypertensive reactions with tyramine-containing foods and some medications).

ADVERSE REACTIONS AND SIDE EFFECTS*

CNS: dizziness, lightheadedness, fainting, confusion, hallucinations, vivid dreams.
GI: <u>nausea</u>, abdominal pain, dry mouth.

INTERACTIONS

Drug–Drug: ▪ May initially increase risk of side effects of **levodopa/carbidopa** (dosage of levodopa/carbidopa may need to be decreased by 10–30%) ▪ Concurrent use with **meperidine** or other **narcotic analgesics** may possibly result in a potentially fatal reaction (excitation, sweating, rigidity, and hypertension; or hypotension and coma).
Drug–Food: ▪ Doses >10 mg/day may produce hypertensive reactions with **tyramine-containing foods** (see list in Appendix K).

ROUTE AND DOSAGE

- **PO (Adults):** 5 mg bid (with breakfast and lunch).

PHARMACODYNAMICS (onset of beneficial effects in Parkinson's disease)

	ONSET	PEAK	DURATION
PO	2–3 days	UK	UK

NURSING IMPLICATIONS

Assessment

- Assess patient for signs and symptoms of Parkinson's disease (tremor, muscle weakness and rigidity, ataxic gait) prior to and throughout therapy.
- Assess blood pressure periodically throughout therapy.

Potential Nursing Diagnoses

- Mobility, impaired physical (indications).
- Injury, high risk for (indications, side effects).
- Knowledge deficit related to medication regimen (patient/family teaching).

Implementation

- **General Info:** An attempt to reduce the dose of levodopa/carbidopa by 10–30% may be made after 2–3 days of selegiline therapy.
- **PO:** Administer 5-mg tablet with breakfast and lunch.

Patient/Family Teaching

- Instruct patient to take medication exactly as directed. Caution patient that taking more than the prescribed dose may increase side effects and place patient at risk for hypertensive crisis if foods containing tyramine are consumed (see Appendix K).
- Inform patient and family of the signs and symptoms of MAO inhibitor-induced hypertensive crisis (severe headache, chest pain, nausea, vomiting, photosensitivity, enlarged pupils). Advise patient to notify physician immediately if severe headache or any other unusual symptoms occurs.

*<u>Underlines</u> indicate most frequent; **CAPITALS** indicate life-threatening.

S

Evaluation

Effectiveness of therapy can be demonstrated by: ▪ Improved response to levodopa/carbidopa in patients with Parkinson's disease.

SENNA

(se-na)

Black Draught, Fletcher's Castoria, Senexon, Senokot, Senolax, X-Prep Liquid

CLASSIFICATION(S):

Laxative–stimulant

Pregnancy Category UK

INDICATIONS

▪ Treatment of constipation, particularly when associated with: ▫ Slow transit time ▫ Constipating drugs ▫ Irritable or spastic bowel syndrome ▫ Neurologic constipation.

ACTION

▪ Active components (sennosides) alter water and electrolyte transport in the large intestine, resulting in accumulation of water and increased peristalsis.
Therapeutic Effect: ▪ Laxative action.

PHARMACOKINETICS

Absorption: Minimally absorbed following oral administration.
Distribution: Distribution not known.
Metabolism and Excretion: Converted to active laxative compounds by bacteria in the colon.
Half-life: UK.

CONTRAINDICATIONS AND PRECAUTIONS

Contraindicated in: ▪ Hypersensitivity ▪ Abdominal pain of unknown cause, especially if associated with fever ▪ Rectal fissures ▪ Ulcerated hemorrhoids.
Use Cautiously in: ▪ Chronic use (may lead to laxative dependence) ▪ Pregnancy or lactation (safety not established) ▪ Possible intestinal obstruction.

ADVERSE REACTIONS AND SIDE EFFECTS*

GI: diarrhea, cramping, nausea.
GU: pink-red or brown-black discoloration of urine.
F and E: electrolyte abnormalities (chronic use or dependence).
Misc: laxative dependence.

INTERACTIONS

Drug-Drug: ▪ May decrease absorption of other **orally administered drugs,** due to decreased transit time.

ROUTE AND DOSAGE

Laxative

- **PO (Adults and Children >12 yr):** 0.5–2 g of senna or 12–50 mg of sennosides 1–2 times daily.
- **PO (Children 6–11 yr):** 50% of adult dose.
- **PO (Children 1–5 yr):** 33% of adult dose.

Evacuation of Colon Prior to X-Rays

- **PO (Adults):** 105–157.5 mg of sennosides 12–14 hr prior to examination.

PHARMACODYNAMICS (laxative effect)

	ONSET	PEAK	DURATION
PO	6–12 hr*	UK	3–4 days

*May take as long as 24 hr.

NURSING IMPLICATIONS

Assessment

- ▫ Assess patient for abdominal distention, presence of bowel sounds, and usual pattern of bowel function.
- ▫ Assess color, consistency, and amount of stool produced.

Potential Nursing Diagnoses

- Bowel elimination, altered: constipation (indications).
- Bowel elimination, altered: diarrhea (side effects).
- Knowledge deficit related to medication regimen (patient/family teaching).

*Underlines indicate most frequent; **CAPITALS** indicate life-threatening.

Implementation

- **General Info:** Available in tablets, oral soln, syrup, and granules. Available in combination with docusate and psyllium (see Appendix A).
- **PO:** Take with a full glass of water. Administer at bedtime for evacuation 6–12 hr later. Administer on an empty stomach for more rapid results.
  - Shake oral soln well before administering.
  - Granules should be dissolved or mixed in water or other liquid before administration.

Patient/Family Teaching

- Advise patient that laxatives should be used only for short-term therapy. Long-term therapy may cause electrolyte imbalance and dependence.
- Encourage patient to use other forms of bowel regulation, such as increasing bulk in the diet, increasing fluid intake, increasing mobility. Normal bowel habits are individualized and may vary from 3 times/day to 3 times/wk.
- Inform patient that this medication may cause a change in urine color to pink, red, violet, yellow, or brown.
- Instruct patients with cardiac disease to avoid straining during bowel movements (Valsalva maneuver).
- Advise patient not to use laxatives when abdominal pain, nausea, vomiting, or fever are present.

Evaluation

Effectiveness of therapy can be demonstrated by: ■ A soft, formed bowel movement.

SILVER SULFADIAZINE

(**sil**-ver sul-fa-**dye**-a-zeen)
{Flamazine}, Flint SSD, Silvadene, Thermazene

CLASSIFICATION(S):
Anti-infective—topical
Pregnancy Category C

INDICATIONS

■ Prevention and treatment of infection in patients with 2nd- and 3rd-degree burns.

ACTION

■ Splits to produce bactericidal concentrations of silver and sulfadiazine ■ Action is at level of cell membrane and cell wall. **Therapeutic Effect:** ■ Bactericidal action against organisms found in burns. **Spectrum:** ■ Broad spectrum includes activity against many gram-negative and gram-positive pathogens, some fungi, and anaerobes.

PHARMACOKINETICS

Absorption: Small amounts of silver are systemically absorbed following topical application. Up to 10% of sulfadiazine is absorbed.
Distribution: Distribution not known.
Metabolism and Excretion: Absorbed sulfadiazine is excreted unchanged by the kidneys.
Half-life: UK.

CONTRAINDICATIONS AND PRECAUTIONS

Contraindicated in: ■ Infants <2 mon (risk of kernicterus) ■ Pregnancy near term (increased risk of kernicterus in infant) ■ G6-PD deficiency.
Use Cautiously in: ■ Hypersensitivity to sulfonamides, silver, or parabens ■ Cross-sensitivity with thiazides, sulfonylurea oral hypoglycemic agents, or carbonic anhydrase inhibitors may exist ■ Impaired hepatic or renal function ■ Pregnancy (use only if burn area is >20% of BSA).

ADVERSE REACTIONS AND SIDE EFFECTS*

GU: crystalluria.
Derm: pain, burning, itching.
Hemat: leukopenia.

INTERACTIONS

Drug-Drug: ■ Silver may inactivate concurrently applied topical **proteolytic**

{} = Available in Canada only.
*Underlines indicate most frequent; **CAPITALS** indicate life-threatening.

S

enzymes (fibronolysin, desoxyribonuclease).

ROUTE AND DOSAGE

- **Top (Adults and Children):** Apply 1% cream 1–2 times daily in layer 1/16 in thick.

PHARMACODYNAMICS (anti-infective action)

	ONSET	PEAK	DURATION
Top	on contact	UK	as long as applied

NURSING IMPLICATIONS

Assessment

- □ Assess burned tissue for infection (purulent discharge, excessive moisture, odor, and culture results) and sepsis (WBC, fever, or shock) prior to and throughout course of therapy.
- □ Monitor for hypersensitivity reaction (rash, itching, or burning) at and surrounding sites of application.
- **Lab Test Considerations:** Monitor renal function studies and CBC periodically when applied to large area, as systemic absorption may cause nephritis and reversible leukopenia. Decrease in neutrophil count is greatest 4 days after initiation of therapy; levels usually normalize after 2–3 days.

Potential Nursing Diagnoses

- Infection, high risk for (indications).
- Skin integrity, impaired: actual (indications).
- Knowledge deficit related to medication regimen (patient/family teaching).

Implementation

- **General Info:** Generally applied after cleansing and debriding of burn wound. Premedicate with analgesic.
- **Top:** Cream is white; discard if it becomes dark.
- □ Use sterile technique to apply. Cover entire wound at depth of 1/16 in. Reapply on sites where cream rubs off as a result of patient movement; burn should be coated at all times. Burn may be dressed or kept open, depending upon physician's order.

Patient/Family Teaching

- □ Explain purpose of medication to patient and family. This medication will not stain skin.

Evaluation

Effectiveness of therapy can be demonstrated by: ▪ Prevention and treatment of infection in 2nd- and 3rd-degree burns. Therapy is continued until burn is healed or skin graft is performed.

SIMETHICONE

(si-**meth**-i-kone)
Extra Strength Gas-X, Gas-X, Mylicon, {Ovol}, Phazyme

CLASSIFICATION(S):
Antiflatulent
Pregnancy Category UK

INDICATIONS

- Relief of painful symptoms of excess gas in the GI tract that may occur postoperatively or as a consequence of: □ Air swallowing □ Dyspepsia □ Peptic ulcer □ Diverticulitis.

ACTION

- Causes the coalescence of gas bubbles ▪ Does not prevent the formation of gas. **Therapeutic Effect:** ▪ Passage of gas through the GI tract by belching or passing flatus.

PHARMACOKINETICS

Absorption: No systemic absorption occurs.
Distribution: Not systemically distributed.
Metabolism and Excretion: Excreted unchanged in the feces.
Half-life: UK.

CONTRAINDICATIONS AND PRECAUTIONS

Contraindicated in: ▪ Not recommended for infant colic.

Use Cautiously in: ▪ Abdominal pain of unknown cause, especially when accompanied by fever.

ADVERSE REACTIONS AND SIDE EFFECTS*

▪ None significant.

INTERACTIONS

Drug–Drug: ▪ None significant.

ROUTE AND DOSAGE

▪ **PO (Adults):** 40–120 mg qid, after meals and at bedtime.

PHARMACODYNAMICS (antiflatulent effect)

	ONSET	PEAK	DURATION
PO	immediate	UK	3 hr

NURSING IMPLICATIONS

Assessment

□ Assess patient for abdominal pain, distention, and bowel sounds prior to and periodically throughout course of therapy. Frequency of belching and passage of flatus should also be assessed.

Potential Nursing Diagnoses

▪ Comfort, altered: pain (indications).
▪ Knowledge deficit related to medication regimen (patient/family teaching).

Implementation

▪ **General Info:** Available in combination with many other drugs (see Appendix A).
▪ **PO:** Administer after meals and at bedtime for best results. Shake liquid preparations well prior to administration. Chewable tablets should be chewed thoroughly before swallowing for faster and more complete results.

Patient/Family Teaching

□ Explain to patient the importance of diet and exercise in the prevention of gas. Also explain that this medication does not prevent the formation of gas.
□ Advise patient to notify physician if symptoms are persistent.

Evaluation

Effectiveness of therapy can be demonstrated by: ▪ Decrease in abdominal distention and discomfort.

SODIUM BICARBONATE

(**soe**-dee-um bye-**kar**-boe-nate)
Baking Soda, Bell-ans, Citrocarbonate, Neut, Soda Mint

CLASSIFICATION(S):
Electrolyte modifier—alkalinizing agent, Antacid
Pregnancy Category C

INDICATIONS

▪ **PO, IV:** Management of metabolic acidosis ▪ **PO, IV:** Used to alkalinize urine and promote excretion of certain drugs in overdosage situations (phenobarbital, aspirin) ▪ **PO:** Antacid.

ACTION

▪ Acts as an alkalinizing agent by releasing bicarbonate ions ▪ Following oral administration, releases bicarbonate, which is capable of neutralizing gastric acid. **Therapeutic Effects:** ▪ Alkalinization ▪ Neutralization of gastric acid.

PHARMACOKINETICS

Absorption: Following oral administration, excess bicarbonate is absorbed and results in metabolic alkalosis and alkaline urine.
Distribution: Widely distributed into extracellular fluid.
Metabolism and Excretion: Sodium and bicarbonate are excreted by the kidneys.
Half-life: UK.

CONTRAINDICATIONS AND PRECAUTIONS

Contraindicated in: ▪ Metabolic or respiratory alkalosis ▪ Hypocalcemia

*Underlines indicate most frequent; **CAPITALS** indicate life-threatening.

▪ Excessive chloride loss ▪ As an antidote following ingestion of strong mineral acids ▪ Patients on sodium-restricted diets (oral use as an antacid only) ▪ Renal failure (oral use as an antacid only) ▪ Severe abdominal pain of unknown cause, especially if associated with fever (oral use as an antacid only).

Use Cautiously in: ▪ Congestive heart failure ▪ Renal insufficiency ▪ Concurrent glucocorticoid therapy ▪ Chronic use as an antacid (may cause metabolic alkalosis and possible sodium overload).

ADVERSE REACTIONS AND SIDE EFFECTS*

CV: edema.
F and E: sodium and water retention, metabolic alkalosis, hypernatremia, hypokalemia, hypocalcemia.
GI: PO—gastric distention, flatulence.
Local: irritation at IV site.
Neuro: tetany.

INTERACTIONS

Drug-Drug: ▪ Following oral administration may decrease the absorption of **ketoconazole** ▪ Concurrent use with **calcium-containing antacids** may lead to milk-alkali syndrome ▪ Urinary alkalinization may result in decreased **salicylate** or **barbiturate** blood levels or increased blood levels of **quinidine, mexiletine, flecainide,** or **amphetamines.**

ROUTE AND DOSAGE

Note: Contains 12 mEq of sodium/g.

Antacid
- **PO (Adults):** 0.3–4 g qid.

Metabolic Acidosis
Dose should be determined on the basis of frequent lab assessment.
- **PO (Adults):** 20–36 mEq/day in divided doses.
- **IV (Adults and Children >12 yr):** 2–5 mEq/kg as a 4–8-hr infusion.

Cardiopulmonary Resuscitation
Dose should be determined on the basis of frequent lab assessment.
- **IV (Adults):** 1 mEq/kg may repeat 0.5 mEq/kg q 10 min.
- **IV (Neonates and Children):** 1 mEq/kg, may repeat q 10 min.

Alkalinization of Urine
- **PO (Adults):** 48 mEq (4 g) initially. Then 12–24 mEq (1–2 g) q 4 hr (up to 48 mEq q 4 hr).
- **PO (Children):** 1–10 mEq/kg (12–120 mg/kg) per day in divided doses.

PHARMACODYNAMICS (PO = antacid effect, IV = alkalinization)

	ONSET	PEAK	DURATION
PO	immediate	30 min	1–3 hr
IV	immediate	rapid	UK

NURSING IMPLICATIONS

Assessment
- ▫ Assess fluid balance (intake and output, daily weight, edema, lung sounds) throughout course of therapy. Notify physician if symptoms of fluid overload (hypertension, edema, dyspnea, rales/crackles, frothy sputum) occur.
- ▫ Assess patient for signs of acidosis (disorientation, headache, weakness, dyspnea, hyperventilation), alkalosis (confusion, irritability, paresthesia, tetany, altered breathing pattern), hypernatremia (edema, weight gain, hypertension, tachycardia, fever, flushed skin, mental irritability), or hypokalemia (weakness, fatigue, U wave on ECG, arrhythmias, polyuria, polydipsia) throughout therapy.
- ▫ Observe IV site closely. Avoid extravasation, as tissue irritation or cellulitis may occur. If infiltration occurs, confer with physician regarding warm compresses and infiltration of site with lidocaine or hyaluronidase.
- ▪ **Lab Test Considerations:** Monitor se-

*Underlines indicate most frequent; **CAPITALS** indicate life-threatening.

rum sodium, potassium, calcium, bicarbonate concentrations, serum osmolarity, acid/base balance, and renal function prior to and periodically throughout course of therapy.

- Arterial blood gases (ABGs) should be obtained frequently in emergency situations.
- Monitor urine pH frequently when used for urinary alkalinization.
- Antagonizes effects of pentagastrin and histamine during gastric acid secretion test. Avoid administration during the 24 hr preceding the test.

- **Antacid:** Assess patient for epigastric or abdominal pain and frank or occult blood in the stool, emesis, or gastric aspirate.

Potential Nursing Diagnoses

- Gas exchange, impaired (indications).
- Fluid volume excess (side effects).
- Knowledge deficit related to medication regimen (patient/family teaching).

Implementation

- **General Info:** This medication may cause premature dissolution of enteric-coated tablets in the stomach.
- **PO:** Tablets must be thoroughly chewed and taken with a full glass of water. Effervescent tablets should be completely dissolved before drinking.
  - When used in treatment of peptic ulcers, physician may order administration 1 and 3 hr after meals and at bedtime.
- **SC:** Must be diluted to isotonicity to prevent tissue irritation or cellulitis. Dilute 1 ml of 8.4% sodium bicarbonate soln with 4.6 ml of sterile water for injection; 1 ml of 7.5% soln with 4.0 ml of sterile water for injection; or 1 ml of the 4.2% soln with 1.8 ml of sterile water for injection to prepare 1.5% isotonic soln.
- **Direct IV:** Administer direct IV push in arrest situation. Use premeasured ampules or prefilled syringes to assure accurate dosage. Dosages should be based on ABG results. Dosage may be repeated every 10 min.
  - Flush IV line before and after administration to prevent incompatible medications used in arrest management from precipitating.
- **Intermittent/Continuous Infusion:** May be diluted in dextrose, saline, and dextrose/saline combinations.
- **Syringe Compatibility:** pentobarbital.
- **Syringe Incompatibility:** glycopyrrolate, metoclopramide, or thiopental.
- **Y-Site Compatibility:** acyclovir, famotidine, heparin with hydrocortisone sodium succinate, insulin, morphine, potassium chloride, or tolazoline.
- **Y-Site Incompatibility:** amrinone, calcium chloride, or verapamil.
- **Additive Compatibility:** amikacin, aminophylline, amobarbital, amphotericin B, ampicillin, atropine, bretylium, calcium chloride, calcium gluceptate, cefoxitin, cephalothin, cephapirin, chloramphenicol, chlorothiazide, cimetidine, clindamycin, droperidol/fentanyl, ergonovine maleate, erythromycin, heparin, hyaluronidase, hydrocortisone sodium succinate, kanamycin, lidocaine, metaraminol, methotrexate, methyldopate, multivitamins, nafcillin, netilmicin, oxacillin, oxytocin, phenobarbital, phenylephrine, phenytoin, phytonadione, potassium chloride, prochlorperazine, promazine, sodium iodide, thiopental, or verapamil.
- **Additive Incompatibility:** ascorbic acid, carmustine, cefotaxime, cisplatin, codeine, corticotropin, dobutamine, dopamine, epinephrine, hydromorphone, imipenem cilastatin, insulin, isoproterenol, labetalol, magnesium sulfate, meperidine, methadone, morphine, norepinephrine, penicillin G potassium, pentazocine, pentobarbital, procaine, secobarbital, streptomycin, succinylcholine, or tetracycline. Do not add to Ringer's soln, lactated Ringer's soln, or Ionosol

products as compatibility varies with concentration.

Patient/Family Teaching

- **General Info:** Instruct patient to take medication as directed. A missed dose should be taken as soon as remembered unless almost time for next dose.
  - Review symptoms of electrolyte imbalance with patients on chronic therapy; instruct patient to notify physician if these symptoms occur.
  - Advise patient not to take milk products concurrently with this medication. Renal calculi or hypercalcemia (milk-alkali syndrome) may result.
  - Emphasize the importance of regular follow-up examinations to monitor serum electrolyte levels and acid-base balance and to monitor progress.
- **Antacid:** Advise patient to avoid routine use of sodium bicarbonate for indigestion. Dyspepsia that persists >2 wk should be evaluated by a physician.
  - Advise patient on sodium-restricted diet to avoid use of baking soda as a home remedy for indigestion.
  - Instruct patient to notify physician if indigestion is accompanied by chest pain, difficulty breathing, or diaphoresis or if stools become dark and tarry.

Evaluation

Effectiveness of therapy can be demonstrated by: ▪ Increase in urinary pH ▪ Clinical improvement of acidosis ▪ Enhanced excretion of selected overdoses and poisonings ▪ Decreased gastric discomfort.

SODIUM CHLORIDE

(**soe**-dee-um **klor**-ide)
NaCl, Salt

CLASSIFICATION(S):
Electrolyte—replacement soln, Abortifacient
Pregnancy Category UK

INDICATIONS

▪ **IV:** Hydration and provision of sodium chloride in deficiency states ▪ Maintenance of fluid and electrolyte status in situations in which losses may be excessive (excess diuresis or severe salt restriction) ▪ 0.45% ("half-normal saline") soln is most commonly used for hydration and in the treatment of hyperosmolar diabetes ▪ 0.9% ("normal saline") soln is used for: ▫ Replacement ▫ To treat metabolic alkalosis ▫ A priming fluid for hemodialysis ▫ To begin and end blood transfusions ▫ May also be used as an irrigating soln ▪ Small volumes of 0.9% sodium chloride (preservative-free or bacteriostatic) are used to reconstitute or dilute other mediations ▪ Hypertonic soln (3%, 5%) may be required in situations in which rapid replacement of sodium is necessary: ▫ Hyponatremia ▫ Hypochloremia ▫ Renal failure ▫ Heart failure. ▪ **PO:** Used orally to prevent heat prostration when excessive sweating occurs during exposures to high temperatures ▪ **Intra-amniotic:** 20% soln is used as an oxytocic agent to induce abortion.

ACTION

▪ Sodium is a major cation in extracellular fluid and helps maintain water distribution, fluid and electrolyte balance, acid-base equilibrium, and osmotic pressure ▪ Chloride is the major anion in extracellular fluid and is involved in maintaining acid-base balance. Solns of sodium chloride resemble extracellular fluid. **Therapeutic Effects:** ▪ ***IV, PO:*** Replacement in deficiency states and maintenance of homeostasis ▪ ***Intra-amniotic:*** Expulsion of fetus.

PHARMACOKINETICS

Absorption: Well absorbed following oral administration. Replacement solns of sodium chloride are administered IV only. Sodium may be systemically absorbed following intra-amniotic instillation.

Distribution: Rapidly and widely distributed.

Metabolism and Excretion: Excreted primarily by the kidneys.
Half-life: UK.

CONTRAINDICATIONS AND PRECAUTIONS

Contraindicated in: ▪ **IV solns:** no known contraindications ▪ **Intra-amniotic instillation:** contracting or hypertonic uterus, coagulopathies, ruptured membranes.

Use Cautiously in: ▪ Patients prone to metabolic, acid-base, or fluid and electrolyte abnormalities, including: ▫ Geriatric patients ▫ Those with nasogastric suctioning ▫ Vomiting ▫ Diarrhea ▫ Diuretic therapy ▫ Glucocorticoid therapy ▫ Fistulas ▫ Congestive heart failure ▫ Severe renal failure ▫ Severe liver diseases (additional electrolytes may be required) ▪ Sodium chloride preserved with benzyl alcohol should not be used in neonates ▪ **Intra-amniotic instillation:** ▫ Cardiovascular diseases ▫ Impaired renal function ▫ History of previous uterine surgery or adhesions ▫ History of seizures.

ADVERSE REACTIONS AND SIDE EFFECTS*

CV: PULMONARY EMBOLISM (intra-amniotic instillation only), edema, congestive heart failure, pulmonary edema.
Resp: pneumonia (intra-amniotic instillation only).
GU: renal cortical necrosis (intra-amniotic instillation only).
Derm: flushing (intra-amniotic instillation only).
F and E: hypokalemia, hypervolemia, hypernatremia.
Hemat: DISSEMINATED INTRAVASCULAR COAGULATION (intra-amniotic instillation only).
Local: extravasation, irritation at IV site.
Misc: fever, infection at injection site (intra-amniotic instillation only).

INTERACTIONS

Drug-Drug: ▪ Excessive amounts of sodium chloride may partially antagonize the effects of **antihypertensive medications** ▪ Increased risk of hypertonic uterus when intra-amniotic instillation is used concurrently with **oxytocic agents** ▪ Use with **glucocorticoids** may result in excess sodium retention.

ROUTE AND DOSAGE

0.9% Sodium Chloride (isotonic)
- **IV (Adults):** 1 liter (contains 150 mEq sodium per liter).

0.45% Sodium Chloride (hypotonic)
- **IV (Adults):** 1–2 liter (contains 75 mEq sodium per liter).

3%, 5% Sodium Chloride (hypertonic)
- **IV (Adults):** 100 ml over 1 hr (3% contains 50 mEq sodium per 100 ml; 5% contains 83.3 mEq sodium per 100 ml).

Oral Replacement
- **PO (Adults):** 1–2 g 3 times daily.

Intra-Amniotic Instillation
- **Intra-Amniotic (Adults):** Instill volume of 20% soln equal to volume of amniotic fluid removed in tap (up to 200–250 ml). If unsuccessful, may repeat in 48 hr.

PHARMACODYNAMICS (PO, IV = electrolyte effects, intra-amniotic = abortion time)

	ONSET	PEAK	DURATION
PO	UK	UK	UK
IV	rapid (min)	end of infusion	UK
Intra-amniotic	12–24 hr	UK	36 hr

NURSING IMPLICATIONS

Assessment
- ▫ Assess fluid balance (intake and output, daily weight, edema, lung sounds) throughout course of therapy.
- ▫ Assess patient for symptoms of hyponatremia (headache, tachycardia, lassitude, dry mucous membranes, nausea, vomiting, muscle cramps) or

*Underlines indicate most frequent; **CAPITALS** indicate life-threatening.

hypernatremia (edema, weight gain, hypertension, tachycardia, fever, flushed skin, mental irritability) throughout therapy. Sodium is measured in relation to its concentration to fluid in the body, and symptoms may change based on patient's hydration status.

- **Lab Test Considerations:** Monitor serum sodium, potassium, bicarbonate, and chloride concentrations and acid-base balance periodically for patients receiving prolonged therapy with sodium chloride.
- □ Monitor serum osmolarity in patients receiving hypertonic saline solns.

POTENTIAL NURSING DIAGNOSES

- Fluid volume deficit (indications).
- Fluid volume excess (side effects).

IMPLEMENTATION

- **General Info:** Dosage of sodium chloride depends on patient's age, weight, condition, fluid and electrolyte balance, and acid-base balance.
- □ Do not administer bacteriostatic sodium chloride containing benzyl alcohol as a preservative to neonates. This should not be used to reconstitute or to dilute soln or to flush intravascular cathethers in neonates.
- □ Infusion of 0.45% NaCl is hypotonic, 0.9% NaCl is isotonic, and 3% and 5% NaCl are hypertonic.
- □ Also available as a diluent and as a soln for irrigation.
- **Intermittent Infusion:** Administer 3% or 5% NaCl via a large vein and prevent infiltration. After the first 100 ml, sodium, chloride, and bicarbonate concentrations should be re-evaluated to determine the need for further administration.
- □ *Rate:* Rate should not exceed 100 ml/hr.
- **Additive Compatibility:** D5W, D10W, Ringer's and lactated Ringer's injection, dextrose/Ringer's soln combinations, dextrose/lactated Ringer's soln combinations, dextrose/saline combinations, or ⅙ M sodium lactate.
- **Additive Incompatibility:** amphotericin B, mannitol, or streptomycin.

PATIENT/FAMILY TEACHING

- □ Explain to patient the purpose of the infusion.

EVALUATION

Effectiveness of therapy can be demonstrated by: ▪ Prevention or correction of dehydration ▪ Normalization of serum sodium and chloride levels ▪ Prevention of heat prostration during exposure to high temperatures ▪ Induction of abortion.

SODIUM CITRATE AND CITRIC ACID

(**soe**-dee-um **sye**-trate and **sit**-rik **as**-id)

Bicitra, Oracit, Shohl's Solution modified

CLASSIFICATION(S):
Electrolyte modifier—alkalinizing agent, Antiurolithic
Pregnancy Category UK

INDICATIONS

▪ Management of chronic metabolic acidosis associated with chronic renal insufficiency or renal tubular acidosis ▪ Alkalinization of urine ▪ Prevention of cystine and urate urinary calculi ▪ Prevention of aspiration pneumonitis during surgical procedures.

ACTION

▪ Converted to bicarbonate in the body, resulting in increased blood pH ▪ As bicarbonate is renally excreted, urine is also alkalinized, increasing the solubility of cystine and uric acid ▪ Neutralizes gastric acid. **Therapeutic Effects:** ▪ Provision of bicarbonate in metabolic acidosis ▪ Alkalinization of the urine ▪ Prevention of cystine and urate urinary calculi ▪ Prevention of aspiration pneumonitis.

PHARMACOKINETICS

Absorption: Well absorbed following oral administration.

Distribution: Rapidly and widely distributed.

Metabolism and Excretion: Rapidly oxidized to bicarbonate, which is excreted primarily by the kidneys. Small amounts (<5%) excreted unchanged by the lungs.
Half-life: UK.

CONTRAINDICATIONS AND PRECAUTIONS

Contraindicated in: ▪ Severe renal insufficiency ▪ Severe sodium restriction ▪ Congestive heart failure, untreated hypertension, edema, or toxemia of pregnancy.
Use Cautiously in: ▪ Pregnancy or lactation (safety not established).

ADVERSE REACTIONS AND SIDE EFFECTS*

GI: diarrhea.
F and E: fluid overload, hypernatremia (severe renal impairment), metabolic alkalosis (large doses only), hypocalcemia.
MS: tetany.

INTERACTIONS

Drug–Drug: ▪ May partially antagonize the effects of **antihypertensives** ▪ Urinary alkalinization may result in decreased **salicylate** or **barbiturate** blood levels or increased blood levels of **quinidine, flecainide,** or **amphetamines**.

ROUTE AND DOSAGE

Note: Adjust dosage according to urine pH. Contains 1 mEq sodium/ml soln.

Alkalinizer

- **PO (Adults):** 1–3 g (10–30 ml soln) diluted in water qid.
- **PO (Children):** 500 mg–1.5 g (5–15 ml soln) qid.

Antiurolithic

- **PO (Adults):** 1–3 g (10–30 ml soln) diluted in water qid.

Neutralization of Gastric Acid

- **PO (Adults):** 1.5 g (15 ml soln) diluted in 15 ml of water.

PHARMACODYNAMICS (effects on serum pH)

	ONSET	PEAK	DURATION
PO	rapid (min–hr)	UK	4–6 hr

NURSING IMPLICATIONS

Assessment

- □ Assess patient for signs of alkalosis (confusion, irritability, paresthesia, tetany, altered breathing pattern) or hypernatremia (edema, weight gain, hypertension, tachycardia, fever, flushed skin, mental irritability) throughout therapy.
- □ Monitor patients with renal dysfunction for fluid overload (discrepancy in intake and output, weight gain, edema, rales/crackles, and hypertension).
- ▪ **Lab Test Considerations:** Prior to and every 4 mon throughout chronic therapy, monitor hematocrit, hemoglobin, electrolytes, pH, creatinine, urinalysis, and 24-hr urine for citrate.
- □ Monitor urine pH if used to alkalinize urine.

Potential Nursing Diagnoses

- ▪ Knowledge deficit related to medication regimen (patient/family teaching).

Implementation

- ▪ **PO:** Soln is more palatable if chilled. Administer with 30–90 ml of chilled water. Administer 30 min after meals or bedtime snack to minimize saline laxative effect.
- □ When used as preanesthetic, administer 15–30 ml of sodium citrate with 15–30 ml of chilled water.

Patient/Family Teaching

- □ Instruct patient to take as directed. Missed doses should be taken within 2 hr. Do not double doses.
- □ Instruct patients receiving chronic sodium citrate on correct method of monitoring urine pH, maintenance of alkaline urine, and the need to increase fluid intake to 3000 ml/day.

*Underlines indicate most frequent; **CAPITALS** indicate life-threatening.

- ▫ Advise patients receiving long-term therapy on need to avoid salty foods.

Evaluation

Effectiveness of therapy can be demonstrated by: ▪ Correction of metabolic acidosis ▪ Maintenance of alkaline urine with resulting decreased stone formation ▪ Buffering the pH of gastric secretions, thereby preventing aspiration pneumonitis associated with intubation and anesthesia.

SODIUM PHOSPHATE

(**soe**-dee-um **foss**-fate)

CLASSIFICATION(S):
Electroyte—phosphate supplement
Pregnancy Category C

INDICATIONS

▪ Treatment and prevention of phosphate depletion in patients who are unable to ingest adequate dietary phosphates.

ACTION

▪ Phosphate is present in bone and is involved in energy transfer and carbohydrate metabolism ▪ Serves as a buffer for the excretion of hydrogen ions by the kidney. **Therapeutic Effect:** ▪ Replacement of phosphorous in deficiency states.

PHARMACOKINETICS

Absorption: Administered IV only, resulting in complete bioavailability.

Distribution: Phosphates enter extracellular fluids and are then actively transported to sites of action.

Metabolism and Excretion: Excreted mainly (>90%) by the kidneys.

Half-life: UK.

CONTRAINDICATIONS AND PRECAUTIONS

Contraindicated in: ▪ Hyperphosphatemia ▪ Hypocalcemia ▪ Severe renal impairment.

Use Cautiously in: ▪ Hyperparathyroidism ▪ Cardiac disease ▪ Hypernatremia ▪ Hypertension.

ADVERSE REACTIONS AND SIDE EFFECTS*

Note: Related to hyperphosphatemia, unless indicated.

CNS: listlessness, confusion, weakness.

Resp: hypernatremia—shortness of breath.

CV: ARRHYTHMIAS, ECG changes (absent P waves, widening of the QRS complex with biphasic curve), CARDIAC ARREST, hypotension; hypernatremia—edema.

F and E: hypomagnesemia, hyperphosphatemia, hyperkalemia, hypocalcemia, hypernatremia.

GI: diarrhea, nausea, vomiting, abdominal pain.

Local: phlebitis, irritation at IV site.

MS: hypocalcemia—tremors.

Neuro: paresthesias of extremities, flaccid paralysis, heaviness of legs.

INTERACTIONS

Drug-Drug: ▪ Concurrent use of **glucocorticoids** with sodium phosphate may result in hypernatremia.

ROUTE AND DOSAGE

Note: Each ml contains 285 mg phosphate (3 millimoles phosphorus) and 4 mEq sodium.

- **IV (Adults):** 10–15 millimoles phosphorus/day as an infusion.
- **IV (Neonates):** 1.5–2 millimoles/kg/day (infused as part of parenteral nutrition).

PHARMACODYNAMICS (effects on serum phosphate levels)

	ONSET	PEAK	DURATION
IV	rapid (min–hr)	end of infusion	UK

*Underlines indicate most frequent; **CAPITALS** indicate life-threatening.

NURSING IMPLICATIONS

Assessment

- ▫ Assess patient for signs and symptoms of hypophosphatemia (anorexia, weakness, decreased reflexes, bone pain, confusion, blood dyscrasias) throughout course of therapy.
- ▫ Monitor intake and output ratios and daily weight. Report significant discrepancies to physician.
- ■ **Lab Test Considerations:** Monitor serum phosphate, potassium, sodium, and calcium levels prior to and periodically throughout therapy. Increased phosphate may cause hypocalcemia.
- ▫ Monitor renal function studies prior to and periodically throughout course of therapy.
- ■ **Toxcity and Overdose:** Symptoms of toxicity are those of hyperphosphatemia or hypocalcemia (paresthesia, muscle twitching, laryngospasm, colic, cardiac arrhythmias, Chvostek's or Trousseau's signs) or hypernatremia (thirst, dry flushed skin, fever, tachycardia, hypotension, irritability, decreased urine output).

Potential Nursing Diagnoses

- ■ Nutrition, altered: less than body requirements (indications).
- ■ Knowledge deficit related to medication regimen (patient/family teaching).

Implementation

- ■ **General Info:** Available in oral form in combination with potassium phosphate to acidify urine and to prevent formation of renal calculi.
- ■ **IV:** Administer IV only in dilute concentrations and infuse slowly.
- ■ **Additive Incompatibility:** calcium or magnesium.

Patient/Family Teaching

- ▫ Explain purpose of the medication to patient.

Evaluation

Effectiveness of therapy can be demonstrated by: ■ Prevention and correction of serum phosphate deficiency.

SODIUM POLYSTYRENE SULFONATE

(**soe**-dee-um po-lee-**stye**-reen **sul**-fon-ate)
Kayexalate, SPS

CLASSIFICATION(S):
Electrolyte modifier—cation exchange resin
Pregnancy Category UK

INDICATIONS

■ Treatment of mild to moderate hyperkalemia (if severe, more immediate measures such as sodium bicarbonate IV, calcium or glucose/insulin infusion should be instituted).

ACTION

■ Exchanges sodium ions for potassium ions in the intestine (each 1 g is exchanged for 0.5–1 mEq potassium). **Therapeutic Effect:** ■ Reduction of serum potassium levels.

PHARMACOKINETICS

Absorption: Distributed throughout the intestine but is nonabsorbable.
Distribution: Not distributed.
Metabolism and Excretion: Eliminated in the feces.
Half-life: UK.

CONTRAINDICATIONS AND PRECAUTIONS

Contraindicated in: ■ Life-threatening hyperkalemia (other, more immediate measures should be instituted) ■ Hypersensitivity to saccharin or parabens (some products) ■ Ileus.
Use Cautiously in: ■ Elderly patients ■ Congestive heart failure, hypertension, edema ■ Sodium restriction ■ Constipation.

ADVERSE REACTIONS AND SIDE EFFECTS*

GI: <u>constipation</u>, <u>fecal impaction</u>, anorexia, nausea, vomiting, gastric irritation.

*<u>Underlines</u> indicate most frequent; **CAPITALS** indicate life-threatening.

F and E: hypokalemia, hypocalcemia, sodium retention.

INTERACTIONS

Drug–Drug: ▪ Administration with **calcium** or **magnesium-containing antacids** may decrease resin-exchanging ability and increase risk of systemic alkalosis ▪ Hypokalemia may enhance **cardiac glycoside** toxicity.

ROUTE AND DOSAGE

Note: 4 level tsp = 15 g. Each g contains 4.1 mEq sodium.

- **PO (Adults):** 15 g 1–4 times daily in water or sorbitol (up to 160 g/day).
- **PO, Rect (Children):** 1 g/kg/dose.
- **Rect (Adults):** 30–50 g in 100 ml sorbitol q 1–2 hr initially, then q 4–6 hr as a retention enema (range 25–100 g).

PHARMACODYNAMICS (decrease in serum potassium)

	ONSET	PEAK	DURATION
PO	2–12 hr	UK	6–24 hr
Rect	2–12 hr	UK	4–6 hr

NURSING IMPLICATIONS

Assessment

- □ Monitor response of symptoms of hyperkalemia (fatigue, muscle weakness, paresthesia, confusion, dyspnea, peaked T waves, depressed ST segments, prolonged QT segments, widened QRS complexes, loss of P waves, and cardiac arrhythmias). Assess for development of hypokalemia (weakness, fatigue, arrhythmias, flat or inverted T waves, prominent U waves).
- □ Monitor intake and output ratios and daily weight. Assess for symptoms of fluid overload (dyspnea, rales/crackles, jugular venous distention, peripheral edema). Physician may order concurrent low-sodium diet in patients with congestive heart failure (see Appendix K for foods included).
- □ In patients receiving concurrent cardiac glycosides, assess for symptoms of digitalis toxicity (anorexia, nausea, vomiting, visual disturbances, arrhythmias).
- □ Assess abdomen and note character and frequency of stools. Physician may order concurrent sorbitol or laxatives to prevent constipation or impaction. Some products contain sorbitol to prevent constipation. Patient should ideally have 1–2 watery stools each day during course of therapy.
- ▪ **Lab Test Considerations:** Monitor renal function and electrolytes (especially potassium, sodium, calcium, and magnesium) prior to and periodically throughout therapy. Notify physician when potassium decreases to 4–5 mEq/liter.

Potential Nursing Diagnoses

- ▪ Bowel elimination, altered: constipation, diarrhea (side effects).
- ▪ Knowledge deficit related to medication regimen (patient/family teaching).

Implementation

- ▪ **General Info:** Soln is stable for 24 hr when refrigerated.
- ▪ **PO:** An osmotic laxative (sorbitol) is usually administered concurrently to prevent constipation.
- □ For oral administration, add prescribed amount of powder to 3–4 ml water/g of powder. Shake well. Physician may order syrup to improve palatability. Resin cookie or candy recipes are available; discuss with pharmacist or dietician.
- ▪ **Retention Enema:** Precede retention enema with cleansing enema. Administer soln via rectal tube or 28 French foley catheter with 30-ml balloon. Insert tube at least 20 cm and tape in place.
- □ For retention enema, add powder to 100 ml of prescribed soln (usually sorbitol or 20% dextrose in water). Shake well to dissolve powder thoroughly; should be of liquid consistency. Position patient on left side and elevate hips on pillow if soln begins to leak. Follow administration of medication with additional 50–100 ml of diluent to ensure administra-

tion of complete dose. Encourage patient to retain enema as long as possible, at least 30–60 min.

□ After retention period irrigate colon with 1–2 liters of non-sodium-containing soln. Y-connector with tubing may be attached to foley or rectal tube; cleansing soln is administered through one port of the Y and allowed to drain by gravity through the other port.

PATIENT/FAMILY TEACHING

□ Explain purpose and method of administration of medication to patient.

□ Inform patient of need for frequent lab tests to monitor effectiveness.

EVALUATION

Effectiveness of therapy can be demonstrated by: ▪ Normalization of serum potassium levels.

SOMATROPIN
(soe-ma-**troe**-pin)
Humatrope

SOMATREM
(**soe**-ma-trem)
Protropin

CLASSIFICATION(S):
Hormone—growth hormone
Pregnancy Category UK

INDICATIONS

▪ Growth failure in children due to deficiency of growth hormone.

ACTION

▪ Produces growth (skeletal and cellular) ▪ Metabolic actions include: □ Increased protein synthesis □ Increased carbohydrate metabolism □ Lipid mobilization □ Retention of sodium, phosphorus, and potassium ▪ Somatropin has the same amino acid sequence as naturally occurring growth hormone; somatrem has one additional amino acid. Both are produced by recombinant DNA techniques. **Therapeutic Effect:** ▪ Increased skeletal growth in children with growth hormone deficiency.

PHARMACOKINETICS

Absorption: Well absorbed following SC or IM administration.
Distribution: Distribution not known.
Metabolism and Excretion: Metabolism and excretion not known.
Half-life: UK.

CONTRAINDICATIONS AND PRECAUTIONS

Contraindicated in: ▪ Closure of epiphyses ▪ Tumors ▪ Hypersensitivity to m-cresol or glycerin (somatropin) or benzyl alcohol (somatrem).
Use Cautiously in: ▪ Growth hormone deficiency due to intracranial lesion ▪ Coexisting adrenocorticotropic hormone (ACTH) deficiency ▪ Thyroid dysfunction.

ADVERSE REACTIONS AND SIDE EFFECTS*

CV: edema.
Endo: hyperglycemia, insulin resistance, hypothyroidism.
Local: pain at injection site.

INTERACTIONS

Drug-Drug: ▪ Excessive **glucocorticoid** use may decrease response to somatropin.

ROUTE AND DOSAGE

Somatropin

▪ **IM, SC (Children):** Up to 0.06 mg/kg (0.16 IU/kg) 3 times weekly.

Somatrem

▪ **IM, SC (Children):** Up to 0.1 mg/kg (0.26 IU/kg) 3 times weekly.

PHARMACODYNAMICS (growth)

	ONSET	PEAK	DURATION
IM, SC	within 3 mon	UK	UK

NURSING IMPLICATIONS

ASSESSMENT

□ Monitor bone age and height and weight.

*Underlines indicate most frequent; **CAPITALS** indicate life-threatening.

■ **Lab Test Considerations:** Monitor thyroid function prior to and throughout course of therapy. May decrease T_4, radioactive iodine uptake, and thyroxine-binding capacity. Hypothyroidism necessitates concurrent thyroid replacement for growth hormone to be effective.
□ Monitor blood or urine glucose periodically throughout therapy. Diabetic patients may require increased insulin dose.
□ Monitor for development of neutralizing antibodies if growth rate does not exceed 2.5 cm/6 mon.

Potential Nursing Diagnoses
■ Body image disturbance (indications).
■ Knowledge deficit related to medication regimen (patient/family teaching).

Implementation
■ **Somatrem:** Reconstitute 5-mg (10-IU) vial with 10 ml of bacteriostatic water for injection. Do not shake; swirl gently to dissolve. Soln is clear. Discard vial after withdrawing dose.
■ **Somatropin:** Reconstitute 13-IU vial with 1.5–5 ml of water for injection provided by manufacturer (contains preservative m-cresol). Do not shake; swirl gently to dissolve. Soln is clear. Stable for 14 days when refrigerated.

Patient/Family Teaching
□ Instruct patient and parents on correct procedure for reconstituting medication, site selection, and technique for IM or SC injection. Review dosage schedule. Somatropin injections should be at least 48 hr apart. Parents should report persistent pain or edema at injection site.
□ Explain rationale for prohibition of use for increasing athletic performance. Administration to persons without growth hormone deficiency or after epiphyseal closure may result in acromegaly (coarsening of facial features; enlarged hands, feet, and internal organs; increased blood sugars; hypertension).
□ Emphasize need for regular follow-up with endocrinologist to ensure appropriate growth rate, to evaluate lab work, and to determine bone age by x-ray examination.
□ Assure parents and child that these dosage forms are synthetic and therefore not capable of transmitting Creutzfeldt-Jakob disease, as was the original somatropin, which was extracted from human cadavers.

Evaluation
Clinical response can be evaluated by:
■ Child's attainment of adult height in growth failure secondary to pituitary growth hormone deficiency. Therapy is limited to period before closure of epiphyseal plates (approximately up to 14–15 yr in girls, 15–16 yr in boys).

SPECTINOMYCIN
(spek-tin-oh-**mye**-sin)
Trobicin

CLASSIFICATION(S):
Anti-infective—miscellaneous
Pregnancy Category UK

INDICATIONS
■ Treatment of gonorrhea and gonococcal urethritis, cervicitis, or proctitis in patients who are infected with susceptible strains of *Neisseria gonorrhea*.

ACTION
■ Inhibits bacterial protein synthesis at the level of the 30S ribosome. **Therapeutic Effect:** ■ Bactericidal action against susceptible organisms. **Spectrum:** ■ Most notable for activity against *Neisseria gonorrhea*, including penicillinase-producing strains (PPNG) ■ Not active against *Treponema pallidum* or *Chlamydia trachomatis*.

PHARMACOKINETICS
Absorption: Rapidly absorbed from IM sites.

Distribution: Distribution not known.
Metabolism and Excretion: Excreted primarily by the kidneys.
Half-life: 1.2–2.8 hr.

CONTRAINDICATIONS AND PRECAUTIONS

Contraindicated in: ▪ Hypersensitivity.
Use Cautiously in: ▪ Neonates (do not reconstitute with sterile water containing benzyl alcohol) ▪ Concurrent infection with other sexually transmitted disease (additional anti-infectives may be required) ▪ Pregnancy, lactation, or children (safety not established; has been used).

ADVERSE REACTIONS AND SIDE EFFECTS*

CNS: dizziness, headache, nervousness, insomnia.
GI: nausea, vomiting.
Derm: urticaria, transient rashes, pruritus.
Local: <u>pain</u> at IM site.
Misc: hypersensitivity reactions, including ANAPHYLAXIS, chills, fever.

INTERACTIONS

Drug-Drug: ▪ None significant.

ROUTE AND DOSAGE

- **IM (Adults and Children >45 kg):** 2 g.
- **IM (Infants and Children <45 kg):** 40 mg/kg.

PHARMACODYNAMICS (blood levels)

	ONSET	PEAK
IM	rapid	1 hr

NURSING IMPLICATIONS

Assessment

- ▫ Assess patient for gonorrheal infection (dysuria, urethral discharge, vaginal discharge, perianal discomfort).
- ▫ Obtain gram-stain smear and specimens for culture and sensitivity prior to initiating therapy. Dose may be given before receiving results.
- ▫ Monitor patients with history of allergies for hypersensitivity reactions (urticaria, wheezing).
- ▪ **Lab Test Considerations:** Additional serologic testing for syphilis should be conducted at the time of therapy and again 3 mon later. Spectinomycin does not cure syphilis, but it may mask symptom development.
- ▫ When multiple doses are given, increased SGPT (ALT), BUN, and alkaline phosphatase and decreased hemoglobin, hematocrit, and creatinine clearance may occur. Urine output often decreases, but this is not associated with renal toxicity.

Potential Nursing Diagnoses

- ▪ Infection, high risk for (indications).
- ▪ Knowledge deficit related to safe sex practices (patient/family teaching).

Implementation

- ▪ **IM:** Reconstitute 2-g vial with 3.2 ml provided diluent (bacteriostatic water with 0.9% benzol alcohol for injection) and 4-g vial with 6.2 ml diluent. Administer deep into well-developed muscle of dorsogluteal site. The 2-g vial yields 5 ml, which can be injected slowly into one site. The 4-g vial yields 10 ml, which should be divided into two 5-ml injections and administered at separate sites. Suspension is stable for 24 hr.

Patient/Family Teaching

- ▫ Discuss need for all sexual contacts to receive treatment. Patient should abstain from sex until repeat tests confirm resolution of infection. Patient should not share washcloths, towels, or underclothes. Review safe sex practices to prevent reinfection.
- ▫ Inform patient that temporary soreness at injection site, nausea, fever, chills, dizziness, and insomnia may occur.
- ▫ Explain need for repeat smears or culture and sensitivity tests 1 wk after

*<u>Underlines</u> indicate most frequent; **CAPITALS** indicate life-threatening.

S

treatment to ensure effectiveness of treatment.

Evaluation

Clinical response can be evaluated by: ▪ Resolution of the signs and symptoms of gonorrheal urethritis ▫ Recurrence of symptoms is usually indicative of re-exposure, not treatment failure.

SPIRONOLACTONE

(speer-oh-no-**lak**-tone)

Aldactone, {Novospiroton}, {Sincomen}

CLASSIFICATION(S):

Diuretic—potassium-sparing

Pregnancy Category UK

INDICATIONS

▪ Most commonly used to counteract potassium loss induced by other diuretics in the management of edema or hypertension ▪ Treatment of hyperaldosteronism.

ACTION

▪ Acts at distal renal tubule to antagonize the effects of aldosterone, causing excretion of sodium, bicarbonate, and calcium while conserving potassium and hydrogen ions. **Therapeutic Effects:** ▪ Weak diuretic and antihypertensive effects when compared to other diuretics, but without potassium loss ▪ Counteracts the effects of excessive aldosterone.

PHARMACOKINETICS

Absorption: Well absorbed following oral administration.

Distribution: Crosses the placenta and enters breast milk (canrenone).

Metabolism and Excretion: Converted by the liver to its active diuretic compound (canrenone).

Half-life: 13–24 hr (canrenone).

CONTRAINDICATIONS AND PRECAUTIONS

Contraindicated in: ▪ Hypersensitivity ▪ Hyperkalemia ▪ Renal insufficiency ▪ Pregnancy or lactation ▪ Menstrual abnormalities ▪ Breast enlargement.

Use Cautiously in: ▪ Hepatic dysfunction ▪ Elderly or debilitated patients.

ADVERSE REACTIONS AND SIDE EFFECTS*

CNS: headache, dizziness.

CV: arrhythmias.

Derm: hirsutism, rashes.

Endo: gynecomastia.

F and E: <u>hyperkalemia</u>, hyponatremia, hypochloremia, metabolic acidosis, dehydration.

GI: <u>nausea</u>, <u>vomiting</u>, <u>anorexia</u>, <u>diarrhea</u>, cramps, constipation, flatulence.

GU: impotence, menstrual irregularities.

INTERACTIONS

Drug-Drug: ▪ Additive hypotension with other **antihypertensives, nitrates,** or acute ingestion of **alcohol** ▪ Use with **angiotensin converting enzyme (ACE) inhibitors** or **potassium supplements** may lead to hyperkalemia ▪ Decreases **lithium** excretion, may lead to toxicity ▪ **Nonsteroidal anti-inflammatory agents** may decrease the antihypertensive response to spironolactone and increase the risk of adverse renal reactions.

Drug-Food: ▪ Ingesting large amounts of **potassium-rich foods** or **salt substitutes** (see list in Appendix K) may lead to hyperkalemia.

ROUTE AND DOSAGE

Edema

- **PO (Adults):** 25–200 mg/day in 1–2 divided doses.
- **PO (Children):** 1–3 mg/kg/day in 1–2 divided doses.

Hypertension

- **PO (Adults):** 50–100 mg/day in 1–2 divided doses.

{} = Available in Canada only.

*<u>Underlines</u> indicate most frequent; **CAPITALS** indicate life-threatening.

- **PO (Children):** 1–3 mg/kg/day in divided doses.

Prevention of Hypokalemia with Potassium-Losing Diuretics

- **PO (Adults):** 25–100 mg/day in 1–2 divided doses.

Primary Hyperaldosteronism

- **PO (Adults):** 100–400 mg/day in 1–2 divided doses.

PHARMACODYNAMICS (effects on serum potassium)

	ONSET	PEAK	DURATION
PO	1–2 days	5 days	2–3 days

NURSING IMPLICATIONS

Assessment

- Monitor intake and output ratios and daily weight throughout therapy.
- If medication is given as an adjunct to antihypertensive therapy, blood pressure and pulse should be evaluated before administering.
- Monitor response of signs and symptoms of hypokalemia (weakness, fatigue, U wave on ECG, arrhythmias, polyuria, polydipsia). Assess patient frequently for development of hyperkalemia (fatigue, muscle weakness, paresthesia, confusion, dyspnea, cardiac arrhythmias). Patients who have diabetes mellitus or kidney disease and elderly patients are at increased risk of developing these symptoms.
- Periodic ECGs are recommended in patients receiving prolonged therapy.
- **Lab Test Considerations:** Serum potassium levels should be evaluated prior to and routinely during course of therapy. Withhold drug and notify physician if patient becomes hyperkalemic.
- Monitor BUN, serum creatinine, and electrolytes prior to and periodically throughout therapy. May cause increased serum glucose, magnesium, uric acid, BUN, creatinine, potassium, and urinary calcium excretion levels. May also cause decreased sodium levels.
- May cause false elevations of plasma cortisol concentrations. Spironolactone should be withdrawn 4–7 days before test.

Potential Nursing Diagnoses

- Fluid volume excess (indications).
- Knowledge deficit related to medication regimen (patient/family teaching).

Implementation

- **General Info:** Available in combination with hydrochlorothiazide (see Appendix A).
- Administer in AM to avoid interrupting sleep pattern.
- **PO:** Administer with food or milk to minimize GI irritation and to increase bioavailability.

Patient/Family Teaching

- **General Info:** Emphasize the importance of continuing to take this medication, even if feeling well. Instruct patient to take medication at the same time each day. If a dose is missed, take as soon as remembered unless almost time for next dose.
- Caution patient to avoid salt substitutes and foods that contain high levels of potassium or sodium, unless prescribed by physician.
- May cause dizziness. Caution patient to avoid driving or other activities requiring alertness until response to medication is known.
- Advise patient to avoid use of over-the-counter medications without consulting with physician or pharmacist.
- Advise patient to notify physician if muscle weakness or cramps, fatigue, or severe nausea, vomiting, or diarrhea occurs.
- **Hypertension:** Reinforce need to continue additional therapies for hypertension (weight loss, restricted sodium intake, stress reduction, moderation of alcohol intake, regular exercise, and cessation of smoking). Spironolactone helps control but does not cure hypertension.
- Teach patients on antihypertensive therapy how to check blood pressure weekly.

S

Evaluation

Effectiveness of therapy can be demonstrated by: ▪ Prevention of hypokalemia in patients taking diuretics ▪ Treatment of hyperaldosteronism.

STREPTOKINASE
(strep-toe-**kye**-nase)
Kabikinase, Streptase

CLASSIFICATION(S):
Thrombolytic agent
Pregnancy Category C

INDICATIONS

▪ Treatment of coronary thrombosis associated with acute transmural myocardial infarction ▪ Treatment of: ▫ Recent, severe, or massive deep vein thrombosis ▫ Pulmonary emboli ▫ Arterial embolism ▫ Thrombosis ▪ Management of occluded arteriovenous cannulae.

ACTION

▪ Directly activates plasminogen, which subsequently dissolves fibrin deposits, including those required for normal hemostasis. **Therapeutic Effects:** ▪ Preservation of left ventricular function after transmural myocardial infarction ▪ Lysis of thrombi or emboli.

PHARMACOKINETICS

Absorption: Administered IV or directly into coronary arteries or cannulae, resulting in immediate and complete bioavailability.
Distribution: Does not cross the placenta.
Metabolism and Excretion: Rapidly cleared from circulation following IV administration by antibodies and the reticuloendothelial system.
Half-life: 23 min (streptokinase/plasmin complex).

CONTRAINDICATIONS AND PRECAUTIONS

Contraindicated in: ▪ Hypersensitivity ▪ Active internal bleeding ▪ Recent (<2 mon) cerebrovascular accident, intracranial or intraspinal surgery, intracranial neoplasm, thoracic surgery ▪ Uncontrolled severe hypertension.
Use Cautiously in: ▪ Pregnancy, lactation, or children (safety not established) ▪ Recent minor trauma or surgery (<2 mon) ▪ Cerebrovascular disease ▪ Diabetic hemorrhagic retinopathy ▪ Recent streptococcal infection ▪ Recent streptokinase therapy ▪ Patients ≥75 yr (increased risk of CNS bleeding) ▪ Arterial emboli originating in the left side of the heart (increased risk of cerebral emboli).

ADVERSE REACTIONS AND SIDE EFFECTS*

CV: reperfusion arrhythmias.
EENT: periorbital edema.
Derm: urticaria, flushing.
Hemat: BLEEDING.
Local: phlebitis at IV site.
Misc: fever, hypersensitivity reactions, including ANAPHYLAXIS, bronchospasm.

INTERACTIONS

Drug-Drug: ▪ Concurrent use with other **anticoagulants, cefamandole, cefotetan, moxalactam, plicamycin,** or **agents affecting platelet function,** including **aspirin, nonsteroidal anti-inflammatory agents,** and **dipyridamole** increase the risk of bleeding.

ROUTE AND DOSAGE

Myocardial Infarction

- **IV (Adults):** 1,500,000 IU.
- **Intracoronary (Adults):** 20,000-IU bolus, followed by 2000 IU/min infusion.

Deep Vein Thrombosis, Pulmonary Emboli, Arterial Embolism, or Thromboses

- **IV (Adults):** 250,000-IU loading dose, followed by 100,000 IU/hr for 24 hr for pulmonary emboli, 72 hr for recurrent pulmonary emboli or deep vein thrombosis.

Arteriovenous Cannula Occlusion

- **(Adults):** 250,000 IU into each oc-

*Underlines indicate most frequent; **CAPITALS** indicate life-threatening.

cluded limb of cannula, clamp for 2 hr, then aspirate.

PHARMACODYNAMICS (fibrinolysis)

	ONSET	PEAK	DURATION
IV	immediate	rapid	4 hr (up to 12 hr)

NURSING IMPLICATIONS

Assessment

- **General Info:** Monitor vital signs, including temperature, closely during course of therapy.
- Assess patient carefully for bleeding every 15 min during the first hr of therapy, every 15–30 min during the next 8 hr, and at least every 4 hr for the duration of therapy. Frank bleeding may occur from invasive sites or body orifices. Internal bleeding may also occur (decreased neurologic status, abdominal pain with coffee ground emesis or black tarry stools, joint pain). If bleeding occurs, stop medication and notify physician immediately.
- Inquire about previous reaction to streptokinase therapy. Assess patient for hypersensitivity reaction (rash, dyspnea, fever). If these occur, inform physician promptly. Keep epinephrine, an antihistamine, and resuscitation equipment close by in the event of an anaphylactic reaction.
- Inquire about recent streptococcal infection. Streptokinase may not be effective if administered between 5 days and 6 mon of a streptococcal infection.
- **Coronary Thrombosis:** Monitor ECG continuously. Notify physician if significant arrhythmias occur. IV lidocaine or procainamide (Pronestyl) may be ordered prophylactically. Cardiac enzymes should be monitored.
- **Pulmonary Embolism:** Monitor pulse, blood pressure, hemodynamics, and respiratory status (rate, degree of dyspnea, ABGs).
- **Deep Vein Thrombosis/Acute Arterial Occlusion:** Observe extremities and palpate pulses of affected extremities every hr. Notify physician immediately if circulatory impairment occurs.
- **Cannula/Catheter Occlusion:** Monitor ability to aspirate blood as indicator of patency. Ensure that patient exhales and holds breath when connecting and disconnecting IV syringe to prevent air embolism.
- **Lab Test Considerations:** Hematocrit, hemoglobin, platelet count, prothrombin time, thrombin time, and activated partial thromboplastin time should be evaluated prior to and frequently throughout course of therapy. Bleeding time may be assessed prior to therapy if patient has received platelet aggregation inhibitors.
- Obtain type and cross-match and have blood available at all times in case of hemorrhage.
- **Toxicity and Overdose:** If local bleeding occurs, apply pressure to site. If severe or internal bleeding occurs, discontinue infusion. Clotting factors and/or blood volume may be restored through infusions of whole blood, packed red blood cells, fresh frozen plasma, or cryoprecipitate. Do not administer dextran, as it has antiplatelet activity. Aminocaproic acid (Amicar) may be used as an antidote.

Potential Nursing Diagnoses

- Tissue perfusion, altered (indications).
- Injury, high risk for (side effects).

Implementation

- **General Info:** This medication should be used only in settings where hematologic function and clinical response can be adequately monitored.
- Invasive procedures, such as IM injections or arterial punctures, should be avoided with this therapy. If such procedures must be performed, apply pressure to IV puncture sites for at least 15 min and to arterial puncture sites for at least 30 min.
- Systemic anticoagulation with heparin is usually begun several hrs after the completion of thrombolytic therapy.

- □ Acetaminophen may be ordered to control fever.
- ▪ **IV:** Reconstitute with 5 ml of 0.9% NaCl or D5W (direct to sides of vial) and swirl gently; do not shake. Dilute further with 0.9% NaCl for a total volume of 45–500 ml and infuse as directed by physician. Infuse via infusion pump to ensure accurate dosage. Administer through 0.8-micron pore size filter. Use reconstituted soln within 24 hr of preparation.
- ▪ **Y-Site/Additive Incompatibility:** Do not admix or administer via Y-site injection with any other medication.
- ▪ **Cannula/Catheter Clearance:** IV preparations used for clearing occluded AV cannulas or central lines are mixed with 2 ml of 0.9% NaCl, administered slowly into each occluded limb of cannula, and then clamped for at least 2 hr. Aspirate contents carefully and flush line with 0.9% NaCl.

Patient/Family Teaching

- □ Explain purpose of medication. Instruct patient to report hypersensitivity reactions (rash, dyspnea) and bleeding or bruising.
- □ Explain need for bedrest and minimal handling during therapy to avoid injury.

Evaluation

Effectiveness of therapy can be demonstrated by: ▪ Lysis of thrombi and restoration of blood flow ▪ Cannula or catheter patency.

STREPTOMYCIN
(strep-toe-**mye**-sin)

CLASSIFICATION(S):
Anti-infective—aminoglycoside, Antitubercular
Pregnancy Category UK

INDICATIONS

▪ Combination therapy of active tuberculosis ▪ Streptococcal or enterococcal endocarditis (in combination with a penicillin) ▪ Treatment of tularemia and plague ▪ Use in other situations should be reserved for organisms not sensitive to less toxic anti-infectives or when other contraindications to their use exists.

ACTION

▪ Inhibits protein synthesis in bacteria at the level of the 30S ribosome. **Therapeutic Effect:** ▪ Bactericidal action against susceptible bacteria. **Spectrum:** ▪ Despite activity against many gram-negative pathogens, toxicity precludes its use in most situations ▪ Notable for activity against the following other organisms: □ *Mycobacterium tuberculosis* □ *Brucella* □ *Nocardia* □ *Erisypelothrix* □ *Pasturella multocida* □ *Yersinia pestis* ▪ In the treatment of enterococcal infections, synergy with a penicillin is required.

PHARMACOKINETICS

Absorption: Well absorbed following IM administration.
Distribution: Crosses the placenta. Small amounts enter breast milk. Poor penetration into CSF.
Metabolism and Excretion: Excretion is mainly (>90%) renal.
Half-life: 2–3 hr (increased in renal impairment).

CONTRAINDICATIONS AND PRECAUTIONS

Contraindicated in: ▪ Hypersensitivity ▪ Cross-sensitivity with other aminoglycosides may exist.
Use Cautiously in: ▪ Renal impairment of any kind (dosage reduction required) ▪ Pregnancy (may cause irreversible deafness in newborns) ▪ Lactation (safety not established) ▪ Neuromuscular diseases, such as myasthenia gravis ▪ Elderly patients (dosage reduction recommended).

ADVERSE REACTIONS AND SIDE EFFECTS*

EENT: ototoxicity (vestibular and cochlear).

*Underlines indicate most frequent; **CAPITALS** indicate life-threatening.

GU: nephrotoxicity.
Neuro: enhanced neuromuscular blockade.
Misc: hypersensitivity reactions.

INTERACTIONS

Drug-Drug: ▪ May be inactivated by **penicillins** when coadministered to patients with renal insufficiency ▪ Increased risk of respiratory paralysis after **inhalation anesthetics (ether, cyclopropane, halothane,** or **nitrous oxide)** or **neuromusclar blockers (tubocurarine, succinylcholine, decamethonium)** ▪ Increased incidence of ototoxicity with **loop diuretics (ethacrynic acid, bumetanide, furosemide)** ▪ Increased risk of nephrotoxicity with **other nephrotoxic drugs (cisplatin).**

ROUTE AND DOSAGE

Tuberculosis

- **IM (Adults):** 1 g or 15 mg/kg/day or 25 mg/kg 2–3 times/wk.
- **IM (Children):** 20–40 mg/kg/day.

Enterococcal Endocarditis

- **IM (Adults):** 1 g q 12 hr for 2 wk, then 500 mg q 12 hr for 4 wk.

Streptococcal Endocarditis

- **IM (Adults):** 1 g q 12 hr for 1 wk, then 500 mg q 12 hr for 1 wk.

Tularemia

- **IM (Adults):** 1–2 g/day in divided doses.

Plague

- **IM (Adults):** 2–4 g/day in divided doses.

PHARMACODYNAMICS (blood levels)

	ONSET	PEAK
IM	rapid	1–2 hr

NURSING IMPLICATIONS

Assessment

- □ Assess patient for infection (vital signs; appearance of wound, sputum, urine, and stool; WBC) at beginning and throughout course of therapy.
- □ Obtain specimens for culture and sensitivity prior to initiating therapy. First dose may be given before receiving results.
- □ Evaluate eighth cranial nerve function by audiometry prior to and throughout course of therapy. Hearing loss is usually in the high-frequency range. Prompt recognition and intervention is essential in preventing permanent damage. Also monitor for vestibular dysfunction (vertigo, ataxia, nausea, vomiting). Eighth cranial nerve dysfunction is associated with persistently elevated peak streptomycin levels. Caloric stimulation tests may also be performed.
- □ Monitor intake and output and daily weight to assess hydration status and renal function.
- □ Assess patient for signs of superinfection (fever, upper respiratory infection, vaginal itching or discharge, increasing malaise, diarrhea). Report to physician.
- ▪ **Lab Test Considerations:** Monitor renal function by urinalysis, specific gravity, BUN, creatinine, and creatinine clearance prior to and throughout therapy.
- □ May cause increased SGOT (AST), SGPT (ALT), LDH, bilirubin, and serum alkaline phosphatase levels.
- □ May cause decreased serum calcium, magnesium, sodium, and potassium levels.
- ▪ **Toxicity and Overdose:** Blood levels should be monitored periodically during therapy. Timing of blood levels is important in interpreting results. Draw blood for peak levels 30–60 min after IM injection. Acceptable peak level is 5–25 mcg/ml. Trough levels should not be >5 mcg/ml.

Potential Nursing Diagnoses

- ▪ Infection, high risk for (indications).
- ▪ Sensory-perceptual alteration: auditory (side effects).

Implementation

- ▪ **General Info:** Keep patient well hydrated (1500–2000 ml/day) during therapy.
- □ Soln may vary from colorless to yel-

low and may darken on exposure to light. This does not affect potency. Do not use soln that contains a precipitate.

- **IM:** Reconstitute by adding 4.2–4.5 ml of 0.9% NaCl or sterile water for injection to each 1-g vial for a concentration of 200 mg/ml, or add 3.2–3.5 ml of diluent for a concentration of 250 mg/ml. Add 17 ml of diluent to each 5-g vial for a concentration of 250 mg/ml, or add 6.5 ml for a concentration of 500 mg/ml. Do not administer concentrations >500 mg/ml. Soln is stable for 2–28 days at room temperature or for 14 days if refrigerated, depending on manufacturer.
  - □ IM administration should be deep into a well-developed muscle. Alternate injection sites.
- **Syringe Incompatibility:** heparin.

Patient/Family Teaching

- □ Instruct patient to report signs of hypersensitivity, tinnitus, vertigo, or hearing loss.

Evaluation

Clinical response can be evaluated by:

▪ Resolution of the signs and symptoms of infection. Length of time for complete resolution depends on the organism and site of infection.

STREPTOZOCIN

(strep-toe-**zoe**-sin)
Zanosar

CLASSIFICATION(S):
Antineoplastic—antitumor antibiotic
Pregnancy Category C

INDICATIONS

▪ Management of metastatic islet cell carcinoma of the pancreas. **Unlabeled Uses:** ▪ Management of: □ Metastatic carcinoid tumor □ Hodgkin's disease □ Pancreatic adenocarcinoma □ Colorectal cancer.

ACTION

▪ Inhibits DNA synthesis by cross-linking DNA strands (cell cycle-phase nonspecific). **Therapeutic Effect:** ▪ Death of rapidly replicating cells, particularly malignant ones.

PHARMACOKINETICS

Absorption: Administered IV only, resulting in complete bioavailability.
Distribution: Rapidly distributed. High concentrations in liver, pancreas, kidneys, and intestine. Probably crosses the placenta. Active metabolite enters the CSF.
Metabolism and Excretion: Highly metabolized in liver and kidneys. 10–20% excreted unchanged by the kidneys. Small amounts excreted in expired air (5%) and feces (1%).
Half-life: 35–40 min.

CONTRAINDICATIONS AND PRECAUTIONS

Contraindicated in: ▪ Hypersensitivity.
Use Cautiously in: ▪ Underlying or pre-existing renal disease (dosage reduction recommended) ▪ Liver disease ▪ Patients with childbearing potential ▪ Active infections ▪ Decreased bone marrow reserve ▪ Other chronic debilitating illnesses ▪ Pregnancy, lactation, or children (safety not established).

ADVERSE REACTIONS AND SIDE EFFECTS*

CNS: confusion, lethargy, depression.
GI: nausea, vomiting, HEPATITIS, diarrhea, duodenal ulcer.
GU: proteinuria, nephrotoxicity, gonadal suppression.
F and E: hypophosphatemia.
Hemat: leukopenia, thrombocytopenia, anemia.
Metab: HYPOGLYCEMIA (first dose), hyperglycemia, diabetes.
Local: phlebitis at IV site.
Misc: fever.

*Underlines indicate most frequent; **CAPITALS** indicate life-threatening.

INTERACTIONS

Drug–Drug: ▪ Additive myelosuppression with other **antineoplastic agents** ▪ Increased risk of nephrotoxicity with other **nephrotoxic agents (aminoglycoside antibiotics)** ▪ Toxicity may be increased by concurrent **phenytoin** therapy ▪ May increase the toxicity of **doxorubicin** ▪ May decrease antibody response to **live virus vaccines** and increase the risk of adverse reactions.

ROUTE AND DOSAGE

- **IV (Adults):** 500 mg/m²/day for 5 days every 6 wk or 1 g/m²/wk for 4–6 wk (not to exceed 1.5 g/dose).

PHARMACODYNAMICS

	ONSET	PEAK	DURATION
IV (effects on blood counts)	UK	1–2 wk	UK
IV (tumor response)	17 days	35 days	UK

NURSING IMPLICATIONS

Assessment

- ▫ Monitor vital signs prior to and periodically during therapy.
- ▫ Monitor intake and output and daily weight. Notify physician if significant discrepancies or dependent edema occur, as these may indicate nephrotoxicity. Encourage fluids to 3000 ml/day to reduce risk of renal damage.
- ▫ Monitor IV site carefully and ensure patency. Discontinue infusion immediately if severe discomfort, erythema along vein, or infiltration occurs. Streptozocin is a vesicant. Tissue ulceration and necrosis may result from infiltration. Notify physician.
- ▫ Assess for fever, chills, sore throat, and signs of infection. Notify physician if these symptoms occur.
- ▫ Monitor platelet count throughout therapy. Assess for bleeding (bleeding gums, bruising, petechiae; guaiac stools, urine, and emesis). If thrombocytopenia occurs, avoid IM injections and rectal temperatures and apply pressure to venipuncture sites for 10 min.
- ▫ Monitor hydration status, appetite, and nutritional intake. Severe, protracted nausea and vomiting may occur 1–4 hr after beginning infusion. Nausea and vomiting may worsen with subsequent doses. Administration of an antiemetic and adjusting diet as tolerated may help maintain fluid and electrolyte balance and nutritional status.
- ▫ Anemia may occur. Monitor for increased fatigue, dyspnea, and orthostatic hypotension.
- ▪ **Lab Test Considerations:** Monitor renal status prior to and frequently throughout therapy and for 4 wk after course of therapy. Nephrotoxicity is common and may be manifested by elevated BUN and creatinine, decreased creatinine clearance, and presence of protein in urine. Reduction or discontinuation of streptozocin may allow reversal of renal damage.
- ▫ Monitor for hepatotoxicity, evidenced by increased SGOT (AST), SGPT (ALT), LDH, serum bilirubin, and alkaline phosphatase or decreased serum albumen.
- ▫ Monitor serum glucose prior to and after initial dose and periodically during therapy.
- ▫ Monitor serum uric acid prior to and periodically throughout therapy.
- ▫ Monitor CBC and differential prior to and throughout therapy. Notify physician of significant decreases.

Potential Nursing Diagnoses

- ▪ Infection, high risk for (side effects).
- ▪ Fluid volume, altered: high risk for (side effects).
- ▪ Knowledge deficit related to medication regimen (patient/family teaching).

Implementation

- ▪ **General Info:** IV dextrose should be immediately available, as hypoglycemia may occur in response to initial dose.
- ▫ Soln is pale gold. Do not use if dark brown. Stable for 12 hr at room temperature, 96 hr at 2–8°C.

- Soln should be prepared in a biologic cabinet. Wear gloves, gown, and mask while handling medication. Discard equipment in designated containers (see Appendix I).
- **IV:** Reconstitute vial with 9.5 ml of D5W or 0.9% NaCl, for a concentration of 100 mg/ml. May be further diluted in 10–200 ml of D5W or 0.9% NaCl. Do not admix.
- *Rate:* Infuse over 10–15 min. Slower infusion rates (45–60 min) have been used to decrease venous irritation. May also be infused over 6 hr.

Patient/Family Teaching

- Instruct patient to notify nurse immediately if pain or redness develops at IV site.
- Instruct patient to notify nurse immediately if symptoms of hypoglycemia occur (anxiety, chills, cold sweats, confusion, cool pale skin, difficulty in concentration, drowsiness, excessive hunger, headache, irritability, nausea, nervousness, shakiness, unusual tiredness, or weakness).
- Instruct patient to notify physician if decreased urine output, swelling of lower extremities, yellowing of skin, fever, chills, sore throat, signs of infection, bleeding gums, bruising, petechiae, or blood in urine, stool, or emesis occurs. Caution patient to avoid crowds and persons with known infections. Instruct patient to use soft toothbrush and electric razor. Patient should be cautioned not to drink alcoholic beverages or take aspirin-containing products.
- This drug may cause gonadal suppression; however, patient should still practice birth control. Advise patient to inform physician immediately if pregnancy is suspected.
- Instruct patient not to receive any vaccinations without advice of physician.
- Advise patient of need for medical follow-up and frequent lab tests.

Evaluation

Effectiveness of therapy can be demonstrated by: ▪ Decrease in size and spread of tumor.

S

STRONG IODINE SOLUTION (LUGOL'S SOLUTION)

(eye-oh-dine)

CLASSIFICATION(S):
Antithyroid
Pregnancy Category C

INDICATIONS

▪ Adjunct with other antithyroid drugs in preparation for thyroidectomy and to treat thyrotoxic crisis or neonatal thyrotoxicosis.

ACTION

▪ Rapidly inhibits the release and synthesis of thyroid hormones ▪ Decreases the vascularity of the thyroid gland. **Therapeutic Effects:** ▪ Control of hyperthyroidism ▪ Decreased bleeding during thyroid surgery.

PHARMACOKINETICS

Absorption: Converted in the GI tract and enters the circulation as iodine.
Distribution: Concentrates in the thyroid gland. Crosses the placenta and enters breast milk.
Metabolism and Excretion: Taken up by the thyroid gland.
Half-life: UK.

CONTRAINDICATIONS AND PRECAUTIONS

Contraindicated in: ▪ Hypersensitivity.
Use Cautiously in: ▪ Tuberculosis ▪ Bronchitis ▪ Hyperkalemia ▪ Impaired renal function ▪ Pregnancy and lactation (thyroid abnormalities may be seen in the newborn).

ADVERSE REACTIONS AND SIDE EFFECTS*

Derm: acneform eruptions.
Endo: thyroid hyperplasia, hypothyroidism, hyperthyroidism.
GI: GI irritation, diarrhea.
Misc: hypersensitivity, iodism.

INTERACTIONS

Drug–Drug: ▪ Use with **lithium** may cause additive hypothyroidism ▪ Increases the antithyroid effect of **antithyroid agents (methimazole, propylthiouracil)** ▪ Additive hyperkalemia may result from combined use of potassium iodide with **potassium-sparing diuretics, potassium supplements,** or **angiotensin converting enzyme (ACE) inhibitors.**

ROUTE AND DOSAGE

Note: Contains 50 mg iodine/ml plus potassium iodide 100 mg/ml.

Preparation for Thyroidectomy

- **PO (Adults and Children):** Strong iodine soln 0.1–0.3 ml (3–5 drops) tid.

Thyrotoxic Crisis

- **PO (Adults and Children):** Strong iodine soln 1 ml in water tid.

PHARMACODYNAMICS (effects on thyroid function testing)

	ONSET	PEAK	DURATION
PO	24 hr	10–15 days	variable

NURSING IMPLICATIONS

Assessment

- Assess for signs and symptoms of iodism (metallic taste, stomatitis, skin lesions, cold symptoms, severe GI upset). Report these symptoms to physician promptly.
- Monitor response symptoms of hyperthyroidism (tachycardia, palpitations, nervousness, insomnia, diaphoresis, heat intolerance, tremors, weight loss).
- Monitor for hypersensitivity reaction (rash, pruritus, laryngeal edema, wheezing). Discontinue drug and notify physician immediately if these occur.
- **Lab Test Considerations:** Monitor thyroid function tests prior to and periodically during course of therapy.
- Monitor serum potassium periodically during course of therapy.

Potential Nursing Diagnoses

- Knowledge deficit related to medication regimen (patient/family teaching).

Implementation

- **PO:** Mix soln in a glass of fruit juice. Administer after meals to minimize GI irritation.
- Soln is normally clear and colorless. Darkening upon standing does not affect potency of drug.

Patient/Family Teaching

- **Hyperthyroidism:** Instruct patient to take medication exactly as directed. Missing a dose may precipitate hyperthyroidism.
- Instruct patient to report suspected pregnancy to physician before therapy is initiated.
- Advise patient to confer with physician regarding avoidance of foods high in iodine (seafood, iodized salt, cabbage, kale, turnips).
- Advise patient to consult physician or pharmacist prior to using over-the-counter cold remedies. Some cold remedies use iodide as an expectorant.

Evaluation

Effectiveness of therapy can be demonstrated by: ▪ Resolution of the symptoms of thyroid crisis ▪ Decrease in size and vascularity of the gland prior to thyroid surgery. Use of iodides in the treatment of hyperthyroidism is usually limited to 2 wk.

*Underlines indicate most frequent; **CAPITALS** indicate life-threatening.

S

SUCCIMER
(**sux**-i-mer)
Chemet

CLASSIFICATION(S):
Antidote—lead chelator
Pregnancy Category C

INDICATIONS

■ Treatment of lead poisoning in children with blood lead levels >45 mcg/dl.

ACTION

■ Forms a water-soluble compound with lead allowing urinary elimination of excessive amounts of lead. **Therapeutic Effect:** ■ Decreased blood lead levels and decreased target organ damage in lead poisoning.

PHARMACOKINETICS

Absorption: Rapidly but variably absorbed following oral administration.
Distribution: Distribution not known.
Metabolism and Excretion: Extensively metabolized. 10% excreted unchanged by the kidneys.
Half-life: 2 days.

CONTRAINDICATIONS AND PRECAUTIONS

Contraindicated in: ■ Hypersensitivity or allergy to succimer ■ Lactation (should be discouraged during succimer therapy).
Use Cautiously in: ■ Pregnancy or children <1 yr (safety not established) ■ Renal failure (chelates are not dialyzable).

ADVERSE REACTIONS AND SIDE EFFECTS*

CNS: headache, drowsiness, dizziness.
EENT: cloudy film in eye, plugged ears, otitis media, watery eyes.
Resp: sore throat, rhinorrhea, nasal congestion, cough.
CV: arrhythmias.
GI: nausea, vomiting, diarrhea, anorexia, hemorrhoidal symptoms, metallic taste, elevated liver function tests, abdominal cramps.
GU: oliguriua, voiding difficulty, proteinuria.
Derm: rashes, mucocutaneous eruptions, pruritus.
Hemat: thrombocytosis, eosinophilia.
MS: back, rib, flank pain, leg pain.
Neuro: paresthesia, sensorimotor neuropathy.
Misc: chills, fever, flu-like syndrome, moniliasis.

INTERACTIONS

Drug-Drug: ■ Not recommended for use with other **chelating agents**.

ROUTE AND DOSAGE

- **PO (Adults and Children):** 10 mg/kg or 350 mg/m^2 q 8 hr for 5 days, then reduce to 10 mg/kg or 350 mg/m^2 q 12 hr for 2 more wks. Repeated courses should follow a 2-wk rest period.

PHARMACODYNAMICS (urinary lead excretion)

	ONSET	PEAK	DURATION
PO	within 2 hr	2–4 hr	8–12 hr

NURSING IMPLICATIONS

Assessment

□ Assess patient and family members for evidence of lead poisoning prior to and frequently throughout course of therapy. Acute lead poisoning is characterized by a metallic taste, colicky abdominal pain, vomiting, diarrhea, oliguria, and coma. Symptoms of chronic poisoning vary with severity and include anorexia, a blue-black line along the gums, intermittent vomiting, paresthesia, encephalopathy, seizures, and coma.

□ Monitor strict intake and output and daily weight. Notify physician of any discrepancies. Patients undergoing succimer therapy should be adequately hydrated.

□ Monitor neurologic status closely (level of consciousness, pupil re-

*Underlines indicate most frequent; **CAPITALS** indicate life-threatening.

sponse, movement). Notify physician immediately of any changes.
- □ Monitor patient for signs of allergic or other mucocutaneous reactions, especially during repeated courses of succimer therapy.
- ▪ **Lab Test Considerations:** Monitor blood and urine lead levels prior to and periodically throughout therapy. After therapy, monitor patients for rebound of blood levels at least once weekly until stable. Succimer is indicated for treatment of blood lead levels of >45 mcg/dl.
- □ May cause elevated serum transaminases, alkaline phosphatase, and cholesterol; monitor prior to and at least weekly during therapy.
- □ May interfere with serum and urine lab tests.

POTENTIAL NURSING DIAGNOSES
- ▪ Injury, high risk for: poisoning (indications, patient/family teaching).
- ▪ Home maintenance management, impaired (indications).
- ▪ Knowledge deficit related to medication regimen (patient/family teaching).

IMPLEMENTATION
- ▪ **General Info:** Coadministration of succimer with other chelation agents is not recommended. Patients who have received EDTA or BAL may receive subsequent therapy with succimer after 4 wk.
- □ Course of treatment lasts 19 days. Doses are administered every 8 hr for 5 days and then every 12 hr for 14 days. Unless blood levels indicate prompt treatment is needed, a minimum of 2 wk between courses is recommended.
- ▪ **PO:** If patient is unable to swallow the capsule, open capsule and sprinkle medicated beads on a small amount of soft food or place in a spoon and follow with a fruit drink.

PATIENT/FAMILY TEACHING
- □ Discuss need for follow-up appointments to monitor lead levels. Additional treatments may be necessary.
- □ Instruct patient to drink adequate fluids throughout therapy.
- □ Advise patient to notify physician if rash occurs.
- □ Consult public health department regarding potential sources of lead poisoning in the home, workplace, and recreational areas. Chelation therapy cannot be used as prophylaxis for lead poisoning.

EVALUATION

Effectiveness of therapy can be demonstrated by: ▪ Decrease in symptoms of lead poisoning □ Decrease in blood lead levels to below 45 mcg/dl although the normal upper limit is 29 mcg/dl.

SUCCINYLCHOLINE
(sux-sin-il-**koe**-leen)
Anectine, Quelicin, Scoline, Sucostrin, Suxamethonium

CLASSIFICATION(S):
Neuromuscular blocking agent—depolarizing
Pregnancy Category UK

INDICATIONS
▪ Used after induction of anesthesia in surgical procedures to produce skeletal muscle paralysis.

ACTION
▪ Prevents neuromuscular transmission by blocking the effect of acetylcholine at the myoneural junction ▪ Has agonist activity initially, producing fasciculation ▪ Causes the release of histamine ▪ Has no analgesic or anxiolytic effects. **Therapeutic Effect:** ▪ Skeletal muscle paralysis.

PHARMACOKINETICS
Absorption: Well absorbed following deep IM administration.
Distribution: Widely distributed into extracellular fluid. Crosses the placenta in small amounts.
Metabolism and Excretion: 90% me-

S

tabolized by pseudocholinesterase in plasma. 10% excreted unchanged by the kidneys.
Half-life: UK.

CONTRAINDICATIONS AND PRECAUTIONS

Contraindicated in: ▪ Hypersensitivity to succinylcholine or parabens ▪ Plasma pseudocholinesterase deficiency ▪ Children and neonates (continuous infusions).
Use Cautiously in: ▪ History of malignant hyperthermia ▪ History of pulmonary disease, renal or liver impairment ▪ Elderly or debilitated patients ▪ Glaucoma ▪ Electrolyte disturbances ▪ Patients receiving cardiac glycosides ▪ Fractures or muscular spasm ▪ Myasthenia gravis or myasthenic syndromes ▪ Has been used in pregnant women undergoing cesarean section ▪ Neonates and children (increased risk of malignant hyperthermia).

ADVERSE REACTIONS AND SIDE EFFECTS*

Note: Most adverse reactions to succinylcholine are extensions of pharmacologic effects.
CV: hypotension, arrhythmias.
Resp: bronchospasm, apnea.
F and E: hyperkalemia.
MS: muscle fasciculation.
Misc: MALIGNANT HYPERTHERMIA.

INTERACTIONS

Drug-Drug: ▪ Concurrent administration of **cholinesterase inhibitors (ecothiophate, isofluorophate,** and **demecarium eyedrops)** reduces pseudocholinesterase activity and intensifies paralysis ▪ Intensity and duration of paralysis may be prolonged by pretreatment with **general anesthesia, aminoglycoside antibiotics, polymyxin B, colistin, clindamycin, lidocaine, quinidine, procainamide, beta-adrenergic blocking agents, potassium-losing diuretics,** and **magnesium**.

ROUTE AND DOSAGE

Note: IV route is preferred, but deep IM injection may be used in children and patients without vascular access.

Test Dose

- **IV (Adults):** 10 mg (0.1 mg/kg), then assess respiratory function.

Short Procedures

- **IV (Adults):** 0.6 mg/kg (range 0.3–1.1 mg/kg); additional doses depend on response.
- **IV (Children):** 1–2 mg/kg; additional doses depend on response.

Prolonged Procedures

- **IV (Adults):** 2.5 mg/min infusion (range 0.5–10 mg/min) or 0.6 mg/kg (range 0.3–1.1 mg/kg) initially, then 0.04–0.07 mg/kg as necessary.

Intramuscular Dosing

- **IM (Adults and Children):** 2.5–4 mg/kg (total dose not to exceed 150 mg).

PHARMACODYNAMICS (skeletal muscle paralysis)

	ONSET	PEAK	DURATION
IM	up to 3 min	UK	10–30 min
IV	0.5–1 min	1–2 min	4–10 min

NURSING IMPLICATIONS

Assessment

- ▫ Assess respiratory status continuously throughout use of succinylcholine. Succinylcholine should be used only by individuals experienced in endotracheal intubation, and equipment for this procedure should be immediately available.
- ▫ Monitor neuromuscular response to succinylcholine with a peripheral nerve stimulator intraoperatively. Paralysis is initially selective and usually occurs consecutively in the following muscles: levator muscles of eyelids, muscles of mastication, limb muscles, abdominal muscles, muscles of the glottis, intercostal muscles, and the diaphragm.
- ▫ Monitor ECG, heart rate, and blood

*Underlines indicate most frequent; **CAPITALS** indicate life-threatening.

pressure throughout use of succinylcholine.

- □ Assess patient for history of malignant hyperthermia prior to administration. Monitor for signs of malignant hyperthermia (tachycardia, tachypnea, hypercarbia, jaw muscle spasm, lack of laryngeal relaxation, hyperthermia) throughout administration.
- □ Observe patient for residual muscle weakness and respiratory distress during the recovery period.
- ▪ **Lab Test Considerations:** May cause hyperkalemia, especially in patients with severe trauma, burns, or neurologic disorders.
- ▪ **Toxicity and Overdose:** If overdose occurs, use peripheral nerve stimulator to determine degree of neuromuscular blockade. Maintain airway patency and ventilation until recovery of normal respirations occurs.

Potential Nursing Diagnoses

- ▪ Breathing pattern, ineffective (indications).
- ▪ Communication, impaired: verbal (side effects).

Implementation

- ▪ **General Info:** Succinylcholine has no effect on consciousness or the pain threshold. Adequate anesthesia should *always* be used when succinylcholine is used as an adjunct to surgical procedures or when painful procedures are performed. Benzodiazepines and/or analgesics should be administered concurrently when prolonged succinylcholine therapy is used for ventilator patients, as patient is awake and able to feel all sensations.
- □ If eyes remain open throughout prolonged administration, protect corneas with artificial tears.
- □ To prevent excessive salivation, patients may be premedicated with atropine or scopolamine.
- □ A small dose of a nondepolarizing agent may be used prior to succinylcholine to decrease the severity of muscle fasciculations.
- ▪ **IM:** If IM route is used, administer deep into the deltoid muscle.
- ▪ **IV:** A test dose of 5–10 mg or 0.1 mg/kg may be administered to determine patient's sensitivity and recovery time.
- ▪ **Direct IV:** Usual adult dose is administered over 10–30 sec. Dose is titrated to patient response.
- ▪ **Continuous Infusion:** Dilute as a 0.1–0.2% soln (1–2 mg/ml) in dextrose/Ringer's or lactated Ringer's combinations, dextrose/saline combinations, 0.45% NaCl, 0.9% NaCl, D5W, D10W, Ringer's or lactated Ringer's injection. Soln is stable for 24 hr at room temperature. Administer only clear soln. Discard any unused soln.
- □ *Rate:* Administer at a rate of 0.5–10 mg/min. Titrate dose to patient response and degree of relaxation required.
- ▪ **Syringe Compatibility:** heparin.
- ▪ **Y-Site Compatibility:** heparin with hydrocortisone sodium succinate or potassium chloride.
- ▪ **Additive Compatibility:** amikacin, cephapirin, isoproterenol, meperidine, methyldopate, morphine, norepinephrine, or scopolamine.
- ▪ **Additive Incompatibility:** barbiturates, nafcillin, or sodium bicarbonate.

Patient/Family Teaching

- □ Explain all procedures to patient receiving succinylcholine therapy without anesthesia, as consciousness is not affected by succinylcholine alone. Provide emotional support.
- □ Reassure patient that communication abilities will return as the medication wears off.

Evaluation

Effectiveness of therapy can be demonstrated by: ▪ Adequate suppression of the twitch response when tested with peripheral nerve stimulation with subsequent muscle paralysis.

S

SUCRALFATE
(soo-**kral**-fate)
Carafate, {Sulcrate}

CLASSIFICATION(S):
Antiulcer agent—protectant
Pregnancy Category B

INDICATIONS
▪ Short-term management of duodenal ulcers ▪ Maintenance therapy of duodenal ulcer. **Unlabeled Uses:** ▪ Management of gastric ulcer ▪ Prevention of aspirin-induced gastric mucosal injury due to high-dose aspirin or nonsteroidal anti-inflammatory agents in patients with rheumatoid arthritis.

ACTION
▪ Reacts with gastric acid to form a thick paste, which selectively adheres to the ulcer surface. **Therapeutic Effect:** ▪ Protection of ulcers, with subsequent healing.

PHARMACOKINETICS
Absorption: Systemic absorption is minimal (<5%).
Distribution: Distribution not known.
Metabolism and Excretion: >90% is eliminated in the feces.
Half-life: 6–20 hr.

CONTRAINDICATIONS AND PRECAUTIONS
Contraindicated in: ▪ Hypersensitivity.
Use Cautiously in: ▪ Children (safety not established).

ADVERSE REACTIONS AND SIDE EFFECTS*
CNS: dizziness, vertigo, sleepiness.
GI: constipation, diarrhea, nausea, gastric discomfort, indigestion, dry mouth.
Derm: rashes, pruritus.

INTERACTIONS
Drug-Drug: ▪ May decrease the absorption of **phenytoin, fat-soluble vitamins,** or **tetracycline** ▪ Concurrent **antacids** decrease the effectiveness of sucralfate ▪ Decreases absorption of **fluoroquinolones** (avoid concurrent use).

ROUTE AND DOSAGE
▪ **PO (Adults):** 1 g qid, 1 hr before meals and at bedtime.

PHARMACODYNAMICS (mucosal protectant effect)

	ONSET	PEAK	DURATION
PO	30 min	UK	5 hr

NURSING IMPLICATIONS
Assessment
□ Assess patient routinely for abdominal pain and frank or occult blood in the stool.

Potential Nursing Diagnoses
▪ Comfort, altered: pain (indications).
▪ Bowel elimination, altered: constipation (side effects).
▪ Knowledge deficit related to medication regimen (patient/family teaching).

Implementation
▪ **PO:** Administer on an empty stomach, 1 hr before meals and at bedtime. Do not crush or chew tablets. If nasogastric administration is required, consult pharmacist for diluent, as sucralfate is relatively insoluble and may form a bezoar.
□ If antacids are also prescribed, do not administer within 30 min before or 1 hr after sucralfate dosage.

Patient/Family Teaching
□ Advise patient to continue with course of therapy for 4–8 wk, even if feeling better, to ensure ulcer healing. If a dose is missed, take as soon as remembered unless almost time for next dose; do not double doses.
□ Advise patient that increase in fluid intake, dietary bulk, and exercise may prevent drug-induced constipation.

{} = Available in Canada only.
*Underlines indicate most frequent; **CAPITALS** indicate life-threatening.

- Inform patient that cessation of smoking may help prevent recurrence of duodenal ulcers.
- Emphasize the importance of routine examinations to monitor progress.

Evaluation

Effectiveness of therapy can be demonstrated by: ▪ Decrease in abdominal pain ▪ Healing of duodenal ulcers, seen by x-ray examination and endoscopy.

SUFENTANIL

(soo-**fen**-ta-nil)
Sufenta

CLASSIFICATION(S):
Narcotic analgesic—agonist
Schedule II
Pregnancy Category C

INDICATIONS

▪ Analgesic adjunct when given in the maintenance of balanced anethesia with barbiturate/nitrous oxide/oxygen ▪ Analgesic administered by continuous IV infusion with nitrous oxide/oxygen while maintaining general anesthesia ▪ Primary induction of anesthesia with 100% oxygen in major surgical procedures.

ACTION

▪ Binds to opiate receptors in the CNS, altering the response to and perception of pain and causing generalized CNS depression. **Therapeutic Effects:** ▪ Decreased intensity of moderate to severe pain ▪ Anesthesia.

PHARMACOKINETICS

Absorption: Following IV administration absorption is essentially complete.
Distribution: Does not readily penetrate adipose tissue. Crosses the placenta, enters breast milk.
Metabolism and Excretion: Mostly metabolized by the liver. Some metabolism in small intestine.
Half-life: 2.7 hr (increased during cardiopulmonary bypass).

CONTRAINDICATIONS AND PRECAUTIONS

Contraindicated in: ▪ Hypersensitivity ▪ Known intolerance.
Use Cautiously in: ▪ Elderly patients ▪ Debilitated or severely ill patients ▪ Diabetic patients ▪ Severe pulmonary disease ▪ Hepatic disease ▪ CNS tumors ▪ Increased intracranial pressure ▪ Head trauma ▪ Adrenal insufficiency ▪ Undiagnosed abdominal pain ▪ Hypothyroidism ▪ Alcoholism ▪ Cardiac disease (arrhythmias) ▪ Pregnancy (has been used in women undergoing cesarean section—drowsiness may occur in infant) ▪ Lactation (safety not established).

ADVERSE REACTIONS AND SIDE EFFECTS*

CNS: dizziness, sleepiness, drowsiness.
EENT: blurred vision.
Resp: apnea, postoperative respiratory depression.
CV: bradycardia, tachycardia, hypotension, hypertension, arrhythmias.
GI: nausea, vomiting.
Derm: itching, erythema.
MS: thoracic muscle rigidity, intraoperative muscle movement.
Misc: chills.

INTERACTIONS

Drug-Drug: ▪ Concurrent use of **alcohol, antihistamines, antidepressants,** or **sedative/hypnotics** results in additive CNS depression ▪ **MAO inhibitors** should be avoided for 14 days prior to use ▪ **Cimetidine** or **erythromycin** may prolong duration of recovery ▪ Concurrent use of **benzodiazepines** may increase the risk of hypotension ▪ **Nalbuphine** or **pentazocine** may decrease response to sufentanil.

ROUTE AND DOSAGE

Low-Dose Anesthesia Adjunct

▪ **IV (Adults):** 0.5–2 mcg/kg initially,

*Underlines indicate most frequent; **CAPITALS** indicate life-threatening.

supplemental doses of 10–25 mcg may be given as needed (not to exceed 1 mcg/kg/hr when administered with nitrous oxide and oxygen).

Moderate-Dose Anesthesia Adjunct

- **IV (Adults):** 2–8 mcg/kg initially, supplemental doses of 10–50 mcg may be given as needed (not to exceed 1 mcg/kg/hr when administered with nitrous oxide and oxygen).

Primary Anesthesia (with 100% Oxygen)

- **IV (Adults):** 8–30 mcg/kg initially, supplemental doses of 25–50 mcg may be given as needed.
- **IV (Children):** Cardiovascular surgery—10–25 mcg/kg initially, followed by maintenance dose of 25–50 mcg.

PHARMACODYNAMICS (analgesia)

	ONSET	PEAK	DURATION
IV	within 1 min	UK	5 min

NURSING IMPLICATIONS

Assessment

- □ Monitor respiratory rate and blood pressure frequently throughout course of therapy. Notify physician of significant changes immediately. The respiratory depressant effects of sufentanil last longer than the analgesic effects. Subsequent narcotic doses should be reduced by ¼ to ⅓ of the usually recommended dose. Monitor closely.
- **Lab Test Considerations:** May cause elevated serum amylase and lipase concentrations.
- **Toxicity and Overdose:** If overdose occurs, naloxone (Narcan) is the antidote.

Potential Nursing Diagnoses

- Comfort, altered: pain (indications).
- Breathing pattern, ineffective (adverse reactions).
- Injury, high risk for (side effects).

Implementation

- **General Info:** Benzodiazepines may be administered prior to administration of sufentanil to reduce the induction dose requirements and to decrease the time until loss of consciousness. This combination may increase the risk of hypotension.
- □ Narcotic antagonist, oxygen, and resuscitative equipment should be readily available during the administration of sufentanil.
- **Direct IV:** Slow IV administration may reduce the incidence or severity of muscle rigidity, bradycardia, or hypotension.
- □ *Rate:* Administer slowly, over at least 1–2 min.
- **Continuous Infusion:** When used as a primary anesthetic agent, a continuous infusion of sufentanil may be administered with or following the initial loading dose to provide immediate and sustained effects throughout a prolonged surgical procedure.

Patient/Family Teaching

- □ Caution patient to make position changes slowly to minimize orthostatic hypotension.
- □ Medication causes dizziness and drowsiness. Advise patient to call for assistance during ambulation and transfer, and to avoid driving or other activities requiring alertness for at least 24 hr after administration of sufentanil following outpatient surgery and until response to medication is known.
- □ Instruct patient to avoid alcohol or other CNS depressants for 24 hr after administration of sufentanil following outpatient surgery.

Evaluation

Effectiveness of therapy can be demonstrated by: ■ General quiescence □ Reduced motor activity □ Pronounced analgesia.

SULCONAZOLE

(sul-**kon**-a-zole)
Exelderm

CLASSIFICATION(S):
Antifungal—topical
Pregnancy Category C

INDICATIONS

■ Treatment of: □ Tinea pedis (athlete's foot) □ Tinea corporis □ Tinea cruris □ Tinea versicolor.

ACTION

■ Inhibits growth of susceptible fungi (fungistatic action). **Therapeutic Effect:** ■ Eradication of superficial fungal infections. **Spectrum:** ■ Broad spectrum includes fungistatic action against many dermatophytes, including: □ *Trichophyton rubrum* □ *Trichophyton mentagrophytes* □ *Epidermophyton floccosum* □ *Microsporum canis* □ *Malassezia furfur* ■ Also active against *Candida albicans* and some gram-positive organisms.

PHARMACOKINETICS

Absorption: Systemic absorption following topical administration not known.
Distribution: Distribution not known.
Metabolism and Excretion: Metabolism and excretion not known.
Half-life: UK.

CONTRAINDICATIONS AND PRECAUTIONS

Contraindicated in: ■ Hypersensitivity to sulconazole or any component of the vehicle.
Use Cautiously in: ■ Pregnancy, lactation, or children (safety not known).

ADVERSE REACTIONS AND SIDE EFFECTS*

Derm: itching, burning, stinging, redness.

INTERACTIONS

Drug–Drug: ■ None significant.

ROUTE AND DOSAGE

■ **Top (Adults):** Apply small amount of 1% cream or lotion 1–2 times daily (bid for tinea pedis) for 3–4 wk.

PHARMACODYNAMICS (resolution of infection)

	ONSET	PEAK	DURATION
Top	UK	3–4 wk	UK

NURSING IMPLICATIONS

Assessment

□ Inspect involved areas of skin and mucous membranes prior to and frequently throughout course of therapy. Increased skin irritation may indicate need to discontinue medication.

Potential Nursing Diagnoses

■ Skin integrity, impaired: actual (indications).
■ Infection, high risk for (indications).
■ Knowledge deficit related to medication regimen (patient/family teaching).

Implementation

■ **General Info:** Consult physician for proper cleansing technique prior to applying medication.
■ **Top:** Apply small amount to cover affected area completely.

Patient/Family Teaching

□ Instruct patient to apply medication as directed for full course of therapy, even if feeling better.
□ Advise patient to report increased skin irritation or lack of response to therapy to physician.

Evaluation

Effectiveness of therapy can be demonstrated by: ■ Decrease in skin irritation and resolution of infection. For tinea pedis, therapeutic response may take 3–4 wk.

SULFACETAMIDE

(sul-fa-**seet**-a-mide)
Ak-Sulf, Bleph 10, Cetamide, Isopto-Cetamide, I-Sylfacet, Ocu-Sul, Sulamyd, Sulf-10, Sulfair, Sulfar Forte, {Sulfex}, Sulten-10

{} = Available in Canada only.
*Underlines indicate most frequent; **CAPITALS** indicate life-threatening.

S

CLASSIFICATION(S):
Anti-infective—sulfonamide,
Ophthalmic—anti-infective
Pregnancy Category UK

INDICATIONS

▪ Treatment of conjunctivitis due to susceptible organisms ▪ Prophylaxis against infection following removal of foreign bodies from the eye.

ACTION

▪ Interferes with bacterial folic acid synthesis. **Therapeutic Effect:** ▪ Bacteriostatic action against susceptible bacteria. **Spectrum:** ▪ Broad spectrum, including many gram-positive and gram-negative pathogens.

PHARMACOKINETICS

Absorption: Minimal absorption from the eye.
Distribution: No distribution.
Metabolism and Excretion: None.
Half-life: UK.

CONTRAINDICATIONS AND PRECAUTIONS

Contraindicated in: ▪ Previous hypersensitivity reactions to sulfonamides ▪ Cross-sensitivity with thiazide diuretics, sulfonylurea oral hypoglycemic agents, or carbonic anhydrase inhibitors may exist.
Use Cautiously in: ▪ None significant.

ADVERSE REACTIONS AND SIDE EFFECTS*

EENT: local irritation.
Misc: superinfection, hypersensitivity reactions, including STEVENS-JOHNSON SYNDROME.

INTERACTIONS

Drug-Drug: ▪ Antagonism may occur with concurrent use of ophthalmic **gentamicin** ▪ Incompatible with **silver nitrate** or **mild silver protein**.

ROUTE AND DOSAGE

Ointment

▪ **Ophth (Adults):** 1.25–2.5-cm ribbon in conjunctival sac 1–3 times/day and at bedtime, or at bedtime in conjunction with daytime use of soln.

Solution

▪ **Ophth (Adults):** 1–3 drops every 1–3 hr, depending on severity of infection.

PHARMACODYNAMICS (anti-infective effects)

	ONSET	PEAK	DURATION
Ophth	rapid	UK	1–4 hr*

*Longer for ointment.

NURSING IMPLICATIONS

Assessment

□ Assess eyes for signs of infection (redness, purulent discharge, pain) prior to and periodically throughout therapy. Report purulent eye discharge to physician; sulfacetamide is inactivated by purulent exudate.
□ Assess patient for allergy to sulfonamides.

Potential Nursing Diagnoses

▪ Infection, high risk for (indications).
▪ Knowledge deficit related to medication regimen (patient/family teaching).

Implementation

▪ **Ophth:** Instill eyedrops by having patient lie down or tilt head back and look at ceiling, pull down on lower lid, and instill medication into conjunctival sac. Do not use soln if dark brown. Wait 5 min before administering any other eyedrops.
□ Prior to instilling ointment, hold in hand for several mins to warm before use. Have patient lie down or tilt head back and look at ceiling, squeeze small amount of ointment (¼–½ in) inside lower lid. Have patient close eye gently and roll eye in all directions while eye is closed. May cause temporary blurring of vision. Allow 10

*Underlines indicate most frequent; **CAPITALS** indicate life-threatening.

min before administration of any other eye ointments.

Patient/Family Teaching

- ▫ Instruct patient to instill medication exactly as directed for full length of prescription, even if feeling better. Missed doses should be taken as soon as remembered unless almost time for next dose.
- ▫ Instruct patient on correct procedure for instillation of eyedrops or ointment. Advise patient of the importance of not allowing the tip of the container to come in contact with the eye or any other surface. Emphasize the importance of handwashing to prevent the spread of infection.
- ▫ Advise patient to notify physician if improvement is not seen in 7–8 days, if condition worsens, or if pain, itching, or swelling of the eye occurs.
- ▫ Patients with ophthalmic infections should be advised to avoid wearing contact lenses until the infection is resolved and physician approves.

Evaluation

Effectiveness of therapy can be demonstrated by: ▪ Resolution of the signs and symptoms of occular infection.

SULFAMETHOXAZOLE

(sul-fa-meth-**ox**-a-zole)
{Apo-Sulfamethoxazole}, Gantanol, Gantanol DS

CLASSIFICATION(S):
Anti-infective—sulfonamide
Pregnancy Category C

INDICATIONS

▪ Treatment of: ▫ Urinary tract infections ▫ Nocardiosis ▫ Toxoplasmosis and malaria (in combination with other anti-infectives).

ACTION

▪ Interferes with bacterial folic acid synthesis. **Therapeutic Effect:** ▪ Bacteriostatic action against susceptible bacteria. **Spectrum:** ▪ Notable for activity against some gram-positive pathogens, including: ▫ Streptococci and staphylococci ▫ *Clostridium perfringens* ▫ *Clostridium tetani* ▫ *Nocardia asteroides* ▪ Active against some gram-negative pathogens, including: ▫ *Enterobacter* ▫ *Escherichia coli* ▫ *Klebsiella* ▫ *Proteus mirabilis* ▫ *Proteus vulgaris* ▫ *Salmonella* ▫ *Shigella*.

PHARMACOKINETICS

Absorption: Well absorbed following oral administration.
Distribution: Widely distributed. Crosses the placenta and enters breast milk.
Metabolism and Excretion: Mostly metabolized by the liver. 20% excreted unchanged by the kidneys.
Half-life: 7–12 hr.

CONTRAINDICATIONS AND PRECAUTIONS

Contraindicated in: ▪ Hypersensitivity ▪ Glucose-6-phosphate dehydrogenase (G6-PD deficiency) ▪ Porphyria ▪ Pregnancy or lactation ▪ Infants (unless treating congenital toxoplasmosis).
Use Cautiously in: ▪ Severe renal or hepatic impairment.

ADVERSE REACTIONS AND SIDE EFFECTS*

CNS: dizziness, ataxia, depression, confusion, psychosis, ataxia, drowsiness, restlessness.
GI: anorexia, nausea, vomiting, hepatitis.
GU: crystalluria.
Derm: rashes, exfoliative dermatitis, photosensitivity.
Hemat: APLASTIC ANEMIA, thrombocy-

{} = Available in Canada only.
*Underlines indicate most frequent; **CAPITALS** indicate life-threatening.

topenia, AGRANULOCYTOSIS, eosinophilia.
Neuro: peripheral neuropathy.
Misc: superinfection, fever, hypersensitivity reactions, including STEVENS-JOHNSON SYNDROME and serum sickness.

INTERACTIONS

Drug-Drug: ▪ May enhance the action and increase the risk of toxicity from **oral hypoglycemic agents, phenytoin, methotrexate, anticoagulants,** or **zidovudine** ▪ Concurrent use with **methenamine** may increase the risk of crystalluria ▪ Increased risk of drug-induced hepatitis with other **hepatotoxic agents.**

ROUTE AND DOSAGE

- **PO (Adults):** 2 g initially, then 1 g q 8–12 hr.
- **PO (Children):** 50–60 mg/kg initially, then 25–30 mg/kg q 12 hr (not to exceed 75 mg/kg/day).

PHARMACODYNAMICS (blood levels)

	ONSET	PEAK
PO	1 hr	2 hr

NURSING IMPLICATIONS

Assessment

- ▫ Assess patient for infection (vital signs; appearance of wound, sputum, urine, and stool; WBC) at beginning and throughout course of therapy.
- ▫ Obtain specimens for culture and sensitivity prior to initiating therapy. First dose may be given before receiving results.
- ▫ Assess patient for allergy to sulfonamides.
- ▫ Monitor intake and output ratios. Fluid intake should be sufficient to maintain a urine output of at least 1200–1500 ml daily to prevent crystalluria and stone formation.
- ▪ **Lab Test Considerations:** Monitor CBC and urinalysis periodically throughout therapy.
- ▫ May produce elevated serum bilirubin, creatinine, and alkaline phosphatase concentrations.

Potential Nursing Diagnoses

- ▪ Infection, high risk for (indications, side effects).
- ▪ Knowledge deficit related to medication regimen (patient/family teaching).
- ▪ Noncompliance related to medication regimen (patient/family teaching).

Implementation

- ▪ **PO:** Administer around the clock on an empty stomach, at least 1 hr before or 2 hr after meals, with a full glass of water. Tablets may be crushed and taken with fluid of patient's choice for patients with difficulty swallowing. Use calibrated measuring device for liquid preparations.

Patient/Family Teaching

- ▫ Instruct patient to take medication around the clock and to finish the drug completely as directed, even if feeling better. If a dose is missed, it should be taken as soon as remembered. Advise patient that sharing of this medication may be dangerous.
- ▫ May cause dizziness. Caution patient to avoid driving or other activities requiring alertness until response to medication is known.
- ▫ Caution patient to use sunscreen and protective clothing to prevent photosensitivity reactions.
- ▫ Advise patient to notify physician if skin rash, sore throat, fever, mouth sores, or unusual bleeding or bruising occurs.
- ▫ Instruct patient to notify physician if symptoms do not improve within a few days. Emphasize the importance of follow-up examinations to monitor progress and side effects.

Evaluation

Clinical response can be evaluated by:
▪ Resolution of the signs and symptoms of infection. Length of time for complete resolution depends on the organism and site of infection.

SULFASALAZINE
(sul-fa-**sal**-a-zeen)
Azulfidine, {PMS Sulfasalazine}, {Salazopyrin}

CLASSIFICATION(S):
Anti-infective—sulfonamide, Gastrointestinal—anti-inflammatory
Pregnancy Category B

INDICATIONS
▪ Used with other treatment modalities (glucocorticoids, diet) in the management of ulcerative colitis.

ACTION
▪ May have mild local antibacterial and anti-inflammatory properties in the colon. **Therapeutic Effect:** ▪ Reduction in symptoms of ulcerative colitis.

PHARMACOKINETICS
Absorption: 10–15% absorbed following oral administration.
Distribution: Widely distributed. Crosses the placenta and enters breast milk.
Metabolism and Excretion: Split by intestinal bacteria into sulfapyridine and 5-aminosalicylic acid. Some of absorbed sulfasalazine is excreted by bile back into intestine. 15% excreted unchanged by the kidneys. Sulfapyridine also excreted mostly by the kidneys.
Half-life: 6 hr.

CONTRAINDICATIONS AND PRECAUTIONS
Contraindicated in: ▪ Hypersensitivity reactions to sulfonamides or salicylates ▪ Cross-sensitivity with furosemide, sulfonylurea hypoglycemic agents, or carbonic anhydrase inhibitors may exist ▪ G6-PD deficiency ▪ Urinary tract or intestinal obstruction ▪ Children <2 yr ▪ Porphyria.
Use Cautiously in: ▪ Severe hepatic or renal impairment ▪ Pregnancy (has been used safely) ▪ Lactation (safety not established).

ADVERSE REACTIONS AND SIDE EFFECTS*
CNS: headache, dizziness, ataxia, depression, confusion, psychosis, drowsiness, restlessness.
Resp: pneumonitis.
GI: anorexia, nausea, diarrhea, vomiting, hepatitis.
GU: crystalluria, oligospermia, infertility, orange-yellow discoloration of urine.
Derm: rashes, yellow discoloration, exfoliative dermatitis, photosenstivity.
Hemat: megaloblastic anemia, **APLASTIC ANEMIA**, thrombocytopenia, **AGRANULOCYTOSIS**, eosinophilia.
Neuro: peripheral neuropathy.
Misc: fever, hypersensitivity reactions, including **STEVENS-JOHNSON SYNDROME** and serum sickness.

INTERACTIONS
Drug–Drug: ▪ May enhance the action and increase the risk of toxicity from **oral hypoglycemic agents, phenytoin, methotrexate, zidovudine,** or **oral anticoagulants** ▪ Increased risk of drug-induced hepatitis with other **hepatotoxic agents** ▪ Increased risk of crystalluria with **methenamine**.
Drug–Food: ▪ May decrease **iron** and **folic acid** absorption.

ROUTE AND DOSAGE
- **PO (Adults):** 3–4 g/day in 3–4 divided doses (range 1–12 g/day).
- **PO (Children):** 40–60 mg/kg/day in 3–6 divided doses, maintenance dose of 30 mg/kg/day in 4 divided doses.

PHARMACODYNAMICS (blood levels)

	ONSET	PEAK
PO	1 hr	1.5–6 hr

{} = Available in Canada only.
*Underlines indicate most frequent; **CAPITALS** indicate life-threatening.

S

NURSING IMPLICATIONS

Assessment

- Assess frequency, quantity, and consistency of stools and abdominal pain at beginning and throughout course of therapy.
- Assess patient for allergy to sulfonamides and salicylates.
- Monitor intake and output ratios. Fluid intake should be sufficient to maintain a urine output of at least 1200–1500 ml daily to prevent crystalluria and stone formation.
- Proctoscopy and sigmoidoscopy may be required periodically during treatment to determine patient response and dosage adjustments.
- **Lab Test Considerations:** Monitor CBC prior to and monthly during prolonged therapy. Discontinue sulfasalazine if blood dyscrasias occur.
- Monitor urinalysis prior to and periodically throughout therapy for crystalluria and urinary cell calculi formation.

Potential Nursing Diagnoses

- Comfort, altered: pain (indications).
- Bowel elimination, altered: diarrhea (indications).
- Knowledge deficit related to medication regimen (patient/family teaching).

Implementation

- **General Info:** Varying dosing regimens may be used to minimize GI side effects.
- **PO:** Administer after meals or with food to minimize GI irritation, with a full glass of water. Do not crush or chew enteric-coated tablets. Shake oral suspension well prior to administration. Use a calibrated measuring device to measure liquid preparations.

Patient/Family Teaching

- Instruct patient to take medication as directed, even if feeling better. If a dose is missed, it should be taken as soon as remembered unless almost time for next dose.
- May cause dizziness. Caution patient to avoid driving or other activities that require alertness until response to medication is known.
- Caution patient to use sunscreen and protective clothing to prevent photosensitivity reactions.
- Inform patient that this medication may cause orange-yellow discoloration of urine and skin, which is not significant.
- Advise patient to notify physician if skin rash, sore throat, fever, mouth sores, or unusual bleeding or bruising occurs.
- Instruct patient to notify physician if symptoms do not improve after 1–2 mon of therapy.

Evaluation

Clinical response can be evaluated by:
▪ Decrease in diarrhea and abdominal pain ▫ Return to normal bowel habits in inflammatory bowel disease.

SULFINPYRAZONE

(sul-fin-**peer**-a-zone)
{Antazone}, {Anturan}, Anturane, {Apo-Sulfinpyrazone}, {Novo-pyrazone}

CLASSIFICATION(S):
Antigout agent—uricosuric
Pregnancy Category UK

INDICATIONS

▪ Management (long-term) of gout. **Unlabeled Use:** ▪ Used as an antiplatelet agent in the prevention of myocardial infarction.

ACTION

▪ Decreases serum uric acid levels by decreasing renal reabsorption and subsequently increasing urinary excretion ▪ Decreases platelet aggregation ▪ Increases platelet survival. **Therapeutic Effect:** ▪ Prevention of gouty attacks by keeping serum uric acid levels lowered.

PHARMACOKINETICS

Absorption: Well absorbed following oral administration.
Distribution: Distribution to tissues not known.
Metabolism and Excretion: Mostly metabolized by the liver. Converted to compounds with uricosuric (parahydroxy-sulfinpyrazone) and antiplatelet activity (sulfide metabolite).
Half-life: 3 hr (1 hr for parahydroxy-sulfinpyrazone, up to 13 hr for sulfide metabolite).

CONTRAINDICATIONS AND PRECAUTIONS

Contraindicated in: ▪ Hypersensitivity ▪ Cross-sensitivity with oxyphenbutazone and phenylbutazone may exist.
Use Cautiously in: ▪ History of blood dyscrasias ▪ GI bleeding ▪ History of kidney stones ▪ Neoplastic disease or radiation therapy (increased risk of uric acid stone formation) ▪ Acute attacks of gout.

ADVERSE REACTIONS AND SIDE EFFECTS*

GI: GI bleeding, <u>nausea</u>, <u>vomiting</u>, abdominal pain.
GU: uric acid kidney stones.
Derm: <u>rashes</u>.
Hemat: blood dyscrasias.
Misc: fever.

INTERACTIONS

Drug-Drug: ▪ Concurrent use of **antineoplastic agents** (increased risk of uric acid kidney stones) ▪ Increased risk of bleeding with **aspirin, anticoagulants, cefamandole, cefoperazone, moxalactam, cefotetan, plicamycin,** or **thrombolytic agents**.

ROUTE AND DOSAGE

Hypouricemic

▪ **PO (Adults):** 100–200 mg bid, may increase over 1-wk period to maintenance dose of 200–800 mg/day.

PHARMACODYNAMICS (hypouricemic effects)

	ONSET	PEAK	DURATION
PO	UK	UK	4–10 hr

NURSING IMPLICATIONS

Assessment

▪ **Gout:** Assess involved joints for pain, mobility, and edema throughout course of therapy.
□ Monitor intake and output ratios. Fluids should be encouraged, to prevent urate stone formation (2000–3000 ml/day). Alkalinization of the urine with sodium bicarbonate, potassium citrate, or acetazolamide may also be ordered for this purpose.
▪ **Lab Test Considerations:** CBC, serum uric acid levels, and renal function should be monitored routinely during long-term therapy.
□ Serum and urine uric acid determinations may be measured periodically when sulfinpyrazone is used to treat hyperuricemia.

Potential Nursing Diagnoses

▪ Comfort, altered: pain (indications).
▪ Mobility, impaired physical (indications).
▪ Knowledge deficit related to medication regimen (patient/family teaching).

Implementation

▪ **General Info:** Sulfinpyrazone therapy is not used to treat gouty arthritis but rather, to prevent it. If acute attacks occur during therapy, sulfinpyrazone is usually continued at full dose along with treatment with colchicine or nonsteroidal anti-inflammatory agents.
□ Initiation of sulfinpyrazone therapy should not occur within 2–3 wk of an acute gout attack.
▪ **PO:** Administer with food or antacid to minimize gastric irritation.

Patient/Family Teaching

□ Instruct patient to take medication exactly as directed, and not to discon-

*<u>Underlines</u> indicate most frequent; **CAPITALS** indicate life-threatening.

S

tinue without consulting physician. Irregular dosage schedules may cause elevation of uric acid levels and precipitate an acute gout attack. Missed doses should be taken as soon as remembered, unless almost time for next dose.
- ▫ Advise patient to follow physician's recommendations regarding weight loss, diet, and alcohol consumption.
- ▫ Caution patient not to take aspirin or other salicylates, as they decrease the effects of sulfinpyrazone.
- ▫ Instruct patient to report rash, nausea, vomiting, abdominal pain, unusual bleeding or bruising, sore throat, fatigue, or fever to physician promptly.

EVALUATION

Effectiveness of therapy can be demonstrated by: ▪ Decrease in pain and swelling in affected joints and subsequent decrease in frequency of gout attacks. May require several mons of continuous therapy for maximum effects ▪ Prevention of myocardial infarction.

SULFISOXAZOLE
(sul-fi-**sox**-a-zole)
Gantrisin, Lipo Gantrisin, {Novo-soxazole}

CLASSIFICATION(S):
Anti-infective—sulfonamide
Pregnancy Category C

INDICATIONS

▪ **PO:** Treatment of urinary tract infections, nocardiosis, and, in combination with other anti-infectives, malaria, and pelvic inflammatory disease in prepubertal adolescents ▪ **Ophth:** Treatment of superficial eye infections ▪ **PO, Ophth:** Treatment of trachoma and other chlamydial eye infections.

ACTION

▪ Interferes with bacterial folic acid synthesis. **Therapeutic Effect:** ▪ Bacteriostatic action against susceptible bacteria. **Spectrum:** ▪ Notable for activity against some gram-positive pathogens, including: ▫ Streptococci and staphylococci ▫ *Clostridium perfringens* ▫ *Clostridium tetani* ▫ *Nocardia asteroides* ▪ Active against some gram-negative pathogens, including: ▫ *Enterobacter* ▫ *Escherichia coli* ▫ *Klebsiella* ▫ *Proteus mirabilis* ▫ *Proteus vulgaris* ▫ *Salmonella* ▫ *Shigella.*

PHARMACOKINETICS

Absorption: Well absorbed following oral administration.
Distribution: Widely distributed. Crosses the placenta and enters breast milk.
Metabolism and Excretion: Mostly metabolized by the liver.
Half-life: 5–8 hr.

CONTRAINDICATIONS AND PRECAUTIONS

Contraindicated in: ▪ Hypersensitivity to sulfonamides ▪ Cross-sensitivity with furosemide, thiazides, sulfonylurea oral hypoglycemic agents, or carbonic anhydrase inhibitors may exist ▪ Porphyria ▪ Pregnancy or lactation ▪ Glucose-6-phosphate dehydrogenase (G6-PD) deficiency.
Use Cautiously in: ▪ Severe renal or hepatic impairment.

ADVERSE REACTIONS AND SIDE EFFECTS*

CNS: dizziness, ataxia, depression, confusion, psychosis, drowsiness, restlessness.
GI: anorexia, <u>nausea</u>, <u>vomiting</u>, hepatitis.
GU: crystalluria.
Derm: <u>rashes</u>, exfoliative dermatitis, photosensitivity.
Hemat: APLASTIC ANEMIA, thrombo-

{} = Available in Canada only.
*<u>Underlines</u> indicate most frequent; **CAPITALS** indicate life-threatening.

cytopenia, AGRANULOCYTOSIS, eosinophilia.
Neuro: peripheral neuropathy.
Misc: fever, superinfection, hypersensitivity reactions, including STEVENS-JOHNSON SYNDROME and serum sickness.

INTERACTIONS

Drug-Drug: ▪ May enhance the action and increase the risk of toxicity from **oral hypoglycemic agents, methotrexate, phenytoin, zidovudine,** or **oral anticoagulants** ▪ Increased risk of crystalluria with **methenamine** ▪ Increased risk of drug-induced hepatitis with other **hepatotoxic agents** ▪ Ophthalmic form is incompatible with **silver nitrate** or **mild silver protein.**

ROUTE AND DOSAGE

- **PO (Adults):** 2–4 g initially, then 4–8 g/day in divided doses q 4–6 hr or 4–5 g q 12 hr of extended-release suspension (Lipo Gantrisin).
- **PO (Children):** 75 mg/kg initially, then 150 mg/kg/day in divided doses q 4–6 hr or 60–75 mg/kg q 12 hr of extended-release suspension.
- **Ophth (Adults):** 1 drop of 4% soln q 8 hr (may be used more often) or thin strip (1.25–2.5 cm) of 4% ointment q 8–24 hr and at bedtime.

PHARMACODYNAMICS (blood levels)

	ONSET	PEAK
PO	1 hr	2–4 hr
PO-ER	delayed	delayed
Ophth	UK	UK

NURSING IMPLICATIONS

Assessment

- □ Assess patient for infection (vital signs; appearance of wound, sputum, urine, and stool; WBC) at beginning and throughout course of therapy.
- □ Obtain specimens for culture and sensitivity prior to intiating therapy. First dose may be given before receiving results.
- □ Assess patient for allergy to sulfonamides.
- □ Monitor intake and output ratios. Fluid intake should be sufficient to maintain a urine output of at least 1200–1500 ml daily to prevent crystalluria and stone formation.
- ▪ **Lab Test Considerations:** Monitor CBC prior to and monthly during prolonged therapy. Therapy should be discontinued if blood dyscrasias occur.
- □ Monitor urinalysis prior to and periodically throughout therapy for crystalluria and formation of urinary calculi.

Potential Nursing Diagnoses

- ▪ Infection, high risk for (indications, side effects).
- ▪ Knowledge deficit related to medication regimen (patient/family teaching).
- ▪ Noncompliance related to medication regimen (patient/family teaching).

Implementation

- ▪ **General Info:** Available in tablet, oral suspension, extended-release oral suspension, and ophthalmic soln and ointment forms.
- ▪ **PO:** Administer around the clock on an empty stomach, at least 1 hr before or 2 hr after meals, with a full glass of water. Tablets may be crushed and taken with liquids for patients with difficulty swallowing. Use calibrated measuring device for liquid preparations.
- ▪ **Ophth:** See Appendix H for instillation of ophthalmic preparations.

Patient/Family Teaching

- ▪ **General Info:** Instruct patient to take medication around the clock and to finish the drug completely as directed, even if feeling better. If a dose is missed, it should be taken as soon as remembered unless almost time for next dose. Advise patient that sharing of this medication may be dangerous.
- □ May cause dizziness. Caution patient to avoid driving and other activities requiring alertness until response to medication is known.
- □ Caution patient to use sunscreen and

protective clothing to prevent photosensitivity reactions.

- Advise patient to notify physician if skin rash, sore throat, fever, mouth sores, or unusual bleeding or bruising occurs.
- Instruct patient to notify physician if symptoms do not improve within a few days. Emphasize the importance of follow-up examinations to monitor blood counts.

- **Ophth:** Instruct patient in correct technique for instillation of ophthalmic preparations.
  - Advise patient that stinging or burning may occur after instillation of ophthalmic preparations.
  - Ophthalmic ointment may cause blurred vision. Caution patient to avoid driving or other activities requiring visual acuity until response to medication is known.

Evaluation

Clinical response can be evaluated by: ▪ Resolution of the signs and symptoms of infection. Length of time for complete resolution depends on the organism and site of infection.

SULINDAC

(**soo**-lin-dak)

Clinoril

CLASSIFICATION(S):
Nonsteroidal anti-inflammatory agent
Pregnancy Category UK

INDICATIONS

▪ Management of inflammatory disorders, including: ▫ Rheumatoid arthritis ▫ Osteoarthritis ▫ Acute gouty arthritis ▫ Bursitis.

ACTION

▪ Inhibits prostaglandin synthesis. **Therapeutic Effects:** ▪ Suppression of pain and inflammation.

PHARMACOKINETICS

Absorption: Well absorbed from the GI tract following oral administration.

Distribution: Distribution not known. Enters breast milk in small amounts.

Metabolism and Excretion: Converted by the liver to active drug. Minimal amounts excreted unchanged by the kidneys.

Half-life: 7.8 hr (16.4 hr for active metabolite).

CONTRAINDICATIONS AND PRECAUTIONS

Contraindicated in: ▪ Hypersensitivity ▪ Cross-sensitivity may exist with other nonsteroidal anti-inflammatory agents, including aspirin ▪ Active GI bleeding or ulcer disease ▪ Pregnancy.

Use Cautiously in: ▪ Severe cardiovascular, renal, or hepatic disease (dosage modification recommended) ▪ History of ulcer disease ▪ Lactation or children (safety not established).

ADVERSE REACTIONS AND SIDE EFFECTS*

CNS: <u>headache</u>, drowsiness, <u>dizziness</u>.

CV: edema.

EENT: blurred vision, tinnitus.

GI: <u>nausea</u>, <u>dyspepsia</u>, <u>vomiting</u>, <u>diarrhea</u>, <u>constipation</u>, **GI BLEEDING**, <u>discomfort</u>, **HEPATITIS**, flatulence, anorexia, diarrhea.

GU: renal failure.

Derm: <u>rashes</u>, photosensitivity.

Hemat: blood dyscrasias, prolonged bleeding time.

Misc: Allergic reactions, including **ANAPHYLAXIS**.

INTERACTIONS

Drug-Drug: ▪ Concurrent use of **aspirin** may decrease effectiveness ▪ Increased risk of bleeding with **anticoagulants, thrombolytic agents, cefamandole, cefoperazone, cefotetan, moxalactam,** or **plicamycin** ▪ Additive adverse GI side effects with **aspirin, glucocorticoids,** and other **nonsteroidal anti-inflammatory agents** ▪ May de-

*<u>Underlines</u> indicate most frequent; **CAPITALS** indicate life-threatening.

crease response to **antihypertensives** or **diuretics** ▪ May increase serum levels and risk of toxicity from **lithium** ▪ May increase the risk of hematologic toxicity from **antineoplastic agents** or **radiation therapy** ▪ Increased risk of adverse renal effects with **gold compounds** or chronic use of **acetaminophen** ▪ **Antacids** decrease blood levels and decrease effectiveness of sulindac ▪ Increased risk of photosensitivity reactions with other **photosensitizing medications**.

ROUTE AND DOSAGE

- **PO (Adults):** 150–200 mg bid (not to exceed 400 mg/day).

PHARMACODYNAMICS

	ONSET	PEAK	DURATION
PO (analgesic)	1–2 days	UK	UK
PO (anti-inflammatory)	few days–1 wk	2 wk or more	UK

NURSING IMPLICATIONS

Assessment

- □ Patients who have asthma, aspirin-induced allergy, and nasal polyps are at increased risk for developing hypersensitivity reactions. Monitor for rhinitis, asthma, and urticaria.
- □ Assess pain and range of movement prior to and 1–2 hr following administration.
- ▪ **Lab Test Considerations:** BUN, serum creatinine, CBC, and liver function tests should be evaluated periodically in patients receiving prolonged courses of therapy.
- □ Serum potassium, glucose, alkaline phosphatase, SGOT (AST), and SGPT (ALT) may show increased levels.
- □ Bleeding time may be prolonged for 1 day following discontinuation of therapy.

Potential Nursing Diagnoses

- ▪ Comfort, altered: pain (indications).
- ▪ Mobility, impaired physical (indications).
- ▪ Knowledge deficit related to medication regimen (patient/family teaching).

Implementation

- ▪ **PO:** For rapid initial effect, administer 30 min before or 2 hr after meals. May be administered with food, milk, or antacids to decrease GI irritation. Food slows but does not reduce the extent of absorption. Tablets may be crushed and mixed with fluids or food.

Patient/Family Teaching

- □ Advise patient to take this medication with a full glass of water and to remain in an upright position for 15–30 min after administration.
- □ Instruct patient to take medication exactly as directed. If a dose is missed, it should be taken as soon as remembered but not if almost time for the next dose. Do not double doses.
- □ May cause dizziness. Advise patient to avoid driving or other activities requiring alertness until response to the medication is known.
- □ Caution patient to avoid concurrent use of alcohol, aspirin, acetaminophen, or other over-the-counter medications without consulting physician or pharmacist.
- □ Advise patient to notify physician or dentist of medication regimen prior to treatment or surgery.
- □ Advise patient to use sunscreen and protective clothing to prevent photosensitivity reactions.
- □ Instruct patient to notify physician if rash, itching, weight gain, edema, black stools, or persistent headache occurs.

Evaluation

Effectiveness of therapy can be demonstrated by: ▪ Decreased pain and improved joint mobility. Partial arthritic relief may be seen within 7 days, but maximum effectiveness may require 2–3 wk of continuous therapy. Patients who do not respond to one nonsteroidal anti-inflammatory agent may respond to another.

S

SUPROFEN
(soo-**proe**-fen)
Profenal

CLASSIFICATION(S):
Ophthalmic—nonsteroidal anti-inflammatory agent
Pregnancy Category C

INDICATIONS
▪ Prevention of intraoperative miosis.

ACTION
▪ Inhibits prostaglandin synthesis in the eye, resulting in inhibition of miosis. **Therapeutic Effect:** ▪ Prevention of miosis.

PHARMACOKINETICS
Absorption: Small amounts are systemically absorbed.
Distribution: Enters breast milk.
Metabolism and Excretion: Amounts absorbed are mostly metabolized by the liver. 15% excreted unchanged by the kidneys.
Half-life: 1–4 hr.

CONTRAINDICATIONS AND PRECAUTIONS
Contraindicated in: ▪ Hypersensitivity ▪ Cross-sensitivity may exist with other nonsteroidal anti-inflammatory agents, including aspirin.
Use Cautiously in: ▪ Patients with severe cardiovascular, renal, or hepatic disease ▪ Pregnancy, lactation, or children (safety not established) ▪ Bleeding tendencies.

ADVERSE REACTIONS AND SIDE EFFECTS*
EENT: ocular burning, stinging, irritation, itching, photophobia, conjunctival swelling, photophobia, punctate epithelial staining.

INTERACTIONS
Drug–Drug: ▪ Ophthalmic **carbachol** or **acetylcholine** may not be effective when used concurrently with suprofen.

ROUTE AND DOSAGE
▪ **Ophth (Adults):** 2 drops of 1% soln hourly for 3 hr prior to surgery. In addition, 2 drops may be administered q 4 hr during day preceding surgery.

PHARMACODYNAMICS (ophthalmic effects)

	ONSET	PEAK	DURATION
PO	1–2 hr	UK	4–6 hr

NURSING IMPLICATIONS
Assessment
□ Monitor patient for changes in vision, pupil size, and conjunctival irritation periodically throughout therapy.
□ Patients sensitive to aspirin and other nonsteroidal anti-inflammatory agents are at increased risk for developing hypersensitivity reactions. Monitor for rhinitis, asthma, and urticaria.
▪ **Lab Test Considerations:** May prolong bleeding time if systemically absorbed.

Potential Nursing Diagnoses
▪ Knowledge deficit related to medication regimen (patient/family teaching).

Implementation
▪ **General Info:** Instill 2 drops every hr beginning 3 hr prior to surgery. May also be administered during the day preceding surgery.
▪ **Ophth:** Administer ophthalmic soln by having patient tilt head back and look up. Gently depress lower lid with index finger until conjunctival sac is exposed and instill medication. After instillation, maintain gentle pressure on the inner canthus for 1 min to avoid systemic absorption of the drug. Wait at least 5 min before administering other types of eyedrops.

Patient/Family Teaching
□ Instruct patient in proper technique for instillation of ophthalmic medications. Emphasize the importance of

*Underlines indicate most frequent; **CAPITALS** indicate life-threatening.

not touching the applicator tip to any surface.
- Advise patient to take exactly as prescribed. A missed dose should be taken as soon as remembered, unless almost time for next dose.
- Inform patient that temporary stinging or burning may occur. Instruct patient to notify physician if visual changes occur or eye irritation persists.
- Emphasize the importance of regular follow-up examinations to monitor progress and intraocular pressure.

Evaluation

Effectivness of therapy can be demonstrated by: ▪ Inhibition of intraoperative miosis.

TAMOXIFEN

(ta-**mox**-i-fen)
Nolvadex, {Nolvadex-D}, {Tamofen}

CLASSIFICATION(S):
Antineoplastic—estrogen blocker
Pregnancy Category D

INDICATIONS

▪ Palliative or adjunctive treatment of advanced breast cancer.

ACTION

▪ Competes with estrogen for binding sites in breast and other tissues ▪ Reduces DNA synthesis and estrogen response. **Therapeutic Effect:** ▪ Suppression of tumor growth.

PHARMACOKINETICS

Absorption: Absorbed following oral administration.
Distribution: Distribution not known.
Metabolism and Excretion: Mostly metabolized by the liver. Slowly eliminated in the feces. Minimal amounts excreted in the urine.
Half-life: 7 days.

CONTRAINDICATIONS AND PRECAUTIONS

Contraindicated in: ▪ Hypersensitivity ▪ Pregnancy or lactation.
Use Cautiously in: ▪ Women with childbearing potential ▪ Decreased bone marrow reserve.

ADVERSE REACTIONS AND SIDE EFFECTS*

CNS: confusion, depression, headache, weakness.
CV: edema.
EENT: blurred vision.
GI: nausea, vomiting.
GU: vaginal bleeding.
Derm: photosensitivity.
F and E: hypercalcemia.
Hemat: thrombocytopenia, leukopenia.
Metab: hot flashes.
MS: bone pain.
Misc: tumor flare.

INTERACTIONS

Drug-Drug: ▪ **Estrogens** will decrease the effectiveness of concurrently administered tamoxifen.

ROUTE AND DOSAGE

▪ **PO (Adults):** 20–40 mg/day in 2 divided doses.

PHARMACODYNAMICS (tumor response)

	ONSET	PEAK	DURATION
PO	4–10 wk	several mons	UK

NURSING IMPLICATIONS

Assessment

- Assess for an increase in bone or tumor pain. Confer with physician regarding analgesics. This transient pain usually resolves despite continued therapy.
- **Lab Test Considerations:** Monitor CBC, platelets, and calcium levels prior to and throughout course of therapy. May cause transient hypercalcemia in patients with metastases

{} = Available in Canada only.
*Underlines indicate most frequent; **CAPITALS** indicate life-threatening.

to the bone. An estrogen receptor assay should be assessed prior to initiation of therapy.

Potential Nursing Diagnoses

- Knowledge deficit related to medication regimen (patient/family teaching).

Implementation

- **PO:** Administer with food or fluids if GI irritation becomes a problem. Consult physician if patient vomits shortly after administration of medication to determine need for repeat dose.

Patient/Family Teaching

- Instruct patient to take medication exactly as prescribed. If a dose is missed, it should be omitted.
- If skin lesions are present, inform patient that lesions may temporarily increase in size and number and may have increased erythema.
- Advise patient to report bone pain to physician promptly. This pain may be severe. Inform patient that this may be an indication of the drug's effectiveness and will resolve over time. Analgesics should be ordered to control pain.
- Instruct patient to monitor weight weekly. Weight gain or peripheral edema should be reported to physician.
- This medication may induce ovulation and may have teratogenic properties. Advise patient to practice a nonhormonal method of contraception during and for 1 mon after the course of therapy.
- Caution patient to wear sunscreen and protective clothing to prevent photosensitivity reactions.
- Advise patient that medication may cause hot flashes. Notify physician if these become bothersome.
- Instruct patient to notify physician promptly if swelling, shortness of breath, weakness, or blurred vision occurs. Patient should also report vaginal bleeding or confusion.

Evaluation

Effectiveness of therapy can be demonstrated by: ▪ Decrease in the size or spread of breast cancer. Observable effects of therapy may not be seen for 4–10 wk after initiation.

TEARS, ARTIFICIAL

Adsorbotear, Akwa Tears, Artificial Tears Solution, Hypotears, I-Liqui Tears, Isopto Alkaline, Isopto Plain, Isopto Tears, Just Tears, Lacril Artificial Tears, Lacrisert, Liquifilm Forte, Liquifilm Tears, Lyteers, Moisture Drops, Murocel, Muro Tears, Neo-tears, Refresh, Tearisol, Tears Naturale, Tears Plus, Tears Renewed, Ultra Tears

CLASSIFICATION(S):
Ophthalmic—artificial tears
Pregnancy Category UK

INDICATIONS

▪ Replacement of naturally occurring tears with an isotonic preparation in the management of eyes that are dry or irritated due to lack of tears ▪ Lubrication for artificial eyes.

ACTION

▪ Replaces naturally occurring tears ▪ Soln consists of isotonic salt soln, buffers, preservatives, and agents to increase viscosity and prolong ocular contact time ▪ Ocular insert thickens existing tears and prevents their breakdown. **Therapeutic Effect:** ▪ Relief of ocular dryness and irritation due to lack of tears.

PHARMACOKINETICS

Absorption: Minimal absorption of ingredients. Action is primarily local.
Distribution: Distribution not known.
Metabolism and Excretion: None.
Half-life: UK.

CONTRAINDICATIONS AND PRECAUTIONS

Contraindicated in: ▪ Hypersensitivity to: ▫ Various buffers (boric acid) ▫ Viscosity agents (methylcellulose, hydroethylcellulose, hydroxypropylmethylcellulose, propylene glycol, gelatin, dextran, polyvinyl alcohol, polyethylene glycol) ▫ Preservatives (benzalkonium chloride, methyl and propyl parabens, EDTA, chlorobutanol, thimerisol).
Use Cautiously in: ▪ Patients who wear contact lenses (solns may not be compatible with all types of lenses).

ADVERSE REACTIONS AND SIDE EFFECTS*

EENT: photophobia, edema of eyelids, stinging (ocular insert only), temporarily blurred vision.

INTERACTIONS

Drug–Drug: ▪ None significant.

ROUTE AND DOSAGE

Solution

- **Ophth (Adults and Children):** 1–2 drops 3–4 times daily as needed.

Ocular Insert

- **Ophth (Adults):** 1 insert 1–2 times daily.

PHARMACODYNAMICS (relief of ocular dryness)

	ONSET	PEAK	DURATION*
Ophth soln	immediate	UK	6–8 hr
Ophth insert	rapid	UK	12 hr

*Based on frequency of administration.

NURSING IMPLICATIONS

Assessment

▫ Monitor patient for changes in vision and eye irritation and inflammation.

Potential Nursing Diagnoses

- Sensory-perceptual alteration: visual (indications, side effects).
- Knowledge deficit related to medication regimen (patient/family teaching).

Implementation

- **Ophth:** Wash hands. Instruct patient to lie down or tilt head back and look at ceiling. Pull down on lower lid, creating a small pocket. Place prescribed number of drops in pocket. Instruct patient to close lids gently and roll eyes around in all directions to ensure even distribution. Wait 5 min before applying other prescribed eyedrops. Do not touch cap or tip of container to eye, fingers, or any surface. Discard soln if it becomes cloudy.
- **Ocular Insert:** 2 applicators are provided in the box. Place insert deep within the lower conjunctival sac.

Patient/Family Teaching

- **General Info:** Instruct patient in correct method of application of ophthalmic soln or insert. If a dose is missed, it should be instilled as soon as remembered. Patient should confer with physician before wearing contact lenses.

▫ Medication may cause blurred vision. Caution patient to avoid driving until response to medication is known. Increased sensitivity to light may occur; sunglasses may provide relief.

▫ Discuss the possibility of matting of eyelashes. Instruct patient in correct technique for washing lids from inner to outer canthus.

▫ Instruct patient to notify physician if eye irritation or discomfort increases or if blurred vision persists.

▫ Advise patients using over-the-counter preparations to seek medical help if condition does not resolve within 3 days.

- **Insert:** Instruct patient to replace insert with a new one if the original falls out, in order to prevent contamination of eye. Removing the insert a few hrs after instillation may prevent blurred vision in patients prone to this side effect. Another insert may be placed later.

*Underlines indicate most frequent; **CAPITALS** indicate life-threatening.

- □ Advise patient of the need for regular eye examinations to monitor response to treatment.

Evaluation

Effectiveness of therapy can be demonstrated by: ▪ Increased tear film in dry eye conditions.

TEMAZEPAM
(tem-**az**-a-pam)
Razepam, Restoril, Temaz

CLASSIFICATION(S):
Sedative/hypnotic—benzodiazepine
Schedule IV
Pregnancy Category X

INDICATIONS

▪ Management of insomnia (short-term).

ACTION

▪ Acts at many levels in the CNS, producing generalized depression ▪ Effects may be mediated by gamma-aminobutyric acid (GABA), an inhibitory neurotransmitter. **Therapeutic Effect:** ▪ Relief of insomnia.

PHARMACOKINETICS

Absorption: Well absorbed following oral administration.
Distribution: Widely distributed, crosses blood-brain barrier. Probably crosses the placenta and enters breast milk. Accumulation of drug occurs with chronic dosing.
Metabolism and Excretion: Metabolized by the liver.
Half-life: 10–20 hr.

CONTRAINDICATIONS AND PRECAUTIONS

Contraindicated in: ▪ Hypersensitivity ▪ Cross-sensitivity with other benzodiazepines may exist ▪ Pre-existing CNS depression ▪ Severe uncontrolled pain ▪ Narrow-angle glaucoma ▪ Pregnancy or lactation.
Use Cautiously in: ▪ Pre-existing hepatic dysfunction ▪ Patients who may be suicidal or have been addicted to drugs previously ▪ Elderly or debilitated patients (dosage reduction recommended).

ADVERSE REACTIONS AND SIDE EFFECTS*

CNS: dizziness, drowsiness, lethargy, hangover, paradoxical excitation.
EENT: blurred vision.
GI: nausea, vomiting, diarrhea, constipation.
Derm: rashes.
Misc: tolerance, psychological dependence, physical dependence.

INTERACTIONS

Drug-Drug: ▪ Additive CNS depression with **alcohol, antidepressants, antihistamines, narcotic analgesics,** and other **sedative/hypnotics** ▪ May decrease efficacy of **levodopa** ▪ **Smoking** increases metabolism and may decrease effectiveness of temazepam ▪ **Probenecid** may prolong the effects of temazepam.

ROUTE AND DOSAGE

▪ **PO (Adults):** 15–30 mg at bedtime.

PHARMACODYNAMICS (sedation)

	ONSET	PEAK	DURATION
PO	30 min	2–3 hr	UK

NURSING IMPLICATIONS

Assessment

- □ Assess sleep patterns prior to and periodically throughout course of therapy.
- □ Prolonged high-dose therapy may lead to psychological or physical dependence. Restrict amount of drug available to patient, especially if patient is depressed or suicidal or has a history of addiction.

*Underlines indicate most frequent; **CAPITALS** indicate life-threatening.

Potential Nursing Diagnoses
- Sleep pattern disturbance (indications).
- Injury, high risk for (side effects).
- Knowledge deficit related to medication regimen (patient/family teaching).

Implementation
- **PO:** Administer with food if GI irritation becomes a problem.

Patient/Family Teaching
- Instruct patient to take temazepam exactly as directed. Discuss the importance of preparing environment for sleep (dark room, quiet, avoidance of nicotine and caffeine). If less effective after a few wks, consult physician; do not increase dose.
- May cause daytime drowsiness or dizziness. Caution patient to avoid driving or other activities requiring alertness until response to medication is known.
- Advise patient to avoid the use of alcohol and other CNS depressants and to consult the physician or pharmacist prior to the use of over-the-counter preparations that contain antihistamines or alcohol.
- Advise patient to inform physician if pregnancy is planned or suspected.
- Emphasize the importance of follow-up appointments to monitor progress.

Evaluation
Effectiveness of therapy can be demonstrated by: ▪ Improvement in sleep habits, which may not be noticeable until the third day of therapy.

TERAZOSIN
(ter-ay-zoe-sin)
Hytrin

CLASSIFICATION(S):
Antihypertensive—peripherally acting antiadrenergic
Pregnancy Category C

INDICATIONS
- Treatment of mild to moderate hypertension (alone or with other agents, such as diuretics).

ACTION
- Dilates both arteries and veins by blocking postsynaptic $alpha_1$-adrenergic receptors. **Therapeutic Effect:**
- Lowering of blood pressure.

PHARMACOKINETICS
Absorption: Well absorbed following oral administration.
Distribution: Distribution not known.
Metabolism and Excretion: 50% metabolized by the liver. 10% excreted unchanged by the kidneys. 20% excreted unchanged in feces. 40% eliminated in bile.
Half-life: 12 hr.

CONTRAINDICATIONS AND PRECAUTIONS
Contraindicated in: ▪ Hypersensitivity.
Use Cautiously in: ▪ Pregnancy, lactation, or children (safety not established).

ADVERSE REACTIONS AND SIDE EFFECTS*
CNS: dizziness, nervousness, somnolence, weakness, headache.
CV: palpitations, hypotension, tachycardia, arrhythmias, chest pain.
Derm: pruritus, first dose orthostatic hypotensive reaction.
EENT: nasal congestion, blurred vision, conjunctivitis, sinusitis.
F and E: peripheral edema, fever.
GI: nausea, vomiting, diarrhea, dry mouth, abdominal pain.
GU: impotence, urinary frequency.
Metab: weight gain.
MS: extremity pain, back pain, arthralgia.
Neuro: paresthesia.
Resp: dyspnea.

*Underlines indicate most frequent; **CAPITALS** indicate life-threatening.

T

INTERACTIONS

Drug–Drug: ▪ Additive hypotension with other **antihypertensive agents,** acute ingestion of **alcohol,** or **nitrates** ▪ **Nonsteroidal anti-inflammatory agents, sympathomimetics,** or **estrogens** may decrease the effects of antihypertensive therapy.

ROUTE AND DOSAGE

Note: The first dose should be taken at bedtime.

- **PO (Adults):** 1 mg initially, then slowly increase up to 5 mg/day; may be given as single dose or in 2 divided doses (not to exceed 20 mg/day).

PHARMACODYNAMICS (antihypertensive effects)

	ONSET*	PEAK†	DURATION*
PO	15 min	6–8 wk	24 hr

*After single dose.
†After multiple oral dosing.

NURSING IMPLICATIONS

Assessment

- ▫ Monitor blood pressure (lying and standing) and pulse frequently during initial dosage adjustment and periodically throughout course of therapy. Notify physician of significant changes.
- ▫ Assess patient for first dose orthostatic reaction and syncope. May occur 30 min–2 hr following initial dose and occasionally thereafter. Incidence may be dose-related. Volume-depleted or sodium-restricted patients may be more sensitive to this effect.
- ▫ Monitor intake and output ratios and daily weight; assess for edema daily, especially at beginning of therapy.

Potential Nursing Diagnoses

- Injury, high risk for (side effects).
- Knowledge deficit related to medication regimen (patient/family teaching).
- Noncompliance (patient/family teaching).

Implementation

- **General Info:** May be used in combination with diuretic or beta-adrenergic blocker to minimize sodium and water retention. If these are added to terazosin therapy, reduce dose of terazosin initially and titrate to effect.
- **PO:** Administer daily dose at bedtime. If necessary, dosage may be increased to twice daily.

Patient/Family Teaching

- ▫ Emphasize the importance of continuing to take this medication , as directed, even if feeling better. Medication controls but does not cure hypertension. Instruct patient to take medication at the same time each day. If a dose is missed, take as soon as remembered. If not remembered until next day, do not take; do not double doses.
- ▫ Encourage patient to comply with additional interventions for hypertension (weight reduction, low-sodium diet, discontinuation of smoking, moderation of alcohol consumption, regular exercise, and stress management). Instruct patient and family on proper technique for blood pressure monitoring. Advise them to check blood pressure at least weekly and to report significant changes to physician.
- ▫ Advise patient to weigh self twice weekly and assess feet and ankles for fluid retention.
- ▫ Terazosin may cause dizziness or drowsiness. Advise patient to avoid driving or other activities requiring alertness until response to the medication is known.
- ▫ Caution patient to avoid sudden changes in position to decrease orthostatic hypotension. Alcohol, CNS depressants, standing for long periods, hot showers, and exercising in hot weather should be avoided because of enhanced orthostatic effects.
- ▫ Advise patient to consult physician or pharmacist before taking any cough, cold, or allergy remedies. Patient

should also avoid excessive amounts of tea, coffee, and cola.

- Instruct patient to notify physician or dentist of medication regimen prior to any surgery.
- Advise patient to notify physician if frequent dizziness or fainting or swelling of feet or lower legs occurs.
- Emphasize the importance of follow-up examinations to evaluate effectiveness of medication.

Evaluation

Effectiveness of therapy can be demonstrated by: ▪ Decrease in blood pressure without appearance of side effects.

TERBUTALINE

(ter-**byoo**-ta-leen)
Brethaire, Brethine, Bricanyl

CLASSIFICATION(S):
Bronchodilator—beta-adrenergic agonist
Pregnancy Category B

INDICATIONS

▪ Used as a bronchodilator in reversible airway obstruction due to asthma or COPD. **Unlabeled Use:** ▪ Used to arrest preterm labor (tocolytic).

ACTION

▪ A beta-adrenergic agonist that results in the accumulation of cyclic adenosine monophosphate (cAMP) ▪ Results of increased levels of cAMP at beta-adrenergic receptors include: ▫ Bronchodilation ▫ CNS and cardiac stimulation ▫ Diuresis ▫ Gastric acid secretion ▪ Relatively selective for $beta_2$ (pulmonary) receptors. **Therapeutic Effect:** ▪ Bronchodilation.

PHARMACOKINETICS

Absorption: 35–50% absorbed following oral administration, but rapidly undergoes first-pass metabolism. Well absorbed following SC administration. Minimal absorption following inhalation.

Distribution: Distribution not known. Enters breast milk.

Metabolism and Excretion: Partially metabolized by the liver. 60% excreted unchanged by the kidneys following SC administration.

Half-life: UK.

CONTRAINDICATIONS AND PRECAUTIONS

Contraindicated in: ▪ Hypersensitivity to adrenergic amines or any ingredients in preparations (fluorocarbon propellant in inhaler).

Use Cautiously in: ▪ Elderly patients (more susceptible to adverse reactions; may require dosage reduction) ▪ Pregnancy, lactation, or children <12 yr (safety not established—has been used during pregnancy, but may cause hypokalemia, hypoglycemia, or pulmonary edema in the mother and hypoglycemia in the newborn) ▪ Cardiac disease ▪ Hypertension ▪ Hyperthyroidism ▪ Diabetes mellitus ▪ Glaucoma ▪ Pregnancy near term ▪ Excessive use of inhalers (may lead to tolerance and paradoxical bronchospasm).

ADVERSE REACTIONS AND SIDE EFFECTS*

CNS: <u>nervousness</u>, <u>restlessness</u>, insomnia, <u>tremor</u>, headache, anxiety.

CV: hypertension, arrhythmias, angina, tachycardia, palpitations, PULMONARY EDEMA (maternal—during tocolysis).

GI: nausea, vomiting.

F and E: hypokalemia (during tocolysis in mother).

INTERACTIONS

Drug-Drug: ▪ Additive adrenergic effects with other **adrenergic (sympathomimetic) agents,** including **decongestants** and **vasopressors** ▪ Use with **MAO inhibitors** may lead to hypertensive crisis ▪ **Beta-adrenergic blockers** may block therapeutic effect.

*<u>Underlines</u> indicate most frequent; **CAPITALS** indicate life-threatening.

T

ROUTE AND DOSAGE

Bronchodilation

- **PO (Adults):** 2.5–5 mg tid, at 6-hr intervals.
- **PO (Children 12–15 yr):** 2.5 mg tid, at 6-hr intervals.
- **SC (Adults):** 0.25 mg, may repeat in 15–30 min (not to exceed 0.5 mg in 4 hr).
- **Inhaln (Adults and Children >12 yr):** 2 inhalations q 4–6 hr (200 mcg/spray).

Tocolysis (Arrest of Preterm Labor)

- **PO (Adults):** 2.5 mg q 4–6 hr until delivery.
- **IV (Adults):** 10 mcg/min infusion, increase by 5 mcg/min q 10 min until contractions stop (not to exceed 80 mcg/min). After contractions have ceased for 30 min, decrease infusion rate to lowest effective amount and maintain for 4–8 hr after contractions have stopped.

PHARMACODYNAMICS (bronchodilation)

	ONSET	PEAK	DURATION
PO	30 min	1–2 hr	4–8 hr
SC	15 min	30–60 min	1.5–4 hr
Inhaln	5–30 min	1–2 hr	3–6 hr

NURSING IMPLICATIONS

Assessment

- **Bronchospasm:** Assess blood pressure, pulse, respiratory pattern, lung sounds, and character of secretions prior to and after treatment. Cardiovascular effects are increased with parenteral use.
- □ Observe patient for appearance of drug tolerance and rebound bronchospasm.
- **Preterm Labor:** Monitor maternal pulse and blood pressure, frequency and duration of contractions, and fetal heart rate. Notify physician if contractions persist or increase in frequency or duration or if symptoms of maternal or fetal distress occur. Maternal side effects include tachycardia, palpitations, tremor, anxiety, and headache.
- □ Assess maternal respiratory status for symptoms of pulmonary edema (increased rate, dyspnea, rales/crackles, frothy sputum).
- □ Monitor mother and neonate for symptoms of hypoglycemia (anxiety, chills, cold sweats, confusion, cool pale skin, difficulty in concentration, drowsiness, excessive hunger, headache, irritability, nausea, nervousness, rapid pulse, shakiness, unusual tiredness or weakness) and mother for hypokalemia (weakness, fatigue, U wave on ECG, arrhythmias).
- **Lab Test Considerations:** Monitor maternal serum glucose and electrolytes. May cause hypokalemia and hypoglycemia. Monitor neonate's serum glucose, as hypoglycemia may also occur in neonate.

Potential Nursing Diagnoses

- Airway clearance, ineffective (indications).
- Knowledge deficit related to medication regimen (patient/family teaching).
- Noncompliance (patient/family teaching).

Implementation

- **PO:** Tablet may be crushed and mixed with food or fluids for patients with difficulty swallowing.
- **SC:** Administer SC injections in lateral deltoid area. Do not use soln if discolored.
- **IV:** Use infusion pump to ensure accurate dosage. Begin infusion at 10 mcg/min. Increase dosage by 5 mcg every 10 min until contractions cease. Maximal dose is 80 mcg/min. Begin to taper dose in 5-mcg decrements after a 30–60-min contraction-free period is attained. Switch to oral dosage form after patient is contraction-free 4–8 hr on the lowest effective dose.
- **Solution/Additive Compatibility:** May

be diluted in D5W, 0.9% NaCl, or 0.45% NaCl. Compatible with aminophylline.
- **Additive Incompatibility:** bleomycin.

PATIENT/FAMILY TEACHING
- **Bronchospasm:** Instruct patient to take medication exactly as prescribed. If a dose is missed, take if remembered within 1 hr or so, otherwise do not take; do not double doses. Taking more often than prescribed may lead to tolerance.
- Advise patient to maintain adequate fluid intake to help liquify tenacious secretions.
- Advise patient to consult physician if respiratory symptoms are not relieved or worsen after treatment. Patient should also inform physician if chest pain, headache, severe dizziness, palpitations, nervousness, or weakness occur.
- **Metered-dose Inhaler:** Instruct patient to shake inhaler well, clear airways before taking medication, exhale deeply before placing inhaler in mouth, close lips tightly around mouthpiece, inhale deeply while administering medication, and hold breath for several secs after receiving dose. Wait 1–2 min before administering next dose. Mouthpiece should be washed after each use.
- Patients taking inhalation glucocorticoids concurrently with terbutaline should be advised to take terbutaline first and allow 15 min to elapse between using the 2 aerosols, unless directed by physician.
- **Preterm Labor:** Physician should be notified immediately if labor resumes or significant side effects occur.

EVALUATION

Effectiveness of therapy can be demonstrated by: ▪ Decrease in bronchoconstriction and bronchospasm ▫ Increase in ease of breathing ▪ Control of preterm labor in a fetus of 20–36 wk gestational age.

TERCONAZOLE
(ter-**kon**-a-zole)
Terazol 3, Terazol 7

CLASSIFICATION(S):
Antifungal—topical
Pregnancy Category C

INDICATIONS
- Management of vaginal fungal infections due to *Candida* (vulvovaginal moniliasis).

ACTION
- Inhibits fungal growth and weakens fungal cell membrane, resulting in fungicidal or fungistatic action, depending on organism and concentration. **Therapeutic Effect:** ▪ Death or inhibition of susceptible fungi.

PHARMACOKINETICS
Absorption: Small amounts (5–16%) may be absorbed from vaginal mucosa.
Distribution: Small amounts absorbed from vaginal mucosa may cross placenta.
Metabolism and Excretion: Metabolism and excretion not known.
Half-life: UK.

CONTRAINDICATIONS AND PRECAUTIONS
Contraindicated in: ▪ Hypersensitivity ▪ Pregnancy (vaginal applicator only).
Use Cautiously in: ▪ Lactation and children (safety not established).

ADVERSE REACTIONS AND SIDE EFFECTS*
CNS: headache.
GU: vulvovaginal burning, itching, irritation.
MS: body pain.

INTERACTIONS
Drug–Drug: ▪ None known.

ROUTE AND DOSAGE
- **Vag (Adults):** 1 applicatorful (5 g) into vagina at bedtime daily for 7

*Underlines indicate most frequent; **CAPITALS** indicate life-threatening.

nights or one 80-mg suppository at bedtime for 3 nights.

PHARMACODYNAMICS (antifungal effect)

	ONSET	PEAK	DURATION
Vag	upon application	UK	UK

NURSING IMPLICATIONS

Assessment

- Inspect involved areas of skin and mucous membranes prior to and frequently throughout course of therapy. Increased skin irritation may indicate need to discontinue medication.

Potential Nursing Diagnoses

- Skin integrity, impaired: actual (indications).
- Infection, high risk for (indications).
- Knowledge deficit related to medication regimen (patient/family teaching).

Implementation

- **General Info:** Consult physician for proper cleansing technique prior to applying medication. Sitz baths and vaginal douches may be ordered concurrently with this therapy.
- **Vag:** Applicators are supplied for vaginal administration.

Patient/Family Teaching

- Instruct patient to apply medication as directed for full course of therapy, even if feeling better. Therapy should be continued during menstrual period.
- Instruct patient on proper use of vaginal applicator for vaginal cream. Terconazole should be inserted high into the vagina at bedtime. Instruct patient to remain recumbent for at least 30 min following insertion. Advise use of sanitary napkins to prevent staining of clothing or bedding.
- Advise patient to consult physician regarding douching and intercourse during therapy. Vaginal medication may cause minor skin irritation in sexual partner. Advise patient to refrain from sexual contact during therapy or have male partner wear a condom.
- Advise patient to report to physician increased skin irritation or lack of response to therapy.

Evaluation

Effectiveness of therapy can be demonstrated by: ■ Decrease in skin irritation and vaginal discomfort. Therapeutic response is usually seen after 1 wk. Diagnosis should be reconfirmed with smears or cultures prior to a second course of therapy to rule out other pathogens associated with vulvovaginitis.

TERFENADINE

(ter-**fen**-i-deen)
Seldane

CLASSIFICATION(S):
Antihistamine
Pregnancy Category C

INDICATIONS

■ Symptomatic relief of allergic symptoms caused by histamine release, including nasal allergies and allergic dermatoses.

ACTION

■ Blocks the effects of histamine. **Therapeutic Effect:** ■ Relief of symptoms associated with histamine excess usually seen in allergic conditions.

PHARMACOKINETICS

Absorption: Rapidly and completely absorbed following oral administration.
Distribution: Distribution not known. Appears to have minimal penetration of the blood-brain barrier.
Metabolism and Excretion: Mostly metabolized by the liver. Eliminated mostly in the feces, via biliary excretion.
Half-life: 16–23 hr.

CONTRAINDICATIONS AND PRECAUTIONS

Contraindicated in: ■ Hypersensitivity.

Use Cautiously in: ▪ Prostatic hypertrophy ▪ Narrow-angle glaucoma ▪ Pregnancy, lactation, or children <12 yr (safety not established) ▪ Cardiovascular disease.

ADVERSE REACTIONS AND SIDE EFFECTS*

CNS: drowsiness, sedation, headache, dizziness, nervousness, weakness.
CV: palpitations, tachycardia.
EENT: visual disturbances.
GI: nausea, vomiting, abdominal pain, diarrhea, constipaiton, dry mouth, dry lips.
Derm: rashes, dry skin.
MS: musculoskeletal pain.
Misc: allergic reactions.

INTERACTIONS

Drug–Drug: ▪ Additive CNS depression with other **CNS depressants,** including **alcohol, antidepressants, narcotic analgesics,** and **sedative/hypnotics** ▪ Additive anticholinergic effects with other **drugs possessing anticholinergic properties,** including **antidepressants, atropine, haloperidol, phenothiazines, quinidine,** and **disopyramide** ▪ Increased risk of arrhythmias with **ketoconazole.**

ROUTE AND DOSAGE

▪ **PO (Adults):** 60 mg bid.

PHARMACODYNAMICS (antihistaminic effects)

	ONSET	PEAK	DURATION
PO	1–2 hr	3–6 hr	6–12 hr

NURSING IMPLICATIONS

Assessment

□ Assess allergy symptoms (rhinitis, conjunctivitis, hives) prior to and periodically throughout course of therapy.

□ Assess lung sounds and character of bronchial secretions. Maintain fluid intake of 1500–2000 ml/day to decrease viscosity of secretions.

▪ **Lab Test Considerations:** Will cause false-negative reactions on allergy skin tests; discontinue 3 days prior to testing.

Potential Nursing Diagnoses

▪ Airway clearance, ineffective (indications).
▪ Injury, high risk for (adverse reactions).
▪ Knowledge deficit related to medication regimen (patient/family teaching).

Implementation

▪ **General Info:** Available in combination with pseudoephedrine (Seldane-D); see Appendix A.
▪ **PO:** Administer with food or milk to decrease GI irritation.

Patient/Family Teaching

□ Instruct patient to contact physician if symptoms persist.

□ Instruct patient to take medication as directed. If a dose is missed, take as soon as remembered unless almost time for next dose.

□ Inform patient that drug may cause drowsiness, although it is less likely to occur than with other antihistamines. Avoid driving or other activities requiring alertness until response to drug is known.

Evaluation

Effectivness of therapy can be demonstrated by: ▪ Decrease in allergic symptoms.

TESTOSTERONE

(tess-**toss**-te-rone)

testosterone base
Andro, Histerone, {Malogen}, Testaqua

testosterone cypionate
Andro-Cyp, Andronate, dep Andro, Depotest, Duratest, T-Cypionate, Tesionate, Tesred Cypionate, Virilon IM

{} = Available in Canada only.

*Underlines indicate most frequent; **CAPITALS** indicate life-threatening.

T

testosterone enanthate
Andro LA, Delatestryl, Durathate, Everone, {Malogex}, Testone LA, Testrin-PA

testosterone propionate
{Malogen}, Testex

CLASSIFICATION(S):
Hormone—androgen
Schedule III
Pregnancy Category X

INDICATIONS

▪ Treatment of hypogonadism in androgen-deficient males ▪ Treatment of delayed puberty in males ▪ Palliative treatment of androgen-responsive breast cancer.

ACTION

▪ Responsible for the normal growth and development of male sex organs ▪ Maintenance of male secondary sex characteristics: ▫ Growth and maturation of the prostatic, seminal vesicles, penis, scrotum ▫ Development of male hair distribution ▫ Vocal cord thickening ▫ Alterations in body musculature and fat distribution. **Therapeutic Effects:** ▪ Correction of hormone deficiency in male hypogonadism ▫ Initiation of male puberty ▪ Suppression of tumor growth in some forms of breast cancer.

PHARMACOKINETICS

Absorption: Well absorbed from IM sites. Cypionate, decanoate, propionate, and enanthate salts are absorbed slowly.
Distribution: Probably crosses the placenta and enters breast milk.
Metabolism and Excretion: Metabolized by the liver.
Half-life: Base—10–100 min; cypionate—8 days.

CONTRAINDICATIONS AND PRECAUTIONS

Contraindicated in: ▪ Hypersensitivity ▪ Pregnancy and lactation ▪ Male patients with breast or prostate cancer ▪ Hypercalcemia ▪ Severe liver, renal, or cardiac disease.
Use Cautiously in: ▪ Diabetes mellitus ▪ Coronary artery disease ▪ History of liver disease ▪ Prepubertal males.

ADVERSE REACTIONS AND SIDE EFFECTS*

CV: edema.
GI: nausea, vomiting, changes in appetite, hepatitis.
GU: bladder irritability, prostatic enlargement, menstrual irregularities.
EENT: deepening of voice.
Endo: females—clitoral enlargement, change in libido, decreased breast size; males—acne, priapism, facial hair, oligospermia, impotence, gynecomastia.
F and E: hypercalcemia.
Local: pain at injection site.

INTERACTIONS

Drug–Drug: ▪ Decreases metabolism and may enhance the action of **oral anticoagulants, oral hypoglycemic agents,** and **glucocorticoids** ▪ May also enhance the effect of **insulin** ▪ Additive hepatotoxicity with other **hepatotoxic agents.**

ROUTE AND DOSAGE

Hypogonadism

▪ **IM (Adults):** 200–400 mg q 4 wk (cypionate or enanthate) or 10–25 mg 2–5 times/wk (propionate or base).

Replacement Therapy

▪ **IM (Adults):** 25–50 mg 2–3 times/wk (base or propionate) or 50–400 mg q 2–4 wk (enanthate).

Delayed Male Puberty

▪ **IM (Adolescents):** 12.5–25 mg 2–3 times/wk (base) or 25–200 mg cypionate q 2–4 wk (cypionate) or 50–200 mg q 2–4 wk (enanthate).

Palliative Management of Breast Cancer

▪ **IM (Adults):** 50–100 mg 3 times/wk

*Underlines indicate most frequent; **CAPITALS** indicate life-threatening.

(propionate or base) or 200–400 mg q 2–4 wk (cypionate or enanthate).

PHARMACODYNAMICS (androgenic effects)*

	ONSET	PEAK	DURATION
IM—base	UK	UK	1–3 days
IM—cypionate	UK	UK	2–4 wk
IM—enanthate	UK	UK	2–4 wk
IM—propionate	UK	UK	1–3 days

*Response is highly variable among individuals; may take mons.

NURSING IMPLICATIONS

Assessment

- **General Info:** Monitor intake and output ratios, weigh patient twice weekly, and assess patient for edema. Notify physician of significant changes indicative of fluid retention.
- **Males:** Monitor for precocious puberty in boys (acne, darkening of skin, development of male secondary sex characteristics—increase in penis size, frequent erections, growth of body hair).
  - Monitor for breast enlargement, persistent erections, and increased urge to urinate in men. Monitor for difficulty urinating in elderly men, as prostate enlargement may occur.
- **Females:** Assess for virilism (deepening of voice, unusual hair growth or loss, clitoral enlargement, acne, menstrual irregularity).
  - In women with metastatic breast cancer, monitor for symptoms of hypercalcemia (nausea, vomiting, constipation, lethargy, loss of muscle tone, thirst, polyuria).
- **Lab Test Considerations:** Monitor hemoglobin and hematocrit periodically throughout course of therapy; may cause polycythemia.
  - Monitor hepatic function tests and serum cholesterol levels periodically throughout course of therapy. May cause increased SGOT (AST), increased or decreased cholesterol levels, and suppression of clotting factors II, V, VII, and X.
  - Monitor serum and urine calcium levels and serum alkaline phosphatase concentrations in metastatic cancer.
  - May alter results of fasting blood sugar, glucose tolerance tests, thyroid function tests, and metyrapone tests. Decreased creatine and creatinine clearance may last up to 2 wk following discontinuation of therapy. Serum chloride, potassium, phosphate, and sodium levels may be increased.
  - May cause increased levels in 24-hr urine tests for 17-ketosteroid concentrations.

Potential Nursing Diagnoses

- Sexual dysfunction (indications, side effects).
- Knowledge deficit related to medication regimen (patient/family teaching).

Implementation

- **General Info:** Range-of-motion exercises should be done with all bedridden patients to prevent mobilization of calcium from the bone.
- **IM:** Administer IM deep into gluteal muscle. Crystals may form at low temperatures; warming and shaking vial will redissolve crystals. Use of a wet syringe or needle will cause a cloudy soln but will not affect potency.

Patient/Family Teaching

- Advise patient to report the following signs and symptoms to physician promptly: in male patients, priapism (sustained and often painful erections) or gynecomastia; in female patients, virilism (which may be reversible if medication is stopped as soon as changes are noticed); hypercalcemia (nausea, vomiting, constipation, and weakness); edema (unexpected weight gain, swelling of feet); hepatitis (yellowing of skin or eyes and abdominal pain); or unusual bleeding or bruising.
- Explain rationale for prohibitiion of use for increasing athletic performance. Testosterone is neither safe

nor effective for this use and has a potential risk of serious side effects.

- Instruct patient to notify physician immediately if pregnancy is planned or suspected.
- Advise diabetic patients to monitor blood or urine closely for alterations in blood sugar concentrations.
- Emphasize the importance of regular follow-up physical examinations, lab tests, and x-ray examinations to monitor progress.
- Radiologic bone age determinations should be evaluated every 6 mon in prepubertal children to determine rate of bone maturation and effects on epiphyseal centers.

EVALUATION

Effectiveness of therapy can be demonstrated by: ▪ Resolution of the signs of androgen deficiency without side effects ▪ Decrease in the size and spread of breast malignancy in postmenopausal women. In antineoplastic therapy, response may require 3 mon of therapy; if signs of disease progression appear, therapy should be discontinued.

TETRACYCLINE

(te-tra-**sye**-kleen)

Achromycin, Achromycin V, {Apo-Tetra}, Bristacycline, Cyclopar, Kesso-Tetra, {Novotetra}, Panmycin, Retet-S, Robitet, Sumycin, Tetracyn, {Tetralean}, Tetrex-S, Topicycline

CLASSIFICATION(S):
Anti-infective—tetracycline
Pregnancy Category UK

INDICATIONS

▪ **PO, IM, IV:** Treatment of various infections due to unusual organisms, including: ▫ *Mycoplasma* ▫ *Chlamydia* ▫ *Rickettsia* ▪ **PO, IM, IV:** Treatment of gonorrhea and syphilis in penicillin-allergic patients ▪ **PO, Top:** Treatment of acne ▪ Prevention of exacerbations of chronic bronchitis ▪ **Ophth:** Treatment of superificial eye infections and trachoma ▪ **Ophth:** Prevention of ophthalmia neonatorum ▪ **Top:** Treatment and prophylaxis of superficial skin infections.

ACTION

▪ Inhibits bacterial protein synthesis at the level of the 30S bacterial ribosome. **Therapeutic Effect:** ▪ Bacteriostatic action against susceptible bacteria. **Spectrum:** ▪ Includes activity against some gram-positive pathogens: ▫ *Bacillus antracis* ▫ *Clostridium perfringens* ▫ *Clostridium tetani* ▫ *Listeria monocytogenes* ▫ *Nocardia* ▫ *Propionibacterium acnes* ▫ *Actinomyces isrealii* ▪ Active against some gram-negative pathogens: ▫ *Hemophilus influenzae* ▫ *Legionella pneumophila* ▫ *Yersinia entercolitica* ▫ *Yersinia pestis* ▫ *Neisseria gonorrhoeae* ▫ *Neisseria meningitidis.*

PHARMACOKINETICS

Absorption: 60–80% absorbed following oral administration. IM administration produces lower blood levels than oral administration.
Distribution: Widely distributed, some penetration into CSF. Crosses the placenta and enters breast milk.
Metabolism and Excretion: Excreted mostly unchanged by the kidneys.
Half-life: 6–12 hr.

CONTRAINDICATIONS AND PRECAUTIONS

Contraindicated in: ▪ Hypersensitivity ▪ Hypersensitivity to bisulfites (some products) ▪ Children <8 yr (permanent staining of teeth) ▪ Pregnancy (increased risk of fatty liver with IV use; risk of permanent staining of teeth in infant if used during last half of pregnancy) ▪ Lactation.
Use Cautiously in: ▪ Cachectic or debilitated patients ▪ Hepatic or renal disease.

{} = Available in Canada only.

ADVERSE REACTIONS AND SIDE EFFECTS*

GI: nausea, vomiting, diarrhea, pancreatitis, esophagitis, hepatotoxicity (IV).
Derm: rashes, photosensitivity.
Hemat: blood dyscrasias.
Local: phlebitis at IV site, pain at IM site.
Misc: superinfection, hypersensitivity reactions.

INTERACTIONS

Drug–Drug: ▪ May enhance the effect of **oral anticoagulants** ▪ May decrease the effectiveness of **oral contraceptives** ▪ **Antacids, calcium, iron,** and **magnesium** form insoluble compounds (chelates) and decrease absorption of tetracycline ▪ **Sucralfate** may bind to tetracycline and prevent its absorption from the GI tract ▪ **Cholestyramine** or **colestipol** decrease oral absorption of tetracyclines.
Drug–Food: ▪ **Calcium** in foods or **dairy products** decreases absorption by forming insoluble compounds (chelates).

ROUTE AND DOSAGE

- **PO (Adults):** 1–2 g/day in divided doses every 6–12 hr (small doses of 125–500 mg/day for chronic treatment of acne).
- **PO (Children >8 yr):** 25–50 mg/kg/day in divided doses every 6–12 hr.
- **IM (Adults):** 250 mg/day or 300 mg/day in divided doses q 8–12 hr.
- **IM (Children >8 yr):** 15–25 mg/kg/day in divided doses q 8–12 hr (not to exceed 250 mg as a single injection).
- **IV (Adults):** 250–500 mg q 12 hr (not to exceed 500 mg q 6 hr).
- **IV (Children >8 yr):** 10–20 mg/kg/day in divided doses q 12 hr.
- **Ophth (Adults and Children):** Thin strip of ointment q 2–4 hr or 1 drop of 1% suspension q 6–12 hr (may be used more frequently; single dose used for prevention of ophthalmia neonatorum).
- **Top (Adults and Children >8 yr):** Ointment 1–2 times daily for superficial skin infections or soln applied twice daily for acne.

PHARMACODYNAMICS (blood levels)

	ONSET	PEAK
PO	1–2 hr	2–4 hr
IM	rapid	30–60 min
IV	rapid	end of infusion

NURSING IMPLICATIONS

Assessment

- ▫ Assess patient for infection (vital signs; appearance of wound, sputum, urine, and stool; WBC) at beginning and throughout course of therapy.
- ▫ Obtain specimens for culture and sensitivity prior to initiating therapy. First dose may be given before receiving results.
- ▪ **Lab Test Considerations:** Renal and hepatic functions and CBC should be monitored periodically during long-term therapy.
- ▫ May cause increased BUN, SGOT (AST), SGPT (ALT), serum alkaline phosphatase, bilirubin, and amylase concentrations.
- ▫ May cause false elevations in urinary catecholamine levels.

Potential Nursing Diagnoses

- ▪ Infection, high risk for (indications, side effects).
- ▪ Knowledge deficit related to medication regimen (patient/family teaching).
- ▪ Noncompliance related to medication regimen (patient/family teaching).

Implementation

- ▪ **General Info:** May cause yellow-brown discoloration and softening of teeth and bones if administered prenatally or during early childhood. Not recommended for children <8 yr.
- ▫ Available in tablets, capsules, oral suspension, ophthalmic soln and

*Underlines indicate most frequent; **CAPITALS** indicate life-threatening.

T

ointment, topical soln and ointment, and injectable forms.

- **PO:** Administer around the clock. Administer at least 1 hr before or 2 hr after meals. Take with a full glass of liquid and at least 1 hr before going to bed to avoid esophageal ulceration. Use calibrated measuring device for liquid preparations. Shake liquid preparations well. Do not administer within 1–3 hr of other medications.
- □ Avoid administration of milk, calcium, antacids, magnesium-containing medications, or iron supplements within 1–3 hr of oral tetracycline.
- **IM:** Dilute with 2 ml of sterile water or 0.9% NaCl for injection. IM preparation contains 2% or 40 mg of procaine hydrochloride to decrease pain of injection. Stable for 6–24 hr at room temperature, 24 hr if refrigerated.
- □ Do not administer SC. For deep IM use only. May cause intense pain and local irritation at site of injection. Do not administer >2 ml in each site. Rotate injection sites.
- □ Patient should be converted to oral preparations as soon as possible, because IM administration produces lower serum concentrations than oral route.
- **IV:** Reconstitute each 250-mg vial with 5 ml and each 500-mg vial with 10 ml of sterile water, 0.9% NaCl, or D5W for injection, for a concentration of 50 mg/ml.
- **Direct IV:** Dilute further to a concentration of 10 mg/ml.
- □ *Rate:* Administer at a rate of 100 mg over 5 min.
- **Intermittent Infusion:** Dilute in 100–1000 ml of D5W, D10W, 0.9% NaCl, 0.45% NaCl, Ringer's or lactated Ringer's soln, dextrose/saline combinations, or dextrose/Ringer's or lactated Ringer's combinations. Soln is stable for 12 hr at room temperature, 24 hr if refrigerated. May cause thrombophlebitis; avoid extravasation.
- **Syringe Compatibility:** heparin.
- **Syringe Incompatibility:** ampicillin, methicillin, or penicillin G sodium.
- **Y-Site Compatibility:** acyclovir, cyclophosphamide, magnesium sulfate, multivitamins, ondansetron, or perphenazine.
- **Y-Site Incompatibility:** hydromorphone, meperidine, or morphine.
- **Additive Compatibility:** ascorbic acid, cimetidine, colistimethate, corticotropin, diphenhydramine, dopamine, ephedrine, isoproterenol, kanamycin, lidocaine, metaraminol, norepinephrine, oxytocin, plasma protein fraction, potassium chloride, prednisolone sodium phosphate, procaine, or promazine.
- **Additive Incompatibility:** aminophylline, amobarbital, amphotericin, cephalothin, cephapirin, chlorothiazide, dimenhydrinate, erythromycin gluceptate, erythromycin lactobionate, hydrocortisone sodium succinate, methicillin, methohexital, metoclopramide, oxacillin, penicillin G potassium, polymyxin B, secobarbital, sodium bicarbonate, thiopental, or warfarin.
- **Ophth:** See Appendix H for instillation of ophthalmic preparations.
- **Top:** Apply to entire affected area.

Patient/Family Teaching

- **General Info:** Instruct patient to take medication around the clock and to finish the drug completely as directed, even if feeling better. Avoid taking milk, antacids, calcium, magnesium-containing medications, and iron supplements within 1–3 hr of oral tetracycline. Advise patient that sharing of this medication may be dangerous.
- □ Caution patient to use sunscreen and protective clothing to prevent photosensitivity reactions.
- □ Advise patient to report the signs of superinfection (black, furry overgrowth on the tongue, vaginal itching or discharge, loose or foul-smelling stools) and allergy.
- □ Instruct patient to notify physician if symptoms do not improve.
- □ Caution patient to discard outdated or decomposed tetracyclines, as they may be toxic.

- **Ophth:** Instruct patient on correct technique for instillation of ophthalmic preparations. Caution patient not to allow tip of container to come in contact with eye, fingers, or any other surface.
  - Ophthalmic preparations may cause blurred vision. Caution patient to avoid driving or other activities requiring visual acuity until response to medication is known.
- **Top:** Instruct patient in correct technique for application of soln or ointment. Advise patient to avoid frequent washing of affected area and to wait at least 1 hr before applying other topical acne preparations.
  - Advise patient that topical preparations may stain clothing and may cause slight yellowing of skin.
  - Instruct patient to consult physician if no improvement in lesions with 2 wk of treatment with ointment or 6–8 wk with soln.

EVALUATION

Clinical response can be evaluated by: ▪ Resolution of the signs and symptoms of infection. Length of time for complete resolution depends on the organism and site of infection ▪ Decrease in acne lesions.

THEOPHYLLINE

(thee-**off**-i-lin)
Accurbron, Aquaphyllin, Asmalix, Bronkodyl, Elixomin, Elixophyllin, Lanophyllin, Lixolin, PMS Theophylline, Pulmophylline, Slo-phyllin Syrup, Synophylate, Theolair, Theon, Theophyl, Theostat

THEOPHYLLINE EXTENDED RELEASE

Aerolate, Constant-T, Elixophyllin SR, LaBID, Quibron-T/SR, Respbid, Slo-bid Gyrocaps, Slophyllin Gyrocaps, Sustaire, Theo-24, Theobid Duracap, Theobid Jr. Duracap, Theochron, Theoclear LA Cenules, Theo-dur, Theo-dur Sprinkle, Theolair-SR, Theophyl-SR, Theospan-SR, Theo-Time, Theovent Long-Acting, Uniphyl

CLASSIFICATION(S):
Bronchodilator—phosphodiesterase inhibitor
Pregnancy Category C

INDICATIONS

▪ Bronchodilator in reversible airway obstruction due to asthma or COPD. **Unlabeled Use:** ▪ Respiratory and myocardial stimulant in apnea of infancy.

ACTION

▪ Inhibits phosphodiesterase, producing increased tissue concentrations of cyclic adenosine monophosphate (cAMP) ▪ Increased levels of cAMP result in: ▫ Bronchodilation ▫ CNS and cardiac stimulation ▫ Diuresis ▫ Gastric acid secretion. **Therapeutic Effect:** ▪ Bronchodilation.

PHARMACOKINETICS

Absorption: Well absorbed from oral dosage forms. Absorption from extended-release dosage forms is slow but complete.

Distribution: Widely distributed. Crosses the placenta. Breast milk concentrations 70% of plasma levels.

Metabolism and Excretion: Mostly metabolized by the liver to caffeine, which may accumulate in neonates. Metabolites are renally excreted.

Half-life: 3–13 hr. Increased in the elderly (>60 yr), neonates, and patients with CHF or liver disease. Shortened in cigarette smokers and children.

CONTRAINDICATIONS AND PRECAUTIONS

Contraindicated in: ▪ Uncontrolled arrhythmias ▪ Hyperthyroidism.

Use Cautiously in: ▪ Elderly patients >60 yr (dosage reduction required) ▪ CHF, cor pulmonale, or liver disease (dosage reduction required) ▪ Cigarette smokers (larger doses may be required) ▪ Pregnancy (has been used safely) ▪ Children <6 yr (avoid sustained-release preparations).

ADVERSE REACTIONS AND SIDE EFFECTS*

CNS: nervousness, anxiety, headache, insomnia, **SEIZURES**.

CV: tachycardia, palpitations, arrhythmias, angina pectoris.

GI: nausea, vomiting, anorexia, cramps.

Neuro: tremor.

INTERACTIONS

Drug-Drug: ▪ Additive CV and CNS side effects with **adrenergic (sympathomimetic) agents** ▪ May decrease the therapeutic effect of **lithium** ▪ **Smoking, phenobarbital, rifampin, phenytoin** and **ketoconazole** increase metabolism and may decrease effectiveness ▪ **Erythromycin, beta-adrenergic blockers, influenza vaccination, cimetidine, oral contraceptives, glucocorticoids, disulfiram, interferon, mexiletine, fluoroquinolones, thiabendazole,** and large doses of **allopurinol** decrease metabolism and may lead to toxicity ▪ Increased risk of arrhythmias with **halothane** ▪ **Isoniazid, carbamazepine,** or **loop diuretics** may increase or decrease theophylline labels.

Drug-Food: ▪ Additive adverse reactions may occur with excessive ingestion of **xanthine (caffeine)-containing food** or **beverages**. Excess consumption of **charcoal-broiled beef** may decrease effectiveness.

ROUTE AND DOSAGE

Note: Dosage should be determined by plasma level monitoring.

Bronchodilator

- **PO (Adults):** 5–6 mg/kg initially, followed by 3 mg/kg q 8 hr in otherwise healthy patients, 2 mg/kg q 8 hr in older patients or those with cor pulmonale, 4 mg/kg q 8 hr in young adult smokers. Range 400–900 mg/day; total daily dose may be divided and given q 12–24 hr using sustained-release preparations.
- **PO (Children 12–16 yr):** 5–6 mg/kg initially, followed by 12–18 mg/kg/day in divided doses q 6 hr (q 8–12 hr for sustained-release preparations).
- **PO (Children 9–12 yr):** 5–6 mg/kg initially, followed by 16–20 mg/kg/day in divided doses q 6 hr (q 8–12 hr for sustained-release preparations).
- **PO (Children 1–9 yr):** 5–6 mg/kg initially, followed by 20–24 mg/kg/day in divided doses q 6 hr.
- **PO (Children 6 mon–1 yr):** 5–6 mg/kg initially, followed by maintenance dose in mg/kg q 6 hr = (0.05) (age in wks) + 1.25.
- **PO (Children <6 mon):** 5–6 mg/kg initially, followed by maintenance dose in mg/kg/8 hr = (0.07) (age in wks) + 1.7.
- **IV (Adults):** Loading dose of 5 mg/kg infused over 30 min, followed by 0.2–0.8 mg/kg/hr continuous infusion.
- **IV (Children 12–16 yr):** Loading dose of 5 mg/kg, followed by 0.5–0.7 mg/kg/hr continuous infusion.
- **IV (Children 9–12 yrs):** Loading dose of 5 mg/kg, followed by 0.7 mg/kg/hr continuous infusion.
- **IV (Children 1–9 yrs):** Loading dose of 5 mg/kg, followed by 0.8 mg/kg/hr continuous infusion.
- **IV (Children <1 yr):** Loading dose of 5 mg/kg, followed by continuous infusion in mg/kg/hr = (0.008) (age in wks) + 0.21.

Respiratory Stimulant

- **IV (Neonates):** 5 mg/kg initially, then 1 mg/kg q 8–12 hr.

PHARMACODYNAMICS (bronchodilation)

	ONSET*	PEAK	DURATION
PO	rapid	1–2 hr	6 hr
PO-ER	delayed	4–8 hr	8–24 hr
IV	rapid	end of infusion	6–8 hr

*If a loading dose has been given.

NURSING IMPLICATIONS

ASSESSMENT

- ☐ Assess blood pressure, pulse, and respiratory status (rate, lung sounds, use of accessory muscles) prior to and throughout course of therapy. Ensure

*Underlines indicate most frequent; **CAPITALS** indicate life-threatening.

that oxygen therapy is correctly instituted.

- Monitor intake and output ratios for an increase in diuresis or fluid overload due to volume of medication.
- Patients with a history of cardiovascular problems should be monitored for ECG changes.

- **Lab Test Considerations:** Monitor ABGs and serum electrolytes prior to and periodically throughout therapy.
- **Toxicity and Overdose:** Monitor drug levels routinely. Peak levels should be evaluated 1–2 hr after rapid-acting forms and 4–12 hr after extended-release forms. Therapeutic plasma levels range is 10–20 mcg/ml. Drug levels >20 mcg/ml are associated with toxicity. Caffeine ingestion may falsely elevate drug concentration levels.
  - Observe patient closely for the appearance of progressive theophylline toxicity (anorexia, nausea, vomiting, restlessness, insomnia, tachycardia, arrhythmias, seizures). Notify physician immediately if these symptoms occur.

Potential Nursing Diagnoses

- Airway clearance, ineffective (indications).
- Activity intolerance (indications).
- Knowledge deficit related to medication regimen (patient/family teaching).

Implementation

- **General Info:** Give these medications around the clock. Once-a-day doses should be administered in the morning.
  - Do not refrigerate elixirs, solns, syrups, or suspensions, as crystals may form. Crystals should dissolve when liquid is warmed to room temperature.
  - Wait at least 4 hr after discontinuing IV therapy to begin immediate-release oral dosage; for extended-release oral dosage form, administer first oral dose at time of IV discontinuation.
- **PO:** Administer with a full glass of water or food to minimize GI irritation. Food slows but does not reduce the extent of absorption. Use calibrated measuring device to ensure accurate dose of liquid preparations.
  - Do not crush enteric-coated or sustained-release tablets or capsules. Available in a slow-release sprinkle (Theo-dur Sprinkle) for patients who cannot swallow tablets or capsules. Also available in chewable tablets.
- **Continuous Infusion:** IV theophylline and 5% dextrose is packed in a moisture barrier overwrap. Remove immediately before administration and squeeze bag to check for leaks. Discard if soln is not clear.
  - *Loading Dose:* Administer over 20 min. If patient has had another form of theophylline prior to loading dose, serum theophylline level should be obtained and loading dose proportionately reduced. In emergency situations when serum level is not available, half the usual loading dose may be given if no symptoms of theophylline toxicity are present.
  - *Rate:* Do not exceed 20 mg/min. Rapid administration may cause hypotension, arrhythmias, syncope, and death. Administer via infusion pump to ensure accurate dosage. Monitor ECG continuously, as tachyarrythmias may occur.
- **Y-Site Compatibility:** acyclovir or famotidine.
- **Y-Site Incompatibility:** hetastarch.
- **Additive Compatibility:** methylprednisolone or verapamil.
- **Additive Incompatibility:** ascorbic acid, chlorpromazine, codeine, corticotropin, dimenhydrinate, epinephrine, erythromycin gluceptate, hydralazine, insulin, levorphanol, meperidine, methicillin, morphine, norepinephrine, oxytetracycline, papaverine, penicillin G, pentazocine, phenobarbital, phenytoin, prochlorperazine, promazine, promethazine, tetracycline, or vancomycin.

Patient/Family Teaching

- Emphasize the importance of taking

T

only the prescribed dose at the prescribed time intervals. Missed doses should be taken as soon as remembered or omitted if close to next dose.
- Encourage patient to drink adequate liquids (2000 ml/day minimum) to decrease the viscosity of airway secretions.
- Advise patient not to take any over-the-counter cough, cold, or breathing preparations without consulting physician or pharmacist. These medications may increase side effects and cause arrhythmias.
- Advise patient to minimize intake of xanthine-containing foods or beverages (cola, coffee, chocolate) and not to eat charcoal-broiled foods daily.
- Instruct patient not to change brands or dosage forms without consulting physician.
- Encourage patient not to smoke. Instruct patient to inform physician if smoking pattern changes, as dosage adjustment may be necessary.
- Advise patient to contact physician promptly if usual dose of medication fails to produce the desired results, symptoms worsen after treatment, or toxic effects occur.
- Emphasize the importance of having serum levels routinely tested every 6–12 mon.

Evaluation

Effectiveness of therapy can be demonstrated by: ▪ Increased ease in breathing ▫ Clearing of lung fields on auscultation ▪ Effective respiratory patterns in neonatal apnea.

THIAMINE
(thye-a-min)
Betalin S, {Betaxin}, Bewon, Biamine, vitamin B_1

CLASSIFICATION(S):
Vitamin—water-soluble
Pregnancy Category A

INDICATIONS
▪ Treatment of thiamine deficiencies (beriberi) ▪ Prevention of Wernicke's encephalopathy ▪ Dietary supplement in patients with GI disease, alcoholism, or cirrhosis.

ACTION
▪ Required for carbohydrate metabolism. **Therapeutic Effect:** ▪ Replacement in deficiency states.

PHARMACOKINETICS
Absorption: Well absorbed from the GI tract by an active process. Excessive amounts are not absorbed completely. Also well absorbed from IM sites.
Distribution: Widely distributed. Enters breast milk.
Metabolism and Excretion: Metabolized by the liver. Excess amounts are excreted unchanged by the kidneys.
Half-life: UK.

CONTRAINDICATIONS AND PRECAUTIONS
Contraindicated in: ▪ Hypersensitivity.
Use Cautiously in: ▪ Prevention of Wernicke's encephalopathy (condition may be worsened unless glucose is administered before thiamine).

ADVERSE REACTIONS AND SIDE EFFECTS*
Note: Adverse reactions and side effects are extremely rare and are usually associated with IV administration or extremely large doses.
CNS: weakness, restlessness.
EENT: tightness of the throat.
CV: hypotension, VASCULAR COLLAPSE, vasodilation.
Resp: respiratory distress, pulmonary edema.
GI: nausea, GI bleeding.
Derm: warmth, tingling, pruritus, urticaria, sweating, cyanosis.
Misc: angioedema.

{} = Available in Canada only.
*Underlines indicate most frequent; **CAPITALS** indicate life-threatening.

INTERACTIONS

Drug–Drug: ▪ May enchance **neuromuscular blocking agents.**

ROUTE AND DOSAGE

Thiamine Deficiency (Beriberi)

- **PO (Adults):** 5–30 mg/day in single or 3 divided doses.
- **PO (Children):** 10–50 mg/day in divided doses.
- **IM, IV (Adults):** 50–100 mg tid.
- **IM, IV (Children):** 10–25 mg/day.

Dietary Supplement

- **PO (Adults):** 1–2 mg/day.
- **PO (Children):** 0.5–1 mg/day.
- **PO (Infants):** 0.3–0.5 mg/day.

PHARMACODYNAMICS (time for symptoms of deficiency—edema and heart failure—to resolve; confusion and psychosis take longer to respond)

	ONSET	PEAK	DURATION
PO	hr	days	days–wk
IM	hr	days	days–wk
IV	hr	days	days–wk

NURSING IMPLICATIONS

Assessment

- □ Assess patient for signs and symptoms of thiamine deficiency (anorexia, GI distress, irritability, palpitations, tachycardia, edema, paresthesia, muscle weakness and pain, depression, memory loss, confusion, psychosis, visual disturbances, elevated serum pyruvic acid levels).
- □ Assess patient's nutritional status (diet, weight) prior to and throughout course of therapy.
- □ Monitor patients receiving IV thiamine for anaphylaxis (wheezing, urticaria, edema).
- ▪ **Lab Test Considerations:** May interfere with certain methods of testing serum theophylline, uric acid, and urobilinogen concentrations.

Potential Nursing Diagnoses

- ▪ Nutrition, altered: less than body requirements (indications).
- ▪ Knowledge deficit related to diet and medication regimen (patient/family teaching).

Implementation

- ▪ **General Info:** Because of infrequency of single B-vitamin deficiencies, combinations are commonly administered.
- □ Available in tablet, elixir, or parenteral forms.
- ▪ **IM/IV:** Parenteral administration is reserved for patients in whom oral administration is not feasible.
- ▪ **IM:** Administration may cause tenderness and induration at injection site. Cool compresses may decrease discomfort.
- ▪ **IV:** Sensitivity reactions and deaths have occurred from IV administration. An intradermal test dose is recommended in patients with suspected sensitivity. Monitor site for erythema and induration.
- ▪ **Direct IV:** Administer undiluted each 100 mg over at least 5 min.
- ▪ **Continuous Infusion:** May be diluted in dextrose/Ringer's or lactated Ringer's combinations, dextrose/saline combinations, D5W, D10W, Ringer's and lactated Ringer's injection, 0.9% NaCl, or 0.45% NaCl and is usually administered with other vitamins.
- ▪ **Additive Incompatibility:** barbiturates; solns with neutral or alkaline pH, such as carbonates, bicarbonates, citrates, and acetates; erythromycin, kanamycin, or streptomycin.

Patient/Family Teaching

- □ Encourage patient to comply with physician's dietary recommendations. Explain that the best source of vitamins is a well-balanced diet with foods from the 4 basic food groups.
- □ Teach patient that foods high in thiamine include cereals (whole grain and enriched), meats (especially pork), and fresh vegetables; loss is variable during cooking.
- □ Caution patients self-medicating with vitamin supplements not to exceed RDA (see Appendix L). The effectiveness of megadoses of vitamins for

treatment of various medical conditions is unproven and may cause side effects.

Evaluation

Effectiveness of therapy can be demonstrated by: ▪ Prevention of or decrease in the signs and symptoms of vitamin B_1 deficiency ▫ Decrease in the symptoms of neuritis, ocular signs, ataxia, edema, and heart failure may be seen within hrs of administration and may disappear within a few days ▫ Confusion and psychosis may take longer to respond and may persist if nerve damage has occurred.

THIETHYLPERAZINE

(thye-eth-il-**per**-a-zeen)

Torecan

CLASSIFICATION(S):
Antiemetic—phenothiazine
Pregnancy Category UK

INDICATIONS

▪ Management of nausea and vomiting.

ACTION

▪ Alters the effects of dopamine in the CNS ▪ Depresses the chemoreceptive trigger zone (CTZ) and vomiting center in the CNS. **Therapeutic Effect:** ▪ Diminished nausea and vomiting.

PHARMACOKINETICS

Absorption: Well absorbed following oral, rectal, or IM administration.

Distribution: Widely distributed, high concentrations in the CNS. Crosses the placenta and probably enters breast milk.

Metabolism and Excretion: Highly metabolized by the liver and GI mucosa.

Half-life: UK.

CONTRAINDICATIONS AND PRECAUTIONS

Contraindicated in: ▪ Hypersensitivity ▪ Hypersensitivity to bisulfites (IM) ▪ Hypersensitivity to aspirin or tartrazine (tab) ▪ Cross-sensitivity with other phenothiazines may exist ▪ Narrow-angle glaucoma ▪ Bone marrow depression ▪ Severe liver or cardiovascular disease ▪ Pregnancy ▪ Children <12 yr.

Use Cautiously in: ▪ Elderly or debilitated patients (dosage reduction recommended) ▪ Lactation (safety not established) ▪ Diabetes mellitus ▪ Respiratory disease ▪ Prostatic hypertrophy ▪ CNS tumors ▪ Epilepsy ▪ Intestinal obstruction.

ADVERSE REACTIONS AND SIDE EFFECTS*

CNS: <u>sedation</u>, extrapyramidal reactions, tardive dyskinesia, restlessness, headache, cerebral vascular spasm, **NEUROLEPTIC MALIGNANT SYNDROME.**

EENT: <u>dry eyes</u>, blurred vision, lens opacities, tinnitus.

CV: hypotension (following IM use), peripheral edema.

Derm: rashes, photosensitivity, pigment changes.

Endo: galactorrhea.

GI: <u>constipation</u>, <u>dry mouth</u>, ileus, anorexia, hepatitis, altered taste.

GU: urinary retention.

Hemat: **AGRANULOCYTOSIS**, leukopenia.

Metab: hyperthermia.

Neuro: trigeminal neuralgia.

Misc: allergic reactions.

INTERACTIONS

Drug-Drug: ▪ Additive hypotension with **antihypertensive agents**, acute ingestion of **alcohol**, or **nitrates**, ▪ Additive CNS depression with other **CNS depressants**, including **alcohol, antihistamines, narcotic analgesics, sedative/hypnotics**, or **general anesthetics** ▪ Additive anticholinergic effects with other **drugs possessing anticholinergic properties**, including **antihistamines, antidepressants, atropine, disopyramide, haloperidol**, and other **phenothiazines** ▪ May decrease the beneficial effects of **levodopa** ▪ May

*<u>Underlines</u> indicate most frequent; **CAPITALS** indicate life-threatening.

block alpha-adrenergic effects of **epinephrine** resulting in severe hypotension and tachycardia.

ROUTE AND DOSAGE

- **PO, IM, Rect (Adults):** 10 mg 1–3 times daily.

PHARMACODYNAMICS (antiemetic effect)

	ONSET	PEAK	DURATION
PO	30 min	UK	4 hr
IM	UK	UK	UK
Rect	UK	UK	UK

NURSING IMPLICATIONS

Assessment

- Assess patient for nausea and vomiting prior to and 30–60 min following administration.
- Monitor blood pressure (sitting, standing, lying), pulse, and respiratory rate prior to and frequently during initial therapy.
- Assess patient for level of sedation following administration.
- Assess urine output for possible urinary retention.
- Observe patient carefully for extrapyramidal symptoms (pill-rolling motions, drooling, tremors, rigidity, shuffling gait) or tardive dyskinesia (rhythmic movement of mouth, face, and extremities). Notify physician immediately at the onset of these symptoms.
- Monitor for development of neuroleptic malignant syndrome (fever, respiratory distress, tachycardia, convulsions, diaphoresis, hypertension or hypotension, pallor, tiredness). Notify physician immediately if these symptoms occur.
- **Lab Test Considerations:** CBC and liver function tests should be evaluated periodically throughout course of prolonged therapy.
- May cause false-positive or false-negative pregnancy tests.

Potential Nursing Diagnoses

- Fluid volume deficit, (indications).
- Injury, high risk for (side effects).
- Knowledge deficit related to medication regimen (patient/family teaching).

Implementation

- **General Info:** Available in tablet, suppository, and injectable forms.
- **IM:** Inject slowly into deep, well-developed muscle. Administer only clear, colorless soln. Keep patient recumbent for at least 60 min following injection to minimize hypotensive effects.

Patient/Family Teaching

- Advise patient to make position changes slowly to minimize orthostatic hypotension.
- Medication may cause drowsiness. Caution patient to avoid driving or other activities requiring alertness until response to medication is known.
- Caution patient to avoid taking alcohol or other CNS depressants concurrently with this medication.
- Inform patient of possibility of extrapyramidal symptoms and tardive dyskinesia. Caution patient to report these symptoms immediately to physician.
- Advise patient to use sunscreen and protective clothing when exposed to the sun to prevent photosensitivity reactions. Extremes in temperature should also be avoided, as this drug impairs body temperature regulation.
- Instruct patient to use frequent mouth rinses, good oral hygiene, and sugarless gum or candy to minimize dry mouth. Consult physician or dentist if dry mouth continues $>$2 wk.
- Advise patient that increasing bulk and fluids in the diet and exercise may help minimize the constipating effects of this medication.
- Instruct patient to notify physician promptly if sore throat, fever, unusual bleeding or bruising, skin rashes, weakness, tremors, visual disturbances, dark-colored urine, or clay-colored stools are noted.
- Patients on prolonged therapy should

have periodic lab tests and ocular examinations.

Evaluation

Effectiveness of therapy can be demonstrated by: ■ Relief of nausea and vomiting.

THIOGUANINE

(thye-oh-**gwon**-een)
6-thioguanine, {Lanvis}

CLASSIFICATION(S):
Antineoplastic—antimetabolite
Pregnancy Category UK

INDICATIONS

■ Used in combination chemotherapeutic regimens to induce remission in acute myelogenous leukemia ■ Has also been used alone or in combination with other agents in the treatment of acute lymphocytic leukemia and chronic myelogenous leukemia.

ACTION

■ Incorporated into DNA and RNA, subsequently disrupting synthesis (cell cycle—S-phase specific). **Therapeutic Effects:** ■ Death of rapidly replicating cells, especially malignant ones ■ Immunosuppressive properties.

PHARMACOKINETICS

Absorption: Variable and incomplete (30%) following oral administration.
Distribution: Probably does not enter the CSF. Crosses the placenta.
Metabolism and Excretion: Highly metabolized by the liver.
Half-life: 11 hr.

CONTRAINDICATIONS AND PRECAUTIONS

Contraindicated in: ■ Hypersensitivity ■ Pregnancy or lactation ■ Severe liver disease.
Use Cautiously in: ■ Patients with childbearing potential ■ Infections ■ Decreased bone marrow reserve ■ Other chronic debilitating illnesses.

ADVERSE REACTIONS AND SIDE EFFECTS*

EENT: loss of vibratory sense.
GI: jaundice, hepatotoxicity, nausea, vomiting, stomatitis, diarrhea.
GU: gonadal suppression.
Derm: rash, dermatitis.
Hemat: leukopenia, thrombocytopenia, anemia.
Metab: hyperuricemia.
Neuro: unsteady gait.

INTERACTIONS

Drug-Drug: ■ Additive bone marrow depression with other **antineoplastic agents** or **radiation therapy** ■ May decrease antibody response to **live virus vaccines** and increase the risk of adverse reactions.

ROUTE AND DOSAGE

Note: Many other protocols are used.

Induction

- **PO (Adults and Children):** 2 mg/kg (75–100 mg/m^2) per day, rounded off to nearest 20 mg given as single dose. After 4 wk may increase to 3 mg/kg.

Maintenance Dosage

- **PO (Adults and Children):** 2–3 mg/kg (100 mg/m^2) per day.

PHARMACODYNAMICS (effect on blood counts)

	ONSET	PEAK	DURATION
PO	7–10 days	14 days	21 days

NURSING IMPLICATIONS

Assessment

- □ Assess for fever, chills, sore throat, and signs of infection. Notify physician if these symptoms occur.
- □ Monitor platelet count throughout therapy. Assess for bleeding (bleeding gums, bruising, petechiae; guaiac stools, urine, and emesis). If thrombocytopenia occurs, avoid IM injections and rectal temperatures and ap-

{} = Available in Canada only.
*Underlines indicate most frequent; CAPITALS indicate life-threatening.

ply pressure to venipuncture sites for 10 min.

- ▫ Monitor intake and output, appetite, and nutritional intake. Administration of an antiemetic and adjusting diet as tolerated may help maintain fluid and electrolyte balance and nutritional status.
- ▫ Anemia may occur. Monitor for increased fatigue, dyspnea, and orthostatic hypotension.
- ▫ Monitor for symptoms of gout (increased uric acid, joint pain, edema). Encourage patient to drink at least 2 liters of fluids/day. Physician may order allopurinol or alkalinization of urine to decrease uric acid levels.
- ▪ **Lab Test Considerations:** Monitor CBC and differential at least weekly, daily in patients with elevated leukocyte counts. Bone marrow suppression usually occurs in 2–4 wk, but rapid decrease in leukocyte count may occur in 1–2 wk. Notify physician of any rapid or severe drop in blood counts, as therapy may need to be withheld until values stabilize. Bone marrow aspiration may be required to detect thioguanine-induced hypoplasia.
- ▫ Monitor for increased uric acid, creatinine, and BUN.
- ▫ Monitor for hepatotoxicity evidenced by increased SGOT (AST), SGPT (ALT), LDH, serum bilirubin, and alkaline phosphatase.

Potential Nursing Diagnoses

- ▪ Infection, high risk for (side effects).
- ▪ Injury, high risk for (side effects).
- ▪ Knowledge deficit related to medication regimen (patient/family teaching).

Implementation

- ▪ **PO:** Administer daily dose at bedtime. May also be divided into 2 doses and given 12 hr apart.
- ▫ If patient has difficulty swallowing tablets confer with pharmacist regarding preparation of syrup.

Patient/Family Teaching

- ▫ Instruct patient to take thioguanine exactly as directed, even if nausea and vomiting occurs. If vomiting occurs shortly after dose is taken, consult physician. Take combinations of drugs at prescribed times. If a dose is missed, do not take at all.
- ▫ Instruct patient to notify physician if decreased urine output, swelling of lower extremities, yellowing of skin, nausea, vomiting, severe diarrhea, mouth sores, fever, chills, sore throat, signs of infection, bleeding gums, bruising, petechiae, or blood in urine, stool, or emesis occurs.
- ▫ Caution patient to avoid crowds and persons with known infections. Instruct patient to use soft toothbrush and electric razor. Caution patient not to drink alcoholic beverages or take aspirin-containing products.
- ▫ This medication may cause gonadal suppression; however, patient should still use birth control. Advise patient to inform physician immediately if pregnancy is suspected.
- ▫ Instruct patient to inspect oral mucosa for redness and ulceration. If ulceration occurs, advise patient to use sponge brush and rinse mouth with water after eating and drinking. Physician may order viscous lidocaine swishes if pain interferes with eating.
- ▫ Instruct patient not to receive any vaccinations without advice of physician.
- ▫ Advise patient of need for medical follow-up and frequent lab tests.

Evaluation

Effectiveness of therapy can be demonstrated by: ▪ Induction of remission in patients with leukemia.

THIOPENTAL

(thye-oh-**pen**-tal)
Pentothal

CLASSIFICATION(S):
Anesthetic—barbiturate, Anticonvulsant—barbiturate
Schedule III
Pregnancy Category C

T

INDICATIONS

■ Used to provide an unconscious state as part of balanced anesthesia in combination with muscle relaxants and/or analgesics during short surgical procedures ■ Treatment of seizures in patients with increased intracranial pressure ■ Part of narcoanalysis or narcosynthesis in psychiatric patients ■ Management of increased intracranial pressure.

ACTION

■ Produces all levels of CNS depression: □ Depresses the sensory cortex □ Decreases motor activity □ Alters cerebellar function □ Inhibits transmission in the nervous system ■ Raises the seizure threshold. **Therapeutic Effects:** ■ Induction of sleep and anesthesia without analgesia (short-acting) ■ Decreased seizure activity ■ Lowering of intracranial pressure.

PHARMACOKINETICS

Absorption: Readily absorbed from the rectal mucosa.

Distribution: Rapidly distributed to the CNS, then redistributed to viscera (liver, kidneys, heart), then to muscle, and finally to fat. Crosses the placenta readily. Small amounts enter breast milk.

Metabolism and Excretion: Mostly metabolized by the liver. Small amounts are converted to pentobarbital.

Half-life: 12 hr (increased in obese patients and in pregnant patients at term).

CONTRAINDICATIONS AND PRECAUTIONS

Contraindicated in: ■ Hypersensitivity ■ Porphyria ■ Status asthmaticus ■ Inflammatory rectal or lower bowel conditions or patients undergoing rectal surgery (rectal form only).

Use Cautiously in: ■ Severe cardiovascular disease, shock, or hypotension ■ Myxedema ■ Addison's disease ■ Increased intracranial pressure ■ Liver disease ■ Renal disease ■ Myasthenia gravis ■ Pregnancy or lactation (safety not established) ■ Middle-aged, elderly, or debilitated patients (dosage reduction may be required) ■ Repeated use (tolerance may develop) ■ Repeated doses, large doses, or prolonged infusion in 24-hr period (increased risk of excessive somnolence, respiratory or circulatory depression—dosage reduction required).

ADVERSE REACTIONS AND SIDE EFFECTS*

CNS: emergence delerium, headache, prolonged somnolence.

EENT: salivation.

Resp: respiratory depression, APNEA, laryngospasm, bronchospasm, hiccoughs, sneezing, coughing.

CV: hypotension, myocardial depression, arrhythmias.

GI: rectal irritation (after rectal administration), nausea, vomiting.

Derm: erythema, pruritus, urticaria, rashes.

Local: pain, phlebitis at IV site.

MS: skeletal muscle hyperactivity.

Misc: allergic reactions, including ANAPHYLAXIS, shivering.

INTERACTIONS

Drug-Drug: Additive CNS depression with other **CNS depressants,** including **alcohol, antihistamines, antidepressants, narcotic analgesics,** and **sedative/hypnotics** ■ Increased risk of hypotension with **antihypertensives, diuretics,** or **ketamine.**

ROUTE AND DOSAGE

Note: Dosages must be carefully titrated by patient response.

Test Dose

- IV (Adults): 25–75 mg.

Anesthesia

- **IV (Adults):** 50–100 mg initially, followed by 50–100 mg as needed or 3–5 mg/kg as a single dose.
- **IV (Children):** 3–5 mg/kg initially, followed by 1 mg/kg as needed.

*Underlines indicate most frequent; **CAPITALS** indicate life-threatening.

Anticonvulsant

- **IV (Adults):** 50–100 mg (up to 250 mg may be required).

Preanesthetic Sedation (basal anesthesia)

- **Rect (Adults and Children):** 30 mg/kg.

Narcoanalysis

- **IV (Adults):** 100 mg/min until patient becomes confused.

Basal Narcosis

- **Rect (Adults and Children):** Up to 9 mg/kg, not to exceed 1–1.5 g in children weighing more than 75 lb (34 kg) or 3–4 g in adults weighing 200 lb (90 kg) or more.

Increased Intracranial Pressure

- **IV (Adults):** 1.5–3.5 mg/kg as needed.

PHARMACODYNAMICS (anesthetic effects)

	ONSET	PEAK	DURATION
IV	30–60 sec	UK	10–30 min
Rect	8–10 min	UK	UK

NURSING IMPLICATIONS

Assessment

- **General Info:** Assess blood pressure, ECG, heart rate, and respiratory status continuously throughout thiopental therapy. Monitor for apnea immediately after IV injection, especially in the presence of narcotic premedication.
- □ Monitor IV site carefully. Extravasation may cause pain, swelling, ulceration, and necrosis. Intra-arterial injection may cause arteritis, vasospasm, edema, thrombosis, and gangrene of the extremity.
- **Increased Intracranial Pressure:** Assess level of consciousness and intracranial pressure before and throughout therapy.
- **Toxicity and Overdose:** Monitor for signs of overdose, which may occur from too rapid injections (drop in blood pressure, possibly to shock levels) or excessive or repeated injections (respiratory distress, laryngospasm, apnea).

Potential Nursing Diagnoses

- Breathing pattern, ineffective (side effects).
- Injury, high risk for (side effects).

Implementation

- **General Info:** Thiopental should be used only by individuals qualified to administer anesthesia and experienced in endotracheal intubation. Equipment for this procedure should be immediately available.
- □ Administer premedication with anticholinergics (atropine, glycopyrrolate) to decrease mucus secretions. Narcotics may be administered preoperatively because of the lack of analgesic effects of thiopental. Administer preoperative medications so peak effects are attained shortly before induction of anesthesia. Administer muscle relaxants separately.
- □ Concurrent use of nitrous oxide 67% decreases the requirements for thiopental by ⅔.
- **Rect:** May be administered as a rectal suspension. Do not exert excessive pressure on plunger, to prevent overdose. Use a new applicator for each repeat administration. Unless fecal impaction is present, cleansing enema is not usually required prior to administration of rectal thiopental.
- **IV:** Dilute thiopental with sterile water for injection, D5W, or 0.9% NaCl. Soln should be freshly prepared and used within 24 hr of reconstitution. Refrigerate and keep tightly sealed. Do not administer soln containing a precipitate.
- **Direct IV:** A test dose of 25–75 mg (1–3 ml of a 2.5% soln) may be administered to determine tolerance or unusual sensitivity to thiopental. Observe patient for at least 60 sec.
- □ When thiopental is used as the sole anesthetic agent, small repeated doses may be used to maintain desired level of anesthesia.
- □ *Rate:* Administer slowly. Rapid administration may cause overdose.
- **Intermittent Infusion:** 2% or 2.5% concentration of thiopental is used for intermittent infusion.

T

- **Continuous Infusion:** Solns of 0.2–0.4% have been administered by continuous infusion to maintain anesthesia when thiopental is the sole agent. May be diluted in soln with D5/0.45% NaCl, D5W, multiple electrolyte solns, 0.45% NaCl, 0.9% NaCl, and ⅙ M sodium lactate.
- **Syringe Compatibility:** aminophylline, hydrocortisone sodium succinate, neostigmine, pentobarbital, scopolamine, sodium iodide, or tubocurarine.
- **Syringe Incompatibility:** benzquinamide, chlorpromazine, clindamycin, cimetidine, dimenhydrinate, diphenhydramine, doxapram, droperidol, ephedrine, fentanyl, glycopyrrolate, meperidine, morphine, pentazocine, prochlorperazine, promethazine, propiomazine, sodium bicarbonate, or trimethaphan.
- **Additive Compatibility:** chloramphenicol, hydrocortisone sodium succinate, oxytocin, pentobarbital, phenobarbital, potassium chloride, or sodium bicarbonate.
- **Additive Incompatibility:** amikacin, cephapirin, chlorpromazine, cimetidine, clindamycin, codeine, dimenhydrinate, diphenhydramine, droperidol, fentanyl, fibrinolysin, hydromorphone, regular insulin, levorphanol, meperidine, metaraminol, methadone, morphine, norepinephrine, penicillin G potassium, prochlorperazine, promazine, promethazine, succinylcholine, tetracycline, trimethaphan camsylate, dextrose/Ringer's or lactated Ringer's injection combinations, D10/0.9% NaCl, D10W, and Ringer's and lactated Ringer's injection.

PATIENT/FAMILY TEACHING

- ☐ Thiopental may cause psychomotor impairment for 24 hr following administration. Caution patient to avoid driving or other activities requiring alertness for 24 hr.
- ☐ Advise patient to avoid use of alcohol or other CNS depressants for 24 hr following anesthesia, unless directed by physician or dentist.

EVALUATION

Effectiveness of therapy can be demonstrated by: ▪ Loss of consciousness and maintenance of desired level of anesthesia.

THIORIDAZINE

(thye-oh-**rid**-a-zeen)

{Apo-Thioridazine}, Mellaril, Mellaril S, {Novo-Ridazine}, {PMS Thioridazine}

CLASSIFICATION(S):

Antipsychotic—phenothiazine

Pregnancy Category UK

INDICATIONS

▪ Treatment of acute and chronic psychoses ▪ Treatment of severe behavioral problems in children.

ACTION

▪ Alters the effects of dopamine in the CNS ▪ Possesses significant anticholinergic and alpha-adrenergic blocking activity. **Therapeutic Effect:** ▪ Diminished signs and symptoms of psychoses.

PHARMACOKINETICS

Absorption: Absorption from tablets is variable; may be better with oral liquid formulations.

Distribution: Widely distributed, high concentrations in the CNS. Crosses the placenta and enters breast milk.

Metabolism and Excretion: Highly metabolized by the liver and GI mucosa.

Half-life: UK.

CONTRAINDICATIONS AND PRECAUTIONS

Contraindicated in: ▪ Hypersensitivity ▪ Cross-sensitivity with other phenothiazines may exist ▪ Narrow-angle glaucoma ▪ Bone marrow depression ▪ Severe liver or cardiovascular disease.

Use Cautiously in: ▪ Elderly or debilitated patients ▪ Pregnancy or lactation (safety not established) ▪ Diabetes mellitus ▪ Respiratory disease ▪ Prostatic hypertrophy ▪ CNS tumors ▪ Epilepsy ▪ Intestinal obstruction.

ADVERSE REACTIONS AND SIDE EFFECTS*

CNS: sedation, extrapyramidal reactions, tardive dyskinesia, NEUROLEPTIC MALIGNANT SYNDROME.
EENT: dry eyes, blurred vision, lens opacities.
CV: hypotension, tachycardia.
GI: constipation, dry mouth, ileus, anorexia, hepatitis.
GU: urinary retention.
Derm: rashes, photosensitivity, pigment changes.
Endo: galactorrhea.
Hemat: AGRANULOCYTOSIS, leukopenia.
Metab: hyperthermia.
Misc: allergic reactions.

INTERACTIONS

Drug-Drug: ▪ Additive hypotension with other **antihypertensive agents, nitrates,** and acute ingestion of **alcohol** ▪ Additive CNS depression with other **CNS depressants**, including **alcohol, antihistamines, narcotic analgesics, sedative/hypnotics**, and **general anesthetics** ▪ Additive anticholinergic effects with other **drugs possessing anticholinergic properties,** including **antihistamines, antidepressants, atropine, haloperidol,** other **phenothiazines,** and **disopyramide** ▪ **Lithium** decreases blood levels of thioridazine ▪ Thioridazine may mask early signs of **lithium** toxicity and increases the risk of extrapyramidal reactions ▪ Increased risk of agranulocytosis with **antithyroid agents** ▪ Concurrent use with **epinephrine** may result in severe hypotension and tachycardia ▪ May decrease the effectiveness of **levodopa.**

ROUTE AND DOSAGE

Psychoses

- **PO (Adults):** 50–100 mg tid, up to 800 mg/day.

Depressive Neuroses with Anxiety, Fears, Depression; Anxiety in the Elderly

- **PO (Adults):** 25 mg tid (range of 20–200 mg/day).

Behavioral Problems in Children

- **PO (Children >2 yr):** 0.5–3 mg/kg/day in 2–3 divided doses (10 mg 2–3 times daily).

PHARMACODYNAMICS (antipsychotic effects)

	ONSET	PEAK	DURATION
PO	UK	UK	8–12 hr

NURSING IMPLICATIONS

Assessment

- Assess mental status (orientation, mood, behavior) and degree of anxiety prior to and periodically throughout therapy.
- Monitor blood pressure (sitting, standing, lying), pulse, and respiratory rate prior to and frequently during the period of dosage adjustment.
- Observe patient carefully when administering medication to ensure that medication is actually taken and not hoarded.
- Assess patient for level of sedation following administration.
- Monitor intake and output ratios and daily weight. Notify physician if significant discrepancies occur.
- Observe patient carefully for extrapyramidal symptoms (pill-rolling motions, drooling, tremors, rigidity, shuffling gait) and tardive dyskinesia (uncontrolled movements of face, mouth, tongue, or jaw and involuntary movements of extremities). Notify physician immediately at the onset of these symptoms.
- Monitor for development of neurolep-

*Underlines indicate most frequent; **CAPITALS** indicate life-threatening.

tic malignant syndrome (fever, respiratory distress, tachycardia, convulsions, diaphoresis, hypertension or hypotension, pallor, tiredness). Notify physician immediately if these symptoms occur.

- **Lab Test Considerations:** CBC and liver function tests should be evaluated periodically throughout course of therapy. May cause blood dyscrasias, especially between wks 4–10 of therapy.
- May cause false-positive or false-negative pregnancy tests and false-positive urine bilirubin test results.
- May cause increased serum prolactin levels, thereby interfering with gonadorelin test results.
- May cause Q wave and T wave changes in ECG.

Potential Nursing Diagnoses

- Coping, ineffective individual (indications).
- Thought processes, altered (indications).
- Knowledge deficit related to medication regimen (patient/family teaching).

Implementation

- **General Info:** Available in tablet, concentrate, and suspension.
- To prevent contact dermatitis, avoid getting soln on hands.
- Phenothiazines should be discontinued 48 hr before and not resumed for 24 hr following metrizamide myelography, as they lower the seizure threshold.
- **PO:** Administer with food, milk, or a full glass of water to minimize gastric irritation.
- Dilute concentrate in 120 ml of distilled or acidified tap water or fruit juice just prior to administration.

Patient/Family Teaching

- Advise patient to take medication exactly as directed, not to skip doses or double up on missed doses. If a dose is missed, it should be taken as soon as remembered unless almost time for the next dose. If more than 2 doses are scheduled each day, the missed dose should be taken within 1 hr of the scheduled time.
- Abrupt withdrawal may lead to gastritis, nausea, vomiting, dizziness, headache, tachycardia, and insomnia.
- May cause drowsiness. Caution patient to avoid driving or other activities requiring alertness until response to medication is known.
- Advise patient to use sunscreen and protective clothing when exposed to the sun to prevent photosensitivity reactions. Extremes in temperature should also be avoided, as this drug impairs body temperature regulation.
- Instruct patient to use frequent mouth rinses, good oral hygiene, and sugarless gum or candy to minimize dry mouth. Consult physician or dentist if dry mouth continues >2 wk.
- Advise patient that increasing activity and bulk and fluids in the diet help minimize the constipating effects of this medication.
- Caution patient to avoid taking alcohol or other CNS depressants concurrently with this medication.
- Advise patient to notify physician or dentist of medication regimen prior to treatment or surgery.
- Instruct patient to notify physician promptly if sore throat, fever, unusual bleeding or bruising, skin rashes, weakness, tremors, visual disturbances, difficulty urinating, dark-colored urine, or clay-colored stools are noted.
- Emphasize the importance of routine follow-up examinations to monitor response to medication and to detect side effects. Periodic ocular examinations are indicated. Encourage continued participation in psychotherapy as ordered by physician.

Evaluation

Effectiveness of therapy can be demonstrated by: ▪ Decrease in excitable, paranoic, or withdrawn behavior ▪ Decrease in anxiety associated with depression.

THIOTEPA
(thye-oh-**tep**-a)

CLASSIFICATION(S):
Antineoplastic—alkylating agent
Pregnancy Category UK

INDICATIONS
▪ **Bladder Instillation:** Management or prophylaxis of superficial tumors of the bladder following local resection ▪ **IV:** Palliative treatment for breast and ovarian cancer ▪ **Intracavitary Instillation:** Prevention of recurrent malignant effusions in pleura, pericardium, or peritoneum.

ACTION
▪ Disrupts protein, DNA, and RNA synthesis by cross-linking strands of DNA and RNA (cell cycle-phase nonspecific). **Therapeutic Effects:** ▪ Death of rapidly replicating cells, particularly malignant ones ▪ Has immunosuppressive properties.

PHARMACOKINETICS
Absorption: Variably absorbed following instillation (10–100%).
Distribution: Distribution not known.
Metabolism and Excretion: Extensively metabolized.
Half-life: UK.

CONTRAINDICATIONS AND PRECAUTIONS
Contraindicated in: ▪ Hypersensitivity ▪ Pregnancy or lactation.
Use Cautiously in: ▪ Patients with childbearing potential ▪ Active infections ▪ Decreased bone marrow reserve ▪ Other chronic debilitating illnesses ▪ Severe hepatic or renal disease.

ADVERSE REACTIONS AND SIDE EFFECTS*
CNS: headache, dizziness.
EENT: tightness of the throat.
GI: nausea, anorexia, vomiting, stomatitis.
GU: gonadal suppression.
Derm: alopecia, rash, pruritus, hives.
Hemat: thrombocytopenia, leukopenia, anemia.
Local: pain at IV site, pain at site of intracavitary instillation.
Metab: hyperuricemia.
Misc: fever, allergic reactions.

INTERACTIONS
Drug-Drug: ▪ Additive bone marrow depression with other **antineoplastic agents** or **radiation therapy** ▪ May prolong apnea after **succinylcholine** ▪ May decrease antibody response to **live virus vaccines** and increase the risk of adverse reactions.

ROUTE AND DOSAGE
Bladder Instillation
- **Intravesical (Adults):** 30–60 mg retained for 2 hr weekly for 4 wk, then monthly.

Palliative Therapy of Breast, Ovarian Cancer
- **IV (Adults):** 0.3–0.4 mg/kg q 1–4 wk or 0.2 mg/kg (6 mg/m^2) daily for 4–5 days q 2–4 wk.

Malignant Effusions
- **Intracavitary (Adults):** 0.6–0.8 mg/kg q 1–4 wk (range 0.07–0.8 mg/kg).

PHARMACODYNAMICS (noted as effects on blood counts; effects after intracavitary administration are highly variable)

	ONSET	PEAK	DURATION
IV	10 days (up to 30 days)	14 days	21 days

NURSING IMPLICATIONS
Assessment
- ▫ Monitor vital signs prior to and periodically during therapy.
- ▫ Assess for fever, chills, sore throat, and signs of infection. Notify physician if these symptoms occur.
- ▫ Monitor platelet count throughout therapy. Assess for bleeding (bleeding gums, bruising, petechiae; guaiac stools, urine, and emesis). Avoid IM

*Underlines indicate most frequent; **CAPITALS** indicate life-threatening.

injections and rectal temperatures. Apply pressure to venipuncture sites for 10 min.

- Monitor intake and output, appetite, and nutritional intake. Assess for nausea, vomiting, and anorexia. Administration of an antiemetic and adjusting diet as tolerated may help maintain fluid and electrolyte balance and nutritional status.
- Anemia may occur. Monitor for increased fatigue, dyspnea, and orthostatic hypotension.
- Monitor for symptoms of gout (increased uric acid, joint pain, edema). Encourage patient to drink at least 2 liters of fluids/day. Allopurinol or alkalinization of urine may be used to decrease uric acid levels.
- **Lab Test Considerations:** Monitor CBC and differential prior to and weekly throughout therapy and for at least 3 wk after therapy. The nadir of leukopenia occurs after 10–14 days, although it may be delayed up to 1 mon. Notify physician if platelet count <150,000/mm^3 or leukocyte count <3000/mm^3.
- Monitor for increased SGOT (AST), SGPT (ALT), LDH, serum bilirubin, uric acid, creatinine, and BUN.

Potential Nursing Diagnoses

- Infection, high risk for (side effects).
- Injury, high risk for (side effects).
- Knowledge deficit related to medication regimen (patient/family teaching).

Implementation

- **General Info:** Safe for IM or SC administration.
- Soln is clear to slightly opaque. Do not use soln that is cloudy or that contains precipitate. Stable for 5 days if refrigerated after reconstitution.
- Soln should be prepared in a biologic cabinet. Wear gloves, gown, and mask while handling medication. Discard equipment in designated containers (see Appendix I).
- Reconstitute 15 mg of powder with 1.5 ml of sterile water for injection. This concentration is suitable for intratumor injection. May be further diluted for other routes.
- May be administered by physician via several routes.
- **Intracavitary:** Reconstitute soln. Thiotepa is instilled via tube that was used to drain the effusion.
- **Bladder Instillation:** Limit fluids per physican's order for 8–12 hr prior to treatment. Reconstitute soln. Mix 60 mg with 30–60 ml of sterile water and instill in bladder via foley catheter. Reposition patient every 15 min to allow maximal contact of soln with tumors. Soln should be retained for 2 hr. The lesser amount of soln (30 ml) is usually reserved for patients unable to hold 60 ml.
- **Direct IV:** Following reconstitution, may be administered undiluted over 1–3 min.
- **Intermittent Infusion:** Dilute further in 50–100 ml of 0.9% NaCl, D5W, dextrose/saline combinations, Ringer's or lactated Ringer's soln.
- **Syringe Compatibility:** procaine HCl 2% or epinephrine 1:1000.

Patient/Family Teaching

- Instruct patients receiving thiotepa via foley catheter to contact physician if hematuria or dysuria occurs.
- Instruct patient to notify physician if fever, chills, sore throat, signs of infection, bleeding gums, bruising, petechiae, or blood in urine, stool, or emesis occurs. Caution patient to avoid crowds and persons with known infections. Instruct patient to use soft toothbrush and electric razor. Caution patient not to drink alcoholic beverages or take aspirin-containing products.
- Instruct patient to inspect oral mucosa for redness and ulceration. If ulceration occurs, advise patient to use sponge brush and rinse mouth with water after eating and drinking. Physician may order viscous lidocaine swishes if pain interferes with eating.
- This drug may cause gonadal suppression; however, patient should still use birth control. Advise patient

to inform physician immediately if pregnancy is suspected.
- Discuss possibility of hair loss with patient. Explore methods of coping.
- Instruct patient not to receive any vaccinations without advice of physician.
- Advise patient of need for medical follow-up and frequent lab tests.

Evaluation

Effectiveness of therapy can be demonstrated by: ▪ Decrease in size and spread of malignant tissue.

THIOTHIXENE
(thye-oh-**thix**-een)
Navane

CLASSIFICATION(S):
Antipsychotic—thioxanthene
Pregnancy Category UK

INDICATIONS

▪ Management of psychoses, especially in withdrawn, apathetic schizophrenic patients and patients suffering from delusions and hallucinations.

ACTION

▪ Alters the effect of dopamine in the CNS. **Therapeutic Effect:** ▪ Diminished signs and symptoms of psychoses.

PHARMACOKINETICS

Absorption: Well absorbed following oral and IM administration.
Distribution: Widely distributed. Crosses the placenta.
Metabolism and Excretion: Mainly metabolized by the liver.
Half-life: 30 hr.

CONTRAINDICATIONS AND PRECAUTIONS

Contraindicated in: ▪ Hypersensitivity ▪ Cross-sensitivity with other phenothiazines may exist ▪ Narrow-angle glaucoma ▪ Bone marrow depression ▪ Severe liver or cardiac disease.

Use Cautiously in: ▪ Elderly or debilitated patients (dosage reduction may be required) ▪ Diabetes mellitus ▪ Respiratory disease ▪ Prostatic hypertrophy ▪ CNS tumors ▪ Epilepsy ▪ Intestinal obstruction ▪ Pregnancy, lactation, or children (safety not established).

ADVERSE REACTIONS AND SIDE EFFECTS*

CNS: sedation, extrapyramidal reactions, tardive dyskinesia, **NEUROLEPTIC MALIGNANT SYNDROME.**
EENT: dry eyes, blurred vision, lens opacities.
CV: hypotension, tachycardia.
GI: constipation, dry mouth, ileus, anorexia, hepatitis, nausea.
GU: urinary retention.
Derm: rashes, photosensitivity, pigment changes.
Endo: galactorrhea.
Hemat: leukopenia, leukocytosis.
Metab: hyperpyrexia.
Misc: allergic reactions.

INTERACTIONS

Drug-Drug: ▪ Additive hypotension with **antihypertensive agents,** acute ingestion of **alcohol,** and **nitrates** ▪ Additive CNS depression with other **CNS depressants,** including **alcohol, antihistamines, antidepressants, narcotic analgesics,** and **sedative/hypnotics** ▪ Additive anticholinergic effects with other **drugs having anticholinergic properties,** including **antihistamines, antidepressants, quinidine,** or **disopyramide** ▪ May decrease the effectiveness of **levodopa** ▪ Increased risk of cardiac effects with **quinidine.**

ROUTE AND DOSAGE

Mild to Moderate Psychoses

- **PO (Adults):** 2 mg tid, may be increased to 15 mg/day if necessary.

Severe Psychoses

- **PO (Adults):** 5 mg bid, may be increased to 20–30 mg/day (not to exceed 60 mg/day). May be given as a single daily dose.

*Underlines indicate most frequent; **CAPITALS** indicate life-threatening.

T

Acute Agitation

- **IM (Adults):** 4 mg 2–4 times daily, may be increased to 16–20 mg/day (not to exceed 30 mg/day).

PHARMACODYNAMICS (antipsychotic effects)

	ONSET	PEAK	DURATION
PO	day–wk	UK	UK
IM	1–6 hr	UK	UK

NURSING IMPLICATIONS

Assessment

- Monitor patient's mental status (delusions, hallucinations, and behavior) prior to and periodically throughout therapy.
- Observe patient carefully when administering oral medication to ensure that medication is actually taken and not hoarded.
- Assess patient for level of sedation following administration.
- Monitor patient for onset of extrapyramidal side effects (akathisia—restlessness; dystonia—muscle spasms and twisting motions; pseudoparkinsonism—mask facies, rigidity, tremors, drooling, shuffling gait, dysphagia). Notify physician if these symptoms occur, as reduction in dosage or discontinuation of medication may be necessary. Physician may also order antiparkinson agents (trihexyphenidyl, benztropine) to control these symptoms.
- Monitor for tardive dyskinesia (rhythmic movement of mouth, face, and extremities). Notify physician immediately if these symptoms occur, as these side effects may be irreversible.
- Monitor for development of neuroleptic malignant syndrome (fever, respiratory distress, tachycardia, convulsions, diaphoresis, hypertension or hypotension, pallor, tiredness). Notify physician immediately if these symptoms occur.
- **Lab Test Considerations:** Thiothixene increases serum prolactin levels and lowers serum uric acid levels.
- Monitor CBC and differential prior to and periodically throughout therapy. Risk of leukopenia is highest between wks 4 and 10 of therapy.
- Monitor liver function studies prior to and periodically during therapy. Risk of hepatotoxicity is greatest 2–4 wk after beginning therapy.

Potential Nursing Diagnoses

- Thought processes, altered (indications).
- Injury, high risk for (side effects).
- Knowledge deficit related to medication regimen (patient/family teaching).

Implementation

- **General Info:** Available as capsule, oral soln, and parenteral injection.
- All forms of soln may cause dermatitis; avoid skin contact.
- Thiothixene lowers the seizure threshold; institute seizure precautions for patients with history of seizure disorder.
- **PO:** Administer capsules with food or milk to decrease gastric irritation.
- Dilute oral soln with 240 ml of milk, juice, carbonated drink, or soup to decrease gastric irritation. Measure dose with provided dropper.
- **IM:** Dilute each 10-mg vial with 2.2 ml of sterile water for injection, for a concentration of 5 mg/ml. Administer deep into well-developed muscle.

Patient/Family Teaching

- Instruct patients receiving parenteral thiothixene to remain supine for 30 min after administration. Position changes should be made slowly.
- Instruct patient on need to take medication exactly as ordered. If a dose is missed, it should be taken as soon as remembered until 2 hr before next dose. Do not double doses. Patients on long-term high-dose therapy may need to be tapered off to avoid withdrawal symptoms (dyskinesia, tremors, dizziness, nausea, and vomiting).

- ▫ Instruct patients receiving oral soln on correct method of measuring dose with provided dropper.
- ▫ Drowsiness may occur. Caution patient to avoid driving or other activities requiring alertness until response to medication is known.
- ▫ Inform patient of possibility of extrapyramidal symptoms and tardive dyskinesia. Caution patient to report these symptoms immediately to physician.
- ▫ Advise patient that frequent mouth rinses, good oral hygiene, and sugarless gum or candy may decrease mouth dryness. Physician or dentist should be notified if dryness persists >2 wk.
- ▫ Advise patient that increasing bulk and fluids in the diet and exercise may help minimize the constipating effects of this medication.
- ▫ Caution patient to use sunscreen and protective clothing to prevent photosensitivity reactions.
- ▫ Caution patient to avoid concurrent use of alcohol, other CNS depressants, and over-the-counter medications without prior physician approval.
- ▫ Caution patient to avoid exercising in hot weather and taking very hot baths, as this drug impairs temperature regulation.
- ▫ Instruct patient to notify physician promptly if sore throat, fever, skin rashes or discoloration, weakness, tremors, or visual disturbances are noted.
- ▫ Advise patient to notify physician or dentist of medication regimen prior to treatment or surgery.
- ▫ Emphasize the importance of continued medical follow-up for psychotherapy, eye examinations, and laboratory tests.

Evaluation

Effectiveness of therapy can be demonstrated by: ▪ Decrease in psychotic ideation.

THYROID

(**thye**-royd)

Armour Thyroid, Thyrar

CLASSIFICATION(S):
Hormone—thyroid
Pregnancy Category A

INDICATIONS

▪ Replacement or substitution therapy in diminished or absent thyroid function of many causes ▪ Treatment of some types of thyroid cancer.

ACTION

▪ Principal effect is increasing metabolic rate of body tissues: ▫ Promotes gluconeogenesis ▫ Increases utilization and mobilization of glycogen stores ▫ Stimulates protein synthesis ▫ Promotes cell growth and differentiation ▫ Aids in the development of the brain and CNS ▪ Contains T_3 (triiodothyronine) and T_4 (thyroxine) activity. **Therapeutic Effects:** ▪ Replacement in deficiency states with restoration of normal hormonal balance ▪ Suppression of thyrotropin-dependent thyroid cancers.

PHARMACOKINETICS

Absorption: Well absorbed from the GI tract following oral administration.

Distribution: Distributed into most body tissues. Thyroid hormones do not readily cross the placenta; minimal amounts enter breast milk.

Metabolism and Excretion: Metabolized by the liver and other tissues. Undergoes enterohepatic recirculation. Excreted in the feces via the bile.

Half-life: T_3 (liothyronine)—1–2 days; T_4 (thyroxine)—6–7 days.

CONTRAINDICATIONS AND PRECAUTIONS

Contraindicated in: ▪ Hypersensitivity ▪ Recent myocardial infarction ▪ Thyrotoxicosis.

Use Cautiously in: ▪ Cardiovascular disease ▪ Severe renal insufficiency

T

- Uncorrected adrenocortical disorders
- Elderly and myxedematous patients (extremely sensitive to thyroid hormones; initial dosage should be markedly reduced).

ADVERSE REACTIONS AND SIDE EFFECTS*

CNS: irritability, insomnia, nervousness, headache.
CV: tachycardia, arrhythmias, increased cardiac output, angina pectoris, increased blood pressure, CARDIOVASCULAR COLLAPSE, hypotension.
GI: diarrhea, cramps, vomiting.
Derm: increased sweating, hair loss (in children).
Endo: menstrual irregularities.
Metab: weight loss, heat intolerance.
MS: accelerated bone maturation in children.

INTERACTIONS

Drug–Drug: ▪ **Cholestyramine** or **colestipol** decrease oral absorption ▪ May alter the effectiveness of **oral anticoagulants** ▪ May cause an increase in the requirement for **insulin** or **oral hypoglycemic agents** in diabetics ▪ Additive cardiovascular effects with **adrenergic agents (sympathomimetics)** ▪ May decrease response to **beta-adrenergic blockers**.

ROUTE AND DOSAGE

Note: Each 1 g = 60 mg and is equivalent to 100 mcg or less of levothyroxine (T_4) or 25 mcg of liothyronine (T_3).

- **PO (Adults):** 30–60 mg/day, increase at monthly intervals (usual dose 60–180 mg/day). In adults with severe hypothyroidism, initiate therapy with 15 mg/day.
- **PO (Children):** 15 mg/day, increase at 2-wk intervals (may exceed adult dose).

PHARMACODYNAMICS (effects on thyroid function tests)

	ONSET	PEAK	DURATION
PO	days–wk	1–3 wk	days–wk

NURSING IMPLICATIONS

Assessment

- **General Info:** Assess apical pulse and blood pressure prior to and periodically during therapy. Observe patient for signs of myocardial ischemia and tachyarrhythmias.
  - Monitor for symptoms of hyperthyroidism (tachycardia, chest pain, nervousness, insomnia, diaphoresis, tremors, weight loss).
- **Children:** Monitor bone age, height and weight, and psychomotor development.
- **Lab Test Considerations:** Thyroid function tests should be monitored prior to and throughout course of therapy.
  - Monitor blood and urine glucose in diabetics; insulin or oral hypoglycemic dose may need to be increased.

Potential Nursing Diagnoses

- Knowledge deficit related to medication regimen (patient/family teaching).

Implementation

- **General Info:** Administer as a single dose, preferably before breakfast to prevent insomnia.
- **PO:** Do not crush, break, or chew enteric-coated tablets.

Patient/Family Teaching

- **General Info:** Instruct patient to take medication exactly as prescribed, at the same time each day. If a dose is missed, take as soon as remembered unless almost time for next dose. If more than 2 or 3 doses are missed notify physician. Do not discontinue without consulting physician.
  - Instruct patient and family on correct technique for checking pulse. Dose should be withheld and physician notified if resting pulse is >100 beats/min.
  - Explain to patient that thyroid does not cure hypothyroidism, it provides a replacement hormone; therapy may be lifelong.
  - Caution patient not to change brands

*Underlines indicate most frequent; **CAPITALS** indicate life-threatening.

of this medication, as this may effect drug potency.
- □ Advise patient to notify physician if headache, nervousness, diarrhea, excessive sweating, heat intolerance, chest pain, increased pulse rate, palpitations, or any unusual symptoms occur.
- □ Caution patient to avoid taking other medications concurrently with thyroid, without consulting physician or pharmacist.
- □ Instruct patient to inform physician or dentist of thyroid therapy prior to treatment or surgery.
- □ Emphasize importance of follow-up examinations to monitor effectiveness of therapy. Thyroid function tests are performed at least yearly.
- ▪ **Children:** Discuss with parents need for routine follow-up studies to ensure correct development. Inform parents that partial hair loss may be experienced by children on thyroid therapy. This is usually temporary.

EVALUATION

Clinical response can be evaluated by: ▪ Resolution of symptoms of hypothyroidism. Response includes: □ Diuresis □ Weight loss □ Increased sense of well-being □ Increased energy, pulse rate, appetite, psychomotor activity □ Normalization of skin texture and hair □ Correction of constipation □ Increased T_3 and T_4 levels. Sleeping pulse and basal morning temperature may be used to determine effectiveness ▪ In children, effectiveness of therapy is determined by: □ Appropriate physical and psychomotor development.

TICARCILLIN
(tye-kar-**sil**-in)
Ticar

CLASSIFICATION(S):
Anti-infective—extended-spectrum penicillin
Pregnancy Category UK

INDICATIONS

▪ Treatment of serious infections due to susceptible organisms including: □ Skin and skin structure infections □ Bone and joint infections □ Septicemia □ Respiratory tract infections □ Intra-abdominal □ Gynecologic □ Urinary tract infections ▪ Combination with an aminoglycoside may be synergistic against *Pseudomonas* ▪ Has been combined with other anti-infectives in the treatment of infections in immunosuppressed patients.

ACTION

▪ Binds to bacterial cell wall membrane, causing cell death. **Therapeutic Effect:** ▪ Bactericidal action against susceptible bacteria ▪ Spectrum is extended, compared to other penicillins. **Spectrum:** ▪ Similar to penicillin but greatly extended to include several important gram-negative aerobic pathogens, notably: □ *Pseudomonas aeruginosa* □ *Escherichia coli* □ *Proteus mirabilis* □ *Providencia rettgeri* ▪ Active against some anaerobic bacteria, including *Bacteroides* ▪ Not active against penicillinase-producing staphylococci or beta-lactamase-producing Enterobacteriaceae.

PHARMACOKINETICS

Absorption: Well absorbed following IM administration.

Distribution: Widely distributed. Enters CSF well only when meninges are inflammed. Crosses the placenta and enters breast milk in low concentrations.

Metabolism and Excretion: 10% metabolized by the liver, 90% excreted unchanged by the kidneys.

Half-life: 0.9–1.3 hr (increased in renal impairment).

CONTRAINDICATIONS AND PRECAUTIONS

Contraindicated in: ▪ Hypersensitivity to penicillins or cephalosporins.

Use Cautiously in: ▪ Renal impairment (dosage reduction required)

▪ Pregnancy and lactation (safety not established) ▪ History of hypersensitivity ▪ Severe liver disease.

ADVERSE REACTIONS AND SIDE EFFECTS*

CNS: confusion, lethargy, SEIZURES (high doses).
CV: congestive heart failure, arrhythmias.
GI: nausea, diarrhea.
GU: hematuria (children only).
Derm: rashes, urticaria.
F and E: hypokalemia, hypernatremia.
Hemat: bleeding, blood dyscrasias, increased bleeding time.
Local: phlebitis.
Metab: metabolic alkalosis.
Misc: superinfection, hypersensitivity reactions, including ANAPHYLAXIS and serum sickness.

INTERACTIONS

Drug-Drug: ▪ **Probenecid** decreases renal excretion and increases blood levels ▪ May alter excretion of **lithium** ▪ **Diuretics, glucocorticoids,** or **amphotericin B** may increase the risk of hypokalemia ▪ Hypokalemia increases the risk of **cardiac glycoside** toxicity.

ROUTE AND DOSAGE

Note: Contains 4.75 mEq sodium/g.

- **IV (Adults and Children >40 kg):** 1–4 g q 4–6 hr (150–300 mg/kg/day).
- **IV (Children >1 mon and <40 kg):** 50–300 mg/kg/day in divided doses q 4–8 hr.
- **IV (Neonates >2 kg):** 75 mg/kg q 8 hr, increase to 100 mg/kg q 8 hr after first wk of life.
- **IV (Neonates <2 kg):** 75 mg/kg q 12 hr, increase to q 8 hr after first wk of life.
- **IM (Adults and Children >40 kg):** 1 g q 6 hr.
- **IM (Children >1 mon and <40 kg):** 50–100 mg/kg/day in divided doses q 6–8 hr.
- **IM (Neonates >2 kg):** 75 mg/kg q 8 hr, increase to 100 mg/kg q 8 hr after first wk of life.
- **IM (Neonates <2 kg):** 75 mg/kg q 12 hr, increase to q 8 hr after first wk of life.

PHARMACODYNAMICS (blood levels)

	ONSET	PEAK
IM	rapid	30–75 min
IV	rapid	end of infusion

NURSING IMPLICATIONS

Assessment

- □ Assess patient for infection (vital signs; appearance of wound, sputum, urine, and stool; WBC) at beginning and throughout course of therapy.
- □ Obtain a history before initiating therapy to determine previous use of and reactions to penicillins or cephalosporins. Persons with a negative history of penicillin sensitivity may still have an allergic response.
- □ Obtain specimens for culture and sensitivity prior to initiating therapy. First dose may be given before receiving results.
- □ Observe patient for signs and symptoms of anaphylaxis (rash, pruritus, laryngeal edema, wheezing). Discontinue drug and notify physician immediately if these occur. Keep epinephrine, an antihistamine, and resuscitation equipment close by in the event of an anaphylactic reaction.
- ▪ **Lab Test Considerations:** Renal and hepatic function, CBC, serum potassium, and bleeding times should be evaluated prior to and routinely throughout course of therapy.
- □ May cause false-positive urine protein testing and increased BUN, creatinine, SGOT (AST), SGPT (ALT), serum bilirubin, alkaline phosphatase, LDH, and uric acid levels. May also cause increased bleeding time.
- □ May cause hypernatremia and hypokalemia with high doses.

Potential Nursing Diagnoses

- ▪ Infection, high risk for (indications, side effects).

*Underlines indicate most frequent; **CAPITALS** indicate life-threatening.

- Knowledge deficit related to medication regimen (patient/family teaching).

Implementation

- **IM:** Reconstitute 1-g vial with 2 ml of sterile water or bacteriostatic water for injection or 1% lidocaine hydrochloride injection (without epinephrine), for a concentration of 1 g/2.5 ml.
  - Inject deep into a well-developed muscle mass, to minimize discomfort, and massage well. IM injections should not exceed 2 g at each site.
- **IV:** Change IV sites every 48 hr to prevent phlebitis.
  - Add at least 4 ml of sterile water for injection to each 1-g vial. Further dilute to at least 20 ml with 0.9% NaCl, D5W, Ringer's or lactated Ringer's soln. Soln is stable for 48 hr at room temperature, 14 days if refrigerated.
- **Direct IV:** Administer as slowly as possible to minimize vein irritation. Do not administer concentrations >50 mg/ml.
- **Intermittent Infusion:** Administer over 30 min–2 hr, 10–20 min in neonates.
- **Y-Site Compatibility:** acyclovir, cyclophosphamide, famotidine, hydromorphone, magnesium sulfate, meperidine, morphine, ondansetron, perphenazine, or verapamil.
- **Additive Compatibility:** ranitidine or verapamil.
- **Additive Incompatibility:** Incompatible with aminoglycosides; do not admix; administer at least 1 hr apart.

Patient/Family Teaching

- Advise patient to report the signs of superinfection (black, furry overgrowth on the tongue, vaginal itching or discharge, loose or foul-smelling stools) and allergy.

Evaluation

Clinical response can be evaluated by:
- Resolution of the signs and symptoms of infection. Length of time for complete resolution depends on the organism and site of infection.

TICARCILLIN/CLAVULANATE

(tye-kar-**sil**-in/klav-yoo-**la**-nate)
Timentin

CLASSIFICATION(S):
Anti-infective—extended-spectrum penicillin
Pregnancy Category B

INDICATIONS

- Treatment of serious infections due to susceptible organisms including: ▫ Skin and skin structure infections ▫ Bone and joint infections ▫ Septicemia ▫ Respiratory tract infections ▫ Intra-abdominal infections ▫ Gynecologic infections ▫ Urinary tract infections ▪ Combination with an aminoglycoside may be synergistic against *Pseudomonas* ▪ Has been combined with other anti-infectives in the treatment of infections in immunosuppressed patients.

ACTION

- Binds to bacterial cell wall membrane, causing cell death ▪ Addition of clavulanate enhances resistance to beta-lactamase, an enzyme produced by bacteria capable of inactivating some penicillins. **Therapeutic Effect:** ▪ Bactericidal action against susceptible bacteria ▪ Spectrum is extended compared to other penicillins. **Spectrum:** ▪ Similar to penicillin but greatly extended to include several important gram-negative aerobic pathogens, notably: ▫ *Pseudomonas aeruginosa* ▫ *Escherichia coli* ▫ *Proteus mirabilis* ▫ *Providencia rettgeri* ▪ Active against some anaerobic bacteria, including *Bacteroides* ▪ Not active against penicillinase-producing staphylococci or beta-lactamase producing Enterobacteriaceae.

PHARMACOKINETICS

Absorption: Administered IV only, resulting in complete bioavailability.

T

Distribution: Widely distributed. Enters CSF well only when meninges are inflammed. Crosses the placenta and enters breast milk in low concentrations.
Metabolism and Excretion: 10% of ticarcillin is metabolized by the liver, 90% excreted unchanged by the kidneys. Clavulanate is metabolized by the liver.
Half-life: Ticarcillin—0.9–1.3 hr (increased in renal impairment); clavulanate—1.1–1.5 hr.

CONTRAINDICATIONS AND PRECAUTIONS

Contraindicated in: ▪ Hypersensitivity to penicillins or cephalosporins.
Use Cautiously in: ▪ Renal impairment (dosage reduction required) ▪ Pregnancy and lactation (safety not established) ▪ History of hypersensitivity ▪ Severe liver disease.

ADVERSE REACTIONS AND SIDE EFFECTS*

CNS: confusion, lethargy, SEIZURES (high doses).
CV: congestive heart failure, arrhythmias.
GI: nausea, diarrhea.
GU: hematuria (children only).
Derm: rashes, urticaria.
F and E: hypokalemia, hypernatremia.
Hemat: bleeding, blood dyscrasias, increased bleeding time.
Local: phlebitis.
Metab: metabolic alkalosis.
Misc: superinfection, hypersensitivity reactions, including ANAPHYLAXIS and serum sickness.

INTERACTIONS

Drug-Drug: ▪ **Probenecid** decreases renal excretion and increases blood levels ▪ May alter excretion of **lithium** ▪ **Diuretics, glucocorticords,** or **amphotericin B** may increase the risk of hypokalemia ▪ Hypokalemia increases the risk of **cardiac glycoside** toxicity.

ROUTE AND DOSAGE

Note: Ticarcillin contains 4.75 mEq sodium/g; ticarcillin/clavulanate contains 0.15 mEq potassium/100 mg clavulanate. 3 g ticarcillin plus 100 mg clavulanate labeled as 3.1 g combined potency.

- **IV (Adults >60 kg):** 3.1 g q 4–6 hr (q 6–8 hr for urinary tract infections only).
- **IV (Children >12 yr and Adults <60 kg):** 200–300 mg/kg/day of ticarcillin equivalent in divided doses q 4–6 hr.

PHARMACODYNAMICS (blood levels)

	ONSET	PEAK
IV	rapid	end of infusion

NURSING IMPLICATIONS

Assessment

- Assess patient for infection (vital signs; appearance of wound, sputum, urine, and stool; WBC) at beginning and throughout course of therapy.
- Obtain a history before initiating therapy to determine previous use of and reactions to penicillins or cephalosporins. Persons with a negative history of penicillin sensitivity may still have an allergic response.
- Obtain specimens for culture and sensitivity prior to initiating therapy. First dose may be given before receiving results.
- Observe patient for signs and symptoms of anaphylaxis (rash, pruritus, laryngeal edema, wheezing). Discontinue drug and notify physician immediately if these occur. Keep epinephrine, an antihistamine, and resuscitation equipment close by in the event of an anaphylactic reaction.
- **Lab Test Considerations:** Renal and hepatic function, CBC, serum potassium, and bleeding times should be evaluated prior to and routinely throughout course of therapy.

*Underlines indicate most frequent; **CAPITALS** indicate life-threatening.

- May cause false-positive urine protein testing and increased BUN, creatinine, SGOT (AST), SGPT (ALT), serum bilirubin, alkaline phosphatase, LDH, and uric acid levels. May also cause increased bleeding time.
- May cause hypernatremia and hypokalemia with high doses.

POTENTIAL NURSING DIAGNOSES

- Infection, high risk for (indications, side effects).
- Knowledge deficit related to medication regimen (patient/family teaching).

IMPLEMENTATION

- **Intermittent Infusion:** Change IV sites every 48 hr to prevent phlebitis.
- Add 13 ml of sterile water or 0.9% NaCl for injection to each 3.1-g vial, to provide a concentration of ticarcillin 200 mg/ml and clavulanic acid 6.7 mg/ml. Further dilute in 0.9% NaCl, D5W, or Ringer's or lactated Ringer's soln. Stable for 6 hr at room temperature, 72 hr if refrigerated.
- *Rate:* Administer over 30 min via Y-site or direct IV. If Y-site is used, temporarily discontinue primary infusion during ticarcillin/clavulanate administration.
- **Y-Site Compatibility:** cyclophosphamide, famotidine, meperidene, morphine, ondansetron, or perphenazine.
- **Additive Incompatibility:** Incompatible with aminoglycosides; do not admix; administer at least 1 hr apart.

PATIENT/FAMILY TEACHING

- Advise patient to report the signs of superinfection (black, furry overgrowth on the tongue, vaginal itching or discharge, loose or foul-smelling stools) and allergy.

EVALUATION

Clinical response can be evaluated by: ▪ Resolution of the signs and symptoms of infection. Length of time for complete resolution depends on the organism and site of infection.

TICLOPIDINE
(tye-**cloe**-pi-deen)
Ticlid

CLASSIFICATION(S):
Platelet aggregation inhibitor
Pregnancy Category B

INDICATIONS

▪ Prevention of stroke in patients who have had a completed thrombotic stroke or precursors to stroke who are unable to tolerate aspirin.

ACTION

▪ Inhibits platelet aggregation by altering the function of platelet membranes ▪ Prolongs bleeding time. **Therapeutic Effect:** ▪ Decreased incidence of stroke in high risk patients.

PHARMACOKINETICS

Absorption: Well absorbed (>80%) following oral administration.
Distribution: Distribution not known.
Metabolism and Excretion: Extensively metabolized by the liver. Minimal excretion of unchanged drug by the kidneys.
Half-life: Single dose—12.6 hr; multiple dosing—4–5 days.

CONTRAINDICATIONS AND PRECAUTIONS

Contraindicated in: ▪ Hypersensitivity ▪ Bleeding disorders ▪ Active bleeding ▪ Severe liver disease.
Use Cautiously in: ▪ Pregnancy, lactation, or children <18 yrs (safety not established) ▪ Risk of bleeding (trauma, surgery, history of ulcer disease) ▪ Renal or hepatic impairment (dosage adjustments may be necessary) ▪ Elderly patients (increased sensitivity).

ADVERSE REACTIONS AND SIDE EFFECTS*

CNS: headache, weakness, dizziness.
EENT: epistaxis, tinnitus.
GI: diarrhea, nausea, vomiting, GI full-

*Underlines indicate most frequent; **CAPITALS** indicate life-threatening.

T

ness, GI pain, anorexia, abnormal liver function tests.
GU: hematuria.
Derm: urticaria, rashes, ecchymoses, pruritus.
Hemat: neutropenia, INTRACEREBRAL BLEEDING, bleeding.
Metab: hypertriglyceridemia, hypercholesterolemia.

INTERACTIONS

Drug–Drug: ▪ **Aspirin** potentiates the effect of ticlopidine on platelets (concurrent use not recommended) ▪ **Cimetidine** decreases metabolism of ticlopidine and may increase the risk of toxicity ▪ Ticlopidine decreases metabolism of **theophylline** and may increase the risk of toxicity.
Drug–Food: ▪ Absorption of ticlopidine is increased by taking with **food**.

ROUTE AND DOSAGE

- **PO (Adults):** 250 mg bid with food.

PHARMACODYNAMICS (effect on platelet function)

	ONSET	PEAK	DURATION
PO	within 4 days	8–11 days	2 wk

NURSING IMPLICATIONS

Assessment

- □ Assess patient for symptoms of stroke periodically throughout therapy.
- ▪ **Lab Test Considerations:** Causes prolonged bleeding time which is time- and dose-dependent.
- □ Monitor CBC with differential every 2 wk from the second wk to the end of the third mon of therapy; more frequently if absolute neutrophil count (ANC) is declining or <30% of baseline. If neutropenia occurs, ticlopidine should be discontinued.
- □ May cause increased serum total cholesterol and triglyceride levels. Levels usually increase 8%–10% within the first mon and persist at that level.
- □ May cause elevated alkaline phosphatase, SGOT (AST), and SGPT (ALT) levels during the first 4 mon of therapy.
- ▪ **Toxicity and Overdose:** Prolonged bleeding time is normalized within 2 hr after administration of IV methylprednisolone. May also use platelet transfusions to reverse effects of ticlopidine on bleeding time.

Potential Nursing Diagnoses

- ▪ Injury, high risk for (indications, side effects).
- ▪ Knowledge deficit related to medication regimen (patient/family teaching).

Implementation

- ▪ **PO:** Administer with food or immediately after eating to minimize GI discomfort.

Patient/Family Teaching

- □ Instruct patient to take medication exactly as directed.
- □ Advise patient to notify physician promptly if fever, chills, sore throat, unusual bleeding or bruising, severe or persistent diarrhea, skin rash, jaundice, dark-colored urine, or light-colored stools occur.
- □ Advise patient to notify physician or dentist of medication regimen prior to treatment or surgery. Medication may need to be discontinued 10–14 days prior to surgery.

Evaluation

Effectiveness of therapy can be demonstrated by: ▪ Prevention of stroke.

TIMOLOL

(tim-oh-lole)
{Apo-Timol}, Blocadren, Timoptic

CLASSIFICATION(S):
Beta-adrenergic blocker—nonselective, Antihypertensive—beta-adrenergic blocker, Ophthalmic—antiglaucoma
Pregnancy Category C

INDICATIONS

■ **PO:** Used alone or in combination with other agents in the treatment of hypertension ■ **PO:** Prevention of myocardial infarction ■ **Ophth:** Treatment of glaucoma and other forms of elevated intraocular pressure ■ **PO:** Migraine headache prophylaxis. **Unlabeled Uses:** ■ Management of: □ Chronic stable angina pectoris □ Tachyarrhythmias □ Hypertrophic cardiomyopathy □ Pheochromocytoma □ Thyrotoxicosis □ Anxiety □ Tremor □ Mitral valve prolapse.

ACTION

■ Blocks stimulation of $beta_1$ (myocardial) and $beta_2$ (pulmonary, vascular, or uterine) receptor sites. **Therapeutic Effects:** ■ Decreased blood pressure ■ Prevention of myocardial infarction ■ Decreased intraocular pressure ■ Prevention of migraine headaches.

PHARMACOKINETICS

Absorption: Well absorbed following oral administration. Some absorption may occur following ophthalmic use.
Distribution: Distribution not known. Enters breast milk.
Metabolism and Excretion: Extensively metabolized by the liver.
Half-life: 3–4 hr.

CONTRAINDICATIONS AND PRECAUTIONS

Contraindicated in: ■ Uncompensated congestive heart failure ■ Pulmonary edema ■ Cardiogenic shock ■ Bradycardia or heart block ■ Children (safety not established).
Use Cautiously in: ■ Thyrotoxicosis or hypoglycemia (may mask symptoms) ■ Hepatic impairment (dosage reduction may be required) ■ Pregnancy or lactation (may cause apnea, low Apgar scores, bradycardia, and hypoglycemia in the newborn) ■ Ophthalmic use (systemic reactions may occur).

ADVERSE REACTIONS AND SIDE EFFECTS*

CNS: fatigue, weakness, depression, memory loss, mental changes, insomnia, dizziness.
CV: BRADYCARDIA, CONGESTIVE HEART FAILURE, PULMONARY EDEMA, hypotension, edema, peripheral vasoconstriction.
EENT: dry eyes, blurred vision, nasal stuffiness.
Resp: bronchospasm, wheezing.
GI: constipation, diarrhea, nausea, vomiting.
GU: impotence, diminished libido.
Derm: rash.
Endo: hyperglycemia, hypoglycemia.

INTERACTIONS

Drug-Drug: ■ **General anesthesia, IV phenytoin,** and **verapamil** may cause additive myocardial depression ■ Additive bradycardia may occur with concurrent use of **cardiac glycosides** ■ Additive hypotension may occur with other **antihypertensive agents,** acute ingestion of **alcohol,** or **nitrates** ■ Concurrent use with **amphetamines, cocaine, ephedrine, epinephrine, norepinephrine, phenylephrine,** or **pseudoephedrine** may result in excess alpha-adrenergic stimulation, hypertension, and bradycardia ■ May negate the beneficial $beta_1$ cardiac effects of **dopamine** or **dobutamine** ■ Use with **insulin** may result in prolonged hypoglycemia ■ May produce hypertension within 14 days of **MAO inhibitor** therapy ■ **Nonsteroidal anti-inflammatory agents** may decrease antihypertensive effectiveness ■ **Cimetidine** may decrease metabolism and increase effects of timolol ■ May antagonize **beta-adrenergic bronchodilators**.

ROUTE AND DOSAGE

Hypertension

- **PO (Adults):** 10 mg twice daily (range 20–60 mg/day, usual dose 20–40 mg/day).

*Underlines indicate most frequent; **CAPITALS** indicate life-threatening.

T

Prevention of Myocardial Infarction

- **PO (Adults):** 10 mg bid started within 1–4 wk after infarction.

Migraine Prophylaxis

- **PO (Adults):** 10 mg twice daily initially, may be given as 20 mg once daily during maintenance (range 10 mg once daily to 15 mg bid).

Glaucoma

- **Ophth (Adults and Children):** 1 drop of 0.25 or 0.5 soln bid.

PHARMACODYNAMICS (PO = antihypertensive effect; Ophth = effect on intraocular pressure)

	ONSET	PEAK	DURATION
PO	UK	1–2 hr*	12–24 hr
Ophth	15–30 min	1–5 hr	24 hr

*Maximal antihypertensive effects may take several wks.

NURSING IMPLICATIONS

Assessment

- **General Info:** Monitor blood pressure and pulse frequently during period of adjustment and periodically throughout therapy. Confer with physician prior to giving drug if pulse is <50 bpm. Assess for orthostatic hypotension when assisting patient up from supine position.
- Monitor intake and output ratios and daily weight. Assess patient routinely for evidence of congestive heart failure (peripheral edema, dyspnea, rales/crackles, fatigue, weight gain).
- **Ophth:** Intraocular pressure should be monitored periodically during initial therapy and after approximately 4 wk of ophthalmic therapy.
- **Lab Test Considerations:** May cause elevations in serum potassium, uric acid, triglyceride, lipoprotein, LDH, alkaline phosphatase levels, and BUN levels.
- Hepatic and renal function and CBC should be monitored routinely in patients receiving prolonged therapy.

Potential Nursing Diagnoses

- Cardiac output, decreased (indications, adverse reactions).
- Knowledge deficit related to medication regimen (patient/family teaching).
- Noncompliance (patient/family teaching).

Implementation

- **PO:** May be administered without regard to meals. May be crushed and mixed with food or fluid if patient has difficulty swallowing.
- **Ophth:** When instilling eyedrops, have patient tilt head back, pull down on the lower lid, and instill drops into the conjunctival sac. Apply pressure to the inner canthus for 1 min following instillation to prevent systemic absorption.

Patient/Family Teaching

- **General Info:** Instruct patient to take medication exactly as directed, even if feeling well. If a dose is missed it may be taken as soon as remembered up to 4 hr before next dose. Abrupt withdrawal may precipitate life-threatening arrhythmias, hypertension, or myocardial ischemia.
- Teach patient and family how to check pulse and blood pressure, with all dosage forms. Instruct them to take pulse daily and blood pressure at least weekly. Advise patient to withhold dose and contact physician if pulse is <50 bpm or blood pressure changes significantly.
- Reinforce need to continue additional therapies for hypertension (weight loss, restricted sodium intake, stress reduction, regular exercise, moderation of alcohol consumption, cessation of smoking).
- Caution patient that this medication may cause increased sensitivity to cold.
- Advise patient to consult physician or pharmacist before taking any over-the-counter drugs, especially cold remedies, concurrently with this medication. Patient should also avoid ex-

cessive amounts of coffee, tea, and cola.

- □ Diabetics should monitor serum glucose closely, especially if weakness, fatigue, or irritability occurs.
- □ Instruct patient to inform physician or dentist of this therapy prior to treatment or surgery.
- □ Advise patient to carry identification describing medication regimen at all times.
- □ Instruct patient to notify physician if irregular heartbeats, dizziness, depression, or skin rash occur.
- ■ **Ophth:** Instruct patient on correct technique for administration of ophthalmic soln. Emphasize the importance of not touching tip of container to eye, finger, or any other surface and of preventing systemic absorption by placing pressure on the inner canthus.

EVALUATION

Effectiveness of therapy can be demonstrated by: ■ Decrease in blood pressure ■ Prevention of myocardial reinfarction ■ Decreased intraocular pressure ■ Prevention of migraine headaches.

TIOCONAZOLE

(tie-oh-**kon**-a-zole)

Vagistat

CLASSIFICATION(S):
Antifungal—topical
Pregnancy Category C

INDICATIONS

■ Treatment of vaginal candidiasis.

ACTION

■ Inhibits the synthesis of fungal cell membrane, altering permeability. **Therapeutic Effect:** ■ Fungistatic action against susceptible organisms. **Spectrum:** ■ Active against *Candida albicans.*

PHARMACOKINETICS

Absorption: Minimal absorption follows vaginal application.
Distribution: Not known.
Metabolism and Excretion: Not known.
Half-life: UK.

CONTRAINDICATIONS AND PRECAUTIONS

Contraindicated in: ■ Hypersensitivity to tioconazole or components of formulation ■ Cross-sensitivity with other imidazoles may exist.
Use Cautiously in: ■ Lactation or children (safety not established).

ADVERSE REACTIONS AND SIDE EFFECTS*

GU: burning, itching.

INTERACTIONS

Drug–Drug: ■ None significant.

ROUTE AND DOSAGE

- ■ **Vaginal:** 1 applicatorful of 6.5% ointment at bedtime (4.6 g).

PHARMACODYNAMICS

	ONSET	PEAK	DURATION
Vaginal	hrs–days	days	UK

NURSING IMPLICATIONS

ASSESSMENT

- □ Inspect involved areas of skin and mucous membranes prior to and frequently throughout course of therapy. Increased skin irritation may indicate need to discontinue medication.

POTENTIAL NURSING DIAGNOSES

- ■ Skin integrity, impaired (indications).
- ■ Infection, high risk for (indications).
- ■ Knowledge deficit related to medication regimen (patient/family teaching).

IMPLEMENTATION

- □ Consult physician for proper cleansing technique prior to applying medication. Sitz baths and vaginal

*Underlines indicate most frequent; **CAPITALS** indicate life-threatening.

douches may be ordered concurrently with this therapy.
- Applicators are supplied for vaginal administration.

Patient/Family Teaching
- Instruct patient to apply medication as directed for full course of therapy, even if feeling better. Therapy should be continued during menstrual period.
- Instruct patient on proper use of vaginal applicator for vaginal cream. Tioconazole should be inserted high into the vagina at bedtime. Instruct patient to remain in recumbent position for at least 30 min after insertion. Advise use of sanitary napkins to prevent staining of clothing or bedding.
- Advise patient to consult physician regarding douching and intercourse during therapy. Vaginal medication may cause minor skin irritation in sexual partner. Advise patient to refrain from sexual contact during therapy or have partner wear a condom.
- Advise patient to report increased skin irritation or lack of response to therapy to physician.

Evaluation
Effectiveness of therapy can be demonstrated by: ▪ Decrease in skin irritation and vaginal discomfort. Therapeutic response is usually seen after 1 wk. Diagnosis should be reconfirmed with smears or cultures prior to a second course of therapy to rule out other pathogens associated with vulvovaginitis.

TOBRAMYCIN
(toe-bra-**mye**-sin)
Nebcin, Tobrex

CLASSIFICATION(S):
Anti-infective—aminoglycoside
Pregnancy Category D

INDICATIONS
▪ **IM, IV:** Treatment of serious gram-negative bacillary infections and infections due to staphylococci when penicillins or other less toxic drugs are contraindicated or resistance to gentamicin has occurred ▪ **IM, IV:** Treatment of the following infections due to susceptible organisms: ▫ Bone infections ▫ CNS infections (IT administration required) ▫ Respiratory tract infections ▫ Skin and soft tissue infections ▫ Abdominal infections ▫ Complicated urinary tract infections ▫ Endocarditis ▫ Septicemia ▪ **Ophth:** Treatment of superficial eye infections.

ACTION
▪ Inhibits protein synthesis in bacteria at the level of the 30S bacterial ribosome. **Therapeutic Effect:** ▪ Bactericidal action against susceptible bacteria. **Spectrum:** ▪ Notable for activity against important gram-negative pathogens, where resistance to gentamicin has occurred, including: ▫ *Pseudomonas aeruginosa* ▫ *Klebsiella pneumoniae* ▫ *Escherichia coli* ▫ *Proteus* ▫ *Serratia* ▫ *Acenitobacter* ▪ Treatment of enterococcal infections requires synergy with a penicillin.

PHARMACOKINETICS
Absorption: Well absorbed after IM administration. Minimal absorption following topical administration.
Distribution: Widely distributed in extracellular fluids following IM or IV administration. Crosses the placenta. Poor penetration into CSF.
Metabolism and Excretion: Excretion is mainly renal (>90%). Dosage adjustments are required for any decrease in renal function. Minimal amounts metabolized by the liver.
Half-life: 2–3 hr (increased in renal impairment).

CONTRAINDICATIONS AND PRECAUTIONS
Contraindicated in: ▪ Hypersensitivity ▪ Cross-sensitivity with other aminoglycosides may exist.
Use Cautiously in: ▪ Renal impairment of any kind (dosage adjustments required) ▪ Pregnancy (may cause con-

genital deafness) ▪ Lactation (safety not established) ▪ Neuromuscular diseases, such as myasthenia gravis.

ADVERSE REACTIONS AND SIDE EFFECTS*

EENT: ototoxicity (vestibular and cochlear), ocular stinging or burning (ophth).
GU: nephrotoxicity.
Neuro: enhanced neuromuscular blockade.
Misc: hypersensitivity reactions.

INTERACTIONS

Drug–Drug: ▪ Inactivated by **penicillins** when coadministered to patients with renal insufficiency ▪ Possible respiratory paralysis after **inhalation anesthetics (ether, cyclopropane, halothane,** or **nitrous oxide)** or **neuromuscular blockers (tubocurarine, succinylcholine, decamethonium)** ▪ Increased incidence of ototoxicity with **loop diuretics (bumetanide, furosemide)** ▪ Increased incidence of nephrotoxicity with other **nephrotoxic drugs (cisplatin).**

ROUTE AND DOSAGE

Note: All doses after initial loading dose should be determined by renal function/blood levels.

- **IM, IV (Adults):** 3–5 mg/kg/day in divided doses q 8 hr.
- **IM, IV (Children):** 3–5 mg/kg/day in divided doses q 8 hr.
- **IM, IV (Neonates <1 wk):** not to exceed 4 mg/kg/day in divided doses q 12 hr.
- **IT (Adults):** 3–8 mg q 18–48 hr.
- **Ophth (Adults and Children):** 1-cm ribbon of 0.3% ointment 2–3 times daily (q 3–4 hr for severe *Pseudomonas aeruginosa* infections) or 1–2 drops of 0.3% soln q 4 hr (q 30–60 min for severe *Pseudomonas aeruginosa* infections).

PHARMACODYNAMICS (blood levels)

	ONSET	PEAK
IM	rapid	30–90 min
IV	rapid	end of infusion
Ophth oint	rapid	UK
Ophth soln	rapid	UK

NURSING IMPLICATIONS

Assessment

- ▫ Assess patient for infection (vital signs; appearance of wound, sputum, urine, and stool; WBC) at beginning and throughout course of therapy.
- ▫ Obtain specimens for culture and sensitivity prior to initiating therapy. First dose may be given before receiving results.
- ▫ Evaluate eighth cranial nerve function by audiometry prior to and throughout course of therapy. Hearing loss is usually in the high-frequency range. Prompt recognition and intervention is essential in preventing permanent damage. Also monitor for vestibular dysfunction (vertigo, ataxia, nausea, vomiting). Eighth cranial dysfunction is usually associated with persistently elevated peak tobramycin levels.
- ▫ Monitor intake and output and daily weight to assess hydration status and renal function.
- ▫ Assess patient for signs of superinfection (fever, upper respiratory infection, vaginal itching or discharge, increasing malaise, diarrhea). Report to physician.
- ▪ **Lab Test Considerations:** Monitor renal function by urinalysis, specific gravity, BUN, creatinine, and creatinine clearance prior to and throughout therapy.
- ▫ May cause increased SGOT (AST), SGPT (ALT), LDH, bilirubin, and serum alkaline phosphatase levels.
- ▫ May cause decreased serum calcium, magnesium, sodium, and potassium levels.
- ▪ **Toxicity and Overdose:** Blood levels

*Underlines indicate most frequent; **CAPITALS** indicate life-threatening.

should be monitored periodically during therapy. Timing of blood levels is important in interpreting results. Draw blood for peak levels 30–60 min after IM injection and immediately after IV infusion is completed. Trough levels should be drawn just prior to next dose. Acceptable peak level is 4–10 mcg/ml; trough level should not be >2 mcg/ml.

Potential Nursing Diagnoses

- Infection, high risk for (indications).
- Sensory-perceptual alteration: auditory (side effects).

Implementation

- **General Info:** Keep patient well-hydrated (1500–2000 ml/day) during therapy.
- **IM:** Administer deep into a well-developed muscle. SC administration is not recommended and may be painful.
- **Intermittent Infusion:** Dilute each dose of tobramycin in 50–200 ml of D5W, D10W, D5/0.9% NaCl, 0.9% NaCl, Ringer's or lactated Ringer's soln to provide a concentration not >1 mg/ml (0.1%). Pediatric doses may be diluted in proportionately smaller amounts. Stable for 24 hr at room temperature, 96 hr if refrigerated. Also available in commercially mixed piggyback injections.
  - *Rate:* Infuse slowly, over 30–60 min in both adult and pediatric patients. Flush IV line with D5W or 0.9% NaCl following administration.
- **Syringe Incompatibility:** cefamandole, clindamycin, or heparin.
- **Y-Site Compatibility:** acyclovir, ciprofloxacin, cyclophosphamide, enalaprilat, esmolol, foscarnet, furosemide, hydromorphone, labetalol, magnesium sulfate, meperidine, morphine, perphenazine, tolazoline, or zidovudine.
- **Additive Compatibility:** aztreonam, bleomycin, calcium gluconate, cefoxitin, ciprofloxacin, clindamycin, furosemide, metronidazole, ranitidine, or verapamil.
- **Additive Incompatibility:** Administer separately; do not admix. Give aminoglycosides and penicillins at least 1 hr apart to prevent inactivation.
- **Ophth:** Do not touch tip of container to eye, fingers, or any other surface.
  - Ophthalmic soln can be instilled by having patient tilt head back and look up, gently depress lower lid with index finger until conjunctival sac is exposed, and instill medication.
  - Hold ophthalmic ointment tube in hand for several mins to warm. Squeeze ¼ in of ointment onto lower lid. Have patient close eye gently and roll eyeball around in all directions. Wait 10 min before instilling other ophthalmic ointments.

Patient/Family Teaching

- **General Info:** Instruct patient to report signs of hypersensitivity, tinnitus, vertigo, or hearing loss.
- **Ophth:** Patients with ophthalmic infections should be advised to avoid wearing contact lenses until infection is resolved and physician approves.

Evaluation

Clinical response can be evaluated by:

- Resolution of the signs and symptoms of infection. Length of time for complete resolution depends on organism and site of infection.

TOCAINIDE

(toe-**kay**-nide)
Tonocard

CLASSIFICATION(S):
Antiarrhythmic—class IB
Pregnancy Category C

INDICATIONS

- Treatment of ventricular arrhythmias including multifocal and unifocal premature ventricular contractions and ventricular tachycardia.

ACTION

- Suppresses automaticity of conduction tissue and spontaneous depolarization of the ventricles during diastole

■ Has little or no effect on heart rate. **Therapeutic Effect:** ■ Suppression of arrhythmias.

PHARMACOKINETICS

Absorption: Well absorbed following oral administration.
Distribution: Widely distributed. Crosses the blood-brain barrier.
Metabolism and Excretion: Partially metabolized by the liver. 30–50% excreted unchanged by the kidneys.
Half-life: 11–23 hr.

CONTRAINDICATIONS AND PRECAUTIONS

Contraindicated in: ■ Hypersensitivity ■ Advanced heart block.
Use Cautiously in: ■ Congestive heart failure ■ Hepatic or renal impairment (dosage reduction recommended) ■ Pregnancy, lactation, or children (safety not established).

ADVERSE REACTIONS AND SIDE EFFECTS*

CNS: lightheadedness, vertigo, tremor, headache, hallucinations, changes in mood, restlessness, sedation, SEIZURES, coma, depression, paranoia, dizziness.
EENT: blurred vision, tinnitus, thirst.
Resp: pneumonia, pulmonary fibrosis.
CV: hypotension, tachycardia, bradycardia, palpitations, congestive heart failure, arrhythmias, angina, conduction disturbances, hypertension, SINUS ARREST.
GI: nausea, vomiting, anorexia, diarrhea, constipation, dyspepsia, dysphagia, abdominal discomfort, hepatitis.
GU: urinary retention.
Derm: rashes, sweating, flushing, alopecia.
Hemat: blood dyscrasias.
MS: arthralgia, myalgia.
Neuro: myasthenia gravis, numbness.

INTERACTIONS

Drug-Drug: ■ Additive cardiac effects with other **antiarrhythmics** ■ Concurrent use with **beta-adrenergic blocking agents** may precipitate congestive heart failure.

ROUTE AND DOSAGE

- **PO (Adults):** 400 mg q 8 hr initially; usual maintenance dose 1.2–1.8 g/day in divided doses q 8 hr (up to 2.4 g/day may be used). Dosing twice daily may be used in some patients.

PHARMACODYNAMICS (antiarrhythmic effects)

	ONSET	PEAK	DURATION
PO	30–60 min	0.5–2 hr	8–12 hr

NURSING IMPLICATIONS

Assessment

- □ ECG, pulse, and blood pressure should be monitored prior to and periodically throughout therapy.
- □ Assess lungs periodically throughout therapy. Notify physician if cough or shortness of breath occur. Chest x-rays should also be evaluated if signs of pulmonary complications occur.
- ■ **Lab Test Considerations:** CBC should be monitored periodically throughout course of therapy. Leukopenia, agranulocytosis, and thrombocytopenia usually occur after 2–12 wk of therapy and return to normal 1 mon after discontinuation.

Potential Nursing Diagnoses

- ■ Cardiac output, decreased (indications).
- ■ Knowledge deficit related to medication regimen (patient/family teaching).

Implementation

- ■ **PO:** Administer with food or milk to minimize GI irritation.

Patient/Family Teaching

- □ Instruct patient to take medication around the clock, exactly as directed, even if feeling better. If a dose is missed, take as soon as remembered if within 4 hr; do not take if remembered later. Do not double doses.

*Underlines indicate most frequent; **CAPITALS** indicate life-threatening.

T

Consult with physician prior to discontinuing medication, as gradual reduction in dosage may be needed to prevent worsening of condition.

- Instruct patient or family member on how to take pulse. Advise patient to report changes in pulse rate or rhythm to physician.
- Tocainide may cause dizziness or lightheadedness. Caution patient to avoid driving or other activities requiring alertness until response to medication is known.
- Advise patient to inform physician or dentist of medication regimen prior to treatment or surgery.
- Advise patient to carry identification describing disease process and medication regimen at all times.
- Instruct patient to notify physician if trembling, shaking, fever, chills, sore throat, unusual bleeding or bruising, dyspnea, cough, wheezing, or palpitations occur. Physician should also be notified if nausea, vomiting, or diarrhea become severe.
- Emphasize the importance of routine follow-up examinations to monitor progress.

Evaluation

Effectiveness of therapy can be demonstrated by: ▪ Resolution of ventricular arrhythmias without detrimental side effects.

TOLAZAMIDE

(tole-**az**-a-mide)

Ronase, Tolamide, Tolinase

CLASSIFICATION(S):

Oral hypoglycemic agent—sulfonylurea

Pregnancy Category C

INDICATIONS

▪ Used to control blood sugar in adult-onset, noninsulin-dependent (NIDDM, type II, adult-onset, nonketosis-prone) diabetes when dietary therapy alone fails ▪ Requires some pancreatic function.

ACTION

▪ Lowers blood sugar by stimulating the release of insulin from the pancreas and increasing sensitivity to insulin at receptor sites ▪ May also decrease hepatic glucose production. **Therapeutic Effect:** ▪ Lowering of blood sugar in diabetic patients.

PHARMACOKINETICS

Absorption: Slowly but completely absorbed following oral administration.

Distribution: Distribution not known.

Metabolism and Excretion: Metabolized by the liver. Some conversion by the liver to compounds that have hypoglycemic activity.

Half-life: 7 hr.

CONTRAINDICATIONS AND PRECAUTIONS

Contraindicated in: ▪ Hypersensitivity ▪ Cross-sensitivity with sulfonamides may exist ▪ Insulin-dependent (type I, juvenile-onset, ketosis-prone, brittle) diabetics ▪ Severe renal, hepatic, thyroid, or other endocrine disease.

Use Cautiously in: ▪ Severe cardiovascular disease ▪ Elderly patients (dosage reduction may be necessary) ▪ Infection, stress, or changes in diet may alter requirements for control of blood sugar.

ADVERSE REACTIONS AND SIDE EFFECTS*

CNS: headache, weakness, dizziness.

GI: nausea, vomiting, diarrhea, hepatitis, cramps.

Derm: photosensitivity, rashes.

Endo: hypoglycemia.

F and E: hyponatremia.

Hemat: APLASTIC ANEMIA, leukopenia, pancytopenia, thrombocytopenia.

INTERACTIONS

Drug–Drug: ▪ Ingestion of **alcohol** may result in disulfiram-like reaction ▪ **Alcohol, glucocorticoids, rifampin, diclofenac,** and **thiazides** may decrease ef-

*Underlines indicate most frequent; **CAPITALS** indicate life-threatening.

fectiveness ▪ **Androgens (testosterone), chloramphenicol, clofibrate, MAO inhibitors, nonsteroidal anti-inflammatory agents (except for diclofenac), salicylates, sulfonamides,** and **oral anticoagulants** may increase the risk of hypoglycemia ▪ **Beta-adrenergic blockers** may alter the response to oral hypoglycemic agents (increase or decrease requirements).

ROUTE AND DOSAGE

- **PO (Adults):** 100–250 mg/day initially with breakfast, may increase by 50–250 mg/day at weekly intervals (dose range 100–1000 mg/day).

PHARMACODYNAMICS (hypoglycemic effects)

	ONSET	PEAK	DURATION
PO	1 hr	1–6 hr	12–24 hr

NURSING IMPLICATIONS

Assessment

- Observe patient for signs and symptoms of hypoglycemic reactions (sweating, hunger, weakness, dizziness, tremor, tachycardia, anxiety). Monitor patients who experience a hypoglycemic episode closely for 1–2 days.
- Assess patient for allergy to sulfonamides.
- **Lab Test Considerations:** Serum glucose and glycosylated hemoglobin should be monitored periodically throughout therapy to evaluate effectiveness of treatment.
- CBC should be monitored periodically throughout therapy. Notify physician promptly if decrease in blood count occurs.
- Monitor liver function tests periodically. May cause increase in SGOT (AST), SGPT (ALT), bilirubin, and cholesterol. Transient increases in alkaline phosphatase at beginning of therapy are not usually clinically significant.
- **Toxicity and Overdose:** Overdose is manifested by symptoms of hypoglycemia. Mild hypoglycemia may be treated with administration of oral glucose. Severe hypoglycemia should be treated with intravenous D50W followed by continuous intravenous infusion of more dilute dextrose soln at a rate sufficient to keep serum glucose at approximately 100 mg/dl.

Potential Nursing Diagnoses

- Nutrition, altered: more than body requirements (indications).
- Knowledge deficit related to medication regimen (patient/family teaching).
- Noncompliance (patient/family teaching).

Implementation

- **General Info:** May be administered once in the morning or divided into 2 doses.
- Patients stabilized on a diabetic regimen who are exposed to stress, fever, trauma, infection, or surgery may require administration of insulin.
- To convert from insulin dosage of less than 40 units/day, change may be made without gradual dosage adjustments. Patients taking more than 40 units/day should convert gradually—administer tolazamide and 50% of previous insulin dose for first few days, with gradual adjustment of tolazamide as needed. Monitor serum or urine glucose and ketones at least 3 times/day during conversion.
- **PO:** Administer 30 min before meals to ensure best diabetic control.
- Tablets may be crushed and taken with fluids if patient has difficulty swallowing.

Patient/Family Teaching

- Instruct patient to take medication at same time each day. If a dose is missed, take as soon as remembered unless almost time for next dose. Do not take if unable to eat.
- Explain to patient that this medication controls hyperglycemia but does not cure diabetes. Therapy is long-term.
- Review signs of hypoglycemia and hyperglycemia with patient. If hypogly-

cemia occurs, advise patient to take a glass of orange juice or sugar, honey, or corn syrup dissolved in water and notify physician.

- Encourage patient to follow prescribed diet, medication, and exercise regimen to prevent hypoglycemic or hyperglycemia episodes.
- Instruct patient in proper testing of serum glucose or urine glucose and ketones. Stress the importance of double-voided specimens for accuracy. These tests should be closely monitored during periods of stress or illness and physician notified if significant changes occur. During conversion from insulin to oral antidiabetic agents, patient should test urine at least 3 times/day and report results to physician as directed.
- May cause dizziness. Caution patient to avoid driving or other activities requiring alertness until response to medication is known.
- Caution patient to avoid other medications, especially those containing aspirin, and alcohol while on this therapy without consulting physician or pharmacist. Concurrent use of alcohol and tolazamide may cause a disulfiram-like reaction (abdominal cramps, nausea, vomiting, flushing, headache, hypoglycemia).
- This medication should not be used during pregnancy. Counsel patient to use a form of contraception other than oral contraceptives and to notify physician promptly if pregnancy is suspected.
- Caution patient to use sunscreen and protective clothing to prevent photosensitivity reactions.
- Advise patient to carry a form of sugar (sugar packets, candy) and identification describing disease and medication regimen at all times.
- Emphasize the importance of routine follow-up with physician.

Evaluation

Effectiveness of therapy can be demonstrated by: ▪ Control of blood glucose levels without the appearance of hypoglycemic or hyperglycemic episodes.

T

TOLAZOLINE
(tole-**az**-oh-leen)
Priscoline

CLASSIFICATION(S):
Antihypertensive—miscellaneous
Pregnancy Category UK

INDICATIONS

▪ Treatment of pulmonary hypertension in newborns when oxygenation cannot be provided by other methods (oxygen therapy, mechanical ventilation).

ACTION

▪ Direct-acting vasodilator ▪ Also causes vasodilation by alpha-adrenergic blockade. **Therapeutic Effects:** ▪ Decreased pulmonary arterial pressure ▪ Decreased vascular resistance.

PHARMACOKINETICS

Absorption: Administered IV only, resulting in complete bioavailability.
Distribution: Distribution not known.
Metabolism and Excretion: Excreted mostly unchanged by the kidneys.
Half-life: 3–10 hr (neonates).

CONTRAINDICATIONS AND PRECAUTIONS

Contraindicated in: ▪ Hypotension.
Use Cautiously in: ▪ Acidosis ▪ Mitral stenosis (paradoxical response may occur) ▪ Gastritis or history of GI bleeding.

ADVERSE REACTIONS AND SIDE EFFECTS*

EENT: mydriasis.
CV: <u>hypotension</u>, tachycardia, SHOCK.
GI: <u>GI BLEEDING</u>, diarrhea, nausea, vomiting.
GU: <u>acute oliguric renal failure</u>.
Derm: flushing, piloerection.

*<u>Underlines</u> indicate most frequent; **CAPITALS** indicate life-threatening.

F and E: hypochloremic alkalosis.
Hemat: thrombocytopenia.

INTERACTIONS

Drug–Drug: ▪ Concurrent use with **epinephrine** or **norepinephrine** may result in initial hypotension, followed by rebound hypertension ▪ May antagonize the vasopressor effects of **dopamine, ephedrine, metaraminol, methoxamine,** or **phenylephrine**.

ROUTE AND DOSAGE

- **IV (Newborns):** 1–2 mg/kg over 5–10 min through scalp vein or directly into pulmonary artery initially, then 1–2 mg/kg/hr IV infusion, may increase in 1–2 mg/kg/hr increments up to 6–8 mg/kg/hr. Inital bolus dose may be repeated if needed.

PHARMACODYNAMICS (vascular response)

	ONSET	PEAK	DURATION
IV	30 min	UK	UK

NURSING IMPLICATIONS

Assessment

- □ Monitor arterial blood pressure, ECG, and heart rate routinely throughout administration. Tolazoline should be discontinued if systolic blood pressure cannot be maintained at >40–50 mmHg.
- □ Monitor pulmonary artery pressure (PAP) and pulmonary capillary wedge pressure (PCWP) frequently throughout administration.
- □ Monitor intake and output and daily weight throughout therapy.
- □ Assess patient for bleeding, bruising, petechiae, or blood in stools, urine, or emesis throughout therapy.
- ▪ **Lab Test Considerations:** Monitor arterial blood gases (ABGs), CBC, and serum electrolytes, especially potassium and chloride, routinely throughout therapy. If hypochloremic metabolic acidosis occurs, wean patient from tolazoline and administer potassium and chloride.
- □ Hematest gastric aspirate periodically to determine GI bleeding.
- ▪ **Toxicity and Overdose:** If profound hypotension occurs, keep patient's head low and administer IV fluids. Do not administer epinephrine or norepinephrine, as further hypotension followed by rebound hypertension may occur. Dopamine may be infused simultaneously with tolazoline if IV fluids fail to maintain blood pressure.

Potential Nursing Diagnoses

- ▪ Tissue perfusion, altered (indications).
- ▪ Gas exchange, impaired (indications).
- ▪ Knowledge deficit related to medication regimen (patient/family teaching).

Implementation

- ▪ **General Info:** Administer only in a neonatal intensive care area equipped to provide trained personnel and respiratory support.
- □ Antacids may be ordered prior to therapy to minimize GI bleeding.
- ▪ **Direct IV:** Administer initial dose undiluted over 10 min via scalp vein or directly into pulmonary artery. Follow with maintenance infusion. Initial bolus may be repeated during infusion if needed.
- ▪ **Continuous Infusion:** May be diluted in D5W, D10W, 0.45% NaCl, 0.9% NaCl, Ringer's or lactated Ringer's soln, dextrose/saline combinations, dextrose/Ringer's or lactated Ringer's combinations. Do not use diluents containing benzyl alcohol for neonates; fatal reaction may occur.
- □ Administer via infusion pump for accurate dosage.
- ▪ **Y-Site Compatibility:** aminophylline, ampicillin, calcium gluconate, cefotaxime, cimetidine, dobutamine, dopamine, furosemide, gentamicin, phytonadione, sodium bicarbonate, tobramycin, or vancomycin.
- ▪ **Y-Site Incompatibility:** indomethacin.

T

Patient/Family Teaching

□ Explain purpose of medication to parents. Provide emotional support.

Evaluation

Effectiveness of therapy can be determined by: ▪ Decrease in pulmonary artery pressure and vascular resistance. Response should be seen within 30 min of initial dose.

TOLBUTAMIDE

(tole-**byoo**-ta-mide)
{Apo-Tolbutamide}, {Mobenol}, {Novobutamide}, Oramide, Orinase, SK-Tolbutamide

CLASSIFICATION(S):
Oral hypoglycemic agent—sulfonylurea
Pregnancy Category C

INDICATIONS

▪ Used to control blood sugar in adult-onset, noninsulin-dependent (NIDDM, type II, adult-onset, nonketosis-prone) diabetes, when dietary therapy fails ▪ Requires some pancreatic function.

ACTION

▪ Lowers blood sugar by stimulating the release of insulin from the pancreas and increasing sensitivity to insulin at receptor sites ▪ May also decrease hepatic glucose production. **Therapeutic Effect:** ▪ Lowering of blood sugar in diabetic patients.

PHARMACOKINETICS

Absorption: Well absorbed following oral administration.
Distribution: Distribution not known.
Metabolism and Excretion: Mostly metabolized by the liver.
Half-life: 7 hr (range 4–25 hr).

CONTRAINDICATIONS AND PRECAUTIONS

Contraindicated in: ▪ Hypersensitivity ▪ Insulin-dependent (type I, juvenile-onset, ketosis-prone, brittle) diabetics ▪ Severe renal, hepatic, thyroid, or other endocrine disease ▪ Cross-sensitivity with sulfonamides may exist.

Use Cautiously in: ▪ Severe cardiovascular disease ▪ Elderly patients (dosage reduction may be required) ▪ Infection, stress, or changes in diet may alter requirements for control of blood sugar.

ADVERSE REACTIONS AND SIDE EFFECTS*

CNS: headache, weakness, dizziness.
Derm: photosensitivity, rashes.
Endo: hypoglycemia.
F and E: hyponatremia.
GI: nausea, vomiting, diarrhea, hepatitis, cramps.
Hemat: APLASTIC ANEMIA, leukopenia, pancytopenia, thrombocytopenia.

INTERACTIONS

Drug-Drug: ▪ Ingestion of **alcohol** may result in disulfiram-like reaction ▪ **Alcohol, glucocorticoids, rifampin, diclofenac,** and **thiazides** may decrease effectiveness ▪ **Androgens (testosterone), chloramphenicol, clofibrate, MAO inhibitors, nonsteroidal anti-inflammatory agents, salicylates, sulfonamides,** and **oral anticoaglulants** may increase the risk of hypoglycemia ▪ **Beta-adrenergic blockers** may alter the response to oral hypoglycemic agents (increase or decrease requirements).

ROUTE AND DOSAGE

▪ **PO (Adults):** 1–2 g/day in 2–3 divided doses (range 250–2000 mg/day).

PHARMACODYNAMICS (hypoglycemic effects)

	ONSET	PEAK	DURATION
PO	1 hr	4–6 hr	6–12 hr

NURSING IMPLICATIONS

Assessment

□ Observe patient for signs and symptoms of hypoglycemic reactions

{} = Available in Canada only.
*Underlines indicate most frequent; CAPITALS indicate life-threatening.

(sweating, hunger, weakness, dizziness, tremor, tachycardia, anxiety). Monitor patients who experience a hypoglycemic episode closely for 1–2 days.
- Assess patient for allergy to sulfonamides.
- **Lab Test Considerations:** Serum glucose and glycosylated hemoglobin should be monitored periodically throughout theapy to evaluate effectiveness of treatment.
- CBC should be monitored periodically throughout therapy. Notify physician promptly if decrease in blood count occurs.
- May interfere with radioactive iodine uptake tests and urinary albumin measurements.
- **Toxicity and Overdose:** Overdose is manifested by symptoms of hypoglycemia. Mild hypoglycemia may be treated with administration of oral glucose. Severe hypoglycemia should be treated with IV D50W followed by continuous IV infusion of more dilute dextrose soln at a rate sufficient to keep serum glucose at approximately 100 mg/dl.

Potential Nursing Diagnoses
- Nutrition, altered: more than body requirements (indications).
- Knowledge deficit related to medication regimen (patient/family teaching).
- Noncompliance (patient/family teaching).

Implementation
- **General Info:** May be administered once in the morning or divided into 2 doses.
- Patients stabilized on a diabetic regimen who are exposed to stress, fever, trauma, infection, or surgery may require administration of insulin.
- To convert from insulin dosage of 20 units/day, change may be made without gradual dosage adjustment. Patients taking 20–40 units/day should reduce insulin by 30–50% for the first day and adjust dose gradually. Patients taking greater than 40 units/day should reduce insulin by 20% the first day and then gradually as needed. Monitor serum or urine glucose and ketones at least 3 times/day during conversion.
- **PO:** Administer 30 min before meals to ensure best diabetic control.
- Tablets may be crushed and taken with fluids if patient has difficulty swallowing.

Patient/Family Teaching
- Instruct patient to take medication at same time each day. If a dose is missed, take as soon as remembered unless almost time for next dose. Do not take if unable to eat.
- Explain to patient that this medication controls hypoglycemia but does not cure diabetes. Therapy is long-term.
- Review signs of hypoglycemia and hyperglycemia with patient. If hypoglycemia occurs, advise patient to take a glass of orange juice or sugar, honey, or corn syrup dissolved in water and notify physician.
- Encourage patient to follow prescribed diet, medication, and exercise regimen to prevent hypoglycemic or hyperglycemia episodes.
- Instruct patient in proper testing of serum glucose or urine glucose and ketones. Stress the importance of double-voided specimens for accuracy. These tests should be closely monitored during periods of stress or illness and physician notified if significant changes occur. During conversion from insulin to oral antidiabetic agents, patient should test urine at least 3 times/day and report results to physician as directed.
- May cause dizziness. Caution patient to avoid driving or other activities requiring alertness until response to medication is known.
- Caution patient to avoid other medications, especially those containing aspirin, and alcohol while on this therapy without consulting physician or pharmacist. Concurrent use of alcohol and tolbutamide may cause a

T

disulfiram-like reaction (abdominal cramps, nausea, vomiting, flushing, headache, hypoglycemia).

- ▫ This medication should not be used during pregnancy. Counsel patient to use a form of contraception other than oral contraceptives and to notify physician promptly if pregnancy is suspected.
- ▫ Caution patient to use sunscreen and protective clothing to prevent photosensitivity reactions.
- ▫ Advise patient to carry a form of sugar (sugar packets, candy) and identification describing disease and medication regimen at all times.
- ▫ Emphasize the importance of routine follow-up with physician.

EVALUATION

Effectiveness of therapy can be demonstrated by: ▪ Control of blood glucose levels without the appearance of hypoglycemic or hyperglycemic episodes.

TOLMETIN
(tole-met-in)
Tolectin, Tolectin DS

CLASSIFICATION(S):
Nonsteroidal anti-inflammatory agent
Pregnancy Category C

INDICATIONS
▪ Management of inflammatory disorders including: ▫ Rheumatoid arthritis ▫ Juvenile rheumatoid arthritis ▫ Osteoarthritis.

ACTION
▪ Inhibits prostaglandin synthesis. **Therapeutic Effects:** ▪ Suppression of pain and inflammation.

PHARMACOKINETICS
Absorption: Well absorbed from the GI tract following oral administration.
Distribution: Distribution not known.
Metabolism and Excretion: Mostly metabolized by the liver. 20% excreted unchanged by the kidneys.
Half-life: 1 hr.

CONTRAINDICATIONS AND PRECAUTIONS
Contraindicated in: ▪ Hypersensitivity ▪ Cross-sensitivity may exist with other nonsteroidal anti-inflammatory agents, including aspirin ▪ Active GI bleeding or ulcer disease ▪ Pregnancy.
Use Cautiously in: ▪ Severe cardiovascular, renal, or hepatic disease ▪ History of ulcer disease ▪ Lactation (safety not established) ▪ Severe hepatic or renal impairment (dosage reduction recommended).

ADVERSE REACTIONS AND SIDE EFFECTS*
CNS: headache, drowsiness, dizziness, sleep disturbances, depression.
EENT: visual disturbances, tinnitus.
CV: edema, hypertension.
GI: nausea, dyspepsia, vomiting, diarrhea, constipation, **GI BLEEDING**, discomfort, flatulence, **HEPATITIS**.
GU: renal failure.
Derm: rashes.
Hemat: prolonged bleeding time.
MS: muscle weakness.
Misc: allergic reactions, including **ANAPHYLAXIS**.

INTERACTIONS
Drug-Drug: ▪ Increased risk of bleeding with **anticoagulants, cefamandole, cefoperazone, cefotetan, moxalactam, thrombolytic agents,** or **plicamycin** ▪ Additive adverse GI side effects with **aspirin, glucocorticoids,** and other **nonsteroidal anti-inflammatory agents** ▪ May decrease response to **antihypertensives** or **diuretics** ▪ May increase serum levels and risk of toxicity from **lithium** ▪ May increase the risk of hema-

*Underlines indicate most frequent; **CAPITALS** indicate life-threatening.

tologic toxicity from **antineoplastic agents** or **radiation therapy** ▪ Increased risk of adverse renal effects with **gold compounds** or chronic use of **acetaminophen** ▪ May increase the risk of hypoglycemia from **insulin** or **oral hypoglycemic agents**.

ROUTE AND DOSAGE

- **PO (Adults):** 400 mg 3 times daily (range 600–1800 mg/day in 3–4 divided doses, not to exceed 2000 mg/day).
- **PO (Children >2 yr):** 15–30 mg/kg/day in 3–4 divided doses (not to exceed 30 mg/kg/day).

PHARMACODYNAMICS (anti-inflammatory effects)

	ONSET	PEAK	DURATION
PO	within 7 days	1–2 wk	UK

NURSING IMPLICATIONS

Assessment

- □ Patients who have asthma, aspirin-induced allergy, and nasal polyps are at increased risk for developing hypersensitivity reactions. Monitor for rhinitis, asthma, and urticaria.
- □ Assess pain and range of motion prior to and 1 hr following administration.
- ▪ **Lab Test Considerations:** BUN, serum creatinine, CBC, and liver function tests should be evaluated periodically in patients receiving prolonged courses of therapy.
- □ Serum potassium, BUN, SGOT (AST), and SGPT (ALT) may show increased levels.
- □ Hemoglobin and hematocrit may be decreased. Bleeding time may be prolonged for up to 2 days after discontinuation.
- □ May cause false-positive results for urinary protein.

Potential Nursing Diagnoses

- ▪ Comfort, altered: pain (indications).
- ▪ Mobility, impaired physical (indications).
- ▪ Knowledge deficit related to medication regimen (patient/family teaching).

Implementation

- ▪ **General Info:** Available in a double-strength (DS) 400-mg capsule.
- ▪ **PO:** For rapid initial effect, administer 30 min before or 2 hr after meals. May be administered with food, milk, or antacids to decrease GI irritation. Food slows but does not reduce the extent of absorption. Tablets may be crushed and capsules opened and mixed with fluids or food.

Patient/Family Teaching

- □ Advise patient to take this medication with a full glass of water and to remain in an upright position for 15–30 min after administration.
- □ Instruct patient to take medication exactly as prescribed. If a dose is missed, it should be taken as soon as remembered but not if almost time for the next dose. Do not double doses.
- □ This medication may cause drowsiness or dizziness. Advise patient to avoid driving or other activities requiring alertness until response to medication is known.
- □ Caution patient to avoid the concurrent use of alcohol, aspirin, acetaminophen, or other over-the-counter medications without consulting physician.
- □ Instruct patient to notify physician if rash, itching, muscle aches, visual disturbances, weight gain, edema, black stools, or persistent headache occurs.
- □ Advise patient to inform physician or dentist of medication regimen prior to treatment or surgery.

Evaluation

Effectiveness of therapy can be demonstrated by: ▪ Decrease in pain □ Improved joint mobility. Partial arthritic relief is usually seen within 7 days, but maximum effectiveness may require 1–2 wk of continuous therapy. Patients who do not respond to one nonsteroidal anti-inflammatory agent may respond to another.

T

TOPICAL GLUCOCORTICOIDS
(gloo-koe-**kore**-ti-koyds)

alclometasone
Aclovate

amcinonide
Cyclocort

augmented betamethasone dipropionate
Diprolene

betamethasone benzoate
Uticort

betamethasone dipropionate
Alphatrex, Diprosone, Maxivate, Psorion

betamethasone valerate
Betatrex, Beta-Val, Dermabet, Valisone

clobetasol
Temovate

clocortolone
Cloderm

desonide
DesOwen, Tridesilon

desoximetasone
Topicort

dexamethasone
Aeroseb-Dex, Decaderm, Decaspray

diflorasone
Florone, Maxiflor, Psorcon

fluocinolone
Fluonid, Flurosyn, Synalar, Synemol

fluocinonide
Lidex, Vasoderm

flurandrenolide
Cordran

fluticasone
Cutivate

halcinonide
Halog

halobetasol
Ultravate

hydrocortisone
Aeroseb-HC, Ala-Cort, Anusol-HC, CaldeCort Anti-Itch, Cetacort, Cortaid, Cort-Dome, Cortizone, Cortril, Delcort, Dermocort, DermiCort, Gynecort, Hycort, HydroTex, Hytone, LactiCare-HC, Lanacort, Locoid, Nutracort, Penecort, S-T Cort, Synacort, Tega-Cort, Westcort

mometasone
Elocon

triamcinolone acetonide
Aristocort, Flutex, Kenalog, Triderm

CLASSIFICATION(S):
Glucocorticoids
Pregnancy Category C

INDICATIONS

▪ Used in the management of a wide variety of allergic/immunologic reactions.

ACTION

▪ Supresses normal immune response and inflammation. If systemically absorbed for prolonged periods of time may produce adrenal suppression. **Therapeutic Effects:** ▪ Suppression of dermatologic inflammation and immune processes.

PHARMACOKINETICS

Absorption: Minimal if used as directed. Prolonged use on large surface areas or large amounts applied will produce systemic absorption and adrenal suppression.
Distribution: Remains primarily at site of action, unless applied to large areas or in large amounts.
Metabolism and Excretion: Not known following topical administration.
Half-life: UK.

CONTRAINDICATIONS AND PRECAUTIONS

Contraindicated in: ▪ Hypersensitivity to glucocorticoid or components of vehicles (ointment or cream base, preservatives) ▪ Untreated bacterial or viral infections.

Use Cautiously in: ▪ Avoid chronic high-dose usage during pregnancy, lactation, or in children (may result in adrenal suppression in mother, growth suppression in children) ▪ Children may be more susceptible to adrenal and growth suppression ▪ Patients with hepatic dysfunction ▪ Clobetasol not recommended for use in children <12 yr ▪ Desoximetasone not recommended in children <10 yr.

ADVERSE REACTIONS AND SIDE EFFECTS*

Local: burning, irritation, edema, hypopigmentation, maceration, hypertrichosis, perioral dermatitis, allergic contact dermatitis, secondary infection, dryness, folliculitis, atrophy, miliaria, striae, hypersensitivity reactions.
Misc: adrenal suppression.

INTERACTIONS

Drug–Drug: ▪ None significant.

ROUTE AND DOSAGE

- **Top (Adults and Children):** Apply 1–6 times daily (depends on product, preparation, and condition being treated). Available in many strengths as lotions, creams, gels, and aerosols.

PHARMACODYNAMICS (response depends on condition being treated)

	ONSET	PEAK	DURATION
Top	min–hrs	hrs–days	hrs–days

NURSING IMPLICATIONS

Assessment

- Assess affected skin prior to and daily during therapy. Note degree of inflammation and pruritus. Notify physician if symptoms of infection (increased pain, erythema, purulent exudate) develop.
- **Lab Test Considerations:** Periodic adrenal function tests may be ordered to assess degree of hypothalamic-pituitary-adrenal (HPA) axis suppression in chronic topical therapy. Children and patients with dose applied to a large area or using an occlusive dressing are at highest risk for HPA suppression.

Potential Nursing Diagnoses

- Skin integrity, impairment of: actual (indications).
- Infection, high risk for (side effects).
- Knowledge deficit related to medication regimen (patient/family teaching).

Implementation

- Apply as a thin film to clean, slightly moist skin. Wear gloves. Apply occlusive dressing only if specified by physician.

Patient/Family Teaching

- Instruct patient on correct technique of medication administration. Emphasize importance of avoiding the eyes. If a dose is missed it should be applied as soon as remembered unless almost time for the next dose. Do not double doses.
- Instruct patient to inform physician if symptoms of underlying disease return or worsen, or symptoms of infection develop.

Evaluation

Effectiveness of therapy can be demonstrated by: ▪ Resolution of skin inflammation, pruritus, or other dermatologic conditions.

TRACE METAL ADDITIVE

Concentrated Multiple Trace Element, Conte-Pak-4, MTE-4, MTE-4 Concentrated, MTE-5, MTE-5 Concentrated, MTE-6, MTE-7, Multe-Pak-4, Multe-Pak-5, Multiple Trace Element, Neotrace 4, Pedte-Pak-4, Pedtrace-4, PTE-4, PTE-5, Pediatric Multiple Trace Element, TEC

CLASSIFICATION(S):
Nutritional supplement
Pregnancy Category C

*Underlines indicate most frequent; **CAPITALS** indicate life-threatening.

INDICATIONS

■ Administered as a component in total parenteral nutrition (TPN, parenteral hyperalimentation) ■ May contain any or all of the following: □ Chromium □ Copper □ Iodine □ Manganese □ Molybdenum □ Selenium □ Zinc.

ACTION

■ Trace metals serve as cofactors or catalysts for numerous diverse homeostatic processes. **Therapeutic Effect:** ■ Replacement in deficiency states when oral ingestion is not feasible.

PHARMACOKINETICS

Absorption: Administered IV only, resulting in complete bioavailability.
Distribution: Widely distributed.
Metabolism and Excretion: Excretion depends on individual trace element.
Half-life: UK.

CONTRAINDICATIONS AND PRECAUTIONS

Contraindicated in: ■ Hypersensitivity to iodine (iodine-containing products only).
Use Cautiously in: ■ Pregnancy or lactation ■ Nasogastric suction, fistula drainage, prolonged vomiting or diarrhea (may increase requirements) ■ Renal impairment or biliary obstruction (may increase risk of toxicity) ■ Isolated trace element deficiency (other additives may be excessive—use only those required).

ADVERSE REACTIONS AND SIDE EFFECTS*

Note: Listed for individual trace metals—usually associated with toxicity.
Chromium: nausea, vomiting, GI ulceration, renal damage, hepatic damage, SEIZURES, COMA.
Copper: behavioral changes, weakness, diarrhea, photophobia, peripheral edema, progressive marasmus.
Iodine: metallic taste, sore mouth, increased salivation, runny nose, sneezing, headache, swelling of eyelids, headache, parotitis, acneform skin lesions.
Manganese: irritability, speech difficulties, gait disturbances, headache, anorexia, impotence, apathy.
Molybdenum: gout-like syndrome.
Selenium: hair loss, weak nails, mental depression, nervousness, vomiting, garlic-like breath, garlic-like sweat, metallic taste, GI discomfort.
Zinc: toxicitiy poorly defined but may include hypothermia, blurred vision, loss of consciousness, tachycardia, pulmonary edema, jaundice, oliguria, hypotension, vomiting.

INTERACTIONS

Drug–Drug: ■ None significant in replacement doses.

ROUTE AND DOSAGE

■ **IV (Adults and Children):** Amount necessary to maintain normal trace element levels.

PHARMACODYNAMICS (replacement)

	ONSET	PEAK	DURATION
IV	rapid	UK	UK

NURSING IMPLICATIONS

Assessment

□ Assess nutritional status by 24-hr recall prior to therapy.
□ Monitor patient for signs and symptoms of trace metal deficiencies prior to and throughout therapy, as follows:
□ *Chromium:* glucose intolerance, ataxia, peripheral neuropathy, confusion.
□ *Copper:* leukopenia, neutropenia, anemia, iron deficiency, skeletal abnormalities, defective tissue formation.
□ *Iodine:* impaired thyroid function, goiter, cretinism.
□ *Manganese:* nausea, vomiting, weight loss, dermatitis, changes in hair.

*Underlines indicate most frequent; **CAPITALS** indicate life-threatening.

- *Molybdenum:* tachycardia, tachypnea, headache, night blindness, nausea, vomiting, edema, lethargy, disorientation, coma, hypouricemia, hypouricosuria.
- *Selenium:* cardiomyopathy, muscle pain, kwashiorkor, Kershan disease.
- *Zinc:* initially—diarrhea, apathy, depression, anorexia, hypogonadism, growth retardation, anemia, hepatosplenomegaly, impaired wound healing.

- **Lab Test Considerations:** Serum trace metal concentrations should be monitored periodically throughout TPN therapy.

Potential Nursing Diagnoses

- Nutrition, altered: less than body requirements (indications).
- Knowledge deficit related to medication regimen (patient/family teaching).

Implementation

- **IV:** Soln usually does not contain preservatives; discard unused portion.
- **Continuous Infusion:** Must be diluted prior to administration. Dilute each dose in at least 1 liter of IV soln.
  - Administer at prescribed rate for TPN infusion.
- **Additive Compatibility:** Usually compatible with other trace metals, electrolytes, and dextrose/amino acid combinations used for TPN.

Patient/Family Teaching

- Explain purpose of infusion of TPN and components to patient.

Evaluation

Effectiveness of therapy can be demonstrated by: ▪ Prevention or treatment of trace metal deficiencies.

TRAZADONE

(**traz**-oh-done)
Desyrel, Trazon, Trialodine

CLASSIFICATION(S):
Antidepressant—miscellaneous
Pregnancy Category C

INDICATIONS

▪ Treatment of major depression often in conjunction with psychotherapy. **Unlabeled Use:** ▪ Management of chronic pain syndromes, including diabetic neuropathy.

ACTION

▪ Alters the effects of serotonin in the CNS. **Therapeutic Effect:** ▪ Antidepressant action, which may develop only over several wks.

PHARMACOKINETICS

Absorption: Well absorbed following oral administration.
Distribution: Widely distributed.
Metabolism and Excretion: Extensively metabolized by the liver. Minimal excretion of unchanged drug by the kidneys.
Half-life: 5–9 hr.

CONTRAINDICATIONS AND PRECAUTIONS

Contraindicated in: ▪ Hypersensitivity ▪ Recovery period following myocardial infarction ▪ Concurrent electroconvulsive therapy.
Use Cautiously in: ▪ Cardiovascular disease ▪ Suicidal behavior ▪ Pregnancy, lactation, or children (safety not established) ▪ Severe hepatic or renal disease (dosage reduction recommended).

ADVERSE REACTIONS AND SIDE EFFECTS*

CNS: drowsiness, dizziness, lightheadedness, fatigue, weakness, insomnia, confusion, hallucinations, slurred speech, nightmares, syncope, headache.
EENT: blurred vision, tinnitus.
CV: hypotension, chest pain, tachycardia, arrhythmias, palpitations, hypertension.
GI: dry mouth, constipation, nausea, vomiting, bad taste, flatulence, diarrhea, excess salivation.
GU: urinary frequency, impotence, priapism, hematuria.

*Underlines indicate most frequent; **CAPITALS** indicate life-threatening.

T

Derm: rashes.
Hemat: anemia, leukopenia.
MS: myalgia.
Neuro: tremor.

INTERACTIONS

Drug–Drug: ▪ May increase **digoxin** or **phenytoin** serum levels ▪ Additive CNS depression with other **CNS depressants** including **alcohol, antihistamines, narcotic analgesics,** and **sedative/hypnotics** ▪ Additive hypotension with **antihypertensive agents,** acute ingestion of **alcohol,** or **nitrates.**

ROUTE AND DOSAGE

- **PO (Adults):** 150 mg/day in 3 divided doses, increase by 50 mg/day q 3–4 days until desired response (not to exceed 600 mg/day).

PHARMACODYNAMICS (antidepressant effect)

	ONSET	PEAK	DURATION
PO	2 wk	2–4 wk	wks

NURSING IMPLICATIONS

Assessment

- Assess mental status and mood changes frequently. Assess for suicidal tendencies, especially during early therapy. Restrict amount of drug available to patient.
- Monitor blood pressure and pulse rate prior to and during initial therapy. Patients with pre-existing cardiac disease should have ECGs monitored prior to and periodically during therapy to detect arrhythmias.
- **Lab Test Considerations:** Assess CBC and renal and hepatic function prior to and periodically during therapy. Slight, clinically insignificant decrease in leukocyte and neutrophil counts may occur.

Potential Nursing Diagnoses

- Coping, ineffective individual, (indications).
- Knowledge deficit related to medication regimen (patient/family teaching).

Implementation

- **PO:** Administer with or immediately after meals to minimize side effects (nausea, dizziness) and allow maximum absorption of trazadone. A larger portion of the total daily dose may be given at bedtime to decrease daytime drowsiness and dizziness.

Patient/Family Teaching

- Instruct patient to take medication exactly as prescribed. If a dose is missed, take as soon as remembered, not taking if within 4 hr of next scheduled dose; do not double doses. Consult physician prior to discontinuing medication; gradual dosage reduction is necessary to prevent aggravation of condition.
- Trazadone may cause drowsiness and blurred vision. Caution patient to avoid driving and other activities requiring alertness until response to drug is known.
- Caution patient to make position changes slowly to minimize orthostatic hypotension.
- Advise patient to avoid concurrent use of alcohol or other CNS depressant drugs.
- Inform patient that frequent rinses, good oral hygiene, and sugarless candy or gum may diminish dry mouth. Physician or dentist should be notified if this persists >2 wk. An increase in fluid intake, fiber, and exercise may prevent constipation.
- Advise patient to notify physician or dentist of medication regimen prior to treatment or surgery.
- Instruct patient to notify physician if priapism, irregular heartbeat, fainting, confusion, skin rash, or tremors occur. If dry mouth, nausea and vomiting, dizziness, headache, muscle aches, constipation, or diarrhea become pronounced physician should be notified.
- Emphasize the importance of follow-up examinations to evaluate progress.

Evaluation

Effectiveness of therapy can be demonstrated by: ▪ Resolution of depression

□ Increased sense of well-being □ Renewed interest in surroundings □ Increased appetite □ Improved energy level □ Improved sleep ▪ Decrease in severity of pain in chronic pain syndromes. Therapeutic effects are usually seen within 2 wk, although 4 wk may be required to obtain significant therapeutic results.

TRIAMCINOLONE

(trye-am-**sin**-oh-lone)

Amcort, Aristocort, Aristospan, Articulose L.A., Atolone, Cenocort A, Cinonide, Kenacort, Kenaject, Kenalog, Nasacort, Tramacort, Triam-A, Triamonide, Tri-Kort, Trilog, Tristoject

CLASSIFICATION(S):
Glucocorticoid—intermediate-acting, Anti-inflammatory agent
Pregnancy Category UK

INDICATIONS

▪ Used systemically and locally in a wide variety of: □ Chronic inflammatory diseases □ Allergic diseases □ Hematologic diseases □ Neoplastic diseases □ Autoimmune diseases ▪ Not suitable for alternate-day therapy.

ACTION

▪ Suppresses inflammation and the normal immune response ▪ Has numerous intense metabolic effects ▪ Suppresses adrenal function at chronic doses of 4 mg/day ▪ Practically devoid of mineralocorticoid (sodium-retaining) activity. **Therapeutic Effects:** ▪ Suppression of inflammation ▪ Modification of the normal immune response.

PHARMACOKINETICS

Absorption: Well absorbed following oral and IM administration. Chronic high-dose topical application may also lead to systemic absorption. IM acetonide and diacetate salts are long-acting.
Distribution: Widely distributed. Crosses the placenta and probably enters breast milk.
Metabolism and Excretion: Mostly metabolized by the liver and other tissues. Small amounts excreted unchanged by the kidneys.
Half-life: 200 + min; adrenal suppression lasts 2.25 days.

CONTRAINDICATIONS AND PRECAUTIONS

Contraindicated in: ▪ Active untreated infections ▪ Lactation (avoid chronic use).
Use Cautiously in: ▪ Chronic treatment (will lead to adrenal suppression) ▪ Stress (surgery, infection—supplemental doses required) ▪ Chronic use in children (will result in decreased growth) ▪ May mask signs of infections (fever, inflammation) ▪ Children <12 yr (intranasal—safety not established).

ADVERSE REACTIONS AND SIDE EFFECTS*

CNS: headache, restlessness, psychoses, fatigue, depression, euphoria, personality changes; increased intracranial pressure (children only).
EENT: cataracts, increased intraocular pressure; Intranasal—nasal irritation, dry mucous membranes, nasosinus congestion, throat discomfort, sneezing, epistaxis.
CV: hypertension.
GI: nausea, vomiting, anorexia, PEPTIC ULCERATION.
Endo: adrenal suppression, hyperglycemia.
Derm: decreased wound healing, petechiae, ecchymoses, fragility, hirsutism, acne.
F and E: hypokalemia, hypokalemic alkalosis, fluid retention (long-term high doses).
Hemat: thromboembolism, thrombophlebitis.
Metab: weight loss, weight gain.
MS: muscle wasting, muscle pain, aseptic necrosis of joints, osteoporosis.
Misc: increased susceptibility to infec-

*Underlines indicate most frequent; **CAPITALS** indicate life-threatening.

T

tion, cushingoid appearance (moon face, buffalo hump).

INTERACTIONS

Drug-Drug: ▪ Additive hypokalemia with **diuretics, amphotericin B, azlocillin, carbenicillin, mezlocillin, piperacillin,** or **ticarcillin** ▪ Hypokalemia may increase the risk of **cardiac glycoside** toxicity ▪ May increase requirement for **insulin** or **hypoglycemic agents** ▪ Increased risk of adverse GI effects with **nonsteroidal anti-inflammatory agents, alcohol,** or **aspirin.**

ROUTE AND DOSAGE

- **PO (Adults):** 4–48 mg/day in 2–4 divided doses.
- **IM (Adults):** 40 mg (acetonide or diacetate).
- **Intra-Articular (Adults):** 2–40 mg (acetonide or diacetate), 2–20 mg (hexacetonide).
- **Top (Adults and Children):** 0.1–0.5% cream, lotion, ointment 2–3 times daily (acetonide).
- **Intranasal:** 2 sprays in each nostril once daily (55 mcg/spray).

PHARMACODYNAMICS (anti-inflammatory activity)

	ONSET	PEAK	DURATION
PO	UK	1–2 hr	2.25 days
IM—acetonide	24–48 hr	UK	1–6 wk
IM—diacetate	slow	UK	4 days–4 wk
IA—acetonide	UK	UK	several wks
IA—diacetate	UK	UK	1–8 wk
IA—hexacetonide	UK	UK	3–4 wk
Intranasal	12 hr–few days	UK	UK

NURSING IMPLICATIONS

Assessment

- □ This drug is indicated for many conditions. Assess involved systems prior to and periodically throughout course of therapy.
- □ Assess patient for signs of adrenal insufficiency (hypotension, weight loss, weakness, nausea, vomiting, anorexia, lethargy, confusion, restlessness) prior to and periodically throughout course of therapy.
- □ Monitor intake and output ratios and daily weights. Observe patient for the appearance of peripheral edema, steady weight gain, rales/crackles, or dyspnea. Notify physician should these occur.
- □ Children should have periodic evaluations of growth.
- ▪ **Lab Test Considerations:** Patients on prolonged courses of therapy should routinely have hematologic values, serum electrolytes, serum and urine glucose evaluated. May cause decreased WBC counts. May cause hyperglycemia, especially in persons with diabetes. May decrease serum potassium and calcium and increase serum sodium concentrations.
- □ Promptly report presence of guaiac-positive stools.
- □ May suppress reactions to allergy skin tests.
- □ Periodic adrenal function tests may be ordered to assess degree of hypothalamic-pituitary-adrenal axis suppression.

Potential Nursing Diagnoses

- Infection, high risk for (side effects).
- Knowledge deficit related to medication regimen (patient/family teaching).
- Body image disturbance (side effects).

Implementation

- **General Info:** Administer daily dose in the morning to coincide with the body's normal secretion of cortisol.
- **PO:** Administer with meals to minimize gastric irritation. Tablets may be crushed and administered with food or fluids for patients with difficulty swallowing. Use calibrated measuring device to ensure accurate dosage of liquid forms.
- **IM:** Shake suspension well before drawing up. Administer IM deep into well-developed muscle. Do not administer triamcinolone IV.

- **Top:** Wear gloves when applying topical medications.
- **Nasal Spray:** Patients also using topical decongestant should be given decongestant 5–15 min before triamcinolone. Instruct patient to blow nose gently if unable to breathe freely through nasal passages before medication administration.

PATIENT/FAMILY TEACHING

- **General Info:** Instruct patient to take medication exactly as directed, not to skip or double up on missed doses. Stopping the medication suddenly may result in adrenal insufficiency (anorexia, nausea, fatigue, weakness, hypotension, dyspnea, and hypoglycemia). If these signs appear notify physician immediately. This can be life-threatening.
- ▫ Encourage patients on long-term therapy to eat a diet high in protein, calcium, and potassium and low in sodium and carbohydrates (see Appendix K for foods included).
- ▫ This drug causes immunosuppression and may mask symptoms of infection. Instruct patient to avoid people with known contagious illnesses and to report possible infections immediately.
- ▫ Review side effects with patient. Instruct patient to inform physician promptly if severe abdominal pain or tarry stools occur. Patient should also report unusual swelling, weight gain, tiredness, bone pain, bruising, nonhealing sores, visual disturbances, or behavior changes.
- ▫ Instruct patient to inform physician if symptoms of underlying disease return or worsen.
- ▫ Discuss possible effects on body image. Explore coping mechanisms.
- ▫ Advise patient to carry identification in the event of an emergency in which patient cannot relate medical history.
- ▫ Caution patient to avoid vaccinations without consulting physician.
- ▫ Explain need for continued medical follow-up to assess effectiveness and possible side effects of medication. Physician may order periodic lab tests and eye examinations.
- **Top:** Instruct patient on correct technique of administration. Apply topical preparations to skin that is clean and slightly moist. Use occlusive dressing only if ordered by physician; may enhance absorption of medication. Apply with cotton-tipped applicator. Avoid contact with eyes.
- **Nasal Spray:** Instruct patient in correct technique for administering nasal spray. Press gently with finger to occlude one naris. Insert tip of applicator into other naris and spray while gently inhaling. Warn patient that temporary nasal stinging may occur.
- ▫ Instruct patient to notify physician if symptoms do not improve within 1 mon or if nasal discharge becomes purulent.

EVALUATION

Effectiveness of therapy can be demonstrated by: ▪ Suppression of the inflammatory and immune responses in autoimmune disorders, allergic reactions, and neoplasms.

TRIAMTERENE

(trye-**am**-ter-een)
Dyrenium

CLASSIFICATION(S):
Diuretic—potassium-sparing
Pregnancy Category UK

INDICATIONS

- Most commonly used to counteract potassium loss induced by other diuretics in the management of edema or hypertension.

ACTION

- Acts at distal tubule, causing excretion of sodium, bicarbonate, and calcium while conserving potassium

T

and hydrogen ions. **Therapeutic Effects:** ▪ Weak diuretic and antihypertensive response compared to other diuretics ▪ Conservation of potassium.

PHARMACOKINETICS

Absorption: Absorption varies greatly among individuals.
Distribution: Widely distributed.
Metabolism and Excretion: Partially metabolized by the liver. Some excretion of unchanged drug.
Half-life: 100–150 min.

CONTRAINDICATIONS AND PRECAUTIONS

Contraindicated in: ▪ Hypersensitivity ▪ Renal impairment ▪ Pregnancy or lactation ▪ Hyperkalemia.
Use Cautiously in: ▪ Impaired hepatic function ▪ Hyperuricemia ▪ History of nephrolithiasis ▪ Children (safety not established).

ADVERSE REACTIONS AND SIDE EFFECTS*

CNS: dizziness, weakness, headache.
CV: hypotension.
GI: nausea, vomiting, diarrhea.
GU: nephrolithiasis, bluish discoloration of urine.
Derm: rashes, photosensitivity.
F and E: HYPERKALEMIA, hyponatremia.
Hemat: megaloblastic anemia, blood dyscrasias.
MS: muscle cramps.
Misc: hypersensitivity reactions.

INTERACTIONS

Drug-Drug: ▪ Additive hypotension with other **antihypertensives**, acute ingestion of **alcohol**, or **nitrates** ▪ Use with **angiotensin converting enzyme (ACE) inhibitors** or **potassium supplements** may lead to hyperkalemia ▪ Decreases **lithium** excretion, may lead to toxicity.
Drug-Food: ▪ Ingestion of **foods high in potassium content** (see list in Appendix K) may lead to hyperkalemia.

ROUTE AND DOSAGE

- **PO (Adults):** 100 mg bid (up to 300 mg/day). Smaller doses in combination preparations.

PHARMACODYNAMICS (potassium-sparing effects)

	ONSET	PEAK	DURATION
PO	2 hr	6–8 hr	12–16 hr

NURSING IMPLICATIONS

ASSESSMENT

- □ Monitor intake and output ratios and daily weight throughout therapy.
- □ Assess patient routinely for signs of hyperkalemia (fatigue, muscle weakness, paresthesia, confusion, dyspnea, cardiac arrhythmias). Patients who have diabetes mellitus or kidney disease and elderly patients are at increased risk of developing these symptoms.
- □ Periodic ECGs are recommended in patients receiving prolonged therapy.
- ▪ **Lab Test Considerations:** Serum potassium levels should be evaluated prior to and routinely during course of therapy. Withhold drug and notify physician if patient becomes hyperkalemic.
- □ Monitor BUN, serum creatinine, and electrolytes prior to and periodically throughout therapy. CBC and platelet count should also be monitored periodically throughout therapy. May cause increased serum glucose, magnesium, uric acid, BUN, creatinine, potassium, and urinary calcium excretion levels. May also cause decreased sodium levels.

POTENTIAL NURSING DIAGNOSES

- ▪ Fluid volume excess (indications).
- ▪ Knowledge deficit related to medication regimen (patient/family teaching).

*Underlines indicate most frequent; **CAPITALS** indicate life-threatening.

Implementation

- **General Info:** Available in combination with hydrochlorothiazide (Dyazide, Maxzide). Capsules (Dyazide) are not bioequivalent to tablets (Maxzide). When changing brands, dosage may need to be adjusted.
- □ Administer in the morning to avoid interrupting sleep pattern.
- **PO:** Administer with food or milk to minimize GI irritation and increase bioavailability. Capsules may be opened and contents mixed with food or fluids for patients with difficulty swallowing.

Patient/Family Teaching

- □ Emphasize the importance of continuing to take this medication even if feeling better. Instruct patient to take medication at the same time each day. If a dose is missed, take as soon as remembered unless almost time for next dose.
- □ Caution patients to avoid salt substitutes and foods that contain high levels of potassium or sodium, unless physician specifically prescribes them.
- □ Advise patient to use sunscreen and protective clothing to prevent photosensitivity reactions.
- □ May cause dizziness. Caution patient to avoid driving or other activities requiring alertness until response to medication is known.
- □ Advise patient to avoid use of over-the-counter medications without first consulting with physician or pharmacist.
- □ Inform patient that triamterene may cause bluish-colored urine.
- □ Advise patient to notify physician if muscle cramps, fatigue, weakness or severe nausea, vomiting, or diarrhea occurs.

Evaluation

Effectiveness of therapy can be demonstrated by: ▪ Increase in diuresis and a decrease in edema while maintaining serum potassium levels in acceptable ranges.

TRIAZOLAM
(trye-**az**-oh-lam)
Halcion

CLASSIFICATION(S):
Sedative/hypnotic—benzodiazepine
Schedule IV
Pregnancy Category X

INDICATIONS

▪ Short-term management of insomnia.

ACTION

▪ Acts at many levels in the CNS, producing generalized depression ▪ Effects may be mediated by gamma aminobutyric acid (GABA), an inhibitory neurotransmitter. **Therapeutic Effect:** ▪ Relief of insomnia.

PHARMACOKINETICS

Absorption: Well absorbed following oral administration.
Distribution: Widely distributed, crosses blood-brain barrier. Probably crosses the placenta and enters breast milk.
Metabolism and Excretion: Metabolized by the liver.
Half-life: 1.6–5.4 hr.

CONTRAINDICATIONS AND PRECAUTIONS

Contraindicated in: ▪ Hypersensitivity ▪ Cross-sensitivity with other benzodiazepines may exist ▪ Pre-existing CNS depression ▪ Uncontrolled severe pain ▪ Pregnancy, lactation, or children.
Use Cautiously in: ▪ Pre-existing hepatic dysfunction (dosage reduction recommended) ▪ Patients who may be suicidal or have been addicted to drugs previously ▪ Elderly or debilitated patients (dosage reduction recommended).

ADVERSE REACTIONS AND SIDE EFFECTS*

CNS: dizziness, drowsiness, lethargy, hangover, paradoxical excitation, con-

*Underlines indicate most frequent; **CAPITALS** indicate life-threatening.

fusion, mental depression, headache.
Derm: rashes.
EENT: blurred vision.
GI: nausea, vomiting, diarrhea, constipation.
Misc: tolerance, psychological dependence, physical dependence.

INTERACTIONS

Drug–Drug: ▪ Additive CNS depression with **alcohol, antidepressants, antihistamines,** and **narcotic analgesics** ▪ May decrease effectiveness of **levodopa** ▪ May increase toxicity from **zidovudine** ▪ **Isoniazid** may decrease excretion and increase effects of triazolam ▪ **Cimetidine** or **erythromycin** may decrease metabolism and enhance actions of triazolam ▪ Sedative effects may be decreased by **theophylline**.

ROUTE AND DOSAGE

- **PO (Adults):** 0.25–0.5 mg at bedtime.

PHARMACODYNAMICS (sedation)

	ONSET	PEAK	DURATION
PO	15–30 min	3 days*	UK

*Maximum hypnotic response.

NURSING IMPLICATIONS

Assessment

- Assess sleep patterns prior to and periodically throughout course of therapy.
- Prolonged high-dose therapy may lead to psychological or physical dependence. Restrict the amount of drug available to patient, especially if patient is depressed, suicidal, or has a history of addiction.

Potential Nursing Diagnoses

- Sleep pattern disturbance (indications).
- Injury, high risk for (side effects).
- Knowledge deficit related to medication regimen (patient/family teaching).

Implementation

- **PO:** Administer with food if GI irritation becomes a problem.

Patient/Family Teaching

- Instruct patient to take triazolam exactly as directed. Discuss the importance of preparing environment for sleep (dark room, quiet, avoidance of nicotine and caffeine). If less effective after a few wks, consult physician; do not increase dose.
- May cause daytime drowsiness or dizziness. Caution patient to avoid driving or other activities requiring alertness until response to medication is known.
- Advise patient to avoid the use of alcohol and other CNS depressants and to consult physician or pharmacist prior to using over-the-counter preparations that contain antihistamines or alcohol.
- Advise patient to inform physican if pregnancy is planned or suspected or if confusion, depression, or persistent headaches occur.
- Emphasize the importance of follow-up appointments to monitor progress.

Evaluation

Effectiveness of therapy can be demonstrated by: ▪ Improvement in sleep patterns, which may not be noticeable until the third day of therapy.

TRIFLUOPERAZINE

(trye-floo-oh-**pair**-a-zeen)
{Apo-Trifluoperazine}, {Novo-Flurazine}, {Solazine}, Stelazine, Suprazine, {Terfluzine}

CLASSIFICATION(S):
Antipsychotic—phenothiazine
Pregnancy Category UK

INDICATIONS

▪ Treatment of acute and chronic psychoses ▪ Adjunct in the management of anxiety when safer agents are contraindicated.

ACTION

▪ Alters the effects of dopamine in the CNS ▪ Possesses significant anticholinergic and alpha-adrenergic blocking activity. **Therapeutic Effect:** ▪ Diminished signs and symptoms of psychoses.

PHARMACOKINETICS

Absorption: Absorption from tablets is variable; may be better with oral liquid formulations. Well absorbed following IM administration.

Distribution: Widely distributed, high concentrations in the CNS. Crosses the placenta and enters breast milk.

Metabolism and Excretion: Highly metabolized by the liver.

Half-life: UK.

CONTRAINDICATIONS AND PRECAUTIONS

Contraindicated in: ▪ Hypersensitivity ▪ Cross-sensitivity with other phenothiazines may exist ▪ Narrow-angle glaucoma ▪ Bone marrow depression ▪ Severe liver or cardiovascular disease.

Use Cautiously in: ▪ Elderly or debilitated patients (dosage reduction recommended) ▪ Pregnancy or lactation (safety not established; may cause adverse effects in the newborn) ▪ Diabetes mellitus ▪ Respiratory disease ▪ Prostatic hypertrophy ▪ CNS tumors ▪ Epilepsy ▪ Intestinal obstruction.

ADVERSE REACTIONS AND SIDE EFFECTS*

CNS: <u>sedation</u>, <u>extrapyramidal reactions</u>, tardive dyskinesia, NEUROLEPTIC MALIGNANT SYNDROME.

EENT: dry eyes, blurred vision, lens opacities.

CV: hypotension, tachycardia.

GI: <u>constipation</u>, dry mouth, ileus, anorexia, hepatitis.

GU: urinary retention.

Derm: rashes, <u>photosensitivity</u>, pigment changes.

Endo: galactorrhea.

Hemat: AGRANULOCYTOSIS, leukopenia.

Metab: hyperthermia.

Misc: allergic reactions.

INTERACTIONS

Drug-Drug: ▪ Additive hypotension with **antihypertensive agents,** acute ingestion of **alcohol,** or **nitrates** ▪ Additive CNS depression with other **CNS depressants,** including **alcohol, antihistamines, narcotic analgesics, sedative/hypnotics,** and **general anesthetics** ▪ Additive anticholinergic effects with other **drugs having anticholinergic properties,** including **antihistamines, antidepressants,** other **phenothiazines, quinidine,** and **disopyramide** ▪ Acute encephalopathy may occur with **lithium** ▪ May decrease the effectiveness of **levodopa** ▪ Increased risk of agranulocytosis with **antithyroid drugs** ▪ **Lithium** decreases absorption and may increase risk of extrapyramidal reactions.

ROUTE AND DOSAGE

Psychoses

- **PO (Adults):** 1–5 mg bid (up to 40 mg/day).
- **PO (Children 6–12 yr):** 1–2 mg daily or bid (up to 15 mg/day).
- **IM (Adults):** 1–2 mg q 4–6 hr (up to 6 mg/day).

Anxiety

- **PO (Adults):** 1–2 mg bid.

PHARMACODYNAMICS (antipsychotic effects)

	ONSET	PEAK	DURATION
PO	UK	UK	12–24 hr
IM	UK	UK	4–6 hr

NURSING IMPLICATIONS

Assessment

- ▫ Assess mental status (orientation, mood, behavior) and degree of anxiety prior to and periodically throughout therapy.
- ▫ Monitor blood pressure (sitting, standing, lying), pulse, and respiratory rate prior to and frequently during the period of dosage adjustment.

*<u>Underlines</u> indicate most frequent; **CAPITALS** indicate life-threatening.

- □ Observe patient carefully when administering medication to ensure that medication is actually taken and not hoarded.
- □ Monitor intake and output ratios and daily weight. Notify physician if significant discrepancies occur.
- □ Monitor patient for onset of extrapyramidal side effects (akathisia—restlessness; dystonia—muscle spasms and twisting motions; pseudoparkinsonism—mask facies, rigidity, tremors, drooling, shuffling gait, dysphagia). Notify physician if these symptoms occur, as reduction in dosage or discontinuation of medication may be necessary. Physician may also order antiparkinsonian agents (trihexyphenidyl, benztropine) to control these symptoms.
- □ Monitor for tardive dyskinesia (rhythmic movement of mouth, face, and extremities). Notify physician immediately if these symptoms occur, as these side effects may be irreversible.
- □ Monitor for development of neuroleptic malignant syndrome (fever, respiratory distress, tachycardia, convulsions, diaphoresis, hypertension or hypotension, pallor, tiredness). Notify physician immediately if these symptoms occur.
- ▪ **Lab Test Considerations:** CBC and liver function tests should be evaluated periodically throughout course of therapy. May cause blood dyscrasias, especially between wks 4–10 of therapy.
- □ May cause false-positive or false-negative pregnancy tests and false-positive urine bilirubin test results.
- □ May cause increased serum prolactin levels, thereby interfering with gonadorelin test results.
- □ May cause Q Wave and T wave changes in ECG.

Potential Nursing Diagnoses

- ▪ Coping, ineffective individual (indications).
- ▪ Thought processes, altered (indications).
- ▪ Knowledge deficit related to medication regimen (patient/family teaching).

Implementation

- ▪ **General Info:** Available in tablet, concentrate, and injectable forms.
- □ To prevent contact dermatitis, avoid getting soln on hands.
- □ Phenothiazines should be discontinued 48 hr before and not resumed for 24 hr following metrizamide myelography, as they lower the seizure threshold.
- □ Soln may be slightly yellow. Do not use if soln is brown or contains a precipitate. Protect from light.
- ▪ **PO:** Administer oral doses with food, water, or milk to minimize GI irritation. Tablets may be crushed and mixed with food or fluids for patients with difficulty swallowing.
- □ Dilute concentrate just prior to administration, in at least 120 ml of tomato or fruit juice, milk, carbonated beverage, coffee, tea, or water. Semisolid foods (soups, puddings) may also be used.
- ▪ **IM:** Administer deep into well-developed muscle. SC administration may cause tissue necrosis. Keep patient recumbent for at least 30 min following injection to minimize hypotensive effects.

Patient/Family Teaching

- □ Advise patient to take medication exactly as directed, not to skip doses or double up on missed doses. If a dose is missed it should be taken as soon as remembered unless almost time for the next dose. If more than 2 doses are scheduled each day, the missed dose should be taken within about 1 hr of the ordered time.
- □ Abrupt withdrawal may lead to gastritis, nausea, vomiting, dizziness, headache, tachycardia, and insomnia.
- □ May cause drowsiness. Caution patient to avoid driving or other activities requiring alertness until response to medication is known.
- □ Advise patient to make position changes slowly to minimize orthostatic hypotension.

- □ Advise patient to use sunscreen and protective clothing when exposed to the sun to prevent photosensitivity reactions. Extremes in temperature should also be avoided, as this drug impairs body temperature regulation.
- □ Caution patient to avoid taking alcohol or other CNS depressants concurrently with this medication.
- □ Instruct patient to use frequent mouth rinses, good oral hygiene, and sugarless gum or candy to minimize dry mouth. Consult physician or dentist if dry mouth continues >2 wk.
- □ Advise patient that increasing activity and bulk and fluids in the diet helps minimize the constipating effects of this medication.
- □ Advise patient to notify physician or dentist of medication regimen prior to treatment or surgery.
- □ Instruct patient to notify physician promptly if sore throat, fever, unusual bleeding or bruising, skin rashes, weakness, tremors, visual disturbances, difficulty urinating, dark-colored urine, or clay-colored stools are noted.
- □ Emphasize the importance of routine follow-up examinations to monitor response to medication and detect side effects. Periodic ocular examinations are indicated. Encourage continued participation in psychotherapy as ordered by physician.

Evaluation

Effectiveness of therapy can be demonstrated by: ▪ Decrease in excitable, paranoic, or withdrawn behavior ▪ Decrease in anxiety associated with depression. Therapeutic effects of oral doses may not be seen for 2–3 wk.

TRIFLURIDINE

(trye-**flure**-i-deen)
Viroptic

CLASSIFICATION(S):
Ophthalmic—antifungal
Pregnancy Category UK

INDICATIONS

▪ Treatment of herpes simplex type 1 or 2 keratitis or keratoconjunctivitis.

ACTION

▪ Inhibits viral DNA synthesis and subsequent viral replication. **Therapeutic Effect:** ▪ Antiviral action against herpes simplex virus.

PHARMACOKINETICS

Absorption: Systemic absorption does not appear to occur following ophthalmic administration.
Distribution: Penetrates ocular structures (cornea, aqueous humor) following ophthalmic administration. Penetration may be increased in the presence of infection.
Metabolism and Excretion: Metabolism and excretion not known.
Half-life: 12–18 min.

CONTRAINDICATIONS AND PRECAUTIONS

Contraindicated in: ▪ Hypersensitivity to trifluridine or thimerisol.
Use Cautiously in: ▪ Pregnancy or lactation (safety not established).

ADVERSE REACTIONS AND SIDE EFFECTS*

EENT: ocular burning, stinging, palpebral edema, conjunctival irritation.

INTERACTIONS

Drug-Drug: ▪ None significant.

ROUTE AND DOSAGE

- **Ophth (Adults):** 1 drop of 1% soln q 2 hr while awake (not to exceed 9 drops/day) until cornea is re-epithelialized, then decrease to 1 drop q 4 hr while awake (at least 5 drops/day) for 7 more days (not to exceed 21 days of continuous therapy).

PHARMACODYNAMICS (improvement in corneal defects)

	ONSET	PEAK	DURATION
Ophth	7–14 days	14 days	UK

*Underlines indicate most frequent; **CAPITALS** indicate life-threatening.

NURSING IMPLICATIONS

Assessment

- □ Assess eye lesions daily prior to and throughout therapy.

Potential Nursing Diagnoses

- ■ Infection, high risk for (indications).
- ■ Knowledge deficit related to medication regimen (patient/family teaching).

Implementation

- ■ **Ophth Soln:** Instill soln by having patient lie down or tilt head back and look at ceiling. Pull down on lower lid, creating a small pocket, and instill soln in pocket. Gently close eye. Wait 5 min before instilling other ophthalmic medications. Refrigerate soln.

Patient/Family Teaching

- □ Instruct patient in the correct technique for instillation of ophthalmic medications. Emphasize the importance of not touching the cap or tip of tube to eye, fingers, or any other surface.
- □ Instruct patient to instill medication exactly as directed, even if feeling better or if procedure is inconvenient. Herpetic keratitis may recur if trifluridine is discontinued too soon. Missed doses should be instilled as soon as remembered, unless almost time for next dose. Do not use more frequently or for longer than directed.
- □ Advise patient that trifluridine may cause burning or stinging upon instillation.
- □ Advise patient to consult physician if no improvement after 1 wk of therapy, if condition worsens, or if irritation persists.
- □ Emphasize the importance of follow-up examinations to determine progress.

Evaluation

Effectiveness of therapy can be demonstrated by: ■ Resolution of eye lesions in herpetic keratitis. Treatment is usually not continued for more than 21 days or 3–5 days after healing has occurred, except in chronic cases or infections that are difficult to cure.

TRIHEXYPHENIDYL

(trye-hex-ee-**fen**-i-dill)
{Aparkane}, {Apo-Trihex}, Artane, {Novohexidyl}, Trihexane, Trihexy

CLASSIFICATION(S):
Anticholinergic—antimuscarinic, Antiparkinson—anticholinergic
Pregnancy Category C

INDICATIONS

■ Adjunct in the management of parkinsonian syndrome due to many causes, including drug-induced parkinsonism.

ACTION

■ Inhibits the action of acetylcholine, resulting in: □ Decreased sweating and salivation □ Mydriasis (pupillary dilation) □ Increased heart rate ■ Also has spasmolytic action on smooth muscle ■ Inhibits cerebral motor centers and blocks efferent impulses. **Therapeutic Effect:** ■ Diminished signs and symptoms of parkinsonian syndrome (tremors, rigidity).

PHARMACOKINETICS

Absorption: Well absorbed following oral administration.
Distribution: Distribution not known.
Metabolism and Excretion: Metabolism and excretion not known.
Half-life: UK.

CONTRAINDICATIONS AND PRECAUTIONS

Contraindicated in: ■ Hypersensitivity ■ Narrow-angle glaucoma ■ Acute hemorrhage ■ Tachycardia secondary to cardiac insufficiency ■ Thyrotoxicosis.
Use Cautiously in: ■ Elderly and very young patients (increased risk of adverse reactions) ■ Intestinal obstruction or infection ■ Prostatic hypertrophy

▪ Chronic renal, hepatic, pulmonary, or cardiac disease ▪ Pregnancy or lactation (safety not established).

ADVERSE REACTIONS AND SIDE EFFECTS*

CNS: dizziness, nervousness, drowsiness, weakness, headache, confusion.
EENT: blurred vision, mydriasis.
CV: tachycardia, orthostatic hypotension.
GI: dry mouth, nausea, constipation, vomiting.
GU: urinary hesitancy, urinary retention.
Derm: decreased sweating.

INTERACTIONS

Drug–Drug: ▪ Additive anticholinergic effects with other **drugs having anticholinergic properties,** including **phenothiazines, tricyclic antidepressants, quinidine,** and **disopyramide** ▪ Additive CNS depression with other **CNS depressants,** including **alcohol, antihistamines, narcotic analgesics,** and **sedative/hypnotics** ▪ Anticholinergics may alter the absorption of other **orally administered drugs** by slowing motility of the GI tract ▪ **Antacids** may decrease absorption ▪ May increase GI mucosal lesions in patients taking oral **wax-matrix potassium chloride preparations.**

ROUTE AND DOSAGE

- **PO (Adults):** 1 mg/day initially, increase by 2 mg q 3–5 days. Usual maintenance dose is 5–15 mg/day in 3–4 divided doses. Extended-release (Artane Sequels) preparations may be given q 12–24 hr daily after dose has been determined using conventional tablets or liquid.

PHARMACODYNAMICS (antiparkinson effects)

	ONSET	PEAK	DURATION
PO	1 hr	2–3 hr	6–12 hr
PO-ER	UK	UK	12–24 hr

NURSING IMPLICATIONS

Assessment

- □ Assess parkinsonian and extrapyramidal symptoms (akinesia, rigidity, tremors, pill rolling, mask facies, shuffling gait, muscles spasms, twisting motions, and drooling) prior to and throughout course of therapy.
- □ Patients with mental illness are at risk of developing exaggerated symptoms of their disorder during early therapy with this medication. Withhold drug and notify physician if significant behavioral changes occur.

Potential Nursing Diagnoses

- Mobility, impaired physical (indications).
- Injury, high risk for (indications).
- Knowledge deficit related to medication regimen (patient/family teaching).

Implementation

- **General Info:** Sustained-release capsules are not used until dosage is established with shorter-acting forms.
- **PO:** Usually administered after meals. May be administered before meals if patient suffers from dry mouth or with meals if gastric distress is a problem. Sustained-release capsules should be swallowed whole; do not break, crush, or chew. Use calibrated measuring device to ensure accurate dosage of elixir.

Patient/Family Teaching

- □ Instruct patient to take this drug exactly as prescribed. If a dose is missed, take as soon as remembered, unless next scheduled dose is within 2 hr; do not double doses.
- □ Medication should be tapered off gradually when discontinuing, or a withdrawal reaction may occur (anxiety, tachycardia, insomnia, return of parkinsonian or extrapyramidal symptoms).
- □ May cause drowsiness or dizziness. Advise patient to avoid driving or other activities that require alertness

*Underlines indicate most frequent; **CAPITALS** indicate life-threatening.

until response to medication is known.

- □ Caution patient to make position changes slowly to minimize orthostatic hypotension.
- □ Instruct patient that frequent rinsing of mouth, good oral hygiene, and sugarless gum or candy may decrease mouth dryness. Patient should notify physician if dryness persists (saliva substitutes may be used). Also notify dentist if dryness interferes with use of dentures.
- □ Advise patient to consult physician or pharmacist prior to taking over-the-counter medications, especially cold remedies, or drinking alcoholic beverages.
- □ Caution patient that this medication decreases perspiration. Overheating may occur during hot weather. Patient should remain indoors, in an air-conditioned environment, during hot weather.
- □ Advise patient to increase activity and bulk and fluid in diet to minimize constipating effects of medication.
- □ Advise patient to notify physician if confusion, rash, urinary retention, severe constipation, or visual changes occur.

Evaluation

Effectiveness of therapy can be demonstrated by: ▪ Resolution of parkinsonian signs and symptoms ▪ Resolution of drug-induced extrapyramidal symptoms.

TRIMETHAPHAN

(trye-**meth**-a-fan)

Arfonad

CLASSIFICATION(S):
Antihypertensive—ganglionic blocker
Pregnancy Category UK

INDICATIONS

▪ Rapid reduction of blood pressure in the management of hypertensive emergencies ▪ Particularly useful in lowering blood pressure in patients with acute aortic dissection ▪ Controlled hypotension in patients undergoing head and neck surgery.

ACTION

▪ Blocks nerve transmission at sympathetic and autonomic ganglia ▪ Produces vasodilation and histamine release ▪ Increases peripheral blood flow and decreases blood pressure. **Therapeutic Effect:** ▪ Decreased blood pressure.

PHARMACOKINETICS

Absorption: Administered IV only, resulting in complete bioavailability.
Distribution: Crosses the placenta.
Metabolism and Excretion: Mainly excreted unchanged by the kidneys. Small amounts may be metabolized by pseudocholinesterase.
Half-life: UK.

CONTRAINDICATIONS AND PRECAUTIONS

Contraindicated in: ▪ Hypersensitivity ▪ Anemia ▪ Hypovolemia ▪ Shock ▪ Asphyxia ▪ Glaucoma ▪ Respiratory insufficiency ▪ Pregnancy.
Use Cautiously in: ▪ Patients with allergies ▪ Elderly or debilitated patients ▪ Children ▪ Cardiovascular disease ▪ Degenerative CNS disease ▪ Diabetes mellitus ▪ Addison's disease ▪ Safety in lactation not established ▪ Hepatic or renal impairment.

ADVERSE REACTIONS AND SIDE EFFECTS*

CNS: weakness, restlessness.
EENT: cycloplegia, mydriasis.
Resp: apnea, RESPIRATORY ARREST (large doses only).
CV: <u>hypotension</u>, tachycardia, angina.
GI: anorexia, nausea, vomiting, dry mouth, ileus (if therapy >48 hr).
GU: urinary retention.
Derm: urticaria, itching.
Misc: tachyphylaxis.

*<u>Underlines</u> indicate most frequent; **CAPITALS** indicate life-threatening.

INTERACTIONS

Drug–Drug: ▪ Additive hypotension with other **antihypertensives, nitrates, diuretics, anesthetics,** or **procainamide** ▪ May prolong neuromuscular blockade from **succinylcholine** or **tubocurarine**.

ROUTE AND DOSAGE

Severe Hypertension, Hypertensive Emergencies

- **IV (Adults):** 0.5–1 mg/min initially, may be increased gradually to achieve desired response (range 1–5 mg/min).

Aortic Dissection

- **IV (Adults):** 1–2 mg/min initially, increased as needed to maintain systolic blood pressure of 100–200 mm Hg.

Controlled Hypotension During Anesthesia

- **IV (Adults):** 3–4 mg/min initially followed by 0.2–6 mg/min infusion.

PHARMACODYNAMICS (antihypertensive effect)

	ONSET	PEAK	DURATION
IV	immediate	UK	10–15 min

NURSING IMPLICATIONS

Assessment

- Monitor blood pressure, pulse, and respirations at least every 5 min during initial adjustment of dosage and at least every 15 min throughout course of therapy. Titrate infusion rate according to physician's parameters. Patients with cardiac history should be monitored with continuous ECG.
- Monitor intake and output ratios and weight and assess for edema, jugular vein distension, dyspnea, and rales/crackles, especially in patients with pulmonary edema.
- Monitor patients with any allergy history closely for development of tachyphylaxis, because of the effect on histamine release.
- Pupil examination will be inaccurate because of mydriatic (dilating) effect.
- Monitor for nausea and vomiting; protect airway in patients with diminished level of consciousness. Monitor abdominal status (distention, bowel sounds) in patients on therapy >48 hr, as ileus may occur.
- **Lab Test Considerations:** May cause slightly decreased serum potassium and may prevent surgically induced elevation in serum glucose.
- **Toxicity and Overdose:** Toxicity is manifested by severe hypotension. Stop infusion, inform physician, and administer vasopressors.

Potential Nursing Diagnoses

- Cardiac output, altered (indications).
- Tissue perfusion, altered (side effects).

Implementation

- **IV:** Refrigerate prior to reconstitution. Prepare soln immediately prior to use. IV stable for 24 hr after reconstitution.
- **Continuous Infusion:** Dilute 500-mg (10-ml) vial in 500 ml of D5W, 0.9% NaCl, or Ringer's soln, for a final concentration of 1 mg/ml.
  - *Rate:* Infusion rate must be regulated by IV pump or controller and titrated to patient's blood pressure.
- **Y-Site Compatibility:** heparin, hydrocortisone, or potassium chloride.
- **Additive Incompatibility:** alkaline solns, bromides, gallamine triethiodide, thiopental sodium, or tubocurarine. Admixture is not recommended with any medication.

Patient/Family Teaching

- Explain purpose of medication to patient.
- Instruct alert patients to remain supine throughout course of therapy to prevent orthostatic hypotension.

Evaluation

Effectiveness of therapy can be demonstrated by: ▪ Short-term control of blood pressure in hypertensive crisis ▪ Control of intraoperative hypotension.

T

TRIMETHOBENZAMIDE
(trye-meth-oh-**ben**-za-mide)
Tebamide, Tegamide, Ticon, Tigan, Tiject-20

CLASSIFICATION(S):
Antiemetic—miscellaneous
Pregnancy Category UK

INDICATIONS
▪ Management of mild to moderate nausea and vomiting.

ACTION
▪ Inhibits emetic stimulation of the chemoreceptor trigger zone in the medulla. **Therapeutic Effect:** ▪ Decreased nausea and vomiting.

PHARMACOKINETICS
Absorption: Absorption following oral, IM, and rectal administration.
Distribution: Distribution not known.
Metabolism and Excretion: Metabolism and excretion not known. Appears to be mostly metabolized by the liver.
Half-life: UK.

CONTRAINDICATIONS AND PRECAUTIONS
Contraindicated in: ▪ Hypersensitivity ▪ Hypersensitivity to benzocaine (suppositories only).
Use Cautiously in: ▪ Pregnancy or lactation (safety not established) ▪ Children who may have a viral illness (may increase risk of Reye's syndrome).

ADVERSE REACTIONS AND SIDE EFFECTS*
CNS: drowsiness, extrapyramidal reactions, depression, SEIZURES, coma.
CV: hypotension.
GI: diarrhea, hepatitis.
Derm: rashes.
Hemat: blood dyscrasias.
Local: pain at IM injection site, rectal irritation (suppositories).

INTERACTIONS
Drug-Drug: ▪ Additive CNS depression with other **CNS depressants,** including **alcohol, antidepressants, antihistamines, narcotic analgesics,** and **sedative/hypnotics**.

ROUTE AND DOSAGE
- **PO (Adults):** 250 mg 3–4 times daily.
- **PO (Children 13–40 kg):** 100–200 mg 3–4 times daily.
- **IM (Adults):** 200 mg 3–4 times daily.
- **Rect (Adults):** 200 mg 3–4 times daily.
- **Rect (Children 14–45 kg):** 100–200 mg 3–4 times daily.
- **Rect (Children <14 kg):** 100 mg 3–4 times daily.

PHARMACODYNAMICS (antiemetic effect)

	ONSET	PEAK	DURATION
PO	10–40 min	UK	3–4 hr
IM	15–35 min	UK	2–3 hr
Rect	10–40 min	UK	3–4 hr

NURSING IMPLICATIONS
Assessment
- ☐ Assess patient for nausea and vomiting prior to and 30–60 min following administration.
- ☐ Assess blood pressure for hypotension following parenteral administration.

Potential Nursing Diagnoses
- Fluid volume deficit (indications).
- Injury, high risk for (side effects).
- Knowledge deficit related to medication regimen (patient/family teaching).

Implementation
- **General Info:** Available in capsule, suppository, and injectable forms.
- **PO:** Capsules can be opened and contents mixed with food or fluids for patients with difficulty swallowing.
- **IM:** Inject deep into well-developed muscle mass to minimize tissue irritation.

*Underlines indicate most frequent; **CAPITALS** indicate life-threatening.

- **Syringe Compatibility:** glycopyrrolate, hydromorphone, midazolam, or nalbuphine.
- **Y-Site Compatibility:** heparin, hydrocortisone sodium succinate, or potassium chloride.

PATIENT/FAMILY TEACHING

- Instruct patient to take medication exactly as directed. Missed doses should be taken as soon as remembered, unless almost time for next dose; do not double doses.
- Advise patient to make position changes slowly to minimize orthostatic hypotension following parenteral doses.
- May cause drowsiness. Caution patient to avoid driving or other activities requiring alertness until response to medication is known.
- Caution patient to avoid taking alcohol or other CNS depressants concurrently with this medication.
- Instruct patient to notify physician promptly if sore throat, fever, unusual weakness or tiredness, tremors, or yellowing of the skin and eyes occurs.

EVALUATION

Effectiveness of therapy can be demonstrated by: ▪ Prevention and relief of nausea and vomiting.

TRIMETHOPRIM

(trye-**meth**-oh-prim)
Proloprim, Trimpex

CLASSIFICATION(S):
Anti-infective—miscellaneous
Pregnancy Category C

INDICATIONS

▪ Treatment of uncomplicated urinary tract infections. **Unlabeled Use:** ▪ Prophylaxis of chronic recurrent urinary tract infections.

ACTION

▪ Interferes with bacterial folic acid synthesis. **Therapeutic Effect:** ▪ Bactericidal action against susceptible organisms. **Spectrum:** ▪ Some gram-positive pathogens, including: ▫ *Streptococcus pneumoniae* ▫ Group A beta-hemolytic streptococci ▫ Some staphylococci and *Enterococcus* ▪ Gram-negative spectrum includes the following Enterobacteriaceae: ▫ *Acinetobacter* ▫ *Citrobacter* ▫ *Enterobacter* ▫ *Escherichia coli* ▫ *Klebsiella pneumoniae* ▫ *Proteus mirabilis* ▫ *Salmonella* ▫ *Shigella* ▪ Other strains of *Proteus*, some *Provi-dencia*, and some *Serratia* are also susceptible.

PHARMACOKINETICS

Absorption: Well absorbed following oral administration.

Distribution: Widely distributed. Crosses the placenta and is distributed into breast milk in high concentrations.

Metabolism and Excretion: 80% excreted unchanged in the urine. 20% metabolized by the liver.

Half-life: 8–11 hr (increased in renal impairment).

CONTRAINDICATIONS AND PRECAUTIONS

Contraindicated in: ▪ Hypersensitivity ▪ Megaloblastic anemia secondary to folate deficiency.

Use Cautiously in: ▪ Renal impairment (dosage reduction required) ▪ Pregnancy, lactation, or children <12 yr (safety not established) ▪ Debilitated patients ▪ Severe hepatic impairment ▪ Folate deficiency.

ADVERSE REACTIONS AND SIDE EFFECTS*

GI: epigastric discomfort, nausea, vomiting, glossitis, altered taste, hepatitis.

Derm: rash, pruritus.

Hemat: neutropenia, thrombocytopenia, megaloblastic anemia.

Misc: fever.

INTERACTIONS

Drug-Drug: ▪ Increased risk of folate deficiency when used with **phenytoin** or **methotrexate** ▪ Increased risk of bone

*Underlines indicate most frequent; **CAPITALS** indicate life-threatening.

marrow depression when used with **antineoplastic agents** or **radiation therapy** ▪ **Rifampin** may decrease effectiveness by increasing elimination.

ROUTE AND DOSAGE

Treatment of Urinary Tract Infections

- **PO (Adults):** 100 mg q 12 hr or 200 mg as a single daily dose.

Prophylaxis of Chronic Urinary Tract Infections

- **PO (Adults):** 100 mg/day (single dose).

PHARMACODYNAMICS (blood levels)

	ONSET	PEAK
PO	rapid	1–4 hr

NURSING IMPLICATIONS

Assessment

- Assess patient for urinary tract infection (fever, cloudy urine, frequency, urgency, pain and burning on urination) at beginning and throughout course of therapy.
- Obtain specimens for culture and sensitivity prior to initiating therapy. First dose may be given before receiving results.
- Monitor intake and output ratios. Fluid intake should be sufficient to maintain urine output of at least 1200–1500 ml daily.
- **Lab Test Considerations:** May produce elevated serum bilirubin, creatinine, BUN, SGOT (AST), and SGPT (ALT).
- Monitor CBC and urinalysis periodically throughout therapy. Therapy should be discontinued if blood dyscrasias occur.

Potential Nursing Diagnoses

- Infection, high risk for (indications, side effects).
- Knowledge deficit related to medication regimen (patient/family teaching).

Implementation

- **PO:** Administer on an empty stomach, at least 1 hr before or 2 hr after meals, with a full glass of water. May be administered with food if GI irritation occurs.

Patient/Family Teaching

- Instruct patient to take medication and to finish medication completely as directed, even if feeling better. If a dose is missed, it should be taken as soon as remembered, with subsequent doses spaced evenly apart. Advise patient that sharing of this medication may be dangerous.
- Advise patient to notify physician if skin rash, sore throat, fever, mouth sores, or unusual bleeding or bruising occurs. Leucovorin (folinic acid) may be administered if folic acid deficiency occurs.
- Instruct patient to notify physician if symptoms do not improve.
- Emphasize the importance of routine follow-up examinations to evaluate progress.

Evaluation

Clinical response can be evaluated by: ▪ Resolution of the signs and symptoms of infection. Therapy is usually required for 10–14 days for resolution of infection ▪ Decreased incidence of urinary tract infections during prophylactic therapy.

TRIPROLIDINE

(trye-**proe**-li-deen)
Actidil, Alleract, Myidyl

CLASSIFICATION(S):
Antihistamine
Pregnancy Category B

INDICATIONS

▪ Symptomatic relief of allergic symptoms caused by histamine release ▪ Most useful in the management of nasal allergies and allergic dermatoses.

ACTION

▪ Blocks the effects of histamine. **Therapeutic Effect:** ▪ Relief of symptoms associated with histamine excess usually seen in allergic conditions.

PHARMACOKINETICS

Absorption: Well absorbed following oral administration.
Distribution: Widely distributed. Minimal amounts excreted in breast milk. Crosses the blood-brain barrier.
Metabolism and Excretion: Extensively metabolized by the liver.
Half-life: 5 hr.

CONTRAINDICATIONS AND PRECAUTIONS

Contraindicated in: ▪ Hypersensitivity ▪ Acute attacks of asthma ▪ Lactation.
Use Cautiously in: ▪ Elderly patients (increased risk of adverse reactions) ▪ Narrow-angle glaucoma ▪ Liver disease ▪ Pregnancy (safety not established) ▪ Prostatic hypertrophy.

ADVERSE REACTIONS AND SIDE EFFECTS*

CNS: drowsiness, sedation, excitation (in children), dizziness.
EENT: blurred vision.
CV: hypotension, hypertension, palpitations, arrhythmias.
GI: dry mouth, constipation.
GU: urinary hesitancy, retention.

INTERACTIONS

Drug–Drug: ▪ Additive CNS depression with other **CNS depressants,** including **alcohol, narcotic analgesics,** and **sedative/hypnotics** ▪ Additive anticholinergic effects with other **drugs possessing anticholinergic properties,** including **antidepressants, atropine, haloperidol, phenothiazines, quinidine,** and **disopyramide** ▪ **MAO inhibitors** intensify and prolong the anticholinergic effects of antihistamines.

ROUTE AND DOSAGE

- **PO (Adults):** 2.5 mg q 4–6 hr (not to exceed 10 mg/24 hr) or 5 mg of extended-release preparation q 12 hr (not to exceed 10 mg/24 hr).
- **PO (Children 6–12 yr):** 1.25 mg q 6–8 hr (not to exceed 5 mg/24 hr).
- **PO (Children 4–6 yr):** 0.937 mg q 6–8 hr (not ot exceed 3.75 mg/24 hr).
- **PO (Children 2–4 yr):** 0.625 mg q 6–8 hr (not to exceed 2.5 mg/24 hr).
- **PO (Children 4 mon–2 yr):** 0.312 mg q 6–8 hr (not to exceed 1.25 mg/24 hr).

PHARMACODYNAMICS (antihistaminic effects)

	ONSET	PEAK	DURATION
PO	15–60 min	1–2 hr	6–8 hr*

*Up to 12 hr with extended-release preparations.

NURSING IMPLICATIONS

Assessment

- □ Assess allergy symptoms (rhinitis, conjunctivitis, hives) prior to and periodically throughout course of therapy.
- □ Assess lung sounds and character of bronchial secretions. Maintain fluid intake of 1500–2000 ml/day to decrease viscosity of secretions.
- ▪ **Lab Test Considerations:** May cause false-negative reactions on allergy skin tests; discontinue 3 days prior to testing.

Potential Nursing Diagnoses

- ▪ Airway clearance, ineffective (indications).
- ▪ Injury, high risk for (adverse reactions).
- ▪ Knowledge deficit related to medication regimen (patient/family teaching).

Implementation

- ▪ **General Info:** Available in tablet or syrup form. Also available in combination with decongestants and cough syrups (see Appendix A).
- ▪ **PO:** Administer oral doses with food or milk to decrease GI irritation. Use calibrated measuring device to ensure accurate dose of syrup.

*Underlines indicate most frequent; **CAPITALS** indicate life-threatening.

T

PATIENT/FAMILY TEACHING

- □ If a dose is missed, it should be taken as soon as remembered unless almost time for next dose.
- □ Instruct patient to contact physician if symptoms persist.
- □ Triprolidine may cause drowsiness. Caution patient to avoid driving or other activities requiring alertness until response to drug is known.
- □ Caution patient against using alcohol or other CNS depressants concurrently with this drug.
- □ Advise patient that good oral hygiene, frequent mouth rinses, and sugarless gum or candy may help relieve mouth dryness. Physician or dentist should be notified if mouth dryness persists >2 wk.

EVALUATION

Effectiveness of therapy can be demonstrated by: ▪ Decrease in allergic symptoms.

TUBOCURARINE

(too-boh-**cure**-a-reen)
{Tubarine}

CLASSIFICATION(S):
Neuromuscular blocking agent—nondepolarizing
Pregnancy Category C

INDICATIONS

▪ Production of skeletal muscle paralysis after induction of anesthesia in surgical procedures ▪ Used during mechanical ventilation to improve pulmonary compliance ▪ Adjunct to electroconvulsive therapy ▪ Diagnostic agent in myasthenia gravis.

ACTION

▪ Prevents neuromuscular transmission by blocking the effect of acetylcholine at the myoneural junction ▪ Has no anxiolytic or analgesic effects. **Therapeutic Effect:** ▪ Skeletal muscle paralysis.

PHARMACOKINETICS

Absorption: Although well absorbed following IM administration, effect is delayed as compared to IV administration.

Distribution: Extensively distributed and subsequently redistributed to various tissue compartments. Saturation of compartments occurs, explaining prolonged duration of action following repeated doses.

Metabolism and Excretion: 30–75% excreted unchanged by the kidneys. 11% excreted in bile. Small amounts are metabolized by the liver.

Half-life: 2 hr.

CONTRAINDICATIONS AND PRECAUTIONS

Contraindicated in: ▪ Hypersensitivity to tubocurarine ▪ Some products contain chlorobutanol, benzyl alcohol, or bisulfite (avoid use in patients with hypersensitivity to these ingredients).

Use Cautiously in: ▪ History of pulmonary disease, renal or liver impairment ▪ Elderly or debilitated patients ▪ Electrolyte disturbances ▪ Myasthenia gravis or myasthenic syndromes.

ADVERSE REACTIONS AND SIDE EFFECTS*

CV: hypotension, arrhythmias.
EENT: excess salivation.
Resp: bronchospasm, APNEA.
GI: decreased GI tone, decreased GI motility.
MS: muscle weakness.
Misc: allergic reactions.

INTERACTIONS

Drug-Drug: ▪ Intensity and duration of paralysis may be prolonged by pretreatment with **succinylcholine, general anesthesia, aminoglycoside antibiotics, polymyxin B, colistin, clindamycin, lidocaine, quinidine, procainamide, beta-adrenergic blocking agents, potassium-losing diuretics,** and **magnesium** ▪ Dosage should be reduced by ⅔ if concurrent **ether** is used, ⅓ if **meth-**

{} = Available in Canada only.
*Underlines indicate most frequent; **CAPITALS** indicate life-threatening.

oxyflurane is used, and ⅕ if **halothane** or **cyclopropane** is used ▪ **Doxapram** masks residual effects.

ROUTE AND DOSAGE

Note: Preferred route is IV, but IM may be used in infants or other patients without venous access.

Adjunct to General Anesthesia

- **IM, IV (Adults):** 6–9 mg initially, followed by 3–4.5 mg in 3–5 min if needed. Additional doses of 3 mg (0.165 mg/kg) may be given as need is determined.
- **IV (Infants and Children):** 0.5 mg/kg.
- **IV (Neonates–4 wk):** 0.25–0.5 mg/kg.

Adjunct to Electroconvulsive Therapy

- **IV (Adults):** 0.165 mg/kg (initial doses should be 3 mg less than calculated dose).

Aid to Mechanical Ventilation

- **IV (Adults):** 1 mg (0.0165 mg/kg), subsequent doses may be given as necessary.

Diagnoses of Myasthenia Gravis

- **IV (Adults):** 0.004–0.033 mg/kg. Note: profound myasthenic symptoms may occur.

PHARMACODYNAMICS (skeletal muscle paralysis)

	ONSET	PEAK	DURATION*
IV	1 min	2–5 min	20–90 min
IM	15–25 min	UK	UK

*Duration increases with repeated doses.

NURSING IMPLICATIONS

Assessment

- □ Assess respiratory status continuously throughout use of tubocurarine. Notify physician of significant changes immediately.
- □ Neuromuscular response to tubocurarine should be monitored intraoperatively with a peripheral nerve stimulator. Paralysis is intially selective and usually occurs consecutively in the following muscles: levator muscles of eyelids, muscles of mastication, limb muscles, abdominal muscles, muscles of the glottis, intercostal muscles, and the diaphragm. Recovery of muscle function usually occurs in reverse order.
- □ Monitor ECG, heart rate, and blood pressure throughout use of tubocurarine.
- □ Observe patient for residual weakness and respiratory distress during the recovery period.
- ▪ **Toxicity and Overdose:** If overdose occurs use peripheral nerve stimulator to determine the degree of neuromuscular blockade. Maintain airway patency and ventilation until recovery of normal respiration occurs.
- □ Administer anticholinesterase agents (edrophonium, neostigmine, pyridostigmine) to antagonize the action of tubocurarine. Atropine is usually administered prior to or concurrently with anticholinesterase agents to counteract the muscarinic effects.
- □ Administration of fluids and vasopressors may be necessary to treat severe hypotension or shock.

Potential Nursing Diagnoses

- Breathing pattern, ineffective (indications).
- Communication, impaired: verbal (side effects).
- Fear (patient/family teaching).

Implementation

- ▪ **General Info:** Tubocurarine should be used only by individuals experienced in endotracheal intubation, and equipment for this procedure should be immediately available.
- □ Tubocurarine has no effect on consciousness or the pain threshold. Adequate anesthesia should *always* be used when tubocurarine is used as an adjunct to surgical procedures or when painful procedures are performed. Benzodiazepines and/or analgesics should be administered concurrently when prolonged tubocurarine therapy is used for ventilator patients, as patient is awake and able to feel all sensations.

- ◻ If eyes remain open throughout prolonged administration, protect corneas with artificial tears.
- ▪ **Direct IV:** Administer IV dose undiluted over 1–1.5 min. Rapid injection or large doses cause histamine release, resulting in hypotension and bronchospasm. Titrate dose to patient response.
- ▪ **Syringe Compatibility:** pentobarbital or thiopental.
- ▪ **Solution Compatibility:** dextrose in Ringer's or lactated Ringer's combinations, dextrose in saline combinations, D5W, D10W, 0.45% NaCl, 0.9% NaCl, or Ringer's and lactated Ringer's injection.
- ▪ **Additive Incompatibility:** Incompatible with most barbiturates, sodium bicarbonate, and trimethaphan.

PATIENT/FAMILY TEACHING

- ◻ Explain all procedures to patient receiving tubocurarine therapy without anesthesia, as consciousness is not affected by tubocurarine alone. Provide emotional support.
- ◻ Reassure patient that communication abilities will return as the medication wears off.

EVALUATION

Effectiveness of therapy can be demonstrated by: ▪ Adequate suppression of the twitch response when tested with peripheral nerve stimulation and subsequent muscle paralysis ▪ Diagnosis of myasthenia gravis.

UROKINASE
(yoor-oh-**kye**-nase)
Abbokinase, Abbokinase Open-Cath

CLASSIFICATION(S):
Thrombolytic agent
Pregnancy Category B

INDICATIONS

▪ Treatment of acute, massive pulmonary emboli ▪ Lysis of coronary artery thrombi ▪ Management of occluded of IV catheters.

ACTION

▪ Directly activates plasminogen. **Therapeutic Effect:** ▪ Lysis of thrombi or emboli.

PHARMACOKINETICS

Absorption: Administered IV only, resulting in complete bioavailability.
Distribution: Distribution not known.
Metabolism and Excretion: Metabolized by the liver.
Half-life: 10–20 min.

CONTRAINDICATIONS AND PRECAUTIONS

Contraindicated in: ▪ Hypersensitivity ▪ Active internal bleeding ▪ Recent (<2 mon) cerebrovascular accident ▪ Intracranial or intraspinal surgery or intracranial neoplasm.

Use Cautiously in: ▪ Recent (<2 mon) minor trauma or surgery ▪ Patients who are at risk of left heart thrombus ▪ Cerebrovascular disease ▪ Diabetic hemorrhagic retinopathy ▪ Pregnancy, lactation, or children (safety not established) ▪ Elderly patients (increased risk of intracranial bleeding).

ADVERSE REACTIONS AND SIDE EFFECTS*

Resp: bronchospasm.
Derm: rash.
Hemat: BLEEDING.
Misc: fever, hypersensitivity reactions, including ANAPHYLAXIS.

INTERACTIONS

Drug-Drug: ▪ Concurrent use with other **anticoagulants, cefamandole, cefotetan, moxalactam, plicamycin,** or **agents affecting platelet function,** including **aspirin, nonsteroidal anti-inflammatory agents,** or **dipyridamole** increases the risk of bleeding.

*Underlines indicate most frequent; **CAPITALS** indicate life-threatening.

ROUTE AND DOSAGE

Lysis of Coronary Thrombi, Myocardial Infarction

- **Intracoronary (Adults):** (preceded by 2500–10,000 units of heparin IV) 6000 IU/min for up to 2 hr.

Pulmonary Emboli, Deep Vein Thrombosis

- **IV (Adults):** 4400 IU/kg loading dose over 10 min followed by 4400 IU/kg/hr for 12 hr.

Occluded IV Catheters

- **Into Catheter (Adults):** 1–1.8 ml of 5000 IU/ml soln injected into catheter, then aspirated; may repeat q 5 min for 30 min; if no result may cap and leave in catheter for 30–60 min, then aspirate.

PHARMACODYNAMICS (thrombolysis)

	ONSET	PEAK	DURATION
IV	immediate	rapid	up to 12 hr

NURSING IMPLICATIONS

Assessment

- Monitor vital signs, including temperature, closely during course of therapy.
- Assess patient carefully for bleeding every 15 min during the first hr of therapy, every 15–30 min during the next 8 hr, and at least every 4 hr for the duration of therapy. Frank bleeding may occur from invasive sites or body orifices. Internal bleeding may also occur (decreased neurologic status, abdominal pain with coffee ground emesis or black tarry stools, joint pain). If bleeding occurs, stop medication and notify physician immediately.
- Inquire about previous reaction to urokinase therapy. Assess patient for hypersensitivity reaction (rash, dyspnea) or fever. If these occur, inform physician promptly. Keep epinephrine, an antihistamine, and resuscitation equipment close by in the event of an anaphylactic reaction.
- **Coronary Thrombosis:** Monitor ECG continuously. Notify physician if significant arrhythmias occur. IV lidocaine or procainamide (Pronestyl) may be ordered prophylactically. Cardiac enzymes should be monitored.
- **Pulmonary Embolism:** Monitor pulse, blood pressure, hemodynamics, and respiratory status (rate, degree of dyspnea, ABGs).
- **Deep Vein Thrombosis/Acute Arterial Occlusion:** Observe extremities and palpate pulses of affected extremities every hr. Notify physician immediately if circulatory impairment occurs.
- **Cannula/Catheter Occlusion:** Assess ability to aspirate blood as indicator of patency. Ensure that patient exhales and holds breath when connecting and disconnecting IV syringe, to prevent air embolism.
- **Lab Test Considerations:** Hematocrit, hemoglobin, platelet count, prothrombin time, thrombin time, and activated partial thromboplastin time should be evaluated prior to and frequently throughout course of therapy. Bleeding time may be assessed prior to therapy if patient has received platelet aggregation inhibitors.
- Obtain type and cross-match and have blood available at all times in case of hemorrhage.
- **Toxicity and Overdose:** If local bleeding occurs, apply pressure to site. If severe or internal bleeding occurs, discontinue infusion. Clotting factors and/or blood volume may be restored through infusions of whole blood, packed red blood cells, fresh frozen plasma, or cryoprecipitate. Do not administer dextran, as it has antiplatelet activity. Aminocaproic acid (Amicar) may be used as an antidote.

Potential Nursing Diagnoses

- Tissue perfusion, altered (indications).
- Injury, high risk for (side effects).

Implementation

- **General Info:** This medication should

be used only in settings where hematologic function and clinical response can be adequately monitored.

- Invasive procedures, such as IM injections or arterial punctures, should be avoided with this therapy. If such procedures must be performed, apply pressure to IV puncture sites for at least 15 min and to arterial puncture sites for at least 30 min.
- Systemic anticoagulation with heparin is usually begun several hrs after the completion of thrombolytic therapy.
- **Intermittent Infusion:** Reconstitute each vial with 5.2 of ml sterile water for injection without preservatives (direct to sides of vial) and swirl gently; do not shake. Dilute further with 190 ml of 0.9% NaCl or D5W. Use reconstituted soln immediately after preparation.
- *Rate:* Infuse as directed by physician through a 0.22- or 0.45-micron filter. Administer via infusion pump to ensure accurate dosage.
- **Additive Incompatibility:** Manufacturer recommends not admixing with any medications.
- **Cannula/Catheter Clearance:** Add 1 ml of the previously reconstituted drug to 9 ml of sterile water for injection without preservatives. Inject 1 ml slowly and gently into occluded cannula, and then clamp for 5 min. Aspirate contents carefully to remove clot. If unsuccessful, reclamp for 5 min. Repeat aspiration every 5 min until clot clears or for 30 min. If still unsuccessful, clamp for 30–60 min and attempt to aspirate again. A second dose of urokinase may be needed.
- Available in a dual-chamber vial, which reconstitutes to 5000 IU/ml concentration for clearance of occluded cannulae and catheters.

Patient/Family Teaching

- Explain purpose of medication to patient. Instruct patient to report hypersensitivity reactions (rash, dyspnea), bleeding or bruising.
- Explain need for bed rest and minimal handling during therapy to avoid injury.

Evaluation

Effectiveness of therapy can be demonstrated by: ▪ Lysis of thrombi and restoration of blood flow ▪ Cannula or catheter patency.

VALPROIC ACID

(val-**pro**-ik **as**-id)
Dalpro, Depakene, Deproic, Myproic Acid

DIVALPROEX SODIUM

(dye-val-**pro**-ex **soe**-dee-um)
Depakote, {Epival}

CLASSIFICATION(S):
Anticonvulsant—miscellaneous
Pregnancy Category D

INDICATIONS

▪ Treatment of simple and complex absence seizures. **Unlabeled Uses:** ▪ Treatment of partial seizures with complex symptomatology ▪ Myoclonic seizures ▪ Tonic-clonic seizures.

ACTION

▪ Increases levels of gamma aminobutyric acid (GABA), an inhibitory neurotransmitter in the CNS. **Therapeutic Effect:** ▪ Suppression of absence seizures.

PHARMACOKINETICS

Absorption: Well absorbed from the GI tract following oral administration. Divalproex is enteric-coated and absorption is delayed by 1 hr.

Distribution: Rapidly distributed into plasma and extracellular water. Crosses blood-brain barrier and placenta and enters breast milk.

Metabolism and Excretion: Mostly metabolized by the liver, minimal amounts excreted unchanged in the urine.

Half-life: 5–20 hr.

{} = Available in Canada only.

CONTRAINDICATIONS AND PRECAUTIONS

Contraindicated in: ▪ Hypersensitivity ▪ Hepatic impairment.

Use Cautiously in: ▪ Bleeding disorders ▪ Pregnancy and lactation (safety not established) ▪ History of liver disease ▪ Organic brain disease ▪ Bone marrow depression ▪ Renal impairment ▪ Children (increased risk of hepatotoxicity).

ADVERSE REACTIONS AND SIDE EFFECTS*

CNS: drowsiness, sedation, headache, dizziness, ataxia, confusion.

EENT: visual disturbances.

GI: nausea, vomiting, indigestion, HEPATOTOXICITY, pancreatitis, hypersalivation, anorexia, increased appetite, diarrhea, constipation.

Derm: rashes.

Hemat: prolonged bleeding time, leukopenia, thrombocytopenia.

Metab: hyperammonemia.

Neuro: paresthesia.

INTERACTIONS

Drug-Drug: ▪ Increased risk of bleeding with **antiplatelet agents** (including **aspirin** and **nonsteroidal anti-inflammatory agents**), **heparin, thrombolytic agents,** or **warfarin** ▪ Decreases the metabolism of **barbiturates** and **primidone**, increasing risk of toxicity ▪ Additive CNS depression with other **CNS depressants**, including **alcohol, antihistamines, antidepressants, narcotic analgesics, MAO inhibitors,** and **sedative/hypnotics** ▪ May increase or decrease the effects and toxicity of **phenytoin** ▪ **MAO inhibitors** and other **antidepressants** may lower seizure threshold and decrease effectiveness of valproates ▪ **Carbamazepine** may decrease valproic acid blood levels ▪ Valproic acid may increase toxicity of **carbamazepine**.

ROUTE AND DOSAGE

Note: Doses expressed in mg of valproic acid.

▪ **PO (Adults and Children):** Initial dose of 15 mg/kg/day, increase by 5–10 mg/kg/day at weekly intervals until therapeutic levels are reached (not to exceed 60 mg/kg/day). When daily dosage exceeds 250 mg, give in 2 divided doses.

PHARMACODYNAMICS (onset = anticonvulsant effect; peak = blood levels)

	ONSET	PEAK	DURATION
PO—liquid	2–4 days	15–120 min	24 hr
PO—capsules	2–4 days	1–4 hr	24 hr
PO—enteric-coated tab	2–4 days	3–5 hr	24 hr

NURSING IMPLICATIONS

Assessment

- Assess location, duration, and characteristics of seizure activity. Institute seizure precautions.
- **Lab Test Considerations:** Monitor CBC prior to and periodically throughout course of therapy. May cause leukopenia and thrombocytopenia.
- Monitor hepatic function (LDH, SGPT [ALT], SGOT [AST], and bilirubin) prior to and periodically throughout course of therapy. May cause hepatotoxicity; monitor closely, especially during initial 6 mon of therapy.
- May interfere with accuracy of thyroid function tests. May cause false-positive results in urine ketone tests.

Potential Nursing Diagnoses

- Injury, high risk for (indications).
- Knowledge deficit related to medication regimen (patient/family teaching).

Implementation

- **General Info:** Single daily doses are usually administered at bedtime because of sedation.
- **PO:** Administer with or immediately after meals to minimize GI irritation.

*Underlines indicate most frequent; **CAPITALS** indicate life-threatening.

Swallow capsules and enteric-coated tablets whole; do not break or chew, as this will cause irritation of the mouth or throat. Do not administer tablets with milk, to prevent premature dissolution.

- Shake liquid preparations well before pouring. Use calibrated measuring device to ensure accurate dosage. Syrup may be mixed with food or other liquids to improve taste.

Patient/Family Teaching

- Instruct patient to take medication exactly as directed. If a dose is missed on a once-a-day schedule it should be taken as soon as remembered that day. If on a multiple-dose schedule, take within 6 hr of the scheduled time; then space remaining doses throughout the remainder of the day. Abrupt withdrawal may lead to status epilepticus.
- May cause drowsiness or dizziness. Caution patient to avoid driving or other activities requiring alertness until effects of medication are known.
- Caution patient to avoid taking alcohol, CNS depressants, or over-the-counter medications concurrently with valproates without consulting physician or pharmacist.
- Instruct patient to notify physician or dentist of medication regimen prior to treatment or surgery. Patient should also carry identification describing medication regimen at all times.
- Advise patient to notify physician if anorexia, severe nausea and vomiting, yellow skin or eyes, fever, sore throat, malaise, weakness, facial edema, lethargy, unusual bleeding or bruising, pregnancy, or loss of seizure control occur. Children <2 yrs of age are especially at risk for fatal hepatotoxicity.
- Emphasize the importance of routine examinations to monitor progress.

Evaluation

Effectiveness of therapy can be demonstrated by: ▪ Decrease or cessation of seizures without excessive sedation.

VANCOMYCIN

(van-koe-**mye**-sin)
Vancocin

CLASSIFICATION(S):
Anti-infective—miscellaneous
Pregnancy Category C

INDICATIONS

▪ **IV:** Treatment of potentially life-threatening infections when less toxic anti-infectives are contraindicated. Particularly useful in staphylococcal infections, including: ▫ Endocarditis ▫ Osteomyelitis ▫ Pneumonia ▫ Septicemia ▫ Soft tissue infections in patients who have allergies to penicillin or its derivatives or where sensitivity testing demonstrates resistance to methicillin ▪ **PO:** Treatment of pseudomembranous colitis due to *Clostridium difficile* ▪ **IV:** Part of endocarditis prophylaxis in high-risk patients who are allergic to penicillin.

ACTION

▪ Binds to bacterial cell wall, resulting in cell death. **Therapeutic Effect:** ▪ Bactericidal action against susceptible organisms. **Spectrum:** ▪ Active against gram-positive pathogens, including: ▫ Staphylococci (including methicillin-resistant strains of *Staphylococcus aureus*) ▫ Group A beta-hemolytic streptococci ▫ *Streptococcus pneumoniae* ▫ *Corynebacterium* ▫ *Clostridium*.

PHARMACOKINETICS

Absorption: Poorly absorbed from the GI tract.

Distribution: Widely distributed. Some penetration (20–30%) of CSF. Crosses placenta.

Metabolism and Excretion: Oral doses excreted primarily in the feces. IV vancomycin eliminated almost entirely by the kidneys.

Half-life: 6 hr (increased in renal impairment).

CONTRAINDICATIONS AND PRECAUTIONS

Contraindicated in: ▪ Hypersensitivity.

Use Cautiously in: ▪ Renal impairment (dosage reduction required) ▪ Pregnancy and lactation (safety not established) ▪ Hearing impairment ▪ Intestinal obstruction or inflammation (increased systemic absorption when given orally).

ADVERSE REACTIONS AND SIDE EFFECTS*

Note: Associated with IV administration unless otherwise indicated.

EENT: IV and PO—ototoxicity.

CV: hypotension.

GI: nausea, PO—vomiting, unpleasant taste.

GU: nephrotoxicity.

Derm: rashes.

Hemat: leukopenia, eosinophilia.

Local: phlebitis.

MS: back and neck pain.

Misc: hypersensitivity reactions, including **ANAPHYLAXIS**; fever, chills, red man syndrome, superinfection.

INTERACTIONS

Drug-Drug: ▪ May cause additive ototoxicity and nephrotoxicity with other **ototoxic** and **nephrotoxic drugs (aspirin, aminoglycosides, cyclosporine, cisplatin, loop diuretics)**.

ROUTE AND DOSAGE

Serious Systemic Infections

- **IV (Adults):** 500 mg q 6 hr or 1 g q 12 hr.
- **IV (Children):** 40 mg/kg/day in divided doses q 6–12 hr.
- **IV (Neonates 1 wk–1 mon):** 15 mg/kg initially, then 10 kg/kg q 8 hr.
- **IV (Neonates <1 wk):** 15 mg/kg initially, then 10 mg/kg q 12 hr.

Endocarditis Prophylaxis in Penicillin-Allergic Patients

- **IV (Adults and Children >27 kg):** 1 g single dose 1 hr preprocedure.
- **IV (Children <27 kg):** 20 mg/kg single dose 1 hr preprocedure.

Pseudomembranous Colitis

- **PO (Adults):** 0.5–2 g/day in divided doses q 6–8 hr.
- **PO (Children):** 40 mg/kg/day in divided doses q 6–8 hr (not to exceed 2 g/day).

PHARMACODYNAMICS (blood levels)

	ONSET	PEAK
IV	rapid	end of infusion

NURSING IMPLICATIONS

Assessment

- Assess patient for infection (vital signs; appearance of wound, sputum, urine, and stool; WBC) at beginning and throughout course of therapy.
- Obtain specimens for culture and sensitivity prior to initiating therapy. First dose may be given before receiving results.
- Monitor IV site closely. Vancomycin is irritating to tissues and causes necrosis and severe pain with extravasation. Rotate infusion site.
- Monitor blood pressure throughout IV infusion.
- Evaluate eighth cranial nerve function by audiometry and serum vancomycin levels prior to and throughout course of therapy in patients with borderline renal function or those >60 yr. Prompt recognition and intervention is essential in preventing permanent damage.
- Monitor intake and output ratios and daily weight. Cloudy or pink urine may be a sign of nephrotoxicity.
- Assess patient for signs of superinfection (black, furry overgrowth on tongue, vaginal itching or discharge, loose or foul-smelling stools). Report occurrence to physician.
- ▪ **Pseudomembranous Colitis:** Assess bowel status (bowel sounds, frequency and consistency of stools,

*Underlines indicate most frequent; **CAPITALS** indicate life-threatening.

presence of blood in stools) throughout therapy.

- **Lab Test Considerations:** Monitor for casts, albumin, or cells in the urine or decreased specific gravity, CBC, and renal function periodically throughout course of therapy.
- May cause increased BUN levels.
- **Toxicity and Overdose:** Peak serum vancomycin levels should not exceed 5–40 mcg/ml. Trough concentrations should not exceed 5–10 mcg/ml.

Potential Nursing Diagnoses

- Infection, high risk for (indications).
- Sensory-perceptual alteration: auditory (side effects).
- Knowledge deficit related to medication regimen (patient/family teaching).

Implementation

- **General Info:** Available in capsule, oral soln, and injectable forms.
- **PO:** Use calibrated measuring device for liquid preparations. IV dosage form may be diluted in 30 ml of water for oral or nasogastric tube administration. Resulting soln has a bitter, unpleasant taste. Stable for 14 days if refrigerated.
- **Intermittent Infusion:** Dilute each 500-mg vial with 10 ml of sterile water for injection. Dilute further with 100–200 ml of 0.9% NaCl, D5W, D10W, or lactated Ringer's soln. Soln is stable for 14 days after initial reconstitution if refrigerated. After further dilution, soln is stable for 96 hr if refrigerated.
- *Rate:* Administer over 60 min. Do not administer rapidly or as a bolus to minimize risk of thrombophlebitis, hypotension, and red man or red neck syndrome (sudden severe hypotension, flushing and/or maculopapular rash of face, neck, chest, upper extremities).
- **Continuous Infusion:** Should be used only if intermittent infusion is not feasible.
- *Rate:* May also be prepared as a continuous infusion with 1–2 g in sufficient volume to infuse over 24 hr.
- **Syringe Incompatibility:** heparin.
- **Y-Site Compatibility:** acyclovir, atracurium, cyclophosphamide, enalaprilat, esmolol, hydromorphone, labetalol, magnesium sulfate, meperidine, morphine, ondonsetron, pancuronium, perphenazine, tolazoline, vecuronium, or zidovudine.
- **Y-Site Incompatibility:** foscarnet.
- **Additive Compatibility:** amikacin, calcium gluconate, cimetidine, corticotroprin, dimenhydrinate, hydrocortisone sodium succinate, potassium chloride, ranitidine, or verapamil.
- **Additive Incompatibility:** amobarbital, chloramphenicol, chlorothiazide, dexamethasone, heparin, methicillin, pentobarbital, phenobarbital, secobarbital, or warfarin.

Patient/Family Teaching

- Advise patients on oral vancomycin to take exactly as directed. Missed doses should be taken as soon as remembered, unless almost time for next dose; do not double doses.
- Instruct patient to report signs of hypersensitivity, tinnitus, vertigo, or hearing loss.
- Advise patient to notify physician if no improvement is seen in a few days.
- Patients with a history of rheumatic heart disease or valve replacement need to be taught the importance of using antimicrobial prophylaxis prior to invasive dental or medical procedures.

Evaluation

Clinical response can be evaluated by:
- Resolution of the signs and symptoms of infection. Length of time for complete resolution depends on organism and site of infection ▪ Endocarditis prophylaxis.

VASOPRESSIN

(vay-soe-**press**-in)
Pitressin

CLASSIFICATION(S):
Hormone—antidiuretic
Pregnancy Category UK

INDICATIONS

▪ Treatment of central diabetes insipidus due to deficient antidiuretic hormone ▪ Management of abdominal distention ▪ Used to eliminate gas shadows during abdominal x-rays. **Unlabeled Use:** ▪ Management of GI bleeding (IV or by selective intra-arterial infusion).

ACTION

▪ Alters the permeability of the renal collecting ducts, allowing reabsorption of water ▪ Direct stimulant effect on musculature of the GI tract ▪ Vasoconstriction (large doses). **Therapeutic Effects:** ▪ Decreased urine output and increased urine osmolality in diabetes insipidus ▪ Relief of abdominal distention ▪ Decreased GI bleeding.

PHARMACOKINETICS

Absorption: IM absorption may be unpredictable.
Distribution: Widely distributed throughout extracellular fluid.
Metabolism and Excretion: Rapidly degraded by the liver and kidneys. Small amounts (<5%) excreted unchanged by the kidneys.
Half-life: 10–20 min.

CONTRAINDICATIONS AND PRECAUTIONS

Contraindicated in: ▪ Chronic renal failure with increased BUN ▪ Hypersensitivity to beef or pork proteins.
Use Cautiously in: ▪ Perioperative polyuria (increased sensitivity to vasopressin) ▪ Comatose patients ▪ Seizures ▪ Migraine headaches ▪ Asthma ▪ Heart failure ▪ Cardiovascular disease ▪ Elderly patients and children (increased sensitivity to vasopressin) ▪ Renal impairment.

ADVERSE REACTIONS AND SIDE EFFECTS*

CNS: dizziness, "pounding" sensation in head.
CV: chest pain, MYOCARDIAL INFARCTION, angina.
GI: abdominal cramps, belching, diarrhea, nausea, vomiting, flatulence, heartburn.
Derm: sweating, paleness, perioral blanching.
Neuro: trembling.
Misc: water intoxication (high doses only), fever, allergic reactions.

INTERACTIONS

Drug-Drug: ▪ Antidiuretic effect may be decreased by concurrent administration of **alcohol, lithium, demeclocycline, heparin,** or **norepinephrine** ▪ Antidiuretic effect may be increased by concurrent administration of **carbamazepine, chlorpropamide, clofibrate,** or **fludrocortisone** ▪ Vasopressor effect may be increased by concurrent administration of **ganglionic blocking agents.**

ROUTE AND DOSAGE

Central Diabetes Insipidus

- **IM, SC (Adults):** 5–10 units 2–3 times daily.
- **IM, SC (Children):** 2.5–10 units 3–4 times daily.

Abdominal Distention

- **IM (Adults):** 5 units initially, may increase to 10 units if needed q 3–4 hr.

Preparation for GI X-Rays

- **IM, SC (Adults):** 10 units at 2 hr and again at 30 min prior to x-rays.

GI Bleeding

- **IV (Adults):** 0.2–0.4 units/min, may be increased up to 0.9 units/min.
- **Intra-arterial (Adults):** 0.1–0.5 units/min.

PHARMACODYNAMICS (antidiuretic effect)

	ONSET	PEAK	DURATION
IM	UK	UK	2–8 hr

NURSING IMPLICATIONS

ASSESSMENT

- **General Info:** Monitor ECG periodically throughout therapy.
- **Diabetes Insipidus:** Monitor urine osmolality and urine volume frequently

*Underlines indicate most frequent; CAPITALS indicate life-threatening.

to determine effects of medication. Assess patient for symptoms of dehydration (excessive thirst, dry skin and mucous membranes, tachycardia, poor skin turgor). Weigh patient daily, monitor intake and output, and assess for edema.

- **GI Hemorrhage:** Monitor abdominal status (distension, bowel sounds, presence of blood in nasogastric aspirate or stool). Also monitor for signs and symptoms of hypovolemia leading to shock (decreased blood pressure, tachycardia, diaphoresis).
- **Lab Test Considerations:** Monitor urine specific gravity throughout course of therapy.
- □ Monitor serum electrolyte concentrations periodically throughout therapy.
- **Toxicity and Overdose:** Signs and symptoms of water intoxication include confusion, drowsiness, headache, weight gain, difficulty urinating, seizures, and coma.
- □ Treatment of overdose includes water restriction and temporary discontinuation of vasopressin until polyuria occurs. If symptoms are severe, administration of mannitol, hypertonic dextrose, urea, and/or furosemide may be used.

Potential Nursing Diagnoses

- Fluid volume deficit (indications).
- Fluid volume excess (adverse reactions).
- Knowledge deficit related to medication regimen (patient/family teaching).

Implementation

- **General Info:** Aqueous vasopressin injection may be administered SC or IM for diabetes insipidus, or IV or intra-arterially for GI hemorrhage.
- □ Administer 1–2 glasses of water at the time of administration to minimize side effects (blanching of skin, abdominal cramps, nausea).
- **Continuous Infusion:** Vasopressin injection may be diluted to a concentration of 0.1–1 unit/ml with 0.9% NaCl or D5W.
- □ *Rate:* Titrate dose according to patient response. Administer via infusion pump for accurate dosage.

Patient/Family Teaching

- □ Instruct patient to take medication exactly as directed. Do not use more than the prescribed amount. Missed doses should be taken as soon as remembered, unless almost time for next dose.
- □ Advise patient to drink 1–2 glasses of water at the time of administration to minimize side effects (blanching of skin, abdominal cramps, nausea). Inform patient that these side effects are not serious and usually disappear in a few mins.
- □ Caution patient to avoid concurrent use of alcohol while taking vasopressin.
- □ Patients with diabetes insipidus should carry identification describing disease process and medication regimen at all times.

Evaluation

Effectiveness of therapy can be demonstrated by: ▪ Decrease in urine volume □ Relief of polydipsia □ Increased urine osmolality in patients with central diabetes insipidus ▪ Prevention and treatment of abdominal distention ▪ Control of GI hemorrhage.

VECURONIUM

(ve-kure-**oh**-nee-yum)
Norcuron

CLASSIFICATION(S):
Neuromuscular blocking agent—nondepolarizing
Pregnancy Category C

INDICATIONS

▪ Production of skeletal muscle paralysis and facilitation of intubation after induction of anesthesia in surgical procedures ▪ Used during mechanical ventilation to increase pulmonary compliance.

ACTION

▪ Prevents neuromuscular transmission by blocking the effect of acetylcholine at the myoneural junction ▪ Has no analgesic or anxiolytic effects. **Therapeutic Effect:** ▪ Skeletal muscle paralysis.

PHARMACOKINETICS

Absorption: Administered IV only, resulting in complete bioavailability.
Distribution: Rapidly distributed in extracellular fluid. Minimal penetration of the CNS.
Metabolism and Excretion: Some metabolism by the liver (20%), with conversion to at least one active metabolite. 35% excreted unchanged by the kidneys.
Half-life: 31–80 min (decreased near term in pregnant patients, increased in patients with hepatic impairment).

CONTRAINDICATIONS AND PRECAUTIONS

Contraindicated in: ▪ Hypersensitivity to vecuronium or bromides.
Use Cautiously in: ▪ Patients with any history of pulmonary or cardiovascular disease or renal or liver impairment ▪ Elderly or debilitated patients ▪ Electrolyte disturbances ▪ Myasthenia gravis or myasthenic syndromes (extreme caution) ▪ Pregnancy or lactation (safety not estblished) ▪ Infants <7 wk (safety not established) ▪ Children 7 wk–1 yr (increased sensitivity resulting in prolonged recovery time).

ADVERSE REACTIONS AND SIDE EFFECTS*

Note: Most adverse reactions to vecuronium are extensions of pharmacologic effects.
Resp: APNEA, respiratory insufficiency.
MS: muscle weakness.
Misc: allergic reactions.

INTERACTIONS

Drug-Drug: ▪ Intensity and duration of paralysis may be prolonged by pretreatment with **succinylcholine, general anesthesia, aminoglycoside antibiotics, polymyxin B, colistin, clindamycin, lidocaine, quinidine, procainamide, beta-adrenergic blocking agents, potassium-losing diuretics,** and **magnesium** ▪ Additive neuromuscular blockade with **inhalation anesthetics**—decrease vecuronium dose by 15% when used with **enflurane** or **isoflurane,** and decrease dose of anesthetic by 30–50%.

ROUTE AND DOSAGE

- **IV (Adults):** Initial dose 80–100 mcg/kg after steady-state anesthesia achieved or 40–60 mcg/kg after succinylcholine-assisted intubation and anesthesia (wait for disappearance of succinylcholine effects). Up to 150–280 mcg/kg as been used in some patients. Then maintenance dose of 10–15 mcg/kg 25–40 min after initial dose, then q 12–15 min as needed or as a continuous infusion at 1 mcg/kg/min (range 0.8–1.2 mcg/kg/min).

PHARMACODYNAMICS (skeletal muscle paralysis)

	ONSET	PEAK	DURATION
IV	1 min	3–5 min	15–25 min

NURSING IMPLICATIONS

Assessment

- Assess respiratory status continuously throughout use of vecuronium. Notify physician of significant changes immediately.
- Neuromuscular response to vecuronium should be monitored intraoperatively with a peripheral nerve stimulator. Paralysis is initially selective and usually occurs consecutively in the following muscles: levator muscles of eyelids, muscles of mastication, limb muscles, abdominal muscles, muscles of the glottis, intercostal muscles, and the diaphragm. Recovery of muscle function usually occurs in reverse order.
- Monitor ECG, heart rate, and blood

*Underlines indicate most frequent; **CAPITALS** indicate life-threatening.

pressure throughout use of vecuronium.

- □ Observe patient for residual muscle weakness and respiratory distress during the recovery period.
- ■ **Toxicity and Overdose:** If overdose occurs use peripheral nerve stimulator to determine the degree of neuromuscular blockade. Maintain airway patency and ventilation until recovery of normal respiration occurs.
- □ Administer anticholinesterase agents (edrophonium, neostigmine, pyridostigmine) to antagonize the action of vecuronium. Atropine is usually administered prior to or concurrently with anticholinesterase agents to counteract the muscarinic effects.
- □ Administration of fluids and vasopressors may be necessary to treat severe hypotension or shock.

Potential Nursing Diagnoses

- ■ Breathing pattern, ineffective (indications).
- ■ Communication, impaired: verbal (side effects).
- ■ Fear (patient/family teaching).

Implementation

- ■ **General Info:** Vecuronium should be used only by individuals experienced in endotracheal intubation, and equipment for this procedure should be immediately available.
- □ Vecuronium has no effect on consciousness or the pain threshold. Adequate anesthesia should *always* be used when vecuronium is used as an adjunct to surgical procedures or when painful procedures are performed. Benzodiazepines and/or analgesics should be administered concurrently when prolonged vecuronium therapy is used for ventilator patients, as patient is awake and able to feel all sensations.
- □ If eyes remain open throughout prolonged administration, protect corneas with artificial tears.
- ■ **IV:** Reconstitute vecuronium with bacteriostatic water (may be provided by manufacturer), D5W, 0.9% NaCl, D5/0.9% NaCl, or lactated Ringer's injection. Soln reconstituted with bacteriostatic water is stable if refrigerated for 5 days. If other diluents are used, soln is stable for 24 hr if refrigerated. Discard all unused soln.
- ■ **Direct IV:** Reconstitute each dose in 5–10 ml. Titrate dose according to patient response.
- ■ **Continuous Infusion:** Dilute vecuronium to a concentration of 10–20 mg/100 ml.
- □ *Rate:* Titrate rate of infusion according to patient response.
- ■ **Syringe/Y-Site Incompatibility:** Incompatible in syringe or via Y-site injection with most barbiturates.

Patient/Family Teaching

- □ Explain all procedures to patient receiving vecuronium therapy without anesthesia, as consciousness is not affected by vecuronium alone. Provide emotional support.
- □ Reassure patient that communication abilities will return as the medication wears off.

Evaluation

Effectiveness of therapy can be demonstrated by: ■ Adequate suppression of the twitch response when tested with peripheral nerve stimulation and subsequent muscle paralysis.

VERAPAMIL

(ver-**ap**-a-mil)
Calan, Calan SR, Isoptin, Isoptin SR, Verelan

CLASSIFICATION(S):
Calcium channel blocker, Antianginal, Antihypertensive—calcium channel blocker, Antiarrhythmic—class IV, Coronary vasodilator
Pregnancy Category C

INDICATIONS

■ **PO:** Treatment of angina pectoris ■ **PO:** Management of hypertension ■ **PO, IV:** Control of supraventricular tachyarrhythmias and rapid ventricular rates in atrial flutter or fibrillation. **Unlabeled Uses:** ▪ Relief of ventricular outflow obstruction in the management of hypertrophic cardiomyopathy ▪ Prevention of migraine headaches.

ACTION

▪ Inhibits calcium transport into myocardial and vascular smooth muscle cells, resulting in inhibition of excitation-contraction coupling and subsequent contraction ▪ Decreases SA and AV conduction and prolongs the AV node refractory periods in cardiac conduction tissue. **Therapeutic Effects:** ▪ Coronary vasodilation, resulting in decreased frequency and severity of angina pectoris ▪ Decreased blood pressure ▪ Suppression of supraventricular tachyarrhythmias.

PHARMACOKINETICS

Absorption: Well absorbed following oral administration.
Distribution: Distribution not known. Small amounts enter breast milk.
Metabolism and Excretion: Mostly metabolized by the liver, much of it on first pass through the liver.
Half-life: 4.5–12 hr.

CONTRAINDICATIONS AND PRECAUTIONS

Contraindicated in: ▪ Hypersensitivity ▪ Sinus bradycardia ▪ Advanced heart block ▪ Severe congestive heart failure.
Use Cautiously in: ▪ Liver disease (dosage reduction recommended) ▪ Pregnancy, lactation, or children (safety not established) ▪ Hypertrophic cardiomyopathy (when accompanied by paroxysmal nocturnal dyspnea, orthopnea, left ventricular obstruction, SA node dysfunction, heart block, or elevated pulmonary wedge pressure) ▪ Congestive heart failure ▪ Sick-sinus syndrome ▪ Duchenne's muscular dystrophy (may precipitate respiratory muscle failure).

ADVERSE REACTIONS AND SIDE EFFECTS*

CNS: <u>dizziness</u>, headache, fatigue.
CV: <u>bradycardia</u>, <u>hypotension</u>, <u>edema</u>, heart block, congestive heart failure, SINUS ARREST, ASYSTOLE.
GI: <u>constipation</u>, nausea, abdominal discomfort.
Resp: pulmonary edema.

INTERACTIONS

Drug-Drug: ▪ Increases serum **digoxin** levels and may cause toxicity ▪ Increased risk of bradycardia, congestive heart failure, and arrhythmias when used with **beta-adrenergic blocking agents** or **disopyramide** ▪ Additive hypotension with **antihypertensive agents,** acute ingestion of **alcohol, nitrates,** or **quinidine** ▪ Decreases effectiveness of oral **rifampin** ▪ Increases muscle relaxant effects of **nondepolarizing neuromuscular blockers** ▪ Coadministration with **calcium** and **vitamin D** may result in decreased effectivenes of verapamil ▪ May increase or decrease **lithium** blood levels ▪ Verapamil may decrease metabolism of and increase risk of toxicity from **carbamazepine, cyclosporine, prazosin,** or **quinidine** ▪ Increases anesthetic effect of **etodimate** ▪ Severe hypotension may occur with **fentanyl** ▪ May increase risk of toxicity from **theophylline.**

ROUTE AND DOSAGE

- **PO (Adults):** 80 mg 3–4 times daily, increased in daily or weekly intervals as needed, or 120–240 mg/day as a single dose of extended-release preparation increased in daily or weekly intervals as needed (range 240–480 mg/day).
- **IV (Adults):** 5–10 mg over 2 min, may repeat in 30 min.
- **IV (Children 1–16 yr):** 0.1–0.3 mg/kg over 2 min (with ECG monitoring), may repeat in 30 min. Initial dose not to exceed 5 mg, repeat dose not to exceed 10 mg.

*<u>Underlines</u> indicate most frequent; **CAPITALS** indicate life-threatening.

- **IV (Children <1 yr):** 0.1–0.2 mg/kg over 2 min (with ECG monitoring), may repeat in 30 min.

PHARMACODYNAMICS (cardiovascular effects)

	ONSET	PEAK	DURATION
PO	1–2 hr	30–90 min*	3–7 hr
PO-ER	UK	5–7 hr	24 hr
IV	1–5 min†	3–5 min	2 hr†

*Single dose; effects from multiple doses may not be evident for 24–48 hr.
†Antiarrhythmic effects; hemodynamic effects begin 3–5 min following injection and persist for 10–20 min.

NURSING IMPLICATIONS

Assessment

- **General Info:** Monitor blood pressure and pulse before and frequently during parenteral administration and periodically throughout therapy.
  - Monitor intake and output ratios and daily weight. Assess patient for signs of congestive heart failure (peripheral edema, rales/crackles, dyspnea, weight gain, jugular venous distention).
  - Patients receiving cardiac glycosides concurrently with verapamil should have routine serum digitalis levels and be monitored for signs and symptoms of cardiac glycoside toxicity.
  - Monitor ECG periodically in patients receiving long-term therapy.
- **Angina:** Assess location, duration, intensity, and precipitating factors of patient's anginal pain.
- **Arrhythmias:** ECG should be monitored continuously during IV administration. Notify physician of symptomatic bradycardia or prolonged hypotension promptly. Emergency equipment and medication should be available.
- **Lab Test Considerations:** May cause elevated alkaline phosphatase, CPK, LDH, SGOT (AST), and SGPT (ALT) levels.

Potential Nursing Diagnoses

- Cardiac output, decreased (indications).
- Comfort, altered: pain (indications).
- Knowledge deficit related to medication regimen (patient/family teaching).

Implementation

- **PO:** Administer with meals or milk to minimize gastric irritation.
  - Extended-release tablets should be swallowed whole or broken in half; do not crush or chew.
- **IV:** Patients should remain recumbent for at least 1 hr following IV administration to minimize hypotensive effects.
- **Direct IV:** Administer IV undiluted through Y-site or 3-way stopcock over 2 min for each single dose. Administer over 3 min in elderly patients.
- **Syringe Compatibility:** heparin.
- **Y-Site Compatibility:** amrinone, dobutamine, dopamine, famotidine, methicillin, penicillin G potassium, piperacillin, or ticarcillin.
- **Y-Site Incompatibility:** albumin, ampicillin, mezlocillin, nafcillin, oxacillin, or sodium bicarbonate.

Patient/Family Teaching

- **General Info:** Advise patient to take medication exactly as directed, even if feeling well. Missed doses should be taken as soon as remembered, unless almost time for next dose; do not double doses. Do not discontinue therapy without consulting physician, as gradual dosage reduction may be necessary.
  - Instruct patient or family members to take pulse each day before taking verapamil. Advise patient to notify physician if pulse is irregular or <50 bpm.
  - Caution patient to make position changes slowly to minimize orthostatic hypotension.
  - Verapamil may cause dizziness. Advise patient to avoid driving or other activities requiring alertness until response to the medication is known.
  - Instruct patient to avoid concurrent use of alcohol or over-the-counter medications without consulting physician or pharmacist.

- □ Instruct patient to notify physician if headache is severe or persistent.
- ▪ **Angina:** Instruct patients on concurrent nitrate therapy to continue taking both medications as ordered and using SL nitroglycerin as needed for anginal attacks.
- □ Advise patient to contact physician if chest pain worsens or does not improve after therapy, or is accompanied by diaphoresis or shortness of breath, or if severe, persistent headache occurs.
- □ Advise patient to discuss activity limitations with physician.
- ▪ **Hypertension:** Instruct patient and family on correct method for monitoring blood pressure weekly. Advise patient to notify physician if significant changes occur.
- □ Encourage patient to comply with additional interventions for hypertension (low-sodium diet, regular exercise, weight reduction, stress management, moderation of alcohol consumption, discontinuation of smoking). Verapamil controls but does not cure hypertension.

EVALUATION

Effectiveness of therapy can be demonstrated by: ▪ Decrease in frequency and severity of anginal attacks □ Decreased need for nitrate therapy □ Increase in activity tolerance and sense of well-being ▪ Decrease in blood pressure to normal limits ▪ Resolution and prevention of supraventricular tachyarrhythmias.

VIDARABINE

(vye-**dare**-a-been)
adenine arabinoside, Ara-A, Vira-A

CLASSIFICATION(S):
Antiviral
Pregnancy Category C

INDICATIONS

▪ **IV:** Treatment of: □ Herpes simplex encephalitis □ Serious herpes simplex infections in neonates □ Herpes zoster due to reactivated varicella-zoster inimmunosuppressed patients ▪ **Ophth:** Treatment of herpes simplex keratitis and keratoconjunctivitis. **Unlabeled Use:** ▪ Treatment of varicella-zoster infections in immunosuppressed patients.

ACTION

▪ Appears to inhibit viral DNA synthesis. **Therapeutic Effect:** ▪ Decreased viral replication.

PHARMACOKINETICS

Absorption: Complete bioavailability follows IV administration. No apparent systemic absorption following ophthalmic administration.

Distribution: Widely distributed. Crosses the blood-brain barrier well.

Metabolism and Excretion: 75–90% converted to another active antiviral compound (ara-HX). Both are excreted by the kidneys.

Half-life: Vidarabine—1.5 hr; ara-HX—3.3 hr (both increased in renal impairment).

CONTRAINDICATIONS AND PRECAUTIONS

Contraindicated in: ▪ Hypersensitivity.

Use Cautiously in: ▪ Impaired renal function (dosage reduction required) ▪ Impaired hepatic function ▪ Patients susceptible to fluid overload or cerebral edema.

ADVERSE REACTIONS AND SIDE EFFECTS*

CNS: malaise, weakness, tremors, ataxia, hallucinations, psychoses, confusion, headache, encephalopathy.

Derm: pruritus, rash.

EENT: Ophth—ocular burning, itching, irritation, blurred vision, photophobia.

F and E: hyponatremia, fluid overload.

GI: <u>nausea</u>, <u>vomiting</u>, <u>anorexia</u>, <u>weight loss</u>, <u>diarrhea</u>, <u>GI bleeding</u>, hepatitis.

*<u>Underlines</u> indicate most frequent; **CAPITALS** indicate life-threatening.

Hemat: anemia, leukopenia, thrombocytopenia.
Local: phlebitis at IV site.

INTERACTIONS

Drug–Drug: ▪ Concurrent use with **allopurinol** may increase the risk of adverse reactions (tremors, anemia, nausea, pain, and pruritus).

ROUTE AND DOSAGE

Herpes Simplex Encephalitis

- **IV (Adults and Children):** 15 mg/kg/day for 10 days.

Herpes Simplex Keratitis or Keratoconjunctivitis

- **Ophth (Adults and Children):** 1 cm of 3% ointment in lower conjunctival sac 5 times daily, (q 3 hr).

Herpes Zoster in Immunosuppressed Patients

- **IV (Adults and Children):** 10 mg/kg/day for 5 days.

Varicella-Zoster in Immunosuppressed Patients

- **IV (Adults and Children):** 10 mg/kg/day for 5–7 days.

Herpes Simplex Virus Infections in Neonates

- **IV (Neonates):** 15 mg/kg/day for 10–14 days.

PHARMACODYNAMICS (blood levels)

	ONSET	PEAK	DURATION
IV	rapid	end of infusion	UK

NURSING IMPLICATIONS

Assessment

- **Ophth:** Assess eye lesions prior to and daily during therapy.
- **Encephalitis:** Assess level of consciousness and neurologic status frequently throughout therapy.
- ▫ Assess patient for fluid overload (rales/crackles, dyspnea, weight gain, peripheral edema, jugular venous distention) during IV infusions.
- **Lab Test Considerations:** May cause elevation of SGOT (AST) and total bilirubin.
- ▫ Monitor CBC, WBC, and platelet count periodically throughout therapy.
- ▫ May cause decreased leukocytes, platelets, reticulocytes, hemoglobin, and hematocrit. These effects are usually reversible 3–5 days after discontinuation of therapy.

Potential Nursing Diagnoses

- Infection, high risk for (indications).
- Skin integrity, impaired: actual (indications).
- Knowledge deficit related to medication regimen (patient/family teaching).

Implementation

- **Intermittent Infusion:** Any IV soln is suitable as a diluent, except for blood products or protein soln. Prewarm the IV soln to 35–40°C (95–100°F) to facilitate dilution of the suspension. Shake until completely clear and in soln. Use an in-line filter (0.45-micron pore size or smaller) for final filtration. Dilute just prior to administration and use within 48 hr. Do not refrigerate soln.
- ▫ For adults, dilute each 1 mg of vidarabine in 2.22 ml of soln (450 mg requires 1 liter). Depending on dose, may require more than 1 liter of solution.
- ▫ For neonates, dilute each 200 mg (1 ml) of vidarabine in 9 ml of 0.9% NaCl or sterile water for injection, for a concentration of 20 mg/ml. Withdraw dose from diluted suspension and dilute further in minimum volume (2.22 ml IV fluid per mg of vidarabine).
- ▫ *Rate:* Administer total daily dose for both adults and neonates over 12–24 hr using an infusion pump for accurate regulation.

Patient/Family Teaching

- **Ophth:** Instruct patient on correct application technique for ophthalmic vidarabine. Hold tube in hand for several mins to warm. Lie down or tilt head back and look at ceiling, squeeze a small amount of ointment (¼–½ in) inside lower lid. Do not touch cap or tip of tube to eye, fingers,

or any surface. Close eye gently and roll eyeball around in all directions with eye closed. Wait 10 min before applying any other ointment.
□ Instruct patient to instill vidarabine as directed and not to use more frequently or longer than prescribed. Missed doses should be instilled as soon as remembered, unless almost time for next dose. Advise patient not to discontinue use of ointment without consulting physician. Patient should also contact physician if no improvement is seen in 7 days, condition worsens, or pain, burning, or irritation of the eye occurs.
□ Ointment may cause blurred vision. Caution patient to avoid driving or other activities requiring visual acuity until vision has cleared.
□ Advise patient to wear dark glasses and avoid bright lights to prevent photophobic reactions.
□ Patients with ophthalmic infections should be advised to avoid wearing contact lenses until the infection is resolved and physician approves.
□ Emphasize the importance of follow-up ophthalmic examinations to determine progress.

Evaluation

Effectiveness of therapy can be demonstrated by: ▪ Re-epithelialization of the cornea in herpetic keratitis. Treatment is not usually continued for more than 21 days or 3–5 days after healing has occurred, except in chronic cases or infections that are difficult to cure ▪ Resolution of the signs and symptoms of herpetic encephalitis.

VINBLASTINE

(vin-**blass**-teen)
Velban, {Velbe}

CLASSIFICATION(S):
Antineoplastic agent—vinca alkaloid
Pregnancy Category UK

INDICATIONS

▪ Combination chemotherapy of: □ Lymphomas □ Nonseminomatous testicular carcinoma □ Advanced breast cancer □ Other tumors.

ACTION

▪ Binds to proteins of mitotic spindle, causing metaphase arrest. Cell replication is stopped as a result (cell cycle-specific for M phase). **Therapeutic Effects:** ▪ Death of rapidly replicating cells, particularly malignant ones ▪ Has immunosuppressive properties.

PHARMACOKINETICS

Absorption: Administered IV only, resulting in complete bioavailability.
Distribution: Does not cross the blood-brain barrier well.
Metabolism and Excretion: Converted by the liver to an active antineoplastic compound. Excreted in the feces via biliary excretion, some renal elimination.
Half-life: 24 hr.

CONTRAINDICATIONS AND PRECAUTIONS

Contraindicated in: ▪ Hypersensitivity ▪ Pregnancy or lactation.
Use Cautiously in: ▪ Patients with childbearing potential ▪ Infections ▪ Decreased bone marrow reserve ▪ Other chronic debilitating illnesses.

ADVERSE REACTIONS AND SIDE EFFECTS*

CNS: neurotoxicity, depression, weakness, seizures.
Resp: BRONCHOSPASM.
GI: nausea, vomiting, anorexia, diarrhea, stomatitis, constipation.
GU: gonadal suppression.
Derm: dermatitis, vesiculation, alopecia.
Hemat: anemia, leukopenia, thrombocytopenia.
Local: phlebitis at IV site.
Metab: hyperuricemia.

{} = Available in Canada only.
*Underlines indicate most frequent; **CAPITALS** indicate life-threatening.

Neuro: peripheral neuropathy, paresthesia, neuritis.

INTERACTIONS

Drug–Drug: ▪ Additive bone marrow depression with other **antineoplastic agents** or **radiation therapy** ▪ Bronchospasm may occur in patients who have been previously treated with **mitomycin** ▪ May decrease antibody response to **live virus vaccines** and increase the risk of adverse reactions.

ROUTE AND DOSAGE

Note: Doses may vary greatly depending on tumor, schedule, condition of patient, and blood counts.

- **IV (Adults):** 3.7 mg/m^2, single dose; increase at weekly intervals as tolerated by 1.8 mg/m^2 to a maximum of 18.5 mg/m^2 (usual maintenance dose is 5.5–7.4 mg/m^2).
- **IV (Children):** 2.5 mg/m^2, single dose; increase as tolerated at weekly intervals by 1.25 mg/m^2 to a maximum of 12.5 mg/m^2.

PHARMACODYNAMICS (effects on white blood cell counts)

	ONSET	PEAK	DURATION
IV	5–7 days	10 days	7–14 days

NURSING IMPLICATIONS

Assessment

- Monitor blood pressure, pulse, and respiratory rate during course of therapy. Notify physician immediately if respiratory distress occurs. Bronchospasm can be life-threatening and may occur at time of infusion or several hrs later.
- Assess for fever, sore throat, and signs of infection. Notify physician if these symptoms occur.
- Assess for bleeding (bleeding gums, bruising, petechiae; guaiac stools, urine, and emesis). Avoid IM injections and rectal temperatures. Apply pressure to venipuncture sites for 10 min.
- May cause nausea and vomiting. Monitor intake and output, appetite, and nutritional intake. Confer with physician regarding prophylactic use of an antiemetic. Adjust diet as tolerated.
- Assess injection site frequently for redness, irritation, or inflammation. If extravasation occurs infusion must be stopped and restarted elsewhere to avoid damage to SC tissue. Standard treatment includes application of heat.
- Monitor for symptoms of gout (increased uric acid, joint pain, edema). Encourage patient to drink at least 2 liters of fluid per day. Physician may order allopurinol or alkalinization of urine to decrease uric acid levels.
- Anemia may occur. Monitor for increased fatigue and dyspnea.
- **Lab Test Considerations:** Monitor CBC prior to and routinely throughout course of therapy. Notify physician if WBC <2000; subsequent doses are usually withheld until WBC is at least 4000. The nadir of leukopenia occurs in 5–10 days and recovery usually occurs 7–14 days later. Thrombocytopenia may also occur in patients who have received radiation or other chemotherapy agents.
- Monitor liver function studies (SGOT [AST], SGPT [ALT], LDH, bilirubin) and renal function studies (BUN, creatinine) prior to and periodically throughout therapy.
- May cause increased uric acid. Monitor periodically during therapy.

Potential Nursing Diagnoses

- Infection, high risk for (adverse reactions).
- Nutrition, altered: less than body requirements (adverse reactions).
- Knowledge deficit related to medication regimen (patient/family teaching).

Implementation

- **General Info:** Soln should be prepared in a biologic cabinet. Wear gloves, gown, and mask while handling medication. Discard IV equipment in specially designated containers (see Appendix I).

- **Direct IV:** Dilute each 10 mg with 10 ml of 0.9% NaCl for injection with phenol or benzyl alcohol. Reconstituted medication is stable for 30 days if refrigerated.
  - *Rate:* Administer each single dose over 1 min through Y-site injection or 3-way stopcock of a free-flowing infusion of 0.9% NaCl or D5W.
- **Intermittent Infusion:** May be further diluted with 50–100 ml of 0.9% NaCl.
  - Manufacturer recommends not mixing vinblastine with any other medication in soln or syringe.
  - *Rate:* Administer over 15–30 min. Administering medication over a longer period or with more diluent may increase irritation of vein.
- **Syringe Compatibility:** bleomycin, cisplatin, cyclophosphamide, droperidol, fluorouracil, leucovorin calcium, methotrexate, metoclopramide, mitomycin, ondansetron, or vincristine.
- **Y-Site Compatibility:** bleomycin, cisplatin, cyclophosphamide, doxorubicin, droperidol, fluorouracil, heparin, leucovorin calcium, methotrexate, metoclopramide, mitomycin, or vincristine.
- **Y-Site Incompatibility:** furosemide.

Patient/Family Teaching

- Advise patient to notify physician if fever, chills, sore throat, signs of infection, bleeding gums, bruising, petechiae, or blood in urine, stool, or emesis occurs. Caution patient to avoid crowds and persons with known infections. Instruct patient to use soft toothbrush and electric razor. Caution patient not to drink alcoholic beverages or take products containing aspirin.
- Instruct patient to inspect oral mucosa for redness and ulceration. If ulceration occurs advise patient to avoid spicy foods, use sponge brush, and rinse mouth with water after eating and drinking. Physician may order viscous lidocaine swishes if mouth pain interferes with eating.
- Instruct patient to report symptoms of neurotoxicity (paresthesia, pain, difficulty walking, persistent constipation).
- Advise patient that this medication may have teratogenic effects. Contraception should be used during and for at least 2 mon after therapy is concluded.
- Discuss the possibility of hair loss with patient. Explore coping strategies.
- Instruct patient not to receive any vaccinations without advice of physician.
- Emphasize need for periodic lab tests to monitor for side effects.

Evaluation

Effectiveness of therapy can be demonstrated by: ▪ Regression of malignancy without the appearance of detrimental side effects.

VINCRISTINE

(vin-**kriss**-teen)

Oncovin, Vincasar PFS

CLASSIFICATION(S):

Antineoplastic agent—vinca alkaloid

Pregnancy Category D

INDICATIONS

▪ Used alone and in combination with other treatment modalities (antineoplastic agents, surgery, or radiation therapy) in the treatment of: ▫ Hodgkin's disease ▫ Leukemias ▫ Neuroblastoma ▫ Malignant lymphomas ▫ Rhabdomyosarcoma ▫ Wilms' tumor ▫ Other tumors.

ACTION

▪ Binds to proteins of mitotic spindle, causing metaphase arrest ▪ Cell replication is stopped as a result (cell cycle-specific for M phase) ▪ Has little or no effect on bone marrow. **Therapeutic Effects:** ▪ Death of rapidly replicating cells, particularly malignant ones ▪ Has immunosuppressive properties.

PHARMACOKINETICS

Absorption: Administered IV only, resulting in complete bioavailability.

Distribution: Rapidly and widely distributed.

Metabolism and Excretion: Metabolized by the liver and eliminated in the feces via biliary excretion.

Half-life: 10.5–37.5 hr.

CONTRAINDICATIONS AND PRECAUTIONS

Contraindicated in: ▪ Hypersensitivity ▪ Pregnancy or lactation.

Use Cautiously in: ▪ Patients with childbearing potential ▪ Infections ▪ Decreased bone marrow reserve ▪ Other chronic debilitating illnesses ▪ Hepatic impairment (dosage reduction recommended).

ADVERSE REACTIONS AND SIDE EFFECTS*

CNS: mental status changes, depression, agitation, insomnia.

Resp: bronchospasm.

GI: <u>nausea</u>, <u>vomiting</u>, anorexia, stomatitis, constipation, ileus, abdominal cramps.

GU: urinary retention, nocturia, oliguria, gonadal suppression.

Derm: <u>alopecia</u>.

Endo: syndrome of inappropriate secretion of antidiuretic hormone (SIADH).

Hemat: anemia, leukopenia, thrombocytopenia (mild and brief).

Local: <u>phlebitis</u> at IV site.

Metab: hyperuricemia.

Neuro: <u>neurotoxicity</u> (ascending peripheral neuropathy).

INTERACTIONS

Drug-Drug: ▪ Bronchospasm may occur in patients who have been previously treated with **mitomycin** ▪ **L-asparaginase** may decrease hepatic metabolism of vincristine (give vincristine 12–24 hr prior to asparaginase) ▪ May decrease antibody response to **live virus vaccines** and increase the risk of adverse reactions.

ROUTE AND DOSAGE

Note: Many other protocols are used.

- **IV (Adults):** 10–30 mcg/kg or 0.4–1.4 mg/m^2, may repeat q week (not to exceed 2 mg each dose).
- **IV (Children >10 kg):** 1.5–2 mg/m^2 single dose, may repeat q week.
- **IV (Children <10 kg):** 50 mcg/kg (0.05 mg/kg) single dose, may repeat q week.

PHARMACODYNAMICS (effects on blood counts, which are usually mild)

	ONSET	PEAK	DURATION
IV	UK	UK	7 days

NURSING IMPLICATIONS

Assessment

- ☐ Monitor blood pressure, pulse, and respiratory rate during course of therapy. Notify physician of significant changes.
- ☐ Monitor neurologic status. Assess for paresthesia (numbness, tingling, pain), loss of deep tendon reflexes (Achilles reflex is usually first involved), weakness (wrist or foot drop, gait disturbances), cranial nerves palsies (jaw pain, hoarseness, ptosis, visual changes), autonomic dysfunction (ileus, difficulty voiding, orthostatic hypotension, impaired sweating), and CNS dysfunction (decreased level of consciousness, agitation, hallucinations). Notify physician if these symptoms develop, as they may persist for mons.
- ☐ Monitor intake and output ratios and weight; inform physician if significant discrepancies occur. Decreased urine output with concurrent hyponatremia may indicate SIADH, which usually responds to fluid restriction.
- ☐ Assess infusion site frequently for redness, irritation, or inflammation. If extravasation occurs infusion must be stopped and restarted elsewhere to avoid damage to SC tissue. Standard

*<u>Underlines</u> indicate most frequent; **CAPITALS** indicate life-threatening.

treatment includes application of heat.

- Assess nutritional status. An antiemetic may be ordered to minimize nausea and vomiting.
- Monitor for symptoms of gout (increased uric acid, joint pain, edema). Encourage patient to drink at least 2 liters of fluid per day. Physician may order allopurinol or alkalinization of urine to decrease uric acid levels.
- **Lab Test Considerations:** Monitor CBC prior to and periodically throughout course of therapy. May cause slight leukopenia 4 days after therapy, which resolves within 7 days. Platelet count may increase or decrease.
- Monitor liver function studies (SGOT [AST], SGPT [ALT], LDH, bilirubin) and renal function studies (BUN, creatinine) prior to and periodically throughout therapy.
- May cause increased uric acid. Monitor periodically during therapy.

Potential Nursing Diagnoses

- Injury, high risk for (adverse reactions).
- Nutrition, altered: less than body requirements (adverse reactions).
- Knowledge deficit related to medication regimen (patient/family teaching).

Implementation

- **General Info:** Soln should be prepared in a biologic cabinet. Wear gloves, gown, and mask while handling medication. Discard IV equipment in specially designated containers (see Appendix I).
- Do not administer SC, IM, or IT. Intrathecal administration is fatal.
- **Direct IV:** Manufacturer does not recommend admixture.
- *Rate:* Administer each single dose direct IV push over 1 min through Y-site injection or 3-way stopcock of a free-flowing infusion of 0.9% NaCl or D5W.
- **Syringe Compatibility:** bleomycin, cisplatin, cyclophosphamide, doxapram, doxorubicin, droperidol, fluorouracil, heparin, leucovorin calcium, methotrexate, metoclopramide, mitomycin, or vinblastine.
- **Syringe Incompatibility:** furosemide.
- **Y-Site Compatibility:** bleomycin, cisplatin, cyclophosphamide, doxorubicin, droperidol, fluorouracil, heparin, leucovorin calcium, methotrexate, metoclopramide, mitomycin, or vinblastine.
- **Y-Site Incompatibility:** furosemide.

Patient/Family Teaching

- Instruct patient to report symptoms of neurotoxicity (paresthesia, pain, difficulty walking, persistent constipation).
- Inform patient that increased fluid intake, dietary fiber, and exercise may minimize constipation. Physician may order stool softeners or laxatives. Patient should inform physician if severe constipation or abdominal discomfort occur, as this may be a sign of neuropathy.
- Advise patient to notify physician if fever, chills, sore throat, signs of infection, bleeding gums, bruising, petechiae; or blood in urine, stool, or emesis; or mouth sores occur. Caution patient to avoid crowds and persons with known infections.
- Advise patient that this medication may have teratogenic effects. Contraception should be used during and for at least 2 mon after therapy is concluded.
- Discuss the possibility of hair loss with patient. Explore coping strategies.
- Instruct patient not to receive any vaccinations without advice of physician.
- Emphasize need for periodic lab tests to monitor for side effects.

Evaluation

Effectiveness of therapy can be demonstrated by: ▪ Regression of malignancy without the appearance of detrimental side effects.

VITAMIN A
(vye-ta-min A)
Aquasol A, Del-Vi-A

CLASSIFICATION(S):
Vitamin—fat-soluble
Pregnancy Category X

INDICATIONS

▪ Treatment and prevention of deficiency states ▪ Prevention of vitamin A deficiency in patients who have fat malabsorption or are taking bile acid sequestrants.

ACTION

▪ Serves as a cofactor in many biochemical processes ▪ Necessary for growth, bone development, vision, reproduction and integrity of mucosal and epithelial surfaces, and formation of visual pigment. **Therapeutic Effects:** ▪ Resolution of signs of deficiency ▪ Prevention of deficiency.

PHARMACOKINETICS

Absorption: GI absorption requires bile acids, fat, lipase, and protein. Aqueous preparations are absorbed more readily than emulsions.
Distribution: Stored primarily in the liver (2-yr supply), small amounts stored in kidneys and lungs. Does not cross the placenta but enters breast milk.
Metabolism and Excretion: Mostly metabolized by the liver.
Half-life: UK.

CONTRAINDICATIONS AND PRECAUTIONS

Contraindicated in: ▪ Hypervitaminosis A ▪ Malabsorption ▪ Hypersensitivity to ingredients in preparations (chlorobutanol, polysorbate 80, butylated hydroxyanisole, butylated hydroxytoluene).
Use Cautiously in: ▪ Lactation (supplements to infant necessary) ▪ Pregnancy (avoid amounts greater than RDA; see Appendix L) ▪ Severely impaired renal function.

ADVERSE REACTIONS AND SIDE EFFECTS*

Misc: hypervitaminosis A syndrome.

INTERACTIONS

Drug-Drug: ▪ **Cholestyramine, colestipol,** and **mineral oil** decrease absorption of vitamin A ▪ **Oral contraceptives** increase plasma levels of vitamin A.

ROUTE AND DOSAGE

Severe Deficiency

- **PO (Adults):** 10,000–50,000 units/day.
- **PO (Children):** 5000 units/kg/day for 5 days or until recovery.
- **IM (Adults):** 50,000–100,000 units/day for 3 days, then 50,000 units/day for 2 wk.
- **IM (Children):** 5000–15,000 units/day for 10 days.

Dietary Supplement

- **PO (Adults):** 4000–5000 units/day.
- **PO (Children 7–10 yr):** 3300–3500 units/day.
- **PO (Children 4–6 yr):** 2500 units/day.
- **PO (Children 6 mon–3 yr):** 1500–2000 units/day.
- **PO (Infants <6 mon):** 1500 units/day.

Malabsorption

- **PO (Adults):** 10,000–50,000 units/day.

PHARMACODYNAMICS

	ONSET	PEAK	DURATION
PO	UK	UK	UK
IM	UK	UK	UK

NURSING IMPLICATIONS

Assessment

- Assess patient for signs of vitamin A deficiency (night blindness; frequent eye, ear, sinus, and GU infections; dry mucous membranes; rough scaly skin with goose pimple-like lesions; photophobia; and dry eyes) prior to and periodically throughout therapy.

*Underlines indicate most frequent; **CAPITALS** indicate life-threatening.

- Assess nutritional status through 24-hr diet recall. Determine frequency of consumption of vitamin A-rich foods.
- **Lab Test Considerations:** Chronic toxicity may cause increased blood glucose, calcium, BUN, cholesterol, and triglyceride levels.
- Plasma vitamin A and carotene levels may be evaluated prior to therapy to determine vitamin A deficiency.
- With high doses, erythrocyte and leukocyte counts may be decreased and erythrocyte sedimentation rate (ESR) and prothrombin time (PT) may be increased.

Potential Nursing Diagnoses

- Nutrition, altered: less than body requirements (indications).
- Knowledge deficit related to medication regimen (patient/family teaching).

Implementation

- **General Info:** Available in tablets, capsules, oral soln, and injectable forms. Available in combination with other vitamins.
- Tablets and capsules are water-miscible for patients with malabsorption syndromes.
- **PO:** Administer with or after meals.
- Soln may be dropped directly into mouth or mixed with cereal, fruit juice, or other food. Use calibrated dropper supplied by manufacturer to measure soln accurately.
- **IM:** Parenteral administration is indicated only when oral administration is not possible (because of malabsorption, NPO status, or vomiting or when ocular damage is severe).
- Do not administer vitamin A intravenously, because of the risk of anaphylactic shock and death.

Patient/Family Teaching

- Instruct patient to take medication as directed. If a dose is missed it should be omitted, as fat-soluble vitamins are stored in the body for long periods.
- Encourage patient to comply with physician's diet recommendations. Explain that the best source of vitamins is a well-balanced diet with foods from the 4 basic food groups.
- Foods high in vitamin A include liver, fish liver oils, egg yolks, yellow-orange fruits and vegetables, dark green leafy vegetables, whole milk, vitamin A-fortified skim milk, butter, and margarine. Ordinary cooking does not destroy vitamin A but frozen foods loose 5–10% during storage for 12 mon.
- Patients self-medicating with vitamin supplements should be cautioned not to exceed RDA (see Appendix L). The effectiveness of megadoses for treatment of various medical conditions is unproven and this may cause side effects and toxicity.
- Review symptoms of hypervitaminosis A syndrome (headaches, bulging fontanelles in infants, irritability, yellow-orange discoloration of skin, drying and desquamation of skin and lips, hair loss, anorexia, vomiting, joint and bone pain). Instruct patient to report these promptly to physician.
- Advise patient that mineral oil may interfere with the absorption of fat-soluble vitamins and should not be used concurrently.
- Emphasize the importance of follow-up examinations to evaluate progress. Ophthalmologic examinations may be required prior to and periodically throughout therapy.

Evaluation

Effectiveness of therapy can be demonstrated by: ■ Prevention of or decrease in the symptoms of vitamin A deficiency.

VITAMIN B COMPLEX WITH VITAMIN C

Allbee-T, Allbee with C, Arcobee with C, BC-Vite, Becotin-T, Bee-Forte w/C, Beminal 500, Beminal Forte with Vitamin C, Bexomal-C, C-B Time, Ceebeevim, Cee with Bee, Gen-bee with C, Hi-Bee W/C, Probec-T, Stresscaps, Surbex-T,

Surbex with C, Surbu-Gen-T, Thera-Combex HP, Therapeutic B Complex with Vitamin C, Vari-plex-C, Vita-bee with C

CLASSIFICATION(S):
Vitamin—water-soluble
Pregnancy Category UK

INDICATIONS

▪ Treatment and prevention of vitamin deficiencies.

ACTION

▪ Contains B-complex vitamins (B_1, B_2, B_3, B_5, B_6, B_{12}) and vitamin C, a diverse group of compounds necessary for normal growth and development that act as coenzymes or catalysts in numerous metabolic processes. **Therapeutic Effect:** ▪ Replacement of vitamins in patients who are deficient or at risk of deficiency.

PHARMACOKINETICS

Absorption: Well absorbed following oral administration. Some absorptive processes require cofactors (B_{12}).
Distribution: Widely distributed, crosses the placenta and enters breast milk.
Metabolism and Excretion: Utilized in various biologic processes. Excess amounts are excreted unchanged by the kidneys.
Half-life: UK.

CONTRAINDICATIONS AND PRECAUTIONS

Contraindicated in: ▪ Hypersensitivity to ingredients in preparations (benzyl alcohol, parabens, bisulfites, tartrazine).

ADVERSE REACTIONS AND SIDE EFFECTS*

Note: In recommended doses, adverse reactions are extremely rare.
Misc: allergic reactions to preservatives, ANAPHYLAXIS (thiamine).

INTERACTIONS

Drug-Drug: ▪ Large amounts of vitamin B_6 may interfere with the beneficial effect of **levodopa**.

ROUTE AND DOSAGE

▪ **PO (Adults and Children):** Amount sufficient to meet RDA for age group (see Table in Appendix L).

PHARMACODYNAMICS

	ONSET	PEAK	DURATION
PO	UK	UK	UK

NURSING IMPLICATIONS

Assessment

□ Assess patient for signs of vitamin deficiency prior to and periodically throughout therapy. Assess nutritional status through 24-hr diet recall. Determine frequency of consumption of vitamin-rich foods. Therapy is limited to periods of high physiologic stress when patient is not able to ingest adequate vitamins orally.
□ Monitor patient for anaphylaxis (wheezing, urticaria, edema): contains thiamine.

Potential Nursing Diagnoses

▪ Nutrition, altered: less than body requirements (indications).
▪ Knowledge deficit related to medication regimen (patient/family teaching).

Implementation

▪ **PO:** Available in capsule and tablet form.

Patient/Family Teaching

□ Encourage patient to comply with physician's diet recommendations. Explain that the best source of vitamins is a well-balanced diet with foods from the 4 basic food groups.

Evaluation

Effectiveness of therapy can be demonstrated by: ▪ Prevention of or decrease in the symptoms of vitamin deficiencies.

*Underlines indicate most frequent; **CAPITALS** indicate life-threatening.

VITAMIN E

(**vye**-ta-min E)
alpha-tocopherol, Amino-Opti-E, Aquasol E, Chew-E, E-Ferol, Eprolin, Epsilan-M, Gordo-Vite E, Pheryl-E, Vitec, Viterra E

CLASSIFICATION(S):
Vitamin—fat-soluble
Pregnancy Category UK

INDICATIONS

▪ **PO:** Used as a dietary supplement ▪ **PO:** Used in low-birth-weight infants to prevent and treat hemolysis due to vitamin E deficiency ▪ **Top:** Treatment of irritated, chapped, or dry skin.

ACTION

▪ Prevents the oxidation (antioxidant) of other substances ▪ Protects red blood cell membranes against hemolysis, especially in low-birth-weight neonates. **Therapeutic Effects:** ▪ Prevention and treatment of deficiency in high-risk patients.

PHARMACOKINETICS

Absorption: 20–80% absorbed following oral administration. Absorption requires fat and bile salts.
Distribution: Widely distributed, stored in adipose tissue (4-yr supply).
Metabolism and Excretion: Metabolized by the liver, excreted in bile.
Half-life: UK.

CONTRAINDICATIONS AND PRECAUTIONS

Contraindicated in: ▪ Hypersensitivity to ingredients in preparations (parabens, propylene, glycol).
Use Cautiously in: ▪ Anemia due to iron deficiency ▪ Low-birth-weight infants (oral administration may cause necrotizing enterocolitis) ▪ Vitamin K deficiency (may increase risk of bleeding).

ADVERSE REACTIONS AND SIDE EFFECTS*

Note: Seen primarily with large doses over long periods of time.
CNS: fatigue, weakness, headache.
EENT: blurred vision.
GI: necrotizing enterocolitis (oral administration in low-birth-weight infants), nausea, diarrhea, cramps.
Derm: rash.
Endo: gonadal dysfunction.

INTERACTIONS

Drug-Drug: ▪ **Cholestyramine, colestipol, mineral oil,** and **sucralfate** decrease absorption ▪ May decrease hematologic response to **iron supplements**.

ROUTE AND DOSAGE

- **PO (Adults):** 30–75 units/day.
- **PO (Neonates—Premature, Low-Birth-Weight):** 5 units/day.
- **PO (Neonates—Full-Term):** 5 units/liter of formula.
- **Top (Adults and Children):** Apply to affected areas as needed.

PHARMACODYNAMICS

	ONSET	PEAK	DURATION
PO	UK	UK	UK

NURSING IMPLICATIONS

ASSESSMENT

- □ Assess patient for signs of vitamin E deficiency (neonates—irritability, edema, hemolytic anemia, creatinuria; adults/children (rare)—muscle weakness, ceroid deposits, anemia, creatinuria) prior to and periodically throughout therapy.
- □ Assess nutritional status through 24-hr diet recall. Determine frequency of consumption of vitamin E-rich foods.
- ▪ **Lab Test Considerations:** Large doses may increase cholesterol, triglyceride, and CPK levels.

POTENTIAL NURSING DIAGNOSES

- ▪ Nutrition, altered: less than body requirements (indications).

*Underlines indicate most frequent; **CAPITALS** indicate life-threatening.

W

- Knowledge deficit related to medication regimen (patient/family teaching).

Implementation

- **General Info:** Available in tablets, capsules, and oral soln. Available in combination with other vitamins.
  - ▫ Water-miscible oral forms are available for patients with malabsorption syndromes.
- **PO:** Administer with or after meals.
  - ▫ Chewable tablets should be chewed well or crushed before swallowing. Soln may be dropped directly into mouth or mixed with cereal, fruit juice, or other food. Use calibrated dropper supplied by manufacturer to measure soln accurately.

Patient/Family Teaching

- ▫ Instruct patient to take medication as directed. If a dose is missed it should be omitted, as fat-soluble vitamins are stored in the body for long periods.
- ▫ Encourage patient to comply with physician's diet recommendations. Explain that the best source of vitamins is a well-balanced diet with foods from the 4 basic food groups.
- ▫ Foods high in vitamin E include vegetable oils, wheat germ, whole grain cereals, egg yolk, and liver. Vitamin E content is not markedly affected by cooking.
- ▫ Patients self-medicating with vitamin supplements should be cautioned not to exceed RDA (see Appendix L). The effectiveness of megadoses for treatment of various medical conditions is unproven and this may cause side effects and toxicity.
- ▫ Review symptoms of overdosage (blurred vision, flu-like symptoms, headache, breast enlargement). Instruct patient to report these promptly to physician.
- ▫ Mineral oil may interfere with the absorption of fat-soluble vitamins and should not be used concurrently.

Evaluation

Effectiveness of therapy can be demonstrated by: ▪ Prevention of or decrease in the symptoms of vitamin E deficiency ▪ Control of dry or chapped skin.

WARFARIN

(**war**-fa-in)

{Athrombin-K}, Coumadin, Panwarfin, Sofarin, {Warfilone}

CLASSIFICATION(S):

Anticoagulant

Pregnancy Category UK

INDICATIONS

▪ Prophylaxis and treatment of: ▫ Venous thrombosis ▫ Pulmonary embolism ▫ Atrial fibrillation with embolization ▪ Adjunct in the treatment of coronary occlusion ▪ Prevention of thrombus formation and embolization after prosthetic valve placement.

ACTION

▪ Interferes with hepatic synthesis of vitamin K-dependent clotting factors (II, VII, IX, and X). **Therapeutic Effect:** ▪ Prevention of thromboembolic events.

PHARMACOKINETICS

Absorption: Well absorbed from the GI tract following oral administration.

Distribution: Crosses the placenta but does not enter breast milk.

Metabolism and Excretion: Metabolized by the liver.

Half-life: 0.5–3 days.

CONTRAINDICATIONS AND PRECAUTIONS

Contraindicated in: ▪ Pregnancy ▪ Uncontrolled bleeding ▪ Open wounds ▪ Active ulcer disease ▪ Malignancy ▪ Recent brain, eye, or spinal cord injury or surgery ▪ Severe liver disease ▪ Uncontrolled hypertension.

Use Cautiously in: ▪ Patients with history of ulcer or liver disease ▪ History of poor compliance ▪ Women with childbearing potential.

ADVERSE REACTIONS AND SIDE EFFECTS*

GI: nausea, cramps.
Derm: dermal necrosis.
Hemat: BLEEDING.
Misc: fever.

INTERACTIONS

Drug–Drug: ▪ **Androgens, cefamandole, cefoperazone, cefotetan, chloral hydrate, chloramphenicol, disulfiram, metronidazole, moxalactam, plicamycin, streptokinase, urokinase, sulfonamides, quinidine, nonsteroidal anti-inflammatory agents, valproates,** and **aspirin** may increase the response to warfarin and increase the risk of bleeding ▪ **Alcohol, barbiturates,** and **oral contraceptives containing estrogen** may decrease the anticoagulant response to warfarin.
Drug–Food: ▪ Ingestion of large quantities of **foods high in vitamin K content** (see list in Appendix K) may antagonize the anticoagulant effect of warfarin.

ROUTE AND DOSAGE

- **PO (Adults):** 5–15 mg/day for 2–5 days, then adjust daily dose by results of prothrombin time (usually 2–10 mg/day).
- **IM, IV (Adults):** 10–15 mg/day for 2–5 days, then adjust daily dose by results of prothrombin time (usually 2–10 mg/day).

PHARMACODYNAMICS (effects on coagulation tests)

	ONSET	PEAK	DURATION
PO	several hrs	0.5–3 days	2–5 days
IM	several hrs	0.5–3 days	2–5 days
IV	several hrs	0.5–3 days	2–5 days

NURSING IMPLICATIONS

Assessment

□ Assess patient for signs of bleeding and hemorrhage (bleeding gums, nose bleed, unusual bruising, tarry black stools, hematuria, fall in hematocrit or blood pressure; guaiac-positive stools, urine, or nasogastric aspirate). Notify physician if these occur.

□ Assess patient for evidence of additional or increased thrombosis. Symptoms will depend on area of involvement.

▪ **Lab Test Considerations:** Prothrombin time (PT) and other clotting factors should be monitored frequently during therapy. Therapeutic PT ranges from 1.5 to 2.0 times greater than control. Notify physician if significant discrepancies occur.

□ Hepatic function and CBC should be monitored prior to and periodically throughout course of therapy.

□ Stool and urine should be monitored for occult blood prior to and periodically throughout course of therapy.

▪ **Toxicity and Overdose:** Withholding 1 or more doses of medication is usually sufficient if PT is excessively prolonged or minor bleeding occurs. If overdose occurs or anticoagulation needs to be immediately reversed, the antidote is vitamin K (phytonadione, AquaMEPHYTON). Administration of whole blood or plasma may also be required in severe bleeding because of the delayed onset of vitamin K.

Potential Nursing Diagnoses

- Tissue perfusion, altered (indications).
- Injury, high risk for (side effects).
- Knowledge deficit related to medication regimen (patient/family teaching).

Implementation

▪ **General Info:** Administer medication at same time each day.

□ Protect injectable form from light.

▪ **PO:** Medication requires 3–5 days to reach effective levels. It is usually begun while patient is still on IV heparin.

▪ **Direct IV:** Reconstitute each 50-mg vial with 2 ml of sterile water for injec-

*Underlines indicate most frequent; **CAPITALS** indicate life-threatening.

tion, for a concentration of 25 mg/ml. May be administerd IM or IV. Use immediately after reconstitution.

- Administer direct IV push.

Patient/Family Teaching

- Instruct patient to take medication exactly as directed. If a dose is missed it should be taken as soon as remembered that day. Do not double doses. Physician should be informed of missed doses at time of check-up or lab tests.
- Review foods high in vitamin K (see Appendix K). Patient should have consistent limited intake of these foods, as vitamin K is the antidote for warfarin and alternating intake of these foods will cause PT levels to fluctuate.
- Caution patient to avoid IM injections and activities leading to injury. Instruct patient to use a soft toothbrush, not to floss, and to shave with an electric razor during warfarin therapy. Advise patient that venipunctures and injection sites require application of pressure to prevent bleeding or hematoma formation.
- Advise patient to report any symptoms of unusual bleeding or bruising (bleeding gums, nose bleed, black tarry stools, hematuria, excessive menstrual flow). Notify physician if these occur.
- Instruct patient not to take over-the-counter medications, especially those containing aspirin, or alcohol without advice of physician or pharmacist.
- Emphasize the importance of frequent lab tests to monitor coagulation factors.
- Instruct patient to carry identification describing medication regimen at all times and to inform all health care personnel caring for patient of anticoagulant therapy prior to lab tests, treatment, or surgery.

Evaluation

Clinical respone can be evaluated by: ▪ Prolonged PT (1.5–2 times the control) without signs of hemorrhage.

Z

ZIDOVUDINE

(zye-**doe**-vue-deen)
azidothymidine, AZT, Retrovir

CLASSIFICATION(S):
Antiviral
Pregnancy Category C

INDICATIONS

▪ Management of symptomatic human immunodeficiency virus (HIV, AIDS) and selected patients with AIDS-related complex (ARC).

ACTION

▪ Following intracellular conversion to its active form, inhibits viral RNA synthesis by inhibiting the enzyme DNA polymerase (reverse transcriptase) ▪ Prevents viral replication. **Therapeutic Effects:** ▪ Virustatic action against selected retroviruses ▪ Not curative, but may slow the progression or decrease the severity of the disease and its associated sequelae.

PHARMACOKINETICS

Absorption: Well absorbed following oral administration.
Distribution: Widely distributed. Enters the CNS. Probably crosses the placenta.
Metabolism and Excretion: Mostly (75%) metabolized by the liver. 15–20% excreted unchanged by the kidneys.
Half-life: 1 hr.

CONTRAINDICATIONS AND PRECAUTIONS

Contraindicated in: ▪ Hypersensitivity ▪ Lactation.
Use Cautiously in: ▪ Decreased bone marrow reserve (dosage reduction required for anemia or granulocytopenia) ▪ Severe hepatic or renal disease (dosage modification may be required) ▪ Pregnancy or children (safety not established).

ADVERSE REACTIONS AND SIDE EFFECTS*

CNS: headache, weakness, malaise, somnolence, restlessness, insomnia, anxiety, confusion, depression, decreased mental acuity, dizziness, fainting.

GI: nausea, abdominal pain, diarrhea, dyspepsia, anorexia, vomiting, hepatitis.

Derm: nail pigmentation.

Hemat: anemia, granulocytopenia, thrombocytosis.

MS: back pain, myalgia.

Neuro: tremor.

INTERACTIONS

Drug-Drug: ▪ Additive bone marrow depression with other **agents having bone-marrow-depressing properties (antineoplastic agents** or **radiation therapy)** ▪ Additive neurotoxicity may occur with **acyclovir** ▪ Toxicity may be increased by concurrent administration of **acetaminophen, amphotericin B, aspirin, benzodiazepines, cimetidine, indomethacin, inteferon, morphine, pentamidine, sulfonamides,** or **probenecid**.

ROUTE AND DOSAGE

Symptomatic HIV Infection

- **PO (Adults):** 200 mg q 4 hr (6 times daily) or 2.9 mg/kg q 4 hr (6 times daily for 1 mon, then decrease to 100 mg q 4 hr).
- **PO (Children 3 mon–12 yr):** 180 mg/m^2 every 6 hr (not to exceed 200 mg q 6 hr).
- **IV (Adults and Children):** 1–2 mg/kg infused over 1 hr q 6 hr. Change to oral therapy as soon as possible.

Asymptomatic HIV Infection

- **PO (Adults):** 100 mg q 4 hr while awake (500 mg/day).

PHARMACODYNAMICS (blood levels)

	ONSET	PEAK	DURATION
PO	UK	0.5–1.5 hr	UK

NURSING IMPLICATIONS

Assessment

- ▫ Assess patient for change in severity of symptoms of acquired immunodeficiency syndrome (AIDS) or AIDS-related complex (ARC) and for symptoms of opportunistic infections throughout therapy.
- ▪ **Lab Test Considerations:** Monitor CBC every 2 wk throughout therapy. Commonly causes granulocytopenia and anemia. Anemia may occur 2–4 wk after initiation of therapy. Anemia may respond to epoetin alpha administration. Granulocytopenia usually occurs after 6–8 wk of therapy. Dosage reduction, discontinuation of therapy, or blood transfusions should be considered if hemoglobin is <7.5 g/dl or reduction of >25% from baseline and/or granulocyte count is $<750/mm^3$ or reduction of >50% from baseline. Therapy may be gradually resumed when bone marrow recovery is evident.

Potential Nursing Diagnoses

- ▪ Infection, high risk for (indications, side effects).
- ▪ Knowledge deficit related to medication regimen (patient/family teaching).

Implementation

- ▪ **General Info:** Administer capsules every 4 hr around the clock.
- ▫ Also available as a liquid.
- ▪ **IV:** Patient should receive the IV infusion only until oral therapy can be administered.
- ▪ **Intermittent Infusion:** Remove the calculated dose from the vial and dilute with D5W for a concentration of <4 mg/ml. Stable for 24 hr at room temperature or 48 hr if refrigerated.
- ▫ *Rate:* Infuse at a constant rate over 1 hr. Avoid rapid infusion or bolus injection.
- ▪ **Additive Incompatibility:** blood products or protein solns.

Patient/Family Teaching

- ▫ Instruct patient to take zidovudine ex-

*Underlines indicate most frequent; **CAPITALS** indicate life-threatening.

actly as directed, around the clock, even if sleep is interrupted. Emphasize the importance of compliance with therapy, not taking more than the prescribed amount, and not discontinuing without consulting physician. Missed doses should be taken as soon as remembered, unless almost time for next dose; do not double doses.

- Supply patient with information about zidovudine. Inform patient that drug is shipped from manufacturer and may take several days. Patient should contact pharmacy for prescription refills several days before supply runs out. Instruct patient that zidovudine should not be shared with others.
- Zidovudine may cause dizziness or fainting. Caution patient to avoid driving or other activities requiring alertness until response to medication is known.
- Inform patient that zidovudine does not cure AIDS and does not reduce the risk of transmission of HIV to others through sexual contact or blood contamination. Caution patient to avoid sexual contact, use a condom, and avoid sharing needles or donating blood, to prevent spreading the AIDS virus to others.
- Instruct patient to notify physician promptly if fever, sore throat, or signs of infection occur. Caution patient to avoid crowds and persons with known infections. Instruct patient to use soft toothbrush, to use caution when using toothpicks or dental floss, and to have dental work done prior to therapy or deferred until blood counts return to normal.
- Advise patient to avoid taking any over-the-counter medications without consulting physician or pharmacist.
- Advise patients to bring their own zidovudine if hospitalized, as hospitals may not have this drug in stock.
- Emphasize the importance of regular follow-up examinations and blood counts to determine progress and monitor for side effects.

Evaluation

Effectivness of therapy can be demonstrated by: ▪ Prevention and treatment of AIDS, ARC, and opportunistic infections in patients with human immunodeficiency virus (HIV).

ZINC SULFATE

(zink **sul**-fate)

Orazinc, Scrip-Zinc, Zincate, Zinctrace, Zinkaps

CLASSIFICATION(S):

Nutritional supplement—trace metal

Pregnancy Category UK

INDICATIONS

▪ Replacement and supplementation therapy in patients who are at risk for zinc deficiency, including patients on long-term parenteral nutrition. **Unlabeled Uses:** ▪ Treatment of acrodermatitis enteropathica ▪ Management of impaired wound healing due to zinc deficiency.

ACTION

▪ Serves as a cofacter for many enzymatic reactions ▪ Required for normal growth and tissue repair, wound healing, and senses of taste and smell. **Therapeutic Effect:** ▪ Replacement in deficiency states.

PHARMACOKINETICS

Absorption: Poorly absorbed from the GI tract (20–30%).

Distribution: Widely distributed. Concentrates in muscle, bone, skin, kidney, liver, pancreas, retina, prostate, red blood cells, and white blood cells.

Metabolism and Excretion: 90% excreted in feces, remainder lost in urine and sweat.

Half-life: UK.

CONTRAINDICATIONS AND PRECAUTIONS

Contraindicated in: ▪ Hypersensitivity or allergy to any components in formulation ▪ Pregnancy or lactation (supplemental amounts greater than RDA for pregnant or lactating patients; see list in Appendix L).

Use Cautiously in: ▪ Renal failure.

ADVERSE REACTIONS AND SIDE EFFECTS*

GI: nausea, vomiting, gastric irritation (oral use only).

INTERACTIONS

Drug–Drug: ▪ Oral zinc may decrease the absorption of **tetracyclines,** or **fluoroquinolones.**

Drug–Food: ▪ **Caffeine, dairy products,** and **bran** may decrease the absorption of orally administered zinc.

ROUTE AND DOSAGE

Note: RDA = 15 mg. Doses expressed in mg elemental zinc unless otherwise noted. Zinc sulfate contains 23% zinc.

Dietary Supplement

- **PO (Adults):** 25–50 mg/day.

IV Nutritional Supplementation—Metabolically Stable Patients

- **IV (Adults):** 2.5–4 mg/day, additional 2 mg/day in acute catabolic states.
- **IV (Infants and Children ≤5 yr):** 100 mcg/kg/day.
- **IV (Premature Infants <3000 g):** 300 mcg/kg/day.

Metabolically Stable Adults with Small Bowel Fluid Losses

- **IV (Adults):** Additional 12.2 mg/liter TPN soln.

Acrodermatitis Enteropathica and Decreased Wound Healing

- **PO (Adults):** 220 mg 3 times daily.

PHARMACODYNAMICS

	ONSET	PEAK	DURATION
PO	UK	UK	UK
IV	UK	UK	UK

NURSING IMPLICATIONS

Assessment

- ▫ Monitor progression of symptoms of zinc deficiency (impaired wound healing, growth retardation, decreased sense of taste, decreased sense of smell) throughout course of therapy.
- ▪ **Lab Test Considerations:** Serum zinc levels may not accurately reflect zinc deficiency.

Potential Nursing Diagnoses

- ▪ Nutrition, altered: less than body requirements (indications).
- ▪ Knowledge deficit related to medication regimen (patient/family teaching).

Implementation

- ▪ **General Info:** Available in combination with multiple vitamins and minerals.
- ▪ **PO:** Administer oral doses with food to decrease gastric irritation. Administration with caffeine, dairy products, or bran may impair absorption.
- ▪ **IV:** Zinc is often included as a trace mineral in total parenteral nutrition soln prepared by pharmacist.

Patient/Family Teaching

- ▫ Encourage patient to comply with physician's diet recommendations. Explain that the best source of vitamins is a well-balanced diet with foods from the 4 basic food groups. Foods high in zinc include seafood, organ meats, and wheat germ.
- ▫ Patients self-medicating with vitamin supplements should be cautioned not to exceed RDA (see Appendix L). The effectiveness of megadoses for treatment of various medical conditions is unproven and this may cause side effects.
- ▫ Instruct patients receiving oral zinc to notify physician if severe nausea or vomiting, abdominal pain, or tarry stools occur.
- ▫ Emphasize the importance of follow-up examinations to evaluate progress.

Evaluation

Effectiveness of therapy can be demonstrated by: ▪ Improved wound healing ▪ Improved senses of taste or smell. Six to eight wks of therapy may be required before full effect is seen ▪ Resolution of lesions in acrodermatitis.

*Underlines indicate most frequent; **CAPITALS** indicate life-threatening.

APPENDIX CONTENTS

APPENDIX A
Commonly Used Combination Drugs

Note: The drugs listed in this section are in alphabetical order according to trade names. Following each trade name are the generic names of the active drug ingredients contained in each preparation. For information on these drugs, look up each generic name in the combination, listed separately in the *Drug Guide*. For specific doses and inert ingredients see drug label.

Actifed—pseudoephedrine/triprolidine
Alazide—hydrochlorothiazide/spironolactone
Aldactazide—hydrochlorothiazide/spironolactone
Aldoclor—methyldopa/chlorothiazide
Aldoril—hydrochlorothiazide/methyldopa
Alka Seltzer—aspirin/citric acid/sodium bicarbonate
Alka-Seltzer Plus Cold Medicine—chlorpheniramine/phenylpropanolamine/aspirin
All-Nite Cold Formula Liquid—pseudoephedrine/doxylamine/dextromethorphan/acetaminophen
Alodopa—hydrochlorothiazide/methyldopa
Alphaderm—hydrocortisone/urea
Amacodone—acetaminophen/hydrocodone
Amaphen #3—acetaminophen/butalbital/caffeine/codeine
Ambenyl Cough Syrup—codeine/bromodiphenhydramine/alcohol
Amesec—ephedrine/theophylline
Anacin—aspirin/caffeine
Anacin Maximum Strength—aspirin/caffeine
Anatuss—guaifenesin/dextromethorphan/phenylpropanolamine
Anexsia—hydrocodone/acetaminophen
Anodynos-DHC—hydrocodone/acetaminophen
Antrocol—atropine/phenobarbital
Apresazide—hydralazine/hydrochlorothiazide
Apresodex—hydralazine/hydrochlorothiazide
Apresoline-Esidrix—hydralazine/hydrochlorothiazide
Aprodine Syrup—pseudoephedrine/triprolidine
Aprozide—hydralazine/hydrochlorothiazide
Aralen Phosphate with Primoquine Phosphate Tablets—chloroquine/primoquine
Arthritis Pain Formula—aspirin/aluminum hydroxide/magnesium hydroxide
Ascriptin—aspirin/Maalox
Aspirin-Free St. Joseph Complete Nighttime Cold Relief—pseudoephedrine/chlorpheniramine/dextromethorphan
B and O Supprettes—belladonna extract and powdered opium suppositories
B-A-C #3—aspirin/butalbital/caffeine/codeine/buffers
Bacticort Ophthalmic—hydrocortisone/neomycin/polymyxin B
Bancap HC—acetaminophen/hydrocodone
Banex Capsules—guaifenesin/phenylpropanolamine/phenylephrine
Banex-LA Tablets—guaifenesin/phenylpropanolamine
Bayer Children's Cough Syrup—dextromethorphan/phenylpropanolamine
Bellergal-S—ergotamine/belladonna alkaloids/phenobarbital
Benadryl Decongestant—diphenhydramine/pseudoephedrine
Benylin Decongestant Liquid—diphenhydramine/pseudoephedrine/alcohol
Benylin Expectorant Liquid—guaifenesin/dextromethorphan/alcohol
Biphetamine—amphetamine/dextroamphetamine

Blephamide—prednisolone acetate/sulfacetamide
Bromfed Capsules and Tablets—brompheniramine/pseudoephedrine
Bromophen T.D.—brompheniramine/phenylephrine/phenylpropanolamine
Brompheniramine Compound Elixir—brompheniramine/phenylephrine/phenylpropanolamine/alcohol
Bronkaid Tablets—ephedrine sulfate/theophylline/guaifenesin
Buff-A-Comp—aspirin/caffeine/butalbital
Buff-A-Comp #3—aspirin/caffeine/butalbital/codeine
Bufferin—aspirin/buffers: aluminum glycinate, magnesium carbonate
Cafergot—ergotamine/caffeine
Caladryl Lotion—diphenhydramine/calamine/camphor/alcohol
Calcet—calcium lactate/calcium gluconate/calcium carbonate/vitamin D
Calcidrine Syrup—codeine/calcium iodide
Cam-ap-es—hydralazine hydrochloride/hydrochlorothiazide/reserpine
Capozide—hydrochlorothiazide/captopril
Cetacaine—benzocaine/tetracaine/butyl aminobenzoate
Chloromycetin Hydrocortisone Ophthalmic—hydrocortisone/chloramphenicol
Chloroserp—chlorothiazide/reserpine
Chloroserpine—chlorothiazide/reserpine
Chlor-Trimeton Decongestant—pseudoephedrine/chlorpheniramine
Clindex—chlordiazepoxide/clidinium
Clinoxide—chlordiazepoxide/clidinium
Clipoxide—chlordiazepoxide/clidinium
CoAdvil—ibuprofen/pseudoephedrine
Co-Apap—pseudoephedrine/chlorpheniramine/dextromethorphan/acetaminophen
Codamine—hydrocodone/phenylpropanolamine
Codap Tablets—codeine/acetaminophen
Codaphen—codeine/acetaminophen
Codehist DH Elixir—pseudoephedrine/chlorpheniramine/codeine
Codiclear DH Syrup—hydrocodone/guaifenesin
Codimal DH—hydrocodone/phenylephrine/pyrilamine
Codimal Expectorant—guaifenesin/phenylpropanolamine
Codimal LA—chlorpheniramine/pseudoephedrine
Codimal PH—codeine/phenylephrine/pyrilamine
Co-Gesic—acetaminophen/hydrocodone
Colabid—probenecid/colchicine
ColBENEMID—probenecid/colchicine
Coldrine—pseudoephedrine/acetaminophen
Col-Probenecid—probenecid/colchicine
Coly-Mycin S Otic—hydrocortisone/colistin/neomycin/thonzonium
Combipres—chlorthalidone/clonidine
Comtrex—chlorpheniramine/acetaminophen//dextromethorphan/pseudoephredine
Comtrex, Allergy-Sinus—chlorpheniramine/acetaminophen/pseudoephedrine
Comtrex Liqui-Gels—acetaminophen/phenylpropanolamine/chlorpheniramine/dextromethorphan
Congess—guaifenesin/pseudoephedrine
Congestac—guaifenesin/pseudoephedrine
Contac Cough Formula Liquid—dextromethorphan/guaifenesin
Contac Cough & Sore Throat Formula—dextromethorphan/guaifenesin/acetaminophen
Contac Maximum Strength Sinus—pseudoephedrine/acetaminophen
Contac Nighttime Cold—pseudoephedrine/doxylamine succinate/dextromethorphan

Contac Severe Cold—phenylpropanolamine/chlorpheniramine/dextromethorphan/acetaminophen
Contac-12 Hour—phenylpropanolamine/chlorpheniramine
Cope—aspirin/caffeine/magnesium hydroxide/aluminum hydroxide
Cordamine-PA—brompheniramine/phenylephrine/phenylpropanolamine
Cordran-N—flurandreolide/neomycin
Correctol—docusate sodium/phenolphthalein
Cortisporin—bacitracin zinc/neomycin/polymyxin B/hydrocortisone
Corzide—nadolol/bendroflumethiazide
CoTylenol—chlorpheniramine/acetaminophen/pseudoephedrine/dextromethorphan
Cyclomydril—cyclopentolate/phenylephrine
Dallergy—chlorpheniramine/phenylephrine/methscopolamine
Dallergy-D—pseudoephedrine/chlorpheniramine
Damacet-P—hydrocodone/acetaminophen
Damason-P—hydrocodone/aspirin/caffeine
DayCare—guaifenesin/dextromethorphan/pseudoephedrine
Demerol APAP—acetaminophen/meperidine
Demi-Regroton—chlorthalidone/reserpine
Deprol—meprobamate/benactyzine
Dialose Plus—docusate potassium/casanthranol
Dieutrim T. D. Capsules—benzocaine/phenylpropanolamine/carboxymethylcellulose
Di-Gel—aluminum hydroxide/magnesium hydroxide/simethicone
Dihistine DH—pseudoephedrine/chlorpheniramine/codeine
Dilantin with Phenobarbital Kapseals—phenytoin/phenobarbital
Dilaudid Cough Syrup—guaifenesin/hydromorphone
Dimetane Decongestant—brompheniramine/phenylephrine
Dimetapp—brompheniramine/phenylpropanolamine
Diupres—chlorothiazide/reserpine
Diurigen with Reserpine—reserpine/chlorothiazide
Dolacet—hydrocodone/acetaminophen
Donnagel-PG—powdered opium/kaolin/pectin/hyoscyamine/atropine/scopolamine/alcohol
Donnagel—kaolin/pectin/atropine/hyoscyamine/scopolamine
Donnatal—phenobarbital/hyoscyamine/atropine/scopolamine
Doxidan—docusate calcium/phenolphthalein
Dristan—phenylephrine/chlorpheniramine/acetaminophen
Drixoral Plus—pseudoephedrine/dexbrompheniramine/acetaminophen
Drixoral—pseudoephedrine/dexbrompheniramine
D-S-S Plus—docusate sodium/casanthranol
Duo-Medihaler—phenylephrine/isoproterenol
Duradyne—acetaminophen/aspirin/caffeine
Duradyne DHC—hydrocodone/acetaminophen
Dyazide—hydrochlorothiazide/triamterene
Elase-Chloromycetin Ointment—fibrinolysin/desoxyribonuclease/chloramphenicol
Elixophyllin-GG—guaifenesin/theophylline
Empirin #2, #3, #4—aspirin/codeine phosphate
Envoid—mestranol/norethynodrel
E-Pilo—epinephrine bitartrate/pilocarpine
Equagesic—aspirin/meprobamate
Equazine-M—aspirin/meprobamate
Esimil—guanethidine/hydrochlorothiazide

Etrafon—perphenazine/amitriptyline
Excedrin—aspirin/acetaminophen/caffeine
Excedrin P.M. Tablets and Caplets—acetaminophen/diphenhydramine citrate
Ex-Lax Extra Gentle—docusate sodium/phenolphthalein
Feen-A-Mint—docusate sodium/phenolphthalein
Femcaps—acetaminophen/caffeine/ephedrine/atropine
Feosol Plus—ferrous sulfate/folic acid/ascorbic acid
Fergon Plus—ferrous gluconate/ascorbic acid
Ferro-Sequels—docusate sodium/ferrous fumarate
Fiogesic—pseudoephedrine/acetaminophen
Fiorinal #1, #2, #3—aspirin/caffeine/butalbital/codeine
Four-Way Nasal Spray—phenylephrine/naphazoline/pyrilamine
Gaviscon Tablets—aluminum hydroxide/magnesium trisilicate/alginic acid/sodium bicarbonate
Gelusil—aluminum hydroxide/magnesium hydroxide/simethicone
Genatuss DM Syrup—guaifenesin/dextromethorphan/alcohol
Halotussin-DM—guaifenesin/dextromethorphan/alcohol
Head and Chest Cold Medicine—guaifenesin/phenylpropanolamine
Hemorrhoidal HC—hydrocortisone acetate/bismuth/benzyl/benzoate/balsam peru/zinc oxide
H-H-R Tablets—hydralazine/hydrochlorothiazide/reserpine
Histafed C Cough Syrup—pseudoephedrine/triprolidine/codeine
Histafed LA—chlorpheniramine/pseudoephedrine
Histaminic—chlorpheniramine/phenylephrine/phenylpropanolamine/phenyltoloxamine
Hycomine Compound—chlorpheniramine/acetaminophen/phenylephrine/hydrocodone/caffeine
Hycomine Syrup—hydrocodone/phenylpropanolamine
Hyco-Pap—acetaminophen/hydrocodone
Hycotuss Expectorant—guaifenesin/hydrocodone/alcohol
Hydral—hydrochlorothiazide/hydraline
Hydralazine Plus—hydralazine/hydrochlorothiazide
Hydralazine-Thiazide—hydralazine/hydrochlorothiazide
Hydrazide—hydralazine/hydrochlorothiazide
Hydrocet—hydrocodone/acetaminophen
Hydrogesic—hydrocodone/acetaminophen
Hydropine—hydroflumethiazide/reserpine
Hydropres 50—hydrochlorothiazide/reserpine
Hydro-Reserpine—hydrochlorothiazide/reserpine
Hydro-Serp—hydrochlorothiazide/reserpine
Hydroserpalan—hydrochlorothiazide/reserpine
Hydroserpine—hydrochlorothiazide/reserpine
Hydroserpine Plus—hydralazine/hydrochlorothiazide/reserpine
Hydrosine 50—hydrochlorothiazide/reserpine
Iberet Filmtab—ferrous sulfate/ascorbic acid/calcium pantothenate/B-complex vitamins
Iberet Liquid—ferrous sulfate/ascorbic acid/dexpanthenol/B-complex vitamins
Inderide—hydrochlorothiazide/propranolol
Kank-a—benzocaine/benzoin compound/cetylpyridium/castor oil
Kapectolin Belladonna Mixture—kaolin/pectin/atropine/hyoscyamine/scopolamine
Kapectolin PG—kaolin/pectin/atropine/hyoscyamine/scopolamine/powdered opium/alcohol

Kondremul with Cascara—mineral oil/cascara sagrada extract/Irish moss as an emulsifier
Kondremul with Phenolphthalein—phenophthalein/mineral oil/Irish moss
Librax—chlordiazepoxide/clindinium
Lidox—chlordiazepoxide/clidinium
Limbitrol—chlordiazepoxide/amitriptyline
Lophen-C—iodinated glycerol/codeine
Lophen-DM—iodinated glycerol/dextromethorphan
Lopressor HCT—hydrochlorothiazide/metoprolol
Lorcet—acetaminophen/hydrocodone
Lortab—acetaminophen/hydrocodone
Lortab ASA—aspirin/hydrocodone
Lufyllin-EPG—ephedrine/dyphylline/guaifenesin/phenobarbital
Lufyllin-GG—dyphylline/guaifenesin
Maalox Plus—aluminum hydroxide/magnesium hydroxide/simethicone
Marax—ephedrine/theophylline/hydroxyzine
Maxitrol—neomycin/dexamethasone/polymyxin B
Maxzide—hydrochlorothiazide/triamterene
Mediquell Decongestant Formula—dextromethorphan/pseudoephedrine
Menrium—chlordiazepoxide/esterified estrogens
Mepergan—meperidine/promethazine
Mepro-Analgesic—aspirin/meprobamate
Mepro Compound—aspirin/meprobamate
Minizide—prazosin/polythiazide
Modane Plus—docusate sodium/phenolphthalin
Moduretic—hydrochlorothiazide/amiloride
Myapap with Codeine Elixir—codeine/acetaminophen
Mylanta—aluminum hydroxide/magnesium hydroxide/simethicone
Naldecon—chlorpheniramine/phenylephrine/phenylpropanolamine/phenyltoloxamine
Naldecon CX Liquid—guaifenesin/phenylpropanolamine/codeine
Naldecon DX Syrup—guaifenesin/dextromethorphan/phenylpropanolamine
Naldecon EX Syrup—guaifenesin/phenylpropanolamine
Neo-Cortef—hydrocortisone acetate/neomycin
NeoDecadron—neomycin/dexamethasone
Neosporin—neomycin/bacitracin zinc/polymyxin B
Norcet—hydrocodone/acetaminophen
Norgesic—orphenadrine/aspirin/caffeine
Normozide—labetalol/hydrochlorothiazide
Novafed A—chlorpheniramine/pseudoephedrine
Novahistine DH—chlorpheniramine/pseudoephedrine/codeine
Novahistine DMX—guaifenesin/dextromethorphan/pseudoephedrine
Novahistine Expectorant—guaifenesin/pseudoephedrine/codeine
NyQuil Nighttime Cold Medicine—pseudoephedrine/doxylamine/dextromethorphan/alcohol (may contain tartrazine)
Nytime Cold Medicine—pseudoephedrine/doxylamine/dextromethorphan/alcohol
Octicair—hydrocortisone/neomycin/polymyxin B
Ocu-Cort—hydrocortisone/bacitracin/neomycin/polymyxin B
Ocu-Lone-C—prednisolone acetate/sulfacetamide
Ocumycin—polymyxin/bacitracin
Ocu-Spor-B—neomycin/bacitracin/polymyxin B

Ocu-Spor-G—neomycin/gramicidin/polymyxin B
Ocu-Trol—neomycin/dexamethasone/polymyxin B
Ophthocort—hydrocortisone acetate/chloramphenicol/polymyxin B
Optimyd—prednisolone acetate/sulfacetamide
Optised—phenylephrine/zinc sulfate
Orphengesic—orphenadrine/aspirin/caffeine
Otocort—hydrocortisone/neomycin/polymyxin B
P-A-C Tablets—aspirin/caffeine (contains tartrazine)
Papadeine #3, #4—codeine/acetaminophen
Parapectolin—kaolin/pectin/paregoric/opium/alcohol
PediaCare Cough-Cold Formula—pseudoephedrine/chlorpheniramine/dextromethorphan
Pediacof—codeine/phenylephrine/chlorpheniramine/potassium iodide/alcohol
Pediazole—erythromycin/sulfisoxazole
Penntuss—codeine/chlorpheniramine
Perdiem Granules—senna/psyllium/potassium/sodium
Peri-Colace—docusate sodium/casanthranol
Pertussin AM Liquid—dextromethorphan/pseudoephedrine/guaifenesin
Pertussin PM—pseudoephedrine/doxylamine/dextromethorphan/acetaminophen/alcohol
Phenaphen #2, #3, #4—acetaminophen/codeine
Phenergan-D Tablets—pseudoephedrine/promethazine
Phenergan VC—phenylephrine/promethazine
Pherazine with Dextromethorphan—dextromethorphan/promethazine/alcohol
Phillips' LaxCaps—docusate sodium/phenolphthalein
P-I-N Forte—isoniazid/pyridoxine
PMB—conjugated estrogens/meprobamate
Polaramine Expectorant—guaifenesin/dexchlorpheniramine/pseudoephedrine
Polycillin-PRB—ampicillin/probenecid
Poly-Histine—pheniramine/pyrilamine/phenyltoloxamine/alcohol
Poly-Histine CS—phenylpropanolamine/brompheniramine/codeine
Poly-Histine DM—brompheniramine/phenylpropanolamine/dextromethorplan
Poly-Histine Expectorant—guaifenesin/phenylpropanolamine
Poly-Pred Suspension—prednisolone acetate/neomycin/polymyxin B sulfate
Polysporin—polymyxin B/bacitracin
Probampacin—ampicillin/probenecid
Proben-C—probenecid/colchicine
Propain HC—hydrocodone/acetaminophen
Pseudo-Bid A—guaifenesin/chlorpheniramine/pseudoephedrine
Pseudo-Chlor—pseudoephedrine/chlorpheniramine
Pseudo-gest Plus—pseudoephedrine/chlorpheniramine
P-V-Tussin Tablets—guaifenesin/hydrocodone/phenindamine
Quadrinal Tablets—ephedrine/theophylline/potassium iodide/phenobarbital
Quelidrine Cough Syrup—dextromethorphan/phenylephrine/ephedrine/chlorpheniramine/ammonium/ipecac
Quibron—guaifenesin/theophylline
Quiet Night Liquid—pseudoephedrine/doxylamine/dextromethorphan
Regroton—chlorthalidone/reserpine
Regulace—docusate sodium/casanthranol
Respaire-60 SR—guaifenesin/pseudoephedrine
Respinol-G Tablets—guaifenesin/pseudoephedrine/phenylephrine

Rezide—hydralazine/hydrochlorothiazide/reserpine
Rid-A-Pain with Codeine—codeine/aspirin/acetaminophen/caffeine/salicylamide
Rifamate—isoniazid/rifampin
Riopan Plus—magaldrate/simethicone
Robaxisal—aspirin/methocarbamol
Robitussin A-C Syrup—codeine/guaifenesin/alcohol
Robitussin-CF Syrup—guaifenesin/dextromethorphan/phenylpropanolamine/alcohol
Robitussin-DAC—codeine/guaifenesin/pseudoephedrine/alcohol
Robitussin-DM Syrup—guaifenesin/dextromethorphan
Robitussin Night Relief Cold Formula Liquid—dextromethorphan/pyrilamine/phenylephrine/acetaminophen
Robitussin-PE—guaifenesin/pseudoephedrine/alcohol
Ru-Tuss DE Tablets—pseudoephedrine/guaifenesin
Ru-Tuss Expectorant—guaifenesin/pseudoephedrine/dextromethorphan/alcohol
Ru-Tuss Tablets—phenylephrine/phenylpropanolamine/chlorpheniramine/hyoscyamine/atropine/scopolamine
Ru-Tuss II Capsules—phenylpropanolamine/chlorpheniramine
Ru-Tuss with Hydrocodone—hydrocodone/phenylephrine/pyrilamine/pheniramine/phenylpropanolamine/alcohol
Ryna—pseudoephedrine/chlorpheniramine
Ryna-C—guaifenesin/pseudophedrine
Rynatuss—ephedrine/carbetapentane/chlorpheniramine/phenylephrine
Salazide—reserpine/hydroflumethiazide
Salutensin—reserpine/hydroflumethiazide
Sedapap #3—acetaminophen/butabital/codeine
Seldane-D—terfenadine/pseudoephedrine
Senokap DSS—docusate sodium/sennosides
Senokot-S—standardized senna concentrate/docusate sodium
Ser-A-Gen—hydralazine/hydrochlorothiazide/reserpine
Ser-Ap-ES—hydralazine/hydrochlorothiazide/reserpine
Seralazide—hydrochlorothiazide/reserpine/hydralazine
Serathide—hydralazine/hydrochlorothiazide/reserpine
Serpasil-Apresoline—hydralazine/reserpine
Serpasil-Esidrix—hydrochlorothiazide/reserpine
Serpazide—hydralazine/hydrochlorothiazide/reserpine
Sinarest No-Drowsiness Tablets—pseudoephedrine/acetaminophen
Sine-Aid—pseudoephedrine/acetaminophen
Sine-Off Maximum Strength Allergy/Sinus Caplets—pseudoephedrine/chlorpheniramine/acetaminophen
Sine-Off Maximum Strength No Drowsiness Formula Caplets—pseudoephedrine/acetaminophen
Sinutab—acetaminophen/chlorpheniramine/pseudoephedrine
Slo-Phyllin GG Capsules—guaifenesin/theophylline
Soma Compound—aspirin/carisoprodol
Spironazide—hydrochlorothiazide/spironolactone
Sudafed Cough Syrup—guaifenesin/dextromethorphan/pseudoephedrine
Sudafed Plus Tablets—pseudoephedrine/chlorpheniramine
Sulfacort ophthalmic—prednisolone acetate/sulfacetamide
Sulfamide—prednisolone acetate/sulfacetamide
Sulpred—prednisolone/sulfacetamide
Synalgos DC—aspirin/caffeine/dihydrocodeine
Talacen—acetaminophen/pentazocine

Talwin Compound—aspirin/pentazocine
Talwin NX—pentazocine/naloxone
Tavist-D—clemastine/phenylpropanolamine
Tedral—ephedrine/theophylline/phenobarbital
Tedrigen—ephedrine/theophylline/phenobarbital
Tega-Tussin Syrup—hydrocodone/chlorpheniramine/phenylephrine
T.E.H. Tablets—ephedrine/theophylline/hydroxyzine
Tenoretic—chlorthalidone/atenolol
Terphan Elixir—dextromethorphan/terpin hydrate
Terpin-Dex Elixir—dextromethorphan/terpin hydrate/alcohol
Terra-Cortril Suspension—hydrocortisone acetate/oxytetracycline
Terramycin with Polymyxin B Sulfate Ophthalmic Ointment—polymyxin B/oxytetracycline
T-Gesic—hydrocodone/acetaminophen
Theodrine—ephedrine/theophylline/phenobarbital
Timolide—hydrochlorothiazide/timolol
Trandate HCT—hydrochlorothazide/labetalol
Triacin-C Cough Syrup—codeine/pseudoephedrine/triprolidine
Triaminic Allergy—phenylpropanolamine/chlorpheniramine
Triaminic-DM—dextromethorphan/phenylephrine
Triaminic Expectorant—guaifenesin/phenylpropanolamine
Triaminic Expectorant DH—guaifenesin/hydrocodone/phenylpropanolamine/pheniramine/pyrilamine/alcohol
Triaminic Nite Light Liquid—pseudoephedrine/chlorpheniramine/dextromethorphan
Triaminic TR Tablets—phenylpropanolamine/pyrilamine/pheniramine
Triavil—perphenazine/amitriptyline
Trigesic—acetaminophen/aspirin/caffeine
Tri-Hydroserpine—hydralazine/hydrochlorothiazide/reserpine
Trimedine—dextromethorpan/chlorpheniramine/phenylephrine
Triminol Cough Syrup—dextromethorphan/chlorpheniramine/phenylpropanolamine
Trinalin Repetabs—azatadine maleate/pseudoephedrine
Tuinal—amobarbital/secobarbital
Tums Liquid Extra Strength with Simethicone—simethicone/calcium carbonate
Tums Plus—simethicone/calcium carbonate
Tussionex—chlorpheniramine (as polistrix)/hydrocodone polistirix
Ty-Cold Tablets—pseudoephedrine/chlorpheniramine/dextromethorphan/acetaminophen
Tycolet—hydrocodone/acetaminophen
Tylenol #1, #2, #3, #4—acetaminophen/codeine
Tylenol Allergy Sinus—acetaminophen/chlorpheniramine/pseudoephedrine
Tylenol Cold & Flu—acetaminophen/chlorpheniramine/pseudoephedrine/dextromethorphan
Tylenol Cold Medication—acetaminophen/chlorpheniramine/pseudoephedrine/dextromethorphan
Tylenol Maximum Strength Sinus Tablets—pseudoephedrine/acetaminophen
Ty-Pap with Codeine Elixir—codeine/acetaminophen
Ty-Tab #3, #4 Tablets—codeine/acetaminophen
Unipres—hydralazine/hydrochlorothiaizide/reserpine
Vanquish—aspirin/acetaminophen/caffeine/aluminum hydroxide/magnesium hydroxide

Vaseretic—enalapril/hydrochlorothiazide
Veltap Elixir—brompheniramine/phenylephrine/phenylpropanolamine/alcohol
Vicks Children's Cough Syrup—guaifenesin/dextromethorphan
Vicks Children's Nyquil—dextromethorphan/pseudoephedrine/chlorpheniramine
Vicks Cough Silencers—dextromethorphan/benzocaine
Vicks Formula 44 Cough Control Disc—benzocaine/dextromethorphan
Vicks Formula 44 Cough Medicine—dextromethorphan/chlorpheniramine/alcohol
Vicks Formula 44D Liquid—dextromethorphan/pseudoephedrine
Vicks Formula 44M Cough and Cold Medication Liquid—guaifenesin/dextromethorphan/pseudoephedrine
Vicodin—acetaminophen/hydrocodone
Wigraine—ergotamine/caffeine
Zestoretic—lisinopril/hydrochlorthiazide
Zydone—hydrocodone/acetaminophen

APPENDIX B
Equianalgesic Doses of Narcotic Analgesics

EQUIANALGESIC DOSES OF NARCOTIC ANALGESICS

	ROUTE*	EQUI-ANALGESIC DOSE (mg)†	DURATION (hr)	PLASMA HALF-LIFE (hr)	COMMENTS
Narcotic Agonists					
Morphine sulfate	IM PO	10 30	4–6 4–7	2–3.5	Standard for comparison; also available in slow-release tablets and as rectal suppositories
Codeine	IM PO	130 200	4–6 4–6	3	Useful as initial narcotic analgesic
Oxycodone HCl	IM PO	15 30	 3–5	—	Short-acting; available as 5-mg dose in combination with aspirin and acetaminophen and as a soln
Heroin	IM PO	5 60	4–5 4–5	0.5	Illegal in US; high solubility for parenteral administration
Levorphanol tartrate (Levo-Dromoran)	IM PO	2 4	4–6 4–7	12–16	Good oral potency; requires careful titration in initial dosing because of drug accumulation
Hydromorphone HCl (Dilaudid)	IM PO	1.5 7.5	4–5 4–6	2–3	Available in high-potency injectable form (10 mg/ml) for cachectic patients and as rectal suppositories; more soluble than morphine
Oxymorphone HCl (Numorphan)	IM PR	1 10	4–6 4–6	2–3	Available in parenteral and rectal suppository forms only
Meperidine HCl (Demerol HCl, et al)	IM PO	75 300	2–4 4–6	3–8 12–16	Contraindicated in patients with renal disease; accumulation of active toxic metabolite normeperidine produces CNS excitation; also available as a syrup
Methadone HCl (Dolophine HCl)	IM PO	10 20	4–6	15–30	Good oral potency; requires careful titration of the initial dose to avoid drug accumulation
Mixed Agonist-Antagonist Drugs					
Pentazocine (Talwin)	IM PO	60 180	4–6 4–7	2–3	Limited use for cancer pain; psychotomimetic effects with dose escalation; PO form available only in combination with naloxone, aspirin, or acetaminophen; may precipitate withdrawal in physically dependent patients
Nalbuphine HCl (Nubain)	IM PO	10 —	4–6	5	Not available orally; less severe psychotomimetic effects than pentazocine; may precipitate withdrawal in physically dependent patients

EQUIANALGESIC DOSES OF NARCOTIC ANALGESICS

	ROUTE*	EQUI-ANALGESIC DOSE (mg)†	DURA-TION (hr)	PLASMA HALF-LIFE (hr)	COMMENTS
Butorphanol tartrate (Stadol)	IM PO	2 —	3–4	2.5–3.5	Not available orally; produces psychotomimetic effects; may precipitate withdrawal in physically dependent patients
Partial Agonists					
Buprenorphine HCl (Buprenex)	IM SL	0.4 0.8	4–6 5–6	2–3	SL form not available in US; no psychotomimetic effects; may precipitate withdrawal in tolerant patients
Dezocine (Dalgan)	IM	10	3–6	2.4	Not available orally; negligible psychotomimetic effects; may precipitate withdrawal in physically dependent patients

* IM denotes intramuscular; PO, oral; PR, rectal; and SL, sublingual.

† Based on single-dose studies in which an intramuscular dose of each drug listed was compared with morphine to establish the relative potency. Oral doses are those recommended when changing from a parenteral to an oral route. For patients without prior narcotic exposure, the recommended oral starting dose is 30 mg for morphine, 5 mg for methadone, 2 mg for levorphanol, and 4 mg for hydromorphone.

‡ From Fine, PG: Cancer pain: Assessment and management. Hospital Formulary. 22:936, 1987, with permission.

APPENDIX C
Schedules of Controlled Substances

Classes or schedules are determined by the Drug Enforcement Agency (DEA), which is an arm of the United States Justice Department, and are based on the potential for abuse and dependence liability (physical and psychological) of the medication.

Schedule I (C-I): Potential for abuse is so high as to be unacceptable. May be used for research with appropriate limitations. Examples are LSD and heroin.

Schedule II (C-II): High potential for abuse and extreme liability for physical and psychological dependence (amphetamines, narcotic analgesics, dronabinol, certain barbiturates). Outpatient prescriptions must be in writing. In emergencies, telephone orders may be acceptable if a written prescription is provided within 72 hr. No refills are allowed.

Schedule II Drugs Included in Davis's Drug Guide for Nurses

alfentanil
amobarbital
codeine (single entity; solid dosage form or injectable
dronabinol
droperidol/fentanyl
fentanyl
glutethimide
hydromorphone
levorphanol
meperidine
methadone
methylphenidate
morphine
oxycodone
oxymorphone
pentobarbital (oral and parenteral)
secobarbital (oral and parenteral)
sufentanil

Schedule III (C-III): Intermediate potential for abuse (less than C-II) and intermediate liability for physical and psychological dependence (certain nonbarbiturate sedatives, certain nonamphetamine CNS stimulants, and limited dosages of certain narcotic analgesics). Outpatient prescriptions can be refilled five times within 6 mon from date of issue if authorized by prescriber. Telephone orders are acceptable.

Schedule III Drugs Included in Davis's Drug Guide for Nurses

anabolic steroids (testosterone, nandrolone)
butalbital compound (in combination with non-narcotic analgesics)
codeine (in combination with non-narcotic analgesics; solid oral dosage forms)
hydrocodone (in combination with non-narcotic analgesics)
pentobarbital (rectal)
secobarbital (rectal)
thiopental

Schedule IV (C-IV): Less abuse potential than Schedule III with minimal liability for physical or psychological dependence (certain sedative/hypnotics, certain antianxiety agents, some barbiturates, benzodiazepines, chloral hydrate, pentazocine, and propoxyphene). Outpatient prescriptions can be refilled five times within 6 mon from date of issue if authorized by prescriber. Telephone orders are acceptable.

Schedule IV Drugs Included in Davis's Drug Guide for Nurses

alprazolam
chloral hydrate
chlordiazepoxide
clonazepam
clorazepate
codeine (elixir or oral suspension with acetaminophen)
diazepam
estazolam
ethchlorvynol

flurazepam
halazepam
lorazepam
meprobamate
midazolam
oxazepam
paraldehyde
pemoline
pentazocine
phenobarbital
prazepam
propoxyphene
quazepam
temazepam
triazolam

Schedule V (C-V): Minimal abuse potential. Number of outpatients refills determined by prescriber. Some products (cough suppressants with small amounts of codeine, and antidiarrheals containing paregoric) may be available without prescription to patients >18 yrs of age.

Schedule V Drugs Included in Davis's Drug Guide for Nurses

buprenorphine
codeine (in cough preparations; ≤10 mg/5 ml or dosage unit)
diphenoxylate/atropine
paregoric

Some states may have prescription regulations which are stricter.

APPENDIX D
Infusion Rate Tables

ALTEPLASE (Activase)

Dilution: 20 mg vial with 20 ml diluent or 50 mg vial with 50 ml diluent = 1 mg/ml.

Alteplase	dose (vol)	dose (vol)	dose (vol)
1 mg/ml	*1st hr**	*2nd hr*	*3rd hr*
pt >65 kg	60 mg (60 ml)	20 mg (20 ml)	20 mg (20 ml)
Alteplase	dose (mg/kg)	dose (mg/kg)	dose (mg/kg)
1 mg/ml	*1st hr***	*2nd hr*	*3rd hr*
pt <65 kg	0.75 mg/kg	0.25 mg/kg	0.25 mg/kg

* Give 6–10 mg (6–10 ml) as a bolus over first 1–2 min.
** 0.075–0.125 mg/kg of this given as a bolus over the first 1–2 min.

AMINOPHYLLINE

Dilution: 250 mg in 250 ml or 500 mg in 500 ml or 1000 mg in 1000 ml = 1 mg/ml.
Loading dose in patients who have not received aminophylline in preceeding 24 hr = 5.6 mg/kg (5.6 ml/kg) of above dilution administered over 20 min.

Aminophylline Infusion Rates (ml/hr)
Concentration = 1 mg/ml

	Patient Weight					
Dose	**50 kg**	**60 kg**	**70 kg**	**80 kg**	**90 kg**	**100 kg**
loading dose (mg)*	**280 mg**	**336 mg**	**392 mg**	**448 mg**	**504 mg**	**560 mg**
0.9 mg/kg/hr	45 ml/hr	54 ml/hr	63 ml/hr	72 ml/hr	81 ml/hr	90 ml/hr
0.8 mg/kg/hr	40 ml/hr	48 ml/hr	56 ml/hr	64 ml/hr	72 ml/hr	80 ml/hr
0.7 mg/kg/hr	35 ml/hr	42 ml/hr	49 ml/hr	56 ml/hr	63 ml/hr	70 ml/hr
0.6 mg/kg/hr	30 ml/hr	36 ml/hr	42 ml/hr	48 ml/hr	54 ml/hr	60 ml/hr
0.5 mg/kg/hr	25 ml/hr	30 ml/hr	35 ml/hr	40 ml/hr	45 ml/hr	50 ml/hr
0.4 mg/kg/hr	20 ml/hr	24 ml/hr	28 ml/hr	32 ml/hr	36 ml/hr	40 ml/hr
0.3 mg/kg/hr	15 ml/hr	18 ml/hr	21 ml/hr	24 ml/hr	27 ml/hr	30 ml/hr
0.2 mg/kg/hr	10 ml/hr	12 ml/hr	14 ml/hr	16 ml/hr	18 ml/hr	20 ml/hr
0.1 mg/kg/hr	5 ml/hr	6 ml/hr	7 ml/hr	8 ml/hr	9 ml/hr	10 ml/hr

*Loading dose administered over 20 min.

AMRINONE (Inocor)

Dilution: 100 mg/100 ml = 1 mg/ml.
Dilute with 0.45% or 0.9% sodium chloride.
Loading dose: 0.75 mg/kg (0.75 ml/kg) over 2–3 min.
To calculate infusion rate (ml/min), multiply patient's weight (kg) by dose in ml/kg/min.
To calculate infusion rate (ml/hr), multiply patient's weight (kg) by dose in mg/kg/min × 60.

Amrinone Infusion Rates
(ml/hr)
Concentration = 1 mg/ml

	Patient Weight					
Dose	**50 kg**	**60 kg**	**70 kg**	**80 kg**	**90 kg**	**100 kg**
loading dose (mg)*	**37.5 mg**	**45 mg**	**52.5 mg**	**60 mg**	**67.5 mg**	**75 mg**
5 mcg/kg/min	15 ml/hr	18 ml/hr	21 ml/hr	24 ml/hr	27 ml/hr	30 ml/hr
6 mcg/kg/min	18 ml/hr	21.6 ml/hr	25.5 ml/hr	28.8 ml/hr	32.4 ml/hr	36 ml/hr
7 mcg/kg/min	21 ml/hr	25.2 ml/hr	29.4 ml/hr	33.6 ml/hr	37.8 ml/hr	42 ml/hr
8 mcg/kg/min	24 ml/hr	28.8 ml/hr	33.6 ml/hr	38.4 ml/hr	43.2 ml/hr	48 ml/hr
9 mcg/kg/min	27 ml/hr	32.4 ml/hr	37.8 ml/hr	43.2 ml/hr	48.6 ml/hr	54 ml/hr
10 mcg/kg/min	30 ml/hr	36 ml/hr	42 ml/hr	48 ml/hr	54 ml/hr	60 ml/hr

BRETYLIUM (Bretylol)

A. For life-threatening ventricular arrhythmias: (V Fib. or hemodynamically unstable V Tach). Administer 5 mg/kg (0.1 ml/kg) of *undiluted* drug by rapid IV injection. *Undiluted* drug concentration = 50 mg/1 ml.

Rapid IV Injection of Undiluted Bretylium
Doses given in volume of undiluted bretylium injection
50 mg/1 ml

	Patient Weight					
Dose	**50 kg**	**60 kg**	**70 kg**	**80 kg**	**90 kg**	**100 kg**
5 mg/kg	5 ml	6 ml	7 ml	8 ml	9 ml	10 ml

B. For other ventricular arrhythmias: Dilution: 2 g/500 ml = 4 mg/ml. Administer as 5–10 mg/kg (1.25–2.5 ml/kg) IV over 10–30 min, may be repeated q 6 hr or administered as a continuous infusion at 1–2 mg/min.

Bretylium Intermittent Infusion Rates
Volume of diluted bretylium
to infuse over 10–30 min
Concentration = 4 mg/ml

	Patient Weight					
Dose	**50 kg**	**60 kg**	**70 kg**	**80 kg**	**90 kg**	**100 kg**
5 mg/kg	62.5 ml	75 ml	87.5 ml	100 ml	112.5 ml	125 ml
6 mg/kg	75 ml	90 ml	105 ml	120 ml	135 ml	150 ml
7 mg/kg	87.5 ml	105 ml	122.5 ml	140 ml	157.5 ml	175 ml
8 mg/kg	100 ml	120 ml	140 ml	160 ml	180 ml	200 ml
9 mg/kg	112.5 ml	135 ml	157.5 ml	180 ml	202.5 ml	225 ml
10 mg/kg	125 ml	150 ml	175 ml	200 ml	225 ml	250 ml

Bretylium Continuous Infusion Rates
Concentration = 4 mg/ml

Dose mg/min	**Dose ml/hr**
1.0 mg/min	15 ml/hr
1.5 mg/min	23 ml/hr
2.0 mg/min	30 ml/hr

DOBUTAMINE (Dobutrex)

Dilution: May be prepared as 250 mg/1000 ml = 250 mcg/ml.
500 mg/1000 ml = 500 mcg/ml.
1000 mg/1000 ml = 1000 mcg/ml.

To calculate infusion rate (ml/min), multiply patient's weight (kg) by dose in ml/kg/min.
To calculate infusion rate (ml/hr), multiply patient's weight (kg) by dose in ml/kg/min × 60.

Dobutamine Infusion Rates (ml/hr)
Concentration = 250 mcg/ml

	Patient Weight					
Dose	**50 kg**	**60 kg**	**70 kg**	**80 kg**	**90 kg**	**100 kg**
2.5 mcg/kg/min	30 ml/hr	36 ml/hr	42 ml/hr	48 ml/hr	54 ml/hr	60 ml/hr
5 mcg/kg/min	60 ml/hr	72 ml/hr	84 ml/hr	96 ml/hr	108 ml/hr	120 ml/hr
7.5 mcg/kg/min	90 ml/hr	108 ml/hr	126 ml/hr	144 ml/hr	162 ml/hr	180 ml/hr
10 mcg/kg/min	120 ml/hr	144 ml/hr	168 ml/hr	192 ml/hr	216 ml/hr	240 ml/hr

Dobutamine Infusion Rates (ml/hr)
Concentration = 500 mcg/ml

	Patient Weight					
Dose	**50 kg**	**60 kg**	**70 kg**	**80 kg**	**90 kg**	**100 kg**
2.5 mcg/kg/min	15 ml/hr	18 ml/hr	21 ml/hr	24 ml/hr	22.5 ml/hr	30 ml/hr
5 mcg/kg/min	30 ml/hr	36 ml/hr	42 ml/hr	48 ml/hr	54 ml/hr	60 ml/hr
7.5 mcg/kg/min	45 ml/hr	54 ml/hr	63 ml/hr	72 ml/hr	81 ml/hr	90 ml/hr
10 mcg/kg/min	60 ml/hr	72 ml/hr	84 ml/hr	96 ml/hr	108 ml/hr	120 ml/hr

Dobutamine Infusion Rates (ml/hr)
Concentration = 1000 mcg/ml

	Patient Weight					
Dose	**50 kg**	**60 kg**	**70 kg**	**80 kg**	**90 kg**	**100 kg**
2.5 mcg/kg/min	7.5 ml/hr	9 ml/hr	10.5 ml/hr	12 ml/hr	11.3 ml/hr	15 ml/hr
5 mcg/kg/min	15 ml/hr	18 ml/hr	21 ml/hr	24 ml/hr	27 ml/hr	30 ml/hr
7.5 mcg/kg/min	22.3 ml/hr	27 ml/hr	31.5 ml/hr	36 ml/hr	40.5 ml/hr	45 ml/hr
10 mcg/kg/min	30 ml/hr	36 ml/hr	41 ml/hr	48 ml/hr	54 ml/hr	60 ml/hr

DOPAMINE (Intropin)

Dilution: May be prepared as 200 mg/500 ml = 400 mcg/ml.
400 mg/500 ml = 800 mcg/ml.
800 mg/500 ml = 1600 mcg/ml†.

To calculate infusion rate (ml/min), multiply patient's weight (kg) by dose in ml/kg/min.
To calculate infusion rate (ml/hr), multiply patient's weight (kg) by dose in ml/kg/min × 60.

Dopamine Infusion Rates (ml/hr)
400 mcg/ml Concentration

	Patient Weight					
Dose	**50 kg**	**60 kg**	**70 kg**	**80 kg**	**90 kg**	**100 kg**
2 mcg/kg/min	15 ml/hr	18 ml/hr	21 ml/hr	24 ml/hr	27 ml/hr	30 ml/hr
5 mcg/kg/min	37.5 ml/hr	45 ml/hr	52.5 ml/hr	60 ml/hr	67.5 ml/hr	75 ml/hr
10 mcg/kg/min	75 ml/hr	90 ml/hr	105 ml/hr	120 ml/hr	135 ml/hr	150 ml/hr
20 mcg/kg/min	150 ml/hr	180 ml/hr	210 ml/hr	240 ml/hr	270 ml/hr	300 ml/hr
30 mcg/kg/min	225 ml/hr	270 ml/hr	315 ml/hr	360 ml/hr	405 ml/hr	450 ml/hr
40 mcg/kg/min	300 ml/hr	360 ml/hr	420 ml/hr	480 ml/hr	540 ml/hr	600 ml/hr
50 mcg/kg/min	375 ml/hr	450 ml/hr	525 ml/hr	600 ml/hr	675 ml/hr	750 ml/hr

Dopamine Infusion Rates (ml/hr)
800 mcg/ml Concentration

	Patient Weight					
Dose	**50 kg**	**60 kg**	**70 kg**	**80 kg**	**90 kg**	**100 kg**
2 mcg/kg/min	7.5 ml/hr	9 ml/hr	10.5 ml/hr	12 ml/hr	13.5 ml/hr	15 ml/hr
5 mcg/kg/min	18.8 ml/hr	22.5 ml/hr	26.3 ml/hr	30 ml/hr	33.8 ml/hr	37.5 ml/hr
10 mcg/kg/min	37.5 ml/hr	45 ml/hr	52.5 ml/hr	60 ml/hr	67.5 ml/hr	75 ml/hr
20 mcg/kg/min	75 ml/hr	90 ml/hr	105 ml/hr	120 ml/hr	135 ml/hr	150 ml/hr
30 mcg/kg/min	112.5 ml/hr	135 ml/hr	157.5 ml/hr	180 ml/hr	202.5 ml/hr	225 ml/hr
40 mcg/kg/min	150 ml/hr	180 ml/hr	210 ml/hr	240 ml/hr	270 ml/hr	300 ml/hr
50 mcg/kg/min	187.5 ml/hr	225 ml/hr	262.5 ml/hr	300 ml/hr	337.5 ml/hr	375 ml/hr

Dopamine Infusion Rates (ml/hr)
1600 mcg/ml Concentration†

	Patient Weight					
Dose	**50 kg**	**60 kg**	**70 kg**	**80 kg**	**90 kg**	**100 kg**
2 mcg/kg/min	3.8 ml/hr	4.5 ml/hr	5.3 ml/hr	6 ml/hr	6.8 ml/hr	7.5 ml/hr
5 mcg/kg/min	9.4 ml/hr	11.2 ml/hr	13.1 ml/hr	15.0 ml/hr	16.9 ml/hr	18.7 ml/hr
10 mcg/kg/min	18.8 ml/hr	22.5 ml/hr	26.3 ml/hr	30 ml/hr	33.8 ml/hr	37.5 ml/hr
20 mcg/kg/min	37.5 ml/hr	45 ml/hr	52.5 ml/hr	60 ml/hr	67.5 ml/hr	75 ml/hr
30 mcg/kg/min	56.3 ml/hr	67.5 ml/hr	78.8 ml/hr	90 ml/hr	101.3 ml/hr	112.5 ml/hr
40 mcg/kg/min	75 ml/hr	90 ml/hr	105 ml/hr	120 ml/hr	135 ml/hr	150 ml/hr
50 mcg/kg/min	93.8 ml/hr	112.5 ml/hr	131.3 ml/hr	150 ml/hr	168.8 ml/hr	187.5 ml/hr

† Appropriate concentration for patients with fluid restriction.

EPINEPHRINE

Dilution: 1 mg/250 ml = 4 mcg/ml.

Epinephrine Infusion Rates (ml/hr)
Concentration = 4 mcg/ml

Dose (mcg/ml)	Dose (ml/hr)
1 mcg/min	15 ml/hr
2 mcg/min	30 ml/hr
3 mcg/min	45 ml/hr
4 mcg/min	60 ml/hr

ESMOLOL (Brevibloc)

Dilution: 5 g/500 ml = 10 mg/ml.
Loading regimen = 500 mcg/kg (0.05 ml/kg) loading dose over 1 min, followed by 50 mcg/kg/min (0.005 ml/kg/min) infusion over 4 min. If no response, repeat loading dose over 1 min and increase infusion rate to 100 mcg/kg/min for 4–10 min. If no response, loading dose may be repeated before increasing infusion rates in 50 mcg/kg/min increments.

Esmolol Infusion Rates
Concentration = 10 mg/ml

	Patient Weight					
Dose	**50 kg**	**60 kg**	**70 kg**	**80 kg**	**90 kg**	**100 kg**
loading dose (ml)*	**2.5 ml**	**3 ml**	**3.5 ml**	**4 ml**	**4.5 ml**	**5 ml**
50 mcg/kg/min	15 ml/hr	18 ml/hr	21 ml/hr	24 ml/hr	27 ml/hr	30 ml/hr
75 mcg/kg/min	22.5 ml/hr	27 ml/hr	31.5 ml/hr	36 ml/hr	40.5 ml/hr	45 ml/hr
100 mcg/kg/min	30 ml/hr	36 ml/hr	42 ml/hr	48 ml/hr	54 ml/hr	60 ml/hr
125 mcg/kg/min	37.5 ml/hr	45 ml/hr	52.5 ml/hr	60 ml/hr	67.5 ml/hr	75 ml/hr
150 mcg/kg/min	38 ml/hr	54 ml/hr	63 ml/hr	72 ml/hr	81 ml/hr	90 ml/hr
175 mcg/kg/min	52.5 ml/hr	63 ml/hr	73.5 ml/hr	84 ml/hr	94.5 ml/hr	105 ml/hr
200 mcg/kg/min	60 ml/hr	72 ml/hr	84 ml/hr	96 ml/hr	108 ml/hr	120 ml/hr

* Loading dose given over 1 min.

HEPARIN

Dilution: 20,000 units/1000 ml = 20 units/ml.
Loading dose: 1000–2000 units as a bolus.

Heparin Infusion Rates (ml/hr)
Concentration = 20 units/ml

Dose (units/hr)	Dose (ml/hr)
500 units/hr	25 ml/hr
750 units/hr	37.5 ml/hr
1000 units/hr	50 ml/hr
1250 units/hr	62.5 ml/hr
1500 units/hr	75 ml/hr
1750 units/hr	87.5 ml/hr
2000 units/hr	100 ml/hr

ISOPROTERENOL (Isuprel)

Dilution: 2 mg/500 ml.

Isoproterenol Infusion Rates (ml/hr)
Concentration = 4 mcg/ml

Dose (mcg/min)	Dose (ml/hr)
2 mcg/min	30 ml/hr
5 mcg/min	75 ml/hr
10 mcg/min	150 ml/hr
15 mcg/min	225 ml/hr
20 mcg/min	300 ml/hr

LIDOCAINE (Xylocaine)

Dilution: May be prepared as 1 g/1000 ml = 1 mg/ml.
2 g/1000 ml = 2 mg/ml.
4 g/1000 ml = 4 mg/ml.
8 g/1000 ml = 8 mg/ml.
Loading dose: 50–100 mg at 25–50 mg/min.

	Lidocaine Infusion Rates (ml/hr)			
Dose (mg/min)	**1 mg/ml concentration**	**2 mg/ml concentration**	**4 mg/ml concentration**	**8 mg/ml concentration**
1 mg/min	60 ml/hr	30 ml/hr	15 ml/hr	7.5 ml/hr
2 mg/min	120 ml/hr	60 ml/hr	30 ml/hr	15 ml/hr
3 mg/min	180 ml/hr	90 ml/hr	45 ml/hr	22.5 ml/hr
4 mg/min	240 ml/hr	120 ml/hr	60 ml/hr	30 ml/hr

NITROGLYCERIN (Nitro-bid, Nitrol, Nitrostat, and Tridil)

Dilution: May be prepared as 5 mg/100 ml (25 mg/500 ml, 50 mg/1000 ml) = 50 mcg/ml.
25 mg/250 ml (50 mg/500 ml, 100 mg/1000 ml) = 100 mcg/ml.
50 mg/250 ml (100 mg/500 ml, 200 mg/1000 ml = 200 mcg/ml.
Note that different products are available in different concentrated solutions and should be used with appropriate infusion tubing. Changes in tubing may result in altered response to a given dose.

	Nitroglycerin Infusion Rates (ml/hr)		
Dose (mcg/min)	**50 mcg/ml concentration**	**100 mcg/ml concentration**	**200 mcg/ml concentration**
2.5 mcg/min	3 ml/hr	1.5 ml/hr	0.75 ml/hr
5 mcg/min	6 ml/hr	3 ml/hr	1.5 ml/hr
10 mcg/min	12 ml/hr	6 ml/hr	3 ml/hr
15 mcg/min	18 ml/hr	9 ml/hr	4.5 ml/hr
20 mcg/min	24 ml/hr	12 ml/hr	6 ml/hr
30 mcg/min	36 ml/hr	18 ml/hr	9 ml/hr
40 mcg/min	48 ml/hr	24 ml/hr	12 ml/hr
50 mcg/min	60 ml/hr	30 ml/hr	15 ml/hr
60 mcg/min	72 ml/hr	36 ml/hr	18 ml/hr

NITROPRUSSIDE (Nipride, Nitropress)

Dilution: May be prepared as 50 mg/1000 ml = 50 mcg/ml.
100 mg/1000 ml = 100 mg/ml.
200 mg/1000 ml = 200 mcg/ml.
To calculate infusion rate (ml/min), multiply patient's weight (kg) by dose in ml/kg/min.
To calculate infusion rate (ml/hr), multiply patient's weight (kg) by dose in ml/kg/min × 60.

Dose (mcg/kg/min)	Nitroprusside Infusion Rates (ml/kg/min) 50 mcg/ml concentration	100 mcg/ml concentration	200 mcg/ml concentration
0.5 mcg/kg/min	0.01 ml/kg/min	—	—
1 mcg/kg/min	0.02 ml/kg/min	0.01 ml/kg/min	—
2 mcg/kg/min	0.04 ml/kg/min	0.02 ml/kg/min	0.01 ml/kg/min
3 mcg/kg/min	0.06 ml/kg/min	0.03 ml/kg/min	0.015 ml/kg/min
4 mcg/kg/min	0.08 ml/kg/min	0.04 ml/kg/min	0.02 ml/kg/min
5 mcg/kg/min	0.1 ml/kg/min	0.05 ml/kg/min	0.025 ml/kg/min
6 mcg/kg/min	0.12 ml/kg/min	0.06 ml/kg/min	0.03 ml/kg/min
7 mcg/kg/min	0.14 ml/kg/min	0.07 ml/kg/min	0.035 ml/kg/min
8 mcg/kg/min	0.16 ml/kg/min	0.08 ml/kg/min	0.04 ml/kg/min
9 mcg/kg/min	0.18 ml/kg/min	0.09 ml/kg/min	0.045 ml/kg/min
10 mcg/kg/min	0.2 ml/kg/min	0.1 ml/kg/min	0.05 ml/kg/min

Nitroprusside Infusion Rates (ml/hr)
50 mcg/ml Concentration

	Patient Weight					
Dose	50 kg	60 kg	70 kg	80 kg	90 kg	100 kg
0.5 mcg/kg/min	30 ml/hr	36 ml/hr	42 ml/hr	48 ml/hr	54 ml/hr	60 ml/hr
1 mcg/kg/min	60 ml/hr	72 ml/hr	84 ml/hr	96 ml/hr	108 ml/hr	120 ml/hr
2 mcg/kg/min	120 ml/hr	144 ml/hr	168 ml/hr	192 ml/hr	216 ml/hr	240 ml/hr
3 mcg/kg/min	180 ml/hr	216 ml/hr	252 ml/hr	288 ml/hr	324 ml/hr	360 ml/hr
4 mcg/kg/min	240 ml/hr	288 ml/hr	336 ml/hr	384 ml/hr	432 ml/hr	480 ml/hr
5 mcg/kg/min	300 ml/hr	360 ml/hr	420 ml/hr	480 ml/hr	540 ml/hr	600 ml/hr
6 mcg/kg/min	360 ml/hr	432 ml/hr	504 ml/hr	576 ml/hr	648 ml/hr	720 ml/hr
7 mcg/kg/min	420 ml/hr	504 ml/hr	588 ml/hr	672 ml/hr	756 ml/hr	840 ml/hr
8 mcg/kg/min	480 ml/hr	576 ml/hr	672 ml/hr	768 ml/hr	864 ml/hr	960 ml/hr
9 mcg/kg/min	540 ml/hr	648 ml/hr	672 ml/hr	864 ml/hr	972 ml/hr	1080 ml/hr
10 mcg/kg/min	600 ml/hr	720 ml/hr	840 ml/hr	960 ml/hr	1080 ml/hr	1200 ml/hr

Nitroprusside Infusion Rates (ml/hr)
100 mcg/ml Concentration

	Patient Weight					
Dose	50 kg	60 kg	70 kg	80 kg	90 kg	100 kg
0.5 mcg/kg/min	15 ml/hr	18 ml/hr	21 ml/hr	24 ml/hr	27 ml/hr	30 ml/hr
1 mcg/kg/min	30 ml/hr	36 ml/hr	42 ml/hr	48 ml/hr	54 ml/hr	60 ml/hr
2 mcg/kg/min	60 ml/hr	72 ml/hr	84 ml/hr	96 ml/hr	108 ml/hr	120 ml/hr
3 mcg/kg/min	90 ml/hr	108 ml/hr	126 ml/hr	144 ml/hr	162 ml/hr	180 ml/hr
4 mcg/kg/min	120 ml/hr	144 ml/hr	168 ml/hr	192 ml/hr	216 ml/hr	240 ml/hr
5 mcg/kg/min	150 ml/hr	180 ml/hr	210 ml/hr	240 ml/hr	270 ml/hr	300 ml/hr
6 mcg/kg/min	180 ml/hr	216 ml/hr	252 ml/hr	288 ml/hr	324 ml/hr	360 ml/hr
7 mcg/kg/min	210 ml/hr	252 ml/hr	294 ml/hr	336 ml/hr	378 ml/hr	420 ml/hr
8 mcg/kg/min	240 ml/hr	288 ml/hr	336 ml/hr	384 ml/hr	432 ml/hr	480 ml/hr
9 mcg/kg/min	270 ml/hr	324 ml/hr	336 ml/hr	432 ml/hr	486 ml/hr	540 ml/hr
10 mcg/kg/min	300 ml/hr	360 ml/hr	420 ml/hr	480 ml/hr	540 ml/hr	600 ml/hr

Nitroprusside Infusion Rates (ml/hr)
200 mcg/ml Concentration

	Patient Weight					
Dose	**50 kg**	**60 kg**	**70 kg**	**80 kg**	**90 kg**	**100 kg**
0.5 mcg/kg/min	7.5 ml/hr	9 ml/hr	10.5 ml/hr	12 ml/hr	13.5 ml/hr	15 ml/hr
1 mcg/kg/min	15 ml/hr	18 ml/hr	21 ml/hr	24 ml/hr	27 ml/hr	30 ml/hr
2 mcg/kg/min	30 ml/hr	36 ml/hr	42 ml/hr	48 ml/hr	54 ml/hr	60 ml/hr
3 mcg/kg/min	45 ml/hr	54 ml/hr	63 ml/hr	72 ml/hr	81 ml/hr	90 ml/hr
4 mcg/kg/min	60 ml/hr	72 ml/hr	84 ml/hr	96 ml/hr	108 ml/hr	120 ml/hr
5 mcg/kg/min	75 ml/hr	90 ml/hr	105 ml/hr	120 ml/hr	135 ml/hr	150 ml/hr
6 mcg/kg/min	90 ml/hr	108 ml/hr	126 ml/hr	144 ml/hr	162 ml/hr	180 ml/hr
7 mcg/kg/min	105 ml/hr	126 ml/hr	147 ml/hr	168 ml/hr	189 ml/hr	210 ml/hr
8 mcg/kg/min	120 ml/hr	144 ml/hr	168 ml/hr	192 ml/hr	216 ml/hr	240 ml/hr
9 mcg/kg/min	135 ml/hr	162 ml/hr	168 ml/hr	216 ml/hr	243 ml/hr	270 ml/hr
10 mcg/kg/min	150 ml/hr	180 ml/hr	210 ml/hr	240 ml/hr	270 ml/hr	300 ml/hr

NOREPINEPHRINE (Levophed)

Dilution: May be prepared as 1 mg/250 = 4 mcg/ml.
To calculate infusion rate (ml/hr), multiply infusion rate in ml/min × 60.

Norepinephrine Infusion Rates (ml/hr)
Concentration = 4 mcg/ml

Dose (mcg/min)	Dose (ml/hr)
8 mcg/min	120 ml/hr
9 mcg/min	135 ml/hr
10 mcg/min	150 ml/hr
11 mcg/min	165 ml/hr
12 mcg/min	180 ml/hr

PHENYLEPHRINE (Neo-Synephrine)

Dilution: 10 mg/500 ml = 20 mcg/ml.

Phenylephrine Infusion Rates (ml/hr)
Concentration = 20 mcg/ml

Dose (mg/min)	Dose (ml/hr)
0.04 mg/min	120 ml/hr
0.06 mg/min	180 ml/hr
0.08 mg/min	240 ml/hr
0.10 mg/min	300 ml/hr
0.12 mg/min	360 ml/hr
0.14 mg/min	420 ml/hr
0.16 mg/min	480 ml/hr
0.18 mg/min	540 ml/hr

PROCAINAMIDE (Pronestyl)

Dilution: May be prepared as 1000 mg/500 ml = 2 mg/ml.

Loading dose: 50–100 mg q 5 min until arrhythmia is controlled; adverse reaction occurs, or 500 mg has been given, *or* 500–600 mg as a loading infusion over 25–30 min.

Procainamide Infusion Rates (ml/hr)
Concentration = 2 mg/ml

Dose (mg/min)	Dose (ml/hr)
1 mg/min	30 ml/hr
2 mg/min	60 ml/hr
3 mg/min	90 ml/hr
4 mg/min	120 ml/hr
5 mg/min	150 ml/hr
6 mg/min	180 ml/hr

APPENDIX E
Food and Drug Administration Pregnancy Categories

Category A
As demonstrated by studies that are adequate and well controlled, no risk to the fetus in the first trimester has been demonstrated. In addition, there does not appear to be risk in the second or third trimester.

Category B
Studies in animals may or may not have shown risk. If risk has been shown in animals, no risk has been shown in human studies. If risk has not been seen in animals, there are insufficient data in pregnant women.

Category C
Adverse effects have been demonstrated in animals, but there are insufficient data in pregnant women. In certain clinical situations, the benefits of use of the medication could outweigh possible risks.

Category D
Based on information collected in clinical investigations or post-marketing surveillance, human fetal risk has been demonstrated. In certain clinical situations, the benefits of use of the medication could outweigh possible risks.

Category X
Human fetal risk has been clearly documented in human studies, animal studies, clinical investigation, or post-marketing surveillance. Possible risks to the fetus outweigh potential benefits to the pregnant women. Avoid use during pregnancy.

APPENDIX F
Formulas for Calculations

Ratio and Proportion

A ratio is the same as a fraction and can be expressed as a fraction ($\frac{1}{2}$) or in the algebraic form (1:2). This relationship is stated as "one is to two."

A proportion is an equation of equal fractions or ratios.

$$\frac{1}{2} = \frac{4}{8}$$

To calculate doses, begin each proportion with the two known values, for example 15 grains = 1 gram (known equivalent) or 10 milligrams = 2 milliliters (dosage available) on one side of the equation. Next, make certain that the units of measure on the opposite side of the equation are the same as the units of the known values and are placed on the same level of the equation.

Problem A $$\frac{15\ gr}{1\ g} = \frac{10\ gr}{x\ g}$$

Problem B $$\frac{10\ mg}{2\ ml} = \frac{5\ mg}{x\ ml}$$

Once the proportion is set up correctly, cross-multiply the opposing values of the proportion.

Problem A $$\frac{15\ gr}{1\ g} \times \frac{10\ gr}{x\ g}$$

$$15x = 10$$

Problem B $$\frac{10\ mg}{2\ ml} \times \frac{5\ mg}{x\ ml}$$

$$10x = 10$$

Next, divide each side of the equation by the number with the x to determine the answer. Then, add the unit of measure corresponding to x in the original equation.

Problem A $$\frac{15x}{15} = \frac{10}{15}$$

$$x = \frac{2}{3} \text{ or } 0.6\ g$$

Problem B $$\frac{10x}{10} = \frac{10}{10}$$

$$x = 1\ ml$$

Calculation of IV Drip Rate

To calculate the drip rate for an intravenous infusion, three values are needed.

A. The amount of solution and corresponding time for infusion. May be ordered as:

1000 ml over 8 hr

or

125 ml/hr

B. The equivalent in time to convert hours to minutes.

1 hr = 60 min

C. The drop factor or number of drops that equal 1 ml of fluid. (This information can be found on the IV tubing box.)

10 gtt = 1 ml

Set up the problem by placing each of the three values in a proportion.

$$\frac{125\text{ ml}}{1\text{ hr}} \times \frac{1\text{ hr}}{60\text{ min}} \times \frac{10\text{ gtt}}{1\text{ ml}}$$

Numbers and units of measure can be cancelled out from the upper and lower levels of this equation.

The numbers cancel, leaving:

$$\frac{125\text{ ml}}{1\text{ hr}} \times \frac{1\text{ hr}}{\underset{6}{\cancel{60}}\text{ min}} \times \frac{\overset{1}{\cancel{10}}\text{ gtt}}{1\text{ ml}}$$

The units cancel, leaving:

$$\frac{125\ \cancel{\text{ml}}}{1\ \cancel{\text{hr}}} \times \frac{1\ \cancel{\text{hr}}}{6\text{ min}} \times \frac{1\text{ gtt}}{1\ \cancel{\text{ml}}}$$

Next, multiply each level across and divide the numerator by the denominator for the answer.

$$\frac{125\ \cancel{\text{ml}}}{1\ \cancel{\text{hr}}} \times \frac{1\ \cancel{\text{hr}}}{6\text{ min}} \times \frac{1\text{ gtt}}{1\ \cancel{\text{ml}}} = \frac{125\text{ gtt}}{6\text{ min}}$$

$$125 \div 6 = 20.8 \text{ or } 21\text{ gtt/min}$$

APPENDIX G
Body Surface Area Nomograms

ESTIMATING BODY SURFACE AREA IN CHILDREN

For pediatric patients of average size, body surface area may be estimated with the scale on the left. Match weight to corresponding surface area. For other pediatric patients, use the scale on the right. Lay a straightedge on the correct height and weight points for your patient, and observe the point where it intersects on the surface area scale at center.

FOR CHILDREN OF NORMAL HEIGHT AND WEIGHT

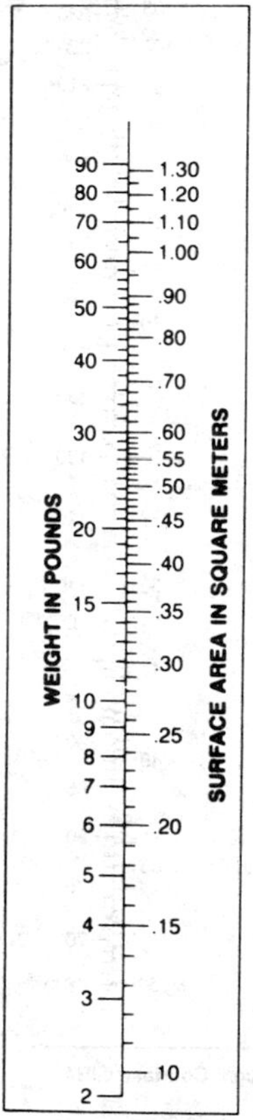

FOR OTHER CHILDREN

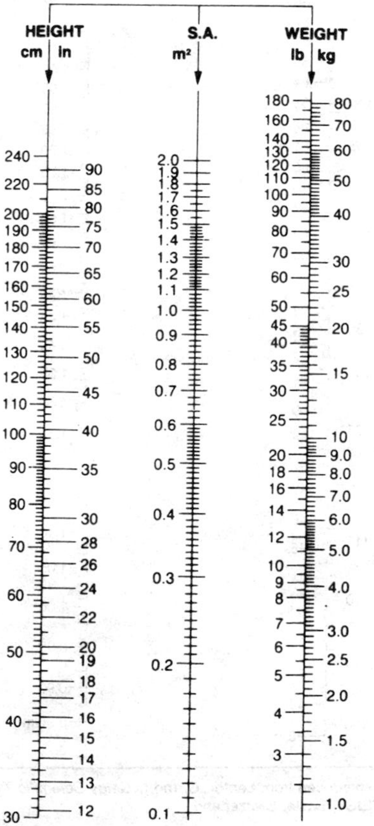

Reproduced from *Nelson Textbook of Pediatrics*, 13th edition. Courtesy W.B. Saunders Co., Philadelphia, Pa.

ESTIMATING BODY SURFACE AREA IN ADULTS

Use a straightedge to connect the patient's height in the left-hand column to weight in the right-hand column. The intersection of this line with the center scale estimates the body surface area.

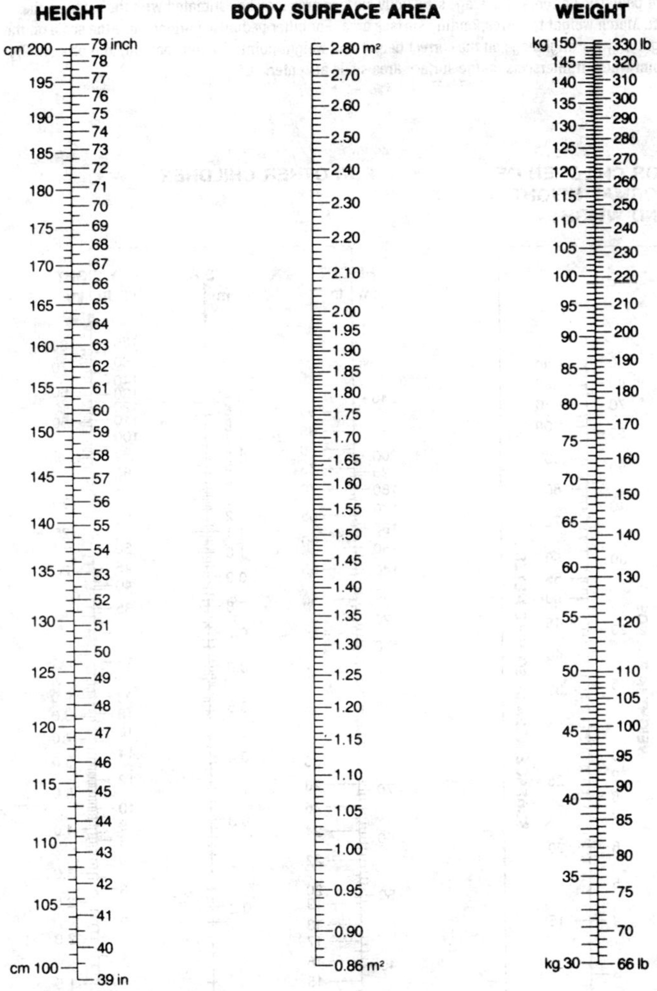

Reproduced from Lenter, C. (ed.), *Geigy Scientific Tables*, 8th edition. Courtesy CIBA-GEIGY, Basle, Switzerland.

Administration Techniques

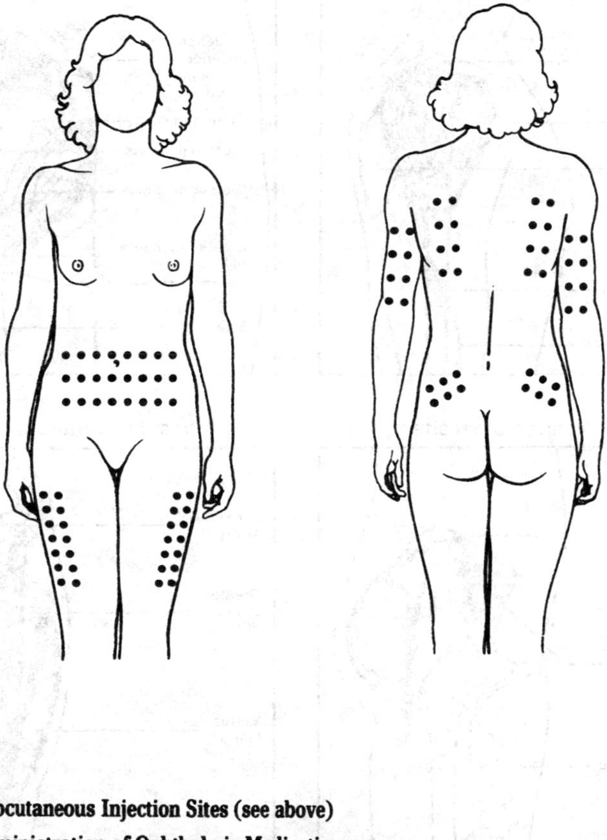

Subcutaneous Injection Sites (see above)

Administration of Ophthalmic Medications

For instillation of ophthalmic solutions, instruct patient to lie down or tilt head back and look at ceiling. Pull down on lower lid, creating a small pocket, and instill solution into pocket. With systemically acting drugs apply pressure to the inner canthus for 1–2 min to minimize systemic absorption. Instruct patient to gently close eye. Wait 5 min before instilling second drop or any other ophthalmic solutions.

For instillation of ophthalmic ointment, instruct patient to hold tube in hand for several minutes to warm. Squeeze a small amount of ointment (¼–½ inch) inside lower lid. Instruct patient to close eye gently and roll eyeball around in all directions with eye closed. Wait 10 min before instilling any other ophthalmic ointments.

Do not touch cap or tip of container to eye, fingers, or any surface.

Intramuscular Injection Sites (see below)

Deltoid site

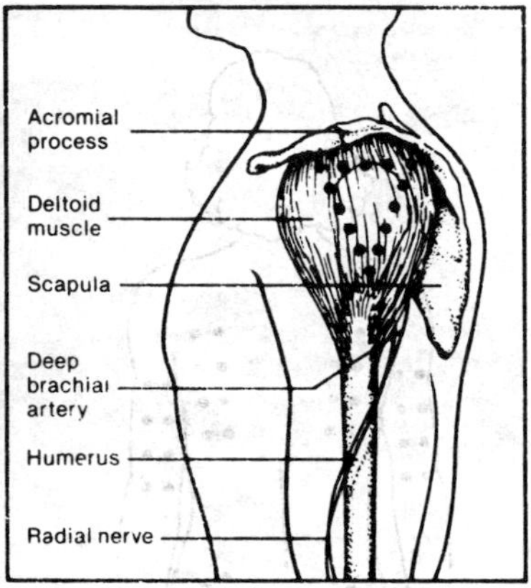

Dorsogluteal site

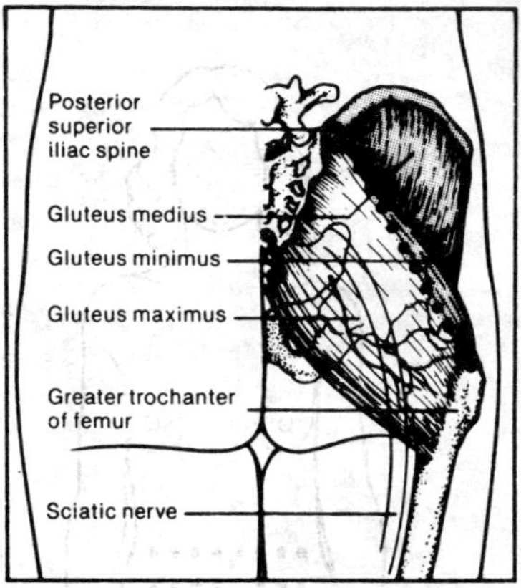

Ventrogluteal site

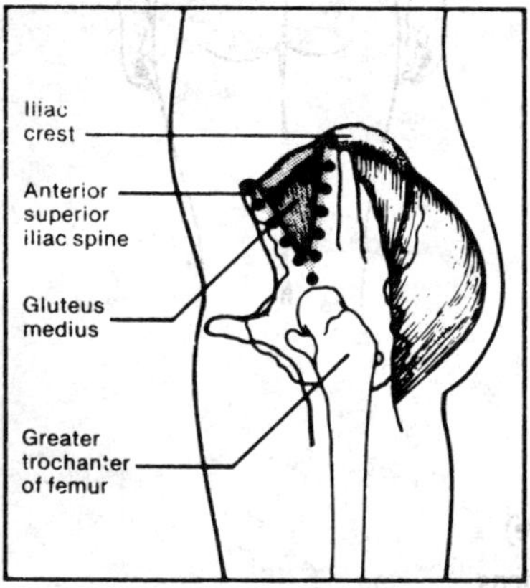

Vastus lateralis site

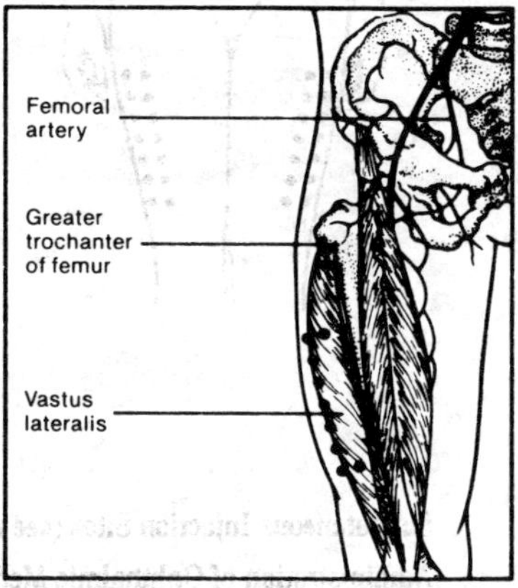

APPENDIX I
Guidelines for Personnel Dealing with Cytotoxic (Antineoplastic Drugs)*

PREAMBLE

The mutagenic, teratogenic, carcinogenic, and local irritant properties of many cytotoxic agents are well established and pose a possible hazard to the health of occupationally exposed individuals. These potential hazards necessitate special attention to the procedures utilized in the handling, preparation and administration of these drugs, and the proper disposal of residues and wastes. These recommendations are intended to provide information for the protection of personnel participating in the clinical process of chemotherapy. It is the responsibility of institutional and private health care providers to adopt and use appropriate procedures for protection and safety.

I. Enrivonmental Protection

1. Preparation of cytotoxic agents should be performed in a Class II biological safety cabinet located in an area with minimal traffic and air turbulence. Class II Type A cabinets are the minimal requirement. Class II cabinets which are exhausted to the outside are preferred.
2. The biological safety cabinet must be certified by qualified personnel at least annually or any time the cabinet is physically moved.

II. Operator Protection

1. Disposable surgical latex gloves are recommended for all procedures involving cytotoxic agents.
2. Gloves should routinely be changed approximately every 30 minutes when working steadily with cytotoxic agents. Gloves should be removed immediately after overt contamination.
3. Protective barrier garments should be worn for all procedures involving the preparation and disposal of cytotoxic agents. These garments should have a closed front, long sleeves and closed cuff (either elastic or knit).
4. Protective garments must not be worn outside the work area.

III. Techniques and Precautions for Use in the Class II Biological Safety Cabinet

1. Special techniques and precautions must be utilized because of the vertical (downward) laminar airflow.
2. Clean surfaces of the cabinet using 70% alcohol and a disposal towel before and after preparation. Discard towel into a hazardous chemical waste container.
3. Prepare the work surface of the biological safety cabinet by covering it with a plastic-backed absorbent pad. This pad should be changed when the cabinet is cleaned or after a spill.
4. The biological safety cabinet should be operated with the blower on, 24 hours per day—seven days a week. Where the biological safety cabinet is utilized infrequently (e.g., 1 or 2 times weekly) it may be turned off after thoroughly cleaning all interior surfaces. Turn on the blower 15 minutes before beginning work in the cabinet.

*From Recommendations for Handling Cytotoxic Agents, National Study Commission on Cytotoxic Exposure, September 1987. For additional information, contact the Commission's Chairman.

5. Drug preparations must be performed only with the view screen at the recommended access opening. Professionally accepted practices concerning the aseptic preparation of injectable products should be followed.
6. All materials needed to complete the procedure should be placed into the biological safety cabinet before beginning work to avoid interruptions of cabinet airflow. Allow a two to three minute period before beginning work for the unit to purge itself of airborne contaminants.
7. The proper procedures for use in the biological safety cabinet differ from those used in the horizontal laminar hood because of the nature of the airflow pattern. Clean air descends through the work zone from the top of the cabinet toward the work surface. As it descends, the air is split, with some leaving through the rear perforation and some leaving through the front perforation.
8. The least efficient area of the cabinet in terms of product and personnel protection is within three inches of the sides near the front operning, and work should not be performed in these areas.
9. Entry into and exit from the cabinet should be in a direct manner perpendicular to the face of the cabinet. Rapid movements of the hands in the cabinet and laterally through the protective air barrier should be avoided.

IV. Compounding Procedures and Techniques

1. Hands must be washed thoroughly before gloving and after gloves are removed.
2. Care must be taken to avoid puncturing of glvoes and possible self-innoculation.
3. Syringes and I.V. sets with Luer-lock fittings should be used whenever possible to avoid spills due to disconnection.
4. To minimize aerosolization, vials containing cytotoxic agents should be vented with a hydrophobic filter to equalize internal pressure, or utilize negative pressure technique.
5. Before opening ampules, care should be taken to insure that no liquid remains in the tip of the ampule. A sterile disposable sponge should be wrapped around the neck of the ampule to reduce aerosolization. Ampules should be broken in a direction away from the body.
6. For sealed vials, final drug measurement should be performed prior to removing the needle from the stopper of the vial and after the pressure has been equalized.
7. A closed collection vessel should be available in the biological safety cabinet or the original vial may be used to hold discarded excess drug solutions.
8. Cytotoxic agents should be properly labeled to identify the need for caution in handling (e.g., "Chemotherapy: Dispose of Properly").
9. The final prepared dosage form should be protected from leakage or breakage by being sealed in a transparent plastic container labeled "Do Not Open if Contents Appear to be Broken".

V. Precautions for Administration

1. Disposable surgical latex gloves should be worn during administration of cytotoxic agents. Hands must be washed thoroughly before gloving and after gloves are removed.
2. Protective barrier garments may be worn. Such garments should have a closed front, long sleeves, and closed cuff (either elastic or knit).
3. Syringes and I.V. sets with Luer-lock fittings should be used whenever possible.

4. Special care must be taken in priming I.V. sets. The distal tip or needle cover must be removed before priming. Priming can be performed into a sterile, alcohol-dampened gauze sponge. Other acceptable methods of priming such as closed receptacles (e.g., evacuated containers) or back-filling of I.V. sets may be utilized. Do not prime sets or syringes into the sink or any open receptacle.

VI. Disposal Procedures

1. Place contaminated materials in a leakproof, puncture-proof container appropriately marked as hazardous chemical waster. These containers should be suitable to collect bottles, vials, gloves, disposable gowns and other materials used in the preparation and administration of cytotoxic agents.
2. Contaminated needles, syringes, sets and tubing should be disposed of intact. In order to prevent aerosolization, needles and syringes should not be clipped.
3. Cytotoxic drug waste should be transported according to the institutional procedures for hazardous material.
4. There is insufficient information to recommend any preferred method for disposal of cytotoxic drug waste.
   - 4.1 One acceptable method for disposal of hazardous waste is by incineration in an Environmental Protection Agency (EPA) permitted hazardous water incinerator.
   - 4.2 Another acceptable method of disposal is by burial at an EPA permitted hazardous waste site.
   - 4.3 A licensed hazardous waste disposal company may be consulted for information concerning available methods of disposal in the local area.

VII. Personnel Policy Recommendations

1. Personnel involved in any aspect of the handling of cytotoxic agents must receive an orientation to the agents, including their known risks, and special training in safe handling procedures.
2. Access to the compounding area must be limited to authorized personnel.
3. Personnel working with these agents should be supervised regularly to insure compliance with procedures.
4. Acute exposures must be documented, and the employee referred for medical examination.
5. Personnel should refrain from applying cosmetics in the work area. Cosmetics may provide a source of prolonged exposure if contaminated.
6. Eating, drinking, chewing gum, smoking or storing food in areas where cytotoxic agents are handled should be prohibited. Each of these can be a source of ingestion if they are accidentally contaminated.

VIII. Monitoring Procedures

1. Policies and procedures to monitor the equipment and operating techniques of personnel handling cytotoxic agents should be implemented and performed on a regular basis with appropriate documentation. Specific methods of monitoring should be developed to meet the complexities of the function.
2. It is recommended that personnel involved in the preparation of cytotoxic agents be given periodic health examinations in accordance with institutional policy.

IX. Procedures for Acute Exposure or Spills

1. ACUTE EXPOSURE
   1.1 Overtly contaminated gloves or outer garments should be removed immediately.
   1.2 Hands must be washed after removing gloves. Some cytotoxic agents have been documented to penetrate gloves.
   1.3 In case of skin contact with a cytotoxic drug product, the affected area should be washed thoroughly with soap and water. Refer for medical attention as soon as possible.
   1.4 For eye exposure, flush affected eye with copious amounts of water, and refer for medical attention immediately.
2. SPILLS
   2.1 All personnel involved in the clean-up of a spill should wear protective barrier garments (e.g. gloves, gowns, etc.). These garments and other material used in the process should be disposed of properly.
   2.2 Double gloving is recommended for cleaning up spills.

POSITION STATEMENT

The Handling of Cytotoxic Agents by Women Who Are Pregnant, Attempting to Conceive, or Breast Feeding

There are substantial data regarding the mutagenic, teratogenic and abortifacient properties of certain cytotoxic agents both in animals and humans who have received therapeutic doses of these agents. Additionally, the scientific literature suggests a possible association of occupational exposure to certain cytotoxic agents during the first trimester of pregnancy with fetal loss or malformation. These data suggest the need for caution when women who are pregnant, or attempting to conceive, handle cytotoxic agents. Incidentally, there is no evidence relating male exposure to cytotoxic agents with adverse fetal outcome. There are no studies which address the possible risk associated with the occupational exposure to cytotoxic agents and the passage of these agents into breast milk. Nevertheless, it is prudent that women who are breast feeding should exercise caution in handling cytotoxic agents.

If all procedures for safe handling, such as those recommended by the Commission are complied with, the potential for exposure will be minimized.

Personnal should be provided with information to make an individual decision. This information should be provided in written form and it is advisable that a statement of understanding be signed.

It is essential to refer to individual state right-to-know laws to insure compliance.

NATIONAL STUDY COMMISSION ON CYTOTOXIC EXPOSURE

Chairman

Louis P. Jeffrey, ScD
President, Massachusetts College of Pharmacy and Allied Health Services
Boston, Massachusetts 02114

Commissioners

Roger W. Anderson, MS
Director of Pharmacy
University of Texas System Cancer Center
M.D. Anderson Hospital and Tumor Institute

Thomas H. Connor, PhD
Assistant Professor of Environmental Sciences
Houston School of Public Health
University of Texas Health Sciences Center at Houston

William E. Evans, PharmD
Director, Pharmaceutical Division
St. Jude Children's Research Hospital

Clarence L. Fortner, MDS
Head, Drug Management and Authorization Section, IDB, CTEP
Division of Cancer Treatment
National Cancer Institute

Joseph F. Gallelli, PhD
Chief, Pharmacy Department
The Clinical Center
National Institutes of Health

Joseph N. Gallina, PharmD
Director of Pharmacy Services
University of Maryland Medical System Hospital

Dennis M. Hoffman, PharmD
Director of Pharmacy Services
University of New York at Stony Brook

Louis A. Leone, MD
Director of Medical Oncology
Rhode Island Hospital

Suzanne A. Miller, RN
Oncology Nurse Consultant

Robert M. O'Bryan, MD
Division Head, Medical Oncology
Henry Ford Hospital

For additional information contact:

Louis P. Jeffrey, ScD,
Chairman
National Study Commission on Cytotoxic Exposure
Massachusetts College of Pharmacy and Allied Health Sciences
179 Longwood Avenue
Boston, Massachusetts 02115

APPENDIX J
Normal Values of Common Laboratory Tests

SERUM TESTS

HEMATOLOGIC	MALE	♂/♀	FEMALE
Hemoglobin	13.5–18 g/dl		12–16 g/dl
Hematocrit	40–54%		38–47%
Red Blood Cells (RBC)	4.6–6.2 million/mm^3		4.2–5.4 million/mm^3
Leukocytes (WBC)		5,000–10,000/mm^3	
Neutrophils		54–75% (3,000–7,500/mm^3)	
Bands		3–8% (150–700/mm^3)	
Eosinophils		1–4% (50–400/mm^3)	
Basophils		0–1% (25–100/mm^3)	
Monocytes		2–8% (100–500/mm^3)	
Lymphocytes		25–40% (1,500–4,500/mm^3)	
T-lymphocytes		60–80% of lymphocytes	
B-lymphocytes		10–20% of lymphocytes	
Platelets		150,000–450,000/mm^3	
Prothrombin Time (PT)	9.6–11.8 sec		9.5–11.3 sec
Partial Thromboplastin Time (PTT)		30–45 sec	
Bleeding Time (Duke)		1–3 min	
(Ivy)		3–6 min	
(Template)		3–6 min	
Clotting Time (Lee-White)		4–8 min	

CHEMISTRY	MALE	♂/♀	FEMALE
Sodium		135–145 mEq/L	
Potassium		3.5–5.0 mEq/L	
Chloride		95–105 mEq/L	
Bicarbonate (HCO_3)		19–25 mEq/L	
Total Calcium		9–11 mg/dl or 4.5–5.5 mEq/L	
Ionized Calcium		4.2–5.4 mg/dl or 2.1–2.6 mEq/L	
Phosphorous/Phosphate		2.4–4.7 mg/dl	
Magnesium		1.8–3.0 mg/dl or 1.5–2.5 mEq/L	
Glucose		70–110 mg/dl	
Osmolality		285–310 mOsm/kg	

HEPATIC	MALE	♂/♀	FEMALE
SGOT (AST)	8–46 U/L		7–34 U/L
SGPT (ALT)		10–30 IU/ml	
Total Bilirubin		0.3–1.2 mg/dl	
Conjugated Bilirubin		0.0–0.2 mg/dl	
Unconjugated (Indirect) Bilirubin		0.2–0.8 mg/dl	
Alkaline Phosphatase		20–90 U/L	

RENAL	MALE	♂/♀	FEMALE
BUN		6–20 mg/dl	
Creatinine	0.6–1.3 mg/dl		0.5–1.0 mg/dl
Uric Acid	4.0–8.5 mg/dl		2.7–7.3 mg/dl

ARTERIAL BLOOD GASES	MALE	♂/♀	FEMALE
pH		7.35–7.45	
pO_2		80–100 mmHg	
pCO_2		35–45 mmHg	
O_2 Saturation		95–97%	
Base Excess		+2–(−2)	
Bicarbonate (HCO_3)		22–26 mEq/L	

Continued

URINE TESTS

URINE	MALE	♂/♀	FEMALE
pH		4.5–8.0	
Specific Gravity		1.010–1.025	

APPENDIX K
Dietary Guidelines for Food Sources

Potassium-Rich Foods

avocados	grapefruit	oranges	rhubarb
bananas	lima beans	peaches	sunflower seeds
broccoli	nuts	potatoes	spinach
cantaloupe	navy beans	prunes	tomatoes
dried fruits			

Sodium-Rich Foods

baking mixes (pancakes, muffins)	canned soups	Parmesan cheese
	canned spaghetti sauce	pickles
barbecue sauce	cured meats	potato salad
buttermilk	dry onion soup mix	pretzels, potato chips
butter/margarine	"fast" foods	sauerkraut
canned chili	macaroni and cheese	tomato ketchup
canned seafood	microwave dinners	TV dinners

Calcium-Rich Foods

bok choy	cream soups	oysters
broccoli	milk and dairy products	spinach
canned salmon/sardines	molasses (blackstrap)	tofu
clams		

Vitamin K-Rich Foods

asparagus	cabbage	fish	rice
beans	cauliflower	milk	spinach
broccoli	cheeses	mustard greens	turnips
brussel sprouts	collards	pork	yogurt

Low-Sodium Foods

baked or broiled poultry	grits (not instant)	potatoes
	honey	puffed wheat and rice
canned pumpkin	jams and jellies	red kidney and lima beans
cooked turnips	lean meats	sherbet
egg yolk	low-calorie mayonnaise	unsalted nuts
fresh vegetables	macaroons	whiskey
fruit		

Foods that Acidify Urine

cheeses	fish	meats	poultry
cranberries	grains (breads and cereals)	plums	prunes
eggs			

Foods that Alkalinize Urine

all fruits except cranberries, prunes, plums
all vegetables
milk

Foods Containing Tyramine

aged cheeses
avocados
bananas
beer
caffeine-containing beverages
chocolate
fermented sausage (bologna, salami, pepperoni)
liver
over-ripe fruit
red wine
smoked or pickled fish
yeasts
yogurt

Iron-Rich Foods

cereals
dried beans and peas
dried fruit
leafy-green vegetables
organ meats

APPENDIX L
Recommended Dietary Allowances (RDAs),[a] revised 1989

AGE (YEARS) AND SEX GROUP	WEIGHT[b]		HEIGHT[b]		PROTEIN	FAT-SOLUBLE VITAMINS			
	kg	lb	cm	in		VITAMIN A	VITAMIN D	VITAMIN E	VITAMIN K
					gm	μg RE[c]	μg[d]	mg α-TE[e]	μg
Infants									
0.0–0.5	6	13	60	24	13	375	7.5	3	5
0.5–1.0	9	20	71	28	14	375	10	4	10
Children									
1–3	13	29	90	35	16	400	10	6	15
4–6	20	44	112	44	24	500	10	7	20
7–10	28	62	132	52	28	700	10	7	30
Males									
11–14	45	99	157	62	45	1,000	10	10	45
15–18	66	145	176	69	59	1,000	10	10	65
19–24	72	160	177	70	58	1,000	10	10	70
25–50	79	174	176	70	63	1,000	5	10	80
51+	77	170	173	68	63	1,000	5	10	80
Females									
11–14	46	101	157	62	46	800	10	8	45
15–18	55	120	163	64	44	800	10	8	55
19–24	58	128	164	65	46	800	10	8	60
25–50	63	138	163	64	50	800	5	8	65
51+	65	143	160	63	50	800	5	8	65
Pregnant					60	800	10	10	65
Lactating									
1st 6 months					65	1,300	10	12	65
2nd 6 months					62	1,200	10	11	65

RECOMMENDED DIETARY ALLOWANCES (RDAs),[a] REVISED 1989 (CONTINUED)

AGE (YEARS) AND SEX GROUP	WATER-SOLUBLE VITAMINS							MINERALS						
	VITAMIN C	THIAMIN	RIBOFLAVIN	NIACIN	VITAMIN B_6	FOLATE	VITAMIN B_{12}	CALCIUM	PHOSPHORUS	MAGNESIUM	IRON	ZINC	IODINE	SELENIUM
	mg			mg NE[f]	mg	µg		mg					µg	
Infants														
0.0–0.5	30	0.3	0.4	5	0.3	25	0.3	400	300	40	6	5	40	10
0.5–1.0	35	0.4	0.5	6	0.6	35	0.5	600	500	60	10	5	50	15
Children														
1–3	40	0.7	0.8	9	1.0	50	0.7	800	800	80	10	10	70	20
4–6	45	0.9	1.1	12	1.1	75	1.0	800	800	120	10	10	90	20
7–10	45	1.0	1.2	13	1.4	100	1.4	800	800	170	10	10	120	30
Males														
11–14	50	1.3	1.5	17	1.7	150	2.0	1,200	1,200	270	12	15	150	40
15–18	60	1.5	1.8	20	2.0	200	2.0	1,200	1,200	400	12	15	150	50
19–24	60	1.5	1.7	19	2.0	200	2.0	1,200	1,200	350	10	15	150	70
25–50	60	1.5	1.7	19	2.0	200	2.0	800	800	350	10	15	150	70
51 +	60	1.2	1.4	15	2.0	200	2.0	800	800	350	10	15	150	70

RECOMMENDED DIETARY ALLOWANCES (RDAs),[a] REVISED 1989 (CONTINUED)

	WATER-SOLUBLE VITAMINS							MINERALS						
AGE (YEARS) AND SEX GROUP	VITAMIN C	THIA-MIN	RIBO-FLAVIN	NIACIN	VITAMIN B_6	FOLATE	VITAMIN B_{12}	CAL-CIUM	PHOS-PHORUS	MAG-NESIUM	IRON	ZINC	IODINE	SELE-NIUM
	mg			mg NE[f]	mg	µg		mg					µg	
Females														
11–14	50	1.1	1.3	15	1.4	150	2.0	1,200	1,200	280	15	12	150	45
15–18	60	1.1	1.3	15	1.5	180	2.0	1,200	1,200	300	15	12	150	50
19–24	60	1.1	1.3	15	1.6	180	2.0	1,200	1,200	280	15	12	150	55
25–50	60	1.1	1.3	15	1.6	180	2.0	800	800	280	15	12	150	55
51+	60	1.0	1.2	13	1.6	180	2.0	800	800	280	10	12	150	55
Pregnant	70	1.5	1.6	17	2.2	400	2.2	1,200	1,200	320	30	15	175	65
Lactating														
1st 6 months	95	1.6	1.8	20	2.1	280	2.6	1,200	1,200	355	15	19	200	75
2nd 6 months	90	1.6	1.7	20	2.1	260	2.6	1,200	1,200	340	15	16	200	75

[a] The allowances, expressed as average daily intakes over time, are intended to provide for individual variations among most normal persons as they live in the United States under usual environmental stresses. Diets should be based on a variety of common foods in order to provide other nutrients for which human requirements have been less well defined. See text for detailed discussion of allowances and of nutrients not tabulated.

[b] Weights and heights of Reference Adults are actual medians for the U.S. population of the designated age, as reported by NHANES II. The median weights and heights of those under 19 years of age were taken from Hamill P.V.V., Drizd, T.A., Johnson, C.L., Reed, R.B., Roche, A.F., and Moore, W.M.: Physical growth. National Center for Health Statistics Percentiles. Am J Clin Nutr 32:607, 1979. The use of these figures does not imply that the height-to-weight ratios are ideal.

[c] Retinol equivalents. 1 retinol equivalent = 1 µg retinol or 6 µg β-carotene. See text for calculation of vitamin A activity of diets as retinol equivalents.

[d] As cholecalciferol. 10 µg cholecalciferol = 400 IU of vitamin D.

[e] α-Tocopherol equivalents. 1 mg d-α tocopherol = 1 α-TE. See text for variation in allowances and calculation of vitamin E activity of the diet as α-tocopherol equivalents.

[f] NE (niacin equivalent) is equal to 1 mg of niacin or 60 mg of dietary tryptophan.

APPENDIX M

Electrolyte Equivalents and Caloric Values of Commonly Used Large-Volume Parenterals

	mEq/LITER							CALORIES/ LITER
	Na	K	Ca	Mg	Cl	Acetate	Lactate	
Solution								
D5W	—	—	—	—	—	—	—	170
D10W	—	—	—	—	—	—	—	340
0.9% NaCl	154	—	—	—	154	—	—	—
D5/0.9% NaCl	154	—	—	—	154	—	—	170
D5/0.45% NaCl	77	—	—	—	77	—	—	170
D5/0.2% NaCl	38.5	—	—	—	38.5	—	—	170
D5/LR	130	4	3	—	109	—	28	170–180
D5/Ringer's	147.5	4	4.5	—	156	—	—	170
LR	130	4	3	—	109	—	28	9
Ringer's Injection	147	4	4.5	—	156	—	—	—

D5W = 5% dextrose in water.
D10W = 10% dextrose in water.
0.9% NaCl = 0.9% sodium chloride = normal saline.
D5/0.9% NaCl = 5% dextrose in water with 0.9% sodium chloride = D5 with normal saline.
D5/0.45% NaCl = 5% dextrose in water with 0.45% sodium chloride = D5 with half normal saline.
D5/0.2% NaCl = 5% dextrose in water with 0.2% sodium chloride = D5 with quarter normal saline.
D5/LR = 5% dextrose in water with lactated Ringer's solution.
D5/Ringer's = 5% dextrose in water with Ringer's solution.
LR = Lactated Ringer's solution.

APPENDIX N
Routine Pediatric and Adult Immunizations

ROUTINE PEDIATRIC IMMUNIZATIONS

GENERIC NAME (TRADE NAMES)	ROUTE AND DOSAGE	CONTRAINDICATIONS AND PRECAUTIONS	ADVERSE REACTIONS AND SIDE EFFECTS	NOTES
Diphtheria toxoid, tetanus toxoid, and pertussis vaccine (Tri-Immunol)	0.5 ml IM at 2 mon, 4 mon, 6 mon, and 15–18 mon; booster at 4–yr	Acute infection, immunosuppressive therapy, previous CNS damage or convulsions	Redness, tenderness, induration at injection site, fever, malaise, myalgia, urticaria, hypotension, neurologic reactions, allergic reactions	If unusual reactions occur, individual components may be given as separate injections. Tetanus booster should be repeated every 10 yrs.
Trivalent oral polio vaccine (Orimune)	0.5 ml PO at 2 mon, 4 mon, and 15–18 mon; booster at 4–6 yr	Vomiting, diarrhea, allergy to streptomycin or neomycin, acute illness, immunosuppression	Vaccine-associated paralysis	Additional dose may be given at 6 mon
Measles, mumps, and rubella vaccines (M-M-R II)	Single dose SC at 15 mon	Allergy to egg or neomycin, active infection, immunosuppression	Burning, stinging, pain at injection site, arthritis/arthralgia (40%), fever, encephalitis, allergic reactions	If usual reactions occur, individual components may be given as separate injections. In adults unimmunized against measles 2 doses of measles vaccine 0.5 ml SC (Attenuvax) may be given 2 mon apart; if previously immunized give a single dose. In adults unimmunized against rubella, a single dose of rubella vaccine 0.5 ml SC (Meruvax II) may be given.
Hemophilus b conjugate vaccine (HibTiter, PedvaxHIB, ProHIBit)	0.5 ml IM at 2 mon, 4 mon, and 15–18 mon	Allergy to diphtheria toxoid or thimerisol	Induration, erythema, tenderness at injection site, fever	(ProHIBit only for single immunization in children 15–59 mon, HibTiter not for this use.)

Nursing Implications:

ASSESSMENT

- Assess previous immunization history and history of hypersensitivity.

POTENTIAL NURSING DIAGNOSES

- Infection, high risk for (indications)
- Knowledge deficit related to medication regimen (patient/family teaching).

IMPLEMENTATION

- Measles, mumps, and rubella vaccine, trivalent oral polio virus vaccine, and diphtheria toxoid, tetanus toxoid, and pertussis vaccine may be given concomitantly.
- Administer each immunization by appropriate route: □ **PO:** Polio □ **SC:** measles, mumps, rubella □ **IM:** diphtheria, tetanus toxoid, pertussis.

PATIENT/FAMILY TEACHING

- Inform parent of potential and reportable side effects of immunization. Physician should be notified if patient develops fever over 39.4°C (103°F); difficulty breathing; hives; itching; swelling of eyes, face, or inside of nose; sudden, severe tiredness or weakness; or convulsions occur.
- Review next scheduled immunization with parent.

EVALUATION

Effectiveness of therapy can be demonstrated by: ▪ Prevention of diseases through active immunity.

ROUTINE ADULT IMMUNIZATIONS

GENERIC NAME (TRADE NAMES)	INDICATIONS	ROUTE AND DOSAGE	CONTRAINDICATIONS	ADVERSE REACTIONS AND SIDE EFFECTS
Hepatitis B vaccine (Engerix B, Recombivax HB)	High risk patients, health care workers	3 doses of 0.5 ml IM, given at 0, 1, and 6 mon	Hypersensitivity to yeast (Recombivax) or thimerisol	Local soreness
Influenza vaccine (Flu-Imune, Fluogen, Fluzone, Influenza virus vaccine [trivalent])	Everyone >65 yr, high risk patients, health care workers	0.5 ml IM every yr (new strain developed yearly)	Allergy to eggs, egg protein, chicken, bisulfites, or thimerisol	Fever, chills, myalgia, malaise

ROUTINE ADULT IMMUNIZATIONS *(Continued)*

GENERIC NAME (TRADE NAMES)	INDICATIONS	ROUTE AND DOSAGE	CONTRAINDICATIONS	ADVERSE REACTIONS AND SIDE EFFECTS
Measles vaccine (Attenuvax)	Unimmunized patients born after 1956	2 doses 0.5 ml SC at least one mon apart	Pregnancy, immunosuppression; allergy to eggs, egg protein, chickens, neomycin	Low-grade fever
	Patients previously immunized with single dose (for college entry, health care workers, or foreign travel)	1 dose 0.5 ml SC		
Pneumococcal vaccine, polyvalent (Pneumovax 23, Pnu-Imune 23)	Everyone >65 yr, high risk patients	0.5 ml IM	Hypersensitivity to phenol or thimerisol	Local soreness
Rubella vaccine (Meruvax II)	Unimmunized young women, health care workers	0.5 ml SC	Pregnancy, immunosuppression, allergy to neomycin	Low-grade fever, lymphadenopathy, sore throat; arthralgia and arthritis are common in non-immune adults
Tetanus-diphtheria (Adult Td)	Unimmunized	2 doses 0.5 ml IM 1–2 mon apart, then a 3rd dose 6–12 mon later	Hypersensitivity to previous dose, thimerisol; neurological reaction	Local pain and swelling
	Everyone	Booster every 10 yr		

APPENDIX O
NANDA Nursing Diagnoses

Activity intolerance
Activity intolerance, high risk for
Adjustment impaired
Airway clearance, ineffective
Anxiety [specify level]
Aspiration, high risk for

Body image disturbance
Body temperature, altered, high risk for
Breastfeeding, effective
Breastfeeding, ineffective
Breathing pattern, ineffective

Cardiac output, decreased
Communication, impaired verbal
Constipation
Constipation, colonic
Constipation, perceived
Coping, defensive
Coping, individual, ineffective

Decisional conflict [specify]
Denial, ineffective
Diarrhea
Disuse syndrome, high risk for
Diversional activity deficit
Dysreflexia

Family coping, compromised
Family coping, disabling
Family coping, potential for growth
Family processes, altered
Fatigue
Fear
Fluid volume deficit [active loss]
Fluid volume deficit [regulatory failure]
Fluid volume deficit, high risk for
Fluid volume excess

Gas exchange, impaired
Grieving, anticipatory
Grieving, dysfunctional
Growth and development, altered

Health maintenance, altered
Health-seeking behaviors [specify]
Home maintenance management, impaired
Hopelessness
Hyperthermia
Hypothermia

Incontinence, bowel
Incontinence, functional
Incontinence, reflex
Incontinence, stress
Incontinence, total
Incontinence, urge
Infection, high risk for
Injury, high risk for

Knowledge deficit [learning need, specify]

Mobility, impaired physical

Noncompliance, [compliance, altered, specify]
Nutrition, altered: less than body requirements
Nutrition, altered: more than body requirements
Nutrition, altered, high risk for more than body requirements

Oral mucous membrane, altered

Pain
Pain, chronic
Parental role conflict
Parenting, altered
Parenting, altered, high risk for
Personal identity disturbance
Poisoning, high risk for
Post-trauma response
Powerlessness
Protection, altered

Rape-trauma syndrome
Rape-trauma syndrome: compound reaction
Rape-trauma syndrome: silent reaction
Role performance, altered

Self-care deficit, feeding,
bathing/hygiene,
dressing/grooming,
toileting
Self-esteem, chronic low
Self-esteem disturbance
Self-esteem, situational low

Sensory-perceptual alterations [specify: visual, auditory, kinesthetic, gustatory, tactile, olfactory]
Sexual dysfunction
Sexuality patterns, altered
Skin integrity, impaired
Skin integrity, impaired: high risk for
Sleep pattern disturbance
Social interaction, impaired
Social isolation
Spiritual distress
Suffocation, high risk for
Swallowing, impaired

Thermoregulation, ineffective
Thought processes, altered
Tissue integrity, impaired
Tissue perfusion, altered [specify: cerebral, cardiopulmonary, renal, gastrointestinal, peripheral]
Trauma, high risk for

Unilateral neglect
Urinary elimination, altered patterns
Urinary retention [acute/chronic]

Violence, high risk for: directed at self/others

APPENDIX P
Recent Drug Release Update

GENERIC NAME (BRAND NAME)	CLASSIFICATION	USE(S)	FDA APPROVAL STATUS
amlodipine (Norvasc)	Calcium channel blocker	Hypertension, angina pectoris	Recommended for FDA approval 6/91
azithromycin (Zithromax)	Anti-infective—macrolide	Respiratory tract infections, skin infections, chlamydia	Approved by FDA 11/91
butorphanol intranasal (Stadol NS)	Narcotic analgesic—agonist/antagonist	Analgesia	Approved by FDA
cefprozil (Cefzil)	Anti-infective—cephalosporin	Respiratory tract, skin and skin structure infections	Approved by FDA
chickenpox vaccine (Varivax)	Vaccine	Prevention of chickenpox	UK
diltiazem IV (Cardizem)	Calcium channel blocker	Atrial fibrillation, atrial flutter, conversion of PSVT	Approved by FDA 12/91
enoxacin (Penetrex)	Anti-infective—fluoroquinolone	Skin, genitourinary, and respiratory tract infections	Recommended for FDA approval 12/90
finasteride (Proscar)	Enzyme inhibitor	Benign prostatic hypertrophy	Recommended for FDA approval 2/92
flumazenil (Mazicon)	Benzodiazepine antagonist	Reversal of benzodiazepine effects	Approved by FDA
isosorbide mononitrate (Ismo)	Vasodilator—nitrate	Management of angina pectoris	Approved by FDA
ketorolac oral (Toradol)	Non-narcotic analgesic—nonsteroidal anti-inflammatory agent	Analgesia (short-term)	Approved by FDA
loracarbef (Lorabid)	Anti-infective—cephalosporin	Skin, urinary and respiratory tract infections	Approved by FDA
MAb (Xomazyme CD5 Plus)	Monoclonal antibody	Graft versus host disease	UK
nabumetone (Relafen)	Nonsteroidal anti-inflammatory agent	Rheumatoid arthritis, osteoarthritis	Approved by FDA
nedocromil (Tilade)	Mast cell stabilizer	Reversible airway disease	Recommended for FDA approval 6/90
nicotine transdermal (Habitrol, Nicoderm, Prostep)	Smoking deterrent	Cessation therapy for smokers	Approved by FDA 1/92
pamidronate (Aredia)	Electrolyte modifier—hypocalcemic	Hypercalcemia of malignancy	Approved by FDA 10/91
sertraline (Zoloft)	Antidepressant	Depression	Recommended for approval 9/91
simvastatin (Zocor)	Lipid-lowering agent	Hyperlipidemia	UK
sumatriptan (Sumatrex)	Serotonin agonist	Migraine and cluster headache	UK
temafloxacin (Omniflox)	Anti-infective—fluoroquinolone	Respiratory and urinary tract infections	UK

Drug Compatibility Charts

IV Admixture Compatibility

KEY
C =Compatible
L =Compatible for a limited period of time
I =Incompatible
* =Conflicting data
– =Data unavailable
■ =Identical drug

	1. amikacin	2. aminophylline	3. amphotericin B	4. ampicillin	5. calcium chloride	6. calcium gluconate	7. cefamandole	8. cefazolin	9. cefoxitin	10. chloramphenicol	11. cimetidine	12. clindamycin	13. dexamethasone	14. diphenhydramine	15. gentamicin
1. amikacin	■	*	I	I	C	C	–	I	C	C	C	C	*	C	–
2. aminophylline	*	■	–	–	–	C	–	–	–	C	I	I	C	C	–
3. amphotericin B	I	–	■	I	I	I	–	–	–	–	I	–	–	I	I
4. ampicillin	I	–	I	■	–	I	–	–	–	–	*	*	–	–	I
5. calcium chloride	C	–	I	–	■	–	–	–	–	C	–	–	–	–	–
6. calcium gluconate	C	C	I	I	–	■	I	I	–	C	–	I	C	C	I
7. cefamandole	–	–	–	–	–	I	■	–	–	–	*	C	–	–	I
8. cefazolin	I	–	–	–	–	I	–	■	–	L	I	C	C	–	I
9. cefoxitin	C	–	–	–	–	–	–	–	■	–	C	C	–	–	I
10. chloramphenicol	C	C	–	–	C	C	–	L	–	■	–	–	C	C	I
11. cimetidine	C	I	I	*	–	–	*	*	C	–	■	C	C	–	C
12. clindamycin	C	I	–	*	–	I	C	C	C	–	C	■	–	–	C
13. dexamethasone	*	C	–	–	–	C	–	C	–	C	C	–	■	I	I
14. diphenhydramine	C	C	I	–	–	C	–	–	–	C	–	–	I	■	I
15. gentamicin	–	–	I	I	–	I	I	I	I	I	C	C	I	I	■
16. heparin	I	C	C	*	–	C	–	–	L	C	–	C	L	–	I
17. hydrocortisone	C	C	C	*	C	C	–	–	–	C	–	C	L	I	I
18. insulin, regular	–	I	–	–	–	–	–	–	C	–	C	–	–	–	I
19. lidocaine	–	C	–	*	C	C	C	–	–	C	C	–	C	C	C
20. methicillin	I	C	–	I	C	C	–	–	–	I	–	–	C	C	I
21. methylprednisolone	–	*	–	–	–	I	–	–	–	C	–	C	–	–	–
22. metoclopramide	–	–	–	–	–	I	–	–	–	–	C	C	C	–	–
23. metronidazole	C	C	–	*	–	–	*	C	*	C	–	C	–	–	C
24. mezlocillin	–	–	–	–	–	–	–	–	–	–	–	–	–	–	I
25. multivitamin infusion	–	–	–	–	–	–	–	–	C	–	–	–	–	–	–
26. nafcillin	–	*	–	–	–	–	–	–	–	C	–	–	C	C	–
27. oxacillin	*	–	–	–	–	–	–	–	–	C	–	–	–	–	–
28. oxytocin	–	–	–	–	–	–	–	–	–	C	–	–	–	–	–
29. penicillin G	*	I	I	–	C	C	–	–	–	C	C	C	–	C	*
30. piperacillin	–	–	–	–	–	–	–	–	–	–	–	C	–	–	–
31. potassium chloride	*	C	I	–	–	C	–	–	–	C	C	C	–	–	–
32. procainamide	–	–	–	–	–	–	–	–	–	–	–	–	–	–	–
33. ranitidine	C	–	I	*	–	–	–	*	–	C	–	I	C	–	C
34. ticarcillin	–	–	–	–	–	–	–	–	–	–	–	–	–	–	–
35. tobramycin	–	–	–	–	–	C	I	–	C	–	–	*	–	–	–
36. vancomycin	C	*	–	–	–	C	–	–	–	I	C	–	I	–	–
37. verapamil	C	C	I	*	C	C	C	C	C	C	C	C	C	–	C

	16. heparin	17. hydrocortisone	18. insulin, regular	19. lidocaine	20. methicillin	21. methylprednisolone	22. metoclopramide	23. metronidazole	24. mezlocillin	25. multivitamin infusion	26. nafcillin	27. oxacillin	28. oxytocin	29. penicillin G	30. piperacillin	31. potassium chloride	32. procainamide	33. ranitidine	34. ticarcillin	35. tobramycin	36. vancomycin	37. verapamil
1.	I	C	–	–	I	–	–	C	–	–	–	*	–	*	–	*	–	C	–	–	C	C
2.	C	C	I	C	C	*	–	C	–	–	*	–	–	I	–	C	–	–	–	–	*	C
3.	C	C	–	–	–	–	–	–	–	–	–	–	–	I	–	I	–	I	–	–	–	I
4.	*	*	–	*	I	–	–	*	–	–	–	–	–	–	–	–	–	*	–	–	–	*
5.	–	C	–	C	I	–	–	–	–	–	–	–	–	C	–	–	–	–	–	–	–	C
6.	C	L	–	C	C	I	I	–	–	–	–	–	–	C	–	C	–	–	–	C	C	C
7.	–	–	–	C	–	–	–	*	–	–	–	–	–	–	–	–	–	–	–	I	–	C
8.	–	–	–	–	–	–	–	C	–	–	–	–	–	–	–	–	–	*	–	–	–	C
9.	L	C	–	–	–	–	–	*	–	C	–	–	–	–	–	–	–	–	–	C	–	C
10.	C	C	–	C	I	C	–	C	–	–	C	C	C	C	–	C	–	C	–	–	I	C
11.	–	–	C	C	–	C	C	–	–	–	–	–	–	C	–	C	–	–	–	–	C	C
12.	C	C	–	–	–	C	C	C	–	–	–	–	–	C	C	C	–	I	–	*	–	C
13.	L	L	–	C	C	–	C	–	–	–	C	–	–	–	–	–	–	C	–	–	I	C
14.	–	I	–	C	C	–	–	–	–	–	C	–	–	C	–	–	–	–	–	–	–	–
15.	I	I	I	C	I	–	–	C	I	–	–	–	–	*	–	–	–	C	–	–	–	C
16.		*	I	C	*	C	–	C	–	–	C	–	–	*	–	C	–	–	–	–	I	C
17.	*		L	C	*	–	–	*	–	–	I	–	–	C	C	C	–	–	–	–	C	C
18.	I	L		C	–	I	–	–	–	–	–	–	–	–	–	–	–	–	–	–	–	C
19.	C	C	C		–	–	–	–	–	–	–	–	–	C	–	C	C	–	–	–	–	C
20.	*	*	–	–		–	–	–	–	–	–	–	–	C	–	C	–	–	–	–	I	C
21.	C	–	I	–	–		C	–	–	–	I	–	–	*	–	–	–	–	–	–	–	C
22.	–	–	–	–	–	C		–	–	C	–	–	–	–	–	C	–	–	–	–	–	–
23.	C	*	–	–	–	–	–		–	C	–	–	–	C	–	–	–	–	–	C	–	–
24.	–	–	–	–	–	–	–	–		–	–	–	–	–	–	–	–	–	–	–	–	*
25.	–	–	–	–	–	–	C	C	–		–	–	–	L	–	–	–	–	–	–	–	C
26.	C	I	–	–	–	I	–	–	–	–		–	–	–	–	C	–	–	–	–	–	*
27.	–	–	–	–	–	–	–	–	–	–	–		–	–	–	C	–	–	–	–	–	*
28.	–	–	–	–	–	–	–	–	–	–	–	–		–	–	–	–	–	–	–	–	C
29.	*	C	–	C	C	*	–	*	–	L	–	–	–		–	*	–	C	–	–	–	C
30.	–	C	–	–	–	–	–	–	–	–	–	–	–	–		C	–	–	–	–	–	C
31.	C	C	–	C	C	–	C	–	–	–	C	C	–	*	C		–	–	–	–	C	C
32.	–	–	–	C	–	–	–	–	–	–	–	–	–	–	–	–		–	–	–	–	C
33.	–	–	–	–	–	–	–	–	–	–	–	–	–	C	–	–	–		C	C	C	–
34.	–	–	–	–	–	–	–	–	–	–	–	–	–	–	–	–	–	C		–	–	C
35.	–	–	–	–	–	–	–	C	–	–	–	–	–	–	–	–	–	C	–		–	C
36.	I	C	–	–	I	–	–	–	–	–	–	–	–	–	–	C	–	C	–	–		C
37.	C	C	C	C	C	C	–	–	*	C	*	*	C	C	C	C	C	–	C	C	C	

BIBLIOGRAPHY

American Hospital Formulary Service: Drug Information 92. American Society of Hospital Pharmacists, Bethesda, 1992.

Cella, JH and Watson, J: *Nurse's Manual of Laboratory Tests,* FA Davis, Philadelphia, 1989.

Doenges, ME and Moorhouse, MF: *Nurse's Pocket Guide: Nursing Diagnoses with Interventions,* ed 3. FA Davis, Philadelphia, 1991.

Facts and Comparisons. JB Lippincott, St. Louis, 1992.

Fischbach, FT: *A Manual of Laboratory Diagnostic Tests,* ed 3. JB Lippincott, Philadelphia, 1988.

Mathewson, MK: *Pharmacotherapeutics: A Nursing Process Approach,* ed 2. FA Davis, Philadelphia, 1991.

Physicians' Desk Reference (PDR). Medical Economics, Oradell, 1992.

Trissel, LA: *Handbook of Injectable Drugs,* ed 6. American Society of Hospital Pharmacists, Bethesda, 1990.

Trissel, LA: *Supplement to Handbook of Injectable Drugs,* ed 6. American Society of Hospital Pharmacists, Bethesda, 1991.

USP Dispensing Information (USP-DI)-Drug Information for the Health Care Provider Volume 1. United States Pharmacopeial Convention, Rockville, 1991.

Whitney, E and Boyle M: *Understanding Nutrition,* ed 3. West Publishing Company, St. Paul, 1984.

NOTES

NOTES

NOTES

NOTES

COMPREHENSIVE INDEX
generic/Trade/CLASSIFICATION

*Entries for **generic** names appear in **boldface type,** trade names appear in regular type, **CLASSIFICATIONS** appear in **BOLDFACE SMALL CAPS**, and *Combination Drugs* appear in *italics*. A "**C**" and a **boldface** page number following a generic name identify the page in the "Classification" section on which that drug is listed.

*Entries for **generic** names appear in **boldface type,** trade names appear in regular type, **CLASSIFICATIONS** appear in **BOLDFACE SMALL CAPS**, and *Combination Drugs* appear in *italics*. A "C" and a **boldface** page number following a generic name identify the page in the "Classification" section on which that drug is listed.

*Entries for **generic** names appear in **boldface type,** trade names appear in regular type, **CLASSIFICATIONS** appear in **BOLDFACE SMALL CAPS**, and *Combination Drugs* appear in *italics.* A "**C**" and a **boldface** page number following a generic name identify the page in the "Classification" section on which that drug is listed.

*Entries for **generic** names appear in **boldface type,** trade names appear in regular type, **CLASSIFICATIONS** appear in **BOLDFACE SMALL CAPS**, and *Combination Drugs* appear in *italics.* A "**C**" and a **boldface** page number following a generic name identify the page in the "Classification" section on which that drug is listed.

*Entries for **generic** names appear in **boldface type,** trade names appear in regular type, **CLASSIFICATIONS** appear in **BOLDFACE SMALL CAPS,** and *Combination Drugs* appear in *italics.* A "**C**" and a **boldface** page number following a generic name identify the page in the "Classification" section on which that drug is listed.

*Entries for **generic** names appear in **boldface type,** trade names appear in regular type, **CLASSIFICATIONS** appear in **BOLDFACE SMALL CAPS**, and *Combination Drugs* appear in *italics.* A "**C**" and a **boldface** page number following a generic name identify the page in the "Classification" section on which that drug is listed.

*Entries for **generic** names appear in **boldface type,** trade names appear in regular type, CLASSIFICATIONS appear in **BOLDFACE SMALL CAPS**, and *Combination Drugs* appear in *italics.* A "C" and a **boldface** page number following a generic name identify the page in the "Classification" section on which that drug is listed.

*Entries for **generic** names appear in **boldface type,** trade names appear in regular type, **CLASSIFICATIONS** appear in **BOLDFACE SMALL CAPS**, and *Combination Drugs* appear in *italics.* A "**C**" and a **boldface** page number following a generic name identify the page in the "Classification" section on which that drug is listed.

*Entries for **generic** names appear in **boldface type,** trade names appear in regular type, CLASSIFICATIONS appear in **BOLDFACE SMALL CAPS**, and *Combination Drugs* appear in *italics.* A "**C**" and a **boldface** page number following a generic name identify the page in the "Classification" section on which that drug is listed.

*Entries for **generic** names appear in **boldface type,** trade names appear in regular type, CLASSIFICATIONS appear in **BOLDFACE SMALL CAPS**, and *Combination Drugs* appear in *italics.* A "**C**" and a **boldface** page number following a generic name identify the page in the "Classification" section on which that drug is listed.

—J—

—K—

*Entries for **generic** names appear in **boldface type,** trade names appear in regular type, **CLASSIFICATIONS** appear in **BOLDFACE SMALL CAPS**, and *Combination Drugs* appear in *italics*. A "**C**" and a **boldface** page number following a generic name identify the page in the "Classification" section on which that drug is listed.

*Entries for **generic** names appear in **boldface type,** trade names appear in regular type, **CLASSIFICATIONS** appear in **BOLDFACE SMALL CAPS**, and *Combination Drugs* appear in *italics.* A "C" and a **boldface** page number following a generic name identify the page in the "Classification" section on which that drug is listed.

*Entries for **generic** names appear in **boldface type,** trade names appear in regular type, **CLASSIFICATIONS** appear in **BOLDFACE SMALL CAPS**, and *Combination Drugs* appear in *italics.* A "**C**" and a **boldface** page number following a generic name identify the page in the "Classification" section on which that drug is listed.

*Entries for **generic** names appear in **boldface type,** trade names appear in regular type, **CLASSIFICATIONS** appear in **BOLDFACE SMALL CAPS**, and *Combination Drugs* appear in *italics.* A "C" and a **boldface** page number following a generic name identify the page in the "Classification" section on which that drug is listed.

*Entries for **generic** names appear in **boldface type,** trade names appear in regular type, **CLASSIFICATIONS** appear in **BOLDFACE SMALL CAPS**, and *Combination Drugs* appear in *italics.* A "**C**" and a **boldface** page number following a generic name identify the page in the "Classification" section on which that drug is listed.

*Entries for **generic** names appear in **boldface type,** trade names appear in regular type, **CLASSIFICATIONS** appear in **BOLDFACE SMALL CAPS**, and *Combination Drugs* appear in *italics.* A "C" and a **boldface** page number following a generic name identify the page in the "Classification" section on which that drug is listed.

*Entries for **generic** names appear in **boldface type,** trade names appear in regular type, CLASSIFICATIONS appear in BOLDFACE SMALL CAPS, and *Combination Drugs* appear in *italics.* A "**C**" and a **boldface** page number following a generic name identify the page in the "Classification" section on which that drug is listed.

*Entries for **generic** names appear in **boldface type**, trade names appear in regular type, **CLASSIFICATIONS** appear in **BOLDFACE SMALL CAPS**, and *Combination Drugs* appear in *italics*. A "C" and a **boldface** page number following a generic name identify the page in the "Classification" section on which that drug is listed.

*Entries for **generic** names appear in **boldface type,** trade names appear in regular type, **CLASSIFICATIONS** appear in **BOLDFACE SMALL CAPS**, and *Combination Drugs* appear in *italics.* A "**C**" and a **boldface** page number following a generic name identify the page in the "Classification" section on which that drug is listed.

*Entries for **generic** names appear in **boldface type,** trade names appear in regular type, **CLASSIFICATIONS** appear in **BOLDFACE SMALL CAPS**, and *Combination Drugs* appear in *italics.* A "**C**" and a **boldface** page number following a generic name identify the page in the "Classification" section on which that drug is listed.

*Entries for **generic** names appear in **boldface type,** trade names appear in regular type, **CLASSIFICATIONS** appear in **BOLDFACE SMALL CAPS**, and *Combination Drugs* appear in *italics.* A "**C**" and a **boldface** page number following a generic name identify the page in the "Classification" section on which that drug is listed.

NOTES

NOTES

NOTES

NOTES